P9-DVS-408

Diagnostic Gynecologic and Obstetric PATHOLOGY

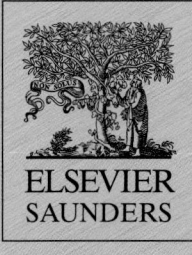

ELSEVIER
SAUNDERS

Commissioning Editor: Michael Houston
Project Development Manager: Belinda Kuhn
Editorial Assistant: Elizabeth Brown
Project Manager: Alan Nicholson
Design Manager: Sarah Russell
Illustration Manager: Mick Ruddy
Marketing Managers: Ethel Cathers (USA); Leontine Treur (EMEA)

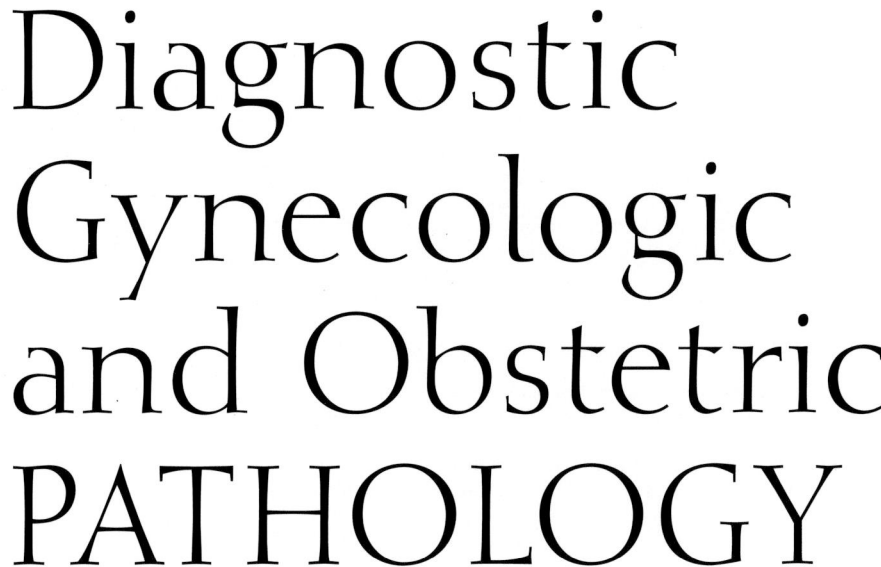

Diagnostic Gynecologic and Obstetric PATHOLOGY

Christopher P. Crum MD
Professor of Pathology
Harvard Medical School
Director
Division of Women's and Perinatal
Pathology
Department of Pathology
Brigham and Women's Hospital
Boston, MA
USA

Kenneth R. Lee MD
Associate Professor of Pathology
Harvard Medical School
Division of Women's and Perinatal
Pathology
Department of Pathology
Brigham and Women's Hospital
Boston, MA
USA

ASSOCIATE EDITORS

David R. Genest MD
Associate Professor of Pathology
Harvard Medical School
Division of Women's and Perinatal
Pathology
Department of Pathology
Brigham and Women's Hospital
Boston, MA, USA

Scott R. Granter MD
Associate Professor of Pathology
Harvard Medical School
Division of Dermatopathology
Department of Pathology
Brigham and Women's Hospital
Boston, MA, USA

Hope K. Haefner MD
Associate Professor of Obstetrics and
Gynecology
University of Michigan Medical School
Department of Obstetrics and
Gynecology
University of Michigan Hospital
Ann Arbor, MI, USA

George L. Mutter MD
Associate Professor of Pathology
Harvard Medical School
Division of Women's and Perinatal
Pathology
Department of Pathology
Brigham and Women's Hospital
Boston, MA, USA

Marisa R. Nucci MD
Assistant Professor of Pathology
Harvard Medical School
Division of Women's and Perinatal
Pathology
Department of Pathology
Brigham and Women's Hospital
Boston, MA, USA

Bradley J. Quade MD
Assistant Professor of Pathology
Harvard Medical School
Division of Women's and Perinatal
Pathology
Department of Pathology
Brigham and Women's Hospital
Boston, MA, USA

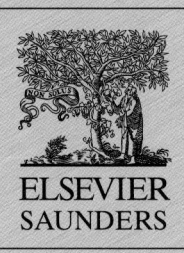

ELSEVIER
SAUNDERS

ELSEVIER
SAUNDERS

An imprint of Elsevier Inc.

ISBN 0 7216 0005 0

British Library Cataloguing in Publication Data
A catalogue record for this book is available from the British Library

Library of Congress Cataloging in Publication Data
A catalog record for this book is available from the Library of Congress

Printed in China

Last digit is the print number: 9 8 7 6 5 4 3 2 1

Contributors

Theonia K. Boyd MD
Assistant Professor of Pathology
Harvard Medical School
Department of Pathology
Children's Hospital
Boston, MA
USA

Priscilla S. Chang MD PhD
Clinical Fellow in Pathology
Harvard Medical School
Department of Pathology
Brigham and Women's Hospital
Boston, MA
USA

Christopher P. Crum, MD
Professor of Pathology
Harvard Medical School
Director
Division of Women's and
Perinatal Pathology
Department of Pathology
Brigham and Women's Hospital
Boston, MA
USA

Ronny L. Drapkin MD PhD
Instructor in Pathology
Harvard Medical School
Associate Pathologist
Department of Pathology
Brigham and Women's Hospital
and Dana Farber Cancer Institute
Boston, MA
USA

Linda R. Duska MD
Assistant Professor of Obstetrics
and Gynecology
Harvard Medical School
Assistant in Gynecology and
Obstetrics
Massachusetts General Hospital
Cancer Center
Boston, MA
USA

Julia A. Elvin MD
Clinical Fellow in Pathology
Harvard Medical School
Fellow in Women's and Perinatal
Pathology
Department of Pathology
Brigham and Women's Hospital
Boston, MA
USA

David R. Genest MD
Associate Professor of Pathology
Harvard Medical School
Division of Women's and
Perinatal Pathology
Department of Pathology
Brigham and Women's Hospital
Boston, MA
USA

Scott R. Granter MD
Associate Professor of Pathology
Harvard Medical School
Division of Dermatopathology
Department of Pathology
Brigham and Women's Hospital
Boston, MA
USA

Hope K. Haefner MD
Associate Professor of Obstetrics
and Gynecology
University of Michigan Medical
School
Department of Obstetrics and
Gynecology
University of Michigan Hospital
Ann Arbor, MI
USA

Jonathan L. Hecht MD PhD
Assistant Professor of Pathology
Harvard Medical School
Department of Pathology
Beth Israel Deaconess Medical
Center
Boston, MA
USA

Michelle S. Hirsch MD PhD
Instructor in Pathology
Harvard Medical School
Division of Women's and
Perinatal Pathology
Department of Pathology
Brigham and Women's Hospital
Boston, MA
USA

Mark D. Hornstein MD
Associate Professor of Obstetrics,
Gynecology and Reproductive
Medicine
Harvard Medical School
Director, Division of
Reproductive Endocrinology
Department of Obstetrics and
Gynaecology
Brigham and Women's Hospital
Boston, MA
USA

David W. Kindelberger MD
Clinical Fellow in Pathology
Harvard Medical School
Fellow in Women's and Perinatal
Pathology
Department of Pathology
Brigham and Women's Hospital
Boston, MA
USA

Alexander J. F. Lazar MD PhD
Assistant Professor of Pathology
and Dermatology
Department of Pathology
University of Texas
M.D. Anderson Cancer Center
Houston, TX
USA

Kenneth R. Lee MD
Associate Professor of Pathology
Harvard Medical School
Division of Women's and
Perinatal Pathology
Department of Pathology
Brigham and Women's Hospital
Boston, MA
USA

Phillip H. McKee MD FRCPath
Associate Professor of Pathology
Harvard Medical School
Formerly Director
Division of Dermatopathology
Department of Pathology
Brigham and Women's Hospital
Boston, MA
USA

Fabiola Medeiros MD
Clinical Fellow in Pathology
Harvard Medical School
Fellow in Women's and Perinatal
Pathology
Department of Pathology
Brigham and Women's Hospital
Boston, MA
USA

Michael G. Muto MD
Associate Professor of Obstetrics
Gynecology and Reproductive
Biology
Harvard Medical School
Division of Gynecologic
Oncology
Department of Obstetrics and
Gynecology
Brigham and Women's Hospital
Boston, MA
USA

George L. Mutter MD
Associate Professor of Pathology
Harvard Medical School
Division of Women's and
Perinatal Pathology
Department of Pathology
Brigham and Women's Hospital
Boston, MA
USA

Alessandra F. Nascimento MD
Instructor of Pathology
Harvard Medical School
Associate Pathologist
Brigham and Women's Hospital
Department of Pathology
Brigham and Women's Hospital
Boston, MA
USA

Marisa R. Nucci MD
Assistant Professor of Pathology
Harvard Medical School
Division of Women's and
Perinatal Pathology
Department of Pathology
Brigham and Women's Hospital
Boston, MA
USA

Kirstine Y-T. Oh MD
Clinical Fellow in Pathology
Harvard Medical School
Department of Pathology
Brigham and Women's Hospital
Boston, MA
USA

Joel M. Palefsky MD
Professor, Laboratory Medicine,
Medicine and Stomatology
University of California
at San Francisco
Director
UCSF General Clinical Research
University of California
at San Francisco
San Francisco, CA
USA

Mana M. Parast MD PhD
Clinical Fellow in Pathology
Harvard Medical School
Fellow
Division of Women's and
Perinatal Pathology
Department of Pathology
Brigham and Women's Hospital
Boston, MA
USA

Bradley J. Quade MD PhD
Assistant Professor of Pathology
Harvard Medical School
Division of Women's and
Perinatal Pathology
Department of Pathology
Brigham and Women's Hospital
Boston, MA
USA

Peter G. Rose MD
Professor and Director of
Gynecologic Oncology
Cleveland Clinic Foundation
Cleveland, OH
USA

Kathleen F. Sirois
Laboratory Specialist
Placental–Perinatal Service
Division of Women's and
Perinatal Pathology
Department of Pathology
Brigham and Women's Hospital
Boston, MA
USA

Elizabeth A. Stewart MD
Associate Professor of Obstetrics
and Gynecology
Harvard Medical School
Clinical Director
Center for Uterine Fibroids
Department of Obstetrics and
Gynecology
Brigham and Women's Hospital
Boston, MA
USA

Preface

Any comprehensive textbook on obstetric and gynecologic pathology should fulfil at least three goals. The first is to provide general or introductory information to the medical student or clinical resident with limited experience in pathology. The second is to school the pathology resident or practicing pathologist in the pathologic diagnosis of common disorders. The third is to assist both in managing diagnostically difficult or rare cases. The degree to which a single book accomplishes these tasks depends on both its mission and the expectations of the reader.

Both academic and practice-based pathologists face increasing demands. In this pressurized setting, the ideal book would deliver a formula to solve the complex problems that characterize modern day practice. Unfortunately, simplicity is a thing of the past. The influx of emerging knowledge has taken diagnostic pathology from a purely descriptive field of 'diagnosis by decree' to one in which visually-based assumptions by both general pathologists and subspecialists are constantly challenged by emerging data. We still have the 'Aunt Minnies', those rare but familiar pathologic disorders that can be recognized instantly in a hematoxylin and eosin-stained section. But we also encounter conditions that vex us daily and for which an objective marker is essential for proper management. For example, an inquiring pathologist who orders an immunohistochemical stain to confirm the diagnosis in a problematic cervical biopsy can make the difference between surgery and a simple follow-up Papanicolaou smear. The wary pathologist who performs a p53 immunostain on an unusual-appearing gland in an endometrial curetting from a postmenopausal woman might ultimately diagnose a potentially lethal serous carcinoma. The pathologist learns to address these challenges in daily practice by constantly sorting through many diagnostic options, thus gaining experience that is not the product of assumption but of repeated self assessment, and by never taking an authoritative opinion at face value if it can be tested by more objective means.

This book is written and edited by members of the Women's and Perinatal Pathology Division at Brigham and Women's Hospital with the assistance of their colleagues and leading authorities in clinical obstetrics and gynecology.

Its goal is to provide a comprehensive review of gynecologic and gestational pathology. To assist readers from different backgrounds, the approach to most of the topics is practice-oriented, each beginning with the patient at risk and ending with management. This sequence varies in its makeup depending on the subject. For example, endometrial carcinoma (Chapter 19) may require pathologic interpretation at four junctures; evaluation of cervical cytology, endometrial biopsy or curettage, intra-operative consultation, and post-operative evaluation of the uterus. Each segment in this evaluation process has its demands and pitfalls. The pathologist makes his or her most important contributions to the management of ovarian neoplasia in the frozen section room. Thus, Chapter 26 is written specifically for the challenges faced there. Sex cord-stromal tumors include the rarest and most confusing entities, and thus are organized in decision-tree algorithms in Chapter 29. Gestational trophoblastic diseases (Chapter 32) are included with early pregnancy, because most are now encountered in this setting. A placenta may be received in the absence of a recognized clinical disorder, and Chapter 33 outlines a systematic approach to placental examination. Conversely, the placenta may arrive in the setting of a known disease, where the purpose of the exam is to quickly narrow the search to a list of relevant pathologic variables, as depicted in Chapter 34. Throughout the book, the reader is introduced to considerable pathologic detail, on the premise that everyone, medical student, clinical resident, pathologist in training and practicing pathologist, must be fully aware of the degrees of certainty and pitfalls of pathologic diagnosis if they are going to care for women with reproductive tract diseases. Diagnostic pathology can be simplified only by confronting its myriad complexities, using a wide range of tools. We begin by seeking order, like librarians who carefully catalogue and organize texts according to conventions. However, in order to evolve, we must periodically rearrange the volumes in our library of medical knowledge, a tribute to the fact that the texts are constantly re-written.

Christopher P. Crum, MD
Kenneth R. Lee, MD

Acknowledgments

We are indebted to our predecessors and mentors, who introduced us to the field of obstetric and gynecologic pathology and expanded our horizons, including Kurt Benirschke, Shirley Driscoll, Cecilia Fenoglio, Alex Ferenczy, Yao-Shi Fu, Arthur Hertig, Ralph M. Richart, Robert E. Scully, and Saul J. Silverstein, and to our many trainees and colleagues whose knowledge and expertise ultimately have contributed to this book.

Dedication
To Tucker and Kathleen

Contents

Contributors

Preface

Acknowledgments

Dedication

1. **Female genital tract development and disorders of childhood** 1
   Theonia K. Boyd, Julia A. Elvin and Christopher P. Crum

2. **Non-infectious inflammatory disorders of the vulva** 23
   Alexander J.F. Lazar, Phillip H. McKee, Hope K. Haefner and Scott R. Granter

3. **Localized vulvodynia** 57
   Hope K. Haefner

4. **Infectious disorders of the lower genital tract** 65
   Alexander J.F. Lazar, Scott R. Granter, Phillip H. McKee and Hope K. Haefner

5. **Benign cysts, rests and adnexal tumors of the vulva** 99
   Alexander J.F. Lazar, Scott R. Granter and Hope K. Haefner

6. **Squamous neoplasia of the vulva** 109
   Christopher P. Crum and Scott R. Granter

7. **Glandular and other malignancies of the vulva** 149
   Christopher P. Crum

8. **Melanocytic lesions of the vulva** 163
   Scott R. Granter, Alexander J.F. Lazar, Hope K. Haefner and Phillip H. McKee

9. **Soft tissue lesions of the vulva and vagina** 179
   Marisa R. Nucci

10. **Diseases of the anus** 199
    Kirstine Y-T. Oh and Joel M. Palefsky

11. **Benign conditions of the vagina** 229
    Hope K. Haefner and Christopher P. Crum

12. **Epithelial and mixed epithelial–stromal neoplasms of the vagina** 245
    Christopher P. Crum and Hope K. Haefner

13. **Cervical squamous neoplasia** 267
Christopher P. Crum and
Peter G. Rose

14. **Glandular neoplasia of the cervix** 355
Kenneth R. Lee and Peter G. Rose

15. **Neuroendocrine carcinoma, mixed epithelial/ mesenchymal and mesenchymal tumors and miscellaneous lesions of the cervix** 411
Marisa R. Nucci and
Christopher P. Crum

16. **Evaluation of cyclic endometrium and benign endometrial disorders** 441
Christopher P. Crum, Mark D. Hornstein and Elizabeth A. Stewart

17. **Endometrial intraepithelial neoplasia** 493
George L. Mutter, Linda R. Duska and Christopher P. Crum

18. **Altered endometrial differentiation (metaplasia)** 519
Christopher P. Crum, Marisa R. Nucci and George L. Mutter

19. **Adenocarcinoma, carcinosarcoma and other epithelial tumors of the endometrium** 545
Christopher P. Crum,
Linda R. Duska, Kenneth R. Lee and George L. Mutter

20. **Uterine mesenchymal tumors** 611
Marisa R. Nucci and
Bradley J. Quade

21. **The fallopian tube and broad ligament** 675
Priscilla S. Chang and
Christopher P. Crum

22. **Benign conditions of the ovary** 713
Alessandra F. Nascimento,
Mark D. Hornstein and
Christopher P. Crum

23. **Disorders of the peritoneum** 753
Alessandra F. Nascimento and
Marisa R. Nucci

24. **Pathogenesis of ovarian cancer** 793
Ronny L. Drapkin and
Jonathan L. Hecht

25. **The patient at risk of ovarian cancer** 811
Michael G. Muto

26. **Intraoperative evaluation of ovarian tumors** 821
Christopher P. Crum, Marisa R. Nucci and Kenneth R. Lee

27. **The pathology of surface epithelial–stromal tumors of the ovary** 839
Kenneth R. Lee

28. **Pathology-based management and outcome of epithelial tumors of the ovary** 905
Michael G. Muto

29. **Germ cell tumors of the ovary** 913
Fabiola Medeiros, Marisa R. Nucci and Christopher P. Crum

30. **Sex cord-stromal and miscellaneous tumors of the ovary** 945
Christopher P. Crum and
Kenneth R. Lee

31. **Metastatic tumors to the ovary** 977
Michelle S. Hirsch and
Kenneth R. Lee

32. **Complications of early pregnancy, including trophoblastic neoplasia** 995
Julia A. Elvin, Christopher P. Crum and David R. Genest

33. **Evaluation of the placenta** 1041
David W. Kindelberger, Kathleen F. Sirois and David R. Genest

34. **Gestational diseases and the placenta** 1083
Mana M. Parast and David R. Genest

Appendix
TNM and FIGO Staging
Diagnostic Terminology
Diagnostic Reporting

Index

1

Female genital tract development and disorders of childhood

Theonia K. Boyd,

Julia A. Elvin and

Christopher P. Crum

Overview of reproductive tract development

The genital ridge
Ovary development and sex
   determination
The uterus and vagina
The external genitalia

Common disorders of gonadal and genital tract development

Ovary and fallopian tube
Uterus and cervix
Vagina
Other lower genital tract and
   vulvar anomalies

Overview of reproductive tract development

The female genital tract is formed by a complex series of events beginning in the 4th week of development. This process involves the formation of the gonads following germ cell migration from the yolk sac to the dorsal mesentery, formation and fusion of the Müllerian ducts to create the uterine corpus and tubes, induction of squamous mucosa in the vagina and cervix and a series of epithelial-mesenchymal interactions in the introitus and external genital region to model the clitoris and labia. Successful completion of these sequential developmental tasks requires, by definition, the cooperation of concurrent events taking place to form the abdominal wall, separate the rectum from the urogenital sinus, induce urothelial differentiation and complete rectal and urethral development (Table 1.1, Figs 1.1–1.5).[1,2]

The above events can be subdivided into four segments, including development of the genital ridge, ovary, uterus and vagina and external genitalia. Each of these is influenced, directly or indirectly, by the expression of a range of transcription factors, X chromosome integrity, germ cell development and secretion of sex steroid hormones. Relative input from these influencing factors ultimately determines the internal and external sexual organ phenotype.

THE GENITAL RIDGE

The genitourinary system begins to develop by the 5th week of gestation (post coital) as a longitudinal ridge of undifferentiated mesenchymal cells that extend bilaterally flanking the mesenteric root (Fig. 1.2). Excluding the bladder and external genitalia, the remainder of the genitourinary system ultimately evolves from this mesenchymal thickening. The undifferentiated mesenchyme in this area comprises the genital ridge and will ultimately give rise to the medulla of the ovary, whereas the coelomic epithelium becomes the ovarian cortex and the ovarian surface epithelium (Fig. 1.3). Genital ridge development is under the control of the homeobox gene family, the expression of which stabilize the intermediate mesoderm.[3] A series of transcription factors are integral to genital ridge development and mouse knockouts affecting these genes will nullify genital ridge development and that of the adjacent kidneys and adrenals.[4] Several genes (Lhx1, Emx2 and Pax2) are integral to the formation of urogenital mesenchyme (Fig. 1.4).[5–7]

Table 1.1 Time line of important milestones in genital tract development

Postconception period	Ovaries	Fallopian tubes/ uterus/vagina	Vulva
3rd week	Primordial germ cells appear in the hindgut yolk sac wall		Primitive streak mesenchyme forms midline genital tubercle, paired cloacal folds
4th–6th weeks	Germ cells migrate along the dorsal mesentery to invade the urogenital ridge	Genital ridge mesenchyme folds into columns which cavitate to form paramesonephric (Müllerian) ducts	Cloacal folds differentiate into urethral and anal folds; labioscrotal swellings form lateral to cloacal folds
7th–8th weeks	Surface coelomic epithelium penetrates mesenchyme to form cortical cords; stromal estradiol production determines ovarian fate	Cephalad ducts differentiate into paired fallopian tubes, caudal fused ducts differentiate into the uterus, cervix and vagina; merged uterine and upper vaginal ducts cavitate to form single uterine and vaginal lumens	Genitalia is indifferent
4th–5th months	Cortical cord cells surround oogonia as granulosa cells; primordial follicles reach maximal number (>7 million)	Lower vaginal canal remains solid until the end of the 5th month, then canalizes except for the hymen, which demarcates the junction between superior Müllerian/inferior urogenital sinus origins	Genitalia is definitive: (1) Genital tubercle→Clitoris (2) Urethral folds→Labia minora (3) Labioscrotal swellings→Labia majora
7th month	Oogonia cease proliferation, enter meiotic prophase		
Term	Germ cell numbers reduced ~70%		

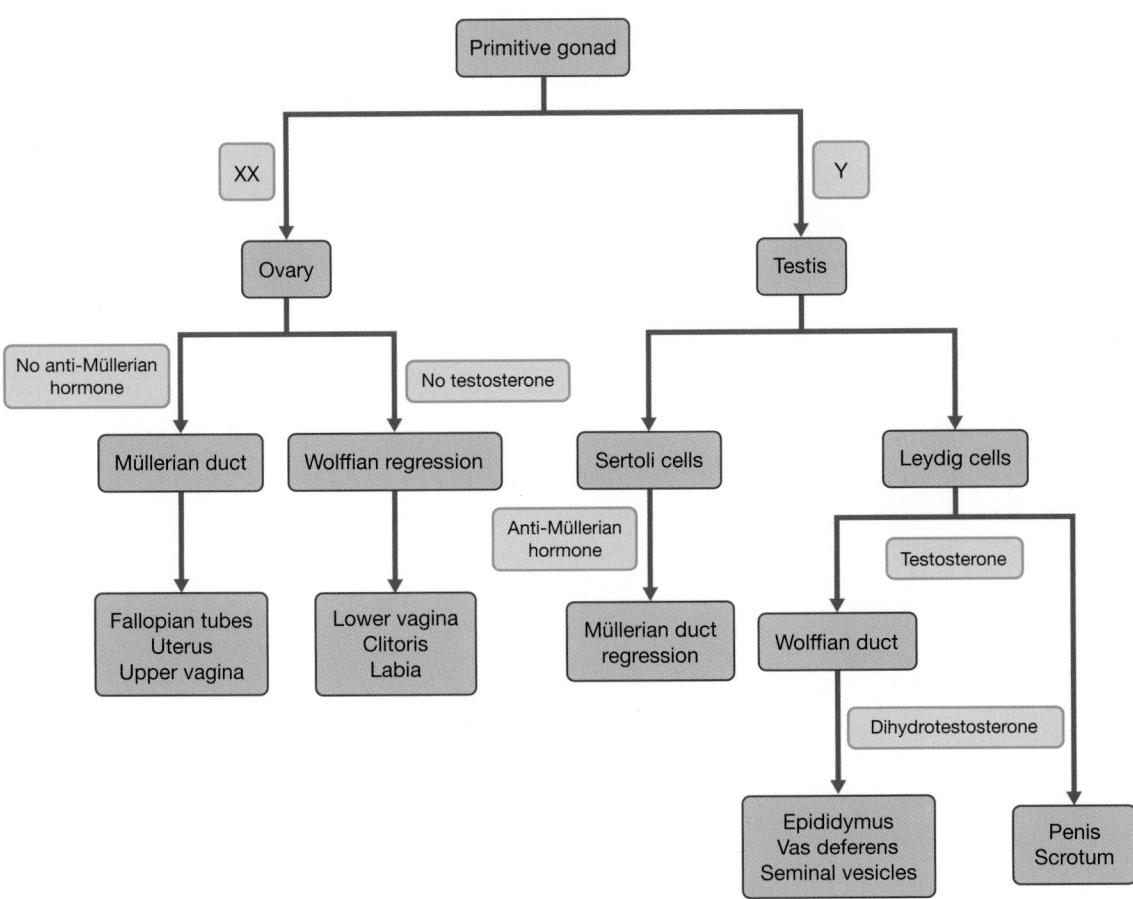

Fig. 1.1 Overview of pathways of Müllerian (female) versus Wolffian (male) development. (From Holm,[8] with permission.)

OVARY DEVELOPMENT AND SEX DETERMINATION

Germ cells in the human enter the genital ridges between 4 and 6 weeks gestation. In the presence of a male genotype containing the sex determining region (SRY) on the Y chromosome, or in the event of an XX genotype in which the SRY region has been retained via translocation, the embryo will develop into a male. The presumed – if not confirmed – target of SRY is SOX9, an HMG box gene that has been shown to 'rescue' the male phenotype in some XX individuals.[8,9] In the absence of SRY, the supporting stromal cells develop into granulosa cells, forming single layers investing the primitive oocytes. These primordial follicles rapidly multiply to over 7 million by the 22nd week. At this point, cell division ceases and the cell population drops by over two-thirds at birth and by another 90% by puberty, when the average number of oocytes in the ovary stands at approximately 300 000.[10] In the genetically female fetus, the gonad is distinguished by the end of the second month due to estradiol production from the stroma.[11] The primitive germ cells proliferate and differentiate to oogonia, beginning in the center of the ovary and moving toward the periphery over time (Fig. 1.5). The oogonia become invested with a single layer of follicular cells derived from coelomic epithelium of mesonephric origin,[12] become oocytes and form primordial follicles. The earliest follicles develop by 15 weeks. By the end of the 7th month of gestation, all of the germ cells have ceased to proliferate and have entered meiotic prophase where they will remain until ovulation. In contrast to the testis, germ cells in the ovary are critical to the development of their supporting stromal cells. In their absence the pre-follicular cells are not sustained and a streak gonad will form.[13]

Germ cells exhibit high levels of proliferative activity in weeks 15–20, with high levels of Ki-67 expression in both the cortex and medulla (Fig. 1.6a). Concurrent with this proliferative activity is the expression of Oct 4, a transcription factor that is expressed early in embryogenesis and has been demonstrated to be integral to maintaining the viability of the primordial germ cell mass (Fig. 1.6b).[14] Oct 4 staining is concentrated primarily along the outer rim of the primitive

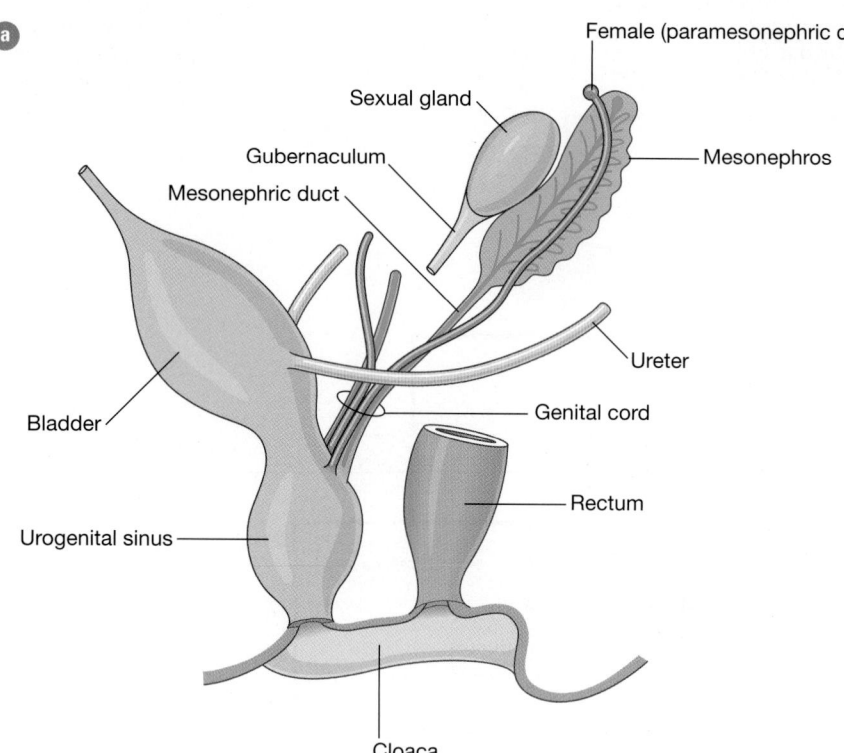

Female (paramesonephric duct)

Sexual gland

Gubernaculum

Mesonephric duct

Mesonephros

Ureter

Bladder

Genital cord

Urogenital sinus

Rectum

Cloaca

Fig. 1.2 Lower genital tract development (a) prior to and (b) following initiation of Müllerian tract development. (Redrawn from *Grays Anatomy*,[2] Fig. 2.158A,B, with permission).

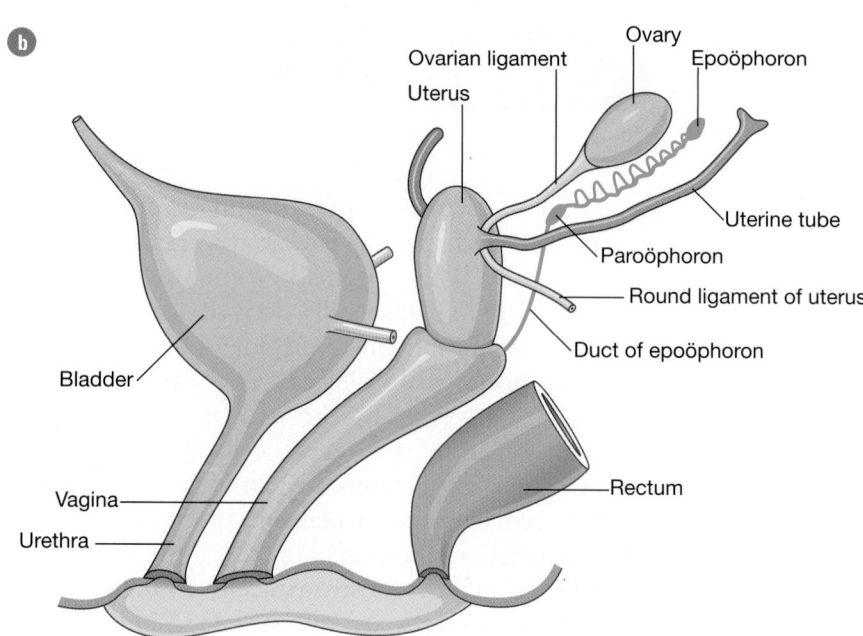

Ovary

Ovarian ligament

Epoöphoron

Uterus

Uterine tube

Paroöphoron

Round ligament of uterus

Duct of epoöphoron

Bladder

Vagina

Rectum

Urethra

ovary at this point. In the center, a gradually increasing population of enlarged oocytes is seen and these cells display strong nuclear staining for p63 (Fig. 1.6c). Between week 20 and term, the percentage of germ cells staining for Oct 4 progressively declines at the periphery and, as germ cells decline in number, a progressively increasing proportion become p63-positive.

Postnatally, all identifiable oocytes show intense p63 nuclear positivity (Fig. 1.6d).

The above sequence of immunostaining patterns is consistent with the role of Oct 4 in maintaining primordial germ cells through the proliferative phase in the first two trimesters of pregnancy. Unknown factors result in programmed cell death of a large

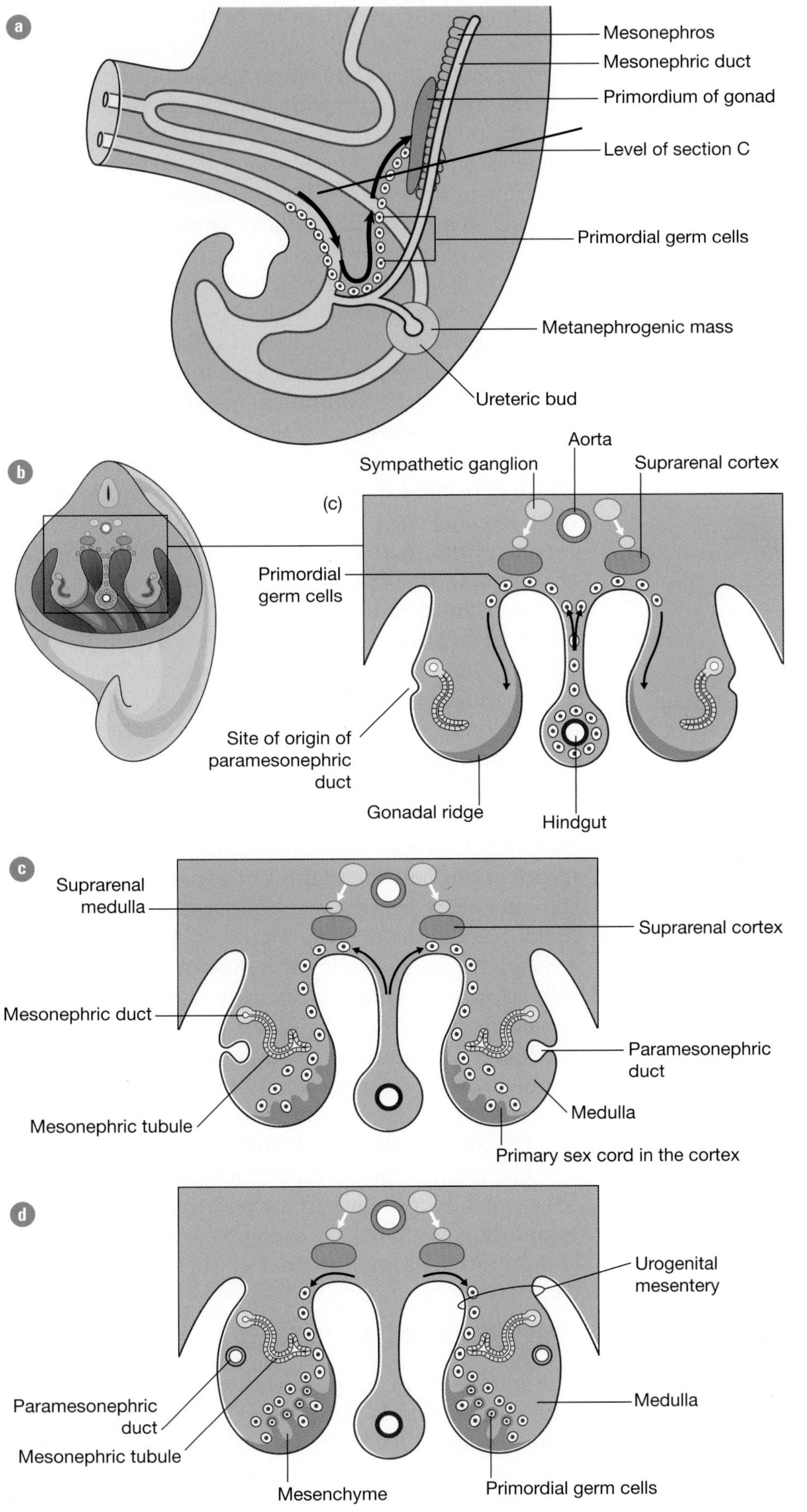

a

Mesonephros

Mesonephric duct

Primordium of gonad

Level of section C

Primordial germ cells

Metanephrogenic mass

Ureteric bud

Fig. 1.3 Development of the genital ridge and early ovarian development. (Redrawn from Moore.[9])

b

(c)

Aorta

Sympathetic ganglion

Suprarenal cortex

Primordial germ cells

Site of origin of paramesonephric duct

Gonadal ridge

Hindgut

c

Suprarenal medulla

Suprarenal cortex

Mesonephric duct

Paramesonephric duct

Mesonephric tubule

Medulla

Primary sex cord in the cortex

d

Urogenital mesentery

Paramesonephric duct

Medulla

Mesonephric tubule

Mesenchyme

Primordial germ cells

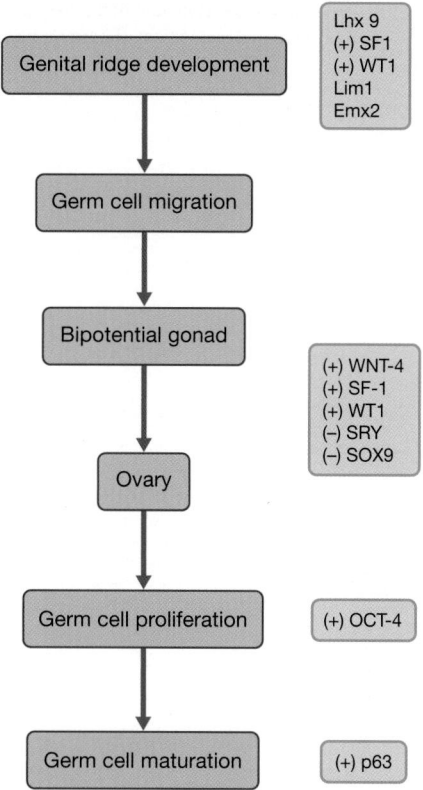

Fig. 1.4 Schematic of genes involved in forming the genital ridge, gonadal development and sex determination.

number of the remaining germ cells in the last trimester. The preservation of a discrete subset is coincident with the expression of p63, which is expressed subsequently throughout the life of the oocyte in the ovarian cortex.

The above process is under control of several genes at critical points. Expression of Lhx9 appears necessary for the development of the supporting stroma. In mouse models lacking this gene, germ cell migration is normal but the somatic cells of the genital ridge fail to proliferate, with failure of gonad formation.[15–18] Lhx9 mutants do not display other disorders, making this gene an attractive candidate for isolated gonadal dysgenesis. However, mutations in this gene have yet to be identified in humans.[19]

Maintenance of the germ cells in the ovary is dependent on an intact X chromosome. X chromosomal abnormalities are associated with accelerated follicular atresia. These include deletions of Xp11, Xq13 and specific genes such as Zfxa and Dazla.[20]

THE UTERUS AND VAGINA

Concurrent with the formation of the genital ridge and germ cell migration during the 4th week is an

infolding of the mesenchyme of the genital ridges to form columns that will become the paramesonephric (Müllerian) ducts. The columns, which extend caudally toward the cloacal opening, cavitate by the 5th week of gestation to form ducts. Cranially, the paramesonephric ducts lie lateral to the mesonephric (Wolffian) ducts; caudally their paths cross the mesonephric ducts ventrolaterally to meet in the midline, where they fuse by the 8th week of gestation. Following this midline fusion, the ducts merge and cavitate to form the uterovaginal cavity. The more caudal vaginal portion remains solid and merges with an ingrowth of solid endoderm from the urogenital sinus. These solid formations undergo canalization by the 20th week, with the hymen demarcating the junction of paramesonephric (cephalad) and endodermal (caudad) tissue origins. The vagina, which is derived from the distal end of the Müllerian duct, is flanked at its superior pole by recesses of mesonephric duct origin, which will eventually form the vaginal fornices (Fig. 1.7).

The eventual epithelialization of the vagina and cervix could be explained by two theories. The first would resolve the presence of squamous mucosa by the ingrowth of squamous epithelium from the introitus. The second holds that the squamous mucosa of the vagina and cervix emerges via induction of basal cells in the Müllerian epithelium of the cervix and vagina. This latter hypothesis is supported by several lines of evidence.[21,22] First, p63 expression is seen in the full length of not only the vagina but also the urethra during this interval, indicating that both urothelium and squamous epithelium develop via the same process (Fig. 1.8a–c). Secondly, while the newborn human vagina is fully covered by squamous epithelium, the vagina of the newborn mouse is lined by mucous-secreting endocervical-type columnar epithelium beneath which lies a single row of reserve cells. With the onset of estrus, the reserve cells expand and undergo squamous differentiation, after which the vagina is permanently lined by mature squamous epithelium. This process of basal cell induction fails in the p63-null mouse and the vagina remains lined by a combination of Müllerian and primitive urogenital sinus epithelium.[21]

THE EXTERNAL GENITALIA

The hindgut and urogenital sinus open into a common cloaca prior to the 7th week of gestation. At this point a ridge of mesenchyme – the urorectal septum – migrates caudad toward the cloacal membrane and separates the genitourinary system from the rectum.

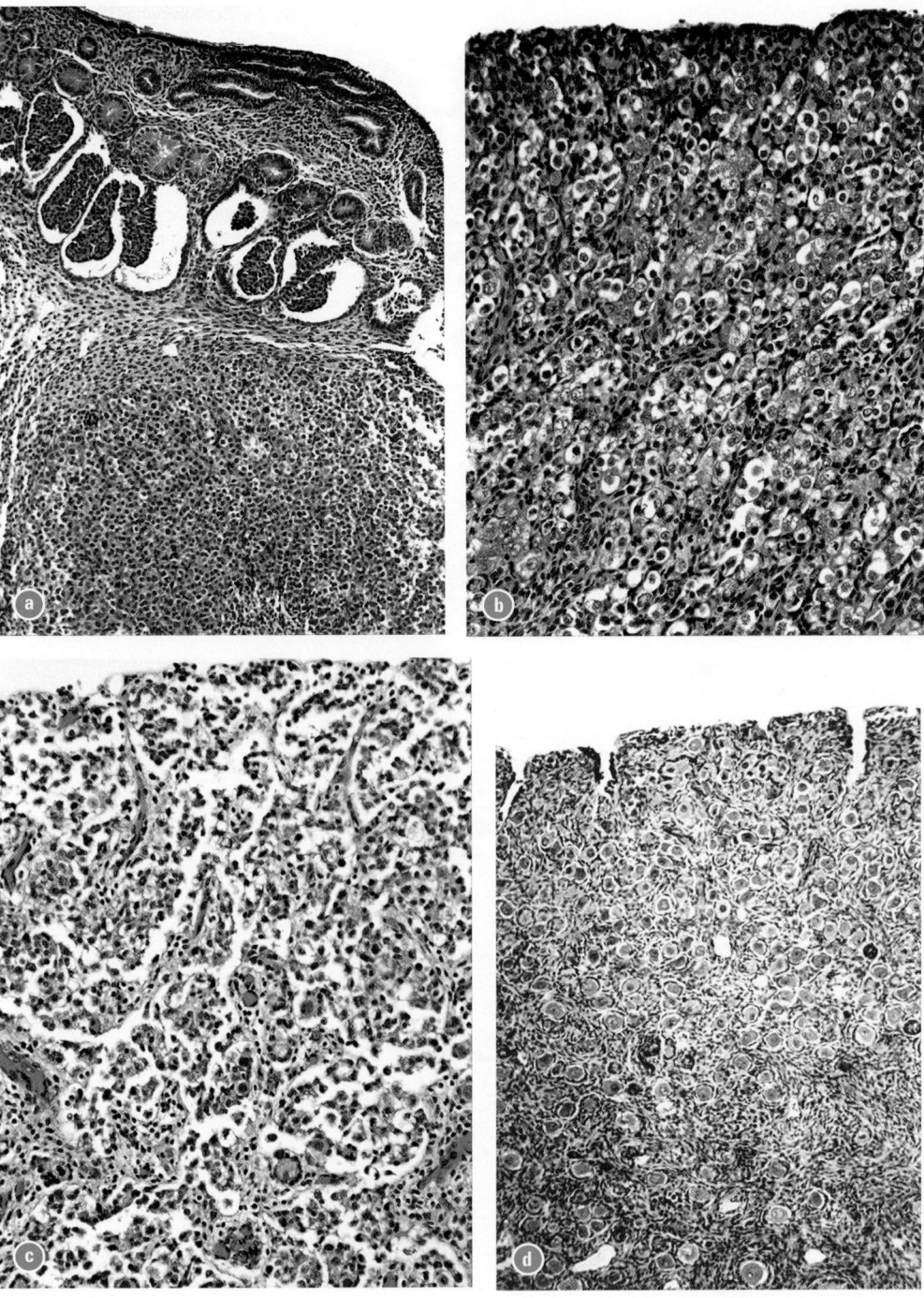

Fig. 1.5 Human ovarian development. (a) Indifferent gonad at 6 weeks with primitive germ cells (lower). The metanephros is above. (b) Germ cells at 19 weeks. Primordial follicles are not yet conspicuous. (c) At 22 weeks a few primordial follicles are seen in the medulla. (d) At term, the cortex is filled with primordial follicles.

An external midline protuberance develops at this point – the genital tubercle – which is flanked dorsolaterally by the genital folds, which are in turn laterally cuffed by the labioscrotal swellings. The genital tubercle ultimately becomes the clitoris, the genital folds eventually form the labia minora and the labioscrotal swellings differentiate into the labia majora (Fig. 1.9).

The factors involved in the modeling of the external genitalia are multiple and involve sequential expression of regulatory genes and the induction of gene expression by specific epithelial-stromal interactions. The sonic hedgehog gene (Shh) has been shown to regulate genes expressed in mesenchyme, including patched 1 (Ptch1), bone morphogenetic protein (Bmp4), Hoxd13 and fibroblastic growth factor

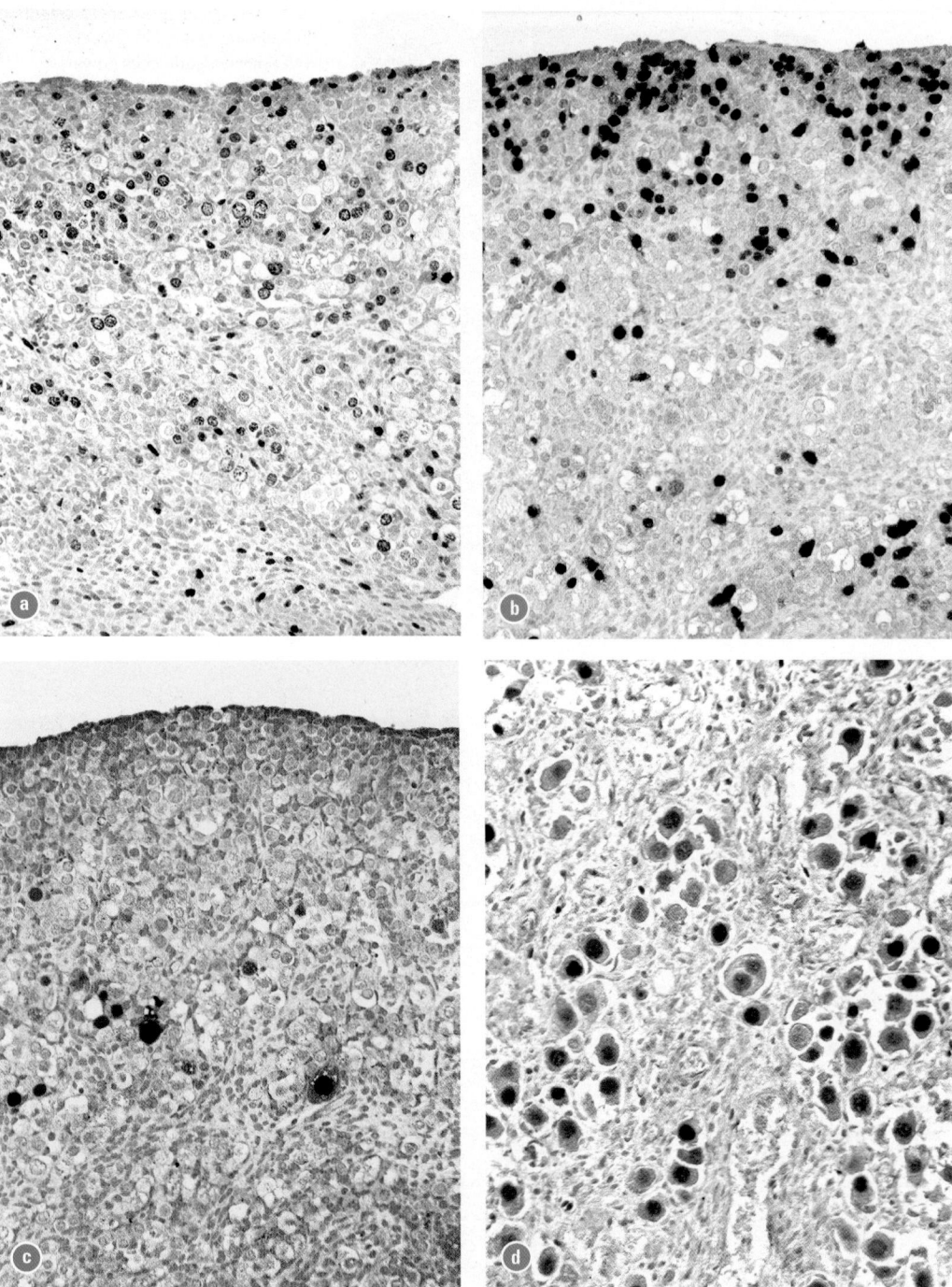

Fig. 1.6 Expression of Oct 3/4, Ki-67 and p63TA at 19 weeks gestation. (a) Ki-67 is expressed in both immature germ cells and stromal cells, predominately in the cortex. (b) Expression of Oct 4 predominates in the immature cortical germ cells. (c) Expression of p63TA is limited to the maturing oocytes in the primordial follicles. (d) At birth, p63TA identifies a high percentage of oocytes in the ovarian cortex. Ki-67 and Oct 3/4 are not expressed at this stage. (From McKeon F and Crum CP, unpublished.)

(Fgf10). Absence of Shh (in Shh-null mice) is associated with agenesis of the genital tubercle, increased cell death, reduced cell growth and an abnormal shift in expression of Bmp4 from the mesenchyme to the epithelium. Thus Shh is considered to increase both outgrowth and differentiation of the genital tubercle.[23] Predictably, maintenance of the mucocutaneous genital mucosal epithelium is critical to the development of the appropriate mesenchymal response. P63-null mice, which are devoid of skin and squamous mucosa, fail to complete the urorectal septum, exhibit abnormalities in both bladder and phallic development and are born with a common cloaca.[21] Humans with p63 mutations have defects in the growth of hair, teeth and distal limb development. They exhibit less conspicuous genital anomalies but exhibit genital hypoplasia, similar to that seen in external genitalia of the p63-null mouse. The conclusion from these models is that the integrity

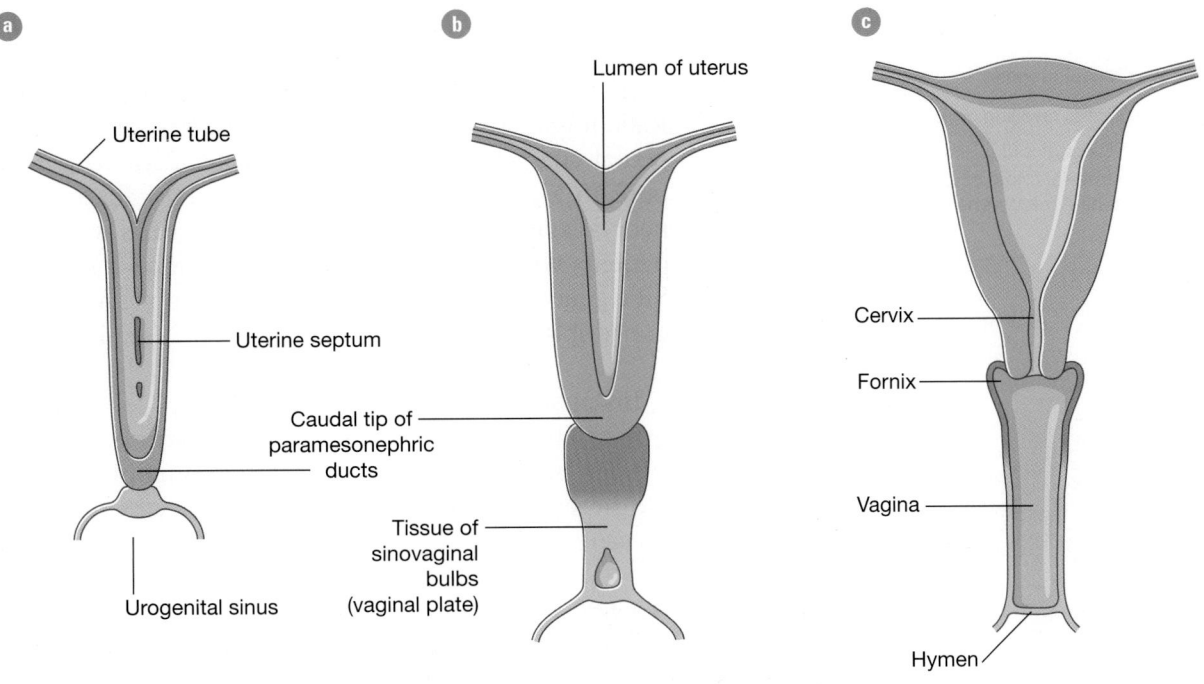

Fig. 1.7 Schematic of uterine and vaginal development. (Redrawn from Sadler,[1] with permission.)

of the squamous mucosa is also critical to normal caudal urogenital mesenchymal development.

The female genital phenotype was once considered a 'default' phenotype, resulting from the absence of

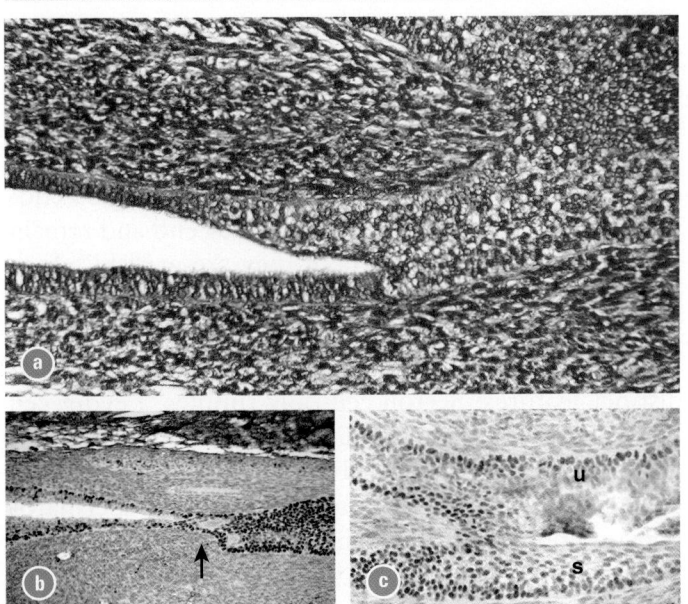

Fig. 1.8 (a) Junction of Müllerian (left) and vaginal squamous (right) epithelium in the mouse embryo. (b) p63 expression highlights the induction of squamous differentiation in the latter (right). (c) At high power both the urethra (upper left) and vagina (lower left and right) in the fetal mouse express p63 during urothelial(u) and squamous(s) differentiation, respectively.

interference by androgenic hormones despite inactivated estrogen receptor proteins or aromatases.[24,25] SRY, the sex-determining gene located on the short arm of the Y chromosome, is critical in gonadal sex differentiation, such that the absence of SRY confers or 'permits' female gonadal differentiation. However, current evidence also indicates generation of the female phenotype occurs actively, via autosomal genes such as WNT4 on chromosome 1p, which functions in the pathway of DAX-1, an X chromosome gene, to antagonize SRY expression.[26] Alternative pathways independent of the genetic gonadal regulation, as with *in utero* DES exposure, lead to inappropriate expression of estrogens, resulting in vaginal adenosis and structural malformations of the uterus and cervix.[27]

Common disorders of gonadal and genital tract development

OVARY AND FALLOPIAN TUBE

Developmental abnormalities

Developmental abnormalities of the fallopian tubes and ovaries arise via three mechanisms, including disturbances in Müllerian duct and gonadal development and abnormalities in the sex chromosomes.

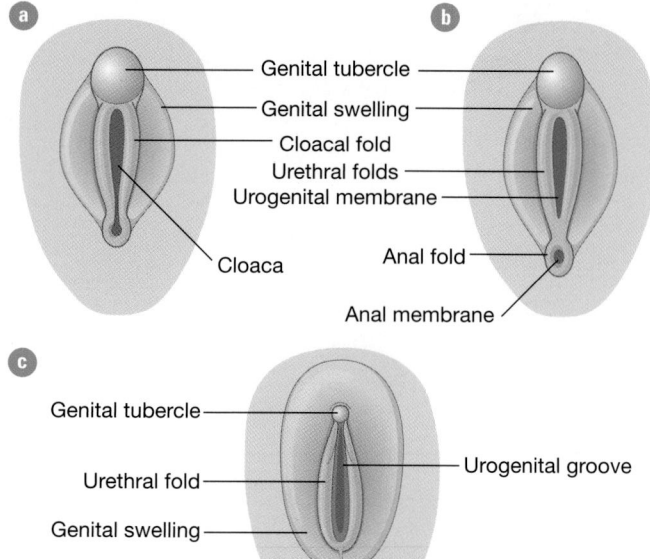

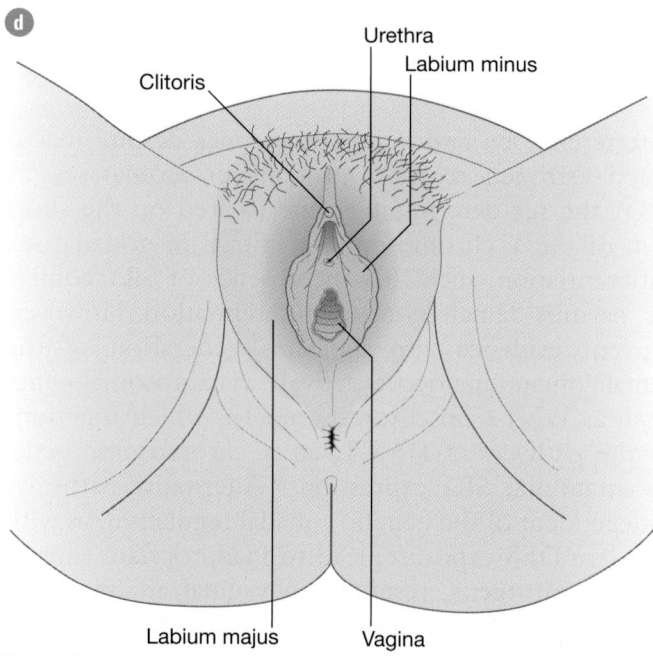

Fig. 1.9 Schematic of the development of the external genitalia. (a) Early development prior to completion of the urorectal septum. (b) Separation of the anus from the urogenital sinus lined by the urethral folds. (c) Development of the genital swelling. (d) Completion of the vagina, labia and clitoris.

Ovarian hypoplasia

Pathogenesis The classic example of ovarian hypoplasia is associated with Turner's syndrome (45,X karyotype, also designated 45,XO or monosomy X). The primordial germ cells make their way to the genital ridge but fail to induce follicle development and degenerate, producing an ovary with no germ cells by 6 months of age. Because the Y chromosome is absent, normal genito-uterine development takes place. However, because the ovary is not capable of promoting folliculogenesis and producing estrogens, the external sexual characteristics remain infantile. Patients with a pure 45,X genotype are not at increased risk for gonadal neoplasia; it is the phenotypic female Turner's syndrome patients with a Y chromosome constitution harboring SRY gene who are at risk for gonadal neoplasia, namely gonadoblastoma and later, dysgerminoma (seminoma).[28]

Histopathology The typical XO ovary is a streak ovary. The ovary is small and consists principally of a small amount of cortical stroma containing a few indifferent sex cord structures. Oocytes are not present (Fig. 1.10a–c).

Agenesis and dysgenesis of the ovary

Pathogenesis This disorder is not associated with a chromosomal anomaly; patients are thus karyotypically normal (46,XX). The primordial germ cells neither develop nor migrate and the gonad does not develop. Maternal–placental estrogens complete the development of the external genitalia and the Müllerian ducts, but none of the features of Turner's syndrome are seen.

Histopathology The ovaries are indistinguishable from the Turner ovarian histologic phenotype.

Testicular feminization syndrome

Pathogenesis These patients have a normal 46,XY male karyotype, do not respond to testosterone and externally are phenotypically female. However, the paramesonephric duct system is suppressed, uterine development is blunted or absent and the vagina ends in a blind pouch. The testes do not descend and remain in the inguinal region, where they are at risk, which increases over time, of germ cell tumorigenesis.[29]

Histopathology The testes may exhibit at least four distinct features: Sertoli cell-only tubules, Leydig cell hyperplasia, nodular Sertoli cell masses and germ cell atypia/neoplasia (Figs 1.11–1.13). The 'background' pattern consists of Sertoli tubules devoid of spermatogonia, admixed with abundant Leydig cells (Fig. 1.12a,b). Within this background, discrete nodular masses of Sertoli tubules are often seen, which are variably and inconclusively described as hyperplastic, neoplastic, or hamartomatous (Fig. 1.11). Scattered enlarged, hyperchromatic intratubular germ cells may be present, with positive immunostaining for placental alkaline

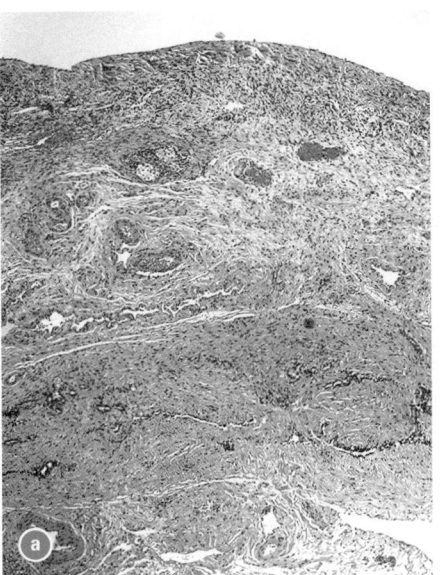 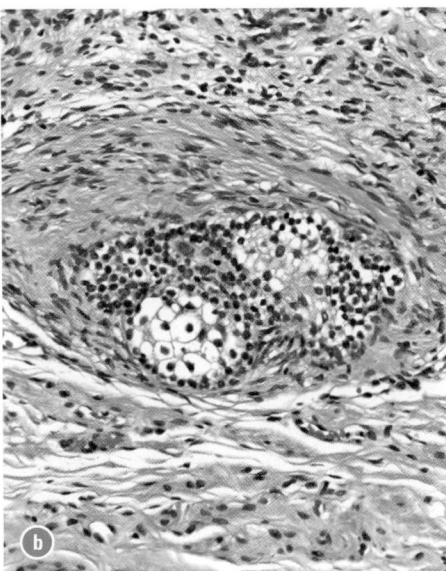 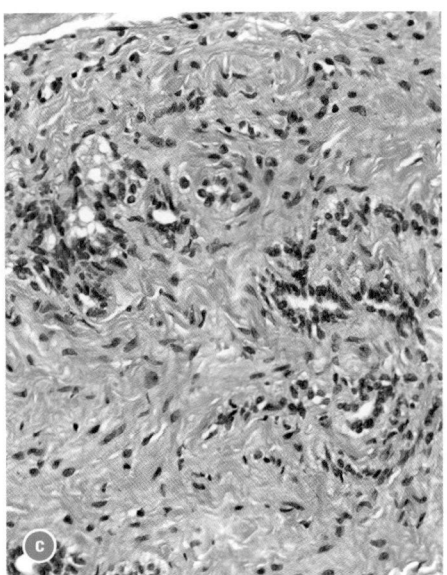

Fig. 1.10 Streak gonad from an XO genotype. (a) Rudimentary cortex with (b) focal islands of sex cord derivatives. (c) Attenuated Wolffian remnants.

phosphatase (Fig. 1.13a–c), suggesting early germ cell neoplasia (gonadoblastoma) that may evolve to or be associated with germ cell tumors, particularly seminoma.[30]

Abnormalities in sex determination (disorders of intersex)[31,32]

Hermaphrodites and pseudohermaphrodites (Table 1.2). By definition, true hermaphrodites have external

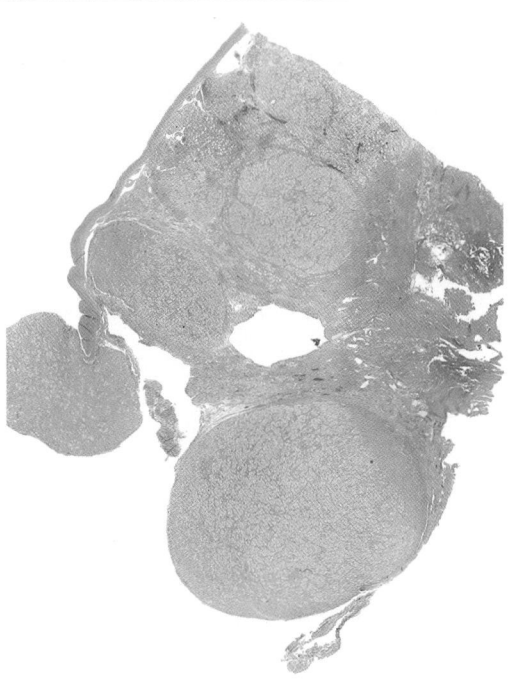

Fig. 1.11 Testis from a case of testicular feminization syndrome, containing nodular masses of Sertoli tubules.

Table 1.2 Ambiguous genitalia and their causes

Female pseudohermaphrodism
  Congenital adrenal hyperplasia (excess fetal androgens)
    21 hydroxylase deficiency
    11β-hydroxylase deficiency
    3β-hydroxysteroid dehydrogenase deficiency
  Exogenous androgens
    Maternal ingestion of androgens, progestogens
    Maternal congenital adrenal hyperplasia
    Virilizing adrenal or ovarian tumor
  Excess placental androgen production
    Placental P450 aromatase deficiency
  Iatrogenic fetal virilization
  Female pseudohermaphrodism with associated congenital malformations
  Idiopathic
Male pseudohermaphrodism
  Impaired Leydig cell activity
    Defects in testosterone biosynthesis
    Leydig cell hypoplasia; LH receptor defect
    20,22-desmolase (congenital lipoid adrenal hyperplasia)
    3β-hydroxysteroid dehydrogenase
    17,20-hydroxlyase (17,20-desmolase)
    17β-hydroxysteroid dehydrogenase (17-ketosteroid reductase)
  Defects of testis development or maintenance
    XY gonadal dysgenesis
    Mixed gonadal dysgenesis
    Rudimentary testis syndromes
  End-organ resistance to androgens (androgen insensitivity syndrome)
    Complete
    Partial
    Defects in the intracellular metabolism of testosterone (5α-reductase deficiency)
  Others
    Persistent Müllerian duct syndrome
    Iatrogenic male pseudohermaphrodism
    Idiopathic male pseudohermaphrodism
    True hermaphrodism

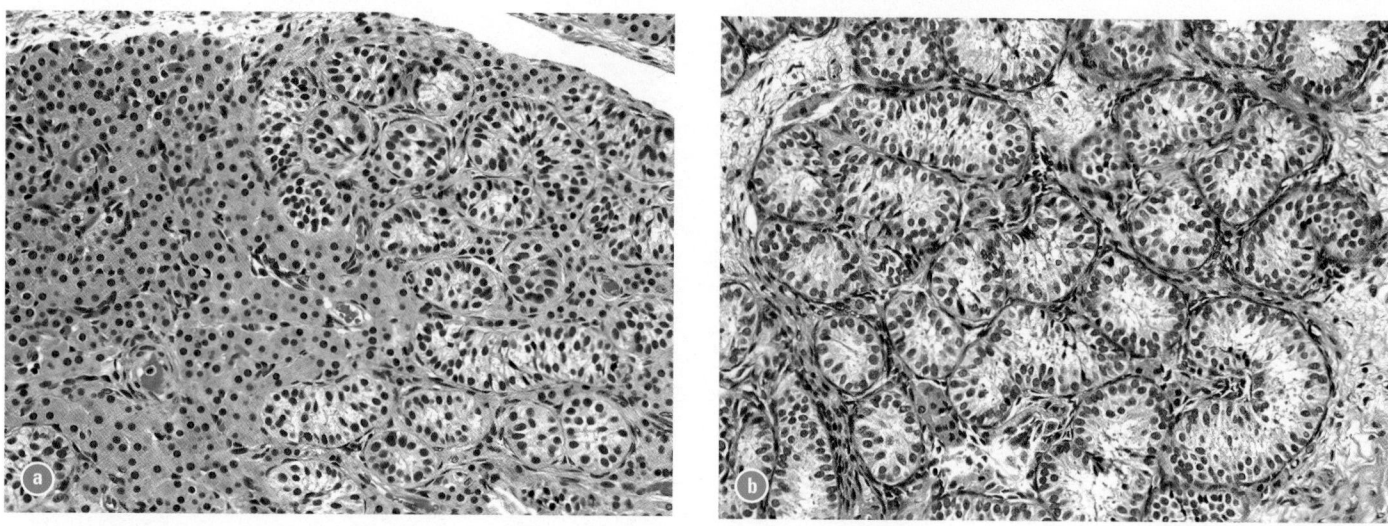

Fig. 1.12 Testicular feminization syndrome. (a) Mixture of Sertoli tubules (right) and Leydig cell hyperplasia (left). (b) Pure Sertoli cell differentiation within a discrete nodule.

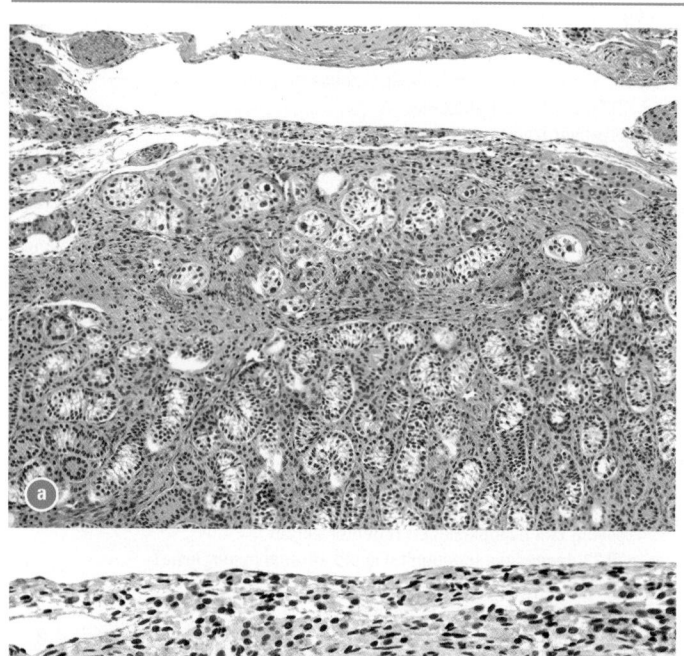

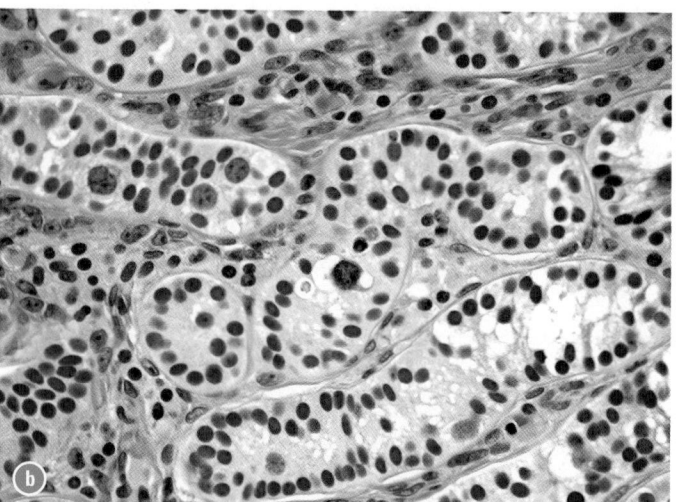

Fig. 1.13 Testicular feminization syndrome with germ cells. (a) Focus of germ cells with atypia (gonadoblastoma; upper) adjacent to uninvolved Sertoli tubules (lower). (b) Discrete nuclear enlargement in the Sertoli tubules characterizes germ cell differentiation (c) Following staining for placental alkaline phosphatase.

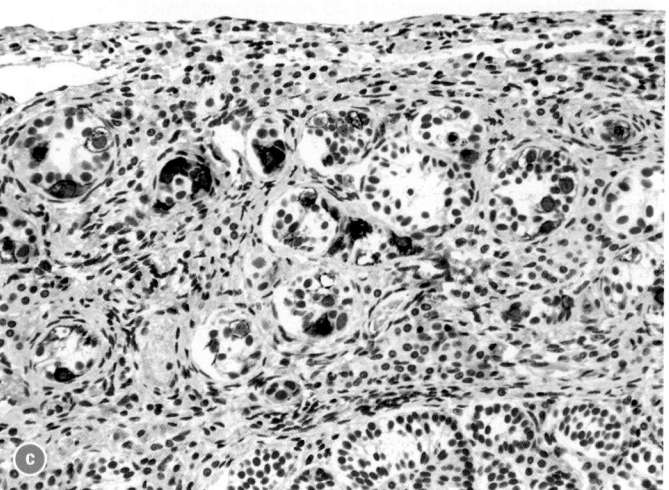

genitalia and gonads of both sexes, whereas pseudo-hermaphrodites have either ovaries or testes and exhibit a genital organ phenotype that belies the genetic sex. Hermaphrodites are much rarer and present with one of the following types of gonad(s): bilateral ovotestes, an ovotestis paired with an ovary or testis and a unilateral ovary/contralateral testis. The diagnosis of hermaphroditism is based entirely on the gonads; the sexual organ phenotype is variable and ranges from entirely female (Bergman type 1) to entirely male (type 5). Intermediate phenotypes characterize ambiguous genitalia.

The gonads of hermaphrodites vary widely in their appearance. Ovary and testis may be juxtaposed, or admixed in a single organ, the latter represented by Sertoli cells arranged in tubules within an ovarian cortex, accompanied by Leydig cells and Wolffian remnants (Fig. 1.14a–c). In general, the ovary is more prominent and Graafian follicles with corpora lutea may develop. In contrast, the testicular tissue is usually less developed, and spermatogenesis is rare. However, based on external phenotype, two-thirds of true hermaphrodites are raised as males, despite the presence of an XX karyotype in at least one-half.

Pseudohermaphrodites exhibit ambiguous genitalia and possess one type of gonad, either testis (male pseudohermaphrodite) or ovary (female pseudo-hermaphrodite). Examples of the latter include adrenogenital syndrome, in which genotypically female (46,XX) individuals present with masculinized external genitalia ranging from clitoral hypertrophy to labial fusion. Male pseudohermaphrodites have a male genotype (46,XY) and variably feminized external sex characteristics depending on the strength of androgenic hormone stimulation. Types of ambiguous genitalia are illustrated in Figure 1.15, the differential diagnosis is outlined in Figure 1.16 and an example of a male pseudohermaphrodite is shown in Figure 1.17.[33,34]

Acquired disorders of childhood associated with gonadal abnormalities

Precocious puberty

Precocious puberty is defined as acquisition of the following characteristics at 8 years of age or younger: (a) breast development, (b) pubic or axillary hair, (c) onset of menstruation, (d) acne and (e) body odor. The incidence is between one and five per 10 000 children.[35,36]

Precocious puberty can be stratified into the following etiologic categories: gonadotropin-dependent, gonadotropin-independent and the consequence of estrogen ingestion (precocious pseudopuberty). Gonadotropin-dependent precocious puberty in young girls is largely idiopathic (95%), associated with premature activation of gonadotropin releasing hormone (GnRH) pulse generator in the hypothalamus, result-

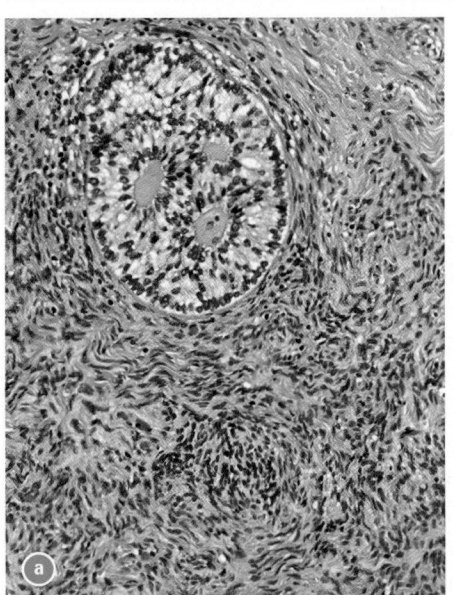 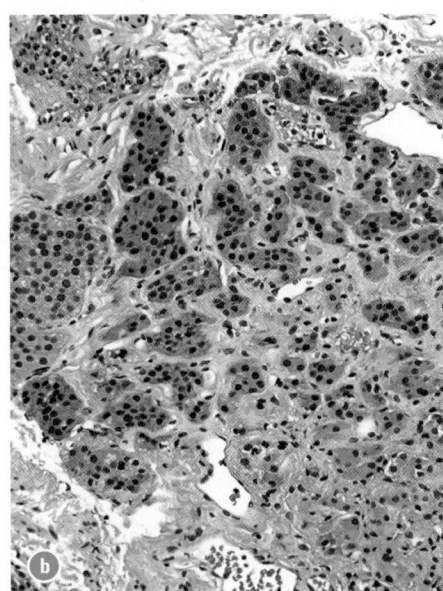 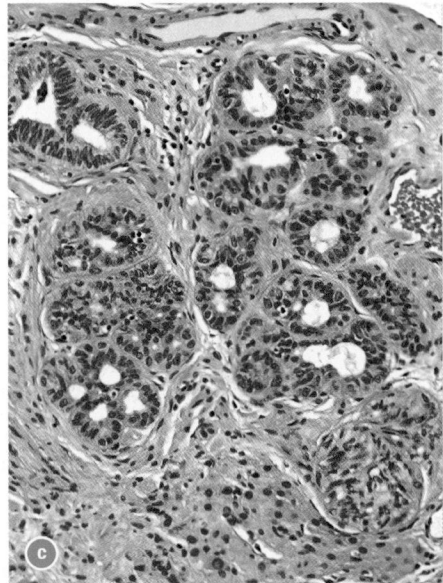

Fig. 1.14 Gonad from a true hermaphrodite. (a) Sertoli cell differentiation is present within ovarian cortical stroma. (b) Leydig cell hyperplasia in the ovarian hilus. (c) Well-developed Wolffian remnants.

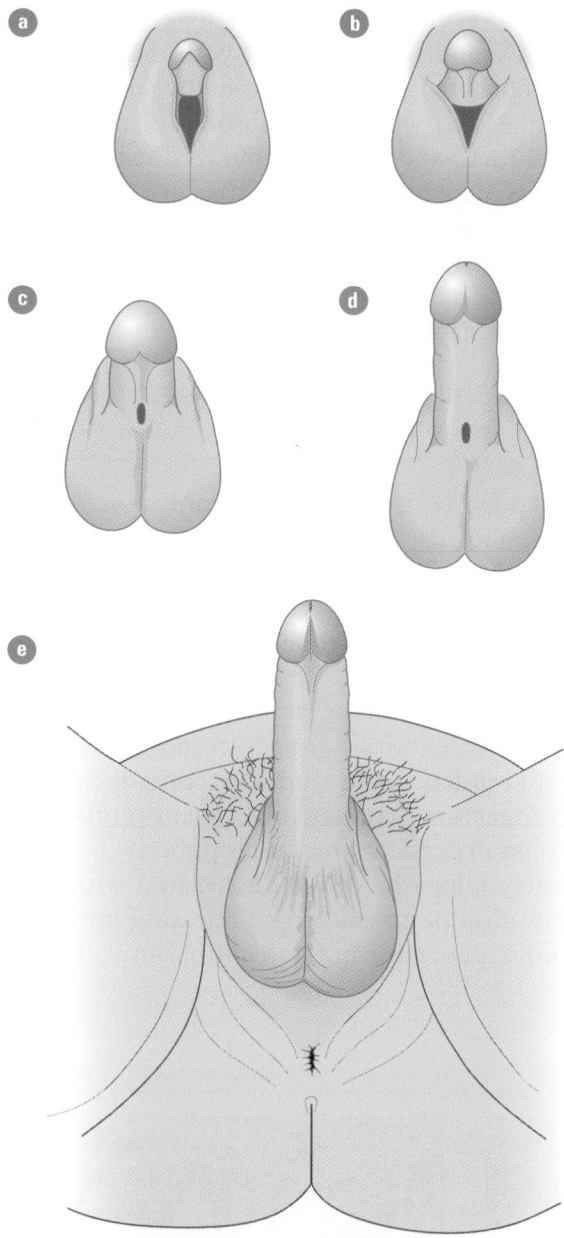

Fig. 1.15 Five stages of ambiguous genitalia, comprising (a) clitoromegaly, (b) clitoromegaly with labial fusion, (c) further phallic enlargement with complete labioscrotal fusion and urogenital sinus, (d) complete scrotal fusion with urogenital sinus at the base of the phallus and (e) normal male genitalia.[33] (Redrawn from *Neonatal Handbook*, copyright 1999 Lippincott, Williams and Wilkins.[34])

ing in pituitary hormone release of follicle stimulating hormone and luteinizing hormones.[34] Less commonly, a range of central nervous system disorders or tumors will initiate premature GnRH secretion. Rarely, gonadotropin-dependent precocious puberty will be triggered following treatment for a sex steroid-producing tumor, with GnRH release initiated as hormone levels fall.

Hormone-producing ovarian neoplasms play a role in gonadotropin-independent precocious puberty, also termed 'pseudopuberty'. These are summarized in Table 1.3 and include the full range of sex steroid- and gonadotropin-producing tumors. Other mechanisms include adrenal cortical tumors and exogenous ingestion of estrogens. The significance of repetitive low levels of exposure to internalized estrogens in accelerating puberty, such as occur in food or other topically applied products, is controversial but supported by epidemiologic studies.

Ovarian neoplasia

Ovarian masses in children are generally benign (Tables 1.4 and 1.5). In a study of 134 records, over 60% were benign functional cysts. Neoplasms were more likely for tumors exceeding 10 cm. Most tumors are germ cell tumors (about two-thirds).[37,38] In one study, 27 of 44 pediatric ovarian tumors were benign cystic teratomas; another six were malignant germ cell tumors.[39] Considered alternatively, a significant percentage of ovarian tumors developing in the pediatric age group are malignant. In a study of 67 tumors, Schultz et al. found 55% were malignant.[40]

Germ cell tumors occurring in infancy are typically extragonadal, whereas after puberty the overwhelming majority are of gonadal origin.[41] A minority of ovarian tumors in children are epithelial (16%). Of these, most are benign or borderline cystadenomas. A few mucinous cystadenocarcinomas have been reported.[36]

UTERUS AND CERVIX

Developmental anomalies

Uterine maldevelopment is subdivided into seven categories, which yield a wide spectrum of anomalies (Fig. 1.18).

Hypoplasia/agenesis

This is a profound anomaly characterized by absence or hypoplasia of Müllerian duct development, which influences the entire genital tract, from vagina to fallopian tubes, with varying severity. Typically, coexisting urinary tract anomalies are present, due to the proximity of the urogenital sinus to the Müllerian and mesonephric ducts.

Unicornuate uterus

This results from the failure of one of the Müllerian ducts to form, resulting in a single uterine tube. However, in about two-thirds of affected females, a rudi-

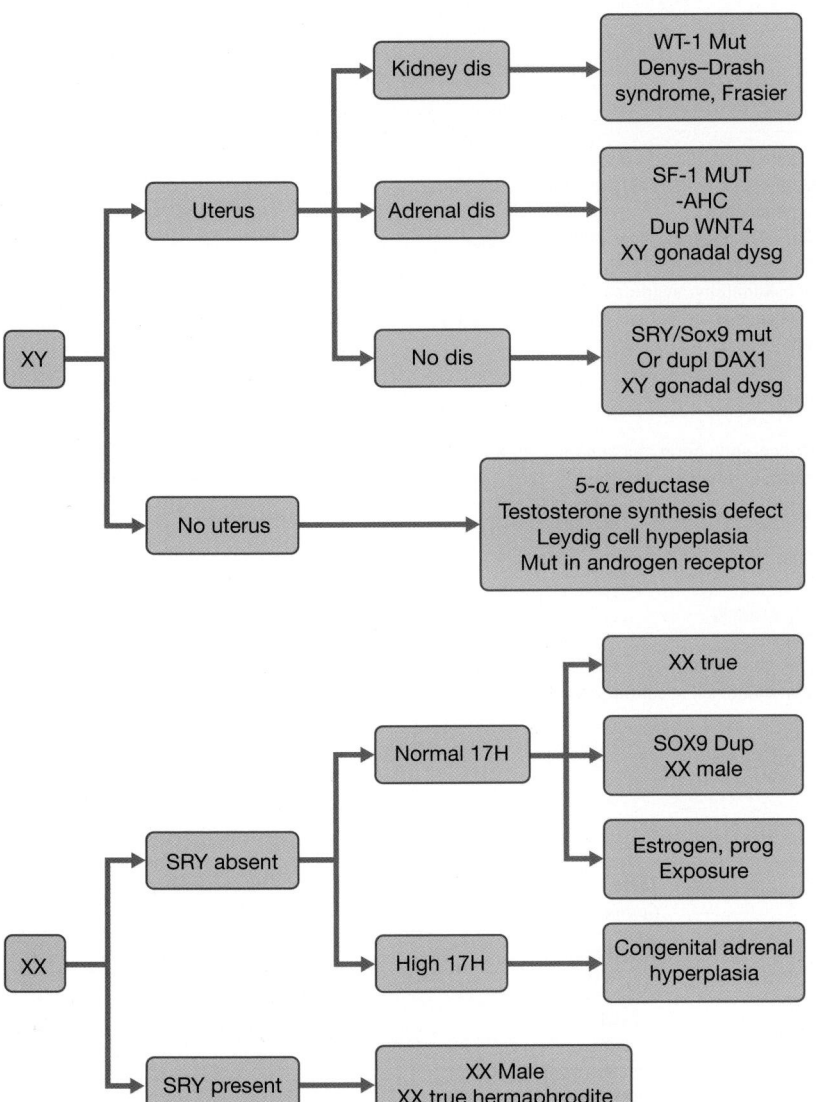

Fig. 1.16 Schematic of the differential diagnosis of intersex. (From Dewing et al, copyright 2002 Thieme Medical Publishers.[36])

mentary horn emerges from the maldeveloped Müllerian duct. The latter may be incompletely cavitated or obstructed, resulting in episodic pain during menstruation. The most serious sequela is embryo implantation and growth resulting in uterine rupture, which occurs in 90% of pregnancies involving the abnormal horn (Fig. 1.19).[42]

Uterus didelphys

A didelphic uterus is the consequence of failed Müllerian duct fusion. The resulting horns may or may not share a common cervix (Fig. 1.20). In the majority of cases, paired cervices continue into a septate vagina.

Bicornuate uterus

Bicornuate uterus is the most common anomaly, comprising nearly one-half of congenital uterine defects. Failure of Müllerian duct fusion at the apex of the uterus results in two uterine horns terminating in a single cervix. The degree of division will vary. In some defects, two separate uterine horns fuse at the cervix; in others, the caudal portion of the uterus forms a single lumen, which branches into horns near the fundus.

Septate uterus

In a septate uterus, the Müllerian ducts fuse but the septum created by apposition of the two ducts fails to

Table 1.3 *Causes of precocious puberty*

Gonadotropin-dependent
  Idiopathic (95%)
  Familial (rare)
  Central nervous system disorders — Inflammatory, infectious, radiation, chemotherapy, trauma
  Central nervous system tumors — Hypothalamic hamartoma, gliomas, craniopharyngioma, ependymoma, LH-secreting adenoma, pinealoma
  Congenital malformations — Arachnoid cyst, suprasellar cyst, phakomatosis, hydrocephalus, septo-optic dysplasia
  Dysmorphic syndromes — Williams–Beuren syndrome, Klinefelter syndrome
  CNS 'priming' by peripheral — Congenital adrenal hyperplasia, sex steroid sex hormone producing disorder producing tumor
Gonadotropin-independent
  Ovarian disorders — Granulosa-theca cell tumors
    Theca cell tumor
    Estrogen- or gonadotropin-secreting germ cell tumors (dysgerminoma, choriocarcinoma, teratoma, embryonal carcinoma)
    Steroid-producing tumors
    SCTAT
    McCune–Albright syndrome
  Other neoplasms — Adrenal adenoma
    Adrenal carcinoma (usually virilizing)
    Congenital adrenal hyperplasia
    Pinealoma, hepatoblastoma, choriocarcinoma, teratoma (HCG)
  Exogenous source — Steroid-producing pills, food additives, cosmetic creams
  Transient — Transient follicle cysts

Adapted from Partsch and Sippell.[35]

Table 1.4 *Causes of ovarian masses in children*

Type	Number	(%)
Functional cyst	81	60.4
Neoplastic	44	32.8
Benign cystic teratoma	27	
Malignant germ cell tumor	5	
Epithelial neoplasm	6	
Other	9	
Total	134	

From de Silva et al.[39]

Table 1.5 *Primary ovarian tumors treated at Children's Hospital Medical Center (1928–1982)*

Classification	Number	(%)
Mature cystic teratoma	78	47
Cystic	76	
Solid	2	
Common epithelial tumors	27	16
Mucinous	12	
Serous	14	
Mixed	1	
Sex-cord stromal tumors	21	13
Granulosa cell	10	
Thecoma	2	
Fibroma	1	
Sertoli–Leydig	7	
Unclassified	1	
Immature teratoma	17	10
Yolk sac carcinoma	14	8
Dysgerminoma	8	5
Choriocarcinoma	1	–
Total	166	100

From Lack and Goldstein.[38]

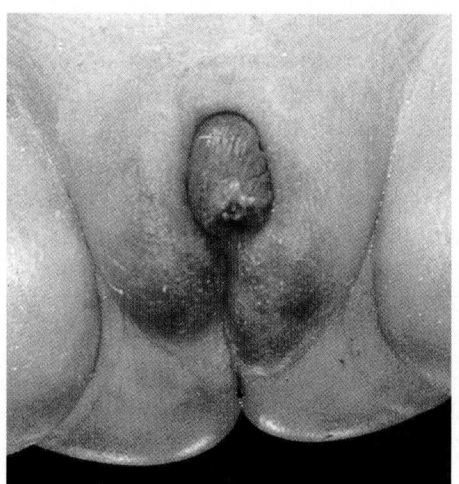

Fig. 1.17 Ambiguous genitalia in a neonate. This phenotype depicts a micropenis with partially fused labioscrotal folds associated with an XY genotype.

degenerate. The degree of septal persistence determines whether the septum is partial or complete.

Arcuate uterus

The arcuate uterus is essentially normal in shape with a small, midline indentation in the uterine fundus,

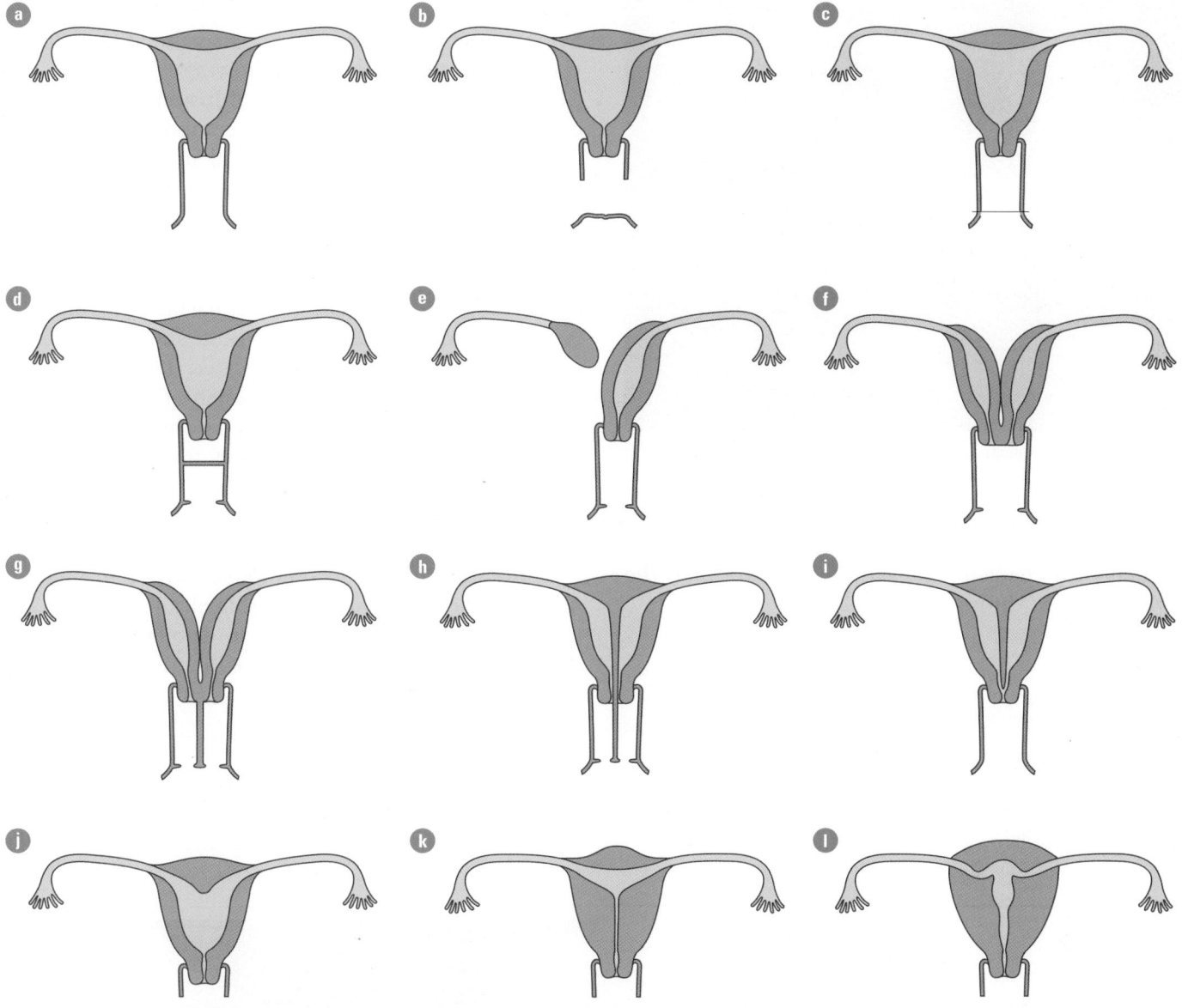

Fig. 1.18 Schematic of abnormal uterine development. (a) Normal anatomy. (b) Vaginal agenesis. (c) Imperforate hymen. (d) Transverse vaginal septum. (e) Unicornuate uterus with rudimentary horn. (f) Uterus didelphys with common vagina. (g) Uterine didelphys with septate vagina. (h) Complete septation of uterus and vagina. (i) Septate uterus. (j) Arcuate uterus. (k) T-shaped uterus in DES exposure. (l) T-shaped uterus with dilatation of horns in DES exposure. (Redrawn from Laufer et al.,[44] with permission.)

which results from failure to completely dissolve the median septum. This is given a distinct classification because it does not seem to have any untoward effects on pregnancy.[43]

Diethylstilbestrol

The cervicovaginal abnormalities seen with DES are discussed below. Two-thirds of daughters of mothers exposed to DES have abnormalities in uterine development, including generalized uterine hypoplasia, an irregular T-shaped uterine cavity and, in 50% of exposed women, an incompletely formed cervix. The major consequence of uterine anomalies is impairment of normal pregnancy.[44] For DES-exposed women with three or more consecutive pregnancy losses, the likelihood of having a uterine anomaly is 8–10%.[45]

Acquired disorders of childhood

In the absence of congenital anatomic defects and botryoid embryonal rhabdomyosarcomas, there are

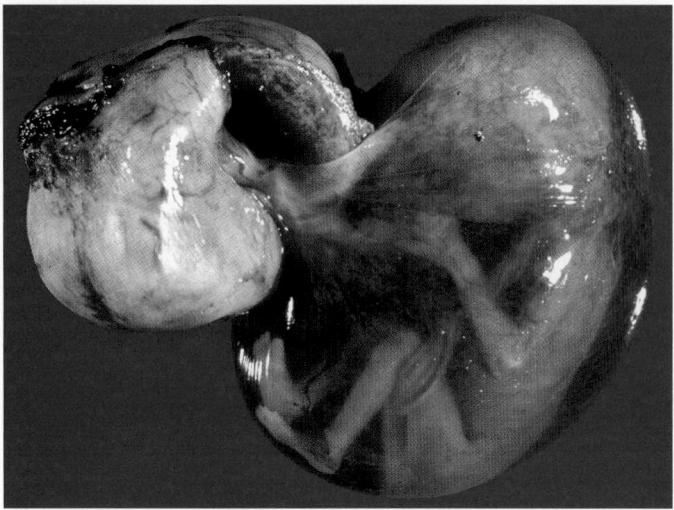

Fig. 1.19 Rupture of a unicornuate uterus during pregnancy.

essentially no characteristic acquired disorders of the uterus or cervix during childhood.

VAGINA

Developmental anomalies

Absent vagina

Vaginal agenesis, presumably due to absence of Müllerian duct formation, is a rare disorder that is often associated with absence of the cervix and uterus.[46]

Septate vagina

Septate vaginal abnormalities are assumed to develop via failure of cavitation following fusion of the Müllerian ducts. Theoretically, if fusion proceeds in a caudal to cephalad direction, combined anomalies, such as duplicated uterine, cervical and vaginal canals, should be most severe when the vagina is involved.[47] More recent studies have described exceptions to this rule and have postulated that Müllerian duct fusion initiates in the region of the uterus, with cavitation proceeding both caudally and cephalad to this site.[48–50] A duplicated vaginal canal almost always occurs in conjunction with other duplicated (septate) lower Müllerian tract derivatives, namely the cervix and uterus. Some disorders, such as trisomy 13, are associated with failed Müllerian duct fusion, leading to septate or duplicated internal Müllerian duct structures.

Imperforate hymen

Imperforate hymen is uncommon, occurring in approximately 1 per 1000 newborn females. It is typically sporadic, but has been seen in families with both dominant and recessive modes of inheritance; multiple genes may thus be involved.[51,52]

Adenosis

Vaginal adenosis, an abnormal proliferation or perhaps persistence of mucus-secreting cervicovaginal glands, has been reported exclusively in the setting of DES

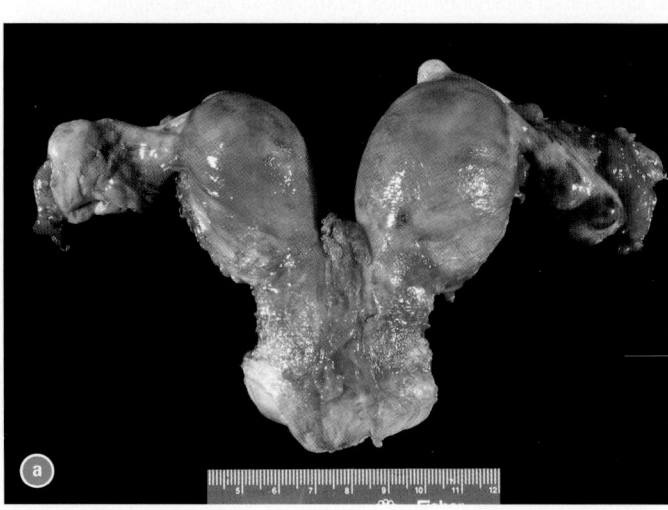

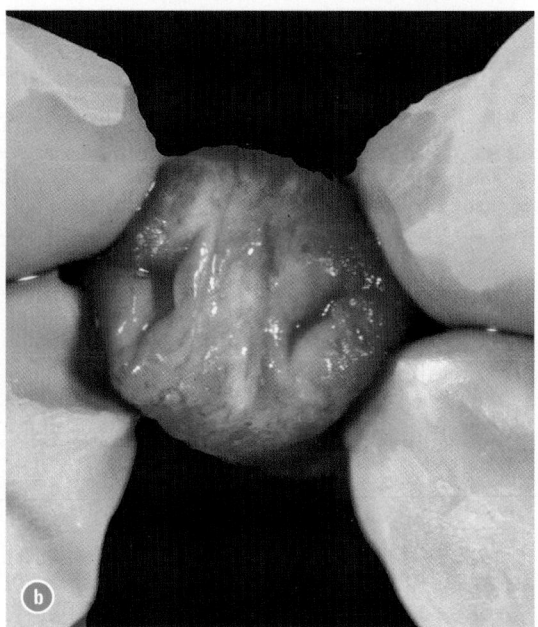

Fig. 1.20 (a) Uterus didelphys, associated with a double cervix and single vagina. (b) Double cervix.

exposure *in utero*. Recent experimental evidence indicates that, under normal circumstances, p63 induces cervicovaginal epithelium to undergo differentiation to a squamous phenotype. Under the experimental influence of DES, p63 induction is suppressed, resulting in a columnar (i.e. persistent uterine) cervicovaginal phenotype.[20] Mechanism(s) which then promulgate progression of adenotic epithelium to neoplasia require subsequent molecular events, since not all DES-exposed women with vaginal adenosis will progress to adenocarcinoma.

Acquired vaginal disorders of childhood

1 Genital warts (see Ch. 6)
2 Neoplasms:
  a Müllerian papilloma[53–55] (see also Ch. 12)
  b Yolk sac carcinoma[56–58] (see Ch. 12)
  c Embryonal rhabdomyosarcoma (see Ch. 11)
  d Clear cell carcinoma (see Ch. 12).

OTHER LOWER GENITAL TRACT AND VULVAR ANOMALIES

Developmental anomalies

Ambiguous genitalia

The most common reported external genital anomaly of either gender is hypospadias, seen in 1:125 live male births.[59] With the exception of ambiguous genitalia, developmental anomalies of the vulva are rare. Ambiguous genitalia are probably most frequently seen in congenital adrenal hyperplasia, an autosomal recessive adrenal and gonadal steroidogenic pathway defect due to a deficiency of 17-alpha-hydroxylase, mapped to gene locus 10q24.3.[60] However, ambiguous genitalia can also occur as a component of multiple malformation syndromes of varying etiologies. In the majority of these cases, the molecular pathway(s) resulting in ambiguous genitalia are unknown.

Genital hypoplasia

Genital hypoplasia has been reported in association with p63 mutations along with the more common defects in skin, hair, teeth, facial and distal limb development. Another disorder with a similar array of anomalies, including genital hypoplasia, is tibial aplasia.[61] Genital anomalies are also associated with facial abnormalities in the Cenani–Lenz syndrome.[62] These various associations suggest that similar genes may be responsible for modeling facial, distal limb and genital mesenchyme, a portion of which are linked to epithelial-stromal interactions, including those along apical ectodermal ridges.

Anorectal and cloacal malformations

Not unexpectedly, genital anomalies are reported in association with other anatomically related disorders, including anorectal malformations and cloacal anomalies.[63] Cloacal anomalies are characterized by a confluence of the urethra, vagina and rectum into a single channel or persistent cloaca with a solitary opening onto the perineum. This abnormality accounts for 10% of anorectal malformations in females and occurs in one of every 50 000 births. It occurs as a consequence of incomplete urorectal septum development and is coupled with maldevelopment of the Müllerian tubercle, sinovaginal bulbs, vaginal plate and urogenital sinus (see also Ch. 10). Approximately 60% of these patients have septate uterovaginal canals, which range in extent from partial to complete duplication of the uterus, cervix and vagina.[64,65]

Acquired vulvar anomalies

Lymphovascular malformations

Benign vulvar lesions acquired in childhood, while uncommon, are probably more frequent than congenital anomalies. These include lymphatic and vascular malformations, such as the vulvar venous malformation, which manifests in late childhood and does not regress (Table 1.6).[66,67]

Prepubertal fibroma

A recently described vulvar mass, composed of collagenous to myxoid fibrous tissue and also occurring in late childhood, has been termed prepubertal vulval fibroma.[68] An histologically similar or identical lesion, which may recur following attempted surgical extir-

Table 1.6 *Vulvo-vaginal masses in children*

Mass	Comment
Benign	
Müllerian papilloma	
Labial hypertrophy	
Urethral prolapse	
Ectopic ureter	Rare clear cell carcinoma
Ureterocele	
Hymenal skin tag	Confusion with condyloma
Condyloma	
Vaginal inclusion cysts	Usually epidermal
Imperforate hymen	
Bartholin duct cyst	Adolescents
Malignant	
Embryonal rhabdomyosarcoma	
Yolk sac carcinoma	
Clear cell adenocarcinoma	DES-related

From Emans.[66]

pation, has been coined CALME (Childhood Asymmetric Labium Majus Enlargement).[69] Whether these lesions represent neoplasms or hormonally stimulated enlargement of native vulvar soft tissue is presently unclear.

Labial hypertrophy

Pre- and post-pubertal girls can present for unilateral or bilateral cosmetic reduction of labium minus hypertrophy, comprising redundant, rugated labial tissue. Although patient histories vary, in some cases these lesions may be congenital but become accentuated as childhood progresses. In contrast to the previously described prepubertal fibroma, which predominantly involves the labium majus, this lesion is restricted to the labium minus.

References

1 Sadler TW. Langman's medical embryology, 5th edn. London: Williams and Wilkins; 1985.

2 Warwick R, Williams PL, eds. Grays anatomy, 35th edn. Philadelphia: WB Saunders; 1973:87.

3 Josso N, Rey R, Gonzalès J. Sexual differentiation, Ch. 7. Pediatric endocrinology. Online. Available: http://www.endotext.org/pediatrics/index.htm.

4 Cotinot C, Pailhoux E, Jaubert F, Fellous M. Molecular genetics of sex determination. Semin Reprod Med 2002; 20:157–166.

5 Shawlot W, Behringer RR. Requirement for Lim1 in head organizer function. Nature 1995; 374:425–430.

6 Miyamoto N, Yoshida M, Kuratani S, Matsuo I, Aizawa S. Defects of urogenital development in mice lacking Emx2. Development 1997; 124:1653–1664.

7 Torres M, Gomez-Pardo E, Dressler GR, Gruss P. Pax-2 controls multiple steps of urogenital development. Development 1995; 121:4057–4065.

8 Holm I. Ambiguous genitalia in the newborn. In: Emans SJ, Laufer MR, Goldstein DP, eds. Pediatric and adolescent gynecology, 5th edn. Philadelphia: Lippincott, Williams and Wilkins; 2005:58.

9 Moore, KL. Before we are born. Basic embryology and birth defects. Philadelphia: WB Saunders; 1974:149.

10 Himelstein-Braw R, Byuskov AG, Peters H, Faber M. Follicular atresia in the infant human ovary. J Reprod Fertil 1976; 46:55–59.

11 George FW, Wilson JD. Conversion of androgen to estrogen by the human fetal ovary. J Clin Endocrinol Metab 1978; 47:550–555.

12 Mackay S. Gonadal development in mammals at the cellular and molecular levels. Int Rev Cytol 2000; 200:47–99.

13 McLaren A. Development of the mammalian gonad: the fate of the supporting cell lineage. Bioessays 1991; 13:151–156.

14 Kehler J, Tolkunova E, Koschorz B, et al. Oct4 is required for primordial germ cell survival. EMBO Rep 2004; 5:1078–1083.

15 Failli V, Rogard M, Mattei MG, Vernier P, Rétaux S. Lhx9 and Lhx9alpha LIM homeodomain factors: genomic structure, expression patterns, chromosomal localization and phylogenetic analysis. Genomics 2000; 64:307–317.

16 Birk OS, Casiano DE, Wassif CA, et al. The LIM homeobox gene Lhx9 is essential for mouse gonad formation. Nature 200; 403:909–913.

17 Gecz J, Gaunt SJ, Passage E, et al. Assignment of a Polycomb-like chromobox gene (CBX2) to human chromosome 17q25. Genomics 1995; 26:130–133.

18 Katoh-Fukui Y, Tsuchiya R, Shiroishi T, et al. Male to female sex reversal in M33 mutant mice. Nature 1998; 393:688–692.

19 Ottolenghi C, Moreira-Filho C, Mendonca BB, et al. Absence of mutations involving the LIM homeobox domain gene LHX9 in 46,XY gonadal agenesis and dysgenesis. J Clin Endocrinol Metabol 2001; 86:2465–2469.

20 Elvin JA, Matzuk MM. Mouse models of ovarian failure. Rev Reprod 1998; 3:183–195.

21 Kurita T, Cunha GR. Roles of p63 in differentiation of Müllerian duct epithelial cells. Ann N Y Acad Sci 2001; 948:9–12.

22 Ince TA, Cviko AP, Quade BJ, et al. p63 Coordinates anogenital modeling and epithelial cell differentiation in the developing female urogenital tract. Am J Pathol 2002; 161:1111–1117.

23 Haraguchi R, Mo R, Hui C, et al. Unique functions of Sonic hedgehog signaling during external genitalia development. Development 2001; 128(21):4241–4250.

24 Lemmen JG, Broekhof JLM, Kuiper GGJM, et al. Expression of estrogen receptor alpha and beta during mouse embryogenesis. Mech Develop 1999; 81:163–167.

25 Simpson ER, Clyne C, Rubin G, et al. Aromatase – a brief overview. Annu Rev Physiol 2002; 64:93–127.

26 Mizusaki H, Kawabe K, Mukai T, et al. Dax-1 (dosage-sensitive sex reversal-adrenal hypoplasia congenita critical region on the X chromosome, gene 1) gene transcription is regulated by wnt4 in the female developing gonad. Mol Endocrinol 2003; 17:507–519.

27 Miller C, Degenhardt K, Sassoon DA. Fetal exposure to DES results in de-regulation of Wnt7a during uterine morphogenesis. Nat Genet 1998; 20:228–230.

28 Canto P, Kofman-Alfaro S, Jimenez AL, et al. Gonadoblastoma in Turner syndrome patients with nonmosaic 45, X Karotype and Y chromosome sequences. Cancer Genet Cytogenet 2004; 150:70–72.

29 Warkany J. Congenital malformations. Chicago: Year Book Medical Publishers; 1971:1105–1145.

30 Verp MS, Simpson JL. Abnormal sex differentiation and neoplasia. Cancer Genet Cytogenet 1987; 25:191–218.

31 Sultan C, Paris F, Jeandel C, Lumbroso S, Galifer RB. Ambiguous genitalia in the newborn. Semin Reprod Med 2002; 20:181–188.

32 Hughes IA. Congenital adrenal hyperplasia: 21-hydroxylase deficiency in the newborn and during infancy. Semin Reprod Med 2002; 20:229–242.

33 Prader Von A. Der genitalbefund beim Pseudohermaproditismus femininus des kongenitalen adrenogenitalen Syndroms. Morphologie, Hausfigkeit, Entwicklung und Vererbung der

verschiedenen Genitalformen. Helv Pediatr Acta 1954; 9:231–248.

34 Reiner WG. Assignment of sex in neonates with ambiguous genitalia. Curr Opin Pediatr 1999; 11(4):363–365.

35 Partsch CJ, Sippell WG. Treatment of central precocious puberty. Best Pract Res Clin Endocrinol Metab 2002; 16:165–189.

36 Dewing P, Bernard P, Vilain E. Disorders of gonadal development. Sem Reprod Med 2002; 20:189–197.

37 Morowitz M, Huff D, von Allmen D. Epithelial ovarian tumors in children: a retrospective analysis. J Pediatr Surg 2003; 38:331–335.

38 Lack E, Goldstein DP. Primary ovarian tumors in childhood and adolescence. Curr Prob Obstet Gynecol 1984; 7:8.

39 de Silva KS, Kanumakala S, Grover SR, Chow CW, Warne GL. Ovarian lesions in children and adolescents – an 11-year review. J Pediatr Endocrinol Metab 2004; 17:951–957.

40 Schultz KA, Sencer SF, Messinger Y, Neglia JP, Steiner ME. Pediatric ovarian tumors: a review of 67 cases. Pediatr Blood Cancer 2005; 44:167–173.

41 Schneider DT, Calaminus G, Koch S, et al. Epidemiologic analysis of 1,442 children and adolescents registered in the German germ cell tumor protocols. Pediatr Blood Cancer 2004; 42:169–175.

42 Patton PE, Novy MJ, Lee DM, Hickok LR. The diagnosis and reproductive outcome after surgical treatment of the complete septate uterus, duplicated cervix and vaginal septum. Am J Obstet Gynecol 2004; 190:1669–1675.

43 Raga F, Bauset C, Remohi J, et al. Reproductive impact of congenital Müllerian anomalies. Hum Reprod 1997; 12:2277–2281.

44 Laufer MR, Goldstein DP, Hendren WH. Structural anomalies of the female reproductive tract. In: Emans SJ, Laufer MR, Goldstein DP, eds. Pediatric and adolescent gynecology, 5th edn. Philadelphia: Williams and Wilkins; 2005:334–416.

45 Propst AM, Hill JA 3rd. Anatomic factors associated with recurrent pregnancy loss. Semin Reprod Med 2000; 18:341–350.

46 Robson S, Oliver GD. Management of vaginal agenesis: review of 10 years practice at a tertiary referral centre. Aust N Z J Obstet Gynaecol 2000; 40:430–433.

47 Crosby WM, Hill EC. Embryology of the müllerian duct system. Obstet Gynecol 1962; 20:507–515.

48 Hundley AF, Fielding JR, Hoyte L. Double cervix and vagina with septate uterus: an uncommon müllerian malformation. Obstet Gynecol 2001; 98:982–985.

49 Musset R, Muller P, Netter A, et al. Study of the upper urinary tract in patients with uterine malformations. Study of 133 cases. Presse Med 1967; 75:1331–1336. [in French]

50 McBean JH, Brumsted JR. Septate uterus with cervical duplication: a rare malformation. Fertil Steril 1994; 62:415–417.

51 Hyatt SW. Imperforate hymen: review of the literature and report of four additional cases. Am Pract Dig Treat 1960; 11:1016–1021.

52 Lim YH, Ng SP, Jamil MA. Imperforate hymen: report of an unusual familial occurrence. J Obstet Gynaecol Res 2003; 29:399–401.

53 Ulbright TM, Alexander RW, Kraus FT. Related intramural papilloma of the vagina: evidence of Müllerian histogenesis. Cancer 1981; 48:2260–2266.

54 McCluggage WG, O'Rourke D, McElhenney C, Crooks M. Müllerian papilloma-like proliferation arising in cystic pelvic endosalpingiosis. Hum Pathol 2002; 33(9):944–946.

55 Abu J, Nunns D, Ireland D, Brown L. Malignant progression through borderline changes in recurrent Müllerian papilloma of the vagina. Histopathology 2003; 42:510–511.

56 Arora M, Shrivastav RK, Jaiprakash MP. A rare germ-cell tumor site: vaginal endodermal sinus tumor. Pediatr Surg Int 2002; 18(5–6):521–523.

57 Copeland LJ, Sneige N, Ordonez NG, et al. Endodermal sinus tumor of the vagina and cervix. Cancer 1985; 55(11):2558–2565.

58 Young RH, Scully RE. Endodermal sinus tumor of the vagina: a report of nine cases and review of the literature. Gynecol Oncol 1984; 18(3):380–392.

59 Stokowski LA. Hypospadias in the neonate. Adv Neonatal Care 2004; 4(4):206–215.

60 Lin D, Harikrishna JA, Moore CC, Jones KL, Miller WL. Missense mutation serine106 proline causes 17 alpha-hydroxylase deficiency. J Biol Chem 1991; 266:15992–15998.

61 Wechsler SB, Lehoczky JA, Hall JG, Innis JW. Tibial aplasia, lower extremity mirror image polydactyly, brachyphalangy, craniofacial dysmorphism and genital hypoplasia: further delineation and mutational analysis. Clin Dysmorphol 2004; 13(2):63–69.

62 Temtamy SA, Ismail S, Nemat A. Mild facial dysmorphism and quasidominant inheritance in Cenani-Lenz syndrome. Clin Dysmorphol 2003; 12(2):77–83.

63 Mittal A, Airon RK, Magu S, Rattan KN, Ratan SK. Associated anomalies with anorectal malformation (ARM). Indian J Pediatr 2004; 71(6):509–514.

64 Warne SA, Wilcox DT, Creighton S, Ransley PG. Long-term gynecological outcome of patients with persistent cloaca. J Urol 2003; 170:1493–1496.

65 Pena A, Levitt MA, Hong A, Midulla P. Surgical management of cloacal malformations: a review of 339 patients. J Pediatr Surg 2004; 39:470–479.

66 Emans SJ. Vulvovaginal problems in the prepubertal child. In: Emans SJ, Laufer MR, Goldstein DP, eds. Pediatric and adolescent gynecology, 5th edn. Philadelphia: Lippincott, Williams and Wilkins; 2005:83–120.

67 Herman AR, Morello F, Strickland JL. Vulvar venous malformations in an 11-year-old girl: a case report. J Pediatr Adolesc Gynecol 2004; 17:179–181.

68 Iwasa Y, Fletcher CD. Distinctive prepubertal vulval fibroma: a hitherto unrecognized mesenchymal tumor of prepubertal girls: analysis of 11 cases. Am J Surg Pathol 2004; 28:1601–1608.

69 Vargas SO, Kozakewich HPW, Boyd TK, et al. Childhood asymmetric labium majus enlargement: mimicking a neoplasm. Am J Surg Pathol 2005; in press.

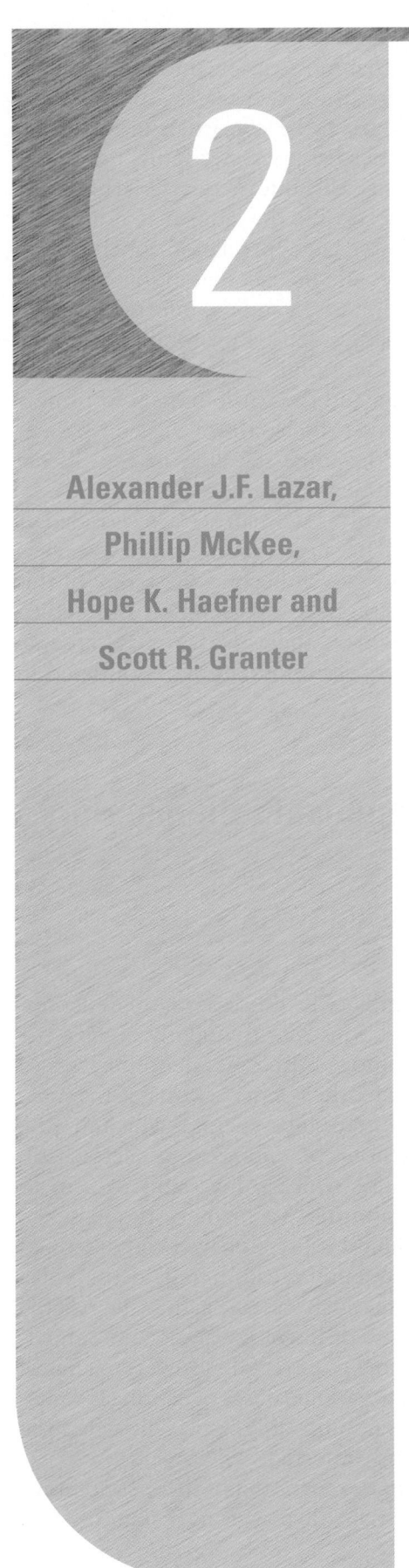

2

Non-infectious inflammatory disorders of the vulva

Alexander J.F. Lazar,

Phillip McKee,

Hope K. Haefner and

Scott R. Granter

Introduction

Localized mucosal inflammatory disorders

Eczematous dermatitis
Lichen simplex chronicus
Psoriasis
Seborrheic dermatitis
Lichen sclerosus
Lichen planus
Zoon's vulvitis (plasma cell vulvitis)
Bullous and cicatricial pemphigoid

Pemphigus vulgaris and pemphigus vegetans
Hailey–Hailey disease
Darier's disease
Acantholytic dermatosis of the vulvocrural area
Fox–Fordyce disease
Hidradenitis suppurativa
Reiter's syndrome
Behçet's disease
Pyoderma gangrenosum
Crohn's disease of the vulva

Summary

Introduction

Diagnostic dermatopathology of the vulva is a field that may be practiced on a multitude of levels. Patients may be seen by either gynecologists, family practitioners, internists or dermatologists. The biopsy may be read by a dermatopathologist, gynecologic pathologist or general pathologist. Thus any chapter addressing diagnostic vulvar dermatopathology must serve a multitude of audiences. This chapter is designed to provide an organized approach to inflammatory vulvar dermatoses and educate the reader on the potential pitfalls in not only the interpretation but also the adherence to concepts that may hinder correct diagnosis and therapy. The reader is referred to more extensive works if a more comprehensive discussion of these entities is desired.[1–3]

For years, a diagnostic schism has existed between dermatopathologists and general surgical and gynecologic pathologists.[4,5] Although there is virtually no form of dermatitis that has not been reported to involve the vulva, separate formal and informal classification schemes for inflammatory dermatoses of the vulva have been used for years. Classification of inflammatory dermatoses of the vulva using the same terminology applied to dermatoses affecting non-vulvar skin is advised for several reasons. In the past, there has been a tendency for general pathologists to lump groups of disorders into 'wastebasket' diagnoses such as 'dystrophy' or 'hyperplasia'. The diagnostic term 'squamous cell hyperplasia' appears in the classification scheme proposed by the International Society for the Study of Vulvovaginal Disease.[6] Although squamous cell hyperplasia is appropriate as a histologic descriptor, to many, it does not connote a specific entity and conceivably could be misused as a label for a more severe epithelial proliferation.[4] The possibility of misclassification is real. One study which reviewed vulvar biopsies diagnosed by general pathologists found that a diagnosis of 'squamous cell hyperplasia' had been applied to cases of lichen simplex chronicus, contact dermatitis, psoriasis, lichen planus and hypertrophic lichen sclerosus.[6]

Notwithstanding the above concerns, a clinician who is comfortable with managing vulvar dermatoses can probably function under any diagnostic terminology, as long as the limitations of some terms (such as hyperplasia) are understood. However, the fact that many non-specific epithelial changes in the vulva are managed as much on clinical as histologic grounds and the use of terminology that most closely mirrors the histologic findings are useful for two reasons. First, it will prompt the pathologist to be consistent in his or her approach to vulvar dermatitides. Secondly, the use of these diagnostic terms will educate the clinician on the nuances of pathology. While the latter may not always be mandatory, it fosters an appreciation for the range of pathologic changes and the fact that in some circumstances (such as psoriasis, candida infection, lichen planus) the diagnosis can have a profound impact on management and patient outcome. An understanding between the clinician and the pathologist is of utmost importance. Continued discussion of difficult patient scenarios enhances the understanding of the disease process and the treatment required.

In the following, vulvar dermatoses are classified as for non-vulvar skin. Because a comprehensive review of dermatopathology is well beyond the scope of this chapter, it will focus on the most common and significant dermatoses seen on the vulva. The differential diagnosis of the more common entities is outlined in Table 2.1.

Localized mucosal inflammatory disorders

ECZEMATOUS DERMATITIS

Introduction

Eczematous dermatitis (ED) is a commonly encountered group of conditions that frequently involve the vulva.[7–10] The common histologic denominator of diseases classified under the rubric 'eczema' is the presence of spongiosis (intercellular edema), which may be mediated by exogenous or endogenous factors. An inflammatory response, which is invariably present, is at least partially responsible for many of the patient's symptoms. Many clinical subtypes have been described and those most frequently encountered in the vulva will be discussed here. Such variants cannot be reliably separated on the basis of histology alone and clinicopathologic correlation is essential. However, clinical distinction among the various causes of eczema is sometimes difficult or even impossible, especially when the vulva is predominantly affected.[11]

To further challenge recognition of these conditions, eczematous dermatitis evolves through stages, often

Table 2.1 Differential diagnosis of common vulvar mucocutaneous disorders

Acan	PK	Spong	HK	LI	ID	IEN	Sclerosis	Atroph	TTR	Diagnosis	Exclude
+		+/−	+							Lichen simplex chronicus (LSC)	Candida
				+/−	+/−		+	+/−		Lichen sclerosus (LS)	Differentiated VIN
+/−		+	+/−	+						Eczema	Seborrheic dermatitis
+/−			+/−		+					Lichen planus	Early LS
+			+/−	+			+			LSC + LS	Differentiated VIN
+		+	+							Eczema + LSC	Candida
				+						Zoon's	Syphilis
+	+					+			+	Psoriasis	LSC, candida

Acan, acanthosis; Pk, parakeratosis; Spong, spongiosis; HK, hyperkeratosis; LI, lichenoid infiltrate; ID, interface dermatitis; IEN, intraepithelial neutrophils; TTR, test tube rete; VIN, vulvar intraepithelia neoplasia. '+/−' indicates 'may be present'.

rapidly, resulting in clinical and histologic patterns that can be strikingly similar regardless of etiology. Many patients are simply designated as having 'eczema'. In some cases, only with specialized investigation, such as patch testing, is the disease precisely characterized. It is the pathologist's role to evaluate for the presence of spongiotic dermatitis and its stage of development, accepting the fact that elucidation of the specific clinical subtype or etiology based on histologic findings is, in most cases, impossible. In this section, the natural history of eczematous dermatitis will be discussed, followed by a discussion of the major clinical subtypes of ED affecting the vulva.

Clinical presentation

Eczematous dermatitis can be seen in all ages, including infants.[12,13] The earliest detectable feature is erythema, most commonly associated with pruritus, dryness or burning. The last two symptoms are more commonly reported with mucosal involvement.[7] Pain upon palpation and dyspareunia can be present.[8] Less commonly, the condition may be asymptomatic. Tiny, delicate vesicles develop and, with time, coalesce to form larger vesicles and even bullae. The epidermal edema will often give the skin surface a 'weepy', wet appearance, but this is not always a prominent feature. A superficial, pale, yellowish scale-crust is a frequent finding. Rubbing and scratching in response to pruritus leads to development of superimposed changes of lichen simplex chronicus (LSC) and often to excoriation. LSC is characterized by a thickening of the skin imparting a leathery quality with accentuation of the skin markings (see LSC, p. 28). Superinfection with either fungal or bacterial organisms may occur. The chronic lesions of all forms of eczematous dermatitis are strikingly similar in appearance.

Major clinical subtypes of eczematous dermatitis

Exogenous dermatitis

Exogenous dermatitis results from direct application of a substance to skin. Two main types of exogenous dermatitis are seen in the vulva: irritant contact dermatitis and allergic contact dermatitis. The distinction between exogenous and endogenous dermatitis can be blurred as contact with irritants can promote or accentuate the latter condition.

Irritant contact dermatitis

Irritant contact dermatitis results from direct damage to the epithelium by exogenous agents. This variant is much more common than allergic contact dermatitis.[14] The dermatitis is typically localized to the area where the offending substance has been applied and the response is usually initiated within minutes to hours of exposure. A secondary inflammatory response develops in response to the injury. Visible vesicles are usually not a feature. Diaper rash is a common irritant contact dermatitis in infants or the elderly where urine and/or stool combine with the friction of the diaper to produce eczematous dermatitis. Irritant contact dermatitis can be localized to the vulva when exposure is limited to this site or because the vulvar region is more sensitive to the offending substance when compared with other areas.[15] Common causes are urine, sweat, friction, topical products such as lotions, soaps, perfumes or cleansers and a variety of topical over-the-counter and prescription medications. Attempts at treatment may exacerbate the disease. In particular, dermatitis in this area is often perceived by the patient as a lack of cleanliness. This can incite an urge to cleanse the area increasing the severity of the dermatitis. Secondary infection is often a problem.[8,16] The cycle is further exacerbated by a reluctance to discuss symptoms with healthcare providers. Treatment mainly involves avoiding inciting and exacerbating substances and in some patients topical steroids are also required.[7]

Allergic contact dermatitis

Allergic contact dermatitis is less often encountered than irritant contact dermatitis and is distinctly uncommon in both the very young and elderly. It represents a type IV hypersensitivity reaction to a specific antigen to which the patient has been previously exposed.[17] Lesions tend to develop significant erythema, often with subsequent bulla formation. The condition usually arises within 48 h after exposure in the sensitized patient and is generally confined to the area of exposure, but can become generalized. Lesions can persist for several weeks. This type of reaction is exemplified by the well-known response to poison ivy. The list of causes in the vulva is similar to contact dermatitis elsewhere and includes specific ingredients in substances such as soaps, lotions, perfumes and cosmetics. Topical medication is also a common cause.[8] Allergic dermatitis in response to semen and constituents of latex condoms has been described.[18]

Allergic contact dermatitis is confirmed by skin patch testing, which involves placing small pieces of material containing the substance to be tested on the skin and measuring the inflammatory response. Such methodology can identify the specific substance causing the dermatitis in a significant portion of appropriately selected patients.[11] Constituents of topical medications are quite commonly identified as the allergen. Allergic contact dermatitis is often seen in patients with a history of atopy (see below) and thus likely involves inheritance of a propensity for its later development. Complete avoidance of the contactant is recommended. The use of topical products should be minimized. If medications are required, an ointment base is recommended, since creams contain many additives.

Atopic dermatitis

Atopic dermatitis (AD) is a hypersensitivity condition with familial clustering that involves skin and mucosal sites and is associated with respiratory conditions such as asthma and allergic rhinitis. It is seen in 10–20% of children and its incidence may be increasing.[19] The most common allergen inciting AD is from the common household dust-mite, *Dermatophagoides pteronyssinus*. AD can be conceptualized as an exaggerated response to common cutaneous antigens.[20] It usually involves the face, scalp and the extensor surfaces of the arms and legs. Atopic dermatitis is believed to be an IgE-mediated immune reaction with pathogenic similar-

ities to asthma. However, the precise mechanisms of the hypersensitivity are poorly understood.[21] Although atopic dermatitis often resolves by puberty, predisposition to eczematous dermatitis with irritation of the skin from a variety of sources can endure for life.[21] Some authorities believe this to be the most common form of eczematous dermatitis involving the vulva.[7,8] In patients with a history of atopic dermatitis, eczematous dermatitis is often attributed to atopy when other causes are excluded. Treatment consists of eliminating inflammation and infection. Emollients and antipruritic agents are used to reduce the self-inflicted damage to the involved skin and to control exacerbating factors. The majority of patients can be brought under adequate control in less than 3 weeks. Reasons for failure include: poor patient compliance, the simultaneous occurrence of asthma or hay fever, inadequate sedation and continued emotional stress. Allergic contact dermatitis is found to be more common in patients with a history of atopy.[19]

Nummular dermatitis

Nummular dermatitis is generally seen more often in men than women with peak incidence in those greater than 55 years of age. However, a predominantly female incidence is found from ages 15 to 25. The characteristic lesions start as erythema with tiny vesicles that quickly coalesce to form discrete 'coin-shaped' plaques that given rise to the alternative designation, 'discoid' eczematous dermatitis. These lesions can be single or multiple and are usually less than 10 cm in diameter. They are intensely pruritic and commonly present in the upper extremities (dorsum of the hand is a classic site) and trunk, but can be seen in a wider distribution. The vulva is rarely involved. With time, the lesions can show central clearing and may be mistaken for a fungal infection. The lesions can persist and will often recur in a previous site of involvement. Topical steroids are commonly used in the treatment of this condition.[22]

Histopathology

Histologically, eczematous dermatitis is defined by epidermal spongiosis – intercellular epidermal edema that splays keratinocytes apart, rendering their spinous processes more prominent (Fig. 2.1). A spectrum of histologic changes corresponding to the duration of lesions is well-recognized and has been traditionally divided into acute, subacute and chronic phases. As with all stages of eczematous dermatitis, the composition and amount of inflammation is variable. Often in

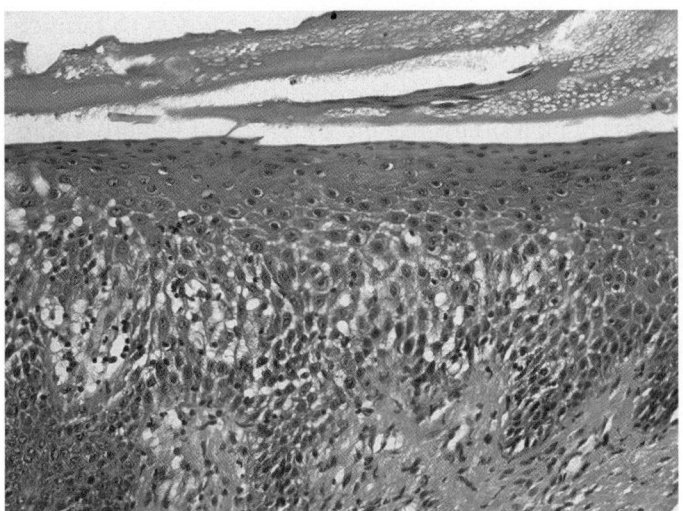

Fig. 2.1 Eczematous dermatitis, showing a spongiosis and intra-epithelial mononuclear cell infiltrate.

the acute phase, there is a variable superficial papillary dermal inflammatory cell infiltrate consisting primarily of lymphocytes, sometimes with eosinophils. Scattered lymphocytes, eosinophils and even neutrophils can be seen in the epidermis. With increasing spongiosis, the cell-to-cell junctions of the epidermal keratinocytes are compromised and small intraepidermal vesicles form. These can eventually coalesce to form larger vesicles and even bullae. With severe edema, focal separations at the dermal–epidermal junction may also occur. With time, secondary keratinocyte necrosis may be seen in severe cases. The intraepidermal vesicles empty onto the epidermal surface and give rise to the 'weepy' appearance and may dry to form a scale-crust. Incited by the pruritic nature of the vesicles, rubbing and scratching usually accelerate the uncapping of vesicles and produces erosions. Significant hyperkeratosis or epidermal acanthosis are not seen in the acute phase.

In the subacute phase – in addition to spongiosis – acanthosis or hyperplasia of the epidermis is seen. Often, the acanthosis occurs in a psoriasiform pattern (i.e. resembling psoriasis) and at least in part is a response to scratching or rubbing. A dermal inflammatory infiltrate of variable density and composition is seen. Mild hyperkeratosis and hypergranulosis are often present in subacute lesions of eczematous dermatitis.

In the chronic phase, spongiosis may be more difficult to identify and the epidermal hyperplasia becomes more pronounced. Marked hyperkeratosis and hyper-

granulosis are regular features. The changes come to resemble the microscopic appearance of acral skin (which is determined by constant exposure to friction). When the features of epidermal acanthosis, hyperkeratosis and hypergranulosis are sufficiently pronounced due to rubbing and scratching, the lesion is designated chronic eczematous dermatitis with superimposed lichen simplex chronicus (Fig. 2.2). However, it should be understood that, while eczematous dermatitis is a frequent underlying cause of LSC, other associations are well-documented. Therefore, the changes of LSC should not be viewed as synonymous with chronic eczematous dermatitis (see LSC, p. 28); however, debate continues on this issue.

Differential diagnosis

There is considerable histologic overlap between the various types and causes of eczematous dermatitis in the vulva. The role of the pathologist is to recognize eczematous dermatitis and be able to distinguish it from other dermatitis. Once a diagnosis of spongiotic dermatitis is reached, it is then the clinician's responsibility to search for the cause and precisely classify the reaction. It is especially important for the pathologist to be aware that all the histologic features of eczematous dermatitis can be precisely mimicked by fungal infection. Therefore, a diagnosis of spongiotic dermatitis or eczematous dermatitis should never be rendered until a periodic acid–Schiff (PAS) or silver stain has been performed to exclude the possibility of a fungal infection. This is particularly important since a fungal infection misdiagnosed as eczematous dermatitis and treated with topical steroids will exacerbate the infection (Fig. 2.3).

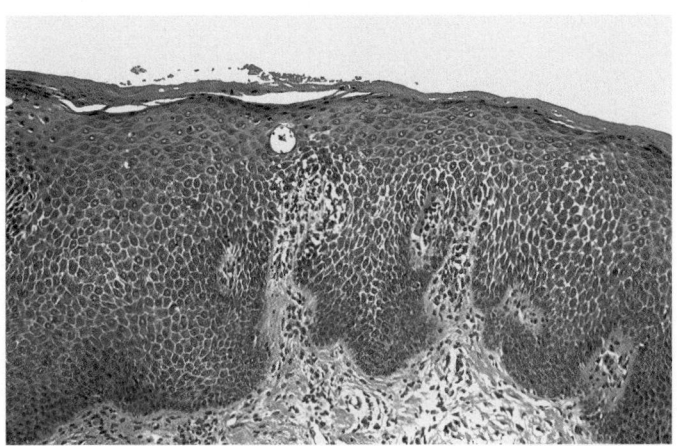

Fig. 2.2 Eczematous dermatitis with superimposed lichen simplex chronicus.

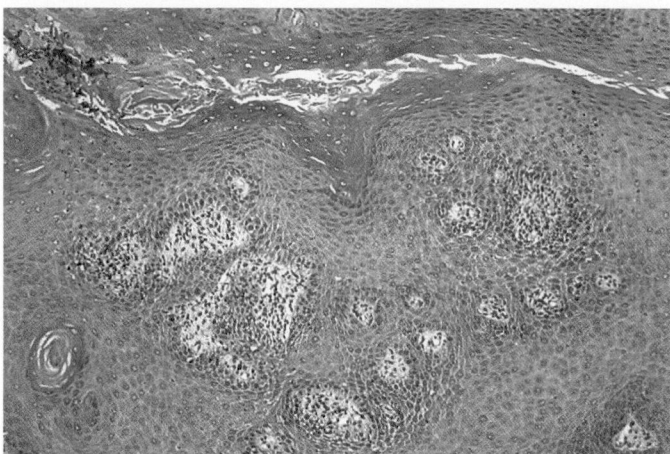

Fig. 2.3 Candida infection may mimic chronic eczematous dermatitis.

LICHEN SIMPLEX CHRONICUS

Clinical presentation

Lichen simplex chronicus (LSC) is not a distinctive condition, but rather denotes a characteristic clinical and pathologic, response of skin to repeated physical trauma such as rubbing or scratching, often superimposed on a pruritic lesion such as eczematous dermatitis. LSC is commonly seen in patients who habitually scratch, but have no identifiable underlying dermatoses. When no underlying etiology is discovered, this process has sometimes been referred to as neurodermatitis. The vulva is a frequently involved site.[23,24]

LSC presents as thickened skin that has erythema and scaling that is plaque-like, often with overlying excoriation. Physiological skin markings are exaggerated and visual excoriations are present (Fig. 2.4). Hyperpigmentation may also be seen. Patients usually present with complaints of pruritus of weeks to months' duration, often with nocturnal accentuation. Scratching of the lesion can become habitual and subconscious. The lesion is usually solitary and the most common vulvar site is the labium majus. There is usually an erythematous hue to the skin. Postinflammatory hyperpigmentation may develop. Patches of hypopigmentation or depigmentation may occur.

Histopathology

Biopsy is usually not necessary in LSC. However, when it is required, it should not be attempted until the itch–scratch cycle is stopped. LSC is characterized by thickening of the skin. The epidermis shows hyperkeratosis and hypergranulosis (Figs 2.5, 2.6). Superimposed excoriation and scale-crust may be seen following vigorous scratching. The rete ridges are elongated and thickened in an irregular psoriasiform

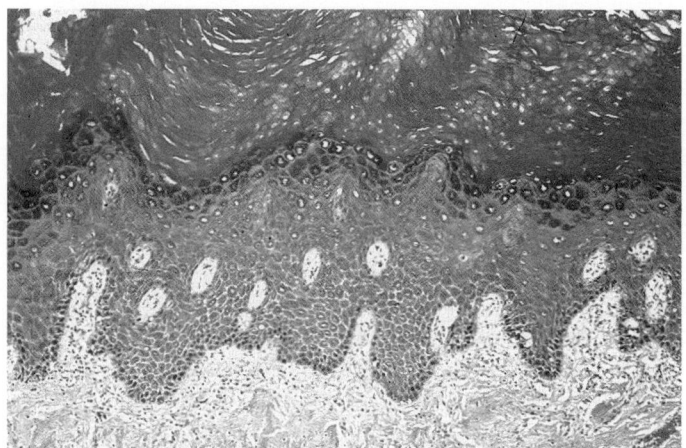

Fig. 2.5 Lichen simplex chronicus, with acanthosis, hyperkeratosis and hypergranulosis.

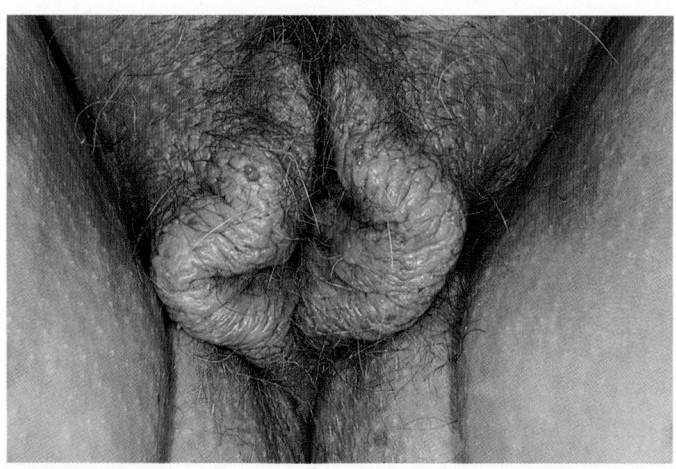

Fig. 2.4 Lichen simplex chronicus with pronounced changes associated with itch–scratch cycle.

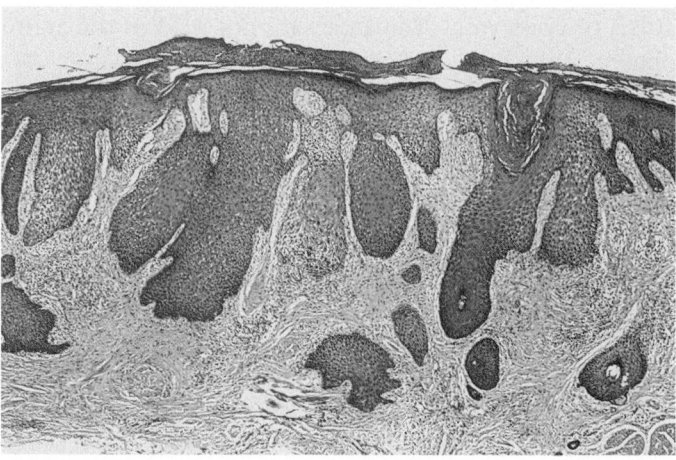

Fig. 2.6 Marked acanthosis associated with scratching (prurigo nodularis).

pattern. In non-vulvar skin, vertically streaked coarse collagen and small vessels are often present, but these features are less prominent in the vulva.[24] A sparse mononuclear infiltrate is often found in the dermis and epidermal mononuclear cells can be seen. Neutrophils may be present in the epidermis if there is excoriation.

Differential diagnosis

Since LSC is often superimposed on another, typically pruritic, lesion it is important not to diagnose LSC without pursuing the underlying 'cause'. Conditions that can be confused with LSC include fungal infection, tinea cruris, chronic eczematous dermatitis (Fig. 2.2) and psoriasis. Fungal infections are often pruritic and chronic infections may be associated with superimposed features of LSC (Fig. 2.3). It is important to exclude fungi with a periodic acid–Schiff or silver stain, particularly if neutrophils are seen in the epidermis or stratum corneum. Chronic eczematous dermatitis is often associated with LSC (see chronic eczematous dermatitis, p. 25). In fact, chronic eczematous dermatitis forms a spectrum with LSC and precise designation is somewhat arbitrary. However, if spongiosis is identified, it is important to indicate this in the diagnostic report. In our experience, eczematous dermatitis is the most common specific dermatosis associated with LSC. To help differentiate chronic eczematous dermatitis from isolated LSC, it is necessary to identify epidermal spongiosis, which can be focal (Fig. 2.2). Finally, psoriasis can be differentiated from LSC by virtue of its narrow, deep rete peg, more regular hyperplasia of the rete pegs, plaque-like parakeratosis often associated with neutrophils and hypogranulosis (see Psoriasis, below).

When not associated with other epithelial changes LSC is not considered a precursor to vulvar squamous carcinoma. However, certain patterns, such as verruciform LSC, verruciform LSC with altered squamous differentiation, LSC associated with lichen sclerosus and LSC complicated by differentiated vulvar intraepithelial neoplasia (VIN), may increase the risk of squamous cell carcinoma of the vulva. These patterns are discussed in Chapter 6.

Treatment

For successful treatment, it is imperative to interrupt the 'itch–scratch' cycle. A severe case of this condition is seen in Figures 2.4 and 2.6. The labia are thickened and have many areas of tissue denudation from the constant scratching. Treatment involves topical steroids and the wearing of cotton gloves at night to prevent skin damage from scratching.[23]

For severe disease, high-dose (Class 1) topical steroids may be required for a 2–4-week period and then decreased to a mid-dose (Class 4) topical steroid. If the skin is not significantly thickened, a Class 4 steroid is the first line of treatment. Generally short-term use is all that is required.

Other considerations for the itch–scratch cycle include:
1 Night-time sedation initially (low-dose amitriptyline or hydroxyzine).
2 Minimize irritation:
   * Eliminate contactants, overwashing.
   * Rule out infection as precipitating or driving factor – for recalcitrant disease, perform an aerobic and yeast culture. For women on a topical corticosteroid and an antibiotic, cover with an oral antifungal agent every 3 to 7 days during the antibiotic therapy. Minimize the potential for additional irritation by treating infections orally.
3 Provide patient education regarding therapy, possible chronicity and recurrence.

Resolution of the dermatitis after the cause has been removed confirms the diagnosis. Since LSC is commonly superimposed on specific dermatoses, treatment of any associated disorder is also required.

PSORIASIS

Introduction

Psoriasis is a chronic, relapsing hyperproliferative papulosquamous disorder that affects 1–2% of the Caucasian population. Approximately one-third of patients have a first-degree relative with the disease. The mean age of onset is in the late twenties. The male to female ratio is equal in adults, but there is a female predominance in pediatric cases. The disease commonly affects the vulva (up to one-third of cases), which can be involved at presentation.[25] Isolated vulvar involvement is occasionally seen, but is uncommon.[16] The pathogenesis of psoriasis is complex,[26] but appears to involve immune dysfunction. Linkage to certain HLA class I haplotypes is seen. This may help explain the familial clustering of psoriasis. Aberrant activities of both CD4- and CD8-positive T-lymphocytes, which appear to help initiate and sustain the lesions, are likely involved.[27] The antigen or antigens inciting this response have not been elucidated. There are also epidermal abnormalities leading to hyperproliferation with abnormal maturation. Up to one-third of patients with psoriasis have a first-degree relative with psoriasis.[26]

Clinical presentation

Psoriasis has a wide and variable spectrum of clinical presentations. Classic plaque (psoriasis vulgaris), inverse (or flexural), guttate and pustular forms will be discussed in detail. These forms commonly involve the vulva.

Classic plaque-type psoriasis presents with symmetrically distributed erythematous, often indurated, plaques that are well-circumscribed. This is most common variant of psoriasis to involve the vulva (Fig. 2.7a). The lesions are often covered by a silvery scale, but this finding is less frequently seen on the vulva.[25] When present, the scale tends to be present at the border of the plaque. Vulvar lesions often have a shiny erythematous appearance and are well-demarcated. Removal of the scale may produce pinpoint bleeding referred to as the Auspitz sign. While probably not diagnostic of psoriasis, this is a characteristic finding. The extensor surfaces of the upper and lower extremities are most often involved. The pretibial, umbilical, intragluteal and lumbosacral regions may also be affected. Psoriasis is associated the Koebner phenomenon (lesions arising in areas of prior trauma).

Inverse or flexural psoriasis shows an alternative distribution in which moist flexural surfaces such as the inframammary, inguinal and abdominal pannus areas are involved. This pattern is more commonly found in obese individuals. The involved areas are erythematous, but generally do not show the silvery micaceous scale of classic plaque psoriasis. Given their location, these lesions may become macerated or fissured (Fig. 2.7b)

Guttate psoriasis preferentially affects children, adolescents and young adults. The condition often arises after a beta-hemolytic streptococcal infection. Guttate lesions may herald the onset of plaque-type psoriasis. It presents as crops of small (< 1 cm) pink to erythematous lesions usually without prominent scale. The trunk, buttocks and periphery of the extremities are most commonly affected. Vulvar involvement is rare and lesions limited to the vulva would be exceptional.[16,25]

The lesions of pustular psoriasis are typically red, crusted plaques with superimposed pustules. The crust is often more prominent than in other variants. Patients with pustular psoriasis usually show systemic symptoms such as fever that may become severe enough to warrant hospitalization.[28]

Psoriasis may be associated with a debilitating form of arthritis. Usually psoriasis precedes the onset of arthritis by many years. The arthritis is most often asymmetric, but can also be symmetrical in distribution. Psoriatic spondylitis is also present in the occasional patient.[29]

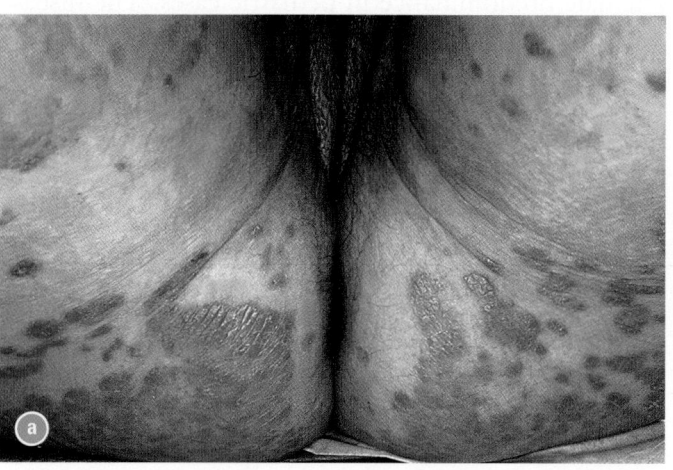
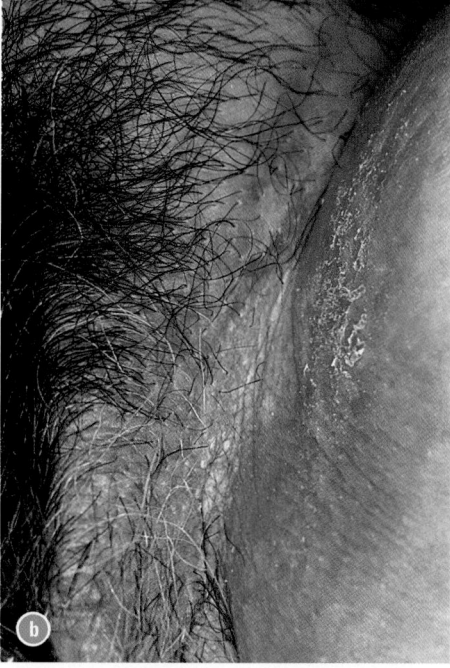

Fig. 2.7 (a) Plaque-like psoriasis involving the buttocks and thighs. (b) Flexural psoriasis.

Histopathology

The classic lesion of plaque-type psoriasis is characterized by regular acanthosis or hyperplasia of the epidermis with the rete pegs elongated to a similar extent. This pattern of epidermal hyperplasia, termed psoriasiform hyperplasia, resembles test tubes in a test tube rack. The tips of the rete may be widened or 'clubbed' and can fuse in longstanding lesions (Fig. 2.8). Parakeratosis is frequently associated with neutrophils and intraepidermal pustules are often present. Munro microabscesses are intracorneal collections of neutrophils with pyknotic nuclei. The spinous layer can contain collections of neutrophils with spongiosis referred to as spongiform pustules of Kogoj (Fig. 2.9). The superficial dermal papillae contain tortuous vessels and marked attenuation of the suprapapillary plate. Trauma to the thinned epidermis above the expanded highly vascular papillae accounts for the Auspitz sign. Extravasated red blood cells are seen in the superficial dermis, particularly in early lesions. A variable superficial interstitial mixed inflammatory infiltrate is usually present.

The lesions of psoriasis evolve with time.[30,31] The earliest recognizable changes in psoriasis are dilation of the vessels of the superficial vascular plexus with a mild lymphocytic perivascular and interstitial infiltrate. Over time, acanthosis and parakeratosis develop with increased mitotic activity in the epidermis. Guttate lesions show a more subtle, irregular psoriasiform hyperplasia and may maintain a granular cell layer. Distinct foci of parakeratosis with associated neutrophils are typically seen.

Pustular psoriasis typically has more prominent Munro microabscesses which often merge to form macropustules and conspicuous spongiform pustules of Kogoj.

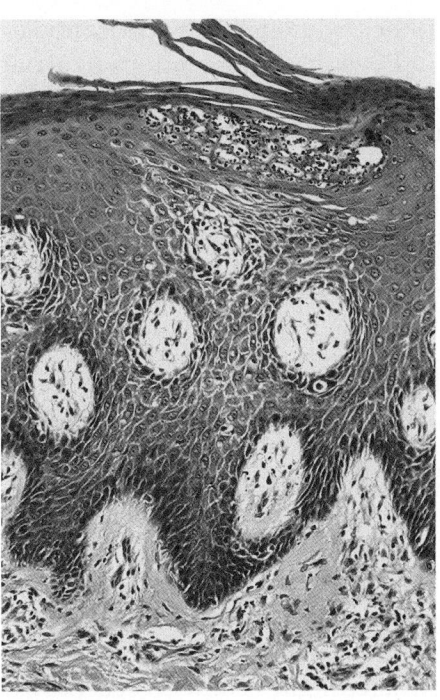

Fig. 2.9 Psoriasis. A superficial intraepidermal neutrophil-rich microabscess (spongiform pustule of Kogoj).

Differential diagnosis

The differential diagnosis of psoriasis includes fungal infection. Thus, it is important to perform a PAS stain to rule out fungal infection. Although focal spongiosis is not uncommon in psoriasis, eczematous lesions exhibit more diffuse spongiosis and are not associated with thinning of the suprapapillary plate and parakeratosis, when present, is typically focal. Hypergranulosis and hyperkeratosis, in the setting of spongiosis, suggests a diagnosis of subacute to chronic eczematous dermatitis. Psoriasiform drug reactions are common and can closely mimic psoriasis. Eosinophils in the inflammatory cell infiltrate favors a psoriasiform drug reaction. Clinical history is paramount in differentiating these two possibilities. Lichen simplex chronicus shows marked acanthosis, often in an irregular pattern associated with hyperkeratosis and hypergranulosis. The lesions of Reiter's syndrome can appear identical to psoriasis, particularly the pustular variant, and clinical information is required to make the distinction (see Reiter's syndrome, p. 46).

Treatment

Treatment for psoriasis depends on the severity of the disease and includes topical antiproliferative agents, steroids and methotrexate and cyclosporine in severe cases.

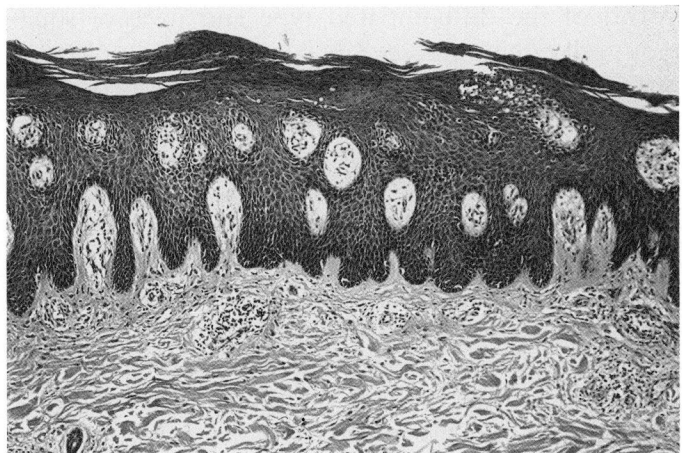

Fig. 2.8 Psoriasis. The rete ridges show regular elongation with fusion at their bases. Note the confluent parakeratosis typical of psoriasis.

When considering the traditional therapeutic modalities for management of psoriasis, be cautious to avoid irritating the sensitive genital skin. Treatment can lead to apparent remission of lesions, but the propensity to develop plaques remains, and psoriasis is thus usually a chronic and frustrating problem. A new generation of biological therapies is currently being introduced that may radically alter the manner in which psoriasis is treated.[32,33]

SEBORRHEIC DERMATITIS

Risk factors and clinical presentation

Seborrheic dermatitis (SD) is a predominately chronic condition dermatosis of unknown etiology. Some evidence suggests an association with *Malassezia* (formerly *Pityrosporum*) *ovalis*; however, the mechanism and significance of this association is controversial.[34] SD is characterized by an ill-defined area of erythema that is pruritic and has associated light yellow to red-brown plaques with a dry to greasy scale. Mild involvement of the scalp is commonly referred to as 'dandruff'. Intraepidermal edema and surface weeping are not prominent features. It is most commonly seen in flexural areas with significant sebaceous activity such as upper trunk, scalp, face (especially the eyebrows and nasolabial folds) and the ears (particularly the external auditory meatus).

The vulva is less often affected and is often accompanied by concurrent involvement of one of the more common sites.[7,10] When the vulva is involved, it usually presents on the labia majora with extension onto the mons pubis and crural folds of the groin.[35,36] Mucosal involvement is not seen.

Mild SD is frequently evident in the general population (1–3%), but is present in greater than three-quarters of those infected by HIV. In immunocompetent patients, seborrheic dermatitis is limited to the areas mentioned above. However, in patients with acquired immune deficiency syndrome (AIDS), the disease is often more severe and can have a wide distribution involving much of the skin surface.[37] It can be seen early in HIV infection and is the most prevalent skin condition in this population.[38] Seborrheic dermatitis has also been associated with Parkinson's disease.

Histopathology

The biopsy findings in SD are often subtle and nonspecific. Usually acanthosis of the epidermis is present, often in a psoriasiform pattern. Parakeratosis is typically present and may be accentuated around follicular ostia where small numbers of neutrophils are commonly present. Variable spongiosis and dermal lymphocytic infiltrate may be seen.

Differential diagnosis

Distinction from psoriasis is often difficult. Well-developed parakeratotic mounds associated with neutrophils and uniform 'test-tube' epidermal hyperplasia favor psoriasis. SD often shows significant spongiosis and, indeed, is sometimes classified under the rubric of eczematous dermatitis. Distinction from other forms of eczema requires clinical correlation. It is important to exclude a candidal fungal infection before diagnosing seborrheic dermatitis or other eczematous dermatitides. This is commonly done by the clinician with a KOH preparation from the skin scale, or an aerobic culture swab sent to microbiology for fungal culture, but is also readily accomplished by a diastase-PAS stain. SD is not commonly biopsied on the vulva, since characteristic lesions are commonly seen elsewhere in the body, most often the scalp and face.[10]

Treatment

Topical steroids should be considered for symptomatic seborrheic dermatitis. Antifungals may also be required. At times, Burow's solution is utilized. It is recommended that topical medications be applied immediately after bathing when keratin is softer to maximize dermal penetration.

LICHEN SCLEROSUS

Introduction

Lichen sclerosus (LS) is a common chronic inflammatory dermatosis that frequently involves the vulva and causes considerable tissue destruction. It is occasionally associated with vulvar intraepithelial neoplasia (VIN) of the differentiated type and invasive squamous cell carcinoma (see Ch. 6). While the etiology of this condition is not known, it is seen in association with autoimmune diseases[39] that also involve the skin (alopecia areata) and other organs (pernicious anemia and thyroid disorders).[40] Certain HLA types are more common in patients with LS underscoring its presumed autoimmune etiology or predisposition.[11] Women with this condition have also been reported to have a deficiency of androgens[41] and a subset of LS cases respond to androgen therapy. However, numerous studies emphasize the lack of efficacy of testosterone and support the use of steroids.[42–51] Infectious and environmental etiologies have also been considered.[52] Rare familial cases have been reported.[53–56]

Clinical presentation

The incidence of LS is not known, as many cases are asymptomatic and the disease is under-reported by those suffering with it. The use of numerous different names for this condition has led to confusion in its diagnosis and treatment. The term 'lichen sclerosus' is now preferred over other terms such as kraurosis, mixed dystrophy, leukoplakia and sclerotic dermatosis.[4,6,57] The suffix 'et atrophicus' is no longer used since atrophy is often absent or inconspicuous. While LS most commonly presents in peri- and post-menopausal women, it can be seen in women of reproductive age and children.[58,59] The most common presenting complaint is vulvar pruritus, but a burning sensation and dyspareunia can also be experienced. In some patients, the lesion is asymptomatic and may only be detected during a routine examination.

Clinically, LS most often presents with white scaly lesions that infrequently form symmetrical plaques. The skin surface in these areas is frequently described as having an appearance similar to wrinkled parchment or cigarette paper (Fig. 2.10). The lesion can extend to involve the perianal region in what is often described as a 'figure of eight' or hourglass pattern (Fig. 2.11). Other regions of the body, such as the arms or trunk, are involved in ~20% of cases.[57] These cutaneous lesions are very rarely seen in the absence of anogenital involvement. LS does not involve the vagina. With time, this disease can cause disruption of the normal vulvar architecture with effacement of both the labia majora

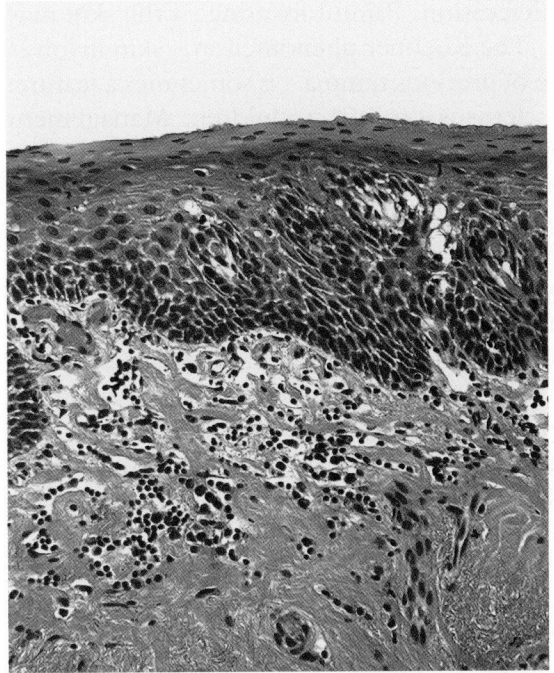

Fig. 2.11 Early lichen sclerosus. The dominant findings are a mononuclear infiltrate at the epidermal–stromal interface with subtle sclerosis. At this stage the inflammatory cells are not separated by the sclerotic stroma.

and minora. Lichen sclerosus can occur on the clitoral hood. At times the labia minora adhere to one another, resulting in stenosis. The diameter of the introitus may become so narrow that intercourse is not possible. Stenosis around the anus can also occur, leading to

Fig. 2.10 (a) Lichen sclerosus with a prominent hourglass appearance. (b) Clinical appearance of lichen sclerosus. Note the atrophy of the labium minus.

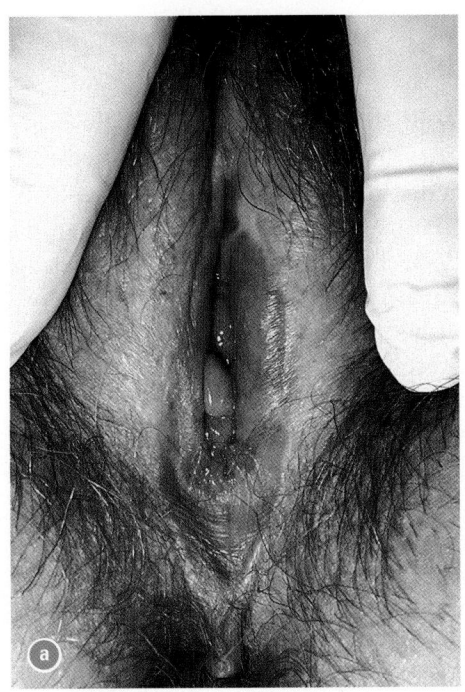

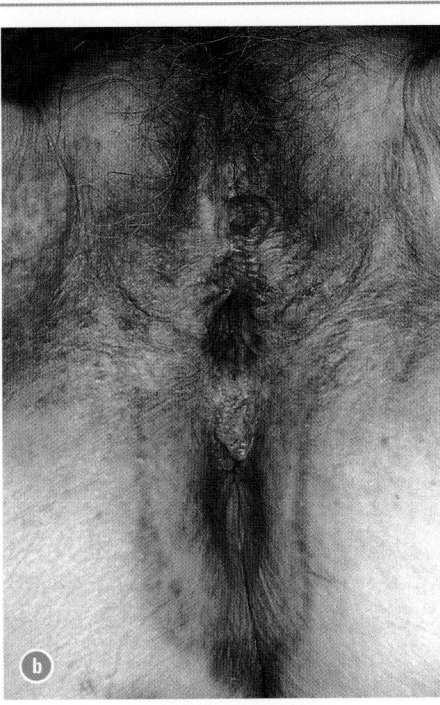

pain with defecation. Painful fissuring of the skin may be present. The Koebner phenomenon – skin involvement at site of previous trauma – is sometimes a feature.

Lichen sclerosus can affect children. Management in this population is similar to the adult population. There is an increased incidence of extra-anogenital lesions in children.[60] The characteristic involvement in the anogenital distribution can be mistaken for sexual abuse in younger children.[39] Because of the intense pruritic nature of this lesion, changes of lichen simplex chronicus are often superimposed. Similarly, attempts to medicate the lesion can cause concomitant contact irritant dermatitis. Such changes, when present, can make diagnosis challenging to both the clinician and pathologist.

Histopathology

Like most inflammatory dermatoses, the biopsy appearance of LS is dependent on the age of the lesion and the area biopsied. Biopsies taken at the edge of an established lesion may show features of early LS, while a biopsy taken from the center of the lesion may show more chronic features. The most common site biopsied in a large published series is the labium majus.[24] If an ulcer or erosion is present, it is important to biopsy the tissue at the edge of the lesion.

Very early lesions may be very difficult, and sometimes impossible, to diagnose with certainty. Biopsies from early lesions show vacuolar-type interface dermatitis at the epidermal–dermal junction with scattered lymphocytes and occasional necrotic keratinocytes (Fig. 2.12). Alternatively, biopsies of early lesions may also show a dense lichenoid band of lymphocytes associated with interface dermatitis. The inflammatory infiltrate is composed mainly of lymphocytes and a few histiocytes (some laden with melanin – 'melanophages'); however, occasional eosinophils or plasma cells may be seen in lesions involving the mucosa.

Even in early lesions, some degree of superficial dermal (submucosal) edema or sclerosis is usually present (Fig. 2.12). Sclerosis takes the form of hyalinization involving the superficial reticular dermis and papillary dermis in skin and superficial submucosa in lesions of the labia minora. The superficial hyalinized or sclerotic collagen has an amorphous quality and contrasts with the fibrillary texture of normal collagen. Interestingly, the extent or thickness of this band may not correlate with the age of the lesion although this is almost certainly due to sampling bias. Large biopsies often show a spectrum of change from early interface dermatitis to areas of well-established sclerosis. As

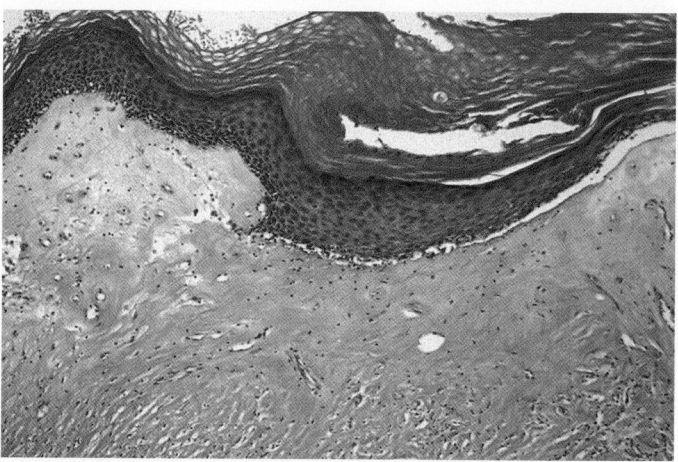

Fig. 2.12 Low-power of established lesion with extensive dermal sclerosis and minimal inflammation.

sclerosis becomes better developed, the inflammatory infiltrate becomes less apparent in the superficial layers of dermis/submucosa and becomes more prominent below the zone of sclerosis, sometimes forming a prominent band. In longstanding lesions, a complete absence of inflammatory cells may be noted.

The epidermal surface often shows loss of rete pegs and thinning; hence, the synonym lichen sclerosus et atrophicus (Figs 2.13, 2.14). However, hyperkeratosis and/or acanthosis due to superimposed lichen simplex chronicus secondary to the trauma of scratching and rubbing is also commonly present (Fig. 2.15). This hyperkeratotic pattern is common in the vulva in contrast to the much more common atrophic epidermis seen in extra-anogenital LS.[61,62]

Differential diagnosis

Established lesions of lichen sclerosus are usually easily recognized. Early lesions, as noted above, are not always associated with specific histologic findings and distinction from lichen planus, in particular, may be quite difficult. In a study by Fung and LeBoit[63] comparing early LS and lichen planus, they found that the following features favored lichen sclerosus: psoriasiform epidermal changes, presence of lymphocytes within the epidermis (exotropism), decreased elastic fibers and basement membrane thickening. Features that favored lichen planus included basal layer squamatization (loss of the basal layer), wedge-shaped hypergranulosis, the presence of numerous necrotic keratinocytes and pointed ('saw-tooth') rete ridges. (See also p.000 for a more detailed discussion of lichen planus.)

Vitiligo may be confused on gross evaluation with LS. Lichen sclerosus is characterized by hypopigmen-

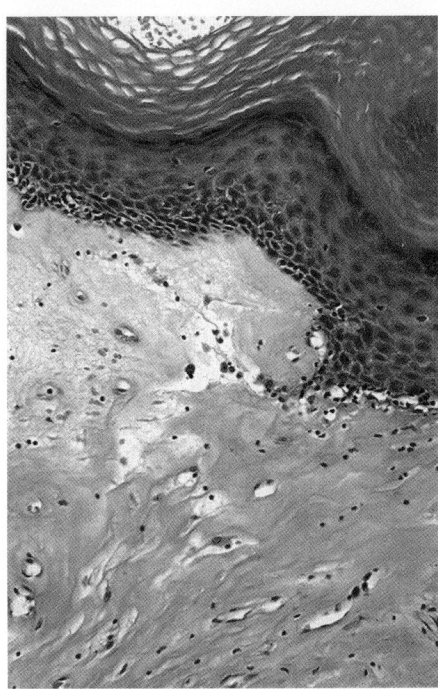

Fig. 2.13 Vulval lichen sclerosus: in this view, there is marked hyperkeratosis, hypergranulosis and acanthosis. The dermis shows severe sclerosis.

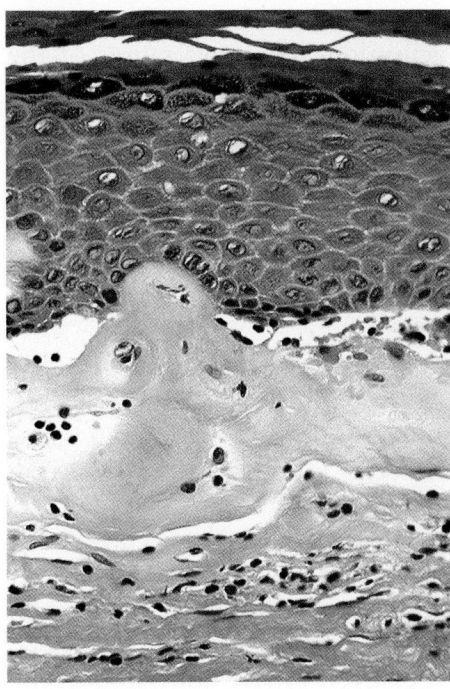

Fig. 2.15 Lichen sclerosus with superimposed lichen simplex chronicus.

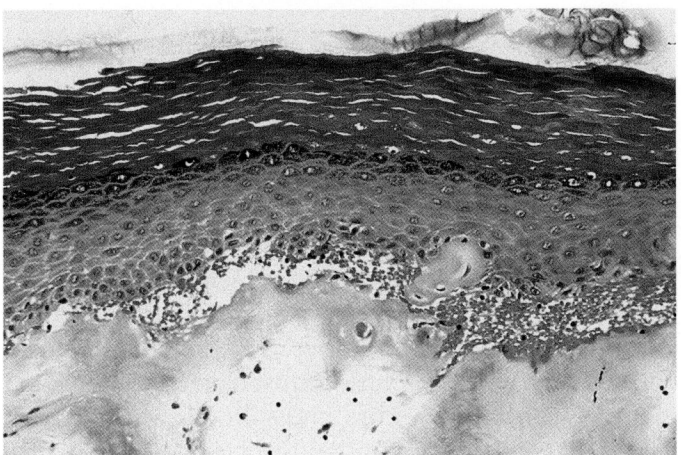

Fig. 2.14 Higher power of Figure 2.12 shows prominent basal cell hydropic degeneration (interface change).

tation and loss of melanocytes. It is not associated with sclerosis of the dermis/submucosa. This differential diagnosis is usually a clinical, rather than histologic, dilemma. In vitiligo, the whitened area is usually flat and symmetrical.

Radiation change, like LS, is associated with sclerosis of the dermis/submucosa but the sclerosis is not limited to a well-defined superficial band as is the case in LS. Also, bizarre 'radiation fibroblasts' and thick-walled vessels that are characteristic of radiation damage are not seen in LS. Clinical correlation is important when radiation change is suspected.

Cancer risk

LS may be associated with squamous cell carcinoma, which is estimated to occur in ~5% of women with LS.[61,64] This figure is difficult to verify as lesions adjacent to squamous cell carcinoma are often overlooked.[64] Women with concomitant squamous cell carcinoma and LS seem to be significantly older compared with women with uncomplicated LS.[61] The association of LS with vulvar cancer and additional patterns that may increase the risk of vulvar cancer (such as coexisting lichen simplex chronicus in older women and differentiated VIN) are discussed in Chapter 6.

Therapy of lichen sclerosus

The treatment of choice is an ultra-potent, topical corticosteroid ointment (clobetasol propionate 0.05% – Temovate®) b.i.d. × 1 month, then q.d. × 2 months. Follow with a Class 4 steroid, then gradually decrease the steroid dose. (There is debate regarding whether or not long-term steroids are required. Some health-care providers prescribe clobetasol propionate 0.05% to be used p.r.n. after completing the first 3 months of treatment.) Scarring is not reversible by any medical therapy.

For severe lichen sclerosus, night-time sedation for the first week or two may be required to enhance comfort and healing. Recently, it has been reported that tacrolimus ointment has been used for the treatment of vulvar lichen sclerosus. Tacrolimus inhibits the production of interleukin IL-2 by helper T-cells, thereby blocking activation and proliferation of the immune response.

Surgery is rarely required; however, patients with vulvar changes affecting the vaginal diameter, such as labial adhesions, may require surgical intervention.

LICHEN PLANUS

Clinical presentation

Lichen planus (LP) is a chronic inflammatory dermatosis that can involve both skin and mucosal sites. A clinical spectrum ranging from a self-limited papulosquamous disorder (Fig. 2.16) to an erosive form (Fig. 2.17) associated with significant tissue destruction is recognized.[65] The prevalence is not known, but it is commonly seen in dermatology clinics. Vulvar involvement is significantly less common than extra-genital disease.

The pathogenesis of LP is poorly understood. The disease is probably related to T-cell autoimmunity. LP appears to be slightly more common in women. This female predilection is more pronounced in the oral erosive form. Occasionally, LP has been seen in association with vulvar squamous cell carcinoma[66,67] and vulvar intraepithelial neoplasia 3 (VIN 3),[68] but the relationship between these conditions is unclear. LP, mainly the erosive form, appears to be a minor risk factor for development of subsequent squamous cell carcinoma. Vulvar lichen planus occurs in women primarily between the ages of 30 and 60. While the cutaneous and oral mucosal lesions of lichen planus (Fig. 2.16) are well-documented, vulvar involvement by lichen planus has received much less attention. As more healthcare providers become aware of this condition, it is recognized more frequently. LP has several appearances in the vulva. Lesions of the labia majora (true hair-bearing skin) are characterized as small, often violaceous, polygonal papules that are usually intensively pruritic. While these lesions are usually quite well-demarcated on non-vulvar skin, this is often not the case in the vulva. Lesions commonly resolve within 2 years and can leave residual hyperpigmented areas. However, chronic erosive LP is much more refractory to therapy and may persist for years. LP characteristically exhibits the Koebner phenomenon – development of lesions at sites of previous trauma. For example, a linear arrangement of lesions often follows scratching. A variant designated hypertrophic LP has a marked papular appearance with a scaly surface (lichenification).[69] Hypertrophic

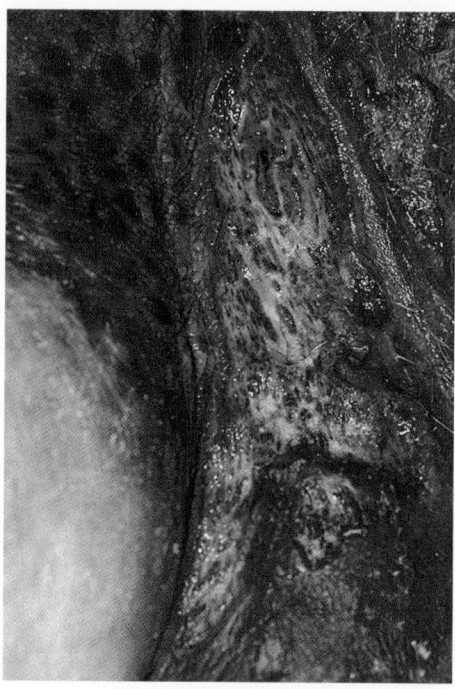

Fig. 2.16 Non-erosive lichen planus of the vulva.

LP represents lichen simplex chronicus secondary to rubbing and scratching superimposed on LP.

Erosive LP is the most common type, as well as the most challenging form for both the healthcare provider and patient. Erosive LP[70,71] may present as a desquamative disease with ulceration that often extends into the vagina and can also involve the labia majora to a limited extent. This form often presents with dyspareunia. The edges of these lesions appear similar to the classic lesions described above. Erosive LP is usually chronic and can cause considerable damage with effacement of the labia minora and clitoral areas, loss of vaginal space by adhesions and stenosis.

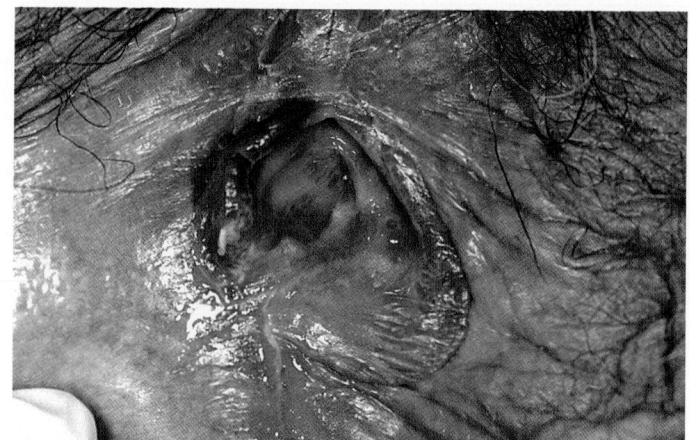

Fig. 2.17 Erosive lichen planus.

A syndrome of involvement by LP of the oral/ buccal, vulvar and vaginal mucosa has been termed the vulvovaginal-gingival syndrome (Fig. 2.18).[70,72] It may be associated with a desquamative vaginitis (with or without adhesions), erythematous vestibulitis (with or without erosions) and erosive gingivitis of the desquamative or bullous type. While likely representing a variant of erosive LP, this syndrome illustrates the importance of examination of the oral mucosa and vulvar areas when the lesions of LP are found at either site. A substantial proportion of patients with vulvar LP have extravulvar lesions and their recognition can aid in the diagnosis. It is also important to examine the vulva in all cases of LP as vulvar involvement may be seen in up to half of the cases with cutaneous disease and is sometimes asymptomatic.[73] Topical steroids are the mainstay of treatment for LP.

Histopathology

The classic changes of LP are of an interface dermatitis consisting primarily of a band-like infiltrate of lymphocytes in the papillary dermis/submucosa associated with necrotic keratinocytes in the lower layers of the epidermis/mucosa (Fig. 2.19). As a response to the interface changes, there is often loss of the basal layer of the epithelium, a change referred to as 'squamatization'. The epithelium may be thickened or thinned. A wedge-shaped zone of hypergranulosis is characteristic of lesions involving the skin, but not mucosa. Hyperkeratosis is more characteristic of skin lesions while parakeratosis is often present in mucosal sites. Frequently, the rete pegs become elongated with sharpened or pointed tips referred to as a 'saw-tooth'

pattern, a finding that again is more pronounced in skin lesions.

The inflammatory infiltrate in lesions involving skin is composed of lymphocytes and a few histiocytes. Some histiocytes contain intracytoplasmic melanin ('melanophages') as a result of pigment incontinence, a non-specific feature encountered in many inflammatory dermatoses. In non-mucosal sites, plasma cells and eosinophils are generally not seen (Fig. 2.20). In contrast, plasma cells and the occasional eosinophil may be encountered in mucosal LP.[69] Thus, it is imperative to determine the site of biopsy (skin versus mucosa) since the composition of the inflammatory infiltrate broadens or narrows the histologic differential diagnosis (see below).

Erosive LP in the mucosa shows non-specific changes of chronic inflammation with loss of the epidermal layer in the ulcerated areas. It is important in such cases to biopsy the edge of the lesion to see the classic and pathognomonic changes described above. Direct immunofluorescence of erosive LP lesions reveals an irregular deposition of fibrin at the dermal–epidermal junction without immunoglobulin deposition.[74] It is important to have the clinician biopsy the suspicious area at the edge of the lesion and send this biopsy to histopathology. An additional biopsy should be obtained from the adjacent normal tissue and this should be sent for immunofluorescent testing.

Differential diagnosis

Early lichen sclerosus (LS) can present as an interface dermatitis and may exhibit both a psoriasiform and saw-toothed epithelial growth pattern. The most

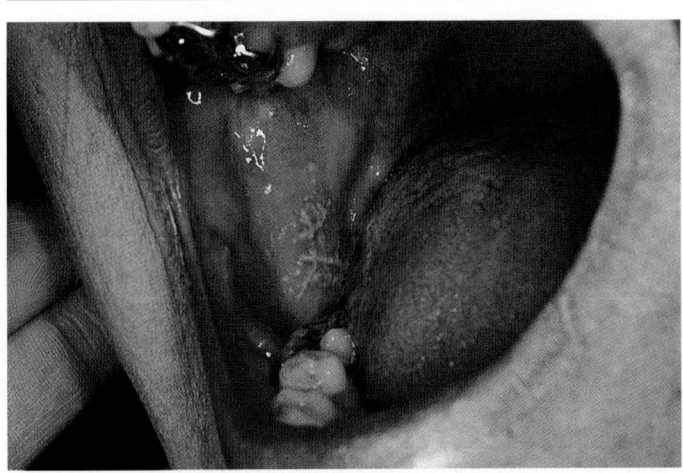

Fig. 2.18 Oral lichen planus.

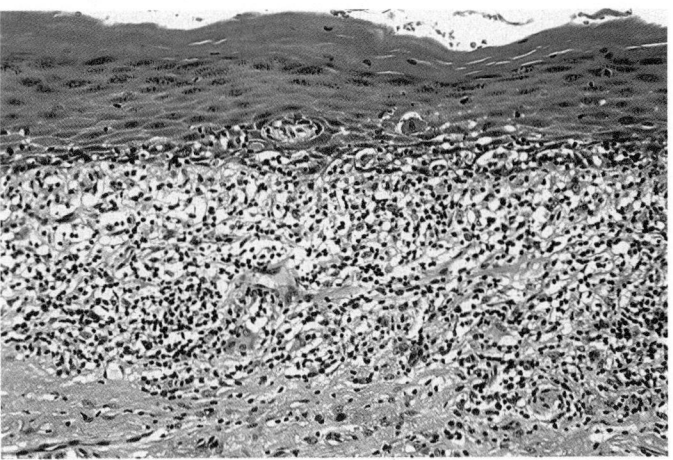

Fig. 2.19 Vulval lichen planus. There is hyperkeratosis, hypergranulosis, apoptosis, basal cell hydropic change and a superficial band-like infiltrate.

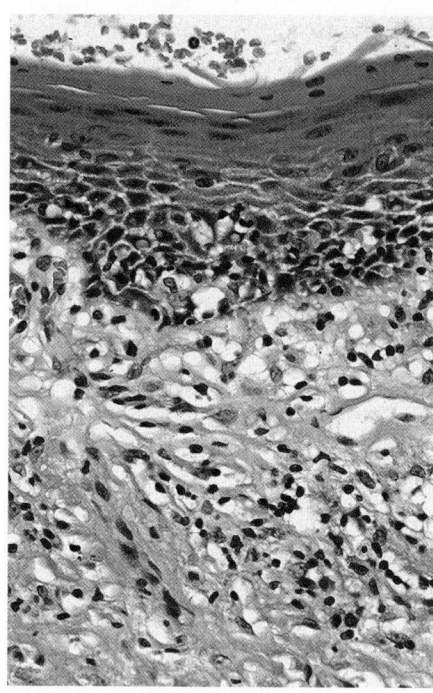

Fig. 2.20 Vulval lichen planus. In addition to lymphocytes and histiocytes, scattered eosinophils are present.

important distinguishing feature is hyalinization of the papillary dermis in LS (Fig. 2.11). In some cases, however, it is impossible to make the distinction on histologic grounds.

Erosive LP brings to bear the differential diagnosis of all desquamating dermatoses. Biopsies from the ulcer bed will show non-specific inflammatory changes, so it is important to obtain a biopsy from the edge of an erosive lesion to differentiate these entities. LP can occasionally form bullous lesions and, in difficult cases, immunofluorescence studies should readily distinguish immunobullous disorders from LP. When significant numbers of plasma cells and eosinophils are present in mucosal biopsies, other dermatoses such as hypersensitivity reactions (i.e. lichenoid drug eruption) must be considered. Zoon's vulvitis is distinguished by the presence of a heavy plasma cell-rich infiltrate and absence of interface changes Additional conditions to consider in the differential diagnosis include genital warts, psoriasis, VIN and candidiasis. White lesions can mimic lichen sclerosus. Erosive lesions mimic cicatricial pemphigoid and pemphigus vulgaris. At times, squamous dysplasia may be in the differential diagnosis.

Treatment

Success of treatment varies, dependent on the extent of the disease. Papular disease responds well to topical steroids. Erosive disease is much more difficult to treat. Potent steroids will produce improvement, but cures are rare. The most recent treatment for lichen planus is tacrolimus.

Regular follow-up is required in patients with vulvo-vaginal lichen planus, including evaluation for any suspicious changes that could represent cancer. Additionally, emotional support is of utmost importance for this often devastating condition.

ZOON'S VULVITIS (PLASMA CELL VULVITIS)

Clinical presentation

Zoon's vulvitis (ZV), also known as vulvitis circumscripta plasmacellularis or plasma cell vulvitis, is a rare vulvar condition, with less than 70 cases reported. It is characterized, as the latter name implies, by a sharply defined, red-to-brown macule (Fig. 2.21). These lesions are often solitary and can be asymptomatic, but soreness, pruritus and burning are occasional complaints.[75,76] This condition can also affect the lips and other mucosal sites. Penile lesions were first described by Zoon in 1952 as balanitis chronica circumscripta plasmacellularis[77] and are usually seen in uncircumcised men.[78] The vulvar form was first described in 1954[79] and most often affects middle-aged women. The age range is 25–70 years. It has not been reported in prepubescent females. While penile involvement can be associated with development of carcinoma,[80] this has not been reported in Zoon's vulvitis.

Histopathology

Biopsy of ZV reveals a dense lichenoid (or band-like) infiltrate in the upper submucosa or lamina propria in the absence of interface change (Fig. 2.22). In addi-

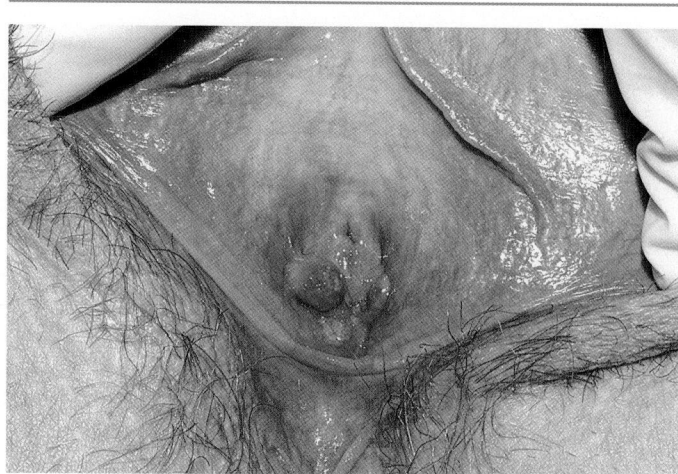

Fig. 2.21 Zoon's vulvitis gross exam.

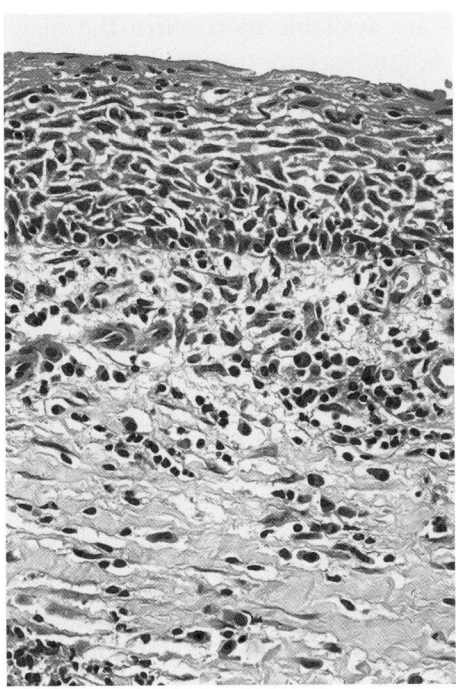

Fig. 2.22 Zoon's balanitis of the penile mucosa. Note the heavy plasma cell infiltrate and spongiosis.

tion, the infiltrate may also involve the deeper connective tissue as well. Plasma cells comprise the majority of the infiltrate, admixed with lymphocytes, mast cells and occasional eosinophils. Lymphoid follicles are unusual. Increased vascularity is sometimes seen with extravasated red cells and hemosiderin deposition. Longer-standing lesions may show dermal fibrosis. The overlying epidermis varies from thin and attenuated to hyperplastic. Spongiosis is often present. Due to the non-specific nature of this constellation of features, clinical correlation is necessary to establish the diagnosis. It is also important to rule out infection. Some authors feel that this condition may be an unusual reaction to injury rather than an inflammatory disorder sui generis.[81]

Differential diagnosis

Excluding syphilis is critical before rendering a diagnosis of ZV. Appropriate serology (rapid plasma reagent (RPR) or venereal disease research laboratory, VDRL tests) or a histochemical stain identifies syphilis. It should be remembered that spirochetes may not be identified in the later stages of disease and, therefore, their absence on histochemical stains does not exclude syphilis. Lichen planus can be distinguished from ZV by the presence of interface change. The band-like lymphocytic infiltrate in lichen planus may contain plasma cells when involving mucosal sites. The lack of blistering in ZV allows differentiation from cicatricial pemphigoid.

Treatment

Treatment involves the use of corticosteroids. The steroids are given topically, intravaginally or as intralesional steroid injections.

BULLOUS AND CICATRICIAL PEMPHIGOID

Introduction

Pemphigoid is an autoimmune bullous disorder that usually occurs in older adults. It has been seen in the setting of other autoimmune diseases such as systemic lupus erythematosus, primary biliary cirrhosis, ulcerative colitis, alopecia areata and diabetes.[82] While a number of variants have been described, two are of particular importance in the vulva. Cicatricial pemphigoid (CP) is associated with mucosal involvement and scarring while bullous pemphigoid (BP) is not associated with scarring.

BP is the most common subepidermal autoimmune bullous disorder, representing the majority of cases. It is caused by autoantibodies against a 230 kD intracellular plakin (known as BPAg1) that is a component of the hemidesmosome and a 180 kD transmembrane glycoprotein (BPAg2) that is a component of type XVII collagen and seen in the lamina lucida.[82] The presence of these autoantibodies leads to deposition of IgG and complement in the basement membrane with subsequent damage and loss of adhesion between the dermal and epidermal layers. CP has a similar pathogenic mechanism.

Bullous pemphigoid

The lesions of BP initially arise as tense intact vesicles. There is no gender predilection. Nikolsky's sign is usually negative. Prodromal changes include erythema and urticaria, though preceding skin changes may not be seen. The most commonly affected areas are the lower abdomen, groin and flexural surfaces of the arms and legs. Mucosal involvement is not commonly seen. BP is a chronic disease, but patients experience periods of remission. It usually carries a good prognosis, but can be associated with considerable morbidity if it becomes widespread and unresponsive to treatment. Isolated vulvar involvement and presentation in the vulva have been described for both BP and CP, but are uncommon.[83,84] While pemphigoid usually occurs in older adults, younger adults and children may also be affected, including patients with vulvar involvement.[85–87] Of the approximately 50 reported cases of childhood BP, the vulva was the primary site of involvement in 10 patients.[87] BP rarely involves the vagina.

The degree of involvement and the rate of disease progression guide the treatment of bullous pemphigoid. Hydroxyzine is used to control pruritus. Steroids (topical, systemic) are common treatment. Antibiotics (tetracycline, minocycline, or erythromycin, with or without niacinamide) and dapsone are also used for some patients. Adjuvant immunosuppression with azathioprine may be considered if dapsone and oral steroids fail. Cyclophosphamide is also used as a steroid-sparing drug. It is more toxic than azathioprine and is reserved for elderly patients who have extensive disease and who do not tolerate azathioprine. Methotrexate has also been utilized for this condition. Other treatments that have been used in patients with severe progressive disease include cyclosporine, chlorambucil, mycophenolate mofetil, plasmapheresis and intravenous immunoglobulins.[4]

Cicatricial pemphigoid

Cicatricial pemphigoid has a predilection for mucous membrane surfaces (conjunctivae and oral mucosa). The lesions of CP are quite similar to those of BP, except that scarring is common and mucosal surfaces are more often involved.[88,89] It more commonly involves the vulva than bullous pemphigoid. There appears to be a female predominance and the average age of onset is somewhat younger[90] than for BP. CP may be more common than BP in the vulva. CP can also be associated with vaginal desquamation. Smaller blisters and erosions sometimes lead to severe scarring and disfigurement, including labial fusion. In CP, the erosion occurs at a deep area within the basement membrane, resulting in scarring. The presence of scarring is critical to separate CP from BP. Cases of drug-induced vulvar CP have also been described.[91]

Histopathology

Pemphigoid is characterized by subepidermal, unilocular bullae (Fig. 2.23). It is one of several acantholytic lesions of the vulva that are summarized in Table 2.2. Early lesions and lesions involving non-inflamed skin may be cell-poor, but most bullae contain a prominent inflammatory infiltrate with conspicuous eosinophils and variable numbers of neutrophils in a background of serum and fibrin (Fig. 2.24). While these bullae are subepithelial, care must be taken in older lesions not to interpret re-epithelialization as an intraepidermal split. In some cases, the lesions of BP and CP are identical, as scarring may not be prominent in some cases of CP. However, scarring is usually seen in older CP lesions.

Several methods are available to confirm the diagnosis. Direct immunofluorescence usually demonstrates a linear, homogenous pattern of IgG and often C3 at the basement membrane for both bullous and cicatricial pemphigoid, while a reticular or intercellular pattern of IgG and C3 deposition is demonstrated in pemphigus vulgaris and vegetans. A salt split skin preparation usually demonstrates that autoantibodies from the patient's serum are associated with the epidermal side of the split in the test sample. Serum autoantibodies to the 230 kD BPAg1 and 180 kD BPAg2 can be demonstrated by immunoblotting, but serum autoantibody testing is usually not necessary[82,92] to make the diagnosis.

Differential diagnosis

CP is distinguished from BP by the clinical history of scarring. Pemphigus is differentiated by the presence of suprabasilar blistering on histology. Pemphigus also shows intermembranous staining for IgG and C3 on immunofluorescence. CP lesions with scarring may mimic lichen sclerosus.[11] Immunofluorescence staining will readily differentiate lichen sclerosus from CP. Lichen planus may show atrophic scarring in the vulva and may also be associated with mucosal erosions, but the direct immunofluorescence findings of CP will not be present.

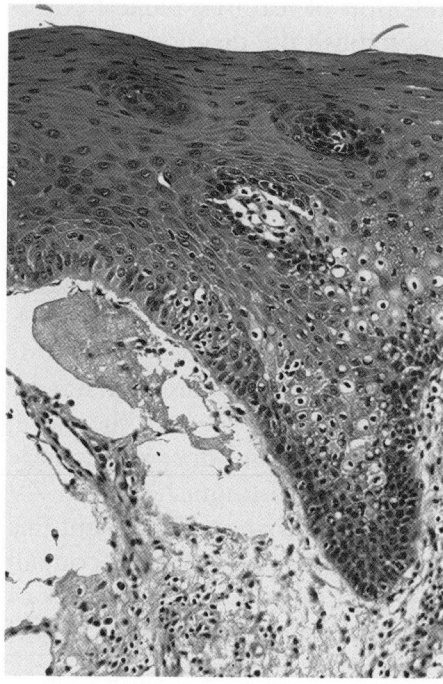

Fig. 2.23 Mucosal cicatricial pemphigoid. Part of a cell-poor subepidermal blister is evident.

Table 2.2 *Differential diagnosis of acantholytic disorders of the vulva*

Disorder	Familial	Truncal involvement	Solitary versus multiple	Other
Pemphigus vulgaris	No	Sometimes	Multiple	IgG oral involvement
Hailey–Hailey disease (benign familial pemphigus)	Yes; onset in 3rd or 4th decade	Intertriginous areas	Multiple	
Darier's disease	Family history; onset in 2nd and 3rd decade	Seborrheic (face, scalp, chest, back)	Multiple	
Acantholytic dermatosis	No	No	Multiple	Limited to vulva by definition
Grover disease (transient acantholytic dermatosis)	No	Yes	Multiple	Extremely pruritic
Warty dyskeratoma	No	No	Solitary	
VIN, differentiated type	No	No	Solitary	Atypia

VIN, vulvar intraepithelial neoplasia.

Treatment

Patients with CP are treated like those with BP (see Treatment section for bullous pemphigoid). Patients with genital involvement are treated aggressively. Other treatments include labial separation (gentle manual separation) and vaginal dilation to prevent adhesions.

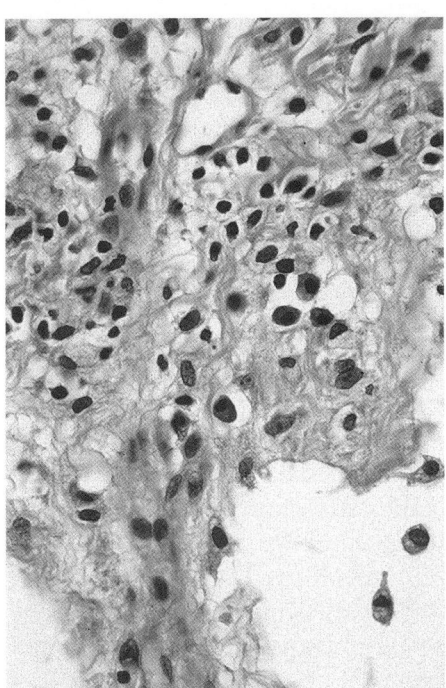

Fig. 2.24 Mucosal cicatricial pemphigoid. The adjacent lamina propria shows a plasma cell-rich infiltrate.

PEMPHIGUS VULGARIS AND PEMPHIGUS VEGETANS

Clinical presentation

Pemphigus vulgaris is a rare acquired autoimmune blistering disorder associated with mucosal erosions and flaccid bullae on the skin. It is caused by autoantibodies against desmoglein 3, a 130 kD glycoprotein representing a component of the desmosome that forms tight junctions in the epidermis.[93,94] The 160 kD desmoglein 1 may also be involved,[94] although its role in pemphigus foliaceus is more fully understood.

Patients often present with painful mucosal erosions involving the mouth, nasal or anogenital mucosa; however, bullae can be seen at any site. They are rarely pruritic, but can be painful. Intact bullae are positive for Nikolsky's sign: the borders of a blister can be extended with pressure. Intact blisters may be few, or absent, due to fragility. While pemphigus vulgaris is not associated with scarring at other sites, vulvar involvement sometimes leads to local scarring and disfigurement.[95] Vaginal adhesions and discharge can also be present.[96]

The pemphigus vegetans variant can arise in the setting of pemphigus vulgaris. In this condition, hypertrophic or warty vegetations develop in association with the bullae.

Histopathology

Acantholysis leads to suprabasilar blistering with basilar cells aligned at the dermal–epidermal junction resembling a 'row of tombstones' in well-developed blisters

(Fig. 2.25). Immunofluorescence studies reveal IgG and C3 decorating the cell surface or intercellular regions of the epidermis. The lesions of pemphigus vegetans show similar immunofluorescence findings, but are associated with extreme acanthosis, hyperkeratosis and an inflammatory infiltrate consisting primarily of lymphocytes and eosinophils which often masks the acantholysis.

Differential diagnosis

The differential diagnosis of vulvar pemphigus vulgaris includes other blistering and ulcerative disorders. Pemphigus can be distinguished from pemphigoid (both the bullous and cicatricial types) by the location at which the blisters occur. Bullous pemphigoid is associated with a subepidermal split and linear deposition of IgG and usually C3 along the basement membrane on immunofluorescence. The blisters of pemphigoid are more tense and do not erode as readily. Since the blisters of pemphigus have often been eroded by the time they are biopsied, obtaining tissue from the edge of the lesion combined with the characteristic immunofluorescence findings of intercellular IgG and C3 is often critical.

Pemphigus must be distinguished from Hailey–Hailey disease, Darier's disease, acantholysis of the vulvocrural area and warty dyskeratoma.[97,98] Hailey–Hailey disease (autosomal dominant disorder) is often associated with a positive family history. Immunofluorescence is negative in Hailey–Hailey disease. In contrast to pemphigus, dyskeratosis involving all levels of the epidermis is seen in Darier's disease, warty dyskeratoma and acantholysis of the vulvocrural area. These diseases are not immunobullous disorders and, therefore, have negative immunofluorescence findings.

Treatment

The primary treatment for pemphigus consists of corticosteroids. Potent topical corticosteroids, intralesional as well as oral steroids are used as treatments. At times, steroid-sparing agents (cyclophosphamide, azathioprine) are required. Rarely, methotrexate may be required. It is important to treat any superinfection that may occur.

HAILEY–HAILEY DISEASE

Clinical presentation

Hailey–Hailey disease (HHD) is an acantholytic genodermatosis with predilection for moist body creases such as flexural or intertriginous areas (neck, axillae and inguinal areas).[97] It may also occur in the inframammary folds. HHD is a rare autosomal dominant disorder. The pathogenesis of HHD is not fully understood but involves mutations in a calcium pump, ATP2C1. Of interest, Darier's disease (see p. 43), another acantholytic dermatosis, is also associated with mutations in a gene encoding a different, but related, calcium pump. Dysregulation of calcium metabolism is thought to weaken intracellular junctions. Approximately 70% of cases are familial.[97]

In the past, this disease has been referred to as benign familial pemphigus, a name that caused confusion, as this disease bears no relationship to pemphigus. Inguinal involvement often extends to the vulva and isolated vulvar involvement has been described.[98–101] The lesions begin as pruritic erosions that spread centrifugally to involve the surrounding skin. They tend to form a crust centrally and are often associated with a foul odor. Resolution, usually over several months, can result in hypopigmentation, but scarring is not a feature. Maceration is common in the intertriginous areas as is superinfection with *Candida albicans*, *Staphylococcus aureus* and herpesvirus. HHD cases clinically masquerading as candidiasis or leukoplakia have been described.[98,99] Rarely, squamous cell carcinoma (SCC) can arise in association with vulvar or non-vulvar HHD.[102,103] One vulvar SCC in this setting was associated with human papillomavirus infection.[104]

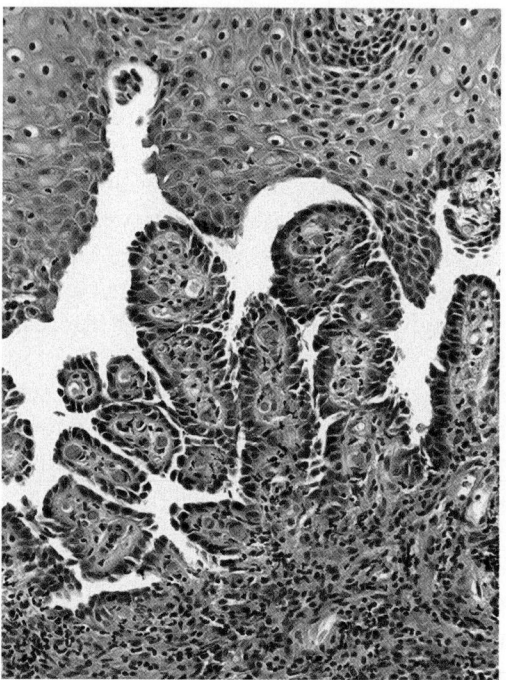

Fig. 2.25 Pemphigus vulgaris: supra-basal acantholysis and 'pseudo villi' ('tombstone effect').

Histopathology

Histologic examination of HHD reveals intraepidermal acantholytic vesicles and bullae. The acantholytic keratinocytes in the blister maintain a somewhat ordered appearance sometimes described as a 'dilapidated brick wall' (Fig. 2.26). Early lesions may show only suprabasilar lacunae, similar to Darier's disease or pemphigus. Dyskeratotic cells similar to the corps ronds and grains of Darier can be seen, but are usually not conspicuous. Immunofluorescence staining is negative in HHD.

Differential diagnosis

HHD may show histologic findings that closely resemble pemphigus vulgaris. In fact, before the advent of immunofluorescence, these two orders were considered related due to their histologic similarities. Fortunately, immunofluorescence easily distinguishes them. Pemphigus vulgaris is associated with intercellular immunoreactants, usually IgG and C3. HHD should be distinguished from bullous pemphigoid and cicatricial pemphigoid, which can also involve the vulva.[84,105,106] In contrast to HHD, the blisters of pemphigoid are subepidermal and tend to be rich in inflammatory cells, particularly eosinophils. Cicatricial pemphigoid involves mucosal sites (including the modified mucosa of the vulvar labia) and often results in scarring. The blisters of cicatricial pemphigoid are similar to those of bullous pemphigoid. Positive immunofluorescence

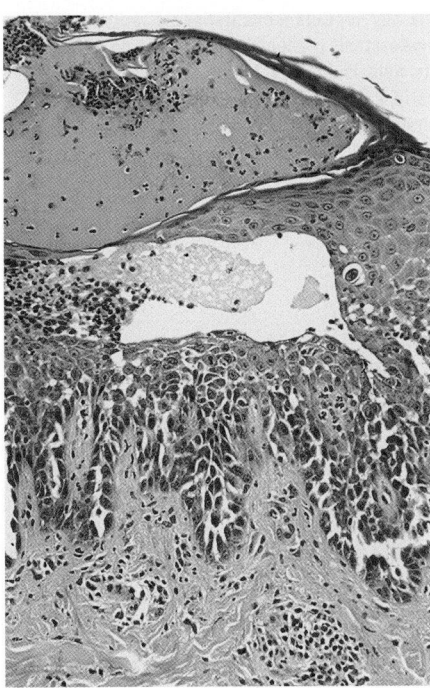

Fig. 2.26 Cutaneous Hailey–Hailey disease: the dilapidated brick wall appearance as shown in this field is a characteristic finding.

staining (often IgG and C3 along the basement membrane) is seen in bullous pemphigoid. HHD is distinguished from Darier's disease by its more uniform acantholysis. In addition, dyskeratosis is a more prominent feature in Darier's disease.

Because HHD is associated with marked acantholysis, it may be confused with vulvar intraepithelial neoplasia, which may contain acantholysis. In the latter, acantholysis is usually focal and the diagnosis of VIN is easily made. However, this may explain occasional associations between HHD and vulvar cancer (see Ch. 6).

Treatment

Currently, there is no cure for Hailey–Hailey disease. Patients should avoid triggers such as sunburn, sweating and friction. Aluminum acetate compresses, mild corticosteroid preparations and topical antibiotics may result in transient improvement.

DARIER'S DISEASE

Clinical presentation

Darier's disease is an uncommon genodermatosis in which patents present with numerous hyperkeratotic papules usually distributed over the trunk. It can be inherited in an autosomal dominant fashion, although only about one-half of the cases reported in a large series have a positive family history.[107] The gene linked to this condition has been isolated and codes for ATP2A2, a calcium pump protein.[108] Despite this discovery, the precise pathogenic mechanism remains poorly understood. A localized form that does not appear to be inherited has also been described.

Lesions usually present around puberty, but can occur later in life. The gender distribution is equal, although males appear to be more severely affected.[109] Skin lesions are warty and pruritic and can be associated with a foul odor, resulting in considerable embarrassment to the patient. Nails tend be thin, brittle and dystrophic. Superinfection with bacteria, virus or fungus is common and superficial wounds resulting from scratching to relieve pruritus are often evident. Isolated vulvar disease is rare, but has occasionally been documented.[110–112] The presentation can be subtle. Heat, sweating and maceration, which are common conditions in the vulvar region, can induce or exacerbate lesions.[109] A case of squamous cell carcinoma of the vulva found incidentally in association with Darier's disease has been described.[112]

Histopathology

Histologic examination reveals acanthosis, columns of parakeratosis and acantholysis with suprabasilar clefts or lacunae. The surrounding epidermis often shows hyperkeratosis. Characteristic dyskeratotic cells termed corps ronds and grains of Darier are usually present (Fig. 2.27a,b). Corps ronds occur in the stratum spinosum and have irregular nuclei that are eccentrically placed. The cytoplasm is clear but surrounded by a dense keratotic shell. Grains of Darier are found in the stratum corneum and are elongated cells with conspicuous keratohyaline granules representing premature keratinization.

Differential diagnosis

Darier's disease should be distinguished from Hailey–Hailey disease which commonly involves the genital region. Early lesions in Hailey–Hailey disease can show more limited suprabasilar acantholysis, but extensive acantholysis is seen in fully developed lesions. Extensive dyskeratosis is not a feature of Hailey–Hailey disease. Warty dyskeratoma can occur in the vulva[113] and, while it can be histologically similar to a lesion of Darier's disease, it is typically solitary and usually has a distinct papillary architecture. Acantholysis of the vulvocrural area has a similar histologic appearance to Darier's disease, but does not occur in a familial setting.

Corp rond-like structures may also be seen in classic vulvar intraepithelial neoplasia and pseudo-Bowenoid papulosis (a variant of condyloma). These are discussed in Chapter 6.

Treatment

Patients should be advised to use high-factor sunscreens and to avoid from sunlight as much as possible. Treatment with oral retinoids, such as isotretinoin, have been the most effective medical treatment for Darier's disease; however, prolonged remissions are not seen.

ACANTHOLYTIC DERMATOSIS OF THE VULVOCRURAL AREA

Clinical presentation

Acantholytic dermatosis of the vulvocrural area (ADV) was first proposed as a distinct entity in 1984.[114] The condition presents as discrete flesh-colored to white papules that are less than 1 cm in diameter and may be solitary or grouped and can become confluent. The involved skin is sometimes erythematous and pruritic. The lesions involve the labia and/or the inguinal crease.[115] Similar lesions in males have been described.[116] The lesions tend to be chronic and treatment is problematic.[116,117]

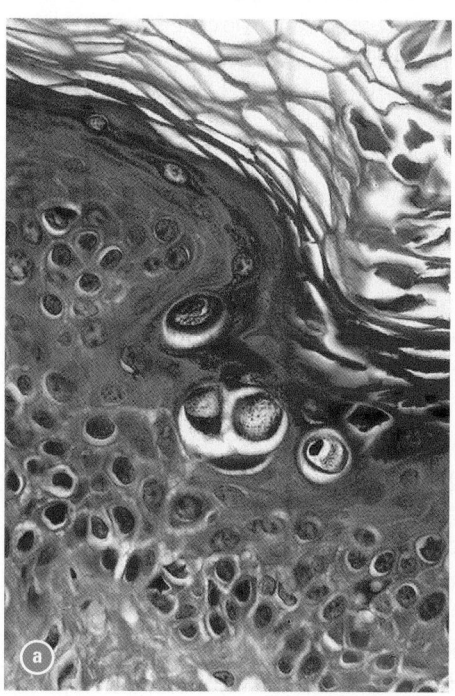
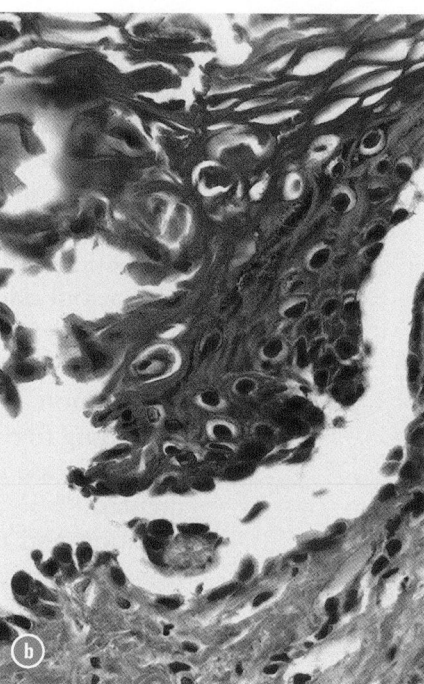

Fig. 2.27 (a) Cutaneous Darier's disease. Dyskeratosis presenting as corps rond, as seen in this field, is a typical feature. (b) Cutaneous Darier's disease. Parakeratosis with large retained nuclei (grains of Darier) is commonly present.

Histopathology

On biopsy, these lesions resemble Darier's or Hailey–Hailey disease. The involved skin may exhibit hyperkeratosis. Acantholysis is prominent and scattered dyskeratotic cells including corps ronds and grains of Darier can be seen. ADV is consistently negative when analyzed by immunofluorescence.

Differential diagnosis

ADV is a sporadic disease and is thus distinguished from cases of Darier's and Hailey–Hailey disease that are associated with a family history. Grover's disease or transient acantholytic disease can have a similar histologic appearance, but involves the trunk and usually resolves within weeks to months. Warty dyskeratoma usually affects the head and neck but may rarely present in the vulva[113] and histologically shows overlap with ADV,[96] although it typically has a papillary structure. Focal acantholytic dermatosis is differentiated by its very localized involvement and frequent association with another cutaneous lesion such a melanocytic nevus, dermatofibroma or scar. Pemphigus vegetans shows characteristic immunofluorescence findings that are lacking in ADV.

Treatment

Acantholytic dermatosis of the vulvocrural area is a difficult condition to treat. The lesions persist long term. Topical treatments generally have not proven to be effective. Some patients have responded to surgical excisions.[111] Electrocautery has also been used to remove some papules.[114]

FOX–FORDYCE DISEASE

Clinical

Fox–Fordyce disease (FFD), alternatively designated apocrine miliaris, is characterized by pruritic papules confined to skin-bearing apocrine glands. FFD most commonly affects the axillae, but is also seen in the apocrine-rich genital, perianal and mammary regions. Women represent the vast majority of the reported cases.[118,119] Papular eruptions are associated with severe paroxysmal pruritus. The vulva can be affected due to the presence of numerous apocrine glands in this region. Symptoms at this site can be accentuated by emotional or physical stimuli. FFD has been described to coexist with hidradenitis suppurativa,[120] but the relationship between these two conditions is not clear. Keratolytic agents are sometimes effective treatment. The pathogenesis is not understood. Apocrine duct

plugging results in complete apocrine anhidrosis, though eccrine sweating is intact.

Histopathology

The findings in FFD are not specific, but hyperkeratosis with plugging and surrounding spongiosis is often present. Involvement of the apocrine duct as it enters infundibular epithelium is a more specific marker, but can be difficult to demonstrate in histologic sections. Some authors have suggested that transverse sectioning of a punch biopsy aids in this distinction.[121] The apocrine plugging results in cystic ducts that can rupture and form retention cysts. Mild chronic inflammation surrounding the adnexal glands and follicles is sometimes a feature.[122]

Differential diagnosis

Eczematous dermatitis may occasionally show follicular involvement in a pattern that may be very difficult or impossible to distinguish from FFD. Clinical correlation should help in most cases since FFD shows a predilection for apocrine-rich areas of the body. Hyperkeratotic plugging of hair follicles is not a feature of eczematous dermatitis.

It is important to differentiate FFD from the yellow papules of Fordyce spots that can be demonstrated on normal inner labia majora and minora. Fordyce spots represent sebaceous glands unassociated with hair follicles that communicate directly with the epithelium. They are an incidental finding not associated with any symptoms.

Treatment

Retinoids, topical steroids, antibiotics, hormonal therapy, ultraviolet light, dermabrasion and surgical excision may provide symptomatic relief but are not curative.

HIDRADENITIS SUPPURATIVA

Clinical

Hidradenitis suppurativa (HS) is a chronic suppurative inflammatory process associated with abscess and sinus tract formation that occurs in apocrine-rich areas of the skin. Severe scarring and disfigurement can result. A recent study has questioned the strict apocrine association.[123]

HS presents in young adults and is more frequently seen in females. Presentation before puberty is exceptional. The majority of cases show axillary involvement, but groin or genital involvement is also common. Other sites include perineal and perianal regions and, more rarely, the breast. It has a wide range of severity. Patients with mild cases have recurrent isolated nodules. Patients with severe disease have involvement of the mons pubis and the disease may extend out to the thighs (Fig. 2.28). The disease presents as a single warm, erythematous papule that can be painful. With time, ulceration and sinus tract formation associated with abscesses develop. Secondary infection with cutaneous commensal bacteria such as staphylococci and streptococci may be seen. Infection with anaerobic bacteria can cause the exudates to be malodorous and result in considerable social discomfort in addition to the physical discomfort of these lesions. Severe local scarring and disfigurement is seen in some cases.[124] Polypoid lesions associated with more advanced disease have been described.[125,126] Squamous cell carcinoma is an uncommon late complication.[127,128] Antibiotics and local hygiene can be palliative, but severe involvement may require surgical intervention.[124] HS sometimes represents part of the so-called follicular occlusion tetrad that also includes the pathologically similar conditions acne vulgaris, dissecting cellulitis[129] and pilonidal sinus.[130] Hyperkeratotic plugging of sweat glands is believed to be the underlying cause of HS, but this is controversial and often difficult to demonstrate in more well-established lesions. There is no evidence (despite its name) that the condition results from a primary hidradenitis.

Histopathology

The microscopic features of HS are not specific, but when combined with a proper clinical context, the diagnosis is rarely a challenge.[124] Early lesions show follicular hyperkeratosis. Other findings include abscesses and sinus tracts that are often at least focally lined by squamous epithelium, fibrosis and granuloma formation (Fig. 2.29a,b). Pseudoepitheliomatous hyperplasia of the squamous epithelium can be seen and must be distinguished from squamous cell carcinoma arising in the setting of HS.

Differential diagnosis

The differential includes other causes of destructive inflammation and scarring of the vulva. Metastatic Crohn's disease is usually associated with granulomatous inflammation. An enterocutaneous fistula in Crohn's disease could mimic HS, but a clinical history of preceding bowel symptoms should aid in differentiation. Fox–Fordyce disease is associated with apocrine hyperkeratotic plugging and does not form sinus tracts. Lymphogranuloma venereum can result in

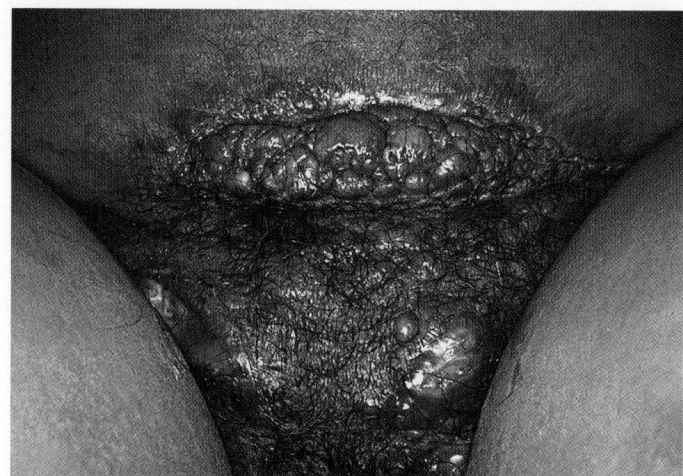
Fig. 2.28 Hidradenitis suppurativa.

appearances similar to HS, but chlamydia serology will aid in differentiation.

Treatment

Early hidradenitis suppurativa is treated with systemic antibiotics, topical antiseptics and compresses. In patients with isolated symptomatic lesions, intralesional corticosteroids may be beneficial. Retinoids have been used in the disease management.[131]

Other treatments utilized include systemic corticosteroids, azathioprine and cyclosporine. Hormonal therapy has been reported with some success. Surgery is utilized for patients with extensive hidradenitis suppurativa. A limited surgical approach is to de-floor or marsupialize troublesome lesions or sinus tracts. Most often a wide local excision with skin graft or flaps if indicated is the treatment of choice for advanced disease. Additionally CO_2 laser treatment has been reported as a successful treatment.[132,133]

REITER'S SYNDROME

Clinical presentation

Reiter's syndrome is classified as a seronegative spondyloarthropathy with clinical presentation of erythematous plaques combined with urethritis or cervicitis that occur following a bacterial infection. The cutaneous lesions of Reiter's syndrome have been referred to as 'keratoderma blennorrhagicum' and begin as small vesicles or erythematous macules that eventually coalesce to form erythematous plaques with scale-crust. Clinically these lesions are similar, if not identical to, those of pustular psoriasis and most frequently involve the hands and feet. These cutaneous lesions occur as

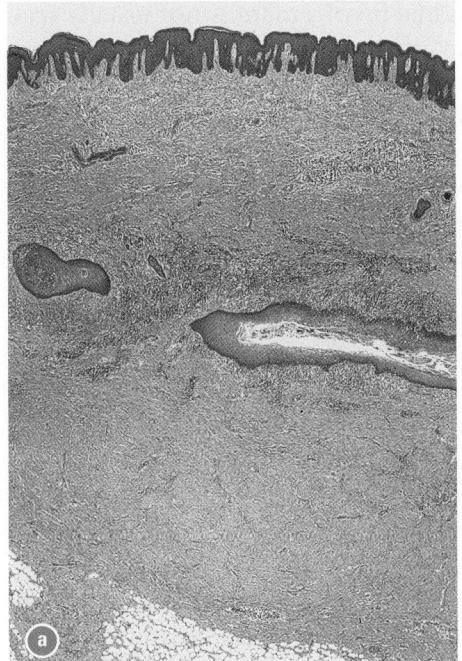 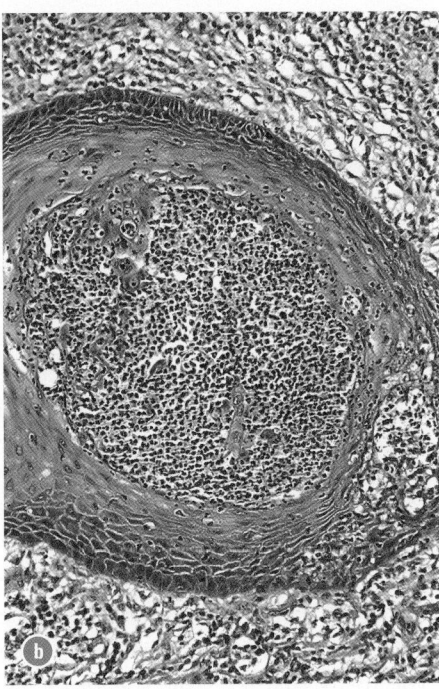

Fig. 2.29 Hidradenitis suppurativa. (a) There is dermal scarring, chronic inflammation and squamous epithelial-lined sinus. (b) High-power view of a sinus showing abscess formation.

part of a post-infectious syndrome. Two broad types of infection predispose to Reiter's syndrome and are designated 'endemic' and 'epidemic'.[134]

Endemic infections are often caused by *Chlamydia trachomatis*, commonly present as urethritis and show a striking predilection for males (> 80%). The epidemic form occurs in small subsets of people following outbreaks of enteric infections. Gastroenteritis is most commonly due to *Shigella dysenteriae*, *Salmonella typhimurium* or *Yersinia enterocolitica*.[134] There is no gender predilection in epidemic outbreaks, but such outbreaks are a very rare cause of Reiter's syndrome in Western countries.

The pathogenesis of Reiter's syndrome is poorly understood. The major histocompatibility HLA-B27 haplotype is greatly over-represented in patients with Reiter's syndrome, making immune dysregulation a plausible explanation. Dysregulation of CD8-positive T-cells has been proposed as a mechanism. Predisposition to the disease appears inherited and tends to run in families with other seronegative spondyloarthropathies and also pustular psoriasis. That these diseases occur in families and coexist in individuals with Reiter's syndrome complicates the study of pathogenesis, but also indicates probable shared pathogenic mechanisms.

Vulvar involvement is rare as exemplified by the paucity of reports in the English medical literature.[135] Within approximately 1 month of infection, urethritis (or more often cervicitis in women) occurs. With time,

arthritis, usually asymmetrical and involving the large joints of the lower limbs, ensues. The cutaneous lesions can occur at any time during this course. Other symptoms include onychodystrophy, enthesopathy (tendon or ligament inflammation at its insertion; the Achilles' tendon is most commonly involved), mouth ulcers, iritis and conjunctivitis. The syndrome is often chronic and relapsing and can be quite debilitating and even fatal. Among the most serious complications are heart block and mitral or aortic valve incompetence due to involvement of these sites. Reiter's syndrome appears to be particularly serious in the setting of patients with AIDS.[136]

Vulvar disease appears strikingly similar to vulvar pustular psoriasis with red crusted plaques involving the skin of the vulva and perineum.[135] Well-defined ulcerations within areas of erythema may be seen.[137,138] Small white papules on the mucosal surfaces of the vulva have been noted.[136] Vaginal and cervical discharges can be present.[137,139] The timing and severity of the symptoms varies greatly from case to case, making a high index of suspicion necessary to make this diagnosis, especially when it involves a less common site such as the vulva.

Histopathology

The vulvar lesions of Reiter's syndrome show all the features of pustular psoriasis including uniform elongation of the rete pegs with thinning of the suprapapillary plate, epidermal hyperplasia and parakeratosis. The granular cell layer is often greatly diminished or absent. Neutrophils can be found in the parakeratotic areas. The spinous layer often contains conspicuous collections of neutrophils and micro- or macro-abscesses can be seen in the corneal layer.

Differential diagnosis

The major histologic differential diagnoses include psoriasis, mainly the pustular type and infection. Histologically, psoriasis may show identical features. Clinical information is, therefore, required for discrimination. Nevertheless, there appears to be significant overlap between these conditions and classification may be somewhat artificial. Clinical presentations that favor Reiter's syndrome include cervicitis, iritis, conjunctivitis, mouth ulcers and presence of the HLA-B27 haplotype.[135] While arthritis can be a feature of either disease, asymmetrical involvement of the larger joints of the lower extremities (rather than in the more distal joints of the hand as seen in psoriasiform arthritis) favors Reiter's syndrome. It should be kept in mind that Reiter's syndrome uncommonly involves the vulva, while psoriasis is often seen at this site. As with psoriasis, a PAS stain should be performed to exclude a fungal infection, which can mimic the histologic features of Reiter's syndrome.

Treatment

Domeboro's soaks (aluminum acetate) and topical triamcinolone acetonide are often used for vulvar lesions. Oral acitretin, methotrexate, azathioprine and cyclosporine have also been suggested. Tacrolimus ointment has been utilized with limited benefit.[138]

BEHÇET'S DISEASE

Clinical presentation

Behçet's disease classically consists of the clinical triad of oral and genital ulcers with uveitis. The pathogenesis of Behçet's disease is not clearly understood, but appears to be due to an immunologically mediated vasculitis. Familial cases of Behçet's disease are not common.[140] Behçet's disease is not common among American and Northern European populations, but is more common in Middle Eastern countries, Asia and Turkey, where it was originally described.[140] Patients usually present with painful aphthous ulcers of the oral mucosa. Not uncommonly, they will have a long history of such lesions before developing the other characteristic manifestations of Behçet's disease. Vulvar ulceration is com-

mon; however, vaginal involvement is not usually seen (Fig. 2.30). Vulvar ulceration can be deep and result in scarring; severe cases sometimes appear gangrenous. Occasionally, the distribution of lesions will be herpetiform. Chronic involvement, with cycles of resolution and subsequent recurrence, is characteristic. Presentation in the vulva is rare.[141]

Systemic disease involves the eyes, skin, joints, brain, bowel, heart, lung and kidneys; in fact, virtually any organ may be affected. The most common serious consequence of this disease is progression of posterior uveitis to blindness. The involvement of these organs appears to be due to vasculitis often complicated by thrombophlebitis. Criteria for the diagnosis of Behçet's disease are outlined in Table 2.3.[142] It is important to note that these criteria should apply only when other causes have been excluded. One of the diagnostic criteria, pathergy, is defined by the formation of sterile cutaneous pustules 24–48 h after an intradermal needle prick. This response may be largely due to an exaggerated response to injury in Behçet's disease.[143] Non-vulvar cutaneous involvement shows differing patterns including papular pustules and lesions similar to erythema nodosum, pyoderma gangrenosum and Sweet's syndrome.[144–146]

Histopathology

The vulva is usually involved by ulceration that can be either shallow or extend deeply into the dermis. The histologic features are not specific. A mixed inflammatory infiltrate in the superficial and often deep dermis is seen and neutrophils or lymphocytes can predominate. Plasma cells and eosinophils are often present. There may be associated endothelial swelling with perivascular inflammation. Leukocytoclastic vasculitis is sometimes seen, but in many cases it is unclear whether this represents the cause or is a result of the ulceration.

Differential diagnosis

It is important to recognize that Behçet's disease is a syndrome for which criteria are somewhat controversial. Furthermore, patients may have some, but not all, of the manifestations of Behçet's disease for years before fulfilling the formal criteria for this diagnosis. The differential diagnosis of vulvar involvement by Behçet's disease includes a variety of conditions that ultimately lead to ulceration. These include herpes virus infection, syphilis, lymphogranuloma venereum, pyoderma gangrenosum and blistering disorders such as pemphigus and pemphigoid. Clinical correlation

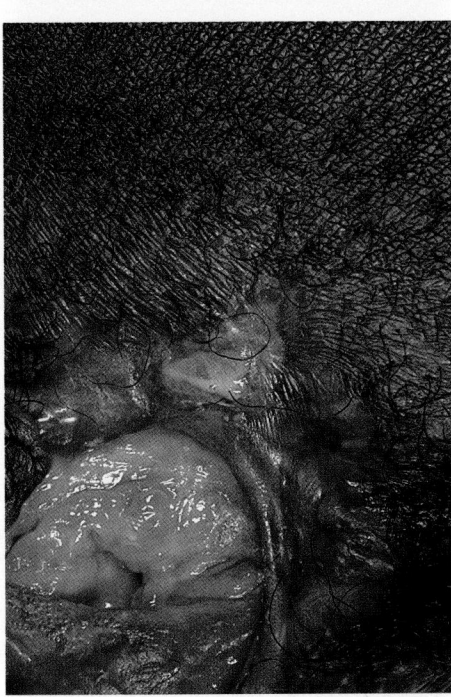

Fig. 2.30 Behçet's disease of the vulva.

Table 2.3 Behçet's disease – criteria for diagnosis (adapted from Magro and Crowson, 1995 with permission)[142]

Recurrent oral ulceration
  Minor aphthous, major aphthous or herpetiform ulcers observed or reported reliably by patient, occurring
Plus 2 of the following
Recurrent genital aphthous ulcers or scars observed by physician or reliably reported by patient
  Eye lesions:
    Anterior uveitis
    Posterior uveitis
    Cell in vitreous on slit lamp examination or retinal vasculitis observed by ophthalmologist
  Skin lesions:
    Erythema nodosum-like lesions observed by physician or reliably reported by patient
    Pseudofolliculitis
    Papulopustular lesions or acneiform nodules observed by physician in post-adolescent patient not receiving corticosteroids.
  Positive pathergy test:
    Performed by oblique insertion of 20-gauge or smaller needle (blunt is ideal) under sterile conditions and read by a healthcare provider after 24–48 h. Occurrence of a small red bump or pustule at the site of needle insertion constitutes a positive test. Only a minority of Behçet's patients demonstrate the pathergy phenomenon. Patients from the Mediterranean region are more likely to demonstrate a positive pathergy test.

and, when indicated, the use of immunofluorescence tests, infectious serologies, histochemical and immunohistochemical stains and culture are required. It is important, when doing immunofluorescent studies, to biopsy the normal tissue adjacent to the ulcer and send it in the proper media. Mucocutaneous involvement by Crohn's disease (see p. 50) is also considered in the histologic differential diagnosis. Clinical history such as the presence of oral ulceration can be helpful for differentiation. Involvement by Crohn's disease frequently involves the more lateral extents of the vulva and may extend even to the medial thighs whereas the ulceration of Behçet's disease tends to occur in the more central portions of the vulva. Compared with the ulcers seen in Behçet's disease, the lesions of Crohn's disease may be deeper, frequently forming sinus tracts. As both these diseases can involve the bowel, vulvar biopsy may be important for differentiation. Vulvar involvement by Crohn's disease is characterized by granulomatous inflammation and is usually easily distinguished from Behçet's disease.

Treatment

Topical steroids are used early in the disease course. Oral antibiotics and oral steroids are often required in the treatment of Behçet's disease. At times, admissions for intravenous steroids and pain control are needed. Intralesional steroid injections are also used for this patient population. Other treatments include azathioprine, methotrexate, colchicine, thalidomide and infliximab (Remicade®, Centocor Inc.).

PYODERMA GANGRENOSUM

Clinical presentation

Pyoderma gangrenosum (PG) is an uncommon ulcerating condition that is often seen in association with systemic disease. The etiology is unknown. PG is usually seen in young to middle-aged adults, but can present at any age. A female predominance has been noted in several large case studies.[147–149] The lesions are usually large ulcerations with characteristic ragged red to purple 'overhanging' edges. These can be single or multiple and tend to occur in the lower extremities. They may begin as erythematous nodules or pustules that subsequently expand and ulcerate. Extensive scarring and disfigurement can be seen. The surface sometimes has a cribriform appearance from coalescence of the ulcers with subsequent re-epithelialization. Lesions have a tendency to occur at sites of previous trauma, a process known as pathergy. Recurrence is not uncommon.

Early recognition is critical as surgical debridement, a common treatment for ulceration, tends to exacerbate this condition and is generally contraindicated. Spontaneous regression is rare.

Approximately half of the cases of PG are associated with systemic disease. Those most commonly reported are inflammatory bowel disease (Crohn's and ulcerative colitis), arthritis (rheumatoid and seronegative types), hematological malignancies, myeloproliferative disorders and monoclonal gammopathies.[149] Association with underlying malignancy, hepatitis and Behçet's syndrome has also been described.[147,148] The ulcers of PG may be seen preceding, concurrent with, or during an inactive phase of these conditions.[150] The diagnosis of PG is one of exclusion; all other causes of ulceration must be excluded before rendering this diagnosis.

Primary vulvar involvement by PG is rare, but has been described as single case reports.[151-157] Genital involvement was present in 9% of the cases in a large series, but the gender and exact site are not indicated.[158] The appearances of the vulvar ulcers vary in size and number and can extend to involve the mons pubis, lower abdomen, perineum and thighs.[157]

Histopathology

The histologic findings in PG are non-specific and diagnosis requires careful clinicopathologic correlation. Early lesions reveal an intense neutrophilic infiltrate that may be perifollicular. A typical, but probably not specific feature, is that of an ulcer with an 'overhanging' border.[155] Later lesions are rich in mononuclear cells and reveal marked necrosis. Pseudoepitheliomatous hyperplasia and marked dermal fibrosis or scarring are usually present at the edge of the lesion where biopsies are often taken.

Differential diagnosis

The differential diagnosis for PG is broad and includes other causes of cutaneous ulceration. Because the ulcers in PG show non-specific changes, a high index of suspicion is critical when a biopsy of a large ulcerated lesion is received. Clinical information is essential when evaluating such specimens. Infectious etiologies should be excluded by culture and use of special stains. It is particularly important that debridement specimens from pyoderma gangrenosum are not mistaken for necrotizing fasciitis. Gram stain and clinical information should establish the diagnosis in the majority of cases.

Treatment

Corticosteroids are the preferred treatment for pyoderma gangrenosum, occasionally other agents are used.[150]

CROHN'S DISEASE OF THE VULVA

Clinical presentation

Crohn's disease (CD) is a granulomatous inflammatory disease of the bowel that may also involve other sites, including skin and mucosa. The etiology is unknown. Crohn's disease has no gender predilection and usually presents in the second to third decades. Pediatric cases are also seen.[159] Gastrointestinal symptoms are the most common complaint. Crohn's disease shows discontinuous ulceration of the bowel, separating it from the more uniform involvement of ulcerative colitis. Crohn's disease of the vulva (Fig. 2.31) may be contiguous (bowel and vulva are both involved and sinuses or fistulae occur between them), metastatic or noncontiguous.[160,161] Cutaneous manifestations with significant edema and drainage present are shown in Figure 2.32. Some lesions have direct extension from the bowel to the vulva, in the form of a fistulous tract (Fig. 2.33). Occasionally, the development of mucocutaneous lesions, including vulvar involvement, precedes evidence of bowel disease.[162-165] Cutaneous involvement limited to the vulva has also been reported, but it is very rare.[162,163] Ulcerative and, less commonly, mass lesions[164] have been described. Cutaneous involvement may be associated with extensive scarring and destruction of vulvar anatomy. Involvement may be severe, requiring radical excisions, though conservative medical treatment is often

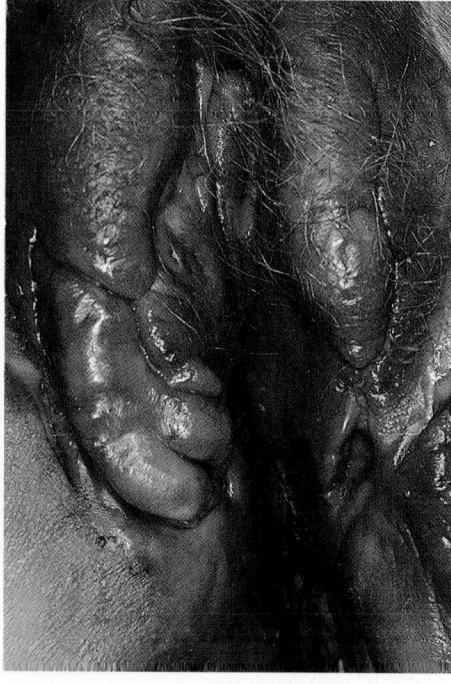

Fig. 2.31 Crohn's disease of the vulva with edema and disturbance of normal vulvar anatomy.

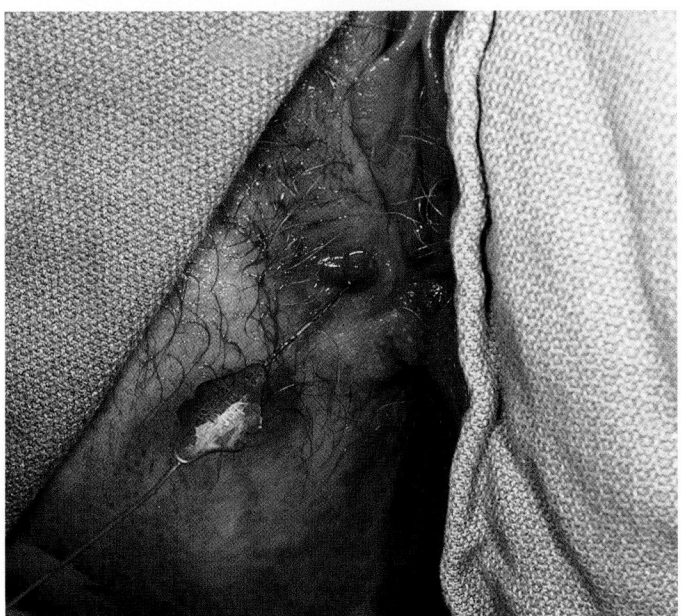

Fig. 2.32 Crohn's with a fistula tract (probe) extending into the perineum.

histiocytes, giant cells and plasma cells is seen. Sterile, non-caseating granulomata composed of epithelioid cells, often with Langerhans-type giant cells, can be seen, but are not an invariable feature (Fig. 2.33).[163] The granulomata and histiocytic giant cells are often sparsely distributed and easily overlooked.

Differential diagnosis

As noted above, the histologic findings are non-specific and a strong index of clinical suspicion is required to make a diagnosis of CD. It is important to exclude other causes of granulomatous disease, particularly infectious processes. As noted above, mucocutaneous involvement may precede gastrointestinal symptoms. Therefore, patients should be evaluated for subclinical evidence of bowel disease with a colonoscopy. Patients with granulomatous vulvitis should be followed carefully since some of these patients may eventually develop gastrointestinal involvement. The term vulvitis granulomatosa has been applied to rare patients with lesions histologically identical to metastatic Crohn's disease but who do not have evidence of gastrointestinal disease. However, some patients have developed Crohn's disease subsequent to a biopsy showing granulomatous vulvitis.[167] More experience is required to determine if vulvitis granulomatosa is a genuine entity or form fruste of Crohn's disease. Regardless, all patients with unexplained granulomatous vulvitis need to be followed closely for evidence of inflammatory bowel disease.

sufficient. The ulcerative lesions are usually non-specific, but may mimic the findings of genital herpes virus infection.[166]

Histopathology

The histologic findings of vulvar CD are non-specific. A polymorphous infiltrate with variable numbers of

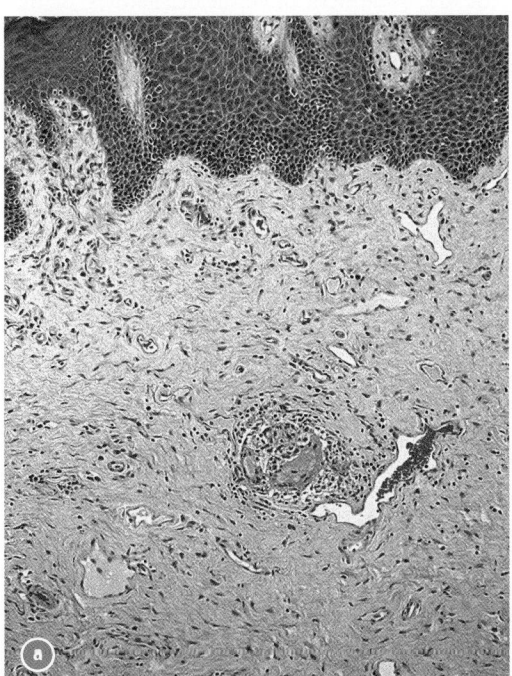

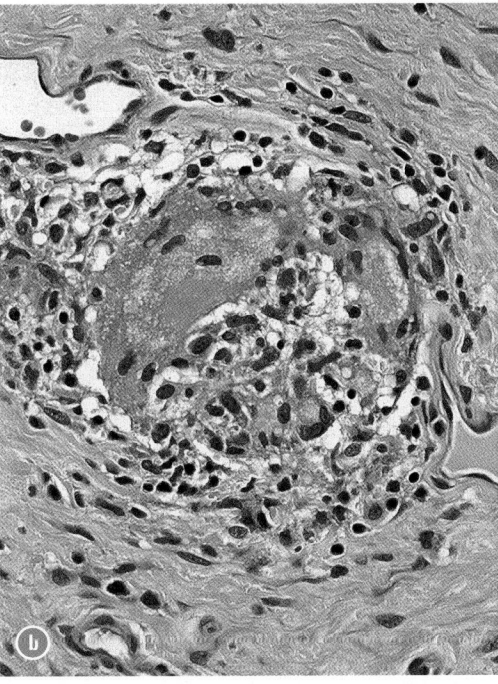

Fig. 2.33 Histopathology of vulvar Crohn's disease. (a) Note the presence of granulomas in the dermis. (b) Higher power of (a).

Treatment of vulvar Crohn's disease

The treatment of vulvar Crohn's disease varies from the usual gastrointestinal treatment regimen. Steroids and the 5-ASA drugs are generally effective only for bowel disease rather than for perineal disease; however, some clinicians feel that should be tried initially in some patients. Many patients with vulvar Crohn's disease have symptomatic bowel disease and require these drugs. Immunosuppressants such as 6-mercaptopurine and a related drug, azathioprine, may also be required at times.

Generally for initial treatment of vulvar Crohn's disease, metronidazole is used. Ciprofloxacin may also be used as a single drug. Metronidazole and ciprofloxacin may be combined if needed for better response. For resistant disease as well as for the treatment of open, draining fistulas, infliximab (Remicade®) may be used. It is an anti-tumor necrosis factor (TNF) substance. TNF is a protein produced by the immune system that may cause the inflammation associated with Crohn's disease.[168]

Summary

The vulva plays host to a wide range of vulvar inflammatory conditions. It is important to understand the disease process, both clinically and histologically, to optimize patient care. When examining these patients, the clinician should identify and exclude affected non-genital sites (eye, oral and axillary examination) that may provide clues to the nature of the vulvar lesion. This information should be made available to the pathologist to maximize the yield from the histologic analysis. Interpretation of tissue specimens may be difficult and the pathologist must be aware of not only the clinical impact of his interpretation but also the fact that the treatments for many of these conditions are similar. Above all, the terminology used must be understood by the clinician. When more complex-appearing dermatological terms are used, particularly if they convey information that may influence therapy, the pathologist must ensure that these terms are understood by his clinical colleagues.

References

1 McKee P, Callonje E, Granter S. Pathology of the skin. Philadelphia: WB Saunders; 2005.

2 Wilkinson EJ, Stone IK. Atlas of vulvar disease. Baltimore: Williams & Wilkins; 1995.

3 Habif TP. Clinical dermatology: a color guide to diagnosis and therapy. 4th edn. Philadelphia: Mosby; 2004:570.

4 Ambros RA, Malfetano JH, Carlson JA, Mihm MC. Non-neoplastic epithelial alterations of the vulva: recognition assessment and comparisons of terminologies used among various specialties. Mod Pathol 1997; 10:401–408.

5 Kiru H, Ackerman AB. Critique of current classification of vulvar disease. Am J Derm 1990; 12:377–392.

6 Ridley CM. Nomenclature of non-neoplastic vulvar conditions. Br J Derm 1986; 115:647–651.

7 Fischer G, Spurrett B, Fischer A. The chronically symptomatic vulva: aetiology and management. Br J Obstet Gynaecol 1995; 102:773–779.

8 Fischer GO. The commonest causes of symptomatic vulvar disease: a dermatologist's perspective. Australas J Derm 1996; 37:12–18.

9 Heller DS, Randolph P, Young A, Tancer ML, Fromer D. The cutaneous-vulvar clinic revisited: a 5-year experience of the Columbia Presbyterian Medical Center Cutaneous-Vulvar Service. Dermatology 1997; 195:26–29.

10 O'Hare PM, Sherertz EF. Vulvodynia: a dermatologist's perspective with emphasis on an irritant contact dermatitis component. J Women's Health Gend Based Med 2000; 9:565–569.

11 Marren P, Wojnarowska F. Dermatitis of the vulva. Semin Derm 1996; 15(1):36–41.

12 Fivozinsky KB, Laufer MR. Vulvar disorders in prepubertal girls. A literature review. J Reprod Med 1998; 43:763–773.

13 Williams TS, Callen JP, Owen LG. Vulvar disorders in the prepubertal female. Pediatr Ann 1986; 15:588–589, 592–601, 604–605.

14 McKay M. Vulvitis and vulvovaginitis: cutaneous considerations. Am J Obstet Gynecol 1991; 165:1176–1182.

15 Elsner P, Wilhelm D, Maibach HI. Multiple parameter assessment of vulvar irritant contact dermatitis. Contact Dermatitis 1990; 23:20–26.

16 Zellis S, Pincus SH. Treatment of vulvar dermatoses. Semin Derm 1996; 15:71–76.

17 Grabbe S, Schwarz T. Immunoregulatory mechanisms involved in elicitation of allergic contact hypersensitivity. Immunol Today 1998; 19(1):37–44.

18 Kint B, Degreef H, Dooms-Goossens A. Combined allergy to human seminal plasma and latex: case report and review of the literature. Contact Dermatitis 1994; 30:7–11.

19 Leung DYM. Pathogenesis of atopic dermatitis. J Allergy Clin Immunol 1999; 104(3):S99–S108.

20 Robert C, Kupper TS. Inflammatory skin diseases, T cells and immune surveillance. N Engl J Med 1999; 24:1817–1828.

21 Leung DYM. Cellular and immunologic mechanisms in atopic dermatitis. J Am Acad Derm 2001; 44(1):S1–S12.

22 Soter NA. Nummular eczematous dermatitis. In: Freedberg IM, Eisen AZ, Wolff K, et al., eds. Fitzpatrick's dermatology in general medicine. New York: McGraw-Hill; 1999: 1480–1482.

23 Virgili A, Bacilieri S, Corazza M. Managing vulvar lichen simplex chronicus. J Reprod Med 2001; 46:343–346.

24 O'Keefe RJ, Scurry JP, Dennerstein G, Sfameni S, Brenan J. Audit of 114 non-neoplastic vulvar biopsies. Br J Obstet Gynaecol 1995; 102:780–786.

25 Farber EM, Nall L. Genital psoriasis. Cutis 1992; 50:263–266.

26 Gottlieb AB. Psoriasis. Immunopathology and immunomodulation. Derm Clin 2001; 19:649–657.

27 Robert C, Kupper TS. Inflammatory skin diseases, T cells, and immune surveillance. N Engl J Med 1999; 341(24): 1817–1828.

28 Prystowsky JH, Corn PR. Pustular and erythrodermic psoriasis. Derm Clin 1995; 13(4):757–770.

29 Khan MA. Update on spondyloarthropathies. Ann Intern Med 2002; 136(12):896–907.

30 Cox AJ, Watson W. Histologic variations in lesions of psoriasis. Arch Dermatol 1972; 106:503–506.

31 Ragaz A, Ackerman AB. Evolution, maturation and regression of lesions of psoriasis: new observations and correlation of clinical and histologic findings. Am J Derm 1979; 1(3):199–214.

32 Lebwohl M. Psoriasis. Lancet 2003; 361(9364):1997–1204.

33 Kupper TS. Immunologic targets in psoriasis. N Engl J Med 2003; 349(21):1987–1990.

34 Bergbrandt I-M. Seborrheic dermatitis and Pityrosporum yeasts. Curr Top Med Mycol 1995; 6:95–112.

35 Larrabee R, Kylander DJ. Benign vulvar disorders. Identifying features, practical management of non-neoplastic conditions and tumors. Postgrad Med 2001; 109:151–154, 157–159, 163–164.

36 Wilkinson EJ, Stone IK. Seborrhea. Atlas of vulvar disease. Baltimore: Williams & Wilkins; 1995:96–97.

37 Myskowski PL, Ahkami R. Dermatologic complications of HIV infection. Med Clin North Am 1996; 80(6): 1415–1435.

38 Gelfand JM, Rudikoff D. Evaluation and treatment of itching in HIV-infected patients. Mt Sinai J Med 2001; 68(4,5):298–308.

39 Handfield-Jones SE, Hinde FRJ, Kennedy CTC. Lichen sclerosus et atrophicus in children misdiagnosed as sexual abuse. Br Med J 1987; 294:1404–1405.

40 Meyrick Thomas RH, Ridley CM, McGibbon DH, Black MM. Lichen sclerosus et atrophicus and autoimmunity – a study of 350 women. Br J Derm 1988; 118(43):41–46.

41 Friedrich EG Jr, Kalra PS. Serum levels of sex hormones in vulvar lichen sclerosus and the effect of topical testosterone. N Engl J Med 1984; 310(8):488–491.

42 Smith YR, Quint EH. Clobetasol propionate in the treatment of premenarchal vulvar lichen sclerosus. Obstetric Gynecol 2001; 98(4):588–591.

43 Bornstein J, Heifetz S, Kellner Y, et al. Clobetasol dipropionate 0.05% versus testosterone propionate 2% topical application for severe vulvar lichen sclerosus. Am J Obstet Gynecol 1998; 178:80–84.

44 Sinha P, Sorinola O, Luesley D. Lichen sclerosus of the vulva. Long-term steroid maintenance therapy. J Reprod Med 1999; 44:621–624.

45 Cattaneo A, Carli P, Marco A De, et al. Testosterone maintenance therapy. Effects on vulvar lichen sclerosus treated with clobetasol propionate. J Reprod Med 1996; 41:99–102.

46 Sideri M, Origoni M, Spinaci L, et al. Topical testosterone in the treatment of vulvar lichen sclerosus. Intl J Gynaecol Obstet 1994; 46:53–56.

47 Carli P, Bracco G, Taddei G, et al. Vulvar lichen sclerosus immunohistologic evaluation before and after therapy. J Reprod Med 1994; 39:110–114.

48 Bracco GL, Carli P, Sonni L, et al. Clinical and histologic effects of topical treatments of vulvar lichen sclerosus. A critical evaluation. J Reprod Med 1993; 38:37–40.

49 Dalziel KL, Millard PRP, Wojnarowska F. The treatment of vulvar lichen sclerosus with a very potent topical steroid (clobetasol propionate 0.05%) cream. Br J Derm 1991; 124:461–464.

50 Cattaneo A, Marco A De, Sonni L, et al. Clobetasol vs. testosterone in the treatment of lichen sclerosus of the vulvar region. Minerva Gynecol 1992; 44:567–571.

51 Dalziel KL, Wojnarowska F. Long-term control of vulvar lichen sclerosus after treatment with a potent topical steroid cream. J Reprod Med 1993; 38:25–27.

52 Ball SB, Wojnarowska. Vulvar dermatoses: lichen sclerosus, lichen planus and vulval dermatitis/lichen simplex chronicus. Sem Cutan Med Surg 1998; 17:182–188.

53 Sahn EE, Bluestein EL, Oliva S. Familial lichen sclerosus et atrophicus in childhood. Pediatr Derm 1994; 11: 160–163.

54 Meyrick Thomas RH, Kennedy CT. The development of lichen sclerosus et atrophicus in monozygotic twin girls. Br J Derm 1986; 108:41–46.

55 Cox NH, Mitchell JHS, Morley WN. Lichen sclerosus et atrophicus in non-identical female twins. Br J Derm 1986; 115:743–746.

56 Shirer J, Ray M. Familial occurrence of lichen sclerosus et atrophicus. Arch Derm 1987; 123:485–488.

57 Smith YR, Haefner HK. Vulvar lichen sclerosus: pathophysiology and treatment. Am J Clin Derm 2004: 5(2):105–125.

58 Berth-Jones J, Graham-Brown RAC, Burns DA. Lichen sclerosus et atrophicus – a review of 15 cases in young girls. Clin Exp Derm 1991; 16:14–17.

59 Loening-Baucke V. Lichen sclerosus et atrophicus in children. Am J Dis Child 1991; 42:1058–1061.

60 Powell J, Wojnarowska F. Childhood vulvar lichen sclerosus: an increasingly common problem. J Am Acad Derm 2001; 44:803–806.

61 Zaki I, Dalziel KL, Solomonsz FA, Stevens A. The under-reporting of skin disease in association with squamous cell carcinoma of the vulva. Clin Exp Derm 1996; 21(5): 334–337.

62 Carlson JA, Lamb P, Malfetano J, Ambros RA, Mihm MC Jr. Clinicopathologic comparison of vulvar and extragenital lichen sclerosus: histologic variants, evolving lesions and etiology of 141 cases. Mod Pathol 1998a; 11:844–854.

63 Fung MA, LeBoit PE. Light microscopic criteria for the diagnosis of early vulvar lichen sclerosis: a comparison with lichen planus. Am J Surg Pathol 1998; 22(4):473–478.

64 Carlson JA, Ambros R, Malfetano J, et al. Vulvar lichen sclerosus and squamous cell carcinoma: a cohort, case control and investigational study with historical perspective; implications for chronic inflammation and sclerosis in the development of neoplasia. Hum Pathol 1998; 29(9): 932–948.

65 Edwards L. Vulvar lichen planus. Arch Derm 1989; 125:1677–1680.

66 Dwyer CM, Kerr REI, Millan DWM. Squamous carcinoma following lichen planus of the vulva. Clin Exp Derm 1995; 20:171–172.

67 Lewis FM, Harrington CI. Squamous cell carcinoma arising in vulval lichen planus. Br J Derm 1994; 131:703–705.

68 Franck JM, Young AW. Squamous cell carcinoma in situ arising within lichen planus of the vulva. Derm Surg 1995; 21:890–894.

69 Lewis FM. Vulval lichen planus. Br J Derm 1998; 138:569–575.

70 Pelisse M. Erosive vulvar lichen planus and desquamative vaginitis. Sem Derm 1996; 15:47–50.

71 Mann MS, Kaufman RH. Erosive lichen planus of the vulva. Clin Obstet Gynecol 1991; 34:605–613.

72 Eisen D. The vulvovaginal-gingival syndrome of lichen planus. The clinical characteristics of 22 patients. Arch Derm 1994; 130:1379–1382.

73 Lewis FM, Shah M, Harrington CI. Vulval involvement in lichen planus: a study of 37 women. Br J Derm 1996; 135:89–91.

74 Taaffe A. Current concepts in lichen planus [Review]. Int J Derm 1979; 18:533–538.

75 McCreedy CA, Melski JW. Vulvar erythema. Vulvitis chronica plasmacellularis (Zoon's vulvitis). Arch Derm 1990; 126(10):352–353.

76 Yoganathan S, Bohl TG, Mason G. Plasma cell balanitis and vulvitis (of Zoon). A study of 10 cases. J Reprod Med 1994; 39(12):939–944.

77 Zoon JJ. Balanoposthite chronique circonscrite benigne a plasmocytes. Dermatologica 1952; 105:1–7.

78 Weyers W, Ende Y, Schalla W, Diaz-Cascajo C. Balanitis of Zoon: a clinicopathologic study of 45 cases. Am J Derm 2002; 24(6):459–467.

79 Garnier G. Vulvite erythemateuse circonscrite benigne a type erythroplasique. Bull Soc Fr Derm Syphilol 1954; 61:102–104.

80 Joshi UY. Carcinoma of the penis preceded by Zoon's balanitis. Int J STD AIDS 1999; 10(12):823–825.

81 Neri I, Patrizi A, Marzaduri S, Marini R, Negosanti M. Vulvitis plasmacellularis: two new cases. Genitourin Med 1995; 71(5):311–313.

82 Liu Z, Diaz LA. Bullous pemphigoid: end of the century overview. J Derm 2001; 28(11):647–650.

83 Marren P, Wojnarowska F, Venning VA, et al. Vulvar involvement in the auto-immune bullous diseases. J Reprod Med 1993; 38:101–108.

84 Urano S. Localized bullous pemphigoid of the vulva. J Derm 1996; 23(8):580–582.

85 Guenther LC, Shum D. Localized childhood vulvar pemphigoid. J Am Acad Derm 1990; 22(1):762–764.

86 Farrell AM, Kirtschig G, Dalziel KL, et al. Childhood vulval pemphigoid: a clinical and immunopathological study of five patients. Br J Derm 1999; 140(2):308–312.

87 Fisler RE, Saeb M, Liang MG, Howard RM, McKee PH. Childhood bullous pemphigoid: a clinicopathologic study and review of the literature. Am J Dermatopathol 2003; 25(3):183–189.

88 Frith P, Charnock M, Wojnarowski F. Cicatricial pemphigoid diagnosed from ocular features in recurrent severe vulval scarring. Two case reports. Br J Obstet Gynaecol 1991; 98(5):482–484.

89 Chan LS, Ahmed AR, Anhalt GJ, et al. The first international consensus on mucous membrane pemphigoid: definition, diagnostic criteria, pathogenic factors, medical treatment and prognostic indicators. Arch Derm 2002; 138:370–379.

90 Bickle KM, Roark TR, Hsu S. Autoimmune bullous dermatoses: a review. Am Fam Physician 2002; 65(9):1861–1870.

91 Joost T Van, Faber WR, Manuel HR. Drug-induced cicatricial pemphigoid. Br J Derm 1980; 102(6):715–718.

92 Lim HW, Bystryn JC. Evaluation and management of disease of the vulva: bullous diseases. Clin Obstet Gynecol 1978; 21(4):1007–1022.

93 Amagai M. Pemphigus: Autoimmunity to epidermal cell adhesion molecules. Adv Derm 1996; 11:319–352.

94 Ding X, Diaz LA, Fairley JA, Giudice GJ, Liu Z. The anti-desmoglein 1 autoantibodies in pemphigus vulgaris sera are pathogenic. J Invest Derm 1999; 112:739–743.

95 Batta K, Munday PE, Tatnall FM. Pemphigus vulgaris localized to the vagina presenting as chronic vaginal discharge. Br J Derm 1999; 140(5):945–947.

96 Amagai M, Klaus-Kovtun V, Stanley JR. Autoantibodies against a novel epithelial cadherin in pemphigus vulgaris, a disease of cell adhesion. Cell 1991; 67:869–877.

97 Burge SM. Hailey-Hailey disease: the clinical presentation, response to treatment and prognosis. Br J Derm 1992; 126:275–282.

98 Evron S, Leviatan A, Okon E. Familial benign chronic pemphigus appearing as leukoplakia of the vulva. Int J Derm 1984; 23(8):445–557.

99 Misra R, Raman M, Singh N, Agarwal. Hailey-Hailey disease masquerading as candidiasis. Int J Gynecol Obstet 1993; 42:51–52.

100 King DT, Hirose FM, King LA. Simultaneous occurrence of familial benign chronic pemphigus (Hailey-Hailey disease) and syringoma on the vulva. Arch Dermatol 1978; 114(5):801.

101 Wieselthier JS, Pincus SH. Hailey-Hailey disease of the vulva. Arch Derm 1993; 129(10):1344–1345.

102 Cockayne SE, Rassl DM, Thomas SE. Squamous cell carcinoma arising in Hailey-Hailey disease of the vulva. Br J Derm 2000; 142(3):540–542.

103 Holst VA, Fair KP, Wilson BB, Patterson JW. Squamous cell carcinoma arising in Hailey-Hailey disease. J Am Acad Derm 2000; 43(2):368–371.

104 Ochiai T, Honda A, Morishima T, Sata T, Satoh K. Human papillomavirus types 16 and 39 in a vulval carcinoma occurring in a woman with Hailey-Hailey disease. Br J Derm 1999; 140(3):509–513.

105 Ridley CM. Cicatricial pemphigoid of the vulva. Am J Obstet Gynecol 1985; 152(7):916–917.

106 Burge SM. Hailey-Hailey disease: the clinical presentation, response to treatment and prognosis. Br J Derm 1992; 126:275–282.

107 Burge SM, Wilkinson JD. Darier-White disease: a review of the clinical presentation in 163 patients. J Am Acad Derm 1992; 27:40–50.

108 Sakuntabhai A, Ruiz-Perez V, Carter S, et al. Mutation in ATP2A2, encoding a Ca^{2+} pump, cause Darier disease. Nat Genet 1999; 21:271–277.

109 Barrett JFR, Murray LA, MacDonald HN. Darier's disease localized to the vulva. Case report. Br J Obstet Gynecol 1989; 96:997–999.

110 Ridley CM, Buckley CH. Darier's disease localized to the vulva (correspondence). Br J Obstet Gynecol 1991; 98(1):112.

111 Cooper PH. Acantholytic dermatosis localized to the vulvocrural area. J Cutan Pathol 1989; 16:81–84.

112 Vazquez J, Morales C, Gonzales LO, Lamelas ML, Ribas A. Vulval squamous cell carcinoma arising in localized Darier's disease. Eur J Obstet Gynecol Reprod Biol 2002; 102:206–208.

113 Duray PH, Merino MJ, Axiotis C. Warty dyskeratoma of the vulva. Int J Gynecol Pathol 1983; 2(3):286–293.

114 Chorzelski TP, Kudejko J, Jablonska S. Is papular acantholytic dyskeratosis of the vulva a new entity? Arch Derm 1984; 106:702–706.

115 Wong T-Y, Mihm MC Jr. Acantholytic dermatosis localized to genitalia and crural areas of male patients: a report of three cases. J Cutan Pathol 1994; 21(1):27–32.

116 Krishnan RS, Ledbetter LS, Reed JA, Hsu S. Acantholytic dermatosis of the vulvocrural area. Cutis 2001; 67:217–220.

117 Hsu S, Ledbetter LS, Krishnan RS, Reed JA. Acantholytic dermatosis of the vulvocrural area. J Am Acad Derm 2003; 48(4):638–639.

118 Macmillan DC, Vickers HR. Fox-Fordyce disease. Br J Derm 1971; 84(2):181.

119 Helm TN, Chen PW. Fox-Fordyce disease. Cutis 2002; 69(5):335, 342.

120 Spiller RF, Knox JM. Fox-Fordyce disease with hidradenitis suppurativa. J Invest Derm 1958; 31:127–135.

121 Stashower ME, Krivda SJ, Turiansky GW. Fox-Fordyce Disease: diagnosis with transverse histologic sections. Acad Derm 2000; 42:89–91.

122 Hobbs JE. Tumors of the vulva and vagina. Sweat gland tumors. Clin Obstet Gynecol 1965; 8(4):946–952.

123 Heller DS, Haefner HK, Hameed M, Lieberman RW. Vulvar hidradenitis suppurativa. Immunohistochemical evaluation of apocrine and eccrine involvement. J Reprod Med 2002; 47(9):695–700.

124 Mitchell KM, Beck DE. Hidradenitis suppurativa. Surg Clin North Am 2002; 82(6):1187–1197.

125 Goldberg JM, Buchler DA, Dibbell DG. Advanced hidradenitis suppurativa presenting with bilateral vulvar masses. Gynecol Oncol 1996; 60:494–497.

126 Wrone DA, Landeck A, Dibbell DG, Xie H, Warner TF. Hidradenitis suppurativa polyposa. Pathol Res Pr 2000; 196(8):589–592.

127 Manolitsas T, Blankin S, Jaworski R, et al. Vulval squamous cell carcinoma arising in chronic hidradenitis suppurativa. Gynecol Oncol 1999; 75:285–288.

128 Lapins J, Ye W, Nyren O. Incidence of cancer among patients with hidradenitis suppurativa. Arch Derm 2001; 137:730–734.

129 Chicarelli ZN. Follicular occlusion triad: hidradenitis suppurativa, acne conglobata and dissecting cellulitis of the scalp. Ann Plast Surg 1987; 18(3):230–237.

130 Wiseman MC. Hidradenitis suppurativa: a review. Dermatol Ther 2004; 17:50–54.

131 Brown CF, Gallup DG, Brown VM. Hidradenitis suppurativa of the anogenital region: response to isotretinoin. Case Reports. Am J Obstet Gynecol 1988; 158(1):12–15.

132 Haefner HK. A patient with hidradenitis suppurativa. International Correspondence Society of Obstetricians & Gynecologists. Collect Lett 1997; 38:6–7.

133 Wiseman MC. Hidradenitis suppurativa: a review. Dermatol Ther 2004; 17:50–54.

134 Armor B. Reiter's syndrome: diagnosis and clinical presentation. Rheumatol Clin North Am 1998; 24(4):677–695.

135 Edwards L, Hansen RC. Reiter's syndrome of the vulva: the psoriasis spectrum. Arch Derm 1992; 128:811–814.

136 Winchester R, Bernstein DH, Fischer HD, Enlow R, Solomon G. The co-occurrence of Reiter's syndrome and acquired immunodeficiency. Ann Intern Med 1987; 106(1):19–26.

137 Thambar IV, Dunlop R, Thin RN, Huskisson EC. Circuate vulvitis in Reiter's syndrome. Br J Vener Dis 1977; 53:260–262.

138 Lotery HE, Galask RP, Stone MS, Sontheimer RD. Ulcerative vulvitis in atypical Reiter's syndrome. J Am Acad Derm 2003; 48(4):613–616.

139 O'N Daunt S, Kotowski KE, O'Reilly, Richardson AT. Ulcerative vulvitis in Reiter's syndrome: a case report. Br J Vener Dis 1982; 58:405–407.

140 Yazici H, Fresko I, Tunc R, Melikoglu M. Behçet's syndrome: pathogenesis, clinical manifestations and treatment. In: Ball GV, Bridges, Jr. SL, eds. Vasculitis. Oxford: Oxford University Press; 2002:406–432.

141 Haidopolous D, Rodolakis A, Stefanidis K, et al. Behçet's disease: part of the differential diagnosis of the ulcerative vulva. Clin Exp Obstet Gynecol 2002; 29(3):219–221.

142 Magro CM, Crowson AN. Cutaneous manifestations of Behçet's disease. Int J Derm 1995; 34(3):159–165.

143 Ergun T, Gurbuz O, Dogusoy, Mat C, Yazici H. Histopathologic features of the spontaneous pustular lesions of Behçet's syndrome. Int J Derm 1998; 37:194–196.

144 Mangelsdorf HC, White WL, Jorizzo JL. Behçet's disease: report of twenty-five patients from the United States with prominent mucocutaneous involvement. J Am Acad Derm 34(5):745–750.

145 Jorizzo JL, Abernethy JL, White WL, et al. Mucocutaneous criteria for the diagnosis of Behçet's disease: an analysis of clinicopathologic data from multiple international centers. J Am Acad Derm 1995; 32:968–976.

146 Balabanova M, Calamia KT, Perniciaro C, O'Duffy JD. A study of the cutaneous manifestations of Behçet's disease in patients from the United States. J Am Acad Derm 1999; 41:540–545.

147 Powell FC, Schroeter AL, Su WPD, Perry HO. Pyoderma gangrenosum: a review of 86 patients. Q J Med (NS) 1985; 55:173–186.

148 Prystowsky JH, Kahn SN, Lazarus GS. Present status of pyoderma gangrenosum: a review of 21 cases. Arch Derm 1989; 125:57–64.

149 Bennett ML, Jackson JM, Jorizzo JL, et al. Pyoderma gangrenosum. A comparison of typical and atypical forms with and emphasis on time to remission. Case review of 86 patients from 2 institutions. Medicine 2000; 86:37–46.

150 Crowson AN, Mihm MC Jr, Magro C. Pyoderma gangrenosum: a review. J Cutan Pathol 2003; 30:97–107.

151 Borum ML, Cannava M, Myrie-Williams C. Refractory, disfiguring vulvar pyoderma gangrenosum and Crohn's disease. Dig Dis Sci 1998; 43(4):720–722.

152 Grant P, Beischer A. Pyoderma gangrenosum of the vulva. Aust N Z J Obstet Gynaecol 1989; 29(3):360–362.

153 Lebbe C, Moulonguet-Michau I, Perrin P, et al. Steroid-responsive pyoderma gangrenosum with vulvar and pulmonary involvement. J Am Acad Derm 1992; 27(4):623–625.

154 McCalmont CS, Leshin B, White WL, Greiss FC Jr, Jorizzo JL. Vulvar pyoderma gangrenosum. Int J Gynaecol Obstet 1991; 35(2):175–178.

155 Segal I, Tim LO, Rubin A, et al. Rare and unusual manifestations of Crohn's disease with pyoderma gangrenosum and sclerosing cholangitis. S Afr Med J 1979; 55(15):596–599.

156 Valmadre S, Gee A, Dalrymple C. Pyoderma gangrenosum of the vulva. Aust N Z J Obstet Gynaecol 2002; 42(5):548–549.

157 Work BA. Pyoderma gangrenosum of the perineum. Obstet Gynecol 1980; 55:126–128.

158 Bennett ML, Jackson JM, Jorizzo JL, et al. Pyoderma gangrenosum. A comparison of typical and atypical forms with an emphasis on time to remission. Case review of 86 patients from 2 institutions. Medicine (Baltimore) 2000; 79(1):37–46.

159 Tuffnell D, Buchan PC. Crohn's disease of the vulva in childhood. Br J Clin Pr 1991; 45:159–160.

160 Bohl TG. Vulvar ulcers and erosions – a dermatologist's viewpoint. Dermatol Ther 2004;17(1):55–67.

161 Burgdorf W. Cutaneous manifestations of Crohn's disease. J Am Acad Derm 1981; 5(6):689–695.

162 Virgili A, Corazzo M. Crohn's disease of the vulva. A case report. J Reprod Med 1994; 39:115–117.

163 Urbanek M, Neill SM, McKee PH. Vulval Crohn's disease: difficulties in diagnosis. Clin Exp Derm 1996; 21:211–214.

164 Mould TAJ, Rodgers ME, Burnham WR, Weekes ARL. Metastatic Crohn's disease causing a vulval mass and involving the cervix. Int J STD AIDS 1997; 8:461–463.

165 Holohan M, Coughlan M, O'Loghlin S, Dervan P. Crohn's disease of the vulva. BJOG 1988; 95:943–945.

166 Shen RN, Cybulska BA, Thin RN, McKee PH. Vulval Crohn's disease mimicking genital herpes. Int J STD AIDS 1993; 4:54–56.

167 Guerrieri C, Ohlsson E, Ryden G, Westermark P. Vulvitis granulomatosa: a cryptogenic chronic inflammatory hypertrophy of vulvar labia related to cheilitis granulomatosa and Crohn's disease. Int J Gynecol Pathol 1995; 14(4):352–359.

168 Haefner HK, Elta GH. Home study course. Vulvar case presentation. J Lower Genital Tract Dis 2001; 5:105–108.

3

Hope K. Haefner

Localized vulvodynia

Introduction

Historical information on vulvar pain terminology

Etiologic theories on vulvodynia

Embryologic development
Infection
Inflammation

Genetic/immune factors
Neuropathways
Association with human
  papillomavirus

Histopathology

Treatment of localized vulvodynia

Introduction

Vulvodynia, once believed to be a rare condition, is now known to affect millions of women. However, the exact number of women experiencing pain localized to the vulvar vestibule is unknown. What is known is that the number of women previously afflicted with vulvar pain has been underestimated and that improved communication with patients has revealed a higher incidence. The pain can be generalized (diffuse vulvar burning or irritation) or localized (pain at a specific area such as the vestibule or clitoris). The localized vulvodynia that was previously termed vulvar vestibulitis is currently known as vestibulodynia. The vestibule is defined as the area between the hymen and Hart's line (Fig. 3.1).

Historical information on vulvar pain terminology

Vulvar pain discussion first appeared in the literature in the late 1800s. Thomas described the condition as 'excessive hypersensibility of the nerves supplying the mucous membrane of some portion of the vulva…'.[1] In 1889, Skene depicted a condition 'characterized by a supersensitiveness of the vulva… .When, however, the examining finger comes in contact with the hyperaes-

thetic part, the patient complains of pain, which is sometimes so great as to cause her to cry out…'.[2] In the same year, Kellogg wrote about a patient with 'sensitive points about the mouth of the vagina'.[3] The topic was not readdressed until 1928, when Howard Kelly saw a woman with 'exquisitely sensitive deep red spots' that were a 'fruitful source of dyspareunia'.[4] In 1983, Friedrich reported on 13 patients with 'vestibular adenitis'.[5] Terminology continues to change throughout time. The International Society for the Study of Vulvovaginal Disease (ISSVD) popularized a definition of vulvar pain in the 1980s (essential or dysesthetic vulvodynia) describing patients with a chronic discomfort, burning, stinging, irritation and rawness of the vulva. In 1987, Friedrich developed the term 'vulvar vestibulitis syndrome'.[6] There are two major forms of vulvar pain: hyperalgesia (low pain thresholds) and allodynia (pain to light touch).

Table 3.1 demonstrates the recent terminology changes for vulvar pain. The terminology of pain localized to the vulvar vestibule continues to undergo change.[7] The debate regarding the terminology continues.

Patients with vulvar pain localized to the vestibule have a normal-appearing vulva, other than erythema at times (Fig. 3.2). The erythema tends to be most prominent at the Bartholin's, Skene's and vestibular duct openings. Pain associated with an abnormal vulvar appearance does not qualify for the diagnosis of localized vulvodynia (Table 3.2).

Etiologic theories on vulvodynia

Many theories have been proposed for the etiology of vulvodynia, including abnormalities of embryologic development, infection, inflammation, genetic and immune factors and nerve sensitization. The exact etiology of vulvodynia is unknown. There may not be one single etiology.

EMBRYOLOGIC DEVELOPMENT

McCormack[8] and Fitzpatrick et al.[9] have linked vestibular pain with interstitial cystitis, another idiopathic inflammatory syndrome of the urogenital tract. These authors speculated that the tissues from these distinct anatomic sites had a common embryologic origin and therefore were predisposed to similar pathologic responses when challenged.

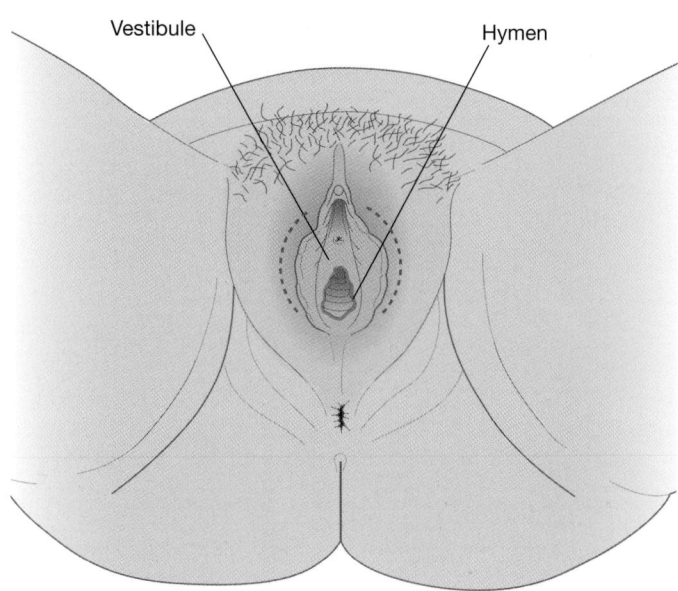

Fig. 3.1 Diagram of the vulvar vestibule. Hart's line is delineated by the dotted lines (see text)

Table 3.1 *ISSVD terminology and classification for vulvodynia*

Vulvar dysesthesia (1999)	Vulvar dysesthesia (2001)	Vulvodynia (2003)
New Mexico, USA, ISSVD World Congress	Lisbon, Portugal, ISSVD World Congress (Note: this was a provisional terminology system)	Salvador, Brazil, ISSVD World Congress

Generalized vulvar dysesthesia	Provoked vulvar dysesthesia
	    Generalized
	    Localized (vestibule, clitoris, other)
		Vulvodynia, generalized
		    Provoked (sexual, nonsexual or both)
		    Unprovoked
		    Mixed (provoked and unprovoked)

Localized vulvar dysesthesia
 	
    Vestibulodynia (formerly vulvar vestibulitis)
    Clitorodynia
    Other localized forms of vulvar dysesthesia
	Spontaneous vulvar dysesthesia
	
	    Generalized
	    Localized (vestibule, clitoris, other)
		Vulvodynia, localized (vestibulodynia, clitorodynia, hemivulvodynia, etc.)
		    Provoked (sexual, nonsexual or both)
		    Unprovoked
		    Mixed (provoked and unprovoked)

ISSVD, The International Society for the Study of Vulvovaginal Disease.

INFECTION

Infection with candidiasis has been suggested to be associated with vestibular pain. Frequently, patients with vulvar pain mention a history of recurrent Candida infections. Two specific studies have compared the frequency of Candida infections in patients with vestibular pain to a control population.[10,11] Both studies found that patients with pain reported more Candida infections than normal controls. Yet, this association is based on patient self-reports of past infections, not culture tests. Meana et al. and Bazin et al. did not find a high prevalence of culture-documented Candida infection.[10,12] Additionally, Marinoff and Turner did not demonstrate a hypersensitivity to Candida in patients with vestibular pain.[13] Bazin et al. assessed the prevalence of genital bacterial infection among women with localized vestibu-

Table 3.2 *Diseases associated with vulvar pain, not qualifying for the diagnosis of vulvodynia*

Podophyllin overdose	Pemphigus
Condylox (podofilox) overdose	Pemphigoid
Behçet's disease	Atrophy
Aphthous ulcers	Lichen sclerosus
Herpes (simplex and zoster)	Lichen planus
Candidiasis	Crohn's disease
Trichomonas	Bartholin's abscess
Chancroid	Trauma
Sjögren's disease	Imperforate hymen
Contact dermatitis	Prolapsed urethra
Endometriosis	Vulvar intraepithelial neoplasia Carcinoma

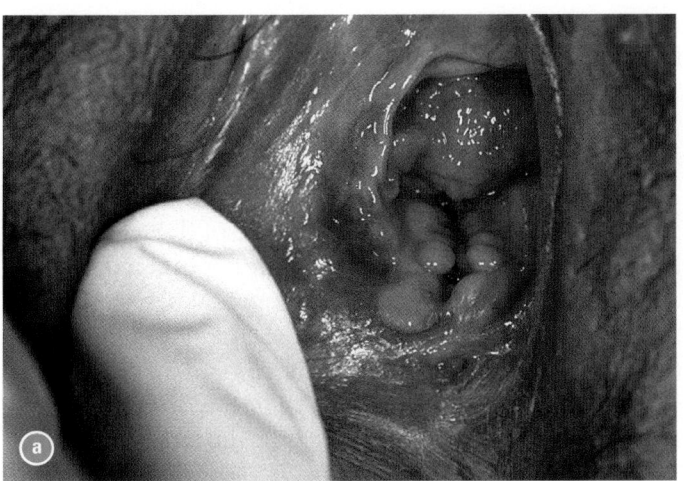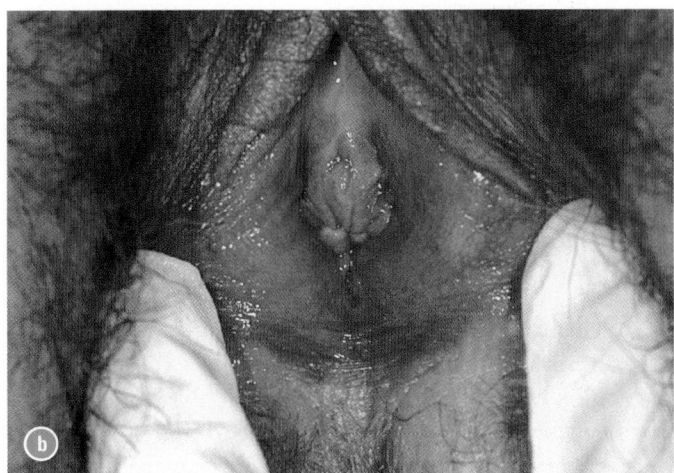

Fig. 3.2 (a,b) Clinical photos of localized vulvodynia (vestibulodynia) showing introital erythema.

lar pain. They found little for the idea that infection causes pain on the vestibule.[12]

INFLAMMATION

The role that inflammation plays in the development of localized vulvodynia is unclear. Various papers that mention inflammation and inflammatory cytokines show inconsistent results.[14–22] Currently, the suffix 'itis' (as in vestibulitis) has been excluded from the recent ISSVD terminology, since studies found a lack of association between excised tissue and inflammation. Bohm-Starke et al. found a low expression of the inflammatory markers cyclo-oxygenase 2 and inducible nitric oxide synthase in the vestibular mucosa of women with localized vestibular pain as well as in healthy control subjects.[23]

GENETIC/IMMUNE FACTORS

Goetsch was one of the first researchers to question a genetic association of localized vulvar pain.[24] A total of 31 gynecology patients (15%) questioned over a 6-month period were found to have localized vestibular pain. A total of 32% had a female relative with dyspareunia or tampon intolerance, raising the issue of a genetic predisposition. Another genetic connection has been suggested.[25] Allele 2 in the interleukin-1beta gene was found to be more common in women with vestibulodynia than in other women. Allele 2 of the interleukin-1beta gene was identified in 27 (46%) women with vestibulodynia as opposed to 12 (25%) control women ($P = 0.03$). Susceptibility to vestibulodynia might be influenced by carriage of this polymorphism.[25] Persons homozygous for allele 2 of the IL-1RA gene (IL1RN*2) have a more prolonged and more severe proinflammatory immune response than persons with other IL-1RA genotypes.[26] A role for defective immune regulation in this patient population has also been proposed.[27] In summary, a relative inability to down-regulate pro-inflammatory interleukin-1 beta activity by interleukin-1 receptor antagonist may contribute to the pathophysiologic features of localized vulvodynia.

NEUROPATHWAYS

Kermit Krantz was instrumental in examining the nerve characteristics of the vulva and vagina.[28] In this study, the region of the hymeneal ring was richly supplied with free nerve endings. No corpuscular endings of any form were observed. Only free nerve endings were observed in the fossa navicularis. A sparsity of nerve endings was noted in the vagina as compared to the region of the fourchette, fossa navicul009aris and hymeneal ring. Additionally, an association with age was noted. Interestingly, there were more free nerve endings in the genitalia of young patients than in older patients.

More recent studies have analyzed the nerve factors in women with vulvar pain. Westrom and Willen utilized S-100 stains for neural tissue protein and found that 44 out of 47 patients with localized pain to the vestibule had more nerve fibers than the control patients.[29] Vessels in this patient population were found to have a proliferation of nerve bundles around the vessels, thus possibly contributing to the erythema that often occurs in this patient population. Women suffering from vestibular pain have also demonstrated lowered tactile detection and pain thresholds in the vulvar vestibule than a control population.[14] Patients with vulvar pain localized to the vestibule have an increased innervation and/or sensitization of thermoreceptors and nociceptors in their vestibular mucosa.[30]

ASSOCIATION WITH HUMAN PAPILLOMAVIRUS

A further area of confusion has been the emphasis on the human papillomavirus (HPV) in the causation of symptoms of vulvar pain. The debate continues as to whether or not HPV is associated with vulvar pain. Several studies have been found to support the association of HPV with vulvar pain.[11,31–36] However, the majority of recent studies do not find an association of HPV and vulvar pain, particularly in pain that is localized to the vestibule.[12,19,21,24,37–41] Some studies have found the presence of HPV and vulvar pain localized to the vestibule, yet an association with response to treatment has not been noted. It appears to be unrelated to the presentation or response to surgical therapy or interferon.[35,42]

Histopathology

The epithelium covering the vestibule of the vulva differs from extra-genital skin as it is non-keratinized, with a non-pigmented surface and consequently has more similarity to mucosal surfaces than to skin at an ultrastructural level. The vestibular surface has an epithelium of several layers of closely packed cells. These cells mature and differentiate as they approach the surface. Unlike keratinized skin, appendages such as hair follicles and sweat glands and the characteristic granular and cornified cells are absent from vestibular epithelium. The surface of the vestibular epithelium is characterized by microridges. The surface cells of perineum, a keratinized epithelial surface, do not show this type of microridge.[43]

Vestibulectomy specimens in patients with vulvar pain have been analyzed and have revealed several findings. On occasion, vestibular gland adenomas have been associated with pain.[44] Glomus tumors have also been reported to cause pain on the vulva.[45–47] The focus of this discussion, though, is on pain localized to the vestibule, with a normal appearance, excluding erythema. Findings described in vestibulectomy specimens include a mixed population of T-lymphocytes, variable numbers of monocytes and rare plasma cells (Fig. 3.3). The microscopic findings are entirely non-specific inflammatory infiltrate,[15] sometimes present around the minor vestibular gland (Fig. 3.4). Squamous metaplasia in the vestibular glands and their ducts has been reported[15,19] (Fig. 3.5). Epidermal hyperkeratosis and parakeratosis have also been described but may represent lichenification due to rubbing of the underlying condition.[37] White blood cells may be seen in all layers of the epithelium. Small surface erosions (ulcers) may be seen, either acute or healing (Fig. 3.6). These findings are not specific and can be seen in unaffected women. Many studies support the association of inflammation to the disease of the vestibule,[15,17,48–50] while other studies lack support for

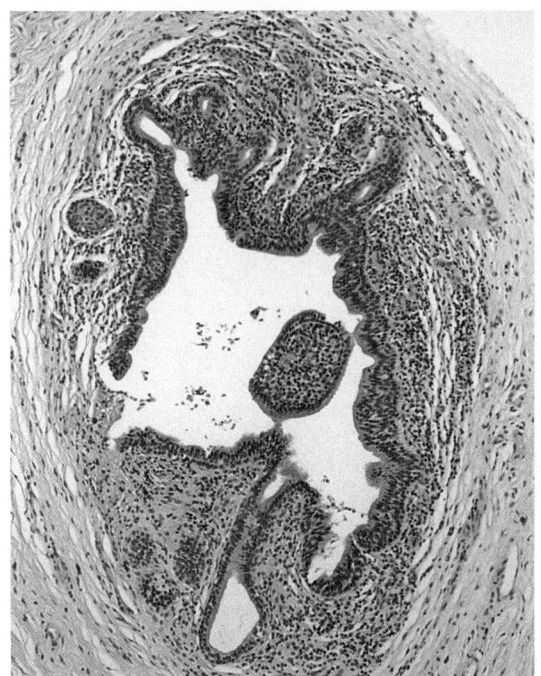

Fig. 3.4 Inflammation in minor vestibular glands.

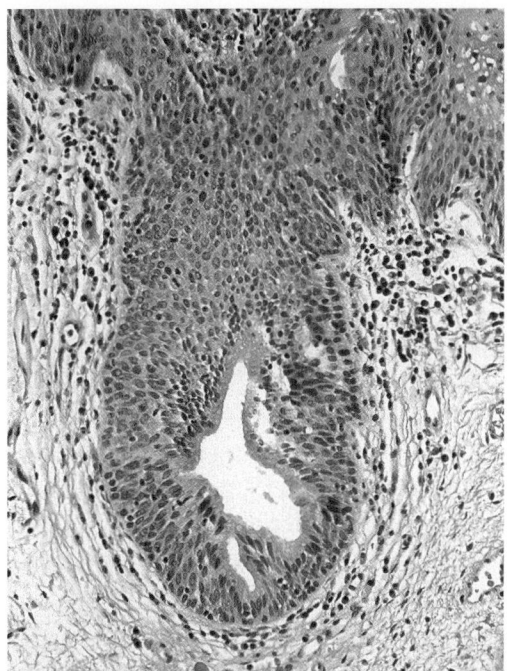

Fig. 3.5 Squamous metaplasia of vestibular glands.

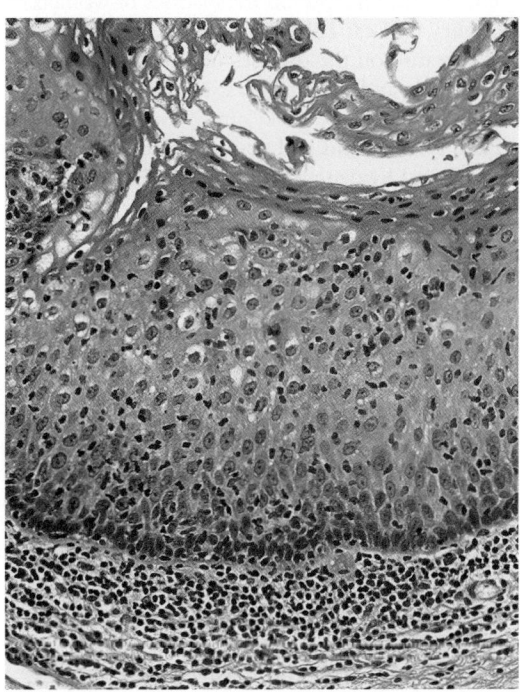

Fig. 3.3 Histopathology of vestibulectomy specimens from patient with vestibulodynia ('vestibulitis') showing inflammatory cells in the epithelium and lamina propria.

this concept, having found inflammation to be present in the control population also.[21] Whether localized vulvodynia can be distinguished from the more generalized form by pathologic parameters remains to be determined. Conceivably, a more discrete inflammatory response may co-segregate with the localized form,

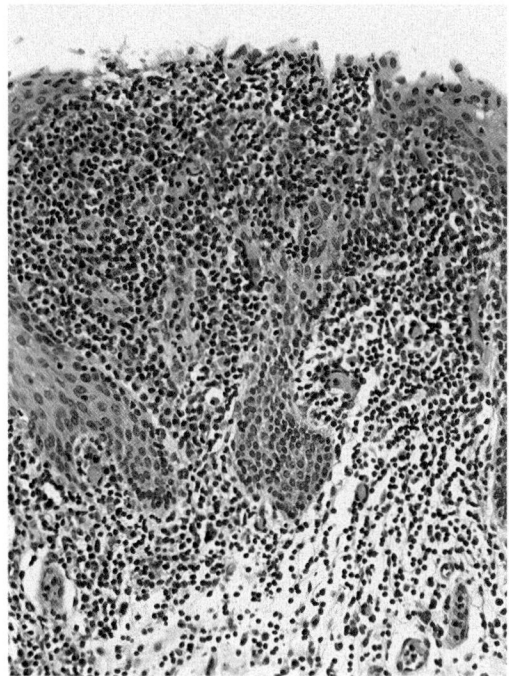

Fig. 3.6 Small surface ulcerations from a vestibulectomy specimen.

providing a morphologic correlate for the discomfort that is produced by point pressure. However, until this is proven, the pathologist is reminded that the above histologic findings found in the setting of vulvar pain may or may not correlate with the clinical diagnosis of vestibulodynia (vestibulitis). A format for pathologic reporting is outlined in Table 3.3.

Treatment of localized vulvodynia

The complex and mysterious nature of vulvodynia is exemplified by the diversity of therapeutic approaches.
1 General vulvar care measures focus on avoidance of detergents, synthetic undergarments and tight fitting clothing and the use of adequate lubrication.
2 Topical application of 5% lidocaine ointment, ELA-Max®, amitriptyline and baclofen and estrogens.

Table 3.3 Reporting of pathology in the setting of vulvodynia

Descriptive terminology	Comment
Surface epithelial erosion Submucosal acute and chronic inflammation Perivestibular adenitis Squamous metaplasia of vestibular ductal epithelium	These features have been reported in association with vestibulodynia (vestibular adenitis). However, their pathogenetic significance is unclear. Clinical correlation is advised

3 In severe cases, intralesional injections of anesthetics at pain trigger points. Interferon, which was advocated when it first became available, is not used frequently.
4 Dietary regimens that include low oxalate intake and calcium citrate supplementation.
5 Approaches targeting neural pathways, including psychotropic drugs (amitriptyline, gabapentin, carbamazepine), physical therapy and biofeedback, acupuncture and hypnosis.

Notwithstanding the value of the above therapies for some patients, controlled trials of new treatments for vulvodynia are few.[51,52] Vestibulodynia is a complex disorder that can be a difficult process to treat and intractable or severe cases may require excision of the vestibule (vestibulectomy). Gaunt et al. reported significant improvement of symptoms in 90% of 42 women with what was termed 'pure vestibulitis';[53] however, many other studies report less improvement with surgery. Given the mysterious nature of vestibulodynia and the broad and diverse range of entities that may fall under this term, surgical approaches should be explored in carefully selected patients after other therapies have failed to provide adequate relief.

References

1 Thomas TG, ed. Practical treatise on the diseases of women. Philadelphia: Henry C. Lea; 1880:145–147.
2 Skene AJC, ed. Treatise on the diseases of women: for the use of students and practitioners. New York: Appleton; 1889:93–94.
3 Kellogg JH. Plain facts for old and young: embracing the natural history and hygiene of organic life. Burlington: IF Segner; 1889.
4 Kelly HA. Gynecology. New York: D. Appleton; 1928:235–239.
5 Friedrich EG Jr. The vulvar vestibule. J Reprod Med 1983; 28(11):773–777.
6 Friedrich EG Jr. Vulvar vestibulitis syndrome. J Reprod Med 1987; 32(2):110–114.
7 International Society for the Study of Vulvovaginal Disease. Summary of meeting discussions for the International Society for the Study of Vulvovaginal Disease 1999, 2001, 2003.
8 McCormack WM. Two urogenital sinus syndromes. Interstitial cystitis and focal vulvitis. J Reprod Med 1990; 35(9):873–876.
9 Fitzpatrick CC, DeLancey JO, Elkins TE, McGuire EJ. Vulvar vestibulitis and interstitial cystitis: a disorder of urogenital sinus-derived epithelium? Obstet Gynecol 1993; 81(5):860–862.
10 Meana M, Binik YM, Khalif S, Cohen DR. Deconstructing dyspareunia: description, classification and biopsychosocial

correlates of a pain disorder (Thesis), McGill University, Montreal, Canada, 1995.

11 Mann MS, Kaufman RH, Brown D Jr, Adam E. Vulvar vestibulitis: significant clinical variables and treatment outcome. Obstet Gynecol 1992; 79(1):122–125.

12 Bazin S, Bouchard C, Brisson J, et al. Vulvar vestibulitis syndrome: an exploratory case-control study. Obstet Gynecol 1994; 83(1):47–50.

13 Marinoff SC, Turner ML. Hypersensitivity to vaginal candidiasis or treatment vehicles in the pathogenesis of minor vestibular gland syndrome. J Reprod Med 1986; 31(9):796–799.

14 Pukall CF, Binik YM, Khalifé S, Amsel R, Abbott FV. Vestibular tactile and pain thresholds in women with vulvar vestibulitis syndrome. Pain 2002; 96(1–2):163–175.

15 Pyka RE, Wilkinson EJ, Friedrich EG Jr, Croker BP. The histopathology of vulvar vestibulitis syndrome. Int J Gynecol Pathol 1988; 7(3):249–257.

16 Michlewitz H, Kennison RD, Turksoy RN, Fertitta LC. Vulvar vestibulitis – subgroup with Bartholin gland duct inflammation. Obstet Gynecol 1989; 73(3):410–413.

17 Furlonge CB, Thin RN, Evans BE, McKee PH. Vulvar vestibulitis syndrome: a clinico-pathological study. Br J Obstet Gynaecol 1991; 98(7):703–706.

18 Friedman M. Understanding vaginal vestibulum dyspareunia syndrome. Cerv Lower Female Genital Tract 1995; 13:135–140.

19 Prayson RA, Stoler MH, Hart WR. Vulvar vestibulitis. A histopathologic study of 36 cases, including human papillomavirus in situ hybridization analysis. Am J Surg Pathol 1995; 19(2):154–160.

20 Foster DC, Hasday JD. Elevated tissue levels of interleukin-1 beta and tumor necrosis factor-alpha in vulvar vestibulitis. Obstet Gynecol 1997; 89(2):291–296.

21 Lundqvist EN, Hofer PA, Olofsson JI, Sjoberg I. Is vulvar vestibulitis an inflammatory condition? A comparison of histological findings in affected and healthy women. Acta Derm Venereol 1997; 77(4):319–322.

22 Slone S, Reynolds L, Gall S, et al. Localization of chromogranin, synaptophysin, serotonin and CXCR2 in neuroendocrine cells of the minor vestibular glands: an immunohistochemical study. Int J Gynecol Pathol 1999; 18(4):360–365.

23 Bohm-Starke N, Falconer C, Rylander E, Hilliges M. The expression of cyclooxygenase 2 and inducible nitric oxide synthase indicates no active inflammation in vulvar vestibulitis. Acta Obstet Gynecol Scand 2001; 80(7):638–644.

24 Goetsch MF. Vulvar vestibulitis: prevalence and historic features in a general gynecologic practice population. Am J Obstet Gynecol 1991; 164(6):1609–1616.

25 Gerber S, Bongiovanni AM, Ledger WJ, Witkin SS. Interleukin-1beta gene polymorphism in women with vulvar vestibulitis syndrome. Eur J Obstet Gynecol Reprod Biol 2003; 107(1):74–77.

26 Gerber S, Bongiovanni AM, Ledger WJ, Witkin SS. Defective regulation of the proinflammatory immune response in women with vulvar vestibulitis syndrome. Am J Obstet Gynecol 2002; 186(4):696–700.

27 Witkin SS, Gerber S, Ledger WJ. Influence of interleukin 1 receptor antagonist gene polymorphism on disease. Clin Infect Dis 2002; 34(2):204–209.

28 Krantz KE. Innervation of the human vulva and vagina. Obstet Gynecol 1958; 12(2):382–396.

29 Westrom LV, Willen R. Vestibular nerve fiber proliferation in vulvar vestibulitis syndrome. Obstet Gynecol 1998; 91(4):572–576.

30 Bohm-Starke N, Hilliges M, Brodda-Jansen G, Rylander E, Torebjork E. Psychophysical evidence of nociceptor sensitization in vulvar vestibulitis syndrome. Pain 2001; 94(2):177–183.

31 Growdon WA, Fu YS, Lebherz TB, et al. Pruritic vulvar squamous papillomatosis: evidence for human papillomavirus etiology. Obstet Gynecol 1985; 66(4):564–568.

32 di Paola GR, Rueda NG. Deceptive vulvar papillomavirus infection. A possible explanation for certain cases of vulvodynia. J Reprod Med 1986; 31(10):966–970.

33 Reid R, Greenberg MD, Daoud Y, et al. Colposcopic findings in women with vulvar pain syndromes. A preliminary report. J Reprod Med 1988; 33(6):523–532.

34 Turner ML, Marinoff SC. Association of human papillomavirus with vulvodynia and the vulvar vestibulitis syndrome. J Reprod Med 1988; 33(6):533–537.

35 Umpierre SA, Kaufman RH, Adam E, Woods KV, Adler-Storthz K. Human papillomavirus DNA in tissue biopsy specimens of vulvar vestibulitis patients treated with interferon. Obstet Gynecol 1991; 78(4):693–695.

36 Bornstein J, Shapiro S, Rahat M, et al. Polymerase chain reaction search for viral etiology of vulvar vestibulitis syndrome. Am J Obstet Gynecol 1996; 175(1):139–144.

37 Wilkinson EJ, Guerrero E, Daniel R, et al. Vulvar vestibulitis is rarely associated with human papillomavirus infection types 6, 11, 16, or 18. Int J Gynecol Pathol 1993; 12(4):344–349.

38 Bergeron C, Moyal-Barracco M, Pelisse M, Lewin P. Vulvar vestibulitis. Lack of evidence for a human papillomavirus etiology. J Reprod Med 1994; 39(12):936–938.

39 Chadha S, Gianotten WL, Drogendijk AC, et al. Histopathologic features of vulvar vestibulitis. Int J Gynecol Pathol 1998; 17(1):7–11.

40 Origoni M, Rossi M, Ferrari D, Lillo F, Ferrari AG. Human papillomavirus with co-existing vulvar vestibulitis syndrome and vestibular papillomatosis. Int J Gynaecol Obstet 1999; 64(3):259–263.

41 Morin C, Bouchard C, Brisson J, et al. Human papillomaviruses and vulvar vestibulitis. Obstet Gynecol 2000; 95(5):683–687.

42 Bornstein J, Shapiro S, Goldshmid N, et al. Severe vulvar vestibulitis. Relation to HPV infection. J Reprod Med 1997; 42(8):514–518.

43 Sargeant P, Moate R, Harris JE, Morrison GD. Ultrastructural study of the epithelium of the normal human vulva. J Submicrosc Cytol Pathol 1996; 28(2):161–170.

44 Axe S, Parmley T, Woodruff JD, Hlopak B. Adenomas in minor vestibular glands. Obstet Gynecol 1986; 68(1):16–18.

45 Kohorn EI, Merino MJ, Goldenhersh M. Vulvar pain and dyspareunia due to glomus tumor. Obstet Gynecol 1986; 67(3):41S–42S.

46 Jacobsen JC. Glomangioma of the vulva. A painful benign tumor in the vulva. Ugeskr Laeg 1973; 135(11):594.

47 Katz VL, Askin FB, Bosch BD. Glomus tumor of the vulva: a case report. Obstet Gynecol 1986; 67(3):43S–45S.

48 Friedrich EG Jr. Therapeutic studies on vulvar vestibulitis. J Reprod Med 1988; 33(6):514–518.

49 Woodruff JD, Parmley TH. Infection of the minor vestibular gland. Obstet Gynecol 1983; 62(5):609–612.

50 Chaim W, Meriwether C, Gonik B, Qureshi F, Sobel JD. Vulvar vestibulitis subjects undergoing surgical intervention: a descriptive analysis and histopathological correlates. Eur J Obstet Gynecol Reprod Biol 1996; 68(1–2):165–168.

51 Edwards L. New concepts in vulvodynia. Am J Obstet Gynecol 2003; 189:S24–S30.

52 Reed BD, Haefner HK, Cantor L. Vulvar dysesthesia (vulvodynia). A follow-up study. J Reprod Med 2003; 48(6):409–416.

53 Gaunt G, Good A, Stanhope CR. Vestibulectomy for vulvar vestibulitis. J Reprod Med 2003; 48(8):591–595.

4

Infectious disorders of the lower genital tract

Alexander J.F. Lazar,

Scott R. Granter,

Phillip H. McKee and

Hope K. Haefner

Introduction

Common parasites

Pediculosis pubis (crab lice)
Scabies

Common infections not typically linked to sexually transmitted diseases

Vulvovaginal candidiasis
Tinea cruris
Bacterial vaginosis
Folliculitis

Common sexually transmitted infections

Trichomonas
Molluscum contagiosum
Herpes simplex infections
Neisseria gonorrhea

Uncommon sexually transmitted diseases

Syphilis
Chancroid

Granuloma inguinale
Lymphogranuloma venereum

Other rare infections

Periclitoral abscess
Schistosomiasis
Epstein–Barr virus

Common and rare vulvar infections associated with immune suppression

Introduction
Tuberculosis
Bacillary angiomatosis
Necrotizing fasciitis of the vulva
Chronic erosive genital herpes
Varicella zoster
Extensive genital warts in the
    immunosuppressed patient
Disseminated molluscum
Norwegian scabies

Introduction

A variety of organisms can infect the female genital tract, accounting for considerable suffering and morbidity (Table 4.1). Some, such as candidal infections, trichomoniasis and bacterial vaginosis, are extremely common and may cause significant discomfort with no serious sequelae. Others, such as gonorrhea and chlamydial infection, are major causes of female infertility. Viruses, principally the human papillomaviruses (HPV), are involved in the pathogenesis of vulvar, vaginal and cervical cancer. Many infections are sexually transmitted, including trichomoniasis, gonorrhea, chancroid, granuloma inguinale, lymphogranuloma venereum, syphilis, chlamydia, herpes and HPV. This chapter will focus on pathogens encountered principally in the lower genital tract (vulva, vagina and cervix). Those involving the upper genital tract will be discussed under the fallopian tube (pelvic inflammatory disease). Papillomavirus infections (condylomata) are discussed in Chapters 6 and 13.

Many of the common infections discussed below are 'clinician's diseases', meaning the diagnosis is made exclusively by the clinician or the role of the pathologist is largely confirmatory. Many disorders, such as candidiasis, bacterial vaginosis and common sexually transmitted diseases, do not require the expertise of a diagnostic pathologist. Thus, the reader will appreciate a bias towards clinical diagnosis and treatment. For others, such as clinically unsuspected candidiasis, syphilis, or other rare sexually transmitted diseases (STDs) such as tuberculosis and bacillary angiomatosis, recognition by the pathologist may be key to diagnosis and treatment (Table 4.1).

Treatment of these disorders will be summarized where appropriate. For treatment specifics of sexually transmitted diseases, the Centers for Disease Control and Prevention (CDC) has developed an STD treatment guideline (accessible on the internet at http://www.cdc.gov/STD/treatment/), which can be used to expand on particular treatment regimens discussed in this chapter.

Common parasites

PEDICULOSIS PUBIS (CRAB LICE)

Clinical presentation

Pediculosis pubis is caused by an ectoparasite, *Phthirus pubis*, also known as the crab louse. Patients present with pruritus in the pubic area. Transmission is by direct

Table 4.1 Infections of the lower female genital tract

Common infections
Pediculosis pubis (crab lice)
Scabies
Vulvovaginal candidiasis
Tinea cruris (jock itch)
Bacterial vaginosis
Folliculitis

Sexually transmitted diseases
Trichomonas
Molluscum contagiosum
Herpes simplex
Gonorrhea
Syphilis
Chancroid
Granuloma inguinale
Lymphogranuloma venereum

Rare infections
Periclitoral abscess (less common)
Schistosomiasis
Epstein–Barr virus

Infections seen in the immunosuppressed patient (including HIV)
Tuberculosis
Bacillary angiomatosis
Necrotizing fasciitis
Chronic erosive herpes simplex virus infections
Extensive genital warts
Varicella zoster
Disseminated molluscum
Norwegian scabies

intimate contact. The lice appear as brown gray circular specks attached to the pubic hair base. The parasites are 1–3 mm long and have three pairs of legs.[1] They can be seen with the naked eye. They infest hair in the pubic area and occasionally other body areas that contain terminal hairs. The life cycle of the female is 1–3 months. The adult female lays eggs that adhere to hair at the skin–hair junction. A nit may be seen as a small opalescent gray speck connected to the hairs (Fig. 4.1).[2] These eggs or nits hatch in 6–10 days. Nymphs then mature to adults within 10 to 14 days. Pediculosis pubis is diagnosed by the identification of live lice and/or viable nits. Physical examination reveals visible opalescent nits or live lice and blue macules (maculae caeruleae) at feeding sites. All patients with pediculosis pubis should have a thorough investigation for other sexually transmitted diseases (30% of patients will have another concurrent STD). Screening for HIV, syphilis, gonorrhea, chlamydia infection, herpes, warts and trichomoniasis should be considered in this patient population.[3]

Diagnosis

Patients who have pediculosis pubis (i.e. pubic lice) usually seek medical attention because of pruritus or

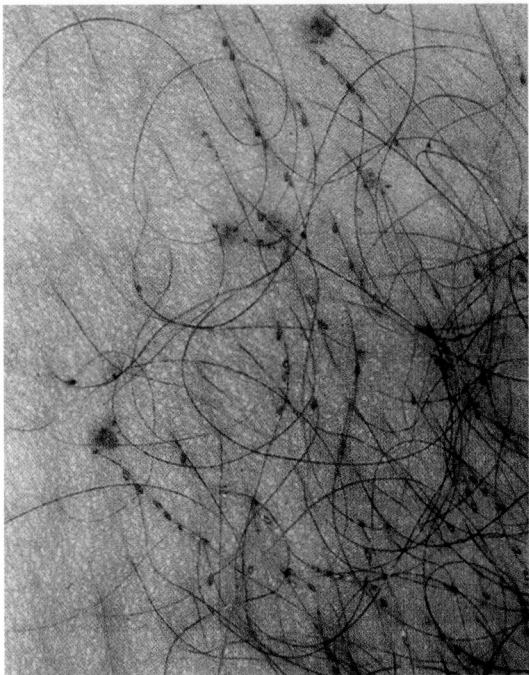

Fig. 4.1 Pediculosis pubis (crab lice) attached to hair shafts. (From Sidhu-Malik and Rein. Ectoparasitic infections. In: Rein M, ed. Atlas of Infectious Diseases, Vol. V: Sexually Transmitted Diseases. Philadelphia: Churchill Livingstone; 1996:13.3, Fig. 13.7.)

because they notice lice or nits on their pubic hair. The vulvar lesions can be scraped onto a slide and the contents viewed under a microscope. The entire crab is visualized, containing three pairs of legs. In contrast to the oval shape of head and body lice, the crab louse is almost as wide as it is long, allowing it to grasp widely spaced pubic hairs.[4]

Clinical differential diagnosis

The clinical differential diagnosis of pediculosis pubis includes dermatophyte infection, folliculitis and contact dermatitis.

Treatment for vulvar pediculosis pubis

Several options exist for the treatment of pediculosis pubis. These include permethrin 1% creme rinse, lindane 1% shampoo or pyrethrins with piperonyl butoxide. Pregnant and lactating women should be treated with either permethrin or pyrethrins with piperonyl butoxide. Lindane is contraindicated in pregnancy. Bedding and clothing should be decontaminated but fumigation of living areas is not necessary.[5] Patients should (1) avoid contact with their sexual partner, (2) be evaluated after 1 week if symptoms persist and (3) encourage their partner to be treated if exposed within the past month.

SCABIES

Clinical presentation

Scabies is an infection caused by *Sarcoptes scabiei* var *hominis* (itch mite). Its mode of transmission is from skin contact. It can also be transmitted from bed linens or intimate clothing. Scabies in adults is often sexually acquired. However, scabies in children is not usually sexually acquired. A small burrow occurs on the skin. The mite may be visualized in early disease as a tiny dot at the end of the burrow. The predominant symptom of scabies is pruritus (generally worse at night) and scratching will produce excoriation and a maculopapular rash (Fig. 4.2). Sensitization to *S. scabiei* must occur before pruritus begins. The first time a person is infected with *S. scabiei*, sensitization takes up to several weeks to develop. However, pruritus might occur within 24 hours after a subsequent reinfestation.

Diagnosis

Diagnosis can be confirmed by scraping the lesion onto a slide and viewing it with a microscope. When scraping, select papules or burrows that have not been scratched or disturbed. Crusted scabies (i.e. Norwegian scabies) is an aggressive infestation that usually occurs in immunodeficient, debilitated or malnourished persons (see infections associated with immunosuppression or systemic disorders section).

The lesions of scabies are occasionally biopsied and usually reveal acanthosis with variable hyperkeratosis and spongiosis sometimes with exocytosis of eosinophils and/or neutrophils. Superficial and deep perivascular nodules of lymphocytes are seen often admixed with histiocytes and eosinophils. In persistent nodular scabies, the density of the infiltrate and scattered atypical lymphoid cells can create concern for lymphoma. Serial sections can be performed to search for a burrow through the stratum corneum and mite body parts, eggs or fecal deposits (scybala) in the stratum granulosum or spongiosum, but this effort is often fruitless. The female mite body is rounded and less than 0.5 mm in diameter. A definitive histologic diagnosis requires such demonstration. However, scabies infestation can be suggested to the clinician when this pattern of lymphocytic infiltration is seen. The Norwegian variant of scabies shows exuberant hyperkeratosis with parakeratosis and mites and their eggs are usually numerous and prominent.

Clinical differential diagnosis

The differential diagnosis for scabies includes: insect bites, atopic or contact dermatitis, psoriasis, lichen planus,

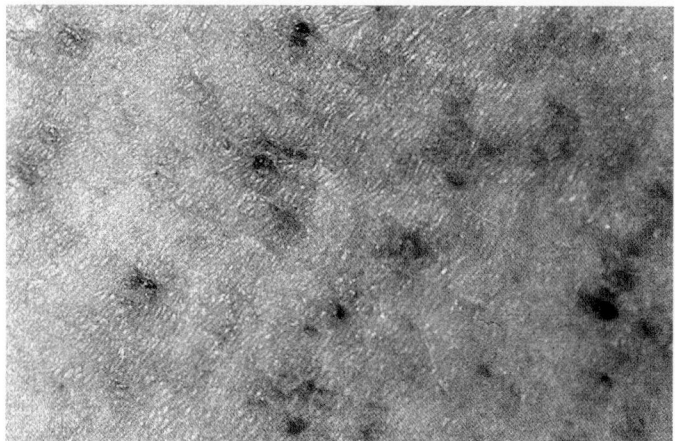

Fig. 4.2 Rash associated with scabies (buttock). (From Sidhu-Malik and Rein. Ectoparasitic infections. In: Rein M, ed. Atlas of Infectious Diseases, Vol. V: Sexually Transmitted Diseases. Philadelphia: Churchill Livingstone; 1996:13.7, Fig. 13.24.)

impetigo, pediculosis pubis, lichen simplex chronicus, prurigo nodularis, seabather's eruption and drug reactions.

Treatment of scabies

Treatments for scabies include permethrin, lindane and ivermectin. As discussed previously, pregnant or lactating women or children aged <2 years should not use lindane and lindane should not be used in the presence of extensive dermatitis. Bedding and clothing should be decontaminated. Patients who do not respond to the recommended treatment should be retreated with an alternative regimen. Both sexual and close personal or household contacts within the preceding month should be examined and treated.

Common infections not typically linked to sexually transmitted diseases

VULVOVAGINAL CANDIDIASIS

Clinical presentation

Vulvovaginal candidiasis (VVC) is a common and vexing problem. In North America, three out of four women will experience at least one episode of VVC and half of women will experience more than one episode. For a smaller percentage of women, the condition will become chronic with multiple relapses over several years.[6] VVC is uncommon before menarche with a rapidly increasing incidence late in the second decade, peaking in the third and fourth decades.[7] Predisposing factors include: uncontrolled diabetes mellitus, immunosuppressed state, steroid and antibiotic use and oral contraceptives. The most common symptoms and signs are intense vulvar pruritus, dysuria, erythema, edema and a white vaginal discharge with a 'curd-like' appearance (Fig. 4.3a).[8] While the most common causative organism is *Candida (C.) albicans*, the incidence of non-albicans species such as *C. glabrata, C. parapsilosis, C. tropicalis, C. lipolytica, Saccharomyces cerevisiae* and others, appear to be rising.[7,8] Recognition of these species is important since they can be more resistant to the traditionally used azole antimycotics. It should be noted that up to 20% of women are asymptomatic carriers of candidal species.[8] Vulvar involvement in the absence of vaginal infection is rare. Diagnosis is usually established by assay of vaginal pH, a potassium hydroxide (KOH) prep and/or fungal cultures (Fig. 4.3b)[9]. When clinicians obtain the fungal cultures, the vulva as well as the vagina should be swabbed. A yeast culture with identification of species is often helpful in treating patients with recurrent vulvovaginitis.

Histologic features

Candida infections are usually associated with hyperkeratosis and/or parakeratosis, epidermal hyperplasia (often psoriasiform) and neutrophil infiltration of the squamous epithelium typically forming microabscesses (Fig. 4.4a,b). The pseudohyphal and budding forms of *Candida* can be demonstrated in the epidermis using either PAS or silver stains (Fig. 4.4c). The various species of *Candida* cannot be reliably differentiated by light microscopy. It is important to note that fungal infections may have been previously treated by antifungals, steroids, or both, at the time of biopsy and may affect the histologic features. In particular, steroid use may reduce the neutrophilic infiltrate.

Histologic differential diagnosis

The differential diagnosis of candidal infection includes eczematous dermatitis, lichen simplex chronicus, intertrigo and psoriasis (Ch. 2 and Table 4.2). Before making any of these diagnoses, PAS and/or silver stains should be examined to exclude a fungal infection. Lichen simplex chronicus may also be superimposed on a candidal infection due to rubbing to relieve the pruritus. It is important to note that fungal superinfection may occur in many other lesions. In such a case, it is wise to advise the physician to treat the fungal infection and repeat the biopsy if the lesion persists.

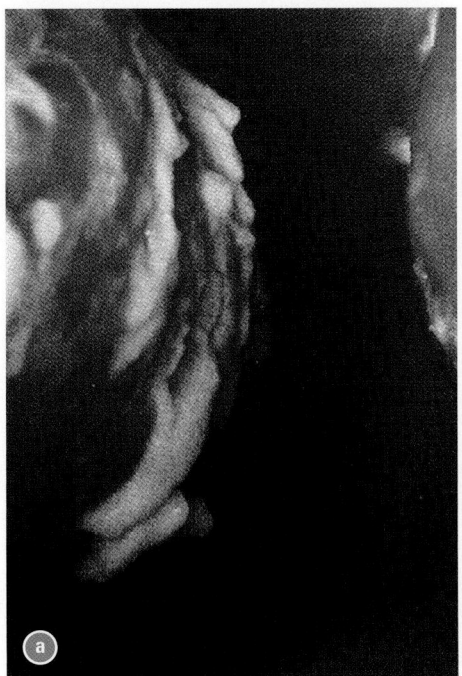
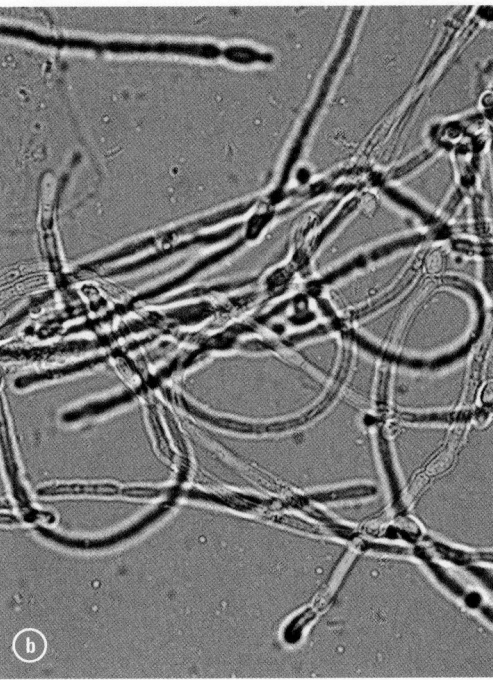

Fig. 4.3 (a) Clinical presentation of candidiasis, with white curd-like deposits on the vaginal wall. (From Sobel JD. Vulvovaginal candidiasis. In: Rein M, ed. Atlas of Infectious Diseases, Vol. V: Sexually Transmitted Diseases. Philadelphia: Churchill Livingstone; 1996:7.10, Fig. 7.34.) (b) Candida hyphae, seen on a KOH prep.

Treatment

It is necessary to consider removal or improvement of predisposing factors in the treatment of candidiasis. Numerous antifungal preparations are available. With failure of topical therapies, oral preparations should be considered, including fluconazole (Diflucan). Other oral medications utilized in recurrent yeast infections are ketoconazole and itraconazole, flucytosine and gentian violet, with attention to potential toxicities.[9]

TINEA CRURIS

Clinical presentation

Tinea cruris is a dermatophytic infection of the groin and pubic region. The lesions are erythematous with central clearing and raised borders. It is more common in men than in women. It is not often seen on the vulva or around the anus.

The signs and symptoms of tinea cruris include itching and erythema in the groin, vulva, inner thighs, anus and buttocks. The skin may flake, crack and peel. A burning sensation may be present. The dermatophyte species that is most prevalent is dependent on geographic location. *Trichophyton rubrum*, *T. tonsurans* and *T. mentagrophytes* are some of the species that cause this condition Other organisms, including *Epidermophyton floccosum* and *Trichophyton verrucosum*, cause an identical clinical condition.

Diagnosis

The diagnosis of tinea cruris is generally confirmed by culture and microscopy of skin scrapings treated with potassium hydroxide to visualize hyphae.

Histologic findings

The epidermis exhibits spongiosis or a psoriasiform pattern of hyperplasia. A granulomatous dermatitis may accompany folliculitis. A diagnostic clue is the presence of neutrophils in the cornified cell layer and fungal elements can be sandwiched between two zones of differing structure within the cornified cell layer; this is sometimes referred to as the sandwich sign. The upper zone of the cornified cell layer has a typical basket-weave pattern of orthokeratosis, while the lower zone consists of more compact orthokeratosis and parakeratosis. The presence of spores and branching hyphae can be confirmed using periodic acid-Schiff or methenamine silver stains, but histologic examination provides no clues regarding the dermatophyte species.[10]

Clinical differential diagnosis

The following conditions should be considered in the differential diagnosis of tinea cruris: acanthosis nigricans, contact dermatitis (allergic and irritant), erythrasma folliculitis, psoriasis, candidal infection and seborrheic dermatitis.

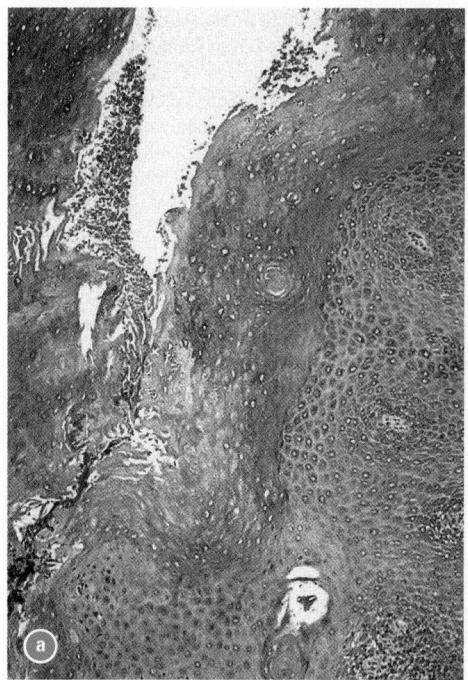

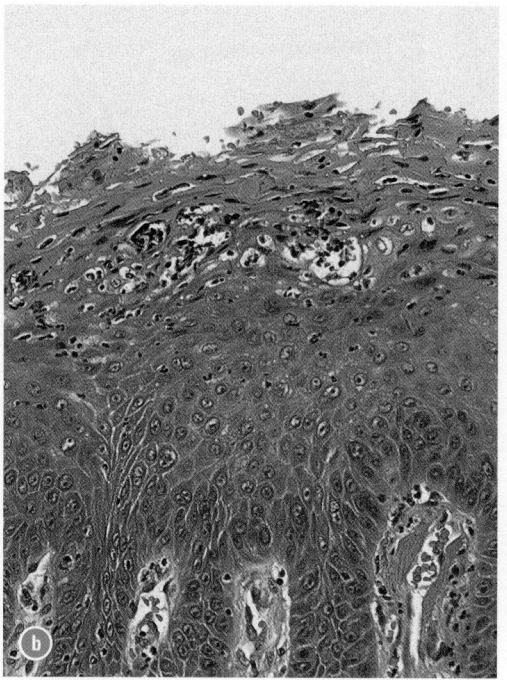

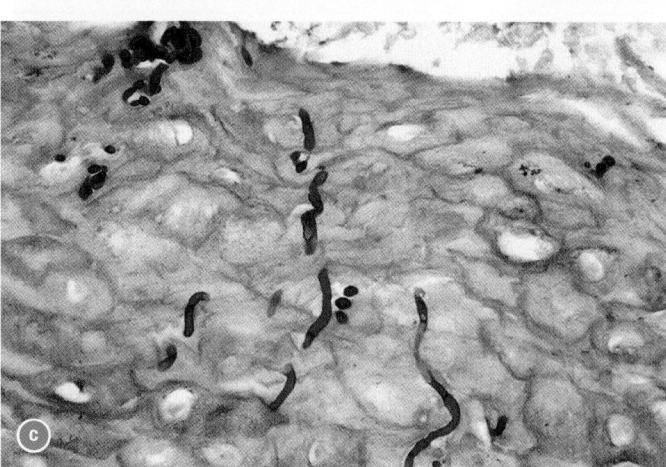

Fig. 4.4 (a) Biopsy of candidiasis at low power, illustrating acanthosis. (b) Superficial microabscess within the surface keratinocytes, containing acute inflammatory cells, should prompt a search for organisms. (c) Pseudohyphae from a surface microabscess.

Treatment

Topical antifungal agents of the imidazole or allylamine family are generally utilized for treatment of tinea cruris. At times, systemic administration of antifungals is needed for patients unable to use topical treatments consistently or those with extensive or recalcitrant infections.[10]

Table 4.2 *Differential diagnosis of candida vulvitis*

Eczematous dermatitis
Lichen simplex chronicus
Intertrigo
Psoriasis
Intraepithelial neoplasia

BACTERIAL VAGINOSIS

Clinical presentation

Various terms have been used for bacterial vaginosis (BV). These include non-specific vaginitis, *Hemophilus* vaginitis, *Corynebacterium* vaginitis, *Gardnerella vaginalis* vaginitis and anaerobic vaginosis. Bacterial vaginosis represents a complex change in the normal vaginal flora. It is characterized by a reduction in the prevalence and concentration of hydrogen-peroxide producing lactobacilli and an increase in the prevalence and concentration of *Gardnerella vaginalis*, *Mobiluncus* species, *Mycoplasma hominis*, anaerobic Gram-negative rods belonging to the genera *Prevotella*, *Porphyromonas*, *Bacteroides* and *Peptostreptococcus* species. The patient presents with a foul, 'fishy' odor, more noticeable following intercourse and during menses. Vaginal discharge is increased. Vulvar itching and/or irritation are present.

Diagnosis

A vaginal pH and wet prep are the usual diagnostic methods. The wet prep or Papanicolaou smear contains clue cells (Fig. 4.5a,b) with an absence of lactobacilli and white blood cells. When KOH is added to the wet prep, an odor is present, due to the anaerobic bacteria. Their concentrations increase 100–1000× with BV. The anaerobic metabolism produces amines (cadaverine, putrescine, trimethylamine). Bacterial vaginosis may also be diagnosed with other laboratory methods such as the use of DNA probes. These are expensive, but may be useful to practitioners unable to perform microscopy. Cultures have been used at times, but they are not useful since they are positive in 40–60% of asymptomatic females. A new technique that includes nucleic acid probes for high concentrations of *G. vaginalis* has recently become available (Affirm™ VPIII Microbial Identification Test).

Clinical differential diagnosis

The differential diagnosis for BV includes: candidiasis, cervicitis, *Chlamydia*, gonorrhea, herpes, *Trichomonas* and desquamative vaginitis. These disorders are typically distinguished by appropriate analysis of the discharge and cultures.

Treatment

Recommended regimens include: metronidazole, metronidazole gel and clindamycin cream 2% (one full applicator (5 g) intravaginally at bedtime for 7 days). The recommended metronidazole regimens are equally efficacious. Studies are currently underway to evaluate the efficacy of vaginal lactobacilli suppositories in addition to oral metronidazole for the treatment of BV. Bacteriotherapy, using harmless bacteria to displace pathogenic organisms, is considered 'natural' and without any side-effects, but is yet to be supported by randomized controlled trials.[11]

Recurrent/resistant bacterial vaginosis

Some 30% of patients have BV recurrence within 3 months. For recurrent/resistant BV, a longer treatment period of 10–14 days is required.[5] Research is currently focusing on the use of *Lactobacillus* and treatment of BV.

FOLLICULITIS

Clinical presentation

Folliculitis is a common condition on the buttock and vulva. The hair follicles can become inflamed by physical injury and chemical irritation. The most common form is superficial folliculitis, which manifests as a tender or painless pustule that heals without scarring.[12] The hair shaft is frequently in the center of the pustule. The most common pathogen associated with

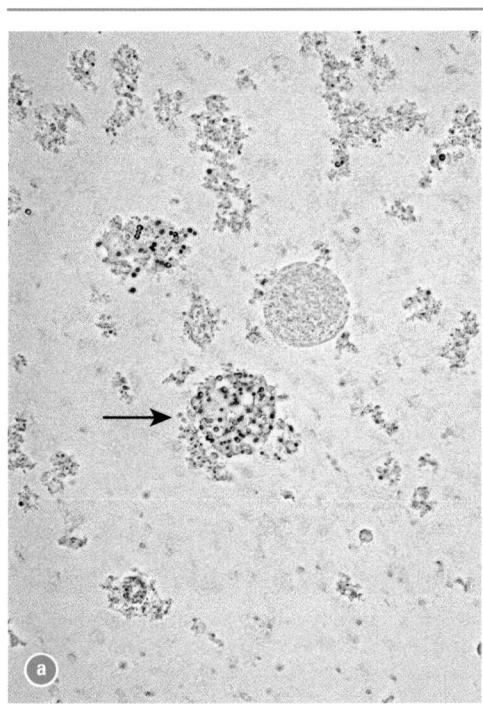
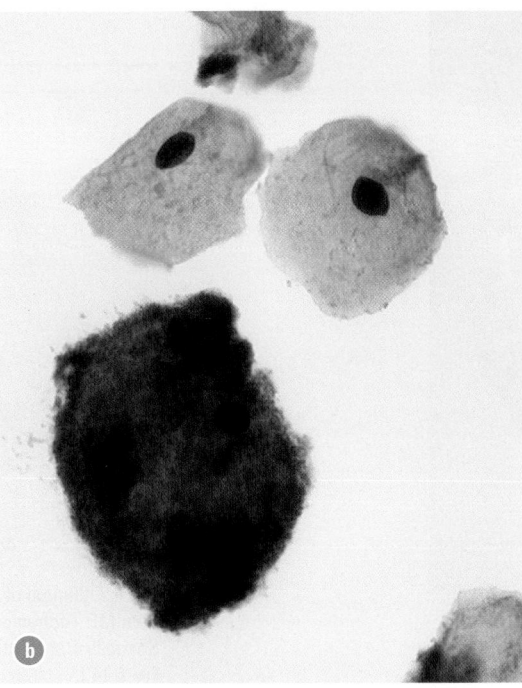

Fig. 4.5 Bacterial vaginosis, seen as dense evenly distributed collections of bacterial rod-like forms in the squamous cells as seen on wet prep (a) or Papanicolaou stain (b).

folliculitis is *Staphylococcus aureus*, but commensal organisms such as yeast and fungi occasionally appear (particularly in the immunosuppressed patient). These lesions typically resolve spontaneously. Staphylococci will occasionally invade the deeper portion of the follicle, causing swelling and erythema with or without a pustule at the skin surface (Fig. 4.6). This inflammation of the entire follicle or the deeper portion of the hair follicle (isthmus and below) is called deep folliculitis.

Diagnosis and histopathology

Visualization of erythema surrounding the hair follicles provides the clinical diagnosis of folliculitis. Folliculitis is characterized by inflammation of the follicle or perifollicular stroma, which may be composed of acute or chronic inflammation. A granulomatous response can be seen with follicular rupture.

Clinical differential diagnosis

The differential diagnosis of folliculitis includes: acne vulgaris, candidiasis, irritant contact dermatitis, insect bites, keratosis pilaris, milia, miliaria, rosacea, scabies, seabather's eruption, tinea and transient acantholytic dermatosis. Fungal folliculitis should be excluded with a PAS stain.

Treatment

Topical therapy with erythromycin, clindamycin, mupirocin or benzoyl peroxide can be administered to accelerate the healing process of superficial follicultis.[13] Oral antibiotics are generally used in the treatment of deep folliculitis (first-generation cephalosporins, penicillinase-resistant penicillins, macrolides and fluoroquinolones).

Common sexually transmitted infections

TRICHOMONAS

Clinical presentation

Trichomonas vaginalis is a large, flagellated ovoid protozoan that can be identified in wet mounts of vaginal discharge in infected patients. Infections may occur at any age and are seen in about 15% of women in sexually transmitted disease clinics. They are associated with a purulent yellow-green vaginal discharge and discomfort; the underlying vaginal and cervical mucosa typically has a fiery red appearance, called strawberry cervix (Fig. 4.7). The vulva may be erythematous and edematous. It is commonly associated with other sexually transmitted diseases. *Trichomonas* is associated with pregnancy complications such as preterm labor.

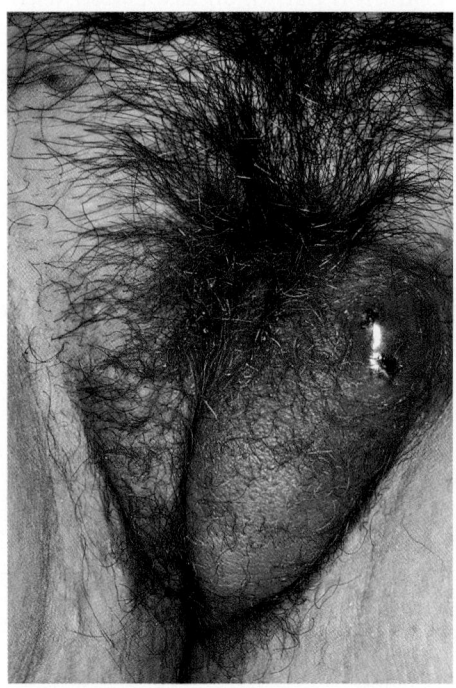

Fig. 4.6 Clinical picture of folliculitis, illustrating diffuse induration produced by dermal follicular inflammation.

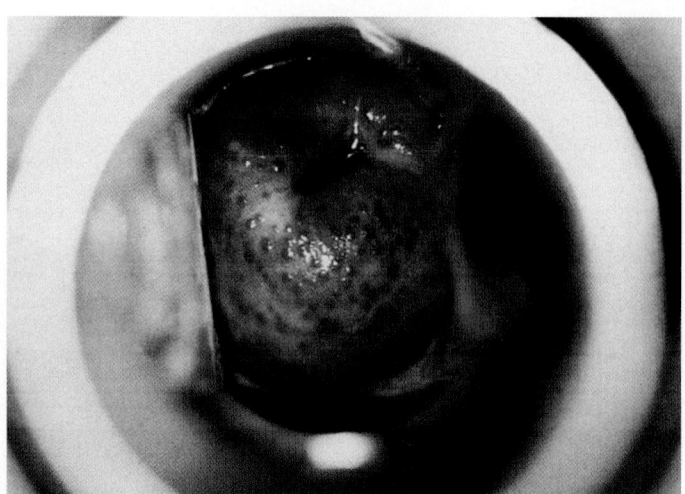

Fig. 4.7 Clinical of *Trichomonas* (strawberry cervix). (From Krieger JN and Rein MF. Trichomoniasis. In: Rein M, ed. Atlas of Infectious Diseases, Vol. V: Sexually Transmitted Diseases. Philadelphia: Churchill Livingstone; 1996:6.5, Fig. 6.14.)

Diagnosis

The vaginal pH is alkaline (>4.5) in patients with *Trichomonas*. Diagnosis of vaginal trichomoniasis is generally performed by microscopy of vaginal secretions, but this method has a sensitivity of only about 60–70%. On histologic examination, the inflammatory reaction is usually limited to the mucosa and immediately subjacent lamina propria. At times, Diamond's media may be used in patients suspected to have trichomoniasis, when the wet prep is negative. Culture is the most sensitive commercially available method of diagnosis. The polymerase chain reaction (PCR) test for *T. vaginalis* is being utilized in some laboratories.

Clinical differential diagnosis

The differential diagnosis of *Trichomonas* includes: candidiasis, bacterial vaginosis, desquamative vaginitis, gonococcal infections, pelvic inflammatory disease and urethritis.

Treatment

Oral metronidazole is the usual treatment for *Trichomonas* infections. It can be given in a single dose or over a week. Treatment of patients as well as their sex partners results in relief of symptoms, microbiologic cure and reduction of transmission. It is important to make sure neither the patient nor the partner(s) have allergies to metronidazole.

The majority of patients who return with recurrence of symptoms are either reinfections due to failure to treat all partners and, less commonly, a strain of *T. vaginalis* resistant to metronidazole. The latter may require an increase in drug dose. The CDC guidelines state that patients with laboratory-documented infection who do not respond to the 3–5 day treatment regimen and who have not been reinfected should be managed in consultation with a specialist; evaluation of such cases should ideally include determination of the susceptibility of *T. vaginalis* to metronidazole. (Consultation is available from CDC: Tel: 770-488-4115; website: http://www.cdc.gov/std/.)

In patients who have an allergy to metronidazole an incremental dosing protocol (oral or intravenous desensitization) may be considered.[14]

MOLLUSCUM CONTAGIOSUM

Clinical presentation

Molluscum contagiosum is an often sexually transmitted viral disease of the skin caused by a poxvirus (Molluscipoxvirus genus).[15] There are four main sub-types of molluscum contagiosum: MCV I, II, III and IV.[16,17] Direct contact with infected hosts or contaminated fomites is required for transmission. It is seen often in young sexually active populations. It affects primarily the genital area, is associated with a variety of other venereal diseases and molluscum increasing in incidence.[18,19] It also occurs in children and in this population is generally not sexually transmitted. Molluscum infection is also seen in the immunodeficient population. It is spread by direct contact with a variable incubation time, typically presenting within a few weeks of inoculation. The characteristic lesion with MC is a discrete flesh-colored papule (Fig. 4.8). Some will contain a dimple beneath which is a core of cheesy material (umbilicated lesion). The size of the papule ranges from 2 to 6 mm. Less commonly, the molluscum will consist of numerous small confluent papules, mimicking the herpes simplex virus infection. The lesions are usually painless except when traumatized.

Histopathology

The clinical appearance of molluscum is in most cases diagnostic.[15] The diagnosis of MC can be confirmed either by excision of the lesion or by cytologic inspection of the debris that is expressed from the center of the lesion and visualized on an hematoxylin and eosin

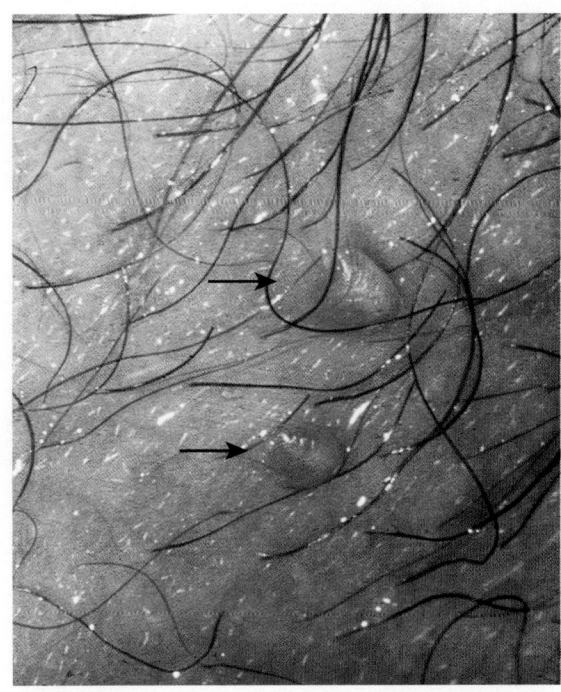

Fig. 4.8 Clinical presentation of molluscum, with discrete flesh-colored papules.

(H&E) or Papanicolaou stain. The infection produces an epithelial hyperplasia with formation of a cup-shaped lesion (Fig. 4.9a). The periphery of the cup contains several layers of basal cells which mature centrally, shedding kerati-nous debris into the lumen or cavity that connects to the surface. Diagnostic viral inclusion bodies (Henderson–Patterson bodies) become visible several layers above the basement membrane and as the cells mature, the eosinophilic or cyanophilic oval viral inclusions (molluscum bodies) completely replace the cytoplasm and marginate the nucleus (Fig. 4.9b). The underlying dermis often contains extensive chronic inflammation. In-situ hybridization for MCV DNA has also been performed, but is not necessary for diagnosis.

Clinical differential diagnosis

The diseases that are in the differential diagnosis of molluscum contagiosum include: acrochordon, epidermal inclusion cyst, dermatitis herpetiformis, keratoacanthoma, neurofibroma, condyloma, pyogenic granuloma, herpes and basal cell carcinoma. Virtually all of the confusion generated by these entities occurs during clinical examination. In our experience, some difficulty may be encountered in the histologic diagnosis if the inclusions are not in the plane of section. For this reason any inverted or cup-shaped lesion that does not contain sufficient atypia to verify condyloma, keratoacanthoma or other keratoses should be sectioned thoroughly to exclude molluscum.

Treatment of molluscum contagiosum

Molluscum contagiosum is a self-limited disease, but can cause discomfort, scarring with persistent scratching and in some schools and day care centers, exclusion until treatment.[15] The most prudent management is sharp curettage with a scalpel or curette. This procedure will usually be followed by disappearance of the lesion.[20] A variety of other methods (cryosurgery, etc.) can be used but are usually not required.

HERPES SIMPLEX INFECTIONS

Clinical presentation

Genital herpes is an ulcerative sexually transmitted disease that is caused by infection with the herpes simplex virus (HSV), a double-stranded DNA virus. It is the most common ulcerative disease in developed countries with approximately 750 000 new cases per year and a prevalence of over 20 million cases in the USA.[21] In clinically apparent cases, the primary lesion appears approximately 3 days to 2 weeks after exposure. In primary herpes, the vulva is red and swollen with numerous vesicles, typical of a more generalized infection. They rapidly become pustular with open tender erosions lasting 2 weeks (Fig. 4.10).[22] In addition, a vaginal discharge may sometimes be noted. With progression, the condition peaks by 7–10 days following initial presentation and usually resolves without scarring within 3 weeks. The lesions are highly

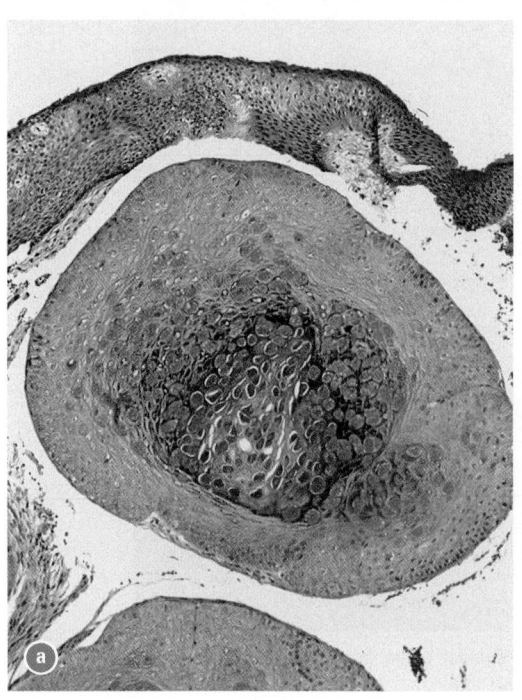

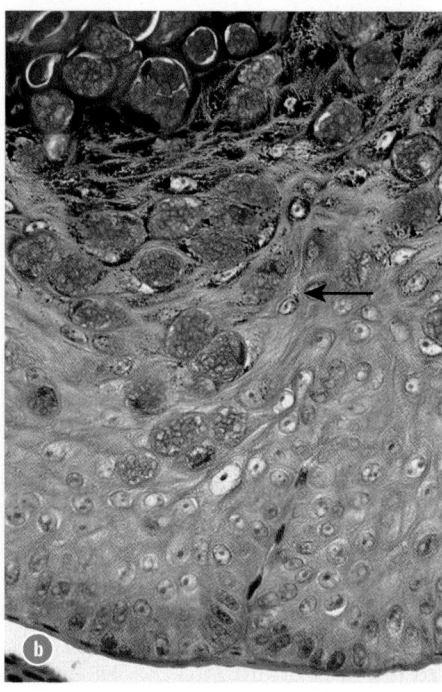

Fig. 4.9 (a) Low-power photomicrograph of molluscum illustrating the cup-shaped architecture; (b) A higher-power view of cytoplasmic inclusions, which become more distinct as a function of keratinocyte maturation (arrows).

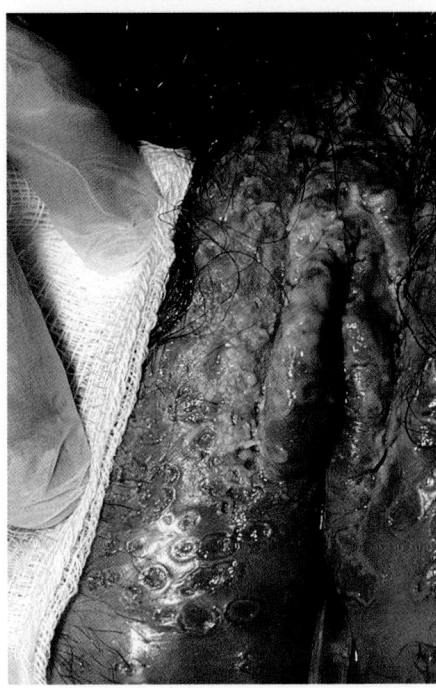

Fig. 4.10 Primary herpes simplex virus infection of the vulva, with a broader distribution of mucosal ulceration and edema. (Courtesy of Mark Pearlman.)

Virologic testing

Herpes simplex virus can be very difficult to confirm. One method for diagnosing HSV it to take a culture of the lesion (ideal if not more than 3 days old). The sensitivity of culture declines rapidly as lesions begin to heal, usually within a few days of onset. Material needed for testing is in the base of the lesion, so aggressive scraping of the base is required. The scraping is placed into the media for culture.

Some HSV antigen detection tests, unlike culture and the direct fluorescent antibody test, do not distinguish HSV-1 from HSV-2. Polymerase chain reaction (PCR) assays for HSV DNA are highly sensitive, but their role in the diagnosis of genital ulcer disease has not been well-defined. However, PCR is available in some laboratories and is the test of choice for detecting HSV in spinal fluid for diagnosis of HSV infection of the central nervous system (CNS).[25] Cytologic detection of cellular changes of herpes virus infection is insensitive and interpretation is not always correct, both in genital lesions (Tzanck preparation) and cervical Pap smears. According to current guidelines, it should not be exclusively relied on for diagnosis or exclusion of HSV infection when the interpretation has clinical or therapeutic consequences.[5]

Both type-specific and nonspecific antibodies to HSV develop during the first several weeks following infection and persist indefinitely. Because almost all HSV-2

infective until they begin to crust over during the healing phase after ulceration (usually about 10 days after their first appearance). However, even asymptomatic individuals may shed virus and most infections appear to result from contact with clinically asymptomatic individuals.[20] Importantly, many people infected by herpes do not develop clinical features of the disease and have not been diagnosed with the disease.[23]

In the USA, approximately one out of five adults is serologically positive for HSV-2. More than one-half of individuals who are seropositive do not experience clinically apparent outbreaks, but these individuals still have episodes of viral shedding and transmit the virus.[24] Lesions on the genitals can spread to other sites such as fingers, buttocks and oral or labial areas, presumably by direct contact.

Recurrence occurs in about half of the women infected, usually within 8 months of the initial infection. In recurrent infection, the lesions are less extensive and are clear in 5–7 days, generally with only mild swelling (Fig. 4.11). Recurrent lesions are usually due to infection with HSV-2 (HSV-2 recurs in 89% of cases while HSV I recurs in 25% of cases) and are often multiple developing approximately 3–4 times per year. Herpes virus can be associated with life-threatening systemic disease in immunosuppressed individuals. Transmission to the fetus during childbirth or intrauterine cases can be a source of significant morbidity.[22]

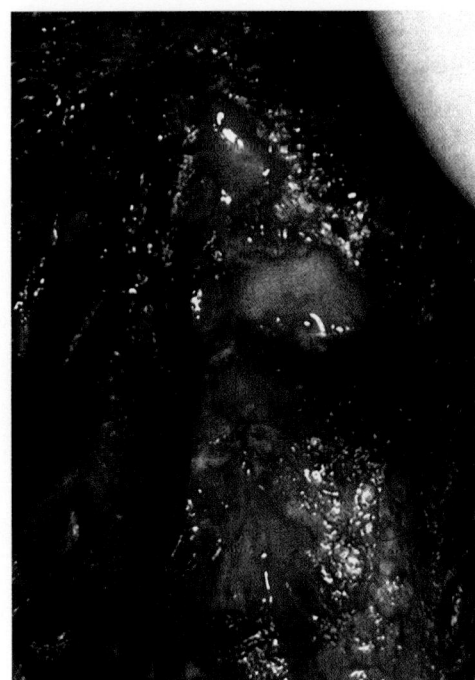

Fig. 4.11 Recurrent herpetic ulcer. (From Corey L. Herpes simplex infections. In: Rein M, ed. Atlas of Infectious Diseases, Vol. V: Sexually Transmitted Diseases. Philadelphia: Churchill Livingstone; 1996:15.12, Fig. 15.33.)

infections are sexually acquired, type-specific HSV-2 antibody generally indicates anogenital infection, but the presence of HSV-1 antibody does not distinguish anogenital from orolabial infection. Accurate type-specific assays for HSV antibodies must be based on the HSV-specific glycoprotein G2 for the diagnosis of infection with HSV-2 and glycoprotein G1 for diagnosis of infection with HSV-1. Such assays are preferable to older assays that do not accurately distinguish HSV-1 from HSV-2 antibody. Therefore, the serologic type-specific IgG-based assays should be specifically requested when serology is performed.

The sensitivities of tests for detection of HSV-2 antibody vary from 80% to 98% and false-negative results may occur, especially at early stages of infection. The specificities of these assays are >96%. False-positive results can occur, especially in patients with low likelihood of HSV infection. Therefore, repeat testing or a confirmatory test (e.g. an immunoblot assay if the initial test was an ELISA) may be indicated in some settings.

Because false-negative HSV cultures are common, especially in patients with recurrent infection or with healing lesions, type-specific serologic tests may be useful in confirming a clinical diagnosis of genital herpes. Additionally, such tests can be used to diagnose persons with unrecognized infection and to manage sex partners of persons with genital herpes.[5]

Histologic features

Lesions initially show vesicles followed by superficial ulceration. The most telling aspect of a herpetic ulcer is the presence of diffuse epithelial necrosis, present as an eosinophilic aggregate of dead and degenerating epithelial cells (Fig. 4.12a). Early in the infection, scattered nuclei may have a homogeneous ground-glass appearance and may be surrounded by a halo. With time, multinucleated keratinocytes will be apparent with eosinophilic and/or basophilic nuclear inclusions, which should be identified in the viable epithelium, or at the interface with the ulcer (Fig. 4.12b). Viral cytopathic effects can also involve hair follicles. An underlying dermal inflammatory component is present and neutrophils may be seen when the lesion ulcerates.[26] Viral inclusions may not be demonstrated in some ulcerated lesions; therefore, it is important to obtain a biopsy from the edge of ulcerative lesions with intact epithelium.

Differential diagnosis

A wide range of disorders are associated with genital ulcers (Table 4.3). In the absence of diagnostic viral cytopathic inclusions, the histologic features are those of a nonspecific erosion or ulceration. A high index of suspicion is required to recognize early infections. Immunohistochemical stains for HSV-1 and HSV-2 are extremely helpful in establishing the correct diag-

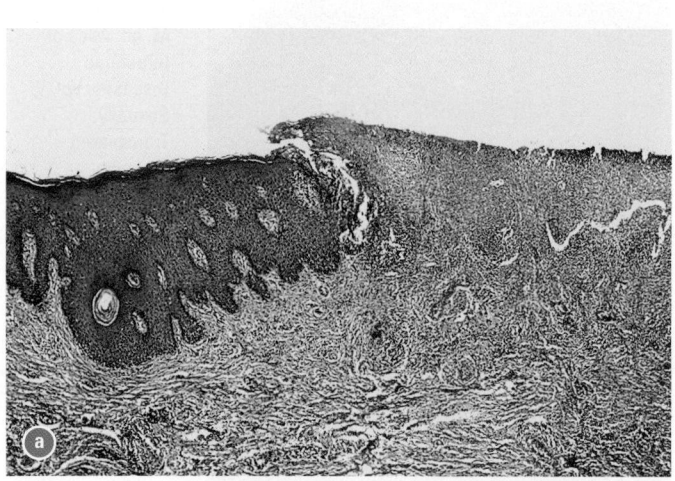

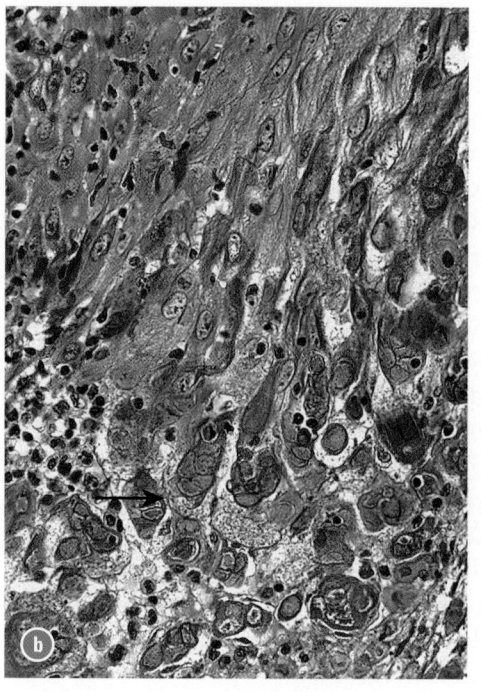

Fig. 4.12 (a) Low-power view of herpetic ulcer, characterized by an eosinophilic zone of epithelial necrosis (right). (b) Higher power demonstrates intranuclear inclusions at the edge of the ulcer.

Table 4.3 *Differential diagnosis of ulcerative lesions*

EBV
HIV
CMV
Herpes simplex
Herpes zoster
Syphilis
Erosive candidiasis
Mycobacterial infection
Chancroid
Lymphogranuloma venereum
Behçet's disease
Excoriation
Aphthous (idiopathic) ulcer
Erythema multiforme
Carcinoma

nosis when unequivocal viral inclusions are not identified on routine light microscopy (Fig. 4.13).

Diseases in the clinical differential diagnosis with herpes infection are syphilis, chancroid, Epstein–Barr virus, herpes zoster, HIV, cytomegalovirus infection, Behçet's disease, erythema multiforme, aphthous ulcers and extensive erosive candidiasis.

Management of genital herpes

Systemic antiviral drugs partially control the symptoms and signs of herpes episodes when used to treat first clinical episodes and recurrent episodes or when used as daily suppressive therapy. However, these drugs neither eradicate latent virus nor affect the risk, frequency or severity of recurrences after the drug is discontinued. Topical therapy with antiviral drugs offers minimal clinical benefit and its use is not recommended. Because many patients with first-episode herpes eventually develop severe or prolonged symptoms, antiviral therapy with acyclovir, famciclovir or valacyclovir should be considered. Antiviral therapy for recurrent genital herpes can be administered either episodically, to ameliorate or shorten the duration

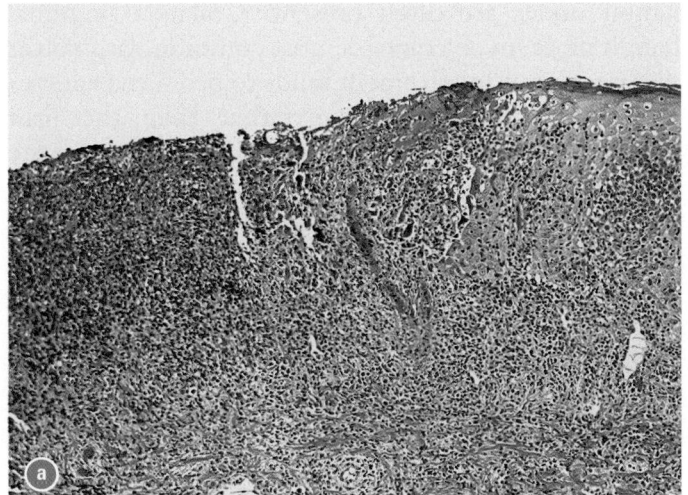

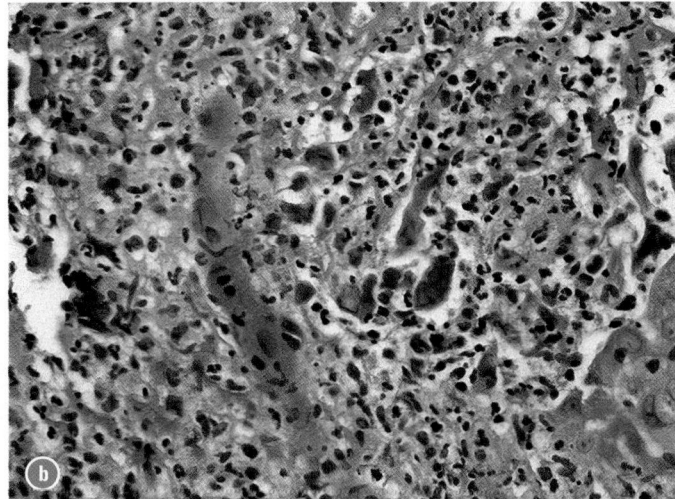

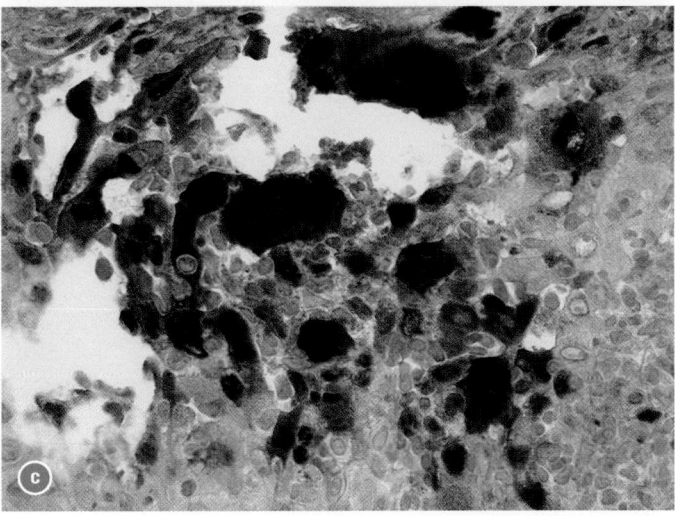

Fig. 4.13 (a) Herpetic ulcer. (b) At higher power, rare cells at the ulcer/epithelial interface contain the characteristic inclusions. (c) Immunostaining highlights a much higher than expected proportion of infected cells.

of lesions, or continuously as suppressive therapy to reduce the frequency of recurrences.[5]

NEISSERIA GONORRHEA

Clinical presentation

Gonorrhea is caused by infection with the Gram-negative diplococcus *Neisseria gonorrhoeae*. There is a high disease rate of gonorrhea in less-developed countries. The incidence of gonorrhea in developed countries is again rising. In the USA, an estimated 600 000 new *N. gonorrhoeae* infections occur each year. In the heterosexual population, concurrent *Chlamydia trachomatis* may also be present in 1 in 3 of these patients.[27,28] Vaginal discharge in women is a sign of this infection. If gonorrhea is left untreated in women, it can lead to pelvic inflammatory disease (PID), with possible infertility and rarely, gonococcal perihepatitis. It is important to screen women at high risk for STDs for gonorrhea.

Differential diagnosis

Conditions to consider in the clinical differential diagnosis include: *Chlamydia*, urinary tract infection and vaginitis.

Treatment

Because there is a high rate of coinfection of *N. gonorrhoeae* with *C. trachomatis*, gonococcal infections are routinely treated with a regimen effective against uncomplicated genital *C. trachomatis* infection. Some specialists believe that the routine use of dual therapy has resulted in substantial decreases in the prevalence of chlamydial infection. Regimens to cover both infections include cefixime, ceftriaxone, ciprofloxacin or comparable class antibiotics; azithromycin and doxycycline may be used if *Chlamydia* is ruled out.[5]

Uncommon sexually transmitted diseases

SYPHILIS

Clinical presentation

Background

Syphilis is a sexually transmitted infectious disease caused by the spirochete *Treponema pallidum*. The disease usually follows a natural history of primary, secondary and tertiary phases. The incidence of this disease declined precipitously after the introduction of penicillin; however, there has been a more recent increase in incidence.[29]

Primary syphilis

The initial manifestation, during the primary phase of infection, is a chancre at the site of exposure. Approximately one-third of exposures to *Treponema pallidum* will result in a chancre, which occurs 10–90 days following exposure (Fig. 4.14). While a single lesion is typical, primary syphilis can occasionally present with multiple lesions.[30] The chancre develops as a round to oval macule that becomes papular with a sharply defined edge and central ulceration. Chancres are painless unless traumatized or superinfected. Vulvar lesions also have a tendency to become superinfected resulting in more painful chancres.[22] Numerous treponemal organisms are shed during the chancre stage and these lesions are highly infective. Treated lesions resolve in 1–2 weeks. The chancre heals in a few weeks, without scarring, even when untreated. Palpable, enlarged, firm lymph nodes are often present. Unilateral inguinal lymph node involvement is most common with vulvar disease. Vulvar involvement tends to produce chancres with edematous induration rather than the firm lesions seen at other sites. In addition, mirror-image or 'kissing' chancres can be seen in the vulva due to skin-to-skin contact at this site.

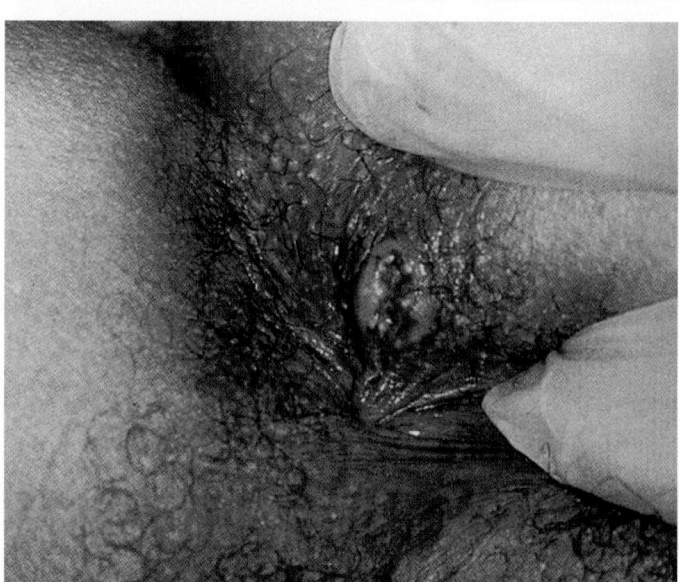

Fig. 4.14 Syphilitic chancre in the perianal region. (From Fiumara NJ. Primary and secondary syphilis. In: Rein M, ed. Atlas of Infectious Diseases, Vol. V: Sexually Transmitted Diseases. Philadelphia: Churchill Livingstone; 1996:9.7, Fig. 9.19.)

Secondary syphilis

Untreated primary syphilis will evolve to secondary syphilis over weeks to months. Most commonly, this occurs after the initial chancre has resolved, but the lesions of primary and secondary syphilis can be simultaneous. Secondary lesions usually resolve within 2 weeks to 3 months without treatment. Scarring is not a feature. Systemic symptoms include fever, malaise and arthralgias. Presentation at this stage is notoriously variable and includes rashes that may be overlooked and severe manifestations that can require hospitalization. The cutaneous lesions of secondary syphilis include macular, papular and mixed maculopapular lesions. Distribution is widespread and is often symmetrical. Initially, the lesions of secondary syphilis are rich in treponemal organisms but the number of organisms declines as the lesions resolve. Relapses of untreated secondary syphilis occur with some frequency. Other organs systems may be involved as well. Another important manifestation of secondary syphilis is condyloma lata of the vulva, a verrucoid lesion that may be mistaken for condyloma acuminata.[22]

Tertiary syphilis

Tertiary syphilis will develop in approximately one-third of patients with untreated syphilis. The remainder results in latency. The three classic clinical presentations of tertiary syphilis are late benign syphilis, cardiovascular syphilis and neurosyphilis. Cutaneous involvement by tertiary syphilis falls within the late benign syphilis category. The lesions of tertiary syphilis can be granulomatous or result in gummas. Granulomatous lesions can be either nodular or plaque-like and are erythematous and often scaly.[31] Gummas are nodules that sometimes ulcerate and have a soft consistency due to central necrosis. Lesions of tertiary syphilis can be quite destructive and heal with scarring.

Histologic features

The primary chancre is the initial manifestation of syphilis and is often limited to the vulva. It is characterized by an intense dermal infiltrate of lymphocytes, histiocytes and neutrophils with overlying epidermal hyperplasia.[32] Plasma cells may not be conspicuous at this time. The epidermal thickening at the edges of the ulcer often becomes pseudoepitheliomatous. Capillaries and small vessels within the lesion often show marked endothelial swelling accompanied by perivascular plasma cells. The histologic findings are not specific, but the diagnosis may be confirmed with Warthin–Starry or Steiner silver stains which typically reveal spirochetes, often in a perivascular distribution. Darkfield examination of secretions also demonstrates spirochetes and this test may be useful during the early stages of infection since confirmatory serologic tests may not be positive.[33] In all cases, serologic testing should be performed to confirm or support the diagnosis as both darkfield examination and silver stains are somewhat insensitive and can also give false-positive results. Among the serologic tests are Venereal Disease Research Laboratory (VDRL), rapid plasma reagin (RPR), fluorescent treponemal antibody absorption (FTA-ABS), microhemagglutination-*Treponema pallidum* (MHA-TP).

The histologic features of lesions of secondary syphilis vary, consistent with the myriad of clinical presentations associated with this stage. Classic lesions of secondary syphilis show psoriasiform epidermal hyperplasia and a superficial and deep perivascular, and often lichenoid, infiltrate of histiocytes and plasma cells (Fig. 4.15a). While perivascular plasma cells with endothelial swelling and injury (so-called plasma cell endarteritis) is considered a classic finding, this feature is often not seen and is nonspecific (Fig. 4.15b).[32,34] Neutrophils may be present in earlier lesions, but are less frequent as the spirochetes diminish in number. Late lesions often have a granulomatous appearance. Genital condyloma lata do not ulcerate and typically show a markedly hyperplastic epidermis with hyperkeratosis. The mixed chronic inflammatory infiltrate in the dermis is rich in perivascular plasma cells and, in this setting, plasma cell endarteritis is more frequently seen (Fig. 4.15c,d).[32] Spirochetes can be visualized with Steiner stain (Fig. 4.16).

The lesions of tertiary syphilis are granulomatous. Plasma cells are present and organisms can be difficult to demonstrate. Gummas show central areas of necrosis bound by a fibrous lymphohistiocytic infiltrate rich in plasma cells. Closer inspection of the necrotic areas will reveal eosinophilic outlines of dead cells.

Differential diagnosis

As mentioned above, the biopsy findings in syphilis (other than direct visualization of spirochetes) are not specific and, thus, confirmatory serologic testing is required. In all cases, this should be performed to confirm or support the diagnosis. Condyloma lata may be mistaken for condyloma acuminata, but the absence of HPV-related viral cytopathic effects in the former should prevent this error.

Zoon's or plasma cell vulvitis (plasmacytosis mucosae) is a rare cause of a plasma cell-rich infiltrate in the vulva. A silver stain is always advised before accepting

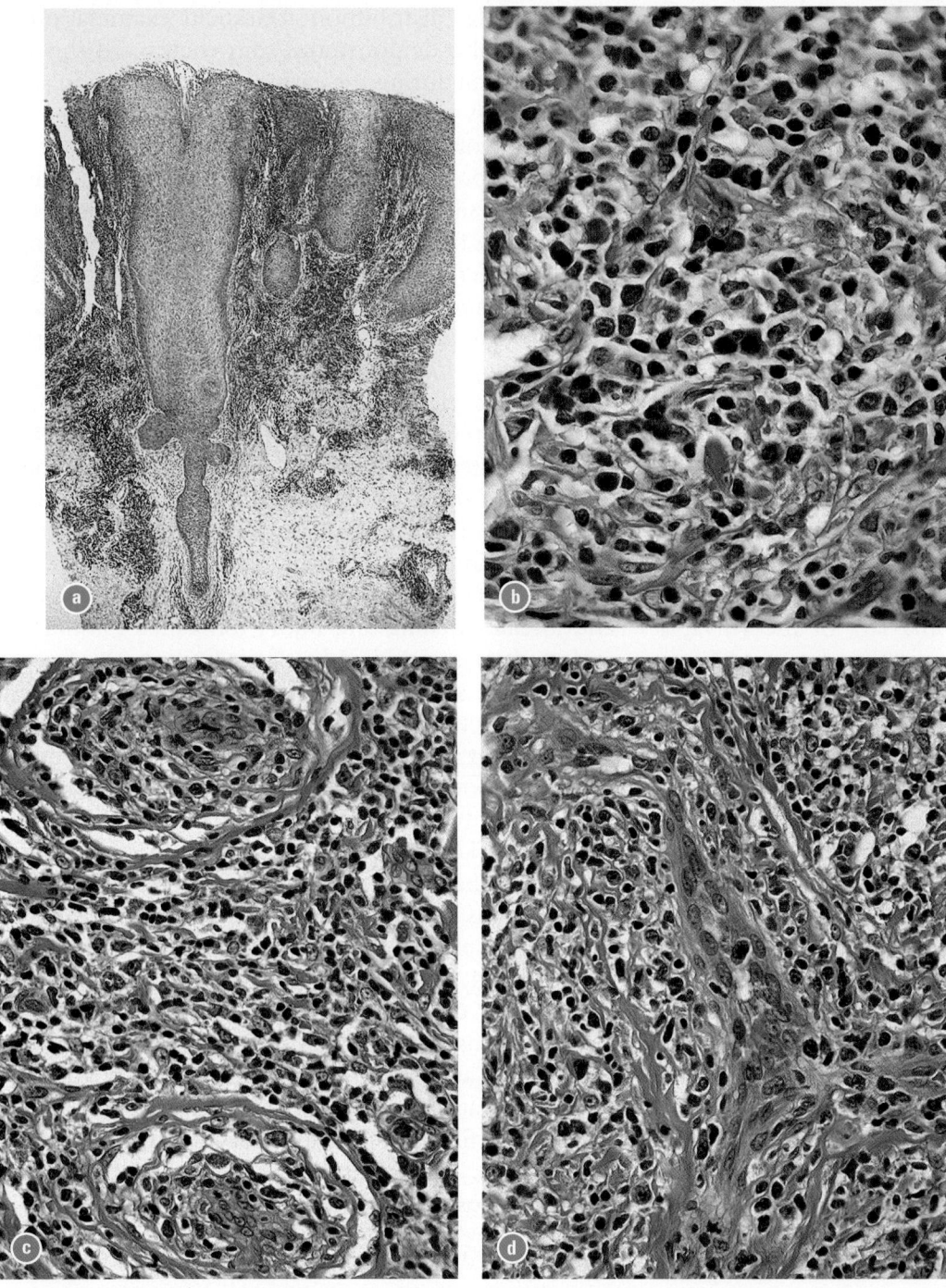

Fig. 4.15 (a) Secondary syphilis at low power, with pseudoepitheliomatous hyperplasia and intense submucosal inflammatory infiltrate. (b) Higher power demonstrates numerous plasma cells. (c,d) Perivascular inflammation (endarteritis) with endothelial hyperplasia is commonly seen in syphilis but is not specific.

this diagnosis. Clinical history is often helpful since the lesions tend to occur in elderly patients, a population in which new presentations of syphilis are uncommon. In difficult cases, serologic testing is advised. Other conditions to consider in the differential diagnosis of syphilis include: herpes (generally painful, but at times the ulcer is painless), staphylococcal or streptococcal pyoderma, chancroid, granuloma inguinale, lymphogranuloma venereum, scabies and tinea corporis.

Clinical management of syphilis

Antibiotics are the main treatment for all forms of syphilis. Penicillin G, administered parenterally, is the preferred drug for treatment of all stages of syphilis. The preparation(s) used (i.e. benzathine, aqueous procaine or aqueous crystalline), the dosage and the length of treatment depend on the stage and clinical manifestations of disease (see CDC STD Treatment Guidelines).[5]

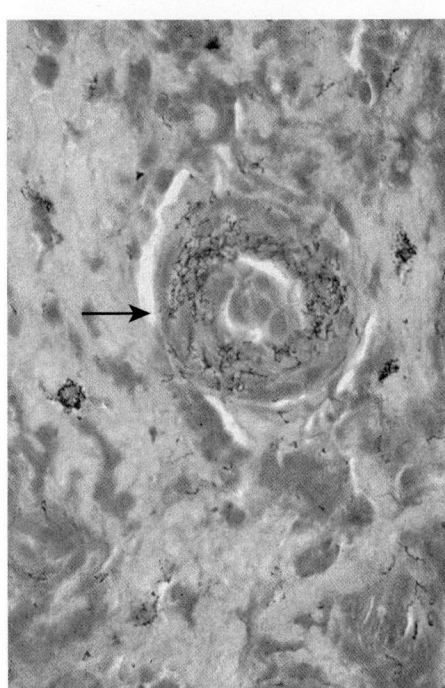

Fig. 4.16 A Steiner stain illustrates numerous filamentous spirochetes.

that ulcerate due to rubbing and scratching. The ulcerated lesions are painful and exhibit ragged edges with a dusky, gray base composed of granulation tissue that bleeds when manipulated. The ulcers often enlarge and have irregular borders with an erythematous surrounding halo (Fig. 4.17). Several lesions can coalesce to form larger areas of ulceration.[37–39] The lesions are not indurated and thus are described as 'soft chancres'. They can also be associated with unilateral or bilateral inguinal lymphadenopathy that develops 1–2 weeks following the appearance of genital lesions. The overlying skin is usually erythematous and, if untreated, these suppurative lesions (bubos) can ulcerate and result in a sinus draining from which a creamy white exudate.[33] Bubos are more common in men than women. Vulvar lesions that are untreated can also result in draining fistulous tracts. The lesions rarely subside without treatment, but when this occurs scarring is typically present and recurrence common at the same site. Extragenital lesions can occur, but are believed to be the result of direct cutaneous spread through damaged skin.[37]

Histopathology

Tissue biopsy is not a common means to confirm a diagnosis of chancroid, although biopsies may be obtained to exclude other conditions.[35] In endemic areas, this

Patients should be reexamined clinically and serologically 6 months and 12 months following treatment, with attention to persistence in signs or symptoms and increases in test titer that may signify reinfection or treatment failure. Testing for HIV is recommended and, in geographic areas in which the prevalence of HIV is high, patients who have primary syphilis should be retested for HIV after 3 months if the first HIV test result was negative.[5]

CHANCROID

Background

Chancroid is caused by the organism *Haemophilus ducreyi*. A painful ulcer is present which is soft and friable. It is also associated with inguinal lymphadenopathy (painful and unilateral). *H. ducreyi* is a Gram-negative bacillus and facultative anaerobe with fastidious culture requirements.[35] Chancroid is most common in developing countries, particularly those with tropical and subtropical climates. Infection is often encountered in the setting of HIV-infected individuals and is itself a risk factor for heterosexual transmission of HIV.[36] Males are more often affected than females.

Clinical presentation

Exposed individuals experience an incubation period of 3–5 days (rarely more than 10 days) with lesions initially appearing as small groups of papules or pustules

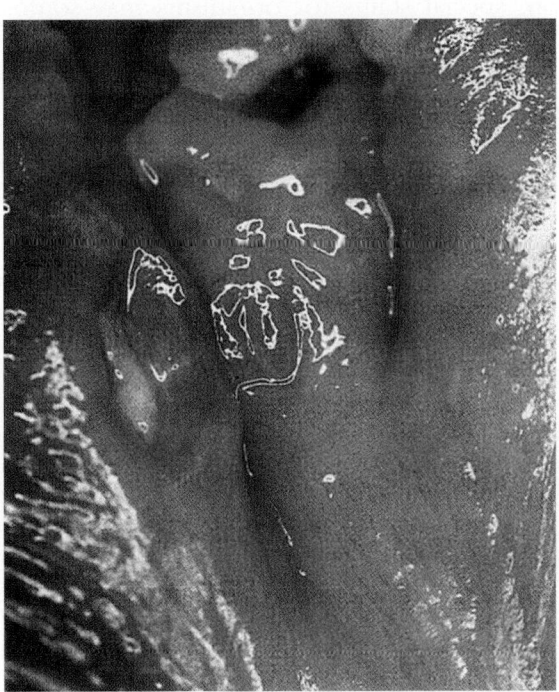

Fig. 4.17 Chancroid. (From Allen R. Chancroid. In: Rein M, ed. Atlas of Infectious Diseases, Vol. V: Sexually Transmitted Diseases. Philadelphia: Churchill Livingstone; 1996:16.7, Fig. 16.18.).

disease is often diagnosed by its characteristic clinical presentation. Traditionally, in-vitro culture has been the mainstay for confirmation of diagnosis, but this method lacks sensitivity.[21] More rapid and sensitive PCR-based methods are now available.[39]

The lesions have a characteristic 'zoned' configuration. The surface of the ulcer is composed of a neutrophilic infiltrate associated with fibrin and red blood cells. Beneath this layer is a band of granulation tissue (Fig. 4.18). Finally, the deepest layer is composed of a mixed chronic inflammatory infiltrate including plasma cells, lymphocytes and histiocytes. Gram stain is not reliable for the demonstration of *Haemophilus* organisms since the ulcers tend to be superinfected with skin commensural bacteria.[33]

Differential diagnosis

The differential diagnosis includes other ulcerative diseases of the vulva such as herpes and syphilis. Herpes usually presents as crops of small vesicles that may subsequently form erosions and ulcers associated with a mixed inflammatory infiltrate. Chancroid ulcers lack viral cytopathic effects. HSV immunohistochemistry can also aid in the differential diagnosis. Syphilis more commonly presents as a single lesion and is generally not painful at presentation. However, the presence of plasma cells in both conditions should elicit a comprehensive historical, clinical and serologic evaluation. In addition, special stains for organisms may some-

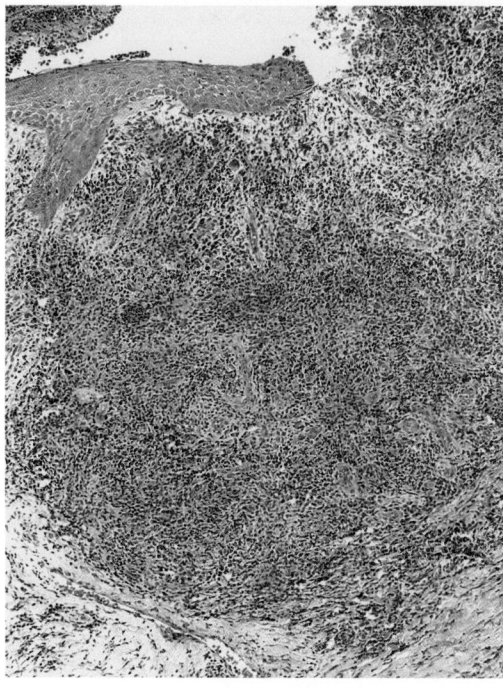

Fig. 4.18 Histopathologic features of chancroid are not specific, but exhibit ulceration and dense inflammatory infiltrate.

times be helpful. Importantly, genital ulcers can be infected with multiple organisms, e.g. chancroid with herpes superinfection. In complex cases, DNA hybridization or PCR-based methods may be helpful in establishing the diagnosis of chancroid.[38]

Clinical management

Antibiotic treatment (azithromycin, ceftriaxone, ciprofloxacin) is curative, resolves the clinical symptoms and prevents transmission to others. If treatment is successful, ulcers usually improve symptomatically within 3 days and objectively within 7 days after therapy. As with other sexually transmitted diseases, patients should be tested for HIV infection at the time chancroid is diagnosed and sexual partners should be examined and treated, regardless of whether symptoms of the disease are present, if they had sexual contact with the patient during the 10 days preceding the patient's onset of symptoms.[5] In advanced cases, scarring can result despite successful therapy.

GRANULOMA INGUINALE

Background

Granuloma inguinale (GI), also known as donovanosis, is an ulcerative sexually transmitted disease caused by the intracellular Gram-negative rod *Calymmatobacterium granulomatis*. GI is endemic in tropical and subtropical countries with only sporadic cases or small isolated epidemics occurring in Western countries.[39]

Clinical presentation

The disease presents as an erythematous papule or small nodule that ulcerates and is typically painless. The incubation period is variable and ranges from weeks to a few months. The lesions expand to form irregular 'beefy red' ulcers which bleed easily on contact (Fig. 4.19). Multiple different clinical presentations and courses have been described including ulcerative and scarring forms.[40] Rarely, a hypertrophic variant characterized by large vegetating masses is encountered.[21] Vulvar involvement can be destructive and may result in pseudoelephantiasis.[41] Very rarely, squamous cell carcinoma can arise in association with GI.[42] The condition is sometimes more aggressive in pregnant women.[43]

Histopathology

Histologic sections reveal an exuberant inflammatory infiltrate consisting of neutrophils, plasma cells, macrophages and scattered lymphocytes (Fig. 4.20a).

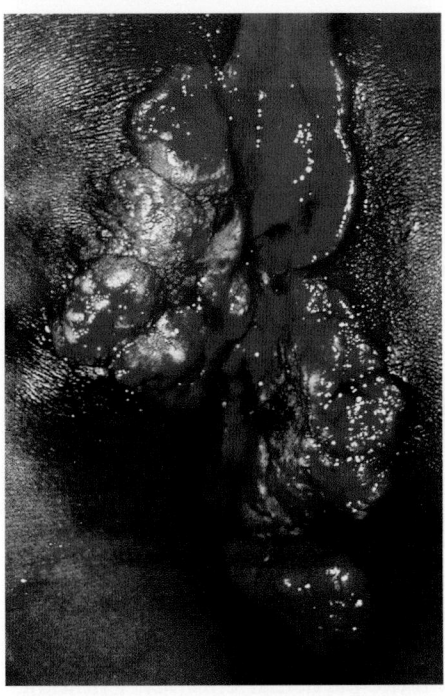

Fig. 4.19 Granuloma inguinale, presenting as a combination of hypertrophic mucosa with submucosal edema and focal ulceration. (From Hart G. Donovanosis. Granuloma inguinale. In: Rein M, ed. Atlas of Infectious Diseases, Vol. V: Sexually Transmitted Diseases. Philadelphia: Churchill Livingstone; 1996:17.8, Fig. 17.21.).

While the pattern of inflammation is nonspecific, some of the macrophages have conspicuous vacuoles containing rod-shaped organisms (Donovan bodies) that can be seen by conventional staining or with Warthin–Starry or Giemsa stains.[21] (Fig. 4.20b). Extracellular organisms may also be seen and they can be identified in scrapings from the ulcer bed.[43] The edges of the ulcer, where biopsies are often obtained, invariably show acanthosis. Pseudoepitheliomatous hyperplasia can also be seen which, in some cases, may be difficult to distinguish from squamous cell carcinoma. Culture conditions for the organism have not been defined.

Clinical differential diagnosis

The differential diagnosis includes lymphogranuloma venereum, syphilis, chancroid, herpes virus infection, candidiasis and genital amoebiasis. While less common in the United States, it is still important to consider GI and LGV in the differential diagnosis. Demonstration of Donovan bodies is diagnostic for GI. Darkfield examination and serology will help exclude syphilis. The characteristic ballooning degeneration, nuclear viral inclusions and multinucleated cells identify herpes. A complement fixation text is used to diagnose LGV. It is important to remember that the sexually transmitted diseases can also coexist.

Treatment

Treatment (doxycycline or trimethoprim-sulfamethoxazole and others) generally halts the disease progression of granuloma inguinale, but prolonged therapy may be required to permit granulation and reepithelialization of the ulcers. Relapses may occur within 18 months and patients should be followed clinically until signs and symptoms have resolved. Sexual partner(s) of a patient

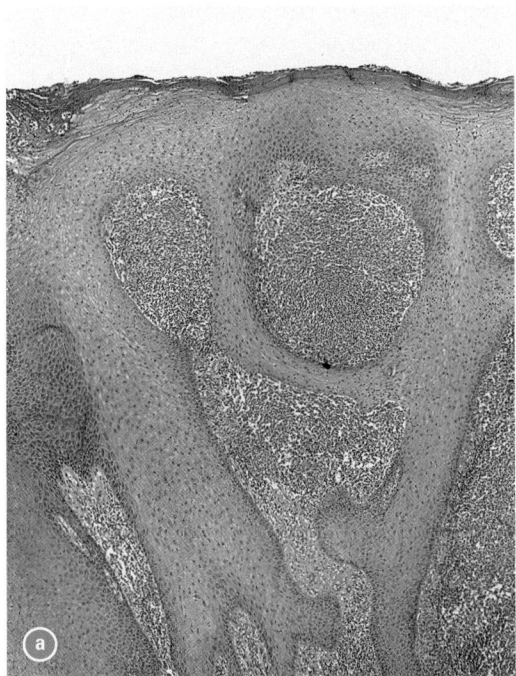

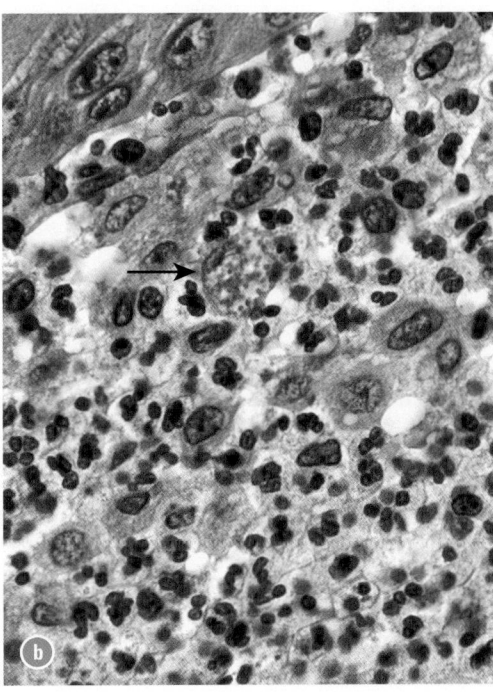

Fig. 4.20 (a) Low power of inflammation in granuloma inguinale exhibits both pseudoepitheliomatous hyperplasia and intense submucosal inflammation, corresponding to the clinical presentation (see Fig. 4.19). (b) Donovan bodies are discrete cytoplasmic vacuoles containing organisms (arrow) seen here on hematoxylin and eosin staining.

who has granuloma inguinale within the 60 days before onset of the patient's symptoms should be examined and offered therapy.

LYMPHOGRANULOMA VENEREUM

Clinical presentation

Lymphogranuloma venereum (LGV) is caused by *Chlamydia trachomatis* serovars L1, L2 or L3. LGV is a rare disease in industrialized countries, but is endemic in parts of Africa, Asia, South America and the Caribbean. A self-limited genital ulcer sometimes occurs at the site of inoculation. However, by the time patients seek care, the ulcer usually has disappeared. It is characterized by inguinal and/or femoral lymphadenopathy (commonly unilateral). The clinical course can be divided into three stages: the primary stage involves the site of inoculation; the secondary stage, the regional lymph nodes and sometimes the anorectum; and the late sequelae, affecting the genitals and/or rectum, comprise the tertiary stage. Women and homosexually active men may have proctocolitis or inflammatory involvement of perirectal or perianal lymphatic tissues resulting in fistulas and strictures. The diagnosis of LGV is usually made serologically. Complement fixation titers >1:64 are consistent with the diagnosis of LGV.

The MIF (microimmunofluorescence) test can distinguish between infections with the different chlamydial species, but it has not been much used in routine clinical practice.[44]

Histopathology

Skin lesions may show ulceration associated with mixed chronic and granulomatous inflammation. Biopsy of lymph nodes can reveal a characteristic stellate area of necrotizing inflammation surrounded by granulomatous and chronic inflammation. Acute inflammation with abscess formation is also associated with the stellate granulomatous area.

Clinical differential diagnosis

Many conditions are in the differential diagnosis of LGV. These include: incarcerated inguinal hernia, Hodgkin's disease, herpes, granuloma inguinale, mycobacterial disease, schistosomiasis, chancroid, syphilis, HIV, amoebiasis and Crohn's disease.

Treatment

Fistulas, sinus tracts and ulcerations may occur if treatment is not given. Lymphedema may occur, occasionally resulting in elephantiasis. Antibiotic therapy (doxycycline, erythromycin) cures infection and prevents ongoing tissue damage, although tissue reaction can result in scarring. Buboes may require aspiration through intact skin or incision and drainage to prevent the formation of inguinal/femoral ulcerations. Persons who have had sexual contact with the patient within the 30 days before onset of the patient's symptoms should be examined and tested.

Other rare infections

PERICLITORAL ABSCESS

Clinical presentation

Periclitoral abscesses are rare. The abscesses can be unilateral or encompass the entire periclitoral area (Fig. 4.21). They have many different causes and treatment is dependent on the particular etiology. Etiologies include: infection, entrapped hair, Crohn's disease and complications from female circumcision.[45–47] Ectopic breast tissue on the vulva has mimicked a periclitoral abscess.[48]

Diagnosis

Diagnosis is confirmed by physical examination. The periclitoral tissues appear inflamed. At times it may be difficult to distinguish the clitoral tissue from the prepuce. Histopathologic examination reveals acute inflammation with abscess formation and or granulomatous inflammation, depending on the etiology.

Differential diagnosis

The clinical differential diagnosis includes ectopic breast tissue, inclusion cyst, angiofibroma, clitoromegaly, lipoma, epidermoid cyst and dermoid cyst.

Treatment

For early infections, antibiotics may be successful for adequate treatment. The abscesses can be unilateral or encompass the entire periclitoral area. Generally, marsupialization is the preferred treatment.[49;50] When infection is present, the etiology of the infection is not always identifiable. Any purulent drainage should be cultured.

SCHISTOSOMIASIS

Clinical presentation

Schistosomiasis is the infection of humans by trematodes (a class of helminths) belonging to the superfamily

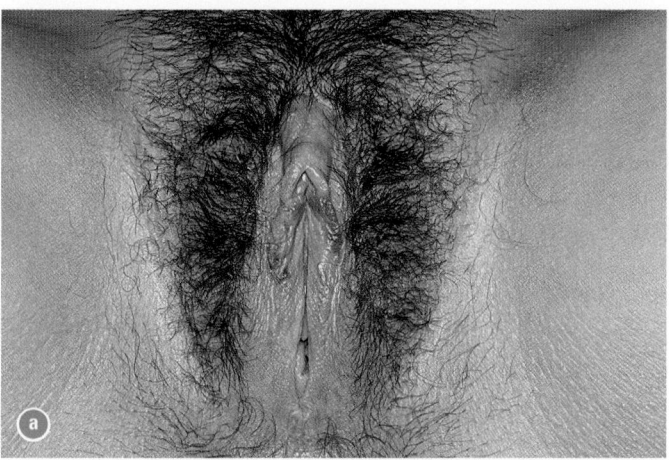
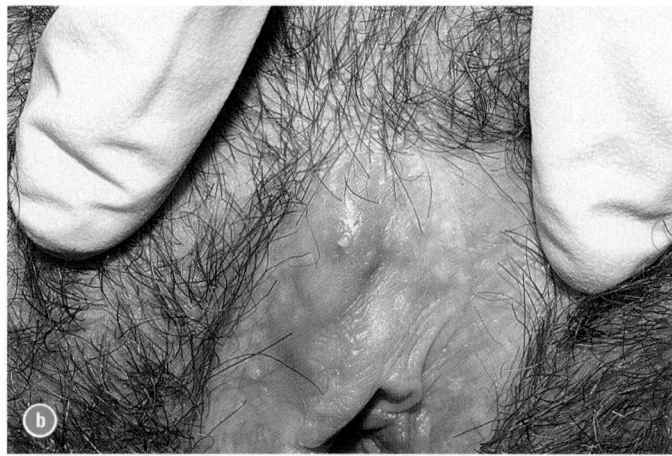

Fig. 4.21 (a) Periclitoral abscess, seen as a discrete swelling on the upper right labium minus. (b) At higher power, exudate delineates an area of epithelial rupture.

Schistosomatoidea.[51] There are three major species of schistosomes that are pathogenic to humans: *Schistosoma haematobium*, *S. japonicum* and *S. mansoni*.[52,53] Schistosomiasis affects approximately 200 million people worldwide. It can affect many organ systems. It is estimated that 9–13 million women are affected by genital lesions due to schistosomiasis.[54] It is endemic in Egypt and occurs in most parts of the Middle East. Female genital schistosomiasis is typically not encountered in immunocompetent American women, without a significant travel history. Infection occurs after bathing in infected fresh water containing cercariae, are the infective form of the parasite that is liberated into fresh water by the specific intermediate snail host. They penetrate unbroken skin and migrate as schistosomals through the venous circulation to the liver where the adult worms mature (Fig. 4.22). Symptoms may not appear until many months, sometimes years, after infection with the helminth.

The vulva is more commonly affected in younger women. *S. haematobium* is the most common species involved. Symptoms and signs of vulvar schistosomiasis are swelling, ulceration (painful or painless), a nodular surface, pruritus and a hypertrophic clitoris with an eroded granular surface. Papules or warts are seen in patients from non-endemic areas. Masses or tumors, ulceration and pain, clitoral hypertrophy and vulvar swelling tend to occur in patients with more chronic infection (Fig. 4.23).[55] It can lead to destruction of the hymen and/or clitoris, incontinence and vesicovaginal fistulae. Involvement of the labia majora rather than

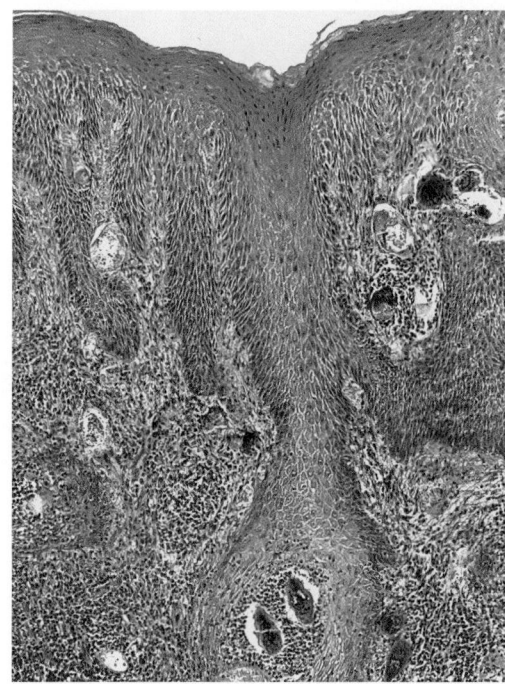

Fig. 4.23 Low-power view of schistosomiasis showing epithelial hyperplasia, marked chronic inflammation and a few ova in this section.

Fig. 4.22 Vaginal schistosomiasis. The mature organism burrows into the skin and is established within a vessel, from which the eggs are discharged.

minora is more frequently seen since easier access is gained by the ova via the veins of the labia majora.[52]

Diagnosis

Direct visualization of schistosome eggs is the diagnostic gold standard. Microscopic examination is performed on fresh, crushed biopsies or histologic sections of formalin-fixed tissue (Fig. 4.24).[56,57] *S. haematobium* eggs are ovoid, average 150 μm × 50 μm in greatest dimensions, and have a delicate terminal spine (as opposed to the pronounced lateral spine of *S. mansoni* or *S. japonicum* that lacks a spine).

Immunodiagnosis by detection of antibody or antigens may be more cost-effective. ELISA has a sensitivity of 76% for *S. haematobium* but it has some disadvantages. These disadvantages are that the antibody titers do not reflect the intensity of infection; the antibody will remain positive despite treatment and the antibody will not become positive for 6–12 weeks after initial infection.

Histology

On histologic evaluation, immature schistosome eggs have a basophilic internal structure.[53] The vulvar and vaginal polypoid or papillary lesions are composed of an acute, florid inflammatory reaction to clusters of viable-appearing eggs.[57] Granulomata and eosinophils are often seen. A noncaseating granulomatous lesion with epithelioid histiocytes and giant cells surrounded by a

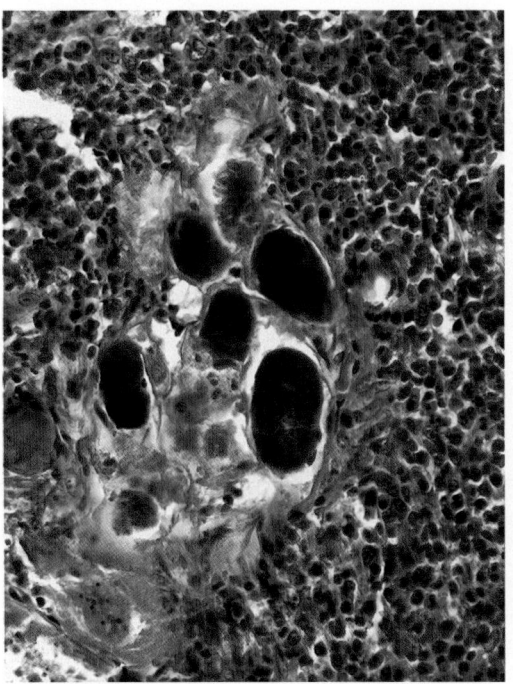

Fig. 4.24 At higher power, schistosome trophozoites are admixed with marked inflammatory infiltrate. They may also be calcified.

thin rim of lymphocytes may be seen. A PAS stain will stain the chitin in the shell of the ova.

Clinical differential diagnosis

Condyloma, typhoid fever, strongyloidosis, trichuriasis and carcinoma are diseases considered in the differential diagnosis of schistosomiasis.

Treatment

Praziquantel is the antihelminthic drug of choice for schistosomiasis, giving high cure rates for cutaneous and systemic infections caused by all species of *Schistosoma*.[58] Lesions heal a few weeks after administration.[59] Follow-up urine or stool examination within 3 months is advised to assess efficacy of therapy.

EPSTEIN–BARR VIRUS

Clinical presentation

Epstein–Barr virus (EBV) is a human herpesvirus and has only rarely been described as a cause of genital ulceration.[60–66] Generally, these are patients in their teens to early twenties. An acute infection is associated with a sore throat, painful punched-out ulcers (purple-red edges) on the vulva with lymphadenopathy distant from the site of ulceration and fever.

Genital contact is not a prerequisite for the development of these ulcers. In many of the cases reported, the ulcers occurred in young females before the onset of genital or oral sexual activity. Interestingly, the acutely painful genital ulcers often presented before the onset of any other features of infectious mononucleosis, in many of the studies.

Diagnosis

Confirmation of the diagnosis of EBV can be made by serology (the presence of IgM to EBV viral capsid antigen) or detection of EBV DNA by PCR examination of vulvar swabs. A culture of EBV can take more than 4 weeks to become positive. This is not a test performed routinely. The histopathologic findings are not specific. Ulcerated lesions will reveal acute and chronic inflammation while non-ulcerated areas associated with rash clinically show a mild superficial perivascular chronic inflammatory infiltrate.

Clinical differential diagnosis and management

The differential diagnosis includes: aphthous ulcers, Behçet's disease, HIV, chancroid, herpes, Crohn's disease, syphilis and a drug reaction. In the child or adolescent, once the above are excluded, EBV should be considered.[66] The infection is not reported to recur and ulcers normally resolve in 2 weeks. Thus, therapy is supportive.

Common and rare vulvar infections associated with immune suppression

INTRODUCTION

Patients may be immunosuppressed for many different reasons and they are a population that is at risk for infectious diseases, including the more common infections that affect immunocompetent individuals (Table 4.4).[67–74] A classic condition for immunosuppression is found with HIV. HIV, or HIV-induced immunosuppression, may modify the presentation and course of selected STDs. The HIV epidemic has altered the field of STDs.[75] In particular, multiple STDs have been found in HIV-positive patients. An increasing recognition of the ways in which STDs influence HIV transmission has underscored the importance of early detection and treatment of all STDs.[75] Many common conditions are seen in association with HIV-infected women including bacterial vaginosis and *Trichomonas* vaginitis.[76] Human papillomavirus (HPV) infection is also more commonly detected and more likely to be persistent in HIV-infected compared with uninfected women. (Guidelines for specific infections and HIV are in the CDC STD Treatment Guidelines.)[5]

The association between HIV infection and vaginal candidiasis is controversial.[77,78] A prospective study of cohorts of HIV-infected and uninfected women showed no difference in the prevalence of vaginal *C. albicans* colonization unless there was immunosuppression, in which case, the rates of colonization and symptomatic infection tripled.[79] The proportion of non-albicans isolates did not differ among groups. In this study, *Candida* colonization was not associated with antibiotic or oral contraceptive use. In contrast, in a cross-sectional study of patients referred to a vaginitis clinic, HIV was associated with non-albicans *Candida* infection.[80] Data from large cross-sectional studies showed a similar prevalence of *T. vaginalis* and bacterial vaginosis among the HIV-infected and uninfected participants and no association with CD4+ cell counts.[81,82] Vulvar, vaginal and anal intraepithelial neoplasia appear to be prevalent among women infected with HIV.

Table 4.4 Infections altered by immunosuppression

Infectious disease	Special concerns for HIV population
Chancroid	Large lesions Extragenital lesions Delayed healing[67] Treatment failure
Granuloma inguinale	Persistent ulcers Higher antibiotic requirement[68]
Lymphogranuloma venereum	A cluster of LGV among homosexual men in Rotterdam has been reported[69]
Syphilis	Rapid progression Refractory to therapy (Czelusta) Atypical serology including false-positive responses to the rapid plasma reagin card test and the Venereal Disease Research Laboratory (VDRL) test[70]
Chlamydia	Increased transmission[71,72]
Gonorrhea	Increased transmission
Bacterial vaginosis	Refractory to treatment. Enhances HIV transmission[73]
Trichomoniasis	Proposed co-factor in amplifying HIV transmission[74]
Vulvovaginal candidiasis	Higher vaginal *Candida* colonization rates, proportional to the level of immunosuppression
Folliculitis (eosinophilic pustular folliculitis)	Occurs in the more advanced stages of HIV infection, usually when the CD4 count is less than 200 cells/mm³

TUBERCULOSIS

Background

Tuberculosis (TB) results from infection with *Mycobacterium tuberculosis* or *M. bovis*. While the incidence of tuberculosis has declined greatly over the last century in developed countries, it is not uncommon and still results in considerable morbidity, particularly in the setting of immunosuppression. The most common site of infection is the lung. Involvement of the female genitalia is seen in endemic areas where fallopian tube involvement is an important cause of sterility. Vulvar involvement is much less frequently seen. HIV-1 infection remains the most common risk factor for developing active TB.

Clinical presentation

Cutaneous tuberculosis is categorized as primary or secondary.[83] Primary lesions are due to direct inoculation of mycobacteria. In the unexposed host, small papules develop into painless ulcers that may heal, but become indurated with time – a process referred to as primary inoculation tuberculosis and the lesions are sometimes called tuberculous chancres. In a previously exposed host, inoculation results in tuberculosis verrucosa cutis, also called warty tuberculosis. In this condition, papules become hyperkeratotic and eventually involute with scarring over a period of years. This form of disease can be seen in patients who have been inoculated with BCG vaccine and then retested for exposure to tuberculosis.[83] These lesions are quite rare in the vulva, although cases of 'venereal' transmission have been documented.[84]

Secondary cutaneous tuberculosis is more prevalent and shows two forms of disease: lupus vulgaris and scrofuloderma.[83] Lupus vulgaris is seen in the setting of pulmonary tuberculosis with hematogenous spread and presents as expanding hyperkeratotic papules with an ulcerated center. The lesions persist indefinitely with slow expansion. In scrofuloderma, skin involvement is by direct extension from underlying infected bone or lymph nodes. Firm, painless, subcutaneous nodules emerge that eventually ulcerate. Ultimately, sinusoidal tracts undermine the skin as the lesion spreads, resulting in scarring. Vulvar involvement appears to be primarily of the lupus vulgaris type.[85,86]

Histologic features

The hallmark of involvement by tuberculosis is the presence of necrotizing granulomata – collections of epithelioid histiocytes and Langerhans' type giant cells that are associated with an inflammatory cell infiltrate composed of variable numbers of lymphocytes and neutrophils. Central (caseation) necrosis is a frequent feature but not invariable and other causes of granulomatous inflammation must be considered (Table 4.5). Acid-fast bacilli may be demonstrated using a Ziehl–Neelsen (AFB) stain. PCR-based molecular testing is also available.[83,87] Organisms can be difficult to demonstrate and an extensive search is often required. Pseudoepitheliomatous hyperplasia can be seen at the edge of the tuberculous ulcers.

Clinical differential diagnosis

While vulvar tuberculosis is rare, it is sometimes encountered in endemic areas.[86] It is important to differentiate vulvar tuberculosis from other ulcerative conditions, particularly venereal diseases, since treatments differ widely for these conditions.[84] Serologic investigations and special stains can be used to demonstrate the various organisms causing herpes, syphilis or chancroid. The

Table 4.5 Differential diagnosis of granulomatous vulvitis

Syphilis
Lymphogranuloma venereum
Mycobacteria
Fungus
Bacillary angiomatosis
Folliculitis
Ruptured pilosebaceous unit
Ruptured cyst
Crohn's disease
Vulvitis granulomatosa

presence of caseating granulomata is highly suggestive of tuberculosis. Caseating granulomatous inflammation differentiates tuberculosis from metastatic Crohn's disease, another granulomatous and ulcerating condition of the vulva that is characterized by noncaseating granulomas.

The clinical differential diagnosis also includes: schistosomiasis, fungal infections, vulvar intraepithelial neoplasia, dermatitis herpetiformis, erythema nodosum, lichen planus, lupus erythematosus, pustular psoriasis, pyoderma gangrenosum, squamous cell carcinoma, syphilis and hidradenitis suppurativa.

Treatment of tuberculosis

Treatment involves long-term administration of combinations of isoniazid, rifampin, ethambutol and pyrazinamide, which are the first-line drugs for the treatment of tuberculosis. (Current treatment recommendations can be viewed at: http://www.cdc.gov/mmwr/preview/mmwrhtml/rr 5211a1 .htm.) Multidrug resistant stains are emerging and are a source of great concern.[83] While medical therapy is sufficient for early disease in vulvar tuberculosis, surgical removal may be needed if there is extensive disease.[88]

BACILLARY ANGIOMATOSIS

Background

Bacillary angiomatosis (BA) is an opportunistic infection that occurs in the setting of immunosuppression and was first recognized in patients with HIV/AIDS.[89] The causative organism is *Bartonella henselae* or *B. quintana*. Both of these bacteria also cause cat-scratch disease in immunocompetent hosts. Cases of BA are often associated with recent contact with a cat.[90] Rare cases have been documented in immunocompetent individuals.[91]

Clinical features

The mucocutaneous lesions present as minute, red papules with a smooth surface that increase in size. Lesions can be single or numerous and sometimes ulcerate. Deeper subcutaneous lesions may also be seen and tend to be pink or flesh-colored. If not treated with appropriate antibiotics, the disease can become widely disseminated with significant morbidity and mortality. Vulvar involvement is rare, but has been reported.[92,93]

Histopathology

In immunocompetent individuals, a suppurative granulomatous response is mounted, particularly in draining lymph nodes, resulting in the characteristic necrotizing granulomatous response. In immunocompromised individuals, this response does not occur and instead a unique vascular proliferation develops. Capillaries with plump 'histiocytoid' endothelial cells that protrude into the luminal space are seen. In addition, endothelial cells, not associated with vascular lumina, are present in an edematous stroma. Conspicuous neutrophils and karyorrhectic debris are invariably present throughout the lesion (Fig. 4.25). Clusters of bacilli can sometimes be seen on H&E, but are much better visualized using a modified Warthin–Starry or other silver stain. Bacillary angiomatosis may involve extracutaneous sites including liver, spleen, lymph nodes, gastrointestinal tract, peritoneum, diaphragm, brain, soft tissue and bone marrow. Involvement of the liver is characterized by peliosis.

Differential diagnosis

Differentiation from Kaposi's sarcoma (KS) is important, as this condition often occurs in a similar patient population. However, KS is extremely uncommon in women. Although slit-like vessels may be seen in BA, this is a focal finding (Fig. 4.26a,b). The abundant neutrophils and karyorrhexis in an edematous background argue against KS. Nuclear staining for herpes virus type 8 (HHV-8) associated proteins can be demonstrated in cases of KS (Fig. 4.26c). An ulcerated pyogenic granuloma (lobular capillary hemangioma) may also be confused with BA (Fig. 4.27a,b); however, the neutrophilic infiltrate only occurs near the ulcerated surface in PG whereas it is more diffuse in BA. Furthermore, bacillary angiomatosis lacks the well-developed lobular architecture of pyogenic granuloma. In difficult cases, a silver stain to look for organisms may be necessary. Angiosarcoma is readily excluded by the lack of both marked cytologic atypia and an infiltrative growth pattern.

Treatment

Antibiotic therapy (erythromycin and others) will typically result in significant clinical improvement after 4–7 days of therapy, with complete resolution within 3–4 weeks.[94] Patients with extensive skin or mucosal

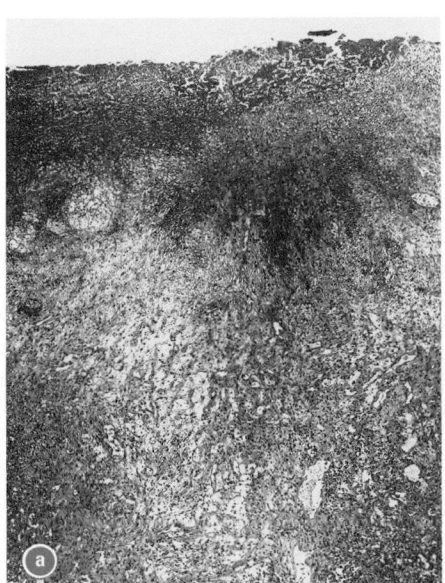 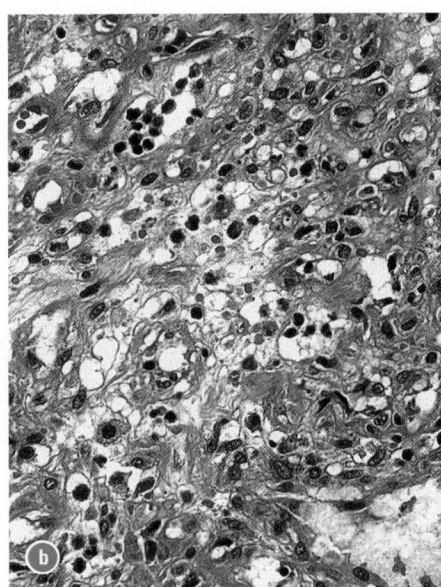 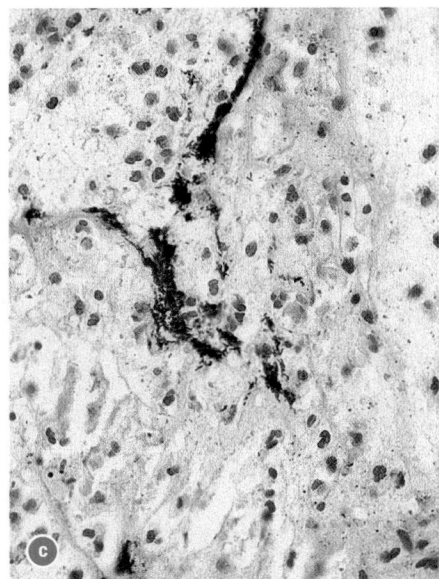

Fig. 4.25 (a) Bacillary angiomatosis, seen as a mucosal ulcer with underlying inflammation. (b) Neutrophils and debris are characteristic features. (c) A Gram stain highlights the organisms.

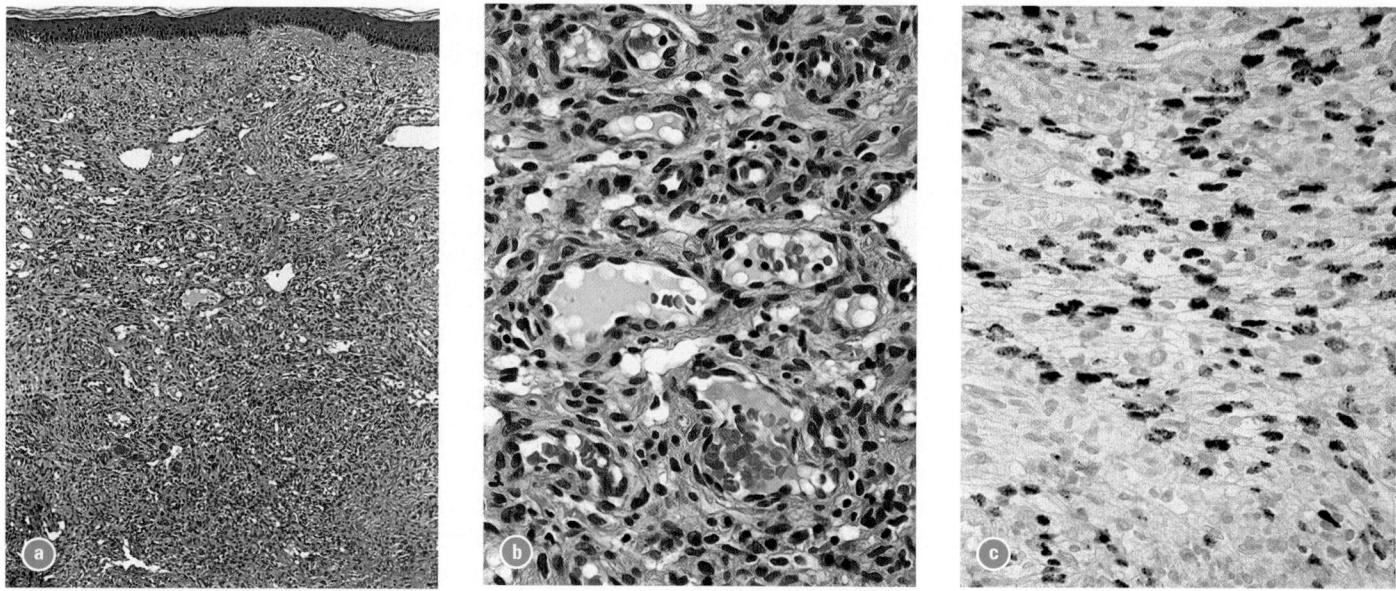

Fig. 4.26 (a) Low-power histology of Kaposi's sarcoma, showing prominent vascular organization. (b) At higher power, the endothelial atypia is accentuated. (c) An HHV-8 staining is strongly positive.

lesions, lytic bone lesions or visceral disease may require prolonged treatment.[95]

NECROTIZING FASCIITIS OF THE VULVA

Background

Necrotizing fasciitis (NF) is an aggressive, rapidly progressive infection of the subcutis and underlying fascia. NF may develop after skin biopsy; at needle puncture sites in illicit drug use; sites of traumatic puncture wounds; after episodes of frostbite; in chronic venous leg ulcers; open bone fractures; insect bites; surgical wounds and skin abscesses. However, in many cases, no association with such factors can be made. Necrotizing fasciitis may occur in the setting of diabetes mellitus, surgery, trauma or infectious processes.[96] NF of the vulva is most commonly seen in the setting of diabetes.[97,98] Obesity, peripheral vascular disease, hypertension and immune compromise are also often associated. A history of prior radiation to the site or a local infection is sometimes elicited. Unlike NF at other sites, prior trauma is rarely noted in cases involving the

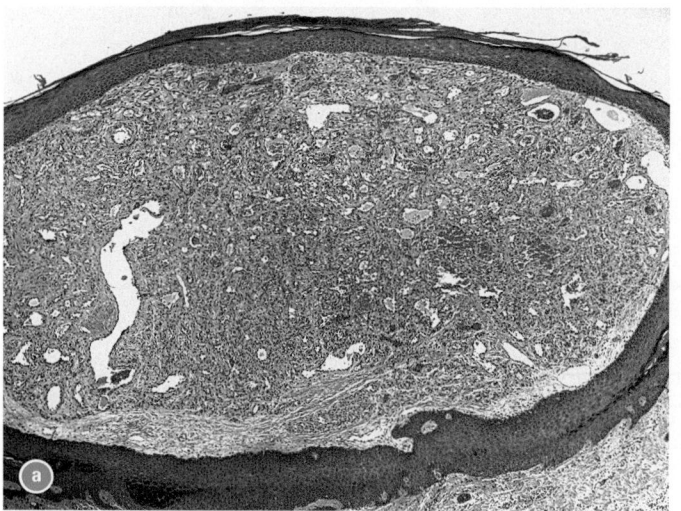

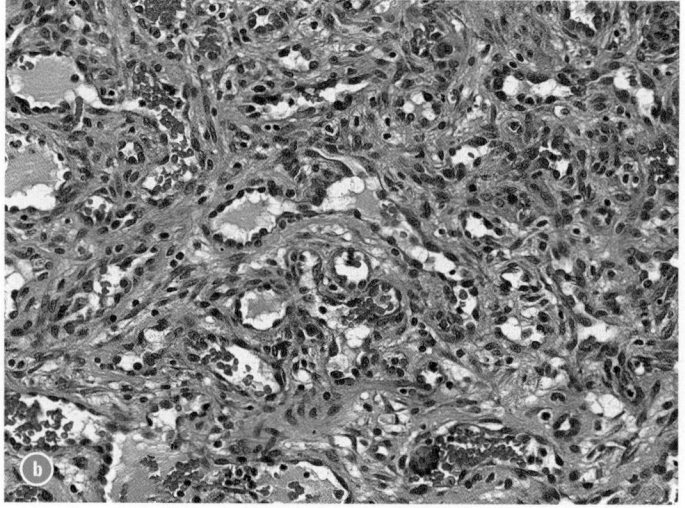

Fig. 4.27 (a) Lobular capillary hemangioma (LCH) closely resembles granulation tissue at low power, forming a discrete unit fed by a single vessel. (b) Uniform vascular network devoid of inflammation seen in LCH.

vulva.[97–100] Extragenital NF is often caused by either streptococcus or staphylococcus. In contrast, vulvar NF is commonly caused by a polymicrobial bacterial infection. Frequently implicated organisms include group B hemolytic streptococcus, *Enterococcus faecalis*, *E. coli*, *Bacteroides* species, *Klebsiella*, *S. aureus* and mixed anerobes.[98]

Clinical presentation

This disease can have an insidious onset with localized erythema, pain and edema often forming a rapidly advancing front. Marking the border with a pen and following its advance will assist in demonstrating its rapid progression and may be a helpful diagnostic exercise. Initially the skin is intact. With time, the skin will break down with ulceration, expression of a gray to clear exudate, necrosis and sloughing of the skin (Fig. 4.28). Crepitation can sometimes be demonstrated. Systemic signs and symptoms such as fever, malaise and confusion are present only late in the disease process.[101] A high index of suspicion is necessary for timely diagnosis of this disease. Early radical treatment appears to improve outcome. Mortality ranges from 25 to 75%.[97–100,102] Recently, a lower mortality rate of 0–40% has been reported.[103] NF has been documented following caesarean section. Cases have also been reported following episiotomy and tend to involve the perineum.[98]

Histopathology

Because early recognition of necrotizing fasciitis is critical for improving outcome in this disease, histologic examination of frozen section material is often used to aid diagnosis and to justify prompt radical surgery. Since

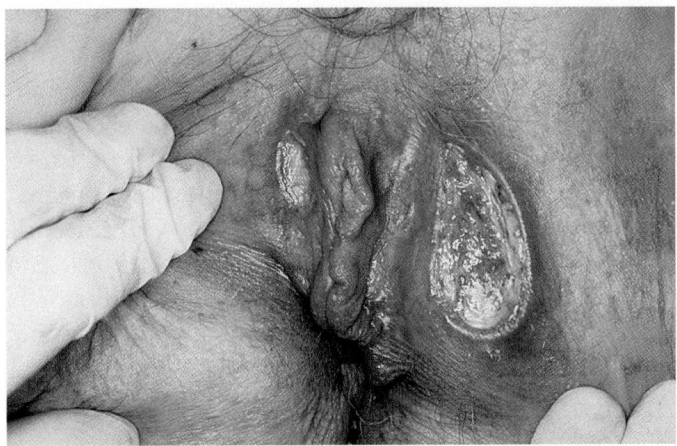

Fig. 4.28 Necrotizing fasciitis, ulcerative and associated with pseudomonas infection.

the histologic findings are nonspecific, clinicopathological correlation is necessary to establish the diagnosis. The histologic findings may vary from area to area. The advancing front may show scant acute inflammation. Sometimes sheets of bacteria with little or no associated inflammation are present in the subcutaneous tissue (Fig. 4.29a). In such biopsies, a Gram stain may assist in diagnosis, particularly at frozen section (Fig. 4.29b). Other areas may show suppurative acute inflammation with abscess formation extending along fascia and septae between fat lobules. In addition, acute inflammation may also spill over to involve fat lobules. Eccrine glands and ducts may show necrosis. Skeletal muscle, when present, may also be involved. Vessels with fibrin thrombi are a common secondary phenomenon.

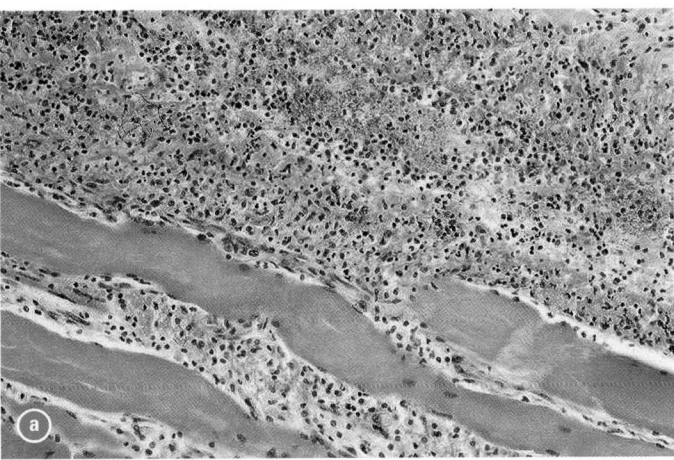

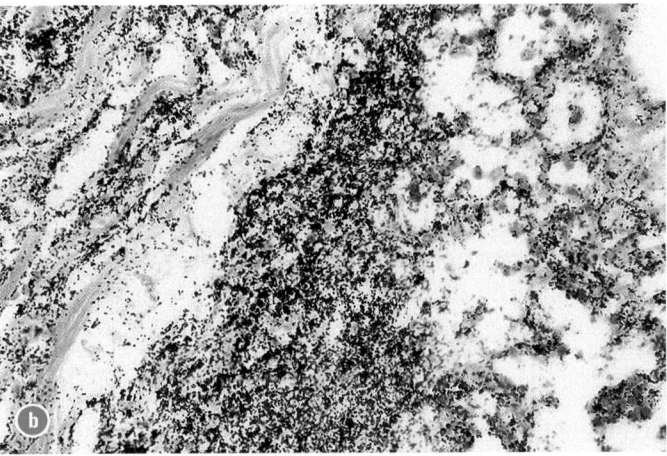

Fig. 4.29 (a) Histopathology of necrotizing fasciitis, showing necrosis of skeletal muscle and collagen with acute inflammatory exudate. (b) A Gram stain depicts many Gram-positive cocci.

Differential diagnosis

As discussed above, it is important to remember that there are no pathognomonic features of NF. Certain histologic features are suggestive, but ultimately clinical correlation is required. It is important not to mistake superficial cellulitis or pyoderma gangrenosum for necrotizing fasciitis. However, knowledge that NF extends to involve fascia in contrast to cellulitis and pyoderma gangrenosum (in which the epicenter of the disease is dermal) should prevent this potentially catastrophic mistake.

Management

The mortality rate can be as high as 25%, so early diagnosis and aggressive surgical management is ideal for treating necrotizing fasciitis. Cases of NF with sepsis and renal failure have a mortality rate as high as 70%. Once the diagnosis of NF is confirmed, treatment should be initiated without delay and includes antibiotic coverage for both aerobic and anaerobic organisms, surgical debridement and intensive supportive care.[104]

CHRONIC EROSIVE GENITAL HERPES

Clinical presentation

Herpes and HIV may be found in association with one another.[75] The association with HIV and genital herpes was noticed as early as 1981.[105] Chronic HSV-2 ulcers of more than 1 month in duration are an AIDS-defining illness in HIV-infected patients.[106,107] Several case reports describe HSV-2 presenting as hyperkeratotic verrucous lesions resembling condyloma in severely immuno-compromised patients.[108–111]

Although genital herpes is most commonly caused by HSV-2, an increasing number of cases are suspected to be caused by HSV-1.[5,112] In HIV-infected patients, severe, atypical clinical presentations often occur. Interaction between HIV and herpes may be associated with an increased size and number of lesions as well as chronic and highly infectious herpes ulcerations.[113] These may persist for several months.[114] They are likely to occur on a frequent basis. The vesicles and ulcers are more painful and heal slower than those experienced by an immunocompetent host.[115] As CD4 cell counts drop and immunosuppression worsens, recurrent outbreaks increase in frequency and severity.[116,117]

Treatment

Treatment in the HIV-positive patient is similar to non-HIV infected patients, but may require increased doses of antiviral medications. Suppressive therapy for HSV appears to significantly improve survival in HIV-positive patients.[5]

If lesions persist or recur in a patient receiving antiviral treatment, HSV resistance should be suspected and a viral isolate should be obtained for sensitivity testing. Management of these patients should be with a specialist and alternate therapy should be administered.[5]

VARICELLA ZOSTER

Clinical presentation

Primary varicella or chickenpox is a common childhood infection. In the USA and Europe, most adults who have HIV disease have previously been infected with varicella-zoster virus (VZV). In primary VZV infection, the rash appears 10–21 days after exposure. Lesions progress from small erythematous macules to papules and vesicles. These vesicles later ulcerate, dry and form crusts. The infection may be recurrent, severe, with more than one dermatome involved in the patient infected with HIV. A lengthened course associated with residual postherpetic neuralgia and scarring may occur. The infection can be more severe in this population and the disease can be fatal.[58]

Histopathology

Zoster and HSV cannot be reliably distinguished by routine light microscopy, as both have similar nuclear inclusions and degenerative changes (Fig. 4.30a,b). Immunohistochemistry can be used to distinguish these infections (Fig. 4.30c).

Treatment of varicella zoster infection in HIV-infected patients

Higher concentrations of acyclovir are required to inhibit replication of VZV than of HSV. Acyclovir (10 mg/kg q. 8 h i.v.) is utilized for disseminated/visceral VZV infection. It is important to monitor renal function. For acyclovir-resistant VZV infection, foscarnet (60 mg/kg q. 12 h i.v.) is utilized. The treatment for VZV is usually for 5–10 days or until resolution of symptoms.

Herpes zoster (shingles) is an acute vesiculobullous infection caused by varicella-zoster virus. Symptoms include pain or paresthesia, itching, burning, tingling, with or without headache and fever. There may be long-term post-herpetic neuralgia with chronic pain in that dermatome, resulting in long-term vulvar pain, clitorodynia, etc. This can be very confusing if the pri-

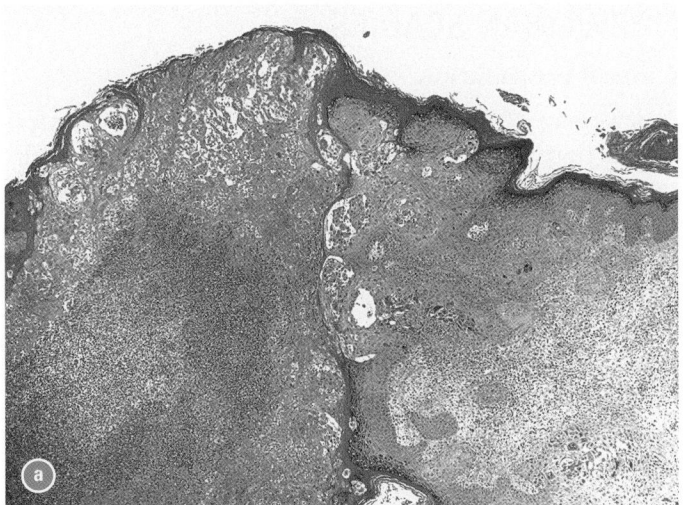

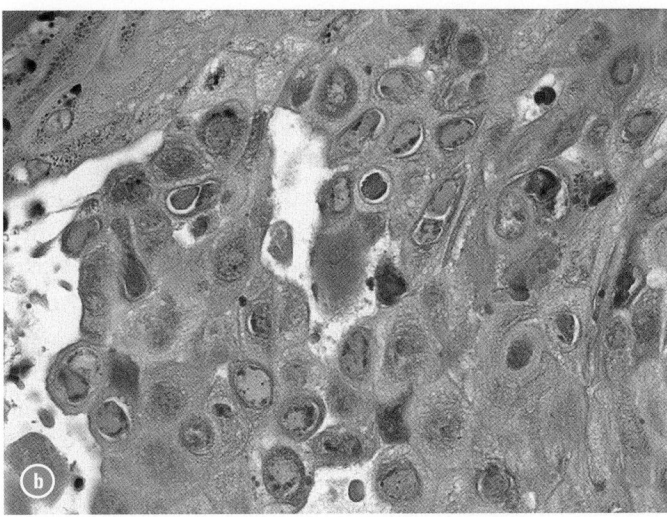

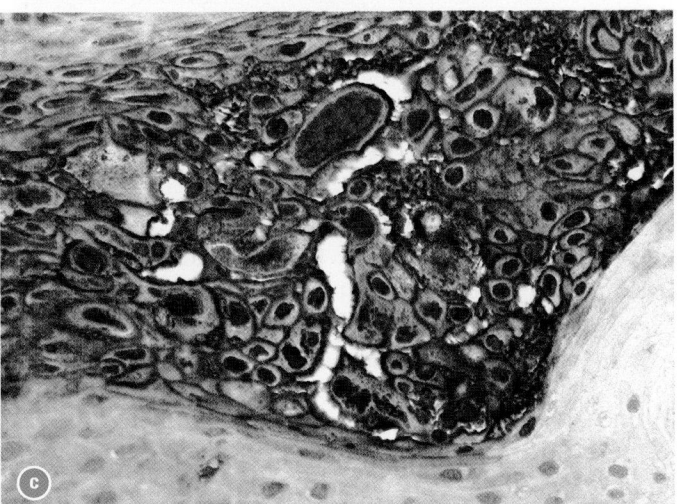

Fig. 4.30 Varicella zoster. (a) At low power, there is pronounced submucosal edema and epithelial hyperplasia. Ulceration is inconspicuous. (b) Inclusions are conspicuous at higher power, similar in appearance to herpes simplex. (c) Immunohistochemical staining for zoster will discriminate this from herpes simplex.

mary condition has been missed. The histopathologic features are similar to those seen with primary herpes infection, although the degree of inflammation is sometimes less profuse.

EXTENSIVE GENITAL WARTS IN THE IMMUNOSUPPRESSED PATIENT

Clinical presentation

Genital HPV infections occur more commonly in immunosuppressed patients when compared with control populations. In the HIV patient, the lesions tend to be diffuse, dysplastic and subclinical.[118] Additionally, HIV-positive patients tend to be infected with more HPV types than control populations.[119,120] The shedding of HPV and the extent of disease increases as CD4 cell counts decrease.[121] HIV-infected patients' condylomas are associated with a significant risk of transformation into squamous cell carcinoma. Thus, these patients require close follow-up and biopsy of any suspicious areas. It is recommended that as part of every gynecologic examination, these women have a thorough inspection of the vulva and perianal region and any abnormalities other than the classic exophytic condylomata acuminata should undergo colposcopy and biopsy.[122]

Treatment

The treatment for vulvar condyloma in the immunosuppressed patient does not differ from the normal population. HIV-positive patients may have more extensive disease than HIV-negative patients. Often, they have a delayed response to treatment, as well as more frequent recurrences are noted.

Treatment options available to the HIV-infected host do not differ from those available to the immunocompetent host previously discussed. Many different considerations exist in treating this patient population.[75] Some clinicians recommend treatment by excision and electrodesiccation because of the poor response and frequent recurrences after topical treatments[123] However, others feel that surgery alone is the treatment indicated, secondary to the association between HPV and cancer in this population.[124–126] Other studies have evaluated nonsurgical treatment modalities for genital warts in the immunocompromised host. Podophyllotoxin has been studied for genital warts in HIV-positive Tanzanian patients.[127] Interferon and imiquimod have also been studied.[128,129] Although both have some efficacy in treating HPV infection in HIV patients, neither appears to be effective as monotherapy in completely clearing clinical lesions from the most severely immunocompromised patients. However, the use of imiquimod as adjunctive therapy after surgical or cytodestructive treatment of condyloma acuminatum does appear effective in HIV-seropositive and in other immunocompromised patients in terms of significant delays or prevention of recurrences.[75] The better the HIV control, the more successful is the condyloma treatment.

DISSEMINATED MOLLUSCUM

Clinical presentation

Over the last 30 years, the incidence of molluscum contagiosum has been increasing, mainly as a sexually transmitted disease and it is particularly rampant as a result of concurrent human immunodeficiency virus (HIV) infection.[130] In the HIV patient population, molluscum contagiosum manifests itself most commonly when immune function has been dramatically reduced. Several studies document that molluscum contagiosum infection is a clinical sign of marked HIV progression and very low CD4 cell counts.[131,132] Numerous lesions on a patient who is not yet diagnosed with HIV disease should prompt discussion of an HIV test.[133] The molluscum presentation in the HIV-positive patient may be quite atypical, so diagnosis of a suspicious vulvar lesion is in large part dependent on biopsy.[75]

Treatment

Molluscum contagiosum in HIV-positive patients is notoriously difficult to treat.[134] Unlike otherwise healthy hosts, there is no evidence that lesions spontaneously resolve and will require one of a variety of traditional methods with varied success.[126,135–142] Success is ultimately linked to optimal treatment of the underlying HIV infection.

NORWEGIAN SCABIES

Clinical presentation

Norwegian scabies (crusted scabies) is a florid infestation that usually occurs in immunodeficient, debilitated or malnourished patients. Patients who are receiving systemic or potent topical glucocorticoids, organ transplant recipients, mentally retarded or physically incapacitated persons, HIV-infected or human T-lymphotropic virus-1 (HTLV-1)-infected persons and persons with various hematologic malignancies are at risk for developing crusted scabies.[5,75,143–145] Patients with crusted scabies have pruritus associated with skin lesions containing thick, friable plaques that are often associated with fissuring. As the lesions become more crusted, the pruritus decreases. As the CD4 cell counts decline, more severe and unusual infestations occur.[146–148] The differential diagnosis consists of eczema, psoriasis, contact dermatitis, drug reactions, seborrheic dermatitis, Darier's disease or dermatophytosis.

The crusted scabies infestations in the HIV-infected patient contain a high mite burden. An immunocompetent host is estimated to have 10–15 live female mites during an infestation,[149] while individual crusts in crusted scabies may harbor thousands of mites.

Treatment

The CDC recommendation for HIV-infected patients with crusted or papular scabies is for 'consultation with an expert' as the disease will invariably require a range of topical and oral medications.[150,151] No controlled therapeutic studies for crusted scabies have been conducted and the appropriate treatment remains unclear. Substantial treatment failure might occur with a single topical scabicide or oral ivermectin treatment and require aggressive therapy.[75]

References

1 Chosidow O. Scabies and pediculosis. Lancet 2000; 355:819–826.
2 Martin DH, Mroczkowski TF. Dermatologic manifestations of sexually transmitted diseases other than HIV. Infect Dis Clin North Am 1994; 8(3):533–582.
3 Lyon WF. Human lice HYG-209. http:ohioline.osu.edu/hyg-fact/2000/2094.html.
4 Ko CJ, Elston DM. Pediculosis. J Am Acad Derm 2004; 50:1–12.
5 CDC. STD Treatment Guidelines. Morbidity and Mortality Weekly Report 2002. http://www.cdc.gov/std/treatment/TOC2002TG.htm.

6 Nyirjesy P. Chronic vulvovaginal candidiasis. Am Fam Physician 2001; 63(4):697–702.

7 Sobel JD, Faro S, Force RW, et al. Vulvovaginal candidiasis: epidemiologic, diagnostic and therapeutic considerations. Am J Obstet Gynecol 1998; 178:203–211.

8 Eckhert LO, Hawes SE, Stevens CE, et al. Vulvovaginal candidiasis: clinical manifestations, risk factors, management algorithm. Obstet Gynecol 1998; 92:757–765.

9 Haefner HK. Current evaluation and management of vulvovaginitis. Clin Obstet Gynecol 1999; 42(2):184–195.

10 Wiederkehr M, Schwartz RA. Tinea cruris. E Medicine. http://www.emedicine.com/derm/topic471.htm.

11 Wilson J. Managing recurrent bacterial vaginosis. Sex Transm Infect 2004; 80(1):8–11.

12 Jaworsky C, Gilliam AC. Immunopathology of the human hair follicle. Derm Clin 1999; 17:561–568.

13 Sadick NS. Current aspects of bacterial infections of the skin. Derm Clin 1997; 15:341–349.

14 Pearlman MD, Yashar C, Ernst S, Solomon W. An incremental dosing protocol for women with severe vaginal trichomoniasis and adverse reaction to metronidazole. Am J Obstet Gynecol 1996; 174(3):934–936.

15 Hanson D, Diven DG. Molluscum contagiosum. Dermatol Online J 2003; 9:2.

16 Scholz J, Rosen-Wolff A, Burgert K, et al. Epidemiology of molluscum contagiosum using genetic analysis of the viral DNA. J Med Virol 1989; 27:87–90.

17 Porter CD, Archard LC. Characterisation by restriction mapping of three subtypes of molluscum contagiosum virus. J Med Virol 1992; 38:1–6.

18 Lynch PJ. Molluscum contagiosum venereum. Clin Obstet Gynecol 1972; 15:966–975.

19 Wilkin JK. Molluscum contagiosum venereum in a women's outpatient clinic: a venereally transmitted disease. Am J Obstet Gynecol 1977; 128:531–535.

20 Carson WE. Molluscum contagiosum. Cutis 1976; 17(4):701–703.

21 Brown TJ, Yen-Moore A, Tyring SK. An overview of sexually transmitted diseases. Part I. J Am Acad Derm 1999; 41:511–532.

22 Moreland AA. Vulvar manifestations of sexually transmitted diseases. Semin Derm 1994; 13(4):262–268.

23 Fleming DT, McQuillan GM, Johnson RE, et al. Herpes simplex virus type 2 in the United States, 1976 to 1994. N Engl J Med 1997; 337:1105–1111.

24 Torres G, Schinstine M, Krusinski P, Tyring SK. Herpes simplex. E Medicine. http://www.emedicine.com/derm/topic179.htm.

25 Kimberlin DW. Herpes simplex virus infections of the central nervous system. Semin Pediatr Infect Dis 2003; 14:83–89.

26 McSorley J, Shapiro L, Brownstein MH, Hsu KC. Herpes simplex and varicella-zoster: comparative histopathology of 77 cases. Int J Dermatol 1974; 13(2):69–75.

27 GRASP. The gonococcal resistance to antimicrobials surveillance program annual report. Year 2001 collection. London: Public Health Laboratory Service; 2002:3–16.

28 Waugh M. Update on gonorrhea. Skinmed 2003; 2(3):188–189.

29 Doherty L, Fenton KA, Jones J, et al. Syphilis: old problem, new strategy. BMJ 2002; 325:153–156.

30 LaGuardia KD, White MH, Saigo PE, et al. Genital ulcer disease in women infected with human immunodeficiency virus. Am J Obstet Gynecol 1995; 172:553–562.

31 Pembroke AC, Michell PA, McKee PH. Nodulosquamous tertiary syphilide. Clin Exp Derm 1980; 5:361–364.

32 Pandhi RK, Singh N, Ramam M. Secondary syphilis: a clinicopathologic study. Int J Derm 1995; 34:240–243.

33 Mroczkowski TF, Martin DH. Genital ulcer disease. Derm Clin 1994; 12(4):753–764.

34 Abell E, Marks R, Wilson Jones E. Secondary syphilis: a clinico-pathological review. Br J Derm 1975; 93:53–61.

35 Lewis DA. Diagnostic tests for chancroid. Sex Transm Infect 2000; 76(2):137–141.

36 Lewis DA. Chancroid: from clinical practice to basic science. AIDS Patient Care STDS 2000; 14(1):19–36.

37 Lewis DA. Chancroid: clinical manifestations, diagnosis and management. Sex Transm Infect 2003; 79(1):68–71.

38 Steen R, Dallabetta G. Genital ulcer disease control and HIV prevention. J Clin Virol 2004; 29(3):143–151.

39 Niemel PLA, Engelkens HJH, Meijden WI van der, et al. Donovanosis (granuloma inguinale) still exists. Int J Derm 1992; 31:244–246.

40 Goens JL, Schwartz RA, De Wolf K. Mucocutaneous manifestations of chancroid, lymphogranuloma venereum and granuloma inguinale. Am Fam Physician 1994; 49:415–418, 423–425.

41 Sehgal VN, Jain MK, Sharma VK. Pseudoelephantiasis induced by donovanosis. Genitourin Med 1987; 63:54–56.

42 MacKay CR, Bunch WL Jr. Carcinoma of the vulva following granuloma inguinale. Am J Syph, Gonorrh, Vener Dis 1952; 36:511–514.

43 O'Farrell N. Donovanosis: an update. Int J STD AIDS 2001; 12:423–427.

44 Mabey D, Peeling RW. Lymphogranuloma venereum. Sex Transm Infect 2002; 78:90–92.

45 Radman HM, Bhagavan BS. Pilonidal disease of the female genitals. Am J Obstet Gynecol 1972; 114(2):271–272.

46 Dirie MA, Lindmark G. A hospital study of the complications of female circumcision. Trop Doct 1991; 21(4):146–148.

47 Chinnock B. Periclitoral abscess. Am J Emerg Med 2003; 21(1):86.

48 Reeves KO, Kaufman RH. Vulvar ectopic breast tissue mimicking periclitoral abscess. Am J Obstet Gynecol 1980; 137(4):509–511.

49 Kent SW, Taxiarchis LN. Recurrent periclitoral abscess. Am J Obstet Gynecol 1982; 142(3):355–356.

50 Sur S. Recurrent periclitoral abscess treated by marsupialization. Am J Obstet Gynecol 1983; 147(3):340.

51 Kameh D, Smith A, Brock MS, Ndubisi B, Masood S. Female genital schistosomiasis. South Med J 2004; 97(5):525–527.

52 Koneman EW, Allen SD, Janda WM, et al. Color atlas and textbook of diagnostic microbiology. Philadelphia: Lippincott, Williams & Wilkins; 1997:1111–1119.

53 Connor DH, Chandler FW, Schwartz DA, et al. Pathology of infectious diseases. Stamford: Appleton and Lange; 1997:1537–1551.

54 Feldmeier H, Helling-Giese G, Poggensee G. Unreliability of PAP smears to diagnose female genital schistosomiasis. Trop Med Int Health 2001; 6(1):31–33.

55 Poggensee G, Feldmeier H, Krantz I. Schistosomiasis of the female genital tract: public health aspects. Parasitol Today 1999; 5(9):378–381.

56 Poggensee G, Kiwelu I, Saria M, et al. Schistosomiasis of the lower reproductive tract without egg excretion in urine. Am J Trop Med Hyg 1998; 59:782–783.

57 Helling-Giese G, Sjaastad A, Poggensee G, et al. Female genital schistosomiasis (FGS): relationship between gynecological and histopathological findings. Acta Trop 1996; 62(4):257–267.

58 Cohen J, Powderly W. Infectious diseases, 2nd edn. Philadelphia: Mosby; 2004:2150.

59 Mawad NM, Hassanein OM, Mahmoud OM, Taylor MG. Schistosomal vulval granuloma in a 12 year old Sudanese girl. Trans R Soc Trop Med Hyg 1992; 86:644.

60 McKenna G, Edwards S, Cleland H. Genital ulceration secondary to Epstein-Barr virus infection. Genitourin Med 1994; 70:356–357.

61 Brown ZA, Stenchever MA. Genital ulceration and infectious mononucleosis: report of a case. Am J Obstet Gynec 1977; 127:673–674.

62 Wilson RW. Genital ulcers and mononucleosis. Pediatr Infect Dis J 1993; 12:418.

63 Portnoy J, Ahronheim GA, Ghibu F, et al. Recovery of Epstein-Barr virus from genital ulcers. N Engl J Med 1984; 311:966–968.

64 Hudson LB, Perlman SE. Necrotizing genital ulcerations in a premenarcheal female with mononucleosis. Obstet Gynecol 1998; 92(4):642–644.

65 Sisson BA, Glick L. Genital ulceration as a presenting manifestation of infectious mononucleosis. J Pediatr Adolesc Gynecol 1998; 11(4):185–187.

66 Taylor S, Drake SM, Dedicoat M, Wood MJ. Genital ulcers associated with acute Epstein-Barr virus infection. Sex Transm Infect 1998; 74(4):296–297.

67 Quale J, Teplitz E, Augenbraun M. Atypical presentation of chancroid in a patient infected with the human immunodeficiency virus. Am J Med 1990; 88(5):43–44.

68 Jamkhedkar PP, Hira SK, Shroff HJ, Lanjewar DN. Clinico-epidemiologic features of granuloma inguinale in the era of acquired immune deficiency syndrome. Sex Transm Dis 1998; 25:196–200.

69 Gotz HM, Ossewaarde JM, Nieuwenhuis RF, et al. A cluster of lymphogranuloma venereum among homosexual men in Rotterdam with implications for other countries in Western Europe. Ned Tijdschr Geneeskd (Dutch) 2004; 148(9):441–442.

70 Rompalo AM, Cannon RO, Quinn TC, Hook EW. Association of biologic false-positive reactions for syphilis with human immunodeficiency virus infection. J Infect Dis 1992; 165:1124–1126.

71 Farley TA, Cohen DA, Wu SY, Besch CL. The value of screening for sexually transmitted diseases in an HIV clinic. J AIDS 2003; 33(5):642–648.

72 Wasserheit JN. Epidemiological synergy: interrelationships between human immunodeficiency virus infection and other sexually transmitted diseases. Sex Transm Dis 1992; 19:61–77.

73 Moodley P, Wilkinson D, Connolly C, Sturm AW. Influence of HIV-1 coinfection on effective management of abnormal vaginal discharge. Sex Transm Dis 2003; 30(1):1–5.

74 Sorvillo F, Smith L, Kerndt P, Ash L. Trichomonas vaginalis. HIV and African-Americans (http://www.cdc.gov/ncidod/eid/vol7no6/sorvillo.htm).

75 Czelusta A, Yen-Moore A, Straten M Van der, Carrasco D, Tyring SK. An overview of sexually transmitted diseases. Part III. Sexually transmitted diseases in HIV-infected patients. J Am Acad Dermatol 2000; 43(3):409–432.

76 Cohn SE, Clark RA. Sexually transmitted diseases, HIV and AIDS in women. Med Clin North Am 2003; 87(5):971–995.

77 White MH. Is vulvovaginal candidiasis an AIDS-related illness? Clin Infect Dis 1996; 22(2):124–127.

78 Korn AP. Gynecologic care of women infected with HIV. Clin Obstet Gynecol 2001; 44(2):226–242.

79 Duerr A, Sierra MF, Feldman J, et al. Immune compromise and prevalence of Candida vulvovaginitis in human immunodeficiency virus-infected women. Obstet Gynecol 1997; 90:252–256.

80 Spinillo A, Capuzzo E, Gulminetti R, et al. Prevalence of and risk factors for fungal vaginitis caused by nonalbicans species. Am J Obstet Gynecol 1997; 176:138–141.

81 Cu-Uvin S, Hogan JW, Warren D, et al. Prevalence of lower genital tract infections among human immunodeficiency virus (HIV)-seropositive and high-risk HIV-seronegative women. HIV Epidemiol Res Study Group Clin Infect Dis 1999; 29:1145–1150.

82 Greenblatt RM, Bacchetti P, Barkan S, et al. Lower genital tract infections among HIV-infected and high-risk uninfected women: findings of the Women's Interagency HIV Study (WIHS). Sex Transm Dis 1999; 26:143–151.

83 Barbagallo J, Tager P, Ingleton R, Hirsch RJ, Weinberg JM. Cutaneous tuberculosis: diagnosis and treatment. Am J Clin Derm 2002; 3(5):319–328.

84 Sardana K, Koranne RV, Sharma RC, Mahajan S. Tuberculosis of the vulva masquerading as a sexually transmitted disease. J Derm 2001; 28(9):505–507.

85 Millar JW, Holt S, Gilmour HM, Roberston DH. Vulvar tuberculosis. Tubercle 1979; 60(3):173–176.

86 Nogales-Ortiz F, Tarancon I, Nogales FF Jr. The pathology of female genital tuberculosis. A 31-year study of 1436 cases. Obstet Gynecol 1979; 53:422–428.

87 Hsiao PF, Tzen CY, Chen HC, Su HY. Polymerase chain reaction based detection of *Mycobacterium tuberculosis* in tissues showing granulomatous inflammation without demonstrable acid-fast bacilli. Int J Derm 2003; 42(4):281–286.

88 Bhattacharya B, Karak K, Ghosal AG, et al. Development of a new sensitive and efficient multiplex polymerase chain reaction (PCR) for identification and differentiation of different mycobacterial species. Trop Med Int Health 2003; 8:150–157.

89 Wong R, Tappero J, Cockerell CJ. Bacillary angiomatosis and other *Bartonella* species infections. Semin Cutan Med Surg 1997; 16(3):188–199.

90 Chian CA, Arrese JE, Pierard GE. Skin manifestations of *Bartonella* infections. Int J Derm 2002; 41(8):461–466.

91 Tappero JW, Koehler JE, Berger TG, et al. Bacillary angiomatosis and bacillary splenitis in immunocompetent adults. Ann Intern Med 1993; 118(5):363–365.

92 Long SR, Whitfield MJ, Eades C, et al. Bacillary angiomatosis of the cervix and vulva in a patient with AIDS. Obstet Gynecol 1996; 88(4):709–711.

93 Tappero JW, Koehler JE. Images in clinical medicine. Bacillary angiomatosis or Kaposi's sarcoma? N Engl J Med 1997; 337:1888.

94 Koehler JE. HIV and Bartonella: bacillary angiomatosis and peliosis. HIV InSite,1977. http://hivinsite.ucsf.edu/InSite?page=kb-05-01-03

95 Cockerell CJ, Whitlow MA, Webster GF, Friedman-Kien AE. Epithelioid angiomatosis: a distinct vascular disorder in patients with the acquired immunodeficiency syndrome or AIDS-related complex. Lancet 1987; 2(8560): 654–656.

96 Schwarts RA, Kapila R. Necrotizing fasciitis. E Medicine. 2004:http://www.emedicine.com/derm/topic743.htm.

97 Addison WA, Livengood CH 3rd, Hill GB, et al. Necrotizing fasciitis of vulvar origin in diabetic patients. Obstet Gynecol 1984; 63(4):473–479.

98 Schorge JO, Granter SR, Lerner LH, Feldman S. Postpartum and vulvar necrotizing fasciitis. Early clinical diagnosis and histopathologic correlation. J Reprod Med 1998; 43:586–590.

99 Stephenson H, Dotters DJ, Katz V, Droegemueller W. Necrotizing fasciitis of the vulva. Am J Obstet Gynecol 1992; 166:1324–1327.

100 Roberts DB. Necrotizing fasciitis of the vulva. Am J Obstet Gynecol 1987; 157:568–571.

101 Fisher JR, Conway MJ, Takeshita RT, Sandoval MR. Necrotizing fasciitis. Importance of roentgenographic studies for soft-tissue gas. JAMA 1979; 241:803–806.

102 Clayton MD, Fowler JE Jr, Sharifi R, Pearl RK. Causes, presentation and survival of fifty-seven patients with necrotizing fasciitis of the male genitalia. Surg Gynecol Obstet 1990; 170(1):49–55.

103 Yaghan RJ, Al-Jaberi TM, Bani-Hani I. Fournier's gangrene: changing face of the disease. Dis Colon Rectum 2000; 43(9):1300–1308.

104 Schwartz RA, Kapila R. Necrotizing fasciitis, E Medicine. 2004: http://www.emedicine.com/derm/topic743.htm

105 Siegal FP, Lopez C, Hammer GS, et al. Severe acquired immunodeficiency in male homosexuals, manifested by chronic perianal ulcerative herpes simplex lesions. N Engl J Med 1981; 305(24):1439–1444.

106 Tayal SC, Pattman RS, Mclelland J, Sviland L, Snow MH. An indolent penile herpetic ulcer in a patient with previously undiagnosed human immunodeficiency virus infection. Br J Derm 1998; 138(2):334–336.

107 Centers for Disease Control. Revised classification system for HIV infection and expanded surveillance case definition for AIDS among adolescents and adults. Centers for Disease Control; 1993.

108 Gretzula J, Penneys NS. Complex viral and fungal skin lesions of patients with acquired immunodeficiency syndrome. J Am Acad Dermatol 1987; 16(6):1151–1154.

109 Smith KJ, Skelton HG 3rd, Frissman DM, Angritt P. Verrucous lesions secondary to DNA viruses in patients infected with the human immunodeficiency virus in association with increased factor XIIIa-positive dermal dendritic cells. The Military Medical Consortium of Applied Retroviral Research Washington, D.C. [erratum appears in J Am Acad Dermatol 1993; 28(3):411]. J Am Acad Dermatol 1992; 27(6):943–950.

110 Tong P, Mutasim D. Herpes simplex virus infection masquerading as condyloma acuminata in a patient with HIV disease. Br J Derm 1996; 134:797–800.

111 Smith K, Skelton H, James W, Angritt P. Concurrent epidermal involvement of cytomegalovirus and herpes simplex virus in two HIV-infected patients. J Am Acad Derm 1991; 25:500–506.

112 Schomogyi M, Wald A, Corey L. Herpes simplex virus-2 infection: an emerging disease? Infect Dis Clin North Am 1998; 12:47–61.

113 Maier J, Bergman A, Ross M. Acquired immunodeficiency syndrome manifested by chronic primary genital herpes. Am J Obstet Gynecol 1986; 155:756–758.

114 Aral SO, Holmes KK. Sexually transmitted diseases in the AIDS era. Sci Am 1991; 264(2):62–69.

115 Skinhoj P. Herpesvirus infections in the immunocompromised patient. Scand J Infect Dis 1985; 47 (Suppl):121–127.

116 Bagdades E, Pillay D, Squire S, et al. Relationship between herpes simplex virus ulceration and CD4+ cell counts in patients with HIV infection. AIDS 1992; 6:1317–1320.

117 Augenbraun M, Feldman J, Chirgwin K, et al. Increased genital shedding of herpes simplex virus type 2 in HIV-seropositive women. Ann Intern Med 1995; 123(11):845–847.

118 Aynaud O, Piron D, Barrasso R, Poveda JD. Comparison of clinical, histological and virological symptoms of HPV in HIV-1 infected men and immunocompetent subjects. Sex Transm Infect 1998; 74:32–34.

119 Williams AB, Darragh TM, Vranizan K, et al. Anal and cervical human papillomavirus infection and risk of anal and cervical epithelial abnormalities in human immunodeficiency virus-infected women. Obstet Gynecol 1994; 83:205–211.

120 Vernon SD, Reeves WC, Clancy KA, et al. A longitudinal study of human papillomavirus DNA detection in human immunodeficiency virus type 1-seropositive and seronegative women. J Infect Dis 1994; 169:1108–1112.

121 Palefsky JM. Cutaneous and genital HPV-associated lesions in HIV-infected patients. Clin Derm 1997; 15:439–447.

122 Conley LJ, Ellerbrock TV, Bush TJ, et al. HIV-1 infection and risk of vulvovaginal and perianal condylomata acuminata and intraepithelial neoplasia: a prospective cohort study. Lancet 2002; 359(9301):108–113.

123 Modesto VL, Gottesman L. Sexually transmitted diseases and anal manifestations of AIDS. Surg Clin North Am 1994; 74(6):1433–1464.

124 Weiss EG, Wexner SD. Surgery for anal lesions in HIV-infected patients. Ann Med 1995; 27(4):467–475.

125 Bryan JT, Stoler MH, Tyring SK, et al. High-grade dysplasia in genital warts from two patients infected with the human immunodeficiency virus. J Med Virol 1998; 54(1):69–73.

126 Petersen CS, Weismann K. Quercetin and kaempherol: an argument against the use of podophyllin? Genitourin Med 1995; 71(2):92–93.

127 Kilewo CD, Urassa WK, Pallangyo K, et al. Response to podophyllotoxin treatment of genital warts in relation

to HIV-1 infection among patients in Dar es Salaam, Tanzania. Int J STD AIDS 1995; 6(2):114–116.

128 Zarcone R, Addonizio D, Voto RI, et al. Therapeutic prospects of natural alpha interferon from normal human leucocytes in the treatment of genital condylomata in HIV positive women. Clin Exp Obstet Gynecol 1994; 21(3):173–176.

129 Frega A. di Renzi F, Stentella P, Pachi A. Management of human papilloma virus vulvo-perineal infection with systemic beta-interferon and thymostimulin in HIV-positive patients. Int J Gynaecol Obstet 1994; 44(3):255–258.

130 Becker TM, Blout JH, Douglas J, Judson FN. Trends in molluscum contagiosum in the United States, 1966–1983. Sex Transm Dis 1986; 13:88–92.

131 Husak R, Garbe C, Orfanos CE. Mollusca contagiosa in HIV infection: clinical manifestations in relation to immune status and prognostic value in 39 patients. Hautarzt 1997; 48:103–109.

132 Jung AC, Paauw DS. Diagnosing HIV-related disease: using the CD4 count as a guide. J Gen Intern Med 1998; 13:131–136.

133 Delescluse J, Goens J. Multiple mollusca contagiosa revealing HTLV-III infection. Dermatologica 1986; 172:283–285.

134 Cronin TA, Resnik BI, Elgart G, Kerdel FA. Recalcitrant giant molluscum contagiosum in a patient with AIDS. J Am Acad Derm 1996; 35:266–267.

135 de Waard-van der Spek FB, Oranje AP, Lillieborg S, Hop WCJ, Stolz E. Treatment of molluscum contagiosum using a lidocaine/prilocaine cream (EMLA) for analgesia. J Am Acad Derm 1990; 23:685–688.

136 Redfield RR, James WD, Wright DC, et al. Severe molluscum contagiosum infection in a patient with human T-cell lymphotrophic (HTLV-III) disease. J Am Acad Derm 1985; 13:821–824.

137 Garrett SJ, Robinson JK, Roenogk HH. Trichloroacetic acid peel of molluscum contagiosum in immunocompromised patients. J Derm Surg Oncol 1992; 18:855–858.

138 Nelson MR, Chard S, Barton SE. Intralesional interferon for the treatment of recalcitrant molluscum contagiosum in HIV-antibody positive individuals, a preliminary report. Int J STD AIDS 1995; 6:351–352.

139 Mayumi H, Yamaoka K, Tsutsui T, et al. Selective immunoglobulin M deficiency associated with disseminated molluscum contagiosum. Eur J Pediatr 1986; 145:99–103.

140 Hengge UR, Cusini M. Topical immunomodulators for the treatment of external genital warts, cutaneous warts and molluscum contagiosum. Br J Derm 2003; 149:15–19.

141 Zabawski EJ, Cockerell CJ. Topical and intralesional cidofovir: a review of pharmacology and therapeutic effects. J Am Acad Derm 1998; 39:741–745.

142 Meadows KP, Tyring SK, Pavia AT, Rallis TM. Resolution of recalcitrant molluscum contagiosum lesions in HIV-infected patients treated with cidofovir. Arch Derm 1997; 133:987–990.

143 Rau RC, Baird IM. Crusted scabies in a patient with acquired immunodeficiency syndrome. J Am Acad Derm 1986; 15:1058–1059.

144 Drabick JJ, Lupton GP, Tompkins K. Crusted scabies in human immunodeficiency virus infection. J Am Acad Derm 1987; 17:142.

145 Guggisberg D, Viragh PA de, Constantin C, Panizzon RG. Norwegian scabies in a patient with acquired immunodeficiency syndrome. Dermatology 1998; 197:306–308.

146 Sadick N, Kaplan MH, Pahwa SG, Sarngadharan MG. Unusual features of scabies complicating human T-lymphotrophic virus type III infection. J Am Acad Derm 1986; 15:482–486.

147 Jucowics P, Ramon ME, Don PC, Stone RK, Barnji M. Norwegian scabies in an infant with acquired immunodeficiency syndrome. Arch Derm 1989; 125:1670–1676.

148 Sirera J, Ruis F, Romeu J, et al. Hospital outbreak of scabies stemming from two AIDS patients with Norwegian scabies. Lancet 1990; 335:1227.

149 Mellanby K. Scabies in 1976. R Soc Health J 1977; 97:32–36.

150 Taplin D, Meinking TL. Treatment of HIV-related scabies with emphasis on the efficacy of ivermectin. Semin Cutan Med Surg 1997; 16:235–240.

151 Meinking TL, Taplin D, Hermida J, Pardo R, Kerdel FA. The treatment of scabies with ivermectin. N Engl J Med 1995; 333:26–30.

5

Benign cysts, rests and adnexal tumors of the vulva

Alexander J.F. Lazar,

Scott R. Granter and

Hope K. Haefner

Introduction

Benign cysts

Bartholin duct cyst
Skene's duct cyst
Vulvar cysts of urogenital sinus
    origin (mucous and ciliated
    cysts)
Epidermal inclusion cyst
Urethral prolapse
Hydrocele of canal of Nuck

Benign rests

Ectopic breast tissue
    of the vulva
Endometriosis

Benign adnexal tumors

Hidradenoma papilliferum
Syringoma
Nodular hyperplasia and
    adenomas of Bartholin gland

Introduction

The clinician and pathologist must recognize benign cysts and adnexal lesions of the vulva to exclude more serious conditions and avoid misclassifying these benign conditions as malignancies. They typically do not pose a diagnostic problem with the exception of (1) ectopic breast tissue, particularly when containing fibroadenomas; (2) endometriosis, particularly if it is gland-poor (stromatosis); and (3) hidradenoma papilliferum, which to the uninitiated, may be interpreted as a malignancy.

Benign cysts

Benign vulvar cysts generally fall into four categories, comprising Bartholin duct cyst, epidermal inclusion cysts, mesonephric remnants and mucous cysts. Additional rare cysts include Skene's duct and prolapsed urethral tissue.

BARTHOLIN DUCT CYST

Cysts in the region of Bartholin gland involve the duct and are termed Bartholin duct cysts. They are typically located in the posterior introitus in the region of the draining ducts of Bartholin gland. Bartholin duct cysts

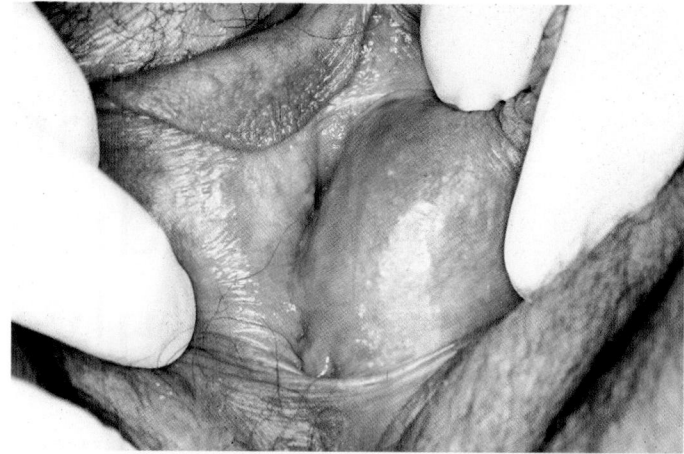

Fig. 5.1 Clinical appearance of Bartholin duct cyst. Reproduced from Marzano DA, Haefner HK. The Barthelin Gland Cyst: Past, Present and Future. Journal of Lower Genital Tract Disease. 2004; 8(3):195–204 Copyright Lippincott Williams and Wilkins, with permission.

presumably follow obstruction of the duct and may be accompanied by infection and a Bartholin gland abscess (Fig. 5.1).[1]

Histologically, a Bartholin duct cyst is lined by a transitional or squamous epithelium and the specimen often contains associated Bartholin gland and skeletal muscle. The diagnosis is made by identification of the transitional epithelium and gland. Its distinction from a Skene's duct cyst is based principally on its posterior rather than periurethral location (Fig. 5.2).[1] The clinical differential diagnosis also includes mucous cysts, epider-

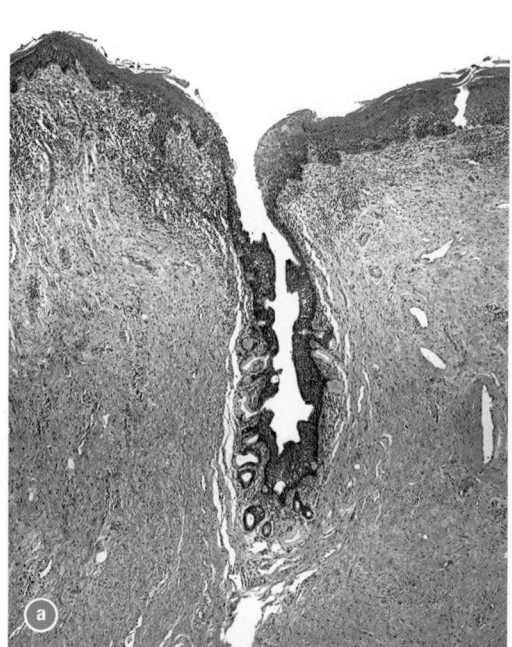

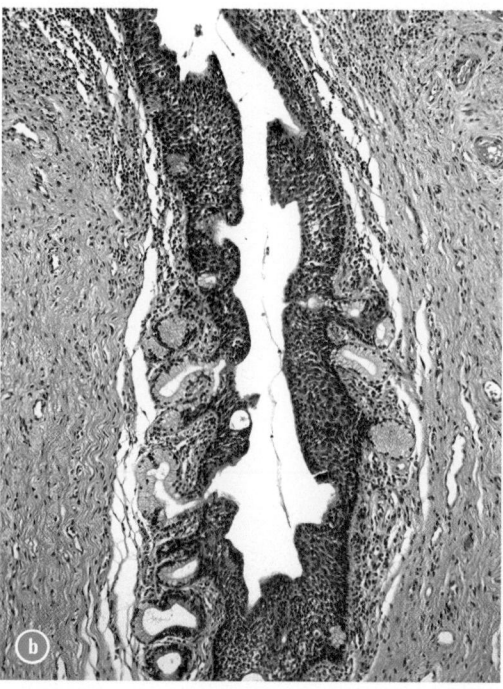

Fig. 5.2 (a) Microscopic view of Bartholin duct at the junction of the skin. (b) Bartholin duct cyst with squamous metaplasia.

mal inclusion cyst, benign adnexal tumors (hidradenoma) and soft tissue tumors such as lipomas.

Management of a Bartholin duct cyst includes insertion of a Word catheter for a duct cyst or gland abscess, and marsupialization.[2] Marsupialization is not recommended for abscesses. Antibiotic therapy is recommended in the setting of cellulitis.[2] As with all cysts, other vulvar neoplasms must be excluded, specifically carcinomas arising in Bartholin gland (see Ch. 7). The latter are, however, extremely rare.

SKENE'S DUCT CYST

Skene's duct cysts are extremely rare and, when seen, are more common in newborns, where they present as discrete periurethral pea-size swellings (Fig. 5.3).[3,4] In adults, they are occasionally reported in association with dyspareunia.[5]

The most important distinction is between Skene's duct cyst and other entities such as ectopic ureterocele, urethrocele, urethral diverticula, and benign or malignant urethral and paraurethral tumors. Management consists of marsupialization.[6]

VULVAR CYSTS OF UROGENITAL SINUS ORIGIN (MUCOUS AND CILIATED CYSTS)

Mucous cysts occur over a wide age range but are usually seen in multiparous women in the third and fourth decades. They present exclusively in the region of the vulvar vestibule and in the majority are solitary lesions of 1–2 cm in diameter. They are usually asymptomatic, but patients may complain of pain if the cysts

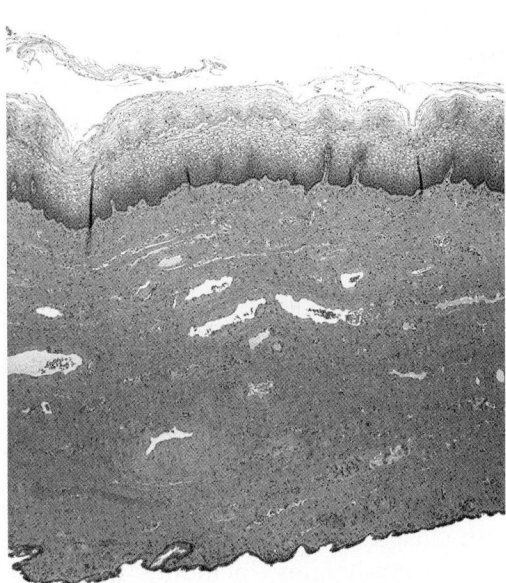

Fig. 5.4 Mucous cyst (bottom) beneath the squamous mucosa.

have recently enlarged or impinge on the urethra, where they may cause dysuria.[7]

Histologically, mucous cysts contain mucinous epithelium identical in appearance to that lining the endocervix or vaginal adenosis (Figs 5.4, 5.5). Less commonly, they will contain squamous metaplasia. Ciliated cells have been reported in some cases and may be mixed with the mucinous epithelium.

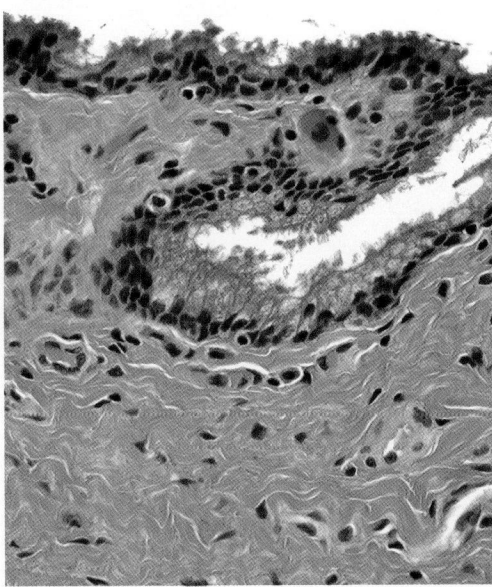

Fig. 5.5 Higher power of mucinous lining.

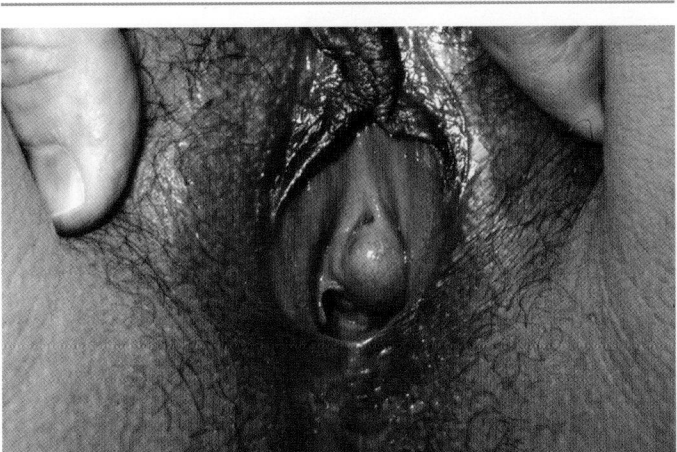

Fig. 5.3 Skene's duct cyst on gross examination (Photo courtesy of John Delancey, MD.)

The origin of mucous cysts has been debated in the past. Theories of origin include invagination of overlying squamous epithelium with mucoid metaplasia, paramesonephric (Müllerian) origin and origin in urogenital sinus epithelium.[8,9] The first is unlikely, as most mucous cysts do not communicate with the overlying squamous epithelium and the squamous differentiation in these cysts is of a metaplastic nature. The paramesonephric origin has been challenged by others who emphasize that the Müllerian ducts terminate in the region of the hymen and play no part in the development of the vulvar vestibule. Moreover, the most caudal extension of Müllerian epithelium seen in diethylstilbestrol exposure is cephalad to the hymen. Finally, clear cell carcinoma, a tumor arising in Müllerian epithelium, has not been reported in the vulvar vestibule. Urogenital sinus epithelium remains the most plausible, inasmuch as both ciliated and mucous cells have been observed in derived epithelium, including Bartholin gland. The differential diagnosis of mucous cysts includes mesonephric remnants (cuboidal epithelium and a fibromuscular wall) and Bartholin duct cysts (transitional epithelium). The latter are typically found in the medial or ventral portion of the labium majus.[7]

The development of mucous cysts appears to be hormone related in that the lesions occur most frequently in the reproductive years, including during pregnancy.

EPIDERMAL INCLUSION CYST

Epidermal inclusion cysts (EICs) occasionally occur in the vulvar region, but are most commonly associated with prior trauma or circumcision.[10,11] Vulvar EICs may become infected and management is similar to that of cutaneous EICs. The characteristic histopathologic features are similar to EICs elsewhere (Fig. 5.6).

URETHRAL PROLAPSE

Prolapse of the urethral mucosa through the urethral meatus may mimic a neoplasm clinically and present with abnormal bleeding. This condition occurs primarily in childhood but may be seen after menopause.[12,13] It has been linked to lack of estrogen and/or congenital redundancy of urologic mucosa and loss of support in the urethral tissues. It is often aggravated by increased intra-abdominal pressure. The majority of young patients are under 8 years of age with a preponderance of black patients in some series. A clinical diagnosis can usually be made, a malignancy excluded and biopsy avoided by careful inspection of the location of the lesion and the soft consistency to palpation. If biopsy is performed, histologic examination will disclose benign-appearing transitional epithelium, with nonspecific inflammation, edema and vascular thrombosis. Ulceration may be present.

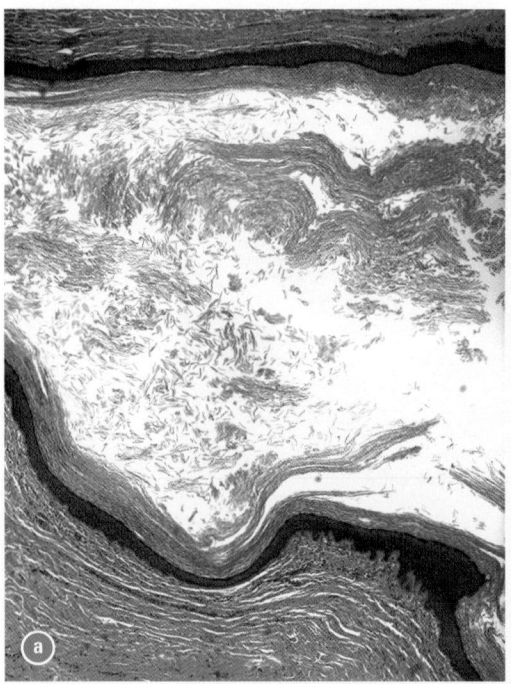
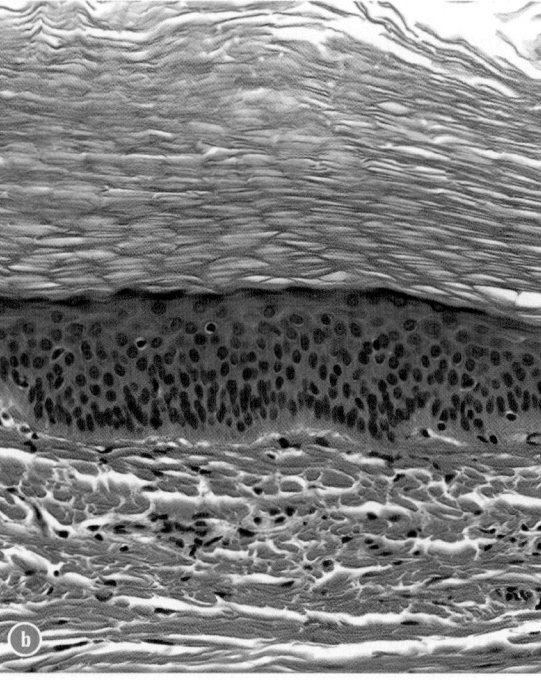

Fig. 5.6 (a) Epidermal inclusion cyst. (b) Higher power shows the squamous epithelium.

The most widely accepted therapy at present is simple excision of the prolapsed mucosa with careful re-approximation.

HYDROCELE OF CANAL OF NUCK

A hydrocele of the canal of Nuck is analogous to encysted hydrocele of the spermatic cord. These hydroceles are derived from the processus vaginalis and their extent is determined by the degree to which the processus vaginalis remains after birth.[14,15] Hence, a cyst of the canal of Nuck may present either as a small discrete cystic mass on the labia majus, extending into the femoral region, or present as an indirect inguinal hernia, which, in extreme cases, may contain adnexa or other pelvic organs. The persistence of the canal of Nuck may also be responsible for unilateral labial swelling in response to intra-abdominal ascites.[15]

Hydroceles can usually be distinguished from soft tissue neoplasms such as lipomas or leiomyomas by their tendency to transilluminate. Bartholin duct cysts can usually be distinguished by their location in the middle and lower third of the labium majus. Malignant soft tissue masses typically form larger masses and may ulcerate. The most appropriate approach to the persistent canal of Nuck is removal of the peritoneal-lined sac by ligation-excision.

Benign rests

ECTOPIC BREAST TISSUE OF THE VULVA

Ectopic breast tissue has long been recognized along the so-called 'milk-line' extending from the nipples to the groin. In the embryo, this line is characterized by a series of paired linear rudimentary 'buds', which are the rudiments of future mammary glands in certain mammals. In the human, all but the most cephalad pair disappear by the 20 mm embryo stage. The appearance of breast tissue in the vulva presumably reflects incomplete regression of this tissue. Association of ectopic breast tissue with a nipple in the vulva is exceedingly rare.[16,17]

The traditional concept of ectopic breast tissue has been challenged. Mammary-like anogenital glands concentrated in the labial sulcus of the vulva and resembling breast tissue have been described and may give rise to 'ectopic breast tissue'. These glands have ducts that open to the surface and lead to deeper coiled structures. The glands are lined by simple columnar epithelium associated with myoepithelial cells. However, acceptance of this source of vulvar ectopic breast tissue lesions is far from universal.[16,17]

Vulvar ectopic breast tissue is rare – less than 50 cases have been described. The significance of this tissue lies in the possibility that it may be misdiagnosed clinically or histologically as a neoplasm. Clinically, ectopic breast tissue appears as a smooth, well-circumscribed mass and is unlikely to be confused with a malignant tumor. The differential diagnosis is Bartholin duct cyst, hidradenoma, and other benign soft tissue neoplasms (Ch. 9). Rare cases have been reported during pregnancy which mimicked abscess by their expanding nature and coexisting pain.[16,17]

Histologically, the classic case of ectopic breast tissue will not be confused with a malignancy. Ectopic breast tissue in the vulva resembles normal breast tissue with glandular epithelium forming ducts and lobules within a fibrous stroma (Fig. 5.7). However, many of the pathologies of the breast have also been described in association with vulvar ectopic breast tissue, including fibroadenomas, cysts, lactational change, papillomas and malignant change, including ductal carcinoma *in situ*, invasive ductal carcinoma, lobular carcinoma and mucinous carcinoma.[18–22] Fibroadenoma in the vulva shows cystic change with a more cellular stroma sometimes resembling that seen in phylloides tumors of the breast, but atypia and mitoses are lacking (Figs 5.8, 5.9).[21] Mammary-type carcinomas, including *in situ* tumors, show morphology similar to those seen in the breast.[22–24]

Diagnostic pitfalls can be avoided by the pathologist who recognizes glandular carcinomas as rare and carefully excludes variants of lactating breast, hidradenoma

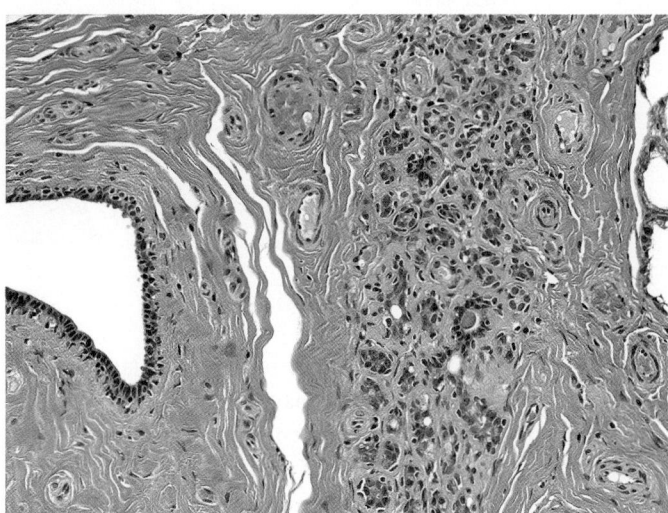

Fig. 5.7 Ectopic breast tissue in the vulva.

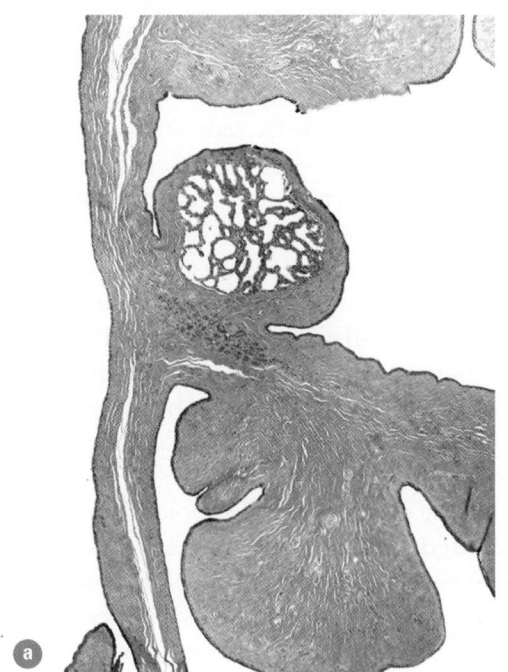

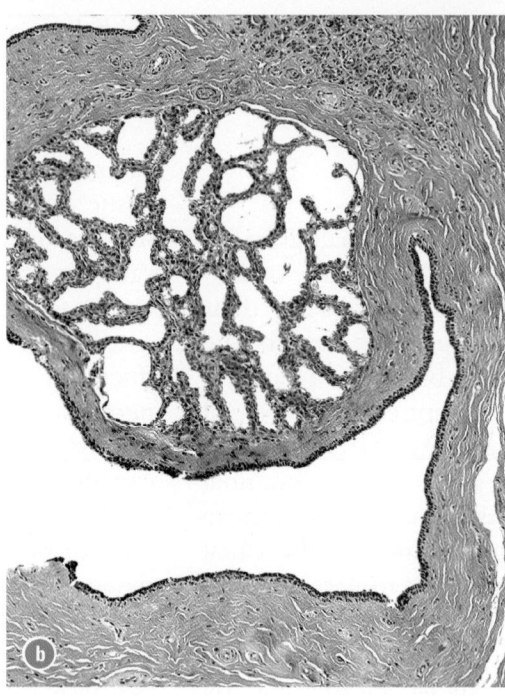

Fig. 5.8 (a) Fibroadenoma of ectopic breast tissue. (b) Note the associated secretory hyperplasia.

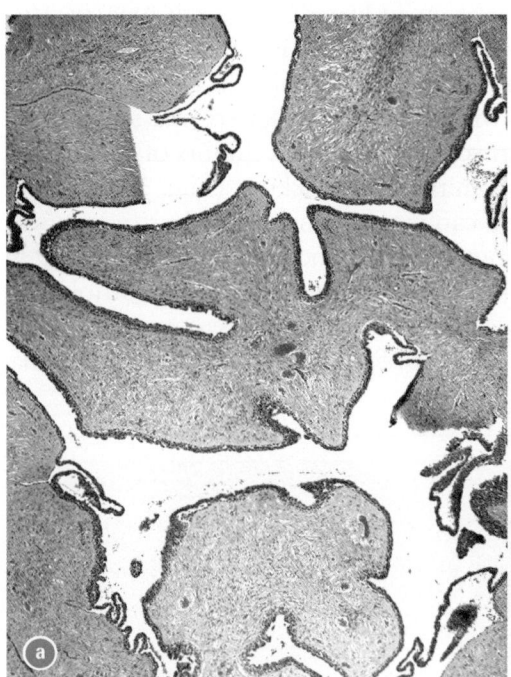

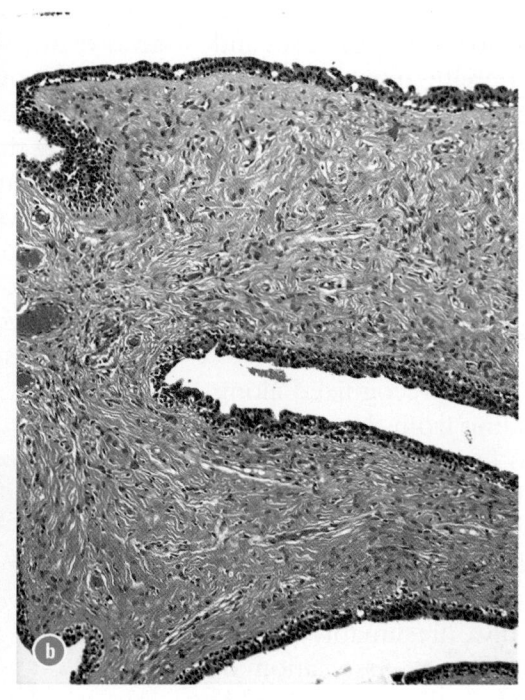

Fig. 5.9 (a) Fibroadenoma with a more complex architecture. (b) At higher power, note the bland stroma.

and fibroadenomas before considering a diagnosis of malignancy. Hidradenoma papilliferum is a well-circumscribed proliferation of papillary glandular epithelium with associated myoepithelial cells and a fibrovascular core forming true papillae. This lesion often has a cribriform appearance due to the highly complex papillary architecture. Cytologic atypia is not a feature. Sweat gland carcinomas are not associated with tissue resembling benign breast. Mammary-type carcinoma of the vulva should also be differentiated from a rare occurrence of metastatic breast carcinoma.[22–24]

ENDOMETRIOSIS

As with other genital sites, the vulva plays host to occasional endometriosis. The origin in all cases is not clear, but the detection of endometriosis following trauma suggests that, like the cervix, the vulva will permit implantation of endometriotic tissue under the appropriate conditions.[25] Endometriosis has also been reported to arise from the Bartholin gland, suggesting that the Bartholin duct may conduct cells from the endometrium into a protected environment where they can grow.[26] The diagnosis is not difficult, provided the practitioner is aware that endometriosis can occur at this site (Fig. 5.10).

Similar to other sites, endometriosis can give rise to carcinomas or sarcomas derived from the glandular or stromal components. A high index of suspicion is important when faced with these rare neoplasms.[27,28]

Benign adnexal tumors

HIDRADENOMA PAPILLIFERUM

Hidradenoma papilliferum (HP) is an uncommon benign adnexal tumor that occurs almost exclusively in the vulva and presumably arises from anogenital glands.[29] These tumors exhibit both eccrine and apocrine differentiation. HP usually presents as a discrete nodule (typically less than 2 cm diameter) in the sulcus between the labium majus and minus, most often in Caucasian women (Figs 5.11, 5.12). Nearly all reported cases are in post-pubertal women, usually adults, and less commonly in the aged. The lesion is painless unless it has ulcerated. Less often, HP presents in the perineal or perianal regions.[30–33] HP is thought to arise from anogenital glands. These show mixed eccrine and apocrine features and their function is not understood.[16,17]

HP is characterized by a well-circumscribed proliferation of papillary glandular epithelium showing 'decapitation secretion' with associated myoepithelial cells and a fibrovascular core forming true papillae (Figs. 5.12, 5.13). The lesions may have a cribriform-like appearance due to the highly complex papillary architecture.[33–35] Overlying acanthosis may be present

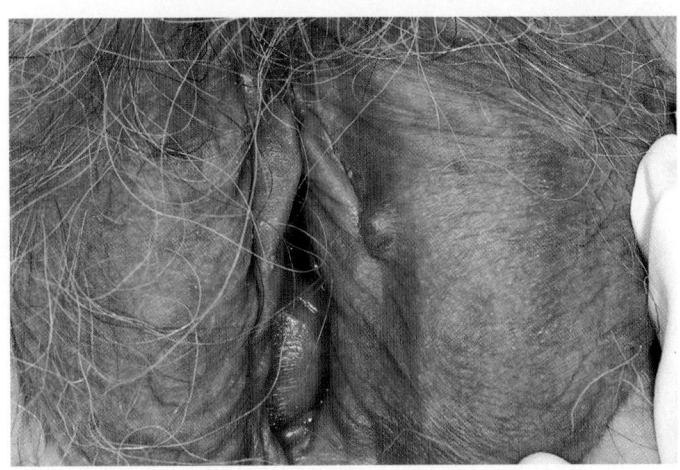

Fig. 5.11 Clinical appearance of hidradenoma papilliferum.

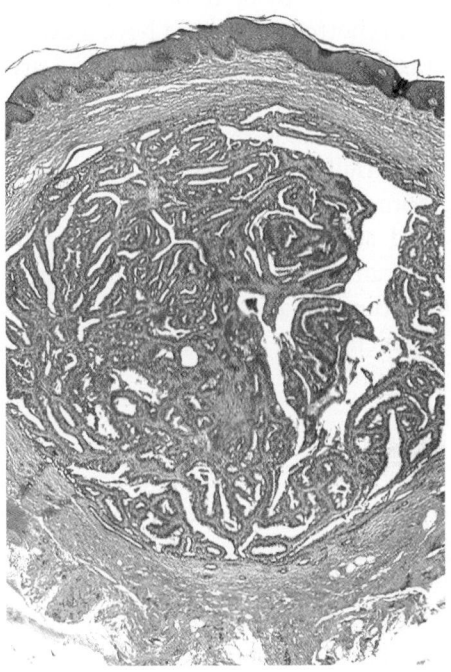

Fig. 5.12 Low power of hidradenoma.

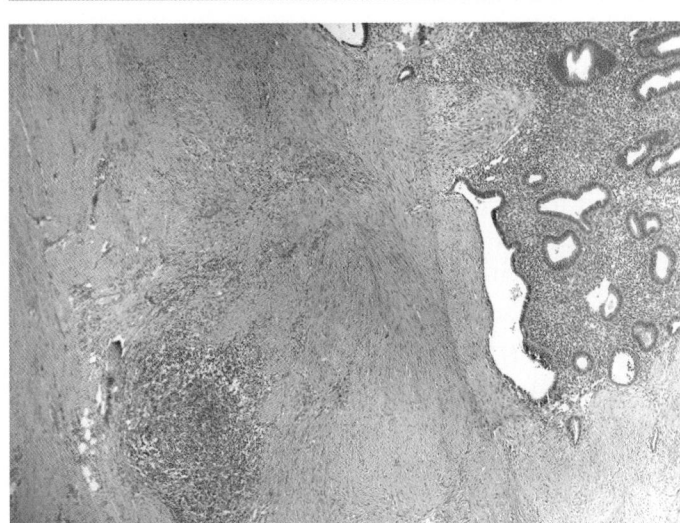

Fig. 5.10 Endometriosis of the vulva.

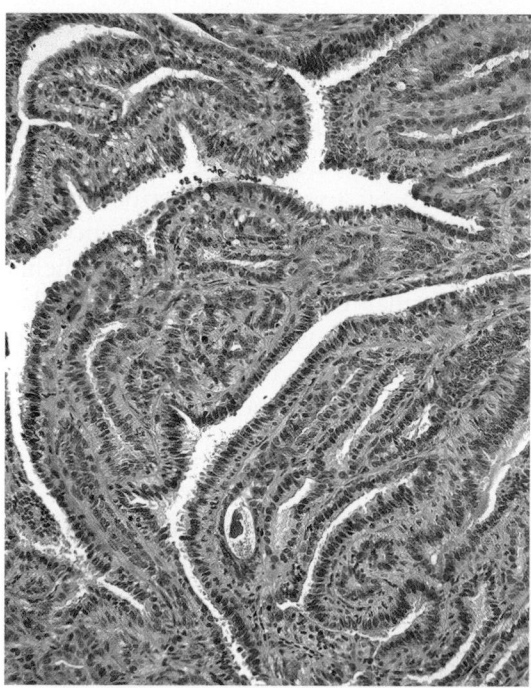

Fig. 5.13 Higher power of hidradenoma.

and the lesion may occasionally extend to the surface epithelium.

At higher magnification, the architectural features of HP are distinctive and diagnostic. The lining cell nuclei are uniform in appearance, and are accompanied by the second cell layer that distinguishes these and their counterparts in the breast as benign lesions.

On clinical grounds, HP must be distinguished from Bartholin duct cysts, lipomas and other mesenchymal neoplasms. Bartholin duct cysts by definition are located in the region of the fourchette and should have a cystic consistency in contrast to hidradenoma. Lipomas are softer and more moveable. Soft tissue tumors are easily distinguished following histologic examination. Histologically, the primary pitfall is misclassifying hidradenoma as adenocarcinoma, specifically metastatic endometrial carcinoma and adenocarcinoma of Bartholin gland. However, these can be excluded by their distinctive morphology–including a lack of two cell layers–and an index of suspicion for hidradenoma when confronted by any glandular lesion.

SYRINGOMA

Syringomas are benign adnexal tumors containing eccrine differentiation. They present as 1–4 mm flesh-colored papules, most commonly on the lower eyelid. The lesions are frequently multiple and usually symmetrically distributed. The chest, face, neck and vulva can also be affected.[36] Widespread involvement has been described, but is rare. Uncommonly, an eruptive form can occur with waves of new lesions. This variant appears to be more common in women and perhaps Asians.[37] There is a marked female predominance and the lesions commonly appear at puberty or earlier. Vulvar lesions have been documented in early childhood.[38] They appear with increased frequency in Down's syndrome. Isolated vulvar involvement is uncommon but, when present, is usually symmetrical in distribution.[39] Lesions in the vulva may be associated with pruritus[40] and symptoms may be exacerbated during pregnancy, warm weather, or menstruation.[41–43] Laser ablation has been used as treatment for pruritic lesions or for cosmetic purposes.[40]

Syringomas are characterized by a proliferation of eccrine epithelium forming duct-like structures lined by a double layer of cells typically dispersed in a fibrous stroma (syringoma) (Fig. 5.14). The nuclei are bland and mitoses are not a feature. Characteristically, the epithelial strands intersect with the ducts, forming short tails creating the impression of a comet or tadpole. Glycogen accumulation can lead to clear cell variants that are more common in diabetics.[43]

The clinical differential diagnosis of syringomas in the vulva includes Fox–Fordyce disease and, more remotely, steatocystoma multiplex and lymphangioma circumscriptum.[44,45] Fox–Fordyce disease is characterized by hyperkeratotic plugging of apocrine ducts with resultant cystic change. The characteristic comma-like acrosyringial proliferations seen in syringomas are absent. Steatocystoma multiplex is a hereditary condition that presents with multiple small flesh-colored papules and, rarely, involves the vulva.[45] Histologically, this lesion is composed of cysts often filled with sebum that connect directly with the pilosebaceous unit. Lymphangioma circumscription can occur as a congenital abnormality or arise later in life. Clinically, it is characterized by numerous small cutaneous vesicles or blebs that correspond to dilated lymphatics. Both the congenital and acquired forms can involve the vulva.[44] Histologically, lymphangioma circumscriptum consists of cystically dilated lymphatic vessels.

NODULAR HYPERPLASIA AND ADENOMAS OF BARTHOLIN GLAND

These lesions are rare. The largest series defined two types of glandular lesions of the Bartholin gland, adenoma and nodular hyperplasia.[46] Both are seen over a wide age range although hyperplasias predo-

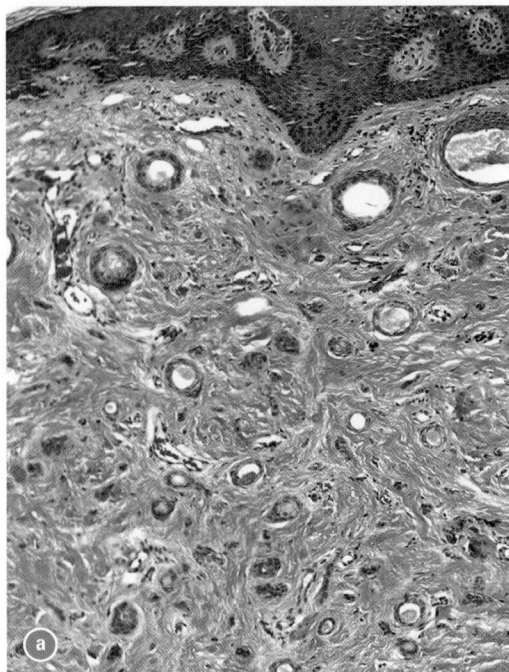 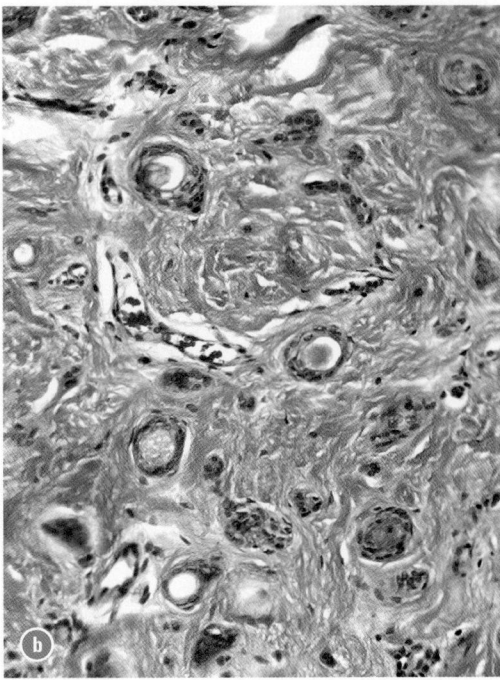

Fig. 5.14 Syringoma at (a) low and (b) high power, with multiple small cysts.

minate in younger adults. Both are often misdiagnosed as Bartholin's cysts. The distinction between adenoma and hyperplasia is based on the preservation of ductal and acinar relationships in hyperplasias, often with coexisting inflammation and ductal squamous metaplasia. Adenomas display a more haphazard growth, with absence of normal gland architecture.[46]

References

1 Marzano DA, Haefner HK. The Bartholin gland cyst: past present and future. J Lower Genital Tract Dis 2004; 8(3):195–204.

2 Downs MC, Randall HW Jr. The ambulatory surgical management of Bartholin duct cysts. J Emerg Med 1989; 7(6):623–626.

3 Kimbrough HM Jr, Vaughan ED Jr. Skene's duct cyst in a newborn: case report and review of the literature. J Urol 1977; 117(3):387.

4 Fathi K, Pinter A. Paraurethral cysts in female neonates. Case reports. Acta Paediatr 2003; 92(6):758–759.

5 James ST. A large cyst of Skene's duct – a rare cause of superficial dyspareunia. Aust N Z J Obstet Gynaecol 1979; 19(1):61–62.

6 Ishigooka M, Hayami S, Hashimoto T, et al. Skene's duct cyst in adult women: report of two cases. Int Urol Nephrol 1995; 27(6):775–778.

7 Friedrich EG Jr, Wilkinson EJ. Mucous cysts of the vulvar vestibule. Obstet Gynecol 1973; 42(3):407–414.

8 Hart WR. Paramesonephric mucinous cysts of the vulva. Am J Obstet Gynecol 1974; 107; 1079–1084.

9 Robboy SJ, Ross JS, Prat J, et al. Urogenital sinus origin of mucinous and ciliated cysts of the vulva. Obstet Gynecol 1978; 51:347–351.

10 Yoong WC, Shakya R, Sanders BT, Lind J. Clitoral inclusion cyst: a complication of type I female genital mutilation. J Obstet Gynaecol 2004; 24(1):98–99.

11 Ofodile FA, Oluwasanmi JO. Post-circumcision epidermoid inclusion cysts of the clitoris. Plast Reconstr Surg 1979; 63(4):485–486.

12 Kasby CB, Parsons KF. Prolapsed ureterocele presenting as a vulvar mass in a child. Br J Obstet Gynecol 1980; 87:1178–1180.

13 Capraro VJ, Bayonet-Rivera NP, Magoss I. Vulvur tumor in children due to prolapse of urethral mucosa. Am J Obstet Gynecol 1970; 108(4):572–575.

14 Block RE. Hydrocele of the canal of Nuck. A report of five cases. Obstet Gynecol 1975; 45(4):464–466.

15 Cleary RE, Spadoni LR, Herrmann WL. Unilateral labial swelling: patent canal of Nuck and ascites. Gynecologia 1968; 166; 461–465.

16 van der Putte, SCJ. Review: Mammary-like glands of the vulva and their disorders. Int J Gynecol Pathol 1994; 13:150–160.

17 van der Putte SCJ. Anogenital 'sweat' glands: histology and pathology of a gland that may mimic mammary glands. Am J Dermatopathol 1991; 13:557–565.

18 Castro CY, Deavers M. Ductal carcinoma in-situ arising in mammary-like glands of the vulva. Int J Gynecol Pathol 2001; 20(3):277–283.

19 Neuman I, Strauss HG, Buchmann J, Koelbl H. Ectopic lobular breast cancer of the vulva. Anticancer Res 2000; 20:4805–4808.

20 Yin C, Chapman J, Tawfik O. Invasive mucinous (colloid) adenocarcinoma of ectopic breast tissue in the vulva: a case report. Breast J 2003; 9(2):113.

21 Sington JD, Manek S, Hollowood K. Fibroadenoma of the mammary-like glands of the vulva. Histopathology 2002; 41:563–565.

22 Irvin WP, Cathro HP, Grosh WW, et al. Case report: primary breast carcinoma of the vulva: a case report and literature review. Gynecol Oncol 1999; 73:155–159.

23 Curtin WM, Murthy B. Vulvar metastasis of breast carcinoma. A case report. J Reprod Med 1997; 42(1):61–63.

24 Miliaras D. Breast-like cancer of the vulva: primary or metastatic? A case report and review of the literature. Eur J Gynaecol Oncol 2002; 23(4):350–352.

25 Katz Z, Goldchmit R, Blickstein I. Post-traumatic vulvar endometriosis. Eur J Pediatr Surg. 1996; 6(4):241–242.

26 Gocmen A, Inaloz HS, Sari I, Inaloz SS. Endometriosis in the Bartholin gland. Eur J Obstet Gynecol Reprod Biol 2004; 114(1):110–111.

27 Bolis GB, Maccio T. Related clear cell adenocarcinoma of the vulva arising in endometriosis. A case report. Eur J Gynaecol Oncol 2000; 21(4):416–417.

28 Irvin W, Pelkey T, Rice L, Andersen W. Endometrial stromal sarcoma of the vulva arising in extraovarian endometriosis: a case report and literature review. Gynecol Oncol 1998; 71(2):313–316.

29 Meeker JH, Neubecker RD, Helwig EB. Hidradenoma papilliferum. Am J Clin Pathol 1962; 37:182–195.

30 Veraldi S, Schianchi-Veraldi R, Marini D. Hidradenoma papilliferum of the vulva: report of a case characterized by unusual clinical behavior. J Dermatol Surg Oncol 1990; 16:674–676.

31 Virgili A, Marzola A, Corazza M. Vulvar hidradenoma papilliferum. A review of 10.5 years' experience. J Reprod Med 2000; 45(8):616–618.

32 Basta A, Madej JG. Hydradenoma of the vulva: incidence and clinical observations. Eur J Gynaecol Oncol 1990; 11:185–189.

33 Hobbs JE. Tumors of the vulva and vagina. Sweat gland tumors. Clin Obstet Gynecol 1965; 8(4):946–952.

34 Meeker JH, Neubecker, RD, Helwig, EB. Hidradenoma papilliferum. Am J Clin Pathol 1962; 37:182–195.

35 Woodworth H, Dockerty M, Wilson RB, et al. Papillary hidradenoma of the vulva: a clinicopathologic study of 69 cases. Am J Obstet Gynecol 1971; 110:501–508.

36 Weedon D. Eccrine tumors: a selective review. J Cutan Pathol 1984; 11:421–436.

37 Soler-Carrillo J, Estrach T, Mascaro JM. Eruptive syringoma: 27 new cases and review of the literature. J Eur Acad Dermatol Venereol 2001; 15(3):242–246.

38 Di Lernia V, Bisighini G. Localized vulvar syringomas. Pediatr Dermatol 1996; 13(1):80–81.

39 Huang YH, Chuang YH, Kuo TT, Yang LC, Hong HS. Vulvar syringoma: a clinicopathologic and immunohistologic study of 18 patients and results of treatment. J Am Acad Dermatol 2003; 48(5):735–739.

40 Young AW Jr, Herman EW, Tovell HM. Syringoma of the vulva: incidence, diagnosis, and cause of pruritis. Obstet Gynecol 1980; 55(4):515–518.

41 Bal N, Aslan E, Kayaselcuk F, Tarim, Tuncer I. Vulvar syringoma aggravated by pregnancy. Pathol Oncol Res 2003; 9(3):196–197.

42 Turan C, Ugur M, Kutluay, et al. Vulvar syringoma exacerbated during pregnancy. Eur J Obstet Gynecol Reprod Biol 1996; 64(1):141–142.

43 Frurue M, Hori Y, Nakabayashi Y. Clear cell syringoma: association with diabetes mellitus. Am J Dermatopathol 1984; 6:131–138.

44 Vlastos, A-T, Malpica A, Follen M. Lymphangioma circumscriptum of the vulva: a review of the literature. Obstet Gynecol 2003; 101:946–954.

45 Rongioletti F, Cattarini G, Romanelli P. Late onset vulvar steatocystoma multiplex. Clin Exp Dermatol 2002; 27:445–447.

46 Koenig C, Tavassoli FA. Nodular hyperplasia, adenoma, and adenomyoma of Bartholin's gland. Int J Gynecol Pathol 1998; 17(4):289–294.

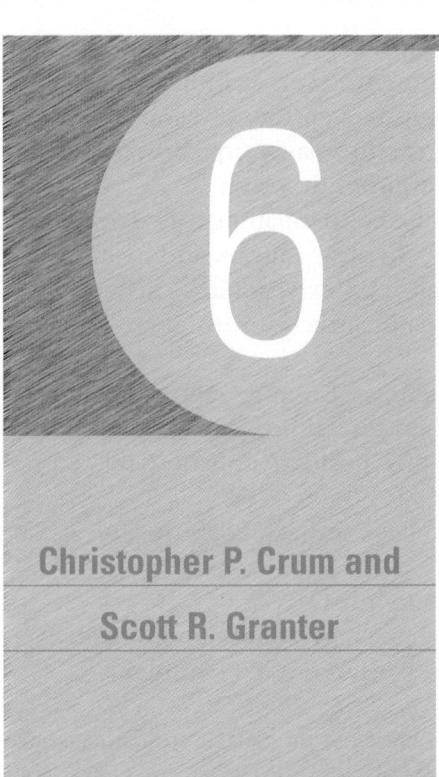

6

Squamous neoplasia of the vulva

Christopher P. Crum and

Scott R. Granter

Introduction

Condyloma acuminatum

Introduction and risk factors
Clinical presentation
Histopathology
Differential diagnosis
Biomarkers and diagnosis of
    condyloma
Natural history and management

**Defining vulvar intraepithelial
neoplasia**

**Classic vulvar intraepithelial
neoplasia**

Introduction
The patient at risk
Clinical presentation
Histopathologic findings
Differential diagnosis
Biomarkers
Natural history and outcome
Clinical management

**Differentiated (simplex) vulvar
intraepithelial neoplasia**

Introduction
Clinical presentation
Pathologic findings

Differential diagnosis
Biomarkers
Natural history and management

**Other intraepithelial alterations
of potential significance**

Introduction
Histologic patterns

**Diagnostic terminology for
preinvasive vulvar disease**

Squamous cell carcinoma

Clinical presentation
Criteria for diagnosis of invasion
Growth patterns of carcinoma
Differential diagnosis of invasive
    squamous carcinoma

**Superficially invasive
(microinvasive) squamous
cell carcinoma**

Introduction
Definition
Other studies of early invasive
    carcinoma
Management

Basal cell carcinoma

Introduction

Squamous cancer of the vulva is a relatively uncommon disease with an incidence of approximately 1.8 per 100 000, increasing significantly after age 75, to 20 per 100 000.[1,2] Approximately 5% occur in women under age 40.[1] In the past 40 years, the incidence of invasive vulvar cancer has remained essentially unchanged, while that of preinvasive disease has increased several-fold.[2,3] This highlights the importance of sexual transmission in the genesis of the latter, while the pathway to invasion entails additional risk factors. These include chronic vulvar inflammatory disorders, smoking, immune status and increasing age.[4–6] This range of risk factors identifies vulvar carcinoma as a disease with at least two major pathogenetic routes which are distinct, yet share certain features (Fig. 6.1).

The first route is strongly linked to human papillomavirus (HPV) infection, associates with 40% of vulvar cancers and includes:

1 Association with HPV exposure or history of STDs[7]
2 Slightly younger age group than HPV-negative tumors (average seventh decade)[7–9]
3 Tendency for multifocality or association with cervical neoplasia[10]
4 Share certain cytogenetic characteristics with cervical carcinomas, including amplification at 3p25-27 and papillomaviral genomic integration[11]
5 Association with smoking[7–9]

6 Preceded by 'classic VIN', which is identical in appearance to high grade cervical intraepithelial neoplasia and comprises entities previously termed Bowen's disease, carcinoma *in situ*, Bowenoid papulosis and Bowenoid dysplasia.[6]

The second route is linked to inflammatory dermatoses, associates with 60% of vulvar cancers and includes:

1 Pre-existing lichen simplex chronicus, lichen sclerosus and other acanthoses with altered differentiation[12]
2 Slightly older mean age (average eighth decade)[8]
3 Lower risk of other genital primary neoplasms[10]
4 Association with p53 positivity, possibly related to mutations[12]
5 Association with allelic imbalance in the vulvar mucosa[13,14]
6 Lack of association with HPV[15]
7 Preceded in many cases by atypias involving the above dermatoses (differentiated (simplex) VIN).[12,16]

Importantly, vulvar cancers in both categories share some common features:

1 Reports of HPV-positive neoplasms associated with lichen sclerosus[13,16,17]
2 Relatively small differences in mean age (10 years), indicating a role for increasing age in the pathogenesis of both
3 Both are uncommon despite the high rate of HPV infection in the population.

Whatever the factors involved, vulvar carcinomas comprise a heterogeneous morphologic group. Figure 6.2 depicts selected fields from several vulvar tumors and illustrates the wide range of epithelial alterations that are associated with or precede invasive carcinoma of the vulva. The reader can appreciate that the subsequent effort to subdivide these tumors into discrete groups will necessarily ignore potential pathways that remain to be more clearly delineated in the future. Table 6.1 lists some of the common findings associated with vulvar cancers, not all of which are specific.

In practice, the management of vulvar squamous neoplasia centers on the following:

1 Identification and removal of genital warts in young women
2 Identification and classification of preinvasive (vulvar intraepithelial neoplasia) disease
3 Classification and management of early invasive squamous cell carcinoma
4 Recognition and proper management of squamous carcinoma variants, including verrucous carcinoma.

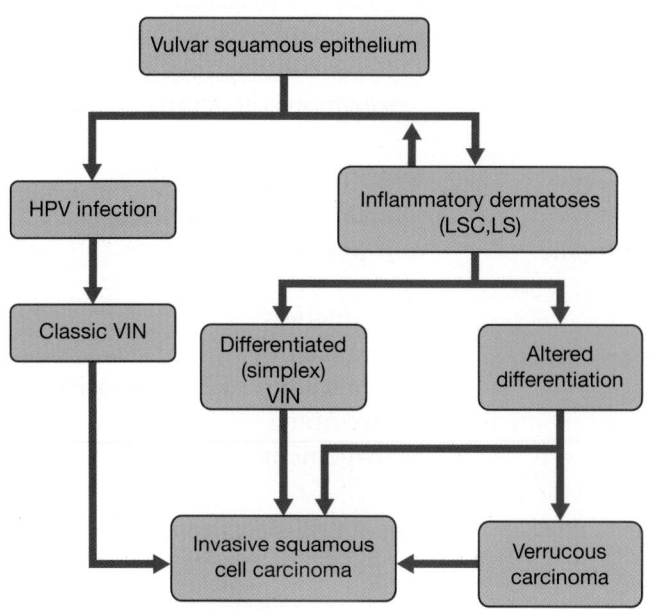

Fig. 6.1 Pathogenetic routes to vulvar cancer.

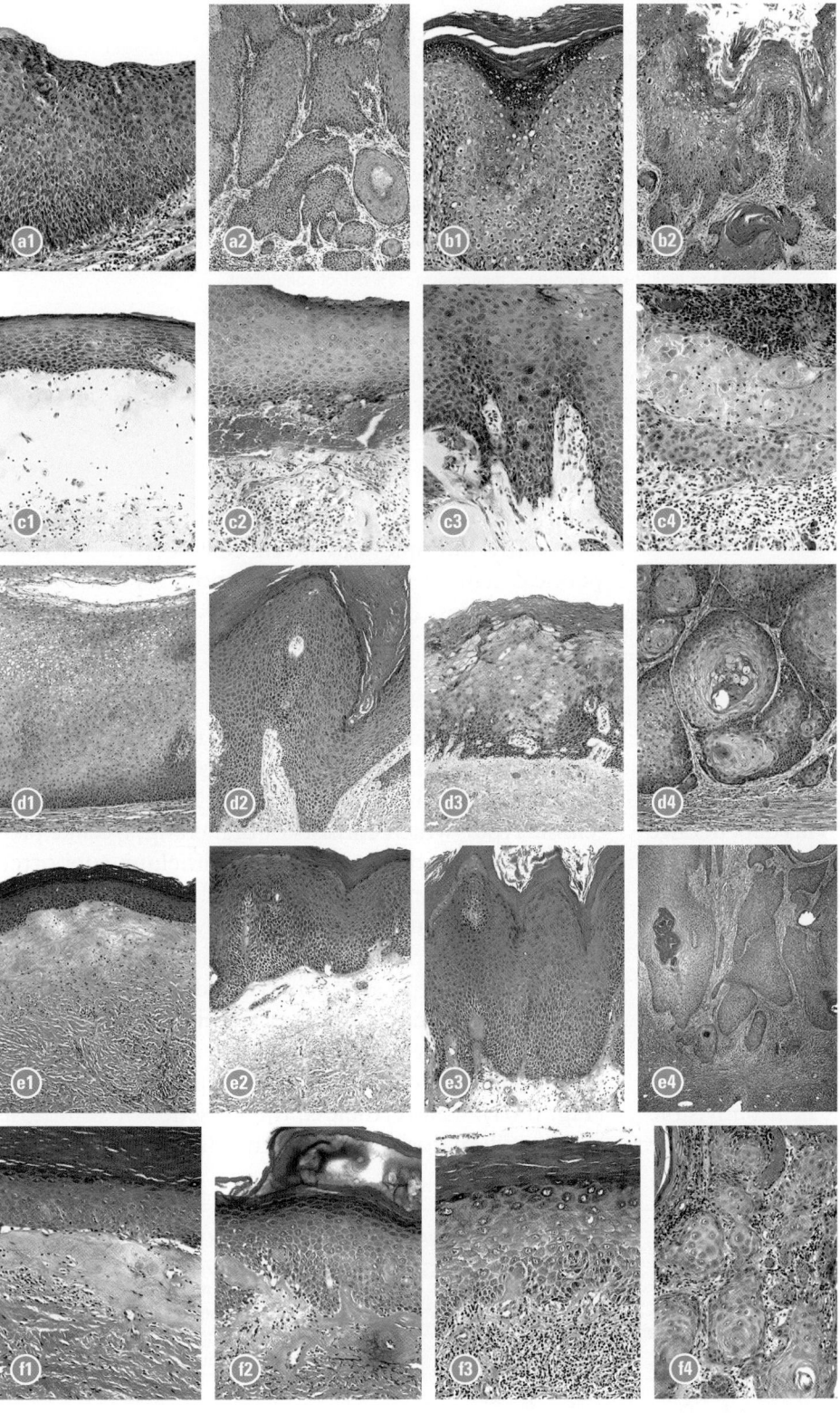

Fig. 6.2 Morphologic spectra seen in vulvar cancer, beginning from non-invasive epithelium (left) to invasive carcinoma (right), are depicted in the following cases and may include the following: (a) Classic VIN (1) and well-differentiated squamous carcinoma (2). (b) Classic VIN (1) and 'warty' carcinoma (2). (c) Lichen sclerosus (1), with superimposed acanthosis (2), classic VIN (3) and keratinizing squamous carcinoma (4). (d) Acanthosis (1), verruciform lichen simplex chronicus (2), acanthosis with altered differentiation (3) and well-differentiated carcinoma (4). (e) Lichen sclerosus (1), with superimposed lichen simplex chronicus (2), verruciform lichen simplex chronicus (3) and well-differentiated carcinoma (4). (f) Lichen sclerosus (1), superimposed lichen simplex chronicus (2), differentiated VIN (3) and invasive carcinoma (4). HPV is associated with a–c, whereas d–f are HPV-negative pathways.

Table 6.1 *Common findings in vulvar neoplasia*

Finding	Fig(s)	Ref(s)	Association with vulvar cancer
Lichen sclerosus (LS)	2	12,15	1–4% risk of vulvar cancer on follow-up, high concurrent association
Lichen simplex chronicus (LSC)	2	15,115	Little prospective data, high concurrent association
LS with LSC	2,23	75	Increased risk
Verrucous LSC	2,23	76	No prospective data, high concurrent association
Differentiated VIN	2,19,20	15	Little prospective data, high concurrent association
Classic VIN	12	61,62	High risk in untreated women at menopause, 19% risk of concurrent invasion
Condyloma	5–8	7	Retrospective association only. Association with regressing VIN
Vulvar acanthoses with altered differentiation	24	76	No prospective data; concurrent association with well-differentiated (including verrucous) carcinomas

Condyloma Acuminatum

INTRODUCTION AND RISK FACTORS

Condylomata acuminata are extremely common sexually transmitted, benign tumors that are most common in the early years of sexual activity and afflict approximately 1 million women yearly. Approximately 80% are associated with HPV type 6 or (less commonly) 11.[18]

The virus life cycle is completed in the epithelium, specifically the mature superficial cells. This dependence of viral growth on squamous maturation is typical of HPV and produces a distinct cytologic change in the mature cells – koilocytotic atypia (nuclear atypia and perinuclear vacuolization) – that is considered a viral 'cytopathic' effect (Fig. 6.3).[19]

CLINICAL PRESENTATION

They may range in presentation from nearly invisible maculopapillary lesions in the introitus to extensive disease involving the entire vulva. They are more frequently multiple and often coalesce; they involve perineal, vulvar and perianal regions as well as the vagina and, less commonly, the cervix (Fig. 6.4).[20]

HISTOPATHOLOGY

Condylomata may present in several forms, several of which may coexist in the same lesion and all of which are associated with HPV types 6/11.[18] The first is the 'classic type', which consists of branching, treelike proliferation of stratified squamous epithelium supported by a fibrous stroma (Fig. 6.5). Acanthosis, parakeratosis, hyperkeratosis and, most specifically, nuclear atypia in the surface cells with perinuclear vacuolization (called koilocytosis) are present. The second presentation, and one that is frequent, consists of the above features without conspicuous cytopathic change. Such lesions may call to mind the diagnosis of 'fibroepithelial papilloma' (Fig. 6.6a).[21] Nevertheless, the presence of acanthosis and papillomatosis warrants the diagnosis of condy-

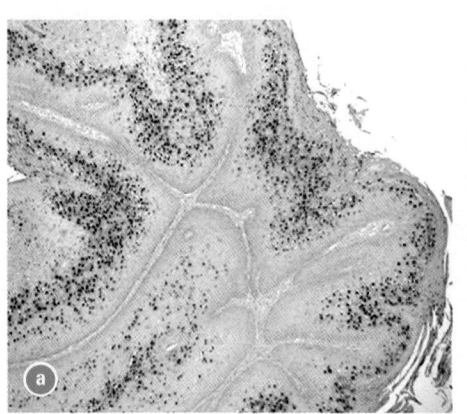 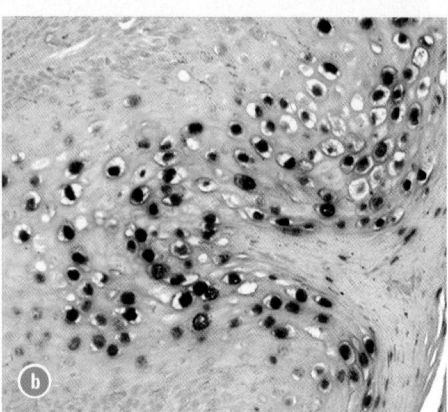

Fig. 6.3 Localization of low-risk HPV nucleic acids in a condyloma. (a) Low-power photomicrograph shows a predominate distribution in upper cell layers. (b) Most intense staining in superficial keratinocytes, including koilocytes. (Courtesy of Lisa Jensen-Long, Ventana Medical Systems.)

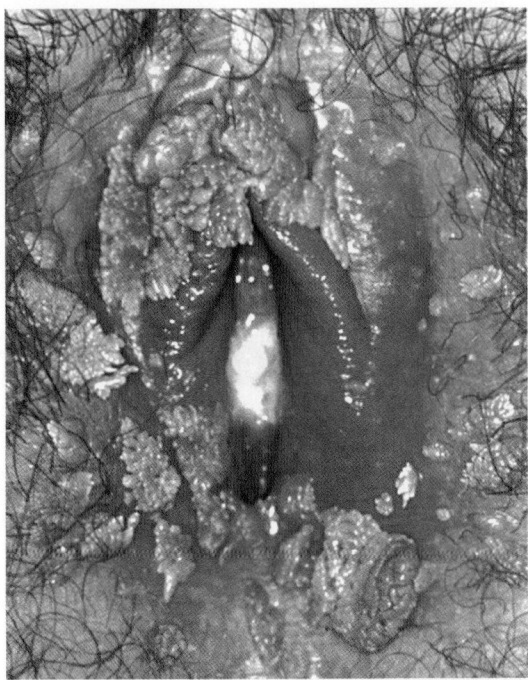

Fig. 6.4 Clinical appearance of vulvar condylomata, including multiple discrete lesions. (Courtesy of Alex Ferenczy.)

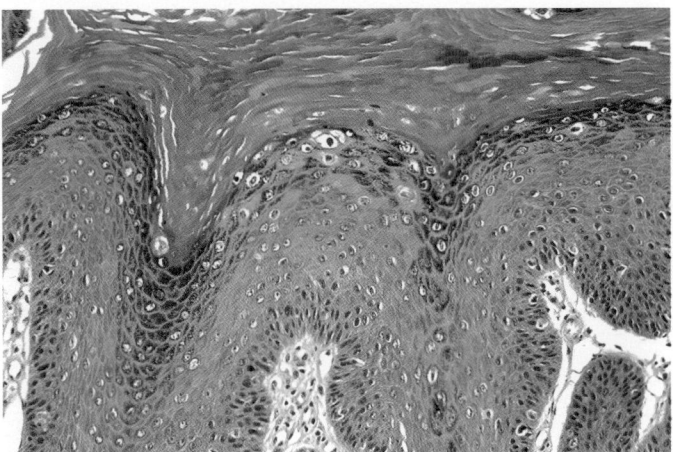

Fig. 6.5 Classic microscopic appearance of condyloma. This image illustrates the papillomatosis, hyperkeratosis and focal koilocytotic atypia that characterizes these lesions. Note the absence of atypia in the lower third of the epithelium.

loma by virtue of the strong association with HPV.[15] The third presentation closely resembles a seborrheic keratosis, with a prominent homogeneous population of basaloid cells, horn cysts and inconspicuous koilocytosis (Fig. 6.6b). This subset differs from cutaneous seborrheic keratosis by the strong association with HPV 6 nucleic acids.[22,23] The fourth category consists of flat lesions, either flat condyloma or discrete foci of mild acanthosis with minimal nuclear atypia (Fig. 6.7).

An unusual variant of condyloma is characterized by a striking increase in apoptosis in the upper epithelial layers, resulting in multiple cells in various stages of degeneration, beginning with chromatin dispersal (pseudomitoses) and ending with small condensed

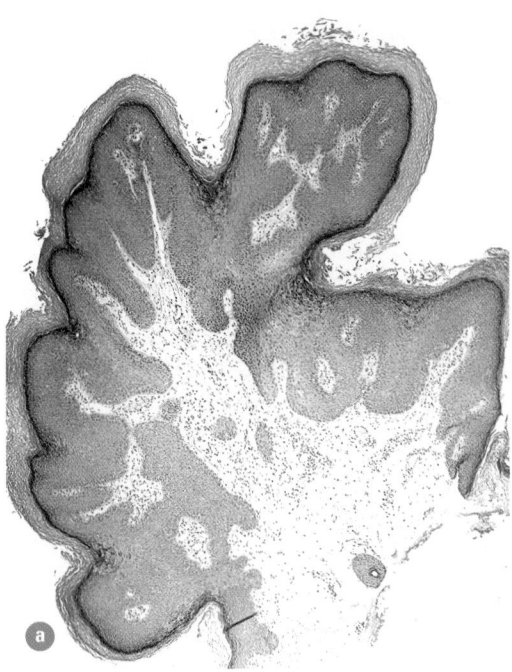

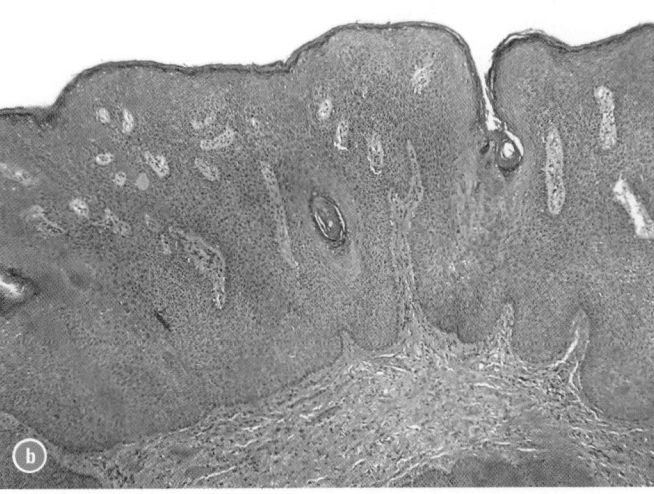

Fig. 6.6 Vulvar condylomata may exhibit a range of appearances, including (a) fibroepithelial papillomas and (b) seborrheic keratosis-like lesions.

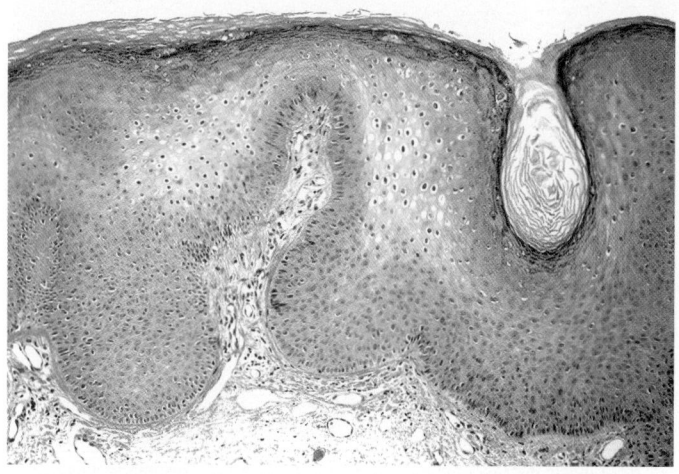

Fig. 6.7 HPV-positive papular lesion. Such lesions are typically discrete and resemble small seborrheic keratoses.

eosinophilic bodies derived from shrunken cytoplasm. This variant closely resembles oral epithelial hyperplasia of Hecht and has been termed 'pseudoBowenoid papulosis' (Fig. 6.8a,b).[24-26] This variant is not associated with the common genital HPV types in our experience and has been associated with HPV 13 and 32 in some reports of cutaneous lesions.[27]

A proportion of genital condylomata may resemble cutaneous warts, raising the question of a cutaneous papillomavirus infection. Although the majority of these lesions will contain genital HPV types, cutaneous HPVs may be present.[21] This will be addressed later under pediatric condylomata.

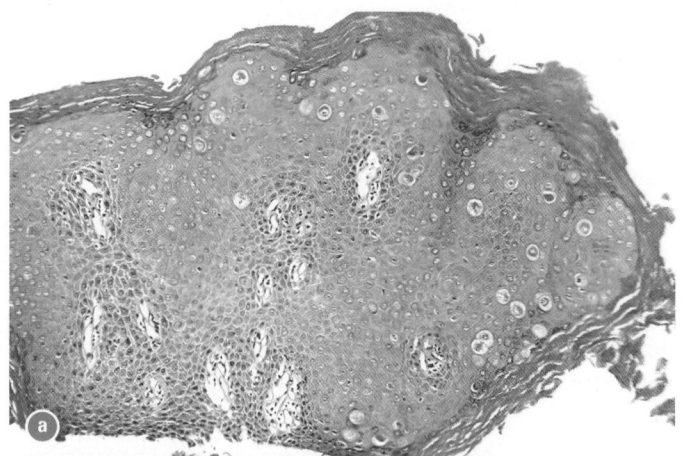

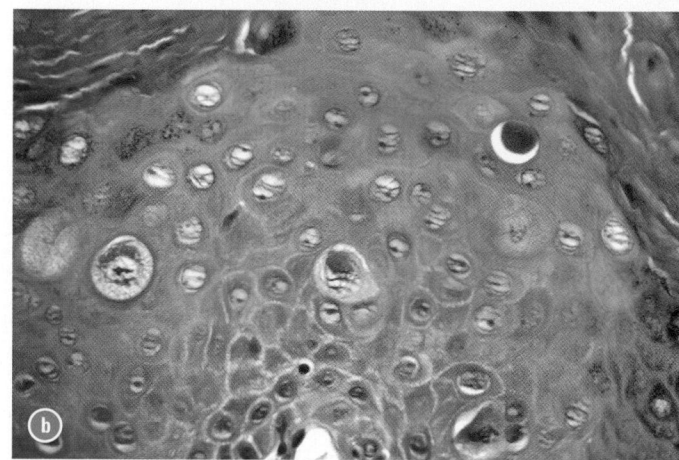

Fig. 6.8 (a,b) PseudoBowenoid papulosis. This variant of condyloma has the characteristic architecture of a condyloma with minimal atypia in the lower epithelium; however, the superficial cells exhibit minimal koilocytosis and are distinguished by various stages of apoptosis, including pseudomitoses (center). (c) Basal epithelial cells exhibit minimal atypia.

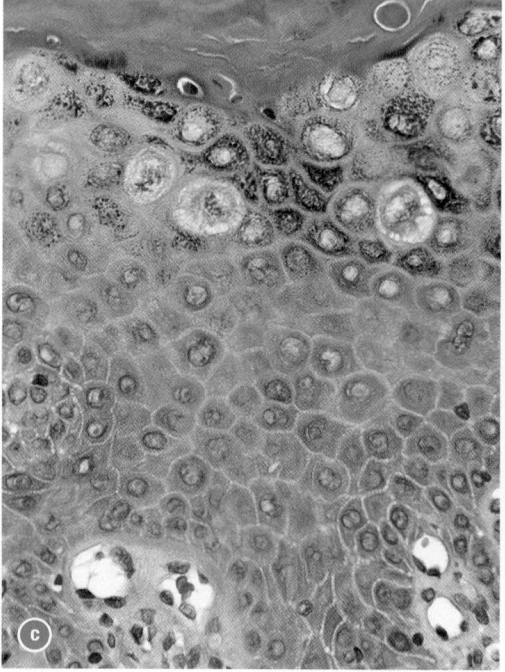

DIFFERENTIAL DIAGNOSIS

The differential diagnosis of condyloma includes a range of verruciform lesions, which is discussed in greater detail below and summarized in Table 6.2. The most common mimic is the fibroepithelial mucosal polyp. In the introitus or distal vagina, these are essentially mucosal folds that are the remnants of the hymenal ring (Fig. 6.9a–c).[28] Vulvar lesions are similar and lesions are distinguished by minimal acanthosis and usually score negative for HPV (Fig. 6.9d). Nonetheless, some of these lesions are HPV positive, underscoring the difficulty in consistently distinguishing condyloma from polyps. Ultimately, with the exception of children, for whom the question of sexual abuse or exposure must be excluded, and the potential stigma of a sexually transmitted disease, the practical distinction of a low-risk HPV infection from a non-infectious polyp is not critical. One exception is the distinction of introital condylomata from hymenal ring, particularly if a misdiagnosis precipitates treatment that is painful and unnecessary (Fig. 6.9).[29,30] For this reason, the management of introital condylomas in young women – most of which will regress spontaneously – should be conducted with care. A third mimic is pronounced polynucleated atypias associated with non-specific vulvar inflammatory changes (see below).[31]

These conditions are characterized by multiple (2–15), normal-sized nuclei associated with mild acanthosis. The atypia may be seen in both the lower and upper epithelial layers and must be distinguished from both condyloma and vulvar intraepithelial neoplasia. The presence of multiple nuclei, their similarity in appearance to the nuclei in adjacent cells and the absence of hyperchromasia and nuclear enlargement support this benign variant, which is analogous to non-specific cutaneous inflammatory changes.[32]

As will be discussed subsequently, the diagnosis of condyloma based on acanthosis, papillomatosis and hyperkeratosis should be made with care if these changes are accompanied by more pronounced nuclear atypia, abnormalities in squamous differentiation and a clinical history of vulvar inflammatory dermatoses. Concerning the latter, particular care must be taken in older women with limited samples, in which case a vulvar neoplasm must be excluded.

BIOMARKERS AND DIAGNOSIS OF CONDYLOMA

Normal squamous mucosa undergoes progressive maturation with cessation of cell cycle activity. The latter concentrates in the cells immediately above the basal layer (transient amplifying cells) and is absent in the

Table 6.2 Differential diagnosis of verruciform lesions of the vulva

Diagnosis	Fig.	Atypia	Comment
Condyloma	5	Variable koilocytosis	No atypia in lower two-thirds of the epithelium
Fibroepithelial papilloma	6	Mild surface karyomegaly	Similar to condyloma but lacks koilocytosis
Seborrheic keratosis	6	None	Resembles cutaneous SK, may have rare koilocytosis.
PseudoBowenoid papulosis	8	0	Prominent apoptosis with 'pseudomitoses'
Fibroepithelial stromal polyp	9	None, except stromal	Minimal acanthosis
Verruciform lichen simplex chronicus	23	None	Preservation of keratohyalin granules
Vulvar acanthosis with altered differentiation	24	None	Surface pallor, parakeratosis
Verrucous carcinoma	29	0–1+	Minimal surface or interface atypia; uniform invasion
Verruciform squamous cell carcinoma	28	1–2+ surface and interface	Atypia may be minimal in some cases but irregular invasive growth should be present
Keratoacanthoma	33	+	Slight interface atypia, pseudoepitheliomatous appearance
Classic vulvar intraepithelial neoplasia	11	+++	High-grade nuclear changes with variable verruciform growth
Papillary squamous carcinoma	30	+++	Uniformly demarcated but disordered epithelial growth (intraepithelial carcinoma)

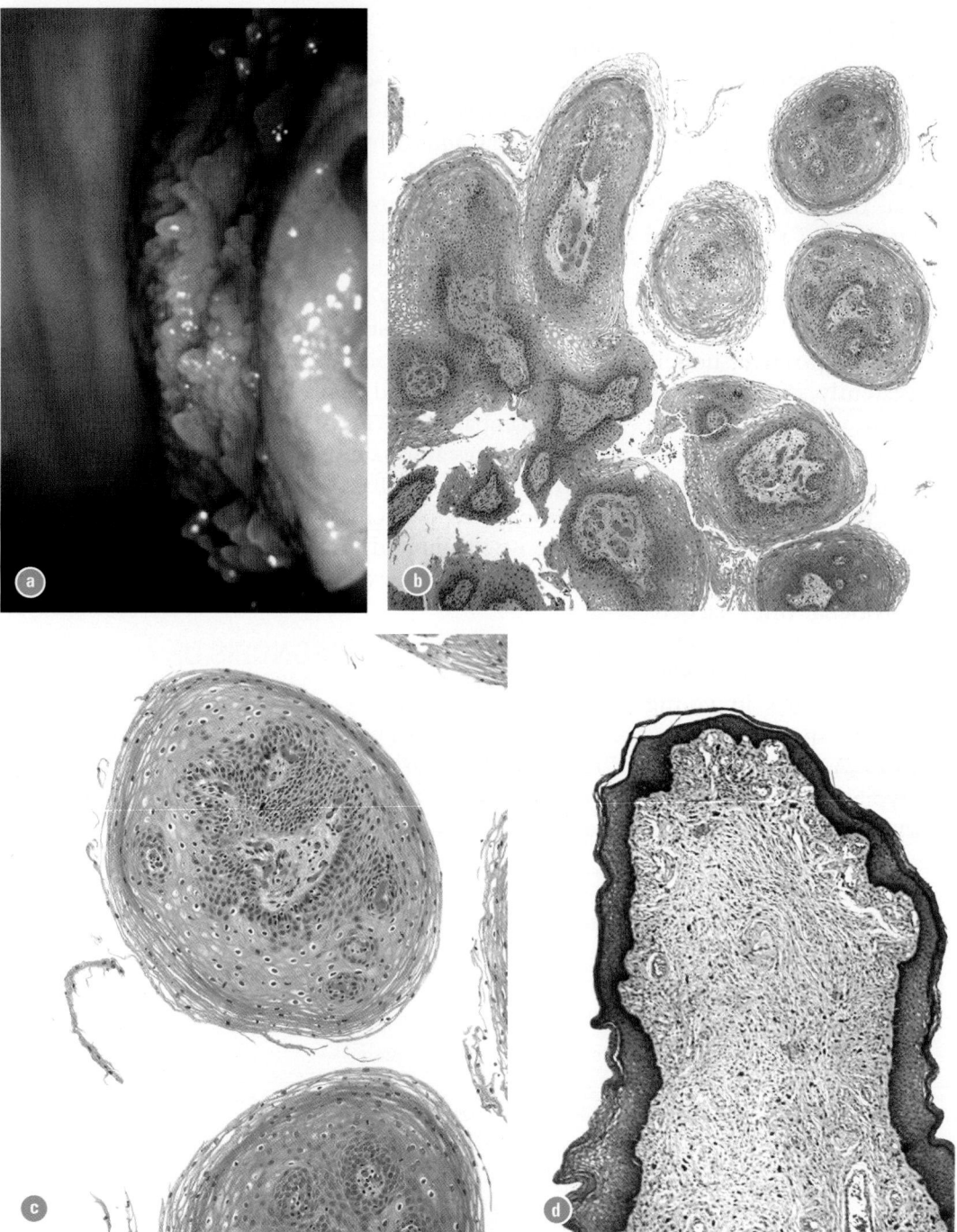

Fig. 6.9 Differential diagnosis of condyloma. (a,b) Introital (hymenal) mucosal folds lack acanthosis or atypia. (c,d) Fibroepithelial stromal polyps.

upper half of the epithelium. Human papillomavirus infections result in the induction of viral replication and reciprocal cell cycle activation as a function of cell maturation. Consequently, markers for proliferation will score positive in the upper cell layers. Several studies have established increased proliferative activity in the upper layers and have proposed the use of Ki-67 (MIB-1) as a marker to distinguish non-HPV from HPV-related lesions (Fig. 6.10).[22,33,34] However, a minority of HPV-positive lesions will score positive.[22] Another option is either HPV *in situ* hybridization or polymerase chain reaction amplification of extracted DNA. It should be emphasized that the demonstration of HPV serves relatively little purpose from the standpoint of management although confirmation of a genital virus may be required to shed light on the cause of genital lesions in children.

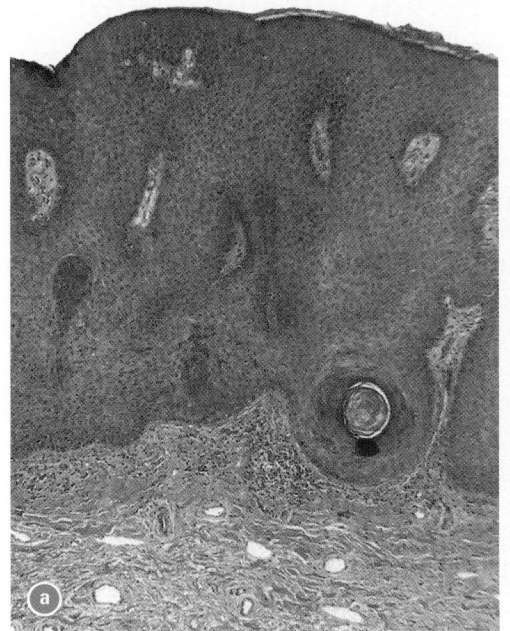
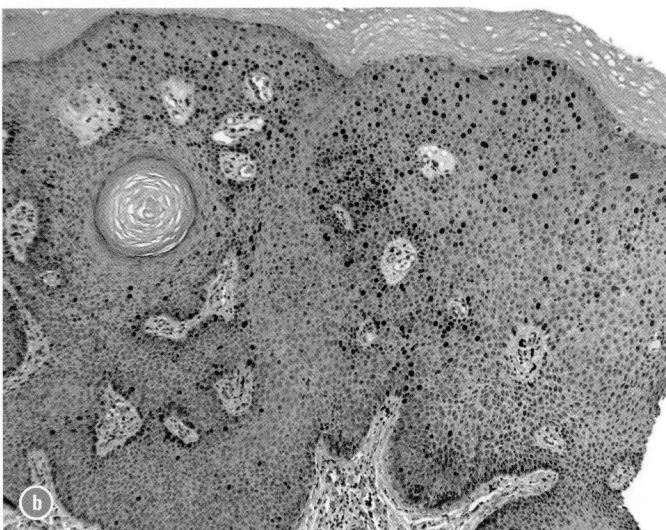

Fig. 6.10
Biomarkers in the diagnosis of condyloma. (a) Seborrheic keratosis-like condyloma. (b) Staining of MIB-1 is distributed in the upper and lower cell layers in contrast to non-infected mucosa.

NATURAL HISTORY AND MANAGEMENT

Condylomata typically fulminate within 6 weeks of infection and regress over the ensuing months.[34,35] In a minority of cases, the lesions will persist. For this reason, immediate treatment may or may not be successful and should be conservative. Small condylomata in teenagers may be best managed by addressing coexisting infections (*Candida*), with follow-up in 3–6 months. Care should be taken in treating small introital lesions, particularly with attention to avoiding treatments (such as 5-fluorouracil (5-FU)) that could produce long-standing irritation and dyspareunia. Larger lesions may be treated by topical agents (Aldara (imiquimod)) or cryotherapy and, if extensive, carbon dioxide laser.[36-38]

Pediatric complications of HPV infection

Genital warts

Genital warts can occur at any point in infancy and childhood. The potential mechanisms of transmission include vertical (during birth), casual contact and sexual abuse. Spontaneous regression occurs in approximately one-half.[39] Although the principal concern imposed by genital wart virus infection in the pediatric population is sexual abuse, HPV infection does not correlate closely with abuse.[40] Moscicki reported that HPV types 16/18 were more commonly seen in infections that were presumed vertical (neonates and infants), whereas genital warts later in childhood were due to HPVs 6/11.[41] Even in the latter case, modes of transmission other than sexual abuse have been proposed.[42]

While the detection of HPV has been reported in the absence of abuse, abused children clearly have a higher frequency of HPV infection than controls. Studies have documented that while the frequency of HPV infection in abused children between 4 and 12 years (those without obvious warts) is low (10–16%), it is significantly higher than in non-abused individuals (0%).[43] Nevertheless, HPV testing is of questionable value unless abuse is highly suspected. A proportion of genital infections have been associated with HPV2 (~15%), with the majority (75%) belonging to the common genital types 6 and 11 (Table 6.3).

Stevens-Simon et al. proposed the following criteria for sexual abuse: (1) The child discloses that abuse has occurred under appropriate interview. (2) A physical examination discloses genital trauma characteristic of

Table 6.3 Percentage of low and high risk HPV types associated with genital lesions[21,33]

Lesion	n	LR	:	HR
Vulvar condyloma	34	97	:	3
VIN 1	11	70	:	30
VAIN 1	19	16	:	84
VIN 3	6	0	:	100

LR = low risk HPV, VIN = vulvar intraepithelial neoplasia, HR = high risk HPV, VAIN = vaginal intraepithelial neoplasia.

abuse. (3) Other sexually transmitted diseases are present. (4) A perpetrator admits to abuse. (5) A credible witness observed abuse to occur. (6) A forensic examination reveals semen, sperm or acid phosphatase from genital fluids.[43]

In summary, a careful history and examination are warranted when children present with genital warts. However, sexual abuse will not always be confirmed and HPV testing alone is unlikely to resolve this question.

Respiratory papillomatosis

Respiratory papillomatosis (laryngeal papillomas) is an uncommon chronic papillomavirus infection in children, associated with HPV 6 or 11 and affecting between 3 and 4 offspring per 100 000 births. It is the most common laryngeal infection in children, associated with voice changes, hoarseness, choking and failure to thrive.[44,45] Approximately 30% extend beyond the larynx, and the risk of malignant transformation is estimated at 5%. Deaths are rare, but the disease is chronic, often necessitating numerous procedures to maintain the airway, including tracheotomy in up to 14% of cases with juvenile onset.[45] The risk factors vary between studies. Shah et al. noted a strong relationship between juvenile papillomatosis and a lower incidence of Cesarean births (4.6-fold less); first-order births (1.6-fold higher) and younger (<20 years) maternal age (2.6-fold greater). The impression from these statistics is that laryngeal papillomas are transmitted at birth via contact with an infected genital canal, particularly in younger women. The latter would suggest a shorter interval between exposure to HPV and birth, implying insufficient time to generate protective antibodies.[46] In a recent study from Denmark, Silverberg et al. observed a strong association between laryngeal papillomas and maternal genital warts during pregnancy, with a risk of 7 per 1000 live births. The authors estimated that the relative risk imposed by concurrent genital warts in the mother was 231-fold.[44] Additional risk factors included a non-cohabiting father and longer delivery time (>10 h). The former was considered to increase the risk of additional exposures during pregnancy and the latter to increase contact between mother and fetus during labor. Despite the latter, Cesarean section offered minimal protection (RR = 0.86). However, it is conceivable that infection can occur in the interval from membrane rupture and surgery. Whether the virus can ascend through intact membranes to infect the fetus is controversial.[44]

Defining vulvar intraepithelial neoplasia

Because cancer of the vulva comprises several pathogenetic routes, it is predictable that a range of precursor lesions exists, each with its own morphologic appearance. In 1965, Kaufmann and Gardner grouped precancers into three categories, corresponding to erythroplasia of Queyrat, Bowenoid carcinoma *in situ* and carcinoma simplex.[47] They were distinguished by the presence of disordered epithelial growth, which usually involved the entire thickness of the epithelium with loss of cellular polarity, enlarged and multinucleated cells, hyperchromatism and dyskeratosis. Carcinoma *in situ* simplex designated lesions in which nuclear atypia was most conspicuous in the lower portions of the epithelium while the surface layers maintained squamous maturation and only minor atypia.[12] The criteria for the first category are relatively well defined and essentially define HPV16 infections of the vulva. However, the reader is cautioned that the second category of preinvasive disease is less well understood. This is in part due to the fact that while HPV induces clear-cut changes in cell biology, the morphologic changes that accompany progressive host gene mutations in the absence of HPV infection are more subtle and may not be associated with pronounced atypia. In the latter instances, more subtle alterations, such as defects in differentiation, or mild alterations in nuclear morphology, may predominate. The changes are analogous to those seen associated with sun exposure (actinic keratosis) or tobacco use (oropharyngeal dysplasias). What follows is a description of these categories and their distinguishing features.

Classic vulvar intraepithelial neoplasia

INTRODUCTION

These lesions are called 'classic' vulvar intraepithelial neoplasia (VIN), inasmuch as they exhibit the features typical of HPV-associated lower genital tract squamous precursor disease. This most common group of VIN lesions is morphologically analogous to high-grade squamous intraepithelial lesions (CINII-III) of the cervix. Although classic VIN is less common than cervical intraepithelial neoplasia (CIN), it is strongly associated with HPV, particularly type 16, which is isolated from nearly 70% of cases.[16,48] Other HPV types include types 31 and 33. HPV 18 is rarely found in VIN.

THE PATIENT AT RISK

Unlike CIN, VIN typically occurs in slightly older women, with a mean age in the mid-to-late 30s, rather than 10 years earlier.[2,49] Whether this reflects a fundamental difference in epithelial–viral interaction common to vulvar mucosa, or the fact that clinically subtle lesions may be missed by younger patients and their caregivers, is unclear. In any event, these lesions are considerably less commonly appreciated relative to CIN, suggesting that the vulva is not as susceptible to infection in the second and third decades. In recent years, the mean age of women with classic VIN has decreased from over 50 years to under age 40.[2,49] This has been attributed to the higher index of sexual activity in young women and the increased exposure during the reproductive years. However, other factors have been implicated. A strong correlation with smoking, both for classic VIN and HPV-positive vulvar carcinomas, has been reported.[7,8] Immunosuppressed patients are also at risk and may exhibit a range of HPV-related lesions affecting younger women.[50] Importantly, the frequency of VIN in older women appears to have remained relatively constant, suggesting that in the older age group, factors other than HPV exposure may be involved.

CLINICAL PRESENTATION

Classic VINs are more likely to present as discrete abnormalities in the vulvar squamous mucosa. They can appear as small pigmented or hyperkeratotic maculopapular plaque-like lesions, or more extensive, confluent lesions (Fig. 6.11). They may closely resemble condylomata, although they tend to be less discrete and more irregular in their distribution. They may coexist with condylomata, a feature more commonly seen in (but not limited to) immunosuppressed individuals.[50]

HISTOPATHOLOGIC FINDINGS

The diagnosis of classic VIN is based on the presence of nuclear atypia in virtually all layers of the epithelium (Fig. 6.12). Characteristic morphologic findings include nuclear enlargement, hyperchromasia and multinucleation in the lower epithelial layers, often with abnormal mitoses.[51,52] Apoptosis with corp ronds are frequently present. The surface often contains atypical parakeratosis with or without koilocytotic atypia. Kurman et al. subdivided classic VINs into warty and basaloid types, the former being associated with a slightly younger age group.[53] Similarly, certain variants of preinvasive disease, termed Bowenoid papulosis or Bowenoid dysplasia, may exhibit more or less of the above features.[54,55] However, all of these categories display nuclear atypia in the lower third of the epithelium, which distinguishes classic VINs from condylomata.

Skin appendage involvement is common in classic VIN and is analogous to crypt involvement in the cervix (Fig. 6.13).[56,57] The significance of this phenomenon is two-fold. First, it may be confused with superficial invasion if sectioned in a tangential manner. Secondly, it may influence the therapeutic success of treatment methods that target removal of the superficial mucosa, such as laser and topical application of 5-FU (Efudex). However, the latter are employed less commonly now and appendage involvement is not a factor in choice of therapy for classic VIN.

Although it is not specific for VIN, a lichenoid inflammatory infiltrate is commonly associated with these lesions and may demarcate them from the surrounding normal mucosa (Fig. 6.14).

A rare variant of classic VIN is termed pagetoid VIN, in which less well-differentiated squamous cells invade the mature squamous epithelium (Fig. 6.15).[58] The neoplastic cells form a discrete nesting pattern interposed with normal keratinocytes.

DIFFERENTIAL DIAGNOSIS (Fig. 6.16)

The differential diagnosis of classic VIN includes the following: (1) Condylomata with apoptosis (pseudo-Bowenoid papulosis) may mimic VIN by the presence of pseudomitoses and apoptosis (corp ronds) (Fig. 6.16e,f). However, the lower epithelial layers are bland in appearance.[24] (2) Multinucleated atypias involving the lower epithelial layers may mimic VIN; however, the lack of atypia in the multinucleated cells distinguishes this from VIN (Fig. 6.16a–c).[31] (3) Seborrheic keratosis-like condylomata are composed of immature squamous cells but lack atypia and are usually easily distinguished from VIN.[22,23] In rare instances, other neoplasms may mimic VIN. Rare reports have described vulvar mucosal involvement by urothelial neoplasia, which may be confused with either VIN or Paget's

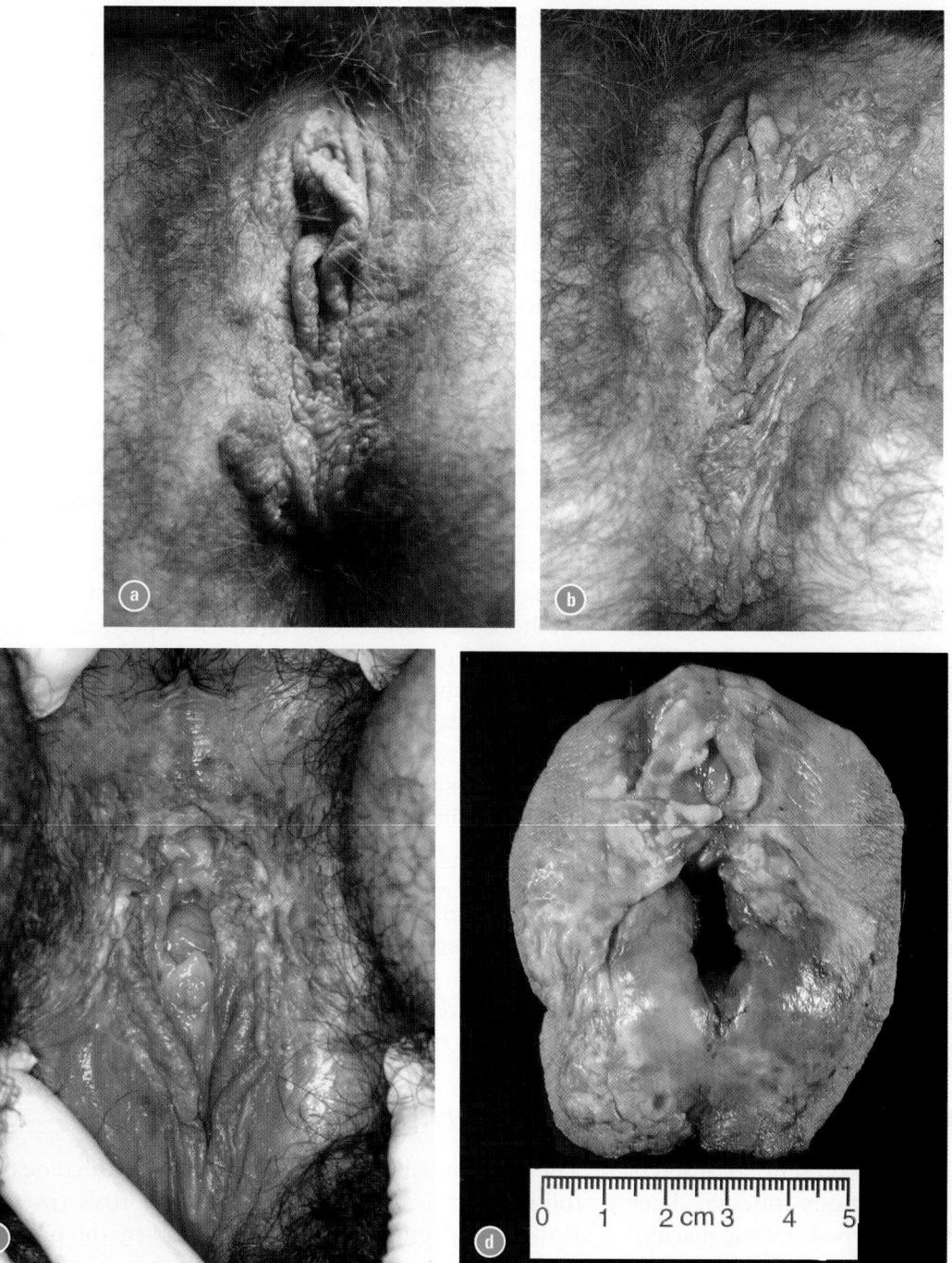

Fig. 6.11 Clinical presentations of classic vulvar intraepithelial neoplasia. (a,b) Raised irregular lesions with variable hyperkeratosis; (c) more macular pigmented VIN. (d) Simple vulvectomy specimen with extensive VIN.

disease (see Chapter 7).[59] (4) Rarely, herpes-zoster-like lesions may mimic VIN, particularly when multinucleated cells are conspicuous but inclusions are not (Fig. 6.16d).

BIOMARKERS

Studies have shown strong staining for p16 and diffuse staining for Ki-67, similar to cervical intraepithelial neoplasia. The former will distinguish classic VIN from most conventional and seborrheic keratosis-like condylomata (Fig. 6.17).[60] However, special stains are generally not required to distinguish classic forms of VIN from their mimics.

NATURAL HISTORY AND OUTCOME

Few reports exist with follow-up data on untreated VIN. Jones et al. followed 31 treated and 5 untreated

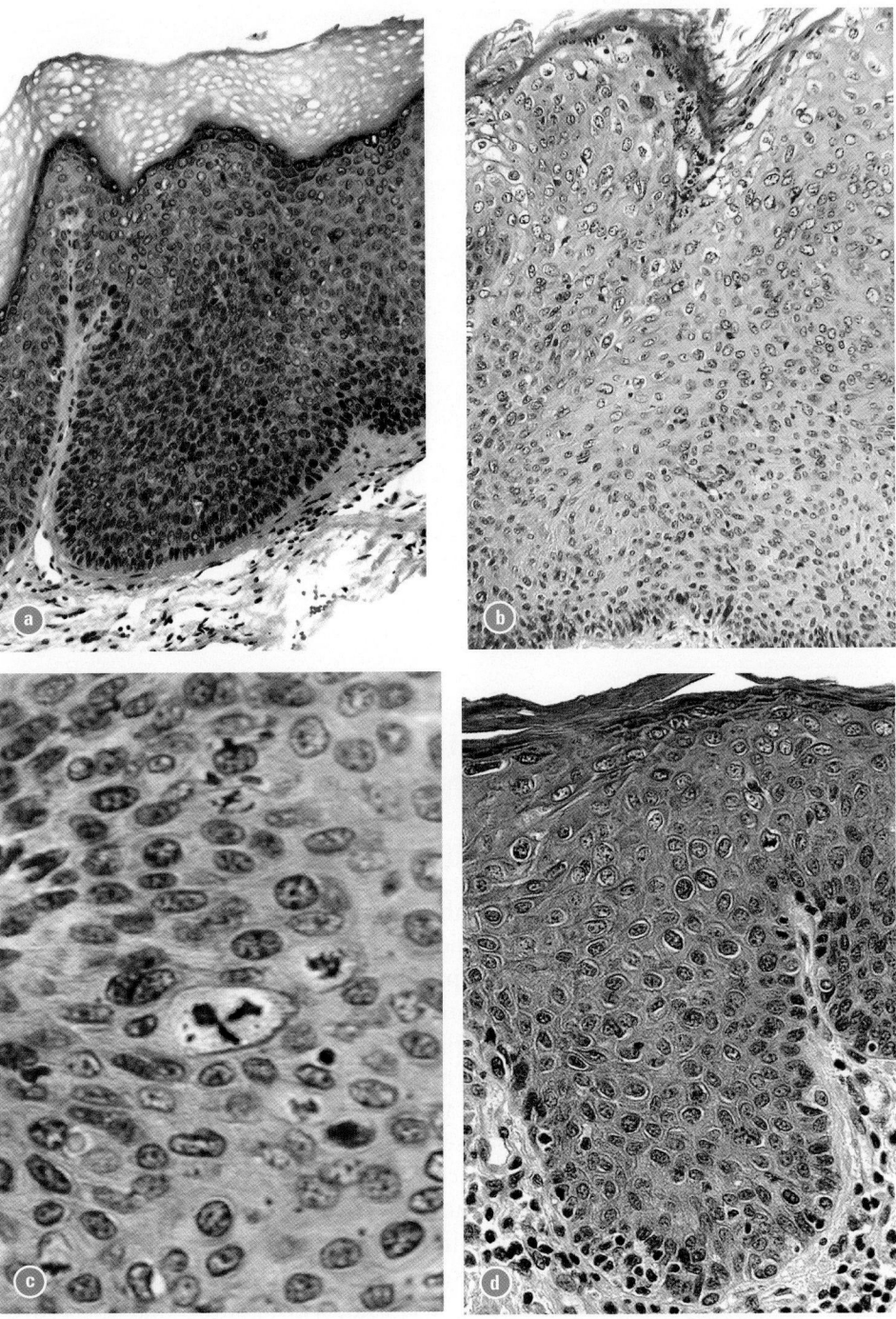

Fig. 6.12 Microscopic features of classic VIN. (a) Full-thickness atypia with minimal maturation, characteristic of carcinoma *in situ* (VIN 3). (b) VIN with koilocytotic atypia (VIN 2). (c) Abnormal (tripolar) mitotic figure in VIN. (d) Milder forms of atypia have been termed Bowenoid dysplasia.

patients with VIN. Four and one of the treated patients developed recurrent VIN and cancer, respectively. All five treated by biopsy or subtotal excision developed invasive carcinoma within 8 years.[61] Importantly, all in the latter group were menopausal. Chafe et al. identified unsuspected invasive carcinoma in 18.8% of patients undergoing surgical treatment for VIN. Again, the mean age of this group was 58 years, in contrast to 39 years for those without invasion.[62] These studies underscore the risk of invasion in women with VIN as a function of increasing age.[2]

Regression of VIN, like its counterpart in the male, has been reported. Features that are associated with regression include younger age (mean 19.5 years), non-white, history of condyloma, concurrent pregnancy in some and absence of symptoms.[63]

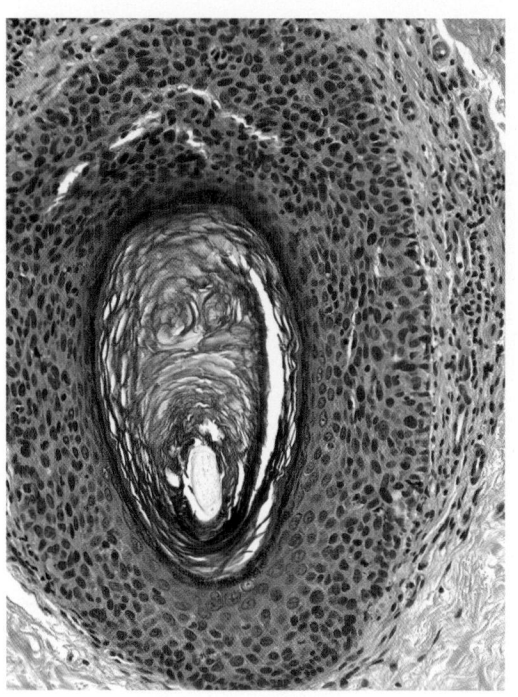

Fig. 6.13 Appendage involvement (hair shaft) by classic VIN.

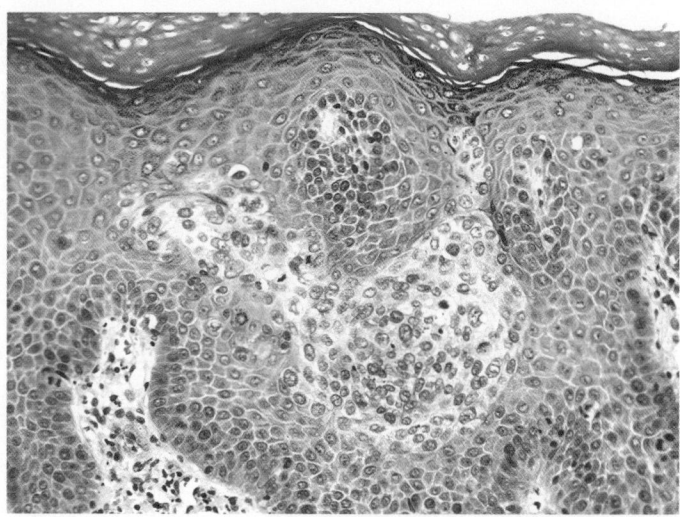

Fig. 6.15 Pagetoid VIN. This biopsy from a patient with a history of classic VIN (Bowenoid papulosis) depicts nests of neoplastic squamous cells within a normal squamous mucosa.

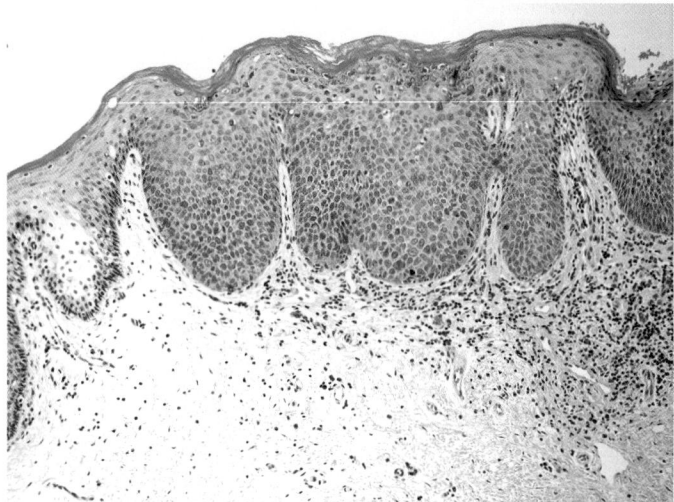

Fig. 6.14 A lichenoid infiltrate distinguishes normal mucosa (right) from classic VIN (left).

CLINICAL MANAGEMENT

The mainstay of management of VIN is local excision, which is the preferred method.[64] Approximately 76% of patients are cured on the initial procedure and over 98% after two treatments.[64] Imiquimod has also been attempted in some small studies, with a 27–50% complete response.[65–67]

Differentiated (simplex) vulvar intraepithelial neoplasia

INTRODUCTION

As discussed above, the pathway to vulvar cancer involves a classic VIN in about 40% of cases. In the majority, the epithelium adjacent to the cancer contains inflammatory dermatoses. The latter may be devoid of atypia, but in approximately one-half, a second subset of VIN can be found. This process likely involves a series of host gene alterations predating the onset of atypia and contributing subsequently to their evolution from non-atypical to frank preinvasive lesions. However, because the invasive cancers associated with this process are often well-differentiated, keratinizing, and often accompanied by minimal atypia, it is logical to assume that these precursors may share some of these features of subtle atypia. Thus, the recognition of these epithelial alterations requires an appreciation of the spectrum normally accompanied by host gene alterations seen with aging or carcinogen exposure. What the pathologist is seeking is a series of cellular changes that distinguish this form of precursor disease. The clinical management is more problematic, inasmuch as these atypias may be indistinguishable from the surrounding dermatoses on gross examination.[68,69]

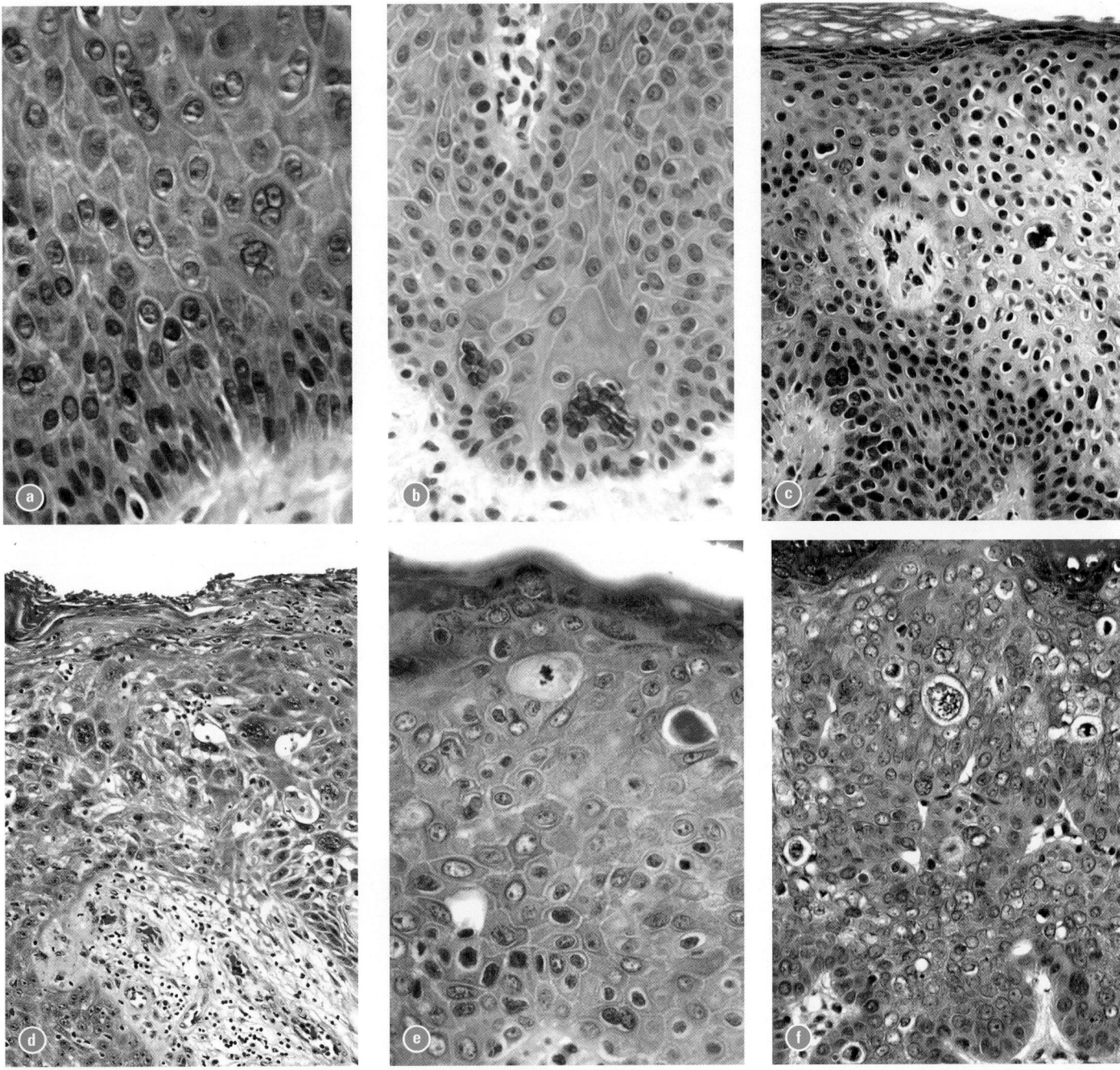

Fig. 6.16 Differential diagnosis of classic VIN. (a,b) Multinuclear atypia, with polynucleation. Note the normal nuclear size and chromasia of the cells and the absence of surrounding atypia. (c) Polynucleation in VIN for comparison. (d) PseudoBowenoid papulosis with (e) prominent apoptosis. Apoptosis (f) in VIN. Herpes zoster with multinucleated cells and inconspicuous inclusions may mimic classic VIN.

CLINICAL PRESENTATION

Unlike classic VINs, the differentiated variant comprises a small proportion (less than 5%) of *prospectively* identified VINs. They typically are identified in older women and in association with clinical presentations associated with vulvar lichen sclerosus and lichen simplex chronicus.[68,69] They are more commonly identified retrospectively, in reviews of epithelium adjacent to vulvar carcinomas, often in continuity with conventional appearing vulvar lichen sclerosus (LSA) or lichen simplex chronicus (LSC) (Fig. 6.18).[12,68,69] Differentiated VINs are less conspicuous clinically and may be impossible to separate from the background changes of lichen simplex chronicus. Epithelial thickening (acanthosis), hyperkeratosis, verruciform changes and ulceration may be present.

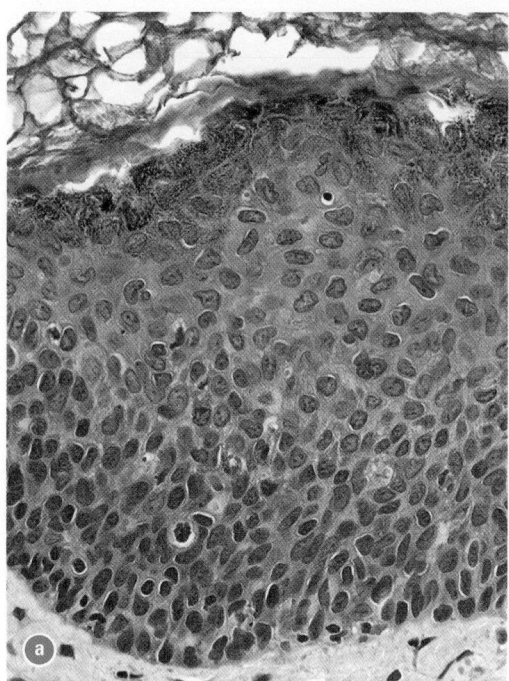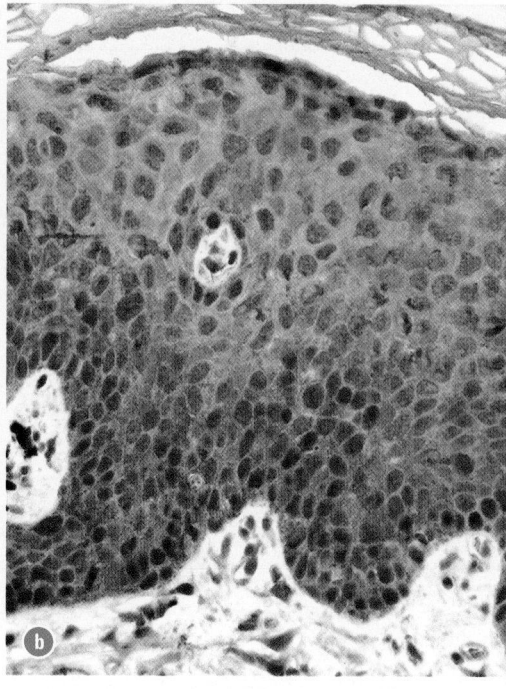

Fig. 6.17 Biomarkers staining of classic VIN. (a) H&E stained VIN. (b) Following staining for p16, with prominent staining of both nucleus and cytoplasm.

PATHOLOGIC FINDINGS

Differentiated (simplex) VINs exhibit one or more of the following features: atypia confined to the first 2–3 cell layers (basal atypia), subtle forms of atypia with hypercellularity or mild hyperchromasia, acantholysis and abnormal cell maturation with abnormal keratinization.[68,69] Because this spectrum is not well defined, it is useful to subdivide it into four categories for recognition (not diagnostic) purposes (Figs 6.19, 6.20):

1 Lichen sclerosus or LSC with prominent basal atypia. The atypia is usually conspicuous, associated with nuclear enlargement and hypercellularity (Fig. 6.19c,d).

2 Actinic-like lesions, with expansile regions of basal cells with mild hypercellularity, associated with LSC (Fig. 6.19a).

3 Acantholytic lesions, in which prominent spongiosis or acantholysis is seen in the lower third of the epithelium. Suprabasal acantholysis may be seen with a host of disorders, including pemphigus, Hailey–Hailey disease, transient acantholytic dermatosis. This condition may also be seen in association with actinic keratoses and squamous cell carcinomas of the skin.[70] These lesions are distinguished from familial conditions (Hailey–Hailey disease and Grover's disease).[71] Again, similar to the previous categories, the nuclear atypia may be subtle (Fig. 6.19b).

4 Defects in cell differentiation. Such cases exhibit individual cells with abnormal cytoplasmic volume and prominent cytoplasmic keratinization. In this variant, nuclear atypia may be present but is subtle. Components of this subtle atypia include loss of polarity, mild irregular clustering of basal cells and prominent nucleoli (Fig. 6.20a,b).

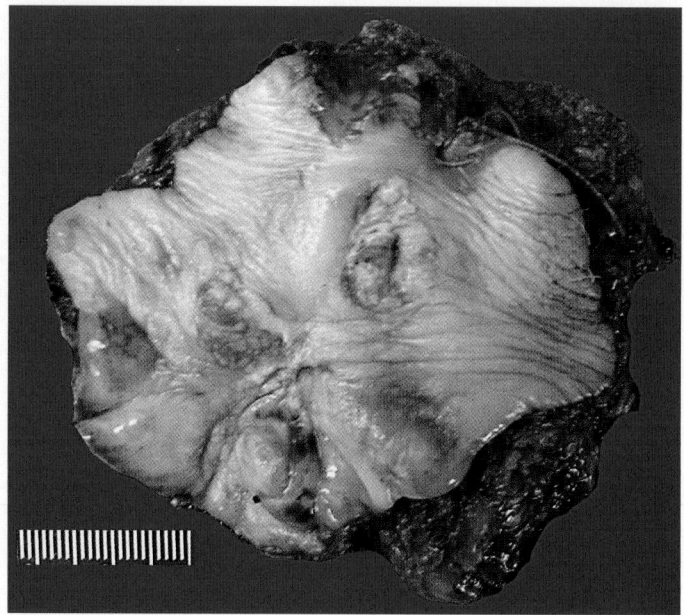

Fig. 6.18 Vulvectomy specimen of differentiated VIN shows indistinct patches of hyperkeratosis and associated superficially invasive squamous cell carcinoma. Compare with Figures 6.11 and 6.25.

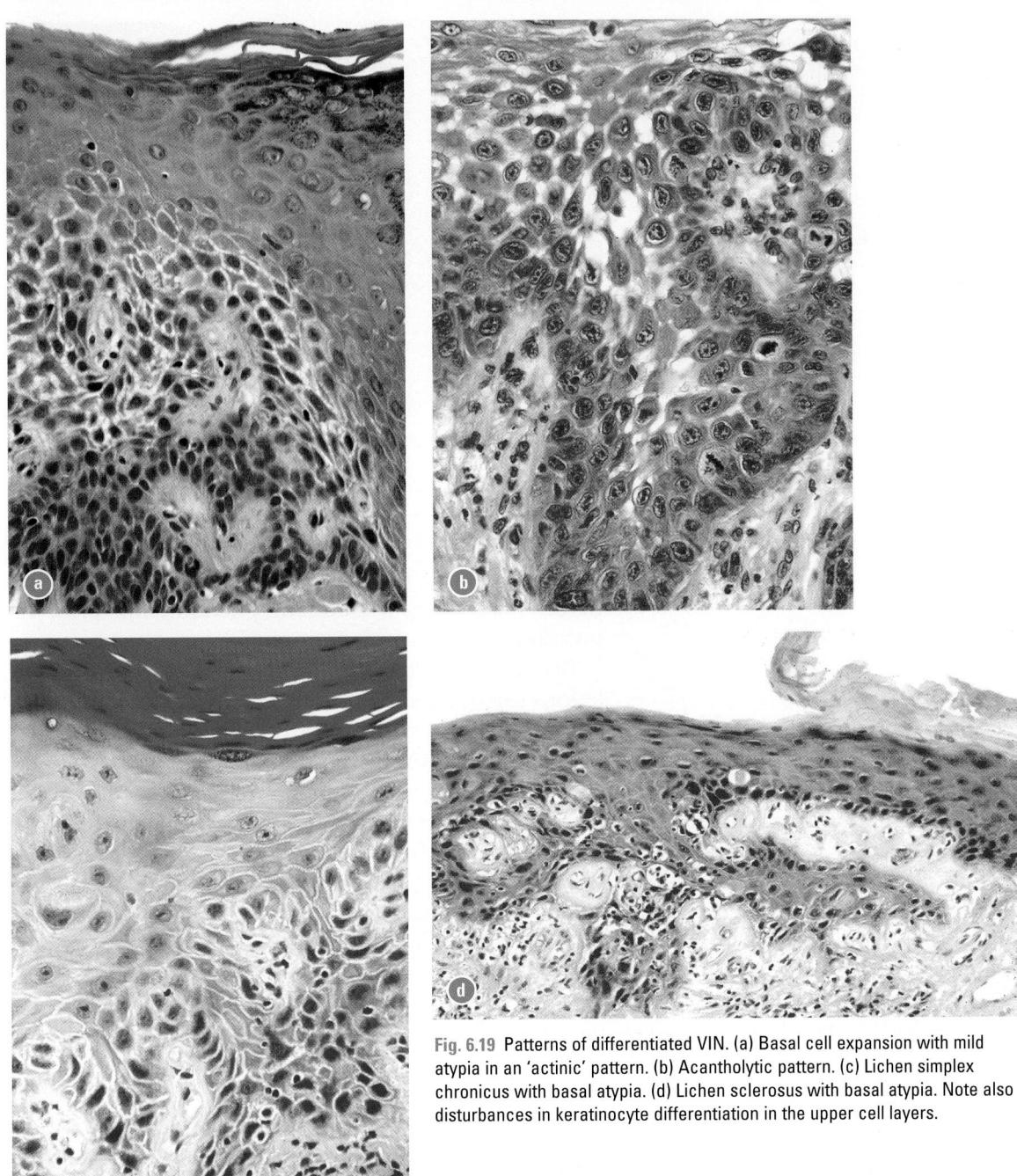

Fig. 6.19 Patterns of differentiated VIN. (a) Basal cell expansion with mild atypia in an 'actinic' pattern. (b) Acantholytic pattern. (c) Lichen simplex chronicus with basal atypia. (d) Lichen sclerosus with basal atypia. Note also disturbances in keratinocyte differentiation in the upper cell layers.

DIFFERENTIAL DIAGNOSIS

The differential diagnosis of simplex VIN includes those entities, that produce prominent acanthosis and/or milder forms of epithelial atypia. Psoriasis exhibits prominent 'test-tube' rete, which may occasionally be interpreted as VIN. However, the absence of either atypia or divergent maturation exclude this entity (Fig. 6.21a). Spongiotic dermatitis may mimic acantholysis and the accompanying eosinophilia may be interpreted as abnormal keratinization (Fig. 6.21b). Similarly, *Candida* vulvitis may produce reactive epithelial changes with hyperkeratosis (Fig. 6.21c). Alternatively, some of the epithelial changes with which differentiated VIN is associated – lichen sclerosus and lichen simplex chronicus – may mimic differentiated VIN (Fig. 6.21d). Both lichen sclerosus and LSC may be inflamed and exhibit reactive epithe-

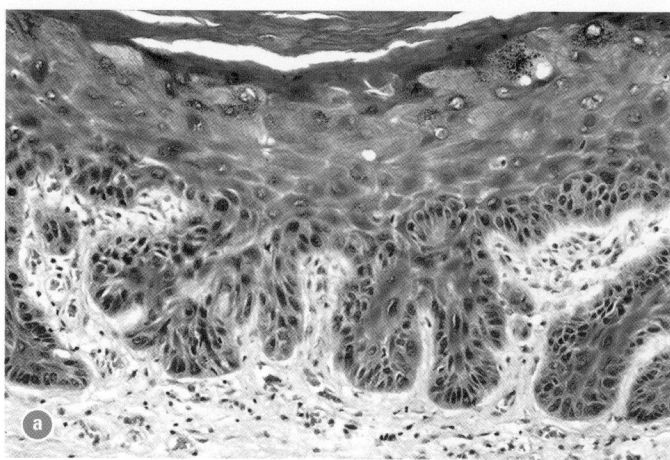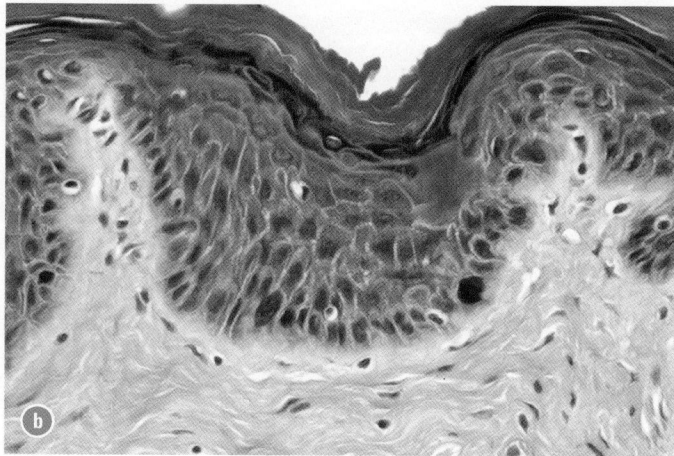

Fig. 6.20 Differentiated VIN with the classic 'simplex' pattern. (a) Basal atypia is accompanied by conspicuous eosinophilia. (b) Lesion with single cells showing marked cytoplasmic eosinophilia.

lial changes, but such features are usually easily distinguished from VIN.

BIOMARKERS

Because the pathogenesis of differentiated (simplex) VIN does not involve HPV, the diagnosis of this entity rests with defining host genetic markers that identify corresponding genomic perturbations. Yang and Hart identified increased staining for p53 in differentiated VIN as a possible marker. p53 stains basal epithelium of normal mucosa, lichen simplex chronicus and lichen sclerosus weakly, while being intense in many differentiated VINs and invasive squamous cell carcinomas (Fig. 6.22).[72] Nascimento et al. recently showed that p16 is also expressed intensely in some of these lesions, although the distribution is less extensive relative to p53; or p16 in classic VIN.[73]

NATURAL HISTORY AND MANAGEMENT

There is little or no information on the natural history of differentiated VIN. An estimated 1–4% of cases of lichen sclerosus eventually develop vulvar cancer.[12] However, the finding of differentiated VIN associated with LS in the absence of cancer is uncommon. For this reason, it can be argued that differentiated VIN does not persist as a precursor for an extended period of time, suggesting that many, if not all, of these lesions will eventually progress to invasion. Because differentiated VIN may coexist with other acanthotic lesions of uncertain malignant potential (such as verruciform lichen sclerosus or LSC), the possibility exists that the

latter may have a longer natural history, with differentiated VIN being a transient phenomenon prior to invasion.

Because most differentiated VINs are not discrete lesions surrounded by normal mucosa, clinical management relies principally on carefully monitoring women with LSC and LSA, by biopsy of suspicious areas. When such areas disclose differentiated VIN, conservative excision and careful follow-up are warranted. Nevertheless, because differentiated VIN exists in a background of other vulvar dermatoses and because vulvar carcinoma may arise from any point in this preinvasive epithelial spectrum, continued follow-up is essential. We and others have encountered cases in which discrete carcinomas arose in the vulvar mucosa of women undergoing follow-up for LSC or LSA, with subsequent fatal outcomes. Thus, vigilance is mandatory.[74]

Other intraepithelial alterations of potential significance

INTRODUCTION

Approximately one-third of HPV-negative vulvar squamous cell carcinomas (SCCs), including verrucous carcinoma, have previously not been associated with a defined non-invasive atypia.[15] There are three potential explanations for the lack of recognizable precursors in these cases. One is that a precursor exists but is obliterated by the tumor as it grows. The second is that the transition from normal to precursor lesion to

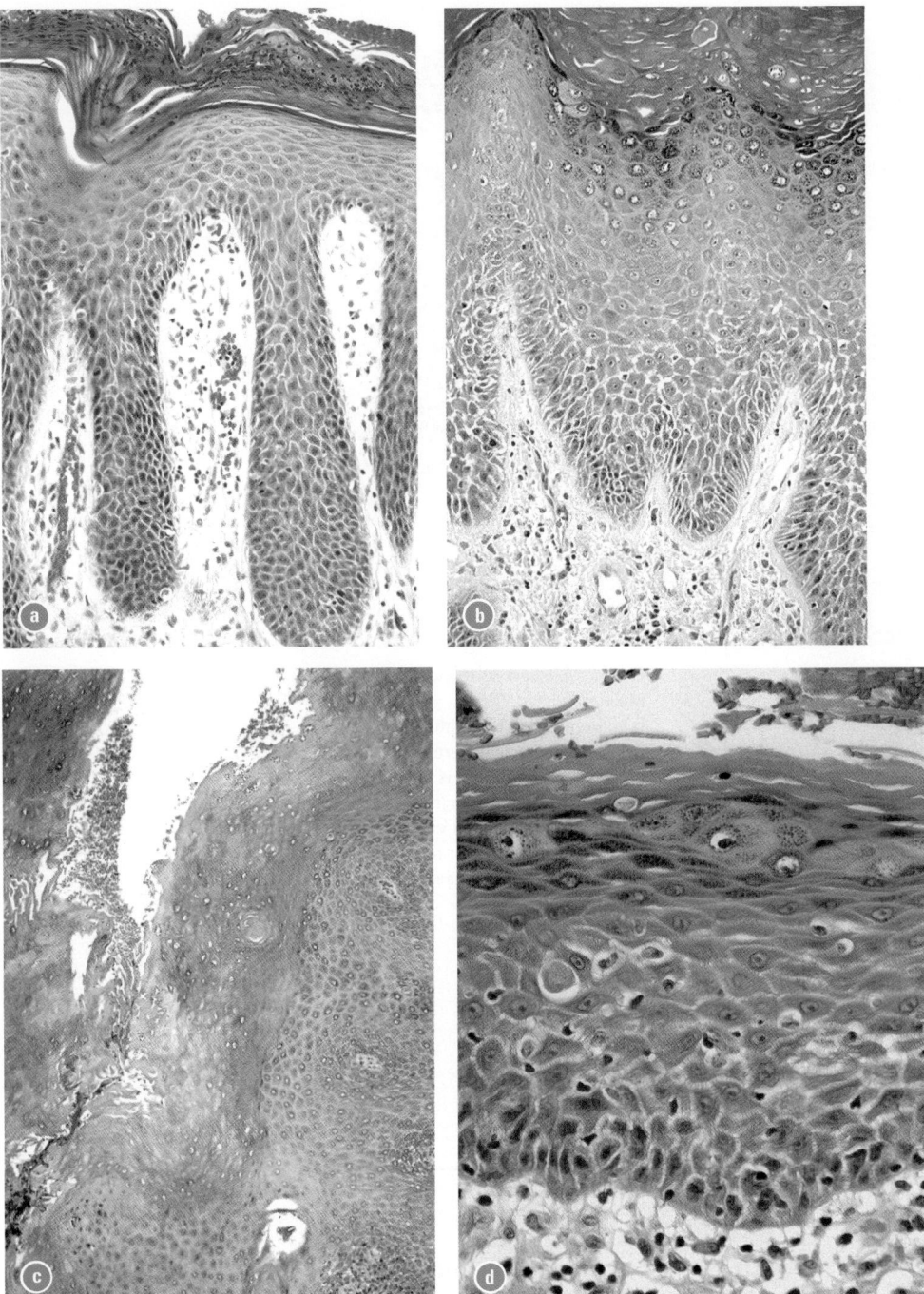

Fig. 6.21 Differential diagnosis of differentiated VIN. (a) Psoriasis exhibits acanthosis with test tube rete and prominent hyperkeratosis. (b) Spongiotic dermatitis may mimic acantholysis. (c) *Candida* vulvitis. There is marked acanthosis and hyperkeratosis, without atypia. (d) Lichen simplex chronicus with focal basal cell hyperchromasia.

cancer proceeds rapidly, in which case the precursor is small and cannot be consistently identified by existing criteria for intraepithelial neoplasia. The third hypothesis is that a precursor exists but is non-conventional (i.e. fails to show conspicuous nuclear atypia). In the case of verrucous carcinoma, such a precursor lesion, if it existed, must by definition differ from those with conspicuous atypia (differentiated (simplex) and classic VIN).

HISTOLOGIC PATTERNS

Three categories of intraepithelial change deserve mention.

1 *Lichen sclerosus with acanthosis* (LSA, also called mixed dystrophy) has been associated with increased risk of vulvar cancer (Fig. 6.23a). Rodke et al. observed that 3 of 15 cases followed developed invasion.[75]

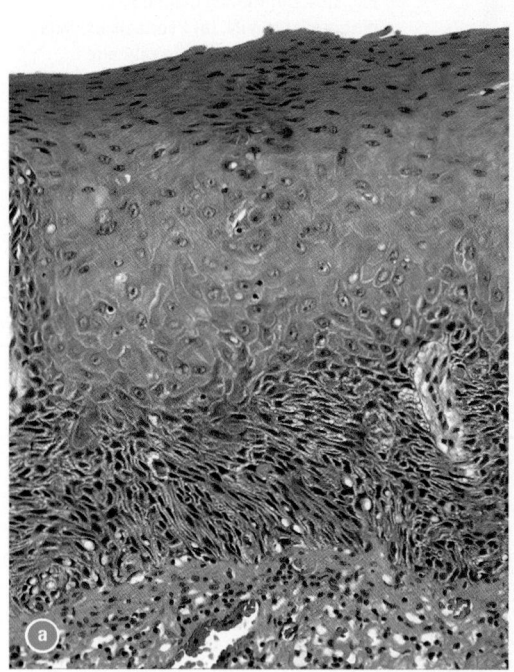

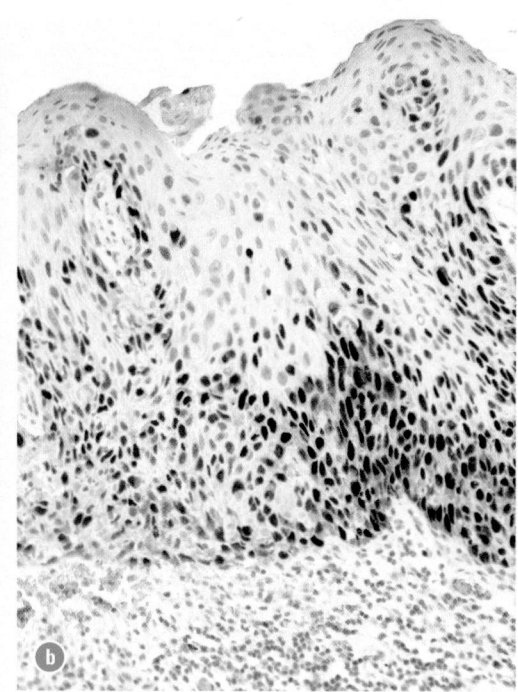

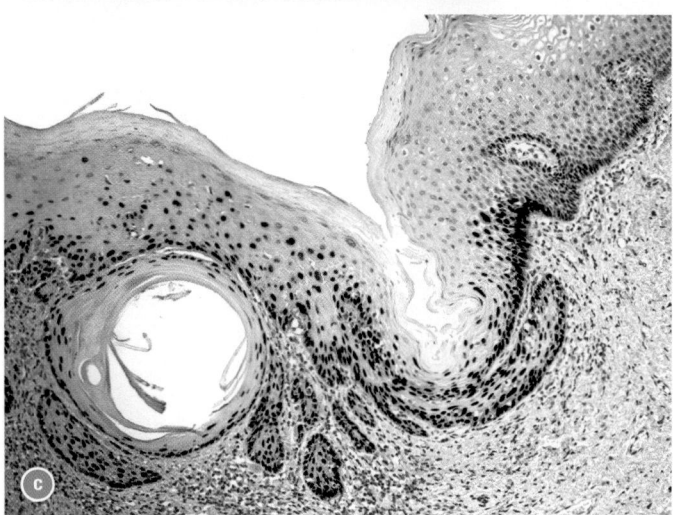

Fig. 6.22 Biomarkers in the diagnosis of differentiated VIN. (a) Differentiated VIN with basal cell expansion and hyperchromasia. (b) Immunostain for p53 is intensely positive. (c) Progression (right to left) of normal, differentiated VIN and early invasion. The latter are highlighted by intense basal p53 staining.

2   *Verruciform lichen simplex chronicus.* LSC with verruciform changes are considered non-specific. However, we have observed these changes in association with vulvar cancer and verrucous carcinomas. Thus, patients with this condition, particularly older women, merit careful follow-up inasmuch as verruciform LSC falls into the category of a chronic hypertrophic dermatosis (Fig. 6.23b,c).[73]

3   *Vulvar acanthosis with altered differentiation (VAAD)* is another epithelial change that has been associated with verrucous carcinoma.[76] This entity is defined by acanthosis with variable verruciform change, plaque-like layers of parakeratosis and an alteration in cytoplasmic differentiation characterized by reduction or loss of granules of the granular cell layer. The latter results in conspicuous cytoplasmic pallor in the upper epithelial layers. It is possible to distinguish VAAD from other neoplastic and non-neoplastic conditions and this distinction is outlined in Tables 6.2 and 6.4 and Figures 6.2 and 6.24.

None of the three entities by themselves contain sufficient cytologic atypia to warrant a diagnosis of VIN. Nonetheless, all should be followed carefully when identified in patients with chronic vulvar disease.

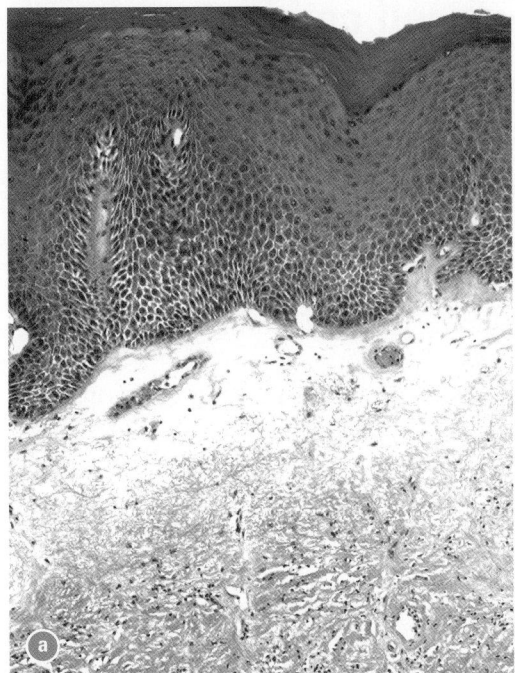

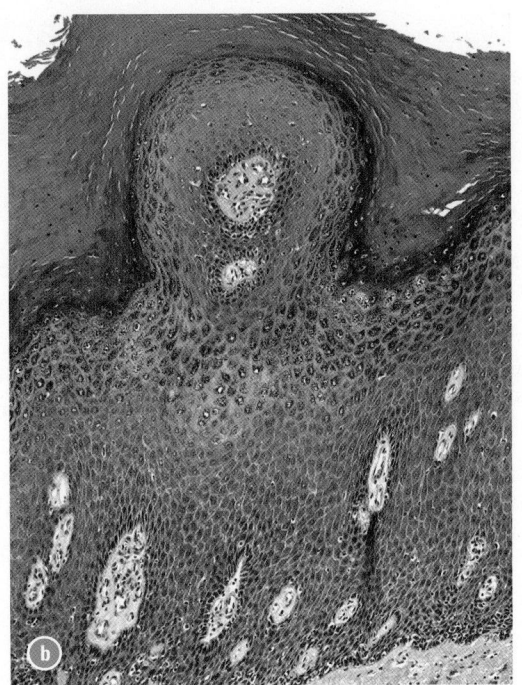

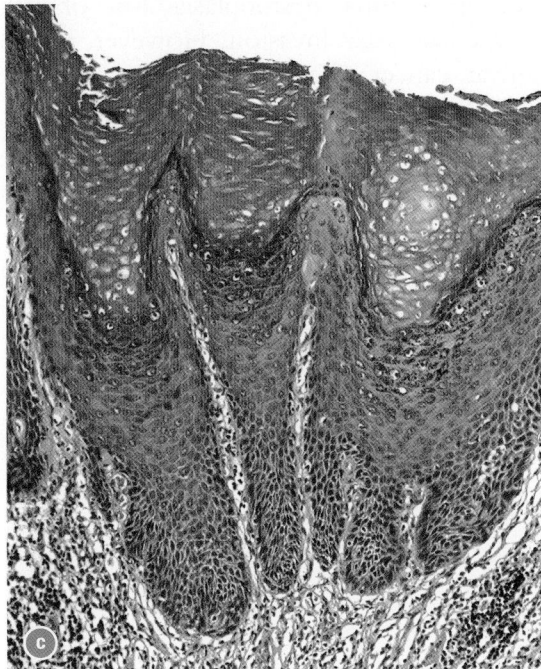

Fig. 6.23 Other epithelial changes that are not classified as neoplastic, but may be associated with squamous cell carcinoma or confer increased risk in the appropriate clinical setting. (a) Lichen sclerosus with superimposed lichen simplex chronicus. (b,c) Verruciform lichen simplex chronicus.

Diagnostic terminology for preinvasive vulvar disease

The selection of terminology should reflect the risk imposed by the condition and convey information that will aid in proper management (Table 6.4). For condylomata and classic VIN lesions, we use the term squamous intraepithelial lesion. Low-grade lesions are synonymous with condyloma/VIN1. VIN1 is poorly defined but includes flat condylomas and acanthotic lesions with mild atypia that do not fall into either the condyloma or classic VIN categories. For simplicity and to avoid confusion, we use the term low-grade squa-

Table 6.4 *Diagnostic terminology for preinvasive vulvar disease*

Condyloma, fibroepithelial papilloma, seborrheic keratosis
  Low-grade squamous intraepithelial lesion (condyloma/VIN1)
Classic VIN:
  High-grade squamous intraepithelial lesion (VIN2/VIN3)
Differentiated VIN:
  High-grade squamous intraepithelial lesion (differentiated or simplex
    VIN, see Comment)
  Comment: Differentiated (simplex) VIN is considered a form of
    preinvasive vulvar disease. Conservative excision and careful
    follow-up are advised
Other vulvar squamous alterations:
  Acanthosis with altered differentiation, see Comment
  Verruciform lichen simplex chronicus, see Comment
  Lichen sclerosus with superimposed lichen simplex chronicus,
    see comment
  Comment: The above changes are not classified as neoplastic, but may
    be associated with an increased risk of vulvar cancer in certain
    clinical settings. Periodic follow-up with biopsy of suspicious
      lesions is advised.

Squamous cell carcinoma

CLINICAL PRESENTATION

Squamous cell carcinomas of the vulva present under two dominant scenarios (Fig. 6.25). The first is in association with a classic VIN, most common in women in the sixth decade. The second presentation is in association with inflammatory dermatoses. Thus, vulvar squamous carcinoma may be found under the following circumstances:

1 Incidentally, upon examination of an excision for VIN
2 As a mass developing in a patient with a history of inflammatory dermatoses
3 With no prior history of vulvar neoplasia.

CRITERIA FOR DIAGNOSIS OF INVASION

The classic features of invasion include irregular epithelial growth in the stroma, desmoplasia, loss of cell polarity and vascular space invasion. However, when evaluating vulvar cancer, the practitioner should be aware of the following patterns, including poorly- and well-differentiated, that are diagnostic of invasion or bear careful scrutiny with additional tissue sampling (Figs 6.25–6.31).

1 Infiltrative moderate to poorly-differentiated invasive tumor associated with classic VIN

mous intraepithelial lesion (condyloma/VIN1). For classic VIN lesions, we use the term high-grade squamous intraepithelial lesion (HSIL; VIN2/VIN3).

Classification of differentiated VIN is more problematic, and here the use of VIN1 must be avoided, despite the well-differentiated appearance of these lesions. We use the term HSIL, differentiated (simplex) type (emphasizing that) these lesions are risk factors for vulvar cancer and should be removed by the most conservative means possible.

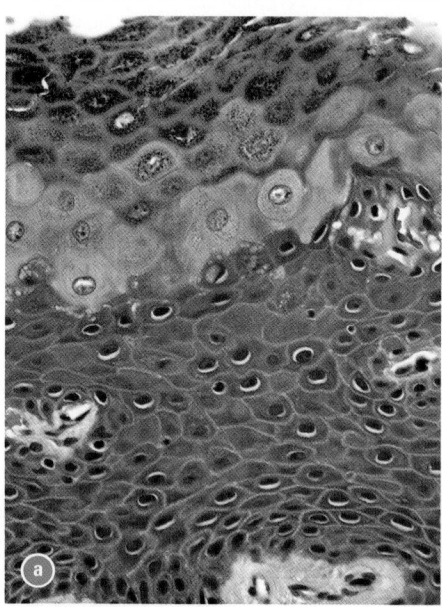 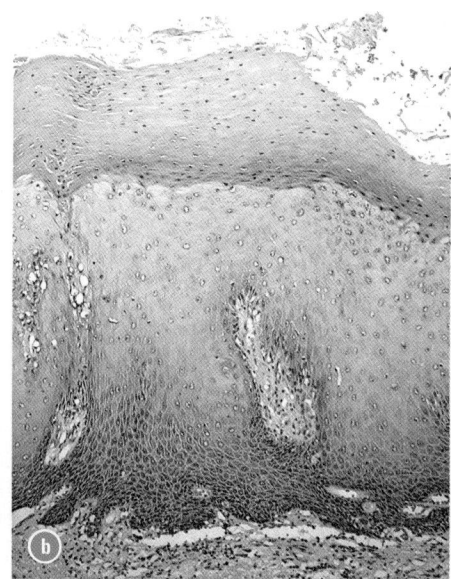 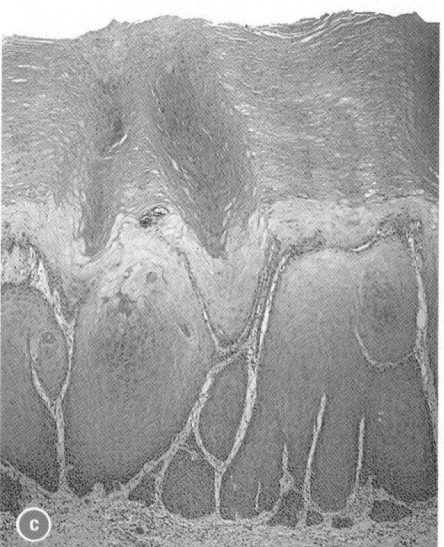

Fig. 6.24 (a) Acanthosis with discrete zone of altered surface cell differentiation with conspicuous cytoplasmic pallor, associated with adjacent well-differentiated carcinoma. (b) Acanthosis with loss of keratohyaline granules, cytoplasmic pallor and conspicuous parakeratosis. (c) Epithelium adjacent to (b) contains features of early verrucous carcinoma, with downward epithelial growth in the form of 'pushing' invasion.

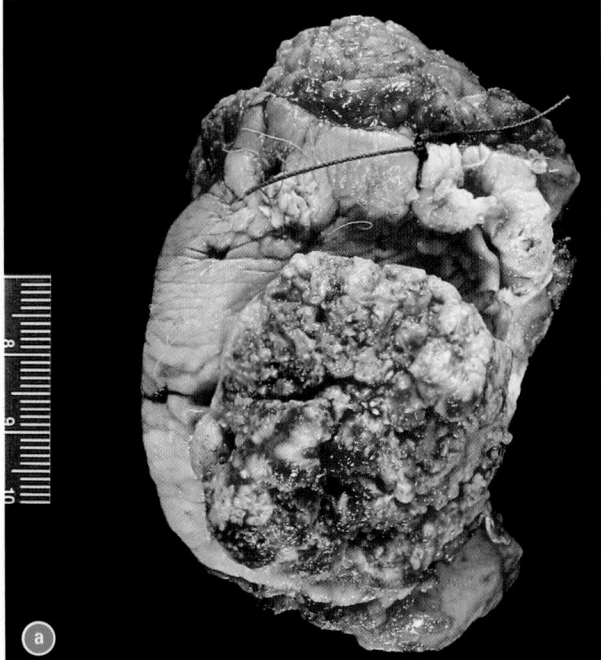

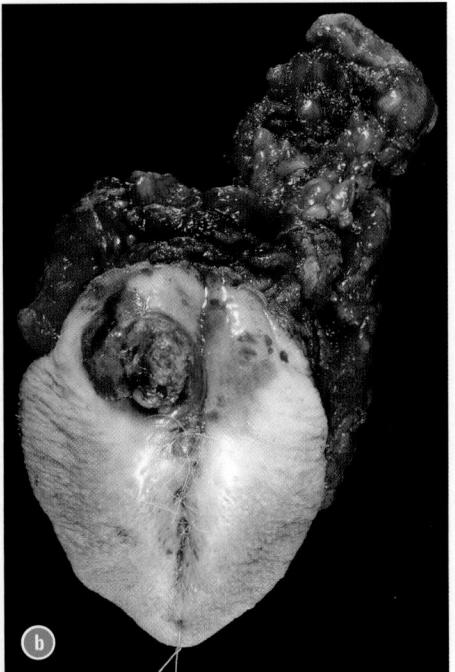

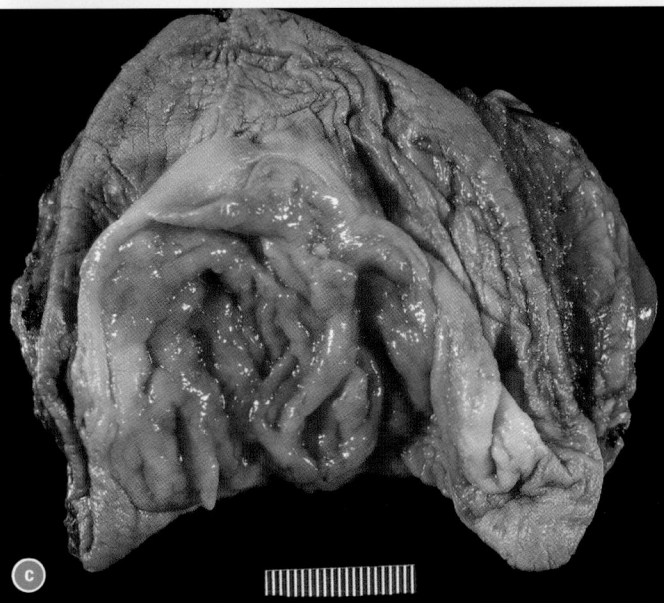

Fig. 6.25 Gross appearances of vulvar cancer. (a) Fungating well-differentiated keratinizing carcinoma. (b) Discrete nodule formed by a moderately differentiated (warty) carcinoma. (c) Smooth homogeneous poorly-differentiated carcinoma with basaloid histology.

2 Cohesive 'intraepithelial-like' invasive patterns alone or in association with classic VIN

3 Linear pavement-like arrangements of poorly differentiated neoplastic epithelium with a discrete epithelial-stromal interface but with sufficient architectural complexity to exceed the criteria for intraepithelial disease

4 Well-differentiated infiltrative patterns with high nuclear grade

5 Well-differentiated cohesive growth patterns with moderate to high nuclear grade

6 Extremely well-differentiated cohesive growth patterns with very low nuclear grade. This group includes rare lesions falling into the category of verrucous carcinoma.

The first three groups are typically associated with HPV-positive tumors, whereas the latter are more commonly associated with the HPV-negative pathway.

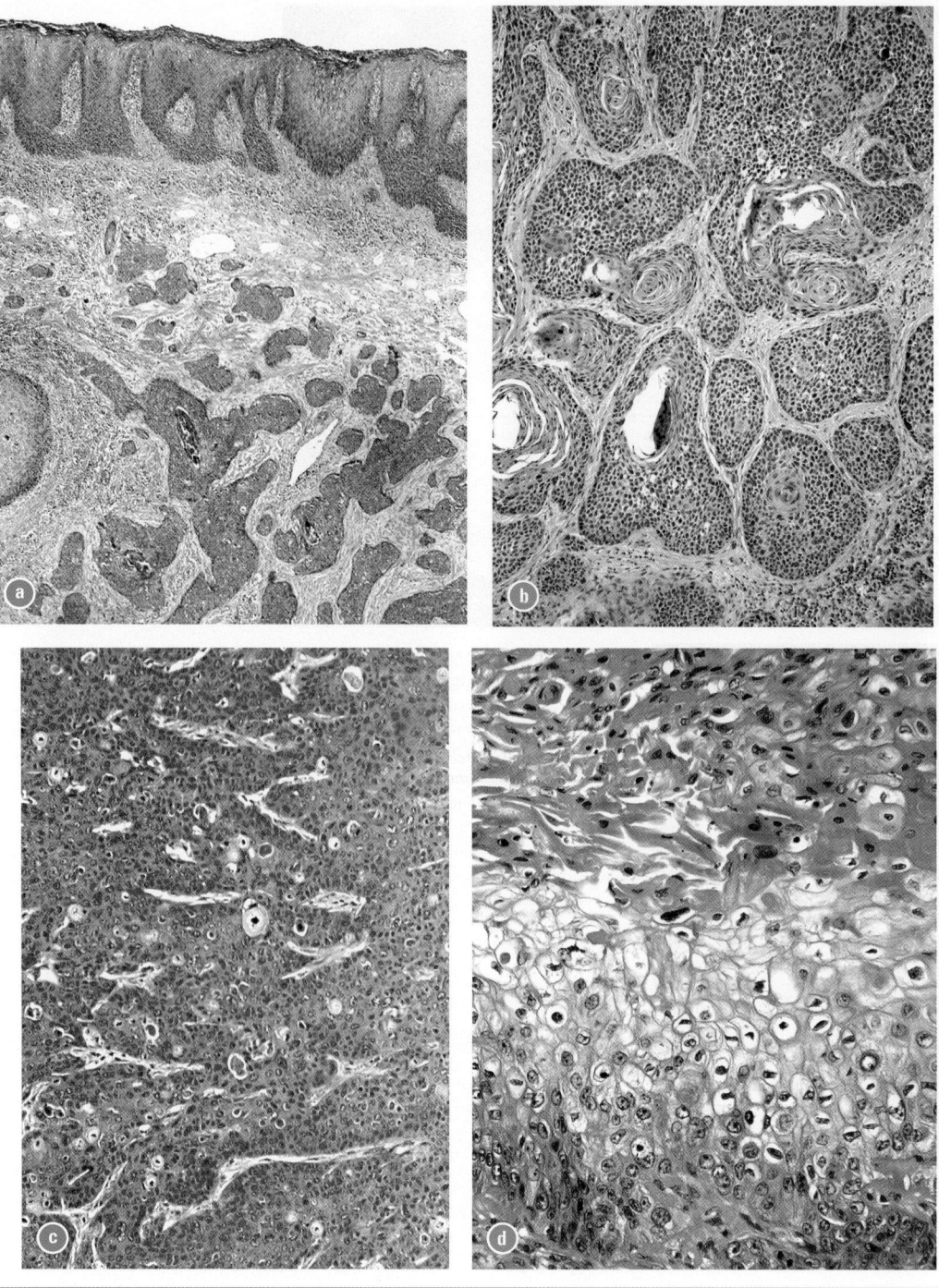

Fig. 6.26 Poorly-differentiated (HPV-associated) carcinomas. (a) Classic VIN with underlying tumor of similar histopathology. (b) Cohesive nesting (intraepithelial-like) in a basaloid carcinoma. (c) Solid poorly-differentiated HPV-positive carcinoma. (d) Warty pattern with pseudokoilocytosis.

GROWTH PATTERNS OF CARCINOMA

Moderate to poorly-differentiated squamous cell carcinoma

This category of carcinoma is frequently associated with HPV nucleic acids and exhibits the following features: (1) sheets of immature neoplastic squamous cells with a high nuclear-cytoplasmic ratio; (2) a tendency for cohesive growth that mimics intraepithelial disease (basaloid or intraepithelial-like); (3) a loss of cell polarity and a tendency to form irregular, interconnecting sheets of tumor cells; and (4) variable maturation, keratinization and pseudokoilocytosis (warty carcinomas). These tumors are often (but not invariably) associated with classic VIN and HPV (Fig. 6.26).[8,53]

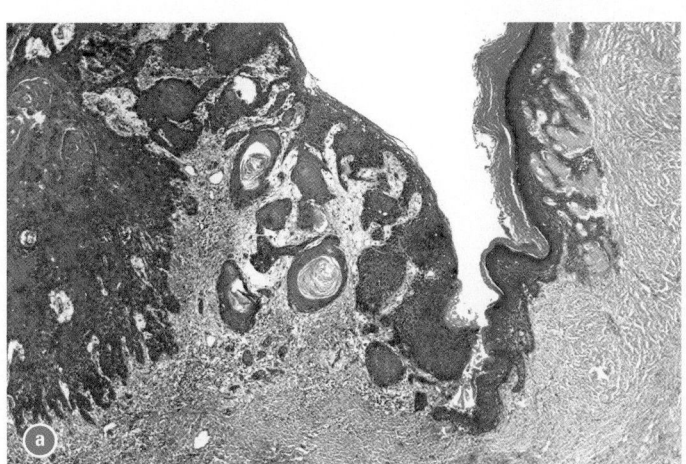

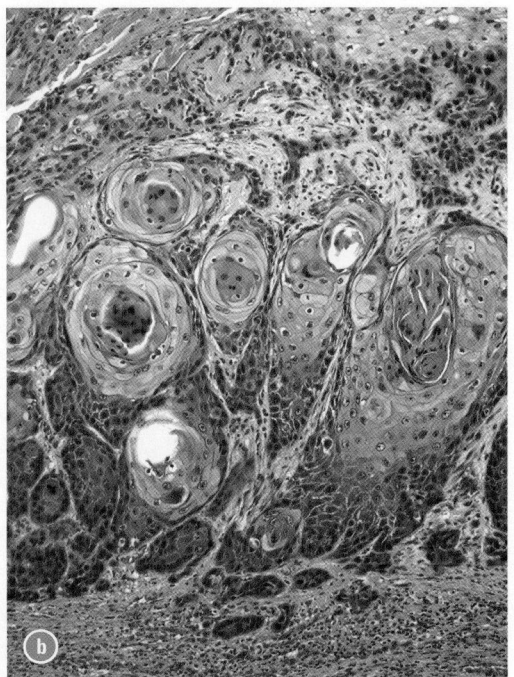

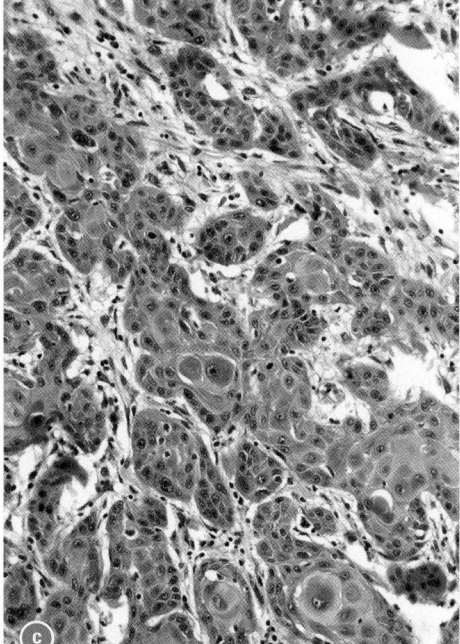

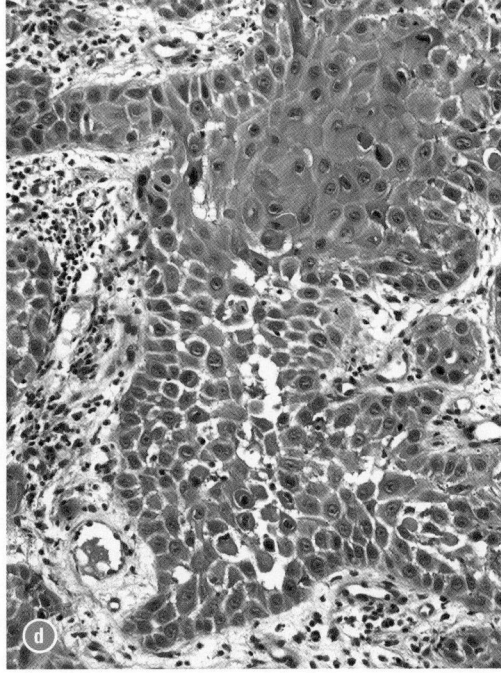

Fig. 6.27 Keratinizing HPV-negative carcinomas. (a) At low power, lichen sclerosus (right) merges with differentiated VIN (center) and invasive carcinoma (left). (b) Keratinizing nests of neoplastic epithelium with prominent interface atypia. (c) Small sinuating cords of neoplasia with focal keratin formation. (d) Acantholytic pattern with disaggregated neoplastic keratinocytes.

Keratinizing squamous carcinoma

These tumors exhibit conspicuous maturation and keratinization. The basal cells typically show mild to moderate atypia, with reduced atypia in the mature cells, which may be seen on the surface or in the centers of the invading tumors nests. These tumors fall into two general subcategories. The first are organized into variably sized cohesive-appearing nests with a tendency toward blunt invasion intermixed with focal frank infiltration of the stroma by small cell clusters. The second is less well organized and infiltrates the stroma with branching tongues and separate small cohesive units of well-differentiated tumor cells. These tumors are frequently associated with differentiated VIN and inflammatory dermatoses and are often HPV negative (Fig. 6.27).[8,53]

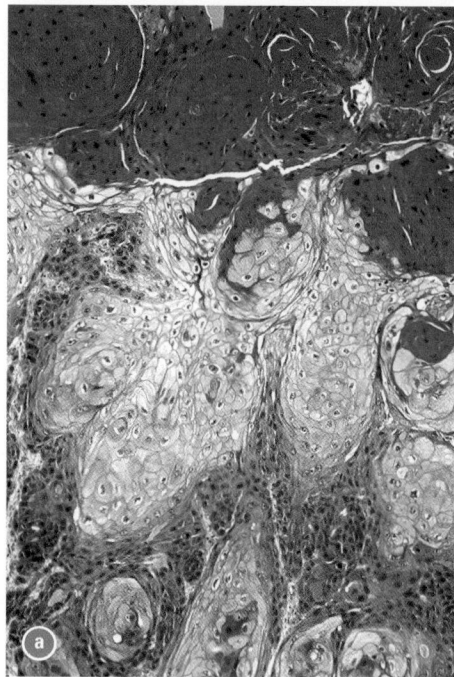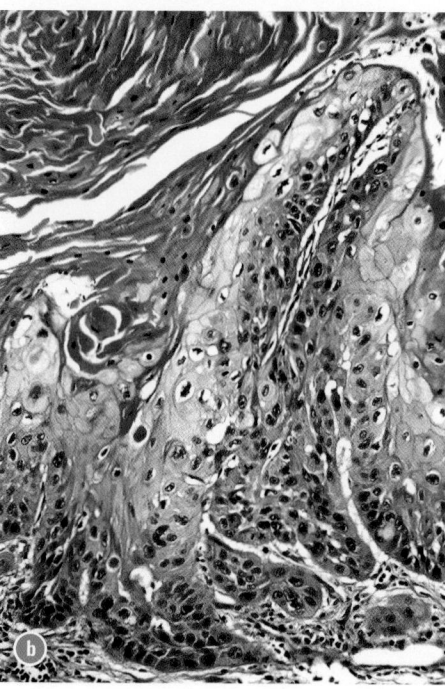

Fig. 6.28 (a,b) Warty-keratinizing patterns. These tumors exhibit both maturation and pseudokoilocytosis and may be HPV negative.

Mixed patterns

As discussed previously, mixtures of the above patterns may occur. Some HPV-negative tumors may have conspicuous surface atypia similar to so-called warty carcinomas, yet be HPV negative (Fig. 6.28). HPV-positive lesions may arise in the setting of lichen sclerosus and classic VINs may be associated with keratinizing carcinomas. For this reason, the precise category of tumor (i.e. keratinizing *vs* poorly-differentiated or HPV positive versus negative) is considered less important than the degree and nature (blunt *vs* infiltrative) of the invasion.

Verrucous carcinoma

Verrucous carcinomas of the genital tract are defined as squamous tumors with characteristics that distinguish them from conventional carcinomas and, by virtue of these differences, possess no risk of nodal metastases.[77–81] The characteristics required to ensure the latter make their classification controversial. At the center of the controversy is the criteria for distinguishing verrucous carcinomas from conventional squamous carcinomas. In fact, studies have shown that the conventional invasive carcinomas may coexist with, or follow, verrucous carcinomas.[82]

The problems in separating verrucous carcinomas from conventional squamous carcinomas are two-fold. The first is inconsistent application of criteria. The diagnosis of verrucous carcinoma requires strict attention to the following parameters: (1) a well-differentiated verrucopapillary carcinoma; (2) minimal or no basal cell (interface) or superficial cell nuclear atypia; (3) a generally blunt epithelial-stromal interface; and (4) absence of coexisting conventional keratinizing squamous cell carcinoma (Fig. 6.29). One report showed uniform staining for AE1 and AE3 in contrast to a more patchy staining pattern in conventional squamous carcinoma.[77] Tumors fulfilling all of these parameters have a negligible risk of lymph node metastases.[78] However, a combination of both verrucous and conventional elements is not uncommon, indicating that the verrucous carcinoma phenotype may be 'unstable', representing one of many morphologic transitions to conventional carcinoma.

Verrucous and other well-differentiated carcinomas are typically associated with inflammatory dermatoses and other parameters linked to HPV-negative tumors. The majority of studies have found verrucous carcinomas to be HPV negative. These tumors may also be associated with verruciform lichen simplex chronicus and other vulvar acanthoses with altered differentiation, characterized by epithelial cell pallor and conspicuous parakeratosis (Fig. 6.24).[76]

Giant condyloma of Buschke–Löwenstein (Fig. 6.29d)

Giant condylomata (of Buschke–Löwenstein) of the anogenital area are extremely uncommon, but the evidence indicates that such lesions are distinct from

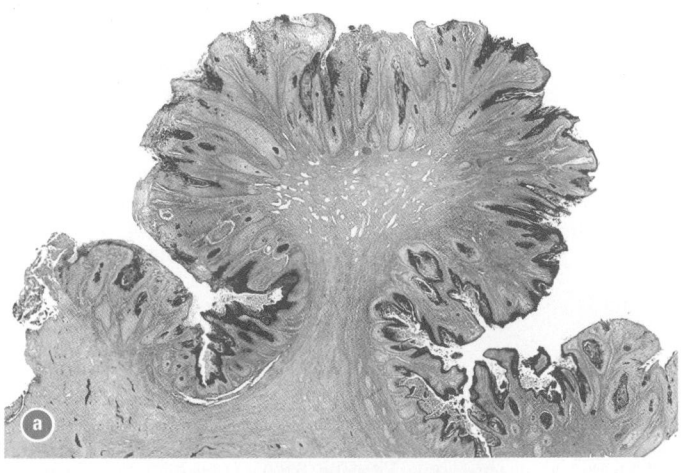

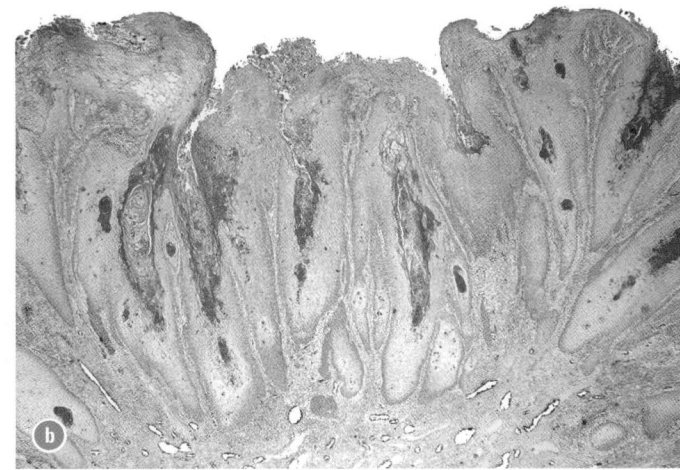

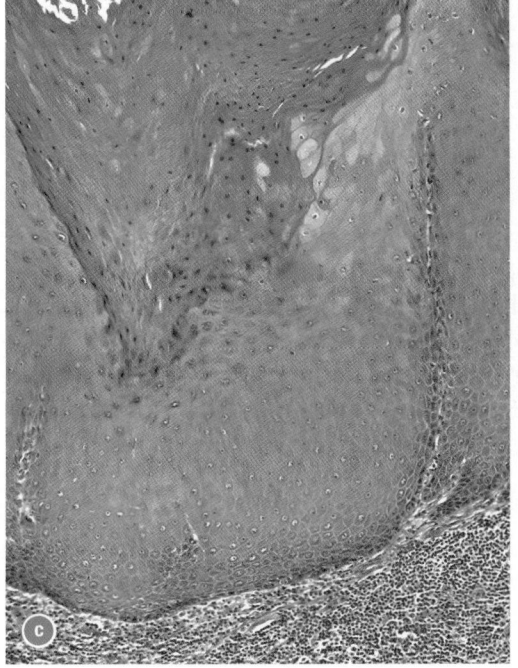

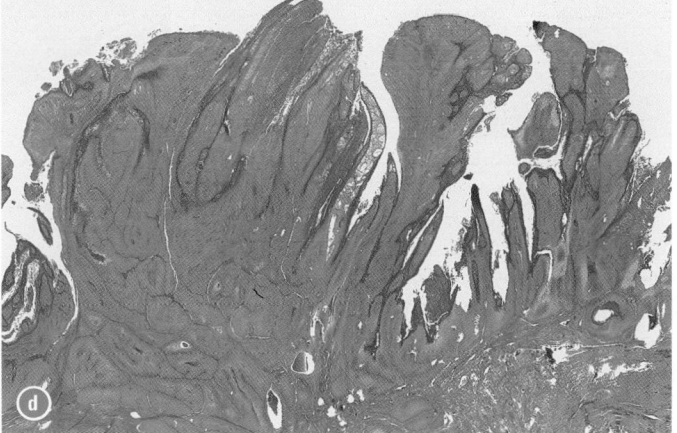

Fig. 6.29 Verrucous carcinoma. (a) The tumor is exophytic and invasive. Invasion (b) takes the form of broad nests of infiltrating tumor. (c) Characteristic features of verrucous carcinoma are a discrete epithelial-stromal interface and minimal to no basal or superficial cell atypia. (d) Giant condyloma of the anus for comparison.

both verrucous carcinomas, which are variably HPV positive, and condylomata.[83,84] These lesions are more commonly found in males, particularly in younger patients, and we have encountered similar lesions in the anogenital region of HIV-infected individuals. The distinction of these lesions from condyloma lies solely in the ease with which the lesions can be excised. Rare cases of coexisting invasive carcinoma have been reported and we have seen similar lesions in the cervix with parametrial extension. Giant condyloma is distinguished from verrucous carcinoma based on the uniform condylomatous architecture, presence of uniform cell maturation with conspicuous koilocytosis and

absence of the more irregular blunt, but finger-like epithelial processes incorporating and fixing the underlying stroma (Fig. 6.29d) (see Ch. 10).

Papillary squamous cell carcinoma

Papillary squamous cell carcinomas of the vulva are extremely rare and have not been reported in detail. These tumors, like their counterparts in the cervix, are exophytic neoplasms composed of filiform papillae lined by a polarized epithelium similar to classic vulvar intraepithelial neoplasia (VIN3)(Fig. 6.30). The papillae may focally coalesce, but maintain their individual architecture and a sharply defined epithelial-stromal

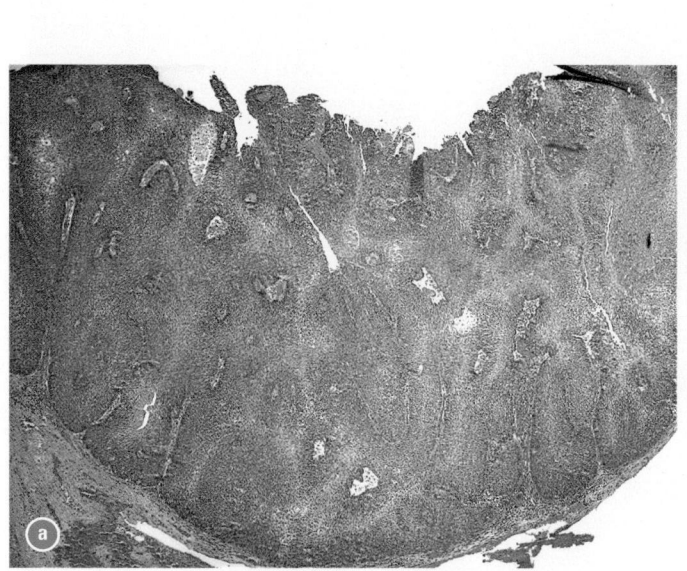 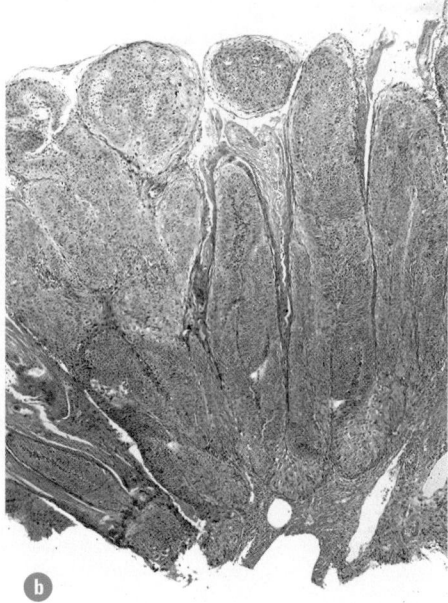

Fig. 6.30 Poorly-differentiated carcinomas with epithelial confluence and expansile growth. (a) Expansile tumor has a discrete epithelial-stromal interface, but is highly complex. (b) Papillary architecture associated with a poorly-differentiated squamous cell carcinoma.

interface. Because of the latter, these tumors may be managed by wide local excision provided there is no invasion and no other parameters (clinical assessment of lymph nodes) suggest metastatic behavior.[85]

Spindle cell (sarcomatoid) squamous carcinoma

A rare variant of squamous carcinoma of the vulva is characterized by a spindle or sarcomatoid cell phenotype. Immunohistochemical and ultrastructural studies support a metaplastic rather than mixed epithelial-mesenchymal origin for these tumors (Fig. 6.31).[86,87]

Other patterns

Additional growth patterns include carcinomas with marked acantholysis and so-called giant cell carcinomas. These have been the subject of sporadic reports. The former is interpreted as a variant of squamous carcinoma, but must be distinguished from warty dyskeratoma, with its characteristic crateriform architecture[70] and rare examples of squamous carcinoma arising in Hailey–Hailey disease.[88]

DIFFERENTIAL DIAGNOSIS OF INVASIVE SQUAMOUS CARCINOMA

Tangential sectioning/adnexal involvement

Classic VIN lesions often exhibit both verruciform architecture and adnexal gland involvement and, when sectioned appropriately or tangentially, may exhibit nests of neoplastic epithelium in the underlying stroma. The distinction of this pattern from invasion is based on the uniformity of the nests, preserved polarity and absence of desmoplasia. Inflammation is often present and is not a distinguishing feature (Fig. 6.32a).

Pseudoepitheliomatous hyperplasia

Pseudoepitheliomatous hyperplasia (PEH) is characterized by acanthosis and irregular epithelial architecture. Characteristically, PEH demonstrates no atypia and the 'invasive' epithelium contains small thin – at times arching – epithelial bridges that are pointed and uncharacteristic of invasion. A known complement to this pattern is an underlying granular cell tumor, but it may be associated with chronic vulvitis (Fig. 6.32b,c).[89]

Artifactual displacement of neoplastic epithelium into spaces by trauma

Neoplastic epithelium may be displaced into the stroma or vascular spaces in the stroma during either anesthetic injection or the pinning of the specimen prior to fixation and sectioning (Fig. 6.32d).

Keratoacanthomas

Keratoacanthomas (KAs) are defined as neoplastic proliferations of keratinocytes arising in follicular epithelium; they rarely evolve into metastatic carcinoma.

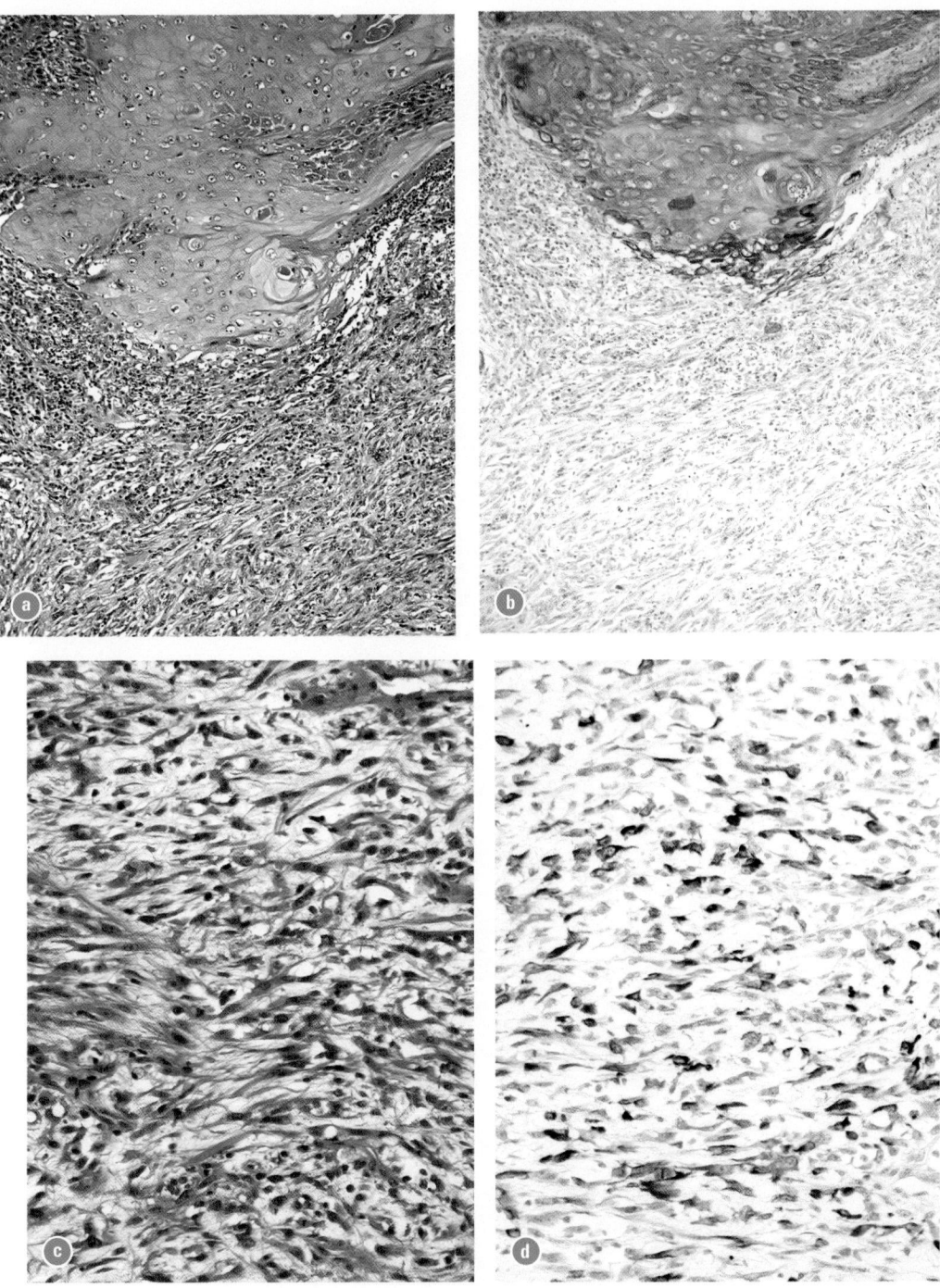

Fig. 6.31 Spindle cell carcinoma. (a) Junction of conventional squamous and spindle cell elements. (b) Keratin positivity in this case is confined to the well-differentiated component. (c) Spindle cell carcinoma. (d) The tumor stains strongly for cytokeratins. (Cases courtesy of Dr Christopher D.M. Fletcher.)

These tumors are known to develop rapidly, spontaneously regress in some instances and occasionally evolve into squamous carcinoma with metastases. Suspected causes in the skin include ultraviolet light, host gene alterations, immunosuppression, chemical carcinogens, viruses and trauma.[90]

Reports of keratoacanthomas in the vulva are extremely rare. Two cases have been reported, both of which were treated by local excision and did not recur.[91,92] Reports of anal KAs have noted an excellent prognosis, notwithstanding the difficulty in distinguishing these tumors from well-differentiated squamous cell carcinomas.[93–95]

Histologically, keratoacanthomas are discrete, inverted and form a crater of well-differentiated neoplastic keratinocytes with central keratin (Fig. 6.33a,b). A pro-

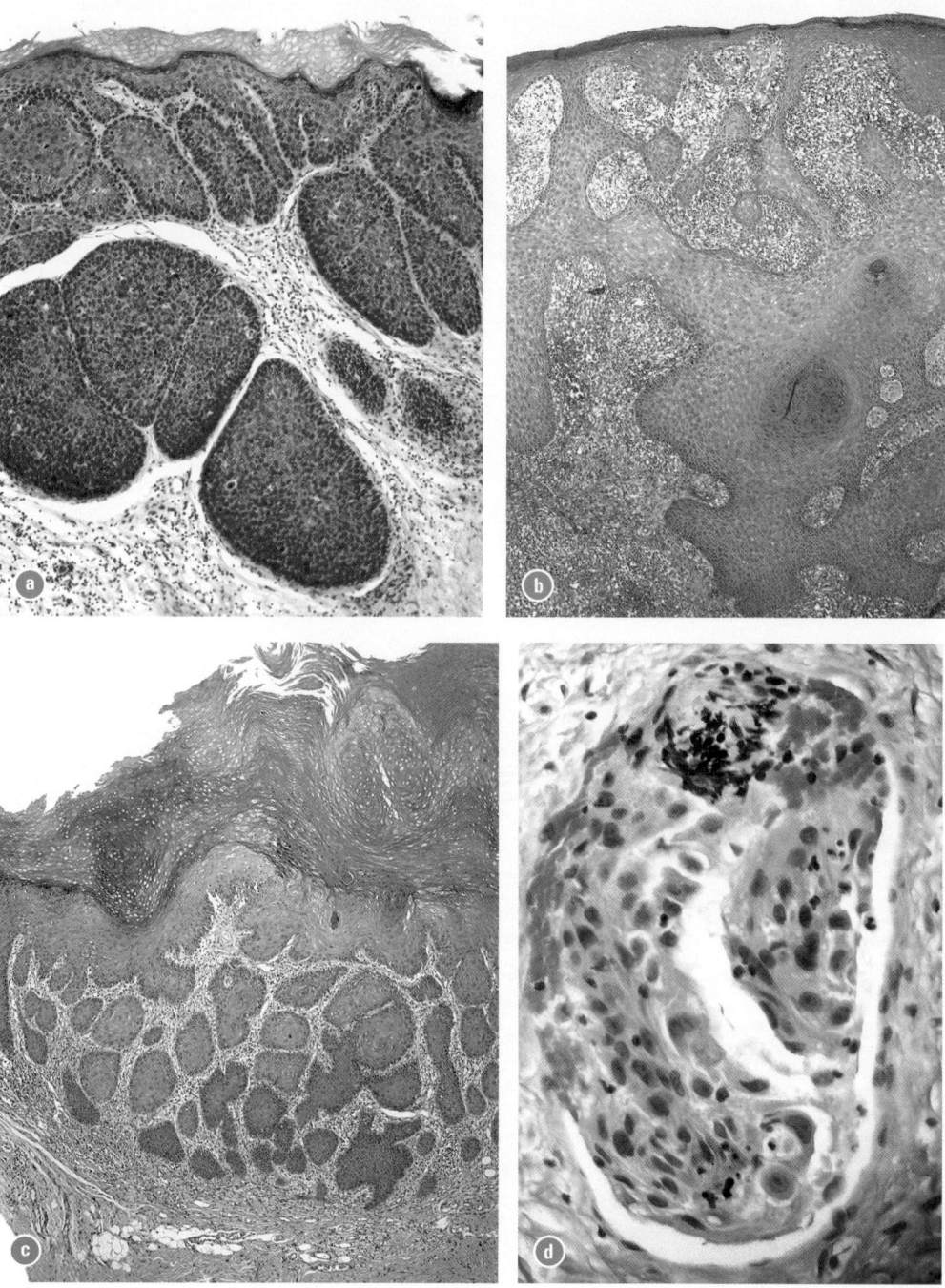

Fig. 6.32 Differential diagnosis of invasion. (a) Tangential section and/or adnexal involvement. In contrast to invasive carcinoma, the nests are discrete, uniform and non-interlacing. (b,c) Pseudoepitheliomatous hyperplasia. (d) Neoplastic epithelium in spaces produced by injection artifact.

portion of these tumors exhibit sufficient atypia to merit a diagnosis of squamous cell carcinoma (Fig. 6.33c). Hence the distinction of KA from SCC is based on careful evaluation of the entire lesion, with an appreciation of the fact that lesions classified as KA may signify an early phase of SCC. Lesions that fulfill the criteria for KA, with rapid onset and classic histologic appearance, may be amenable to conservative excision.

Superficially invasive (microinvasive) squamous cell carcinoma

INTRODUCTION

The designation of microinvasive vulvar squamous carcinoma is based on the assumption that a specific

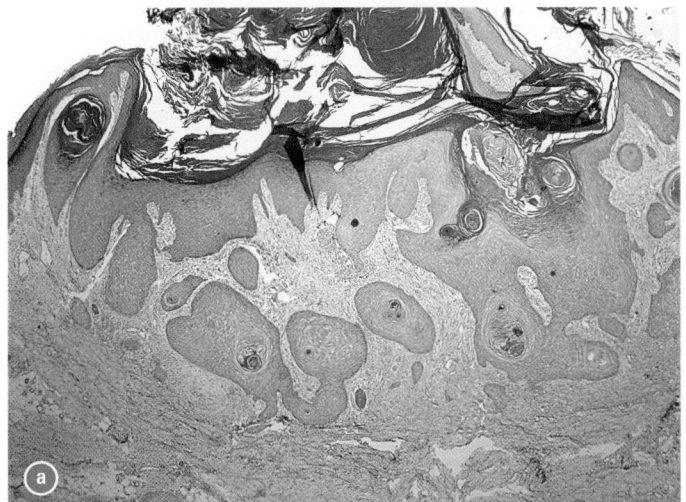

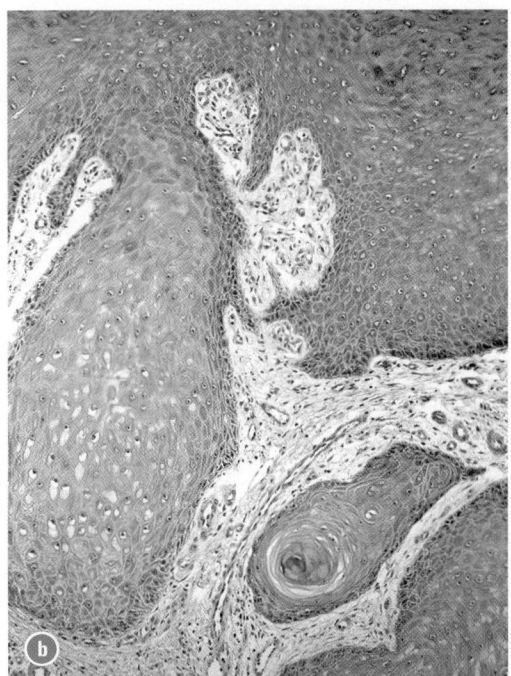

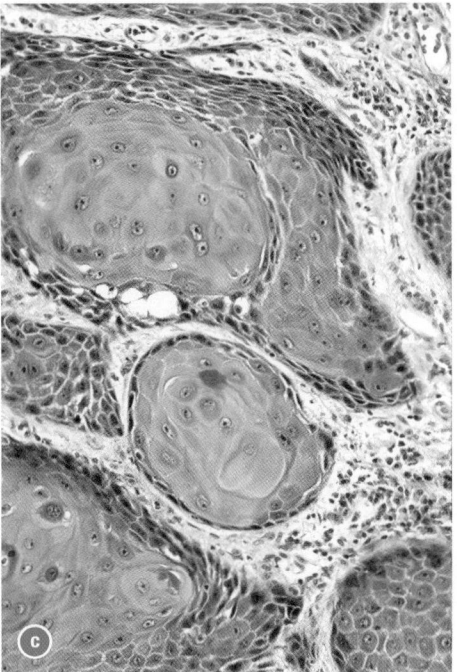

Fig. 6.33 Keratoacanthoma. (a) Cup-shaped lesion. The nesting pattern is non-complex, closely resembling pseudoepitheliomatous hyperplasia (see Fig. 6.32b,c). (b) At higher power, there is no atypia. (c) Well-differentiated carcinoma, with discernible atypia at the epithelial-stromal interface.

cut-off for invasion depth will identify women who do not require lymph node dissection. However, in contrast to the cervix, where the criteria for microinvasion have been defined and are commonly followed in management, the definition of microinvasive vulvar cancer has not always been clear. This is due to the facts that the anatomy of the vulva requires attention to not only size and depth of invasion but also to location of the tumor, inasmuch as the latter may influence the risk of contralateral lymph node involvement. Moreover, the submucosa of the vulva may carry a greater risk of ferrying tumor to the lymph nodes than that of the cervix. Thus, relative to the cervix, the natural history of early vulvar cancer is highly variable. Similar to the cervix, recurrences in untreated nodal fields carry a high risk of mortality. Numerous cases have been reported of conservatively managed early invasive tumors that eventuated in distant failure and loss of life.[96–99]

DEFINITION

In 1984, the ISSVD Task Force on Microinvasive Cancer of the Vulva concluded that the depth of stromal invasion was the critical determinant of prognosis, whereas actual lesion size carried less importance. However, the 3.0 mm cut-off that has been accepted for cervix has not been shown to be a safe threshold. Hoffman et al. found no metastases in 43 patients with 2.0 mm of invasion.[99] Hacker et al. found an unacceptable rate of lymph node involvement with depths of 3.0 mm.[100] Most rejected the term micro-invasion in lieu of simply stage Ia carcinoma and established the criteria as a single lesion less than 1.0 mm in depth and 2.0 cm in diameter (Table 6.5). Multiple sites of invasion did not qualify for this definition.[96]

Additional studies have examined the relationship of depth to risk of nodal metastases, which are summarized in Table 6.6.[101-104] A Gynecologic Oncology Group Study reiterated the importance of thickness, citing the fact that 50% of vulvar carcinomas were less than 5.0 mm thick and that 20% of these tumors metastasized to lymph nodes.[105] Within this range of disease, the most important correlates of lymph node involvement were tumor thickness, histologic grade, capillary-lymphatic space invasion (CLSI), clitoral or perineal involvement and clinically suspicious nodes. In an analysis of 272 women, they identified, retrospectively, two groups of patients who did not exhibit histologic evidence of lymph node metastases. The first had clinically negative nodes, no CLSI and a non mid-line tumor that was grade 1 (well-differentiated) and less than 5 mm thick. The second was the above features and a grade 2 neoplasm that was less than 2 mm thick.[105] Despite the existence of these two general categories, there is sufficient risk of lymph node metastases for tumors exceeding 1 mm that this depth is considered the most appropriate cut-off for the decision regarding lymph nodes dissection (Table 6.6).[106] Moreover, excision of even negative lymph nodes may influence outcome. Magrina et al. observed a lymph node recurrence in one of 30 women with invasion below 1 mm, at

Table 6.6 Lymph node metastases in early invasive vulvar cancer

Depth*	No.	Percent involved
Less than 1 mm	103	0
0–3 mm	277	8.3
3–5 mm	22	41

*For lesions less than 2.0 cm in width.[97,98,100–105]

7.5 years, which was in contrast to no recurrences in 10 of 10 women who underwent lymphadenectomy.[107] However, the above observations establish 1.0 mm as the acceptable cut-off for therapeutic decision making. Examples of early invasive patterns are illustrated in Figure 6.34. Management options will be addressed below.

Like the cervix, the presence or absence of capillary-lymphatic space invasion will influence outcome. In a series of Stage I tumors, Iversen noted the risk of nodal involvement to be 40% for tumors with CLSI versus 3% for those without.[108]

OTHER STUDIES OF EARLY INVASIVE CARCINOMA

Natural history

Squamous cell carcinomas pursue a predictable course, beginning with involvement of the superficial inguinal lymph nodes, followed by spread to the deep inguinal and pelvic lymph nodes (Fig. 6.35).[109] The most important risk factor for death is nodal involvement. Mortality is approximately 10, 60 and 80%, respectively, for tumors with no inguinal and pelvic lymph node involvement. The majority of recurrences manifest within the first year following surgery.[110,111]

Table 6.5 FIGO staging of vulvar carcinoma (1995)

Stage	Description	5-year survival (%) after radical vulvectomy	Actuarial 5-year survival
0	Carcinoma *in situ*		
I	Confined to vulva, ≤2 cm	77.6–87.5	86–97
IA	Invasion ≤1 mm		
IB	Invasion exceeding 1 mm		
II	Confined to vulva/perineum >2 cm	75–87	75–95
III	Involvement of ipsilateral nodes, vagina, anus, lower two-thirds of urethra	39.5–56.3	44–50
IV	Spread beyond the vulva	8.3	–
IVA	Involvement of upper-third of urethra, bladder, rectal mucosa, pelvic bone, bilateral nodal involvement		
IVB	Distant metastases, including pelvic nodes		

American Joint Commission on Cancer staging of vulvar carcinoma.[100,105] Summarized by Fu.[106]

Other risk factors

Additional pathologic risk factors influencing outcome include the following:

1 *Local relapse*: Rouzier et al. showed that relapses in the original surgical site or skin bridge site were significant predictors of poor outcome, with a 71% risk of cancer-related death at 5 years.[112] Interestingly, relapses beyond the surgical site did not influence mortality.

2 *Additional factors* of less significance include older age (73+), obesity, smoking and high parity.[113]

3 *The principal pathologic risk factors* are tumor stage, vascular space invasion and lymph node involvement. The 5-year survival rate was 60% for perineal recurrences, 27% for inguinal and pelvic recurrences, 15% for distant recurrences and 14% for multiple recurrences in a multicenter study.[111]

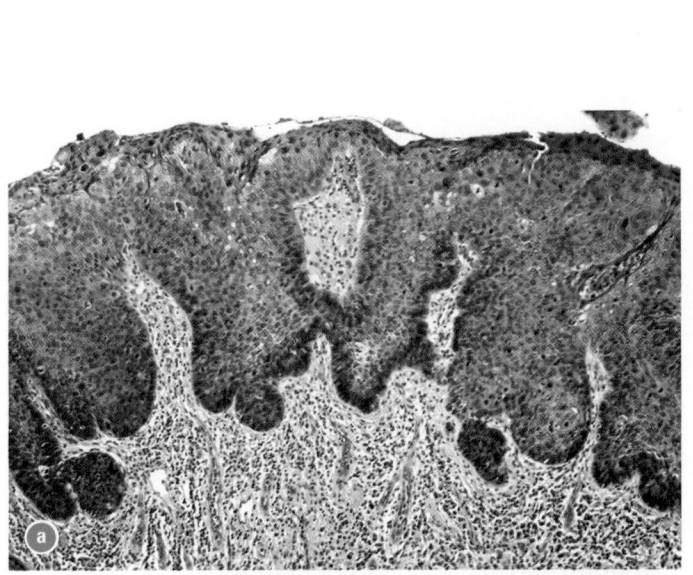
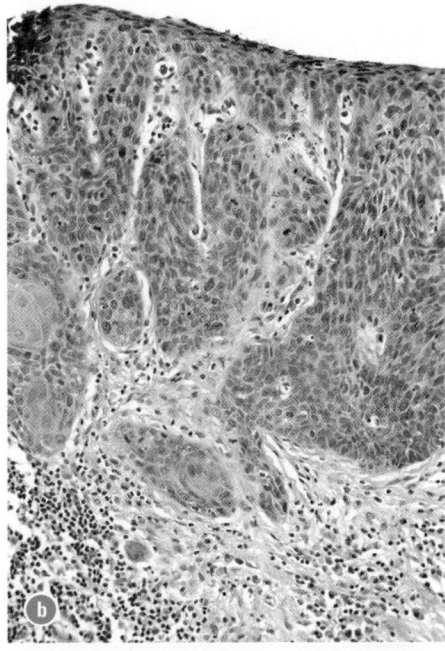
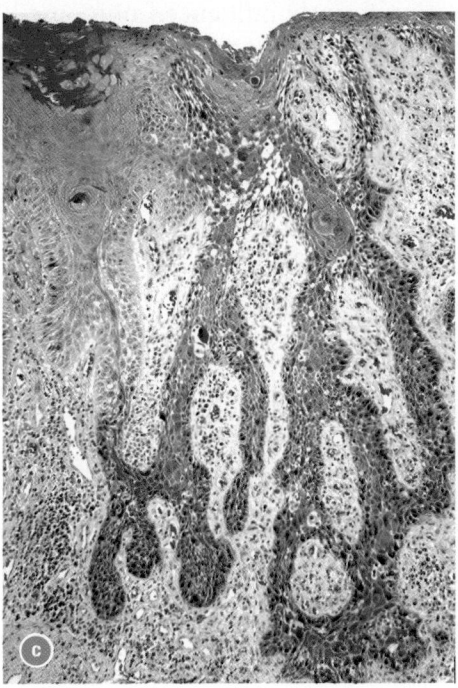
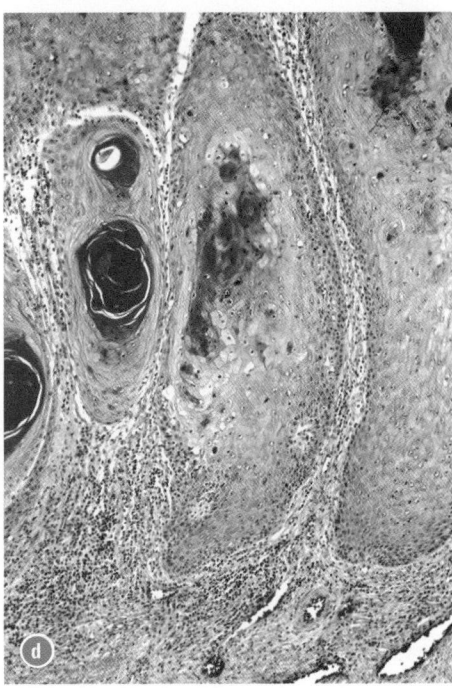

Fig. 6.34 Patterns of superficial invasion. (a) Early budding invasion. (b) Small detached nests from a classic VIN with less than 1.0 mm of invasion. One nest (center below) requires further evaluation to exclude capillary-lymphatic space invasion. (c) Continuous serpentine pattern without detachment, presumably cured by excision. (d) Extremely well-differentiated nests without atypia, characterizing verrucous carcinoma. Local excision was performed.

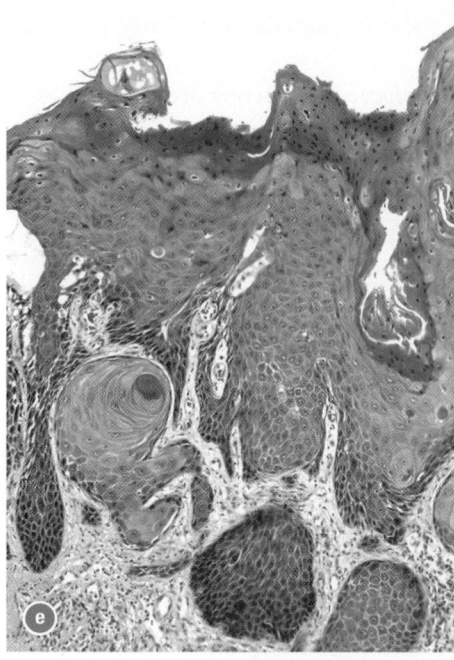 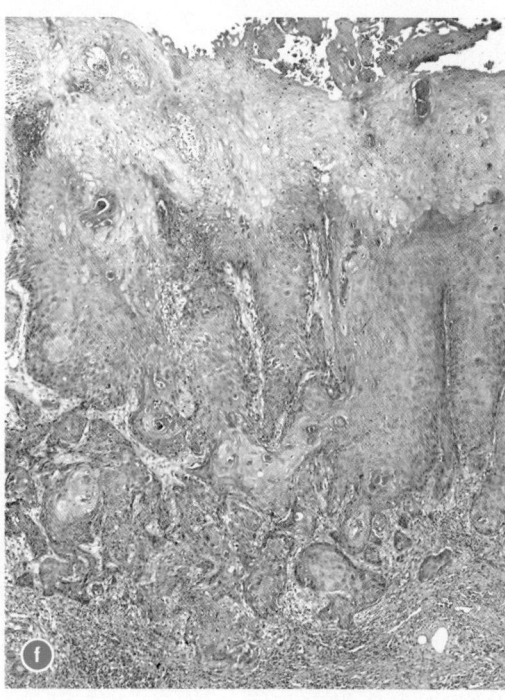

Fig. 6.34 Cont'd (e) Superficial well-differentiated squamous carcinoma. Lymph nodes were dissected and were negative. (f) Invasive squamous cell carcinoma from a tumor measuring 10 mm in length by 3 mm in thickness. This tumor metastasized to the regional lymph nodes, with eventual death of the patient.

4 *Histologic type and HPV status* have both been implicated in prognosis, but there is no consensus. Pinto et al. found that the basaloid pattern (HPV positive) carried a greater than three-fold risk of mortality.[114] Another study showed a higher survival in cases where the adjacent mucosa contained classic VIN versus lichen sclerosus.[112,115] One study found a higher survival in the HPV-positive tumors.[116]

5 *Coexisting VIN.* Rowley et al. showed that the risk of metastases was low (1 of 34) for lesions with a coexisting VIN.[117]

6 *Extent of lymph node metastases.* Hoffman et al. found that size and number of nodal metastases significantly influenced outcome.[118]

7 *Duration from time of surgery.* Some 90% of recurrences develop within 2 years.[111]

8 *Vascular space invasion.* A total of 72% with CLSI metastasize to LN *vs* 34% without.

9 *Clitoral involvement.* A total of 27.4% spread to nodes *vs* 7.4% if confined to the labia.[119–121]

MANAGEMENT

1 *Early invasive carcinoma.* Wide local excision and ipsilateral lymph node dissection are used if the following criteria are met: a lesion less than 2.0 cm, no involvement of midline structures and clinically unsuspicious lymph nodes.

2 *Stage II or greater, or involvement of midline.* Wider excision or vulvectomy with bilateral lymph node dissection is standard management.

3 *Sentinel lymph node in the management of vulvar cancer.* The concept of sentinel node evaluation in

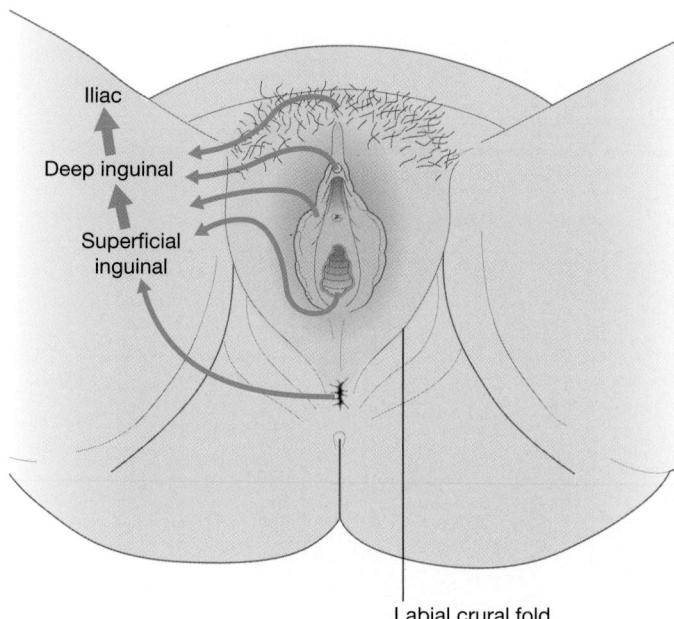

Iliac

Deep inguinal

Superficial inguinal

Labial crural fold

Fig. 6.35 Lymphatic drainage of the vulva. (Modified from Wilkinson et al. (Fig. 4.4), with permission.)[109]

the management of vulvar cancer is particularly attractive because it could conceivably reduce the degree of inguinal dissection required. Moore et al. found that the sentinel node was a reliable indicator of nodal involvement in the inguinal node chain, confirming the consistent pattern of nodal spread that characterizes vulvar cancer.[122,123] In contrast, even micrometastases may require an extensive dissection.[124] The persistent question is whether patients are willing to forgo more extensive surgery based on a single sentinel node determination, which carries a false-negative rate of 5–10%.[125,126] This risk may be reduced by microstaging and step sectioning of these lymph nodes.[126,127] Some authors have also noted a reduction in false negatives with experience and dye-based localization techniques.[128]

Basal cell carcinoma

Basal cell carcinomas of the vulva are rare, with a ratio of approximately 20 squamous carcinomas seen for every basal cell carcinoma at Brigham and Women's Hospital. These tumors are HPV negative and the typical patient is in the seventh or eighth decade.[129] The tumors present clinically as raised discoid or ulcerated neoplasms, although some may be polypoid (Fig. 6.36).[130]

Histologically, basal cell carcinomas are identical to those seen in the skin, exhibiting a uniform population

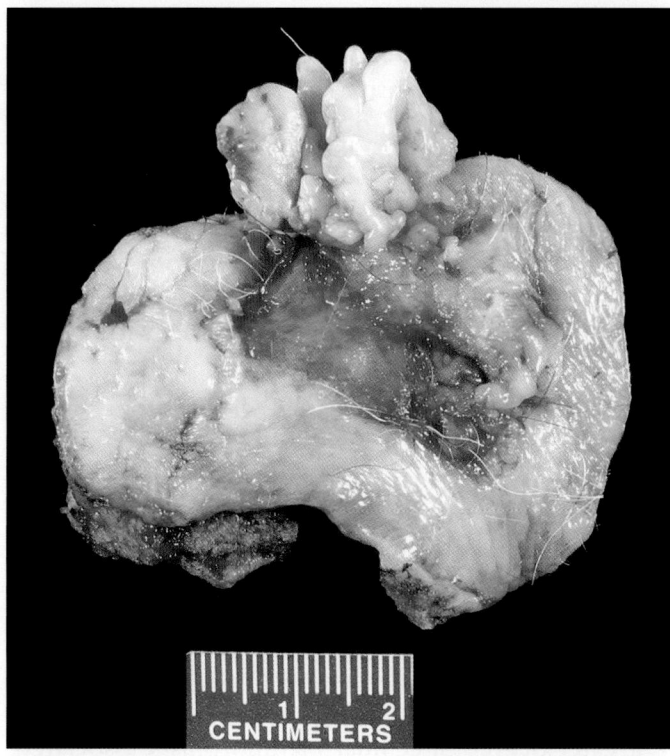

Fig. 6.36 Basal cell carcinoma. This gross photograph depicts an exophytic component adjacent to a shallow ulcer.

of basal cells with peripheral palisaded nuclei, single cell necrosis and absence of the more marked atypia attributed to squamous carcinomas (Fig. 6.37). However, some pathologic features may cause diagnostic confusion and include the following:

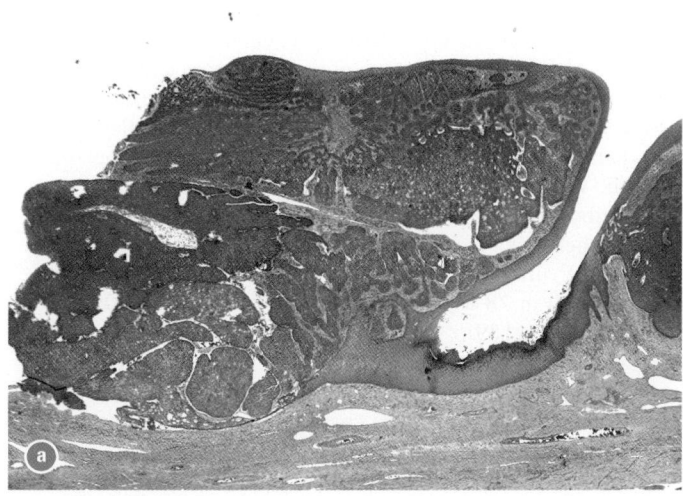
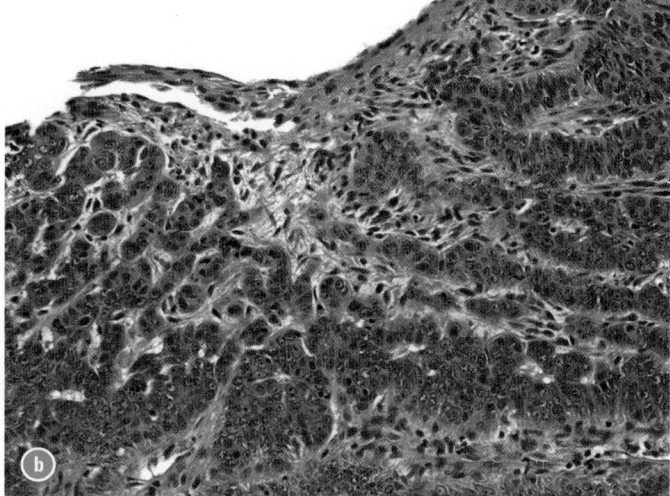

Fig. 6.37 (a) Histology of tumor depicted in Figure 6.36 reveals a combination of fungating tumor with overlying normal mucosa and flat areas with superficial ulceration. (b) A higher power view.

1 *Potential pitfalls of interpretation during intraoperative evaluation.* Because BCC is a non-metastasizing neoplasm, the preoperative or intraoperative recognition of these tumors is critical. Thus, attention must be paid during the frozen section analysis of any vulvar neoplasm for this variant.

2 *Recognition of variants which include the following*: (a) Conventional basal cell carcinomas are composed of cohesive growth patterns with uniform basaloid cells with preservation of polarity, low mitotic index and apoptosis. (b) Metatypical (basosquamous) basal cell carcinomas exhibit conspicuous squamoid differentiation, which may be confused with basaloid patterns seen in conventional squamous cell carcinoma. (c) Adenoid basal cell carcinomas exhibit adenoid differentiation.

3 *Differential diagnosis of basal cell carcinomas includes*: (a) Basaloid variants of squamous carcinoma. These tumors possess a conspicuously greater degree of cellular pleomorphism associated with loss of polarity and prominent desmoplasia. A classic VIN may be seen in the adjacent epithelium. (b) Variants of differentiated VIN, which may exhibit mild basal expansion. Generally the presence of more conspicuous keratinocyte atypia and a more subtle transition from squamous to basal cell phenotype will distinguish this entity from a superficial basal cell carcinoma. (c) The adenoid basal variant may be confused with adenoid cystic carcinoma. However, the latter are more deeply situated and should be easily distinguished. (d) Rare unclassified basaloid neoplasms may be encountered, but are usually more diffusely infiltrative and more poorly differentiated. A diagnosis of basal cell carcinoma must not be made unless the criteria for the entity are strictly met, inasmuch as sparing of lymph nodes is not acceptable in these other forms of carcinoma. (e) Other skin appendage tumors, such as proliferating trichilemmal cysts, may be confused with BCC. The latter present as multiple subcutaneous cystic lesions, however, and would be easily distinguished on clinical grounds.[131]

4 *Management and outcome*: Basal cell carcinomas are considered non-metastasizing and are managed by wide local excision only.[132,133] However, the frequency of metastases may be higher in other populations.[133,134]

References

1 Al Ghamdi A, Freedman D, Miller D, et al. Vulvar squamous cell carcinoma in young women: a clinicopathologic study of 21 cases. Gynecol Oncol 2002; 84:94–101.

2 Crum CP, Liskow A, Petras P, Keng WC, Frick HC. Vulvar intraepithelial neoplasia (severe atypia and carcinoma in situ). A clinicopathologic analysis of 41 cases. Cancer 1984; 54:1429–1434.

3 Sturgeon SR, Brinton LA, Devesa SS, Kurman RJ. In situ and invasive vulvar cancer incidence trends (1973 to 1987). Am J Obstet Gynecol 1992; 166:1482–1485.

4 Chiasson MA, Ellerbrock TV, Bush TJ, Sun XW, Wright TC Jr. Increased prevalence of vulvovaginal condyloma and vulvar intraepithelial neoplasia in women infected with the human immunodeficiency virus. Obstet Gynecol 1997; 89:690–694.

5 Conley LJ, Ellerbrock TV, Bush TJ, et al. HIV-1 infection and risk of vulvovaginal and perianal condylomata acuminata and intraepithelial neoplasia: a prospective cohort study. Lancet 2002; 359:108–113.

6 Crum CP, McLachlin CM, Tate JE, Mutter GL. Pathobiology of vulvar squamous neoplasia. Curr Opin Obstet Gynecol 1997; 9:63–69.

7 Brinton LA, Nasca PC, Mallin K, et al. Case-control study of cancer of the vulva. Obstet Gynecol 1990; 75:859–866.

8 Andersen WA, Franquemont DW, Williams J, Taylor PT, Crum CP. Vulvar squamous cell carcinoma and papillomaviruses: two separate entities? Am J Obstet Gynecol 1991; 165:329–335.

9 Daling JR, Sherman KJ, Hislop TG, et al. Cigarette smoking and the risk of anogenital cancer. Am J Epidemiol 1992; 135:180–189.

10 Mitchell MF, Prasad CJ, Silva EG, et al. Second genital primary squamous neoplasms in vulvar carcinoma: viral and histopathologic correlates. Obstet Gynecol 1993; 81(1):13–18.

11 Worsham MJ, Dyke DL Van, Grenman SE, et al. Consistent chromosome abnormalities in squamous cell carcinoma of the vulva. Genes Chromosomes Cancer 1991; 3(6):420–432.

12 Hart WR. Vulvar intraepithelial neoplasia: historical aspects and current status. Int J Gynecol Pathol 2001; 20(1):16–30.

13 Lin MC, Mutter GL, Trivijisilp P, et al. Patterns of allelic loss (LOH) in vulvar squamous carcinomas and adjacent noninvasive epithelia. Am J Pathol 1998; 152:1313–1318.

14 Pinto AP, Lin MC, Sheets EE, et al. Allelic imbalance in lichen sclerosus, hyperplasia and intraepithelial neoplasia of the vulva. Gynecol Oncol 2000; 77:171–176.

15 Leibowitch M, Neill S, Pelisse M, Moyal-Baracco M. The epithelial changes associated with squamous cell carcinoma of the vulva: a review of the clinical, histological and viral findings in 78 women. Br J Obstet Gynaecol 1990; 97:1135–1139.

16 Haefner HK, Tate JE, McLachlin CM, Crum CP. Vulvar intraepithelial neoplasia: age, morphological phenotype, papillomavirus DNA and coexisting invasive carcinoma. Hum Pathol 1995; 26(2):147–154.

17 Ansink AC, Krul MR, De Weger RA, et al. Human papillomavirus, lichen sclerosus and squamous cell

carcinoma of the vulva: detection and prognostic significance. Gynecol Oncol 1994; 52:180–184.

18 Gissmann L, de Villiers EM, zur Hausen H. Analysis of human genital warts (condylomata acuminata) and other genital tumors for human papillomavirus type 6 DNA. Int J Cancer 1982; 29(2):143–146.

19 Taichman LB, Reilly SS, LaPorta RF. The role of keratinocyte differentiation in the expression of epitheliotropic viruses. J Invest Dermatol 1983; 81:137s–140s.

20 Beutner KR. Human papilloma virus infection of the vulva. Semin Dermatol 1996; 15:2–7.

21 McLachlin CM, Kozakewich H, Craighill M, O'Connell B, Crum CP. Histologic correlates of vulvar human papillomavirus infection in children and young adults. Am J Surg Pathol 1994; 18:728–735.

22 Bai H, Cviko A, Granter S, et al. Immunophenotypic and viral (human papillomavirus) correlates of vulvar seborrheic keratosis. Hum Pathol 2003; 34(6):559–564.

23 Li J, Ackerman AB. 'Seborrheic keratoses' that contain human papillomavirus are condylomata acuminata. Am J Dermatopathol 1994; 16(4):398–408.

24 Nucci MR, Genest DR, Tate JE, Sparks CK, Crum CP. Pseudobowenoid change of the vulva: a histologic variant of untreated condylomata acuminatum. Mod Pathol 1996; 9:375–379.

25 Slater LJ. Correspondence re: Nucci MR, Genest DR, Tate JE, Sparks CK, Crum CP: Pseudobowenoid change of the vulva: a histologic variant of untreated condyloma acuminatum, in Mod Pathol 1996; 9:375. Mod Pathol 1996; 9(8):871.

26 Archard HO, Heck JW, Stanley HR. Focal epithelial hyperplasia: an unusual oral mucosal lesion found in Indian children. Oral Surg Oral Med Oral Pathol 1965; 20:201–212.

27 Bassioukas K, Danielides V, Georgiou I, et al. Oral focal epithelial hyperplasia. Eur J Dermatol 2000; 10(5):395–397.

28 Nucci MR, Young RH, Fletcher CD. Cellular pseudosarcomatous fibroepithelial stromal polyps of the lower female genital tract: an under-recognized lesion often misdiagnosed as sarcoma. Am J Surg Pathol 2000; 24:231–240.

29 Moyal-Barracco M, Leibowitch M, Orth G. Vestibular papillae of the vulva. Lack of evidence for human papillomavirus etiology. Arch Dermatol 1990; 126:1594–1598.

30 Nuovo GJ, Blanco JS, Silverstein SJ, Crum CP. Histologic correlates of papillomavirus infection of the vagina. Obstet Gynecol 1988; 72(5):770–774.

31 McLachlin CM, Mutter GL, Crum CP. Multinucleated atypia of the vulva. Report of a distinct entity not associated with human papillomavirus. Am J Surg Pathol 1994; 18:1233–1239.

32 LeBoit PE. Multinucleated atypia. Am J Surg Pathol 1996; 20(4):507.

33 Logani S, Lu D, Quint WG, Ellenson LH, Pirog EC. Low-grade vulvar and vaginal intraepithelial neoplasia: correlation of histologic features with human papillomavirus DNA detection and MIB-1 immunostaining. Mod Pathol 2003; 16(8):735–741.

34 Mittal K, Palazzo J. Cervical condylomas show higher proliferation than do inflamed or metaplastic cervical squamous epithelium. Mod Pathol 1998; 11(8):780–783.

35 Ferenczy A, Mitao M, Nagai N, Silverstein SJ, Crum CP. Latent papillomavirus and recurring genital warts. N Engl J Med 1985; 313(13):784–788.

36 Ferenczy A. Comparison of 5-fluorouracil and CO_2 laser for treatment of vaginal condylomata. Obstet Gynecol 1984; 64:773–778.

37 Ferenczy A. Treating genital condyloma during pregnancy with the carbon dioxide laser. Am J Obstet Gynecol 1984; 148:9–12.

38 Ferenczy A. Using the laser to treat vulvar condylomata acuminata and intraepidermal neoplasia. Can Med Assoc J 1983; 128:135–137.

39 Allen AL, Siegfried EC. The natural history of condyloma in children. J Am Acad Dermatol 1998; 39(6):951–955.

40 Hammerschlag MR. Sexually transmitted diseases in sexually abused children: medical and legal implications. Sex Transm Infect 1998; 74(3):167–174.

41 Moscicki AB. Genital HPV infections in children and adolescents. Obstet Gynecol Clin North Am 1996; 23(3):675–697.

42 Armstrong DK, Handley JM. Anogenital warts in prepubertal children: pathogenesis, HPV typing and management. Int J STD AIDS 1997; 8(2):78–81.

43 Stevens-Simon C, Nelligan D, Breese P, Jenny C, Douglas JM Jr. The prevalence of genital human papillomavirus infections in abused and nonabused preadolescent girls. Pediatrics 2000; 106(4):645–649.

44 Silverberg MJ, Thorsen P, Lindeberg H, Grant LA, Shah KV. Condyloma in pregnancy is strongly predictive of juvenile-onset recurrent respiratory papillomatosis. Obstet Gynecol 2003; 101(4):645–652.

45 Derkay CS, Darrow DH. Recurrent respiratory papillomatosis of the larynx: current diagnosis and treatment. Otolaryngol Clin North Am 2000; 33(5):1127–1142.

46 Shah K, Kashima H, Polk BF, et al. Rarity of cesarean delivery in cases of juvenile-onset respiratory papillomatosis. Obstet Gynecol 1986; 68(6):795–799.

47 Kaufman RH, Gardner HL. Intraepithelial carcinoma of the vulva. Clin Obstet Gynecol 1965; 8:1035–1050.

48 Ikenberg H, Schworer D, Pfleiderer A. [Detection of human papilloma virus (HPV) DNA in vulvar cancers]. Geburtshilfe Frauenheilkd 1988; 48:776–780. [in German]

49 Friedrich EG Jr. Wilkinson EJ, Fu YS. Carcinoma in situ of the vulva: a continuing challenge. Am J Obstet Gynecol 1980; 136:830–843.

50 Sillman FH, Sentovich S, Shaffer D. Ano-genital neoplasia in renal transplant patients. Ann Transplant 1997; 2(4):59–66.

51 Crum CP, Fu YS, Levine RU, et al. Intraepithelial squamous lesions of the vulva: biologic and histologic criteria for the distinction of condylomas from vulvar intraepithelial neoplasia. Am J Obstet Gynecol 1982; 144:77–83.

52 Crum CP, Braun LA, Shah KV, et al. Vulvar intraepithelial neoplasia: correlation of nuclear DNA content and the presence of a human papilloma virus (HPV) structural antigen. Cancer 1982; 49:468–471.

53 Kurman RJ, Toki T, Schiffman MH. Basaloid and warty carcinomas of the vulva. Distinctive types of squamous cell

carcinoma frequently associated with human papillomaviruses. Am J Surg Pathol 1993; 17:133–145.

54 Ulbright TM, Stehman FB, Roth LM, Ehrlich CE, Ransburg RC. Bowenoid dysplasia of the vulva. Cancer 1982; 50:2910–2919.

55 Wade TR, Kopf AW, Ackerman AB. Bowenoid papulosis of the genitalia. Arch Dermatol 1979; 115(3):306–308.

56 Shatz P, Bergeron C, Wilkinson EJ, Arseneau J, Ferenczy A. Vulvar intraepithelial neoplasia and skin appendage involvement. Obstet Gynecol 1989; 74:769–774.

57 Benedet JL, Wilson PS, Matisic J. Epidermal thickness and skin appendage involvement in vulvar intraepithelial neoplasia. J Reprod Med 1991; 36:608–612.

58 Raju RR, Goldblum JR, Hart WR. Pagetoid squamous cell carcinoma in situ (pagetoid Bowen's disease) of the external genitalia. Int J Gynecol Pathol 2003; 22(2):127–135.

59 Brown HM, Wilkinson EJ. Uroplakin-III to distinguish primary vulvar Paget disease from Paget disease secondary to urothelial carcinoma. Hum Pathol 2002; 33:545–548.

60 Riethdorf S, Neffen EF, Cviko A, et al. p16INK4A expression as biomarker for HPV 16-related vulvar neoplasias. Hum Pathol 2004; 35(12):1477–1483.

61 Jones RW, McLean MR. Carcinoma in situ of the vulva: a review of 31 treated and five untreated cases. Obstet Gynecol 1986; 68:499–503.

62 Chafe W, Richards A, Morgan L, Wilkinson E. Unrecognized invasive carcinoma in vulvar intraepithelial neoplasia (VIN). Gynecol Oncol 1988; 31(1):154–165.

63 Jones RW, Rowan DM. Spontaneous regression of vulvar intraepithelial neoplasia 2–3. Obstet Gynecol 2000; 96:470–472.

64 Penna C, Fallani MG, Fambrini M, Zipoli E, Marchionni M. CO_2 laser surgery for vulvar intraepithelial neoplasia. Excisional, destructive and combined techniques. J Reprod Med 2002; 47(11):913–918.

65 Todd RW, Etherington IJ, Luesley DM. The effects of 5% imiquimod cream on high-grade vulval intraepithelial neoplasia. Gynecol Oncol 2002; 85(1):67–70.

66 Diaz-Arrastia C, Arany I, Robazetti SC, et al. Clinical and molecular responses in high-grade intraepithelial neoplasia treated with topical imiquimod 5%. Clin Cancer Res 2001; 7(10):3031–3033.

67 Seters M van, Fons G, Beurden M van. Imiquimod in the treatment of multifocal vulvar intraepithelial neoplasia 2/3. Results of a pilot study. J Reprod Med 2002; 47:701–705.

68 Hart WR. Simplex (differentiated) VIN: an underappreciated threat. Cont Ob-Gyn 2003; 4:59–83.

69 Crum CP. Vulvar intraepithelial neoplasia: histopathology and associated viral changes. In: Wilkenson E, ed. Pathology of the vulva and vagina. Edinburgh, UK: Churchill Livingstone; 1987:79–102.

70 Duray PH, Merino MJ, Axiotis C. Warty dyskeratoma of the vulva. Int J Gynecol Pathol 1983; 2(3):286–293.

71 Kaddu S, Dong H, Mayer G, Kerl H, Cerroni L. Warty dyskeratoma – "follicular dyskeratoma": analysis of clinicopathologic features of a distinctive follicular adnexal neoplasm. J Am Acad Dermatol 2002; 47(3):423–428.

72 Yang B, Hart WR. Vulvar intraepithelial neoplasia of the simplex (differentiated) type: a clinicopathologic study

73 Nascimento A, Medeiros F, Crum CP. New concepts in preinvasive squamous lesions of the vulva. Adv Anat Pathol 2005; 12:20–26.

74 Jones RW, Joura EA. Analyzing prior clinical events at presentation in 102 women with vulvar carcinoma. Evidence of diagnostic delays. J Reprod Med 1999; 44:766–768.

75 Rodke G, Friedrich EG Jr. Wilkinson EJ. Malignant potential of mixed vulvar dystrophy (lichen sclerosus associated with squamous cell hyperplasia). J Reprod Med 1988; 33:545–550.

76 Nascimento AF, Granter SR, Cviko A, et al. Vulvar acanthosis with altered differentiation: a precursor to verrucous carcinoma? Am J Surg Pathol 2004; 28(5):638–643.

77 Brisigotti M, Moreno A, Murcia C, Matias-Guiu X, Prat J. Verrucous carcinoma of the vulva. A clinicopathologic and immunohistochemical study of five cases. Int J Gynecol Pathol 1989; 8(1):1–7.

78 Andersen ES, Sorensen IM. Verrucous carcinoma of the female genital tract: report of a case and review of the literature. Gynecol Oncol 1988; 30(3):427–434.

79 Dvoretsky PM, Bonfiglio TA. The pathology of vulvar squamous cell carcinoma and verrucous carcinoma. Pathol Annu 1986; 21:23–45.

80 Andreasson B, Bock JE, Strom KV, Visfeldt J. Verrucous carcinoma of the vulval region. Acta Obstet Gynecol Scand 1983; 62(2):183–186.

81 Japaze H, Dinh T Van, Woodruff JD. Verrucous carcinoma of the vulva: study of 24 cases. Obstet Gynecol 1982; 60(4):462–466.

82 Levitan Z, Kaplan AL, Kaufman RH. Advanced squamous cell carcinoma of the vulva after treatment for verrucous carcinoma. A case report. J Reprod Med 1992; 37(10):889–892.

83 Ergun SS, Kural YB, Buyukbabani N, et al. Giant condyloma acuminatum. Dermatol Surg 2003; 29(3):300–303.

84 Trombetta LJ, Place RJ. Giant condyloma acuminatum of the anorectum: trends in epidemiology and management: report of a case and review of the literature. Dis Colon Rectum 2001; 44(12):1878–1886.

85 Lomo L, Crum CP. Papillary carcinoma of the vulva. Mod Pathol 2004; 17:204A.

86 Cooper WA, Valmadre S, Russell P. Sarcomatoid squamous cell carcinoma of the vulva. Pathology 2002; 34(2):197–199.

87 Santeusanio G, Schiaroli S, Anemona L, et al. Carcinoma of the vulva with sarcomatoid features: a case report with immunohistochemical study. Gynecol Oncol 1991; 40(2):160–163.

88 Holst VA, Fair KP, Wilson BB, Patterson JW. Squamous cell carcinoma arising in Hailey-Hailey disease. J Am Acad Derm 2000; 43(2):368–371.

89 Lee ES, Allen D, Scurry J. Pseudoepitheliomatous hyperplasia in lichen sclerosus of the vulva. Int J Gynecol Pathol 2003; 22:57–62.

90 Pattee SF, Silvis NG. Keratoacanthoma developing in sites of previous trauma: a report of two cases and review of the literature. J Am Acad Dermatol 2003; 48(2):S35–S38.

91 Rhatigan RM, Nuss RC. Keratoacanthoma of the vulva. Gynecol Oncol 1985; 21(1):118–123.

92 Gilbey S, Moore DH, Look KY, Sutton GP. Vulvar keratoacanthoma. Obstet Gynecol 1997; 89(5):848–850.

93 Kuppers F, Jongen J, Bock JU, Rabenhorst G. Keratoacanthoma in the differential diagnosis of anal carcinoma: difficult diagnosis, easy therapy. Report of three cases. Dis Colon Rectum 2000; 43(3):427–429.

94 Elliott GB, Fisher BK. Perianal keratoacanthoma. Arch Dermatol 1967; 95(1):81–82.

95 Jensen SL, Sjolin KE. Keratoacanthoma of the anus. Report of three cases. Dis Colon Rectum 1985; 28(10):743–745.

96 Kneale BL. Carcinoma of the vulva then and now. The 1987 ISSVD presidential address. J Reprod Med 1988; 33:496–499.

97 Atamdede F, Hoogerland D. Regional lymph node recurrence following local excision for microinvasive vulvar carcinoma. Gynecol Oncol 1989; 34:125–128.

98 Buckley CH, Butler EB, Fox H. Vulvar intraepithelial neoplasia and microinvasive carcinoma of the vulva. J Clin Pathol 1984; 37:1201–1211.

99 Hoffman JS, Kumar NB, Morley GW. Microinvasive squamous carcinoma of the vulva: search for a definition. Obstet Gynecol 1983; 61:615–618.

100 Hacker NF, Berek JS, Lagasse LD, Nieberg RK. Microinvasive carcinoma of the vulva. Obstet Gynecol 1983; 62:134–135.

101 Heaps JM, Fu YS, Montz FJ, Hacker NF, Berek JS. Surgical-pathologic variables predictive of local recurrence in squamous cell carcinoma of the vulva. Gynecol Oncol 1990; 38(3):309–314.

102 Morley GW. Infiltrative carcinoma of the vulva: results of surgical treatment. Am J Obstet Gynecol 1976; 124(8):874–888.

103 Parker RT, Duncan I, Rampone J, Creasman W. Operative management of early invasive epidermoid carcinoma of the vulva. Am J Obstet Gynecol 1975; 123(4):349–355.

104 DiSaia PJ, Creasman WT, Rich WM. An alternate approach to early cancer of the vulva. Am J Obstet Gynecol 1979; 133(7):825–832.

105 Homesley HD, Bundy BN, Sedlis A, et al. Prognostic factors for groin node metastasis in squamous cell carcinoma of the vulva (a Gynecologic Oncology Group study) Gynecol Oncol 1993; 49(3):279–283.

106 Fu YS, ed. Benign and malignant epithelial tumors of the vulva. In: Pathology of the uterine cervix, vagina and vulva. London: WB Saunders; 2002:168–231.

107 Magrina JF, Gonzalez-Bosquet J, Weaver AL, et al. Squamous cell carcinoma of the vulva stage IA: long-term results. Gynecol Oncol 2000; 76(1):24–27.

108 Iversen T. Squamous cell carcinoma of the vulva. Localization of the primary tumor and lymph node metastases. Acta Obstet Gynecol Scand 1981; 60(2):211–214.

109 Wilkinson EJ, Rico MJ, Pierson KK. Microinvasive carcinoma of the vulva. Int J Gynecol Pathol 1982; 1(1):29–39.

110 Nordin A, Mohammed KA, Naik R, de Barros Lopes A, Monaghan J. Does long-term follow-up have a role for node negative squamous carcinoma of the vulva? The Gateshead experience. Eur J Gynaecol Oncol 2001; 22(1):36–39.

111 Maggino T, Landoni F, Sartori E, et al. Patterns of recurrence in patients with squamous cell carcinoma of the vulva. A multicenter CTF Study. Cancer 2000; 89(1):116–122.

112 Rouzier R, Morice P, Haie-Meder C, et al. Prognostic significance of epithelial disorders adjacent to invasive vulvar carcinomas. Gynecol Oncol 2001; 81(3):414–419.

113 Kouvaris JR, Kouloulias VE, Loghis CD, et al. Minor prognostic factors in squamous cell vulvar carcinoma. Eur J Gynaecol Oncol 2001; 22(4):305–308.

114 Pinto AP, Signorello LB, Crum CP, et al. Squamous cell carcinoma of the vulva in Brazil: prognostic importance of host and viral variables. Gynecol Oncol 1999; 74(1):61–67.

115 Zaino RJ, Husseinzadeh N, Nahhas W, Mortel R. Epithelial alterations in proximity to invasive squamous carcinoma of the vulva. Int J Gynecol Pathol 1982; 1:173–184.

116 Monk BJ, Burger RA, Lin F, et al. Prognostic significance of human papillomavirus DNA in vulvar carcinoma. Obstet Gynecol 1995; 85(5):709–715.

117 Rowley KC, Gallion HH, Donaldson ES, et al. Prognostic factors in early vulvar cancer. Gynecol Oncol 1988; 31(1):43–49.

118 Hoffman JS, Kumar NB, Morley GW. Prognostic significance of groin lymph node metastases in squamous carcinoma of the vulva. Obstet Gynecol 1985; 66:402–405.

119 Rotmensch J, Rubin SJ, Sutton HG, et al. Preoperative radiotherapy followed by radical vulvectomy with inguinal lymphadenectomy for advanced vulvar carcinomas. Gynecol Oncol 1990; 36(2):181–184.

120 Figge DC, Gaudenz R. Related invasive carcinoma of the vulva. Am J Obstet Gynecol 1974; 119(3):382–395.

121 Figge DC, Tamimi HK, Greer BE. Lymphatic spread in carcinoma of the vulva. Am J Obstet Gynecol 1985; 152(4):387–394.

122 Moore RG, DePasquale SE, Steinhoff MM, et al. Sentinel node identification and the ability to detect metastatic tumor to inguinal lymph nodes in squamous cell cancer of the vulva. Gynecol Oncol 2003; 89(3):475–479.

123 Penson RT, Fuller AF Jr. Nodal metastasis is highly consistent in squamous cell carcinoma of the vulva. J Clin Oncol 2001; 19(8):2364–2365.

124 Tamussino KF, Bader AA, Lax SF, Aigner RM, Winter R. Groin recurrence after micrometastasis in a sentinel lymph node in a patient with vulvar cancer. Gynecol Oncol 2002; 86(1):99–101.

125 Hullu JA De, Hollema H, Lolkema S, et al. Vulvar carcinoma. The price of less radical surgery. Cancer 2002; 95(11):2331–2338.

126 Hullu JA de, Hollema H, Piers DA, et al. Sentinel lymph node procedure is highly accurate in squamous cell carcinoma of the vulva. J Clin Oncol 2000; 18(15):2811–2816.

127 Molpus KL, Kelley MC, Johnson JE, Martin WH, Jones HW 3rd. Sentinel lymph node detection and microstaging in vulvar carcinoma. J Reprod Med 2001; 46(10):863–869.

128 Levenback C. Intraoperative lymphatic mapping and sentinel node identification: gynecologic applications. Recent Results Cancer Res 2000; 157:150–158.

129 Gibson GE, Ahmed I. Perianal and genital basal cell carcinoma: a clinicopathologic review of 51 cases. J Am Acad Dermatol 2001; 45(1):68–71.

130 Takahashi H. Non-ulcerative basal cell carcinoma arising on the genitalia. J Dermatol 2000; 27(12):798–801.

131 Ramesh V, Iyengar B. Proliferating trichilemmal cysts over the vulva. Cutis 1990; 45(3):187–189.

132 Mulayim N, Foster Silver D, Tolgay Ocal I, Babalola E. Vulvar basal cell carcinoma: two unusual presentations and review of the literature. Gynecol Oncol 2002; 85(3):532–537.

133 Benedet JL, Miller DM, Ehlen TG, Bertrand MA. Basal cell carcinoma of the vulva: clinical features and treatment results in 28 patients. Obstet Gynecol 1997; 90(5):765–768.

134 Mizushima J, Ohara K. Basal cell carcinoma of the vulva with lymph node and skin metastasis – report of a case and review of 20 Japanese cases. J Dermatol 1995; 22(1):36–42.

7

Glandular and other malignancies of the vulva

Christopher P. Crum

Introduction

Adenosquamous carcinoma

Adenocarcinoma

Paget's disease
Carcinoma arising in ectopic
  breast tissue
Other adnexal carcinomas

Carcinoma of Bartholin gland

Introduction
Tumor categories
Outcome

Merkel cell carcinoma

The patient at risk
Pathologic findings
Biomarkers
Differential diagnosis
Management and outcome

Cloacogenic neoplasms

Metastatic adenocarcinoma

Introduction

By far the most common epithelial malignancies of the vulva are squamous carcinomas and their precursor lesions. The remaining tumors are rarer and include adenosquamous carcinomas, adenocarcinomas, including metastatic (Table 7.1) Bartholin gland and neuroendocrine carcinomas.[1]

Adenosquamous carcinoma

Adenosquamous carcinoma of skin appendages is a well-known variant of squamous cell carcinoma that occurs primarily in sun-exposed areas of the head and neck and rarely metastasizes. In 1974, Lasser et al. described a similar lesion of the vulva that paradoxically was associated with a high rate of metastatic disease.[2] Since their report, an additional series has confirmed the aggressive behavior of this neoplasm and the importance of distinguishing it from conventional squamous carcinoma. Some have been reported in association with hidradenomas although such an occurrence is exceedingly rare.[3]

Adenosquamous carcinoma comprised 18 of 135 cases of vulvar cancer in one study.[4] However, in the author's experience, conspicuous glandular differentiation is present in well under 10% of vulvar squamous carcinomas. Relatively little information is available regarding human papillomavirus (HPV) status, but a minority of cases (1 of 16) scored positive in one study.[5] The relatively older mean age (between 65 and 70 years) and association with chronic vulvar inflammatory disease further supports a pathogenesis that does not include HPV. All tumors involve the labium majus and most also involve the minus.[3] In the majority, glandular differentiation is present in both primary and metastatic tumor. The tumors are usually discovered in an advanced state. Underwood et al. observed that none of their patients presented with T-1 disease and that two-thirds were T-3 or higher when diagnosed.[4]

Histologically, adenosquamous carcinoma exhibits a subtle blend of columnar and squamous differentiation, the former composed of spaces lined by one to two cell layers (Fig. 7.1a,b). The squamous component may exhibit acantholysis and desquamation of dyskaryotic cells into glandular spaces. Based on ultrastructural observations both Johnson and Helwig and Underwood et al. concluded that adenosquamous carcinomas arose from the mucin-producing cells of the hair shafts.[4,6] An alternative explanation is selective re-differentiation within a conventional squamous carcinoma. When entertaining the diagnosis of adenosquamous carcinoma of the vulva, the pathologist should exclude the following: (1) Conventional squamous carcinomas with acantholysis, areas of desquamation or solid components that produce a pseudo-glandular differentiation. (2) Invasive Paget's disease or other adnexal carcinomas that will appear decidedly columnar in origin. (3) Amelanotic malignant melanomas that may mimic adenosquamous tumors, but can usually be distinguished by the presence of melanoma *in situ* and positivity with appropriate immunostains (HMB-45).

The prognosis of adenosquamous carcinoma is considered poorer than conventional squamous carcinoma, although this is based on few reports.[3] Management is similar to that of squamous carcinoma of comparable stage (Ch. 6).

Table 7.1 *Vulvar neoplasms with glandular differentiation*

Adenosquamous carcinoma
Paget's disease
Ectopic breast carcinoma
Adnexal carcinomas
  Microcystic carcinoma
  Adenocystic basal cell carcinoma
  Ductal eccrine carcinomas
  Clear cell hidradenocarcinoma
  Apocrine carcinoma
  Eccrine porocarcinoma
Bartholin gland carcinoma
  Adenoid cystic carcinoma
  Adenocarcinoma
Metastatic adenocarcinoma

Adenocarcinoma

PAGET'S DISEASE

Paget's disease accounts for less than 2% of vulvar neoplasms.[7] The average age in most series is approximately 65 years; the majority of patients are over age 50 when diagnosed. The most common symptom is vulvar pruritus, which predates diagnosis in from 1 to 17 years.[7] The disease may involve the labium majus or minus, perineum, anus and clinically appears as an eczematoid, erythematous, sometimes ulcerated lesion (Fig. 7.2).

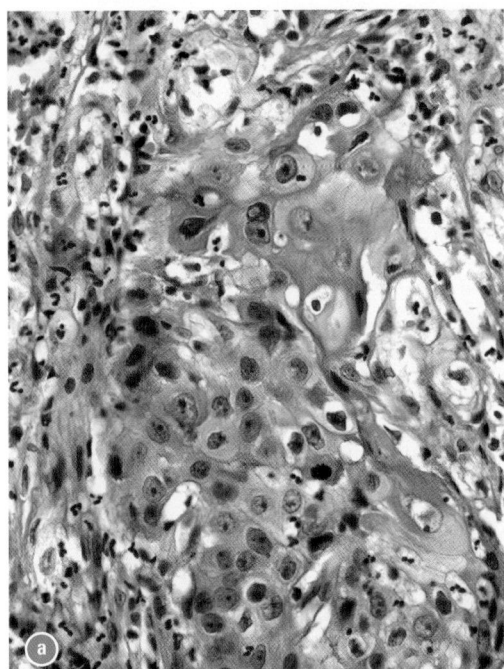 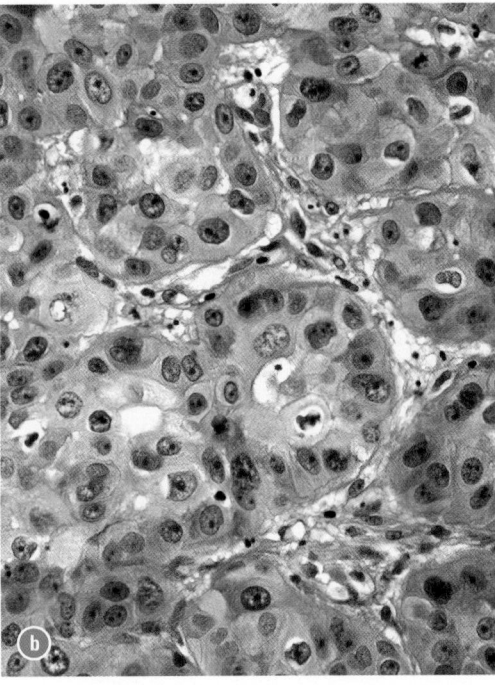

Fig. 7.1 Adenosquamous carcinoma of the vulva. (a) Focus of keratinization, (b) focal acinar formation in the same tumor as (a).

Paget's disease of the vulva, or any site, is characterized by infiltration of the squamous mucosa or adnexae by mucin-producing neoplastic cells. The disease presumably originates in the appendages, and evidence supports both an apocrine and eccrine ductal origin.[8,9] In the breast, this process is usually associated with an underlying intraductal or invasive adenocarcinoma. In the vulva, the majority of cases are *not* associated with invasion; approximately 20% either have a coexisting invasive adenocarcinoma, which is either the source of or sequelae to the intraepithelial lesion.[10,11]

Histologically, vulvar Paget's disease is characterized by large oval to polyhedral cells with pale cytoplasm, large nuclei and small nucleoli. The cells are arranged either singly or in large clusters or nests within the epithelium, where they may be interspersed with normal squamous epithelial cells with or without hyperkeratosis and squamous pearls (Fig. 7.3). Extensive sectioning will virtually always uncover focal involvement of the adnexal glands, and it is this constant feature that further supports an origin in these structures (Fig. 7.4).[9] The tumor cells are characteristically positive for mucin, CEA and her-2-neu (Fig. 7.5).

Important considerations in the laboratory and clinical management of Paget's disease include the following:

Associated squamous lesions. Brainard and Hart reported a diverse array of squamous epithelial alterations associated with Paget's disease of the vulva.[12] Most were benign squamous proliferations, including acanthosis (termed squamous hyperplasia NOS), and mixed stromal epithelial alterations, including 'fibroepithelioma-like hyperplasia' and papillomatous hyperplasia. The authors suggested that these alterations should prompt a search for Paget's disease, although the specificity of these changes is unknown. However, they also observed occasional coexisting squamous neoplasms, including rare HPV-positive squamous carcinomas in association with Paget's disease.[12]

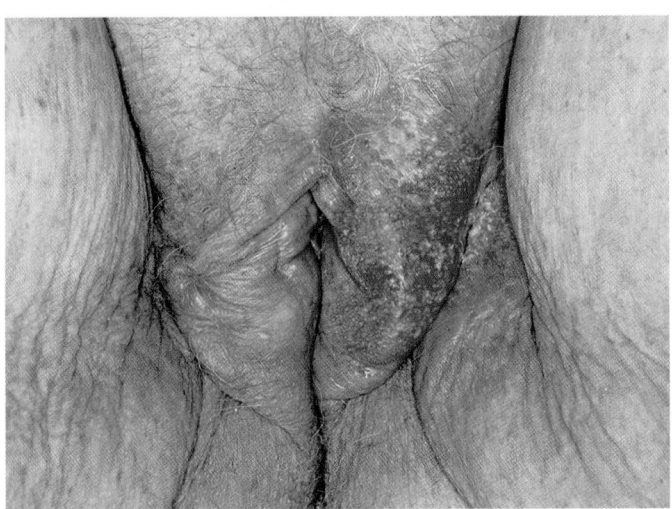

Fig. 7.2 Clinical appearance of Paget's disease of the vulva. The (patient's) left vulva is erythematous and superficially ulcerated.

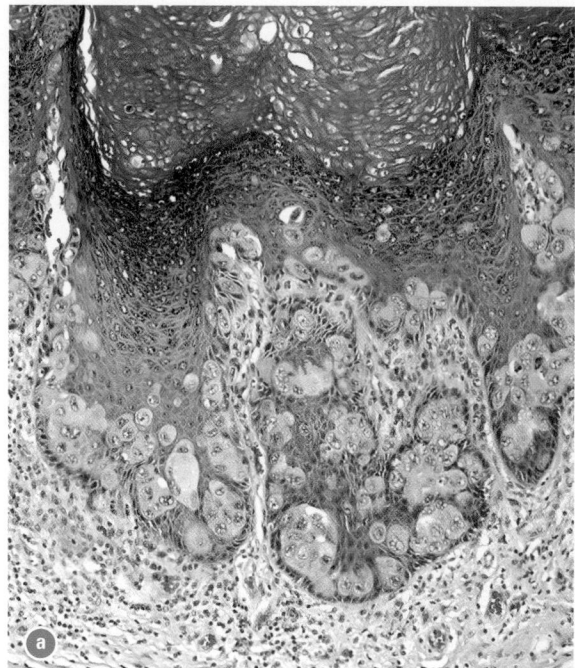

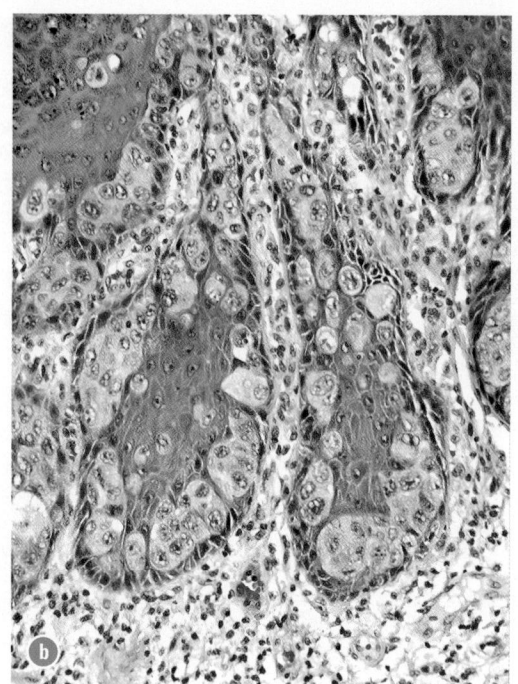

Fig. 7.3 Paget's disease of the vulva. (a) There is replacement of the squamous epithelium by large mucin-filled columnar cells, (b) seen at higher power. (c) In some foci the Paget cells are more scattered and less conspicuous.

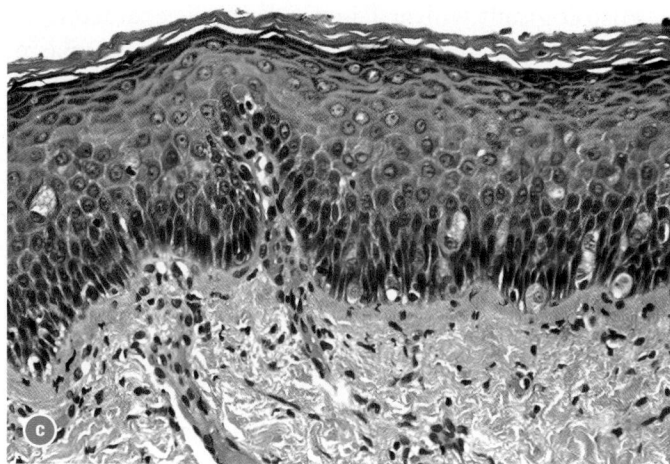

Excluding mimics. Paget's disease must be distinguished from several other entities. The first is malignant melanoma (see Ch. 8, Figs 8.20–8.25). Both Paget's disease and melanoma invade the epidermis, extend into skin appendages, and may even be sloughed in the superficial keratin. Although they can be distinguished by a mucin stain, immunostaining with HMB-45 (melanoma) and CEA (Paget's disease) will confirm the diagnosis. The second is misclassification as an acantholytic dermatosis (Fig. 7.6a). Another mimic is pagetoid vulvar intraepithelial neoplasia of squamous origin

(Fig. 7.6b).[13] This can be distinguished by markers of squamous (p63) differentiation and the absence of mucin. The third is direct extension of a urothelial carcinoma to the vulvar mucosa. This rare disorder may be impossible to distinguish from Paget's disease on first examination. The distinction is made immunohistochemically by a staining profile of GCDFP+ and CK7+/CK20– in vulvar Paget's disease *vs* GDFP– CK7+/CK20+ in urothelial neoplasia (Figs 7.5; 7.6b,c).[12,14]

Excluding invasion on histologic examination. Because Paget's disease develops at the epithelial-stromal interface and extends into adnexal

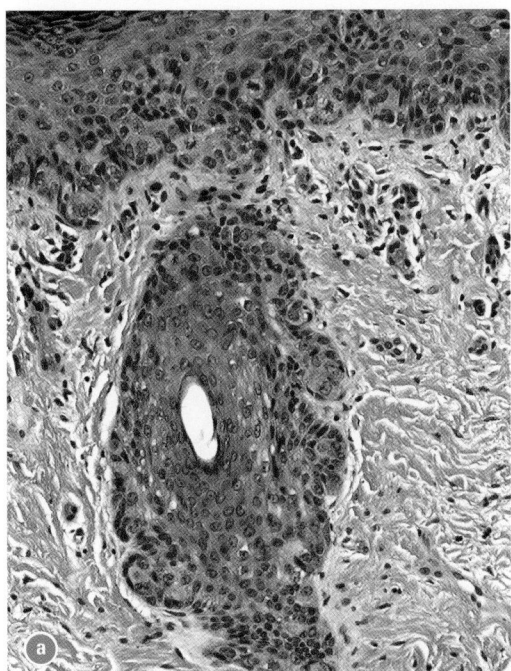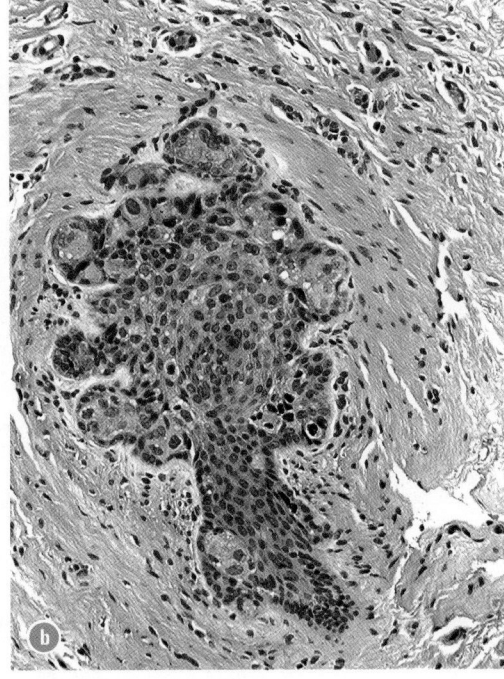

Fig. 7.4 Paget's disease with adnexal involvement. (a) Superficial adnexal extension. (b) Involvement of deeper structures.

structures, the exclusion of invasion may be particularly difficult for the pathologist. This problem is greatest when individual cells are seen in the superficial stroma or when inflammation obscures the tumor cell stromal interface. Invasion is characterized by discohesive groups of tumors cell infiltrating into the underlying dermis or submucosa (Fig. 7.7).[15]

The possibility of an underlying invasive neoplasm. In the majority of cases of Paget's disease associated with cancer, the underlying cancer is diagnosed initially and is of similar histology. Rarely, squamous carcinomas have been reported in association with Paget's disease.[7] One case of primary carcinoma of Bartholin gland with secondary involvement of the overlying epithelium has been reported.[16] Mortality is closely related to the depth of invasion. Crawford et al. correlated outcome with depth of invasion in 10 cases of invasive vulvar Paget's disease. Of seven patients with dermal invasion less than 1.0 mm, none died of their disease. Of three patients with invasion exceeding 1.0 mm, all had nodal metastases.[17]

Extent of epithelial spread. The major problem posed by Paget's disease is the extensive distribution of the lesion. Inasmuch as Paget's disease spreads freely through the network of epithelia, conventional excision will frequently be inadequate and the lesion will recur. Adamson and Reisenfield emphasized this problem in their observation that clinically uninvolved skin frequently contained histologic evidence of neoplasia. Moreover, uninvolved skin adjacent to negative margins could also be involved.[18] However, Taylor et al. noted that if careful histologic examination revealed negative margins, recurrence rates were low.[7] Pierie et al. noted recurrences in 42% and significant association with positive margins requiring up to 6 excisions in some patients.[19]

Risk of subsequent invasion. The risk of subsequent invasion is low once concurrent invasive tumor has been excluded. Hart and McMillan noted a single patient who was followed for nearly 11 years.[10] In these unusual cases, the invasion occurs via disruption of the basement membrane with primary dermal invasion.

Risk of breast or other carcinomas. Friedrich et al. summarized the literature and noted that of 78 reported cases of vulvar Paget's disease, 14 were associated with carcinoma of the breast.[20] In a few, there was coexisting Paget's disease at both sites. Aside from the similarity in embryogenesis and functional anatomy in the two sites, the reason for this frequent association is unknown. It should be stressed that the ratio (14:78) could reflect biased

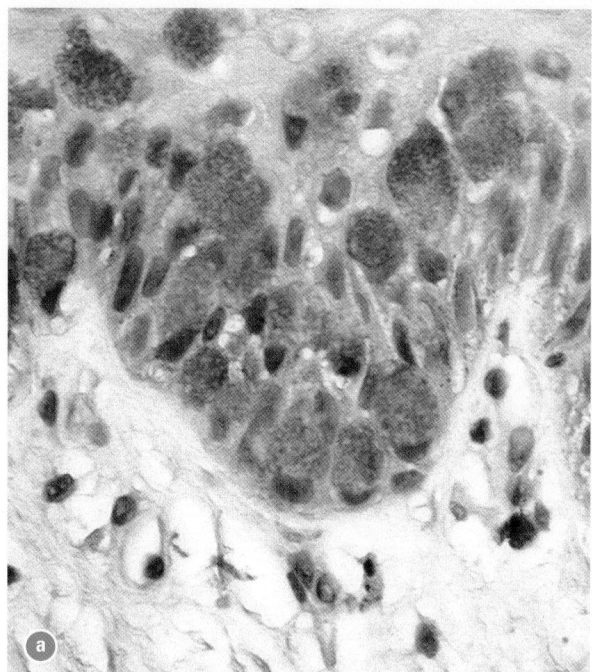
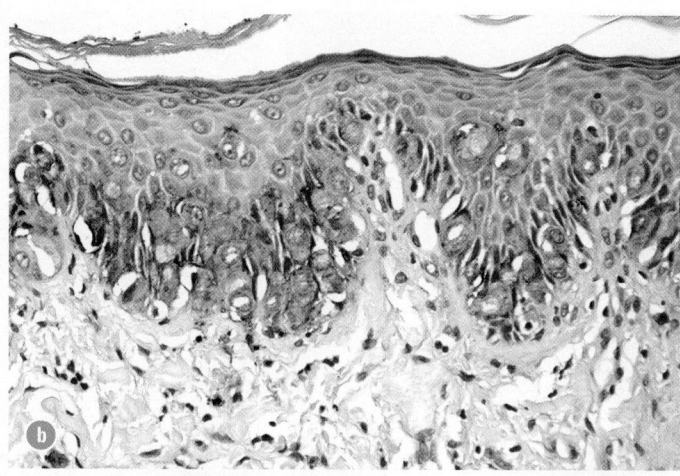
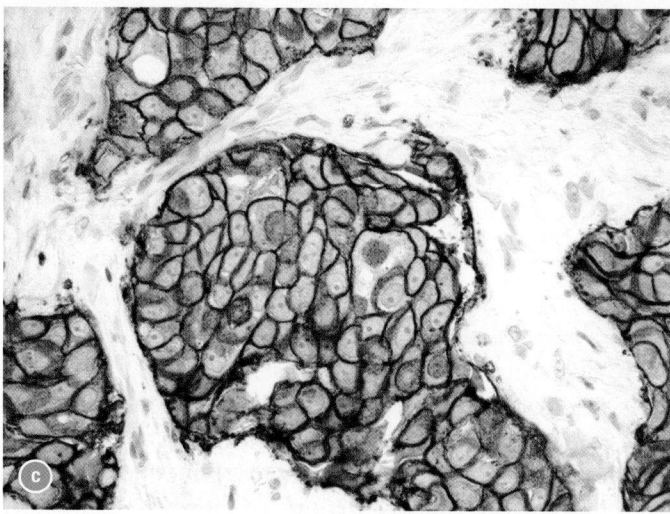

Fig. 7.5 Markers for Paget's disease. (a) A mucicarmine stain highlights individual cells, (b) strong immunopositivity for CEA, (c) staining for her-2-neu.

reporting inasmuch as coexisting breast and vulvar neoplasms may be the subject of case reports.

Pierie et al. noted either breast or other carcinomas in 42% of patients. Overall mortality was not increased over patients of similar age, however.[19] The majority of patients are treated by local excision and reconstruction if necessary but non-surgical approaches with follow-up are also permitted.[21] As mentioned above, Paget's disease may coexist with or mimic squamous CIS.[13,22] Management of vulvar Paget's disease should entail the exclusion of underlying cancer, careful histologic mapping to determine if residual disease is present and careful follow-up with the expectation that the disease will occur.

CARCINOMA ARISING IN ECTOPIC BREAST TISSUE

Supernumerary breast tissue on the vulva is extremely rare, with about 40 cases reported up to 2000.[23]

One review of the literature in 2002 cited only 13 case reports (including their own) of primary mammary carcinoma of the vulva.[24,25] These tumors occur in postmenopausal women, and include mostly ductal and, rarely, colloid carcinomas (Fig. 7.8). Receptors may aid in supporting an ectopic breast origin, although they are not invariably positive.[26,27] Therapy parallels that of breast cancer, with radical excision, lymph node dissection and tamoxifen prophylaxis.[24,28]

In some instances the origin of the vulvar neoplasms may be in question, particularly when a primary carcinoma of the breast is present (see below).

OTHER ADNEXAL CARCINOMAS

Other adnexal tumors of the vulva have been rarely reported. These include microcystic adnexal carcinomas, adenoid cystic carcinomas involving the vestibular glands and other sweat gland tumors.[29–33]

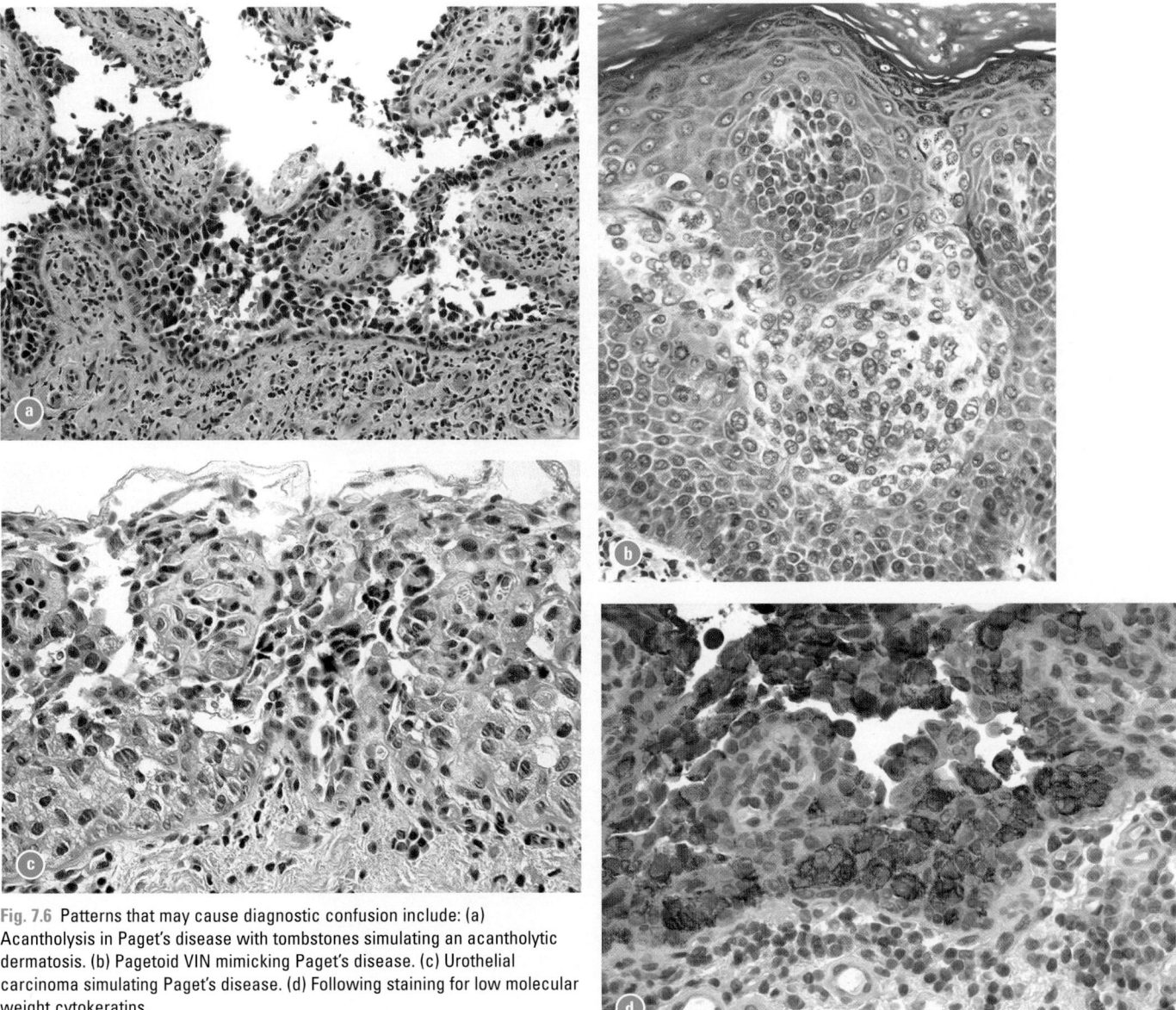

Fig. 7.6 Patterns that may cause diagnostic confusion include: (a) Acantholysis in Paget's disease with tombstones simulating an acantholytic dermatosis. (b) Pagetoid VIN mimicking Paget's disease. (c) Urothelial carcinoma simulating Paget's disease. (d) Following staining for low molecular weight cytokeratins.

Carcinoma of Bartholin gland

INTRODUCTION

Carcinoma of Bartholin gland is rare. In contrast to vulvar squamous carcinoma, which has an incidence of 0.42 and 4.72 per 100 000 woman-years in pre- and postmenopausal women, Bartholin gland carcinoma is approximately 20- and 40-fold less frequent in these populations, respectively. The index of suspicion is so low that Visco and Del Priore recommended drainage rather than surgical excision for primary management of Bartholin gland masses.[34]

TUMOR CATEGORIES

Squamous carcinoma

In the study by Copeland et al., squamous carcinomas comprised nearly three-quarters of Bartholin gland carcinomas.[31] Overall, these tumors are associated with a more favorable outcome than adenocarcinomas and neuroendocrine neoplasms.

Adenoid cystic carcinoma

Adenoid cystic carcinoma of Bartholin gland is a rare tumor of the vulva, accounting for less than 1% of all vulvar carcinomas and only 2 of 36 Bartholin gland tumors in the study by Copeland et al.[31] The rarity of

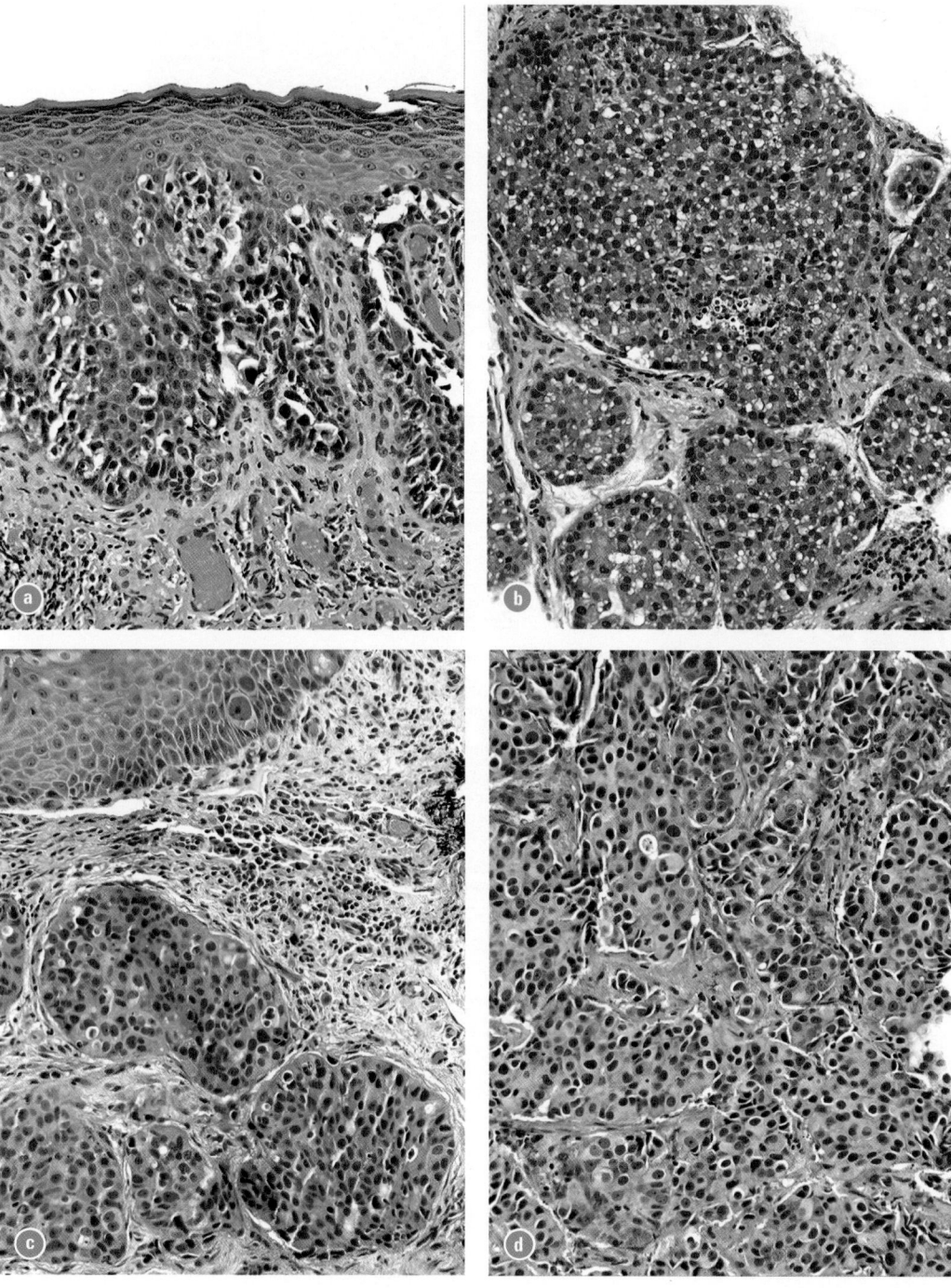

Fig. 7.7 (a) Paget's disease confined to the epithelium. (b) Invasion of the stroma as poorly differentiated cohesive aggregates. (c) Early stromal invasion. (d) Deeply invasive Paget's disease.

this tumor was underscored by Abell et al., who in a series of 719 primary neoplasms and cysts of the vulva, encountered not a single case.[35] Wahlstrom et al. found just 2 in 337 cases of primary vulvar carcinoma.[36] In all, less than 100 have been reported in case reports and short series. The average age is in the fourth decade with a wide age range. Rare cases have been associated with pregnancy. The tumors present as slow-growing masses that may be present for months or years prior to examination.

The histology of adenoid cystic carcinoma is similar to salivary gland, with small uniform tumor cells that may be subdivided into two types. The first are duct-like cells arranged in pseudoglands and containing PAS-positive luminal secretions. The second is the myoepithelial cell, arranged in nests, cords or reticular patterns in which the cells are suspended in a hyaline eosinophilic matrix (Fig. 7.9). Ultrastructurally, this material is composed of replicated basal lamina presumably elaborated by myoepithelial cells.

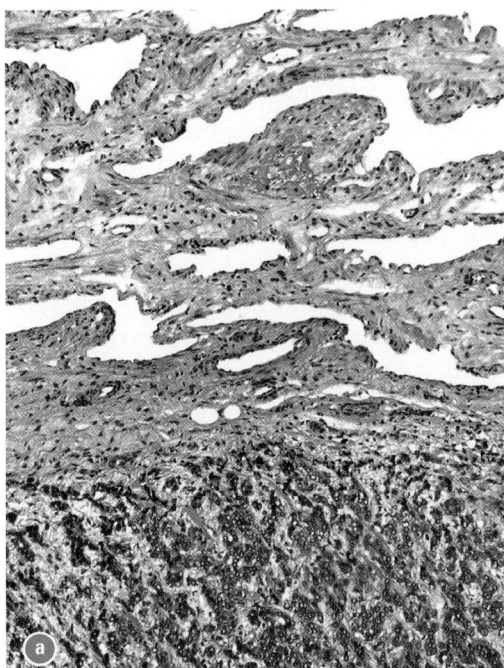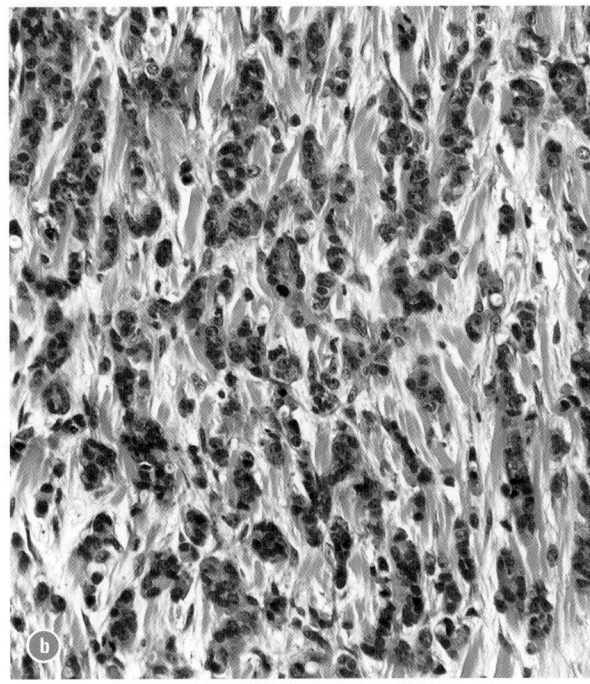

Fig. 7.8 Carcinoma in ectopic breast tissue in the vulva. (a) Erectile tissue is seen in the upper field. (b) The tumor invades as distinct cords of ductal carcinoma.

The differential diagnosis of adenoid cystic carcinoma includes benign hidradenoma (Ch. 5), basal cell carcinoma (Ch. 6), other adenocarcinomas and benign mixed tumors (Ch. 12). Hidradenomas contain the distinctive growth pattern discussed below, with a two-cell layer resembling ductal papilloma of the breast. Adenoid basal cell carcinomas are distinguished by their location in the superficial dermis and palisading nuclei. Benign mixed tumors (pleomorphic adenomas) may contain delicate cyst-like spaces, but are exceedingly rare in the vulva and contain a more subtle blend of epithelial and stromal differentiation. Adenosquamous carcinomas are easily distinguished by their characteristic morphology.

Adenoid cystic carcinomas of the vulva parallel those in the salivary gland by their slow, relentless, destructive and infiltrative growth, propensity for local recurrence and late metastasis to lymph nodes or lung. Perineural infiltration, an important component of salivary gland tumors, has been reported in the vulva and neural sheath involvement likely explains their propensity to recur. Long-term follow-up is required to accurately gauge outcome. Blanck et al. reported a 70% 5-year survival, but this dropped to 13% at 20 years, emphasizing the high risk of recurrence, further spread and death.[37] Radiotherapy is of uncertain benefit, in contrast to salivary gland neoplasms, and experience with chemotherapy is limited.[38]

Adenocarcinoma

Another subset of Bartholin gland carcinomas is adenocarcinoma of conventional type. These are extremely rare.[39,40]

Neuroendocrine carcinoma

Neuroendocrine carcinomas of Bartholin gland are exceedingly rare. Virtually all cases reported in the literature had nodal or distant spread and died within 2 years. This is consistent with the behavior of these tumors in other sites.[38,41–43]

OUTCOME

Copeland et al. have the largest series with outcome data on non-neuroendocrine tumors of Bartholin gland. In a study of 36 cases, 9, 15, 10 and 2 were FIGO Stage I, II, III and IV respectively. The numbers of squamous carcinoma, adenocarcinoma, adenoid cystic carcinoma and adenosquamous cell types were 27, 6, 2, and 1, respectively. A total of 47% with nodal dissections had metastases but 77% of those remained disease free. The authors advised wide excision, ipsilateral inguinal lymphadenectomy and adjunctive irradiation to the vulva and regional lymph nodes for optimal results. They reported a 5-year survival rate of 84%.[39] Wheelock et al. reported a 50% survival in 10 cases, but a poorer outcome for those with nodal metastases.[44] Cardosi et al. reported a 5-year survival of 58%; most were Stage II or greater.[45] They did not perceive a benefit with adjunctive radiotherapy.

Merkel cell carcinoma

THE PATIENT AT RISK

Merkel cell carcinoma of the vulva is a mucocutaneous neuroendocrine neoplasm arising in specialized epithelial cells that morphologically resemble melanocytes and Langerhans cells, but which contain neurosecretory granules. Tumors arising in these cells are exceedingly rare, estimated to be less than one-40th as common as melanomas, for a total of 400 cases per year in the USA. The vulva comprises 3% of Merkel cell carcinomas, bringing the estimated number to about 12 per year (American Cancer Society data). Less than 20 cases have been reported in the vulvar in the English medical literature.[46] The risk factors for cutaneous Merkel cell tumor are sun exposure and older (over 60) age. Patients managed for psoriasis with UV irradiation and Psoriasin are particularly susceptible to this tumor, as well as other cutaneous neoplasms. Exposure to arsenicals and immune suppression have also been associated with increased risk. Rare spontaneous regressions suggest immune factors may modulate behavior in rare cases.

PATHOLOGIC FINDINGS

Merkel cell carcinomas closely resemble other small blue cell tumors of the genital tract, including neuroendocrine (small cell) carcinomas, primitive neuroectodermal tumors and others. The tumors originate as small submucosal papules or nodules. Histologically, the tumors closely resemble other neuroendocrine tumors, composed of undifferentiated epithelial cells with variable nuclear size, high nuclear/cytoplasmic ratio, and oval pale-staining monotonous nuclei. High mitotic index, crush artifact or nuclear molding and geographic necrosis are common features (Fig. 7.10). Some tumors exhibit trabecular architecture seen in other neuroendocrine tumors. In some instances mucosal invasion by the tumor may simulate Paget's disease.[47]

BIOMARKERS

Merkel cell carcinomas express low molecular weight cytokeratins such as Cam5.2, AE1/AE3, and cytokeratin 20, typically in a paranuclear dot or crescent pattern (Fig. 7.11). Neuroendocrine markers such as chromogranin and synaptophysin are present, but S-100 is invariably absent. Ultrastructural studies are not routinely done, but reveal the characteristic 100–250 nm membrane-bound neurosecretory granules.[47]

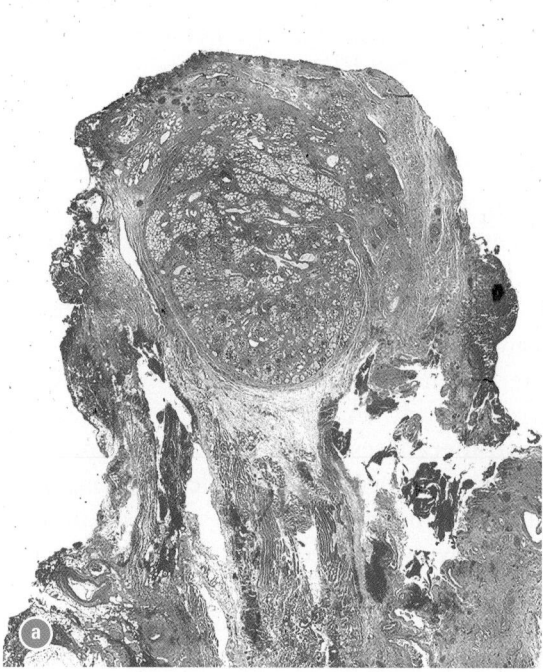

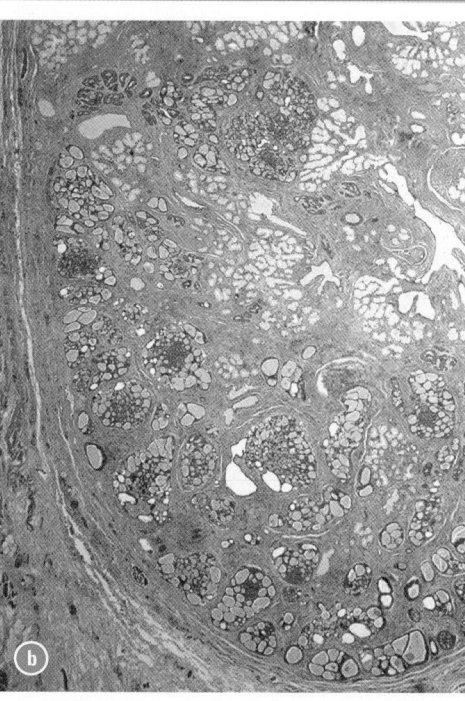

Fig. 7.9 Adenoid cystic carcinoma of Bartholin gland. (a) Resected specimen contains a discrete focus of tumor in the gland (upper center), (b) low power of involved gland,

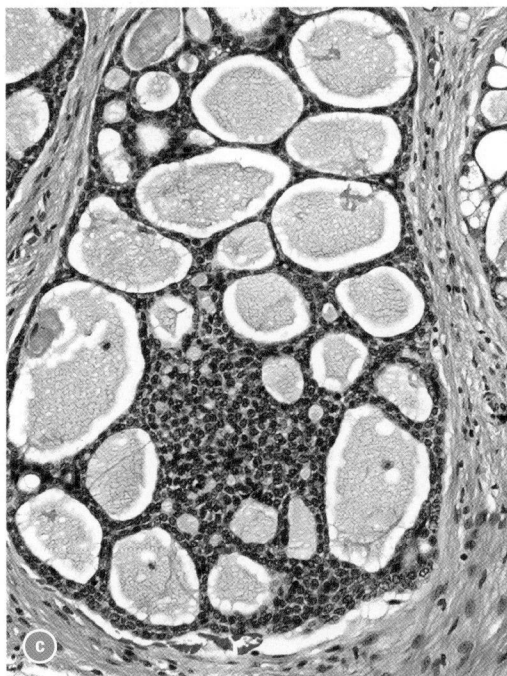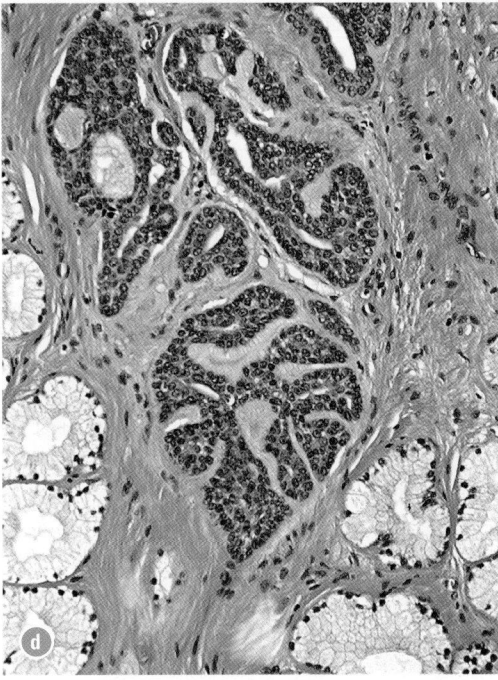

Fig. 7.9 **Cont'd** (c) microcystic growth pattern with delicate gland septae and (d) less well-organized growth with interstitial hyaline changes. Normal glands are below.

DIFFERENTIAL DIAGNOSIS

The differential diagnosis of Merkel cell carcinoma includes metastatic neuroendocrine carcinoma of the lung, PNET, melanoma, basaloid squamous carcinoma and lymphoma. Lung carcinomas are typically CK 7 positive and CK 20 negative. PNETs are negative for the low molecular weight cytokeratins, and melanomas and squamous carcinomas are negative for neuroendocrine markers (melanomas are S-100 positive).

MANAGEMENT AND OUTCOME

Cutaneous Merkel cell carcinomas carry a poor prognosis, with at least a 10% mortality for the earliest-stage lesions. The vulvar tumors are considered to have a higher mortality in that most reported cases have died. Based on what is known about cutaneous tumors, wide margins (at least 2.5) and nodal sampling to exclude regional spread will identify patients with a lower risk of local recurrence and death. Radiation is also recommended and reports have attributed increased survival to its use. The tumors are chemosensitive, but chemotherapy apparently does not extend survival.[48,49]

Fig. 7.10 Merkel cell carcinoma, typically presenting as a poorly-differentiated small cell tumor undermining a normal epithelium.

Cloacogenic Neoplasms

Cloacogenic tumors of the vulva are a curious group of neoplasms that are morphologically identical to colonic neoplasms. They range in appearance from villous tumors closely resembling villous adenomas of

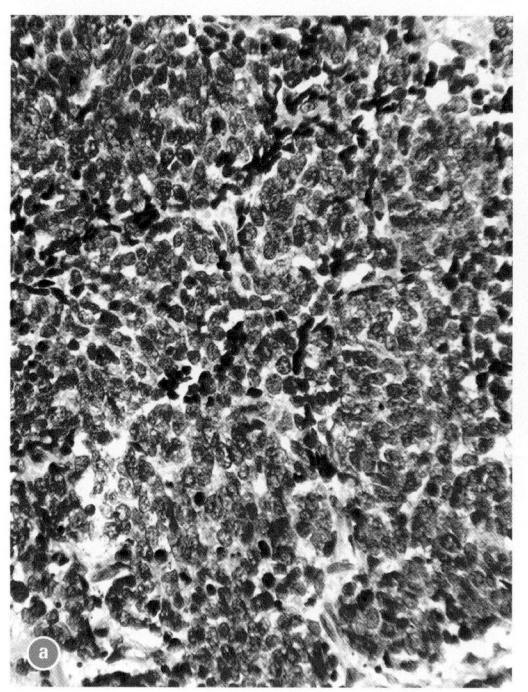
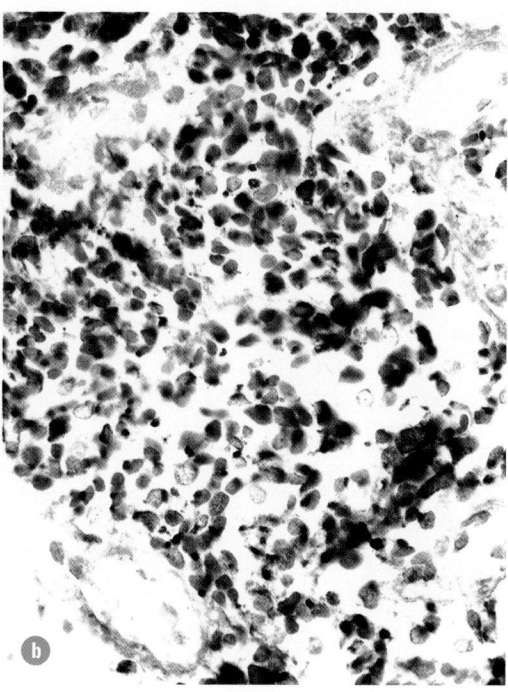

Fig. 7.11 (a) At high power, Merkel cell carcinoma is composed of undifferentiated tumor cells with a high nuclear/cytoplasmic ratio. (b) The tumor stains strongly for CK 20.

the colon to more poorly-differentiated adenocarcinomas (Fig. 7.12). They appear to arise directly from the otherwise-normal mucosa. The more popular theory of histogenesis holds that these tumors arise in some form of embryonic rest that is a hold over from the original cloaca. In the handful of cases reported, positive staining was noted for CEA in one and for both CK 7 and 14 in another. Management of the well-differentiated papillary tumors by excision has been successful in the few cases reported.[50–52] Rare multicentric cases have also been described.[53]

Metastatic adenocarcinoma

Metastatic carcinoma to the vulva is extremely rare, comprising only 5–8% of vulvar malignancies (Fig. 7.13). Reported primary sites include endometrium, lung and breast.[54,55] The two most problematic issues in differential diagnosis are the distinction of primary Paget's disease from metastatic urothelial carcinoma (see discussion of Paget's disease above) and a primary breast carcinoma in ectopic breast tissue *vs* metastatic breast carcinoma.[12,14] The latter has been described in less than 12 cases in

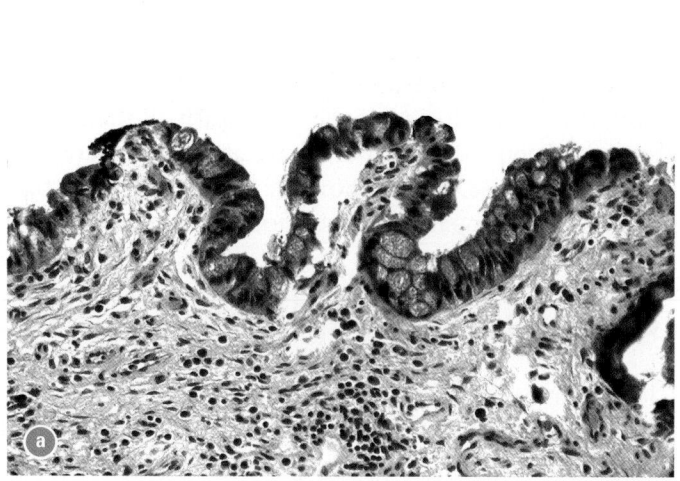
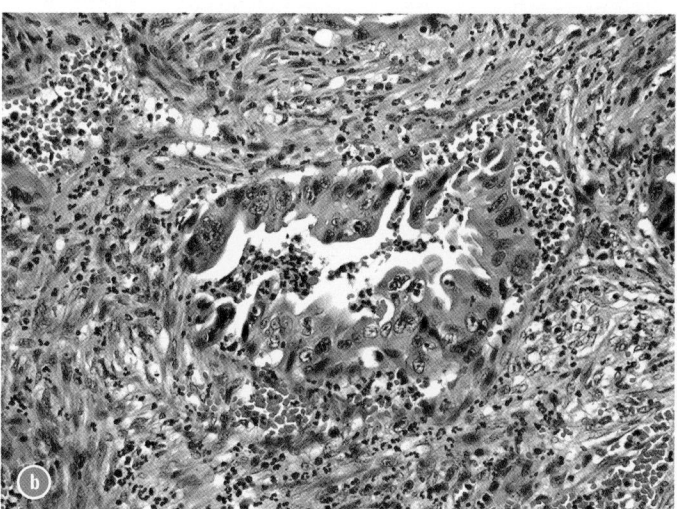

Fig. 7.12 (a) Cloacogenic carcinoma, seen on the mucosa surface as neoplastic goblet cells. (b) An invasive component displays typical colonic differentiation.

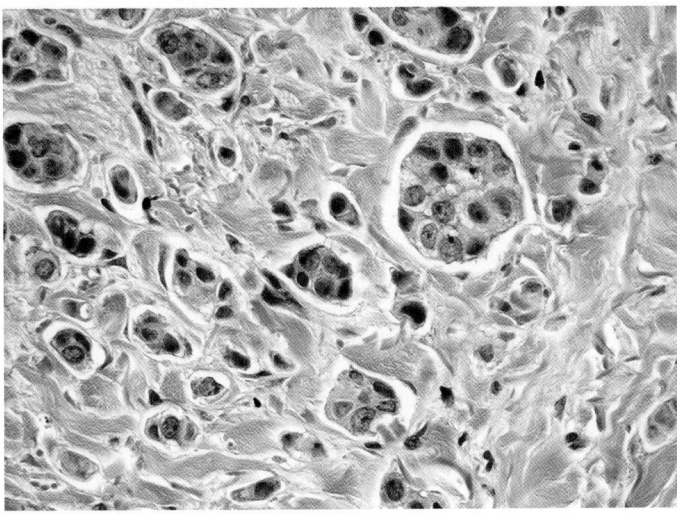

Fig. 7.13 Metastatic carcinoma to the vulva from the breast.

the literature.[56-58] If the tumor closely resembles the original breast carcinoma and normal ectopic breast tissue is not evident, the presumptive diagnosis is metastatic disease.

References

1 Chamlian DL, Taylor HB. Primary carcinoma of Bartholin's gland. A report of 24 patients. Obstet Gynecol 1972; 39(4):489–494.

2 Lasser A, Cornog JL, Morris JM. Adenoid squamous cell carcinoma of the vulva. Cancer 1974; 33(1):224–227.

3 Bannatyne P, Elliott P, Russell P. Vulvar adenosquamous carcinoma arising in a hidradenoma papilliferum, with rapidly fatal outcome: case report. Gynecol Oncol 1989; 35(3):395–398.

4 Underwood JW, Adcock LL, Okagaki T. Adenosquamous carcinoma of skin appendages (adenoid squamous cell carcinoma, pseudoglandular squamous cell carcinoma, adenocanthoma of sweat gland of Lever) of the vulva: a clinical and ultrastructural study. Cancer 1978; 42:1851–1858.

5 Carson LF, Twiggs LB, Okagaki T, et al. Human papillomavirus DNA in adenosquamous carcinoma and squamous cell carcinoma of the vulva. Obstet Gynecol 1988; 72:63–67.

6 Johnson WC, Helwig EB. Adenoid squamous cell carcinoma (adenoacanthoma). A clinicopathologic study of 155 patients. Cancer 1966; 19(11):1639–1650.

7 Taylor PT, Stenwig JT, Klausen H. Paget's disease of the vulva. A report of 18 cases. Gynecol Oncol 1975; 3(1):46–60.

8 Roth LM, Lee SC, Ehrlich CE. Paget's disease of the vulva. A histogenetic study of five cases including ultrastructural observations and review of the literature. Am J Surg Pathol 1977; 1(3):193–206.

9 Lee SC, Roth LM, Ehrlich C, Hall JA. Extramammary Paget's disease of the vulva. A clinicopathologic study of 13 cases. Cancer 1977; 39(6):2540–2549.

10 Hart WR, McMillan JB. Progression of intraepithelial Paget's disease of the vulva to invasive carcinoma. Cancer 1977; 40(5):2333–2337.

11 Baehrendtz H, Einhorn N, Pettersson F, Silfversward C. Paget's disease of the vulva: the Radiumhemmet series 1975–1990. Int J Gynecol Cancer 1994; 4(1):1–6.

12 Brainard JA, Hart WR. Proliferative epidermal lesions associated with anogenital Paget's disease. Am J Surg Pathol 2000; 24:543–552.

13 Raju RR, Goldblum JR, Hart WR. Pagetoid squamous cell carcinoma in situ (Pagetoid Bowen's disease) of the external genitalia. Int J Gynecol Pathol 2003; 22(2):127–135.

14 Wilkinson EJ, Brown HM. Vulvar Paget disease of urothelial origin: a report of three cases and a proposed classification of vulvar Paget disease. Hum Pathol 2002; 33:549–554.

15 Parmley TH, Woodruff JD, Julian CG. Invasive vulvar Paget's disease. Obstet Gynecol 1975; 46:341–346.

16 Tchang F, Okagaki T, Richart RM. Adenocarcinoma of Bartholin's gland associated with Paget's disease of vulvar area. Cancer 1973; 31(1):221–225.

17 Crawford D, Nimmo M, Clement PB, et al. Prognostic factors in Paget's disease of the vulva: a study of 21 cases. Int J Gynecol Pathol 1999; 18(4):351–359.

18 Adamson K, Reisenfield D. Observations on intradermal migration of Paget cells. Am J Obstet Gynecol 1964; 90:1274–1280.

19 Pierie JP, Choudry U, Muzikansky A, Finkelstein DM, Ott MJ. Prognosis and management of extramammary Paget's disease and the association with secondary malignancies. J Am Coll Surg 2003; 196:45–50.

20 Friedrich EG Jr, Wilkinson EJ, Steingraeber PH, Lewis JD. Paget's disease of the vulva and carcinoma of the breast. Obstet Gynecol 1975; 46:130–134.

21 MacLean AB, Makwana M, Ellis PE, Cunnington F. The management of Paget's disease of the vulva. J Obstet Gynaecol 2004; 24:124–128.

22 Quinn AM, Sienko A, Basrawala Z, Campbell SC. Extramammary Paget disease of the scrotum with features of Bowen disease. Arch Pathol Lab Med 2004; 128:84–86.

23 Gorisek B, Zegura B, Kavalar R, But I, Krajnc I. Primary breast cancer of the vulva: a case report and review of the literature. Wien Klin Wochenschr 2000; 112:855–858.

24 Piura B, Gemer O, Rabinovich A, Yanai-Inbar I. Primary breast carcinoma of the vulva: case report and review of literature. Eur J Gynaecol Oncol 2002; 23(1):21–24.

25 Bailey CL, Sankey HZ, Donovan JT, et al. Primary breast cancer of the vulva. Gynecol Oncol 1993; 50:379–383.

26 Yin C, Chapman J, Tawfik O. Invasive mucinous (colloid) adenocarcinoma of ectopic breast tissue in the vulva: a case report. Breast J 2003; 9:113–115.

27 Rose PG, Roman LD, Reale FR, Tak WK, Hunter RE. Primary adenocarcinoma of the breast arising in the vulva. Obstet Gynecol 1990; 76:537–539.

28 Kennedy DA, Hermina MS, Xanos ET, Schink JC, Hafez GR. Infiltrating ductal carcinoma of the vulva. Pathol Res Pract 1997; 193:723–726.

29 Buhl A, Landow S, Lee YC, et al. Microcystic adnexal carcinoma of the vulva. Gynecol Oncol 2001; 82:571–574.

30 Abell MR. Adenocystic basal carcinoma involving vestibular glands. Adenocystic (pseudoadenomatous) basal cell carcinoma of vestibular glands of vulva. Am J Obstet Gynecol 1963; 86:470–482.

31 Copeland LJ, Sneige N, Gershenson DM, et al. Adenoid cystic carcinoma of Bartholin gland. Obstet Gynecol 1986; 67:115–120.

32 Wick MR, Goellner JR, Wolfe JT 3rd, Su WP. Vulvar sweat gland carcinomas. Arch Pathol Lab Med 1985; 109:43–47.

33 DePasquale SE, McGuinness TB, Mangan CE, Husson M, Woodland MB. Adenoid cystic carcinoma of Bartholin's gland: a review of the literature and report of a patient. Gynecol Oncol 1996; 61:122–125.

34 Visco AG, Del Priore G. Postmenopausal Bartholin gland enlargement: a hospital-based cancer risk assessment. Obstet Gynecol 1996; 87:286–290.

35 Abell MR, Behrman SJ, Gosling JR. Carcinoma of the vulva. J Mich State Med Soc 1961; 60:471–479.

36 Wahlstrom T, Vesterinen E, Saksela E. Primary carcinoma of Bartholin's glands: a morphological and clinical study of six cases including a transitional cell carcinoma. Gynecol Oncol 1978; 6:354–362.

37 Blanck C, Eneroth CM, Jacobsson F, Jakobsson PA. Adenoid cystic carcinoma of the parotid gland. Acta Radiol Ther Phys Biol 1967; 6:177–196.

38 Obermair A, Koller S, Crandon AJ, Perrin L, Nicklin JL. Primary Bartholin gland carcinoma: a report of seven cases. Aust N Z J Obstet Gynaecol 2001; 41:78–81.

39 Copeland LJ, Sneige N, Gershenson DM, et al. Bartholin gland carcinoma. Obstet Gynecol 1986; 67:794–801.

40 Mossler JA, Woodard BH, Addison A, McCarty KS Jr. Adenocarcinoma of Bartholin's gland. Arch Pathol Lab Med 1980; 104:523–526.

41 Mirhashemi R, Kratz A, Weir MM, Molpus KL, Goodman AK. Vaginal small cell carcinoma mimicking a Bartholin's gland abscess: a case report. Gynecol Oncol 1998; 68:297–300.

42 Jones MA, Mann EW, Caldwell CL, et al. Small cell neuroendocrine carcinoma of Bartholin's gland. Am J Clin Pathol 1990; 94:439–442.

43 Philippe E, Vetter JM, Dellenbach P, Petit JC. Neuro-endocrine carcinoma of a Bartholin's gland. J Gynecol Obstet Biol Reprod (Paris) 1990; 19:717–719.

44 Wheelock JB, Goplerud DR, Dunn LJ, Oates JF 3rd. Primary carcinoma of the Bartholin gland: a report of ten cases. Obstet Gynecol 1984; 63:820–824.

45 Cardosi RJ, Speights A, Fiorica JV, et al. Bartholin's gland carcinoma: a 15-year experience. Gynecol Oncol 2001; 82(2):247–251.

46 Sober AJ, Haluska FJ. Atlas of clinical oncology: skin cancer. London: BC Decker Inc; 2001:127–141.

47 Hierro I, Blanes A, Matilla A, et al. Merkel cell (neuroendocrine) carcinoma of the vulva. A case report with immunohistochemical and ultrastructural findings and review of the literature. Pathol Res Pract 2000; 196:503–509.

48 Gil-Moreno A, Garcia-Jimenez A, Gonzalez-Bosquet J, et al. Merkel cell carcinoma of the vulva. Gynecol Oncol 1997; 64:526–532.

49 Chen KT. Merkel's cell (neuroendocrine) carcinoma of the vulva. Cancer 1994; 73:2186–2191.

50 Dube V, Veilleux C, Plante M, Tetu B. Primary villoglandular adenocarcinoma of cloacogenic origin of the vulva. Hum Pathol 2004; 35:377–379.

51 Zaidi SN, Conner MG. Primary vulvar adenocarcinoma of cloacogenic origin. South Med J 2001; 94:744–746.

52 Willen R, Bekassy, Carlen B, Bozoky B, Cajander S. Cloacogenic adenocarcinoma of the vulva. Gynecol Oncol 1999; 74:298–301.

53 Lee KC, Su WP, Muller SA. Multicentric cloacogenic carcinoma: report of a case with anogenital pruritus at presentation. J Am Acad Dermatol 1990; 23:1005–1008.

54 Sheen-Chen SM, Eng HL, Huang CC. Breast cancer metastatic to the vulva. Gynecol Oncol 2004; 94:858–860.

55 Rocconi RP, Leath CA 3rd, Johnson WM 3rd, Barnes MN 3rd, Conner MG. Primary lung large cell carcinoma metastatic to the vulva: a case report and review of the literature. Gynecol Oncol 2004; 94:829–831.

56 Curtin WM, Murthy B. Vulvar metastasis of breast carcinoma. A case report. J Reprod Med 1997; 42:61–63.

57 Miliaras D. Breast like cancer of the vulva: primary or metastatic? A case report and review of the literature. Eur J Gynaecol Oncol 2002; 23:350–352.

58 Porzio G, Ficorella C, Calvisi G, et al. Ductal breast carcinoma metastatic to the vulva: a case report. Eur J Gynaecol Oncol 2001; 22:147–148.

Melanocytic lesions of the vulva

Scott R. Granter,

Alexander J.F. Lazar,

Hope K. Haefner and

Philip H. McKee

Introduction

Excisional biopsy

Genital melanosis (genital melanotic macule)

Clinical features
Histopathology

Flexural-type nevus (genital-type nevus, milk-line nevus)

Clinical features
Histologic features

Dysplastic nevi (atypical nevi, nevi with architectural disorder and cytologic atypia)

Clinical features
Histologic features

Melanoma

Clinical features
Histologic features
Differential diagnosis
Management, staging and
    prognosis
Therapy

Summary

Introduction

Pigmented lesions of the vulva are a concern to patients, their healthcare providers and pathologists who interpret the histopathology. Gynecologists are particularly wary of pigmented lesions of the vulva, since the prognosis for vulvar melanoma is poor due to the tendency for increased tumor thickness at the time of presentation. For this reason, gynecologists tend to be liberal about performing biopsies on clinically pigmented lesions.

Familiarity with the range of melanocytic lesions encountered on the vulva is important. Virtually any variant of melanocytic lesion that occurs in non-genital sites may also occur on the vulva. A detailed description of the spectrum of cutaneous melanocytic lesions is beyond the scope of this discussion and the reader is referred to dermatopathology textbooks or monographs on melanocytic lesions to gain a comprehensive understanding of cutaneous melanocytic lesions. The purpose of this chapter is to describe the patterns of melanocytic neoplasia seen in the vulva, acquaint the reader with the terminology used and address the differential diagnosis of this range of entities (Tables 8.1, 8.2).

Excisional biopsy

The initial evaluation of any lesion suspicious for melanoma is a biopsy.

Various methods to perform the biopsy include an elliptical excision or punch biopsy. A superficial shave

Table 8.1 Glossary of terms for pigmented lesions

Term	Definition
Junctional	Refers to melanocytes at the dermal–epidermal junction
Lentiginous	Proliferation of single melanocytes and small clusters of melanocytes along the dermal–epidermal junction
Shoulder	Extension of the junctional component beyond the dermal component of a nevus
Atypia	Increased nuclear size, irregularities in nuclear outline or chromatin and prominent nucleoli. Grading of atypia relies on nuclear size (see text)
Maturation	Constellation of findings, most notably diminution in cell size with depth
Bridging	Nests of melanocytes spanning rete (see Fig. 8.9)
Moth-eaten	Effacement of the dermal–epidermal junction by the dermal component

Table 8.2 Differential diagnosis of melanocytic lesions

Entity	Dominant features	Exclude
Melanosis	Hyperpigmented basal melanocytes	Melanoma in situ
Genital-type nevus	Large, often irregularly placed nests or melanocytes	Melanoma
Dysplastic nevus	Both architectural and cytologic atypia	Melanoma
Melanoma	Monotonous severe cytologic atypia with architectural abnormalities	Dysplastic nevus Genital-type nevus

biopsy should not be performed secondary to the risk of transecting the lesion, which could result in difficulty in histologic evaluation. An incisional biopsy may be performed if the lesion is too large or too close to vital structures to excise completely. Several studies have documented that an incisional biopsy for melanoma does not increase the risk of tumor seeding, metastasis, or decrease survival.[2,3]

Genital melanosis (genital melanotic macule)

CLINICAL FEATURES

Genital melanosis is a benign lesion characterized by macular pigmentation that can involve either cutaneous or mucosal sites.[4–7] Lesions are often clinically concerning, as they are frequently large with irregular borders. The macules may be single or multiple and affect the vulva, vagina or cervix (Fig. 8.1).[8,9] Typically, pigmentation increases slowly over time.

Laugier–Hunziker syndrome (idiopathic lenticular mucocutaneous pigmentation) is a disorder characterized by genital lesions associated with oral pigmentation.[10,11] Rarely, Carney's complex may present with lentigines in genital skin and mucosa.[12–14]

HISTOPATHOLOGY

Biopsy of genital melanosis shows increased pigmentation of basal keratinocytes, predominantly affecting the tips of the rete (Fig. 8.2). In many cases, abundant melanin is present within melanophages in the papillary

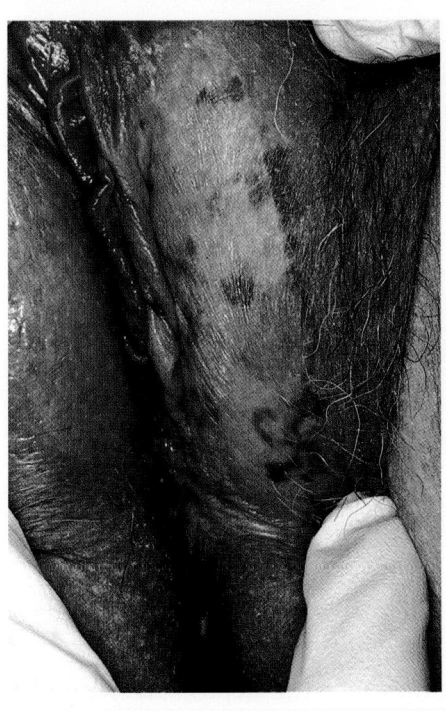

Fig. 8.1 Vulvar melanosis typically presents with multiple macules.

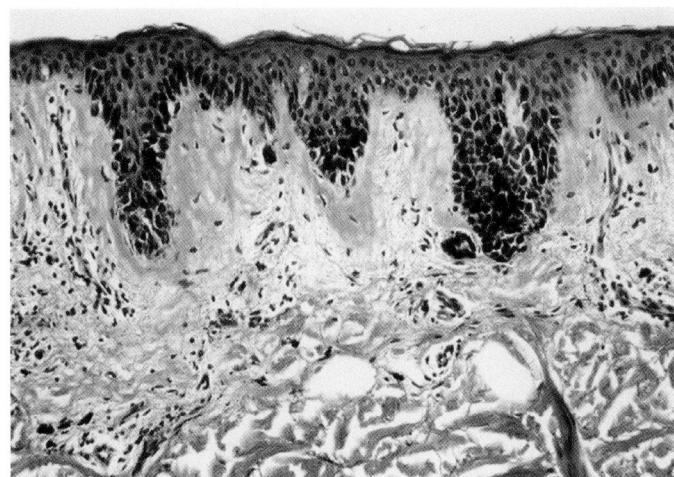

Fig. 8.2 Vulvar lentigo. There is marked basal layer pigmentation and melanocytes are increased in number.

dermis or superficial lamina propria, so-called 'pigment incontinence'. Some authors restrict use of the term genital 'melanosis' to lesions that do not show increased numbers of melanocytes. In contrast, genital 'lentiginosis' is applied to similar lesions that are associated with increased numbers of melanocytes. The terminology used is of nosologic, but not practical, importance. Melanocytic atypia is not a feature and, if present – particularly when accompanied by pagetoid spread of melanocytes – should raise concern for a significant precursor lesion or even melanoma in situ.

Flexural-type nevus (genital-type nevus, milk-line nevus)

CLINICAL FEATURES

The genital-type nevus often shows distinctive histologic features that are also seen in other sites characterized by redundant skin. For this reason, the term flexural-type nevus is sometimes applied to this variant of nevus. Other regions where flexural-type nevi are commonly encountered include the axilla, umbilicus, inguinal creases, scrotum and perianal area.[15]

Familiarity with flexural-type nevi is of great importance since they may be associated with atypical histo-logic features that raise the possibility of, or may be confused with, melanoma.[15–19]

It is estimated that the prevalence of vulvar nevi is approximately 2.3%.[16] They are most common in young women, but may also be seen in young girls and older women. They are often heavily pigmented, irregular, vary in size from a few millimeters to one centimeter in greatest dimension, and may be seen anywhere on the vulva, including the labia majora, labia minora and the clitoris.

HISTOLOGIC FEATURES

As noted above, genital-type nevi can be a source of considerable diagnostic difficulty since they are less frequently encountered than common dermal and compound nevi. Consequently, many general surgical pathologists are not familiar with their unique histo-logic features. When atypical features are present, they may be confused with melanoma.

Genital-type nevi may be junctional or compound. At scanning magnification, they may be symmetrical or asymmetrical and often have a papillomatous appearance (Fig. 8.3). The junctional component is usually lentiginous and nested (Fig. 8.4). The junctional nests are often large, surrounded by a retraction artifact and are frequently irregularly placed at the sides of rete (not a typical feature of nevi at non-flexural sites), as well as rete tips (Fig. 8.5). A common feature is the presence of transepidermal elimination of nests of melanocytes. However, frank intraepidermal pagetoid spread of individual melanocytes is not a prominent

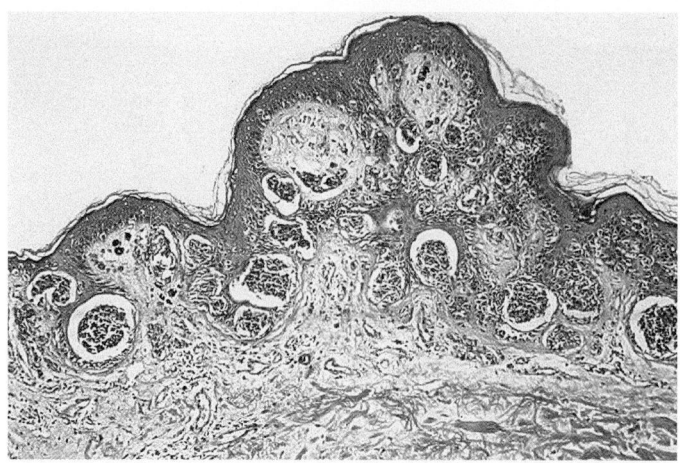

Fig. 8.3 Atypical genital-type nevus. Low-power view showing large junctional nests with a well-developed retraction artifact.

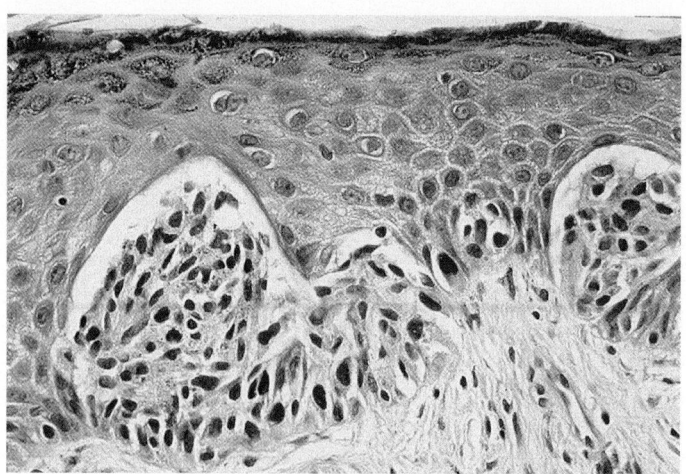

Fig. 8.5 Atypical genital-type nevus. Note the retraction artifact and hyperchromatic irregular nuclei.

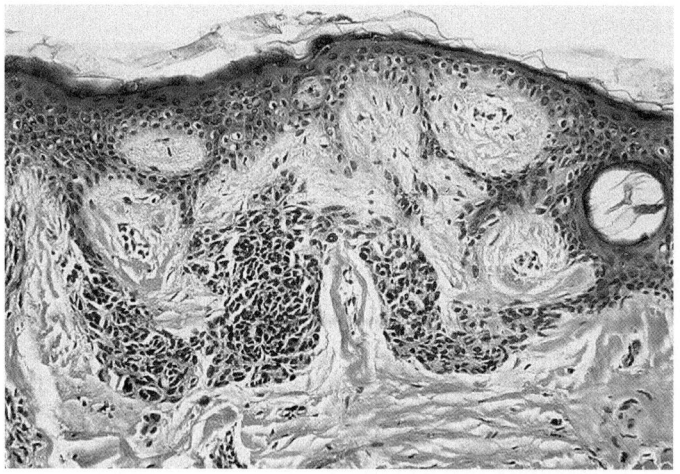

Fig. 8.4 Atypical genital-type nevus. In this lesion, there is bridging and marked cytologic atypia.

feature. When present, it is usually limited to small numbers of cells and restricted to the lower layers of the epidermis.

The composite nevus cells are epithelioid and cytologic atypia, as evidenced by nuclear enlargement and nucleolar prominence, is common. Hyperchromatism is sometimes a feature. Cytologic atypia, if present, is usually seen in only a subpopulation of cells. When it involves a large fraction of melanocytes, concern for melanoma should be raised.

If a dermal component is present, it shows features similar to that of non-genital-type nevi. In other words, it is the architectural features of the junctional component that allows distinction of genital-type nevi from common compound nevi. The dermal component shows maturation with depth. As with the junctional component, however, the dermal component may show cytologic atypia in the superficial component.

Expansile dermal nests with diffuse cytologic atypia, lack of maturation with depth, pagetoid spread of intraepidermal melanocytes, effacement of the epidermis, conspicuous mitoses and asymmetry should all prompt concern for melanoma.[20] It is important to keep in mind that melanoma of the vulva is most often seen in elderly women. Studies have shown that, in contrast to melanoma of non-genital sites that have a peak incidence in early to middle adulthood, vulvar melanoma has a peak incidence around the sixth decade.[21] Therefore, one should approach the diagnosis of melanoma with caution in young patients and, contrariwise, the diagnosis of atypical nevus in the elderly should be rendered with caution. Nevertheless, vulvar melanoma may occur in the young and nevi are certainly encountered in the elderly.[22]

The biological potential of genital-type nevi has not been carefully studied. For this reason, it is recommended that lesions with significant atypia be completely excised.[23]

Although there may be some histologic overlap between dysplastic and vulvar nevi, the former is characterized by elongation of the rete ridges and a more prominent lentiginous growth pattern of junctional melanocytes. Stromal changes that favor dysplastic nevus include eosinophilic and lamellar fibrosis of the papillary dermis and a variable mononuclear inflammatory cell infiltrate.

Dysplastic nevi (atypical nevi, nevi with architectural disorder and cytologic atypia)

CLINICAL FEATURES

Dysplastic nevi are melanocytic proliferations that show clinical or histologic features intermediate between common nevi and melanoma.[24-31] They have also been referred to as atypical nevus, B-K mole, Clark's nevus, and nevus with architectural and cytologic atypia. Patients with dysplastic nevi are at increased risk of developing melanoma; the level of risk is highly dependent on family history. Specifically, patients with dysplastic nevi who also have a family history of melanoma in first-degree relatives have an extremely high risk of developing melanoma compared with patients with dysplastic nevi but who lack a significant family history.

Patients have variable numbers of dysplastic nevi, ranging from a few to hundreds of lesions. They may occur at virtually any site. Although there does not seem to be any particular predilection for the vulva, they can certainly be seen at this site.

Clinically, dysplastic nevi show variation in size, shape and coloration. They tend to be larger than non-dysplastic nevi and typically exhibit some degree of asymmetry and have somewhat irregular ill-defined borders (Figs 8.5, 8.6). These are features that are also seen in melanoma and it is a matter of degree that allows for clinical distinction of dysplastic nevus from common nevus or melanoma. Given this subjectivity and the lack of reliable clinical criteria for the diagnosis of melanocytic lesions, excision or biopsy of these lesions is recommended.

HISTOLOGIC FEATURES

The histologic appearances of dysplastic nevi in both familial and sporadic cases are identical. Architectural features that characterize dysplastic nevi include asymmetry, a prominent lentiginous growth pattern, extension of the intraepidermal component beyond the most lateral extent of the dermal component (the so-called 'shoulder phenomenon') and variation in size, shape and irregular placement of junctional nests. Additional architectural features include discohesion and confluence of junctional nests spanning two or more rete ('bridging') (see Fig. 8.7).

Dysplastic nevi are often associated with stromal changes characterized by lamellar and eosinophilic fibrosis

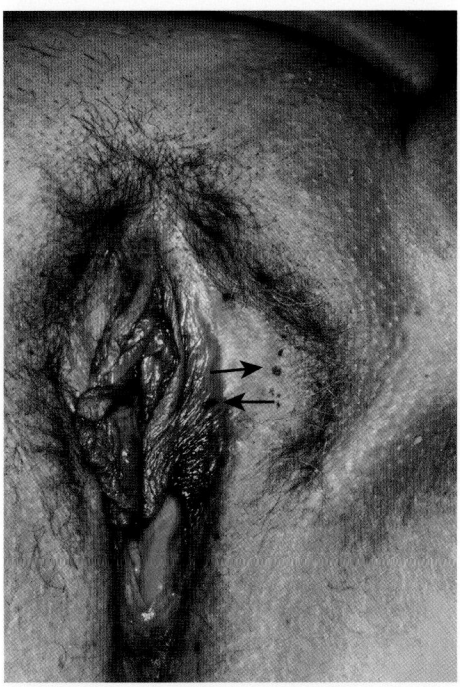

Fig. 8.6 Clinical appearance of dysplastic nevi, seen as small macular lesions on the vulva.

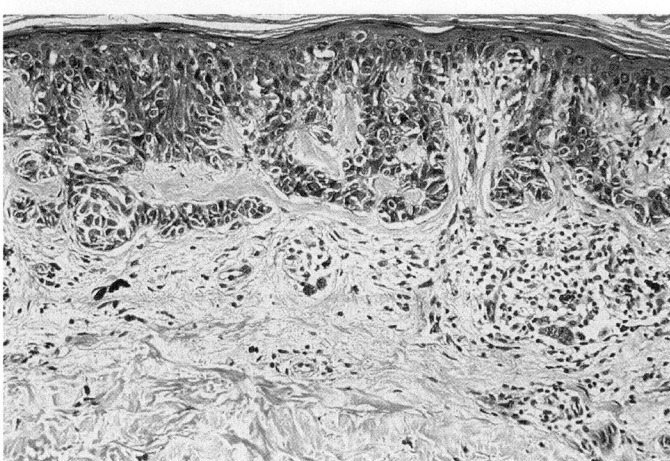

Fig. 8.7 Dysplastic nevus. There is lentiginous hyperplasia. Note the irregularly distributed nevus cells and lymphocytic infiltrate in the upper dermis.

of the papillary dermis, a lymphohistiocytic infiltrate and prominent vascularity of the papillary dermis (Fig. 8.8). Finely dispersed ('dusty') light brown or olive-colored melanin is frequently seen in melanocytes in the junctional component of dysplastic nevi (but is also frequently seen in melanoma).

In addition to architectural abnormalities, cytologic atypia of melanocytes is, by definition, present in dysplastic nevi (Fig. 8.9). It ranges from mild to severe, and atypical cells tend to punctuate a background of bland melanocytes. The finding of monotonous significant atypia should prompt concern for melanoma. Cytologic atypia may be graded by comparing the size of the nuclei

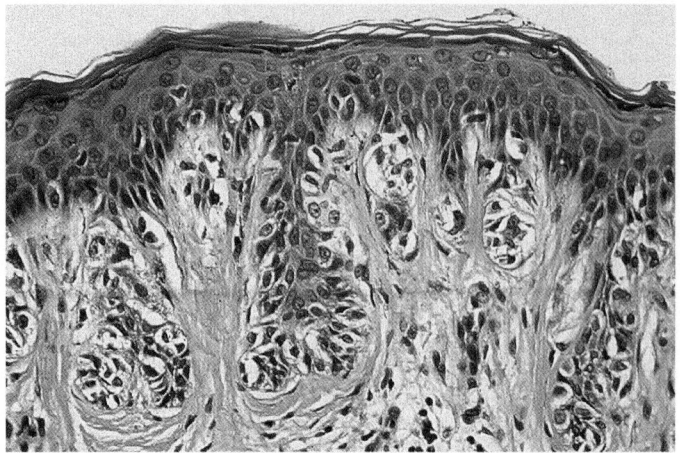

Fig. 8.8 Dysplastic nevus. High-power view showing cytologic atypia and lamellar fibroplasia.

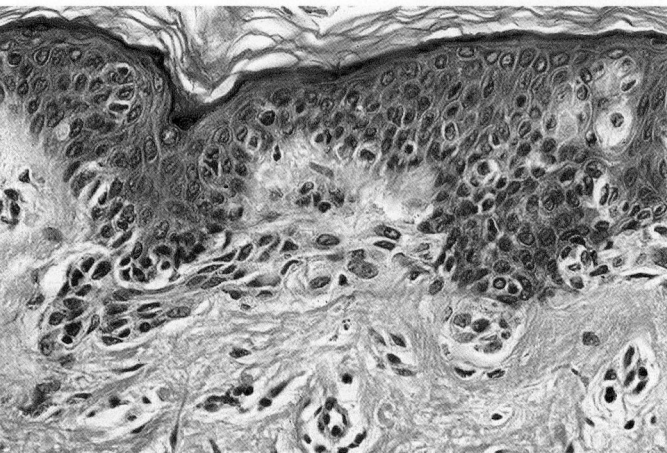

Fig. 8.9 Dysplastic nevus. A high-power view showing bridging and cytologic atypia. Spindle cell melanoma: the tumor cells have elongated nuclei with prominent nucleoli.

of the nevus cells with those of adjacent keratinocytes.[21] With slight atypia, nuclei are similar in size to, or slightly larger than, spinous keratinocyte nuclei. Moderately atypical nuclei are somewhat (1.5 to 2×) larger than those of spinous keratinocytes and have increased hyperchromasia and pleomorphism, and nucleoli are more visible. Melanocytes are considered severely atypical when their nuclei are twice the size of, or larger than, spinous keratinocyte nuclei. In addition, irregular nuclear outlines, course chromatin and prominent nucleoli are often present.[21] In some cases, it is very difficult to distinguish severely atypical dysplastic nevus from early melanoma or melanoma in situ. The presence of diffuse marked cytologic atypia should raise the possibility of melanoma. Dermal mitoses, expansile dermal nests, lack of maturation with depth, pagetoid spread of intraepidermal melanocytes, effacement of the epidermis,

confluence of atypical nests and asymmetry should all raise suspicion for melanoma.

As noted in the section on genital nevi, it is important to keep in mind that melanoma of the vulva is most often seen in elderly women, with a peak incidence around the sixth decade.[32] Therefore, a diagnosis of vulvar melanoma in young patients should be approached with great caution. Likewise, the diagnosis of a vulvar dysplastic nevus in the elderly should be made after careful evaluation of multiple levels and appropriate clinicopathologic correlation.

It is our practice to recommend that dysplastic nevi with significant atypia be completely excised with adequate, clear margins.[21]

Melanoma

INTRODUCTION

Melanoma of the female genital tract is rare; however, it is the second most common vulvar malignancy.[31–47] In contrast to melanoma of non-genital skin, which has a peak incidence in early to middle adulthood, vulvar tumors are most often seen around the sixth decade.[48] Nevertheless, vulvar melanoma is encountered in younger adults and even in children.[49] Using a population-based registry, Weinstock et al. computed an incidence of vulvar and vaginal melanoma of 1.08 and 0.26 per million.[50] Black and white women were at equal risk for vaginal melanomas, but whites had a 2.6 relative risk for vulvar neoplasms.[50] It has been estimated that it accounts for approximately 3% of all melanomas in females, with the vulva being the most frequently site of the genital tract. The vagina and cervix are less commonly affected.[31,35,36,38,40,41]

CLINICAL FEATURES

The majority of vulvar melanomas develop on the labium majus, labium minus and clitoral area (Table 8.3).[50]

Table 8.3 Site distribution of malignant melanoma of the vulva[47]

Site	(%)
Majora	27.3
Minora	19.2
Clitoral	30.8
Periurethral	11.1
Other	11.6

Most lesions are not raised (Fig. 8.10). Approximately one-third present as polypoid masses and one-fifth will contain satellite lesions (Fig. 8.11). Melanomas can be characterized by the 'ABCDs': asymmetrical (A); have irregular or scalloped borders (B); color changes (black, or variegate with shades of red, white or blue) (C) and may have a diameter (D) of more than 6 mm. Most melanomas are pigmented and vary in color from brown to black. However, amelanotic melanomas, which may clinically mimic squamous cell carcinoma or extra-mammary Paget's disease, were seen in nearly one-third of patients in one study.[48,50] The most common presenting complaints are bleeding, noticeable mass lesion and discomfort. Other symptoms and signs include ulceration, discharge, pruritus, burning, foul odor and dysuria. The vast majority of melanomas arise de novo; however, tumors have been shown to arise in association with a pre-existing nevus in approximately 5% of cases.[51]

HISTOLOGIC FEATURES

The microscopic features of genital melanoma are similar to those encountered at extragenital sites. In general, tumors show a proliferation of melanocytes with 'monotonous' severe cytologic atypia in which virtually all of the cells affected show nuclear enlargement, chromatin irregularity and prominent nucleoli. The in-situ component often shows a confluent proliferation of single cells and small clusters of melanocytes in a pattern reminiscent of lentigo maligna melanoma or acral-type melanoma (Fig. 8.12). Effacement of the epidermal rete is common and imparts a 'moth-eaten' appearance to the dermal–epidermal or mucosal–submucosal junction.

The dermal component of invasive tumors is comprised of melanocytes with cytologic features similar to the overlying melanoma in situ (Fig. 8.13). Expansile nests and dermal mitoses are seen in more advanced tumors. Maturation of the dermal component is absent (Fig. 8.14). The dermal component is usually composed of epithelioid melanocytes; however, spindle cell melanomas, including desmoplastic and neurotropic variants, may also be encountered (Fig. 8.15).

Melanomas vary considerably in the degree of melanin deposition, which may range from extensive (Fig. 8.16) to absent (Fig. 8.17). Awareness of the latter is important, as will be discussed below.

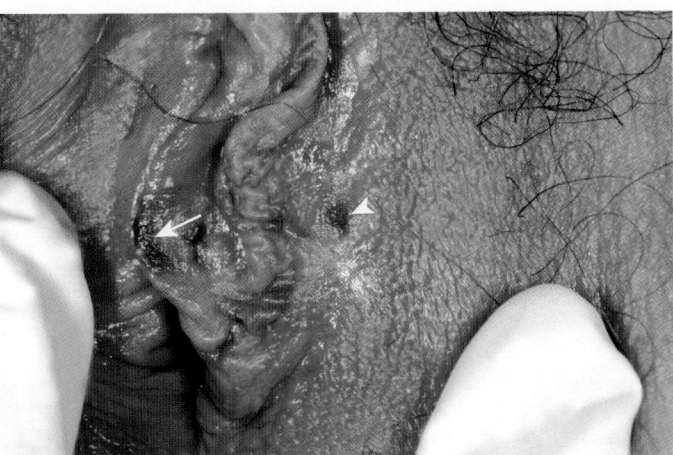

Fig. 8.10 Vulvar melanoma on the labium minus (arrow). Additional lesions are present (arrowhead).

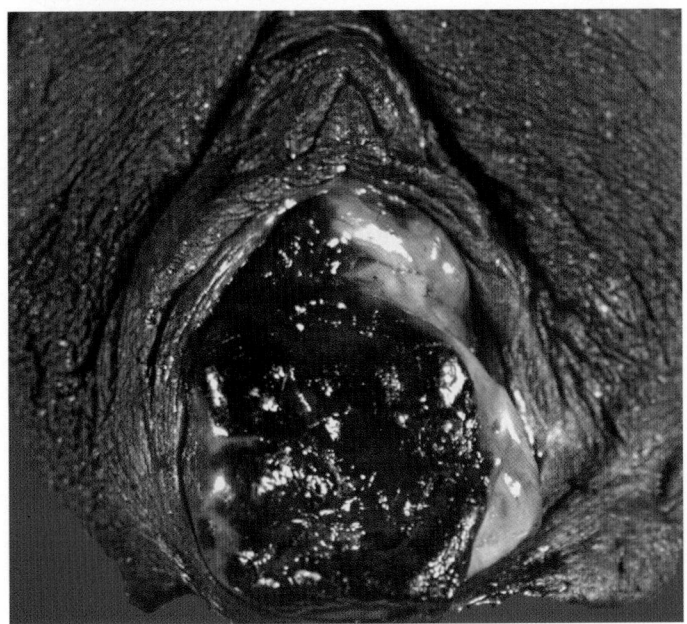

Fig. 8.11 A large vulvar melanoma which extended to regional lymph nodes.

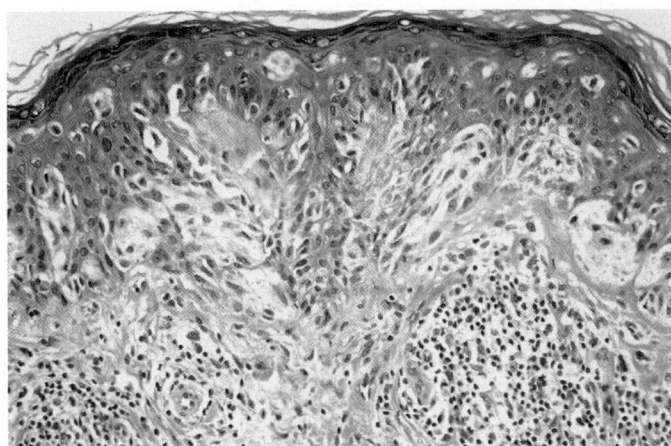

Fig. 8.12 Superficial spreading melanoma: atypical melanocytes are scattered throughout the full thickness of the epidermis.

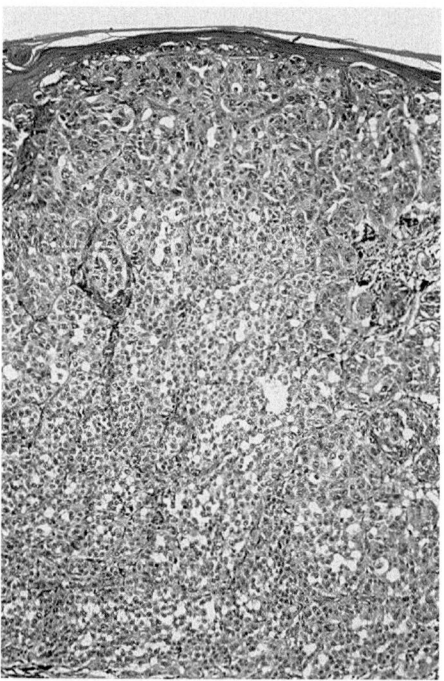

Fig. 8.13 Vertical growth phase melanoma. Large expansile nests fill the reticular dermis (left and right).

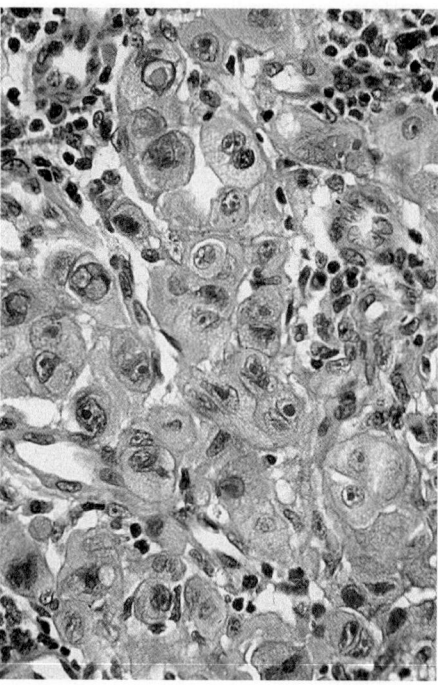

Fig. 8.14 Vertical growth phase melanoma. Dermal component: there is nuclear pleomorphism and eosinophilic nucleoli are prominent.

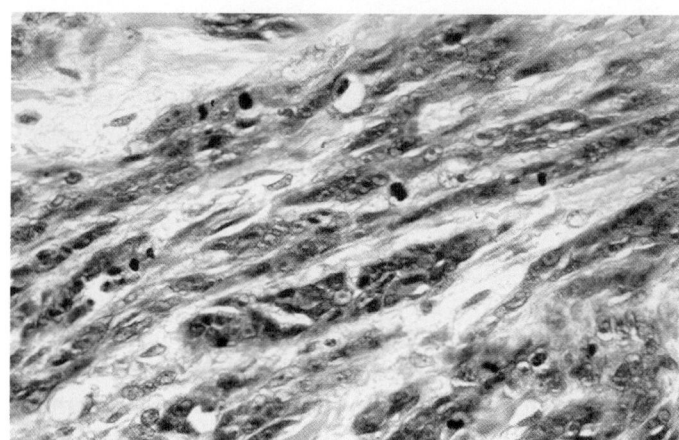

Fig. 8.15 Spindle cell growth pattern in a melanoma.

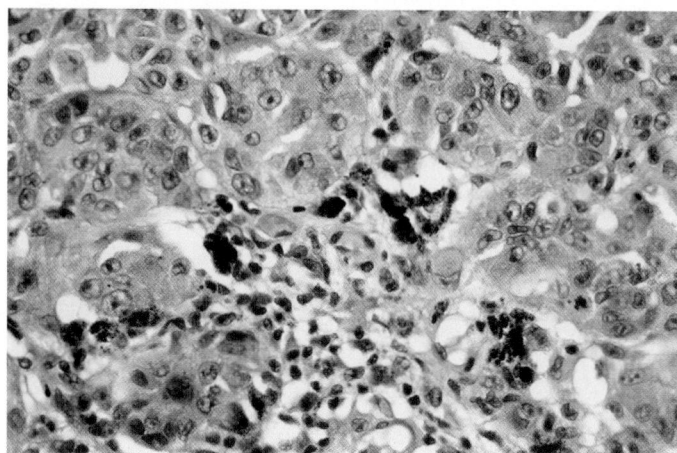

Fig. 8.16 Vulvar melanoma with prominent melanin production.

A list of items to include in the pathology report are summarized below. Important variables include age, gender, anatomic site, thickness, presence or absence of ulceration, histologic pattern, associated nevus, host response, margins, neurotropism, vascular invasion, satellitosis among others.[2,52–54]

The acral mucosal lentiginous pattern is the most common histologic pattern subtype reported for vulvar melanoma. However, for cutaneous melanoma, superficial spreading is the most common pattern.[38,44,48]

The histologic subtype, in general, does not correlate with prognosis or survival after correction for tumor thickness, ulceration and other prognostic parameters.[2,52,53]

Melanocytic lesions may coexist with lichen sclerosus. A recent study found an association between melanocytic lesions and lichen sclerosus, emphasizing the distinction of atypical melanocytic proliferations and melanoma in this setting. The relationship between melanoma and lichen sclerosus, while intriguing, remains to be clarified.[55]

DIFFERENTIAL DIAGNOSIS

The following must be considered in the differential diagnosis of malignant melanoma.

1 Squamous carcinomas. Melanomas with spindle cell morphology may mimic squamous tumors

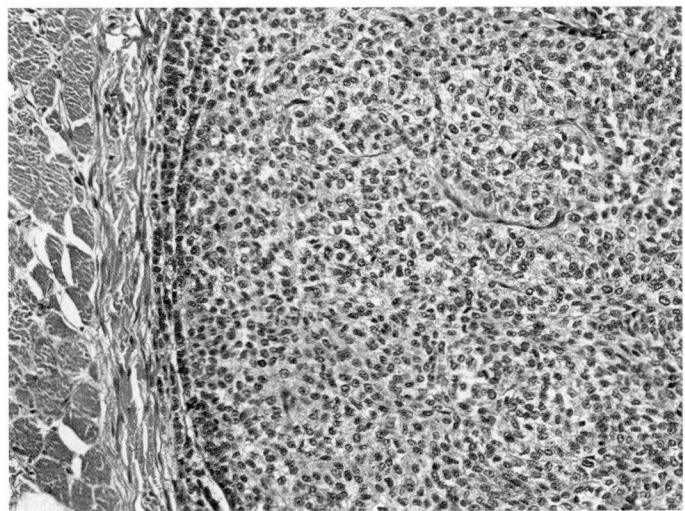

Fig. 8.17 Amelanotic melanoma. This pattern may mimic adenocarcinoma or other malignancies.

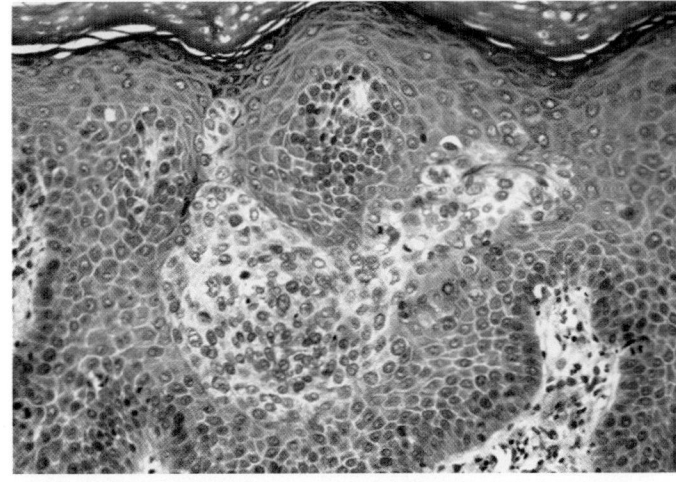

Fig. 8.19 A pagetoid VIN may mimic both Paget's disease and melanoma.

(Fig. 8.18). Rarely, more poorly differentiated vulvar intraepithelial neoplasms may exhibit a pagetoid appearance (Fig. 8.19).[56] Carcinomas are immunoreactive for keratins, helping to distinguish them from melanomas. Melanomas, in contrast, are immunoreactive for S-100 and MART-1. This entity is also discussed in Chapter 6.

2 An important exclusion when considering a diagnosis of vulvar melanoma is extra-mammary Paget's disease. Both melanomas and Paget's disease exhibit intraepithelial nests of tumor cells, including the superficial keratin layers, junctional changes, acantholysis and an invasive component

that may be composed of uniform cells with abundant cytoplasm and prominent nucleoli (Figs 8.20–8.23). The two can be easily distinguished by MART-1 and S-100 staining (melanoma) and CEA, Cam 5.2 and mucicarmine staining (Paget's disease) (Fig. 8.24). A variety of newer biomarkers are currently under study.[57,58]

3 The most important distinction once a diagnosis of melanoma is assured is between in-situ and invasive disease. The potential problems in distinguishing an in-situ from an invasive lesion cannot be overemphasized, and practitioners who are not familiar with the morphologic range of atypical melanocytic lesions should always seek a second opinion from someone familiar with these disorders prior to committing to a diagnosis of melanoma.

MANAGEMENT, STAGING AND PROGNOSIS

General

Survival with vulvar melanoma is dependent almost entirely on the extent of the disease. The American Joint Committee on Cancer developed a staging system in 2001 for cutaneous melanomas. It is applicable to vulvar melanoma.[53]

The treatment for primary melanoma of the vulva is local excision with margin recommendations generally ranging from 1 to 2 cm (dependent on Breslow depth and the proximity of vital structures).[54] Obtaining tumor-free margins is critical to prevent local recurrence.[54,59,60]

Overall, 5-year survival for vulvar melanoma is lower when compared with melanomas at non-genital sites due

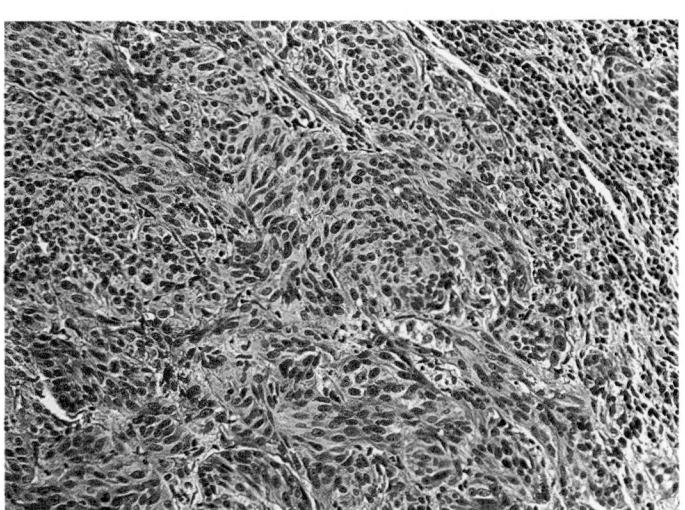

Fig. 8.18 Invasive melanoma with a spindle component, resembling squamous carcinoma.

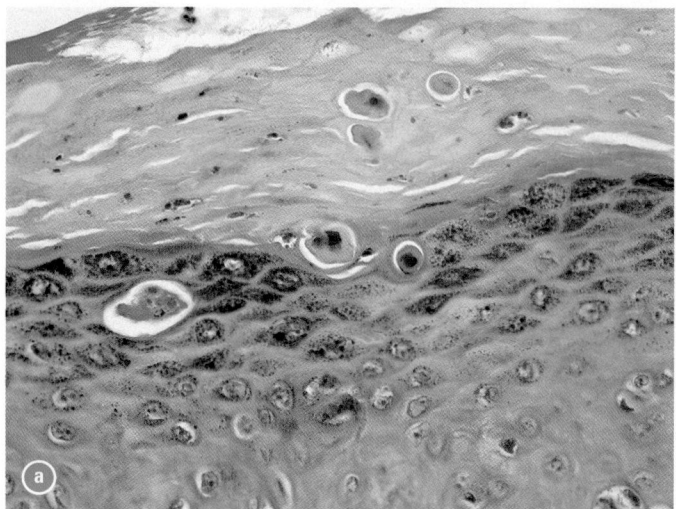

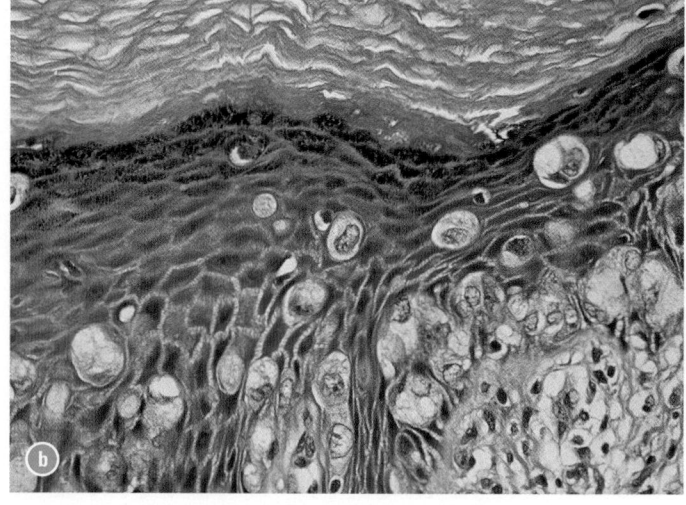

Fig. 8.20 Intraepithelial involvement in (a) melanoma and (b) Paget's disease.

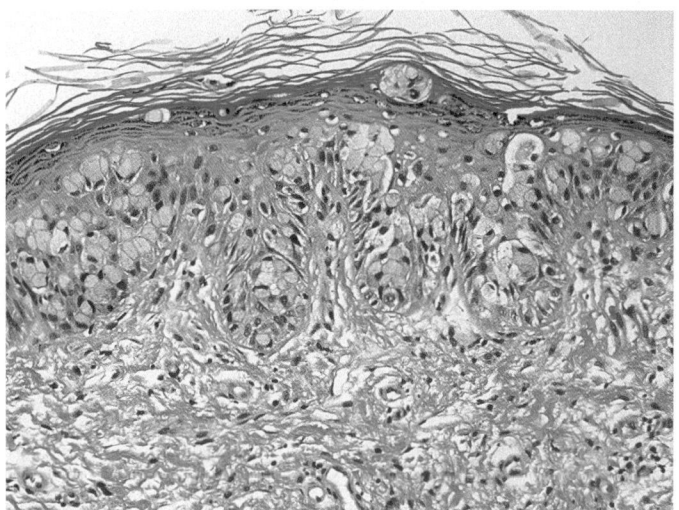

Fig. 8.21 Junctional-type growth patterns in Paget's disease.

to presentation at a later stage and typically greater thickness. The 5-year survival ranges from 15 to 54% in various studies.[34-43,61-63] In a large series of 219 patients, the 5-year survival was 47% (Table 8.4).[63] This is in contrast to vaginal melanomas, which have an even poorer survival (19%). Prognosis of vulvar melanomas is dependent upon tumor thickness which entails the use of Clark's levels (for hair-bearing skin only), measurement of lesion thickness according to Breslow and simple staging. Breslow's measurements are usually employed and performed with a micrometer for small lesions. For cutaneous and vulvar melanoma, the Breslow depth is the single most important independent prognostic factor.[52,53,60,64]

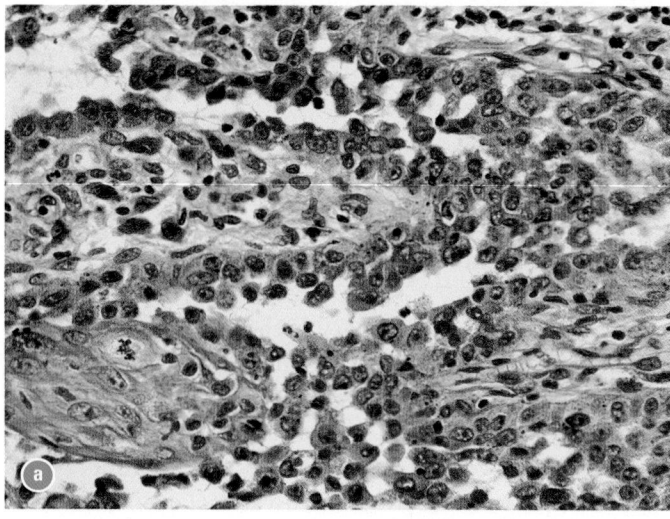

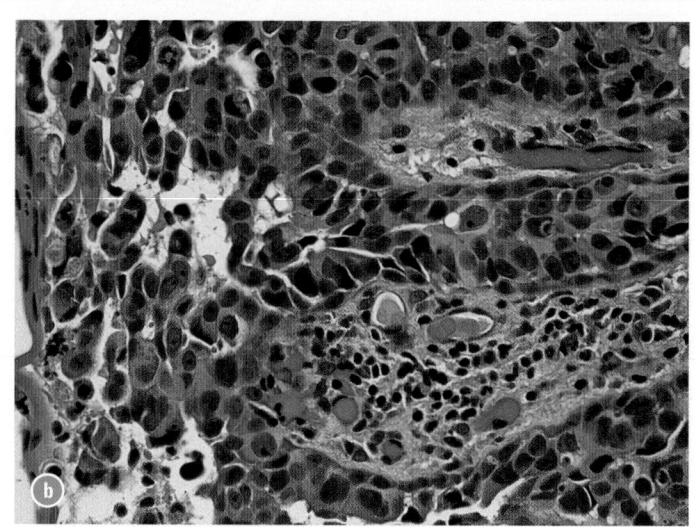

Fig. 8.22 Acantholysis in (a) melanoma and (b) Paget's disease.

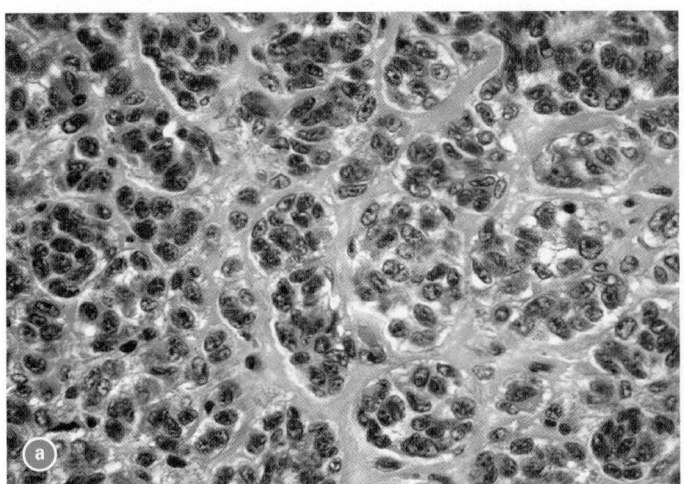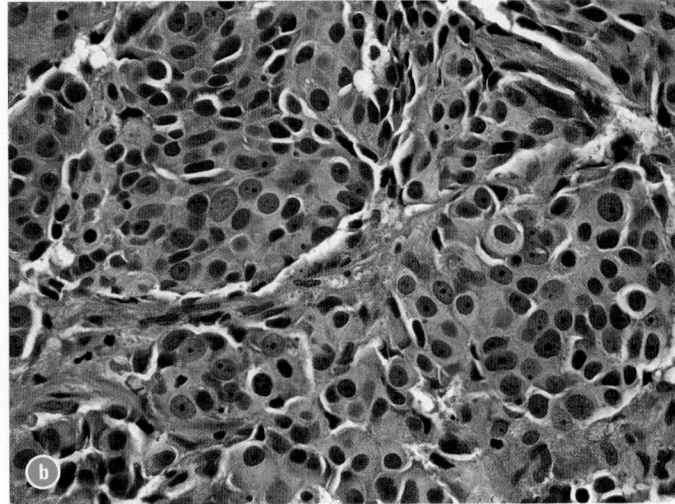

Fig. 8.23 Similarity of cytomorphology between (a) invasive melanoma and (b) Paget's disease.

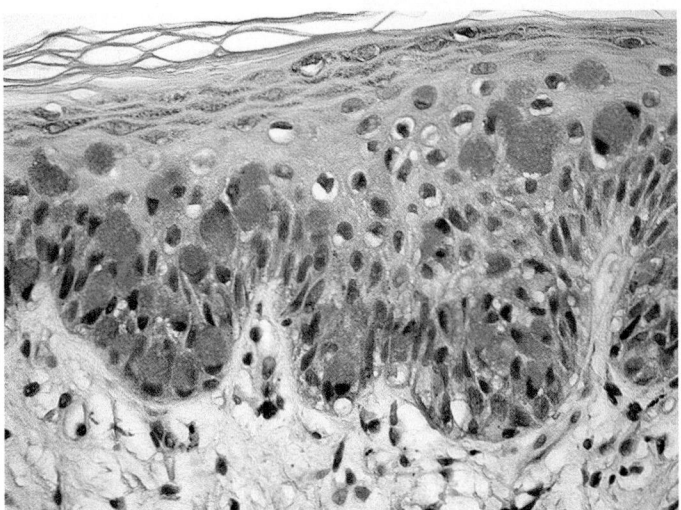

Fig. 8.24 Mucicarmine staining distinguishes vulvar Paget's disease from melanoma.

Depth of invasion

The depth of the lesion is determined by the distance from the surface of the granular layer of the adjacent normal mucosa or the deepest point of the tumor. For ulcerated tumors, the distance is generally computed from the base (surface) of the ulcer to the deepest point (Fig. 8.25).[63] Outcome data are not encouraging. In one study, the death rate for lesions less than 0.9 mm was 26% and was 40–68% for tumors exceeding this depth (Table 8.4). Age (older) and ethnicity (black) are also associated with poor outcome.[31] Overall, the prognosis for vulvar melanoma remains poor relative to other skin areas.[63,65]

Sentinel lymph node biopsy

Figure 8.26 summarizes the parameters of value in work-up of the patient with vulvar melanoma. Nodal metastases correlate highly with mortality (Fig. 8.27). In a limited series of patients culled from a large survey, from 77 to 88% of patients with lesions less than 4.0 mm in thickness with negative lymph nodes survived for 2 years.[66] Sentinel lymph node evaluation may be useful in determining prognosis.[1,67]

The advent of sentinel lymph node biopsy (SLNB) in the 1990s provided a minimally invasive alternative to elective lymph node dissection (ELND) with a lower morbidity and higher sensitivity to stage accurately the entire regional lymph node basin in clinically node-negative patients.[68] The nodal basin contains clusters or groups of nodes (i.e. inguinal, axillary, etc.). Sentinel lymph node biopsy is useful for staging clinically negative regional lymph nodal basins for several solid cancers, including breast, squamous cell carcinoma, thyroid carcinoma, Merkel cell carcinoma and melanoma.[68–70] However, the use of SLNB for gynecologic malignancies until recently, has been reported infrequently.[71–75]

Table 8.4 Distribution of depth of invasion in mucosal melanoma (%)[63]

Depth	All*	Stage I**	Deaths (%)
<0.9 mm	12.2	17.3	5/19 (26)
1.0–1.9	10.0	13.5	8/20 (40)
2.0–2.9	6.7	3.8	5/9 (55)
3.0–3.9	10.0	9.6	9/14 (64)
>4.0	58.9	53.8	36/53 (68)

*n = 90; **n = 52.

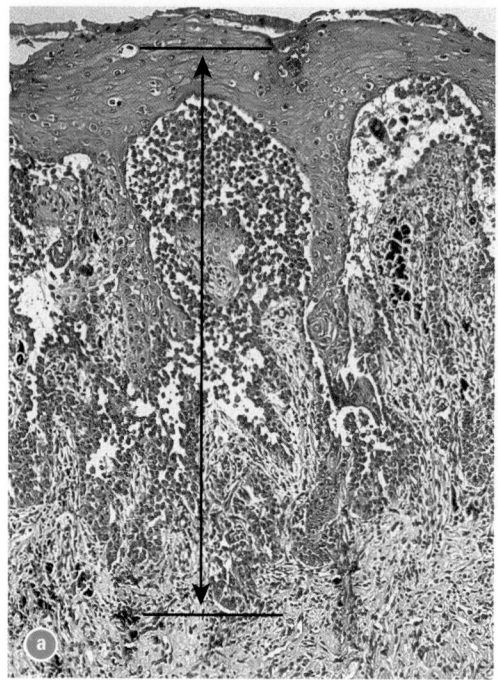 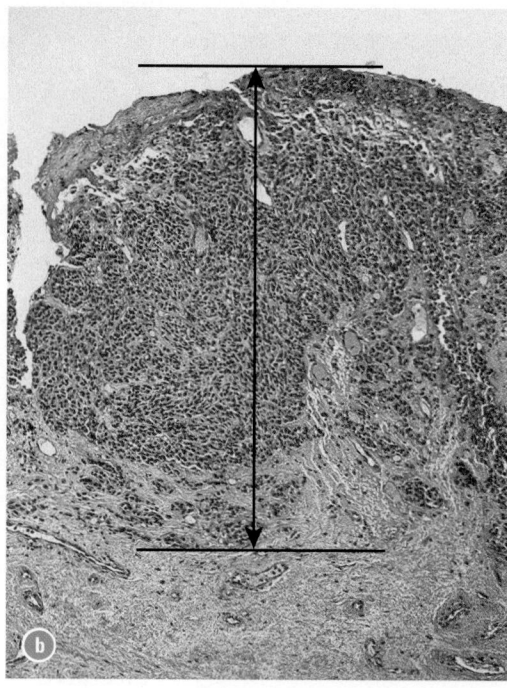

Fig. 8.25 (a) In mucosal melanomas, Breslow's measurements (depth of invasion) are most practical and ideally are measured from the granular layer (if present) to the deepest point of invasion. (b) In ulcerated lesions, the depth is measured from the base of the ulcer to the deepest point of the tumor.

The concurrent injection of radioactive material (technetium 99m-labeled sulfur colloid or albumin) and vital blue dye (isosulfan blue dye) into the primary lesion site leads to the identification of the first node (sentinel node) to which that particular site drains.[75,76] This node is identified by its radioactivity and blue hue and is removed through a small incision and sent for pathologic analysis. The SLNB is performed under general anesthesia in most instances, adding an increased risk in those patients who otherwise could undergo excision simply with local anesthesia. Although an increase in cost occurs, the cost–benefit outcomes analyses are favorable for SLNB. Side-effects from SLNB are rare and include anaphylaxis to blue dye (<2%), lymphedema (exceptionally rare but reported) and permanent blue tattooing.[77]

The SLN is serial sectioned, processed using permanent formalin fixation, and stained with hematoxylin and eosin. At our institution, negative nodes are evaluated further with immunohistochemistry, usually S-100, Melan-A/Mart-1 and/or HMB-45.

Indication for sentinel lymph node mapping

Consideration for SLNB is indicated for melanoma equal to 1.0 mm in tumor thickness, where the risk of nodal metastasis begins to increase. It is not indicated for thinner lesions in general because of low risk of metastasis, although some patients with lesions <1.0 mm with other adverse prognostic factors may be appropriate candidates for SLNB. Other adverse factors are defined variably across melanoma centers and include ulceration, high mitotic rate, microsatellitosis, angiolymphatic invasion, Clark level IV, regression to 1.0 mm and young age. An SLNB may not be indicated for patients not desiring the prognostic information gained or in those with significant comorbidity.[1]

THERAPY

Literally hundreds of adjuvant therapies have been tried for high-risk melanoma, ranging from shark cartilage to chemotherapy during the past several decades. Only one, high-dose interferon α2b (INF), has demonstrated any benefit in randomized controlled trials for surgically resected melanoma at high risk for recurrent disease. The morbidity is significant with the high-dose regimen, and the overall and disease-free survival benefits are small. Adjuvant high-dose INF is associated with significant toxicity, and therefore may not be appropriate for many patients with significant comorbidity.

Summary

The proper and timely management of women with pigmented lesions of the vulva rests with periodic self-examination by the patient, compulsive attention to

Patient Name _____   Surgical No. _____
                                                    Outside Slide No. _____

MELANOMA WORKSHEET

1. Type: _____ Superficial spreading   _____ *in situ*
                   _____ Nodular
                   _____ Lentigo maligna   _____ *in situ*
                   _____ Acral lentiginous   _____ *in situ*
                   _____ Mucosal lentiginous   _____ *in situ*
                   _____ Desmoplastic
                   _____ Neurotropic
                   _____ Type unclassified   _____ *in situ*
                   _____ Other (specify) _____

2. Anatomic level: ___ (for skin; not applicable to mucosal melanomas) _____

3. Greatest thickness: _____ mm

4. Ulceration: _____ Absent   _____ Present _____ mm

5. Radial growth phase: _____ Absent   _____ Present

6. Verticle growth phase: _____ Absent
                            _____ Present _____ Epithelioid _____ Small_____ Spindle

7. Precursor lesion: _____ Not identified
                         _____ Present (specify) _____

8. Margins:
   Biopsies   _____ Extending to the tissue edges
                   _____ Not extending to the tissue edges in the tissue planes examined

Excisions

                   _____ Completely excised
                   _____ Measurement to closest side resecion margin _____ mm
                   _____ Extending to inked   _____ peripheral/radial resection margin
                                                   _____ deep resection margin
                                                   _____ deep and lateral resection margins
                                                   _____ other: _____

9. Mitoses: _____ per mm^2

10. Tumor-infiltrating lymphocytes: _____ Absent
                                       _____ Present, non-brisk
                                       _____ Present, brisk

11. Neural invasion: _____ Absent   _____ Present

12. Vascular invasion: _____ Absent   _____ Present

13. Regression: _____ Absent   _____ Present

14. Microsatellites: _____ Absent   _____ Present

15: Other

Fig. 8.26 Gross and histologic data record for melanoma.

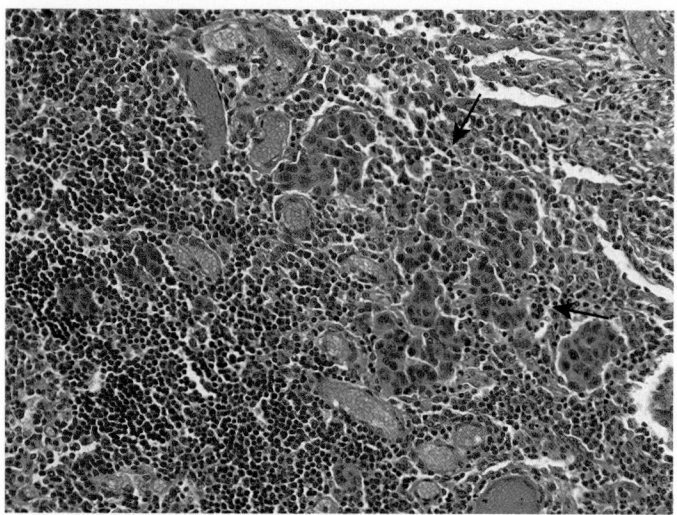

Fig. 8.27 Nodal metastasis in vulvar melanoma (arrows).

pigmented lesions by the clinician and a pathologist who is familiar with the spectrum of melanocytic proliferations of the vulva. The pathologist must be able to distinguish benign melanosis from atypical lesions and be aware that both over- and under-interpretation of melanoma can occur. Whether the natural history of melanomas can be altered by management is uncertain, but careful histologic classification is vital to an informed patient and her clinical caregiver.

References

1 Wechter ME, Reynolds RK, Haefner HK, et al. Vulvar melanoma: review of diagnosis, staging, and therapy. J Lower Genital Tract Dis 2004; 8(1):58–69.

2 Johnson TM, Smith JW 2nd, Nelson BR, Chang A. Current therapy for cutaneous melanoma. J Am Acad Derm 1995; 32:689–707.

3 Arca MJ, Biermann JS, Johnson TM, Chang AE. Biopsy techniques for skin, soft-tissue, and bone neoplasms. Surg Oncol Clin N Am 1995; 4:157–174.

4 Barnhill RL, Alber LS, Shama SK, et al. Genital lentiginosis: a clinical and histopathologic study. J Am Acad Derm 1990; 22:453–460.

5 Estrada R, Kaufman R. Benign vulvar melanosis. J Reprod Med 1993; 38:5–8.

6 Lenane P, Keane CO, Connell BO, et al. Genital melanotic macules: clinical, histologic, immunohistochemical, and ultrastructural features. J Am Acad Derm 2000; 42:640–644.

7 Kanj LF, Rubeiz NG, Mrouett AM, et al. Vulvar melanosis and lentiginosis: a case report. J Am Acad Derm 1992; 27:777–778.

8 Sison-Torre EQ, Ackerman AB. Melanosis of the vagina. Am J Derm 1985; 7:51–60.

9 Karney MY, Cassidy MS, Zahn CM, et al. Melanosis of the vagina. A case report. J Reprod Med 2001; 46:389–391.

10 Lenane P, Sullivan DO, Keane CO, Loughlint SO. The Laugier-Hunziker syndrome. J Eur Acad Derm Venereol 2001; 15:574–577.

11 Gerbig AW, Hunziker T. Idiopathic lenticular mucocutaneous pigmentation of Laugier-Hunziker syndrome with atypical features. Arch Derm 1996; 32:844–845.

12 Reed OM, Mellette JR, Fitzpatrick JE. Cutaneous lentiginosis with atrial myxomas. J Am Acad Derm 1986; 15:398–402.

13 Rhodes AR, Silverman RA, Harrist TJ, et al. Mucocutaneous lentigines, cardiomuco-cutaneous myxomas and multiple blue nevi: the LAMB syndrome. J Am Acad Derm 1986; 10:72–82.

14 Jong E De, Mulder W, Nooitgedacht E, et al. Carney's triad. Eur J Surg Oncol 1998; 24:147–149.

15 Rongioletti F, Ball RA, Marcus R, et al. Histopathological features of flexural melanocytic nevi: a study of 40 cases. J Cutan Pathol 2000; 27:215–217.

16 Rock B, Hood AF, Rock JA. Prospective study of vulvar nevi. J Am Acad Derm 1990; 22:104–106.

17 Christensen WN, Friedman KJ, Woodruff JD, et al. Histologic characteristics of vulvar nevocellular nevi. J Cutan Pathol 1987; 14:87–91.

18 Clark WH Jr, Hood AF, Tucker MA, et al. Atypical melanocytic nevi of the genital type with a discussion of reciprocal parenchymal-stromal interactions in the biology of neoplasia. Hum Pathol 1998; 29(1):S1–S24.

19 Blessing K. Benign atypical naevi: diagnostic difficulties and continued controversy. Histopathology 1999; 34:189–198.

20 Haupt HM, Stern JB. Pagetoid melanocytosis: histologic features in benign and malignant lesions. Am J Surg Pathol 1995; 19:792–797.

21 Dunton CJ, Kautzky M, Hanau C. Malignant melanoma of the vulva: a review. Obstet Gynecol Surv 1995; 50:739–746.

22 Ca E, Bradley RR, Logsdon VK, et al. Vulvar melanoma in childhood. Arch Derm 1997; 133:345–348.

23 Crowson AN, Magro CM, Mihm MC. The melanocytic proliferations. A comprehensive textbook of pigmented lesions. New York: Wiley; 2001.

24 Rhodes AR, Harrist TJ, Day CL, et al. Dysplastic melanocytic nevi in histologic association with 234 primary cutaneous melanomas. J Am Acad Derm 1983; 9:563–574.

25 Rhodes AR, Melski JW, Sober AJ, et al. Increased intraepidermal melanocytic frequency and size in dysplastic melanocytic nevi and cutaneous melanoma. A comparative quantitative study of dysplastic melanocytic nevi, superficial spreading melanoma, nevocellular nevi and solar lentigines. J Invest Derm 1983; 80:452–459.

26 Elder DE, Goldman LI, Goldman SC, Greene MH, Clark WH. Dysplastic nevus syndrome: a phenotypic association of sporadic cutaneous melanoma. Cancer 1980; 46:1787–1794.

27 Clark WH, Reimer RR, Greene M, Ainsworth AM, Mastrangelo MJ. Origin of familial malignant melanomas from heritable melanocytic lesions – the B-K mole syndrome. Arch Derm 1978; 114:732–738.

28 Rhodes AR, Mihm MC Jr, Weinstock MA. Dysplastic melanocytic nevi: a reproducible histologic definition emphasizing cellular morphology. Mod Pathol 1989; 2:306–319.

29 Tong AK, Murphy GF, Mihm MC Jr. Dysplastic nevus: a formal histogenetic precursor of malignant melanoma. In: Mihm MC, Murphy GF, Kaufman N, eds. Pathobiology and recognition of malignant melanoma. Baltimore: Williams & Wilkins; 1988:10–18.

30 Elder DE. The dysplastic nevus. Pathology 1985; 17:291–297.

31 Weinstock MA. Malignant melanoma of the vulva and vagina in the United States: patterns of incidence and population-based estimates of survival. Am J Obstet Gynecol 1994; 171(5):1225–1230.

32 Giles GG, Kneale BL. Vulvar cancer: the Cinderella of gynaecological oncology. Aust N Z J Obstet Gynecol 1995; 35:71–75.

33 Pannizon RG. Vulvar melanoma. Semin Derm 1996; 15:67–70.

34 Raber G, Mempel V, Jackisch C, et al. Malignant melanoma of the vulva. Report of 89 patients. Cancer 1996; 78:2353–2358.

35 Morrow CP, Rutledge FN. Melanoma of the vulva. Obstet Gynecol 1972; 39:745–752.

36 Morrow CP, DiSaia PJ. Malignant melanoma of the female genitalia: a clinical analysis. Obstet Gynecol Surv 1976; 31:233–271.

37 Ariel IM. Malignant melanoma of the female genital system: a report of 48 patients and review of the literature. J Surg Oncol 1981; 16:371–383.

38 Bradgate MG, Rollason TP, McConkey C, et al. Malignant melanoma of the vulva: a clinico-pathological study of 30 women. Br J Obstet Gynaecol 1990; 97:124–133.

39 Ronan SG, Eng AM, Briele HA, et al. Malignant melanoma of the female genitalia. J Am Acad Derm 1990; 22:428–435.

40 Piura B, Egan M, Lopes A, et al. Malignant melanoma of the vulva: a clinicopathologic study of 18 cases. J Surg Oncol 1992; 50:234–240.

41 Ragnarsson-Olding B, Johansson H, Rutqvist LE, et al. Malignant melanoma of the vulva and vagina: trends in incidence and distribution, and long term survival among 245 consecutive cases in Sweden 1960–1984. Cancer 1993; 71:1893–1897.

42 Neven P, Sheperd JH, Masotina A, et al. Malignant melanoma of the vulva and vagina: a report of 23 cases presenting in a 10-year period. Int J Gynecol Cancer 1994; 4:379–383.

43 Konstadoulakis MM, Ricaniadis N, Driscoll DL, et al. Malignant melanoma of the female genital tract. Eur J Surg Oncol 1994; 20:141–145.

44 DeMatos P, Tyler D, Seigler HF. Mucosal melanoma of the female genitalia: a clinicopathologic study of forty-three cases at Duke University Medical Center. Surgery 1998; 124:38–48.

45 Kato T, Takematsu H, Tomita Y, et al. Malignant melanoma of mucous membranes. A clinicopathologic study of 13 cases in Japanese patients. Arch Derm 1987; 123:216–220.

46 Verschraegen CF, Benjapibal M, Supakarapongkul W, et al. Vulvar melanoma at the M.D. Anderson Cancer Center: 25 years later. Int J Gynecol Cancer 2001; 11:359–364.

47 Khoo US, Collins RJ, Ngan HY. Malignant melanoma of the female genital tract. A report of nine cases in the Chinese of Hong Kong. Pathology 1991; 23:312–317.

48 Ragnarsson-Olding BK, Kanter-Lwensohn LR, Lagerlöf B, et al. Malignant melanoma of the vulva in a nationwide, 25-year study of 219 Swedish females: clinical observations and histopathologic features. Cancer 1999; 86(7):1273–1284.

49 Egan CA, Bradley RR, Logsdon VK, et al. Vulvar melanoma in children. Arch Derm 1997; 133:345–348.

50 Heller DS, Moomjy M, Koulos J, et al. Vulvar and vaginal melanoma. A clinicopathologic study. J Reprod Med 1994; 39:945–948.

51 Rigel DS, Carucci JA. Malignant melanoma: prevention, early detection, and treatment in the 21st century. CA Cancer J Clin 2000; 50:215–236.

52 Balch CM, Soong SJ, Gershenwald JE, et al. Prognostic factors analysis of 17,600 melanoma patients: validation of the American Joint Committee on Cancer melanoma staging system. J Clin Oncol 2001; 19:3622–3634.

53 Balch CM, Buzaid AC, Soong SJ, et al. Final version of the American Joint Committee on Cancer staging system for cutaneous melanoma. J Clin Oncol 2001; 19:3635–3648.

54 Sober AJ, Chuang TY, Duvic M, et al. Guidelines of care for primary cutaneous melanoma. J Am Acad Derm 2001; 45:579–586.

55 Carlson JA, Mu XC, Slominski A, et al. Melanocytic proliferations associated with lichen sclerosus. Arch Derm 2002; 138(1):77–87.

56 Raju RR, Goldblum JR, Hart WR. Pagetoid squamous cell carcinoma in situ (pagetoid Bowen's disease) of the external genitalia. Int J Gynecol Pathol 2003; 22(2):127–135.

57 Bacchi CE, Goldfogel GA, Greer BE, Gown AM. Paget's disease and melanoma of the vulva. Use of a panel of monoclonal antibodies to identify cell type and to microscopically define adequacy of surgical margins. Gynecol Oncol 1992; 46(2):216–221.

58 Shah KD, Tabibzadeh SS, Gerber MA. Immunohistochemical distinction of Paget's disease from Bowen's disease and superficial spreading melanoma with the use of monoclonal cytokeratin antibodies. Am J Clin Pathol 1987; 88(6):689–695.

59 Anderson KW, Baker SR, Lowe L, Su L, Johnson TM. Treatment of head and neck melanoma, lentigo maligna subtype: a practical surgical technique. Arch Facial Plast Surg 2001; 3:202–206.

60 Johnson TM, Headington JT, Baker SR, Lowe L. Usefulness of the staged excision for lentigo maligna and lentigo maligna melanoma: the 'square' procedure. J Am Acad Derm 1997; 37:758–764.

61 Blessing K, Kernohan NM, Miller ID, et al. Malignant melanoma of the vulva; clinicopathological features. Int J Gynecol Cancer 1991; 1:81–87.

62 Scheistroen M, Trope C, Kaern J, et al. Malignant melanoma of the vulva: evaluation of prognostic factors with emphasis on DNA ploidy in 75 patients. Cancer 1995; 75:72–80.

63 Ragnarsson-Olding BK, Nilsson BR, Kanter-Lwensohn LR, et al. Malignant melanoma of the vulva in a nationwide, 25 year study of 219 Swedish females: predictors of survival. Cancer 1999; 86:1285–1293.

64 Gershenwald JE, Thompson W, Mansfield PF, et al. Multi-institutional melanoma lymphatic mapping experience: the prognostic value of sentinel lymph node status in 612 stage I or II melanoma patients. J Clin Oncol 1999; 17:976–983.

65 Chang AE, Karnell LH, Menck HR. The National Cancer Data Base report on cutaneous and noncutaneous melanoma: a summary of 84,836 cases from the past decade. The American College of Surgeons Commission on Cancer and the American Cancer Society. Cancer 1998; 83:1664–1678.

66 Creasman WT, Phillips JL, Menck HR. A survey of hospital management practices for vulvar melanoma. J Am Coll Surg 1999; 188(6):670–675.

67 Hullu JA de, Hollema H, Hoekstra HJ, et al. Vulvar melanoma: is there a role for sentinel lymph node biopsy? Cancer 2002; 94(2):486–491.

68 McMasters KM, Reintgen DS, Ross MI, et al. Sentinel lymph node biopsy for melanoma: controversy despite widespread agreement. J Clin Oncol 2001; 19:2851–2855.

69 Morton DL, Wen DR, Wong JH, et al. Technical details of intraoperative lymphatic mapping for early stage melanoma. Arch Surg 1992; 127:392–399.

70 Su LD, Lowe L, Bradford CR, et al. Immunostaining for cytokeratin 20 improves detection of micrometastatic Merkel cell carcinoma in sentinel lymph nodes. J Am Acad Derm 2002; 46:661–666.

71 Levenback C, Burke TW, Gershenson DM, et al. Intraoperative lymphatic mapping for vulvar cancer. Obstet Gynecol 1994; 84:163–167.

72 Ramirez PT, Levenback C. Sentinel nodes in gynecologic malignancies. Curr Opin Oncol 2001; 13:403–407.

73 Levenback C, Coleman RL, Burke TW, et al. Intraoperative lymphatic mapping and sentinel node identification with blue dye in patients with vulvar cancer. Gynecol Oncol 2001; 83:276–281.

74 Cicco C De, Sideri M, Bartolomei M, et al. Sentinel node biopsy in early vulvar cancer. Br J Cancer 2000; 82:295–299.

75 Abramova L, Parekh J, Irvin WP Jr, et al. Sentinel node biopsy in vulvar and vaginal melanoma: presentation of six cases and a literature review. Ann Surg Oncol 2002; 9:840–846.

76 Reintgen DS, Joseph E. Sentinel node localization for cutaneous melanoma. Melanoma Lett 1997; 15:3–4.

77 Cimmino VM, Brown AC, Szocik JF, et al. Allergic reactions to isosulfan blue during sentinel node biopsy – a common event. Surgery 2001; 130:439–442.

9

Soft tissue lesions of the vulva and vagina

Marisa R. Nucci

Introduction

Stromal tumors and tumor-like lesions

Fibroepithelial stromal polyp
Angiomyofibroblastoma
Deep (aggressive) angiomyxoma
Superficial angiomyxoma
Cellular angiofibroma

Fibrohistiocytic tumors

Dermatofibroma (fibrous
    histiocytoma)
Dermatofibrosarcoma
    protuberans

Lipomatous tumors

Lipoma
Liposarcoma

Smooth muscle tumors

Benign, atypical and malignant
    smooth muscle tumors
Leiomyomatosis

Skeletal muscle tumors

Genital rhabdomyoma
Embryonal rhabdomyosarcoma
    (sarcoma botryoides)

Vascular and related lesions

Angiokeratoma
Lymphangioma circumscriptum

Neural tumors

Granular cell tumor

Introduction

Soft tissue lesions of the vulvovaginal region can be separated into two general categories: those that are relatively site-specific[1] and those that occur more commonly at other sites but which may also involve this region.[2] The former group includes aggressive angiomyxoma, angiomyofibroblastoma, cellular angiofibroma and fibroepithelial stromal polyp; the latter group comprises the remainder of entities discussed. The term 'relatively' site-specific is employed since many of the lesions in this group may also be seen, albeit less commonly, at other sites.

Stromal tumors and tumor-like lesions

Differences in clinical presentation and histopathologic features between the entities discussed below are summarized in Table 9.1.

FIBROEPITHELIAL STROMAL POLYP

Clinical presentation

Fibroepithelial stromal polyps are benign lesions that occur in the vagina, vulva and rarely the cervix of young to middle-aged women.[1-12] They generally develop during pregnancy but may also be associated with hormone replacement therapy.[2,7,8] Gross examination reveals lesions that are typically pedunculated/polypoid but may be sessile with a broad base or have a papillary/fronded appearance (Fig. 9.1). Stromal polyps can vary in size, presenting as a solitary lesion or occasionally as multiple polyps, the latter scenario more commonly associated with pregnancy.[5,7]

Histopathologic features

Fibroepithelial stromal polyps are characterized by (1) a central fibrovascular core, (2) stellate and multinucleate stromal cells, which tend to be localized at the stromal–epithelial interface and around blood vessels and (3) overlying squamous epithelium (Fig. 9.2a,b). The most varied aspect of these lesions is the stroma, which can range in appearance from hypocellular and bland to hypercellular and pleomorphic. In particular, polyps that occur during pregnancy tend to exhibit a greater degree of nuclear pleomorphism, cellularity and mitotic activity (including atypical mitotic figures), hence the use of the term 'pseudosarcoma botryoides' by some authors.[2,5-8] Such polyps may raise the possibility of malignancy (Fig. 9.3);[12] however, even in those with these worrisome histologic features, morphologic clues to the diagnosis include (1) lack of an identifiable lesional margin, (2) extension of atypical stromal cells to the stromal–epithelial interface and (3) the frequent presence of individually scattered multinucleate stromal cells (characteristically seen in usual polyps at these sites),

Table 9.1 Differences in clinical presentation and histopathologic features

	Aggressive angiomyxoma	Angiomyo-fibroblastoma	Cellular angiofibroma	Fibroepithelial stromal polyp	Superficial angiomyxoma
Age	Reproductive age	Reproductive age	Reproductive age	Reproductive age	Reproductive age
Location/ configuration	Deep-seated, not polypoid	Subcutaneous	Subcutaneous	Usually polypoid, exophytic	Superficial, subcutaneous, polypoid
Size	Variable	Usually <5 cm	Usually <3 cm	Variable	Usually <3 cm
Margins	Infiltrative	Well circumscribed	Usually well circumscribed	Merges with normal	Lobulated, distinct
Cellularity	Paucicellular	Alternating hyper- and hypocellular	Cellular	Variable	Hypocellular
Vessels	Medium to large, thick-walled, hyalinized	Delicate, capillary-sized, numerous	Small to medium, thick-walled, hyalinized	Variable, usually large, thick-walled central core	Delicate, thin-walled, elongated
Mitotic index	Rare	Usually uncommon	Variable, may be brisk	Variable	Usually uncommon
Biomarkers	Desmin positive, HMGA2 positive	Desmin positive, HMGA2 negative	Desmin variable, HMGA2 negative	Desmin positive, HMGA2 negative	Desmin negative, HMGA2 negative
Clinical course	30% local destructive recurrence	Benign	Benign	Benign, rare recurrence	30% local non-destructive recurrence

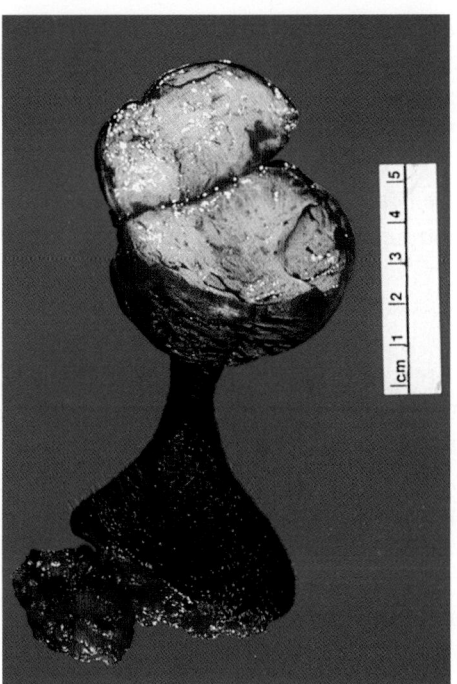

Fig. 9.1
Fibroepithelial
stromal polyp.
A pedunculated
polyp with a thin
stalk and fibrous
core.

since the latter is located more deeply, is more infiltrative, is less polypoid and exhibits a more prominent vascular component that is diffusely present throughout the tumor.

As discussed above, stromal polyps with hypercellular and pleomorphic stroma should not be mistaken for a malignancy, particularly embryonal rhabdomyosarcoma. Fortunately, this differential diagnosis is rarely a problem from a clinical or histopathologic perspective. Clinically, fibroepithelial stromal polyps are rare before puberty, which is the most common age group for embryonal rhabdomyosarcoma. Histologically, cellular stromal polyps tend to exhibit a greater degree of cellularity in the central portion of the polyp, which is in direct contrast to the pattern of cellularity in embryonal rhabdomyosarcoma where the cellularity is greatest beneath the epithelium (so-called cambium layer). The presence in embryonal rhabdomyosarcoma of strap cells with cross striations and skeletal muscle marker positivity further aids in this distinction.

Prognosis and management

Although benign, fibroepithelial stromal polyps do have the potential to locally recur, particularly if incompletely excised.[1,8,12] Multiple stromal polyps may occur during pregnancy, spontaneously regress following delivery and 'recur' during subsequent pregnancies, supporting the concept that these lesions are hormonally responsive and likely represent a reactive or hyperplastic process that involves the cells of the subepithelial zone of the distal female genital tract.

most often located close to the surface epithelium (Fig. 9.2a). The stromal cells may be positive for desmin, actin, vimentin, estrogen receptor and progesterone receptor.[8–10,12]

Differential diagnosis

Occasionally, fibroepithelial stromal polyps may undergo torsion, become edematous and histologically mimic aggressive angiomyxoma (Fig. 9.4). Stromal polyps can be distinguished from aggressive angiomyxoma

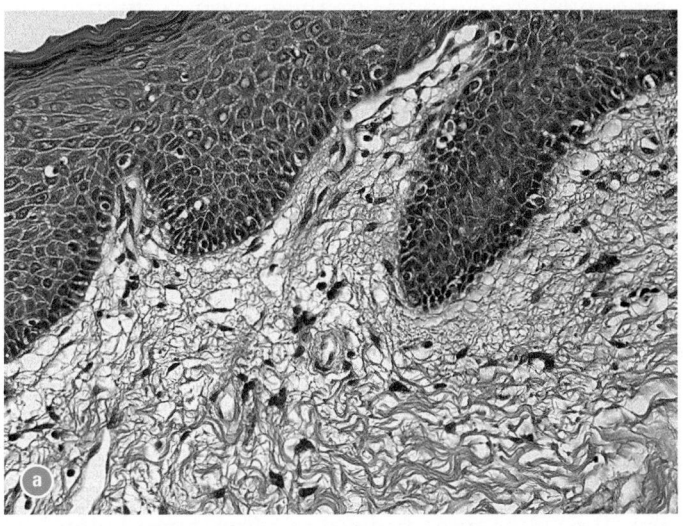

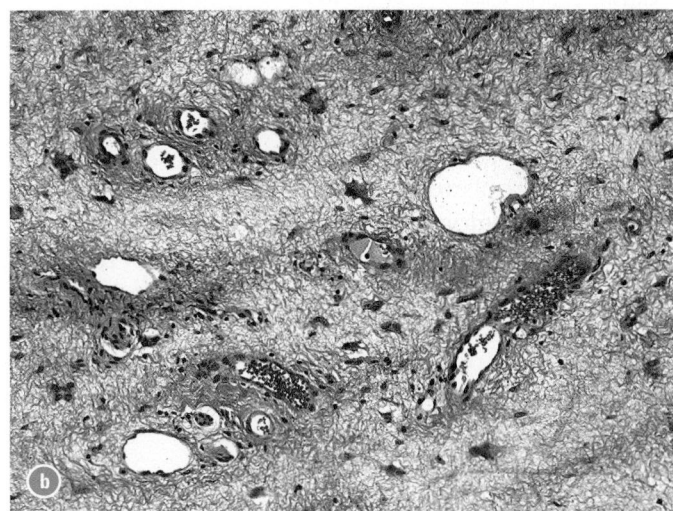

Fig. 9.2 Fibroepithelial stromal polyp. Stellate and multinucleate cells are typically present (a) near the epithelial–stromal interface and (b) around the prominent vascular component.

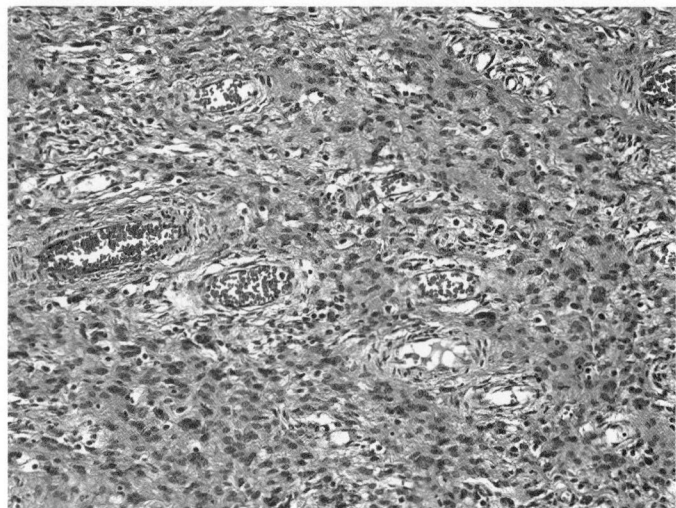

Fig. 9.3 Fibroepithelial stromal polyp. Hypercellularity and nuclear atypia may be present, particularly in those polyps removed during pregnancy.

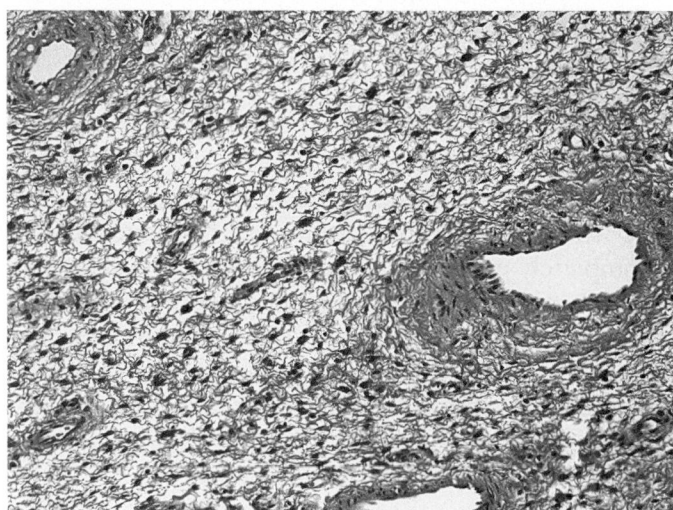

Fig. 9.4 Fibroepithelial stromal polyp. Edematous change may mimic an aggressive angiomyxoma.

ANGIOMYOFIBROBLASTOMA

Clinical presentation

Angiomyofibroblastoma occurs almost exclusively in the vulvovaginal region of reproductive-aged women but may also occur in the inguinal/scrotal region of men.[13–18] Clinically, the tumor is well circumscribed and is often thought to represent a cyst, most commonly a Bartholin's gland cyst. Tumor size is variable, but usually measures less than 5.0 cm.

Histopathologic features

Histologically, angiomyofibroblastoma is a well-circumscribed neoplasm composed of numerous delicate thin-walled capillary-sized vessels and plump, round to spindle-shaped cells. The stromal cells, which are typically clustered around the vessels, are set within a variably edematous to collagenous matrix with alternating zones of cellularity (Fig. 9.5a,b). The tumor cells often appear somewhat epithelioid (except in postmenopausal patients where they are more often spindled), having moderate amounts of eosinophilic cytoplasm and nuclei with fine chromatin and inconspicuous nucleoli. Some of the stromal cells may have eccentrically placed nuclei imparting a plasmacytoid appearance, whereas others are multinucleated. There are typically few mitoses and occasionally intralesional adipose tissue may be present.[17] The stromal cells are typically desmin positive and show variable positivity for actin, although they are usually negative for this marker.

Differential diagnosis

Angiomyofibroblastoma should be distinguished from aggressive angiomyxoma due to differences in biologic behavior (see below). The histologic features that help distinguish between these two entities include the presence in the former of a sharply circumscribed margin and plump epithelioid cells clustered around numerous capillary-sized vessels in contrast to aggressive angiomyxoma, which typically is less cellular, has an infiltrative margin and tends to contain larger, thicker-walled vessels.

Prognosis and management

Angiomyofibroblastoma is a benign, non-recurring neoplasm; local excision with clear margins is adequate treatment. There is one case report of sarcomatous transformation of an angiomyofibroblastoma, which subsequently recurred; in this case areas typical of angiomyofibroblastoma merged with a high-grade sarcoma.[19]

DEEP (AGGRESSIVE) ANGIOMYXOMA

Clinical presentation

Aggressive angiomyxoma is a locally infiltrative, non-metastasizing neoplasm that occurs in the female pelvis and perineum as well as analogous sites in men.[20–25] In women, the median age at presentation is typically in the fourth decade. Similar to other soft tissue tumors that occur at this site, aggressive angiomyxoma is often mistaken for a labial cyst, most commonly a Bartholin's gland cyst. Tumors can be of varying size, but are often relatively large with distortion of normal anatomy (Fig. 9.6). Imaging studies are often quite helpful in assessing extent of disease and for surgical planning,

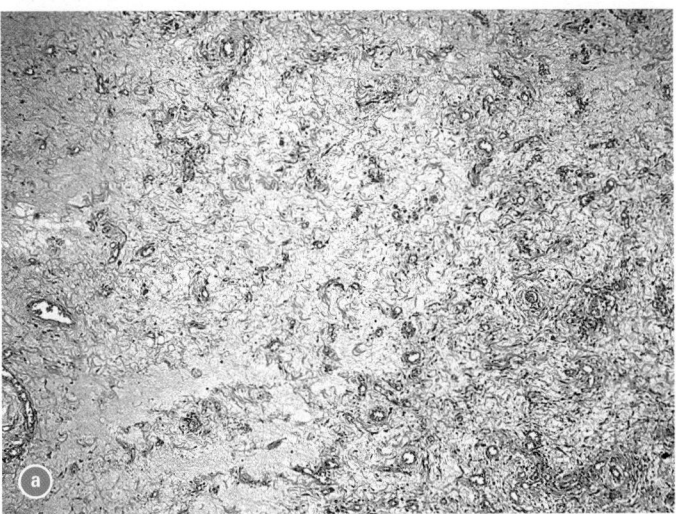
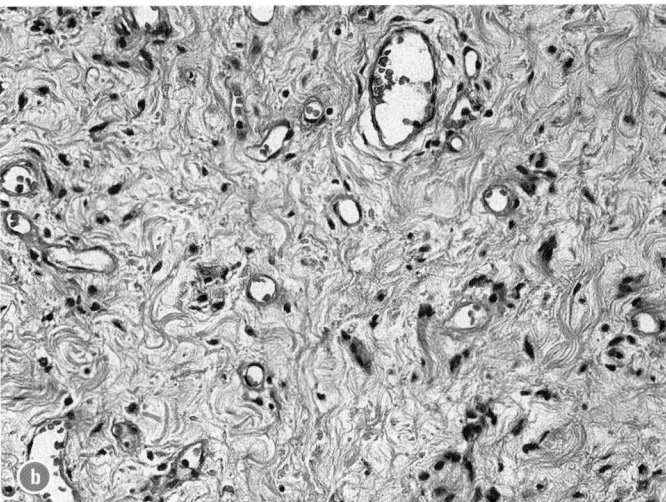

Fig. 9.5 Angiomyofibroblastoma. (a) Alternating zones of cellularity are characteristic. (b) Numerous capillaries are surrounded by lesional spindled cells, some of which are arranged in clusters.

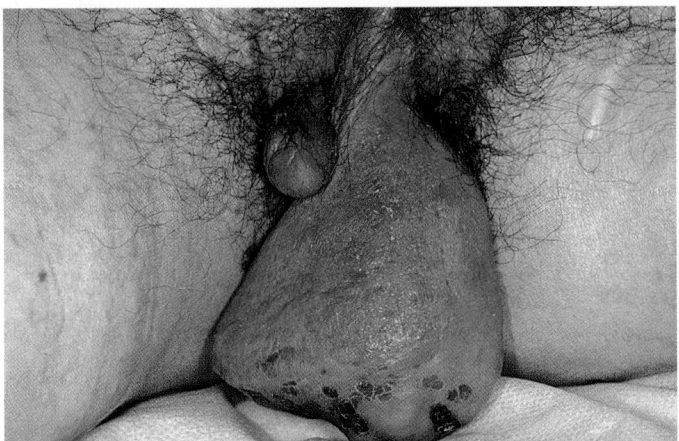

Fig. 9.6 Deep (aggressive) angiomyxoma. Large tumor mass with distortion of normal anatomy.

since tumors may be larger than appreciated on clinical examination alone (Fig. 9.7).[26]

Histopathologic features

Aggressive angiomyxoma typically has a gelatinous appearance on gross examination but may appear more fibrous – a feature mainly seen in recurrent cases (Fig. 9.8). Histologically, it is paucicellular with deceptively infiltrative borders, which accounts for its propensity to recur. Bland spindle-shaped cells with delicate uni- or bipolar cytoplasmic processes are set within a myxoid stroma with interspersed medium-to large-sized vessels that are often thick-walled and hyalinized (Fig. 9.9). Loose fibrillar collagen and collections of smooth muscle cells (so-called 'myoid bundles') are typically arranged in either loose clusters or tight whorls adjacent to blood vessels (Fig. 9.10). The lesional stromal cells of aggres-

sive angiomyxoma may be positive for desmin as well as actin, particularly in the myoid bundles.[27]

Differential diagnosis

The entities that most commonly fall into the differential diagnosis of aggressive angiomyxoma include angiomyofibroblastoma, fibroepithelial stromal polyp and superficial angiomyxoma; the two former lesions and their distinction from aggressive angiomyxoma were discussed in the previous sections. Although more commonly encountered outside of the vulvovaginal region, superficial angiomyxoma can occur in this area and represents a myxoid neoplasm that may be mistaken for aggressive angiomyxoma. Superficial angiomyxoma differs from aggressive angiomyxoma in its tendency to be centered in the dermis and subcutis and by its lobu-

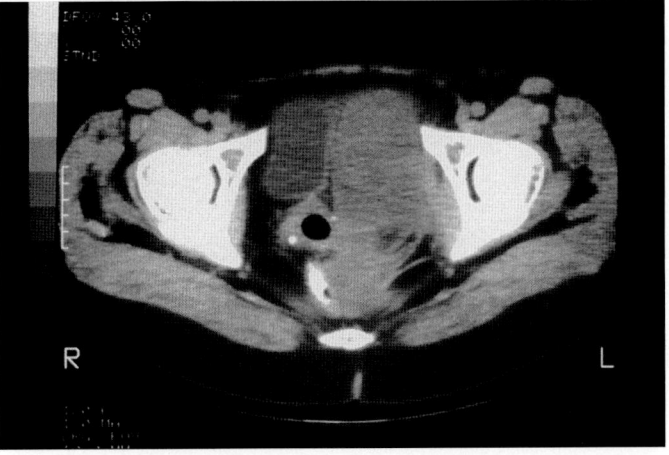

Fig. 9.7 Deep (aggressive) angiomyxoma. Preoperative imaging helps define the extent of the disease, which can extend into the pelvis.

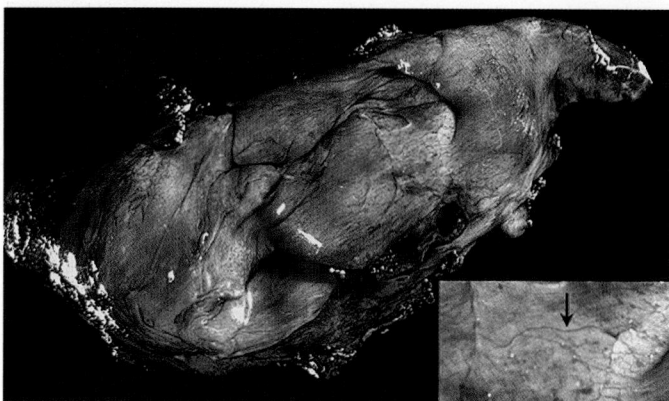

Fig. 9.8 Aggressive angiomyxoma. Ill-defined neoplasm with glistening cut surface. Numerous vessels are discernible (inset, arrow).

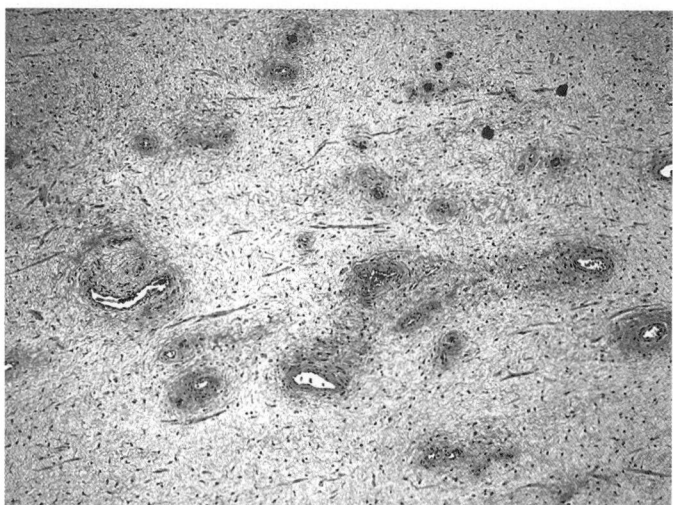

Fig. 9.9 Aggressive angiomyxoma. Paucicellular spindle cell neoplasm punctuated by numerous thick-walled vessels.

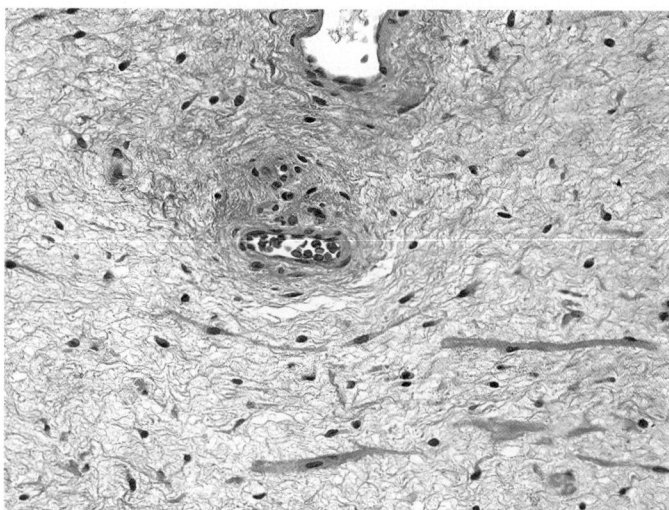

Fig. 9.10 Aggressive angiomyxoma. Bland spindle cells are set within a loosely collagenous and myxoid matrix. Brightly eosinophilic bands of smooth muscle are often present near the vessels.

lated growth pattern. In addition, the lesional stromal cells of superficial angiomyxoma are desmin negative.

Prognosis and management

Aggressive angiomyxoma has a propensity for local destructive recurrence, which occurs in approximately 30–40% of cases, sometimes many years (often decades) after the initial excision, particularly if the tumor is incompletely excised.[20–25] Therefore, wide excision with clear margins of at least 1 cm is optimal.

SUPERFICIAL ANGIOMYXOMA

Clinical presentation

The head and neck region and trunk are the most common sites for superficial angiomyxoma; however, it may also occasionally occur in the genital region. It occurs most commonly in the fourth decade, typically as a slow-growing, painless, polypoid tumor that is usually less than 5 cm.[28–30] The presence of multiple cutaneous myxomas and angiomyxomas that occur at certain sites, such as the external ear or breast, is highly associated with Carney's complex; this association is less clear with superficial angiomyxoma occurring in the genital area.[29]

Histopathologic features

Histologically, superficial angiomyxoma is characteristically multilobulated, superficially located in the dermis and subcutis and has a well-demarcated border (Fig. 9.11). The myxoid nodules are composed of slender spindle and stellate-shaped cells, inflammatory cells

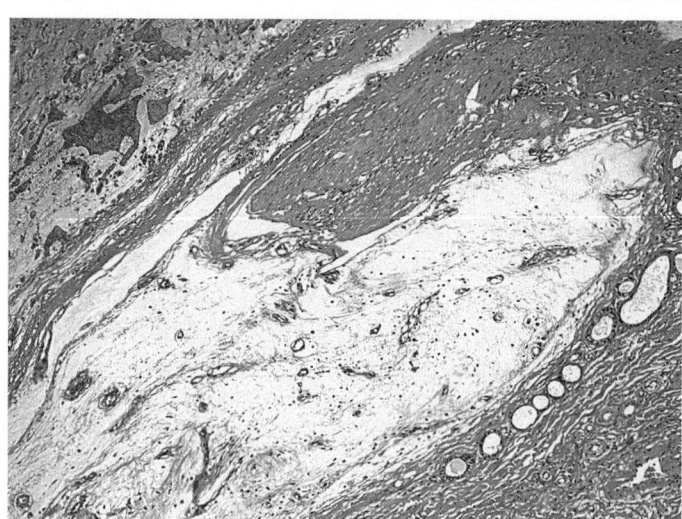

Fig. 9.11 Superficial angiomyxoma. Well-demarcated, multilobulated tumor located in the dermis.

(particularly polymorphonuclear leukocytes) and thin-walled vessels (Fig. 9.12). An epithelial component, usually in the form of a squamous epithelial-lined cyst or basaloid epithelial nests and strands, is present in approximately 30% of the cases (Fig. 9.13).

Differential diagnosis

Superficial angiomyxoma may sometimes be mistaken for aggressive angiomyxoma since both tumors are hypocellular myxoid neoplasms. Unlike aggressive angiomyxoma, which is a deep-seated tumor, superficial angiomyxoma typically involves the dermis and subcutis and lacks the infiltrative borders and thick-walled vessels of aggressive angiomyxoma. In addition

to these histologic differences, the lesional stromal cells of superficial angiomyxoma are typically desmin negative whereas those of aggressive angiomyxoma are usually desmin positive.[29]

Prognosis and management

Superficial angiomyxoma has the potential for local non-destructive recurrence in approximately 30–40% of cases and should be completely excised with clear margins.[27–30]

CELLULAR ANGIOFIBROMA

Clinical presentation

Cellular angiofibroma typically occurs in the vulvo-vaginal region in middle-aged women (but may also occur in men), is characteristically small (< 3 cm) and is usually well-circumscribed.[31–33]

Histopathologic features

Histologically, cellular angiofibroma is a cellular neoplasm composed of uniform, bland spindle cells arranged in short intersecting fascicles, numerous thick-walled, often hyalinized medium-sized vessels, wispy collagen bundles and a scant component of mature adipose tissue (Fig. 9.14). The spindle cells typically have ovoid to fusiform basophilic nuclei and scant, pale staining cytoplasm with ill-defined borders; multinucleate cells may be present. Mitoses may be frequent.

Differential diagnosis

Occasionally, cellular angiofibroma may be edematous and mimic aggressive angiomyxoma; however, the latter

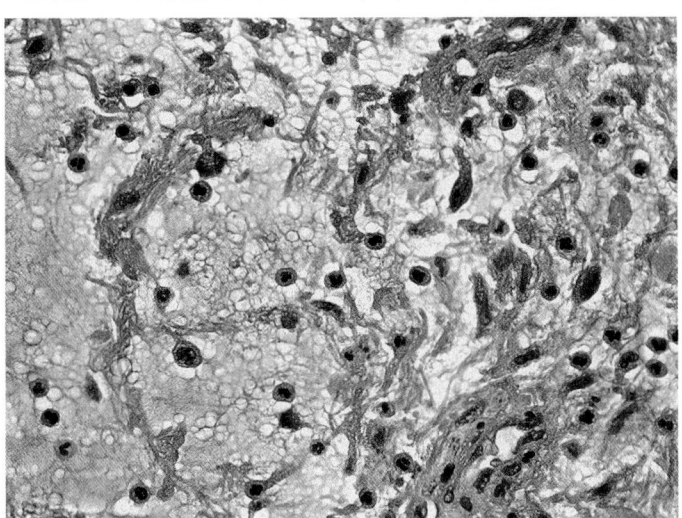

Fig. 9.12 Superficial angiomyxoma. Bland spindle cells are admixed with acute inflammatory cells.

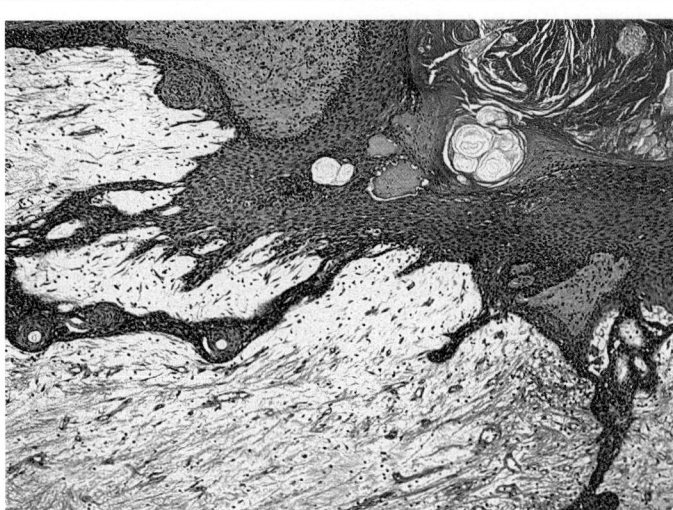

Fig. 9.13 Superficial angiomyxoma. An epithelial component is present in approximately one-third of cases.

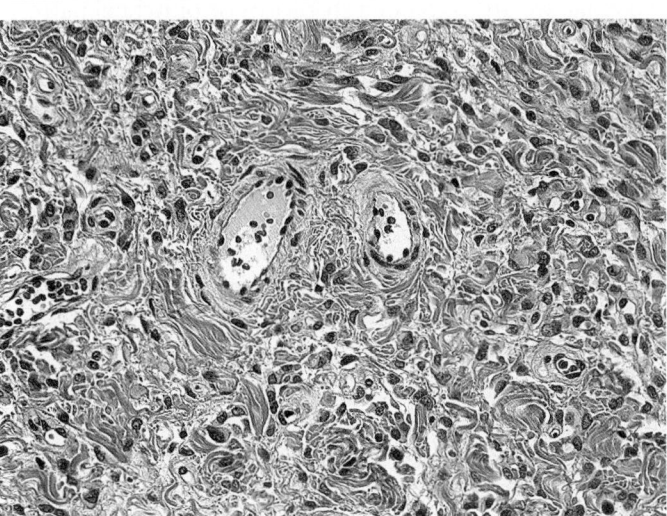

Fig. 9.14 Cellular angiofibroma. Short intersecting fascicles of bland spindle cells are set in a collagenous matrix that is interspersed with medium-sized vessels.

is less cellular, more deeply located, more infiltrative and tends to have larger, thick-walled vessels. Cellular angiofibroma is usually desmin negative and may be CD34 positive, whereas aggressive angiomyxoma is typically CD34 negative and desmin positive.[31,32]

Prognosis and management

Cellular angiofibroma appears to behave in a benign fashion; therefore, local excision with clear margins is adequate treatment.

Fibrohistiocytic tumors

DERMATOFIBROMA (FIBROUS HISTIOCYTOMA)

Clinical presentation

Dermatofibroma, also known as fibrous histiocytoma (as well as nodular subepidermal fibrosis in the older literature) is a tumor of dermal stroma.[34] This tumor most commonly occurs in adults on the limbs and trunk area, but may also rarely involve the vulva. It can have a range of clinical appearances, presenting as flesh-colored or pigmented plaques, nodules or papules. Although non-specific, dermatofibroma can be suspected on clinical examination by the so-called 'dimple' sign: pinching the tumor results in the inward dimpling of the epidermis.

Histopathologic features

Although it can be quite variable, the classic histologic appearance of fibrous histiocytoma is that of a relatively well-circumscribed dermal-based proliferation of spindle cells that are arranged in a storiform or pinwheel pattern (Fig. 9.15). At the edges, the lesional spindle cells wrap around the often-hyalinized dermal collagen bundles in a characteristic fashion (Fig. 9.16). An associated overlying epidermal hyperplasia is often present and, when viewed under polarized light, birefringent collagen is present within the substance of the tumor. A number of variants of dermatofibroma have been described (principally outside of the vulvar region), including (1) hemosiderotic (2) lipidized (cholesterolotic), (3) aneurysmal (angiomatoid), (4) atypical, (5) epithelioid and (6) cellular and deeply penetrating.[35–41] Immunophenotypically, dermatofibroma is usually diffusely positive for factor XIIIa and negative for CD34.[42] One important caveat is that the cellular variant of dermatofibroma may show a 'collar' of positivity for CD34 around the edges of the lesion but typically will not show the diffuse positivity seen in dermatofibrosarcoma protuberans.[41]

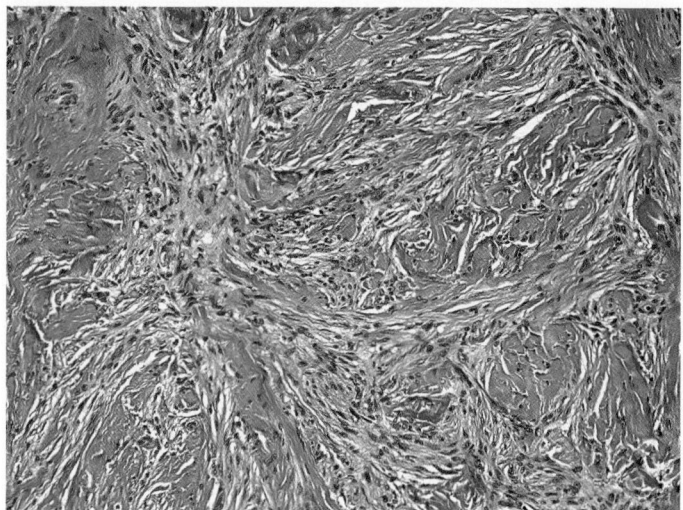

Fig. 9.15 Dermatofibroma. Storiform spindle cell proliferation in a variably hyalinized stroma.

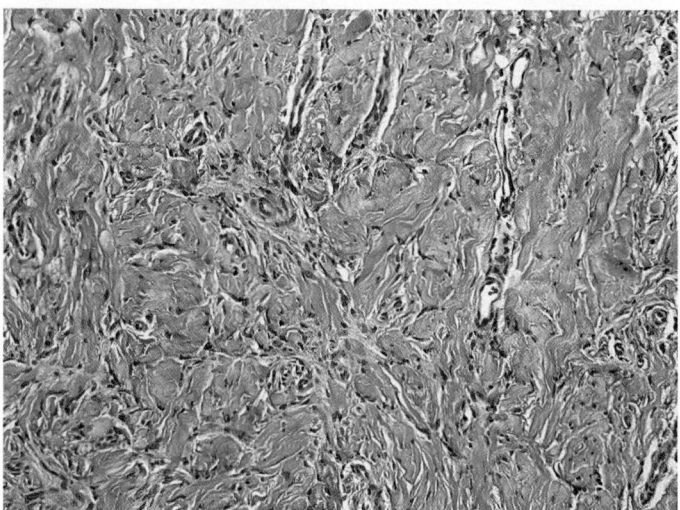

Fig. 9.16 Dermatofibroma. Spindle cells wrapping around collagen bundles at the periphery of the lesion is characteristic.

Differential diagnosis

The principal differential diagnostic consideration is the distinction from dermatofibrosarcoma protuberans (see discussion below).

Prognosis and management

The prognosis and management of patients with dermatofibroma depends upon its histologic appearance. In cases of classic dermatofibroma with typical cytomorphology as described and illustrated above, no further treatment or consideration of re-excision is necessary, as these tumors are benign. The cellular, aneurysmal and atypical variants of dermatofibroma, as well as dermatofibromas that are more deeply infiltrative, have the potential for persistence/local recurrence; therefore, complete excision should be obtained in these cases.[38,39,43] Re-excision should be performed only if the initial tumor was incompletely excised; marginal, but complete, excision is adequate. There are rare cases of dermatofibroma exhibiting features of the cellular, aneurysmal and/or atypical variants that have had distant deposits of tumor to local lymph nodes and lung; in these cases there were no morphologic indicators predictive of this outcome in the primary tumor.[39,44]

DERMATOFIBROSARCOMA PROTUBERANS

Clinical presentation

The groin area is one of the more common sites of dermatofibrosarcoma protuberans (in addition to the trunk and lower extremity). Strictly speaking, however, dermatofibrosarcoma protuberans occurring in the *vulva* is not as common, with only approximately 30 cases or so reported in the literature (predominantly as case reports).[45–53] This tumor can vary in appearance from a plaque or nodule to exophytic, multinodular growths which may be flesh-colored or variably hypo- or hyperpigmented.

Histopathologic features

The characteristic histologic features of dermatofibrosarcoma protuberans include (1) a monomorphous storiform proliferation of spindle cells, (2) poor circumscription with infiltration of subcutaneous adipose tissue in a characteristic lacy or honeycomb pattern, (3) separation of the tumor from the overlying normal-appearing or atrophic epidermis (grenz zone), (4) entrapment of adnexal structures and (5) lack of polarizable collagen (Fig. 9.17). A subset of dermatofibrosarcoma protuberans exhibits fibrosarcomatous change (Fig. 9.18) – a herringbone architectural pattern of growth in combination with increased mitoses and hypercellularity (similar to soft tissue fibrosarcoma);[54] myoid nodules have also been described.[55] This type of fibrosarcomatous change has been described in dermatofibrosarcoma protuberans of the vulva.[45]

Cytogenetic analysis of dermatofibrosarcoma protuberans has shown that these tumors harbor a translocation between chromosomes 17 and 22, which often appears as a supernumerary ring chromosome.[56] The translocation results in the fusion of two genes, collagen type I alpha 1 (*COL1A1*) and platelet-derived growth factor B-chain (*PDGFB*). Similar to dermatofibrosarcoma protuberans at other sites, those that occur in the vulva contain COL1A1-PDGFB chimeric fusion transcripts.[46,47]

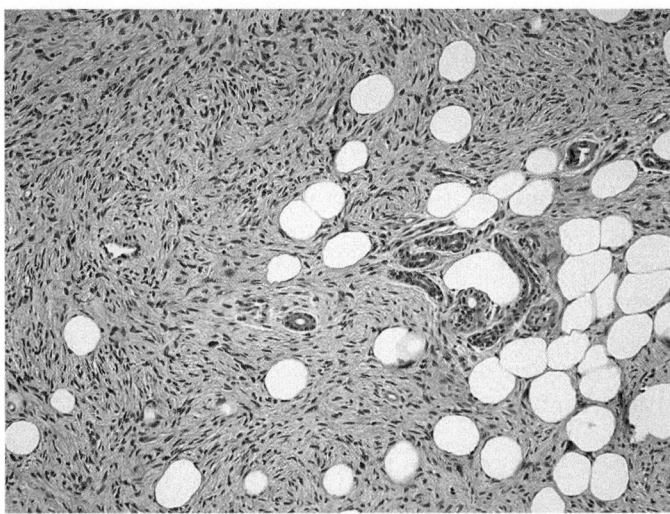

Fig. 9.17 Dermatofibrosarcoma protuberans. Entrapment of adnexal structures and infiltration of adipose tissue.

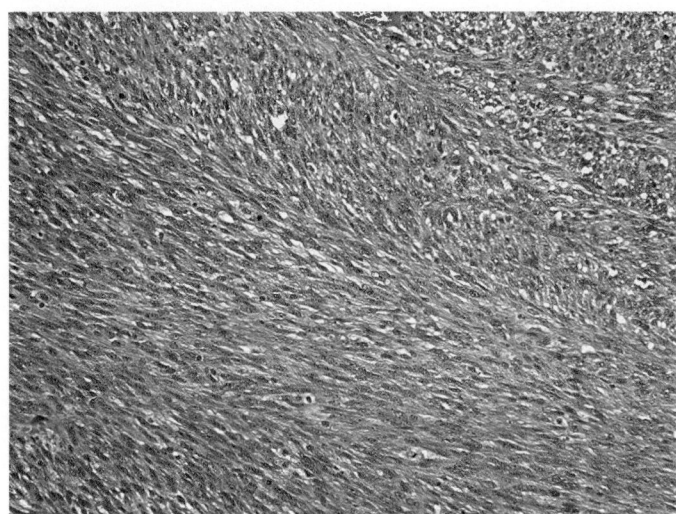

Fig. 9.18 Dermatofibrosarcoma protuberans. Fibrosarcomatous change.

Differential diagnosis

The chief differential diagnostic consideration is the distinction from dermatofibroma. Dermatofibrosarcoma protuberans can be distinguished from dermatofibroma by its (1) tendency to infiltrate subcutaneous tissue in a characteristic lacy pattern, (2) lack of overlying epidermal hyperplasia, (3) lack of birefringent collagen when viewed under polarized light, (4) tendency to infiltrate around and surround adnexal structures, which often can be found within the substance of the tumor and (5) typically diffuse positivity for CD34 and lack of positivity for factor XIIIa (although there can be overlap in staining for these markers in these two entities).

In addition to the above differential diagnostic consideration, any spindle cell proliferation in the vulva showing mitotic activity and/or deep infiltration, particularly in a postmenopausal woman, should always raise the possibility of a spindled invasive squamous cell carcinoma and desmoplastic malignant melanoma. Careful observation of the overlying epidermis for squamous cell carcinoma in situ or melanoma in situ is useful. In addition, immunohistochemistry with a panel of keratins, S100, Mart-1 and HMB-45 will help in this distinction; a panel of keratins is recommended since the spindled variant of squamous cell carcinoma may not show the same degree of positivity with keratin as those tumors with a more conventional appearance.

Management and prognosis

Dermatofibrosarcoma protuberans has a propensity for local recurrence; therefore, wide local excision is recommended. Metastasis in typical cases is infrequent; however, tumors that show fibrosarcomatous change have a higher risk of metastasis (15% in one series).[54]

Lipomatous tumors

LIPOMA

Clinical presentation

Lipomas occur rarely in the vulva and most often present as a slowly growing, soft mass involving the labium majus, which when large can be pedunculated (Fig. 9.19).[57,58]

Histopathologic features

Similar to lipomas at other sites, vulvar lipoma is well circumscribed and composed of mature adipose tissue. A pleomorphic lipoma of the vulva, containing floret-like multinucleated cells, has been described.[59]

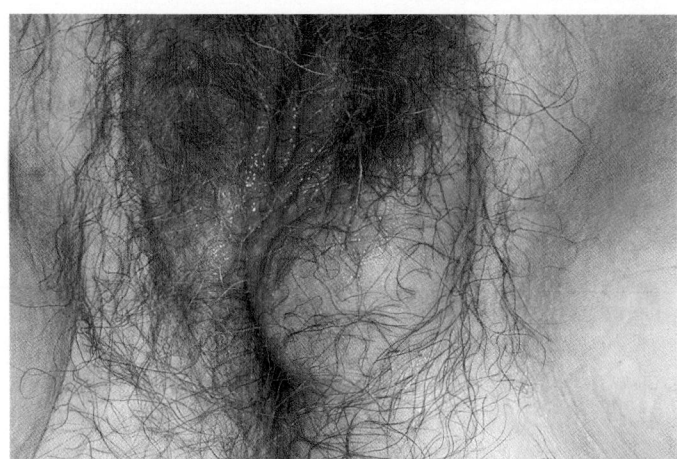

Fig. 9.19 Lipoma.

Differential diagnosis

The principal differential diagnostic consideration is distinction of benign lipoma from well-differentiated liposarcoma (described below).

Prognosis and management

Lipomas are benign neoplasms. Excision is curative.

LIPOSARCOMA

Clinical presentation

Liposarcoma of the vulva is rare, with less than 10 well-documented cases reported in the literature.[60–62] They typically occur in predominantly middle-aged women (median age 52), are variably sized and are most commonly of the well-differentiated histologic subtype. They are often thought to represent benign lesions prior to excision (most commonly a lipoma or cyst).

Histopathologic features

Most cases have the usual appearance of well-differentiated liposarcoma elsewhere, with variation in adipocyte size, adipocytic nuclear atypia and cellular fibrous septa containing atypical stromal cells (Fig. 9.20); similar to well-differentiated liposarcoma at other sites, the presence of lipoblasts is not a prerequisite for the diagnosis. Of note, some cases of liposarcoma that involve the vulva can exhibit a different histologic appearance with the presence of an admixture of bland spindle cells, variable-sized adipocytes and numerous bivacuolated lipoblasts (Fig. 9.21).[62]

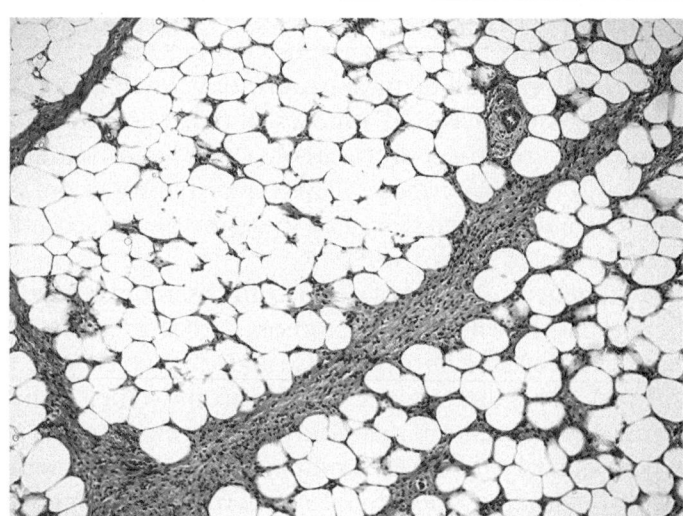

Fig. 9.20 Well differentiated Liposarcoma. Note the presence of cellular fibrous septa and variation in adipocyte size containing atypical stromal cells.

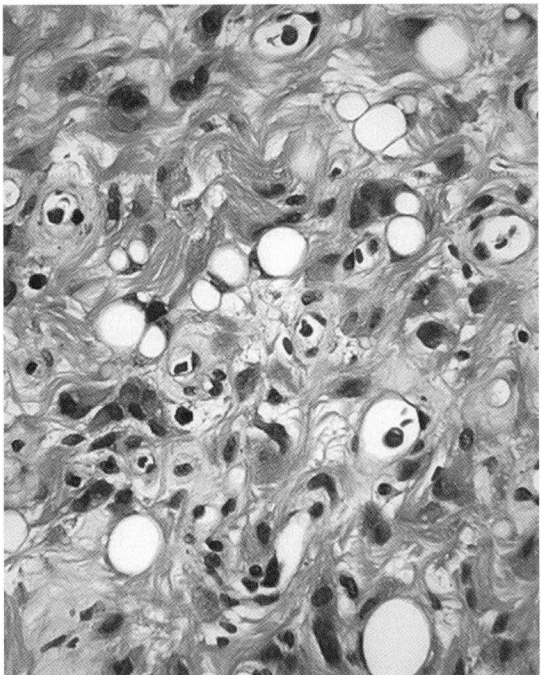

Fig. 9.21 Variant of well-differentiated liposarcoma of vulva. Numerous bivacuolated lipoblasts set within a collagenous matrix.

Differential diagnosis

The principal diagnostic consideration is the distinction of well-differentiated liposarcoma from a lipoma. Liposarcoma can be distinguished from lipoma by its (1) variation in adipocyte size, (2) presence of fibrous septa containing cells with atypical nuclei and (3) lipoblasts. Of note, these diagnostic features may be present only focally; therefore, generous sampling is recommended. Cases that demonstrate the unusual histologic features described above (bland spindle cells admixed with adipocytes) may be confused with spindle cell lipoma. The presence of bivacuolated lipoblasts and the lack of the typical ropy collagen bundles seen in spindle cell lipoma help distinguish between the two. The presence of lipoblasts should also help distinguish this variant from angiomyofibroblastoma, although the lack of numerous capillary-sized vessels in well-differentiated liposarcoma (which is commonly seen in angiomyofibroblastoma), is useful.

Prognosis and management

Well-differentiated liposarcoma, in its pure histologic form, has the potential to recur but not metastasize. It is now generally accepted that tumors previously classified as well-differentiated liposarcoma should be called 'atypical lipomatous tumors' at sites that are amenable to complete excision to reflect this biologic behavior.

Only tumors that have areas of dedifferentiation (which most commonly is seen as an area of high-grade sarcoma within the tumor) have the potential to metastasize.

Wide local excision with clear margins is the optimal treatment in well-differentiated liposarcoma to prevent local recurrence; however, since recurrence may be delayed and the probability of dedifferentiation in the recurrence (and hence metastatic risk) is very low, it is difficult to justify any type of mutilating wide excision in this anatomic location.[62]

Smooth muscle tumors

BENIGN, ATYPICAL AND MALIGNANT SMOOTH MUSCLE TUMORS

Smooth muscle neoplasms are uncommon in the vulvovaginal region, being much more common in the uterine corpus. Uterine smooth muscle tumors have their own distinct criteria for malignancy and recurrent potential, which do not apply to those that occur in the distal female genital tract. Genital smooth muscle tumors were originally considered to be in the category of superficial smooth muscle tumors, which included angioleiomyoma and pilar leiomyoma and were therefore believed to share the same criteria for malignancy. It is now known that smooth muscle tumors of the distal genital tract differ from cutaneous (pilar) smooth muscle tumors both clinically and histologically and should therefore not be considered or classified as such.[63] The vulvovaginal region is not a common site for smooth muscle tumors; therefore, there is difficulty in establishing criteria for recurrent and metastatic potential (as discussed below).

Clinical presentation

Smooth muscle neoplasms occur over a wide age range, but predominantly in the fourth and fifth decade.[63–65] They typically present as a painless subcutaneous mass, first noticed by either the patient or by the physician during routine gynecologic examination; clinical impression is often that of a cyst. These tumors may be of varying size – usually those that are benign or have recurrent potential are well circumscribed and measure less than 3 cm, while malignant tumors usually are infiltrative and are greater than 5 cm.[63–65]

Histopathologic features

There are three main histologic patterns of smooth muscle tumors of the vulvovaginal region, which may be present in mixed or pure form: (1) spindled, (2) epithelioid and (3) myxohyaline. The spindled leiomyoma is comparable with those that occur in the uterine corpus, being composed of intersecting fascicles of spindle-shaped cells with typical smooth muscle morphology. In the epithelioid pattern, there is a combination of spindled cells and round cells; the latter present as either clusters or sheets with the cells having more abundant eosinophilic or clear cytoplasm (Fig. 9.22). The myxohyaline pattern is one that is seen more commonly in smooth muscle tumors at this site than at other sites in the female genital tract. In this pattern, the spindled smooth muscle cells are separated by variable amounts of myxohyaline material, which imparts a lacy or plexiform appearance (Fig. 9.23). Occasionally, prominent mucin pooling may be present.[65]

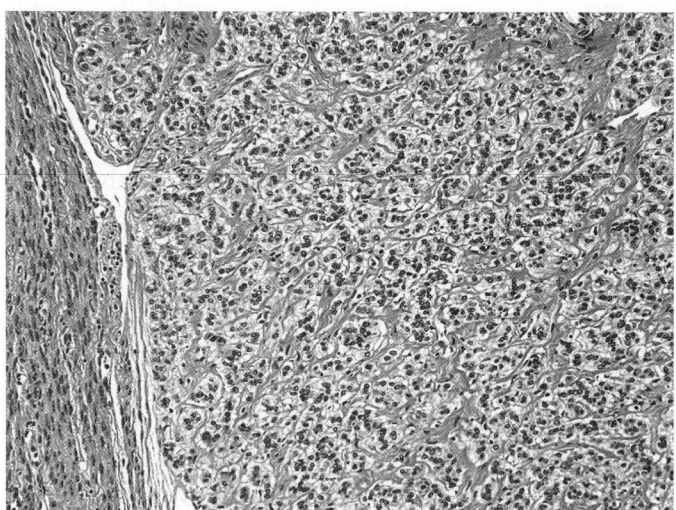

Fig. 9.22 Epithelioid leiomyoma.

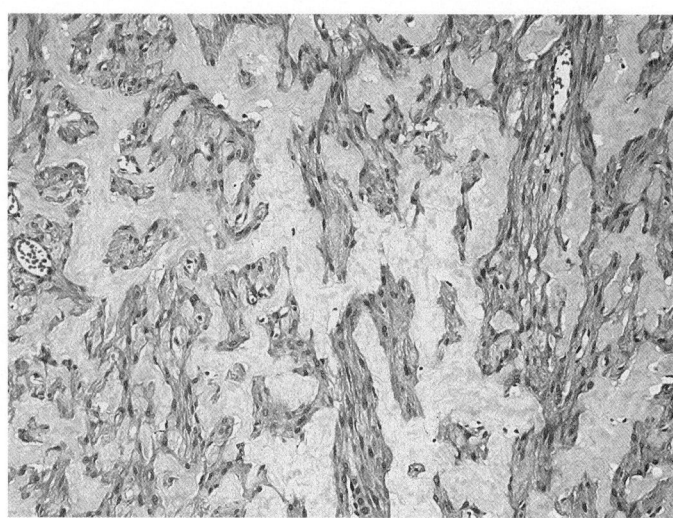

Fig. 9.23 Leiomyoma with myxohyaline change.

Differential diagnosis (criteria for recurrent and metastatic potential)

Recognition of a tumor as being within the category of smooth muscle neoplasia is relatively straightforward. Reliably predicting those tumors that have recurrent or metastatic potential is more difficult, mainly because of the relative infrequency of smooth muscle tumors at this site and therefore the limited series of cases with long-term follow-up. Although a combination of size, circumscription, atypia and mitotic count has been proposed to identify those smooth muscle tumors with recurrent and metastatic potential, it is likely that these currently established criteria probably underdiagnose malignant tumors as well as those that have the potential to recur. Based on personal experience, if a smooth muscle tumor has any mitotic activity, nuclear pleomorphism or evidence of an infiltrative margin, it has the potential for local recurrence.[27] For classification as sarcoma, use of the criteria proposed by Tavassoli and Norris is recommended (which has been validated in other studies).[63–65] Tumors with three or more of the following criteria should be classified as a sarcoma: (1) >5 cm in size, (2) infiltrative margins, (3) >5 mitoses/10 high-power fields and (4) moderate to severe cytologic atypia. Although necrosis is not listed as a criterion, its presence should strongly raise the possibility of sarcoma.

LEIOMYOMATOSIS

Vulvar leiomyomatosis is a rare condition that is characterized by mucosal-based ill-defined multinodular proliferations of smooth muscle. Patients with vulval leiomyomatosis can have synchronous or metachronous esophageal lesions (esophageal leiomyomatosis).[66] Possible pathogenetic mechanisms include altered hormonal responsiveness and familial factors, including an association with Alport's syndrome.[27,66]

Skeletal muscle tumors

GENITAL RHABDOMYOMA

Clinical presentation

Genital rhabdomyoma typically presents as a single, polypoid lesion, usually less than 3 cm, in the vagina (most common site), vulva or cervix of middle-aged women (median age 42).[67–73] Symptoms, if any, are related to the presence of a polyp, most commonly bleeding or dyspareunia.[67]

Histopathologic features

Within the submucosa is a somewhat irregular but vaguely fascicular proliferation of spindle- or-strap shaped rhabdomyoblasts with abundant eosinophilic cytoplasm and easily identifiable cross-striations within the cytoplasm (Fig. 9.24). There is no nuclear atypia and mitotic activity is scarce. These cells are positive for skeletal muscle markers (desmin, myoglobin, MyoD1 and myogenin, myf4).

Differential diagnosis

The principal differential includes embryonal rhabdomyosarcoma (discussed below). Genital rhabdomyoma differs from embryonal rhabdomyosarcoma by its (1) clinical presentation (occurring in an older patient population), (2) lack of nuclear atypia, (3) lack of mitotic activity and (4) lack of a cambium layer characteristic of embryonal rhabdomyosarcoma.

Prognosis and management

Genital rhabdomyoma is a benign tumor that is typically only treated by excision.

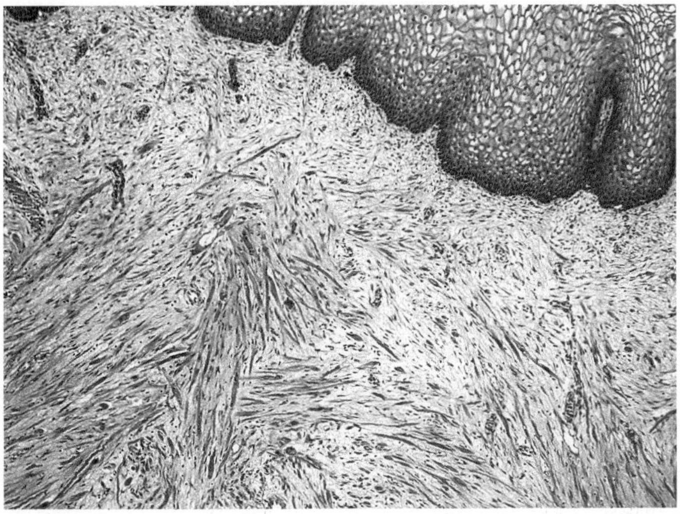

EMBRYONAL RHABDOMYOSARCOMA (SARCOMA BOTRYOIDES)

Clinical presentation

Sarcoma botryoides is a subset of embryonal rhabdomyosarcoma that occurs in a submucosal location in infants and children younger than 5 years. These tumors tend to grow as polyploid, rounded, bulky masses, most commonly in the vagina, the appearance of which has been likened to a cluster of grapes (hence the designation botryoides, meaning grapelike, see Fig. 9.25).

Histopathologic features

Embryonal rhabdomyosarcoma, one of the three main groups of rhabdomyosarcoma (which also includes alveolar and pleomorphic rhabdomyosarcoma), consists predominantly of malignant embryonal rhabdomyoblasts. On histologic examination, the tumor cells are small and have oval nuclei, with small protrusions of brightly eosinophilic cytoplasm from one end (with an overall appearance of the cell somewhat resembling a tennis racket). Striations can sometimes be seen within the cytoplasm. Beneath the vaginal epithelium, the tumor cells are condensed in a so-called cambium layer (Fig. 9.26); but in the deep regions, they lie within a loose fibromyxomatous stroma that is edematous and may contain many inflammatory cells. For this reason, the lesions can be mistaken for benign inflammatory polyps, leading to unfortunate delays in diagnosis and treatment. Immunohistochemistry can be useful in making the diagnosis, as the tumor cells are positive for desmin, actin and skeletal muscle markers (myoglobin, MyoD1 and myogenin, myf4).

Differential diagnosis

The principal differential diagnostic consideration is distinction of embryonal rhabdomyosarcoma from a fibroepithelial stromal polyp, particularly one which is

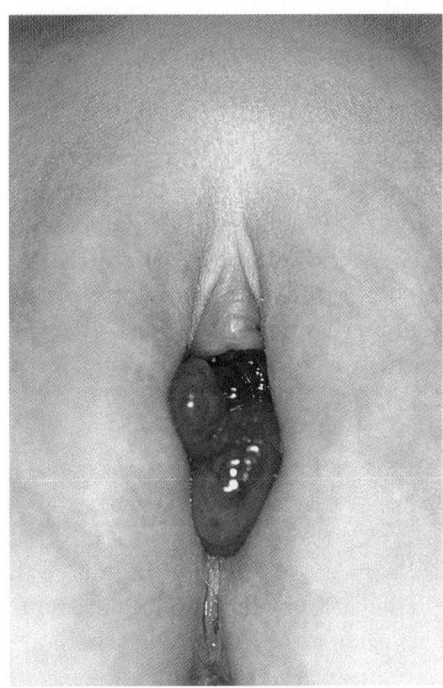

Fig. 9.25 Embryonal rhabdomyosarcoma, botryoid type. Grape-like clusters of tumor project out of the vagina.

Fig. 9.24 Genital rhabdomyoma. Strap-shaped rhabdomyoblasts are present in the submucosa.

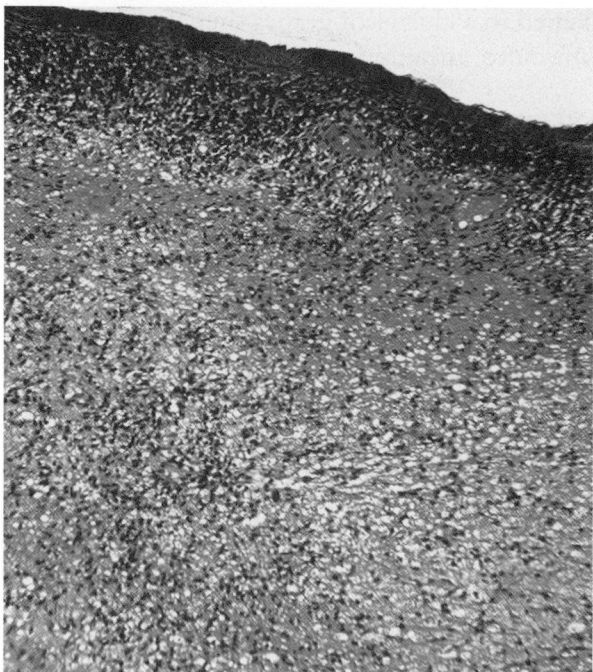

Fig. 9.26 Embryonal rhabdomyosarcoma, botryoid type. Condensation of tumor cells beneath surface epithelium (cambium layer).

hypercellular. Cellular stromal polyps differ from embryonal rhabdomyosarcoma by (1) occurring more commonly postpubertal, (2) showing a greater degree of cellularity in the center of the polyp as opposed to beneath the epithelium (in direct contrast to the cambium layer of botryoid embryonal rhabdomyosarcoma) and (3) lacking rhabdomyoblasts and immunophenotypic evidence of skeletal muscle differentiation.

Prognosis and management

The botryoid (exophytic) variant of embryonal rhabdomyosarcoma has an excellent prognosis in comparison with the usual (non-exophytic) type of embryonal rhabdomyosarcoma and other subtypes, particularly the alveolar subtype, which connotes a much worse prognosis.[74] Conservative surgery with primary chemotherapy and adjunctive radiotherapy can result in long-term disease-free survival.[75]

Vascular and related lesions

A number of vascular tumors and related lesions may occasionally involve the vulvovaginal region, but are typically more common at other sites (e.g. capillary hemangioma, cavernous hemangioma). In contrast, angiokeratoma is a lesion that has a predilection for this site and therefore will be included in this chapter. In addition, lymphangioma circumscriptum will be described since this rare entity has the potential to be misdiagnosed at this site.

ANGIOKERATOMA

Angiokeratoma is considered more likely to represent vascular ectasia with associated overlying epidermal changes rather than a true vascular neoplasm. Angiokeratoma may be seen in association with the following four clinical scenarios: (1) Fabry's disease, a rare X-linked chromosomal lipid disorder (deficiency of lysosomal alpha-galactosidase A) associated with multiple angiokeratomas (angiokeratoma corporis diffusum), (2) multiple angiokeratomas involving fingers and toes (angiokeratoma of Mibelli), (3) angiokeratoma involving the scrotum (angiokeratoma of Fordyce) and (4) solitary angiokeratoma.

Clinical presentation

Angiokeratoma involving the vulva is a papular, sometimes warty-appearing, lesion that may be solitary or multiple, usually measures less than 1 cm and varies in color from red to purple.[76] Lesions typically present before the sixth decade and usually are asymptomatic; symptoms, when present, include bleeding, pain or pruritus.[76]

Histopathologic features

Angiokeratoma is characterized histologically by the presence of dilated, blood-filled vascular spaces in the papillary dermis associated with acanthosis, hyperkeratosis and sometimes papillomatosis. Characteristically, the vascular spaces are closely apposed and partially surrounded by the overlying epithelium (Fig. 9.27).

Prognosis and management

Clinical management depends upon the presence of symptoms. In most women, the lesions are asymptomatic and once a diagnosis is established, whether based on clinical examination or biopsy results, follow-up observation of any remaining lesions is adequate; in symptomatic women, surgical removal or ablation may be considered.[76]

The vast majority of angiokeratomas are not associated with Fabry's disease; however, when multiple angiokeratomas are encountered in a single patient, this possibility should be considered.

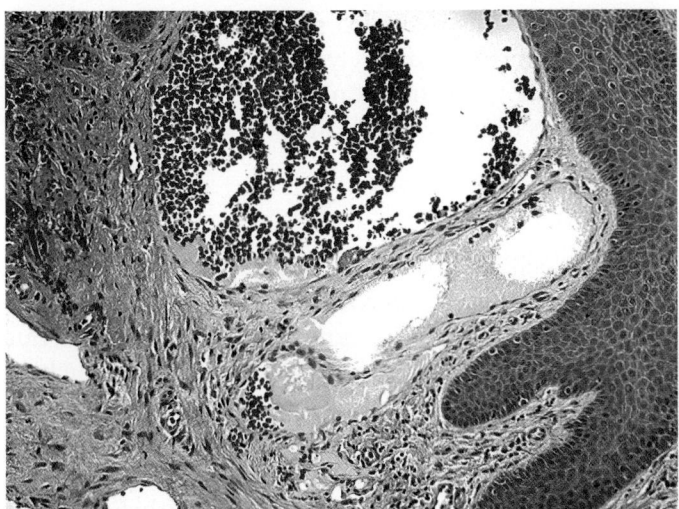

Fig. 9.27 Angiokeratoma. Blood-filled vascular spaces are closely apposed to the epidermis.

LYMPHANGIOMA CIRCUMSCRIPTUM

Clinical presentation

Lymphangioma circumscriptum is a lesion of lymphatic channels that may be either congenital or acquired, the latter scenario in the setting of damage to lymphatic channels. It only rarely involves the vulva, more commonly affecting the skin and subcutaneous tissue of the trunk, thigh and buttock.[77] Characteristically, numerous small vesicles filled with clear fluid are present; symptoms include vulvar swelling, pain and infection secondary to oozing and excoriation.[77] Clinically, these changes may be mistaken for herpetic blisters and when associated epidermal changes are present, such as hyperkeratosis, they also may mimic genital warts.

Histopathologic features

Within the papillary and reticular dermis are numerous dilated lymphatic channels (Fig. 9.28). Many cysts are closely apposed to the epidermis, which may be acanthotic, leading to the clinical impression of a small vesicle.

Prognosis and management

The congenital form is considered a hamartomatous lesion. Management includes observation versus surgical excision.[77]

Neural tumors

Neurofibroma and schwannoma may rarely occur in the vulva and have the typical clinical and histologic

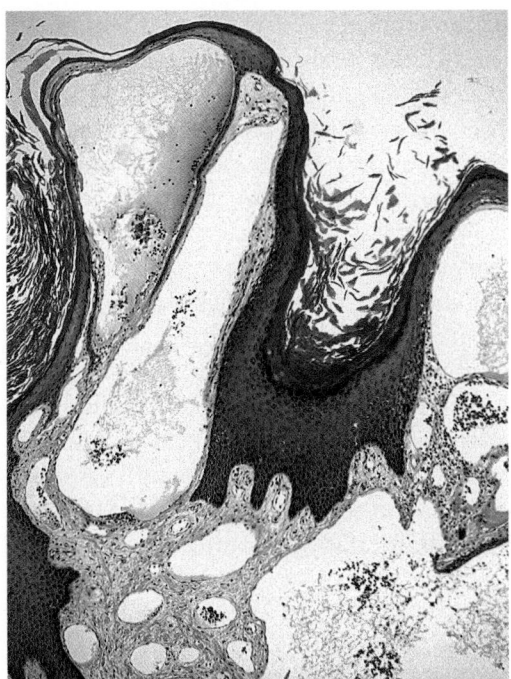

Fig. 9.28 Lymphangioma circumscriptum. Numerous dilated lymphatic channels within papillary dermis.

features of those that occur outside of this site. Rarely, neurofibromatosis involves the female genital tract and may present as clitoromegaly.[78,79]

GRANULAR CELL TUMOR

Clinical presentation

Granular cell tumor is an uncommon lesion that occurs primarily in the head and neck region (particularly the tongue) but may also occur in the vulva, usually involving the labium majora, where from 5 to 15% of all granular cell tumors occur.[80–82] It is more frequent in women and African-Americans and has a wide age distribution, but is less often seen in children. The mean age at presentation in the vulva is approximately 50 years, but granular cell tumor has been described in children as young as 6 years of age.[83] The tumors often present as slowly growing asymptomatic nodules that may be found incidentally during a routine examination. If symptomatic, increased growth, pain and pruritus are common.[81] The size varies from less than 1 cm to 12 cm in diameter. Patients with multiple vulvar granular cell tumors have rarely been reported.[84]

Histopathologic features

The tumors are situated in the dermis or subcutis and consist of polygonal cells with abundant granular eosinophilic cytoplasm and small, centrally located, often hyperchromatic nuclei (Fig. 9.29). The borders of the lesion can be broad and pushing or diffuse with cells infiltrating between collagen bundles. Lesions with an infiltrative border may be more likely to recur even if the surgical margin appears uninvolved.[85] Perineural involvement is extremely common; this feature does not confer a more aggressive behavior. Pseudoepitheliomatous hyperplasia of the overlying squamous epithelium is a frequent and often dramatic feature (Fig. 9.30). In superficial, particularly shave biopsies, prominent pseudoepitheliomatous hyperplasia can easily be confused with well-differentiated squamous cell carcinoma.[86] The granular cytoplasm of the tumor cells is diastase-resistant PAS-positive and contains numerous lysosomes. These tumors are also immunoreactive for S-100 protein, supporting differentiation toward a neural crest lineage. The cells may also stain for NKI-C3, a non-specific antibody against lysosomes. Neuron-specific enolase (NSE), another non-specific marker that reacts with tumors of neural crest differentiation, is frequently positive.

Differential diagnosis

Granular cell tumor is distinctive and usually easily recognized by light microscopy. Smooth muscle neoplasms may also show granular cell change, but immunoreactivity for muscle-specific markers such as desmin or caldesmon readily assist in this distinction. The most important pitfall is misdiagnosing squamous cell carcinoma based on a superficial biopsy of granular cell tumor with extensive pseudoepitheliomatous hyperplasia. This can be particularly problematic when the underlying granular cell tumor is not present in the shave biopsy.

Prognosis and management

Complete surgical excision is the treatment of choice; however, recurrence is uncommon even in incompletely excised tumors.[80] Malignant granular cell tumors are extremely rare, but have been reported in the vulva.[87]

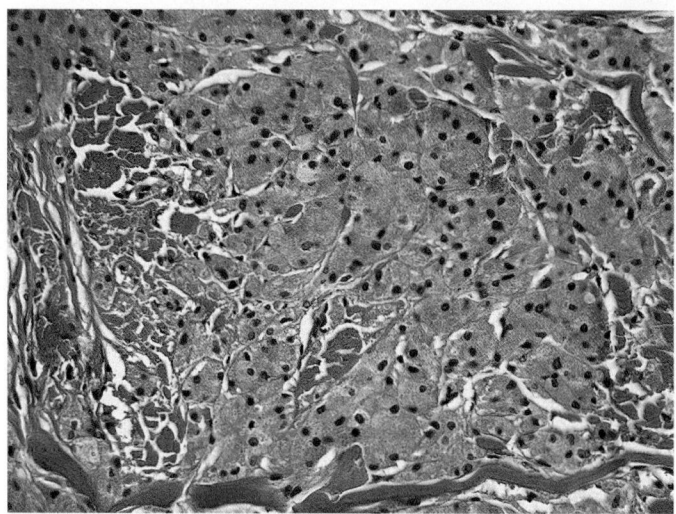

Fig. 9.29 Granular cell tumor. Polygonal cells with abundant granular eosinophilic cytoplasm and small, centrally located nuclei.

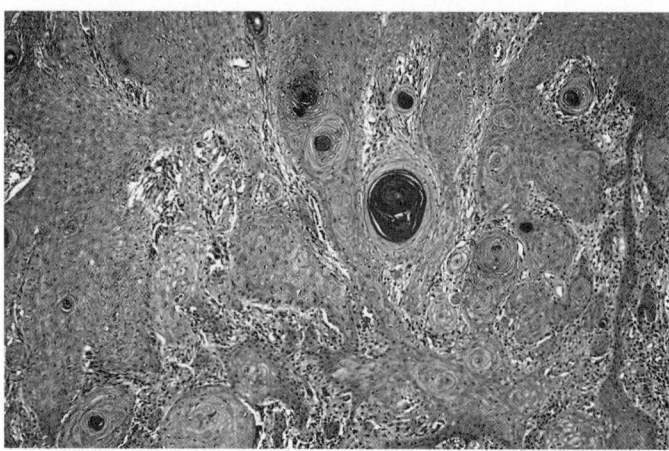

Fig. 9.30 Pseudoepitheliomatous hyperplasia. Dramatic epithelial proliferation associated with underlying granular cell tumor.

References

1 Norris HJ, Taylor HB. Polyps of the vagina. A benign lesion resembling sarcoma botryoides. Cancer 1966; 19:227–232.

2 Elliott GB, Reynolds HA, Fidler HK. Pseudo-sarcoma botryoides of cervix and vagina in pregnancy. J Obstet Gynaecol Br Commonw 1967; 74:728–733.

3 Burt RL, Prichard RW, Kim BS. Fibroepithelial polyp of the vagina. A report of five cases. Obstet Gynecol 1976; 47:52S–54S.

4 Chirayil SJ, Tobon H. Polyps of the vagina: a clinicopathologic study of 18 cases. Cancer 1981; 47:2904–2907.

5 O'Quinn AG, Edwards CL, Gallager HS. Pseudosarcoma botryoides of the vagina in pregnancy. Gynecol Oncol 1982; 13:237–241.

6 Miettinen M, Wahlstrom T, Vesterinen E, Saksela E. Vaginal polyps with pseudosarcomatous features. A clinicopathologic study of seven cases. Cancer 1983; 51:1148–1151.

7 Maenpaa J, Soderstrom KO, Salmi T, Ekblad U. Large atypical polyps of the vagina during pregnancy with concomitant human papilloma virus infection. Eur J Obstet Gynecol Reprod Biol 1988; 27:65–69.

8 Ostor AG, Fortune DW, Riley CB. Fibroepithelial polyps with atypical stromal cells (pseudosarcoma botryoides) of vulva and vagina. A report of 13 cases. Int J Gynecol Pathol 1988; 7:351–360.

9 Hartmann CA, Sperling M, Stein H. So-called fibroepithelial polyps of the vagina exhibiting an unusual but uniform antigen profile characterized by expression of desmin

and steroid hormone receptors but no muscle-specific actin or macrophage markers. Am J Clin Pathol 1990; 93:604–608.

10 Mucitelli DR, Charles EZ, Kraus FT. Vulvovaginal polyps. Histologic appearance, ultrastructure, immunocytochemical characteristics and clinicopathologic correlations. Int J Gynecol Pathol 1990; 9:20–40.

11 Nucci MR, Fletcher CD. Fibroepithelial stromal polyps of vulvovaginal tissue: from the banal to the bizarre. Pathol Case Rev 1998; 3:151–157.

12 Nucci MR, Young RH, Fletcher CD. Cellular pseudosarcomatous fibroepithelial stromal polyps of the lower female genital tract: an underrecognized lesion often misdiagnosed as sarcoma. Am J Surg Pathol 2000; 24:231–240.

13 Fletcher CD, Tsang WY, Fisher C, Lee KC, Chan JK. Angiomyofibroblastoma of the vulva. A benign neoplasm distinct from aggressive angiomyxoma. Am J Surg Pathol 1992; 16:373–382.

14 Nielsen GP, Rosenberg AE, Young RH, et al. Angiomyofibroblastoma of the vulva and vagina. Mod Pathol 1996; 9:284–291.

15 Ockner DM, Sayadi H, Swanson PE, et al. Genital angiomyofibroblastoma. Comparison with aggressive angiomyxoma and other myxoid neoplasms of skin and soft tissue. Am J Clin Pathol 1997; 107:36–44.

16 Fukunaga M, Nomura K, Matsumoto K, et al. Vulval angiomyofibroblastoma. Clinicopathologic analysis of six cases. Am J Clin Pathol 1997; 107:45–51.

17 Laskin WB, Fetsch JF, Tavassoli FA. Angiomyofibroblastoma of the female genital tract: analysis of 17 cases including a lipomatous variant. Hum Pathol 1997; 28:1046–1055.

18 Hisaoka M, Kouho H, Aoki T, et al. Angiomyofibroblastoma of the vulva: a clinicopathologic study of seven cases. Pathol Int 1995; 45:487–492.

19 Nielsen GP, Young RH, Dickersin GR, Rosenberg AE. Angiomyofibroblastoma of the vulva with sarcomatous transformation ('angiomyofibrosarcoma'). Am J Surg Pathol 1997; 21:1104–1108.

20 Steeper TA, Rosai J. Aggressive angiomyxoma of the female pelvis and perineum. Report of nine cases of a distinctive type of gynecologic soft-tissue neoplasm. Am J Surg Pathol 1983; 7:463–475.

21 Begin LR, Clement PB, Kirk ME, et al. Aggressive angiomyxoma of pelvic soft parts: a clinicopathologic study of nine cases. Hum Pathol 1985; 16:621–628.

22 Fetsch JF, Laskin WB, Lefkowitz M, et al. Aggressive angiomyxoma: a clinicopathologic study of 29 female patients. Cancer 1996; 78:79–90.

23 Granter SR, Nucci MR, Fletcher CD. Aggressive angiomyxoma: reappraisal of its relationship to angiomyofibroblastoma in a series of 16 cases. Histopathology 1997; 30:3–10.

24 Tsang WY, Chan JK, Lee KC, et al. Aggressive angiomyxoma. A report of four cases occurring in men. Am J Surg Pathol 1992; 16:1059–1065.

25 Iezzoni JC, Fechner RE, Wong LS, Rosai J. Aggressive angiomyxoma in males. A report of four cases. Am J Clin Pathol 1995; 104:391–396.

26 Hoyte L, Lu K, Muto M, et al. Magnetic resonance imaging based three dimensional modeling of a complex vulvar tumor as a component of presurgical planning. J Women's Imaging 2000; 2:138–140.

27 Nucci MR, Fletcher CD. Vulvovaginal soft tissue tumours: update and review. Histopathology 2000; 36:97–108.

28 Allen PW, Dymock RB, MacCormac LB. Superficial angiomyxomas with and without epithelial components. Report of 30 tumors in 28 patients. Am J Surg Pathol 1988; 12:519–530.

29 Fetsch JF, Laskin WB, Tavassoli FA. Superficial angiomyxoma (cutaneous myxoma): a clinicopathologic study of 17 cases arising in the genital region. Int J Gynecol Pathol 1997; 16:325–334.

30 Calonje E, Guerin D, McCormick D, Fletcher CD. Superficial angiomyxoma: clinicopathologic analysis of a series of distinctive but poorly recognized cutaneous tumors with tendency for recurrence. Am J Surg Pathol 1999; 23:910–917.

31 Nucci MR, Granter SR, Fletcher CD. Cellular angiofibroma: a benign neoplasm distinct from angiomyofibroblastoma and spindle cell lipoma. Am J Surg Pathol 1997; 21:636–644.

32 Laskin WB, Fetsch JF, Mostofi FK. Angiomyofibroblastoma-like tumor of the male genital tract: analysis of 11 cases with comparison to female angiomyofibroblastoma and spindle cell lipoma. Am J Surg Pathol 1998; 22:6–16.

33 Dargent JL, Saint AN de, Galdon MG, et al. Cellular angiofibroma of the vulva: a clinicopathological study of two cases with documentation of some unusual features and review of the literature. J Cutan Pathol 2003; 30:405–411.

34 Gonzalez S, Duarte I. Benign fibrous histiocytoma of the skin. A morphologic study of 290 cases. Pathol Res Pr 1982; 174:379–391.

35 Requena L, Aguilar A, Lopez Redondo MJ, et al. Multinodular hemosiderotic dermatofibroma. Dermatologica 1990; 181:320–323.

36 Iwata J, Fletcher CD. Lipidized fibrous histiocytoma: clinicopathologic analysis of 22 cases. Am J Derm 2000; 22:126–134.

37 Calonje E, Fletcher CD. Aneurysmal benign fibrous histiocytoma: clinicopathological analysis of 40 cases of a tumour frequently misdiagnosed as a vascular neoplasm. Histopathology 1995; 26:323–331.

38 Calonje E, Mentzel T, Fletcher CD. Cellular benign fibrous histiocytoma. Clinicopathologic analysis of 74 cases of a distinctive variant of cutaneous fibrous histiocytoma with frequent recurrence. Am J Surg Pathol 1994; 18:668–676.

39 Kaddu S, McMenamin ME, Fletcher CD. Atypical fibrous histiocytoma of the skin: clinicopathologic analysis of 59 cases with evidence of infrequent metastasis. Am J Surg Pathol 2002; 26:35–46.

40 Singh GC, Calonje E, Fletcher CD. Epithelioid benign fibrous histiocytoma of skin: clinico-pathological analysis of 20 cases of a poorly known variant. Histopathology 1994; 24:123–129.

41 Zelger B, Sidoroff A, Stanzl U, et al. Deep penetrating dermatofibroma versus dermatofibrosarcoma protuberans. A clinicopathologic comparison. Am J Surg Pathol 1994; 18:677–686.

42 Abenoza P, Lillemoe T. CD34 and factor XIIIa in the differential diagnosis of dermatofibroma and dermatofibrosarcoma protuberans. Am J Derm 1993; 15:429–434.

43 Franquemont DW, Cooper PH, Shmookler BM, Wick MR. Benign fibrous histiocytoma of the skin with potential for local recurrence: a tumor to be distinguished from dermatofibroma. Mod Pathol 1990; 3:158–163.

44 Colome-Grimmer MI, Evans HL. Metastasizing cellular dermatofibroma. A report of two cases. Am J Surg Pathol 1996; 20:1361–1367.

45 Ghorbani RP, Malpica A, Ayala AG. Dermatofibrosarcoma protuberans of the vulva: clinicopathologic and immunohistochemical analysis of four cases, one with fibrosarcomatous change and review of the literature. Int J Gynecol Pathol 1999; 18:366–373.

46 Gokden N, Dehner LP, Zhu X, Pfeifer JD. Dermatofibrosarcoma protuberans of the vulva and groin: detection of COL1A1-PDGFB fusion transcripts by RT-PCR. J Cutan Pathol 2003; 30:190–195.

47 Vanni R, Faa G, Dettori T, et al. A case of dermatofibrosarcoma protuberans of the vulva with a COL1A1/PDGFB fusion identical to a case of giant cell fibroblastoma. Virchows Arch 2000; 437:95–100.

48 Moodley M, Moodley J. Dermatofibrosarcoma protuberans of the vulva: a case report and review of the literature. Gynecol Oncol 2000; 78:74–75.

49 Soergel TM, Doering DL, O'connor D. Metastatic dermatofibrosarcoma protuberans of the vulva. Gynecol Oncol 1998; 71:320–324.

50 Davos I, Abell MR. Soft tissue sarcomas of vulva. Gynecol Oncol 1976; 4:70–86.

51 Leake JF, Buscema J, Cho KR, Currie JL. Dermatofibrosarcoma protuberans of the vulva. Gynecol Oncol 1991; 41:245–249.

52 Barnhill DR, Boling R, Nobles W, et al. Vulvar dermatofibrosarcoma protuberans. Gynecol Oncol 1988; 30:149–152.

53 Bock JE, Andreasson B, Thorn A, Holck S. Dermatofibrosarcoma protuberans of the vulva. Gynecol Oncol 1985; 20:129–135.

54 Mentzel T, Beham A, Katenkamp D, et al. Fibrosarcomatous ('high-grade') dermatofibrosarcoma protuberans: clinicopathologic and immunohistochemical study of a series of 41 cases with emphasis on prognostic significance. Am J Surg Pathol 1998; 22:576–587.

55 Calonje E, Fletcher CD. Myoid differentiation in dermatofibrosarcoma protuberans and its fibrosarcomatous variant: clinicopathologic analysis of 5 cases. J Cutan Pathol 1996; 23:30–36.

56 Naeem R, Lux ML, Huang SF, et al. Ring chromosomes in dermatofibrosarcoma protuberans are composed of interspersed sequences from chromosomes 17 and 22. Am J Pathol 1995; 147:1553–1558.

57 Kurman RJ, Norris HJ, Wilkinson E. Atlas of tumor pathology. Tumors of the cervix. Vagina Vulva 1992; 215.

58 Kehagias DT, Smyrniotis VE, Karvounis EE, et al. Large lipoma of the vulva. Eur J Obstet Gynecol Reprod Biol 1999; 84:5–6.

59 Reis-Filho JS, Milanezi F, Soares MF, et al. Intradermal spindle cell/pleomorphic lipoma of the vulva: case report and review of the literature. J Cutan Pathol 2002; 29:59–62.

60 Brooks JJ, LiVolsi VA. Liposarcoma presenting on the vulva. Am J Obstet Gynecol 1987; 156:73–75.

61 Genton CY, Maroni ES. Vulval liposarcoma. Arch Gynecol 1987; 240:63–66.

62 Nucci MR. Fletcher CD. Liposarcoma (atypical lipomatous tumors) of the vulva: a clinicopathologic study of six cases. Int J Gynecol Pathol 1998; 17:17–23.

63 Newman PL, Fletcher CD. Smooth muscle tumours of the external genitalia: clinicopathological analysis of a series. Histopathology 1991; 18:523–529.

64 Tavassoli FA, Norris HJ. Smooth muscle tumors of the vulva. Obstet Gynecol 1979; 53:213–217.

65 Nielsen GP, Rosenberg AE, Koerner FC, et al. Smooth-muscle tumors of the vulva. A clinicopathological study of 25 cases and review of the literature. Am J Surg Pathol 1996; 20:779–793.

66 Faber K, Jones MA, Spratt D, Tarraza HM Jr. Vulvar leiomyomatosis in a patient with esophagogastric leiomyomatosis: review of the syndrome. Gynecol Oncol 1991; 41:92–94.

67 Lin GY, Sun X, Badve S. Pathologic quiz case. Vaginal wall mass in a 47-year-old woman. Vaginal rhabdomyoma. Arch Pathol Lab Med 2002; 126:1241–1242.

68 Iversen UM. Two cases of benign vaginal rhabdomyoma. Case reports. APMIS 1996; 104:575–578.

69 Lopez JI, Brouard I, Eizaguirre B. Rhabdomyoma of the vagina. Eur J Obstet Gynecol Reprod Biol 1992; 45:147–148.

70 Chabrel CM, Beilby JO. Vaginal rhabdomyoma. Histopathology 1980; 4:645–651.

71 Gee DC, Finckh ES. Benign vaginal rhabdomyoma. Pathology 1977; 9:263–267.

72 Gold JH, Bossen EH. Benign vaginal rhabdomyoma: a light and electron microscopic study. Cancer 1976; 37:2283–2294.

73 Gad A, Eusebi V. Rhabdomyoma of the vagina. J Pathol 1975; 115:179–181.

74 Leuschner I, Harms D, Mattke A, et al. Rhabdomyosarcoma of the urinary bladder and vagina: a clinicopathologic study with emphasis on recurrent disease: a report from the Kiel Pediatric Tumor Registry and the German CWS Study. Am J Surg Pathol 2001; 25:856–864.

75 Andrassy RJ, Hays DM, Raney RB, et al. Conservative surgical management of vaginal and vulvar pediatric rhabdomyosarcoma: a report from the Intergroup Rhabdomyosarcoma Study III. J Pediatr Surg 1995; 30:1034–1036.

76 Cohen PR, Young AW Jr, Tovell HM. Angiokeratoma of the vulva: diagnosis and review of the literature. Obstet Gynecol Surv 1989; 44:339–346.

77 Vlastos AT, Malpica A, Follen M. Lymphangioma circumscriptum of the vulva: a review of the literature. Obstet Gynecol 2003; 101:946–954.

78 Sutphen R, Galan-Gomez E, Kousseff BG. Clitoromegaly in neurofibromatosis. Am J Med Genet 1995; 55:325–330.

79 Gersell DJ, Fulling KH. Localized neurofibromatosis of the female genitourinary tract. Am J Surg Pathol 1989; 13:873–878.

80 Lack EE, Worsham GF, Callihan MD, et al. Granular cell tumor: a clinicopathologic study of 110 patients. J Surg Oncol 1980; 13:301–316.

81 Horowitz IR, Copas P, Majmudar B. Granular cell tumors of the vulva. Am J Obstet Gynecol 1995; 173:1710–1713.

82 Haley JC, Mirowski GW, Hood AF. Benign vulvar tumors. Semin Cutan Med Surg 1998; 17:196–204.

83 Cohen Z, Kapuller V, Maor E, Mares AJ. Granular cell tumor (myoblastoma) of the labia major: a rare benign tumor in childhood. J Pediatr Adolesc Gynecol 1999; 12:155–156.

84 Majmudar B, Castellano PZ, Wilson RW, Siegel RJ. Granular cell tumors of the vulva. J Reprod Med 1990; 35:1008–1014.

85 Althausen AM, Kowalski DP, Ludwig ME, et al. Granular cell tumors: a new clinically important histologic finding. Gynecol Oncol 2000; 77:310–313.

86 Wolber RA, Talerman A, Wilkinson EJ, Clement PB. Vulvar granular cell tumors with pseudocarcinomatous hyperplasia: a comparative analysis with well-differentiated squamous carcinoma. Int J Gynecol Pathol 1991; 10:59–66.

87 Schmidt O, Fleckenstein GH, Gunawan B, et al. Recurrence and rapid metastasis formation of a granular cell tumor of the vulva. Eur J Obstet Gynecol Reprod Biol 2003; 106:219–221.

10

Diseases of the anus

Kirstine Y-T. Oh and

Joel M. Palefsky

Introduction

Embryology
Anorectal anomalies
Anatomy

Non-neoplastic lesions

Perianal cysts
Hemorrhoids
Anal tags/fibroepithelial polyps
Inflammatory polyps
Anal fissures and ulcers
Anal abscesses and fistulas

Inflammatory bowel disease
Endometriosis
Infections
Iatrogenic lesions

Neoplasms of the anus

Introduction
Benign adnexal lesions
Squamous intraepithelial lesions
Malignant tumors of the anus and
   anal canal

Introduction

EMBRYOLOGY

The division of the cloaca into separate conduits for the intestinal, urinary and reproductive tracts begins in the 5th week of embryogenesis. At that point, the caudally located cloaca is a common chamber for all three future functioning systems. The urorectal septum, a coronal ridge of mesenchyme, extends caudally to join the urogenital membrane, thereby creating two separate tracts: anteriorly the urogenital sinus and posteriorly the rectum by the end of the 8th week (Fig. 10.1, see Ch. 1). Concurrently, the Müllerian ducts extend caudally toward the cloaca and merge with the posterior wall of the urogenital sinus to form the Müllerian tubercle. The ducts fuse and join with the ligamentum inguinale, to differentiate into the vagina and uterus distally and the fallopian tube proximally.

ANORECTAL ANOMALIES

Defects of anorectal development are rare and range from up to 1:3000 births for anorectal anomalies to 1:50 000 for cloacal malformations.[1] Overall, these developmental disturbances comprise approximately 10% of all anogenital malformations in females.[2] The spectrum of anorectal malformations ranges from the mildly stenotic anus to imperforate anus with a fistula between the urinary and intestinal tracts to the most severe form, persistent cloaca.[3–5] Cloacal defects may affect the gastrointestinal, urinary and reproductive tracts; cases of associated anomalies also have involved the respiratory tract, neural tube, abdominal wall, cardiac

anomalies, hemivertebrae and digits. These anomalies often present in the newborn period, but may not be detected until adulthood. A common urogenital sinus is often present in these patients, which may be the common site of exit for the rectum, urethra and vagina. In approximately 30% of cases, the anal opening is present in the perineum, but is displaced anteriorly.[6,7] The urethra may exit normally or drain into the urogenital sinus or vagina, or is entirely absent. Variably, a neurogenic bladder may be present. The external genitalia in chromosomally female patients often consist of an empty skin sac or phallus-like structure, occasionally with a draining urethra. Vaginal structures may be bifid or duplexed and lead into the urogenital sinus or into the urethra or bladder. Abnormal sacral development is also frequently present.[8,9]

Anorectal anomalies are less rare and may occur in 1 in 3000–5000 births. They are divided into three types, defined by the location of the defect: high (supralevator), low (translevator) and intermediate. A miscellaneous group also exists. High defects are characterized as anorectal agenesis, with fistulization of the rectum to the bladder, urethra or vagina. Intermediate defects include anal agenesis, anorectal stenosis and anorectal membrane. Low defects predominate in female children and include ectopic anus, anal stenosis and membrane-covered anus.[7]

The pathogenesis of many of these anomalies lies in defects in the completion of the urorectal septum, which in turn may reflect abnormalities in signaling, documented in many instances by genetic mutation. One proposed mechanism includes defects in expression of sonic hedgehog, of which experimental mutations lead to a dose-dependent range of anorectal malfor-

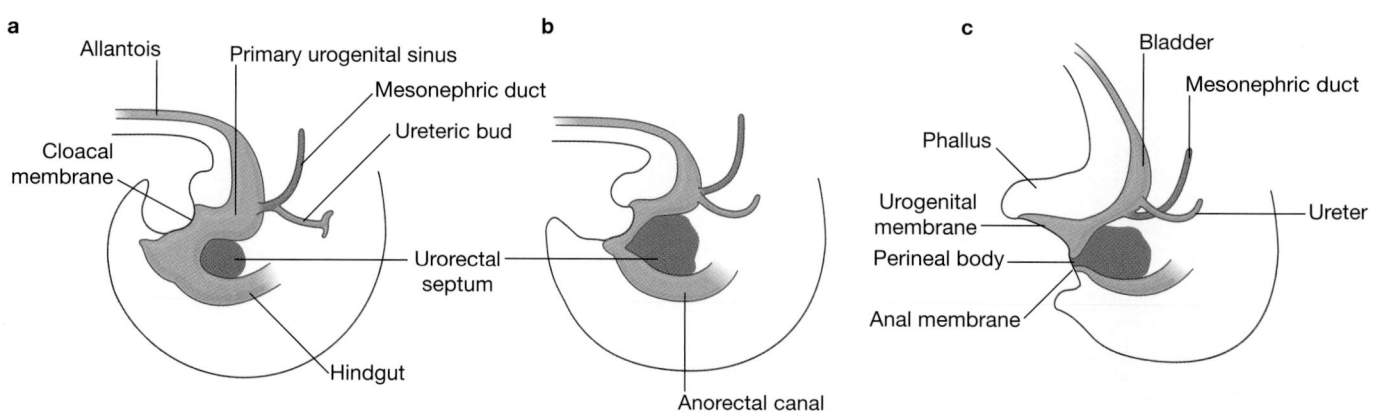

Fig. 10.1 Embryology of anorectal development. (a) The urorectal septum begins as a horizontal shelf of mesenchyme at the 5th week, (b) progressing towards the cloacal membrane by the seventh week and (c) completing the separation of the urogenital sinus and rectum by the 8th week. (Adapted from Sadler TW (ed.) *Langmans Medical Embryology*, 5th edn, p. 242, Fig. 15.10, copyright 1985 Lippincott, Williams and Wilkins, with permission.)

mations including the cloaca.[10] Mice null for p63, a p53 homologue expressed in basal epithelial cells and critical to epithelial development, fail to compete the urorectal septum, leading to a cloaca (Fig. 10.2). Humans with gain of function mutations in this gene also exhibit milder urogenital anomalies (see Ch. 1).

ANATOMY

The anal canal is a grossly and histologically defined anatomic area joining the distal intestinal tract with the external perianal skin. Conceptually, the anal canal is the transition from an absorptive epithelium that samples materials from the external environment to a protective epithelium, which provides a barrier between the body and external environment (Fig. 10.3).

The most important gross landmark is the dentate or pectinate line, formed by the distal edge of the anal columns. The anal columns are separated by grooves known as the anal valves and sinuses. The line grossly defined by the most distal edge of the anal valves and columns is defined as the dentate line. This line defines the histologic zones of the anal canal. Importantly, it also indicates the division of the vascular, lymphatic and neural supply and divides the anal canal into cranial and caudal regions.

The histologic zones of the anal canal are divided into four components, defined loosely by the type of mucosal surface (Fig. 10.4). These include: (1) the

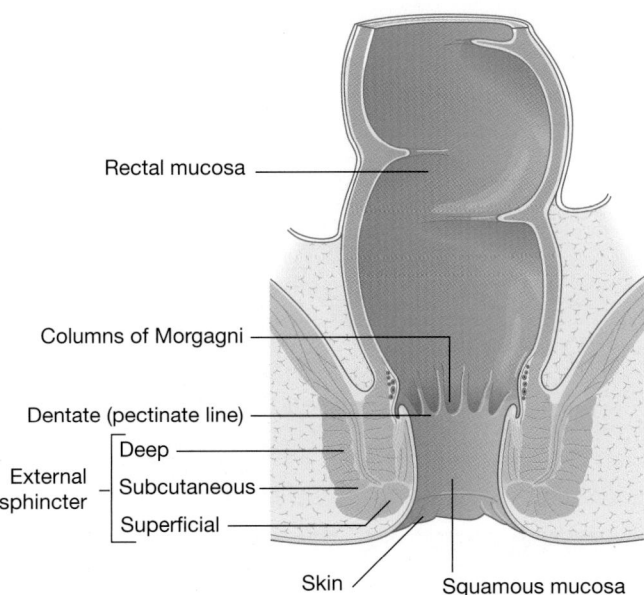

Fig. 10.3 Drawing of the anal canal. (Modified from Ryan DP, et al., Carcinoma of the anal canal. N Engl J Med 2000; 342:792–800, copyright 2000, Massachusetts Medical Society, with permission.)

colorectal zone (Fig. 10.5), which is most cephalad and is the most caudad portion of the colonic mucosa; (2) the anal transitional zone; (3) the non-hair-bearing zone near the anal margin; and (4) the perianal skin with hair-bearing appendages. The colorectal zone is lined by absorptive columnar epithelium and extends

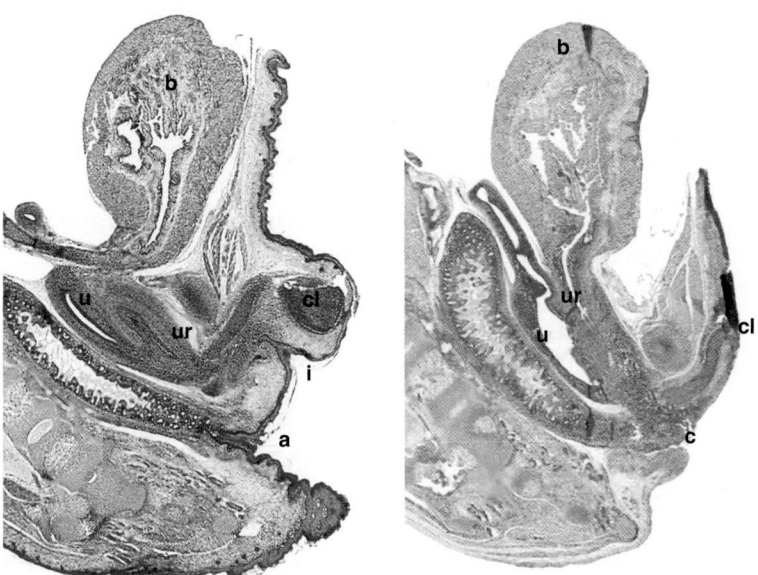

Fig. 10.2 Common opening (cloaca) produced by p63 knockout in the mouse. Presumably the absence of p63, via the loss of the epithelium, interferes with normal induction of the underlying mesenchyme to subdivide the rectum and vagina. (From Ince et al. p63 coordinates anogenital modeling and epithelial cell differentiation in the developing female urogenital tract. Am J Pathol 2002; 161:1111–1117, copyright 2002, American Society for Investigative Pathology, with permission. Ur, urethra; b, bladder; cl, clitoris; a, anus; c, cloaca; i, introitus; u, uterus

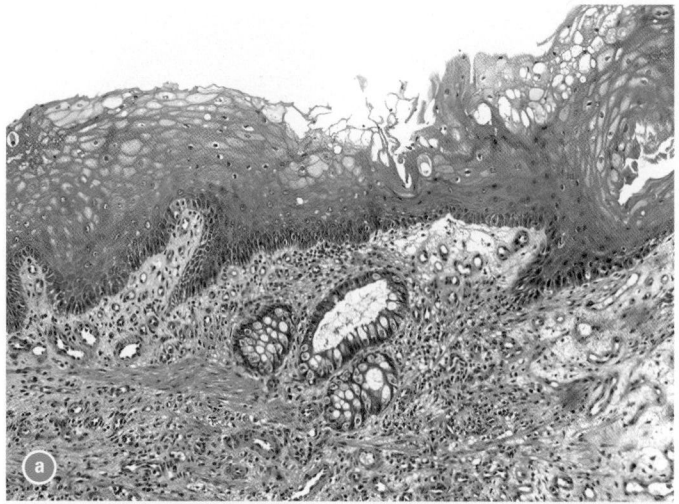

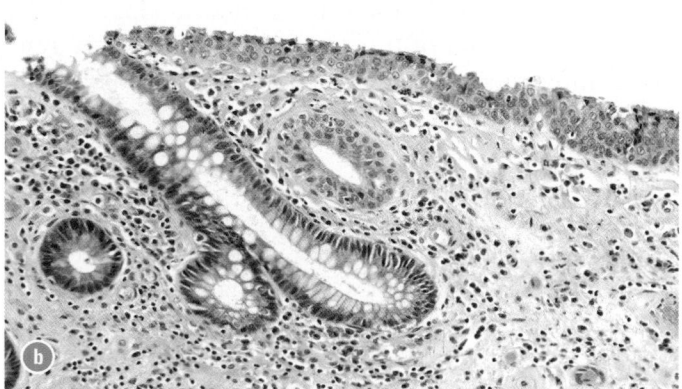

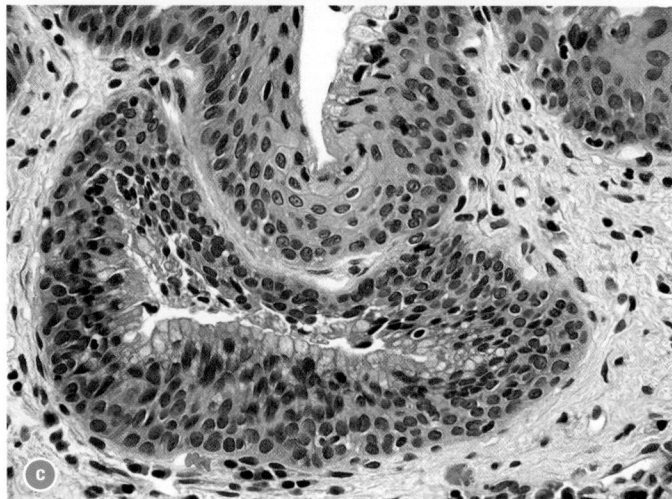

Fig. 10.4 Histologic images of the zones of the anal canal near the squamo-columnar junction. (a) Mature squamous epithelium with underlying glands. (b) A transition from columnar to an immature squamo-transitional epithelium. (c) Adnexal structures with transitional epithelium.

to the proximal extent of the anal columns. The anal transitional zone extends from the colorectal zone caudally to the dentate line for a total distance of approximately 9 cm in most people. Due to normal variation, the transitional zone may end at or around the dentate line, with variably regular borders. The transitional zone is lined by multiple layers of cuboidal or polygonal cells, histologically not unlike the transitional zone found in the cervix. The third zone is lined by squamous mucosa without hair-bearing skin appendages and extends to the anal margin. Finally, the fourth zone is also known as perianal skin, with hair-bearing skin appendages (Fig. 10.3). The region near the transition from squamous to columnar is remarkably similar to the cervix. Both mature (Fig. 10.4a) and immature (Fig. 10.4b) squamous mucosa may be found at the transition, similar to mature and immature squamous metaplasia of the cervix.

Histologic cell types present in the anal canal include the following: (1) melanocytes are present in the epithelium; (2) lymphoid follicles and anal ducts are present in the mucosa and submucosa; (3) anal glands,

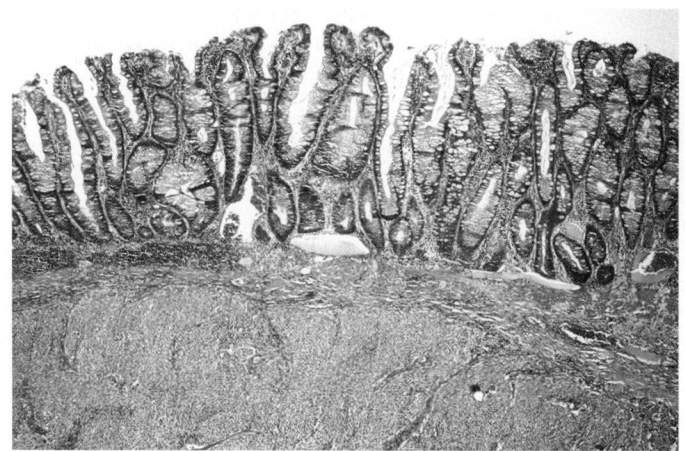

Fig. 10.5 Colorectal zone of the anal canal.

mucus-producing columnar to cuboidal cells similar to apocrine appendages, drain into the anal canal via anal ducts; (4) the ducts are lined by a basal layer of squamoid cells with a variable layer of more cuboidal mucous-type cell and may penetrate the internal sphincter muscles on the way to the anal glands; (5) smooth muscle and nerves are present in the wall of the canal.

Understanding the gross and histologic anatomy of the anal canal is important for understanding the pattern of neoplastic development in this complex site. Knowledge of the presence of these additional cell types is useful for understanding and recalling neoplastic entities that may arise from these cells. Squamous carcinoma commonly arises in the canal and is linked to human papillomavirus (HPV) infection. Adenocarcinoma of the anal canal frequently arises from the distal rectal mucosa and more rarely from anal ducts. Melanoma, lymphoma, leiomyomas, leiomyosarcoma and neural tumors such as schwannomas have also been reported.

The anatomy of the anal canal is also the key to understanding the spread of neoplastic disease and trace its origin to the upper or lower anal canal. This is divided into two components: (1) The upper two-thirds of the anal canal is supplied with blood mainly from the superior rectal artery (itself a branch of the inferior mesenteric artery) and drains into the superior rectal veins. The venous drainage of the superior rectal vein empties into the inferior mesenteric vein, but branches of the superior mesenteric and middle veins may also anastomose in that area. Drainage from the upper two-thirds of the canal leads to the inferior mesenteric lymph nodes. The autonomic nervous system innervates the anal canal above the dentate line, while the somatic nervous system via the pudendal nerve and the sacral plexus innervates the canal below the dentate line. (2) The lower third is supplied by the inferior rectal arteries (branches of the internal pudendal arteries). Venous drainage is provided by the inferior rectal veins leading to the internal iliac veins via the internal pudendal veins. Lymphatics for the lower third of the canal lead to the superficial inguinal lymph nodes. The somatic nervous system via the inferior rectal nerve supplies that area. Understanding of the histologic zones and gross anatomy of the anal canal can provide important clinical clues for clinical disease. For example, lymph node metastases from above the dentate line are frequently seen in adenocarcinomas, while in contrast lymphadenopathy of the superficial iliac nodes is strongly suggestive of a squamous cell carcinoma.

Accordingly, clinical examination of the anal canal should be performed among at-risk individuals to rule out the presence of carcinoma and identify dysplastic lesions that are at risk of future progression to carcinoma. Risk factors for anal carcinoma are described in Table 10.1.[11-14] The clinical examination should begin with a visual inspection of the perianal region for signs of condyloma acuminatum or plaque-like lesions suggestive of Bowen's disease. Fissures and fistulas should also be sought since these are also risk factors for carcinoma. The inguinal region should be palpated for masses. Following the visual inspection, a moistened Dacron swab may be inserted to perform an anal cytology, as described by Chin-Hong et al.[15] After the cytology specimen is obtained, further procedures may be performed with the addition of lubrication. A digital examination of the anal canal with a lubricated gloved finger should be performed to exclude the presence of palpable surface and submucosal masses that could indicate the presence of carcinoma. Digital examination is especially important since cytology and direct visualization of lesions using high-resolution anoscopy (HRA) may not always identify submucosal lesions. In addition, important information such as the degree of firmness of the lesion and its mobility may be obtained with digital examination and may alter the index of suspicion for cancer. Following the digital examination, HRA may be performed as described by Chin-Hong et al.[15]

Non-neoplastic lesions

PERIANAL CYSTS

A variety of developmental anomalies may lead to perianal or anal cysts. It is believed cysts in these areas may arise from remnants of the neuroenteric canal, tailgut or hindgut, but in practice these mucus-producing cysts may be difficult to distinguish from anal duct cysts or anal gland cysts. The cyst lining typically is composed

Table 10.1 Risk factors for squamous carcinoma of the anus

Ref.	Variable	Risk
76	Female gender	2–4×
11,12,13	Anal intercourse	RR = 1.8–2.4, OR = 6.9
	HIV(+)	RR = 3.2
	Abnormal cervical cytology	RR = 1.8–4.13
13	Smoking	RR = 7.7
51	Anal condyloma	SIR = 8.5

OR, odds ratio; RR, risk ratio; SIR = standardized incidence ratio of mucus-producing cuboidal to columnar epithelium. Clinically, these cysts come to attention due to infection and perianal abscess formation.[16]

HEMORRHOIDS

Clinical

Hemorrhoids are characterized by dilations of superficial mucosal vessels accompanied by enlargement or prolapse of connective tissue. Traditionally it was believed that hemorrhoids were caused by the pathologic development of superficial varicosities of the submucosal plexus of venules. However, hemorrhoids are now presumed to result from enlarged or prolapsed fibrovascular and connective 'cushions' in the submucosa, which perform a physiologic protective role during defecation. Portal hypertension does not cause hemorrhoids, but may precipitate bleeding (Fig. 10.6).

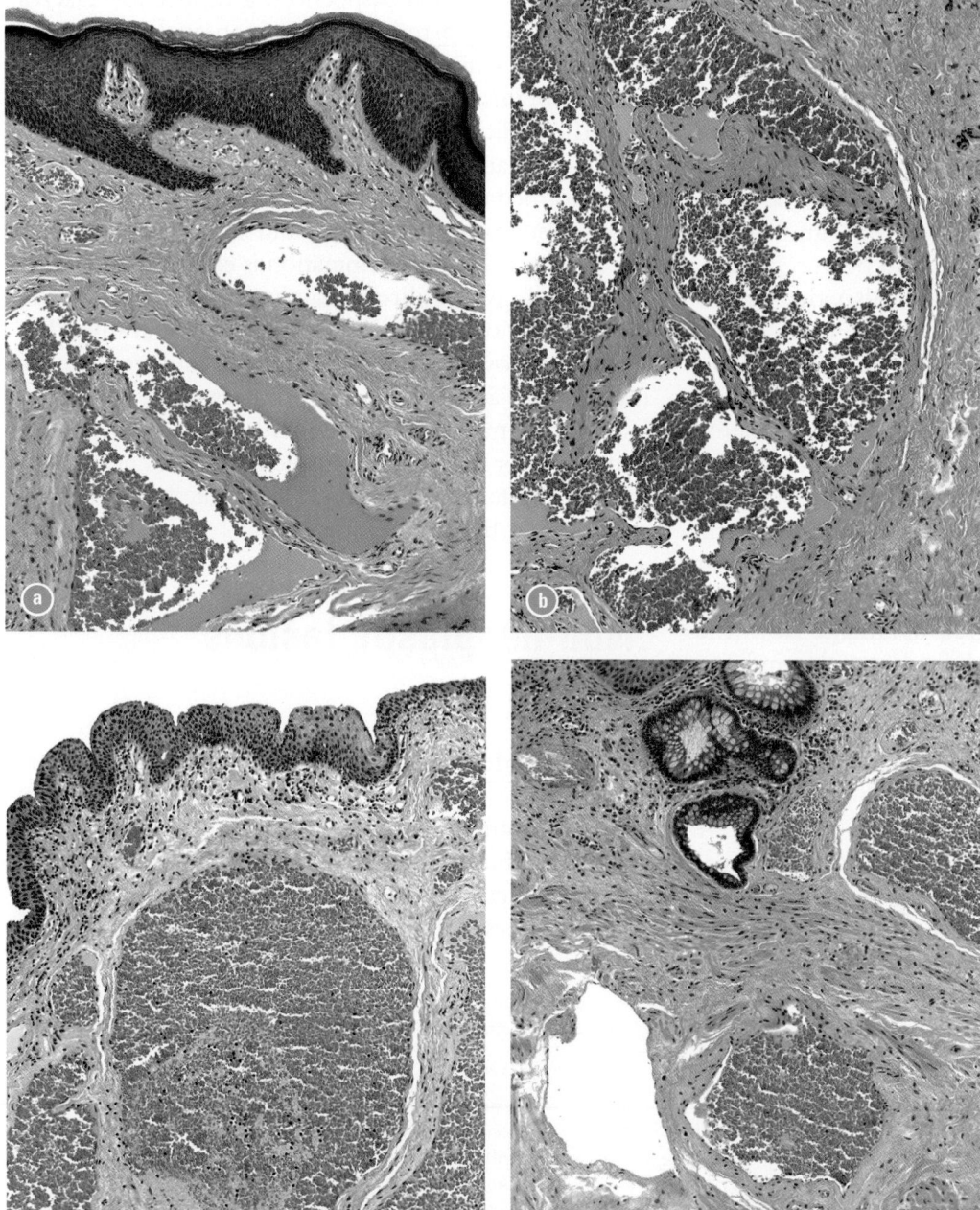

Fig. 10.6 Hemorrhoids. (a) Low-power photomicrograph of external hemorrhoid with accentuated vasculature and acanthosis of the surface squamous mucosa. (b) Recanalized thrombosed vessels. (c,d) Internal hemorrhoids, underlying (c) transitional and (d) rectal mucosa, respectively.

Risk factors for hemorrhoids include low fiber diet, constipation and prolonged intra-abdominal pressure (straining). Other factors implicated in their development include diarrhea, obesity, hypertension, or hereditary tendency. Increased age also predisposes to symptomatic hemorrhoids, as loss of elastic tissue and replacement of muscle with collagen fibers causes instability and venous stasis. Patients with concomitant portal hypertension and/or coagulopathy are then susceptible to bleeding and prolapse.

Hemorrhoids can occur caudal (external) or cephalad (internal) to the sphincter (external) and the location will determine the symptoms. Internal hemorrhoids cause principally painless bleeding, while external hemorrhoids are associated with pain, particularly when thrombosed, strangulated or inflamed. Erosion of the surface of a prolapsed hemorrhoid may also cause pain and/or infection.

Histology

The hemorrhoidal tissue is composed of (1) thick-walled medium-sized vessels in the submucosa and (2) background stroma containing connective tissue and smooth muscle fibers (Fig. 10.6). Additional features include (3) thromboses, (4) neuronal hyperplasia and (5) erosion with inflammatory changes of the mucosal surface. Incidental anal intraepithelial neoplasia (AIN) has been reported with low frequency (2%) of excised hemorrhoids.[17]

ANAL TAGS/FIBROEPITHELIAL POLYPS

Fibroepithelial stromal polyps (FSPs) are polypoid projections of the anal mucosa with stromal hyperplasia in response to mucosal trauma. FSPs are composed of two components, including a squamous mucosa with minimal acanthosis and an underlying loose to compact stromal tissue, often with distinctive stellate or multinucleate cells showing fibroblastic and myofibroblastic differentiation.[18] Various degrees of inflammation are present depending on the degree of trauma to the polyp. Fibroepithelial polyps lack the dilated submucosal vessels of a hemorrhoid and are thought to be the equivalent of acrochordons found in other sites of the body (Fig. 10.7).

INFLAMMATORY POLYPS

Clinical

Inflammatory polyps or *inflammatory cloacogenic polyps* are prolapsed mucosal projections with histologic features suggesting an ischemic or reactive origin. Inflammatory polyps are believed to occur as a component of the solitary rectal ulcer syndrome/mucosal prolapse syndrome. These polyps occur most often in middle-aged patients, though they also occur in children and often present with rectal bleeding. A few case reports of dysplasia found in these polyps are present in the literature. Grossly the lesions are pink/

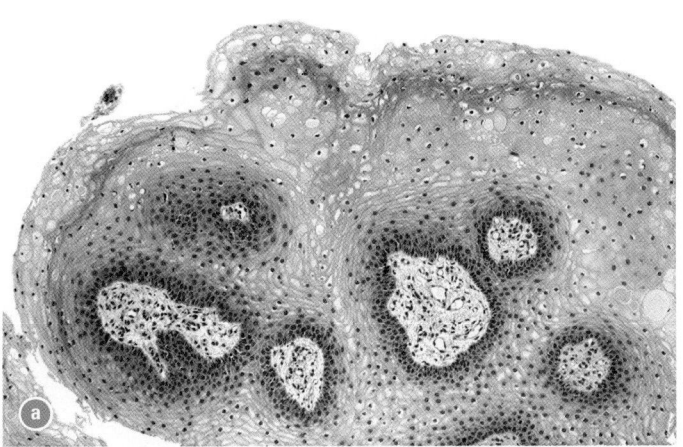
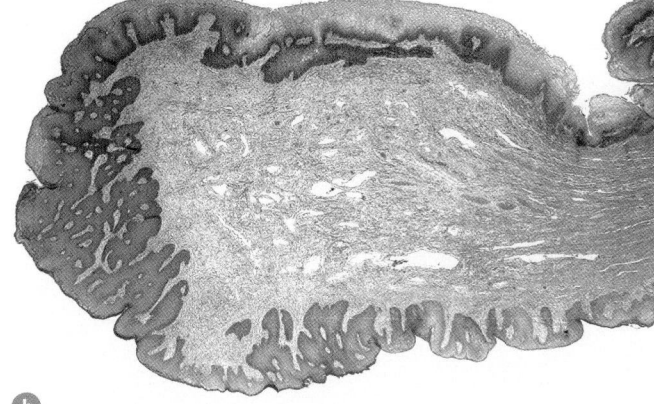

Fig. 10.7 Fibroepithelial stromal lesions. (a) Acrochordon, (b) fibroepithelial stromal polyp.

tan polypoid excrescences of the anal canal mucosa which are varied in size and are typically sessile with a tubulovillous architecture.

Histology

The lesions are lined by a mixture of squamous and colorectal epithelium, often with surface ulceration or erosion. In addition, fibrosis of the lamina propria and thickening of the muscularis propria is present, with some extension of smooth muscle into the lamina propria. Mucosal gland hypertrophy and surface telangiectasia may also be seen. Treatment of the lesions is simple excision, usually with curative results (Fig. 10.8).

ANAL FISSURES AND ULCERS

Clinical

Anal fissures are traumatic erosions of the mucosal surface, primarily caused by the passage of hard stool. These so-called stercoral fissures usually occur in the posterior midline of the anal canal and may develop into chronic ulcers with repeated trauma. A reactive stromal hyperplasia, histologically similar to a fibro-epithelial polyp, can form in chronic cases at the proximal end of the lesion and is called a sentinel tag. Secondary causes of anal fissures include inflammatory bowel disease, particularly Crohn's disease, neoplasm or infectious process. Trauma and anal intercourse are also implicated in the formation of fissures.

Histology

The fissures or ulcers show mucosal erosion with fibrinoid ulcer formation and underlying granulation tissue. Foreign-body giant cells may also be present and should not be mistaken for the granulomas of Crohn's disease.

ANAL ABSCESSES AND FISTULAS

Clinical

The majority of anal fistulous disease is believed to arise from infection of the anal ducts and subsequent tracking into the anal glands. Because of the position of the anal glands deep to the wall of the internal anal sphincter muscle, deep abscesses may result acutely. Fistulous tracts may form in the chronic inflammatory phase. Hidradenitis suppurativa is an associated condition, which is a chronic infection of the apocrine glands and surrounding connective tissue occurring most often in males (Fig. 10.9).[19] Patients present with complaints of pain, purulent discharge and pruritus. Inflammation may involve the distal anus as well as the anal canal and rectum with formation of fistulas (Fig. 10.10). Associated conditions include oily skin, acne, obesity, smoking and diabetes mellitus. Crohn's disease may also result in perianal and anal fistulous disease.

Histology

The characteristic features include ulceration and granulation tissue area present in the tracts, with foreign-body giant cells and fibrosis.

INFLAMMATORY BOWEL DISEASE

Inflammatory bowel disease can manifest in the anal canal in several ways.

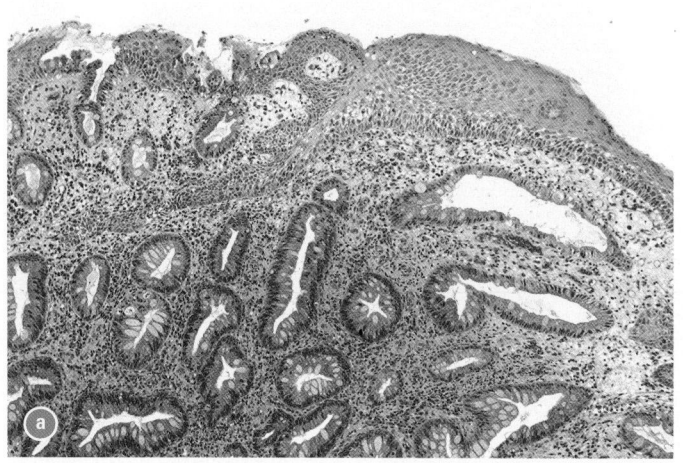
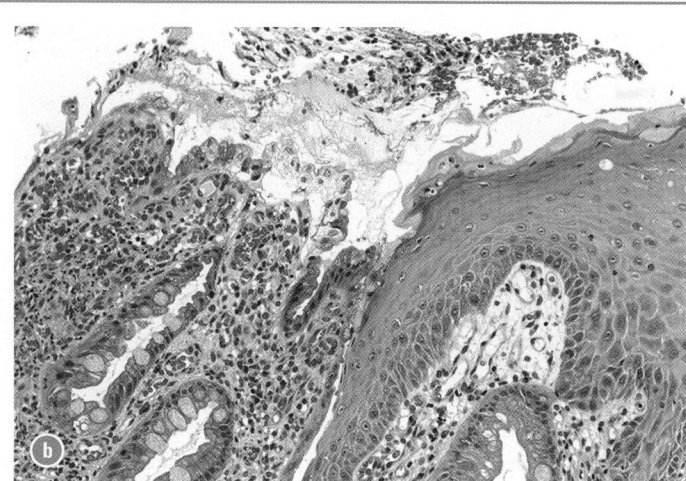

Fig. 10.8 Inflammatory/cloacogenic polyp. (a) Low power, (b) higher power illustrating mixture of intestinal and squamous epithelium.

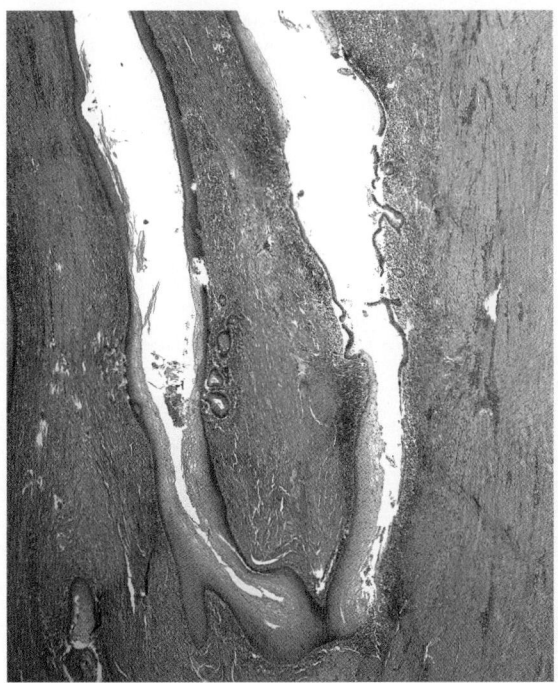

Fig. 10.9 Hidradenitis suppurativa, illustrating inflammation around adnexal structures.

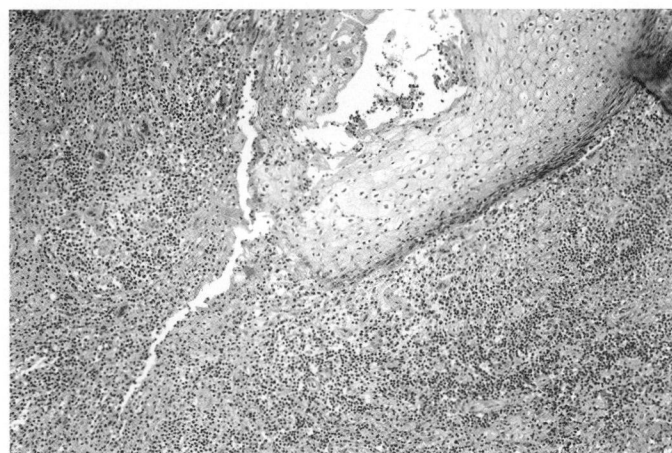

Fig. 10.10 Fistula tract in hidradenitis.

Ulcerative colitis

Ulcerative colitis uncommonly involves the anal region (ulcerative proctitis) and produces non-specific inflammatory changes in the anal canal, restricted to the mucosa of the colorectal zone. Fissures and fistulas are more rare. Of note, however, one study found that the columnar epithelium affected by ulcerative colitis often extended in irregular tongues into the transitional epithelium, occasionally reaching the dentate line.[20] Thus, surgical intervention for ulcerative colitis is a balance between removing all the mucosa of the colorectal zone and preservation of sphincter function.[21,22]

Female fecundity following surgical procedures for ulcerative colitis decreases, specifically following ileal pouch-anal anastomoses (IPAA). Studies have shown that fecundity prior to surgery in patients with ulcerative colitis is equivalent to a control population.[23,24] However, following bowel excision and revision, women had more difficulty getting pregnant. A small study of hysterosalpingography in 21 women after IPAA found abnormalities in two-thirds of patients. Abnormalities included fibrous bands, fallopian tubes adherent to the pelvic sidewall, hydrosalpinx and tubal occlusion.[25]

Crohn's disease

Crohn's disease affects the anus more frequently and with a wider variety of symptoms and pathology. Some

25% of patients with small bowel Crohn's disease have anal canal involvement, compared with involvement of 50–75% of those with small and large bowel disease. Anal tags, fissures, ulcers, fistulas and abscesses may form. Granulomatous inflammation affecting the anal canal mucosa and wall are seen histologically.

Squamous atypia of the anal transition zone may also occur following IPAA for either ulcerative colitis or Crohn's disease.[20] A study from the Cleveland Clinic showed that although no patients in their series (total 210 patients) developed carcinoma of the transitional zone, low- and high-grade squamous intraepithelial lesions emerged in 6 patients and 1 patient, respectively. All patients who developed a lesion had had a prior history of dysplasia or carcinoma, either in the colon or the rectum.[22]

ENDOMETRIOSIS

Endometriosis rarely involves the anus and perianal area. Eight reported cases exist in the literature, with similar clinical presentations. The patients reported cyclical pain that correlated with menses, occasionally with perianal nodule formation.[26–28] Many cases are associated with an episiotomy scar and occasionally may involve the sphincter muscles. The histologic correlate is an endometrioma, composed of a blood-filled cyst containing endometrial glands and stroma and hemosiderin deposition.

INFECTIONS

The anus may be involved in a wide range of infections, including tuberculosis, amebiasis, fungal and yeast infections. Other infections typically associated with the

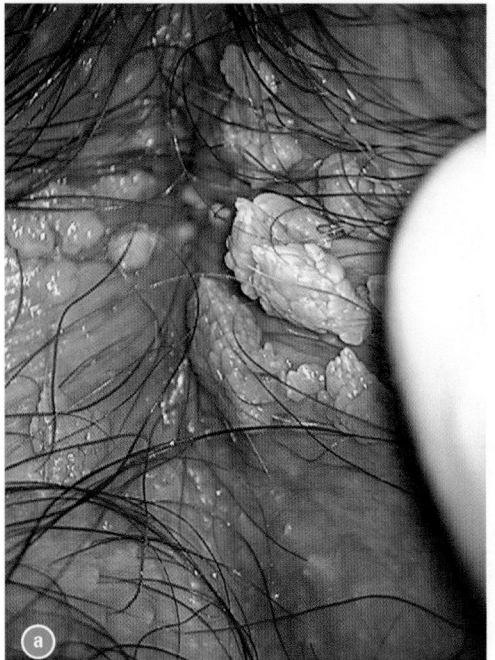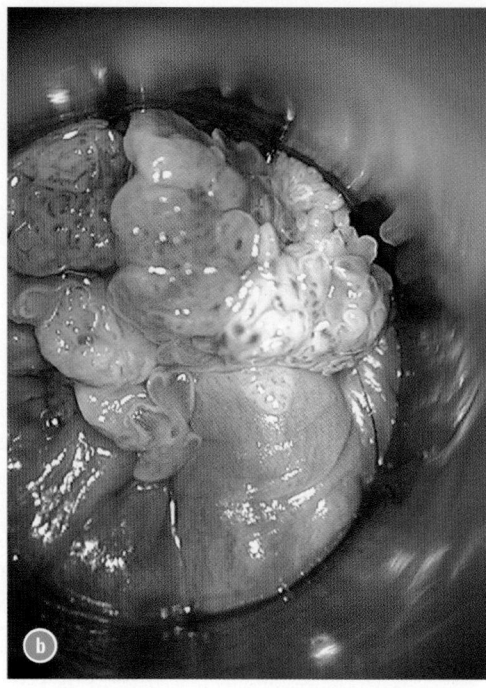

Fig. 10.11 (a) Clinical photo of anal condyloma. (b) Condyloma in the anal canal.

vulva may also involve the anus, including herpes, syphilis and, as discussed below, papillomaviruses (see Ch. 4).

IATROGENIC LESIONS

Various iatrogenic insults to the anal region have been reported in the literature. Irradiation of the anal region following abdominoperineal resection for rectal neoplasia is one of the most common causes of iatrogenic injury. Histologically, the anal sphincter muscle shows increased fibrosis and nerve density.[29] Ergotamine-induced strictures from ergotamine suppositories for migraine treatment have also been reported. In addition to trauma from repeated suppository use, ergotamine toxicity results from the drug's vasoconstrictive properties producing local ischemia. Rectal ulcerations are the most common early manifestation of this disorder, leading to progressive fibrosis and stricture formation.[30]

Neoplasms of the anus

INTRODUCTION

The most recent WHO classification (2000) divides tumors of the anal canal into epithelial tumors, carcinoids, malignant melanoma, non-epithelial tumor and secondary tumors. The epithelial tumors are subdivided into intraepithelial neoplasia (squamous and glandular dysplasia and Paget's disease) and carcinoma. The carcinoma group consists of squamous carcinoma, adenocarcinoma, small cell carcinoma, undifferentiated carcinoma and others.

For practical purposes, neoplastic lesions can be divided into three categories, comprising benign adnexal lesions, squamous intraepithelial lesions and malignancies. Squamous lesions are the most commonly encountered neoplasms in women and will occupy the bulk of the discussion below.

BENIGN ADNEXAL LESIONS

Hidradenoma papilliferum or papillary hidradenoma[31–33]

Clinical presentation

This is a rare neoplasm of the vulvovaginal and perianal skin, primary in women. A few cases have been reported in men and in other sites (breast, eyelid, ear canal) in women. The majority of patients are asymptomatic, though some have reported fluctuation in tumor size during the menstrual cycle.

Histopathology

The tumor is present in the dermis as a well-circumscribed solid or cystic nodule with papillae and glands and is similar to that of the vulva (see Ch. 5, Figs 5.11–5.13). The papillae are arranged in fronds or complex anastomotic patterns, usually completely enclosed in the dermis and without epidermal connection. The papillae are lined by two cell layers: an epithelial and a myoepithelial layer. The epithelial layer is composed of tall cuboidal to columnar cells with pale eosinophilic cytoplasm with regular nuclei. In about 30% of tumors, the epithelium may exhibit brightly eosinophilic cytoplasm and snouting with decapitation secretion may be seen (see Ch. 5). Occasionally, nuclear atypia and mitoses may be present. The myoepithelial cells are small cells with round to ovoid nuclei and clear to pale eosinophilic cytoplasm. Periodic acid–Schiff (PAS)-positive diastase-resistant granules are present in the larger epithelial cells. Immunohistochemical staining has shown the epithelial cells to stain for a variety of receptors, including estrogen and progesterone. The myoepithelial layer has been shown to be immunoreactive with S100 protein and smooth muscle actin. It is speculated that these tumors arise from sweat glands, though some authors believe they arise in ectopic mammary tissue.

Differential diagnosis

The differential diagnosis of these tumors includes syringocystadenoma papilliferum and tubular apocrine adenoma. Hidradenoma papilliferum is distinctive for its occurrence in the anogenital region of women almost exclusively and its disconnection from the epidermis.

Granular cell tumor

Granular cells tumors are relatively common benign tumors that occur at a variety of sites and in a wide age range. They rarely involve the anus.[34] The cells are thought to be of Schwann cell origin. Histologically, the tumours are characterized on low microscope power as a circumscribed nodule of eosinophilic cells in the dermis, with overlying pseudoepitheliomatous hyperplasia (see Ch. 6, Fig. 6.32b,c). The lesion may have a slightly infiltrative appearance, particularly at the edges, which may extend into the papillary dermis. The cells are plump with abundant granular pink cytoplasm, and contain small hyperchromatic round to slightly irregular nuclei. The granular cytoplasm is PAS diastase-resistant and may also be stained immunohistochemically with NKIC3. These tumors have a very low malignant potential. Sometimes marked epithelial hyperplasia may be present, giving the false impression of an invasive malignant lesion (see Ch. 9).

SQUAMOUS INTRAEPITHELIAL LESIONS

Definition

Squamous intraepithelial lesions (SILs) of the anus are defined as a range of HPV infections, leading to morphologic alterations of the squamous mucosa. This spectrum includes classic infections by low-risk (HPVs type 6 or 11) HPVs, which in most instances produce exophytic condylomata. In contrast, a range of flat lesions is more strongly associated with high-risk HPVs, the most common of which is HPV type 16. These have been classified as anal intraepithelial neoplasia or AIN. For the purposes of this chapter, low-grade (LSILs) will correspond to condylomata and flat lesions (AINs) containing milder forms of atypia. High-grade SILs (HSILs) comprise those lesions that correspond to high-grade SILs of the cervix and vulva (see Chs 6 and 13). This definition comes with the caveat that the natural history of both low- and high-grade SILs of the anus is not well understood and with the knowledge that some low-grade SILs may be associated with or progress to high-grade lesions. It is accepted that low-grade exophytic and flat lesions of the anus may contain different HPV types and different risks of progression to high-grade lesions. Nonetheless, for functional purposes, they are combined under the category of low-grade SILs.

Epidemiology

The incidence of anal SILs has increased since the early 1980s in both sexes for at least two reasons: (1) an increased risk and incidence in association with HIV and immune defects and (2) increasing clinical awareness of the connection between human immunodeficiency virus (HIV), lifestyle habits and HPV, leading to increasing screening for anal HPV-related diseases. Historically, the introduction of HIV into the human population and the development of acquired immunodeficiency syndrome (AIDS) may have resulted in a population of patients who were at high risk of developing HPV-related anogenital neoplasms. Generalized immunosuppression for other reasons has also been shown to be associated with a higher risk of anal HPV-related disease.[35,36] Another reason may be changes in sexual habits in the general population relating to the sexual revolution.

Risk factors for anal SIL and other squamous neoplasms include the following:
1. *Receptive anal intercourse*: One study showed that the risk of anal cancer increased up to 18-fold for individuals (men or women) who frequently engage

in receptive anal intercourse.[37] Other studies have shown much lower relative risk estimates, in accord with the frequent detection of HPV in the anal canal of women who do not engage in anal intercourse (Table 10.1).[11–14,38]

2. *HIV infection and immunosuppression:* Anal HPV infections are found in approximately 30–76% of HIV-positive women,[38–40] and in up to 43% of HIV-negative women. In a San Francisco cohort, the relative risk for HIV-positive women of developing abnormal anal cytology findings was 3.2 compared with controls. There was also an increasing risk of abnormal cytology in these patients with decreasing CD4 counts (<500) and increasing HIV viral load.[11] A larger, more comprehensive study from the AIDS-Cancer Match Registry from 1978–1996 found a relative risk of 7.8 and 60.1 for women and men diagnosed with AIDS, for the development of higher grades of AIN (carcinoma *in situ*). In particular, the risk for women who were diagnosed with AIDS between the ages of 30 and 39 years was increased 21-fold compared with controls. Other risk factors for anal HPV infection include younger age (<45 years), intravenous drug use (17-fold risk increase) and white race.[41] It should be emphasized that HIV confers an increased risk of HPV even in the absence of anal intercourse. In one study the risk of anal infection in HIV-infected heterosexual drug users *vs* homosexuals was 46 and 85%, respectively.[14] This underscores the importance of anal examinations for high-risk individuals irrespective of sexual practices. Cervical examinations in patients with anal lesions are particularly important (and vice versa), given the high frequency of concurrent anal and cervical HPV infection in this population.[38]

3. *Role of HPV testing and anal cytology:* HPV testing, particularly of HIV-infected individuals, yields positive rates in up to 85% of men who have sex with men.[42] Similar to findings in other sites, such as the cervix, the presence of HPV does not necessarily indicate a coexisting anal lesion. Even in normal anal cytology specimens it has been shown that HPV DNA may be detected in over 70% of women who are HIV positive.[43] However, HPV testing is highly sensitive and will target those individuals at greatest risk for anal lesions. Moreover, the risk of concomitant infections by *Chlamydia trachomatis*, gonococci, or herpes simplex viruses is higher.[42] Concurrent infection

with cervical HPV infection is common, although in fact infection with anal HPV in women with HIV is more common than cervical infection.[44]

In a study of heterosexual women, Moscicki et al. examined the natural history of abnormal anal cytology in 410 women who underwent both anal HPV testing and anal cytologic examination. Rates of abnormal cytology (3.9%) were low, but correlated strongly with a history of anal sex, cervical lesions and current anal HPV infection.[12]

One compelling study by Goldstone et al. examined the risk of HSIL and cancer outcome in 200 men who had sex with men. Although most (79%) were referred for anal condylomata or other benign conditions, 93% had abnormal cytology, 54% had a cytologic diagnosis of HSIL and 60% had biopsy-proven HSIL. The frequency of anal cancer was 3%.[45]

Examination

Anoscopy and sampling of the cells of the anal epithelium for cytologic preparation has developed in the same model as cervical cytology, particularly in high-risk populations. One study that correlated gross and histologic findings found some differences between low-grade and high-grade lesions.[46] High-grade lesions were significantly more likely to have a flat, smooth, non-papillary surface compared with low-grade lesions. Low-grade lesions were also more likely to have warty vessels, punctation and vascular mosaicism. AIN may also be discovered incidentally on specimens excised for unrelated reasons. For example, 25–40% of patients with newly diagnosed AIN or Bowen's disease are discovered by histologic examination of routine hemorrhoidectomy specimens.[47,48]

Histopathology

Low-grade squamous intraepithelial lesions (condyloma acuminatum/AIN 1)

Definition and clinical presentation Condyloma is an exophytic HPV-related lesion of the perianal skin in which HPV 6/11 is found in up to 85% of these lesions, with less than 5% containing HPV 16 and 18.[49] Clinically, they are warty white, pink or gray excrescences with occasionally filiform fronds (Fig. 10.11). The lesions are typically more extensive in immunosuppressed patients. AIN grade 1 is analogous to CIN 1 and comprises flat acetowhite lesions.

Histology Histologically, condylomata display the characteristic combination of acanthosis, papillomatosis and variable viral cytopathic effect (koilocytosis). Para-

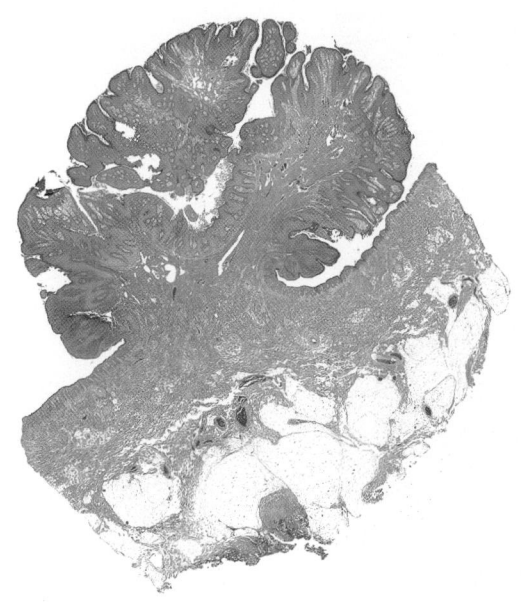

Fig. 10.12 Low-power microphotograph, anal condyloma.

keratosis is often present (Figs. 10.12, 10.13). By definition, the atypia should be confined to the upper epithelial layers with minimal variations in nuclear size or staining in the lower third. AIN 1 is defined as a flat condyloma, possessing the same distribution of cellular atypia seen in the exophytic lesions. Other lesions that may be included in the AIN 1 category are flat lesions that lack koilocytosis but contain insufficient atypia to warrant a diagnosis of a high-grade SIL, as defined below.

Two additional diagnostic pitfalls must be carefully considered when making a diagnosis of LSIL of the anus and both pertain to the HIV-infected or immuno-suppressed individual. First, these patients often have multiple lesions (and multiple HPV infections), which may coexist (Fig. 10.14). Careful histologic examination is mandatory to exclude a coexisting HSIL. Secondly, the risk that a more bland-appearing lesion will progress to a high-grade lesion on follow-up must be taken seriously, as discussed below.

Differential diagnosis and diagnostic pitfalls As in the vulva, the differential diagnosis of condyloma includes fibroepithelial polyps, mucosal tags, non-specific acanthosis and reactive changes with cytoplasmic halos (Fig. 10.15a–d). The most important distinction in such cases is to exclude high-grade squamous intra-

epithelial lesions (AIN 2/3). Hemorrhoids may also be confused with condyloma clinically, but lack the necessary epithelial features.

Natural history of low-grade SIL The natural history of anal condylomata varies and lesions may persist for some time. Giant condylomata, a rare variant, are discussed below. HIV status, anal intercourse, sexually transmitted infections and multiple sexual partners increase the risk of both condylomata and coexisting AIN.[50] Moreover, anal condylomata pose an increased risk for anal carcinoma, as well as vulvar and cervical dysplasia and carcinoma.[45,51] Presumably, this increased risk is due to the sharing of common risk factors for cancer-associated HPV infections.

HSIL has been reported in 6% of condylomata in heterosexual males and from 31 to 60% of condylomata of homosexual males.[45,50] The risk appears higher than would be expected in the non-HIV infected population. Palefsky et al. studied the risk of lesion development and risk of progression from low to high-grade lesions over a 4-year interval in 346 HIV-positive and 262 HIV-negative homosexual or bisexual men. The incidence of HSIL within 4 years was 32% in HIV-positive men and 12% in HIV-negative men who were normal at baseline. However, the rates of progression from LSIL to HSIL were 52% of HIV-positive and 41% of HIV-negative men and correlated with low CD4 counts.[52] Irrespective of whether the HSIL outcomes signify progression or concomitant infection by other high-risk HPVs, they underscore the importance of follow-up of these patients.

High-grade squamous intraepithelial lesions (anal intraepithelial neoplasia grades 2/3)

Definition and clinical presentation AIN is synonymous with high-grade squamous intraepithelial lesions in the cervix (CIN 2/3) and vulva (VIN 2/3). Like the latter, lesions previously classified as Bowen's disease, bowenoid papulosis and carcinoma *in situ* are combined into a single diagnostic entity. The lesions are all HPV related, with infection by the so-called high-risk HPV subgroups with HPV 16 (and others) predominating.

Clinically, different forms of high-grade SIL are somewhat distinct, but histopathologically are the same entity (Fig. 10.16). *Bowenoid papulosis* is an older term describing the syndrome of multiple small pigmented papules on the perianal, penile or vulvar skin of young adults. Frequently, HPV 16 is found in the lesions, have the histologic appearance of squamous carcinoma *in situ*. *Bowen's disease* is a disease of adult men and women

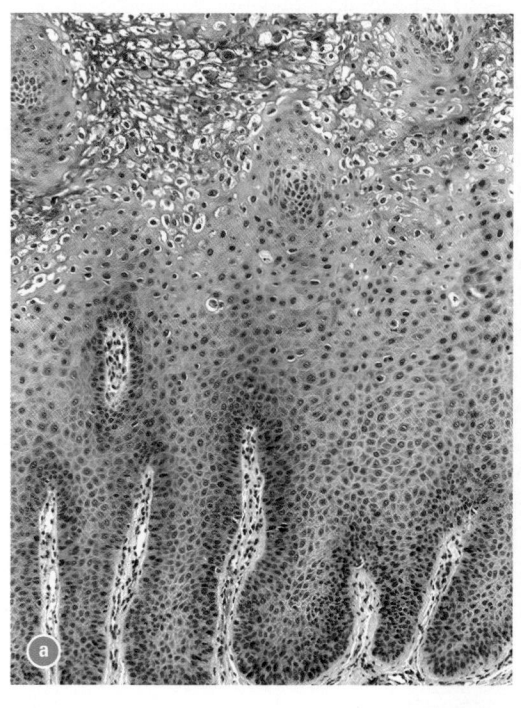

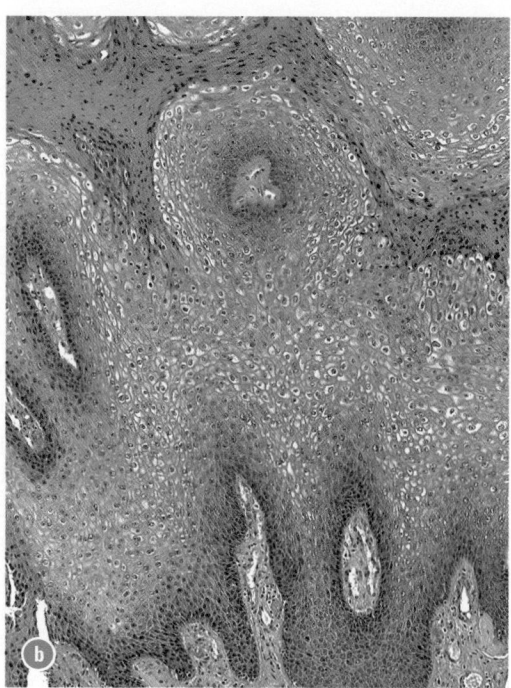

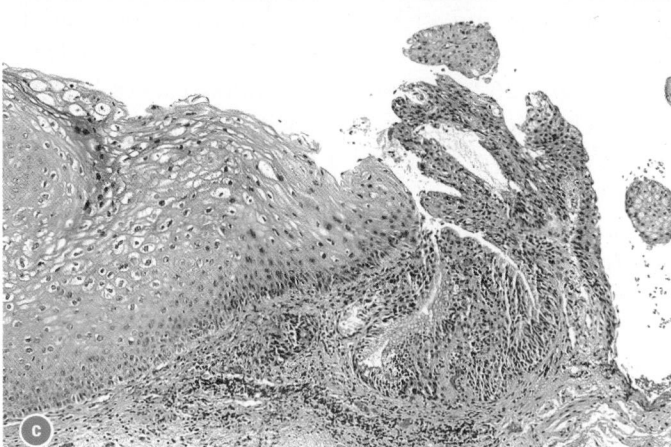

Fig. 10.13 (a–c) Low-grade squamous intraepithelial lesions of the anus. (a,b) Exophytic condyloma, (c) flat condyloma.

that presents as a pruritic scaly red or white patch of perianal skin that may extend into the anal canal. There is a low incidence of associated internal malignancy and a low incidence of neighboring invasive carcinoma in these lesions. Progression to cancer occurs in 2–6% of cases. However, a large minority of female patients (21–36%) have concomitant Bowen's disease of the labia and vulva or cervical intraepithelial neoplasia.[53–55] Histologically, Bowen's disease is squamous cell carcinoma *in situ*. Frequently, the lesions are associated with HPV 16 and 18 infection.

Histology In practice, high-grade SILs of the anus fall within a relatively narrow spectrum of lesions containing full-thickness atypia and variable maturation,

similar to high-grade squamous intraepithelial lesions of the other mucosal sites (Fig. 10.17, Table 10.2). As such, the distinctions between grade 2 and grade 3 become arbitrary and may be difficult to reproduce. Studies have shown the degree of interobserver and intraobserver agreement to be variable, reporting weighted kappa scores varying from 0.17 to 0.64.[56,57] The reader is cautioned that a diagnosis of AIN 1, like that of the vulva, is difficult to reproduce between observers and is best distinguished from AIN 2/3.

All high-grade SILs contain atypia in at least the lower two-thirds of the epithelium, with loss of polarity, increased mitotic index, anisokaryosis, dyskeratosis and abnormal mitotic figures (see Ch. 6, Figs 6.12a–d, for comparison). These disturbances in epithelial growth

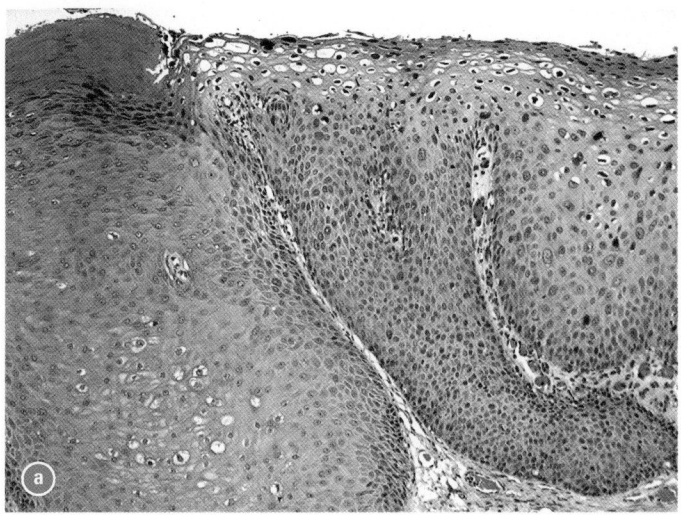 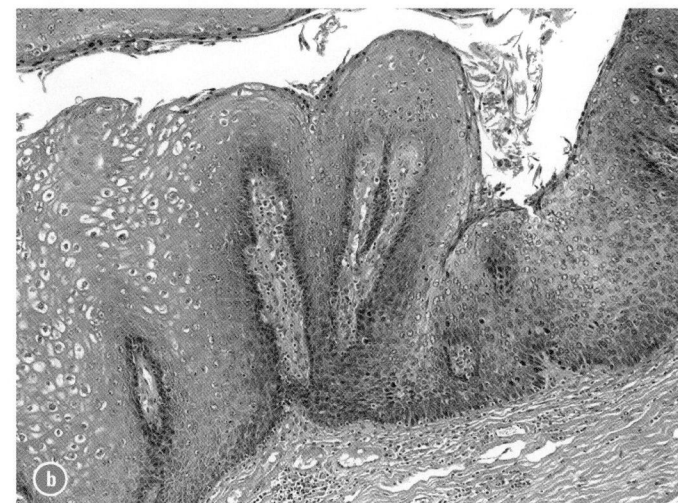

Fig. 10.14 (a) Condyloma (LSIL) in continuity with HSIL (AIN 2). (b) Another condyloma (LSIL) in continuity with AIN 3.

and maturation are the direct consequences of oncogenic HPV (see Ch. 13). A study detecting HPV DNA from paraffin sections by Carter et al. found HPV-16 and HPV-18 DNA in 43% and 67% of AIN 3 lesions in women.[58]

In perianal skin, AIN may involve skin appendages, most commonly hair follicles but also sebaceous glands and sweat glands.[59]

Differential diagnosis HSIL must be distinguished from four other entities. The first is inflamed or reactive changes in the transitional mucosa (Fig. 10.18a). Secondly, pseudoepitheliomatous hyperplasia may mimic LSIL, HSIL or even early carcinoma (Fig. 10.18b). Marked repair may be extremely difficult to distinguish if associated with chronic ulceration. Typically the presence of uniform nuclear morphology, prominent nucleoli and absence of infiltration will distinguish this mimic from either HSIL or invasive carcinoma. Finally,

atypical presentations of Paget's disease may mimic HSIL, but can easily be distinguished with the appropriate special stains (see below and Ch. 6).

Outcome As discussed above, the risk of HSIL outcomes is high with anal HPV infection; however, the natural history of anal HSILs and risk of invasive carcinoma are not well understood. Rates of regression appear low in HIV-infected individuals.[60] The effect of highly active antiretroviral therapy (HAART) on the natural history of AIN has not been extensively studied; however, the literature suggests that the intensive drug regimen has relatively little or no effect on natural history of HPV-related squamous lesions. Palefsky et al.[61] followed 98 males (who had sex with men) for 6 months after the initiation of HAART and found no difference in disease natural history between test patients and controls. Of the men who began therapy with a diagnosis of atypical squamous cells of undetermined significance (ASCUS) or LSIL, 18% progressed and 21% regressed in histologic grade. A small number of control patients developed low-grade lesions. One of the 28 patients who were initially diagnosed with a high-grade lesion regressed. Lillo et al. studied cervical dysplasia in 163 HIV-positive women and likewise found no difference in grade of squamous dysplasia between patients who had or had not received HAART.[62]

Various immunohistological markers have been applied to AIN in an attempt to predict their natural history. Thus far, a high MIB-1 (Ki-67) proliferative index has variably been found to be associated with high-grade

Table 10.2 Classification of anal squamous neoplasia

Terminology	HPV status
Low-grade squamous intraepithelial lesions	
Exophytic condyloma	Low-risk HPV
Anal intraepithelial neoplasia grade 1	High-risk HPV
High-grade squamous intraepithelial lesions	High-risk HPV
Anal intraepithelial neoplasia grade 2	
Anal intraepithelial neoplasia grade 3	
Squamous carcinoma	High-risk HPV
Large cell non-keratinizing	
Basaloid (cloacogenic/transitional)	

HPV, Human papillomavirus.

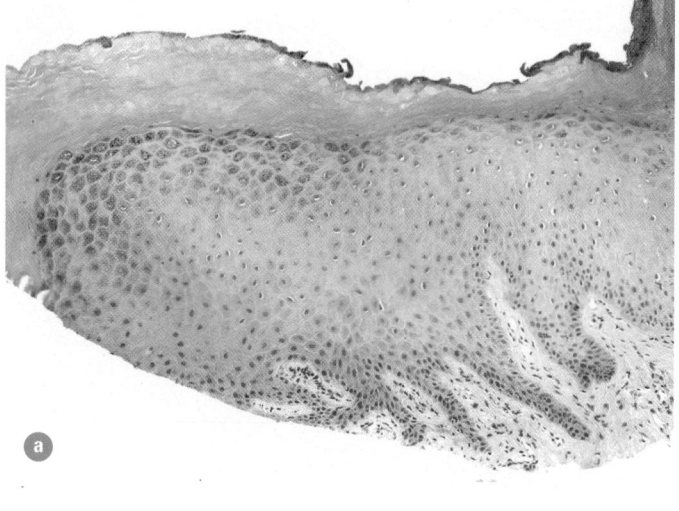

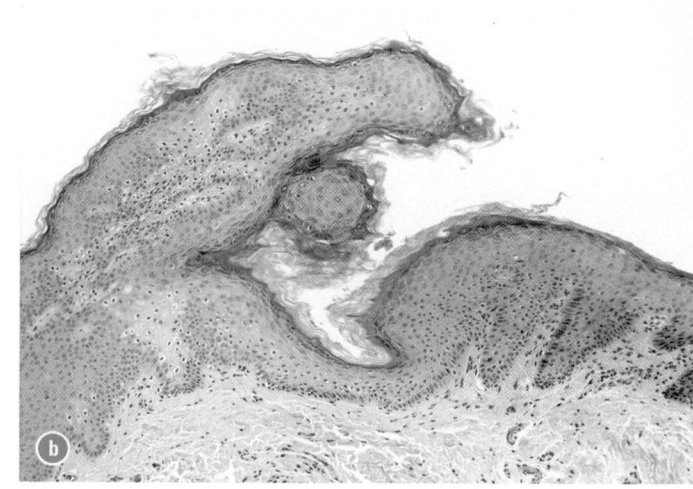

Fig. 10.15 Differential diagnosis of LSIL includes: (a) reactive epithelial changes with acanthosis, (b,c) mild degrees of verruciform change associated with acanthosis seen in prolapse, hemorrhoids, or trauma, (d) reactive epithelium with cytoplasmic halos.

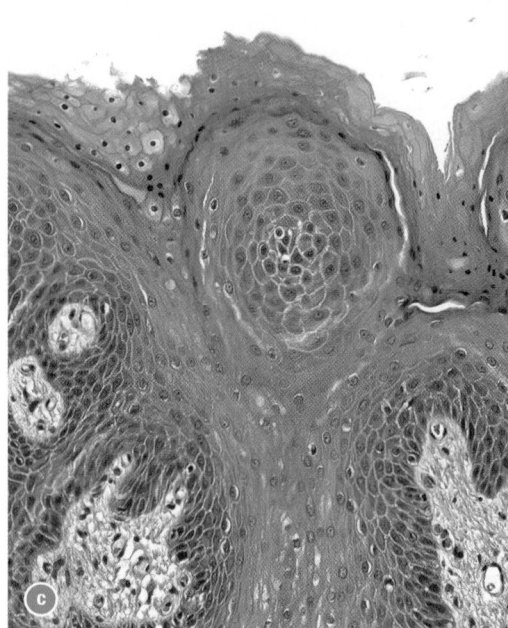

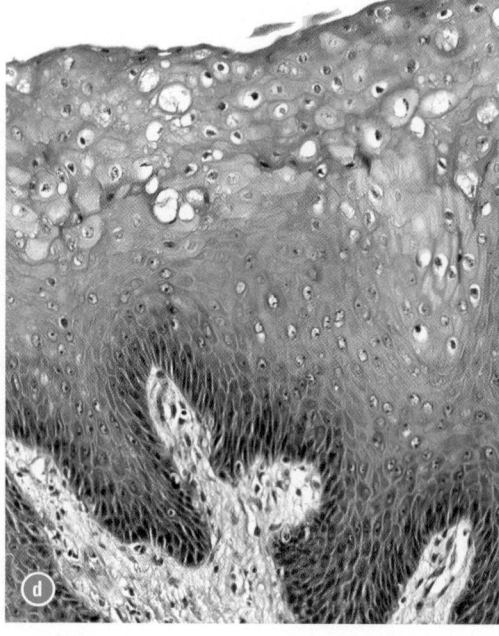

lesion and with recurrence of low-grade lesions.[53,63] Immunohistochemical staining for p53 has shown to be increased with the level of dysplasia and is suggested to be linked to higher risk of invasion.[64–66] In general, AIN lesions show similar histologic features as CIN lesions, including increased angiogenesis and proliferation and decreased apoptosis.[67]

Treatment Treatment of these lesions includes several modalities. Localized low-grade lesions may be treated by trichloroacetic acid (TCA), cryotherapy, liquid nitrogen treatment, or laser surgery. The efficacy or utility of treating low-grade lesions is controversial;

clinicians in the literature usually cite the desire to limit the size of the lesion and to eliminate the possibility of progression to a high-grade lesion.[15,60] High-grade lesions are more often treated surgically, depending on the size of the lesion. Smaller high-grade lesions can be treated with TCA. Both incisional biopsy and electrocautery fulguration are employed on lesions visualized by HRA, with split-thickness skin grafts applied as needed. Persistent or recurrent disease has been reported in approximately 30% of patients with AIN 3 with unknown HIV status.[68] In patients with HIV, approximately 80% of patients with AIN 3 developed recurrent lesions after surgical excision.[55]

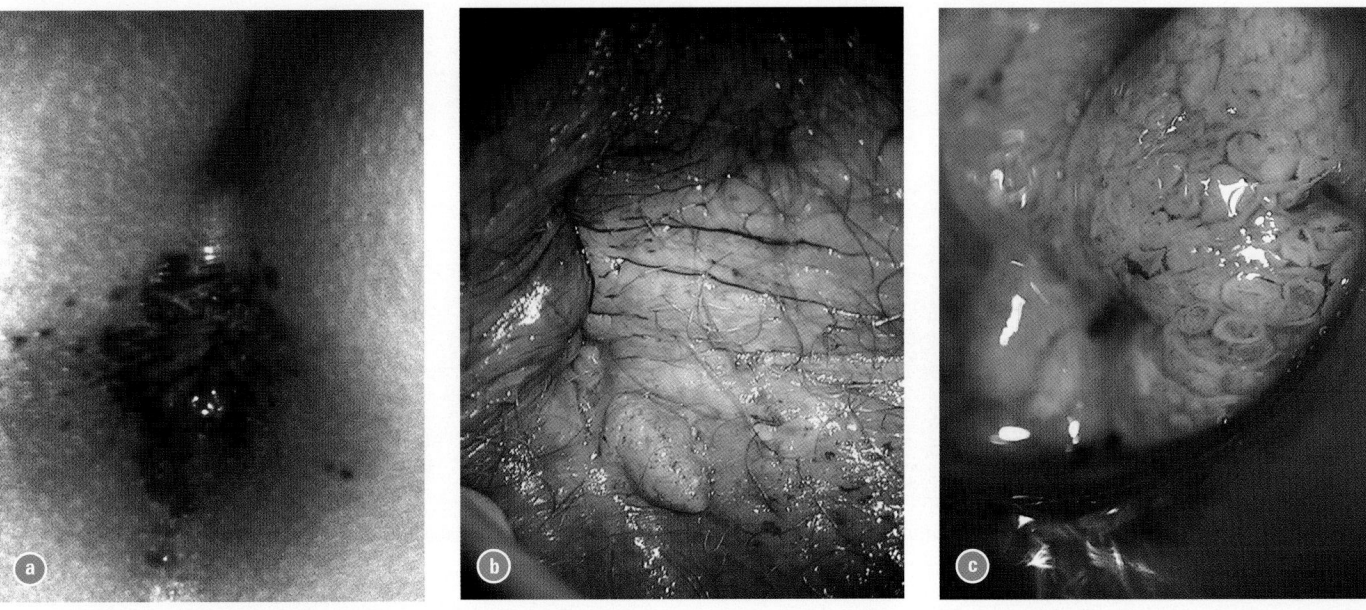

Fig. 10.16 Clinical images of high-grade intraepithelial lesions. (a) Pigmented perianal bowenoid papulosis. (b) Non-pigmented raised lesion at the entrance to the canal. (c) Complex mosaic formed by a high-grade lesion in the canal.

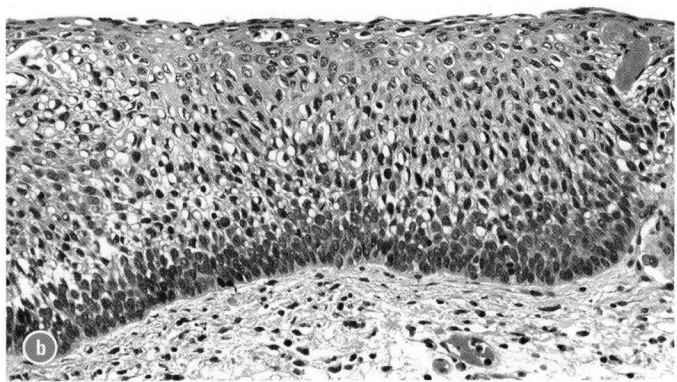

Fig. 10.17 Histology of HSIL of the anus. (a) AIN 2, (b) AIN 3, (c) AIN 3 overlying anal columnar mucosa.

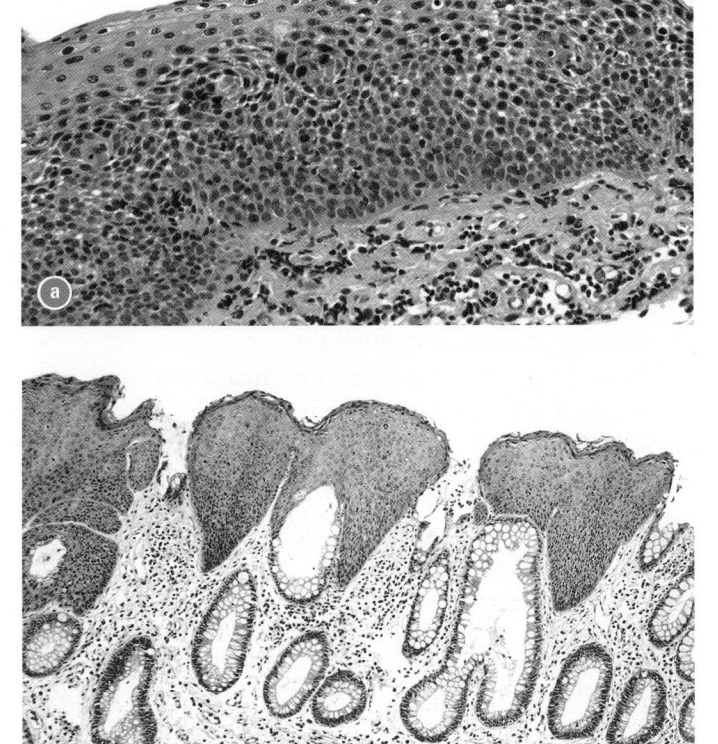

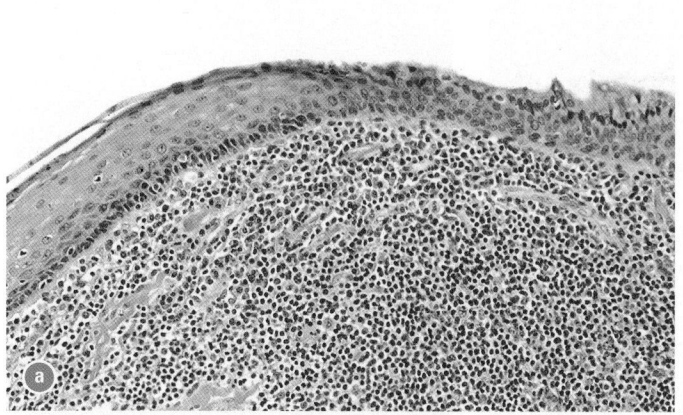
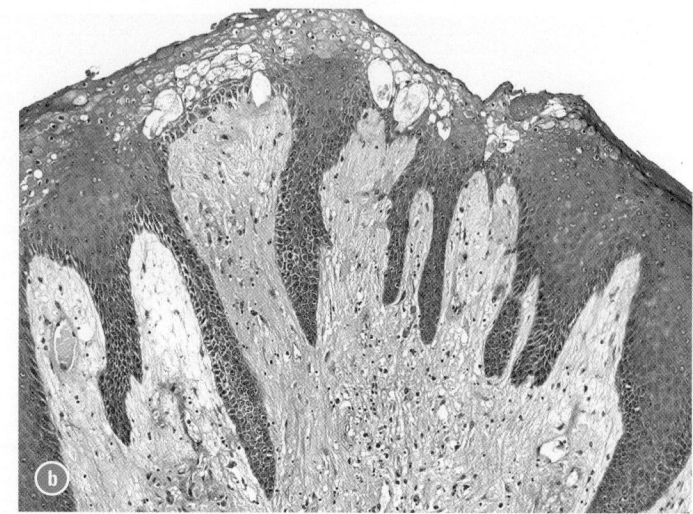

Fig. 10.18 Differential diagnosis of anal HSIL includes (a) inflammatory changes in transitional epithelium; (b) pseudoepithelial hyperplasia may mimic early invasion.

MALIGNANT TUMORS OF THE ANUS AND ANAL CANAL

Introduction

As noted above, the WHO Classification divides anal tumors into the categories of epithelial malignancies, carcinoid tumor, malignant melanoma, non-epithelial/ mesenchymal tumors and secondary tumors. Anal carcinoma is rare; the incidence based on the 1993 SEER data was estimated at 9/1 000 000 women and 7/1 000 000 men. Overall, tumors of the anal canal are rare, comprising 2% of all large bowel tumors.[69] Anal carcinomas arising above the dentate line are three times more common than those arising below.

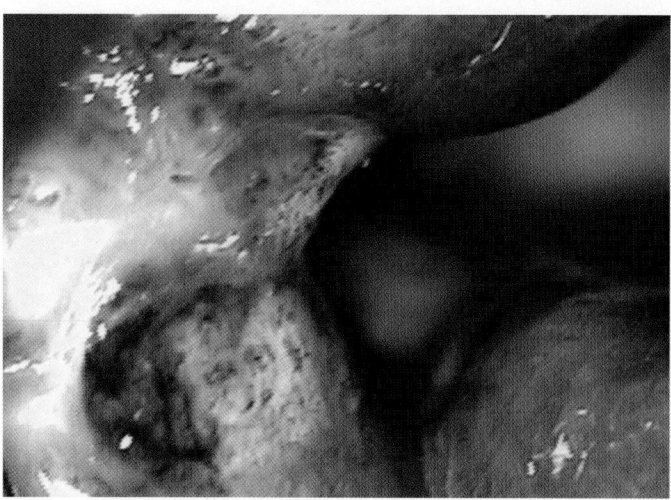

Fig. 10.19 Anoscopic image of anal cancer (lower left).

Tumors from the upper area include adenocarcinomas and 'transitional' tumors, also known as cloacogenic. They are two to three times more common in women than men and occur often during the seventh decade. Metastases from this site spread to the lower rectum and perirectal and lower inguinal lymph nodes. Anal carcinomas from below the dentate line are most often squamous cell carcinomas and have been thought to arise more frequently in men than women. Visceral metastases are rare in these lower carcinomas. The clinical profile stated above is largely derived from studies in the 1970s.[70–73] In practice, currently, it is often difficult to pinpoint the origin of anal cancers in many cases due to tumor overgrowth. The clinical literature frequently does not differentiate tumors from above or below the dentate line and so, particularly with squamous cell carcinoma, epidemiologic studies based on position relative to the dentate line should be performed cautiously.

The majority of anal cancers are squamous carcinomas. In a survey of 204 tumors with sufficient histologic information, 80% were typical squamous cell, 13% basaloid variant of squamous cell, 4% melanomas and 3% anal gland.[74]

Squamous carcinoma

Demographics

Squamous cell carcinoma is the most common anal canal cancer (80% of total). The incidence of anal carcinoma is rising, due in part to the synergistic effects of HIV and HPV infection. From 1973 to 1998 incidence of anal cancer in both sexes in the USA increased from 0.35 per 100 000 to 0.98 per 100 000.[75] The incidence in females rose specifically from 0.44 to 1.07 per 100 000, which was a smaller increase than for men during the same time period. Data from the National Cancer Database noted an increase of number of cases by 31% comparing number of cases of epidermoid carcinoma from 1988 and 1993.[76] The average age of patients is in the sixth–seventh decade, with a female to male predominance of 2:1. Risk factors for development of squamous carcinoma include HPV infection, HIV infection, urban populations, anal intercourse and number of sexual partners. Weaker associations in women with cigarette smoking have been reported.[77] The estimated incidence of anal carcinoma in the male homosexual population was up to 35 per 100 000 before the HIV epidemic and has presumably increased. The white population has the highest incidence rate, followed by the black population and Asian and Hispanic populations. The predominant etiologic agent is HPV. Prior literature had suggested that chronic inflammatory conditions such as fistulas were risk factors for anal squamous carcinoma. However, further case control and cohort studies have not borne this out.[13,77–80] HPV infection, particularly with HPV 16 and 18, is frequently found in anal squamous cell carcinomas, both of the anal canal and perianal skin.[81–84]

Clinical presentation

Clinical signs of anal squamous cell carcinoma are usually non-specific and related to tumor size. Complaints include anal pruritus, pain, sensation of a mass, pelvic pain, local pain, changes in bowel habits including incontinence, discharge or bleeding. Grossly, tumors are varied in appearance depending on size. A small and minimally invasive tumor may appear as a dimpling or ulceration of the mucosa with rolled edges. Thickened and discolored anal mucosa with irregular edges may also be present. As the tumor grows and invades, it appears more as a tan to pink glistening fixed mass with areas of necrosis, hemorrhage and surface ulceration (Fig. 10.19). Verrucous carcinoma, a specialized variant of squamous cell carcinoma, will be discussed separately below.

Histology

Conventional squamous cell carcinomas have been subclassified into the following morphologic variants: large cell keratinizing, large cell non-keratinizing and basaloid (also known as cloacogenic) (Fig. 10.20). None of these histological subtypes associate with a parti-

cularly better or worse outcome and frequently a combination of morphologic features may be found in the same tumor.[69,85] The kappa scores on histologic subtyping by pathologists using the WHO definitions have been reported as 0.47–0.61.[86] Therefore in the current WHO classification of tumors of the anal canal it is recommended that the term 'squamous cell carcinoma' should be generically utilized with the optional mention of additional histologic features. In practice, the patterns seen, ranging from well to moderately differentiated squamous cell carcinoma to basaloid carcinomas, are nearly identical to those seen in the cervix.

Despite the above, recognition of these patterns is important when excluding more (mucin-producing or undifferentiated) or less (basal cell carcinoma of the perianal skin) aggressive variants.[85] Whether HPV testing will distinguish these groups is doubtful. Some studies have not noticed equally high frequencies of HPV positivity between the basaloid/cloacogenic and other squamous carcinomas, in some cases reaching 89% of cases in some studies.[81,87–89] Others have distinguished the basaloid/cloacogenic as a predominately, if not exclusively, HPV-negative tumor.[90,91] Some of these differences in experience between laboratories may reflect evolving changes in assay sensitivity and specificity. However, the sharp difference in the index of HPV positivity observed by some between squamous and cloacogenic (transitional) types deserves further study.[90,91]

The typical large cell carcinomas are composed of irregular infiltrating nests and strands of medium to large cells with pale eosinophilic cytoplasm and vesicular nuclei. Keratinization may occur in lamellar whorls or in single cells, appearing as deeply eosinophilic cytoplasm. The basaloid (previously termed cloacogenic or transitional) variant is composed usually of infiltrating islands and nests of small to medium-sized cells with a high nuclear to cytoplasmic ratio. Intercellular bridges are difficult to find and peripheral retraction artifact may be seen around the islands. Typically, the nuclei are arranged in a palisade around the edges of the islands and central necrosis is present. Mitoses are frequently present in all histologic subtypes. Adjacent HSIL is frequently present. Occasionally, small areas of mucin-producing glands or microcysts may be present in the tumor, which had led some to further define a mucoepidermoid variant of squamous cell carcinoma (Fig. 10.20). Anal duct carcinoma is an extremely rare entity that arises from the basal-squamous cells of the anal ducts and also is included

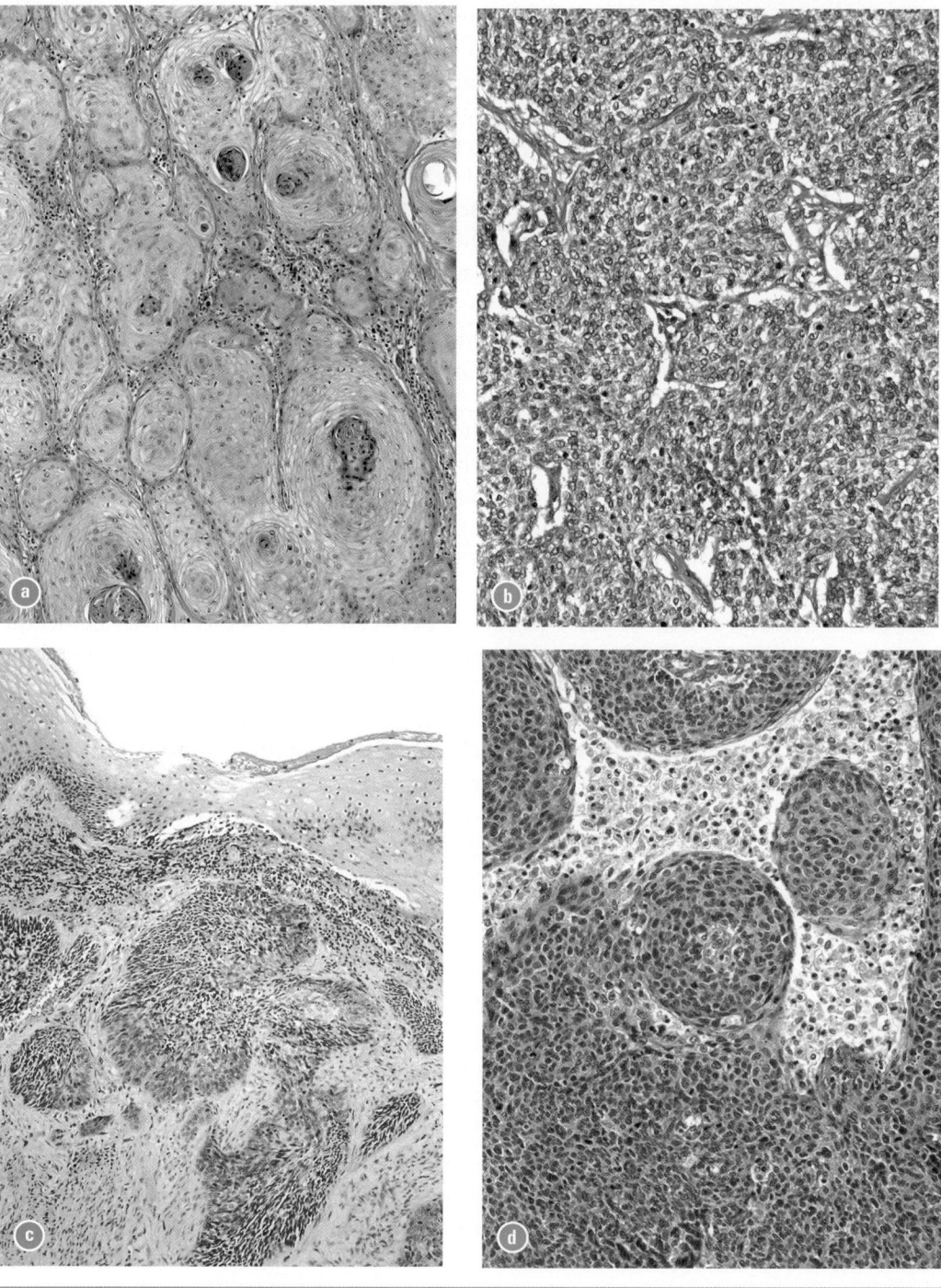

Fig. 10.20 Histology of anal cancer, including: (a) well-differentiated keratinizing, (b) large cell non-keratinizing, (c) poorly-differentiated basaloid (cloacogenic) carcinomas and (d) papillary carcinoma. These histologic patterns are essentially identical to those found in the cervix.

in this classification. Immunohistochemically, tumors of the anal canal have a slightly different cytokeratin staining pattern than those of the anal margin; Behrendt et al. reported a higher proportion of anal canal carcinomas stained positively for cytokeratin 7, 18 and 19.[92] However, the distinction was not significant.

Verrucous carcinoma and giant condyloma of the anus are specialized squamous cell carcinomas with distinct gross and histologic appearances as well as different prognosis (Fig. 10.21). Both are extremely rare and correspond to similar entities in the cervix and vulva. Verrucous carcinoma is a rare entity, with less than 40 reported cases in the literature in the anogenital area. Histologically, the warty fronds are composed of markedly acanthotic epithelium several cell layers thick showing orderly maturation. The cells are medium to large in size with abundant pale eosinophilic cytoplasm showing a smooth texture. The nuclei of the cells are

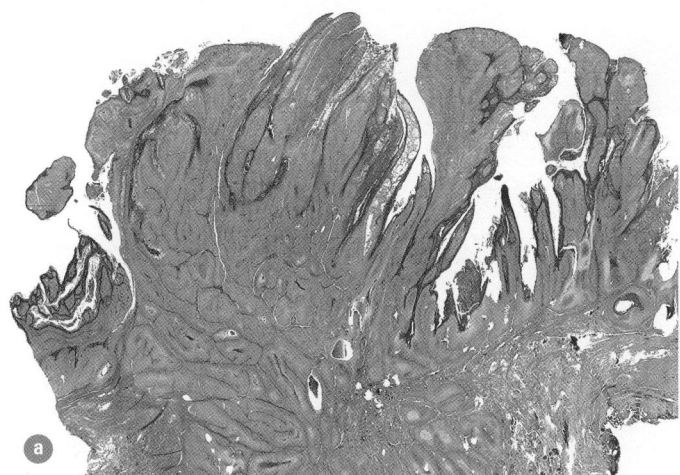

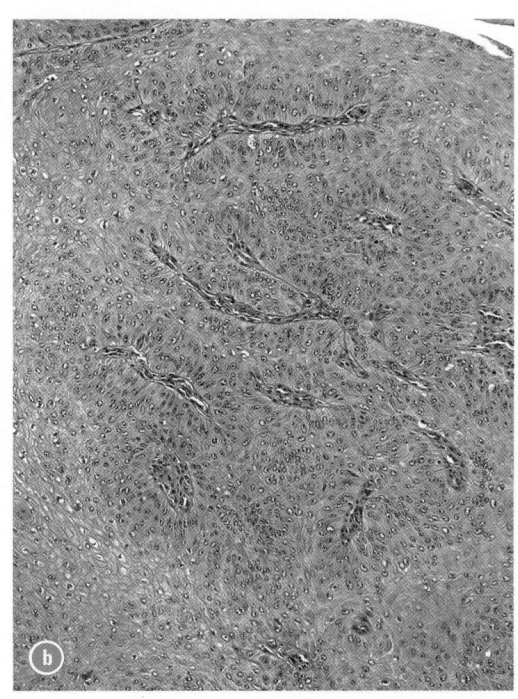

Fig. 10.21 Giant condyloma of the anus, presenting as an exophytic mass (a) with morphologic features identical to condyloma (b). These tumors are identical to condyloma but display expansile behavior characteristic of a well-differentiated carcinoma. This case was positive for HPV type 11. Compare with verrucous carcinoma (Ch. 6).

small to medium in size with vesicular chromatin, occasional small distinct nucleoli and an absolute absence of atypia. Mitoses are present only at the base, and HPV-related changes are not seen. The base of the lesion is defined by invasion with a broad pushing border rather than infiltrating border (see Ch. 6).

It is a subject of some debate whether verrucous carcinoma is in fact the same entity as giant condyloma acuminatum, otherwise known as Buschke–Löwenstein tumor (Fig. 10.21). In the opinion of these authors, the two entities are distinct. Typically, giant condyloma acuminatum present more frequently in males (with a 2.7:1 male to female ratio), with complaints of a mass, inflammation, purulent discharge, pruritus, abscess or fistulas and bleeding.[93] In contrast to the more sessile and broad-based appearance and altered keratinocyte differentiation of verrucous carcinomas, giant condylomas exhibit a combination of exophytic and endophytic growth, may exhibit typical viral cytopathic effect and by definition and cannot be distinguished from condyloma when viewed out of context of the mass. However, foci of invasive cancer have been reported in approximately 50% of cases, with atypia noted in up to 8%. HPV 6 and 11 have been detected in giant condyloma but the association between HPV and verrucous carcinoma is less consistent.

Excepting rare examples with both condyloma and invasive carcinoma, how is giant condyloma distinguished from extensive condyloma? First, the answer lies in subtle differences in growth pattern, extent of disease and, for practical purposes, the surgical procedure required for removal. Giant condylomata prompt aggressive excision methods, both in the cervix and anus. Secondly, on histologic examination: the complexity of epithelial growth is much more pronounced. Although frank invasion of tissues may not be seen, the complexity of epithelial growth incorporates more underlying stroma with an endophytic pattern.

Differential diagnosis

The three most important exclusions that must be made when considering a diagnosis of anal cancer are the following: (1) Pseudoepitheliomatous hyperplasia, associated with fistula formation or other inflammatory conditions (see Ch. 6). (2) Benign condyloma must be distinguished from giant condyloma or verrucous carcinoma; however, the clinical presentation of the latter is usually sufficiently compelling to dispel any doubts about the diagnosis. (3) Basal cell carcinomas of the perianal skin represent an important exclusion, inasmuch as confusion with basaloid differentiation in an anal cancer would prompt overtreatment (see Ch. 6).

Therapy and outcome

Prognostic factors in squamous cell carcinoma include depth of spread, inguinal lymph node involvement and DNA ploidy. Aneuploidy is associated with a

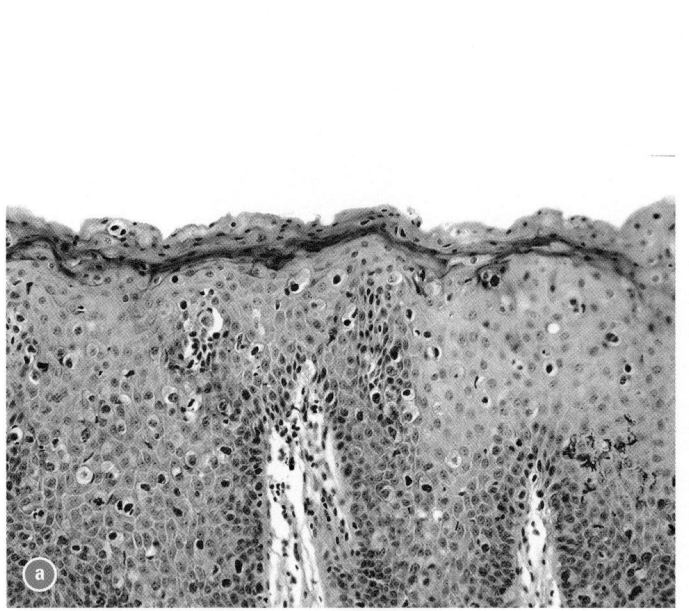

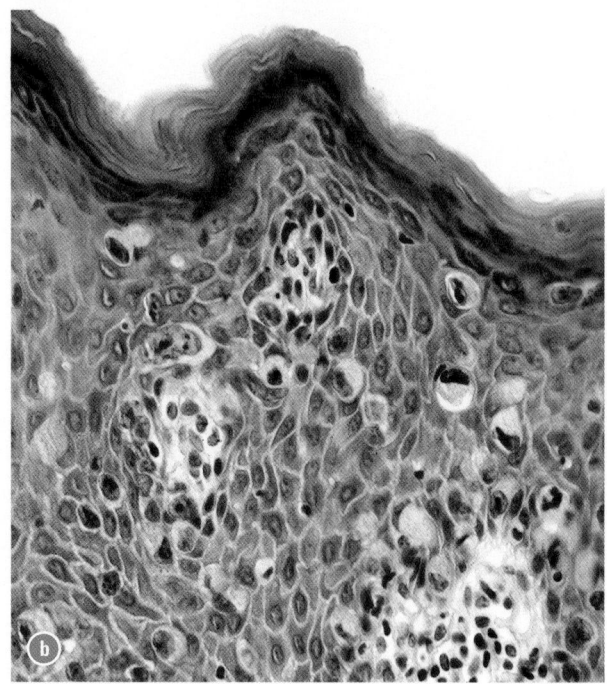

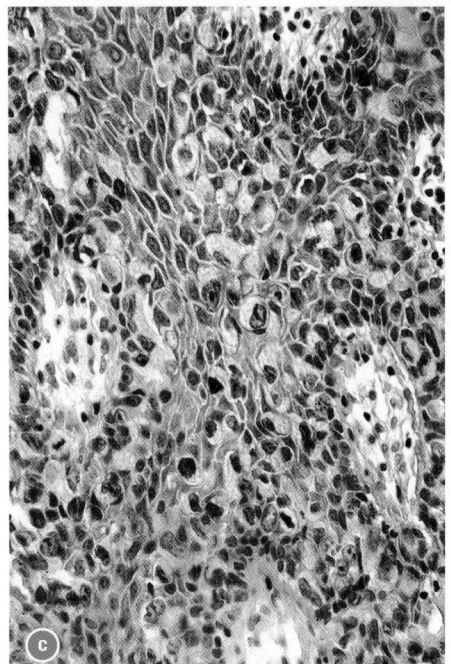

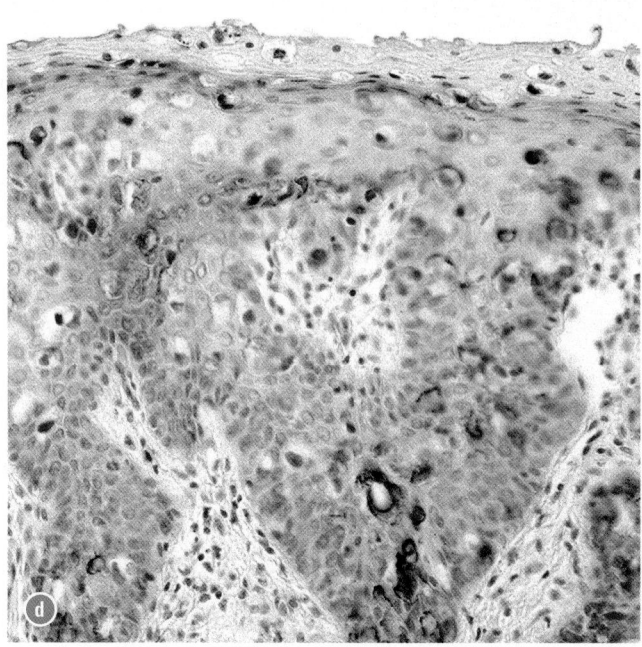

Fig. 10.22 (a) Paget's disease. (b,c) At higher magnification the individual Paget's cells are seen admixed with squamous epithelium. (d) Following staining for CEA.

poorer prognosis and HPV infection (Table 10.3).[94–96] Degree of differentiation also shows some prognostic importance as well, particularly for extremely poorly-differentiated tumors or those with mucinous microcysts. Studies of p53 expression by the tumor have been explored to predict outcome, but the results are conflicting and these markers are not currently used.[97,98] Like most tumors, squamous carcinoma has

a favorable outcome if the nodes are not involved (Table 10.4).[99]

Treatment of squamous cell carcinomas has shifted considerably since the 1970s. While previous therapy included radical excision, a recent survey of the National Cancer Data Base noted that the majority of squamous cell carcinomas in 1993 were treated non-surgically with a combination of chemotherapy (typi-

Table 10.3 *Outcomes of anal HPV infection and morphologic (cytologic/histologic) abnormalities*

Ref.	Baseline	Variable	End point	Comment
96	Normal cytology	HIV+	Abnormal cytology	Risk = 22/100 person years
		+ CD<500		RH = 4.11
		+ HR HPV		RH = 2.54
		+ Smoker		RH = 3.88
96a	LSIL cytology	HIV+	HSIL	62%
		HIV(–)	HSIL	36%
45	H/o Anal Condyloma or benign disease	Homosexual males	HSIL	60% at initial biopsy
			Cancer	3% at initial biopsy

CD, CD5 lymphocytes; HR, high risk; HPV, human papillomavirus, LSIL, low-grade squamous intraepithelial lesion; HSIL, high-grade squamous intraepithelial lesion; RH, relative hazard. H/o, History of
Source: Palefsky et al. (1998)[96a]

cally 5-FU and mitomycin C) and radiotherapy. Combination therapy is recommended by some for tumors exceeding 4.0 cm in size.[100] The rate of colostomy-free survival, disease-free survival and loco-regional control of disease at 5-year follow-up has ranged from mid-60–80% in recent studies, with varied results depending on the stage of tumor. Sparing of the anus and conservation of anal function is achieved in up to 81% of patients.[101–105]

Basal cell carcinoma of the anal margin[32,69]

Basal cell carcinoma (BCC) has been reported in a little over 100 cases in the skin of the anal margin. It has the same histologic appearance as basal cell carcinoma arising in other sides of hair-bearing skin, though it is otherwise thought to arise in areas of sun-exposure (see Ch. 6, Figs 6.36 and 6.37). Less than 1% of BCCs arise in the perianal and genital region. Demographically, a slight male predominance has been reported, with the mean patient age of approximately 70 years. Treatment by wide local excision appears curative in most cases.

The differential diagnosis includes basaloid squamous cell carcinoma, which is clinically a more aggressive disease. Basal cell carcinoma is typically less mitotically active and does not exhibit necrosis, while basaloid squamous cell carcinoma may show less even palisading of cells, more mitoses (including atypical forms) and necrosis. Basal cell carcinoma is reported to stain positively for BerEp4 and negative for epithelial membrane antigen (EMA), carcinoembryonic antigen (CEA) and cytokeratins 13, 19 and 22. Basaloid squamous cell carcinoma has been reported to show the opposite staining pattern.[106]

Adenocarcinoma

Adenocarcinoma of the anal canal is less frequent than squamous cell carcinoma; recent population studies find adenocarcinomas account for approximately 20% of anal cancers.[76,101] The WHO histologic classification subclassifies adenocarcinomas into those arising from the anal canal, anal glands or fistulous tracts.[69]

Table 10.4 *Staging and prognosis for anal squamous carcinomas*

Stage	Definition	Overall 5-year survival (%)
T1/Tx	<2.0 cm	100
T2	2.0–5.0 cm	80
T3	>5.0 cm	85
T4	Invasion of adjacent organs (vagina, urethra, bladder)	92
N0	No nodal metastases	88
N1	Nodal metastases in perirectal lymph node(s)	100
N2	Nodal metastases in unilateral internal iliac and/or inguinal lymph node(s)	67
N3	Nodal metastases in perirectal and inguinal lymph nodes and/or bilateral internal iliac and/or inguinal lymph nodes	83

Source: from Hung et al.[135]

Adenocarcinoma of anal mucosa

Adenocarcinoma of the anal canal most probably represents growth of tumors arising from the columnar absorptive epithelium of the distal rectum. In fact, recent data on the frequency of anal carcinoma note that over half of the adenocarcinomas were found in an area overlapping the anus and rectum so that the true percentage of anal canal adenocarcinomas may be less than the number stated above.[76] Clinically, they may present as a mass, with pain and bleeding. Grossly and histologically they have the appearance of typical colorectal adenocarcinomas.

Anal gland carcinoma

This rare and controversial entity has been postulated to arise from the anal glands and was first proposed in 1934.[107] Since that time, a number of cases have been reported in the literature. Distinct criteria were proposed[108] as (1) location where anal glands are normally present; (2) transition from normal anal gland to carcinoma; (3) interposition of dysplastic epithelium; and (4) a distinctive histologic appearance of small infiltrative glands with scant mucin production. In the two largest series,[109,110] patients had a median age of mid-50s to mid-70s. Patients presented with the sensation of a perianal lump, bleeding, pain, soiling, pruritus, change in bowel habits, prolapse or weight loss. Tumors were present in the ischiorectal space, in the anal canal and in fistula in-ano. Frequently, the tumors were intramuscular in location. Hobbs et al.[111] performed immunohistochemical staining on seven cases of anal gland carcinoma, finding CK7+CK20– in six cases and CK7+CK20+ in one case. These findings strongly suggest that anal gland carcinomas are indeed distinct from colorectal carcinomas. Treatment of anal gland carcinoma includes wide local excision, abdominoperineal resection, radiotherapy and lymph node excision. Epidemiologic and prognostic information is difficult to glean from the limited number of cases, but overall the prognosis of these tumors has been reported to be poor.[109,112–117]

A less well-defined subcategory is extramucosal perianal adenocarcinoma. These tumors do not connect with the anal mucosa; instead, they present usually as perianal or buttock masses. More frequently found in males in their 60s, these tumors are actually slow growing. They are histologically well-differentiated with abundant mucin production. It is believed they may arise from anal ducts, but are also found more in association with chronic fistulas and Crohn's disease.[69]

Adenocarcinoma within a fistula

The development of adenocarcinoma in a fistula is a rare phenomenon.[118] Possible causes of predisposing fistulous disease include anal gland and duct infection, Crohn's disease, or, rarely, infection of congenital abnormalities.[69,110,119–121] Histologically, the tumors are described as arising in the bowel wall with transmural acute and chronic inflammation with granulomata and crypt architectural distortion. Abundant mucin production may be present.

The common theme of adenocarcinomas of the anal region is the difficulty in assigning site of origin. Often it is difficult to demonstrate origin in anal glands and ducts unless an area of transition from normal to dysplastic to frankly malignant epithelium can be found. The anatomy of the anal glands and ducts suggests that the histogenesis of anal gland adenocarcinoma, perianal extramucosal adenocarcinoma and adenocarcinoma within a fistula may find a common route; however, literature on this subject is limited.

Paget's disease

Extramammary Paget's disease (EPD) first appeared in the literature in 1889.[122] It is defined as an intraepithelial adenocarcinoma involving an extramammary squamous epithelium. Paget's disease may be classified as primary (thought to arise from apocrine glands) or secondary (resulting from spread of an underlying adenocarcinoma). The most common extramammary site is the vulva, though cases have been described in the axillae, male external genitalia, perianal skin, external ear canal, eyelid, esophagus and urethra.

Perianal Paget's disease has been described in a few hundred cases, comprising approximately 20% of all cases of extramammary Paget's disease. Patients are usually in their seventh–eighth decade, with no clear gender predilection. Presenting complaints include pruritus, constipation, anal tenderness and rectal bleeding. On physical examination, patients often present with tan to erythematous plaques in the perianal area. Scaling, ulceration or erosion of the skin may be present. The skin lesion may be associated with an underlying mass lesion.

Histologically, the tumor is composed of large malignant cells, varying in size and shape, located in the epidermis. Clustering of malignant cells may occur in the basal portion of the epidermis and invasion of the underlying dermis may be present (Fig. 10.22a–d). The cells contain a large amount of palely eosinophilic grainy or vacuolated cytoplasm, with large vesicular nuclei containing distinct nucleoli. Signet-ring cell morphology and intraepithelial glands have also been described. The tumor often involves the skin appendages. The epidermis often shows changes of hyper-parakeratosis, parakeratosis, acanthosis, papillomatous hyperplasia or fibroepithelioma-like interlacing epidermal lining.[123]

Immunohistochemical staining has been studied to differentiate between primary and secondary Paget's disease.[124–127] Cases that have been reported as primary EPD are generally CK7+CK20–. Cases of secondary EPD, often associated with urothelial and colorectal adenocarcinoma, are usually CK7-CK20. Gross cystic disease fluid protein (GCDFP)-15 positivity has also been reported in primary disease.

The treatment for EPD has been wide local excision with or without skin grafting and abdominoperineal resection. Radiotherapy has also been attempted. Overall survival of patients treated for Paget's disease (both primary and secondary) has been reported to be 59% and 33% at 5 and 10 years, respectively.[128]

Anorectal melanoma

Malignant melanoma of the anorectum is a rare entity that comprises less than 0.5% of colorectal malignancies and 0.4–1.6% of all melanomas. Demographic data from the SEER database from 1973–1992 found the mean age of patients to be 66 years, with a male to female ratio of 1:1.72. A slight trend towards a bimodal age distribution was noted, with an early age peak in young adult males.[129] Patients often present with symptoms of rectal bleeding, pruritus, mass, pain or change in bowel habits. Grossly, the tumor may be at any level of the anal canal, either above or below the dentate line (Fig. 10.23).[130] Histologically, the tumor cells are typical of a melanocytic malignancy, with light gray-blue cytoplasm, large nucleus and often prominent nucleolus. The cells are typically arranged in nests in the squamous mucosa and submucosa, with a variable infiltrate of lymphocytes. Usually, they are acral-lentiginous in type and most commonly epithelioid melanoma, though sarcomatoid and desmoplastic melanoma have also been described. Junctional activity may also be obscured by ulceration. Melanin pigmentation has been noted in one study as present grossly or histologically in 71% of patients.[131]

Immunohistochemically, anorectal melanomas have the same profile as other melanomas, with strong S100 protein positivity and variable staining for HMB-45, Mart-1 (melan-A) and D5. The differential diagnosis of these tumors includes adenocarcinoma with pagetoid spread. Immunohistochemical markers such as cytokeratins may be used in addition to morphology.

The prognosis of these tumors is extremely poor. Presentation with local disease in 37–76%, with loco-regional disease in 11–41% and distant metastases in 15–26% of patients has been reported. Local recurrence does not appear to correlate with gender, size of tumor, depth of invasion, nodal metastases or degree of excision. Distant metastases occur most commonly to the liver, but also to lung, pelvic lymph nodes, bone and brain. The reported 5-year survival rates vary from 0 to 22%.[129–135]

Lymphoma

Extranodal lymphoma of the anorectum is extremely rare, representing 0.1–1.3% of all malignant rectal neoplasms. However, it has become more prevalent with the advent of HIV infection and a number of cases of AIDS-associated anorectal lymphoma have been reported in the literature. Over 40 cases of non-Hodgkin's lymphoma of the anorectum in AIDS patients have been reported in the literature.[69] Most of the patients are male and young to middle-aged adults (27–54 years). The most common presentation is of a painful mass, occasionally as an abscess. Patients often have decreased CD4 counts. Histologically, the tumors are frequently aggressive B-cell tumors; diffuse large B-cell lymphoma or Burkitt's lymphoma. Rare cases of EBV-related Hodgkin's lymphoma have also been reported.

Mesenchymal tumors

Mesenchymal tumors[69] comprise a small percentage of tumors of the anus. Gastrointestinal stromal tumor

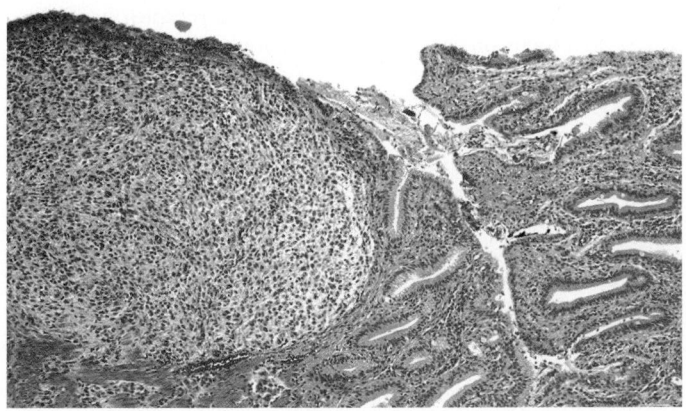

Fig. 10.23 Anal melanoma, left, replacing columnar mucosa, seen on right.

(GIST), leiomyoma, leiomyosarcoma, rhabdomyosarcoma, fibrosarcoma and aggressive angiomyxoma have all been described. In addition, vascular tumors such as hemangioma and lymphangioma have been reported.

References

1 Alexander F, Kay R. Technical considerations in the repair of cloacal vaginal deformities. J Urol 1995; 153:788–791.

2 Pena A. The surgical management of persistent cloaca: results in 54 patients treated with a posterior sagittal approach. J Pediatr Surg 1989; 24:590–598.

3 Warne SA, Wilcox DT, Creighton S, Ransley PG. Long-term gynecological outcome of patients with persistent cloaca. J Urol 2003; 170:1493–1496.

4 Mills PL, Pergament E. Urorectal septal defects in a female and her offspring. Am J Med Genet 1997; 70:250–252.

5 Gale DH, Stocker JT. Cloacal dysgenesis with urethral, vaginal outlet and anal agenesis and functioning internal genitourinary excretion. Pediatr Pathol 1987; 7:457–466.

6 Allen TD, Husmann DA. Cloacal anomalies and other urorectal septal defects in female patients: a spectrum of anatomical abnormalities. J Urol 1991; 145:1034–1039.

7 Hashmi MA, Hashmi S. Anorectal malformations in female children – 10 years experience. J R Coll Surg Edinb 2000; 45:153–158.

8 Escobar LF, Weaver DD, Bixler D, et al. Urorectal septum malformation sequence. Report of six cases and embryological analysis. Am J Dis Child 1987; 141:1021–1024.

9 Currarino G. Large prostatic utricles and related structures, urogenital sinus and other forms of urethrovaginal confluence. J Urol 1986; 136:1270–1279.

10 Mo R, Kim JH, Zhang J, et al. Anorectal malformations caused by defects in sonic hedgehog signaling. Am J Pathol 2001; 159:765–774.

11 Holly EA, Ralston ML, Darragh TM, et al. Prevalence and risk factors for anal squamous intraepithelial lesions in women. J Natl Cancer Inst 2001; 93:843–849.

12 Moscicki AB, Hills NK, Shiboski S, et al. Risk factors for abnormal anal cytology in young heterosexual women. Cancer Epidemiol Biomarkers Prev 1999; 8:173–178.

13 Daling JR, Weiss NS, Hislop TG, et al. Sexual practices, sexually transmitted diseases and the incidence of anal cancer. N Engl J Med 1987; 317:973–977.

14 Piketty C, Darragh TM, Da Costa M, et al. High prevalence of anal human papillomavirus infection and anal cancer precursors among HIV-infected persons in the absence of anal intercourse. Ann Intern Med 2003; 138:453–459.

15 Chin-Hong PV, Palefsky JM. Natural history and clinical management of anal human papillomavirus disease in men and women infected with human immunodeficiency virus. Clin Infect Dis 2002; 35:1127–1134.

16 Kulaylat MN, Doerr RJ, Neuwirth M, Satchidanand SK. Anal duct/gland cyst: report of a case and review of the literature. Dis Colon Rectum 1998; 41:103–110.

17 Cataldo PA, MacKeigan JM. The necessity of routine pathologic evaluation of hemorrhoidectomy specimens. Surg Gynecol Obstet 1992; 174:302–304.

18 Groisman GM, Polak-Charcon S. Fibroepithelial polyps of the anus: a histologic, immunohistochemical and ultrastructural study, including comparison with the normal anal subepithelial layer. Am J Surg Pathol 1998; 22:70–76.

19 Wiltz O, Schoetz DJ Jr, Murray JJ, et al. Perianal hidradenitis suppurativa. The Lahey Clinic experience. Dis Colon Rectum 1990; 33:731–734.

20 Ambroze WL Jr, Pemberton JH, Dozois RR, et al. The histological pattern and pathological involvement of the anal transition zone in patients with ulcerative colitis. Gastroenterology 1993; 104:514–518.

21 Horai T, Kusunoki M, Shoji Y, et al. Clinicopathological study of anorectal mucosa in total colectomy with mucosal proctectomy and ileoanal anastomosis. Eur J Surg 1994; 160:233–238.

22 O'Riordain MG, Fazio VW, Lavery IC, et al. Incidence and natural history of dysplasia of the anal transitional zone after ileal pouch-anal anastomosis: results of a five-year to ten-year follow-up. Dis Colon Rectum 2000; 43:1660–1665.

23 Wax JR, Pinette MG, Cartin A, Blackstone J. Female reproductive health after ileal pouch anal anastomosis for ulcerative colitis. Obstet Gynecol Surv 2003; 58:270–274.

24 Olsen KO, Juul S, Bulow S, et al. Female fecundity before and after operation for familial adenomatous polyposis. Br J Surg 2003; 90:227–231.

25 Oresland T, Palmblad S, Ellstrom M, et al. Gynaecological and sexual function related to anatomical changes in the female pelvis after restorative proctocolectomy. Int J Colorectal Dis 1994; 9:77–81.

26 Hernandez-Magro PM, Villanueva Saenz E, Alvarez-Tostado Fernandez F, et al. Endoanal sonography in the assessment of perianal endometriosis with external anal sphincter involvement. J Clin Ultrasound 2002; 30:245–248.

27 Kanellos I, Kelpis T, Zaraboukas T, Betsis D. Perineal endometriosis in episiotomy scar with anal sphincter involvement. Tech Coloproctol 2001; 5:107–108.

28 Dougherty LS, Hull T. Perineal endometriosis with anal sphincter involvement: report of a case. Dis Colon Rectum 2000; 43:1157–1160.

29 Da Silva GM, Berho M, Wexner SD, et al. Histologic analysis of the irradiated anal sphincter. Dis Colon Rectum 2003; 46:1492–1497.

30 Sayfan J. Ergotamine-induced anorectal strictures: report of five cases. Dis Colon Rectum 2002; 45:271–272.

31 Offidani A, Campanati A. Papillary hidradenoma: immunohistochemical analysis of steroid receptor profile with a focus on apocrine differentiation. J Clin Pathol 1999; 52:829–832.

32 Weedon D. Skin pathology. London: Churchill Livingstone; 2002.

33 Barnhill RL. Textbook of dermatopathology. London: McGraw-Hill Health Professions Division; 1998.

34 Cohen MG, Greenwald ML, Garbus JE, Zager JS. Granular cell tumor – a unique neoplasm of the internal anal sphincter: report of a case. Dis Colon Rectum 2000; 43:1444–1447.

35 Penn I. Cancers of the anogenital region in renal transplant recipients. Analysis of 65 cases. Cancer 1986; 58:611–616.

36 Ogunbiyi OA, Scholefield JH, Robertson G, et al. Anal human papillomavirus infection and squamous

neoplasia in patients with invasive vulvar cancer. Obstet Gynecol 1994; 83:212–216.

37 Tseng HF, Morgenstern H, Mack TM, Peters RK. Risk factors for anal cancer: results of a population-based case – control study. Cancer Causes Control 2003; 14:837–846.

38 Palefsky JM, Holly EA, Ralston ML, et al. Prevalence and risk factors for anal human papillomavirus infection in human immunodeficiency virus (HIV)-positive and high-risk HIV-negative women. J Infect Dis 2001; 183:383–391.

39 Hillemanns P, Ellerbrock TV, McPhillips S, et al. Prevalence of anal human papillomavirus infection and anal cytologic abnormalities in HIV-seropositive women. AIDS 1996; 10:1641–1647.

40 Sun XW, Kuhn L, Ellerbrock TV, et al. Human papillomavirus infection in women infected with the human immunodeficiency virus. N Engl J Med 1997; 337:1343–1349.

41 Frisch M, Biggar RJ, Goedert JJ. Human papillomavirus-associated cancers in patients with human immunodeficiency virus infection and acquired immunodeficiency syndrome. J Nat Can Inst 2000; 92:1500–1510.

42 van der Snoek EM, Niesters HG, Mulder PG, et al. Human papillomavirus infection in men who have sex with men participating in a Dutch gay-cohort study. Sex Transm Dis 2003; 30:639–644.

43 Melbye M, Smith E, Wohlfahrt J, et al. Anal and cervical abnormality in women – prediction by human papillomavirus tests. Int J Cancer 1996; 68:559–564.

44 Williams AB, Darragh TM, Vranizan K, et al. Anal and cervical human papillomavirus infection and risk of anal and cervical epithelial abnormalities in human immunodeficiency virus-infected women. Obstet Gynecol 1994; 83:205–211.

45 Goldstone SE, Winkler B, Ufford LJ, et al. High prevalence of anal squamous intraepithelial lesions and squamous-cell carcinoma in men who have sex with men as seen in a surgical practice. Dis Colon Rectum 2001; 44:690–698.

46 Jay N, Berry JM, Hogeboom CJ, et al. Colposcopic appearance of anal squamous intraepithelial lesions: relationship to histopathology. Dis Colon Rectum 1997; 40:919–928.

47 Beck DE, Fazio VW, Jagelman DG, Lavery IC. Perianal Bowen's disease. Dis Colon Rectum 1988; 31:419–422.

48 Sarmiento JM, Wolff BG, Burgart LJ, et al. Perianal Bowen's disease: associated tumors, human papillomavirus, surgery and other controversies. Dis Colon Rectum 1997; 40:912–918.

49 Rock B, Shah KV, Farmer ER. A morphologic, pathologic, and virologic study of anogenital warts in men. Arch Dermatol 1992; 128:495–500.

50 Metcalf AM, Dean T. Risk of dysplasia in anal condyloma. Surgery 1995; 118:724–726.

51 Friis S, Kjaer SK, Frisch M, et al. Cervical intraepithelial neoplasia, anogenital cancer and other cancer types in women after hospitalization for condylomata acuminata. J Infect Dis 1997; 175:743–748.

52 Palefsky JM, Holly EA, Ralston ML, et al. High incidence of anal high-grade squamous intra-epithelial lesions among HIV-positive and HIV-negative homosexual and bisexual men. AIDS 1998; 12:495–503.

53 Marchesa P, Fazio VW, Oliart S, et al. Perianal Bowen's disease: a clinicopathologic study of 47 patients. Dis Colon Rectum 1997; 40:1286–1293.

54 Cleary RK, Schaldenbrand JD, Fowler JJ, et al. Perianal Bowen's disease and anal intraepithelial neoplasia: review of the literature. Dis Colon Rectum 1999; 42:945–951.

55 Chang GJ, Berry JM, Jay N, et al. Surgical treatment of high-grade anal squamous intraepithelial lesions: a prospective study. Dis Colon Rectum 2002; 45:453–458.

56 Carter PS, Sheffield JP, Shepherd N, et al. Interobserver variation in the reporting of the histopathological grading of anal intraepithelial neoplasia. J Clin Pathol 1994; 47:1032–1034.

57 Colquhoun P, Nogueras JJ, Dipasquale B, et al. Interobserver and intraobserver bias exists in the interpretation of anal dysplasia. Dis Colon Rectum 2003; 46:1332–1338.

58 Carter JJ, Madeleine MM, Shera K, et al. Human papillomavirus 16 and 18 L1 serology compared across anogenital cancer sites. Cancer Res 2001; 61:1934–1940.

59 Skinner PP, Ogunbiyi OA, Scholefield JH, et al. Skin appendage involvement in anal intraepithelial neoplasia. Br J Surg 1997; 84:675–678.

60 Sobhani I, Vuagnat A, Walker F, et al. Prevalence of high-grade dysplasia and cancer in the anal canal in human papillomavirus-infected individuals. Gastroenterology 2001; 120:857–866.

61 Palefsky JM, Holly EA, Ralston ML, et al. Effect of highly active antiretroviral therapy on the natural history of anal squamous intraepithelial lesions and anal human papillomavirus infection. J Acquir Immune Defic Syndr 2001; 28:422–428.

62 Lillo FB, Ferrari D, Veglia F, et al. Human papillomavirus infection and associated cervical disease in human immunodeficiency virus-infected women: effect of highly active antiretroviral therapy. J Infect Dis 2001; 184:547–551.

63 Calore EE, Nadal SR, Manzione CR, et al. Expression of Ki-67 can assist in predicting recurrences of low-grade anal intraepithelial neoplasia in AIDS. Dis Colon Rectum 2001; 44:534–537.

64 Ogunbiyi OA, Scholefield JH, Smith JH, et al. Immunohistochemical analysis of p53 expression in anal squamous neoplasia. J Clin Pathol 1993; 46:507–512.

65 Mullerat J, Deroide F, Winslet MC, Perrett CW. Proliferation and p53 expression in anal cancer precursor lesions. Anticancer Res 2003; 23:2995–2999.

66 Caruso ML, Valentini AM. Localization of p53 protein and human papillomavirus in laryngeal squamous lesions. Anticancer Res 1997; 17:4671–4675.

67 Litle VR, Leavenworth JD, Darragh TM, et al. Angiogenesis, proliferation and apoptosis in anal high-grade squamous intraepithelial lesions. Dis Colon Rectum 2000; 43:346–352.

68 Scholefield JH, Ogunbiyi OA, Smith JH, et al. Treatment of anal intraepithelial neoplasia. Br J Surg 1994; 81:1238–1240.

69 Aaltonen LA, Hamilton SR, World Health Organization. International Agency for Research on Cancer. Pathology and genetics of tumours of the digestive system. Oxford: IARC Press; 2000.

70 Hughes ESR, Cuthbertson AM, Killingback MK. Colorectal surgery. London: Churchill Livingstone; 1983.

71 Wexner SD, Milsom JW, Dailey TH. The demographics of anal cancers are changing. Identification of a high-risk population. Dis Colon Rectum 1987; 30:942–946.

72 Kodner IJ, Fry RD, Roe JP. Colon, rectal and anal surgery: current techniques and controversies. St Louis, MO: Mosby; 1985.

73 Wellman KF. Adenocarcinoma of anal duct origin. Can J Surg 1962; 5:311–318.

74 Longo WE, Vernava AM 3rd, Wade TP, et al. Rare anal canal cancers in the U.S. veteran: patterns of disease and results of treatment. Am Surg 1995; 61:495–500.

75 Maggard MA, Beanes SR, Ko CY. Anal canal cancer: a population-based reappraisal. Dis Colon Rectum 2003; 46:1517–1524.

76 Myerson RJ, Karnell LH, Menck HR. The National Cancer Data Base report on carcinoma of the anus. Cancer 1997; 80:805–815.

77 Holmes F, Borek D, Owen-Kummer M, et al. Anal cancer in women. Gastroenterology 1988; 95:107–111.

78 Frisch M, Glimelius B, van den Brule AJ, et al. Benign anal lesions, inflammatory bowel disease and risk for high-risk human papillomavirus-positive and -negative anal carcinoma. Br J Cancer 1998; 78:1534–1538.

79 Frisch M, Olsen JH, Bautz A, Melbye M. Benign anal lesions and the risk of anal cancer. N Engl J Med 1994; 331:300–302.

80 Lin AY, Gridley G, Tucker M. Benign anal lesions and anal cancer. N Engl J Med 1995; 332:190–191.

81 Vincent-Salomon A, de la Rochefordiere A, Salmon R, et al. Frequent association of human papillomavirus 16 and 18 DNA with anal squamous cell and basaloid carcinoma. Mod Pathol 1996; 9:614–620.

82 Youk EG, Ku JL, Park JG. Detection and typing of human papillomavirus in anal epidermoid carcinomas: sequence variation in the E7 gene of human papillomavirus Type 16. Dis Colon Rectum 2001; 44:236–242.

83 Zaki SR, Judd R, Coffield LM, et al. Human papillomavirus infection and anal carcinoma. Retrospective analysis by in situ hybridization and the polymerase chain reaction. Am J Pathol 1992; 140:1345–1355.

84 Frisch M, Fenger C, van den Brule AJ, et al. Variants of squamous cell carcinoma of the anal canal and perianal skin and their relation to human papillomaviruses. Cancer Res 1999; 59:753–757.

85 Goldman S, Glimelius B, Pahlman L, et al. Anal epidermoid carcinoma: a population-based clinico-pathological study of 164 patients. Int J Colorectal Dis 1988; 3:109–118.

86 Fenger C, Frisch M, Jass JJ, et al. Anal cancer subtype reproducibility study. Virchows Arch 2000; 436:229–233.

87 Beckmann AM, Daling JR, Sherman KJ, et al. Human papillomavirus infection and anal cancer. Int J Cancer 1989; 43:1042–1049.

88 Aparicio-Duque R, Mittal KR, Chan W, Schinella R. Cloacogenic carcinoma of the anal canal and associated viral lesions. An in situ hybridization study for human papilloma virus. Cancer 1991; 68:2422–2425.

89 Higgins GD, Uzelin DM, Phillips GE, et al. Differing characteristics of human papillomavirus RNA-positive and RNA-negative anal carcinomas. Cancer 1991; 68:561–567.

90 Olofinlade O, Adeonigbagbe O, Gualtieri N, et al. Anal carcinoma: a 15-year retrospective analysis. Scand J Gastroenterol 2000; 35:1194–1199.

91 Wolber R, Dupuis B, Thiyagaratnam P, Owen D. Anal cloacogenic and squamous carcinomas. Comparative histologic analysis using in situ hybridization for human papillomavirus DNA. Am J Surg Pathol 1990; 14:176–182.

92 Behrendt GC, Hansmann ML. Carcinomas of the anal canal and anal margin differ in their expression of cadherin, cytokeratins and p53. Virchows Arch 2001; 439:782–786.

93 Trombetta LJ, Place RJ. Giant condyloma acuminatum of the anorectum: trends in epidemiology and management: report of a case and review of the literature. Dis Colon Rectum 2001; 44:1878–1886.

94 Shepherd NA, Scholefield JH, Love SB, et al. Prognostic factors in anal squamous carcinoma: a multivariate analysis of clinical, pathological and flow cytometric parameters in 235 cases. Histopathology 1990; 16:545–555.

95 Noffsinger AE, Hui YZ, Suzuk L, et al. The relationship of human papillomavirus to proliferation and ploidy in carcinoma of the anus. Cancer 1995; 75:958–967.

96 Durante AJ, Williams AB, Da Costa M, et al. Incidence of anal cytological abnormalities in a cohort of human immunodeficiency virus-infected women. Cancer Epidemiol Biomarkers Prev 2003; 12(7):638–642.

96a. Palefsky JM, Holly EA, Hogeboom CJ, et al. Virologic, immunologic, and clinical parameters in the incidence and progression of anal squamous intraepithelial lesions in HIV-positive and HIV-negative homosexual men. J Acquir Immun Defic Syndr Hum Retroviral 1998; 17(4):314–319.

97 Bonin SR, Pajak TF, Russell AH, et al. Overexpression of p53 protein and outcome of patients treated with chemoradiation for carcinoma of the anal canal: a report of randomized trial RTOG 87–04. Radiation Therapy Oncology Group. Cancer 1999; 85:1226–1233.

98 Wong CS, Tsao MS, Sharma V, et al. Prognostic role of p53 protein expression in epidermoid carcinoma of the anal canal. Int J Radiat Oncol Biol Phys 1999; 45:309–314.

99 Schlienger M, Krzisch C, Pene F, et al. Epidermoid carcinoma of the anal canal treatment results and prognostic variables in a series of 242 cases. Int J Radiat Oncol Biol Phys 1989; 17(6):1141–1151.

100 Touboul E, Schlienger M, Buffat L, et al. Epidermoid carcinoma of the anal canal. Results of curative-intent radiation therapy in a series of 270 patients. Cancer 1994; 73:1569–1579.

101 Klas JV, Rothenberger DA, Wong WD, Madoff RD. Malignant tumors of the anal canal: the spectrum of disease, treatment and outcomes. Cancer 1999; 85:1686–1693.

102 Faynsod M, Vargas HI, Tolmos J, et al. Patterns of recurrence in anal canal carcinoma. Arch Surg 2000; 135:1090–1095.

103 Peiffert D, Giovannini M, Ducreux M, et al. High-dose radiation therapy and neoadjuvant plus concomitant chemotherapy with 5-fluorouracil and cisplatin in patients with locally advanced squamous-cell anal canal cancer: final results of a phase II study. Ann Oncol 2001; 12:397–404.

104 Kapp KS, Geyer E, Gebhart FH, et al. Experience with split-course external beam irradiation +/– chemotherapy and integrated Ir-192 high-dose-rate brachytherapy in the

treatment of primary carcinomas of the anal canal. Int J Radiat Oncol Biol Phys 2001; 49:997–1005.

105 Mitchell SE, Mendenhall WM, Zlotecki RA, Carroll RR. Squamous cell carcinoma of the anal canal. Int J Radiat Oncol Biol Phys 2001; 49:1007–1013.

106 Alvarez-Canas MC, Fernandez FA, Rodilla IG, Val-Bernal JF. Perianal basal cell carcinoma: a comparative histologic, immunohistochemical and flow cytometric study with basaloid carcinoma of the anus. Am J Dermatopathol 1996; 18:371–379.

107 Rosser C. The relation of fistula in ano to cancer of the anal canal. Trans Am Proct Soc 1934; 35:65–70.

108 Fenger C, Morson BC. Anal duct carcinoma. Dis Colon Rectum 1989; 32:355–357.

109 Jensen SL, Shokouh-Amiri MH, Hagen K, et al. Adenocarcinoma of the anal ducts. A series of 21 cases. Dis Colon Rectum 1988; 31:268–272.

110 Abel ME, Chiu YS, Russell TR, Volpe PA. Adenocarcinoma of the anal glands. Results of a survey. Dis Colon Rectum 1993; 36:383–387.

111 Hobbs CM, Lowry MA, Owen D, Sobin LH. Anal gland carcinoma. Cancer 2001; 92:2045–2049.

112 Timaran CH, Sangwan YP, Solla JA. Adenocarcinoma in a hemorrhoidectomy specimen: case report and review of the literature. Am Surg 2000; 66:789–792.

113 Hagihara P, Vazquez MD, Parker JC Jr, Griffen WO. Carcinoma of anal-ductal origin: report of a case. Dis Colon Rectum 1976; 19:694–701.

114 Parks TG. Mucus-secreting adenocarcinoma of anal gland origin. Br J Surg 1970; 57:434–436.

115 Winkelman J, Grosfeld J, Bigelow B. Colloid carcinoma of anal-gland origin. Report of a case and review of the literature. Am J Clin Pathol 1964; 42:395–401.

116 Wong AY, Rahilly MA, Adams W, Lee CS. Mucinous anal gland carcinoma with perianal Pagetoid spread. Pathology 1998; 30:1–3.

117 Behan WM, Burnett RA. Adenocarcinoma of the anal glands. J Clin Pathol 1996; 49:1009–1011.

118 Getz SB Jr, Ough YD, Patterson RB, Kovalcik PJ. Mucinous adenocarcinoma developing in chronic anal fistula: report of two cases and review of the literature. Dis Colon Rectum 1981; 24:562–566.

119 Anthony T, Simmang C, Lee EL, Turnage RH. Perianal mucinous adenocarcinoma. J Surg Oncol 1997; 64:218–221.

120 Ky A, Sohn N, Weinstein MA, Korelitz BI. Carcinoma arising in anorectal fistulas of Crohn's disease. Dis Colon Rectum 1998; 41:992–996.

121 Basik M, Rodriguez-Bigas MA, Penetrante R, Petrelli NJ. Prognosis and recurrence patterns of anal adenocarcinoma. Am J Surg 1995; 169:233–237.

122 Crocker HR. Paget's disease affecting the scrotum and penis. Trans Pathol Soc Lond 1888–1889; 40:187–191.

123 Brainard JA, Hart WR. Proliferative epidermal lesions associated with anogenital Paget's disease. Am J Surg Pathol 2000; 24:543–552.

124 Ohnishi T, Watanabe S. The use of cytokeratins 7 and 20 in the diagnosis of primary and secondary extramammary Paget's disease. Br J Dermatol 2000; 142:243–247.

125 Lundquist K, Kohler S, Rouse RV. Intraepidermal cytokeratin 7 expression is not restricted to Paget cells but is also seen in Toker cells and Merkel cells. Am J Surg Pathol 1999; 23:212–219.

126 Nowak MA, Guerriere-Kovach P, Pathan A, et al. Perianal Paget's disease: distinguishing primary and secondary lesions using immunohistochemical studies including gross cystic disease fluid protein-15 and cytokeratin 20 expression. Arch Pathol Lab Med 1998; 122:1077–1081.

127 Miller LR, McCunniff AJ, Randall ME. An immunohistochemical study of perianal Paget's disease. Possible origins and clinical implications. Cancer 1992; 69:2166–2171.

128 McCarter MD, Quan SH, Busam K, et al. Long-term outcome of perianal Paget's disease. Dis Colon Rectum 2003; 46:612–616.

129 Cagir B, Whiteford MH, Topham A, et al. Changing epidemiology of anorectal melanoma. Dis Colon Rectum 1999; 42:1203–1208.

130 Roumen RM. Anorectal melanoma in The Netherlands: a report of 63 patients. Eur J Surg Oncol 1996; 22:598–601.

131 Brady MS, Kavolius JP, Quan SH. Anorectal melanoma. A 64-year experience at Memorial Sloan-Kettering Cancer Center. Dis Colon Rectum 1995; 38:146–151.

132 Weyandt GH, Eggert AO, Houf M, et al. Anorectal melanoma: surgical management guidelines according to tumour thickness. Br J Cancer 2003; 89:2019–2022.

133 Weinstock MA. Epidemiology and prognosis of anorectal melanoma. Gastroenterology 1993; 104:174–178.

134 Thibault C, Sagar P, Nivatvongs S, et al. Anorectal melanoma – an incurable disease? Dis Colon Rectum 1997; 40:661–668.

135 Hung A, Crane C, Delclos M, et al. Cisplatin-based combined modality therapy for anal carcinoma, a wider therapeutic index. Cancer 2003; 97:1195–1202.

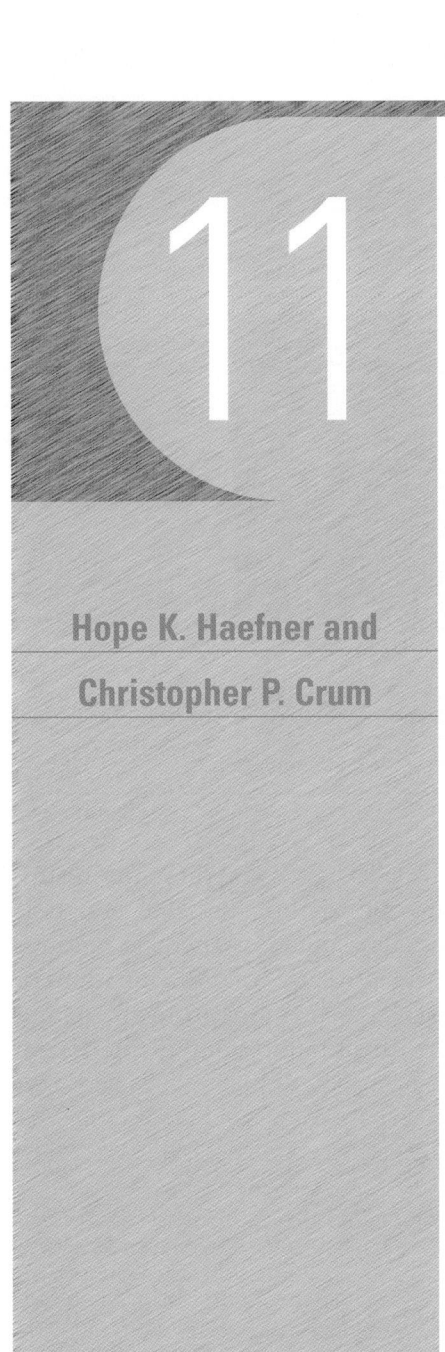

11

Benign conditions of the vagina

Hope K. Haefner and

Christopher P. Crum

Introduction

Benign vaginal epithelial changes occurring in older women

Vaginal prolapse
Atrophic vaginitis
Radiation-induced atrophy

Benign lesions following hysterectomy

Granulation tissue
Prolapse of the fallopian tube

Adenosis and columnar metaplasia

Adenosis
Benign columnar cells in the vagina
Cysts of the vagina

Endometriosis

Fibroepithelial polyps of the lower female genital tract

Traumatic lesions

Traumatic injury
Tampon ulcers
Other traumatic lesions

Infections of systemic importance

Group B streptococcus
Toxic shock syndrome

Rare infections

Malakoplakia
Tuberculosis
Inflammatory lesions of unknown etiology

Emphysematous vaginitis

Introduction

Both the anatomy and histology of the vagina vary throughout life. Traditionally, the vagina is divided into thirds – upper, middle and lower third, utilizing pelvic, fascial and muscular planes. The mucous membrane of the vagina is covered by a stratified, squamous, non-keratinizing epithelium. In the normal reproductive age women with cyclic menses, the superficial epithelium is glycogenized, with maximum amounts of glycogen appearing during ovulation (Fig. 11.1).

The squamous epithelium is composed of four layers.[1] (1) The basal layer is a generative layer with minimal cell turnover, attached to the basement membrane. (2) Above this is the suprabasal layer with larger round cells containing desmosomes. At the interface of this layer and the basal layer, the second layer of cells undergo transient DNA proliferation in preparation, which defines the cell population destined for differentiation (Fig. 11.2). (3) The upper intermediate layer contains large, rounded and somewhat flattened cells with glycogen. (4) The final layer is the superficial layer containing small dense nuclei (Fig. 11.1).

Benign vaginal epithelial changes occurring in older women

VAGINAL PROLAPSE

The most common alterations of the vaginal mucosa occur as a consequence of prolapse and atrophy. Vaginal prolapse is due to loss of support of the ligaments that suspend the vagina, usually as a consequence of prior pregnancies. Signs and symptoms of vaginal prolapse include 'fullness' in the region of the bladder, vagina and rectum, lower abdominal discomfort and backache, vaginal discharge and, most notably, increased frequency of urination and inadequate bladder emptying.

The pathologist usually encounters vaginal specimens from patients with prolapse during the evaluation of routine vaginal hysterectomies. The histopathologic findings in prolapse typically include mild epithelial acanthosis and hyperkeratosis (Fig. 11.3). If epithelial erosion has taken place, reparative changes are also present and can be seen on cytologic evaluation of prolapse.[2] Similar findings are seen in patients that are using pessaries. The pathologist who is familiar with

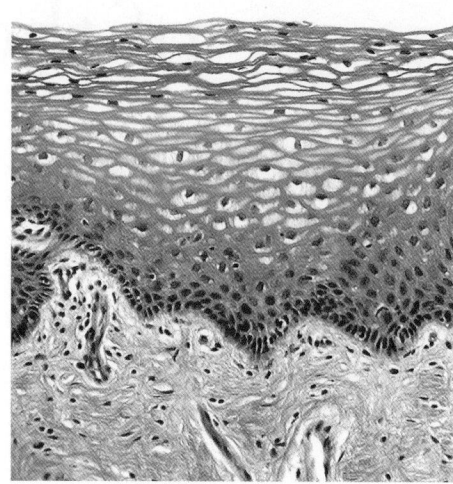

Fig. 11.1 Normal squamous mucosa of the vagina.

these findings will usually have little difficulty distinguishing them from vaginal intraepithelial neoplasia (VAIN) (see Ch. 12), inasmuch as there is minimal nuclear atypia. In the presence of inflammation or repair, excluding VAIN may be more problematic, but can be done easily with immunostaining for p16, if needed.

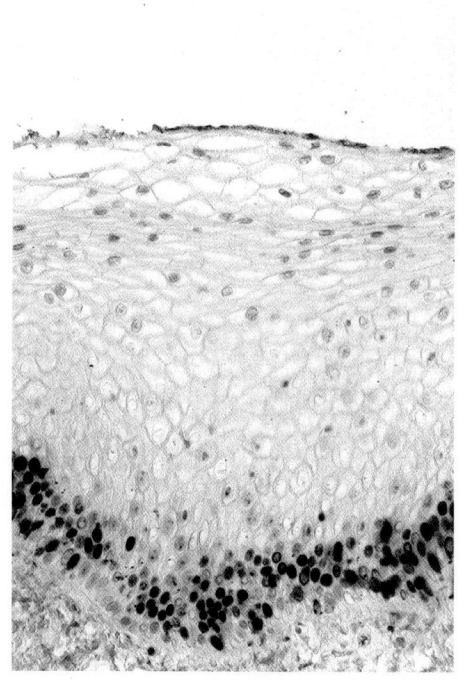

Fig. 11.2 Immunostaining of normal mucosa for Ki-67. Expression highlights nuclei just above the basal layer. This population is destined to undergo maturation.

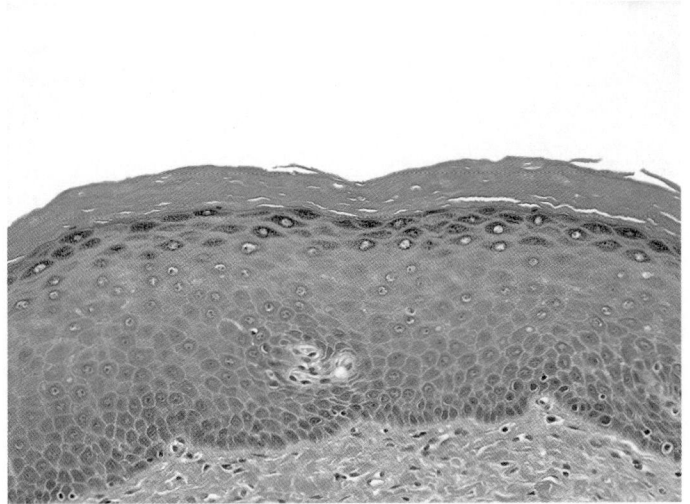

Fig. 11.3 Histologic findings in prolapse. The most prominent are mild thickening of the epithelium (acanthosis) and hyperkeratosis.

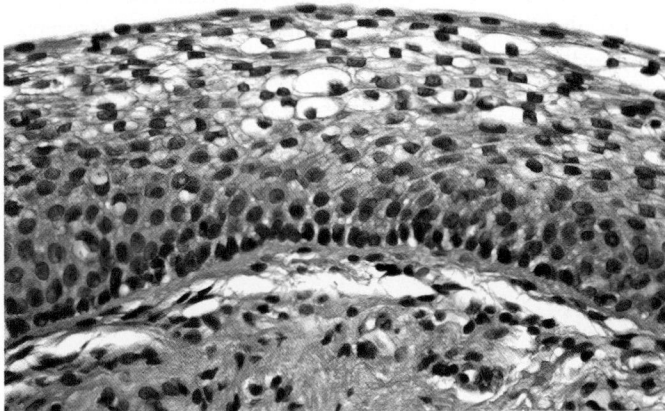

Fig. 11.4 Mucosal atrophy of the vagina. Maturation is delayed, with an increased nuclear/cytoplasmic ratio.

The principal consequence of prolapse is the symptomatic discomfort of the patients. Cancer has been reported in association with vaginal prolapse but is extremely rare and not considered a risk with this disorder.[3]

ATROPHIC VAGINITIS

Atrophic vaginitis occurs most commonly post menopause, when estrogen levels are low and no longer support glycogenization of the vaginal epithelium. However, it is also common in the reproductive years post-partum during breast-feeding. Typically the vaginal pH is weakly acidic or alkaline (most often over 5.0) and the wet prep contains a profuse number of parabasal cells and inflammatory cells. Symptoms include vaginal dryness, itching, and vulvodynia (most often localized vulvodynia).

The classic appearance of atrophic vaginitis on gross examination is small punctuate hemorrhages in the mucosa. A serosanguineous or watery discharge may be present and a wet prep reveals parabasal cells and PMNs. Cytologic smears may be difficult to interpret because parabasal cells with an increased nuclear/cytoplasmic ratio predominate.[4] These patients are often referred for colposcopy, revealing a thin friable vaginal epithelium with enhancement of the underlying vasculature. Lugol's solution uptake is minimal (due to the lack of estrogen-induced glycogen in the epithelium), resulting in a diffuse light brown-to-yellow color.[5]

The histopathology of atrophic vaginitis is characteristic of a non-glycogenized epithelium (Fig. 11.4).

The epithelium may be attenuated, composed of no more than 4–6 cell layers, but may be normal in thickness, with uniform, slightly pale to homogeneous nuclei and smoothly-uniform appearing chromatin. If coexisting inflammation is present, the distinction between atrophic vaginitis and VAIN may be difficult, but can be easily made by immunostaining for a proliferative marker such as Ki-67 (see Ch. 12). In general, atrophic vaginitis is more problematic clini-

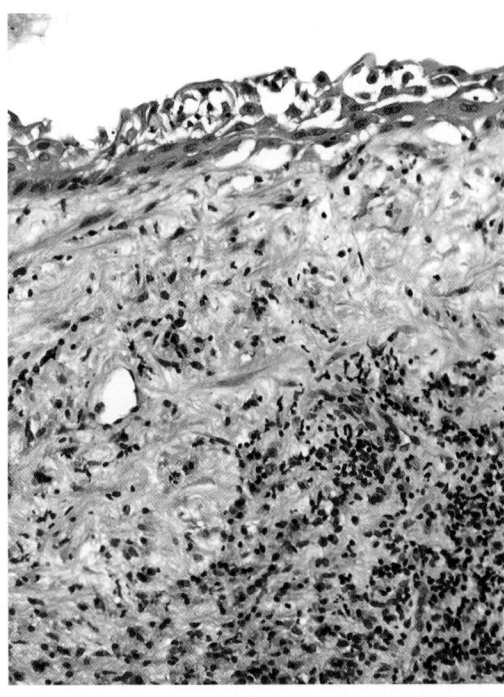

Fig. 11.5 Atrophic vaginitis. The epithelium is attenuated and coexists with a mononuclear submucosal inflammatory infiltrate.

cally, colposcopically and cytologically than histologically (Fig. 11.5)

The treatment of vaginal atrophy is hormone therapy. Many alternatives exist including estrogenic preparations administered vaginally (e.g. creams, tablets and the estradiol-releasing ring)[6] as well as oral hormone therapy. Vaginal moisturizers and lubricants may also be beneficial.[7] Following estrogen replacement, parabasal cells will mature into intermediate and superficial squamous cells, returning to a normal colposcopic appearance.

RADIATION-INDUCED ATROPHY

Radiation therapy for cervical, vaginal, and occasionally endometrial cancers can have serious consequences. The vaginal mucosa tends to be thin and friable, characteristic of atrophy, and colposcopic evaluation can be difficult. Typically, there is minimal uptake of Lugol's solution, a sign of poorly glycogenized epithelium. Irregular vessels may appear, making interpretation difficult. Papanicolaou smear changes of radiation therapy can be confused with either vaginal intra-epithelial neoplasia or cancer on cytologic interpretation. These changes include cytoplasmic vacuolization, nuclear enlargement and multinucleation (Fig. 11.6).[8] However, the nuclear:cytoplasmic ratio remains low and chromatin remains smooth, rather than coarse.

In addition to the atrophic changes, radiation induces ischemic changes via its effects on the vasculature. In severe cases, superficial necrosis and repair are present (Fig. 11.7).

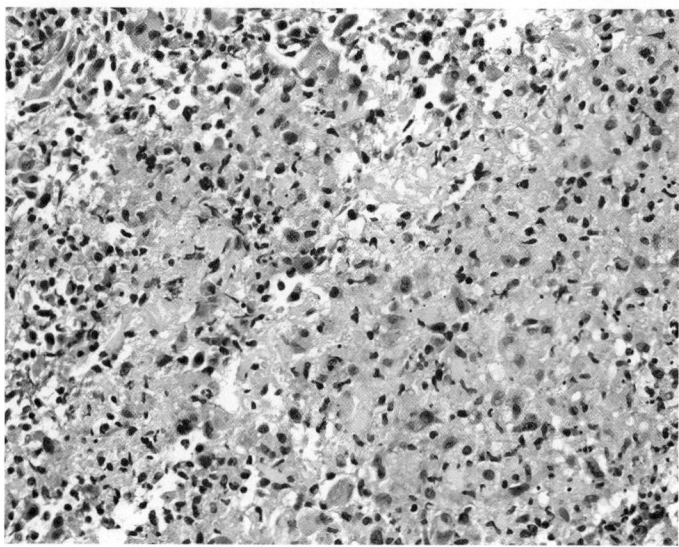

Fig. 11.7 Radiation-induced necrosis.

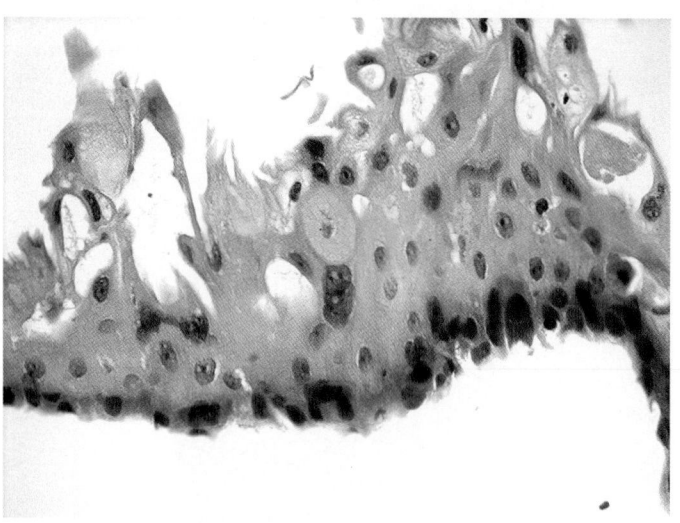

Fig. 11.6 Radiation-induced atypia, characterized by nuclear enlargement, cytoplasmic vacuoles and abundant cytoplasm in the epithelial cells.

Benign lesions following hysterectomy

Benign lesions following hysterectomy include the following, in decreasing order of frequency.

GRANULATION TISSUE

Granulation tissue is a common cause of post-surgery vaginal bleeding and frequently is biopsied, particularly if concerns stem from a prior surgical procedure for a neoplasm. Typically, granulation tissue appears as a raised red, lobular lesion in the upper vagina near or within the sutured cuff. The histologic features are characteristic, with abundant vascular growth, epithelial erosion and intense inflammation (Figs 11.8, 11.9) The process evolves (heals) over time, with a greater proportion of the lesion being occupied by fibrous tissue with less-prominent vessels.

PROLAPSE OF THE FALLOPIAN TUBE

Tubal prolapse occasionally occurs following a hysterectomy, when the tubes are fixed near the apex of the vaginal cuff. It most commonly follows vaginal hysterectomy, but also with an abdominal hysterectomy if the tubes are spared.[9,10] A small nodule resembling granulation tissue is visible at the vaginal apex. The biopsy discloses tubal plicae with a bland tubal epithelial lining

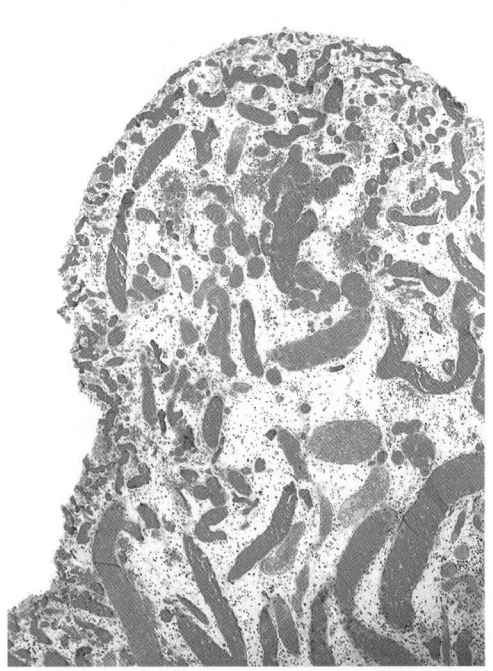

Fig. 11.8 Granulation tissue. In this low-power photomicrograph, the vessels are prominent, but the endothelial cells are less conspicuous.

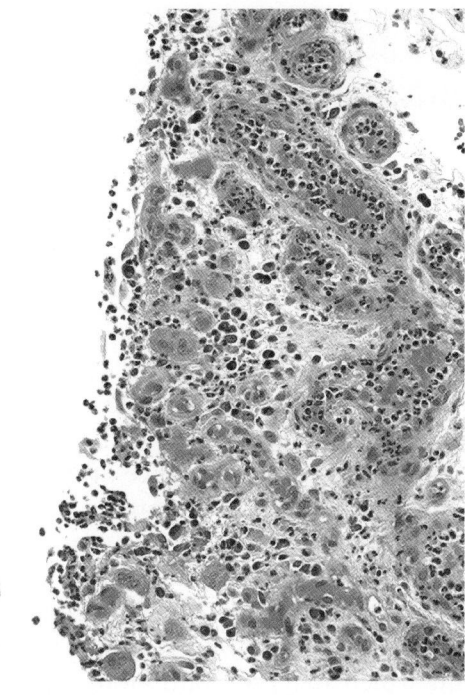

Fig. 11.9 Prominent endothelial cell proliferation with a mixed inflammatory cell infiltrate.

(Fig. 11.10).[11-13] However, misdiagnosis as neoplasia can occur if the tubal epithelium is not recognised. Moreover, fallopian tube prolapse has been associated with an exuberant angiomyofibroblastic stroma response. The richly vascularized stroma is arranged in a retiform pattern with mildly atypical glandular inclusions derived from tubal epithelium.[14] If the tubal glandular component is overlooked, this might be erroneously diagnosed as a mesenchymal lesion of the vagina, such as vaginal fibroepithelial polyp, angiomyofibroblastoma, aggressive angiomyxoma, or superficial myofibroblastoma (see Chapter 9).[14]

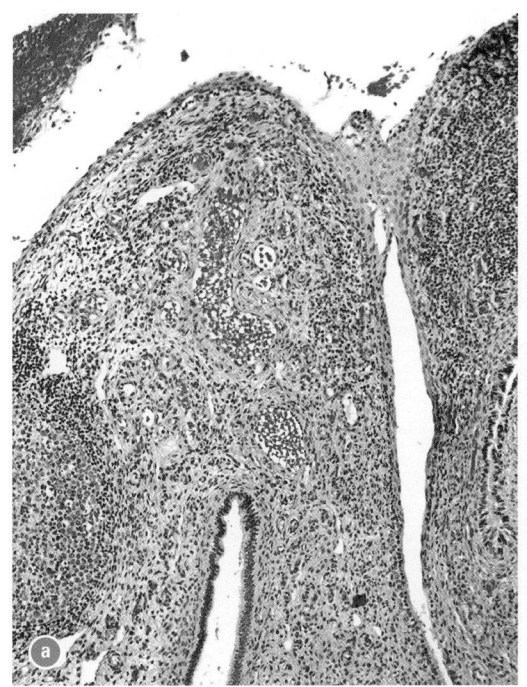

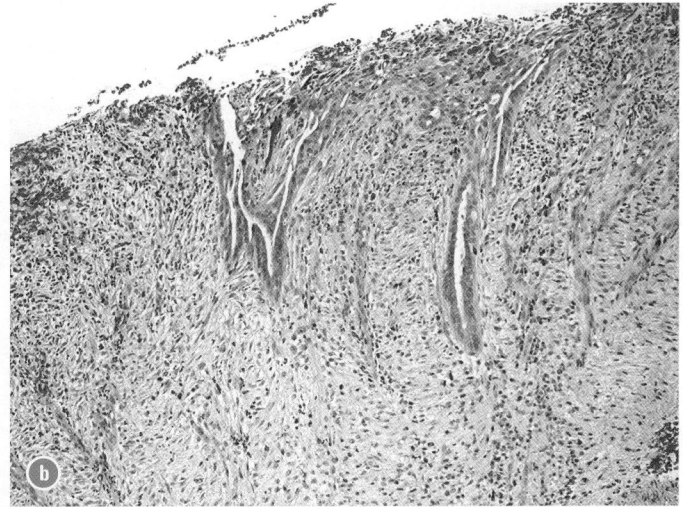

Fig. 11.10 Prolapsed fallopian tube. (a) The salpingeal epithelium is in continuity with the overlying squamous mucosa. (b) Salpingeal epithelium merges with an eroded mucosal surface.

Adenosis and columnar metaplasia

ADENOSIS

The association of *in utero* exposure with diethylstilbestrol (DES), vaginal adenosis and clear cell adenocarcinoma of the vagina was revealed in the early 1970s and is well known.[15] Adenosis is found in about one-third of women exposed to DES *in utero* and is responsible for not only vaginal abnormalities but also uterine structural anomalies (see Ch. 1). The principal defect consists of the congenital presence of columnar epithelium of the endocervical or endometrial type in the vaginal apex. Vaginal adenosis was appreciated prior to the DES era but was extremely rare.

Colposcopic findings in vaginal adenosis consist of a red and granular vaginal lesion, which fails to stain with iodine and which may be continuous with the cervix. The upper one-third of the vagina is almost always affected; the middle third is involved in 10% of cases and the lower third in 2% of cases. The histologic findings include benign endocervical glandular epithelium, endocervical epithelium with squamous metaplasia and an endocervical epithelium with tubal endometrial metaplasia, the latter characterized by ciliated cells (Fig. 11.11a,b). If the glandular lesion is large, additional and less-common findings include papillae (i.e. papillary adenosis), microglandular hyperplasia, particularly if the patient has taken oral contraceptives or been pregnant, Arias-Stella reaction, intestinal metaplasia and varying degrees of glandular atypia.

Adenosis is rarely complicated by the development of vaginal clear cell adenocarcinoma, which historically has occurred in one in 1000 to 5000 exposed individuals.[11]

BENIGN COLUMNAR CELLS IN THE VAGINA

A curious finding in cytologic preparations of postmenopausal women following hysterectomy is benign glandular cells in the vaginal vault (Fig. 11.12).[16,17] Explanations for these cells include the following: (1) an intact cervix (supracervical hysterectomy),[17] (2) vaginal endometriosis,[18] (3) mesonephric duct remnants and cysts, (4) vaginal adenosis, (5) fallopian tube prolapse,[19] (6) reparative fibroblasts in ulcers and granulation tissue, (7) rectovaginal fistulae, (8) adenocarcinoma (recurrent or metastatic), (9) exfoliated reparative squamous parabasal and basal cells resembling columnar-type cells, goblet cell metaplasia,[20] and (10) cytologic effects following the use of 5-fluorouracil (5-FU).[21,22] Most cases of benign columnar cells cannot be explained, and appear to be of little clinical consequence if cytologically banal.

CYSTS OF THE VAGINA

Cysts of the vagina are common and are generally benign.[23] Clinically, they may be single or multiple.[24] At times, imaging (ultrasound, voiding cystourethrogram (VCUG), computed tomography (CT) or magnetic resonance imaging (MRI)) may be required to characterize the lesion further.[23] It is important to rule out cystoceles or enteroceles, which can mimic a vaginal cyst.

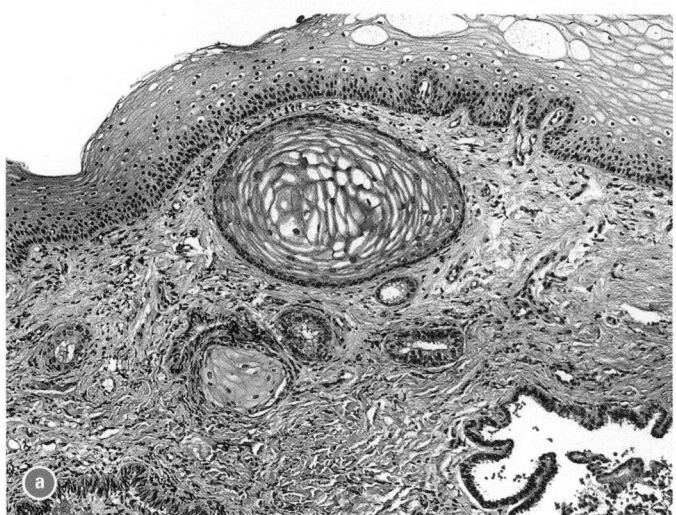 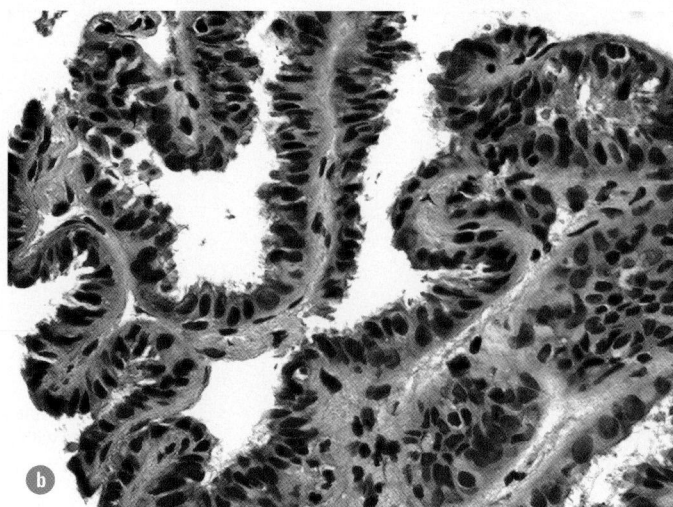

Fig. 11.11 (a) Vaginal adenosis with squamous metaplasia. (b) Tubal–endometrial metaplasia in vaginal adenosis.

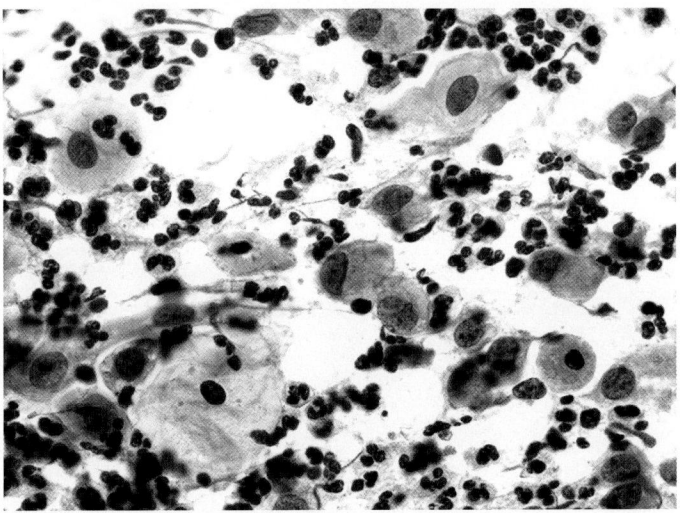

Fig. 11.12 Benign columnar cells (center) in a vaginal smear post hysterectomy.

The principal types of vaginal cysts include the following:

Müllerian cysts

Müllerian (mucous cysts, Figs 11.13, 11.14) derivatives are the most common type of vaginal cyst (Figs 11.1, 11.2), and these vary in size from 1 to 7 cm in diameter.[25] They may be lined by any of the epithelia that derive from the Müllerian ducts (endocervical, endometrial, or endosalpinx); however, endocervical is the most commonly found epithelium.[26] Some arise from adenosis.[11] Also, they may be seen in the DES-exposed patient.

Epithelial inclusion cysts

Epithelial inclusion cysts are lined by squamous epithelium and filled with keratin, as well as sebaceous-appearing material representing desquamated epithelial cells. Many epithelial inclusion cysts arise in sites of episiotomy or lacerations.[11] Deppisch reported 64 cases of vaginal cysts, of which 34 were inclusion cysts.[27] Epithelial inclusion cysts have a wide size range, varying from a few millimeters to several centimeters in diameter.

Mesonephric cysts

Mesonephric cysts of the vagina are the least commonly encountered in practice.[28] Gartner's duct cysts are usually found on the lateral to anterolateral vaginal walls, are 1–2 cm in size and occasionally up to 10 cm in diameter. The majority of women are asymptomatic; however, larger cysts may be symptomatic and produce urinary urgency during intercourse.[5] Histologically, the cysts are lined by a cuboidal to flattened epithelium devoid of cytoplasmic mucin.[11] Gartner's duct cysts were originally believed to be of common mesonephric (Wolffian) duct origin; however, many are derived from the paramesonephric (Müllerian) ducts or remnants of the urogenital sinus. Gartner's duct cysts have been associated with abnormalities of the metanephric urinary system.[29–33]

Although not generally required for clinical management, the distinction between Müllerian and mesonephric cysts can be made by histochemical staining. Paramesonephric epithelium contains both acid

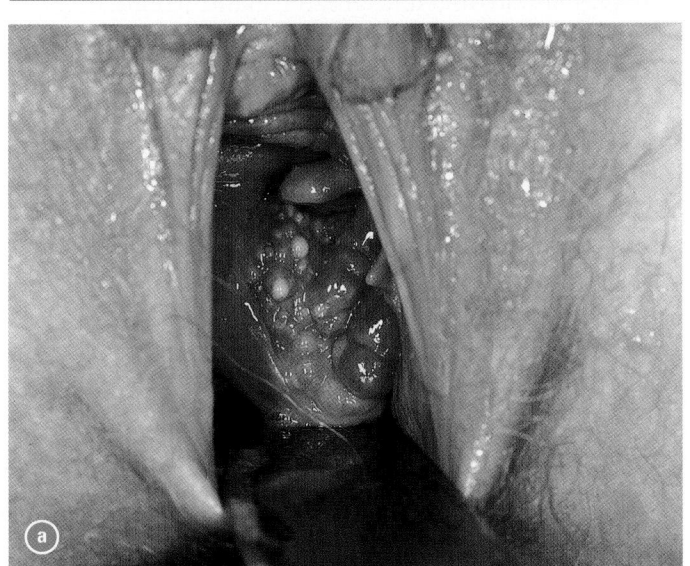

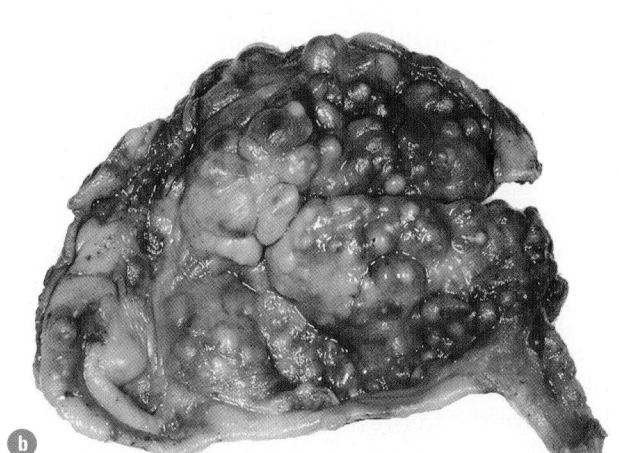

Fig. 11.13 (a) Multiple mucous cysts of the vagina. (b) Excised specimen.

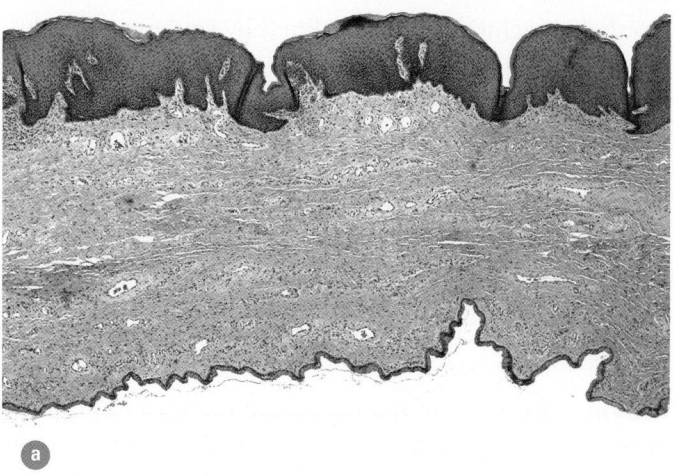
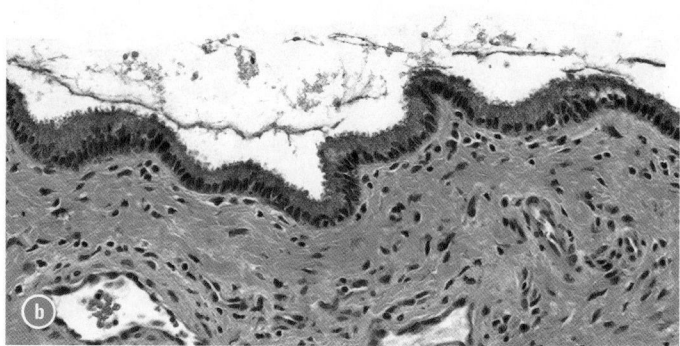

Fig. 11.14 (a) Mucous cyst beneath the vaginal squamous mucosa. (b) Higher magnification illustrating the endocervical-like columnar epithelium.

and neutral mucopolysaccharides and will stain positive with periodic acid–Schiff (PAS) before and after digestion with diastase and with mucicarmine stains. Mesonephric cysts do not contain mucin (PAS and mucicarmine negative).[28]

The majority of vaginal cysts, if asymptomatic, require no treatment. A thorough physical examination evaluating the location, mobility, tenderness and consistency is prudent and biopsy should be performed if neoplasia is suspected, i.e. cysts that are enlarging, are irregular or fixed in place, or if an endometriotic origin is suspected.[23]

Endometriosis

Vaginal endometriosis is an uncommon condition; less than 10% of pelvic endometriosis is found in the vagina.[34–36] Presumably the endometrial tissue gains access to the vagina via three mechanisms. The first is direct implantation of exiting endometrium on the vaginal surface. The second is implantation on, or coelomic metaplasia in, the retro-uterine cul de sac, with subsequent erosion into the vaginal apex. The third mechanism is via retrograde lymphatic spread from the endometrium to the vaginal submucosa.

Like elsewhere in the reproductive tract, vaginal endometriosis develops via three patterns:

1 Isolated subsurface glands with variable stroma. These give the impression of implantation on erosive areas with subsequent covering by the regenerating squamous epithelium (Fig. 11.15).

2 Deeper situated glands, which either form small foci or enlarge to form an endometriotic cyst. Large endometriotic cysts are not as common as smaller 2–3 mm foci.

3 Proliferative lesions that expand and contain abundant endometrial tissue. These lesions are termed 'polypoid endometriosis' and a subset is indistinguishable from an endometrial polyp. The expansive nature of polypoid endometriosis may cause concern, but follow-up studies have validated their benign nature (Figs 11.16, 11.17) The differential diagnosis of polypoid endometriosis is adenosarcoma and metastatic carcinosarcoma. These can be differentiated by the presence of malignant stroma and greater gland irregularity (adenosarcoma) and malignant glands and stroma (carcinosarcoma) (see Ch. 12).[37]

The most common treatment of endometriosis is excision of larger lesions and laser vaporization of smaller foci. Like all endometriosis, vaginal lesions carry a small risk of malignant transformation, including a wide range of neoplasms similar to those in the corpus.[38–43]

Fibroepithelial polyps of the lower female genital tract

Fibroepithelial polyps are discussed in Chapter 9 but will be addressed in terms of the most common, which occur in the introitus. Generally, fibroepithelial polyps are single, but may be multiple. They can be sessile,

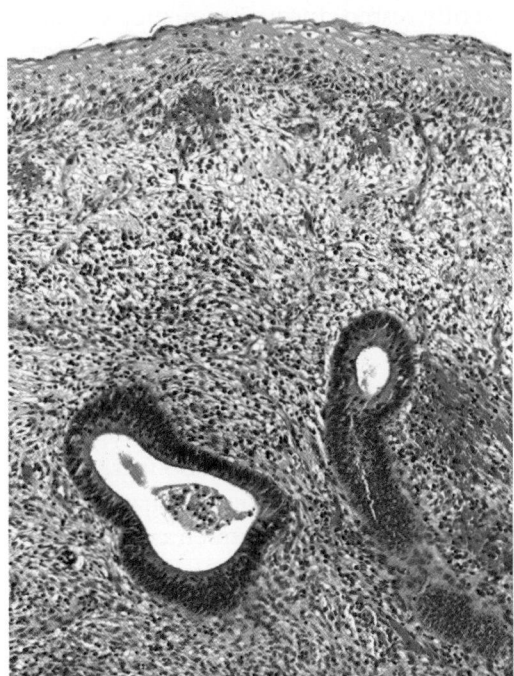

Fig. 11.15 Endometriosis of the vagina, beneath the squamous mucosa.

reactive for vimentin, less commonly for desmin and muscle-specific actin, and in some cases, for estrogen and progesterone receptors. Treatment consists of local excision.[11]

Traumatic lesions

TRAUMATIC INJURY

Excluding trauma from sexual assault, physical trauma is more common in the premenarchal and post-menopausal patient secondary to atrophy; however, it can occur at any age. Trauma from falls onto sharp or blunt objects, such as playground equipment, have been reported. Vaginal lacerations have occurred with water-skiing, water slides as well as with jet-ski accidents.[44–49] Chemical injuries are also reported.[50–53] Foreign bodies can cause vaginal injuries,[54] including ulceration (pessaries),[55] vaginal stenosis,[56] vaginitis,[57] fistulas[58,59] and vaginolithiasis.[60]

TAMPON ULCERS

Tampons were first reported as a cause of vaginal ulcers in 1977.[61] Tampon ulcers are shallow with smooth, rolled edges. They tend to have a clean base of granulation tissue. Tampon use is associated with micro-ulcerations of the vaginal epithelium.[26] Patchy aceto-white areas which stain mustard-yellow after Lugol's iodine application may be noted and confused with low-grade HPV.[5] These micro-ulcerations often heal within 1–2 days; however, they may take as long as 1 week to resolve.[26] Persistent lesions should be biopsied.

pedunculated or villiform, with a soft to rubbery texture. The smallest overlap with mucosal excrescence commonly present at the hymanal ring (Fig. 11.18). They may be associated with post-coital bleeding. Their size tends to be 4 cm or less in greatest dimension, although larger polyps have been reported. Histologic evaluation of fibroepithelial polyps reveals a squamous epithelial covering, dilated, thin-walled vessels, inflammatory cells and widely scattered stromal cells (fibroblasts and myofibroblasts). The stromal cells are typically immuno-

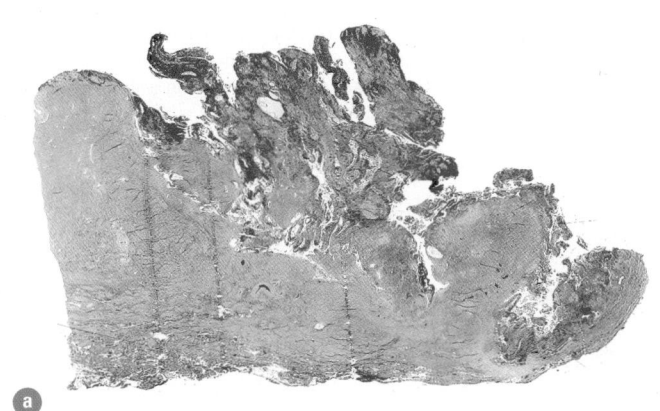

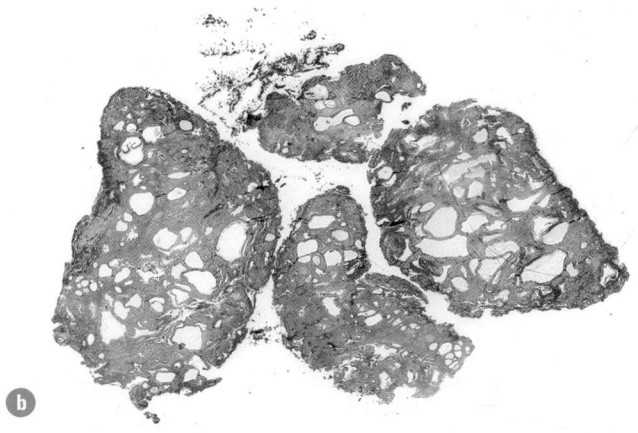

Fig. 11.16 Polypoid endometriosis. (a) The lining of this vaginal cyst contains abundant polypoid endometrial tissue. (b) Contents of a cyst with polypoid endometriosis.

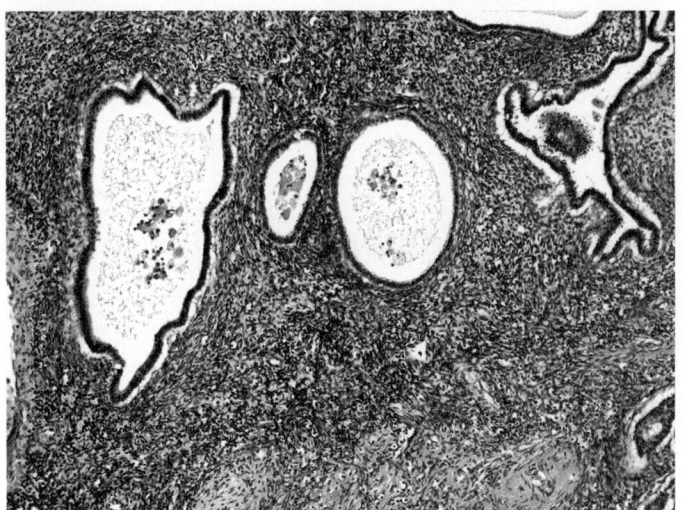

Fig. 11.17 Polypoid endometriosis. At higher power the lesion contains cystic glands and dense stroma similar to endometrial polyp.

OTHER TRAUMATIC LESIONS

Diaphragms and pessaries can also produce ulcers in the vagina; however, it is more common to see thickened tissue around the margin of vaginal tissue in contact with the diaphragm or pessary. Biopsy should be performed on any suspicious ulcerations (Fig. 11.19).

Infections of systemic importance

The following are not associated with specific pathology but are included for completeness.

GROUP B STREPTOCOCCUS

Group B streptococcus (GBS) is a common cause of infections in newborn infants (sepsis and meningitis).

Women are currently tested during pregnancy to determine if they are a carrier for this organism. Approximately 25% of women are carriers of this bacteria. Antibiotics are routinely administered to patients who test positive for this organism during labor. Recent epidemiologic data have resulted in a change in screening policy with a corresponding reduction in disease incidence. Since 1993, over 39 000 cases of GBS are estimated to have been prevented. A large proportion of this is secondary to awareness of recommended screening. A consensus statement for managing GBS was issued in 1996 and the Centers for Disease Control and Prevention also issued universal screening policy guidelines in 2002.[62] (Guidelines for GBS intrapartum antimicrobial prophylaxis and neonatal management are available at http://www.med.umich.edu/obgyn/resdir/protocols/GBS.pdf.)

In the non-pregnant patient, GBS is generally not treated. On occasion, when a patient has recurrent vaginal discharge and irritation, and the aerobic culture of the vagina is positive for GBS, antibiotic treatment is utilized.

TOXIC SHOCK SYNDROME

Toxic shock syndrome (TSS) is a syndrome composed of fever (sudden onset), chills, nausea, vomiting, diarrhea, muscle aches and skin rash. It can progress rapidly to intractable hypotension and multisystem failure. In 1–2 weeks after the illness, the skin can undergo desquamation, particularly on the palms and soles.

Toxic shock syndrome was first described by Todd et al. in 1978 in seven children, aged 8–17 years, with *Staphylococcus aureus* infection.[63] In an epidemic in 1981, TSS was associated with tampon use in healthy

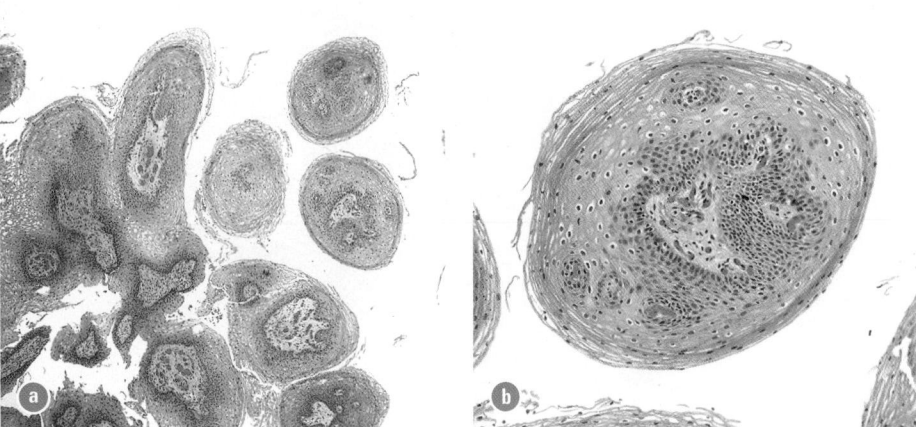

Fig. 11.18 (a) Fibroepithelial excrescences in the vaginal introitus. (b) At higher power, the epithelium is bland-appearing without nuclear atypia.

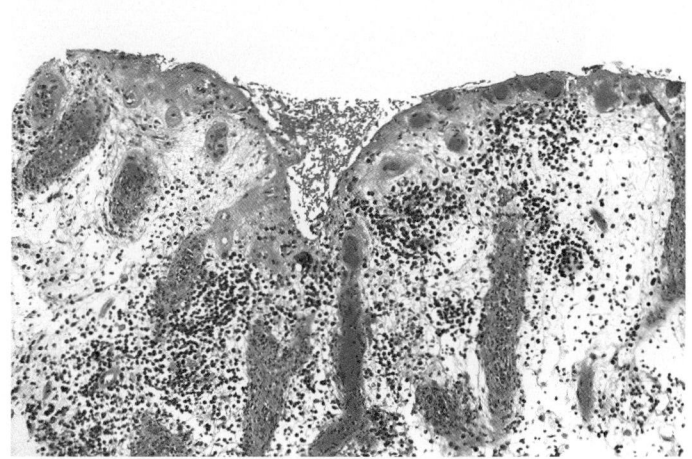

Fig. 11.19 Pessary ulcer. A contact erosion with epithelial denudation and chronic inflammation.

menstruating women. The disease is now known to also occur in men, neonates and non-menstruating women and has been linked to many bacterial infections, including pneumonia, osteomyelitis, sinusitis, skin infections and infections associated with intravaginal contraceptive devices or other gynecologic infections.[64]

TSS is mediated by toxins derived from *staphylococcus aureus* and *Streptococcus pyogenes*. Endotoxin toxic shock syndrome toxin-1 (TSST-1) is the major toxin produced by strains of *Staphylococcus aureus*. *Streptococcus pyogenes* exotoxin A (SPEA) and *Streptococcus pyogenes* exotoxin B (SPEB) are the major toxins produced by group A beta-hemolytic streptococci. These toxins activate production of superantigens, such as tumor necrosis factor, interleukin-1, M protein, and gamma-interferon.[64]

Risk factors from TSS include the use of superabsorbent tampons, postoperative wound infection, post-partum toxic shock, nasal packing, viral infection with influenza A or varicella, diabetes mellitus, infection with HIV, chronic cardiac and/or pulmonary disease.

A leukocytosis, mild anemia with abnormal cells on smears and/or thrombocytopenia are found in TSS. Electrolyte disturbances include hyponatremia, hypokalemia, hypocalcemia, hypoalbuminemia, hypophosphatemia and hypomagnesemia. A urinalysis may reveal sterile pyuria, myoglobinuria and red cell casts. Creatine kinase levels may indicate rhabdomyolysis. It is important to culture all potentially infected sites (including blood), as more than 50% of patients with streptococcal TSS have a positive blood culture results.[64]

The rapid streptococcal test can be performed in 10–15 min and has a sensitivity of 87–95%. Rocky Mountain spotted fever, leptospirosis, measles, hepatitis B surface antigen, antinuclear antibody, VDRL and mononucleosis should be excluded.

TSS has a significant mortality rate that varies depending on whether streptococcal (30–70%) or staphylococcal (<3%) organisms are involved. Aggressive fluid resuscitation and oxygen should be administered, and tampons and packing materials, if present, should be removed. For patients with menstruation-related TSS, irrigation of the vagina with isotonic sodium chloride solution or povidone-iodine solution has been recommended. Drainage, debridement, fasciotomy, or amputation of an infected site may be required. Because of the similarity in the clinical appearances of both staphylococcal and streptococcal TSS adequate antibiotic coverage for both staphylococci and streptococci should be initiated until the organism is isolated.[64]

Rare infections

MALAKOPLAKIA

Malakoplakia is a chronic inflammatory condition associated with a spectrum of bacterial infections. The pathogenesis of malakoplakia is not completely understood. *Escherichia coli* is the most common organism isolated (70–90%) from patients presenting with this disease. However, many other bacteria may be found in this condition.[65] Malakoplakia is often associated with a primary or acquired immunodeficiency. This condition is characterized by soft tissue tumor-like lesions which can mimic a variety of infectious, inflammatory and malignant conditions.[66] Extensive involvement of the abdominal wall and pelvic organs can occur,[67] and extensive disease may be associated with a fatal outcome.[68]

The first case of malakoplakia affecting the female genital tract was reported in 1973[69] in the upper vagina of a 65-year-old patient who had experienced vaginal bleeding for 3 months with a yellow, offensive, vaginal discharge for a slightly longer period of time and dyspareunia for 1 year.

Numerous histiocytes with intracellular and extracellular inclusions (Michaelis–Gutmann bodies) are present on histology. These are spherical structures, ranging from 5 to 10 μm, with concentric laminations that yield a 'bull's eye' or 'target-like' appearance. Treatment with surgery and/or antibiotics is usually curative.[65]

TUBERCULOSIS

The vagina is a rare site for infection with tuberculosis (1% of cases).[70–72] The clinical appearance consists of shallow ulcers with undermined edges. They tend to be small, but may have multiple sinus tracts with scarring. They also may be hypertrophic.[26] At times, they may be associated with vesicovaginal fistulas.[73]

On histologic evaluation, tuberculosis of the vagina contains multiple granulomas or tubercles with central caseation necrosis, epithelioid histiocytes and multinucleated Langhans giant cells are present. Although material is usually obtained for culture or fluorescence microscopy, polymerase chain reaction analysis can now be used for the rapid detection and identification of *Mycobacterium tuberculosis*.[74–77]

INFLAMMATORY LESIONS OF UNKNOWN ETIOLOGY

Desquamative inflammatory vaginitis

Desquamative inflammatory vaginitis (DIV) is an inflammatory vaginitis of unknown etiology. It was first described in the 1950s and considered by some authorities to be a form of erosive lichen planus.[78-81] In some cases, DIV co-exists with gingival mucositis.[79] Signs and symptoms include an excessive vaginal discharge (alkaline vaginal pH), patches (spots) of erythema (diffuse or localized) on the cervix, vagina, or vestibule (Fig. 11.3), an increased vaginal pH, postcoital bleeding and dyspareunia. Occasionally, portions of the vagina will be covered by a gray pseudomembrane.[5] Clinically, the picture is very similar to atrophic vaginitis (Fig. 11.20); however, DIV has been reported in both premenopausal as well as postmenopausal women.[82,83]

On microscopic examination of the wet prep, numerous leukocytes and parabasal cells are present (massive vaginal cell exfoliation). The PMN/epithelial cell ratio is greater than 1:1 in at least four high power fields of the wet prep. There is an absence of lactobacilli. A biopsy from the erythematous portion of the vaginal wall for histology and immunofluorescence is essential to exclude any underlying cause of DIV. However, the pattern of inflammation in the vaginal wall is often non-specific.[84] Histology is significant for a dense infiltrate of PMNs, loss of surface epithelium and thinning of adjacent epithelium, similar to atrophic vaginitis. Gram staining shows an absence of lactobacilli and occasionally increased levels of Gram-positive cocci.[85]

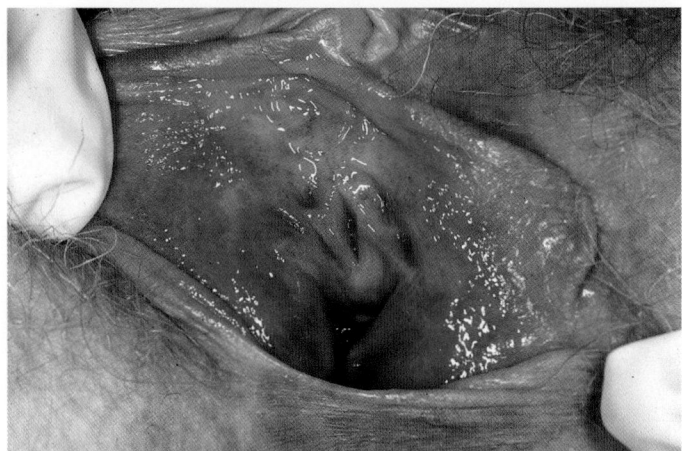

Fig. 11.20 Clinical appearance of desquamative vaginitis.

Various treatments exist for DIV, including clindamycin cream base, hydrocortisone and a third regimen combining the clindamycin and the hydrocortisone per vagina.

Ulcers and other dermatoses of the vagina

Numerous conditions can be associated with vaginal ulcers and dermatoses of the vagina, including bullous dermatoses, contact dermatitis, graft versus host disease, plasma cell vulvitis, lichen planus, aphthous ulcers (Fig. 11.21), pemphigus vulgaris, toxic epidermal necrolysis (TEN), Stevens–Johnson syndrome, systemic lupus erythematosus, herpes, HIV, Behçet's disease and benign familial chronic pemphigus (Hailey–Hailey disease) (see also Chapter 2).

Bullous dermatoses

Bullous pemphigoid affecting the vagina has been reported, even in children.[86,87] In a study by Kirtschig et al., 8 of 19 patients with bullous pemphigoid were found to have split vagina and occasionally split oral mucosa. There was a correlation between autoantibody reactivity with split mucous membrane tissues and clinical mucosal involvement, suggesting heterogeneity of antigens or epitopes expressed between tissues. In both split skin and mucosa, all sera consistently detected an antigen on the epidermal side of the split regardless of the stage of the disease.[88] Similarly, cicatricial pemphigoid, a systemic autoimmune disease with both ocular and extraocular manifestations, may affect the vagina.[89]

Pemphigus vulgaris, a disease which commonly affects mucosal surfaces, may also affect the vagina. Persistent vaginal discharge and extensive vaginal erosions may be present. Abnormal acantholytic cells on Papanicolaou smears may be misinterpreted as evidence of cervical dysplasia or malignancy in smears from this patient population.[90,91] Oral involvement is seen in approximately one-half of patients. Other less commonly involved sites include the esophagus, conjunctiva, nasal mucosa, cervix and anus. Histologic evaluation of vaginal biopsies is often non-diagnostic; however, direct immunofluorescent studies may be helpful. IgG and C3 in the intercellular epidermis support a diagnosis of pemphigus vulgaris.[92]

Vaginal adhesions may be a consequence of Stevens–Johnson syndrome

Stevens–Johnson syndrome[93,94] is a rare, life-threatening condition characterized by epidermal necrosis and involvement of the mucosal surfaces. Hart et al. reported vaginal involvement resulting in adhesions in an 11-year-old girl.[94]

Behçet's disease

Behçet's disease is a rare condition that is found predominantly in Japan, the Middle East and the Mediterranean. Turkey and Iran have reported the highest number of cases. It is more common in males than females. It is considered a multisystem disorder, affecting the oral mucosa, skin, vulva, vagina, joints, cardiovascular system, gastrointestinal tract and central nervous system. The skin lesions tend to be painful, shallow to deep, and have erythematous borders with yellow, fibrinous bases. The mouth is the most common location for ulcer formation. Some 10% of patients, however, develop major aphthous ulcerations. They can persist for weeks to months before completely healing. While Behçet's disease in the genital tract is common on the vulva, involvement of the vagina is less common.

The diagnosis of Behçet's disease is based on clinical symptomatology. Tissue biopsy is generally non-specific; however, at times a prominent vasculitis is present, with capillary and venule involvement. There may be swelling on the vessel walls with a perivascular infiltrate of lymphocytes.

The skin pathergy test is one of the diagnostic criterions for Behçet's disease and consists of development of a small pustule within 24–48 h after the skin has been pricked by a blunt sterile needle. Although helpful if positive, its sensitivity is debatable, with some studies finding it as low as 10%.[95] North American patients rarely test positive with the skin pathergy test.

Many treatments have been used for Behçet's disease, including colchicine, steroids (topical, oral, intravenous),

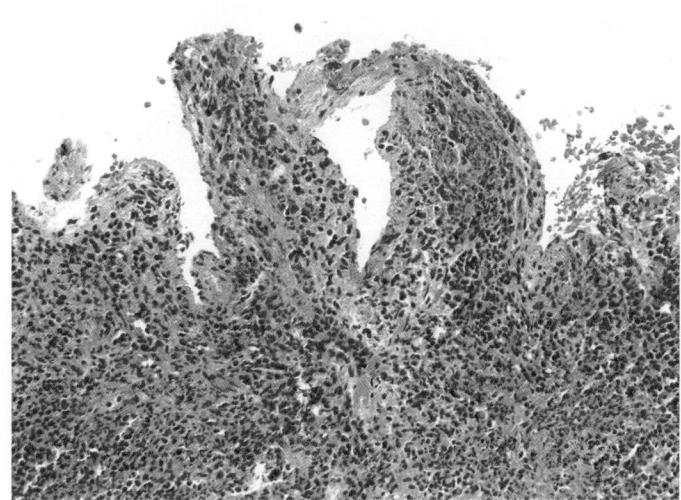

Fig. 11.21 Aphthous ulcer of the vagina. Complete epithelial necrosis has left the dermal papillae suspended, similar to tombstone artifacts seem in desquamative dermatoses (see Ch. 2).

azathioprine, methotrexate, chlorambucil, dapsone, cyclosporine, cyclophosphamide, thalidomide, infliximab, pentoxifylline, sucralfate suspension, and interferon alfa (particularly with ocular disease). The therapeutic decisions are guided by the severity and extent of involvement. An ideal therapeutic regimen does not exist. Often, treatment is given in conjunction with a rheumatologist and are usually symptomatic and palliative, rather than curative. Recurrences are common and unpredictable.[96]

Emphysematous vaginitis

Emphysematous vaginitis is characterized by gas-filled cysts in the vaginal wall producing 'popping' sounds are heard when pressure is applied to the vagina with a speculum, pelvic examination, or with intercourse. The cysts of this condition tend to be a few millimeters in diameter; however, they may be as large as 2 cm. Other manifestations of emphysematous vaginitis include an increased vaginal discharge and postcoital bleeding.[5] The cause of vaginitis emphysematosa is not completely understood. It is often seen in patients who are pregnant or who have impaired immunity.[97,98] The gas-filled cysts have been described in the radiology literature.[99–101]

Histologic evaluation reveals inflammatory cells with cysts in the stroma lined by either multinucleated giant cells, squamous cells or both ((Fig. 11.22). The disease is benign, self-limited and not life-threatening.[101,102]

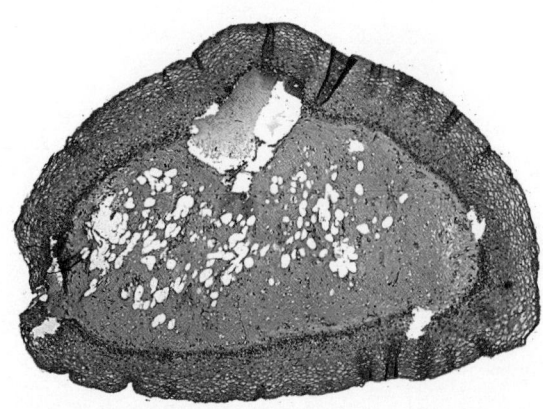

Fig. 11.22 Emphysematous vaginitis. This biopsy depicts the multiple gas-filled cysts in the submucosa that give rise to the crepitants appreciated on palpation.

References

1 Ham AW, Cormack DH. Histology, 8th edn. Philadelphia: JB Lippincott; 1979.

2 Ng WK, Li AS, Cheung LK. Significance of atypical repair in liquid-based gynecologic cytology: a follow-up study with molecular analysis for human papillomavirus. Cancer 2003; 99:141–148.

3 Bardawil T, Mane A. Surgical treatment of vaginal cancer. Online. Available: http://www.emedicine.com/med/topic3330.htm.

4 Selvaggi SM. Atrophic vaginitis versus invasive squamous cell carcinoma on ThinPrep cytology: can the background be reliably distinguished? Diagn Cytopathol 2002; 27:362–364.

5 Ferris DG, Cox JT, O'Connor DM, Wright VC, Foerster J. Modern colposcopy textbook and atlas, 2nd edn. Colposcopy of the vagina. Dubuque, Iowa: Kendall/Hunt Publishing Co.; 2004:1414–1448.

6 Nothnagle M, Taylor JS. Vaginal estrogen preparations for relief of atrophic vaginitis. Am Fam Phys 2004; 69:2111–2112.

7 Bachmann GA, Nevadunsky NS. Diagnosis and treatment of atrophic vaginitis. Am Fam Phys 2000; 61:3090–3096.

8 Shield PW. Chronic radiation effects: a correlative study of smears and biopsies from the cervix and vagina. Diagn Cytopathol 1995; 13:107–119.

9 Aboud E. Prolapse of the fallopian tube into the vaginal vault. Clin Exp Obstet Gynecol 1997; 24:116.

10 Byrne DL, Edmonds DK. Prolapse of the fallopian tube following abdominal hysterectomy. J R Soc Med 1989; 82:764–765.

11 Clement PB, Young RH. Atlas of gynecologic surgical pathology. Philadelphia, PA: WB Saunders; 2000:43–62.

12 Ellsworth HS, Harris JW, McQuarrie HG, et al. Prolapse of the fallopian tube following vaginal hysterectomy. JAMA 1973; 224:891–827.

13 Sapan IP, Solberg NS. Prolapse of the uterine tube after abdominal hysterectomy. Obstet Gynecol 1973; 42: 26–32.

14 Michal M, Rokyta Z, Mejchar B, et al. Prolapse of the fallopian tube after hysterectomy associated with exuberant angiomyofibroblastic stroma response: a diagnostic pitfall. Virchows Archiv 2000; 437:436–439.

15 Robboy SJ, Szyfelbein WM, Goellner JR, et al. Dysplasia and cytologic findings in 4,589 young women enrolled in diethylstilbestrol-adenosis (DESAD) project. Am J Obstet Gynecol 1981; 140:579–586.

16 Ramirez NC, Sastry LK, Pisharodi LR. Benign glandular and squamous metaplastic-like cells seen in vaginal Pap smears of post hysterectomy patients: incidence and patient profile. Eur J Gynaecol Oncol 2000; 21:43–48.

17 Sodhani P, Gupta S, Prakash S, Singh V. Columnar and metaplastic cells in vault smears: cytologic and colposcopic study. Cytopathology 1999; 10:122–126; discussion 131.

18 Frable WJ, Smith JH, Perkins J, Foley C. Vaginal cuff cytology: some difficult diagnostic problems. Acta Cytol 1973; 17:135–140.

19 Wolfendale M. Exfoliative cytology in a case of prolapsed fallopian tube. Acta Cytol 1980; 24:545–548.

20 Bewtra C. Columnar cells in posthysterectomy vaginal smears. Diagn Cytopathol 1992; 8:342–345.

21 Dungar CF, Wilkinson EJ. Vaginal columnar cell metaplasia. An acquired adenosis associated with topical 5-fluorouracil therapy. J Reprod Med 1995; 40:361–366.

22 Koike N, Higuchi T, Sakai Y. Goblet-like cells in atrophic vaginal smears and their histologic correlation. Possible confusion with endocervical cells. Acta Cytol 1990; 34:785–788.

23 Eilber KS, Raz S. Benign cystic lesions of the vagina: a literature review. J Urol 2003; 170:717–722.

24 Wai CY, Corton MM, Miller M, Sailors J, Schaffer JI. Multiple vaginal wall cysts: diagnosis and surgical management. Obstet Gynecol 2004; 103:1099–1102.

25 Wilkinson, EJ. Pathology of the vulva and vagina. New York: Churchill Livingstone; 1987.

26 Brown D. Postmenopausal atropism, atrophic vaginitis, and other vaginitides. In: Kaufman RH, Faro S, Brown D, eds. Benign diseases of the vulva and vagina. Philadelphia, PA: Elsevier Mosby; 2005:391–410.

27 Deppisch LM. Cysts of the vagina: classification and clinical correlations. Obstet Gynecol 1975; 45:632–637.

28 Kaufman RH. Cystic tumors. In: Kaufman RH, Faro S, Brown D, eds. Benign diseases of the vulva and vagina. Philadelphia, PA: Elsevier Mosby; 2005:216–256.

29 Rosenfeld DL, Lis E. Gartner's duct cyst with a single vaginal ectopic ureter and associated renal dysplasia or agenesis. J Ultrasound Med 1993; 12:775–778.

30 Borer JG, Corgan FJ, Krantz R, et al. Unilateral single vaginal ectopic ureter with ipsilateral hypoplastic pelvic kidney and bicornuate uterus. J Urol 1993; 149:1124–1127.

31 Watanabe K, Ogawa A, Inoue Y, Yoneyama T. Single vaginal ectopic ureter via Gartner's duct cyst spontaneously perforating into the bladder. J Urol 1989; 142:1044–1046.

32 Utsunomiya M, Itoh H, Yoshioka T, Okuyama A, Itatani H. Renal dysplasia with a single vaginal ectopic ureter: the role of computerized tomography. J Urol 1984; 132:98–100.

33 Currarino G. Single vaginal ectopic ureter and Gartner's

duct cyst with ipsilateral renal hypoplasia and dysplasia (or agenesis). J Urol 1982; 128:988–993.

34 Gardner HL. Cervical and vaginal endometriosis. Clin Obstet Gynecol 1966; 9:358–372.

35 Sinha AK, Agarwal A, Lakhey M, Mishra A, Sah SP. Incidence of pelvic and extrapelvic endometriosis in Eastern region of Nepal. Indian J Pathol Microbiol 2003; 46:20–23.

36 Azzena A, Ferrara A, Castellan L, Quinticri F, Salmaso R. Vaginal endometriosis. Two case reports and review of the literature on rare urogenital sites. Clin Exp Obstet Gynecol 1996; 23:94–98.

37 Mulvany NJ, Surtees V. Cervical/vaginal endometriosis with atypia: a cytohistopathologic study. Diagn Cytopathol 1999; 21:188–193.

38 Granai CO, Walters MD, Safaii H, et al. Malignant transformation of vaginal endometriosis. Obstet Gynecol 1984; 64:592–595.

39 Berkowitz RS, Ehrmann RL, Knapp RC. Endometrial stromal sarcoma arising from vaginal endometriosis. Obstet Gynecol 1978; 51:34s-7s.

40 Liu L, Davidson S, Singh M. Müllerian adenosarcoma of vagina arising in persistent endometriosis: report of a case and review of the literature. Gynecol Oncol 2003; 90:486–490.

41 Anderson J, Behbakht K, De Geest K, Bitterman P. Adenosarcoma in a patient with vaginal endometriosis. Obstet Gynecol 2001; 98:964–966.

42 Gucer F, Pieber D, Arikan MG. Malignancy arising in extraovarian endometriosis during estrogen stimulation. Eur J Gynaecol Oncol 1998; 19:39–41.

43 Judson PL, Temple AM, Fowler WC Jr, Novotny DB, Funkhouser WK Jr. Vaginal adenosarcoma arising from endometriosis. Gynecol Oncol 2000; 76:123–125.

44 Haefner HK, Andersen HF, Johnson MP. Vaginal laceration following a jet-ski accident. Obstet Gynecol 1991; 78:986–988.

45 Goldberg J, Horan C, O'Brien LM. Severe anorectal and vaginal injuries in a jet ski passenger. J Trauma 2004; 56:440–441.

46 Fauconnier A, Legier JP, Nicoloso E. Vaginal pressure trauma: a complication of jet-skis. J Gynecol Obstet Biol Reprod 1995; 24:604–605.

47 Mushkat Y, Lessing JB, Jedwab GA, David MP. Vaginal trauma occurring while sliding down a water chute. B J Obstet Gynaecol 1995; 102:933–934.

48 Kunkel NC. Vaginal injury from a water slide in a premenarcheal patient. Pediatr Emerg Care 1998; 14:210–211.

49 Niv J, Lessing JB, Hartuv J, Peyser MR. Vaginal injury resulting from sliding down a water chute. Am J Obstet Gynecol 1992; 166:930–931.

50 Clarke J, De Silva PA. Chemical burns in colposcopy; a hazard in GUM clinics? Int J STD AIDS 1994; 5:142–143.

51 Catalani A. [Vulvo-vaginal atresias, caustic pessaries and ritual practices in Nigeria. Medico-social aspects]. Quad Clin Ostet Ginecol 1965; 20:267–277. [in Italian].

52 Aguilar Guerrero JA, Repper Camacho F, Reyes Ceja L. [Considerations on 200 cases of vaginal burns by potassium permanganate]. Ginecol Obstet Mex 1971; 29:275–279. [in Spanish].

53 Zarate Sandoval H, Saldana Garcia R, Samaniego I. [Vaginal burns by caustic substances. A socio-medical problem]. Ginecol Obstet Mex 1970; 27:559–567. [in Spanish]

54 Stricker T, Navratil F, Sennhauser FH. Vaginal foreign bodies. J Paediatr Child Health 2004; 40:205–207.

55 Thornton CA, Harrison RF. Unusually rapid incarceration of a polyvinyl ring pessary. Ir J Med Sci 1977; 146:116.

56 Simon DA, Berry S, Brannian J, Hansen K. Recurrent, purulent vaginal discharge associated with longstanding presence of a foreign body and vaginal stenosis. J Pediatr Adolesc Gynecol 2003; 16:361–363.

57 Dahiya P, Sangwan K, Khosla A, Seth N. Foreign body in vagina – an uncommon cause of vaginitis in children. Indian J Pediatr 1999; 66:466–467.

58 Hoffman MS, Wakeley KE, Cardosi RJ. Risks of rigid dilation for a radiated vaginal cuff: two related rectovaginal fistulas. Obstet Gynecol 2003; 101:1125–1126.

59 Biswas A, Das HS. An unusual foreign body in the vagina producing vesicovaginal fistula. J Indian Med Assoc 2002; 100:257, 259.

60 Dalela D, Agarwal R, Mishra VK. Giant vaginolith around an unusual foreign body – an uncommon cause of urinary incontinence in a girl. Br J Urol 1994; 74:673–674.

61 Barrett KF, Bledsoe S, Greer BE, Droegemueller W. Tampon-induced vaginal or cervical ulceration. Am J Obstet Gynecol 1977; 127:332–333.

62 Cory J, Schrag S, Dinsmoor MJ, Schuchat A. Group B strep: successful model of 'From Science to Action' Emerg Infect Dis [serial on the Internet]. Online. Available: http://www.cdc.gov/ncidod/EID/vol10no11/04–gov/ncidod/EID/vol100623_03.htm, November 2004.

63 Todd J, Fishaut M, Kapral F, Welch T. Toxic-shock syndrome associated with phage-group-I Staphylococci. Lancet 1978; 2:1116–1118.

64 Salandy D, Brenner B, Gaeta T, et al. Toxic shock syndrome. Emedicine. Online. Available: http://www.emedicine.com/emerg/topic600.htm.

65 van der Voort HJ, ten Velden JA, Wassenaar RP, Silberbusch J. Malacoplakia. Two case reports and a comparison of treatment modalities based on a literature review. Arch Intern Med 1996; 156:577–583.

66 Lack EE. Malakoplakia. In: Connor FW, Manz HJ, Schwartz DA, Lack EE, eds. Pathology of infectious disease, 1st edn. Stamford, Connecticut: Appleton & Lange; 1997:1647–1654.

67 Kogulan PK, Smith M, Seidman J, et al. Malakoplakia involving the abdominal wall, urinary bladder, vagina, and vulva: case report and discussion of malakoplakia-associated bacteria. Int J Gynecol Pathol 2001; 20:403–406.

68 Lowitt MH, Kariniemi AL, Niemi KM, Kao GF. Cutaneous malacoplakia: a report of two cases and review of the literature. J Am Acad Dermatol 1996; 34(2 Pt 2):325–332.

69 Van der Walt JJ, Marcus PB, De Wet JJ, Burger AJ. Malacoplakia of the vagina. First case report. S Afr Med J 1973; 47:1342–1344.

70 Coetzee LF. Tuberculous vaginitis. S Afr Med J 1972; 46:1225–1226.

71 Nogales-Ortiz F, Tarancon I, Nogales FF Jr. The pathology of female genital tuberculosis. A 31-year study of 1436 cases. Obstet Gynecol 1979; 53:422–428.

72 Ma YY, Hsu TY, Changchien CC, Chang SY, Lin JW. Vulvovaginal tuberculosis: a case report. Changgeng Yi Xue Za Zhi 1997; 20:66–70.

73 Ba-Thike K, Than-Aye, Nan-Oo. Tuberculous vesicovaginal fistula. Int J Gynaecol Obstet 1992; 37:127–130.

74 Ferrara G, Cannone M, Guadagnino A, Nappi O, Barberis MC. Nested polymerase chain reaction on vaginal smears of tuberculous cervicitis. A case report. Acta Cytol 1999; 43:308–312.

75 Faizal M, Jimenez G, Burgos C, et al. Diagnosis of cutaneous tuberculosis by polymerase chain reaction using a species-specific gene. Int J Dermatol 1996; 35:185–188.

76 Forbes BA, Hicks KE. Direct detection of *Mycobacterium tuberculosis* in respiratory specimens in a clinical laboratory by polymerase chain reaction. J Clin Microbiol 1993; 31:1688–1694.

77 Kim SS, Chung SM, Kim JN, Lee MA, Ha EH. Application of PCR from the fine needle aspirates for the diagnosis of cervical tuberculous lymphadenitis. J Korean Med Sci 1996; 11:127–132.

78 Edwards L, Friedrich EG Jr. Desquamative vaginitis: lichen planus in disguise. Obstet Gynecol 1988; 71:832–836.

79 Pelisse M. The vulvo-vaginal-gingival syndrome. A new form of erosive lichen planus. Int J Dermatol 1989; 28:381–384.

80 Gray LA, Barnes ML. Vaginitis in women, diagnosis and treatment. Am J Obstet Gynecol 1965; 92:125–136.

81 Gardner HL. Desquamative inflammatory vaginitis: a newly defined entity. Obstet Gynecol 1968; 102:1102–1105.

82 Oates JK, Rowen D. Desquamative inflammatory vaginitis. A review. Genitourin Med 1990; 66:275–279.

83 Sobel JD. Desquamative inflammatory vaginitis: a new subgroup of purulent vaginitis responsive to topical 2% clindamycin therapy. Am J Obstet Gynecol 1994; 171: 1215–1230.

84 Edwards L. Desquamative vulvitis. Dermatol Clin 1992; 10:325–337.

85 Jacobson M, Krumholz B, Franks A Jr. Desquamative inflammatory vaginitis. A case report. J Reprod Med 1989; 34:647–650.

86 Fisler RE, Saeb M, Liang MG, Howard RM, McKee PH. Childhood bullous pemphigoid: a clinicopathologic study and review of the literature Am J Dermatopathol 2003; 25:183–189.

87 Haustein UF. Localized nonscarring bullous pemphigoid of the vagina. Dermatologica 1988; 176:200–201.

88 Kirtschig G, Venning VA, Wojnarowska F. Bullous pemphigoid: correlation of mucosal involvement and mucosal expression of autoantigens studied by indirect immunofluorescence and immunoblotting. Clin Exp Dermatol 1999; 24:208–212.

89 Nguyen QD, Foster CS. Cicatricial pemphigoid: diagnosis and treatment. Int Ophthalmol Clin 1996; 36:41–60.

90 Gupta S, Sodhani P, Jain S. Acantholytic cells exfoliated from pemphigus vulgaris of the uterine cervix. A case report. Acta Cytol 2003; 47:795–798.

91 Chan E, Thakur A, Farid L, et al. Pemphigus vulgaris of the cervix and upper vaginal vault: a cause of atypical Papanicolaou smears. Arch Dermatol 1998; 134(11):1485–1486.

92 Batta K, Munday PE, Tatnall FM. Pemphigus vulgaris localized to the vagina presenting as chronic vaginal discharge. Br J Dermatol 1999; 140:945–947.

93 Wilson EE, Malinak LR. Vulvovaginal sequelae of Stevens–Johnson syndrome and their management. Obstet Gynecol 1988; 71:478–480.

94 Hart R, Minto C, Creighton S. Vaginal adhesions caused by Stevens–Johnson syndrome. J Pediatr Adolesc Gynecol 2002; 15:151–152.

95 Davies PG, Fordham JN, Kirwan JR, et al. The pathergy test and Behçet's syndrome in Britain. Ann Rheum Dis 1984; 43:70–73.

96 Haefner HK. Comments on Behcet disease. J Lower Gen Tract Dis 2005: in press.

97 Gardner HL, Fernet P. Etiology of vaginitis emphysematosa. Am J Obstet Gynecol 1964; 88:680–694.

98 Riethdorf L, Nehmzow M, Straube W, Lorenz G. Vaginitis emphysematosa during immunosuppressive therapy. Arch Gynecol Obstet 1995; 256:39–41.

99 Wepfer JF, Sinsky JE. Roentgen manifestations of vaginitis emphysematosa. Am J Roentgenol Radium Ther Nucl Med 1968; 102:946–950.

100 Jaramillo D, Allan NK, Raval B. Computed tomography of vaginitis emphysematosa. J Comput Assist Tomogr 1986; 10:521–523.

101 Leder RA, Paulson EK. Vaginitis emphysematosa: CT and review of the literature. AJR Am J Roentgenol 2001; 176:623–625.

102 Zaino RJ, Robboy SJ, Kurman RJ. Diseases of the vagina. In: Kurman RJ, ed. Blaustein's pathology of the female genital tract, 5th edn. New York: Springer; 2002:165.

12

Epithelial and mixed epithelial–stromal neoplasms of the vagina

Christopher P. Crum and

Hope K. Haefner

Introduction

Vaginal intraepithelial lesions (VAIL; condyloma and VAIN)

Introduction and patient at risk
Natural history of VAIL and
    vaginal cancer
Examination of the patient
Histology of VAIL
Management of vaginal
    intraepithelial lesions
Post-radiation dysplasia (HIVAIL)

Malignant epithelial neoplasms of the vagina

Introduction
Squamous cell carcinoma
Verrucous carcinoma
Squamo-transitional carcinoma
Glandular neoplasia
Vaginal melanoma
Rare tumors

Introduction

This chapter will focus principally on epithelial neoplasms of the vagina (soft tissue tumors are discussed in detail in Ch. 9). The most common lesions in the epithelial group are squamous, specifically vaginal intraepithelial lesions and invasive squamous carcinomas. The most important challenges faced by the pathologist are the classification of vaginal intraepithelial lesions (VAIL), the recognition of potentially serious lesions, including the exclusion of invasion, and recognition of rare entities that could cause diagnostic confusion or inappropriate management.

Table 12.1 *Distribution and comparison of HPV types in vaginal and cervical intraepithelial lesions (%)[1]*

HPV type	LOVAIL	HIVAIL	LSIL	HSIL
Cases (n)	59	16	73	145
6/11[a]	27.1	0.0	21.9	00.0
40,43,54,64,67,71	23.7	25.0	6.8	0.6
16	6.7	18.7	9.6	37.9
18	1.6	–	2.7	0.6
31,33,35,39,51,52,56,58,61,68	28.8	37.5	50.1	52.4
30,53, other	8.5	12.5	4.1	8.3

[a]6/11 was confined to condylomas of the cervix and vagina.
LOVAIL, low-grade vaginal intraepithelial lesion (condyloma/VAIN1); HIVAIL, high-grade vaginal intraepithelial lesion (VAIN2/VAIN3); LSIL, low-grade squamous intraepithelial lesion (condyloma/CIN1) of the cervix; HSIL, high-grade squamous intraepithelial lesion (CIN2/CIN3) of the cervix.

Vaginal intraepithelial lesions (VAIL; condyloma and VAIN)

INTRODUCTION AND PATIENT AT RISK

Vaginal intraepithelial lesions are defined as human papillomavirus-related squamous intraepithelial proliferations. For the purposes of this chapter, the term vaginal intraepithelial lesion, or VAIL, is synonymous with the entire spectrum of both wart virus infections (condylomata) and vaginal intraepithelial neoplasia (VAIN). The risk factors for VAILs are identical to those for cervical and to a lesser degree, vulvar intraepithelial lesions, specifically age at first intercourse and number of sexual partners, as well as conditions that compromise immune function (see Ch. 13). However, there are some slight differences between vaginal intraepithelial lesions and those of the vulva and cervix, related to both differences in sites of origin and the HPV types involved. The vulva is a combination of skin and mucosa and is prone to infections by HPV types 6, 11 and 16. In contrast, the target epithelium in the cervix is the squamocolumnar junction and the area hosting the dynamic remodeling of epithelial phenotypes that characterizes the cervical transformation zone. The vagina is similar to the cervix, in that lesions analyzed from this areas contain a wider range of HPV types than seen in the vulva (Table 12.1).[1] Moreover, the relative frequencies of low- and high-grade preinvasive lesions are similar to the cervix, at approximately 3:1. The age range for different grades of VAIL is more pronounced, however, with a 15-year spread between low- and high-grade disease. The differences in mean age for low- and high-grade SILs of the cervix is less than 10 years.[2]

Approximately 65% of women with VAILs have either concomitant or prior squamous intraepithelial lesion of the cervix.[2,3] Patients who have undergone a prior hysterectomy for dysplasia/carcinoma *in situ* (CIS), radiation therapy to the cervix or vagina, or those on immunosuppressive agents also have an increased risk of VAIL and molecular studies have confirmed that HPV is responsible for these lesions.[4–6] Immunosuppressed women are more likely to have persistent, multifocal lesions.[7]

Another group of patients at risk for abnormal vaginal changes are those with vaginal adenosis secondary to intrauterine exposure to diethylstilbestrol (DES). These patients are known to have an increased risk for vaginal clear cell carcinoma, but also have an increased risk of vaginal and cervical intraepithelial neoplasia.[8]

NATURAL HISTORY OF VAIL AND VAGINAL CANCER

The natural history of VAIL has not been well defined, but the majority of low-grade VAILs (condyloma or VAIN1) regress spontaneously.[9–11] Higher-grade lesions (VAIN grade 2 or 3), multifocal lesions, and those associated with neoplasia in other anogenital sites and in immunosuppressed patients are more likely to persist or recur. Some 5% of VAILs may progress to invasion despite close follow-up. An important variable in cancer risk is the age of the patient. The mean age of VAIL is closer to that of the vulva than cervix. In one study, the mean ages for grades 1, 2 and 3 disease were 39, 49 and 57, fully 10–20 years later than that for comparable grade lesions of the cervix.[11] The peak incidence of vaginal carcinoma is in the seventh decade, over 25 years after lesions begin to develop on the vaginal mucosa.

EXAMINATION OF THE PATIENT

Vaginal inspection is a required component of the pelvic examination, and usually entails rapid inspection of the mucosal surface during speculum placement. The indications for vaginal colposcopy are summarized in Table 12.2.

The entire vagina needs to be closely examined since the appearance of a VAIL can be subtle. Special attention should be given to the upper one-third of the vagina, where the majority of disease is present (Fig. 12.1). Both acetic acid and Lugol's solution can be used in colposcopic evaluation of the vagina provided the patient does not have an allergy to iodine. Lugol's solution stains glycogen-containing tissue, producing a dark mahogany brown color; non-glycogenated epithelium, specifically intraepithelial neoplasia, does not stain, typically appearing mustard-yellow in color (Fig. 12.2). The chief limitation of Lugol's solution is lack of specificity, i.e. atrophic or inflammatory conditions of the vagina accompanied by immature squamous epithelium (and lacking glycogen) will also not stain. This is not as helpful in women with atrophy or inflammation of the vagina.

Table 12.2 *Indications for performing detailed vaginal colposcopy*

1 An abnormal Papanicolaou (Pap) smear following hysterectomy
2 An abnormal Pap smear after apparently successful treatment of cervical neoplasia
3 Any Pap smear unexplained by cervical colposcopy or sampling of the endocervical canal
4 Any palpable or unexplained grossly visible vaginal lesion
5 All women with cervical, vulvar or perianal/anal HPV disease
6 Confirmed cervical neoplasia in an immunosuppressed patient
7 Monitoring all women with a history of *in utero* DES exposure
8 Any woman with abnormal, unexplained, recalcitrant vaginal discharge or bleeding
9 Prior to cervical conization for non-correlating cytology, histology and colposcopic impression

Adapted from Ferris et al.[7]

Abnormal vascular patterns associated with VAIL can be seen with colposcopy, and well-developed vascular patterns of punctuation or mosaicism and atypical irregularly branched vessels are highly suspicious for invasive cancer. However, high-grade VAILs (HIVAIL) may appear simply as flat white epithelium. Thus, any potential lesion should be biopsied.

HISTOLOGY OF VAIL

VAILs are identical to their counterparts in the cervix and fall into a spectrum ranging from flat or exophytic

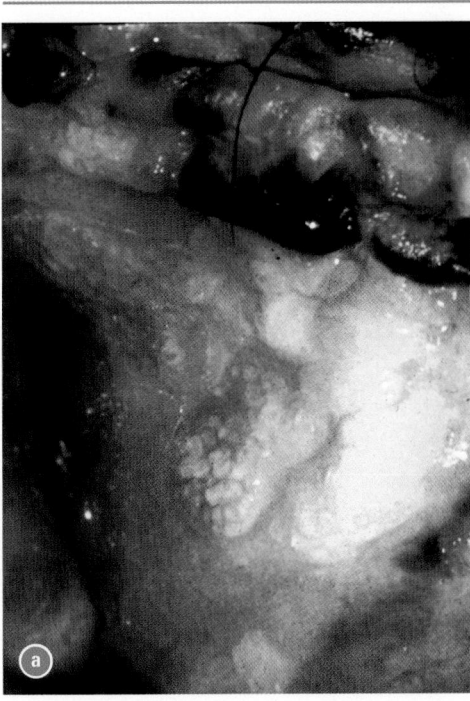 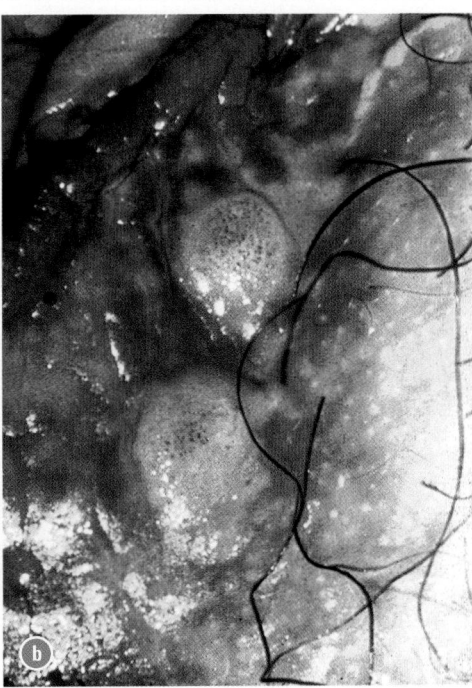

Fig. 12.1 (a) Vaginal intraepithelial lesion with hyperkeratosis (lower right). (b) Acetowhite lesions (center) with punctuation.

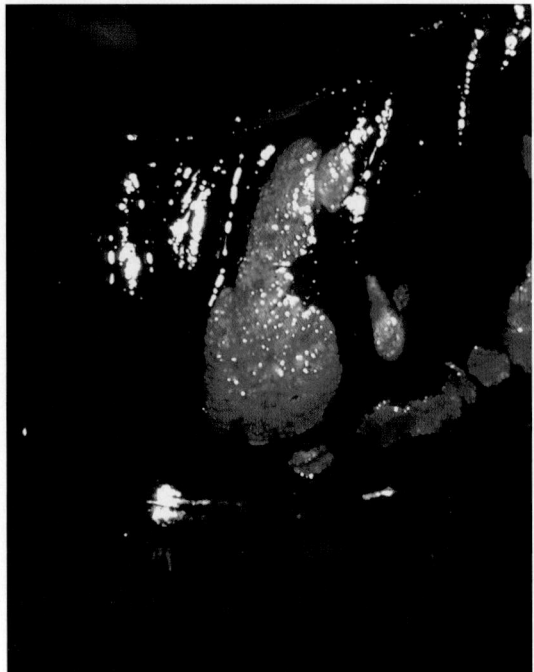

Fig. 12.2 High-grade vaginal intraepithelial lesion (VAIN 3), conspicuous for the absence of Lugol's uptake.

Table 12.3 Classification of vaginal intraepithelial lesions

Term	Term(s) used on the pathology report
LOVAIL	Low-grade squamous intraepithelial lesion (condyloma/VAIN1)
Exophytic condyloma	
Flat condyloma (VAIN1)	
HIVAIL	High-grade squamous intraepithelial lesion (VAIN2/VAIN3)
VAIN2	
VAIN3	
VAIN3 papillary	

the entities that fall into this spectrum and which include the following.

Low-grade vaginal intraepithelial lesions (LOVAILs)

These include exophytic condylomas, which are commonly associated with HPV types 6 and 11. These lesions are discussed in both Chapters 6 and 13 and consist of exophytic verrucopapillary lesions with surface atypia and koilocytosis (Fig. 12.3). The second category is the flat condyloma, which has a similar distribution of cellular atypia, but lacks the exophytic architecture (Fig. 12.4). Central to the diagnosis of these LOVAILs is the absence of conspicuous nuclear atypia in the lower epithelial cell layers.

The epithelial changes most likely to be confused with LOVAIL include non-specific acanthotic changes associated with prolapse (Fig. 12.5a). More likely to

condylomas, in which the atypia manifests as superficial cell nuclear enlargement and koilocytotic atypia, to full-thickness nuclear atypia of variable maturation (vaginal intraepithelial neoplasia). Table 12.3 outlines

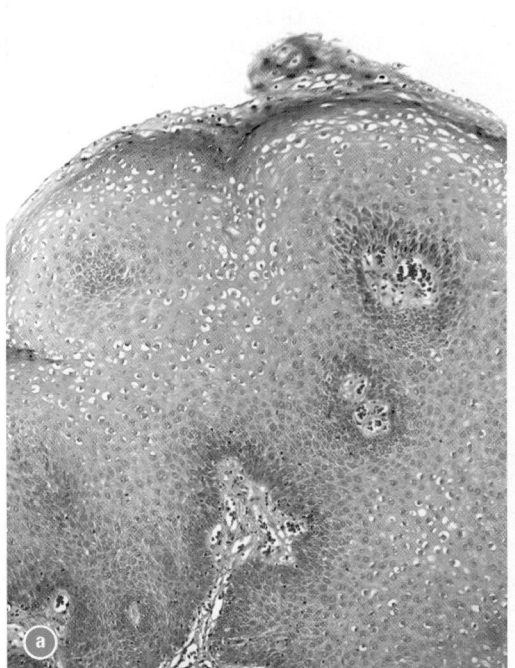
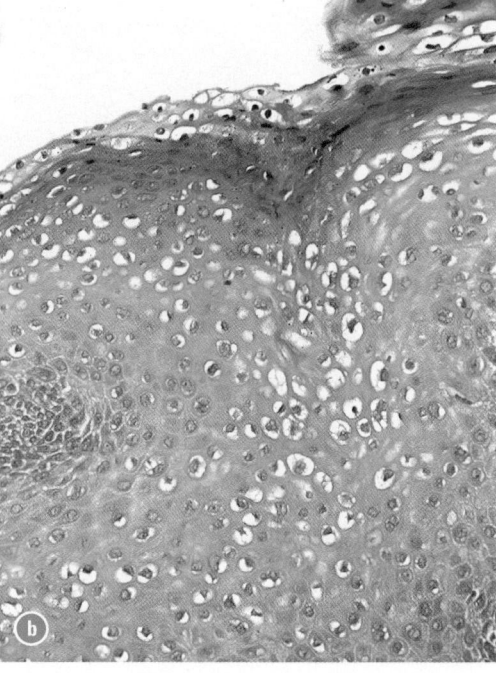

Fig. 12.3 (a,b) Low-grade vaginal intraepithelial lesion (exophytic condyloma).

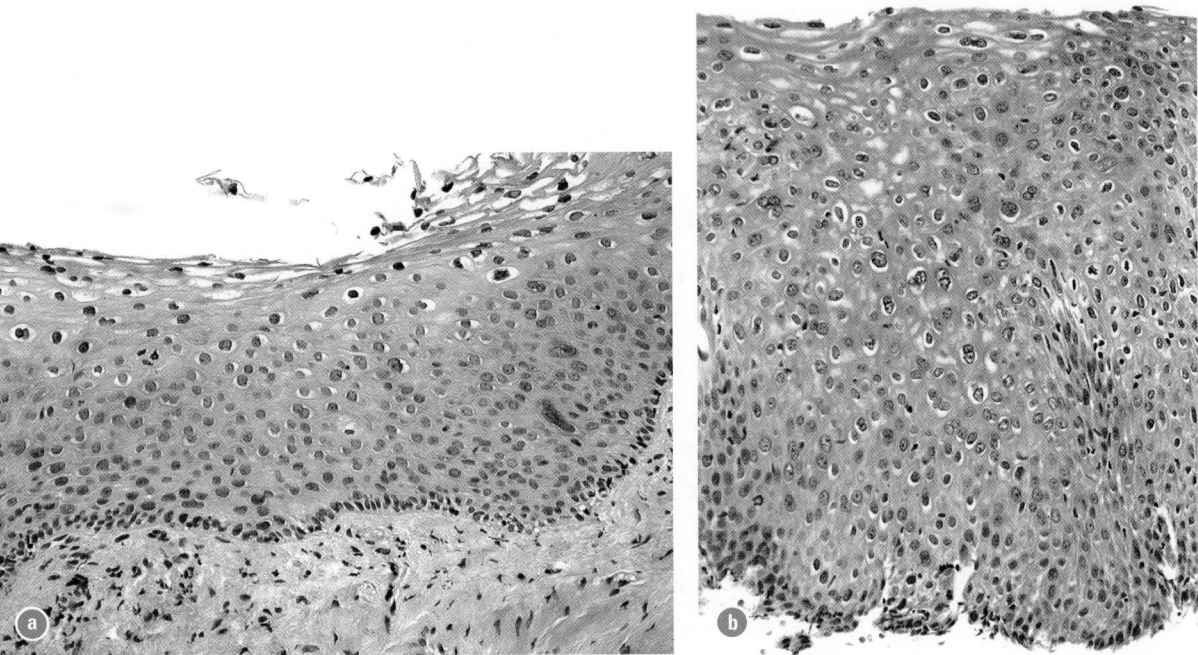

Fig. 12.4 (a,b) Low-grade vaginal intraepithelial lesion (flat condyloma or vaginal intraepithelial neoplasia grade 1).

be confused with LOVAIL, at least historically, are small polyp-like excrescences in the introitus of reproductive age women (see Ch. 11) (Fig. 12.5b). These changes lack cellular atypia and acanthosis and are no longer as likely to be confused with HPV infections as they were in the 1980s.[12] If the pathologist is concerned, he or she can immunostain for a proliferative marker Ki-67 (MIB-1 antibody), which will high-

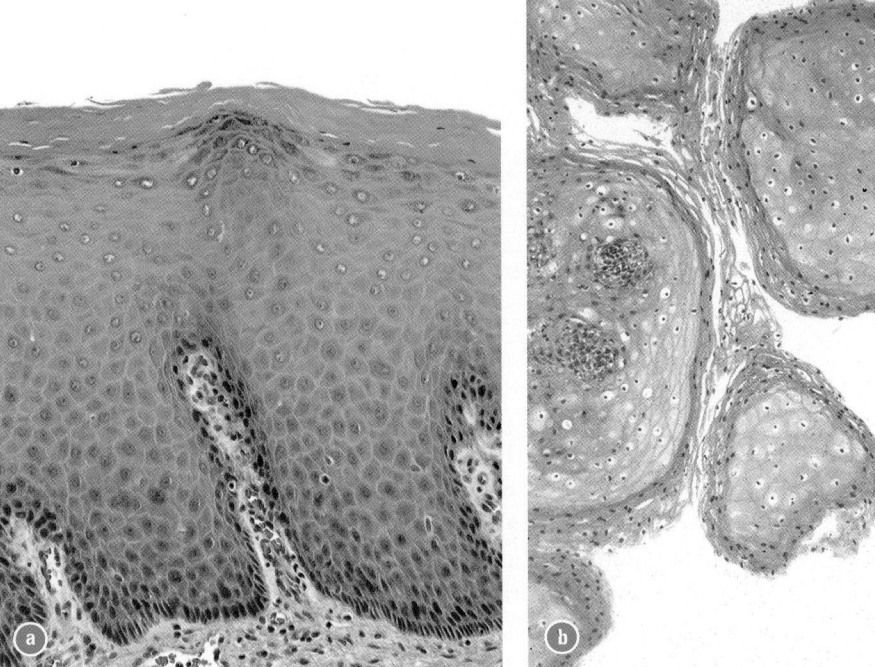

Fig. 12.5 Differential diagnosis of LOVAIL. (a) Non-specific acanthosis. (b) Mucosal excrescences near the hymenal ring.

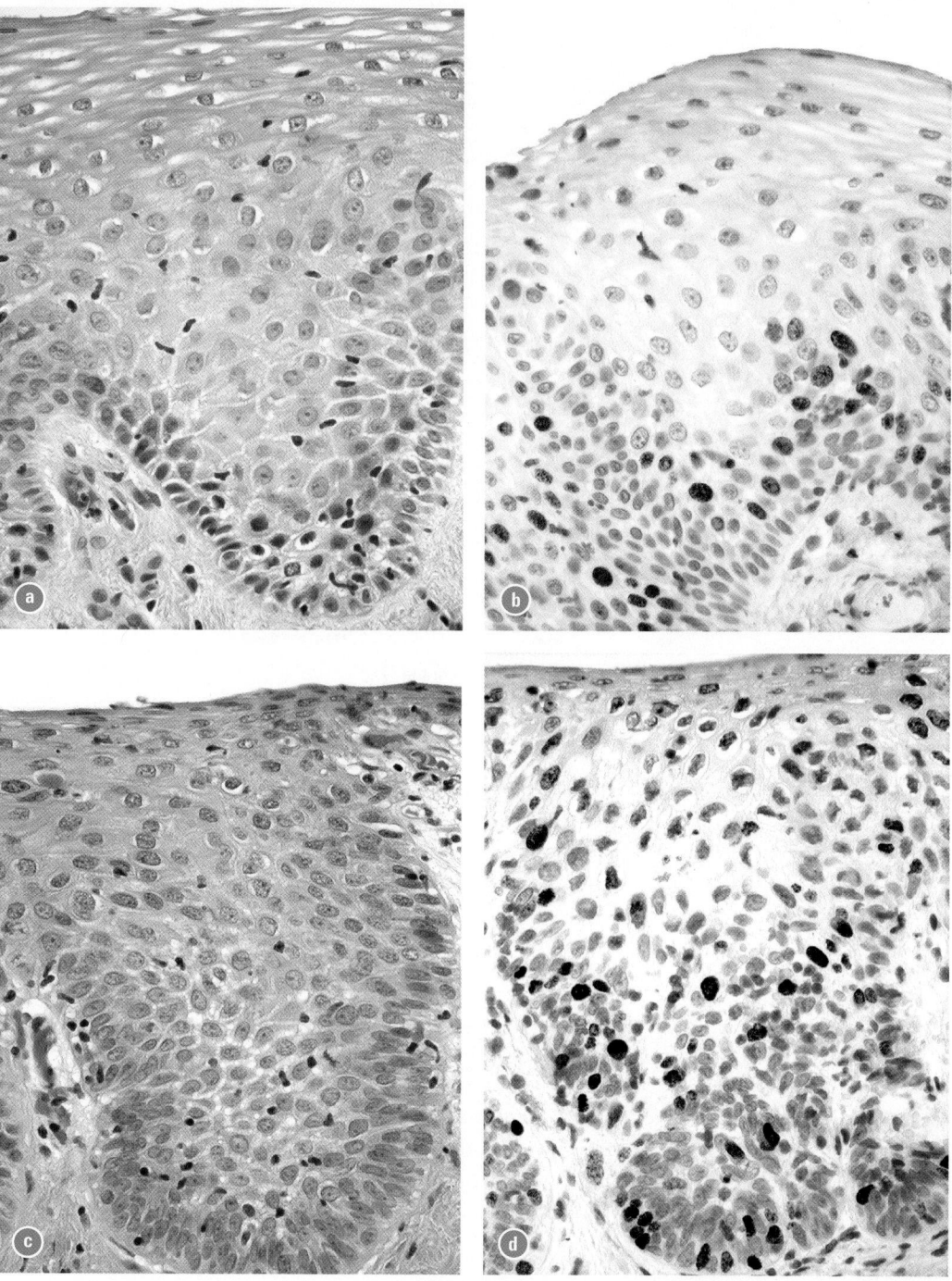

Fig. 12.6 Staining for MIB-1 highlights immunopositive cells in the para basal cells of normal mucosa (a,b). Nuclear staining is seen in the upper cell layer of this LOVAIL (c,d).

light superficial cell nuclei that are undergoing DNA turnover as a consequence of papillomaviral replication (Fig. 12.6). The same cells will harbor HPV nucleic acid (Fig. 12.7).[13,14]

HIVAIL

Criteria for high-grade vaginal intraepithelial lesions (Figs 12.8–12.10) are identical to those of the cervix and vulva. Lesions displaying full-thickness atypia are classified in this category and may be graded as VAIN2 or VAIN3, with increasing loss of maturation. Care should be taken to recognize papillary architecture, which may increase the risk of concomitant invasion (see Chapters 6 and 13) (Fig. 12.11a,b). Conversely, atrophic changes and radiation effect may mimic HIVAIL (Figs 12.12, 12.13).

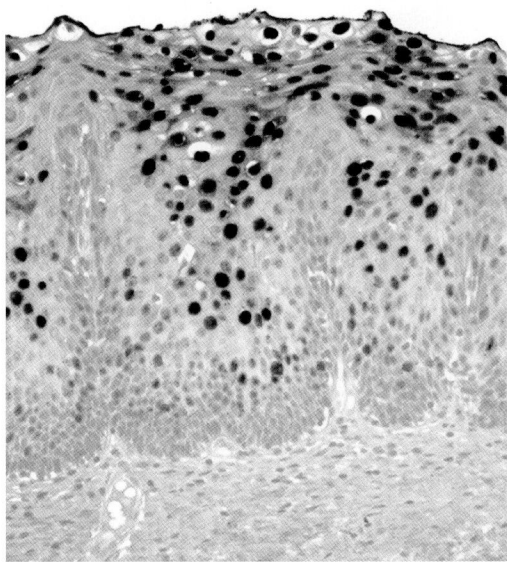

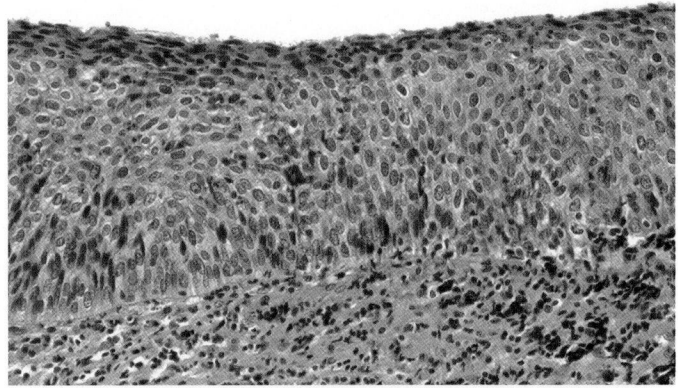

Fig. 12.9 High-grade vaginal intraepithelial lesion (vaginal intraepithelial neoplasia grade 3), containing minimal epithelial maturation.

Fig. 12.7 Localization of HPV nucleic acids in a mucosal condyloma. Note the hybridization signal is strongest in the upper epithelial lesions, similar in distribution to MIB-1 staining (Fig. 12.6). (Compare with Fig. 11.2.)

MANAGEMENT OF VAGINAL INTRAEPITHELIAL LESIONS

The histologic diagnosis of VAIL, age of the patient and available tools for treating the patient will influence management. In young women, who have a high rate of spontaneous regression, the therapeutic option includes simple observation.[15] If treatment is decided upon, treatment, if LOVAIL should not be aggressive, since risk of complications may outweigh the risk of the disease. To avoid post-therapy complications such as adhesions or dyspareunia, the clinician should particularly avoid prolonged topical treatment with 5-fluorouracil or aggressive laser treatment of the vagina, particularly near the introitus. The progression of LOVAIL to a higher grade of cancer is extremely infrequent.[7,16]

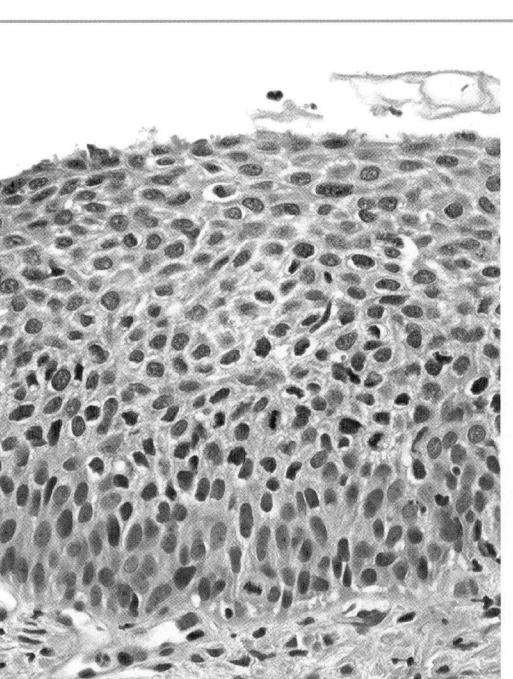

Fig. 12.8 High-grade vaginal intraepithelial lesion (vaginal intraepithelial neoplasia grade 2), exhibiting superficial maturation (center).

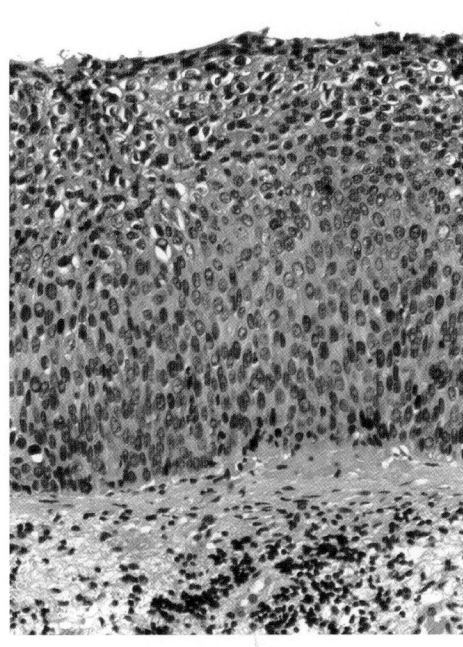

Fig. 12.10 High-grade vaginal intraepithelial lesion (vaginal intraepithelial neoplasia grade 3), similar to classic descriptions of carcinoma in situ.

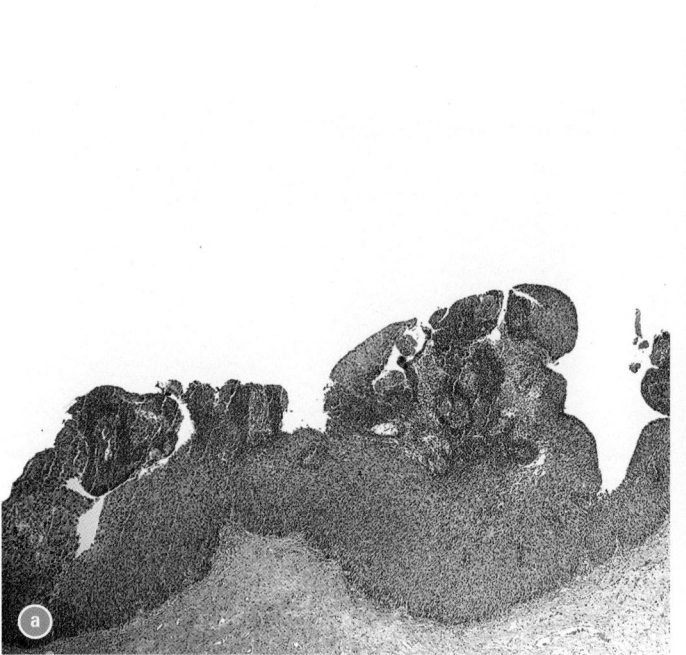
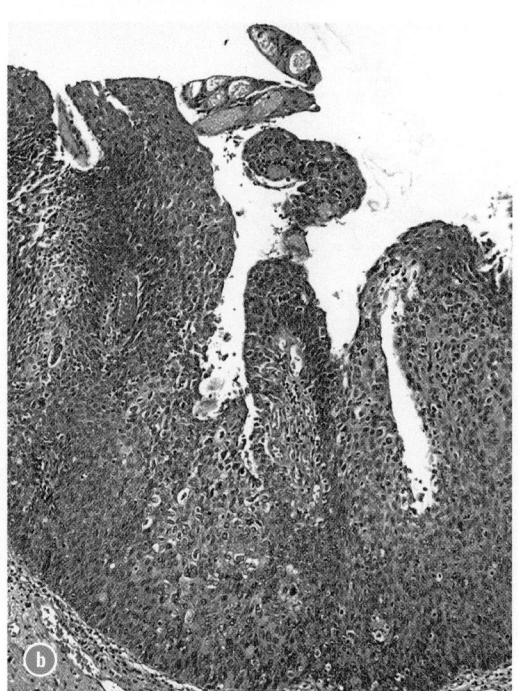

Fig. 12.11 (a) High-grade vaginal intraepithelial lesion with papillary architecture; (b) at higher magnification.

More decisive measures should be reserved for HIVAIL (Figs 12.11–12.14), including vaginal intraepithelial neoplasia grade 2 or 3. Modes of therapy include topical agents (trichloroacetic acid (TCA), 5-fluorouracil[17-22] and imiquimod cream).[23,24] Trichloroacetic acid is only used to very localized low-grade lesions. Imiquimod remains an investigational drug for HIVAIL and is used more frequently for vulvar lesions. Other treatment options include CO_2 laser,[25] loop electroexcision procedure (LEEP) for small discrete lesions, and surgical excision. Treatment failure as well as complications can occur with any

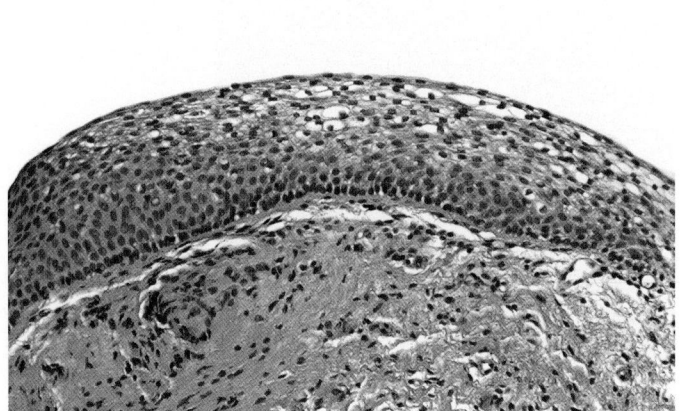

Fig. 12.12 Differential diagnosis of HIVAIL. Atrophic cell changes. Note the uniform nuclear morphology and absence of mitotic activity.

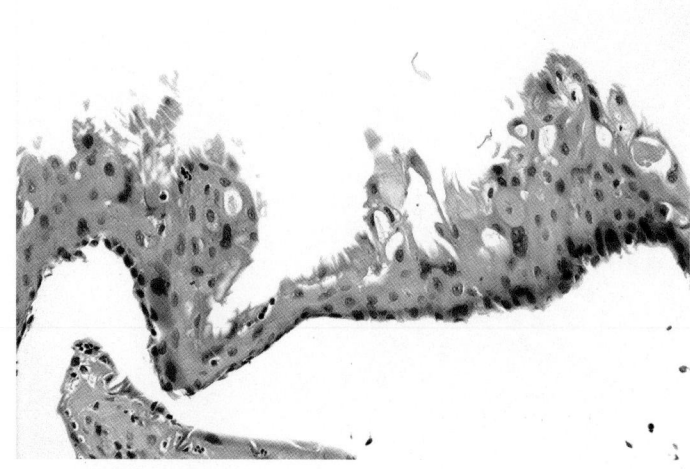

Fig. 12.13 Differential diagnosis of HIVAIL. Radiation effect. Nuclear atypia is present. Note, however, the low nuclear-cytoplasmic ratio and homogeneous chromatin distribution in the abnormal cells.

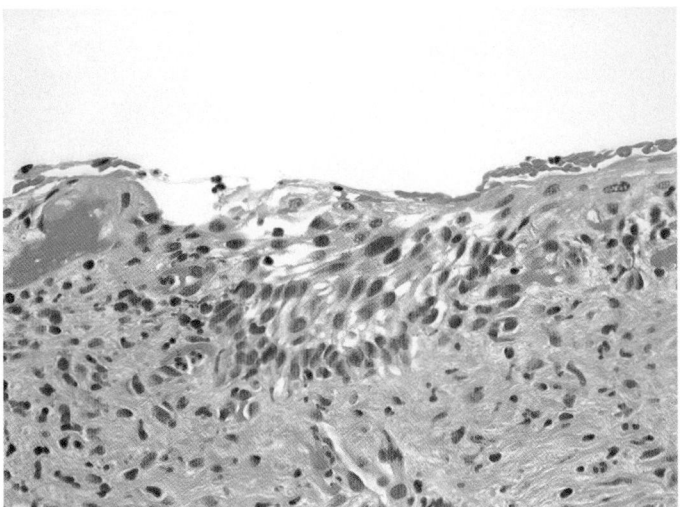
Fig. 12.14 Differential diagnosis of HIVAIL. Marked inflammatory atypia.

Malignant epithelial neoplasms of the vagina

INTRODUCTION

Vaginal cancers constitute approximately 1–4% of all gynecologic cancers. The most common tissue type of carcinoma is squamous cell carcinoma. Rare tumors include adenocarcinoma, melanoma and sarcomas. Non-epithelial tumor types such as endodermal sinus tumor and botryoid embryonal rhabdomyosarcoma are the most common vaginal cancers of children, although rhabdomyosarcomas have been reported in the elderly population.[7,30–34] Several of these tumors will be addressed in the following discussion.

SQUAMOUS CELL CARCINOMA

Introduction and pathogenesis

Squamous cell carcinoma of the vagina is uncommon, and accounts for less than 2% of malignancies in the female genital tract. The following characterize this disorder and distinguish it to some degree from primary cervical cancer:

1 Squamous carcinomas are the most common type, accounting for approximately 85% of vaginal carcinomas.

2 The majority of vaginal squamous carcinomas occur in the sixth to eighth decades, approximately 20 years older than the mean age for squamous carcinoma of the cervix.

3 Vaginal carcinomas in younger (under age 50) women are more closely associated with HPV-related (or cervical) neoplasms, being more commonly linked to location in the upper vagina, vaginal infections and prior cervical intraepithelial neoplasia.

4 Approximately one-fifth have had a prior cervical squamous neoplasm, either preinvasive or invasive.[35]

The above suggest that vaginal carcinomas occurring in older women, like vulvar carcinoma, develop via pathways that require exposure to more than a sexually transmitted agent. The data suggest that vaginal carcinomas in older women are HPV-related, but risk is influenced by other cofactors, including age, lack of estrogen, prior irradiation and vaginal trauma.[35]

Clinical presentation

The patient with vaginal cancer most commonly presents with painless bleeding or a vaginal discharge that is

of these methods. Complications, particularly with 5-fluorouracil, include extensive vaginal ulcerations[26] and difficulty in subsequent healing of these lesions. 5-Fluorouracil is used less frequently today than in previous years. Loop electroexcision has been used for VAIN; however, it can be risky to perform, since surrounding tissue damage may occur. There is a potential for bowel and bladder injury. Laser is best used for extensive persisting LOVAIL or/and HIVAIL.[27,28] Laser is particularly helpful when there is disease extending from the cervix to the superior vagina. Surgery is an excellent alternative in the proper setting. In one study of post-hysterectomy patients with HIVAIL (VAIN3) at the vaginal apex in the region of vaginal cuff scar, upper vaginectomy was found to be the treatment of choice, while multifocal HIVAIL or colposcopically well-defined lesions, involving large areas of vaginal mucosa, were found to be successfully managed by CO_2 laser ablation.[29] Risk factors for persistence or progression of HIVAIL include multifocal lesions and anogenital neoplastic syndrome. Patients should be advised that, with any treatment, there is no guarantee against recurrence, and close follow-up is required.

POST-RADIATION DYSPLASIA (HIVAIL)

As discussed above, preinvasive vaginal disease can occur following radiation therapy, usually within 1 to 10 years. These lesions are typically associated with HPV nucleic acids. There is no evidence for a separate pathway (non-HPV) for these lesions.

malodorous. Urinary symptoms and pain have also been reported. A rectovaginal examination is often helpful in delineating submucosal extension, para-vaginal infiltration and rectal involvement. Tumors may be exophytic, ulcerative, annular, constricting, polypoid, sessile, indurated, or fungating and may be located anywhere in the vagina. Approximately 40% of squamous cell carcinomas of the vagina occur on the anterior, 30% on the posterior and 28% on the lateral walls. From 30 to 50% present as Stage I.[36,37]

Histopathology

The histopathologic findings in vaginal squamous carcinoma are similar to those in other sites. In our experience, two histologic presentations predominate. The first is a typical invasive squamous cell carcinoma (Fig. 12.15). The second is a papillary carcinoma (Fig. 12.16). The latter may or may not demonstrate frank invasion (Fig. 12.11), and often requires a more detailed histologic examination to confirm stromal invasion. A subset of these tumors are often superficial and have a history of prior cervical carcinoma, in which case a secondary implant from the cervix must be considered.

Management of invasive carcinoma of the vagina

Both radiation therapy and surgery are used to treat invasive squamous cell carcinoma of the vagina. Radiation therapy is the primary therapeutic choice for vaginal

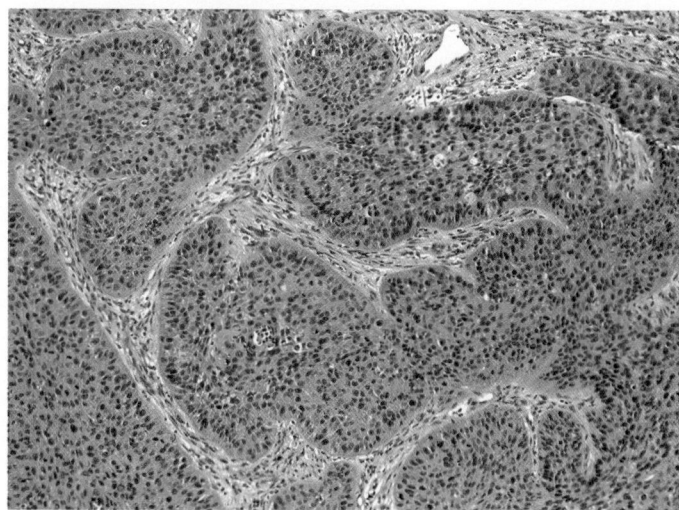

Fig. 12.15 Invasive squamous cell carcinoma with a uniform epithelial stromal interface and basaloid pattern.

cancer. Radiation therapy generally consists of a field pelvic port followed by an interstitial implant. If the lower-third of the vagina is involved, inguinal nodes are also targeted. Patients with large or high-stage lesions may benefit from the addition of radiation sensitizers (hydroxyurea or BUDR). Small Stage I lesions can be treated with brachytherapy alone.

Upper vaginal lesions are treated with radical hysterectomy and vaginectomy. This treatment is better suited

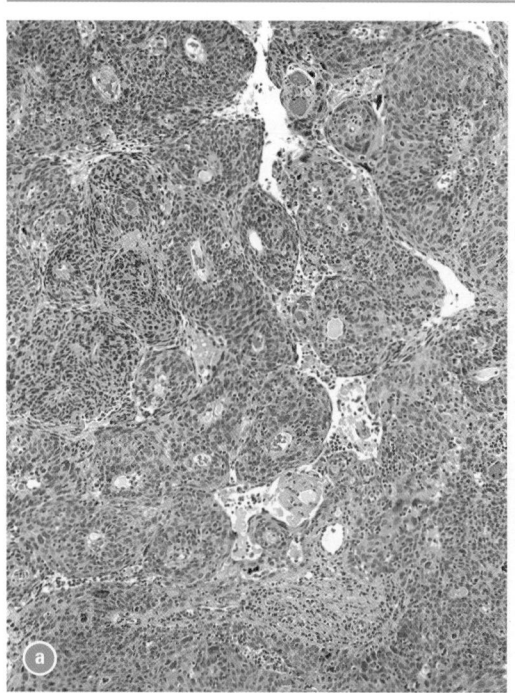
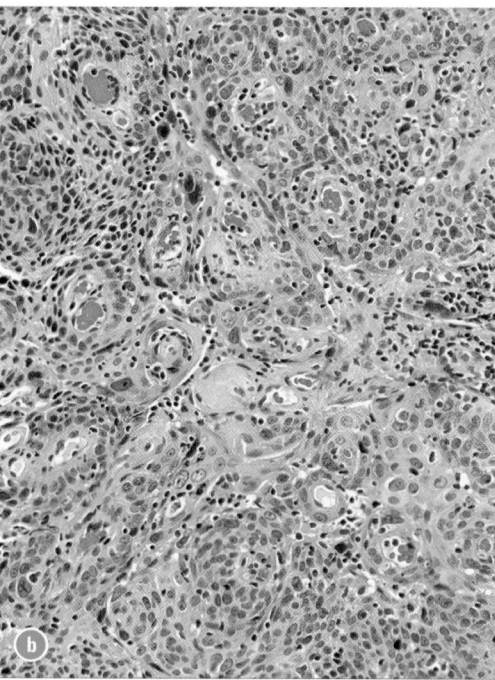

Fig. 12.16 (a) Papillary carcinoma. These tumors often exhibit a regular epithelial contour. Nevertheless, complete removal is necessary to exclude invasion. (b) Surface papillary tumor on the vaginal surface following prior treatment of cervical squamous cell carcinoma. This picture suggests direct implantation of neoplastic epithelium on the mucosal surface.

for superficial, posterior fornix lesions, or for patients who cannot be radiated. Recurrent tumors (after radiation) may be treatable by pelvic exenteration.

Behavior and outcome

The behavior of squamous cell carcinoma is dependent on stage (Table 12.4). Five-year survivals using the above modalities for Stage I, II, III and IV are approximately 75–80%, 45–60%, 31–43% and 20–40%, respectively.[37] These tumors generally spread laterally to the parametrial tissues when located in the upper vagina, and to the paravaginal tissues when originating in the lower vagina. Tumors also invade lymphatics, resulting in metastases to regional lymph nodes and, in some cases, spread to the lungs, liver or brain.

VERRUCOUS CARCINOMA

Verrucous carcinoma, a rare vaginal lesion, is a variant of squamous cell carcinoma.[38] Numerous other terms have been used previously for this condition, including giant condyloma acuminata (Buschke–Löwenstein tumor), squamous papillomatosis, condyloma acuminata with malignant transformation, and well-differentiated squamous cell carcinoma.[39] It is a well-differentiated, slowly growing, locally invasive tumor with a verrucous appearance and 'pushing margin' (Fig. 12.17). It often presents with small wartlike excrescences or larger cauliflower-like masses. The diagnosis of verrucous carcinoma may be difficult, particularly if the biopsy specimen involves only the surface epithelium. Despite macroscopic and microscopic similarities between condyloma acuminata and verrucous carcinoma, the role of human papillomavirus (HPV) in the etiology of verrucous carcinoma is not absolute.[40] Nevertheless, there are numerous case reports of HPV in genital verrucous carcinoma.[40–42]

Treatment consists of surgical excision. Verrucous carcinoma rarely metastasizes to lymph nodes or distant areas. Radiotherapy has been used, but is not the initial treatment.[43] High-dose interferon therapy also has been used both to decrease the tumor size and to prevent recurrences in some reports.[40,44]

Table 12.4 *Carcinoma of the vagina: FIGO nomenclature*

Stage 0	Carcinoma *in situ*, intraepithelial neoplasia grade 3
Stage I	The carcinoma is limited to the vaginal wall
Stage II	The carcinoma has involved the subvaginal tissue but has not extended to the pelvic wall
Stage III	The carcinoma has extended to the pelvic wall
Stage IV	The carcinoma has extended beyond the true pelvis or has involved the mucosa of the bladder or rectum; bullous edema as such does not permit a case to be allotted to Stage IV
IVa	Tumor invades bladder and/or rectal mucosa and/or direct extension beyond the true pelvis
IVb	Spread to distant organs

FIGO, Fédération Internationale de Gynécologie et Obstétrique.

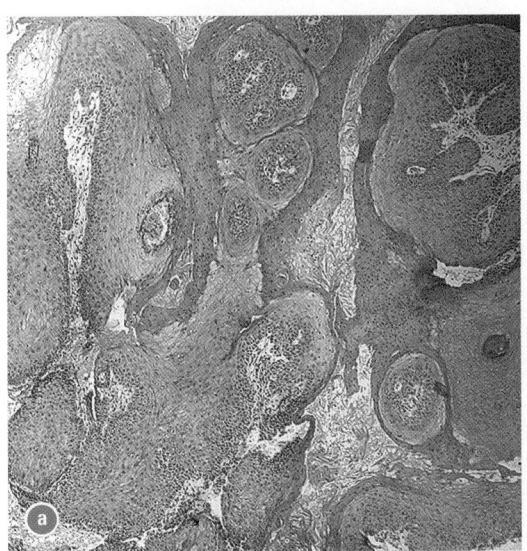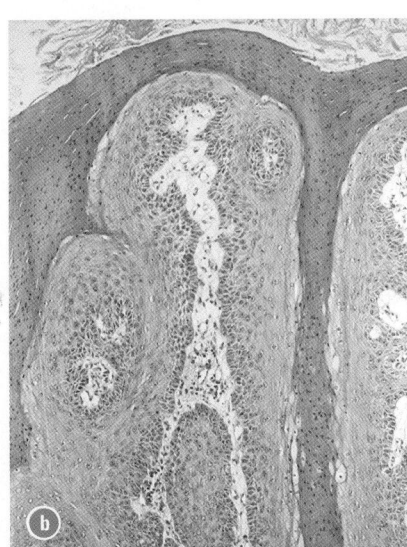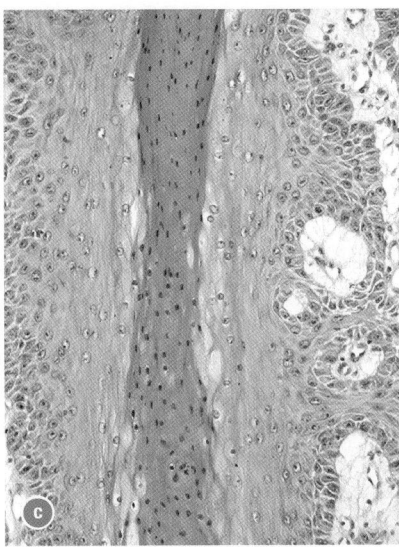

Fig. 12.17 Verrucous carcinoma. (a) The tumor exhibits verruciform architecture and invades along a uniform epithelial-stromal interface with minimal atypia. (b,c) Higher magnification of the epithelium, with pale epithelial cells and minimal surface atypia.

SQUAMO-TRANSITIONAL CARCINOMA

The squamo-transitional carcinoma of the vagina is a rare variant of squamous cell carcinoma. It has been found to be related to human papillomavirus infection, particularly the high-risk types. Rose et al. reported this condition in an 82-year-old patient with a 4 cm mass on the anterior distal vagina and distal urethra. The immunohistochemical profiles (cytokeratin-7 positive and CK-20 negative) and the detection of human papillomavirus 16 support its close relationship to conventional squamous cell carcinoma.[45] Papillary squamo-transitional cell carcinoma can be suspected on Pap smear when high-grade squamous intraepithelial lesion features are found in combination with three-dimensional papillary tissue fragments with prominent fibrovascular cores. It must be distinguished from benign vaginal condylomata, papillary HIVAIL and verrucous carcinoma.[46] In a study by Vesoulis and Erhardt, four criteria were found on a vaginal Pap smear in a patient with squamo-transitional carcinoma of the vagina: (1) large, darkly staining, three-dimensional, branching, papillary epithelial fragments with prominent fibrovascular cores and lined with loosely cohesive epithelial cells; (2) a highly cellular background population of dissociated single epithelial cells with features of severe dysplasia, including hyperchromatic, coarse chromatin; scant, delicate, frayed cytoplasm and karyorrhectic debris; (3) syncytial aggregates of severely dysplastic epithelial cells morphologically similar to the single cells; and (4) lack of a recognizable, morphologically distinct 'transitional cell' population.[46]

GLANDULAR NEOPLASIA

Introduction

Adenocarcinomas may be primary or metastatic (from glandular tumors arising in the endocervix, endometrium, or from distant sites such as breast, ovary, or bowel). Primary adenocarcinomas of the vagina are far less frequent than metastatic spread from local or distant glandular tumors. The diagnosis of adenocarcinoma in the vagina should always raise suspicion of the possibility of a primary elsewhere. The various forms of vaginal adenocarcinomas include endometrioid adenocarcinoma, adenocarcinomas of mucinous or intestinal type, adenosquamous carcinomas, paravaginal mesonephric adenocarcinomas and adnexal (Wolffian) tumors, serous papillary adenocarcinomas and adenoid cystic carcinoma.[47] The treatment of vaginal adenocarcinoma is similar to treatment of squamous cell types.

Primary tumors arising in endometriosis

Endometriosis is uncommon in the vagina but malignant transformation of endometriosis does occur (Fig. 12.18)[48,49]. The criteria for malignancy arising in endometriosis include: (1) demonstration of both cancerous and benign endometrial tissues in the same organ, especially if contiguous; (2) demonstration of cancer arising in the tissue and not invading it from another source; and (3) presence of tissue resembling endometrial stroma surrounding characteristic glands. There are difficulties with the application of these criteria, however. The sampling technique may not be adequate to find a small focus of endometriosis adjacent to a malignant tumor. A tumor may destroy the endometriotic tissue from which it arose, or the endometriosis may be deemed to be a minor component, and in such cases is not reported. These factors may lead to underreporting of the association of malignancy with endometriosis.[50]

Endometriosis-related malignancies generally are associated with a favorable prognosis.[51] Specific malignant tumors arising in endometriosis of the vagina include adenocarcinoma,[52,53] endometrioid adenocarcinoma,[54] Müllerian adenosarcoma[55–57] and stromal sarcoma.[50,58]

Some tumors arising in endometriosis are particularly challenging.[57] In particular, adenosarcomas can be confused with adenofibromas or stromal-rich

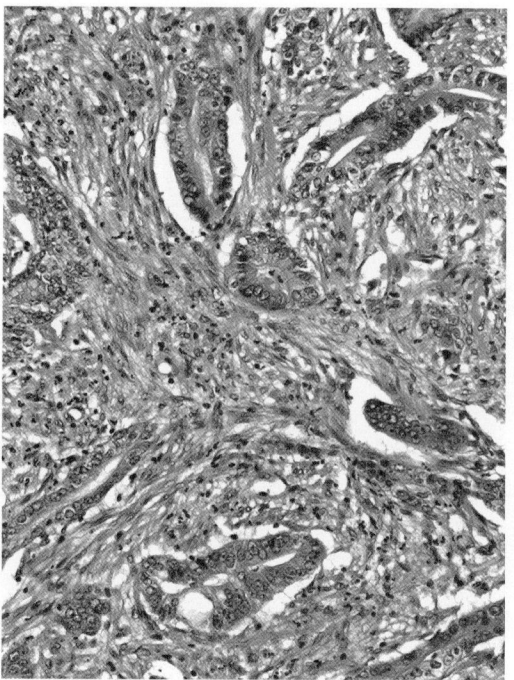

Fig. 12.18 Adenocarcinoma arising in endometriosis.

endometriosis, particularly if they exhibit large areas of low cellularity and infrequent mitoses.[59,60] In these cases, it is important to seek stromal nuclear atypia and periglandular stromal cuffing, which are features that are diagnostic of adenosarcoma. Clement and Scully[61] reported that two or more stromal mitoses per 10 high-power fields, marked stromal cellularity and significant stromal cell atypia are criteria useful in separating Müllerian adenosarcoma from Müllerian adenofibroma. However, these parameters may not resolve the nature of small tissue samples and the pathologist may require additional time to confirm or exclude the diagnosis.

Clear cell adenocarcinoma

Clear cell adenocarcinoma of the vagina and cervix is rare in women without *in utero* DES exposure. In the patient with a clear cell adenocarcinoma who has not been exposed to DES, the cancer usually develops in the postmenopausal period.[62,63]

Clear cell adenocarcinoma of the vagina increased after exposures to diethylstilbestrol (DES).[64,65] Diethylstilbestrol is a synthetic nonsteroidal estrogen that was used to prevent miscarriage and many other pregnancy complications between 1938 and 1971 in the USA. The United States Food and Drug Administration issued a warning in 1971 about the use of diethylstilbestrol during pregnancy secondary to a connection between this synthetic estrogen and the development of clear cell adenocarcinoma of the vagina and cervix. Abnormalities were found in young women whose mothers had taken diethylstilbestrol during pregnancy.

The estimated risk for clear cell adenocarcinoma in DES daughters is approximately 1 per 1000.[66,67] The incidence of adenocarcinoma of the vagina and cervix peaks at age 20 years in this population. It is rare after age 30, but has been reported in a 48-year-old woman. In women not exposed to DES, this cancer occurs much later in life, around the sixth to ninth decade of life. As the age increases in the population of women exposed to DES, these findings are becoming less common. Squamous cell neoplasias have also occurred in this patient population.[68]

The signs of this now rare vaginal adenocarcinoma include bleeding or discharge and a gross lesion on the vagina or cervix. The tumors generally occur in the upper-third of the vagina, on the anterior aspect, which coincides with the most common site of adenosis.[47] Approximately 15% of Stage I tumors and 40% of Stage II tumors have metastasized to lymph nodes at presentation.[47]

Characteristic histologic features of clear cell carcinomas include unbounded tumor cells with prominent nuclear atypia arranged in tubulo-cystic and papillary patterns (Fig. 12.19a,b). These features are similar to clear cell carcinomas elsewhere in the genital tract (see Chapters 19, 27).

Women with a known or suspected intrauterine exposure to DES should undergo regular clinical and cytologic evaluation.[69] Gynecologic examinations should include digital palpation of the vagina and cervix. An initial colposcopic examination should be performed; if the findings are abnormal, colposcopy should be repeated annually and four-quadrant Pap smears are recommended.

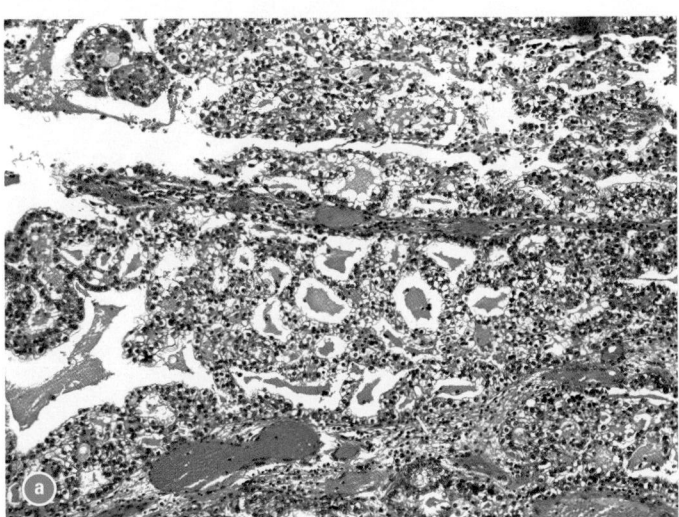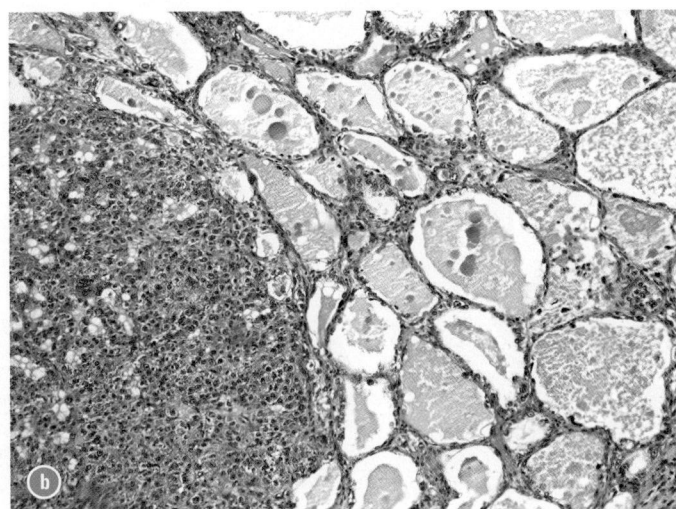

Fig. 12.19 Clear cell carcinoma of the cervix and vagina in a 22-year-old woman. (a) Tubular pattern with characteristic cuboidal epithelial cells, with discrete cell borders, clear cytoplasm and uniform nuclear morphology. (b) Merging of cystic (right) and solid (left) patterns.

A low threshold for biopsy should be present for any new visible or palpable lesions, as well as changes of concern on cytology.[70] Since clear cell adenocarcinoma can occur in postmenopausal women, regular cytologic examinations of DES-exposed women should be continued after menopause.[71] (Additional information on DES exposure is available at: http://www.cdc.gov/des/index.html.)

Both polypoid and ulcerative clear cell adenocarcinomas occur. Atypical vessels predominate as the most identifiable sign in lesions that are less developed. Adenosis is generally located next to the tumor.

Cloacogenic neoplasia

Cloacogenic neoplasia in the vagina is a unique disorder characterized by the presence of colonic-type epithelium, in the absence of a history of a colonic tumor or rectovaginal fistula. These lesions may present as colonic mucosa, colonic-type polyps and, rarely, as invasive adenocarcinomas of colonic type (Fig. 12.20).[72–74]

Müllerian papilloma

Generally, papillary squamous lesions of the vagina are related to the human papillomavirus. However, there is a rare, benign epithelial papilloma of the vagina that is similar to the Müllerian papilloma of the cervix. They are composed of frond-like projections with loose fibrovascular cores. Histologic evaluation reveals flat cuboidal, columnar, or non-keratinizing squamous epithelium (see Ch. 14). Generally, these tumors occur in children,[75] but they have been described the adult.[76] At times they may be pigmented.[77] Treatment is surgical excision of the papilloma. These tumors have been reported to reoccur (see also Chapter 14).[78]

Metastatic tumors to the vagina

Metastatic tumors to the vagina can be divided into two categories. The first and by far most common are metastases from other Müllerian neoplasms. Of these, the most common are of endometrial origin. *Endometrial carcinomas* were the most common primary site (78%) in a study by Mazur et al. (Fig. 12.21, 12.22, 12.23);[79] less common but always deserving consideration in the differential diagnosis are *ovarian and tubal carcinomas* and carcinosarcomas (Figs 12.24, and 12.25). Rarely, trophoblastic tumors, including both *placental site trophoblastic tumors (PSTTs) and choriocarcinomas* may involve the vagina, and we have seen a case of PSTT that presented as a vaginal mass without a prior history.[79–82] Other epithelial neoplasms include urinary bladder,[83,84] breast,[85–87] kidney,[88–90] colorectal carcinomas[91,92] and melanomas.[93,94] Rarely, metastatic mesenchymal lesions such as uterine leiomyosarcomas have been reported in the vagina.[95]

VAGINAL MELANOMA

Primary melanoma of the vagina is an extremely rare condition. It is most often found in postmenopausal women and approximately 40% of the tumors occur in

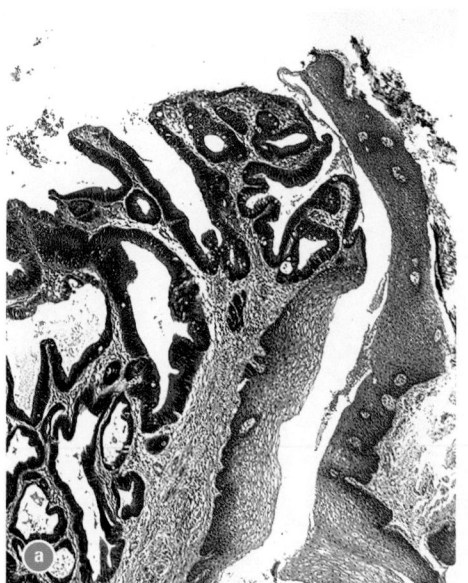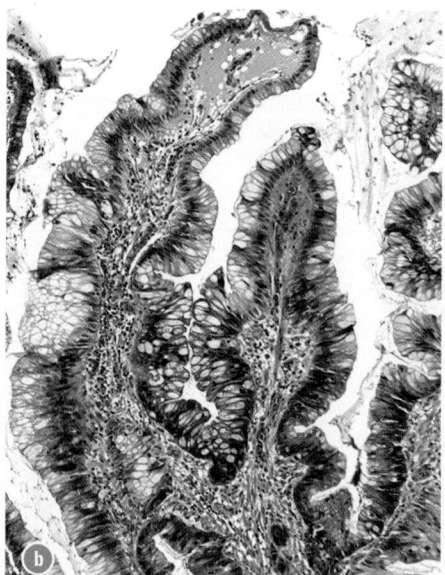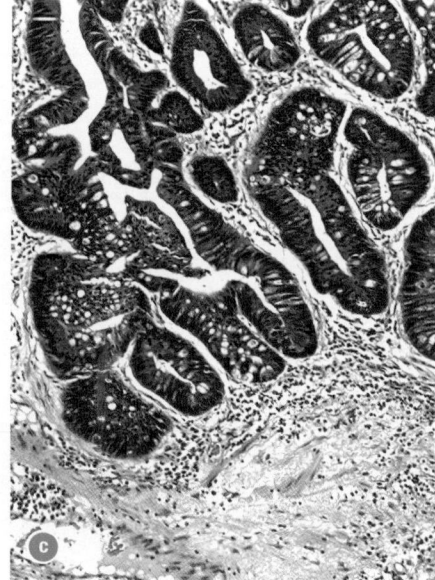

Fig. 12.20 Cloacogenic neoplasia of the vagina. (a) Merging of normal squamous mucosa (right) and a lesion closely resembling a villous adenoma of the colon (left). (b) Well-differentiated villous architecture. (c) Colonic-type glands.

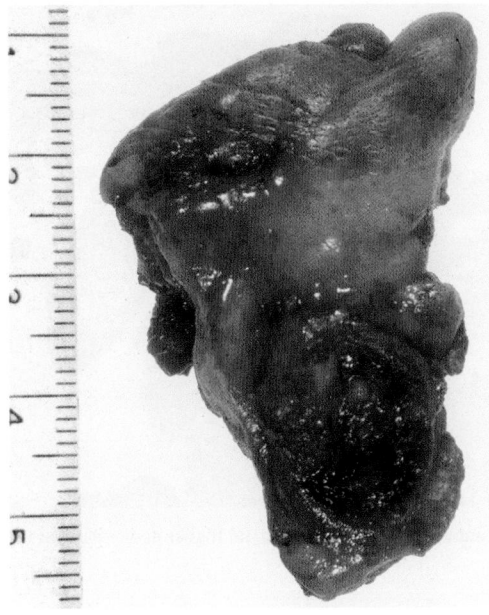

Fig. 12.21 Partial vaginectomy with metastatic endometrial adenocarcinoma. Note the ulcerated tumor at the bottom of the specimen.

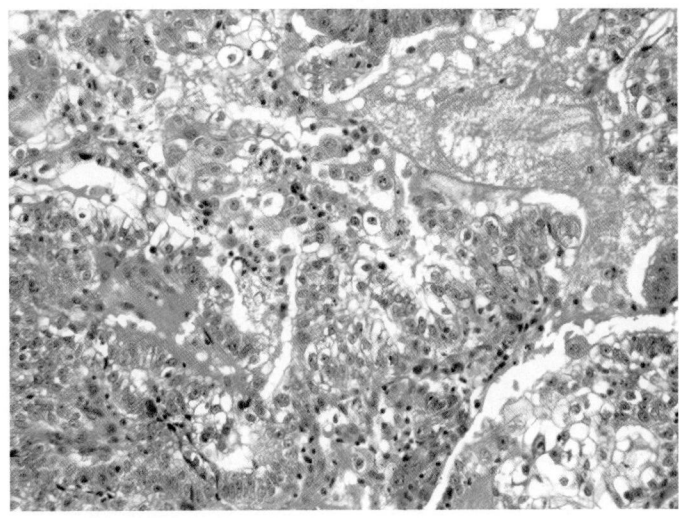

Fig. 12.23 Metastatic endometrial carcinoma; clear cell type.

the lower-third of the vagina.[47] Signs include bleeding, discharge and palpable vaginal mass that may or may not be pigmented.[96] This diagnosis carries a poor prognosis associated with a high rate of recurrences and only rare long-term survivorship.[97,98] Its clinical behavior is notoriously more aggressive than that of cutaneous and vulvar melanoma, with a 5-year survival rate ranging from 5% to 25%.[99] Several clinical subtypes have been described, but the prognosis for all subtypes correlates with the histologic thickness (Breslow depth) of the tumor.

The histologic diagnosis of vaginal melanoma may be difficult in the absence of pigment, but should always be suspected with any poorly differentiated

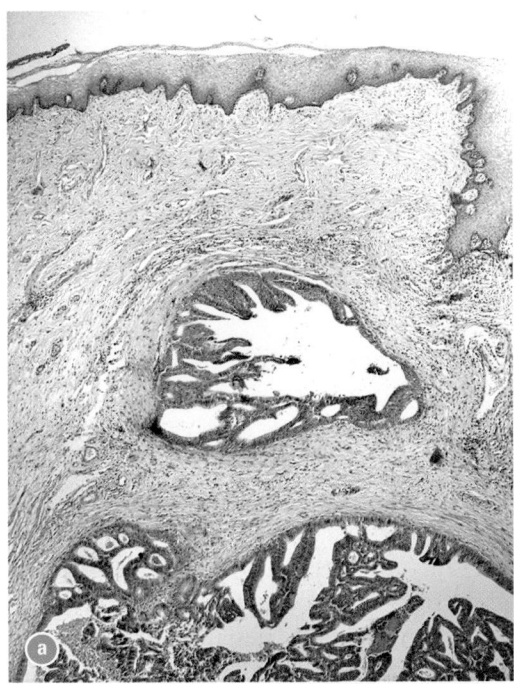

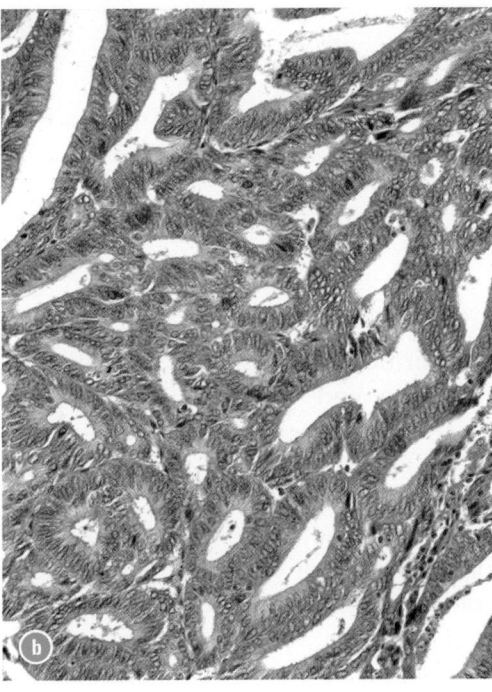

Fig. 12.22 Metastatic endometrial carcinoma, endometrioid type, beneath the mucosa (a) and at higher magnification (b).

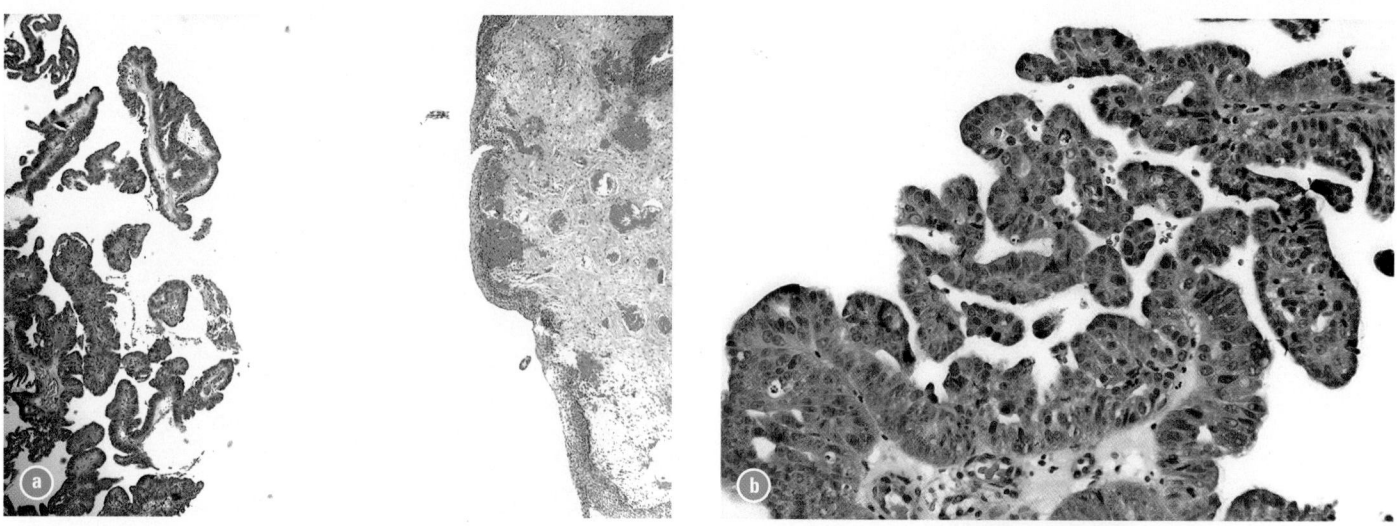

Fig. 12.24 Metastatic carcinoma from the ovary, serous type. (a) Low-power image of tumor (left) and adjacent vaginal mucosa (right). (b) Higher power illustrates the papillary architecture and nuclear atypia of a metastatic serous neoplasm.

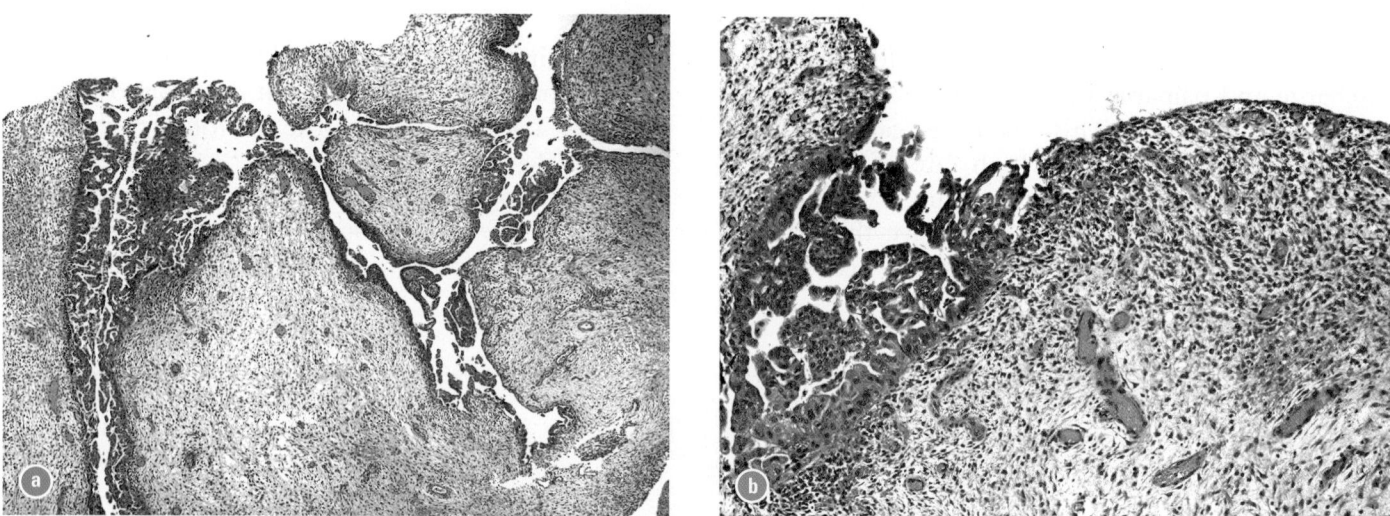

Fig. 12.25 Metastatic carcinoma: carcinosarcoma. (a) Low-power image of glands and stroma. (b) at higher magnification. These tumors might also arise in endometriosis.

epithelial tumor. It can be confirmed by positive immunostaining for S100, vimentin and HMB-45 (Fig. 12.26). The tumors are cytokeratin-negative.[47]

Treatment

Treatment of vaginal melanoma consists of excision when possible. Traditionally, radical surgery has been recommended as the first line of treatment; however, many recent publications have reported that wide local excision has equivalent survival rates.[96,100,101] This tumor tends to have a poor response to radical surgery and adjuvant therapy.[98] Because of the low rate of lymph node metastasis, elective pelvic lymph node dissection is not obligatory. In cases of surgically unresectable disease, primary radiation therapy may be indicated.[102] Adjuvant interferon (INF) is utilized for melanomas at times; however, the use of chemotherapy has not been proven valuable, either as a primary or a salvage therapy.[103,104]

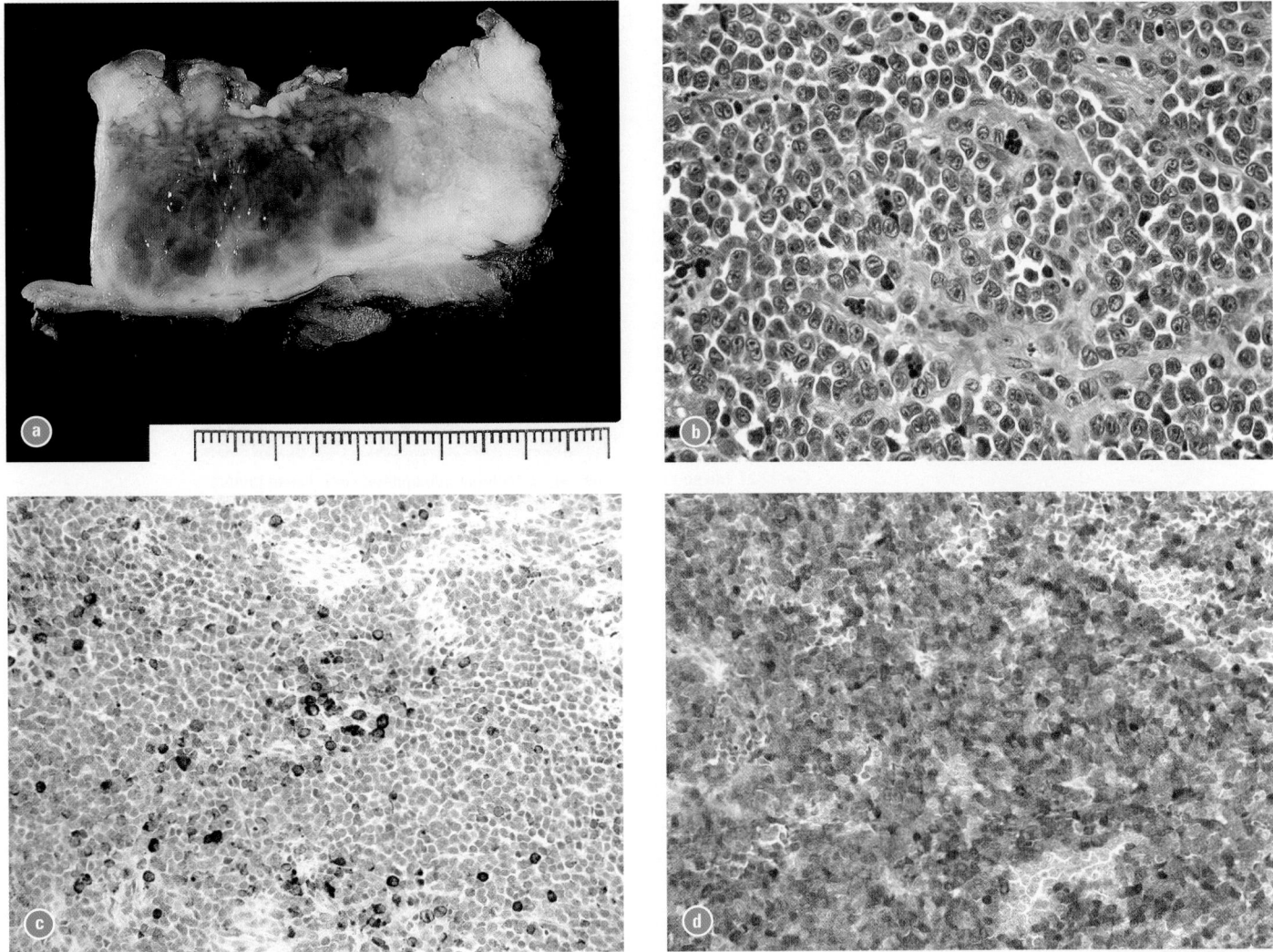

Fig. 12.26 Vaginal melanoma. (a) This section illustrates the mass protruding above the vaginal mucosa (lower). Note the pigmentation, which is variably present. (b) Histologically, the tumor exhibits characteristic vesicular nuclei and prominent nucleoli. Melanin pigment is also present. (c,d) Following staining for HMB-45 and S100, respectively.

RARE TUMORS

Mixed tumors

The uncommon benign mixed tumors ('spindle cell epitheliomas') usually occur near the hymenal ring and tend to not be connected to the surface epithelium.[105] Unlike mixed tumors of other organs vaginal tumors neither immunohistochemically nor ultrastructurally show features of myoepithelial cells.[106] On histologic evaluation, well-circumscribed, non-encapsulated borders are present. They are characterized by a major component of stromal-type cells with scanty cytoplasm, round to spindled nuclei, fine chromatin, indistinct nucleoli and rare to absent mitoses (Fig. 12.27).[47] The stromal cells are typically immunoreactive for cytokeratin, smooth muscle actin and progesterone receptor. The cytokeratin immunoreactivity of the spindle cells and their apparent epithelial nature on ultrastructural examination have led one group of investigators to prefer the designation 'spindle cell epithelioma' for these tumors.[107] A minor component of well-differentiated epithelial elements and squamous metaplasia may be seen. Stainable mucin may be present.[47] Murdoch et al. reported a case with a spindle cell component expressing epithelial markers such as CK7, together with strong CD10, Bcl2, and estrogen and progesterone receptors, favoring a Müllerian-origin.[108]

Recurrence of a benign mixed tumor of the vagina has been reported;[109] thus, careful follow-up of large tumors is recommended

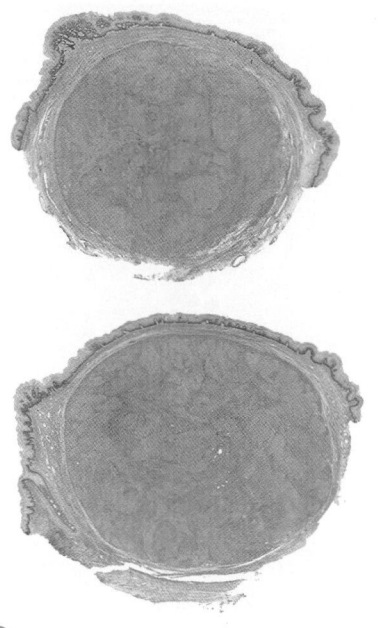

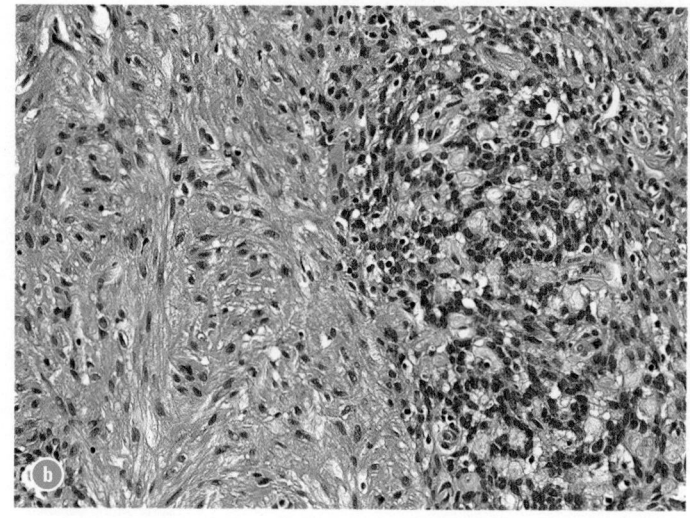

Fig. 12.27 Mixed tumor of the vagina (spindle cell epithelioma). These tumors typically are well circumscribed, keratin-positive and consist of spindle cell foci with epithelioid differentiation (right) admixed with a dominant fibrous component (left).

References

1 Matsukura, Sugase M. Distinct manifestations of human papillomaviruses in the vagina. Int J Cancer 1997; 72:412–415.

2 Audet-Lapointe P, Body G, Vauclair R, Drouin P, Ayoub J. Vaginal intraepithelial neoplasia. Gynecol Oncol 1990; 36:232–239.

3 Lenehan PM, Meffe F, Lickrish GM. Vaginal intraepithelial neoplasia: biologic aspects and management. Obstet Gynecol 1986; 68(3):333–337.

4 Bowen-Simpkins P, Hull MG. Intraepithelial vaginal neoplasia following immunosuppressive therapy treated with topical 5-Fu. Obstet Gynecol 1975; 46:360–362.

5 Fujimura M, Ostrow RS, Okagaki T. Implication of human papillomavirus in postirradiation dysplasia. Cancer 1991; 68(10):2181–2185.

6 Barzon L, Pizzighella S, Corti L, Mengoli C, Palu G. Vaginal dysplastic lesions in women with hysterectomy and receiving radiotherapy are linked to high-risk human papillomavirus. J Med Virol 2002; 67(3):401–405.

7 Ferris DG, Cox JT, O'Connor DM, Wright VC, Foerster J. Modern colposcopy textbook and atlas, 2nd edn. Colposcopy of the vagina. Dubuque, Iowa: Kendall/Hunt Publishing Co; 2004:414–448.

8 Anonymous. Society of Gynecologic Oncologists Clinical Practice Guidelines. Practice guidelines: vaginal cancer. Oncology 1998; 12:449–452.

9 Lopes A, Monaghan JM, Robertson G. Vaginal intraepithelial neoplasia. In: Luesley D, Jordan J, Richart R, eds. Intraepithelial neoplasia of the lower genital tract. New York: Churchill Livingstone; 1995:169–176.

10 Sillman FH, Fruchter RG, Chen YS, et al. Vaginal intraepithelial neoplasia: risk factors for persistence, recurrence, and invasion and its management. Am J Obstet Gynecol 1997; 176:93–99.

11 Micheletti L, Zanotto Valentino MC, Barbero M, et al. Current knowledge about the natural history of intraepithelial neoplasms of the vagina. Minerva Gynecol 1994; 46:195–204.

12 Nuovo GJ, Blanco JS, Silverstein SJ, Crum CP. Histologic correlates of papillomavirus infection of the vagina. Obstet Gynecol 1988; 72:770–774.

13 Turner JR, Odze RD, Crum CP, Resnick MB. MN antigen expression in normal, preneoplastic, and neoplastic esophagus: a clinicopathological study of a new cancer-associated biomarker. Hum Pathol 1997; 28:740–744.

14 Logani S, Lu D, Quint WG, Ellenson LH, Pirog EC. Low-grade vulvar and vaginal intraepithelial neoplasia: correlation of histologic features with human papillomavirus DNA detection and MIB-1 immunostaining. Mod Pathol 2003; 16:735–741.

15 Cardosi RJ, Bomalaski JJ, Hoffman MS. Diagnosis and management of vulvar and vaginal intraepithelial neoplasia. Obstet Gynecol Clin North Am 2001; 28:685–702.

16 Rome RM, England PG. Management of vaginal intraepithelial neoplasia: a series of 132 cases with long-term follow-up. Int J Gynecol Cancer 2000; 10:382–390.

17 Hull MG, Bowen-Simpkins P, Paintin DB. Topical treatment of vaginal intraepithelial neoplasia. Obstet Gynecol 1977; 49:382.

18 Ballon SC, Roberts JA, Lagasse LD. Topical 5-fluorouracil in the treatment of intraepithelial neoplasia of the vagina. Obstet Gynecol 1979; 54:163–166.

19 Petrilli ES, Townsend DE, Morrow CP, Nakao CY. Vaginal intraepithelial neoplasia: biologic aspects and treatment with topical 5-fluorouracil and the carbon dioxide laser. Am J Obstet Gynecol 1980; 138:321–328.

20 Caglar H, Hertzog RW, Hreshchyshyn MM. Topical 5-fluorouracil treatment of vaginal intraepithelial neoplasia. Obstet Gynecol 1981; 58:580–583.

21 Kirwan P, Naftalin NJ. Topical 5-fluorouracil in the treatment of vaginal intraepithelial neoplasia. Br J Obstet Gynaecol 1985; 92:287–291.

22 Gonzalez Sanchez JL, Flores Murrieta G, Chavez Brambila J, Deolarte Manzano JM, Andrade Manzano AF. Topical 5-fluorouracil for treatment of vaginal intraepithelial neoplasms. Gynecol Obstet Mex 2002; 70:244–247.

23 Davis G, Wentworth J, Richard J. Self-administered topical imiquimod treatment of vulvar intraepithelial neoplasia. A report of four cases. J Reprod Med 2000; 45:619–623.

24 Diakomanolis E, Haidopoulos D, Stefanidis K. Treatment of high-grade vaginal intraepithelial neoplasia with imiquimod cream. N Engl J Med 2002; 347:374.

25 Campagnutta E, Parin A, Piero G De, et al. Treatment of vaginal intraepithelial neoplasia (VAIN) with the carbon dioxide laser. Clin Exp Obstet Gynecol 1999; 26:127–130.

26 Krebs HB, Helmkamp BF. Chronic ulcerations following topical therapy with 5-fluorouracil for vaginal human papillomavirus-associated lesions. Obstet Gynecol 1991; 78:205–208.

27 Campagnutta E, Parin A, De Piero G, et al. Treatment of vaginal intraepithelial neoplasia (VAIN) with the carbon dioxide laser. Clin Exp Obstet Gynecol 1999; 26(2):127–130.

28 Yalcin OT, Rutherford TJ, Chambers SK, Chambers JT, Schwartz PE. Vaginal intraepithelial neoplasia: treatment by carbon dioxide laser and risk factors for failure. Eur J Obstet Gynecol Reprod Biol 2003; 106:64–68.

29 Diakomanolis E, Stefanidis K, Rodolakis A, et al. Vaginal intraepithelial neoplasia: report of 102 cases. Eur J Gynaecol Oncol 2002; 23:457–459.

30 Arora M, Shrivastav RK, Jaiprakash MP. A rare germ-cell tumor site: vaginal endodermal sinus tumor. Pediatr Surg Int 2002; 18:521–523.

31 Lopes LF, Chazan R, Sredni ST, de Camargo B. Endodermal sinus tumor of the vagina in children. Med Pediatr Oncol 1999; 32:377–381.

32 Bochner BH, De Filippo RE, Hardy BE. Endodermal sinus tumor of the vagina. J Urol 2000; 163:1293.

33 Hilgers RD, Malkasian GD Jr, Soule EH. Embryonal rhabdomyosarcoma (botryoid type) of the vagina. A clinicopathologic review. Am J Obstet Gynecol 1970; 107:484–502.

34 Leuschner I, Harms D, Mattke A, Koscielniak E, Treuner J. Rhabdomyosarcoma of the urinary bladder and vagina: a clinicopathologic study with emphasis on recurrent disease: a report from the Kiel Pediatric Tumor Registry and the German CWS Study. Am J Surg Pathol 2001; 25:856–864.

35 Hellman K, Silfversward C, Nilsson B, et al. Primary carcinoma of the vagina: factors influencing the age at diagnosis. The Radiumhemmet series 1956–96. Int J Gynecol Cancer 2004; 14:491–501.

36 Stryker JA. Radiotherapy for vaginal carcinoma: a 23-year review. Br J Radiol 2000; 73:1200–1205.

37 Tjalma WA, Monaghan JM, de Barros Lopes A, et al. The role of surgery in invasive squamous carcinoma of the vagina. Gynecol Oncol 2001; 81:360–365.

38 Wood WG, Giustini FG, Sohn S, Aranda RR. Verrucous carcinoma of the vagina. South Med J 1978; 71:368–371.

39 Crowther ME, Lowe DG, Shepherd JH. Verrucous carcinoma of the female genital tract: a review. Obstet Gynecol Surv 1988; 43:263–280.

40 Yorganci A, Serinsoz E, Ensari A, Sertcelik A, Ortac F. A case report of multicentric verrucous carcinoma of the female genital tract. Gynecol Oncol 2003; 90:478–481.

41 Okagaki T, Clark BA, Zachow KR, et al. Presence of human papillomavirus in verrucous carcinoma (Ackerman) of the vagina. Immunocytochemical, ultrastructural, and DNA hybridization studies. Arch Pathol Lab Med 1984; 108:567–570.

42 Nishikawa T, Kobayashi H, Shindoh M, et al. A case of verrucous carcinoma associated with human papillomavirus type 16 DNA. J Dermatol 1993; 20:483–488.

43 Reinecke L, Thornley AL. Case report: radiotherapy – an effective treatment for vaginal verrucous carcinoma. Br J Radiol 1993; 66:375–378.

44 Maiche AG, Pyrhonen S. Verrucous carcinoma of the penis: three cases treated with interferon-alpha. Br J Urol 1997; 79:481–483.

45 Rose PG, Stoler MH, Abdul-Karim FW. Papillary squamotransitional cell carcinoma of the vagina. Int J Gynecol Pathol 1998; 17:372–375.

46 Vesoulis Z, Erhardt CA. Cytologic diagnosis of vaginal papillary squamotransitional cell carcinoma. A case report. Acta Cytol 2001; 45:465–469.

47 Clement PB, Young RH. The vagina. Atlas of gynecological surgical pathology. Philadelphia, PA: WB Saunders; 2000:43–62.

48 Rabinerson D, Avrech O, Kaplan B, et al. Endometrioma of the vagina in menopause. Acta Obstet Gynecol Scand 1996; 75:506–507.

49 Granai CO, Walters MD, Safaii H, et al. Malignant transformation of vaginal endometriosis. Obstet Gynecol 1984; 64:592–595.

50 Berkowitz RS, Ehrmann RL, Knapp RC. Endometrial stromal sarcoma arising from vaginal endometriosis. Obstet Gynecol 1978; 51:34S–37S.

51 Leiserowitz GS, Gumbs JL, Oi R, et al. Endometriosis-related malignancies. Int J Gynecol Cancer 2003; 13:466–471.

52 Kapp DS, Merino M, LiVolsi V. Adenocarcinoma of the vagina arising in endometriosis: long-term survival following radiation therapy. Gynecol Oncol 1982; 14:271–278.

53 Orr JW Jr, Holimon JL, Sisson PF. Vaginal adenocarcinoma developing in residual pelvic endometriosis: a clinical dilemma. Gynecol Oncol 1989; 33:96–98.

54 Haskel S, Chen SS, Spiegel G. Vaginal endometrioid adenocarcinoma arising in vaginal endometriosis: a case report and literature review. Gynecol Oncol 1989; 34:232–236.

55 Judson PL, Temple AM, Fowler WC Jr, Novotny DB, Funkhouser WK Jr. Vaginal adenosarcoma arising from endometriosis. Gynecol Oncol 2000; 76:123–125.

56 Anderson J, Behbakht K, De Geest K, Bitterman P. Adenosarcoma in a patient with vaginal endometriosis. Obstet Gynecol 2001; 98:964–966.

57 Liu L, Davidson S, Singh M. Müllerian adenosarcoma of vagina arising in persistent endometriosis: report of a case and review of the literature. Gynecol Oncol 2003; 90:486–490.

58 Kondi-Paphitis A, Smyrniotis B, Liapis A, Kontoyanni A, Deligeorgi H. Stromal sarcoma arising on endometriosis. A clinicopathological and immunohistochemical study of 4 cases. Eur J Gynaecol Oncol 1998; 19:588–590.

59 Visvalingam S, Jaworski R, Blumenthal N, Chan F. Primary peritoneal mesodermal adenosarcoma: report of a case and review of the literature. Gynecol Oncol 2001; 81:500–505.

60 Inoue M, Fukuda H, Tanizawa O. Adenosarcomas originating from sites other than uterine endometrium. Int J Gynaecol Obstet 1995; 48:299–306.

61 Clement PB, Scully RE. Müllerian adenosarcoma of the uterus: a clinicopathologic analysis of 100 cases with a review of the literature. Hum Pathol 1990; 21:363–381.

62 Kaminski PF, Maier RC. Clear cell adenocarcinoma of the cervix unrelated to diethylstilbestrol exposure. Obstet Gynecol 1983; 62:720–727.

63 Watanabe Y, Ueda H, Nozaki K, et al. Advanced primary clear cell carcinoma of the vagina not associated with diethylstilbestrol. Acta Cytol 2002; 46:577–581.

64 Herbst AL, Ulfelder H, Poskanzer DC. Adenocarcinoma of the vagina. Association of maternal stilbestrol therapy with tumor appearance in young women. N Engl J Med 1971; 284:878–881.

65 Robboy SJ, Noller KL, O'Brien P, et al. Increased incidence of cervical and vaginal dysplasia in 3,980 diethylstilbestrol-exposed young women. Experience of the National Collaborative Diethylstilbestrol Adenosis Project. JAMA 1984; 252:2979–2983.

66 Herbst AL. Behavior of estrogen-associated female genital tract cancer and its relation to neoplasia following intrauterine exposure to diethylstilbestrol (DES). Gynecol Oncol 2000; 76:147–156.

67 Trimble EL. A guest editorial: update on diethylstilbestrol. Obstet Gynecol Surv 2001; 56:187–189.

68 Bornstein J, Adam E, Adler-Storthz K, Kaufman RH. Development of cervical and vaginal squamous cell neoplasia as a late consequence of in utero exposure to diethylstilbestrol. Obstet Gynecol Surv 1988; 43:15–21.

69 Anonymous. Diethylstilbestrol. ACOG Committee Opinion: Committee on Gynecologic Practice. Number 131, December 1993. Int J Gynaecol Obstet 1994; 44:184.

70 Schrager S, Potter BE. Diethylstilbestrol exposure. Am Fam Physician 2004; 69:2395–2400.

71 Hanselaar AG, Boss EA, Massuger LF, Bernheim JL. Cytologic examination to detect clear cell adenocarcinoma of the vagina or cervix. Gynecol Oncol 1999; 75:338–344.

72 Ciano PS, Antoniola DA, Critchlow J, Burke L, Goldman H. Villous adenoma presenting as a vaginal polyp in a rectovaginal tract. Hum Pathol 1987; 18:863–866.

73 Fox H, Wells M, Harris M, McWilliam LJ, Anderson GS. Enteric tumors of the lower female genital tract: a report of three cases. Histopathology 1988; 12:167–176.

74 Mudhar HS, Smith JH, Tidy J. Primary vaginal adenocarcinoma of intestinal type arising from an adenoma: case report and review of the literature. Int J Gynecol Pathol 2001; 20:204–209.

75 Mainkhard K, Raicheva S, Sirakov M. Müllerian papilloma in the vagina of a two year old girl – a case report [Bulgarian]. Akush Ginekol (Sofia) 2002; 41:48–49.

76 McCluggage WG, Nirmala V, Radhakumari K. Intramural Müllerian papilloma of the vagina. Int J Gynecol Pathol 1999; 18:94–95.

77 Cohen M, Pedemonte L, Drut R. Pigmented Müllerian papilloma of the vagina. Histopathology 2001; 39:541–543.

78 Luttges JE, Lubke M. Recurrent benign Müllerian papilloma of the vagina. Immunohistological findings and histogenesis. Arch Gynecol Obstet 1994; 255:157–160.

79 Mazur MT, Hsueh S, Gersell DJ. Metastases to the female genital tract. Analysis of 325 cases. Cancer 1984; 53:1978–1984.

80 Guidozzi F, Sonnendecker EW, Wright C. Ovarian cancer with metastatic deposits in the cervix, vagina, or vulva preceding primary cytoreductive surgery. Gynecol Oncol 1993; 49:225–228.

81 Ohira S, Yamazaki T, Hatano H, et al. Epithelioid trophoblastic tumor metastatic to the vagina: an immunohistochemical and ultrastructural study. Int J Gynecol Pathol 2000; 19:381–386.

82 Yingna S, Yang X, Xiuyu Y, Hongzhao S. Clinical characteristics and treatment of gestational trophoblastic tumor with vaginal metastasis. J Artic Gynecologic Oncol 2002; 84:416–419.

83 Kumar R, Kumar S, Hemal AK. Vaginal and omental metastasis from superficial bladder cancer. Urol Int 2001; 67:117–118.

84 Bulbul MA, Kaspar H, Nasr R, Khalil A. Urothelial carcinoma of the vagina six years following cystectomy for invasive cancer. A case report. Eur J Gynaecol Oncol 1999; 20:233–234.

85 Pineda A, Sall S. Metastasis to the vagina from carcinoma of the breast. J Reprod Med 1978; 20:243–245.

86 Jacobs AJ, Deppe G, Kessinger MA, Newland JR. Breast carcinoma metastatic to the vagina. Acta Obstet Gynecol Scand 1983; 62:83–85.

87 Giacalone PL, Dumontier C, Roger P, Laffargue F, Baldet P. Vaginal metastases of breast cancer [French]. J Gynecol, Obstet Biol Reprod (Paris) 1998; 27:714–717.

88 Allard JE, McBroom JW, Zahn CM, McLeod D, Maxwell GL. Vaginal metastasis and thrombocytopenia from renal cell carcinoma. Gynecol Oncol 2004; 92:970–973.

89 Ovesen H, Gerstenberg T. Vaginal metastasis as the first sign of renal cell carcinoma. A case report and review of the literature. Scand J Urol Nephrol 1990; 24:237–238.

90 Queiroz C, Bacchi CE, Oliveira C, Carvalho M, Santos DR. Cytologic diagnosis of vaginal metastasis from renal cell carcinoma. A case report. Acta Cytol 1999; 43:1098–1100.

91 Chagpar A, Kanthan SC. Vaginal metastasis of colon cancer. Am Surg 2001; 67:171–172.

92 Katsumoto Y, Maruyama K, Furukawa J, et al. A case of metastatic vaginal tumor of rectal cancer [Japanese]. Gan to Kagaku Ryoho [Japanese Journal of Cancer & Chemotherapy] 2002; 29:2406–2409.

93 Gupta D, Neto AG, Deavers MT, Silva EG, Malpica A. Metastatic melanoma to the vagina: clinicopathologic and immunohistochemical study of three cases and literature review. Int J Gynecol Pathol 2003; 22:136–140.

94 Skowronek J, Roszak A. A case of metastatic malignant melanoma of the vagina with a background of primary vaginal melanoma – clinical case [Polish]. Ginekologia Polska 1997; 68:390–393.

95 Cantisani V, Mortele KJ, Kalantari BN, et al. Vaginal metastasis from uterine leiomyosarcoma. Magnetic resonance imaging features with pathological correlation. J Comput Assisted Tomogr 2003; 27:805–809.

96 Buchanan DJ, Schlaerth J, Kurosaki T. Primary vaginal melanoma: thirteen-year disease-free survival after wide local excision and review of recent literature. Am J Obstet Gynecol 1998; 178:1177–1184.

97 Tjalma WA, Monaghan JM, de Barros Lopes A, Naik R, Nordin A. Primary vaginal melanoma and long-term survivors. Eur J Gynaecol Oncol 2001; 22:20–22.

98 Moros ML, Ferrer FP, Mitchell MJ, Romeo JA, Lacruz RL. Primary malignant melanoma of the vagina. Poor response to radical surgery and adjuvant therapy. Eur J Obstet Gynecol Reprod Biol 2004; 113:248–250.

99 Piura B, Rabinovich A, Yanai-Inbar I. Primary malignant melanoma of the vagina: case report and review of literature. Eur J Gynaecol Oncol 2002; 23:195–198.

100 Irvin WP Jr, Bliss SA, Rice LW, Taylor PT Jr, Andersen WA. Malignant melanoma of the vagina and locoregional control: radical surgery revisited. Gynecol Oncol 1998; 71:476–480.

101 DeMatos P, Tyler D, Seigler HF. Mucosal melanoma of the female genitalia: a clinicopathologic study of forty-three cases at Duke University Medical Center. Surgery 1998; 124:38–48.

102 Petru E, Nagele F, Czerwenka K, et al. Primary malignant melanoma of the vagina: long-term remission following radiation therapy. Gynecol Oncol 1998; 70:23–26.

103 Miner TJ, Delgado R, Zeisler J, et al. Primary vaginal melanoma: a critical analysis of therapy. Ann Surg Oncol 2004; 11:34–39.

104 Mishra M, Chawla SC, Chawla S, Basu SM, Tata R. Malignant melanoma of the vagina: report of two cases. Indian J Pathol Microbiol 2003; 46:71–73.

105 Sirota RL, Dickersin GR, Scully RE. Mixed tumors of the vagina. A clinicopathological analysis of eight cases. Am J Surg Pathol 1981; 5:413–422.

106 Skelton H, Smith KJ. Spindle cell epithelioma of the vagina shows immunohistochemical staining supporting its origin from a primitive/progenitor cell population. Arch Pathol Lab Med 2001; 125:547–550.

107 Branton PA, Tavassoli FA. Spindle cell epithelioma, the so-called mixed tumor of the vagina. A clinicopathologic, immunohistochemical, and ultrastructural analysis of 28 cases. Am J Surg Pathol 1993; 17:509–515.

108 Murdoch F, Sharma R, Al-Nafussi A. Benign mixed tumor of the vagina: case report with expanded immunohistochemical profile. Int J Gynecol Cancer 2003; 13:543–547.

109 Wright RG, Buntine DW, Forbes KL. Recurrent benign mixed tumor of the vagina. Gynecol Oncol 1991; 40:84–86.

13

Cervical squamous neoplasia

Christopher P. Crum and

Peter G. Rose

Introduction

Definition
Identifying patients at risk for
cervical neoplasia
Molecular risk factors

Cytology

Expectations from cervical
cytology in cervical cancer
prevention
Non-diagnostic squamous atypia
Management of ASCUS

**Diagnosis and management
of cervical intraepithelial
neoplasia**

Phenotypic changes associated
with HPV infection
Cytologic criteria for squamous
intraepithelial lesions
Histopathologic diagnosis of
preinvasive disease

Biomarkers and the diagnosis and
classification of squamous
lesions
The endocervical curettage
Resolving discordant
Papanicolaou smear and biopsy
results
Therapeutic options

**Diagnosis and management
of invasive squamous cell
carcinoma**

Introduction
Diagnosis of invasion
Defining microinvasive squamous
cell carcinoma
Management of superficially
invasive squamous cell
carcinoma
Pathology of invasive squamous
carcinoma
Treatment and outcome
of squamous carcinoma
Prevention and therapy with
vaccines

Introduction

DEFINITION

Cervical squamous neoplasia is defined as all squamous cell alterations that occur in or near the cervical transformation zone that are causally related to human papillomavirus infections. The terms cervical intraepithelial neoplasia, dysplasia and squamous intraepithelial lesion (SIL) apply to this group of lesions as well. In this chapter, the terms CIN I, flat condyloma and exophytic condyloma will all be used interchangeably with low-grade squamous intraepithelial lesion (LSIL) and the terms CIN II and CIN III/carcinoma *in situ* are synonymous with high-grade squamous intraepithelial lesion (HSIL). The choice of diagnostic terminology (dysplasia, CIN, SIL) is critical only in terms of its impact on clinical care. The impact of this terminology on management will be discussed later in this chapter.

IDENTIFYING PATIENTS AT RISK FOR CERVICAL NEOPLASIA

In clinical practice, there is no algorithm that will decide whether a given reproductive-age woman should or should not have a Papanicolaou smear, short of clinical evidence of human papillomavirus (HPV) infection, lower genital tract symptoms or a prior abnormal Papanicolaou smear. The two risk factors classically associated with cervical cancer – early age of first intercourse and multiple sexual partners – are sufficiently common that a high percentage of women would qualify for Pap smear screening by these criteria. Moreover, timing of sexual activity may be as or more important than absolute number of sexual partners in conferring risk of current HPV infection.[1-3] Conversely, preinvasive disease has even been identified in sexually active women with no prior male sexual partners, indicating that exposure of the cervix to HPV can be mediated by other forms of sexual contact.[4] The following is a series of risk factors associated with cervical neoplasia. These risk factors are summarized in Table 13.1.

Human papillomaviruses

HPV infection is the principal cause of cervical neoplasia. The powerful association between HPV infection and cervical neoplasia has been established, and the accumulated experimental, molecular and clinical evidence has left no doubt that HPV directly influences the pathogenesis of cervical neoplasia. Table 13.2 and Figures 13.1 and 13.2 summarize the frequency of cervical cancer, associations and potential molecular

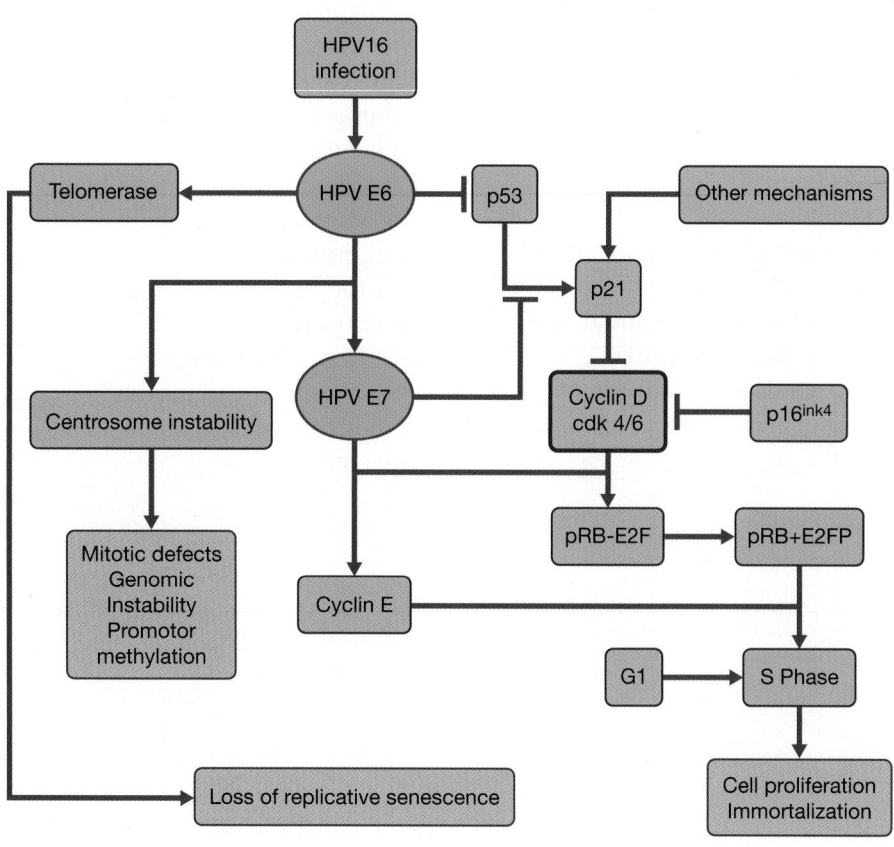

Fig. 13.1 Molecular basis for cervical neoplasia. This composite figure summarizes three pathways involved in HPV-related tumorigenesis with HPV 16 as a model: the cellular functions, including alterations in cell cycle activity induced by E7, upregulation of telomerase via E6 with loss of replicative senescence, and induction of centrosome instability by E6 and E7. Progression is also associated with promotor methylation of tumor suppressor genes, silencing them in the absence of mutation.

Table 13.1 Risk factors for HPV infection and cervical neoplasia

Factor	Outcome variable	Positive/negative	Outcome measure	Reference
Young age of coitarche	HPV + HSIL	Positive	OR 3.2	74
Sex partners >2	HPV infection	Positive	OR 7.5	57
Recent sexual activity	HPV infection	Positive		
Male promiscuity	Carcinoma	Positive	OR 6.9	59
Parity (>7)	Cancer	Positive	OR 6.2	309
Increasing age (> 40 vs <20)	HPV	Negative	10-fold reduction	6, 84
Cervicitis	HSIL	Positive	OR 1.9	76
Genital infections	HPV	Positive		1
C. trachomatis serotype G	Squamous cell carcinoma	Positive	OR 6.6	75
Barrier contraception	HSIL/carcinoma	Negative	OR 0.4	76
Smoking	CIN 2–3	Positive	OR 2.6	67
	CIN 3/cancer	Positive	OR 2.7	76
Oral contraceptives or unopposed estrogens	Adenocarcinoma	Positive	OR 2.0	70
Oral contraceptives	Carcinoma	Positive	OR 3.6	19
High-risk HPV	Cancer	Positive	RR 45–435	13
Persistent infection with high-risk HPVs	HSIL	Positive	OR 11.7	19
	Carcinoma	Positive		210
High viral load (HPV)	HSIL	Positive	OR 35.0	18
HLA B*07+ HLA-DQB1*302	HSIL/carcinoma	Positive	OR 8.2	39
Transplantation	Cervical cancer	Positive	OR 17.0	44
HIV	Index of HPV	Positive	2-fold	18
	Persistent HPV	Positive	6-fold	18
	SIL	Positive	4-fold	50
	Persistent SIL	Positive	4-fold	51
	HSIL/carcinoma	Variable	0–15-fold	51–53

mechanisms. The latter are addressed later in the discussion of biomarkers. What has emerged over the past several years is the realization that: (a) HPV infection is ubiquitous in the young sexually active population, (b) frequency of infection peaks in the early reproductive years, (c) infections are transient, often appearing and disappearing without cytologic abnormality, but (d) persistent infection by the same HPV type is strongly associated with risk of a current or subsequent cervical neoplasm.[5–10] The conclusion to this chapter reiterates the most compelling link between HPV and cervical neoplasia: that immunization with vaccines derived from a high-risk HPV (type 16) will prevent transient infection, persistent infection and finally HPV-16 related squamous intraepithelial lesions with a 91%, 100% and 100% efficacy, respectively.[11]

There is a broad gradient of risk imposed by cancer associated ('high-risk') HPV types, with HPV 16 conferring the greatest risk. Low-risk HPV types may confer risk as surrogate markers of 'at risk behavior'. Over 100 human papillomaviruses have been characterized, and over 25 have been isolated from the genital tract. Genital HPVs have been divided into those with low, intermediate and high association with cervical carcinoma.[12] Currently, those HPVs with any association are termed 'high-risk' HPV types. Tables 13.3 and 13.4 review the types of HPV and the evidence linking them to atypical squamous cells of undeter-

Table 13.2 Incidence of cervical carcinoma worldwide[a]

Locale	Adjusted incidence[b]	Adjusted mortality[b]
Worldwide	16.1	8.0
More developed	11.4	4.1
Less developed	18.7	9.8
East Africa	44.3	24.2
Mid Africa	25.1	14.2
North Africa	16.8	9.1
South Africa	30.3	16.5
West Africa	20.3	10.9
Caribbean	35.8	16.8
Central America	40.3	17.0
South America	30.9	12.0
North America	8.3	3.2
East Asia	6.4	3.2
South-East Asia	18.3	9.7
South-Central Asia	26.5	15.0
Western Asia	4.8	2.5
Eastern Europe	16.8	6.2
Northern Europe	9.8	4.0
Southern Europe	10.2	3.3
Western Europe	10.4	3.7
Australia/NZ	7.7	2.7
Melanesia	43.8	23.8
Micronesia	12.3	6.2
Polynesia	32.9	17.4

[a]Source: http://www-dep.iarc.fr/globocan/globocan.html
[b]Per 100 000 per year.

Table 13.3 Classification of human papillomavirus types

HPV	Cancers (%)	Controls (%)	Odds ratio
16	50.5	3.3	435
18	13.1	1.3	248
45	5.5	0.7	198
31	2.7	0.6	124
52	2.7	0.3	200
33	1.0	0.1	373
58	2.3	0.5	115
35	1.1	0.5	74
59	1.3	0.1	419
51	1.0	0.3	67
56	0.7	0.4	45
39	0.6	0.0	–
73	0.4	0.1	106
68	0.2	0.1	54

High-risk: types 16, 18, 31, 33, 35, 39, 45, 51, 52, 56, 58, 59, 68, 73, 82.
Possibly high-risk: types 26, 53, 66.
Low-risk: types 6, 11, 40, 42, 43, 44, 54, 61, 72, 81, cp6108.
From Munoz et al.[13]

cinomas. Small cell neuroendocrine carcinomas are almost exclusively associated with HPV 18. A fourth group, consisting of newly discovered HPV types, and having uncertain or controversial association with cancer exists and presumably confers a low risk of cancer.[13]

Cervical cancers and high-grade precursor lesions have distinctly different frequencies of certain HPV types than low-grade precancers and non-diagnostic squamous atypias. Less than 10% of these lesions contain HPV types other than the 12 most common types (Table 13.4). In contrast, up to 40% of lower-grade and indeterminate atypias contain viral types in this group.

mined significance (ASCUS), low-grade squamous intraepithelial lesions (LSIL), high-grade squamous intraepithelial lesions (HSIL) and cervical carcinoma. From this information and prior studies, it is possible to ascertain the relative strength of association between certain HPV groups and not only cancer but also pre-invasive atypias.[12]

The relationships between HPVs and cervical neoplasia vary both for lesion grade and cell type. HPVs 6 and 11 are not associated with cervical carcinomas or high-grade squamous intraepithelial lesions. HPV 16 is detected in nearly 50% of HSIL and squamous carcinomas of the cervix and is the 'prototypic' cancer-causing virus. In contrast, HPV 56 is associated with less than 1 in 50 cancers. HPV 18 is associated with less than 15% of squamous carcinomas, predominating in adenocarcinomas *in situ* and invasive adenocar-

Table 13.4 Relative frequencies of higher- and lower-risk HPV types in normal and abnormal cervices

Diagnosis	No.	HPVA (%)[a]	HPVB (%)[b]	UKHPV (%)[c]
ASC[310]	60	36 (60.0)	22(36.7)	2 (3.3)
LSIL[310]	140	76 (54.2)	57(40.7)	7 (5.0)
HSIL[310]	32	28 (87.5)	2 (6.3)	2 (6.3)
Cancer[13]	1739	1578 (90.8)	24 (1.4)	137(6.3)
Adenoca[279]	112	112 (100)	0 (0)	0(0)
NC[252,278]	28	28 (100)	0 (0)	0(0)

LSIL includes cases of LSIL and atypias suggesting LSIL; HSIL, includes cases of HSIL and atypias suggesting HSIL; NC, neuroendocrine carcinoma.
[a]HPVA: types 16, 18, 31, 33, 35, 39, 45, 51, 52, 56, 58, 59.
[b]HPVB: all other classifiable HPV types, including 6, 11, 40, 42, 44, 53, 54, 57, 61, 62, 64, 66, 68, 69, 70, 71 (cp8061), 72, 73 (mm9), 81 (cp8304), 82 (mm4), 83 (mm7), 84, provisional 89 (cp6108), 91, cp141.
[c]Unclassified HPV types, including generic 'high-risk' positives and other multiple infections.

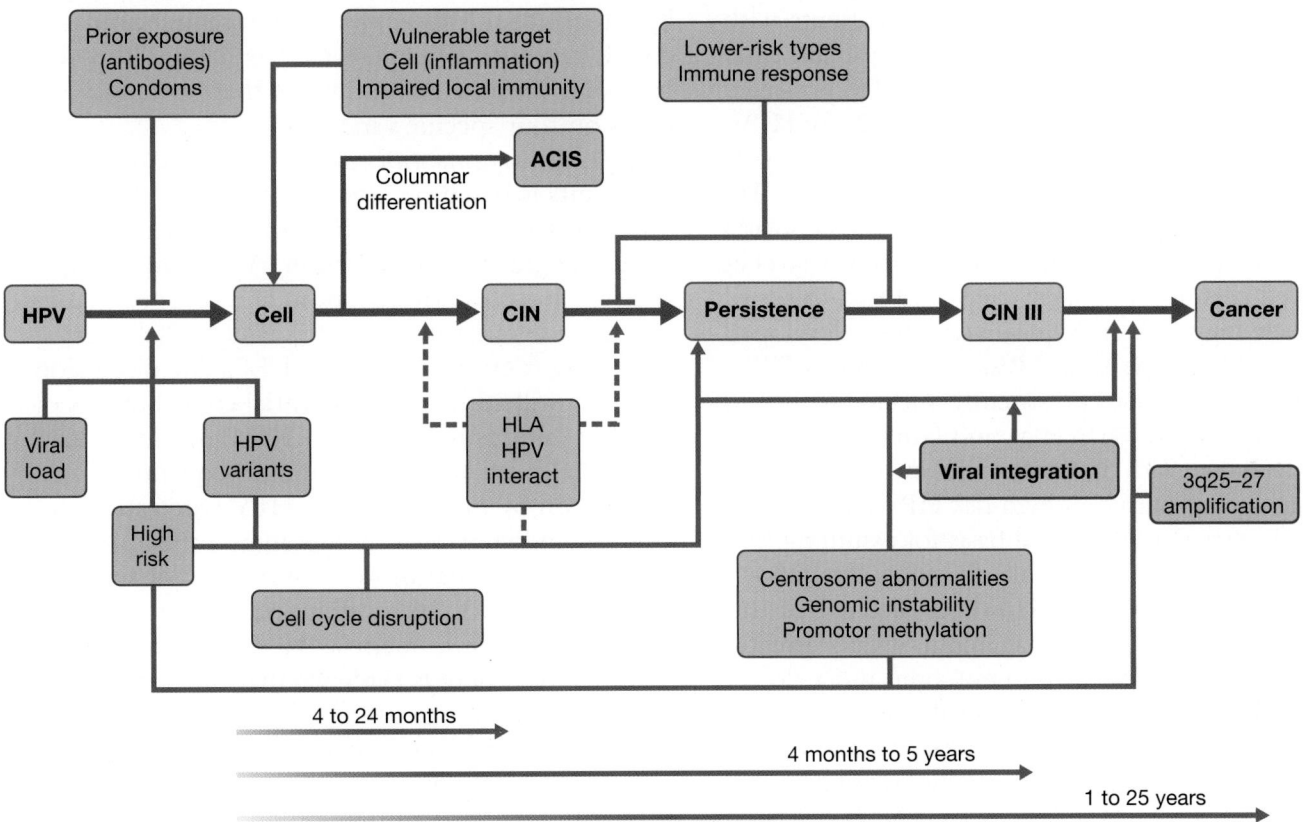

Fig. 13.2 Development and progression of cervical preinvasive neoplasia as a function of multiple factors.

The presence of any HPV, high or low risk, does not exclude the subsequent emergence of another HPV infection of different risk, meaning that infection with one virus may serve as a surrogate marker for subsequent infection by a high-risk HPV.[14] Predictably, many HPVs detected in women with normal Papanicolaou smears have some association with cancer risk, albeit low.[13]

Interestingly, the distribution of HPV types in women with normal Papanicolaou smears closely parallels the frequency of these viruses in cervical neoplasia. For example, HPV 16 is the most common HPV detected in women without abnormality.

If a woman is found to harbor a 'high-risk' HPV in her genital tract, what is her risk of developing a high-grade squamous intraepithelial lesion? In general, approximately 15% of reproductive-age women will score positive for high-risk HPVs. Xi et al. showed that 19 of 123 women infected with HPV 16 developed HSIL.[15] Risk depends upon the actual HPV type (such as type 16 versus other HPV types), the duration of infection (transient versus persistent) and amount of virus present (viral load) (Table 13.1).

Most studies indicate that viral load is strongly associated with risk of developing a biopsy-proven squamous intraepithelial lesion. However, even small amounts of virus may herald the presence of an HSIL. Several studies have shown a direct relationship between the level of the HPV signal (by Hybrid Capture II) and the frequency of biopsy-proven high-grade squamous intraepithelial lesion or persistently abnormal Papanicolaou smears.[16–20] The association between viral load and risk of HSIL is plausible given the strong association between virus infection and neoplasia. However, the association is not consistent in all studies. Others have not demonstrated a significant association between viral load and lesion detection, suggesting that setting too high a threshold for HPV positives will exclude some patients with coincident HSIL.

Persistent infection by the same HPV type is strongly associated with risk of cervical neoplasia. The vast majority of HPV infections are transient. Only a minority of cases score positive for the same HPV type on successive tests. Prospective studies have shown that persistent infections by the same type correlate with increased risk of lesion detection, particularly after cone biopsy.[21] Retrospective studies of patients with cervical cancer have also documented prior infection and an association between persistent HPV positivity and neoplasia.[22] Elfgren et al. found that 92% of HPV-positive women cleared their infection over a 5-year period; persistence of infections, specifically type 16, was associated with cervical intraepithelial neoplasia (CIN) development ($p = 0.03$).[23] Conversely, Clavel et al. showed that approximately one- and two-thirds of persistently high-risk HPV-positive women developed HSIL and LSIL, respectively.[8] Risk of subsequent HSIL for HPV-infected versus persistently infected increased from 7% to 36%. Hopman et al. and Nobbenhuis et al. showed that over 90% of patients who developed smear abnormalities had persistent high-risk HPV infection.[24,25]

There is a strong theoretical basis for assuming that intra-typic sequence variants influence outcome following infections by HPV 16. However, the use of this information in patient management awaits greater consistency in study design and outcome and a clearer understanding of the mechanisms influencing the relationship between intra-typic variants and the risk of developing HSIL or cancer. Clearly the risk of developing high-grade preinvasive lesions or cancers is related to HPV type. HPV types 16 and 18 predominate in cervical cancers and high-grade precursors. HPVs are assigned a different number if they exhibit a greater than 50% difference in sequence make-up from previously classified types.[26] However, within a given type, lesser degrees of sequence variation may exist, producing variants (such as HPV 6a, HPV 6b, etc.). Because the differences in biologic effect (oncogenicity) between HPV types are ultimately influenced by differences in viral sequence, it is logical to presume that sequence alterations within a specific type would produce different – if more subtle – risks of cancer, depending on the location of the sequences involved.

Several studies have exhaustively detailed these sequence variations, focusing on geographic and ethnic differences in sequence make-up for HPV type 16. However, with the exception of a small number of studies, a consistent association between specific variants and cancer or precursor risk has not been established. This may be in part due to the fact that such studies are based on variables that indirectly measure risk, such as short-term follow-up of women to determine development of HSIL, or studies drawing conclusions about 'progression' based on associations of a given variant with normal mucosa or preinvasive lesions versus invasive cancer. Moreover, geography may also influence intra-typic variation. Nevertheless, the

hypothesis that a small variation in sequence make-up could influence oncogenicity has a valid theoretical basis. To simplify the review of these studies we will focus on four specific variables:

1 *Types of variants studied.* The assignment of variants is based on several parameters, including (a) prototypic versus non-prototypic sequence, (b) geographic, as in African, Asian-American, Asian and western European and (c) specific sequence variations in potentially critical open reading frames such as E6 or E7. The discussion below will address the potential contributions of these variants to the risk of HSIL or carcinoma.

2 *Multiple variants.* Concurrent or sequential infection by more than one HPV type variant in a single individual is not uncommon.[27] Sequence data indicate that more than one minor sequence variant of HPV 16 is often present in the cervix, accounting for as many as 10–20% of cases.[28] Moreover, there is evidence that one variant predominates over time.[15] There is also evidence that more than one variant may be isolated from cervical neoplasms, suggesting that co-infection by different variants may persist.

3 *Risk of HSIL as a function of certain HPV 16 variants.* In two studies that provide some of the strongest support for intra-typic variants as risk factors, Xi et al. studied two populations.[29] One studied young women who were HPV 16 positive and identified a relative risk of HSIL of 4.5 in those with variant versus prototypic HPV16 types. In a study of men, histologically confirmed anal carcinoma *in situ* occurred in 6 of 384 (1.6%) consistently HPV16-negative men, 12 of 183 (6.6%) men with HPV16 prototypic-like variants and in 4 of 22 (18.2%) men with HPV16 non-prototypic-like variants, conferring a significantly greater risk for this group.[28] This is some of the most compelling evidence that progression to cervical HSIL or anal CIS is influenced by infection with HPV 16 variant subtypes.

4 *Risk of cancer as a function of HPV variants.* Several studies have examined the risk of cancer associated with specific sequence variants, the premise being that progression from CIN to cancer might be more likely if one were infected by a specific HPV 16 subtype. In one, an HPV 16 E6 variant was identified that segregated more commonly in cancers versus HSIL.[30] This was supported by one study and unconfirmed by another, both from Germany.[31,32] A second

Swedish study did not confirm this observation.[33] Others came to different conclusions, some of which suggested that the differences might signify different frequencies in HLA haplotypes that could act synergistically with these variants to influence risk in different populations.[34,35] Two studies compared sequence variations in HPV 18 between low-grade lesions and adenocarcinomas. McLachlin et al. found no differences in E6 or E7 sequence between LSILs and adenocarcinomas associated with HPV 18.[31,36] Hecht et al. found an association between an E2-E5 sequence variant and cancers.[37] Both studies evaluated relatively small numbers and it remains unresolved whether HPV 18 variants influence the phenotypes (squamous versus glandular) of their respective associated lesions.

HLA type

There is evidence that certain HLA phenotypes confer greater susceptibility to HPV infection and cervical neoplasia. However, as with intra-typic sequence variants, the identification of cogent mechanisms by which these different HLA phenotypes influence risk and the translation of this information into management remain to be accomplished.

Human leukocyte antigen (HLA) molecules regulate immune responses to foreign antigens and discrimination of self from non-self antigens. They are encoded by a series of closely linked genetic loci found on chromosome 6.[38] The purpose of these cell surface histocompatibility antigens is to bind foreign proteins and present them to appropriate antigen-specific T cells. Two HLA classes exist, including class I antigens, present on all nucleated cells, and class II antigens, present on antigen-presenting cells (macrophages). Class II molecules bind foreign (viral) proteins, which are then processed internally by macrophages and presented on the cell surface as a complex for recognition by T cells. HLA class II molecules are divided into three general groups, comprising DP, DQ and DR. The multitude of proteins produced by this highly polymorphic repertoire of genes is genetically diverse and differs between individuals.[38] Given an immune response to a given antigen may be determined by whether an individual possesses a specific group of class II genes, it is conceivable that (1) persons falling into specific HLA sub-classes may have differential risks of infection by certain HPVs and (2) differential binding affinities to intra-typic sequence variations within given HPV types. It is these two concepts that have driven numerous studies exploring the associations between HLA class and cervical cancer risk.

Although the evidence for a link between HLA and cervical cancer has been controversial, it has been recently reported that certain HLA class II haplotypes (linked class II alleles) are positively associated with low- and high-grade SIL or invasive cervical cancer, while other class II haplotypes are negatively associated or protective.[39] Still others have been associated with infection alone versus cancer, or cancers associated with certain HPV types, such as type 16. Some are associated with neoplasia in one study and found to be neutral or protective in another. Some of the more compelling HLA loci are included in Table 13.1. Since HLA associations between human papillomavirus type 16 (HPV16)-mediated cancer cases and non-HPV16-mediated cancer cases have been found to be different, the evidence suggests that specific HLA class II haplotypes may influence HPV antigen presentation and the immune response to HPV infection, in turn influencing the risk of developing invasive cervical carcinoma. It should be emphasized, however, that while a number of associations between HLA class II types and cervical neoplasia or HPV infection have been identified, the precise mechanisms underlying these associations remain to be clarified (Table 13.1).

Age

Young, sexually active women are at greatest risk for HPV infection and preinvasive cervical neoplasia. This risk drops significantly with increasing age, which is associated with increasing risk of cancer (Fig. 13.3). Koutsky et al. showed that women under age 19 had a three-fold higher frequency of developing HSIL (20 vs 7%) during follow-up.[14] Risk drops further with the approach of menopause, paralleling the drop in HPV prevalence with age (Fig. 13.3). The progressive drop in risk with age has been attributed to an effective immune response to the virus that follows the onset of sexual activity and exposure to HPVs. Protection is long lasting, given the low rates of HPV positivity in middle-age women. There is conflicting evidence regarding HPV rates in older women, but some studies support a small but distinct increase in positive rate after menopause.[40,41]

Immunity

Defects in cell-mediated immunity imposed by transplant therapy significantly increase the risk of cervical cancer. HIV-infected individuals are prone to HPV infection, persistent HPV infection and a higher risk

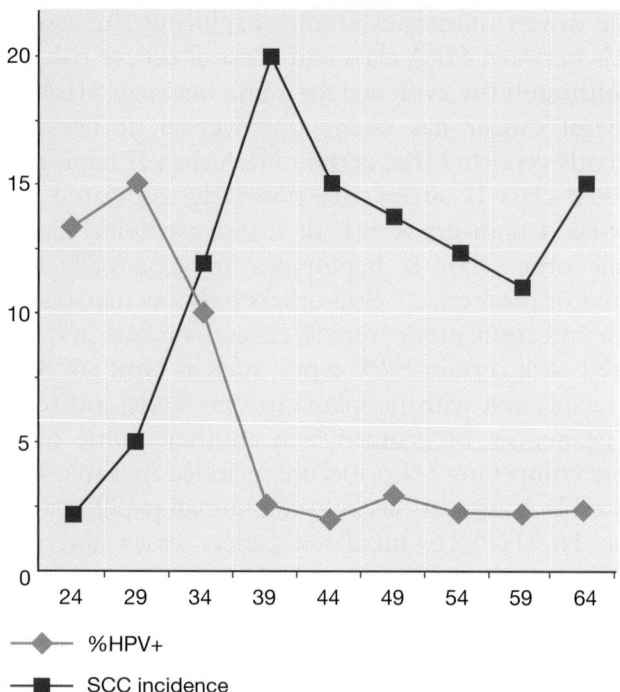

Fig. 13.3 Distribution of human papillomavirus frequency in the population and cervical cancer as a function of age. A progressive decline in HPV index coincides with an increase in cancer risk.

of precursor lesions. The impact of HIV infection on cervical cancer risk is controversial, but prognosis appears worse in patients with severe immunodeficiency.

The risk of cervical neoplasia or HPV infection in immunosuppressed individuals is well documented (Table 13.1). Women post-transplant have higher than normal rates of HPV positivity.[41] Cancer rates are higher in this population, and in general anogenital cancers occur at a younger age. One study suggested a slightly lower incidence in cervical neoplasia following the introduction of cyclosporine.[42,43] One study reported a five-fold increase in risk of HSIL (50% vs 10%) in transplant recipients.[43] In one study, lower genital cytopathology was evaluated in 105 immunosuppressed renal transplant recipients. Evidence of human papillomavirus infection was found in 17.5% and of lower genital neoplasia in 9.5%. The rate of the virus infection in the immunosuppressed was nine times greater than in a general population and 17 times greater than in a matched immunocompetent population.[44] In one-third of patients with human papillomavirus lesions and one-half of patients with neoplastic lesions, multiple lower genital sites were also involved.

Human immunodeficiency virus infection has been the most intensively studied and permits the breakdown of risk according to several outcome measures:

1 The risk of HPV positivity is increased in women who are HIV positive (Table 13.1). Approximately 60% of HIV-infected women vs 36% of uninfected women score positive for HPV, based on testing of cervical samples. Frequencies of HPV16, 18 and multiple infections are also significantly more common in the HIV-infected group.[45,46]

2 The risk of persistent HPV infection is significantly increased in HIV-infected women. Estimates place the risk of high-risk HPV infection at least two-fold of non-HPV infected controls and the risk of persistent infection nearly six times higher.[47] Furthermore, in one study, persistence was 1.9 (95% CI, 1.5–2.3) times greater than normal if the subject had a CD4 cell count <200 cells/μl (vs >500 cells/μl).[48]

3 The risk of a subsequent squamous intraepithelial lesion is significantly higher in HIV-infected women. Ellerbrock et al. showed that 20% vs 5% of HIV-infected and uninfected women developed a squamous intraepithelial lesion (SIL). Cardillo et al. observed that HIV viral load correlated significantly with cytologic abnormalities.[48] Heard et al. found that cervical disease was present in 27% of HIV-infected patients and HPV infection in 53%. High HPV viral load correlated with both low CD4 counts and risk of cervical disease (OR 16.8).[49]

4 The proportion of HSILs appears to be not substantially higher in HIV-infected women. Ellerbrock et al. also showed that 91% and 75% of SILs in the two groups, respectively, were LSILs.[50]

5 The risk of persistent SIL appears higher in women with HIV, being 76% vs 18% in the study by La Ruche et al.[51]

6 The incidence of invasive carcinoma is variably influenced by HIV infection. Fransceschi et al. reported a 15-fold greater risk in HIV-infected women.[52,53] However, Chokunonga et al. and La Ruche et al. did not consider HIV a major factor in cervical cancer incidence in Central Africa.[54,55] Another study from South Africa found no significant difference between stage of presentation and HIV status, although some correlation was observed for patients with CD4 counts of less than 200 cells/μl.[56]

The male partner

Sexual history of the male sexual partner influences risk of cervical neoplasia, but the degree of risk is less than that imposed by the sexual history of the woman. Studies clearly show that the number of lifetime sexual partners increases the risk of HPV infection.[57] Sexual behavior patterns in male consorts also influences risk of both HPV and other sexually transmitted diseases. Thomas et al. linked risk in Thai women with male behavior, specifically unprotected intercourse with prostitutes.[58] Another group showed that monogamous wives of husbands who had sexual relationships both before and during the marriage had a substantial risk of cervical cancer (RR = 6.9 (CI, 2.3–20.7)).[59] However, the degree of risk conferred by extramarital sexual experiences has varied from study to study.[60]

The significance of the male partner may depend in part, on the timing of exposure. For example, Krebs and Helmkamp showed that treating the male partner did not influence risk of recurrent genital warts.[61] The implication of this study is that partners are not re-infected by the same virus, consistent with a functioning immune system. Similarly, there may be a threshold of exposures beyond which further infection is less likely to occur. If this were the case, women with prior exposure to HPV would be less vulnerable to subsequent sexual behavior of the partner. This was shown by Kjaer et al., who found that repeated sexual contacts of the male partner with other women did not increase risk independently, while a history of genital warts and absence of condom use did.[60] Conversely, Agarwal et al. showed that male sexual activity poses the greatest risk to a monogamous female partner with the fewest prior sexual partners.

How is HPV transmitted from male to female? This is a difficult question to answer, but the most likely mechanisms include exfoliation of surface keratinocytes and direct transmission via semen. The former is speculated on the basis of detection of penile mucosal lesions, but a direct connection between male and female infection is difficult to validate. The latter is based on reports identifying HPV in semen, which have ranged widely, from less than 5% to over 50%, and appear to be resistant to sperm washing procedures. Interesting observations of alterations in sperm motility and apoptosis following *in vitro* exposure to HPV DNA have been reported, but one study showed no apparent connection between HPV positivity and fertility rates or pregnancy outcome.[62] The question of whether HPV can be transmitted to the fertilized ovum by sperm remains a matter of speculation.[63]

Will barrier methods of contraception prevent viral spread? Yes and no.

What is the interval from infection by the male partner to a cytologic abnormality? Kreider et al. found that the interval from experimental HPV-11 infection of mucosal epithelium to the development of a morphologically distinct lesion was approximately 4 months.[64] Koutsky et al. showed that the interval from HPV positivity to lesion detection (when lesions developed) ranged from 0 to 24 months.[14]

Oral contraceptives

Oral contraceptive use modestly increases the risk of cervical neoplasia. There is a strong theoretical basis for hormones influencing epithelial growth and susceptibility to neoplasia in the cervical transformation zone.[65] Oral contraceptives use and plasma levels of hormone have been associated with cervical neoplasia;[66] however, Kjellberg et al. and Coker et al. noted an association between OCPs and cervical neoplasia but the association disappeared when HPV was taken into account.[67,68] Others have shown no clear relationship between cervical cancer and oral contraceptives.[69] Lacey et al. showed an association between hormonal replacement and cervical adenocarcinoma.[70]

Smoking

Smoking increases the risk of cervical neoplasia, but the mechanism is unclear. Kjellberg et al. noted a strong (independent of HPV) association between smoking and cervical neoplasia.[67] The theoretical basis is presumably the presence of DNA adducts in the cervical mucus, exposing the transformation zone mucosa to carcinogens.[71] Genetic polymorphisms that theoretically do not reduce adduct formation have also been implicated.[72] Lacey et al. showed a positive relationship to squamous but not adenocarcinoma.[73] Deacon et al. also showed a dose-response relationship.[74]

Chlamydia infections

The association between *Chlamydia* infection and cervical neoplasia is controversial. Anttila et al. found that evidence of infection with *Chlamydia* serotype G conferred a significant risk of cervical cancer (Table 13.1).[75] Several studies have shown a relationship between genital infections and HPV or HSIL.[76] Others, however, have not shown a relationship between antibodies to *Chlamydia* and cervical neoplasia.[77]

Women who have sex with other women

Risk of cervical neoplasia is increased in women who have sex with other women. Studies have shown high rates of sexually transmitted infections in women who have sex predominately with other women, although the rates of genital condylomata were low. However, the risk of developing HSIL was not determined. Two reports have shown that CIN II may occur in lesbians.[4,78,79]

In summary, a multitude of factors, viral and host related, influences risk of cervical neoplasia before, during and following exposure and lesion progression. The schematic outlined in Figure 13.2 attempts to place these factors in their approximate place in the pathway to cervical carcinoma, although the impact of each may vary depending on the individual.

MOLECULAR RISK FACTORS

The Papanicolaou smear and HPV testing are currently approved for cervical cancer screening. Another method under study is detection of other markers of HPV infection (surrogate markers).

Human papillomaviruses

Because HPVs are so strongly associated with cervical cancer, HPV testing is a logical adjunct to the Papanicolaou smear in cancer prevention and precursor diagnosis. The use of HPV testing in the management of the abnormal Papanicolaou smear will be discussed later. This segment will address the utility of HPV testing as a screening tool. The most important issues, including both supportive and negative data, are the following:

1 Unlike Papanicolaou smear and colposcopic analysis, HPV testing combines high sensitivity and an objective measurement of cervical cancer or precursor risk, and the increase in risk attending its presence is approximately 40-fold. If the HPV test is positive, the risk of a high-grade squamous intraepithelial lesion will vary further depending on whether the smear is abnormal (at least 20%) or whether HPV is detected at more than one visit (up to 33%). A single positive Hybrid Capture II test, particularly in young women, has less value. However, the high negative predictive value of this test, combined with a normal Pap smear, virtually assures the patient is free of a cancer precursor. Testing is superior in sensitivity to the Papanicolaou smears and may be a cost-effective alternative.[80–82] However, a significant proportion of women who will not develop a precursor lesion will score positive. Goldie showed that self-testing for HPV was not as sensitive as clinic-testing but was as sensitive as the Papanicolaou smear.[80]

2 Combined negative HPV testing and normal smear may increase the duration of the 'protective effect'. Because HPV is detected prior to the development of a cytologic abnormality, it is likely that patients negative by both HPV testing and smear may be followed at longer intervals than by smear alone. The age of the patient may come into play, with younger sexually active individuals more likely to score positive, and less amenable to a wider screening interval.[83] The index of HPV positivity drops markedly over age 30, suggesting that targeting of specific populations may increase the potential significance of a positive HPV test.[6,84] An important question concerns the specificity of testing in the older age group, where a greater specificity would justify screening this population. In one study, detection of HPV in cytologic negative routine hysterectomies from women in decades 4–6 was extremely low (less than 2%), suggesting that the testing may be cost-effective. However, the increase in specificity of testing in women over 30 is not clear.[20] Clavel et al. showed that the specificities increased modestly, from 85.6% and 87.3%, to 88.4% and 90.1% if HPV testing was reserved for women >30 years old.[8] A recent study suggests that the percentage of women over 30 years of age is sufficiently low that HPV testing is cost-effective for managing smear abnormalities in this population.[85] However, some studies have shown that a sizable fraction of postmenopausal women will score positive for HPV, with the significance of this finding still unclear.[86] A recent study using a very sensitive assay for detecting HPV found two peaks of HPV DNA prevalence, including a first peak of 16.7% in women under 25 years. HPV DNA prevalence declined to 3.7% in the age group 35–44 years, then increased progressively to 23% among women 65 years and older.[87] In all groups, sexual behavior was closely related to HPV positivity, but another study also linked HPV positivity in this group to hormonal therapy.[88] It should be emphasized that not all studies have confirmed the high incidence of HPV in postmenopausal women. Rates calculated by Ferenczy et al. were closer to those of Shen et al. (1%) and were not linked to hormone usage.[89] Another study reported a second peak of HPV positivity in older women but it consisted principally of low-risk HPV types.[87] Overall, low-risk HPVs are more likely to be associated with lesions occurring

in the younger age group, but there is substantial overlap.[90]

3 An increasing proportion of women with invasive carcinoma have had a Papanicolaou smear in the preceding 3 years, many of which were false negatives. This issue has two components. The first is the existence of cervical carcinomas – including adenocarcinomas and adenocarcinomas *in situ* – that occur in young women and are not readily detected by cytologic screening.[91] The second is the concept of rapidly progressive carcinomas, a vague entity that may be attributed as much to difficulties in detection as specific biologic entity.[92] This is one of the more challenging issues in cancer prevention, one which indicates that a specific population of younger women may be at risk for adenocarcinoma, yet be relatively unprotected by conventional screening. It is conceivable that certain demographic factors (such as oral contraceptive use) may be used to identify a patient profile in the younger age group that would benefit from screening for HPV.[93]

4 HPV testing confers a psychological burden pertaining to both the connotations of a sexually transmitted infection and the knowledge that in the absence of an abnormality, there is no treatment for this infection. Some concerns with testing surround not the objectivity of the test but the subjectivity with which it may be managed by the clinician and interpreted by the patient. Because a high percentage of reproductive-age women are HPV positive at a given time, yet only a minority will manifest with a cervical lesion, the success of HPV screening, if it becomes practice, will hinge in part on the success with which the target population can be educated.[94] Unlike the Papanicolaou smear, which in itself imposes considerable psychological burden on the patient if abnormal, HPV testing labels the individual as afflicted with not only a sexually transmitted disease but also an infection that may not be confirmed on examination and may persist for some time with an uncertain outcome.[95] Although an outcome of cancer is highly unlikely in cytologically negative individuals, the uncertainty of the diagnosis requires careful counseling of the patient. Nevertheless, the anxiety provoked by this diagnosis may not exceed that for other sexually transmitted diseases.[96,97]

5 Depending on the testing methods used, HPV testing with 'high-risk' probes is best interpreted as an assessment of risk rather than a marker for high-grade lesions or cancer. The probe cocktails used in some assays, specifically the Hybrid Capture II system, comprise 13 of the most common high- and intermediate-risk types. This cocktail has been demonstrated to detect virtually 100% of infections by these types and to be more sensitive than polymerase chain reaction (Crum, unpublished data). However, to achieve this sensitivity, the test must also detect a range of HPV types that either do not fall within the high-risk group, including, types 6, 11 and 54, or possess debatable oncogenicity such as 66, 53 and others.[13,98] While this is not a significant disadvantage if patients are properly counseled and managed, it emphasizes the importance of viewing the test not as a 'cancer test' but as one that measures relative risk of a preinvasive cervical lesion. Recent epidemiologic studies suggest that some HPVs, such as types 53 and 66, belong in the 'high-risk group', an association that may be controversial when assigning a value of cancer risk to the individual.[99]

6 Are cell-based assays superior to a solution-based technique for detection of HPV? Recent improvements in the sensitivity of *in situ* hybridization have fueled exploration into the use of *in situ*-based methods of HPV detection that could be applied to Papanicolaou smear assessment. The potential advantage of this approach is the direct detection of HPV nucleic acids in abnormal cells, which in turn could be more specific than solution-based methods. The major questions to be answered with this technology include: (a) Is there a substantial lack of direct relationship between a positive solution-based assay and the morphologic changes seen in the cytologic smear? (b) Is the sensitivity of the *in situ* assay sufficient to carry a high negative predictive value? The former theoretically would make an *in situ* assay more specific with a higher positive predictive value. The latter would be essential if clinical decisions were being made from negative assays. If both were answered in the affirmative, it is conceivable that *in situ* hybridization could represent an improvement over solution-based assays.

Other biomarkers

Ultimately, one of the most efficient detection strategies for cervical neoplasia would be a solution-based test that circumvented the need for both cytologic screening yet provided more specific information than HPV testing. The advent of high through-put screening methods for molecular markers linked to cervical neoplasia has and will continue to uncover host cell genes that serve as surrogate markers for cervical neoplasia. As shown in Figure 13.1, the pathways that are positively or negatively influenced by HPV oncoproteins include apoptotic (p53), cell cycle checkpoints (Rb) replicative senescence (telomerase) and mitotic stability (centrosome synthesis). Several biomarkers, including cyclin E, p16[INK4], MN, MCM-2, p55cdc, telomerase and others, are influenced by HPV expression and in variable degrees will identify HPV-infected cells. The potential that these reagents will identify cells generically infected by HPV and serve as surrogates of HPV infection has implications for both solution-based molecular diagnosis and immuno-histochemical screening of cytologic smears. Another strategy is to test for methylation of critical tumor suppressor genes, presumably a result of increasing genomic instability. The potential advantage of this approach is that the detection method targets methylated sequences and would not be hindered by coexisting normal genomes accompanied by normal gene expression in normal cells.[100] The specificity of these biomarkers and their application to routine cytologic screening remains to be resolved and is currently under study.[101–104] Selected biomarkers as adjuncts to histologic diagnosis will be discussed in greater detail later in the chapter.

Cytology

A more comprehensive treatise on the cytopathologic diagnosis of cervical neoplasia can be found in any of several excellent texts addressing this field.[105–108] The purpose of this discussion is to update and integrate several facets of cytologic screening that have been evolving, are directly relevant to patient care, and are thus of interest to anyone involved in the laboratory or clinical management of cervical neoplasia. These include (1) the realistic expectations from cytologic screening, (2) changes in cytologic collection and their significance, (3) two major changes in the terminology for classifying cytologic smears in the past 15 years, based on the Bethesda 1988 and 2001 meetings, (4) cytologic criteria that have emerged and the meaning of the terms employed, (5) purported reasons for recent changes in the classification system and (6) the role

of HPV testing in the management of non-diagnostic squamous atypias.

EXPECTATIONS FROM CERVICAL CYTOLOGY IN CERVICAL CANCER PREVENTION

The conventional Papanicolaou smear

Cervical cancer prevention is both tantalizingly appealing and frustrating. The cervix lies a few centimeters from the external world, is accessible by speculum examination, and preinvasive disease – with its generally protracted natural history – can be detected in a high percentage of cases prior to invasive cancer. Studies of cancer incidence rates have shown an approximately two-thirds reduction in cervical cancer incidence in the past 60 years since the introduction of the Papanicolaou smear. Predictably, the most striking reduction in rates occurs immediately following introduction of screening, where a precipitous reduction (from 28 to 4 cases per 100 000 in the studies by Bryans et al.) occurs simply by removing those with occult cancer.[109] Once this is accomplished, the incidence drops to a steady state of approximately 4 cases per 100 000 and is favorably impacted by screening of women at a young age.[109] According to Miller, the maximum achievable reduction in cancer by conscientious Papanicolaou smear screening is approximately 90%.[110] The success and appeal of this technology is balanced by the fact that the number of women who die of this disease is irreducible beyond a few percentage points due to human variables, such as screening and sampling errors, patient compliance and differences in biologic behavior that in some instances may preclude adequate prevention by proposed screening intervals. The influence of the latter appears to be relatively small. The vast majority of squamous carcinomas of the cervix are preceded by preinvasive abnormalities.

It should be emphasized that the death rate from cervical cancer began to decline in the 1930s prior to widespread use of Papanicolaou smear screening, presumably due to greater patient awareness or more prompt management of women with symptoms. Since that time, the rates of invasive cancer and proportion of invasive carcinomas detected at advance stage has declined greatly.

Changes in population risk over the past 50 years

Since the inception of Papanicolaou smear screening, the incidence of cervical adenocarcinomas has evolved from relatively constant to increasing, implying either that this disease progresses more rapidly from precursor to cancer or that it is less easily detected in its early stages by cytologic screening. This will be discussed in greater detail in the following chapters, but three components of this issue merit concern by the practitioner: (1) the fact that detection errors are common with adenocarcinomas, (2) adenocarcinomas are representing a greater proportion of cancers now detected in reproductive-age women and (3) adenocarcinomas comprise the bulk of the 'surprises' that are being encountered in the 25–35-year-old group. The latter fact has important implications (and a mandate) for cancer detection strategies that augment the Papanicolaou smear in this group of reproductive-age women.

Liquid-based versus conventional preparations for cytology screening

The introduction of liquid-based techniques, including ThinPrep and Autopap has revolutionized the cervical cancer screening industry, with claims of higher rates of precursor detection. Comparisons of these technologies with conventional Papanicolaou smear are summarized in several studies (Michael, Allen, 09-112),[111,112] many of which show an increase in detection of ASCUS and LSIL and either no or a slight increase in detection of HSIL.

Cytologic classification systems

Because the Bethesda System (the 1988 and 2001 Bethesda System for reporting cytologic diagnosis; Bethesda 1988)[113] for reporting cytologic abnormalities is over 15 years old and has been widely adopted, a lengthy discussion of the classic Papanicolaou system is not warranted, other than for comparison. The most important issues addressed in 1988 were: treating the cytology as a medical consult; assigning responsibility to the pathologist for diagnosis; requirements for historical information from the referring physician; statements of adequacy; and recommendations by the cytopathologist regarding follow-up and reclassification of cytologic abnormalities from the Papanicolaou class system to a descriptive system, the latter incorporating specific terms for non-diagnostic atypia (ASCUS) and low- and high-grade squamous intraepithelial lesions. An important area of discussion was selecting appropriate terminology for specimens deemed less than adequate, with the presence or absence of endocervical cells central to this determination. The most recent meetings, in 2001, refined the above system by: (1) eliminating the term 'specimen satisfactory but limited', by (2) combining smears previously termed

Table 13.5 The Bethesda system of cytologic classification (2001)[a]

Specimen type
  Indicate conventional smear (Pap smear) vs liquid based vs other

Specimen adequacy
  Satisfactory for evaluation
  Unsatisfactory for evaluation (specify reason)
  Specimen rejected/not processed (specify reason)
  Specimen processed and examined, but unsatisfactory for evaluation of epithelial abnormality because of (specify reason)

General categorization (optional)
  Negative for intraepithelial lesion or malignancy
  Epithelial cell abnormality: (See Interpretation/Result (specify 'squamous' or 'glandular' as appropriate)
  Other: See Interpretation/Result (e.g. endometrial cells in a woman over 40 years of age)

Automated review (specify)

Ancillary testing (specify)

Interpretation/result

Negative for intraepithelial lesion or malignancy
  Organisms (specify)
  Other non-neoplastic findings (optional to report; list not inclusive)
  Other (specify)

Epithelial cell abnormalities
  Squamous cell
    Atypical squamous cells of undetermined significance (ASCUS) cannot exclude HSIL (ASCH)
    Low-grade squamous intraepithelial lesion (LSIL) encompassing: HPV/mild dysplasia/CIN I
    High-grade squamous intraepithelial lesion (HSIL) encompassing: moderate and severe dysplasia, CIS/CIN II and CIN III (with features suspicious for invasion (if invasion is suspected)
    Squamous cell carcinoma

[a]Modified from http://bethesda2001.cancer.gov/terminology.html

negative and benign cellular changes, (3) contracting ASCUS to ASCUS and ASCUS favor HSIL and (4) similarly contracting AGUS to AGUS NOS and AGUS favor neoplasia. Table 13.5 summarizes the most recent Bethesda classification system for the interpretation of cytologic changes.[114] In the former classification, ASCUS was qualified according to whether the observer suspected a reactive (favor reactive) condition, low- or high-grade squamous intraepithelial lesion (favor LSIL or favor HSIL) or had no opinion as to the possible nature of the atypia present (NOS). This has been refined to two grades of atypical squamous cells 'favor HSIL' and all others, termed 'ASCUS'. This will be discussed further below.

NON-DIAGNOSTIC SQUAMOUS ATYPIA

Introduction

The 1988 Bethesda Conference created the term 'atypical squamous cells of undetermined significance'

(ASCUS) to identify the subset of squamous atypias that cannot be readily designated as benign or pre-invasive.[115] Because the diagnosis of ASCUS is an admission of uncertainty, it can be assumed that the criteria for this process will remain vague and, by definition, much less reproducible than the criteria for squamous intraepithelial lesions. This has been established by numerous studies in which inter-observer reproducibility is poorer for a histologic diagnosis of non-diagnostic squamous atypia than for a diagnosis of SIL.[116,117] Nevertheless, atypical squamous cells on the Papanicolaou smear carry, in aggregate, an approximate 10% risk of a coexisting high-grade squamous intraepithelial lesion.[118]

Efforts to make ASCUS more 'user friendly' initially centered on sub-classifying ASCUS, resulting in marked differences in HSIL risk between ASCUS favor reactive and ASCUS favor HSIL (Table 13.6). Risks for ASCUS NOS and favor LSIL fell between 10% and 15%. Although this strategy provided information useful in triaging patients with ASCUS, the more recent approach, and one that is designed to incorporate HPV testing, has been to contract ASCUS to just two categories, ASCUS and ASCUS favor HSIL. The outcome of studies using HPV testing have demonstrated two important findings, as shown in Table 13.6:

1 The disparity in risk between HPV-positive and HPV-negative ASCUS is approximately 20-fold (20% vs 1.1%) in contrast to an ASCUS sub-classification system, in which the disparity between favor HSIL and favor reactive is only 10-fold.

2 Sub-classification of ASCUS does not add significant value to what is already gained by HPV testing. The role of HPV testing in managing ASCUS will be discussed below.[119]

Cytologic alterations that are best left out of the ASCUS category (Fig. 13.4)

1 Mild superficial cell karyomegaly without hyperchromasia: this applies particularly to the changes seen in association with menopause or women over 40 years of age.
2 Cytoplasmic halos in the absence of nuclear atypia: cytoplasmic halos, which are not accompanied by nuclear enlargement or nuclear hyperchromasia, should not be interpreted as ASCUS. The more problematic are those smears containing mild degrees of nuclear enlargement in association with cytoplasmic halos. In such cases the diagnosis will be subjective.
3 Parakeratosis and anucleated squames: superficial sheets of parakeratotic cells may contain mild degrees of anisokaryosis. In the absence of hyperchromasia, pleomorphic forms or bi-nucleation, these are best interpreted as benign cellular changes.[119]

Cytologic criteria for the diagnosis of ASCUS

The term 'atypia' as defined by the Bethesda System was reserved for cases in which the cellular changes are of uncertain significance.[1] The findings cannot be ascribed with certainty to a benign process such as inflammation or typical repair, and yet they are not sufficient for an unequivocal diagnosis of a squamous intraepithelial lesion. Inevitably, this category has included cases that ultimately proved to be inflammatory, reparative, or atrophic changes, as well as cases that proved to be SIL. If this terminology is to be used, it is critical that alterations such as 'benign atypia', 'inflammatory atypia', or 'reactive atypia' and other recognizably benign alterations be excluded. Whether alterations 'suggestive but not diagnostic of koilocytotic atypia' should be included depends upon whether the diagnosis of ASCUS is based upon cytoplasmic halos alone. In essence, ASCUS is best applied to those alterations that raise the possibility of a cancer precursor. It is unlikely that mild superficial karyomegaly, cytoplasmic halos and normal non-atypical parakeratotic cells qualify as significant cancer risk factors.

The cytologic criteria for ASCUS are designed to identify abnormalities that are intermediate in severity between those of clear-cut reactive or reparative processes

Table 13.6 Risks of high-risk HPV, HSIL or cancer as a function of cytologic diagnosis

Parameter	Reference	Outcome[a]	(%)
ASCUS	114	HPV(+)	30–60
ASCUS	114	HSIL	10
	185	Cancer	0.1
ASCUS (HPV+)	114	HSIL	15–27[b]
	311	Cancer	0.5
ASCUS (HPV–)	114	HSIL	1.1
Follow-up smear (–)	114	HSIL	3.7
LSIL smear	311	HSIL	27.6[c]
LSIL cyt/Colpo (–)	311	HSIL	11.3
LSIL cyt/Biopsy (–)	311	HSIL	11.7
LSIL cyt/Biopsy LSIL	311	HSIL	13.0

[a]Outcomes with follow-up of up to 2 years.
[b]Varies with length of follow-up and cut-off threshold for HPV positive.
[c]2-year follow-up.

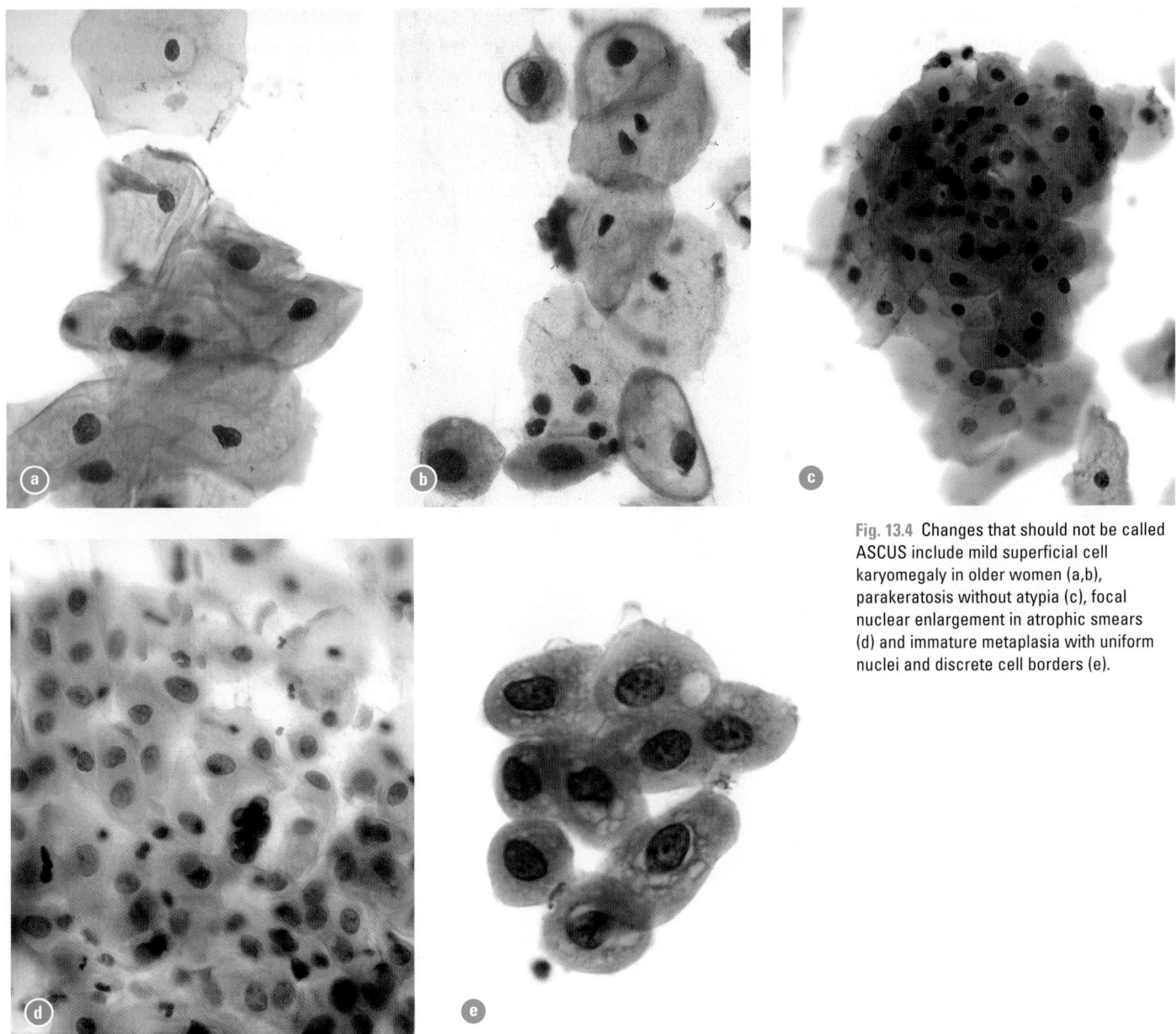

Fig. 13.4 Changes that should not be called ASCUS include mild superficial cell karyomegaly in older women (a,b), parakeratosis without atypia (c), focal nuclear enlargement in atrophic smears (d) and immature metaplasia with uniform nuclei and discrete cell borders (e).

and squamous intraepithelial lesions. Nuclear enlargement exceeds that typically associated with known benign proliferations but falls short of SIL; hence the compromise on 2.5-fold differences in size. Nuclear hyperchromasia may be greater than normal, but the diagnosis of SIL may not be made because the nuclei do not contain coarse chromatin or nuclear membrane irregularity, are associated with a low nuclear/cytoplasmic ratio, appear degenerated, or are arranged in regularly spaced cells more characteristic of a benign process. Alternatively, the cells may be obscured by inflammation, blood or drying artifact, forcing a qualification of the diagnosis. Finally, the number of cells

may be so few that the cytopathologist is uncomfortable with an absolute diagnosis.[120]

ASCUS can be subdivided into several categories, which are illustrated in Figure 13.5. It should be stressed that these groups overlap and may not be reproducible, but their attempted separation may permit a more systematic approach to non-diagnostic squamous atypia. For example, a category such as cells suggesting koilocytosis may be interpreted by one cytopathologist as a mimic of koilocytosis and another as diagnostic of LSIL.

Atypical superficial cells resembling koilocytosis comprise a category of cellular changes which include cytoplasmic halos and minor degrees of nuclear atypia, and is depicted in Figure 13.5. It may be argued that this category of ASCUS is the least supportable, inasmuch as cytoplasmic halos without diagnostic nuclei may warrant a diagnosis of reactive changes only. The spectrum of such changes begins with reactive changes (such as trichomoniasis) and ends with koilocytotic atypia.[121–125] Cells containing the classic irregular densely bordered halos with slight nuclear atypia fall into the category of ASCUS. Cells without any nuclear atypia,

irrespective of the appearance of the cytoplasmic halo, should best be classified as reactive, inasmuch as their contribution to cancer risk is negligible.

Atypical parakeratotic cells may also fall into the realm of ASCUS, but the number of cases designated as ASCUS is small, if non-atypical parakeratosis and minor degrees of atypia (such as that seen with candida infection) are ignored. Once conspicuous atypical parakeratosis is identified, with variations in nuclear size, staining and with binuclear forms, the distinction

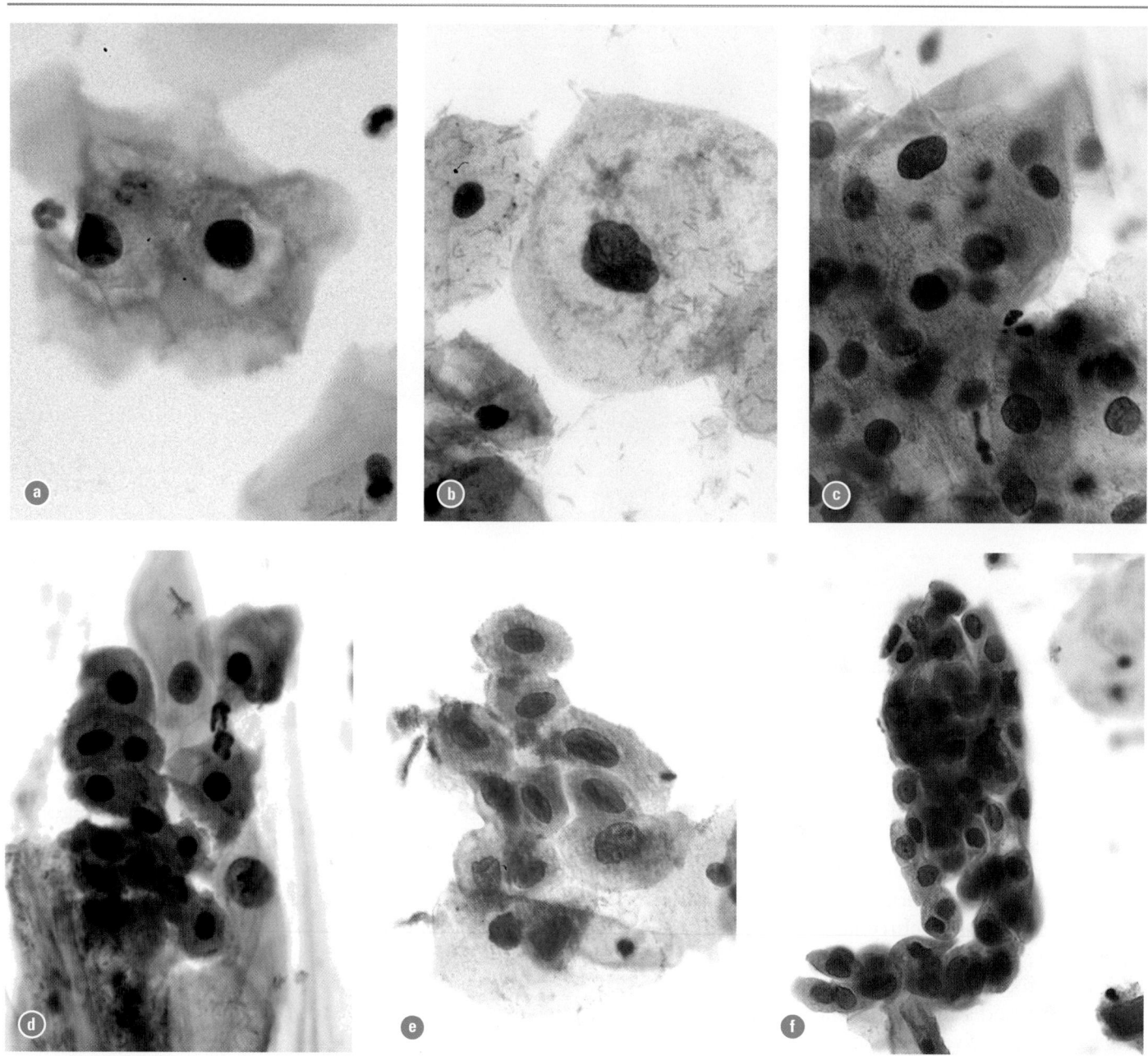

Fig. 13.5 Cytologic patterns often classified as ASCUS include cells bordering on LSIL (a), mildly atypical maturing metaplastic cells (b,c); atypical parakeratotic cells (d); atypical metaplasia (e); atypical immature cells with a metaplastic phenotype (f); hyperchromatic clusters of cells with a high nuclear/cytoplasmic ratio

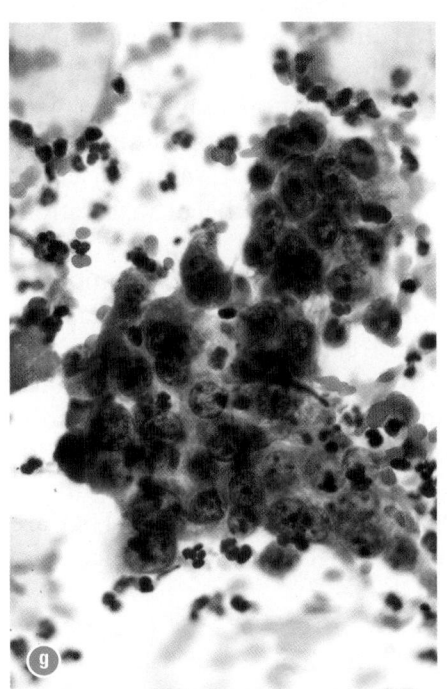

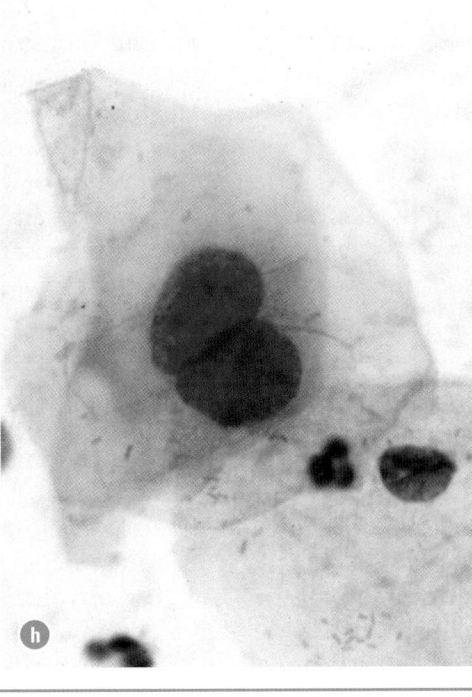

Fig. 13.5 **Cont'd** (g) and degenerated atypical cells (less common with liquid-based preparations (h). (a) and (d) cannot be reproducibly distinguished from LSIL; (b, c and e) are least impressive and might also be classified as reactive changes; (f) and (g) were associated with biopsy-proven HSIL and cervical carcinoma, respectively.

of ASCUS (atypical parakeratosis favor SIL) and SIL, is less clear. Examples are shown in Figure 13.5. Here the decision as to classification will be made upon the extent of the atypical parakeratosis, assuming other superficial cellular changes are absent.

Non-koilocytotic nuclear atypia in mature squamous cells, including squamous metaplasia, is another form of ASCUS, which typically presents with 2–3-fold nuclear enlargement with mild increases in nuclear chromasia and no alterations in nuclear contour (Fig. 13.5). The distinction between this form of ASCUS and SIL is based upon the absence of coarse chromatin or disturbances in cytoplasmic maturation. Depending upon the background changes and degree of nuclear atypia, the diagnosis may be either ASCUS favor reactive or ASCUS; SIL cannot be excluded.

Atypical immature squamous metaplasia (AISM) poses a diagnostic problem as a consequence of the small cell size, and hence, higher nuclear/cytoplasmic ratio of metaplastic cells. If the nuclear changes are interpreted to be those of a SIL, the cytology will be that of a high-grade lesion, almost by definition. For most clinicians, this will result in more aggressive management.

Key features in AISM include nuclear sizes of 35–100 μm, with cyanophilic or granular staining cytoplasm, N/C ratios generally over 60% and irregular nuclear contours. Significant increases in nuclear chromasia are less likely, particularly in liquid-based preparations. The cells tend to occur in strings and small groups and are frequently isolated. Because of their small size, they can be easily overlooked or mistaken for benign histiocytes, small (reserve) squamous cells or endometrial cells. Because of the potential that atypical squamous metaplasia may either accompany, progress to, or represent a HSIL, Papanicolaou smears displaying this abnormality should be carefully scrutinized.

Atypical repair reactions can demonstrate cellular crowding and overlap (as contrasted with typical repair, which is in flat sheets) marked variation in nuclear size, prominent and irregular nucleoli and irregular chromatin distribution. Such cases may be difficult to distinguish from invasive carcinoma and SIL. Carcinomas often have a tumor diathesis and many isolated atypical cells, features that are usually absent in repair reactions.

Atypical squamous cells associated with atrophy may be a diagnostic problem under certain circumstances (Fig. 13.5). Smears obtained from postmenopausal women not receiving hormone replacement often are air-dried with apparent nuclear enlargement, a significant inflammatory component, and clusters of small dark cells, most likely small 'parabasal' cells. In addition, a common finding is the appearance of 'blue blobs' – degenerated nuclear material as well as scattered squamous atypia. A helpful means of assessing atrophy-related atypia is the estrogen test whereby application of estrogen cream results in maturation of the squamous epithelial component and reversal of the atypia. Atypias that persist are investigated further with colposcopy and biopsy. In some cases, atypia persists despite hormonal therapy but the tissue findings are negative.

Two studies seem to indicate that squamous atypia in the postmenopausal population is rarely associated with biopsy-proven SIL in contrast to the situation in the premenopausal group. Symmans et al. correlated cervical cytology and biopsies with HPV DNA detection using *in situ* hybridization.[126] They found that the incidence of a biopsy-proven SIL relative to a concurrent squamous atypia on the Papanicolaou smear was 17% in the postmenopausal group as compared with 46% in the premenopausal group. Further, the rate of HPV detection in the postmenopausal group seen at colposcopy was 10% compared with approximately 50% of premenopausal women seen at colposcopy for an abnormal smear. The authors concluded that squamous atypia in postmenopausal women is rarely associated with either biopsy-proven SIL or HPV DNA detection and may represent atrophic changes.

Kaminski et al. evaluated 115 patients over age 50 with a squamous atypia on cervical cytology using repeat smear and colposcopy.[127] Biopsies were performed at colposcopy when appropriate. Their findings revealed that a single smear with squamous atypia in patients over 50 years of age was associated with CIN or HPV (biopsy diagnoses) in less than 5% of cases. Importantly, abnormal repeat cytology had a significantly lower likelihood of association with pathology on biopsy (9%) when compared with similar data from younger patients (24–45%). Of particular interest to the present discussion were the nine women who had two repeat squamous atypias. One of the nine ultimately had evidence of HPV, yielding a positive rate of HPV detection of 11%, even with three atypical Pap smears. In addition, 37 women with initial diagnoses of squamous atypia and atrophy by colposcopy were placed on estrogen replacement. A total of 31 had negative smears on repeat examination, a proportion that was 'significantly higher' than those not on hormone replacement therapy. Six women persisted with squamous atypia after estrogen administration, with only one showing evidence of HPV in the vagina.[128]

In summary, squamous atypia in the postmenopausal period is associated with significant cervical pathology in a far smaller proportion of cases than in a younger age group. This seems to hold true even in cases with repeated atypias, and the 'estrogen test', while helpful in reversing atrophy atypia for a significant number of women, still resulted in repeat squamous atypia without biopsy-proven disease in 14%.

On a practical level, postmenopausal women with squamous atypia in a setting of atrophy should be offered an estrogen test and repeat smear to check for reversal of the atypia with epithelial maturation. Colposcopy and/or biopsy should be performed in those cases where atypias persist, keeping in mind that some women will continue with persistent squamous atypia, despite estrogen treatment.

Cohesive sheets or clumps of immature cells, so-called 'hyperchromatic clotted groups' (HCGs) may describe a variety of conditions, ranging from benign endocervical, endometrial or lower uterine segment epithelial cells to HSIL, ACIS and invasive carcinomas. They are discussed below and in the chapter on endocervical glandular neoplasia (Ch. 14).[129]

Rare atypical cells falling into the ASCUS category include any cell in which the degree of cytologic atypia exceeds that which can be explained by reactive cellular changes. If the cells are sufficiently rare to exclude categorization, the diagnosis should be left unqualified. If the cells are rare but fall into one of the above categories, a specific diagnosis (such as atypical immature squamous metaplasia) with the qualification of rare cells is appropriate. One study found that the number of atypical cells in the smear was proportional to the rate at which SIL was confirmed on biopsy. However, the role this information should play in management is unclear, excepting cases where degenerative changes are present.

Degenerated atypical cells may produce problems in interpretation, primarily because the degree of nuclear irregularity or hyperchromasia may be marked (Fig. 13.5). In cases where degenerative changes are clearly present, in particular when they occur in small numbers of cells, follow-up smears should be considered. If degeneration appears to be a secondary phenomenon and the numbers of cells in question are plentiful, colposcopy should be performed.

There are relatively few reports which have addressed the risk of subsequent SIL as a function of the type of atypia present. However, certain conclusions can be drawn: (a) virtually all atypias, irrespective of type, confer some risk of SIL; (b) the risk increases with persistent atypia; (c) the risk of high-grade SIL is highest with atypical immature squamous metaplasia; (d) the risk is lowest in atypias associated with atrophy or in women over 35; (e) there is some risk of subsequent SIL in women whose initial follow-up smears are negative; and (f) the role of antibiotic therapy in 'treating' atypical smears remains to be defined.

MANAGEMENT OF ASCUS

Reporting

The 2001 Bethesda reporting recommendations distinguish only 'ASC favor HSIL' and relegate the other three subsets to 'ASCUS' without further classification. The rationale for this approach is the following: (1) Favor reactive should in general not be used as it may be an 'over-call', (2) the HSIL outcomes for NOS and favor LSIL are equivalent (around 15%) and (3) 'favor HSIL' has a significantly higher risk of an HSIL outcome and should be distinguished separately. This strategy has strengths and weaknesses. A strength is that in most studies 'favor-reactive' confers a very low risk of HSIL. Two weaknesses are the following. First, despite its generally low risk of HSIL outcome, ASCUS favor reactive may connote different morphologic changes to different observers. In our experience, 'favor reactive' was no more likely to be reclassified as normal (by other individuals) than to be reclassified as NOS or some other form of ASCUS.[130] Renshaw et al. showed that exclusion of favor reactive would reduce the ASCUS/SIL ratio but also reduced the sensitivity of the diagnosis.[131] Secondly, a recent study showed that efforts to eliminate ASCUS and decisively segregate significant from insignificant cytologic changes nevertheless failed to remove a significant minority of HSIL outcomes from the 'negative' group.[132]

The principal rationale for combining subsets of ASCUS lies in the simplicity of managing all of these subsets equally with reflex HPV testing. While ASCUS favor reactive may be followed by an HSIL outcome in just 4% of instances, an HPV-negative ASCUS of any type carries an HSIL outcome risk of approximately 1%. Thus, HPV testing offers not only an objective measure of risk but also permits distinction of a category with very low risk that can be followed at longer Papanicolaou smear intervals. The balance struck between the sub-classification of ASCUS versus HPV testing with or without ASCUS sub-classification is one that is currently under study.

Clinical management (Fig. 13.6)

Three approaches are currently recommended for management of ASCUS, comprising Papanicolaou smear follow-up, immediate colposcopy and concurrent (reflex) or subsequent HPV testing. These have been detailed in a summary of the ASCCP Consensus Conference held in Bethesda, Maryland in September 2001.[133] In short, Papanicolaou smear follow-up is considered effective but less sensitive and requires continued follow-up. Colposcopic examination and reflex HPV testing are equivalent in sensitivity.[134] A second approach to HPV testing, including the storing of HPV swabs by the clinical practitioner for future testing if an ASCUS is diagnosed, is the more economical, as it can be dovetailed with conventional Papanicolaou smear.[133] It does require, however, a measure of diligence on the part of the practitioner.

Certain questions will likely remain regarding the management of women with HPV testing, particularly if the technology is used 'off label'. For example, how does the practitioner respond to cytologic diagnoses of HSIL or LSIL accompanied by negative HPV tests? The answer is to avoid using the test in these settings where there are no recommendations for management. How is a smear diagnosis of ASCUS favor HSIL managed if the HPV test is negative? The prudent

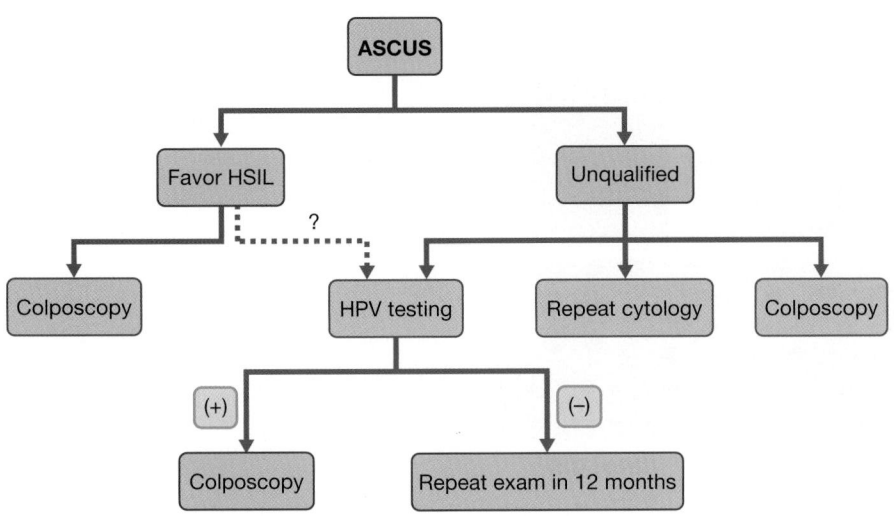

Fig. 13.6 Scheme for clinical management of ASCUS.

approach is to review the smear and manage the patient according to the degree of concern generated by the cytology review. Given the high sensitivity of HPV testing, it is likely that in many instances the cytologic interpretation will be revised.

As discussed previously, the disparity between the number of women scoring positive for HPV and the number manifesting with a significant precursor mandates careful counseling of patients who have access to testing information.

Diagnosis and management of cervical intraepithelial neoplasia

PHENOTYPIC CHANGES ASSOCIATED WITH HPV INFECTION

As will be discussed both here and later in the chapter, the concept of cervical intraepithelial neoplasia has two overlapping components. The first is a traditional view of neoplastic progression in differentiating squamous epithelium, which is depicted schematically as an orderly continuum from normal to carcinoma *in situ* (Fig. 13.7). The second is a view that reflects the influence

of the transformation zone on this continuum. The latter will be discussed later in the chapter (see Fig. 13.13b) and is important for the purpose of navigating the complex morphologies encountered in diagnostic practice. Not all of these morphologic nuances can be translated into cytology, and the cytologic interpretations are typically comparable with the more traditional grading scheme, which will suffice for most preinvasive squamous lesions. This range of morphologic responses following infection by papillomaviruses can be subdivided into two general scenarios shown in the schematic in Figure 13.7. This is analogous to that seen in the vulva in response to prototypic low (HPV 6 or 11) and high (HPV 16) papillomavirus infections. These changes can be correlated with those in the cytologic smear, and a brief review of them is germane to the understanding of the cytologic classification.

1   In the first, basal and parabasal cell morphology is mildly altered, and atypia is most conspicuous in the maturing cell population, giving rise to viral cytopathic effect (koilocytotic atypia), as shown on the left side of Figure 13.7. This may be seen with both high- and low-risk HPVs but is usually more conspicuous in the latter.[135,136] It reflects a close relationship between the onset of vegetative papillomaviral DNA replication and keratinocyte differentiation.

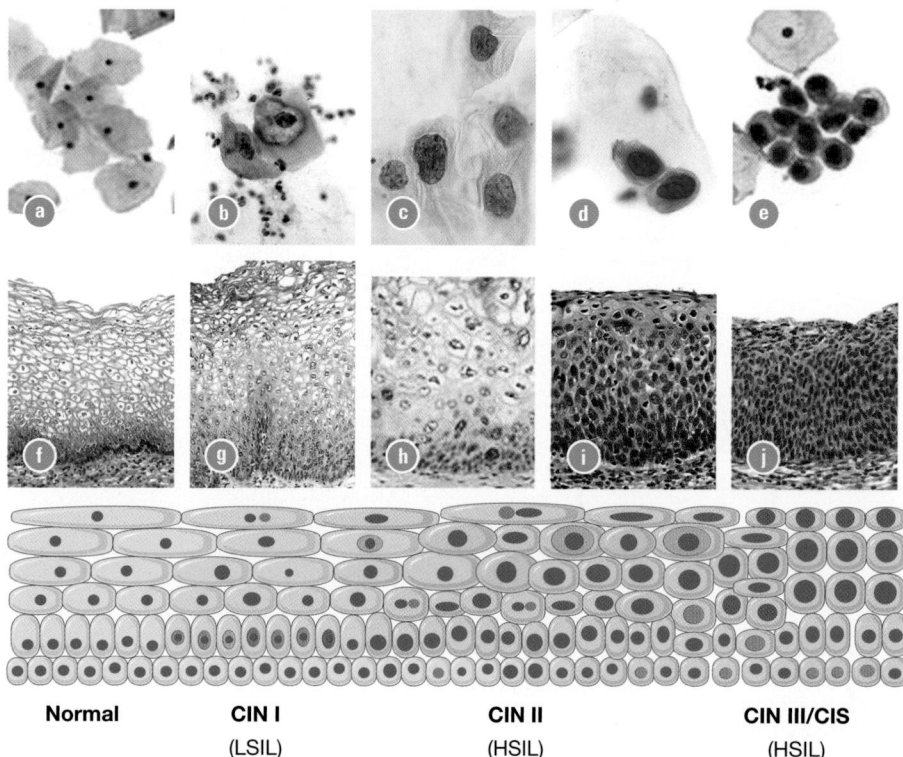

Fig. 13.7 A schematic of cervical intraepithelial neoplasia (lower) defines the cytopathologic (a–e) and histopathologic (f–j) transitions from normal to LSIL (CIN I) to HSIL (CIN II/III). Note that this composite does not take into account nuances of transformation zone differentiation that may further influence morphology (see Fig. 13.13b).

| Normal | CIN I (LSIL) | CIN II (HSIL) | CIN III/CIS (HSIL) |

2 In the second scenario, the immature cells also exhibit nuclear alterations, with loss of cell polarity, increased mitotic index, alterations in nuclear size, staining, chromasia and contour, as shown in the middle of the schematic and superimposed microphotographs in Figure 13.7. These changes presumably reflect important changes in genetic make-up and growth control mediated by the influence of viral oncogenes.[137,138] The atypia is conspicuous in both the immature and mature cells (i.e. full-thickness atypia) and exceeds that seen in prototypic low-risk HPV infections.[139,140] The distinction of CIN II from CIN III is based on the degree of epithelial cell maturation, and to some extent the severity of atypia and is somewhat subjective. Continuity between low- and high-grade epithelial changes often occurs, usually signifying morphologic progression of a single infection and less commonly, coexisting infections by two or more HPV types.[141,142] High-grade lesions may also develop spontaneously with no preceding LSIL. The reproducibility of cytologic and histologic grading systems employing the above strategies will vary. In general, reproducibility of diagnostically difficult (borderline) lesions is poor (as expected, magnitude of uncertainty varies between evaluations separated by time), and distinction of CIN II from CIN III is achieved with less consistency than distinction of CIN I from CIN II, which are based on fundamental albeit subjective differences in the magnitude of atypia in the lower epithelial layers. In the Papanicolaou smear, reproducibility also varies and is generally fair to good.

CYTOLOGIC CRITERIA FOR SQUAMOUS INTRAEPITHELIAL LESIONS

As implied from the above description, cellular changes closely resembling those expected from an epithelium with HPV viral cytopathic effect alone will be classified as LSIL. In contrast, those in which the less mature (including replication competent cells) are altered will be interpreted as HSIL. The following is a guideline for translating this concept into cytologic criteria (see Figs 13.8–13.10).

Low-grade squamous intraepithelial lesions

On cytologic smears, the changes associated with LSIL can be divided into four types:

1 Intermediate or superficial cells with nuclear enlargement (usually three-fold) and hyperchromasia which sharply distinguishes these cells from the adjacent normal cells (Fig. 13.8a,b). As mentioned above under histology, the nuclei exhibit relatively smooth perimeters and small irregularities in nuclear shape and contour. Hyperchromasia is present and

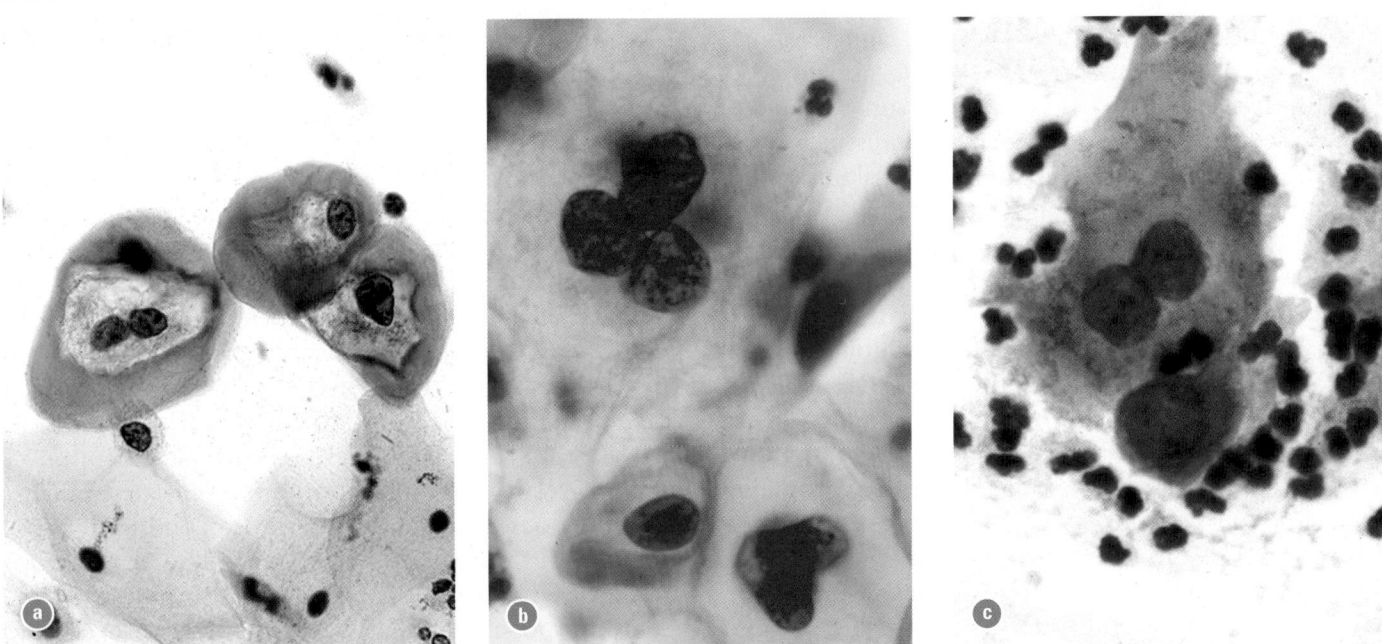

Fig. 13.8 Cytology of low-grade squamous intraepithelial lesions, including koilocytes (a), and superficial cell karyomegaly and binucleation (b,c). The principal features are variation (and increase) in nuclear size and chromatin density.

may take the form of a finely granular chromatin or uniformly increased nuclear density with opaque or smudged appearance. Nucleoli are inconspicuous in both low- and high-grade SILs, excepting those associated with inflammatory change.

2 The classic koilocyte. These cells should have enlarged (2–3×) nuclei and they are usually hyperchromatic (Fig. 13.8a). One defining feature is a sharply etched perinuclear halo with an irregular perimeter of dense cytoplasm.[143,144] Another feature supporting the diagnosis of LSIL is nuclear enlargement and hyperchromasia. Perinuclear halos without any nuclear enlargement, binucleation, or hyperchromasia are not sufficient for a diagnosis of a squamous intraepithelial lesion, inasmuch as perinuclear halos alone have not been shown to correlate independently with the presence of HPV.[145] Binucleation is common in LSIL and is found in intermediate or superficial cells. Just as with the perinuclear halo, binucleation is more specific for the diagnosis of LSIL if it is accompanied by some of the other features such as nuclear enlargement or hyperchromasia.

3 The most subtle manifestation of LSIL is a change confined predominantly in the parabasal-type cells. The degree of parabasal cell atypia may vary and in smears containing LSIL conspicuous atypia is not present. In immature condylomas (see below) cells with a parabasal/intermediate appearance are most prominent and show slight nuclear enlargement, slightly more granular chromatin and binucleation. We have termed a subset of such cells 'abortive koilocytes' inasmuch as they exhibit some features of these cells (nuclear enlargement, indistinct perinuclear halos) but lack the more striking nuclear hyperchromasia and perinuclear clearing.[146]

High-grade squamous intraepithelial lesions

On Papanicolaou smears, the cells of HSIL (Fig. 13.9) are characteristically less mature, and exhibit a higher nuclear/cytoplasmic ratio than those of LSIL. Nuclear enlargement is generally in the same range as in LSILs, but because nuclear/cytoplasmic ratio is increased, the cells appear smaller. Hyperchromasia, coarse chromatin and membrane contour irregularity are all more severe than in LSIL. Architecturally, the cells of HSILs are arranged in two main patterns: as cohesive groups of cells with indistinct cell borders (syncytial-like groupings) or as individual cells arranged in rows or streams. Although usually a lesion of small, immature squamous cells, mature keratinizing cells with marked nuclear atypia are classified as HSIL (Fig. 13.9c,d).

The reader can surmise from the above that it takes more than just an assessment of cell maturity to distinguish low- from high-grade precursors. The nuclear abnormalities associated with high-grade precursors can be appreciated in not only the basal/parabasal cells but also in intermediate and superficial-type cells.[147]

It should be emphasized that a portion of high-grade SILs will be associated with low-grade morphology. As many as three-quarters of SIL lesions of all grades have been reported to contain coexisting koilocytotic.[148] From 10% to 20% of LSILs on Papanicolaou smear are confirmed as HSIL on biopsy.[149,150] Moreover, high-risk HPV types are also associated with low-grade SIL.[136] However, the association between LSIL and HSIL varies depending upon the criteria used to define LSIL. Moreover, at least one-half of high-grade SILs contain some areas of koilocytotic atypia.[151] However, in approximately three-quarters of these cases, the koilocytotic atypia is closely associated with features of HSIL, including nuclear atypia in all epithelial layers. Therefore, the proportion of HSIL cases in which a classic condyloma (LSIL) merges with an HSIL lesion is relatively small. We found that about 14% of HSILs coexist with LSIL as strictly defined. For HSIL lesions associated with HPV 16, the proportion with LSIL in continuity is less than 10%.[135] Higher frequencies of associated LSIL have been reported previously in association with HPV 16, but the areas of LSIL were very focal.[135] In contrast, for HSIL associated with HPV 31, approximately two-thirds contained areas of LSIL, suggesting that for some high-risk HPV infections, an interval of LSIL may be more common. This is in keeping with the concept that HPV 31 is an 'intermediate risk' HPV type. These observations, combined with the relatively low association between koilocytosis on a prior smear and subsequent invasive carcinoma, indicate that lesions with abundant koilocytosis (histologically or cytologically) may belong to a lower risk category. Although this neither justifies conservative therapy of koilocytotic HSILs, nor excludes condyloma predating HSIL, it indicates that the progression of classic LSIL to HSIL to cancer is an uncommon scenario relative to more poorly-differentiated HSILs. When it does occur, it may be more commonly associated with viruses other than HPV 16. At the practical level, the diagnostic pathologist must always consider the possibility that a low-grade SIL, even one which is identical to condyloma, may comprise a portion of a larger lesion which contains high-grade mor-

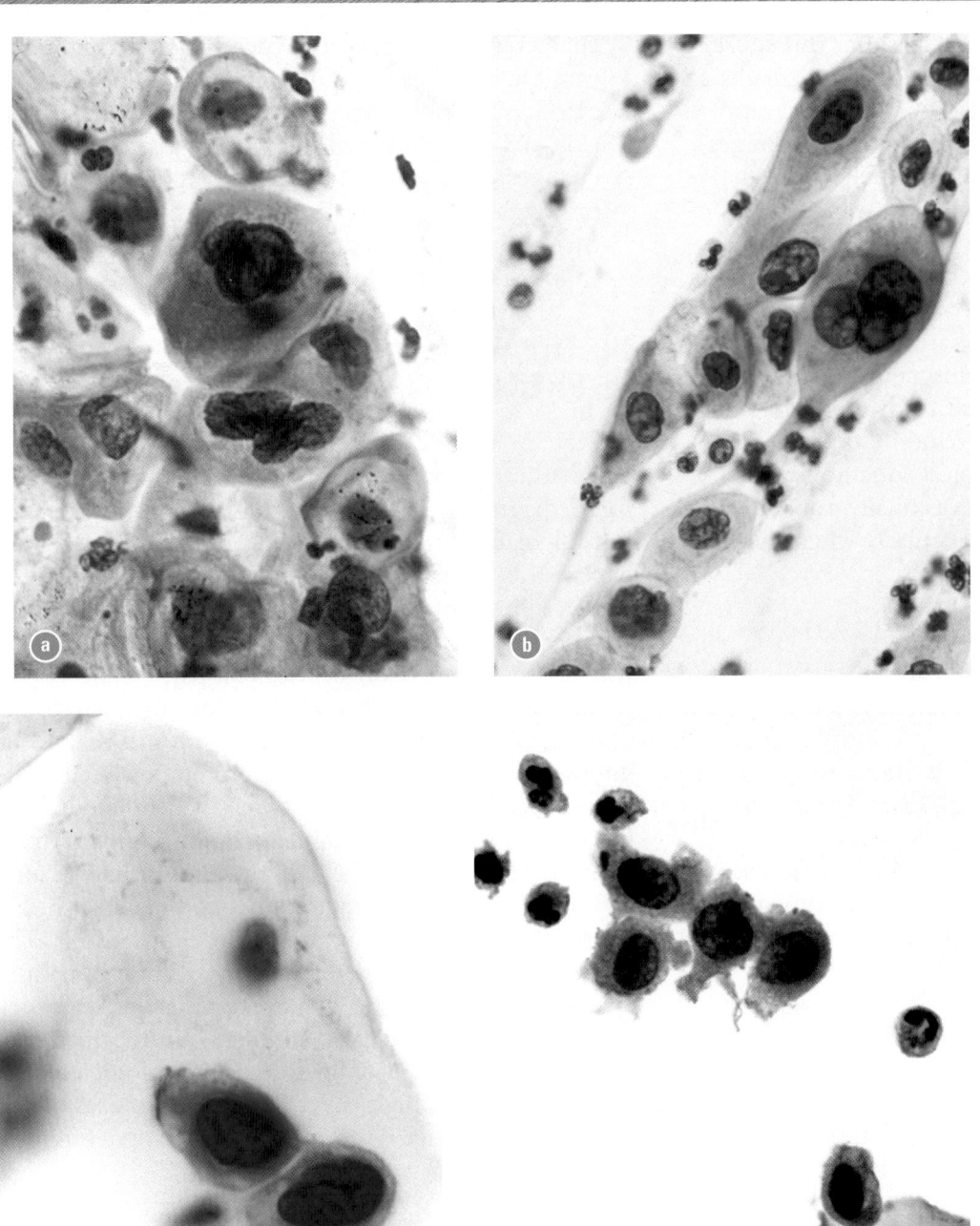

Fig. 13.9 Cytology of high-grade squamous intraepithelial lesions, including abnormal cells with moderate cytoplasm anisokaryosis and coarse-appearing chromatin (a,b); similar nuclear features and a higher nuclear/cytoplasmic ratio (c,d).

phology. In most cases this high-grade morphology will consist of CIN II.[141] Occasionally, a classic LSIL will merge with a CIN III. These facts must be appreciated also when interpreting cytology.

In addition to the above, two other presentations of HSIL may cause diagnostic confusion:

1 HSIL composed of small metaplastic-type cells: some HSILs are composed of exfoliate small metaplastic-type cells with mild to moderate atypia. Because of the relatively mild atypia, the diagnosis of such lesions is poorly reproducible, and they are often diagnosed as atypical squamous metaplasia. Some authors, in fact, prefer to designate these as atypical squamous metaplasia with the proviso that a high-grade SIL cannot be ruled out and a recommendation for a colposcopic examination.[117]

The important features distinguishing this subset of HSIL from benign metaplasia are the small size of the cells, increased nuclear/cytoplasmic ratio and irregularly shaped nuclei. The latter changes may be subtle. Because the extremely course chromatin and bizarre shapes typifying conventional HSIL are not present, a portion of these cases will be diagnosed as atypical squamous metaplasia, or overlooked completely (Fig. 13c,d).

2 Undifferentiated SIL: these are typified by cells arranged primarily in pseudosyncytial groups. Such lesions may be difficult to distinguish cytologically from adenocarcinoma *in situ*, reactive glandular cells atypical squamous metaplasia, atrophy and, occasionally, tubal-endometrial metaplasia, particularly when the latter contains distortion artifact.

Pitfalls in interpretation of LSIL and HSIL

The following are the most common pitfalls in the diagnosis of either LSIL or HSIL on cytologic preparations. The reader should bear in mind that many of the 'pitfalls' of cytologic interpretation are also under the category of non-diagnostic squamous atypias.

1 Mimics of LSIL include the following:
(a) *Trichomonas* infections, with mild perinuclear halos, (b) postmenopausal nuclear karyomegaly (Fig. 13.10a) and (c) non-specific reactive changes leading to mild superficial nuclear atypia (Fig. 13.10d).

2 Mimics of HSIL include (a) atrophic changes, which include a high nuclear/cytoplasmic ratio but greater regularity in nuclear contour, absence of coarse chromatin (Fig. 13.10b,c); (b) sampling of lower uterine segment, in which syncytial groups of LUS may be confused with HSIL and (c) adenocarcinoma *in situ*, which may also be difficult to separate from HSIL (see Ch. 14).
(d) Occasionally immature condylomas may be difficult to distinguish from HSIL on cytology; however, this dilemma is uncommon.

3 Is it LSIL or HSIL? Pitfalls in the diagnosis include keratinizing lesions, including dyskeratosis or atypical parakeratosis (Fig. 13.11a-c). Mild surface binucleation in the absence of hyperchromasia correlates poorly with LSIL (Fig. 13.11a). In general, keratinizing cells consisting of small round to oval hyperchromatic nuclei with uniform chromatin distribution and binucleation and plaque-like clusters correlate with LSIL. Greater disturbances in cellular differentiation,

characterized by densely hyperchromatic nuclei, variable keratinization and increased nuclear/cytoplasmic ratio, are characteristic of HSIL (Fig. 13.11d–f). When the pathologist encounters changes of this magnitude, the diagnosis of HSIL or 'keratinized SIL' is justified, with the disclaimer that a more advanced lesion (such as carcinoma) cannot be excluded.

HISTOPATHOLOGIC DIAGNOSIS OF PREINVASIVE DISEASE

Expectations from the clinical setting

When the clinician sends a biopsy to the pathologist for a diagnosis, it is usually based on an abnormal Papanicolaou smear. Although the practitioner may expect the biopsy to explain the abnormality on the smear, approximately 70%, 45% and 20% of cytologic interpretations of ASCUS, LSIL and HSIL, respectively, will not be verified on cervical biopsy.[147] The colposcopist should expect this. Explanations for such discrepancies include clinical sampling error and diagnostic imprecision, particularly in the interpretation of ASCUS.

In many cases, the colposcopist will not identify a lesion on colposcopic examination and will not perform a biopsy (Fig. 13.12a–d). The pathologist may receive an endocervical curettage only, and again, should approach this specimen with realistic expectations. The pathologist must avoid over-calling minor histologic changes in an effort to achieve consistency between the cytologic and histologic findings. In turn, the colposcopist should be wary of cytologic/histologic correlation rates that are high (over 80%) or diagnoses of SIL that follow negative or equivocal colposcopic findings.

Practical considerations before examining the biopsy

Examination of the cervical specimen requires an understanding of five components germane to interpreting cervical squamous neoplasia:

1 Understanding the transformation zone and the plethora of benign alterations in epithelial differentiation that characterize this region.

2 Excluding non-neoplastic infections, such as herpes, *Chlamydia*, etc.

3 Applying the classic criteria for differentiating grades of CIN as classically described.

4 Understanding the influence of transformation zone epithelial subsets on the morphology of type-specific infections in the transformation zone, producing patterns that do not conform to classic descriptions and less easily classified lesion patterns.

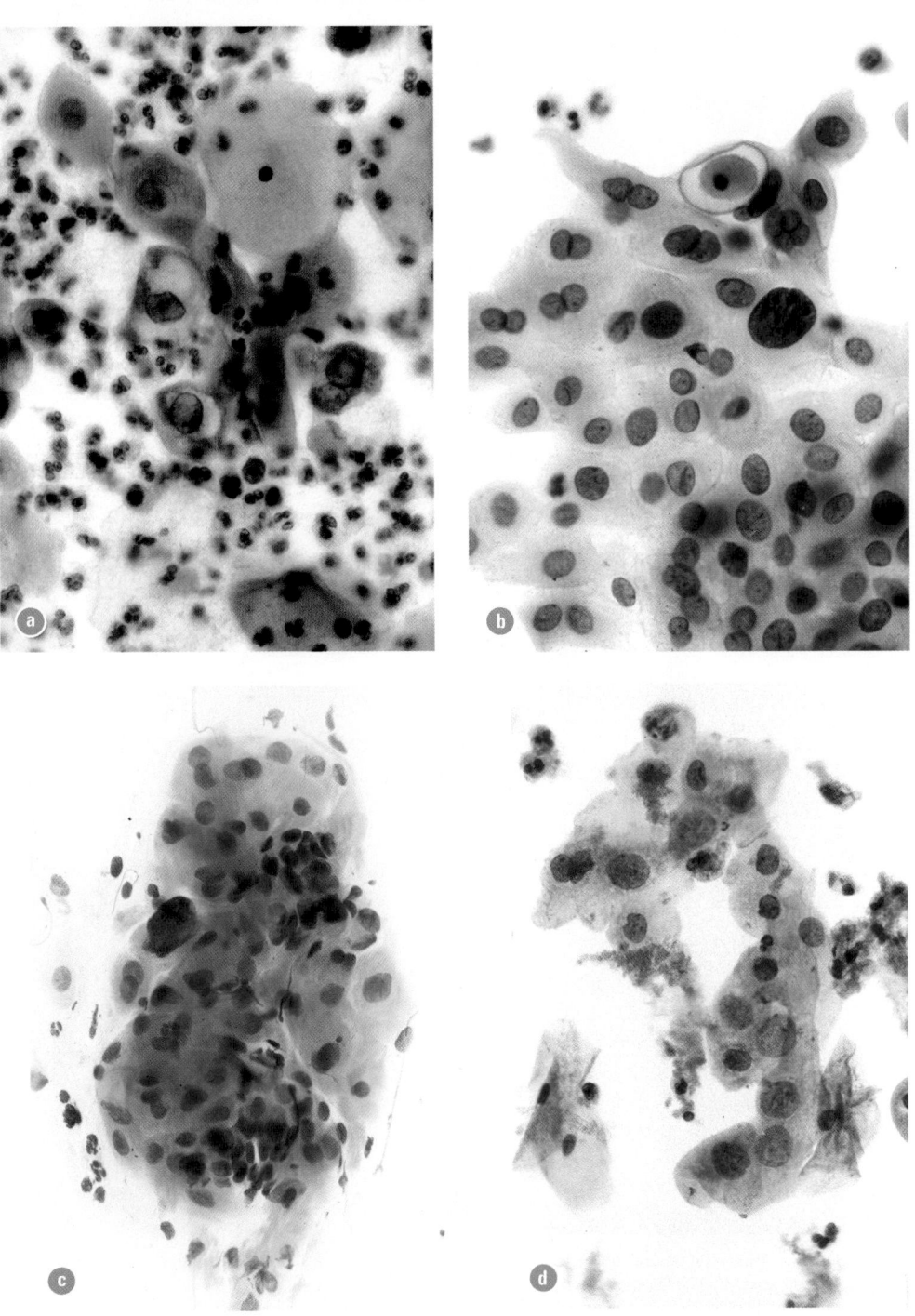

Fig. 13.10 Cytologic mimics of LSIL include menopausal karyomegaly with cytoplasmic halos (a). Mimics of HSIL include atrophic changes (b,c), and rarely immature condyloma (d).

5 Having a working knowledge of the differential diagnosis of classic and variant forms of SIL.

The transformation zone

The cervical transformation zone (Fig. 13.13a,b) is initially formed by immature epithelial cells, located just distal to the squamo-columnar junction at the interface of the vaginal portio and endocervix. During fetal life, immature basal cells emerge in the uterus to form the squamo-columnar junction as well as basal and sub-columnar cells that will comprise the 'multi-potential' component of the transformation zone. This population includes cells destined for both squamous and columnar cell differentiation (metaplasias) that develop in response to inflammatory stimuli and alterations in pH that occur following the onset of menarche.[152,153] They may be identified by basal/reserve cells markers. A generic biomarker that identifies all of

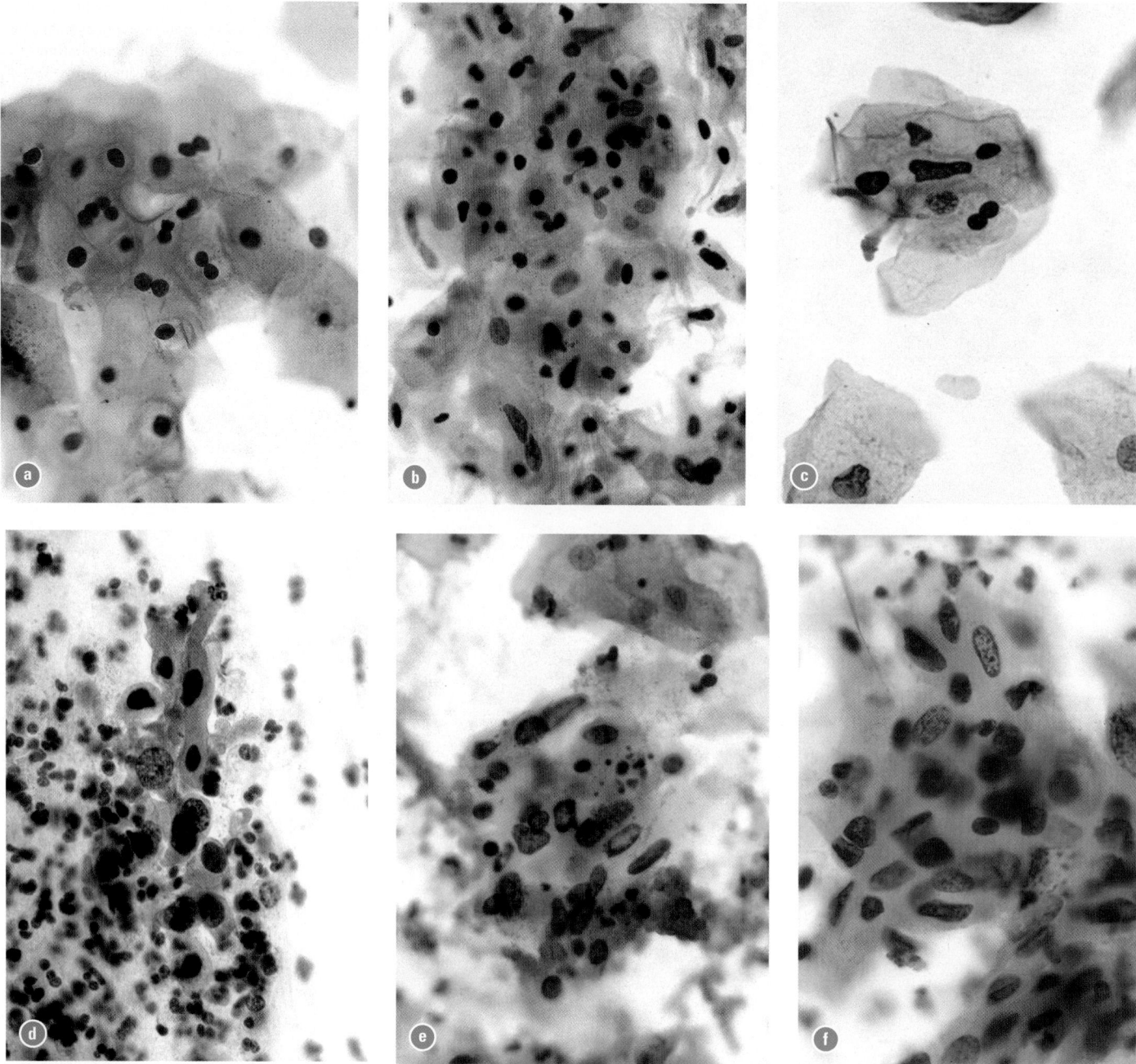

Fig. 13.11 Abnormal parakeratosis and abnormal keratinizing cells. Binucleation and more subtle differences in nuclear size and staining intensity in mature cells are generally more common in LSIL (a,b). More pronounced nuclear disturbances with coarse chromatin raise the possibility of HSIL (c,d) and striking abnormalities in nuclear contour and chromasia coupled with dense cytoplasmic keratinization characterize HSIL, and may be associated with invasive carcinoma (e,f).

these cells – p63– has been identified in basal cells of skin appendages, myoepithelial cells in the breast and salivary gland, and sub-columnar cells in the prostate. Recent studies with this and other markers have discriminated subsets of reserve/basal cells of the cervix that may be subdivided into uncommitted sub-columnar monolayers (p63 positive, CK-14 negative), populations undergoing squamous (p63 positive/CK-14

positive) and columnar cell (p63 positive/CK-14 negative) differentiation. Whether the range of lesion phenotypes seen in the cervix reflects infection of these specific cell types or other factors peculiar to the HPV type involved is unclear. However, the emergence of both glandular and squamous lesions in this region argues for a relationship between this phenotypic plasticity and the multi-potentiality of these cells in the

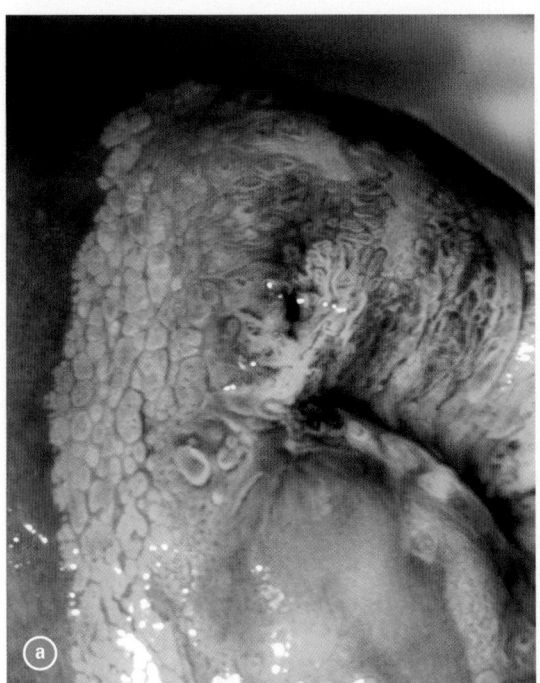

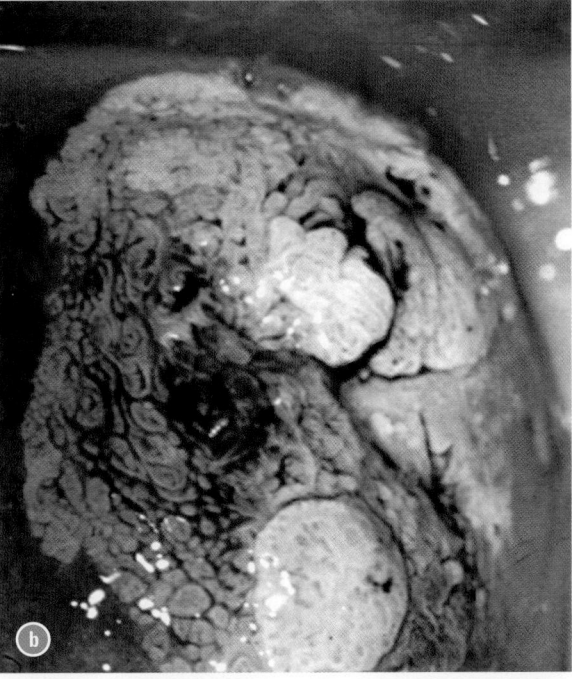

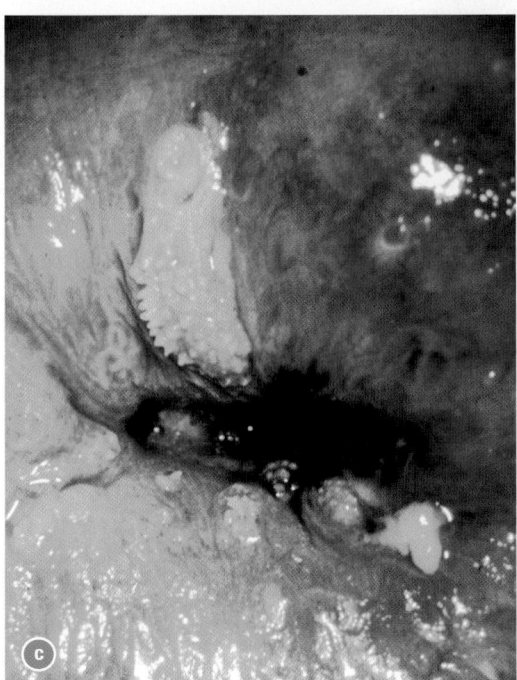

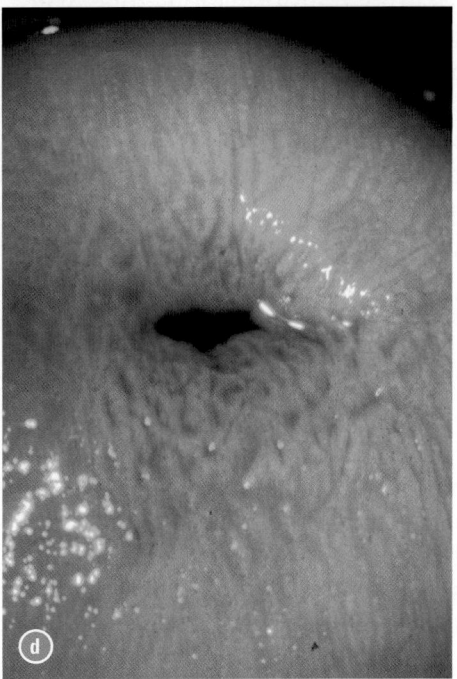

Fig. 13.12 Colposcopy photographs of prominent transformation zone in a diethylstilbestrol-exposed patient (a); low-grade squamous intraepithelial lesions (b,c). Following cryotherapy, the transformation zone is ablated and re-epithelialized with mature squamous mucosa (d). (Photographs courtesy of Richard U. Levine and Alex Ferenczy.)

cervical transformation zone. Basal and columnar cells appear most susceptible to infection, based on the requirement that these cells be exposed to the virus for infection to take place. Presumably these cells contain receptors targeted by the papillomavirus.[138] The range of underlying morphologies on which HPV infection may be superimposed – and the resulting lesions seen – is illustrated in Figure 13.13b.

Understanding the normal transformation zone is important for several reasons, including (1) the range of normal epithelial change is broad and the diagnostician must be familiar with these patterns to avoid the over-diagnosis of squamous and glandular cell neoplasia; (2) in recognizing these components of normal transformation zone activity the diagnostician can subdivide the landscape into individual components and conduct a more orderly and systematic review of the cervix mucosa. Because some of these phenotypes are reflected in the neoplastic spectrum, a systematic approach of examination, recognition and exclusion is germane to diagnostic consistency and precision. Examples of such phenotypes are illustrated at the bottom of Figure 13.13b. (The reader can contrast the complexity of these patterns with the more traditional view of CIN illustrated in Figure 13.7.)

Categories of squamous differentiation include, in order of maturity, reserve cell expansion, early squamous differentiation, squamous maturation and epidermidalization. This process begins in the recesses of the endocervical papillae, expanding to efface and then eventually obliterate the papillae and form a smooth mucosal surface. Columnar differentiation is less conspicuous, consisting of surface proliferations composed of stratified columnar epithelial cells, occasionally showing columnar cell differentiation with mature columnar cells on the surface.

In many instances, the transformation zone will exhibit populations undergoing both squamous and columnar cell differentiation, a phenomenon appreciated in cell cultures of basal transformation zone. Microglandular hyperplasia is an example of a reserve cell proliferation that evolves temporally, beginning as a principally glandular phenotype with small glands, then transforming into a squamous phenotype as the reserve cells emerge from the columnar cell population, expand and undergo squamous differentiation.

Excluding infections other than HPV

Ostensibly, cervical sampling permits the identification and qualification of HPV-related cervical neoplasia. However, the issue of infection by other microbial agents must be considered when evaluating any cervix. Clinically significant infections, which can be identified or suspected by histologic examination of the cervix, include herpes simplex viruses (HSV) (Fig. 13.14a,b), cytomegalovirus (Fig. 13.14c), *Chlamydia trachomatis* (Fig. 13.14d–h) and, rarely, adenovirus.[122,154,155] HSV should be suspected and excluded in any ulcer, particularly if it is accompanied by epithelial cell necrosis and acute inflammatory exudate. The diagnostic cells contain one or multiple nuclei with either discrete inclusions or smudged (ground glass) chromatin and are typically at the periphery of the ulcer, in the spongiotic epithelium or as single desegregated cells. Special stains may be helpful if the diagnosis is uncertain on morphologic grounds alone. *C. trachomatis* infection does not elicit

specific epithelial changes, but is closely associated with severe acute and chronic inflammatory infiltrates, repair and follicular cervicitis.[156,157] The latter is not a very sensitive marker for *Chlamydia* infection, but has been shown to be more commonly associated with positive cultures than not. Thus, if follicular cervicitis is identified in a biopsy, a comment should be made in the report that this finding may be associated with *Chlamydia*, but is not diagnostic. *Chlamydia* is typically identified in small inclusion vacuoles in the endocervical or reparative epithelial cells. It is uncommonly identified in more mature squamous cells.[158] Raising the suspicion of *Chlamydia* based upon cytoplasmic vacuoles alone is not recommended. Morphologic manifestations of other infections such as yeast, *Trichomonas* and *Gardnerella* are not specifically sought for in biopsy specimens and are in the realm of cytologic and clinical evaluation.

Squamous intraepithelial lesions

Introduction

Squamous intraepithelial lesions are defined as squamous alterations in the cervical transformation zone that are induced by human papillomavirus infection. The understanding of this spectrum of changes requires an appreciation of not only the traditional spectrum illustrated in Figure 13.7 and equated with cytology but also the nuances of the transformation zone imposed by the plasticity of the underlying epithelium summarized in Figure 13.13. Differences in the differentiation level or differentiation pathway of the underlying mucosa may influence the morphologic presentation of cervical lesions, leading to additional patterns not accounted for in traditional classifications.

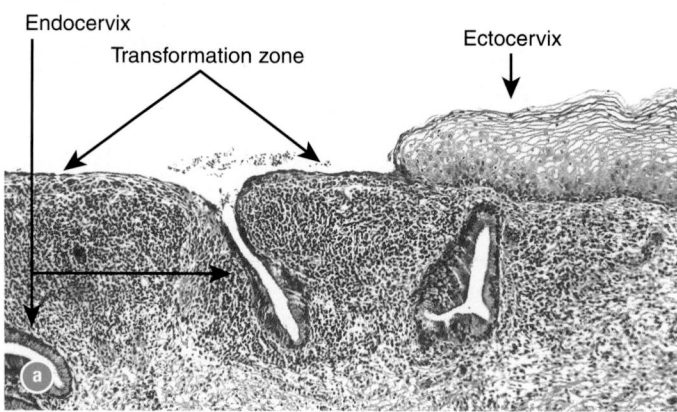

Fig. 13.13 (a) Microphotograph of the transformation zone, depicted here as a thin layer of immature cells of basal type.

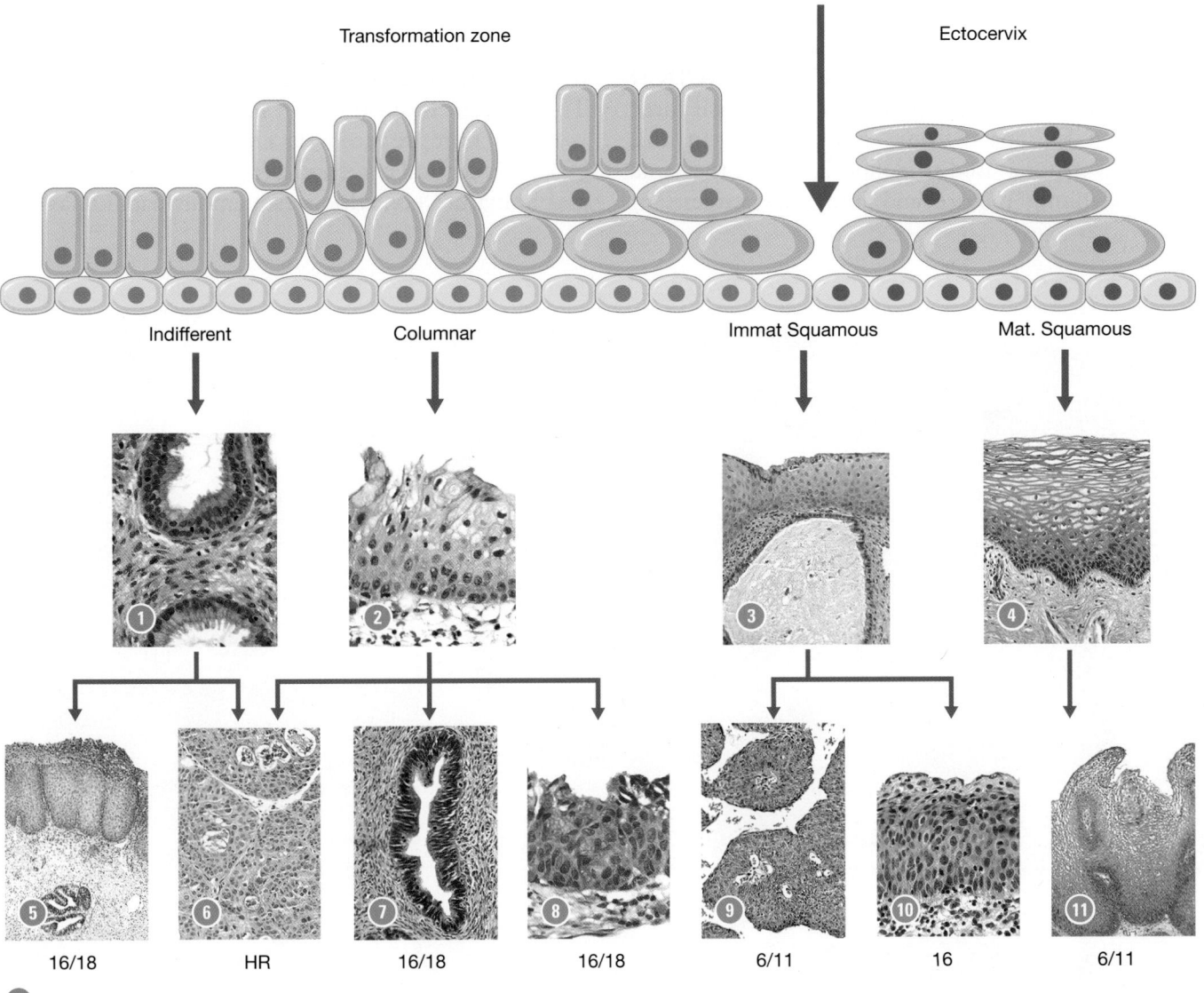

Fig. 13.13 **Cont'd** (b) Schematic of the transformation zone, revealing reserve (indifferent) cells and cells undergoing squamous and columnar differentiation. Middle panel illustrates corresponding photomicrographs of cell types in this region including sub-columnar (1), columnar (2) and squamous (3) metaplasia and portio squamous epithelium (4). Bottom panels depict a similar range of lesions corresponding to these cellular phenotypes, including adenosquamous carcinoma *in situ* (5), SIL in microglandular change (6), ACIS (7), SMILE (8), immature condyloma (9), immature 'metaplastic' HSIL (10) and mature LSIL (condyloma) (11). Below each image are commonly associated HPVs (HR, high-risk).

The classification of squamous intraepithelial lesions has evolved over the past 40 years.[159] Traditional publications either excluded or did not equate flat or exophytic condylomas with cervical dysplasia (CIN), primarily because they did not exhibit the extent of nuclear atypia present in the latter.[159] In the last 25 years, flat and exophytic condylomata of the cervix and CIN have been linked by an association with HPVs, many of them weakly or strongly associated with cancer.[159] The realization that these HPV infections comprise a morphologic continuum has prompted efforts to include them within a single classification system, specifically squamous intraepithelial lesions (SIL).[115] This has been embraced more fully by cyto-pathologists, who do not distinguish the surface keratinocyte atypia of CIN I from the cytopathic effect (koilocytosis) of condyloma and classify both of these changes as low-grade SIL (LSIL) due to the similarity in histologic outcome.[150] Because the diagnosis of CIN historically required full-thickness atypia, the coexistence of both lesions in the histologic CIN classification has required some revision of criteria.[153,159] One response has been a classification in which flat condyloma is equated with CIN I, and lesions traditionally classified as CIN are truncated into two grades (CIN II or III).[159] Others have attempted to distinguish three grades of CIN apart from condyloma.[160] In this chapter, the criteria used to define LSIL are the same as those defining mature and immature variants of

condyloma, both flat (CIN I) and exophytic. Lesions in which the degrees of atypia exceed that characterizing condyloma are classified as CIN II or CIN III. This concept is illustrated in Figure 13.7.

Also of note are recent data demonstrating that both exophytic cervical condyloma (condyloma acuminatum) and immature condyloma (squamous papillomas) are

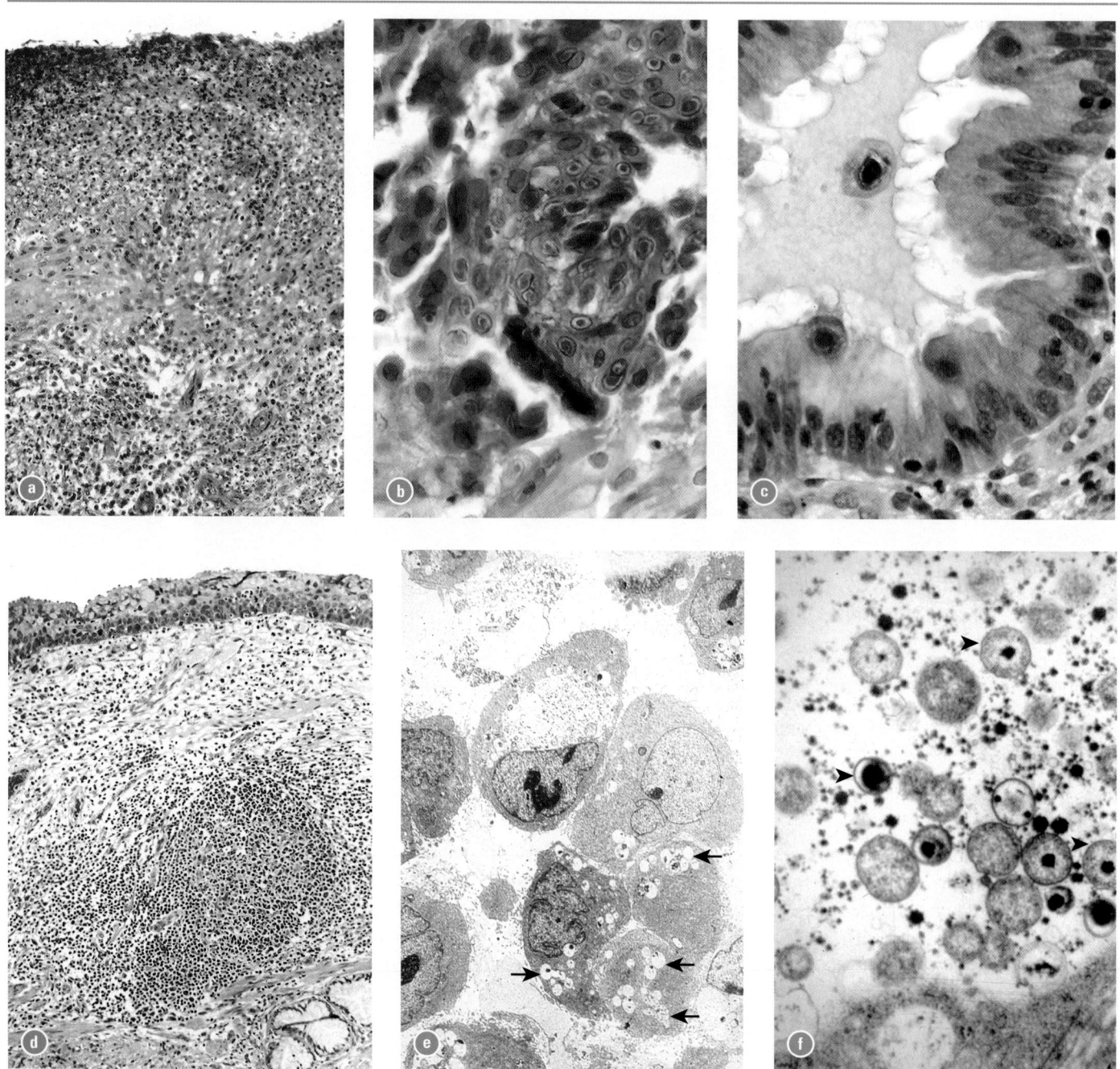

Fig. 13.14 Infections of the cervix that can be identified morphologically include herpes simplex, presenting as an ulcer with epithelial necrosis (a) and intranuclear inclusions (b), cytomegalovirus (c) and *Chlamydia*, which may be associated with follicular cervicitis (d). Inclusions are best seen by electron microscopy (e, arrows) which contain primary and secondary particles (f, small and large arrowheads).

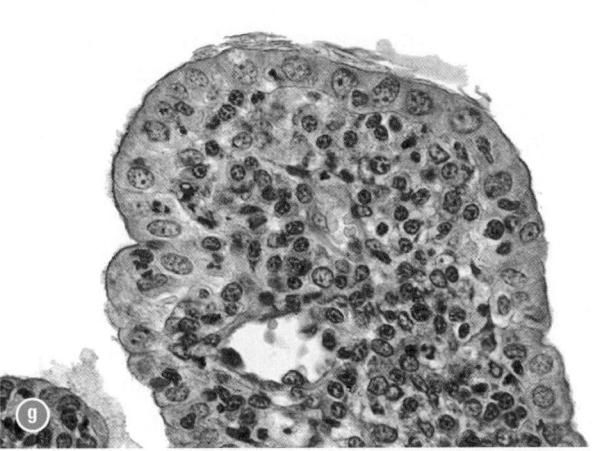
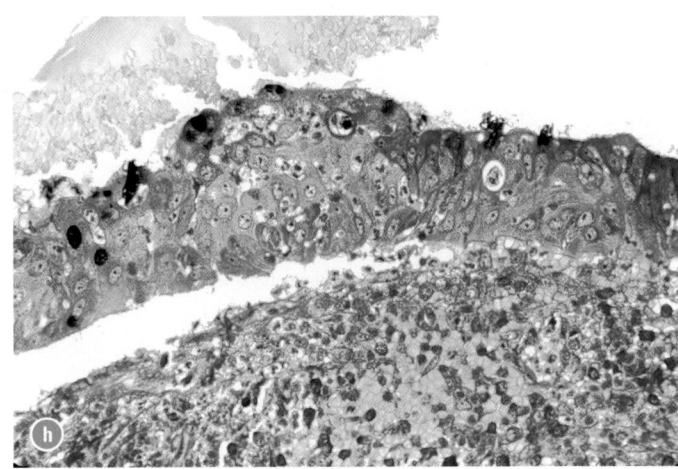

Fig. 13.14 **Cont'd** By light microscopy, inclusions are extremely subtle (g), but may be identified by immunohistochemistry (h).

associated with HPV types 6 and 11 and likely signify different morphologic manifestations of the same infectious process.[161,162] The strong association of these exophytic lesions with defined low-risk HPV types justifies their distinction from CIN I (flat condyloma), but, for purposes of classification, they are included with CIN I within the category of LSIL (Fig. 13.7).

Divisions of SIL and their descriptors are summarized in Table 13.7 and the historical co-evolution of terminology and management is outlined in Figure 13.15. The reader can appreciate that the classification of pre-invasive disease has evolved with the therapeutic options (or opportunities). Colposcopy, cryotherapy and the liberal use of laser or cold knife cone effectively eliminated hysterectomy as a therapeutic option. The recognition that many patients have histologic evidence of mild dysplasia, of which only a minority progress to severe dysplasia, has led to a more conservative management

approach. This is especially important for patients who are interested in further childbearing. This approach is further supported by the persistence of HPV infection following aggressive local or even more radical surgery (hysterectomy). In view of the persistence of the HPV infection, which results in repeated abnormal cervical cytology, the use of cryotherapy has fallen into disfavor. This is due to this modality's thermal damage to the transformation zone, which results in loss of visualization of the squamo-columnar junction. With repeated abnormal cervical cytology and repeat colposcopy, the lack of visualization of the entire squamo-columnar junction by definition results in inadequate colposcopy. Traditionally, in this clinical setting cone biopsy has been suggested; however, with close observation and repeat cervical cytologies, a more conservative approach is possible. This is especially true for patients who have not completed childbearing.

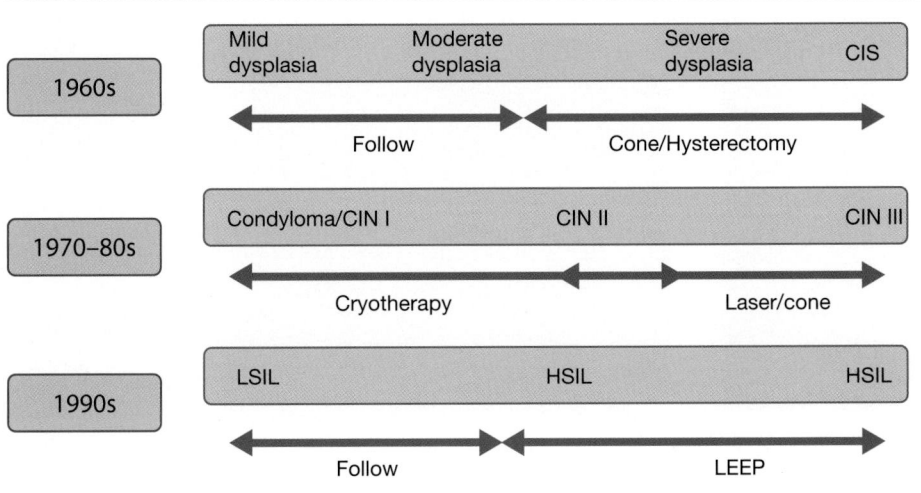

Fig. 13.15 Management of cervical lesions placed in historical perspective. Note that the distinction of moderate from severe dysplasia became less important when the therapeutic options included cryotherapy and laser ablation (middle scheme). In contrast, when the therapeutic options include LEEP vs follow-up, the distinction of CIN 1 (LSIL) from CIN 2 (HSIL) becomes more critical and small differences in interpretation may have significant impact on management.

Table 13.7 Descriptive categories of LSIL and HSIL

Category	Descriptors
LSIL	CIN I
	Flat condyloma
	Mild dysplasia
	Exophytic condyloma
	Immature condyloma (Squamous papilloma[a])
	Transitional papilloma[b]
	Papillary immature metaplasia (synonymous with immature condyloma)
	Flat immature LSIL (rare and controversial)
HSIL	CIN II or moderate dysplasia
	CIN III or severe dysplasia/carcinoma in situ
	Keratinizing SIL
	SIL with immature metaplastic phenotype
	Papillary carcinoma in situ

[a]Presumes papillary lesions with acanthosis (not mucosal polyps).
[b]Data linking transitional papilloma to HPV is non-existent.

The low-risk of high-grade dysplasia or carcinoma occurring following mild dysplasia has led to the binary (Bethesda) system for classification, which separates low- and higher-risk patients, treating only the higher-risk cohort. The development of a binary (Bethesda) system for classification, coupled with a more invasive outpatient management tool (LLETZ), established a sharp cut-off (CIN II or greater) beyond which patients received ablative therapy.

Low-grade squamous intraepithelial lesions

Typically, the diagnosis of a LSIL (condyloma) requires the presence of superficial nuclear atypia. The strong association between atypia and the presence of papillo-mavirus nucleic acids supports establishing a morphologic threshold for the diagnosis of LSIL.[163] However, how this is to be interpreted and separated from non-specific cellular changes can be problematic. A useful approach to the diagnosis of LSIL is to apply several criteria in sequence (Fig. 13.16).

Low-power epithelial organization. In many cases, the diagnosis of a LSIL will be suspected at low magnification (×40–100) based upon the presence of epithelial alterations which are conspicuously different from surrounding epithelium (Fig. 13.16a). These alterations may take the form of changes in epithelial thickness, conspicuous hyperchromasia in the upper cell layers, or more subtle increases in nuclear density, cell arrangement or halo conformation contour in the upper epithelium (Fig. 13.16b).

Major histologic criteria. The next step is to assess the epithelium at higher magnification, and quantify the nuclear atypia. The distinction of a squamous intraepithelial lesion from a non-specific process is based primarily on differences in density, size and staining of the intermediate and superficial cells. Technically, these should be three-fold differences in size with variable staining. Hence the pathologist is searching for large, hyperchromatic nuclei (Fig. 13.16c). Size differences may not be as striking, however, and a combination of nuclear, cytoplasmic and growth pattern alterations may prompt the diagnosis. In some instances the diagnosis may be made on instinct alone, although the reader is warned that instinctive diagnoses (particularly if rendered frequently) may not be reproducible.

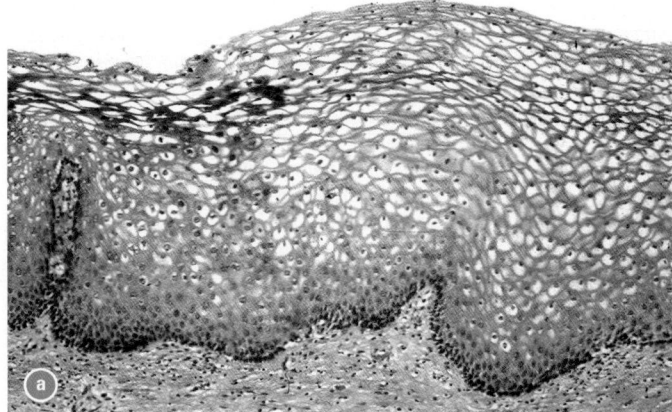
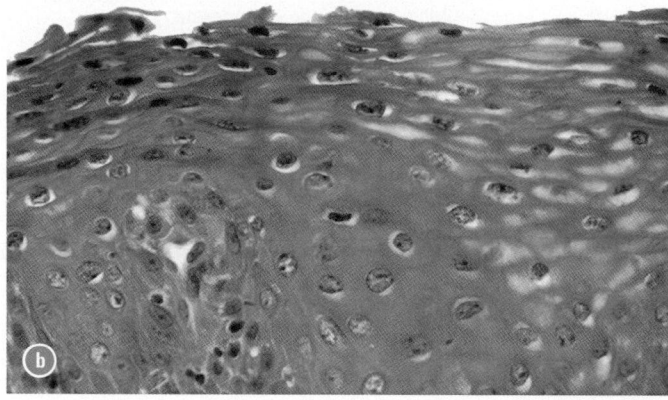

Fig. 13.16 Criteria for the diagnosis of LSIL include discrete alterations in superficial cells with transitions from normal (right) to increased (left) nuclear density (a,b);

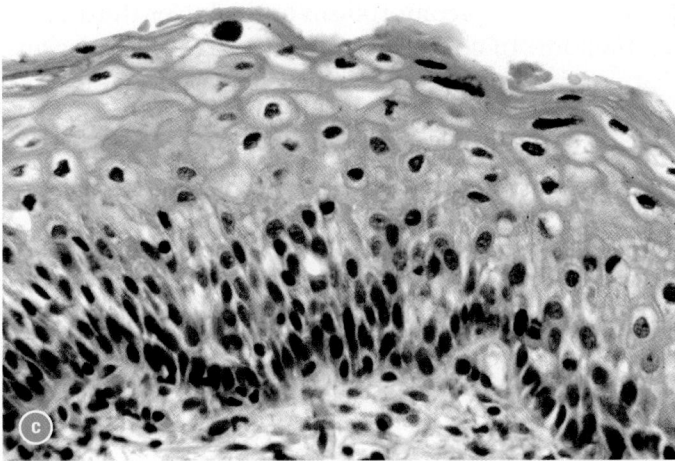

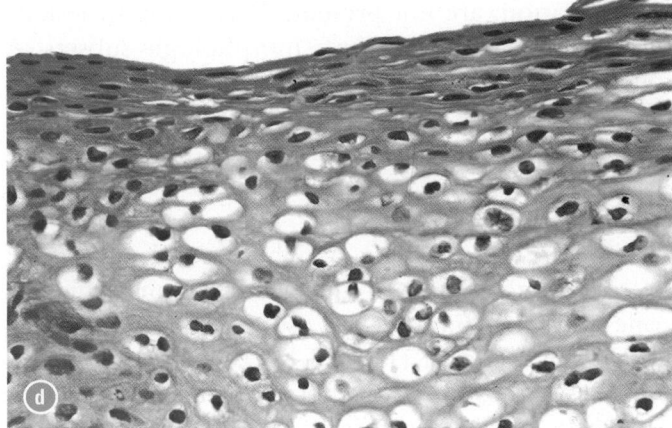

Fig. 13.16 **Cont'd** conspicuous (×3) nuclear enlargement in the superficial cells (c); when present, at least 2 binucleated cells per ×400 field (d). A small atypical parakeratotic plaque with increased nuclear density is seen (e,f).

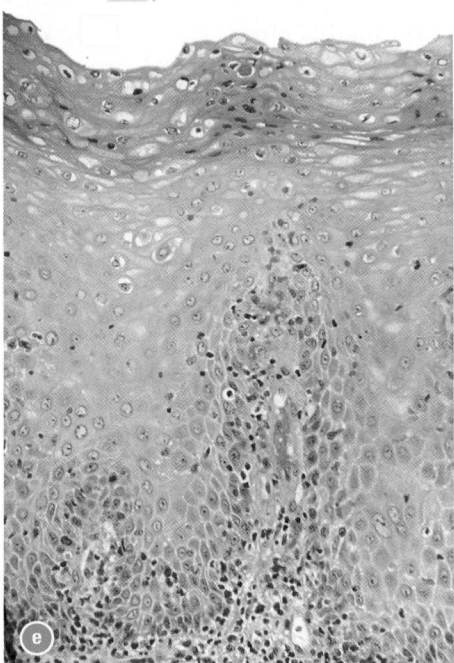

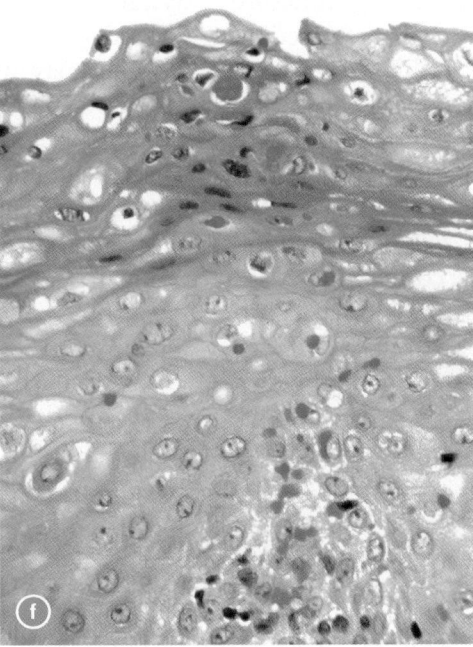

Minor histologic criteria

Once the suspicion of superficial atypia is raised, certain criteria may be useful in confirming the diagnosis. (1) Binucleation is present in approximately 90% of low-grade SIL and condylomata. In our experience, a maximum of two or more binuclear cells in a high power (×400) field strongly supports the diagnosis of an LSIL (Fig. 13.16d), particularly if the binucleated cells are superficial and if the nuclei are enlarged or hyperchromatic. Small, densely hyperkeratotic or parakeratotic binucleated cells also support a diagnosis of a squamous intraepithelial lesion, resembling the atypical parakeratotic cells seen in Papanicolaou smears (see Ch. 4) (Fig. 13.16e,f).[108] It should be emphasized that sporadic binucleation frequently occurs in the setting of reactive epithelial changes (but are usually intermediate or parabasal cells); for this reason, binucleation is used to aid in the diagnosis rather than to make the diagnosis of LSIL *per se*.[145] (2) Irregularly shaped cytoplasmic halos are another useful, if less specific feature. The halos are often punctuated by a rim of dense cytoplasm but with inconspicuous intercellular bridges, forming an interlacing meshwork, or basket weave, in the superficial epithelial layers.[145,164]

As outlined above, the category of low-grade squamous intraepithelial lesions comprises those lesions in which the stigmata of classic precursor lesions, including high mitotic index, parabasal atypia, loss of cell polarity, abnormal mitoses and marked disturbances of maturation, are not present. This group of lesions can be subdivided into three morphologic subsets. A fourth category – lesions falling between low- and high-grade SIL – will also be discussed, inasmuch as they are not uncommonly encountered in practice.

Subtypes of LSIL

Condyloma acuminatum. Exophytic condylomata are relatively uncommon in the cervical transformation zone and when present are associated strongly with HPV types 6 and 11 (Fig. 13.17a). As defined above, these lesions exhibit acanthosis, verruciform growth pattern and viral cytopathic effect (koilocytotic atypia). The verrucous pattern is typified by blunt papillae, in contrast to the slender filiform papillae of immature condyloma (see below). The latter is characterized by karyomegaly, nuclear enlargement with binucleation, irregularities in nuclear membrane and hyperchromasia. These lesions closely resemble vulvar condylomata with the exception of conspicuous cytopathic effect that is not seen commonly in the latter.

Flat condyloma (CIN I) (Fig. 13.17b). The second category of LSIL consists of the flat condyloma (CIN I), which exhibits features similar to condyloma acuminatum but lacks the exophytic or papillary growth pattern. The degree of epithelial maturation and koilo-cytosis may vary, but there is minimal nuclear hyperchromasia and pleomorphism in the lower third of the epithelium. In contrast to exophytic/papillary lesions, flat condylomata are frequently associated with intermediate- and high-risk HPV types.[12] Because exophytic condylomas and papillomas are typically associated with HPV types 6 and 11, they may be segregated from flat condylomas.

Immature condyloma (squamous papilloma, papillary immature metaplasia). Immature condylomas fall into the third category of LSIL variants (Fig. 13.18). Conceptually, immature condylomas may be viewed as an infection of transformation zone epithelium by low-risk HPV types (6 or 11) that fails to mature and maintains a phenotype closely resembling immature metaplasia. Because the atypia in mature condylomas is a function of viral cytopathic effect, and because viral cytopathic effect depends on maturation, immature condylomas will manifest with the degree of atypia usually seen in the immature cell layers of a condyloma, which is mild. Immature condylomas as described are virtually identical to those variously described as squamous papilloma and papillary immature metaplasia.[162] Conceivably, some of these lesions may also be termed 'transitional papillomas'. These lesions present as a spectrum and are illustrated in Figure 13.18a–d. Patterns of immature condyloma include the following: (1) a close similarity to squamous metaplasia, with (a) mild

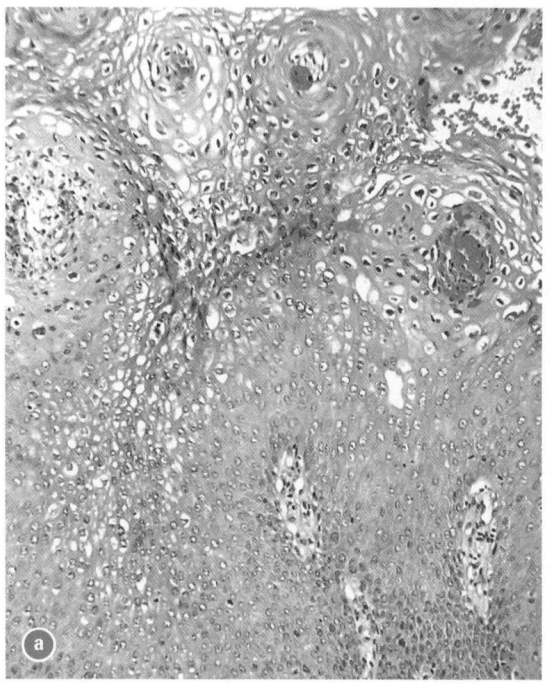
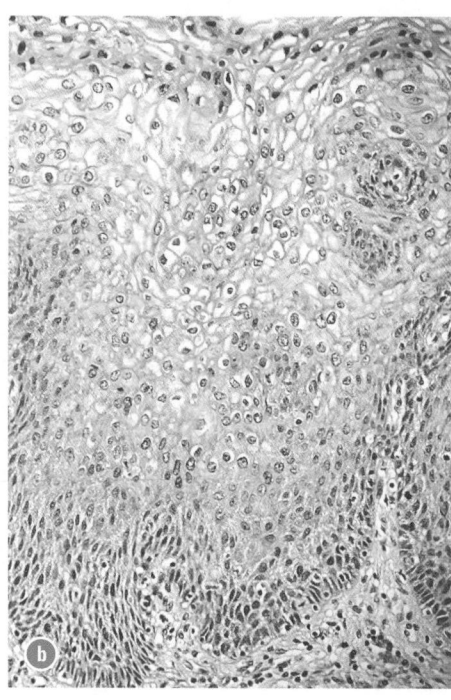

Fig. 13.17 Most common types of LSIL include exophytic (a) and flat (b) condyloma (also termed CIN I). Both forms of LSIL exhibit uniform maturation, preservation of cell polarity, surface (koilocytotic) atypia and uniformity of nuclei in the lower epithelial layers with mild anisokaryosis, hyperchromasia and minimal chromatin irregularity.

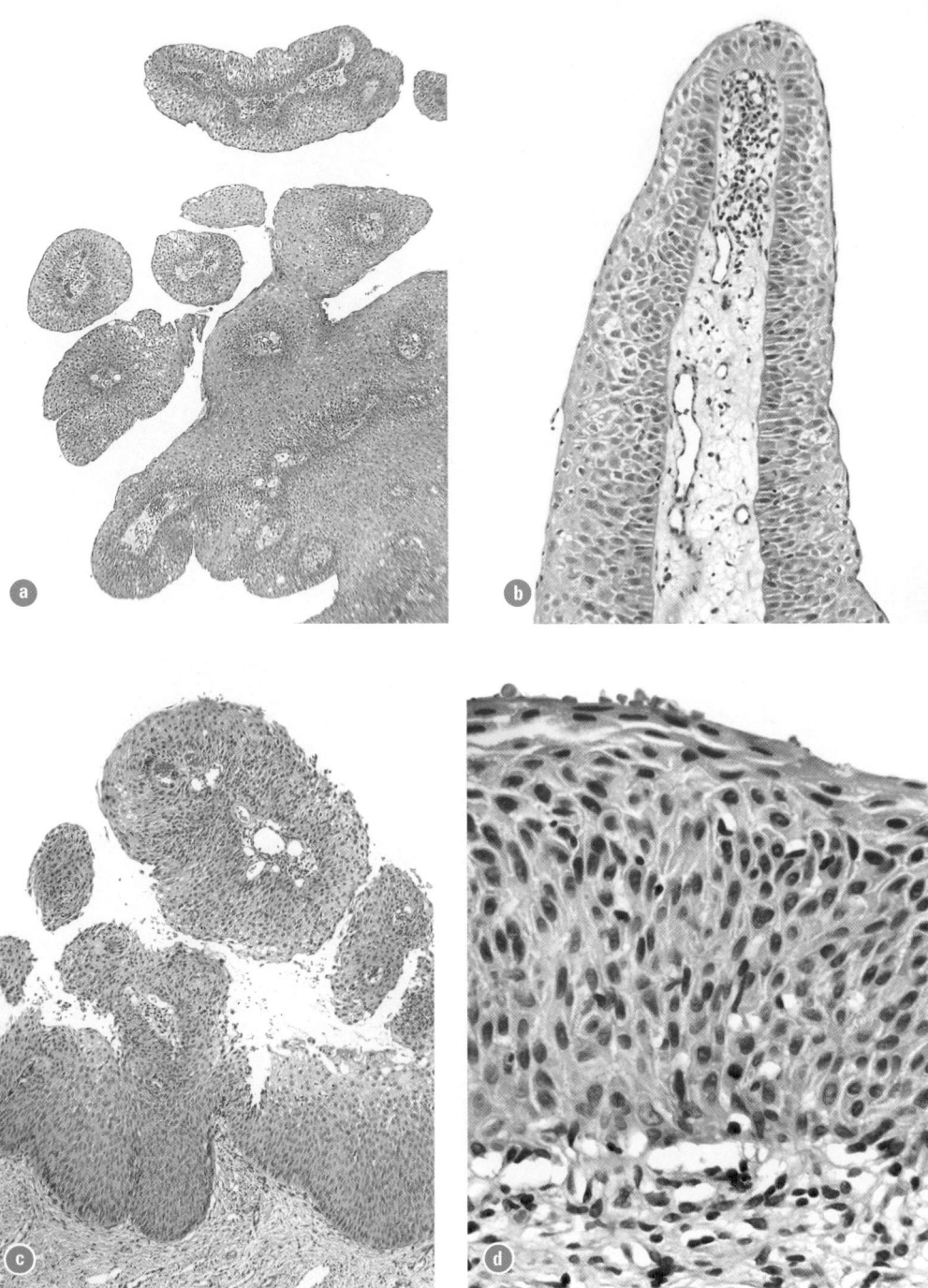

Fig. 13.18 Immature condyloma (LSIL) is characterized by filiform papillary architecture which may be more (a,b) or less (c) mature. Flat areas may mimic HSIL but exhibit uniform nuclear size and spacing, low mitotic index, and prominent chromocenters (d).

increases in nuclear/cytoplasmic ratio, (b) preservation of nucleoli, (c) slight nuclear crowding and (d) a near absence of keratinocyte maturation; (2) the formation of small filiform papillae, which is pathognomonic; and (3) frequent preservation of overlying columnar cell layers, more characteristic with a metaplastic phenotype. Some of these features fall within the descriptive of 'papillary immature metaplasia'. Others may be more florid and at the extreme end are squamous papillomas, with a more well-developed fibrovascular network and containing more mature keratinocytes. Like exophytic condylomas, immature condylomas contain HPV types 6 and 11, meriting definition as immature variants of these lesions.[162,165] Whether they can be distinguished biologically from transitional papillomas is not clear; however, they must be distinguished

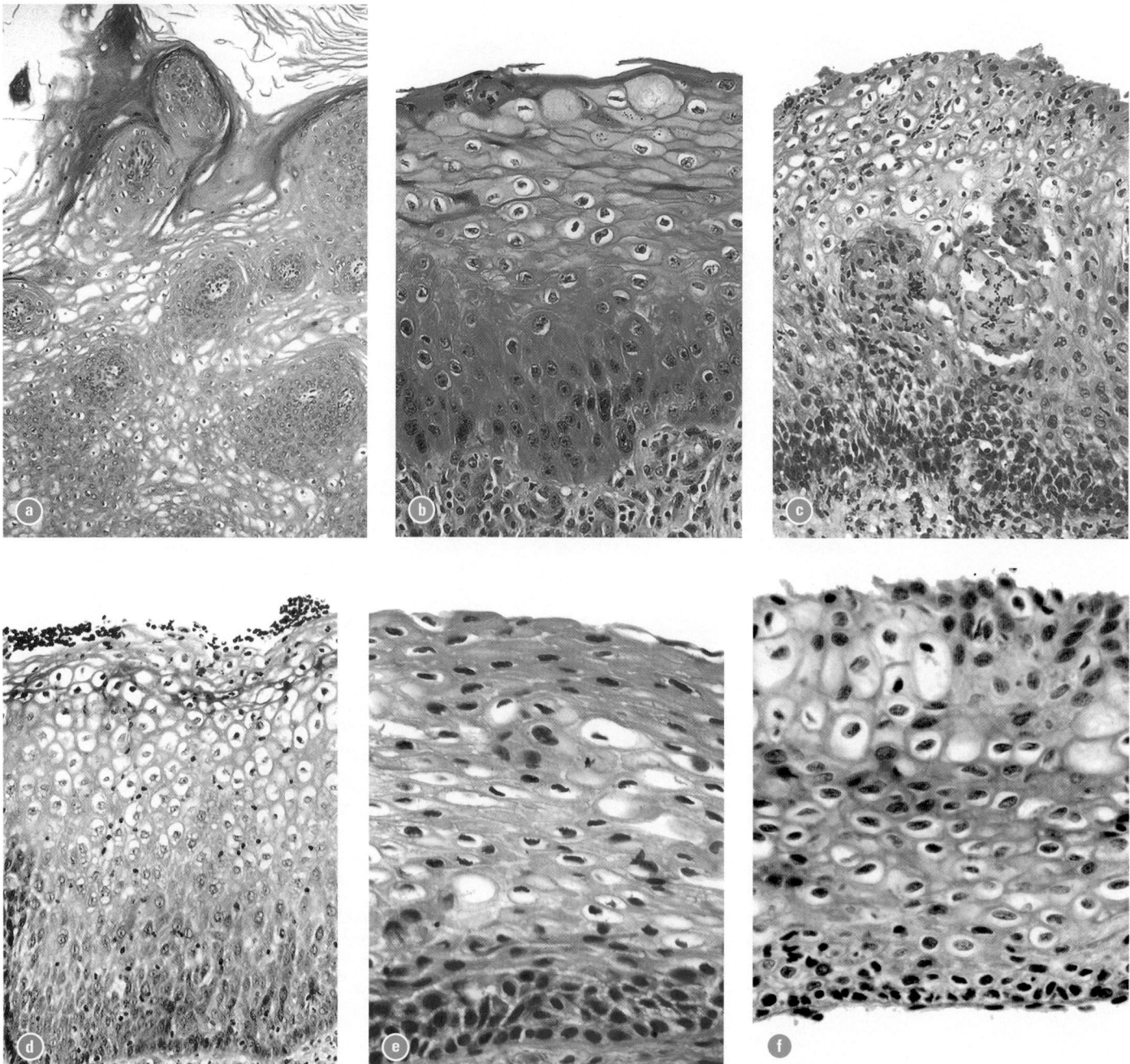

Fig. 13.19 Differential diagnosis of LSIL, including mucosal polyps (vaginal) (a), mild disturbances in maturation (b), mild nuclear irregularity with cytoplasmic halos associated with inflammation (c,d) and menopausal-related changes (e,f).

from papillary carcinomas *in situ* and carcinomas.[166] The latter exhibit a high mitotic index and greater nuclear atypia and will be discussed subsequently.

Differential diagnosis of LSIL

A variety of epithelial alterations may mimic koilocytosis and are illustrated in Figure 13.19a–f and summarized in Table 13.8. They include the following:

Filiform mucosal excrescences of the vagina (Fig. 13.19a). The increased (and at times misplaced) concern over papillomaviruses in the past 10 years has resulted in a higher index of suspicion for lesions in the vaginal mucosa. Because the vagina characteristically contains epithelial folds, excrescences or 'papillae', these may be suspected clinically and sampled. The histologic appearance of such biopsies includes papillo-

Table 13.8 Differential diagnosis of squamous intraepithelial lesions

Category	Mimic	Distinguishing features
LSIL	Mucosal polyp (vaginal)	Minimal acanthosis
	Reactive epithelial changes	Mild superficial karyomegaly, occasional binucleated intermediate cells
	Postmenopausal changes	Superficial cell karyomegaly, cytoplasmic halos
HSIL	Immature repair	Basal hyperchromasia, uniform nuclear spacing and nuclear contour, nucleoli
	Immature metaplasia	Uniform maturation, minimal surface hyperchromasia
	Atrophy	No mitoses, uniform chromasia, nuclear density
	Implantation site	Uniform and wide nuclear spacing, bizarre nuclei
	Endometrial histiocytes	Small indented nuclei, granular cytoplasm, lack of polarity

matosis, parakeratosis and cytoplasmic halos. What are not present are prominent acanthosis, nuclear atypia and atypical parakeratosis. The appropriate diagnosis for biopsies of this type is 'acanthosis, papillomatosis, etc., non-specific'. The term non-specific properly designates these alterations as not associated with HPV nucleic acids. Molecular studies have confirmed that such changes are no more likely to harbor HPV nucleic acids than normal squamous epithelium.[166]

Reactive epithelial changes (non-specific). Prominent cytoplasmic halos may be present in association with any glycogenated epithelium, and mild nuclear atypia will result if the epithelium is either inflamed or associated with underlying inflammation. Occasionally, reparative or reactive epithelial changes will undergo incomplete maturation, in which case, nuclear hyperchromasia will be present in association with the cytoplasmic halos. In such cases, the most important discriminating feature is absence of variation, in either cell size or staining intensity, in the cell population (Fig. 13.19b–d). Binucleated cells may or may not be present, but will usually be inconspicuous.

A second type of reactive epithelial change may exhibit semi-mature metaplasia with prominent binucleation. Such cases should not be confused with condyloma; the binucleated cells are usually not enlarged and appear bland in appearance, occurring in a background pattern of metaplasia.

Postmenopausal squamous atypia (Fig. 13.19e,f). Prior reports have identified cells resembling koilocytes in postmenopausal women.[167] Although LSIL may occur in this age group, a spectrum of epithelial and cellular alterations may exist in menopausal or postmenopausal women, ranging from partial to complete atrophy. This spectrum includes maturation disturbances with 'pseudokoilocytosis', transitional metaplasia and classic atrophic changes. In some instances, all three may be present in the same biopsy. This discussion is limited to the issue of pseudokoilocytosis, which we have observed in biopsies of women in the sixth decade and higher, and occasionally in the late 40s.[168] This phenomenon is characterized by epithelial maturation, cytoplasmic halos and variable (usually mild) nuclear size or staining. The halos are usually round and uniform in appearance, with centrally placed nuclei. The latter are usually slightly hyperchromatic, at times elongated, and occasionally grooved. Occasionally, binucleation is present, and the process may closely mimic koilocytosis. In some cases, peripheral condensation of pale cytoplasm around the uniform halos will give a target-like or 'fried egg' appearance to the cells. This pattern is similar to that produced by navicular cells in pregnancy and post-partum.

Lesions falling between LSIL and HSIL

The distinction of LSIL from HSIL is based primarily on the presence of atypia in the latter that does not fit within the spectrum of a flat or exophytic condyloma. The principal area targeted for this assessment is the lower epithelial layer. Figure 13.20 compares the lower half of the epithelium in six lesions, three LSILs (Fig. 13.20a) and one HSIL (Fig. 13.20d). From these photomicrographs, the two categories can be distinguished with some consistency. However, there exist some variants of SIL that are not amenable to precise grading, and these are illustrated in Figure 13.21. They include the following:

LSILs with increased parabasal hypercellularity (Fig. 13.21a). One of the more difficult tasks in distinguishing LSIL from HSIL lies in the assessment of increased parabasal cellularity. The distinction is made based on the degree of nuclear pleomorphism and coarse chromatin. If the latter are minimal, a diagnosis of LSIL is appropriate.

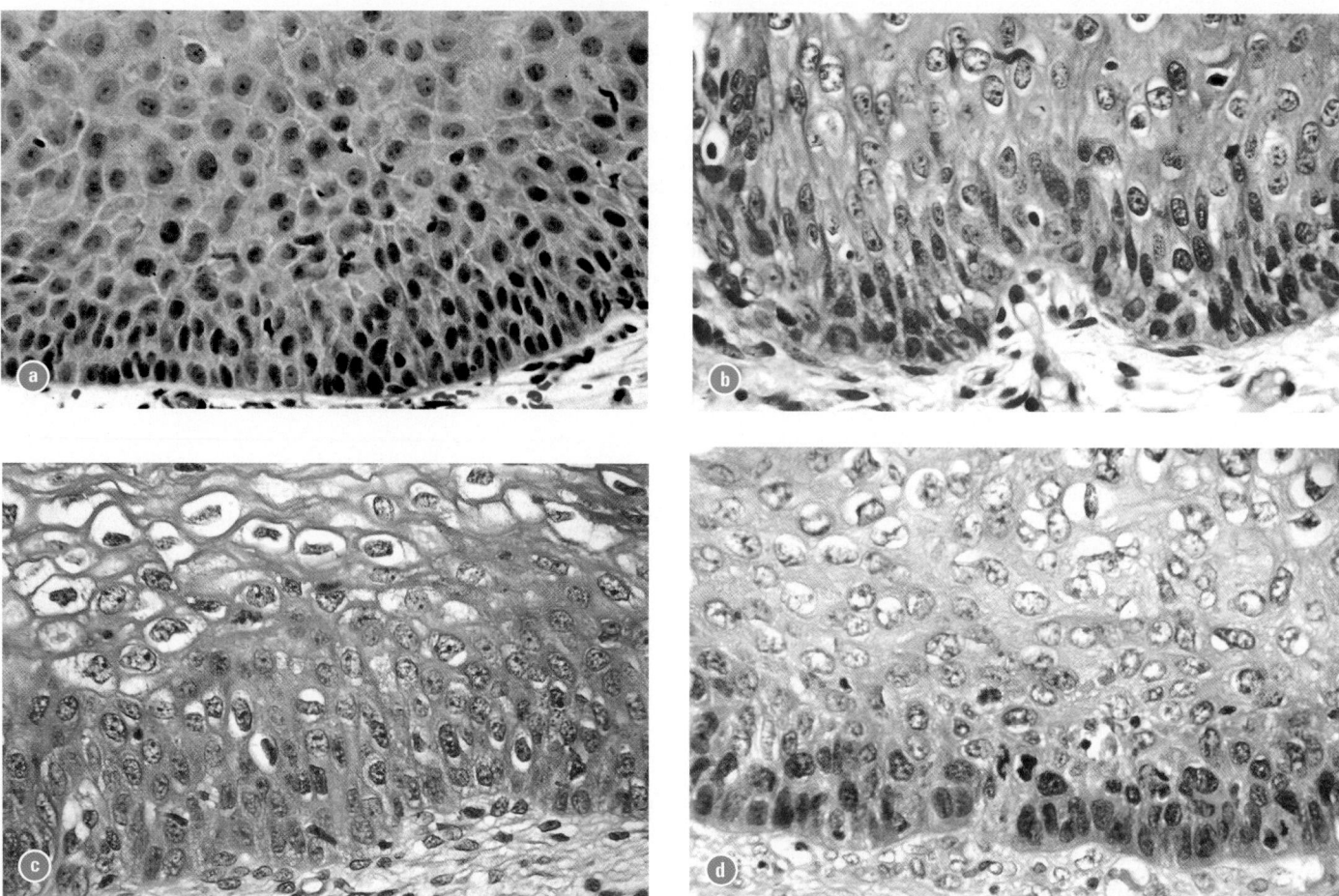

Fig. 13.20• Lower epithelial cell layers of LSIL (a–c) are characterized by preservation of polarity and mild degrees of anisonucleosis and polychromasia. In contrast, HSILs typically exhibit more striking variations in both size and staining intensity and contour and chromatin character in the lower third of the epithelium (d).

Flat immature lesions with minimal nuclear aniso-karyosis (Fig. 13.21b,c). Flat lesions showing an absence of normal maturation fall into the category of 'atypical immature squamous proliferations', which is discussed below under the differential diagnosis of HSIL. This discussion is limited to those occasional flat lesions that exhibit the morphologic features similar to immature condyloma. The most challenging aspect of this subset of precursor lesions is distinguishing them from HSIL and from reactive metaplasias. We classify them as 'SIL, not amenable to precise grading' (CIN 1–CIN 2).

Lesions identical to condyloma but containing abnormal mitoses (Fig. 13.21d) *or single bizarre nuclei* (Fig. 13.21e). Whether these changes justify a diagnosis of CIN II is debatable in the absence of additional nuclear abnormalities in the lower cell layers.

Lesions with atypia in the setting of metaplasia or microglandular change (Fig. 13.21f). This is another very uncommon lesion, but one that can be defined. The pattern closely resembles early squamous meta-plasia in areas of microglandular change, with a lobular or nesting arrangement of immature squamous cells, preservation of cytoplasmic maturation and mucin droplets. The mitotic index is low and the nuclei are evenly spaced with minimal crowding, but exhibit prominent karyomegaly with multinucleation. In the authors' experience, these lesions are usually associated with high-risk HPVs (as many LSILs are). As above, we typically classify these lesions as 'SIL of uncertain grade'.

Papillary cervical lesions exceeding the morphologic limits of immature condyloma. Not all papillary cervical lesions can be readily distinguished as condyloma, immature condyloma or papillary carcinoma (*in situ*). Occasional lesions may not be amenable to being categorized in any of these groups. However, they should be managed as high-grade precursors and removed. The differential diagnosis of verruco-papillary lesions of the cervix is discussed later in this chapter. In practice, lesions falling into the gap between LSIL and HSIL are classified as squamous intraepithelial lesions,

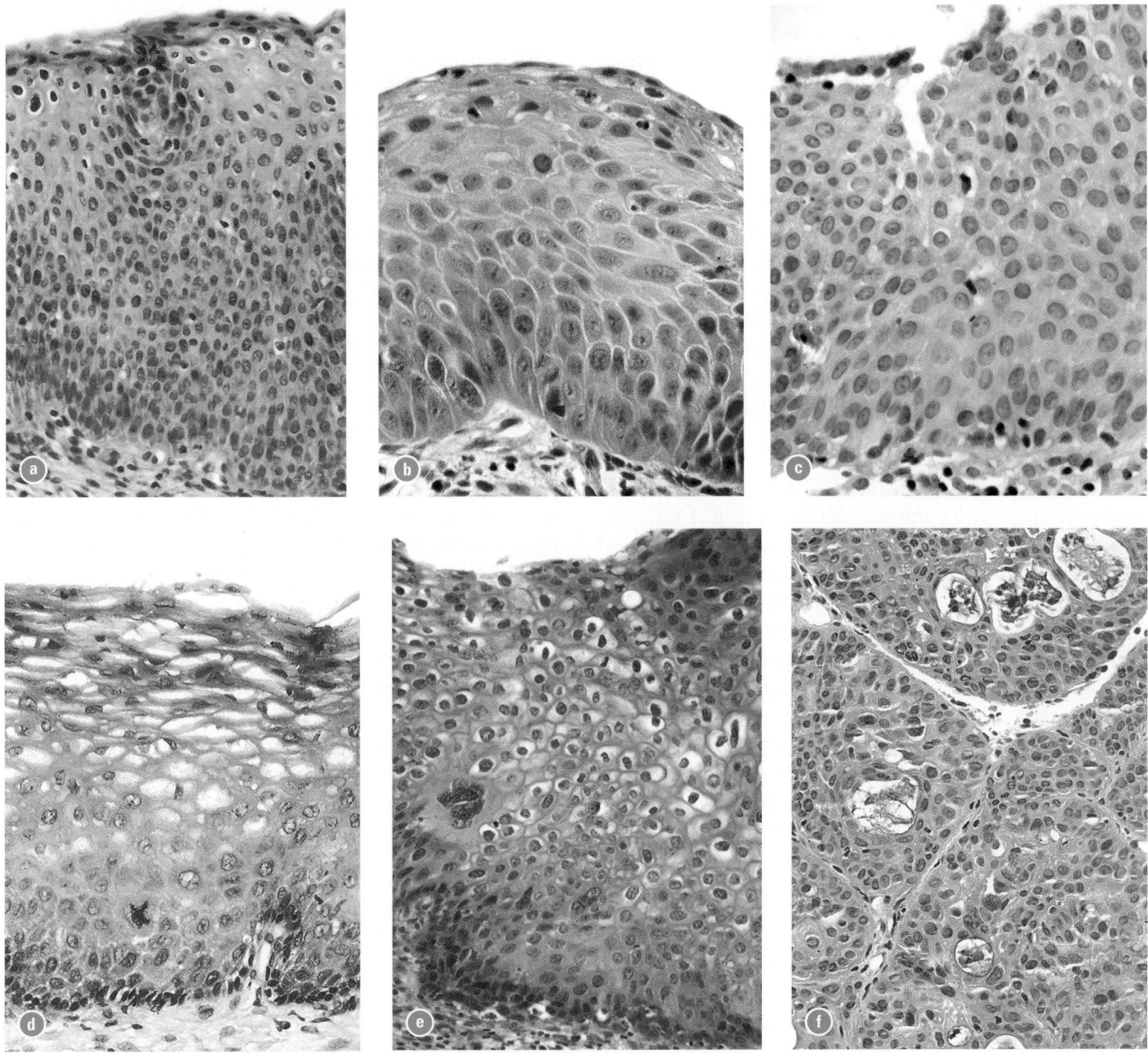

Fig. 13.21 Squamous intraepithelial lesions difficult to classify include lesions with minimal nuclear pleomorphism but parabasal hypercellularity and less maturation (a–c), lesions with abnormal mitoses (d) or occasional bizarre nuclei (e) and, rarely, lesions occurring in areas of microglandular change (f).

not amenable to precise grading. For practical purposes (see below), management of SIL is often keyed to a diagnosis of low or high SIL. Diagnoses of uncertainty invariably occur, but for practical reasons are best used sparingly.

High-grade squamous intraepithelial lesions (HSIL)

Histologic criteria

High-grade squamous intraepithelial lesions (Fig. 13.22a–h) exhibit atypia in all layers of the epithelium

similar to those classically defined as CIN.[153,159] In essence, the extent and degree of nuclear atypia exceeds the limits of that described in flat or exophytic condylomas (LSIL).

As with LSIL, some lesions are easily identified (classic) while certain variants may be less easily recognized. Lesions classified as CIN II exhibit epithelial maturation, often in the form of koilocytosis. Often, but not always, the surface maturation is accompanied by bizarre nuclear forms or abnormal keratinization. In addition to a broader distribution of nuclear atypia, these lesions are distinguished from LSIL by increased mitotic index, loss of cell polarity, abnormal mitotic figures and the presence of occasional bizarre nuclei. CIN IIIs (including carcinomas *in situ*) contain full-thickness nuclear atypia. However, the degree of nuclear atypia may vary in extent, giving rise to variants of CIN III that closely mimic immature metaplastic epithelium, with more subtle degrees of karyomegaly or anisokaryosis. Such cases may be difficult to recognize on both cytologic and histologic examination and other strategies, such as the use of biomarkers, may be required to distinguish them from benign metaplasias.[102,169,170]

HSIL may present in several forms, including the following:

Mature or koilocytotic HSIL (CIN II). These lesions may contain prominent viral cytopathic effect koilocytosis coexisting with parabasal cell atypia (Fig. 13.22a,b).

Keratinizing HSIL. These lesions are characterized by prominent abnormal superficial keratinization with high nuclear density and hyperchromasia (Fig. 13.22c).

HSIL with an immature metaplastic phenotype. This subset is the most difficult to recognize, and must be distinguished from reactive metaplastic changes. The characteristic features include a lack of reduction in nuclear density in the upper layers, the appearance of a syncytium of nuclei in the upper layers and nuclear hyperchromasia (Fig. 13.22d). Occasionally they may undermine intact columnar mucosa (Fig. 13.22e).

Stratified intraepithelial lesions with columnar cell differentiation. Because the transformation zone is composed of multi-potential cells, some HPV infections may give rise to additional variants exhibiting both squamous and columnar cell differentiation (Fig. 13.22f,g). The latter may present as conventional adenocarcinomas *in situ* (ACIS); however, a subset will manifest as stratified neoplastic lesions with prominent mucin droplets, seen also in mucicarmine stains (Fig. 13.22h). These stratified mucin-producing intraepithelial lesions (SMILEs) are typically seen in association with both HSIL and ACIS, suggesting a 'transition' between the two.[171]

Differential diagnosis of HSIL

The diagnosis of HSIL (CIN II or III) is considered when the abnormality in question either does not resemble a condyloma and/or if it does, the atypia under study is not confined strictly to the superficial cell layers (Figs 13.23 and 13.24). Because epithelial immaturity, nuclear atypia and inflammatory cellular changes may be present in both benign and neoplastic squamous proliferations, the distinction of reactive processes from SIL requires careful attention to the growth pattern of the epithelium, the distribution of atypia and degree of nuclear abnormality. Non-neoplastic reactive changes include regularity of nuclear spacing, preservation of nucleoli, absence of marked

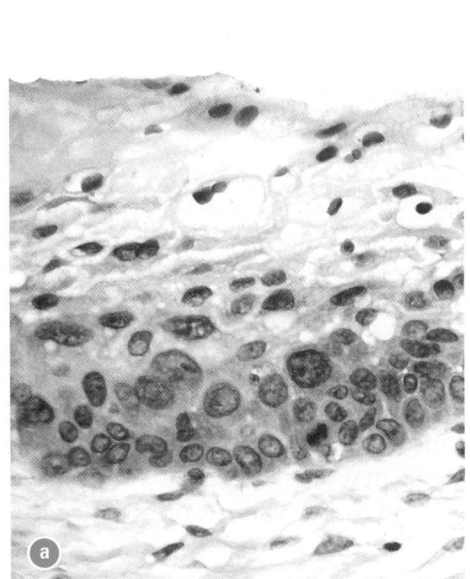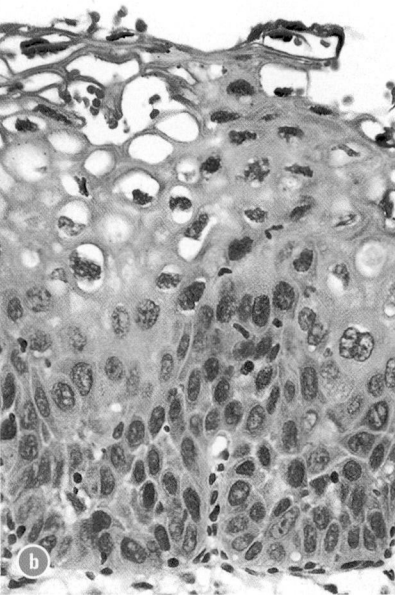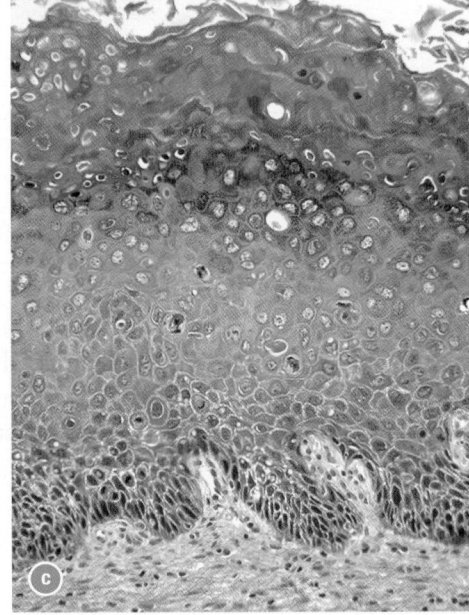

Fig. 13.22 Types of HSIL include well-differentiated or koilocytotic lesions with prominent basal atypia (CIN II, a,b), keratinizing lesions (c)

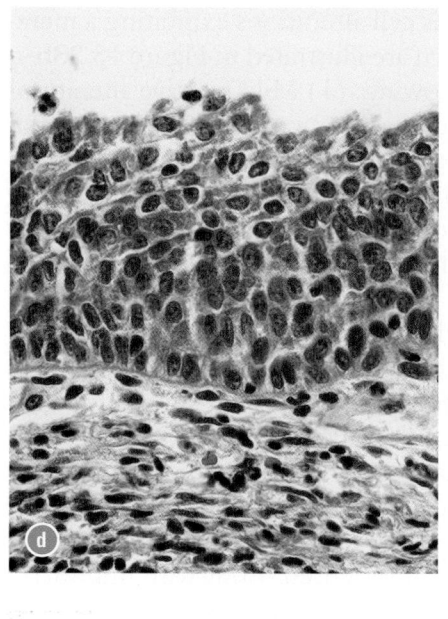

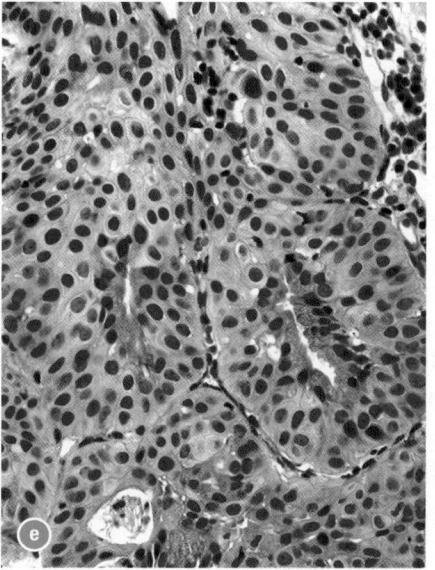

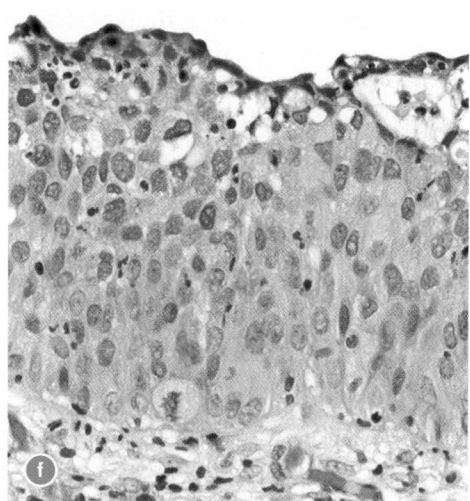

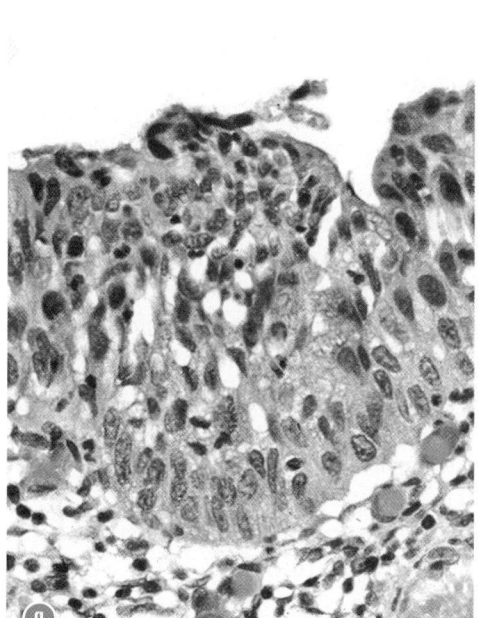

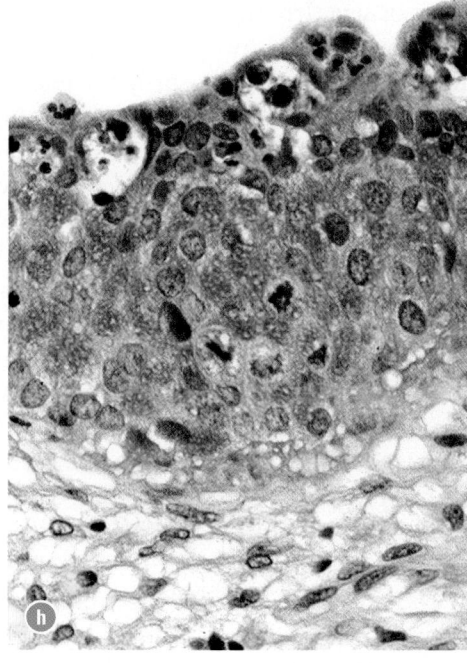

Fig. 13.22 **Cont'd** and immature lesions may resemble metaplastic epithelium (d) and undermine columnar mucosa (e). Rarely, stratified intraepithelial lesions composed of columnar cells may overlap with HSIL (f,g) and are distinguished by diffuse mucicarmine positivity (h). The latter are considered variants of ACIS but are included here because the morphologic patterns closely resemble HSIL.

variation in nuclear size, contour and staining (specifically coarse-appearing hyperchromatic nuclei) and, with minor exceptions, lack of nuclear atypia in the upper epithelial layers. This latter parameter is referred to as 'normalization' of the epithelium with maturation. Nuclear atypia in the upper epithelial cell layers is present in most squamous intraepithelial lesions, irrespective of grade, but the interpretation of this parameter in the context of inflammatory change is subjective. Most reactive/reparative processes, however severe, will mature with spacing of nuclei due to cyto-

plasmic maturation, accompanied by either a reduction in nuclear size or regularity in nuclear morphology (Fig. 13.23). Immature metaplasias and atrophy will usually undergo maturation but in some instances (due to extreme immaturity or partial epithelial denudation) there may be no decrease in nuclear/cytoplasmic ratio in the surface of the epithelium. In such cases, the distinction of benign from neoplastic changes must be made on cytologic grounds, and a diagnosis of uncertainty on cytology (ASCUS) or biopsy (atypical squamous epithelium with a comment) may be necessary if there is atypia present. Occasionally, nuclear enlargement and hyperchromasia may be seen near the surface of inflamed immature metaplasia, in which case the distinction of metaplasia from a SIL is based upon evaluation of the entire epithelium (see below).

Reactive squamous epithelial changes, which may mimic high-grade squamous intraepithelial lesions, include the following:

Reactive/reparative epithelial changes (Fig. 13.23a). Epithelial alterations in this category demonstrate: (1) intercellular edema (spongiosis), (2) evenly spaced nuclei with mild to moderate enlargement but minimal anisokaryosis, (3) prominent nucleoli, (4) intraepithelial neutrophils and (5) a tendency for superficial maturation. Nuclear enlargement may be present, but it is not accompanied by hyperchromasia or changes in nuclear spacing. Incomplete maturation may be present but the nuclei should display regular spacing, distinct cell borders and mild variation in staining or size. Irregularities in the parabasal cell population may accompany inflammation, but normal maturation excludes a SIL. Mild reactive/inflammatory cell changes may produce general nuclear enlargement with binucleation and SIL is excluded by the absence of variation in nuclear staining or contour.

The diagnosis of a SIL, either low- or high-grade, should be considered when features of repair – spongiosis, prominent nucleoli – are accompanied by greater than usual degrees of nuclear enlargement and hyperchromasia and when the abnormalities are present in some superficial epithelial cells. Features that should raise the question of SIL include: (1) irregular nuclear spacing or loss of polarity, (2) discretely enlarged hyperchromatic nuclei or binucleated forms and anisokaryosis and the presence of enlarged hyperchromatic nuclei on the surface. The evaluation of surface atypia is subjective, inasmuch as the number of abnormal cells and the characteristics of the epithelium influence interpretation. In some cases, a diagnosis of uncertainty (atypical squamous epithelium) may be necessary, with a qualifying comment.

Immature squamous metaplasia. It is important here to distinguish metaplasia from HSIL with a metaplastic growth pattern. By definition, epithelial alterations associated with typical squamous metaplasia are usually non-neoplastic and are, particularly if characterized by mucin droplets or endocervical cells, either within the epithelium or on the surface. Surface columnar cells and mucin droplets are uncommonly associated with high-grade precursors; surface columnar cells may be found in association with immature condyloma.

Immature squamous cell alterations exhibiting a metaplastic growth pattern are illustrated in Figure 13.23b–d and include the following: (1) Mild reactive alterations in immature metaplasia characterized by some variation in nuclear staining and size. (2) Acutely inflamed metaplastic epithelia with polynucleation can usually be distinguished from SIL if the nuclei are not densely hyperchromatic and the background cell population displays a uniform nuclear morphology with nucleoli. (3) Occasional surface atypia may be present in association with inflammation, but the general growth pattern of the metaplastic process should not be altered; the lower epithelial cells should exhibit a minimum of nuclear crowding or pleomorphism and display chromocenters or nucleoli (Fig. 13.23b). (4) If extreme degrees of nuclear enlargement and hyperchromasia are present, even in unoriented, otherwise unremarkable metaplastic epithelium, a diagnosis of a squamous intraepithelial lesion should be strongly considered. (5) However, these lesions are typically subtle and the primary features are an immature cell population with consistently high nuclear density from the basal to the surface cells (Fig. 13.23c). When nuclear enlargement and/or hyperchromasia is present in the surface cells, the diagnosis of HSIL is more easily made (Fig. 13.23d). Nevertheless, biomarkers may be particularly helpful when the pathologist is uncertain (see below).

Artifacts may also cause diagnostic confusion, specifically cautery artifacts that induce nuclear enlargement and hyperchromasia as a function of the thermal injury. Importantly, the enlargement is typically uniform and not accompanied by anisonucleosis or nuclear crowding (Fig. 13.23e,f).

Non-epithelial alterations. These include histiocytes (Fig. 13.23g) and implantation site (Fig. 13.23h). Placental implantation site is commonly recognized in the endometrium.[7] It may mimic a neoplasm in cervical biopsies or endocervical curettings, but it is sufficiently distinctive that misdiagnosis is unlikely once the pathologist has some experience with this lesion. Implantation site usually presents as an eosinophilic (by virtue of the abundant keratin-positive matrix) irregularly contoured process in the superficial cervical stroma that is punctuated by scattered hyperchromatic nuclei. On closer examination, the irregular margins of the lesion are composed of a series of small rounded borders and the atypical nuclei are separated by abundant pale to eosinophilic matrix. Occasionally, these lesions may present as plaque-like lesions resembling intraepithelial lesions. Special stains for human chorionic gonadotropin or human placental lactogen are usually not helpful, as these cells often do not stain positive for these markers. Moreover, they will be strongly keratin-positive. Stains for placental alkaline phosphatase (PLAP) will sometimes discriminate these changes from squamous epithelium but the more useful markers are inhibin and HLAG.[172,173] Endometrial macrophages are another phenomenon that may mimic squamous lesions. The distinction from an epithelial neoplasm is based upon the small size of the cells, the small slightly vesicular nuclei, granular cytoplasm without distinct boundaries and a feathering of the peripheral line of demarcation without a sharp basal lamina (Fig. 13.23g). Mitoses may be present and eosinophils

are common. In general, macrophages are commonly encountered in association with inflammatory changes or in smears from postmenopausal women and, in this context, are not related to neoplasia.[3] Keratin (negative) and macrophage (positive) stains may assist in confirming the diagnosis.

Atrophy (Fig. 13.24a–d). The spectrum of squamous epithelial changes associated with older age include the following: (1) conventional atrophy with immature but cytologically bland morphology (Fig. 13.24a); (2) maturation disturbances with pseudokoilocytosis, some of which may resemble transitional metaplasia (Fig. 13.19b); (3) atrophy with partial maturation and

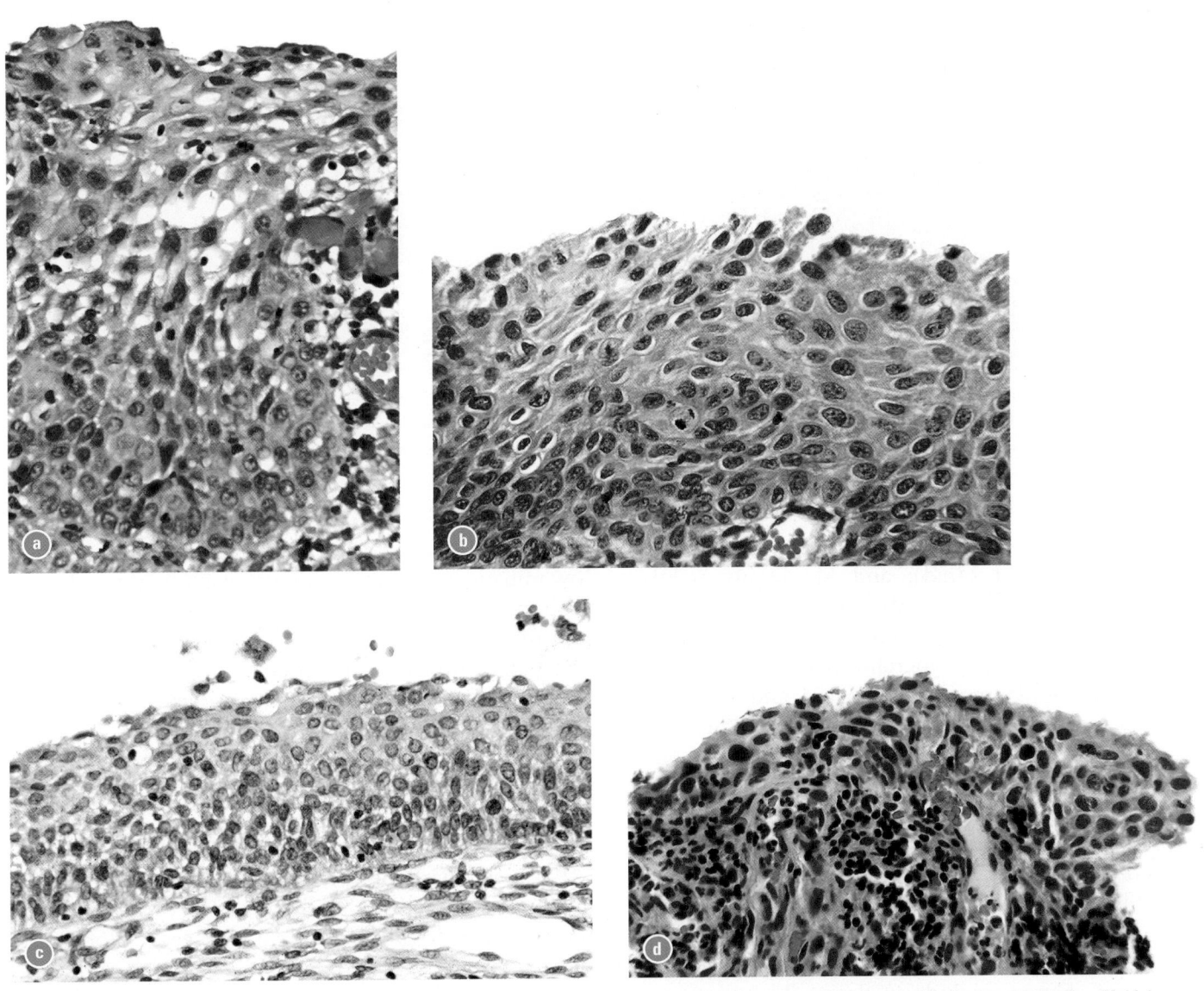

Fig. 13.23 HSIL can usually be distinguished from immature metaplasia with reactive changes (a,b), but should be suspected in immature epithelia with high nuclear density in the superficial epithelial layers or surface nuclear atypia (c,d).

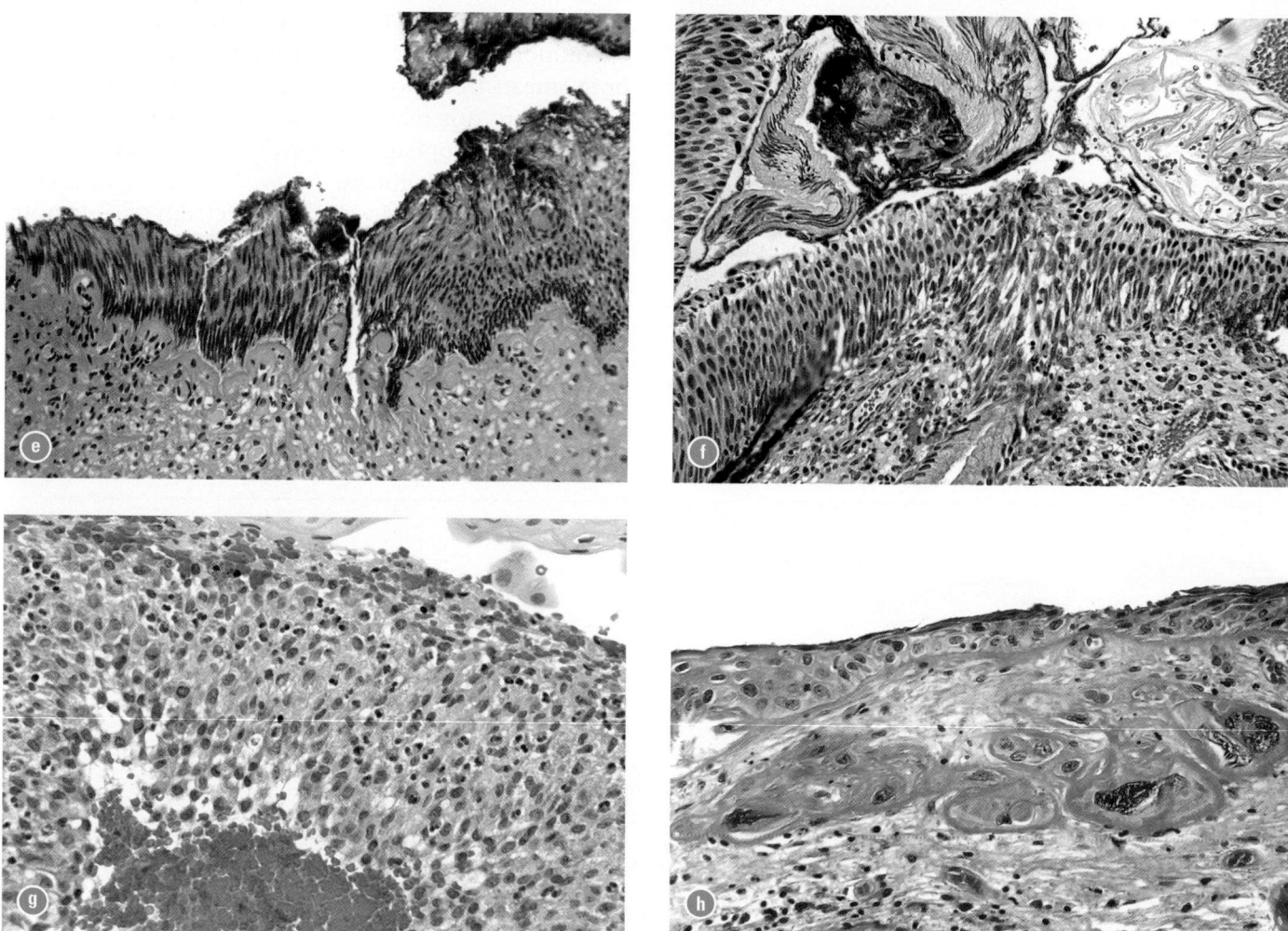

Fig. 13.23 Cont'd Cauterized normal (e) and lesional (f) epithelium can usually be distinguished by greater surface nuclear density and anisokaryosis in the latter. Non-squamous mimics of HSIL include sheets of macrophages from endometrial curettings (g) and implantation site (h).

focal nuclear enlargement or conspicuous nuclear hyperchromasia (Fig. 13.24c,d); and (4) highly cellular lesions with miotic activity that signifies a coexisting HSIL (Fig. 13.24e,f). Features common to atrophic processes include: (1) hyperchromatic but generally uniform nuclei, (2) frequent elongated, and sometimes grooved nuclei, (3) absence of conspicuous atypia in the upper epithelial layers, and importantly, (4) absence of mitotic figures. Atrophic epithelia with partial maturation and enlarged atypical nuclei comprise one of the more difficult categories, and distinction from SIL is based upon even spacing of nuclei with conspicuous intercellular bridges and an absence of mitotic activity.

Radiation effect. Radiation effect can involve both the endocervical and squamous epithelial cells. The prominent changes include nuclear enlargement and hyperchromasia associated with abundant cytoplasm, uniform nuclear spacing with minimal crowding, a low mitotic index, and evidence of cytoplasmic degeneration with vacuoles (see Chapter 11). The nuclear chromatin is often indistinct or smudged in appearance, in contrast to the coarse chromasia associated with neoplasia. Important is the preservation of a low nuclear/cytoplasmic ratio.

BIOMARKERS AND THE DIAGNOSIS AND CLASSIFICATION OF SQUAMOUS LESIONS

HPV, particularly high-risk HPVs, are associated with alterations in cell cycle. Because HPV oncoproteins induce alterations in cell cycle, cell cycle biomarkers may function as surrogate markers of HPV infection and can be used to facilitate the precise diagnosis of cervical precursor lesions (Figs 13.25a–h; Table

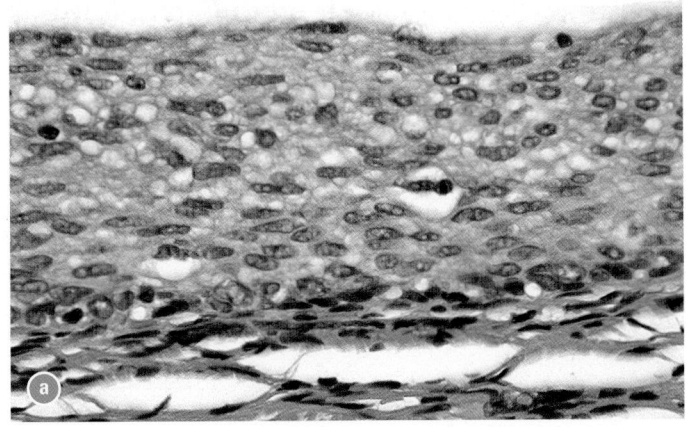

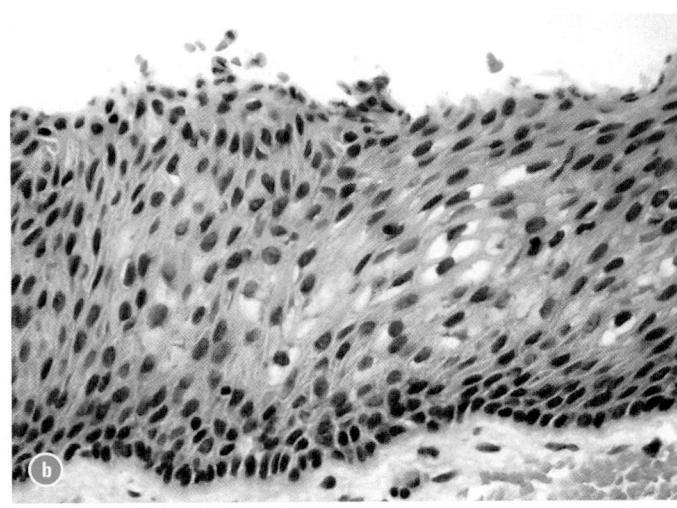

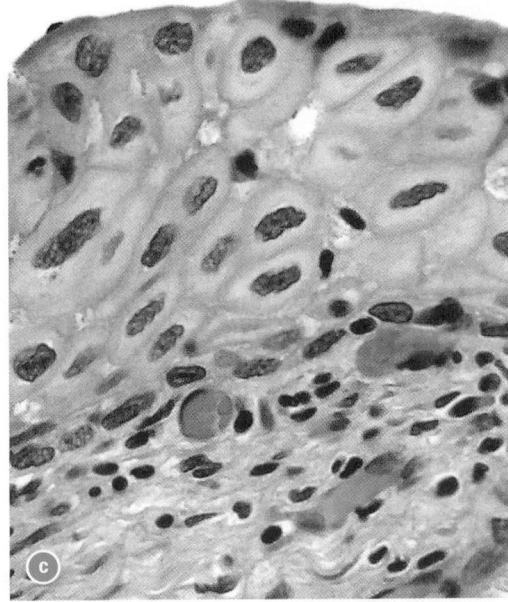

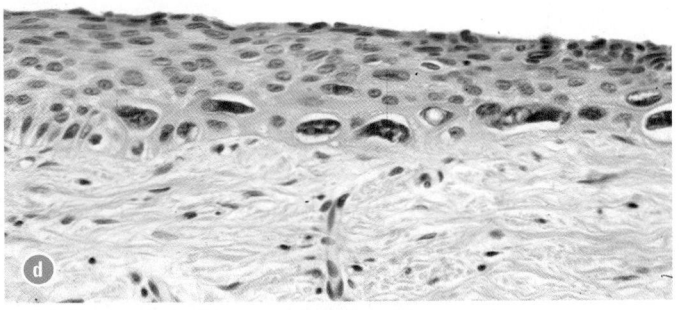

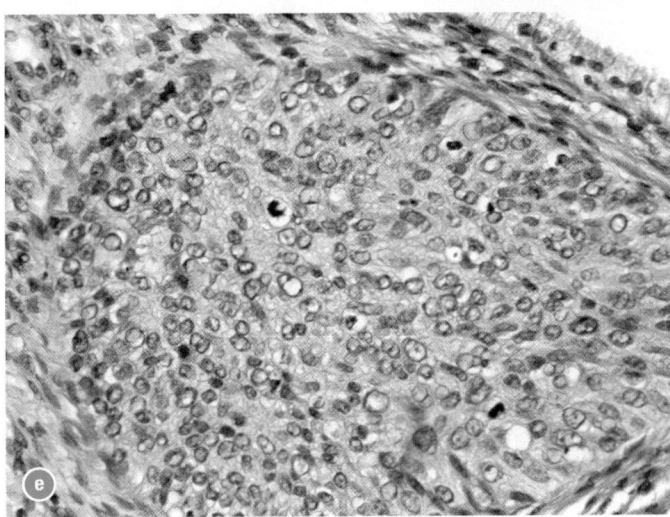

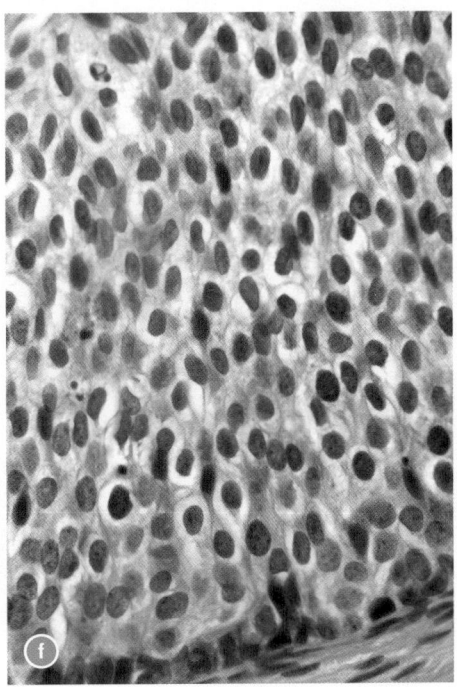

Fig. 13.24 Spectrum of atrophic atypia, including conventional atrophy with variable maturation (a,b), atrophy with sporadic atypia (c,d) and squamous intraepithelial lesions occurring in the setting of atrophy (e,f). The latter exhibit mitotic activity, nuclear crowding and greater (if still subtle) variations in nuclear morphology. MIB-1 and p16 immunohistochemistry is particularly helpful if the pathologist is not confident in making this distinction on morphologic grounds.

13.9).[174–177] The principal value of these markers is to distinguish non-diagnostic atypias from squamous intraepithelial lesions rather than to assign a grade of CIN. Expression of a generic cell cycle proliferative marker (Ki-67) is typically confined to the suprabasal cells of the lower-third of epithelial cells in normal mucosa (Fig. 13.25a). The presence of Ki-67-positive cells in the upper epithelial layers is characteristic of HPV effect, which induces cell cycle activity in these cells (Fig. 13.25b,c,e,f).[174,175] Thus, Ki-67 staining

may be helpful in distinguishing reactive epithelial changes from LSIL or atrophic mucosa from HSIL. Similarly, cyclin E, a nuclear protein upregulated by HPV 16 E7 and also linked to viral replication, is uncommonly expressed in non-infected epithelium and, when conspicuously present in nuclei, will usually discriminate both low- and high-grade lesions.[102,176] p16INK4, a cyclin-dependent kinase inhibitor, is the most promising, being expressed strongly in lesions associated with intermediate- and high-risk HPV types

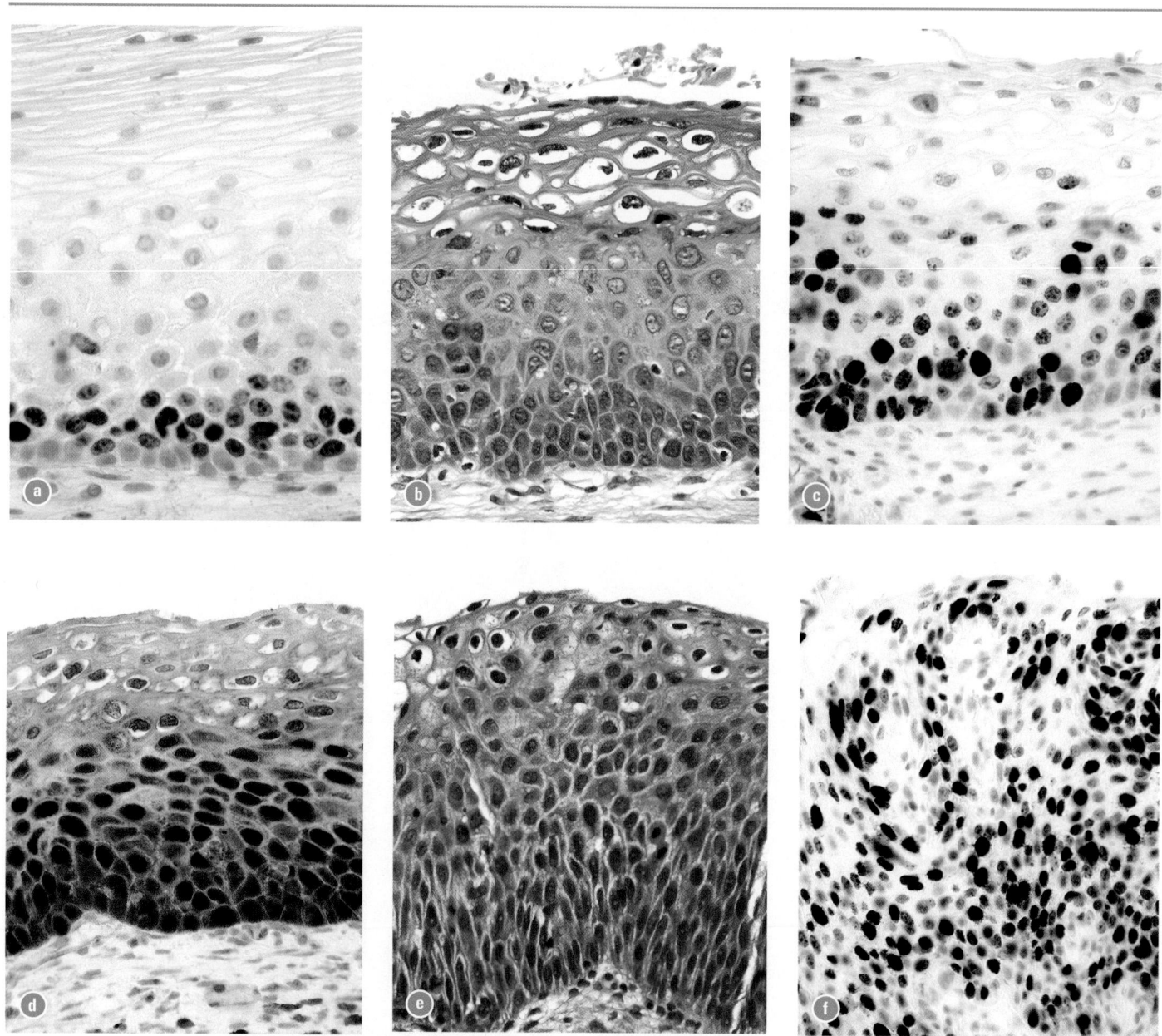

Fig. 13.25 Biomarkers commonly used in the diagnosis of cervical lesions. In contrast to normal mucosa (a), many squamous intraepithelial lesions (b) exhibit Ki-67-positive cells in the upper half of the epithelium (c) and intense p16 staining (d). A mildly atypical reactive metaplasia (e) exhibits diffuse Ki-67 (f)

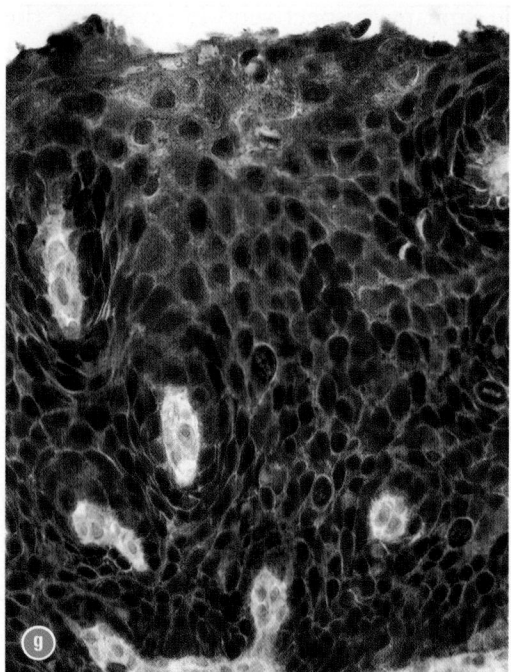
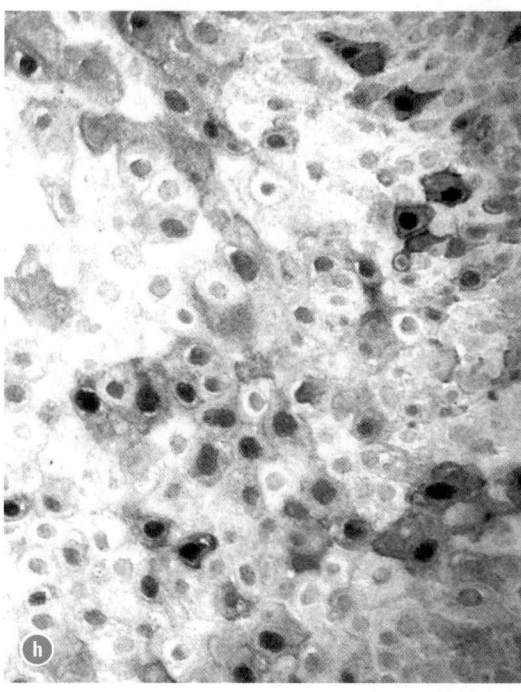

Fig. 13.25 **Cont'd** and p16 (g) staining. Low-risk HPV infections typically exhibit patchy p16 staining in more mature epithelial cells, including koilocytes (h).

(Fig. 13.25d,g), in contrast to low-risk HPV infection (Fig. 13.25h). The reader is reminded that because high-risk HPVs are common in both LSIL and HSIL, p16^{INK4} will not discriminate the two. However, staining for this marker, at least in the cervix, is highly associated with HPV infection. In the vulva and skin, p16 has been associated with non-HPV-related proliferations, a phenomenon that may reflect the relationship between p16 and cell cycle arrest.[177,178] This may be an issue with severely inflamed epithelia or epithelia undergoing repair. Potential misinterpreta-

tion of p16 staining may be reduced by using p16 in conjunction with Ki-67.

THE ENDOCERVICAL CURETTAGE

Endocervical curettage (ECC) is typically used on three occasions: during the initial work-up, at the time of LEEP excision and during follow-up after excisional therapy. Because a diagnosis of HSIL now requires a LEEP or cone biopsy, the precise role of the endocervical curettage in managing women with HSIL is

Table 13.9 Biomarkers in laboratory management of biopsies

Problem	Biomarker	Notes
Atrophy vs SIL	Ki-67	Staining of >30% nuclei or upper layers
Reactive vs SIL	Ki-67	Staining in upper layers; more difficult in unoriented (tangential) sections
Reactive vs LSIL	Cyclin E	2+ nuclear staining; weak diffuse staining not diagnostic
R/0 SIL	p16INK4	Diffuse and often intense staining in immature layers of SIL; good contrast with background but requires titrating positive controls to achieve low background. Lesions associated with low-risk HPVs stain variably
Squamous differentiation vs other	p63	Intense staining of squamous carcinomas; negative/weak in poorly-differentiated adenocarcinomas and small cell neuroendocrine carcinomas
Implantation site vs CIN/carcinoma	HLAG, inhibin	Intense staining of trophoblast, inhibin variable but specific

not clear, particularly when the colposcopic examination is satisfactory. However, the results of the ECC appear to have some prognostic significance.

Endocervical sampling at the initial colposcopy. Kobak et al. found that no patients with negative ECC had invasive disease on the final conization specimen, while all of those with invasion had positive ECC.[179] Other studies have corroborated the value of ECC in ruling out disease in the endocervical canal so that conservative ablation therapy can be considered.[180] Concerning the choice of endobrush versus curettage, the choice is between sensitivity and specificity, respectively. In comparative studies, the sensitivity of the endobrush has been reported as 92% *vs* 74% for ECC.[181] The principal limitation of the endobrush is the higher false-positive rate (62.5%) for endocervical involvement compared with ECC (25%).[182]

RESOLVING DISCORDANT PAPANICOLAOU SMEAR AND BIOPSY RESULTS

As discussed previously, the Papanicolaou smear and biopsy (Fig. 13.26a–g) may not always be concordant, and resolving these discrepancies is important prior to proceeding to LEEP or cone biopsy. Common scenarios are as follows:

The smear is abnormal and the biopsy shows no lesion. This occurs in approximately 15% and 40% of high- and low-grade smears, respectively. If review of the smear confirms the discrepancy, follow-up is necessary. A significant minority of these cases will be proven to have a lesion on a subsequent evaluation. HPV testing is of limited value unless the cytologic diagnosis comes into question.

The smear shows LSIL but the biopsy is HSIL. This occurs in 10–20% of LSIL smears. The cause is usually sampling artifact, which can be 'vertical' (sampling only the surface cells) or 'horizontal' (sampling only a portion of the lesion) (Fig. 13.26a–c). Management is dictated by the severity of the histologic lesion.

In some instances, the cytologic discrepancy is the product of coexisting low- and high-grade lesions. In most instances, when such lesions are present in continuity, they are derived from the same HPV infection. In a minority of cases, two distinct HPV infections may produce two lesions. Figure 13.26d–g illustrate an unusual instance where two HPV infections, one high- and one low-risk, coexist in the same area.

The smear shows HSIL but the biopsy shows LSIL. This is an uncommon discrepancy but one that requires careful review of the cytology and is associated with a substantial risk of subsequent HSIL.[183] If the cytology is confirmed as HSIL, the cervical lesion should be carefully reviewed. Again, a small number of these discrepancies can be attributed to coexisting low- and high-risk HPV infections.[141] It is particularly important

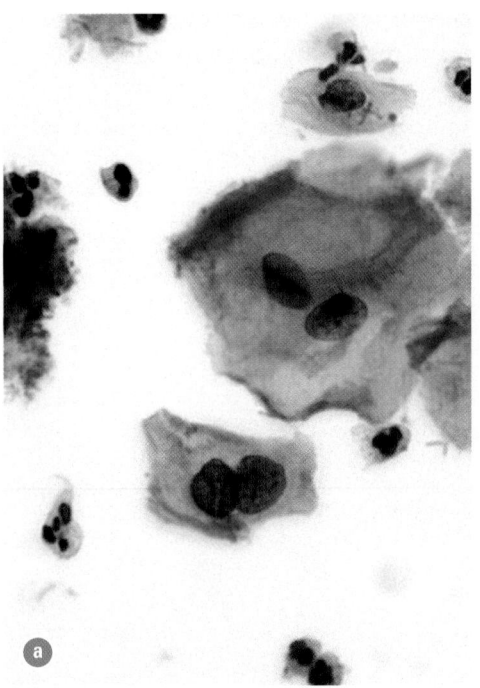
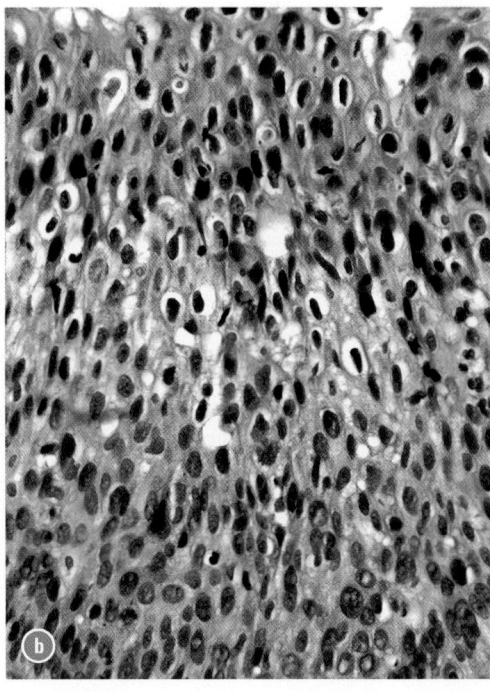

Fig. 13.26 Papanicolaou smear/biopsy discrepancies may be produced by vertical sampling error defined as cytologic sampling (a) of the surface of well-differentiated HSIL (b);

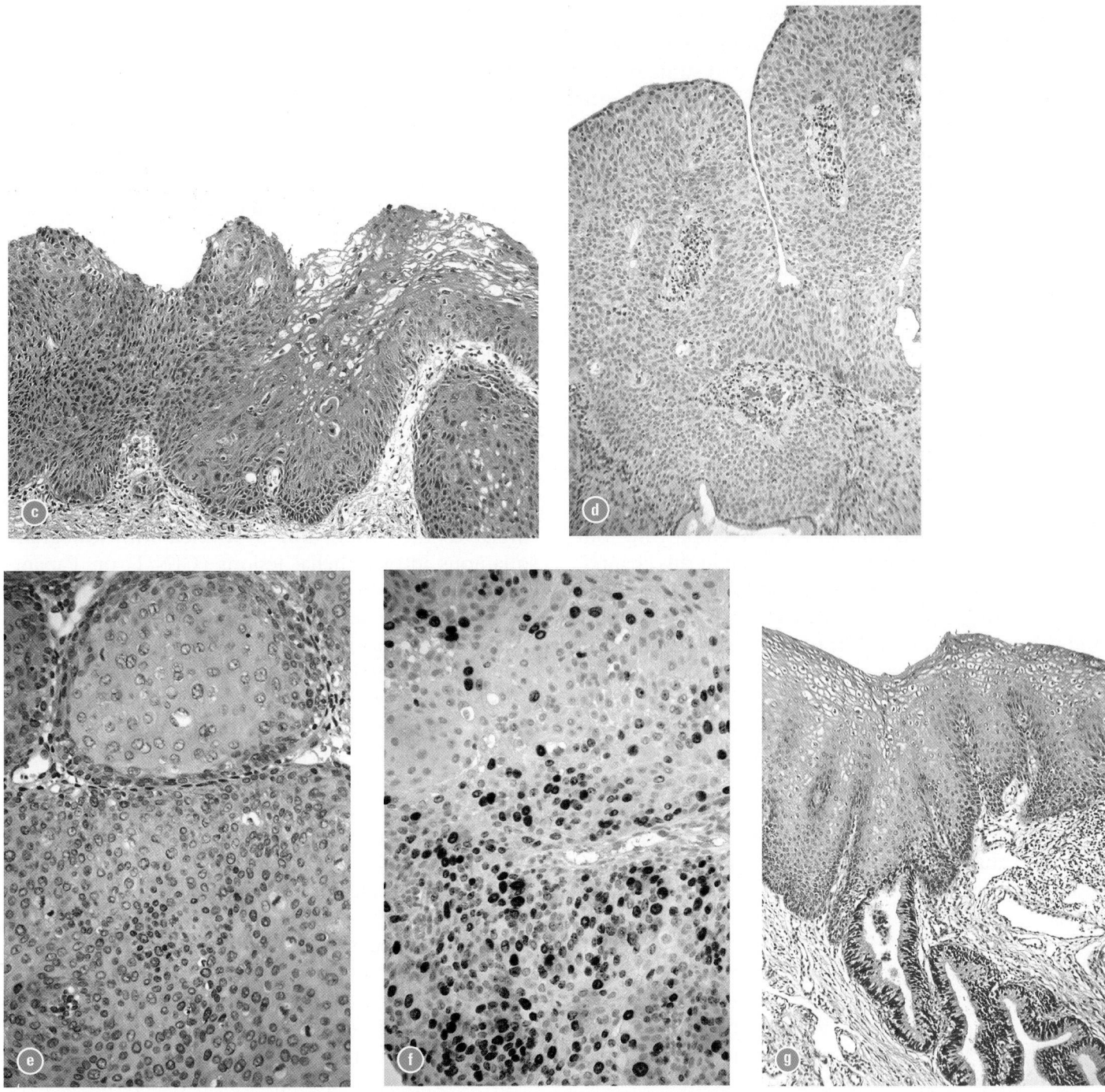

Fig. 13.26 **Cont'd** and horizontal sampling error in which multiple grades are present in the horizontal plane (c). Immature condyloma (LSIL; d) at higher power exhibits both low (e, upper) and high (e, lower) grade nuclei. Note the corresponding disparity of Ki-67 staining nuclei in the same areas (f). This lesion contained both HPV type 6 and 16 nucleic acids. Co-existing LSIL (HPV-II) and adenocarcinoma *in-situ* (lower, HPV-16) (g).

that when faced with a cytologic diagnosis of HSIL the pathologist carefully avoid the *over-diagnosis* of LSIL on histology. Such a diagnosis can be particularly confusing as it may mislead the clinician into assuming LSIL is present, when in fact the HSIL has actually eluded sampling.

THERAPEUTIC OPTIONS

The guidelines for managing women with cytologic and histologic abnormalities are summarized in recent publications based on the ASCCP consensus conference of September 2001 (available: http://consensus.

asccp.org/). Practitioners who do not routinely use cryotherapy are faced with two options, follow-up for LSIL and ablation for HSIL. These two strategies are rooted in the expectation that LSIL will frequently regress and HSIL must be removed and followed. Thus, the clinician must know what to expect if he or she elects not to ablate an LSIL and what factors place a woman at risk following attempted ablation. Three issues that must be understood are the expectations and pitfalls of histologic interpretation, natural history of low-grade squamous intraepithelial lesions and parameters requiring attention following attempted ablation.

Diagnostic reproducibility in histology

There are numerous studies that have addressed the issue of reproducibility in practice:[184] virtually all report between poor and good reproducibility in discriminating three grades of CIN. Relatively few studies exist that examine intra- and interobserver reproducibility with a two-grade system. In a study employing four observers and with the criteria outlined in this chapter, reproducibility was in aggregate good at $k = 0.54$. Some observer pairs had good to excellent reproducibility and others fair to good.[142] Internal reproducibility also varied widely between observers. In an unpublished study focusing on difficult cases, most of which were abnormal, the author had internal reproducibility for normal, non-diagnostic atypia, LSIL and HSIL of $k = 0.85, 0.37, 0.80$ and 0.80, respectively. Reproducibility for HSIL sub-categories of CIN II and CIN III were 0.56, suggesting that the sub-division of CIN II from CIN III cannot be made as consistently, even with the same observer.

Two-grade vs three- or four-grade classification systems

This chapter outlines a two-grade approach to grading squamous intraepithelial lesions that is designed for a management strategy that follows LSIL and ablates HSIL with LEEP, as is currently done in many practices. Practices that use less-traumatic methods of ablation, such as cryotherapy, have the option of treating LSIL and many HSILs with this method, leaving the distinction of CIN I from CIN II moot. However, LEEP is sufficiently traumatic to mandate that at least a portion of patients be spared this option; yet these same patients take the risk, however small, of developing a more serious lesion during follow-up. The dual classification as described here is designed specifically to segregate cervical intraepithelial lesions in such a way that the diagnosis of LSIL will confer minimal risk if the patient were to be lost to follow-up.

Follow-up of biopsy-proven SIL without treatment

How safe is following squamous intraepithelial lesions without treatment? According to the ALTS trial, approximately 1 in 1000 cases of ASCUS had a coexisting invasive carcinoma.[185] Once colposcopic examination and biopsy exclude carcinoma, the issue concerns the safety of follow-up alone after biopsy documentation. In practice, HSIL will be ablated and LSIL will be ablated or followed, but this discussion will address both LSIL and HSIL.

There is a weak relationship between CIN I (or condyloma) and cancer risk, with 1–3% of cases with mild dyskaryosis on the Papanicolaou smear progressing to cancer. The risk of CIN II (moderate dyskaryosis) is similar or slightly higher.[185–188] Regression rates for CIN I range widely, from 30–60%, although a sizable minority will not regress at 1 year.[188] The progression rate to CIN III has been computed up to 35%, with a figure of 11% in Ostor's review.[188] The latter figure is similar to the proportion of women with low-grade squamous intraepithelial lesions (CIN I) on Papanicolaou smears, who prove to have a histologically high-grade precursor lesion (CIN II–III).[149,150] Clearly, a significant proportion of high-risk HPV infections resolve, given the high frequency of such infections in low-grade smears. In a recent study, Cox et al. found that the 2-year outcomes of HSIL following (a) a biopsy diagnosis of LSIL, (b) an LSIL-positive smear with a negative biopsy and (c) an HPV-positive ASCUS that was colposcopically negative, were from 11 to 13%.[189]

Lesions associated with HPV 6 and 11 confer essentially no direct risk of cancer. However, HPV 6 and 11 are surrogate risk factors and identify persons at greater risk for other HPV infections.[14] Low-grade intraepithelial lesions associated with intermediate- and high-risk HPV types have a high rate of spontaneous regression and empirically low risk of progressing to invasive carcinoma.[14] Recent studies are consistent with the fact that many LSILs spontaneously regress.[189]

Invasive cancers are uncommonly associated with LSIL. We have seen three cases of LSIL cytology followed by cancer. One was a keratinizing lesion that was under-diagnosed, the second was a case of koilocytosis accompanied by some cells diagnostic of moderate dysplasia and the last was a CIN I concurrent with invasive carcinoma. Thus, only one of the three was a 'bona fide' LSIL. However, as mentioned above, classic LSILs, including condylomata, may be associated with HSIL as a consequence of either progression or two coexisting HPV infections. Recognizing this, the practitioner should use caution when following LSILs that have been preceded by a cytologic diagnosis of HSIL.

Invasive carcinomas rarely follow LSIL and are almost always preceded by HSIL.[17] Studies investigating the first abnormal smear preceding cervical cancer have found that over 80% contain CIN III (severe dyskaryosis), even as long as 20 years prior to the diagnosis of invasive carcinoma. As mentioned above, koilocytosis uncommonly is present on smears predating cancer and, when present, is associated with younger age, which calls into question its etiologic significance in such cases.[187,190,191]

HPV testing of biopsies is of uncertain value in determining which patients should be treated and which should be followed. Inasmuch as high-risk HPVs are frequently associated with lesions that will not progress, little information of value will be obtained by HPV testing alone. If HPV testing were the driving force behind management, a large proportion of LSILs would be ablated.

In summary, conservative management of women with LSIL diagnosis on biopsy requires that: (1) the biopsy correlates with the Papanicolaou smear; (2) the biopsy findings correlate with the colposcopic impression; and (3) follow-up can be assured. Ablation must be considered if a subsequent smear displays a persisting or higher-grade lesion that is verified by colposcopic examination.

Ablative (electrical excision, LEEP or LLETZ, cone biopsy or cryocautery)

Management of the LEEP specimen

Processing and interpretation: LEEP specimens may come in one or several fragments, well-oriented or impossible to reconstruct. The prosector must identify the mucosal surface and section each fragment perpendicular to the long axis. Margins should be designated only where a cautery artifact can be identified (Fig. 13.27a,b). Thus, there are basically three options in reporting margins: involved, uninvolved, or not amenable to evaluation due to distortion or excessive cautery artifact. If the lesion extends to an edge, but the edge does not contain thermal artifact, margin involvement is not confirmed (Fig. 13.28a–c).

Interpretation of the endocervical curettage. The purpose of performing an immediate post-treatment endocervical evaluation is to assist in determining the risk for recurrent or persistent disease and to delineate endocervical pathology. When performed at the time of excisional surgery, ECC has been shown to have excellent correlation with conization histopathologic results[179,180] and negative predictive value, particularly when conization margins are negative as well.[192] A positive ECC at the time of conization is also predictive of residual disease in the hysterectomy specimen.[193–196] The main limitation of ECC in this application is its potential for contamination with ectocervical cells

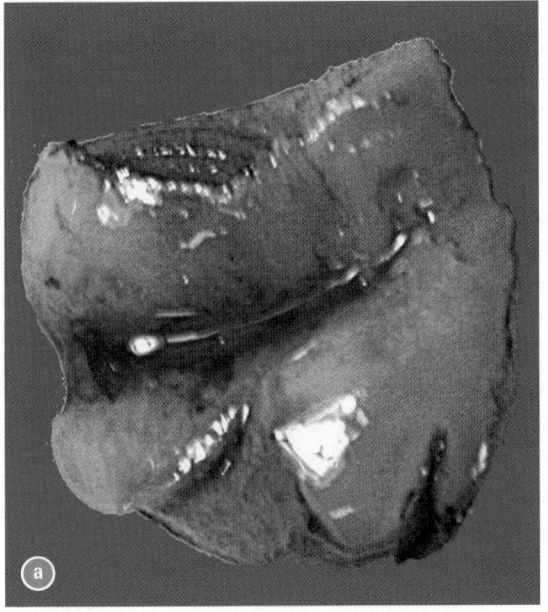

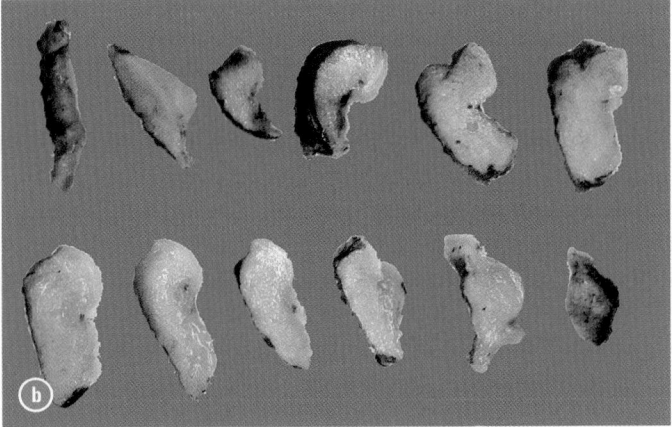

Fig. 13.27 Sectioning of LEEP specimens. Intact specimen (a) and following serial sectioning in a clockwise orientation (b).

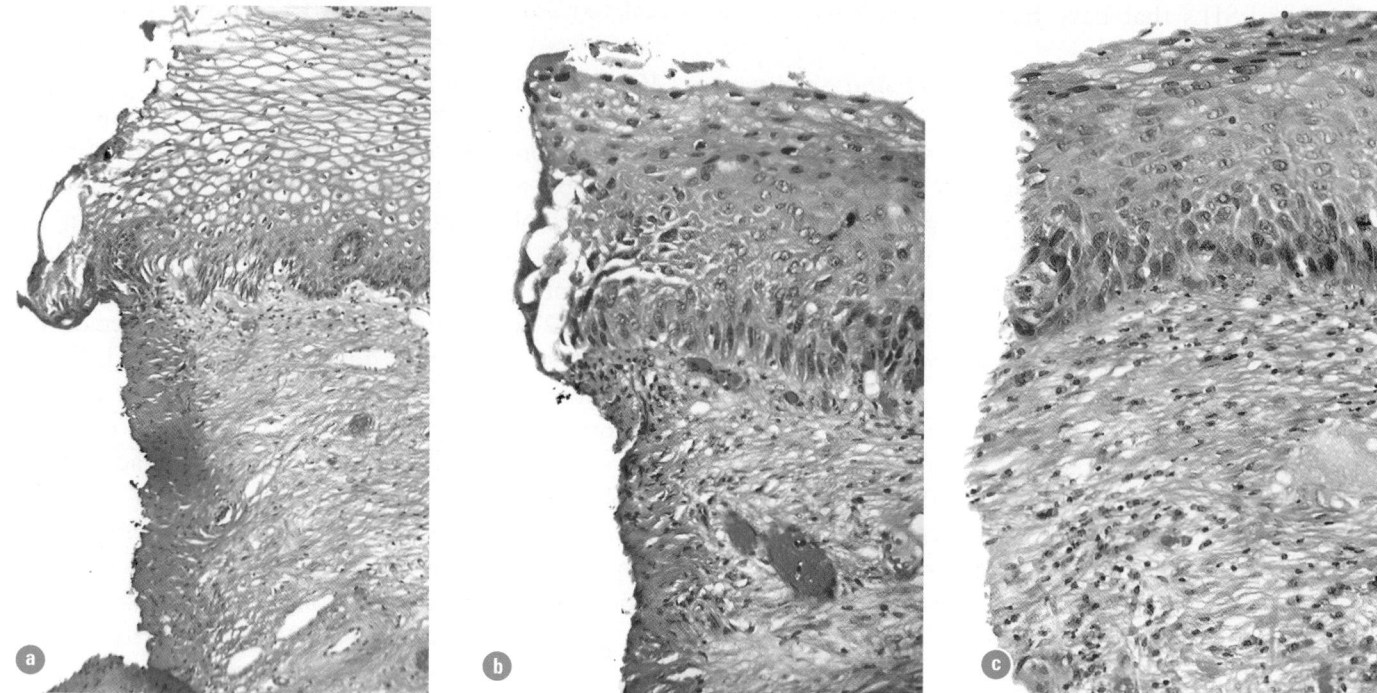

Fig. 13.28 Margins seen in LEEP specimens include normal cauterized edge (a), cauterized edge with HSIL (b) and edge with HSIL that has no cautery present (c). The latter is not interpreted as a margin.

yielding a false-positive result and decreasing its specificity.[197] The endobrush appears to be at least as sensitive if not more sensitive than the endocervical curette.[181,182,198] A positive ECC at conization increases the risk of invasive carcinoma in the residual cervix of patients whose conization revealed high-grade intraepithelial neoplasia at the margin. The risk is greatest in women over 50, or whose colposcopic evaluation is unsatisfactory. When neoplastic epithelium is encountered in the ECC, the pathologist must make the effort to determine if the neoplastic epithelium is derived from an invasive lesion. This is not always easily accomplished, but certain clues, such as poorly-oriented neoplastic epithelium, aberrant differentiation, or papillary architecture, may signify underlying invasion.

The status of the margin is also a predictor for recurrent disease regardless of whether conization was performed.[199,200] There were eight major studies reported in the 1970s and 1980s that encompass 3894 cones. In this group, there were 3066 with cleared margins and an overall 2.9% rate of recurrence or persistence. There were 828 cones (21.3%) with involved margins, with 22% rate of recurrence or persistence. In a review of 20 articles, positive margins varied from 13% to 45%. Recurrences with positive margins ranged from 10% to 69% and from 5% to 38%, with negative margins. Although the presence of involved margins does not necessarily indicate the need for immediate further action other than careful observation in most cases, patients should be counseled on increased risk for persistent or recurrent disease.[201]

In summary, the assessment of surgical margins should be attempted on all specimens sent for pathologic review. Endocervical evaluation and margin status may predict risk for recurrent or persistent disease. For the endocervical evaluation, it is acceptable to use either an ECC or an endobrush, although the latter has limited specificity when employed immediately following excision.[201]

Post excision follow-up

Parameters that influence outcome following excisional or ablative therapy, include: (1) size of lesion treated, (2) presence or absence of a positive endocervical curetting during or following the cone biopsy, (3) presence or absence of positive ecto- or endocervical margins in excised specimens, (4) post-therapy cytology and (5) HPV status post therapy. This discussion addresses risks of recurrence and the role of cytology and HPV testing in managing these patients.

1 The percentage of patients with abnormal histologic outcome that are preceded by an

abnormal cytology. Most if not all positive histologic outcomes are associated with abnormal cytology.[202,203]

2 The percentage of those with normal post-procedural cytology with an abnormal histologic outcome. Buxton et al. found that none of those with normal post-procedural cytology examinations had a histologically confirmed SIL. The study by McIndoe et al., which used cancer as an end-point, found that 1.5% of cases were not preceded by an abnormal cytology.[204] However, Paterson-Brown et al. reported that 45% of cases with persistent SIL post cone had normal cytology.[205]

3 The percentage of those with abnormal cytology who had an abnormal histologic outcome. Buxton et al. and Paterson-Brown et al. showed that 42% and 60% of women with abnormal cytologies had biopsy-proven SIL, respectively.[205,206]

4 Causes of reported abnormalities in Papanicolaou smears following cone biopsy include not only squamous cell abnormalities but also thermal artifacts following LEEP and spurious glandular cell atypias due to sampling of lower uterine segment. The evidence indicates that, for most studies, post-procedural cytology is a sensitive test for recurrent disease, but carries a small false-negative rate. Specificity may vary depending on the experience of the cytopathologist and variables (cautery artifact, changes in anatomy) that alter the nature of the post-procedure cytologic specimen.

Recent studies confirm a high sensitivity for HPV testing in the detection of SIL. In a survey of 1518 unselected women attending routine cytologic screening, Clavel et al. found that 34 of 34 women with biopsy-proven HSIL and 68 of 70 women with positive cone biopsies scored positive for HPV by Hybrid Capture II.[207] In a study of patients with ASCUS, Solomon et al. reported a sensitivity of 95% for HC II. Specificity was lower, with a positive predictive value of approximately 20% for ASCUS. Two studies by Lin et al. and Jain et al. analyzed the relationship between HPV status following cone biopsy and disease detected at hysterectomy.[208,209] Predictably, most of these patients had positive cone margins. The negative predictive value of HPV testing approaches 100%. A third study by Chua and Hjerpe corroborates this conclusion. They found that 25 of 26 women with recurrences scored positive for HPV.[210]

As shown above, in the studies by Lin et al. and Jain et al., specificity of HPV testing was 52 and 14%, indicating that papillomavirus may persist in the absence of recurrence.[208,209] This is in contrast to the study by Chua et al., in which none of the post-cone cytologic specimens from 22 patients with normal follow-up scored HPV positive.[210] Thus, HPV testing, when negative, has a high negative predictive value for HSIL. When combined with a negative cytologic examination, the risk of residual HSIL is negligible. Thus, HPV testing is recommended under circumstances in which exclusion of HSIL is clinically important.

It is important to emphasize that despite the level of sensitivity, the specificity of HPV testing varies as a function of time interval following cone biopsy. Excepting the findings of Chua et al., data from the other two studies indicate that a significant number of women will score positive for HPV immediately following ablative therapy, even if they show no histologic evidence of lesion persistence. This may be explained by transient disease at the cone margins or occult infection, either in normal tissues or vaginal lesions that went unnoticed. Nuovo and Pedemonte showed that additional lesions may develop after cryotherapy and are associated with viruses other than those responsible for the lesion treated initially.[211] Strand et al. found that HPV frequently persisted following therapy for genital HPV infections, similar to the observations by Ferenczy et al., who found occult HPV adjacent to genital warts.[212,213]

Notwithstanding the association of occult HPV infection with active genital warts, studies indicate that, over time, HPV will disappear from the cervix. Other reports have shown that the index of HPV positivity diminishes with age. Tate et al. showed that HPV was uncommonly detected in the normal mucosa adjacent to CIN, suggesting that the virus does not persist indefinitely in the normal mucosa from which lesions develop.[214] Strand et al. found that at 6–12 months following cone biopsy or laser vaporization, only 27 of 30 women were HPV positive.[213] These studies suggest that the time interval between ablation and follow-up testing may influence the index of HPV positivity.

In summary, when considering HPV testing as an adjunct to the Papanicolaou smear, the following can be expected:

1 Repeated Pap smear screening is equivalent to HPV testing in sensitivity for recurrent disease.

2 The sensitivity and negative predictive value of HPV testing is high and can be used either as an adjunct to cytology or – more importantly – as a tool to exclude non-specific atypias developing post ablation.

3 HPV testing done prior to 1 year post-ablation is not recommended unless the patient has a cytologic abnormality.

4 A negative HPV test at 1 year, combined with a negative smear, carries a very high negative predictive value.

The above recommendations for management are guidelines and their adherence will vary considerably between practitioners. McKee et al. demonstrated that a minority of practitioners conformed to published guidelines.[215]

Diagnosis and management of invasive squamous cell carcinoma

INTRODUCTION

Approximately 11 000 women/year develop carcinoma of the cervix. The majority occur between ages 40 and 55 with approximately 10% less than 30 years of age when diagnosed. The predominate histologic type is squamous (80%) and approximately 50% are Stage I when diagnosed. Of Stage I tumors, 10–15% will be less than 5 mm in depth (Stage IA). Survival is close to 100% for Stage IA1 and diminishes significantly with invasion beyond 5 mm and extension beyond the cervix (Stage IIA) (Tables 13.10, 13.11).[216,217]

Colposcopic, cytologic and histologic predictors of malignancy

Sensitivity and specificity of the Papanicolaou smear for invasion

The clinician will either suspect the diagnosis of invasion based on symptomatology, the cytologic report, and on colposcopic examination, or will discover the invasion following pathologic examination. The biopsy will corroborate a smear diagnosis of invasive cancer in nearly 90% of cases.[218] In contrast, when the smear is 'suspicious' for invasion or microinvasion, the predicted value drops to 22% and 17%, respectively.[219] Sensitivity of the smear for microinvasion increases as a function of lesion depth, ranging from 14% to 88% for lesions less than 1 mm, and greater than 2.0 mm in depth.[219,220] The cytologic features of invasive cervical cancer will be discussed in detail later in the chapter. As a rule, approximately 1 in 1000, 650 and 150 ASCUS, LSIL and HSIL smears will be followed by a diagnosis of invasive squamous cell carcinoma on biopsy.[185,221] The frequency will be higher for biopsy-proven HSIL (see below). Clark and Dawson reviewed 13 cases of biopsy-proven cervical cancer and noted that all were preceded by a cytologic diagnosis of carcinoma

Table 13.10 *Staging of cervical squamous carcinoma (FIGO)*[233,234,312]

Stage I	Tumor is strictly confined to cervix
IA	Preclinical carcinomas of cervix diagnosed only by microscopy. All gross lesions even with superficial invasion are Stage IB cancers. Invasion is limited to measured stromal invasion with maximum depth of 5.0 mm and no wider than 7.0 mm
IA1	Stromal invasion no greater than 3.0 mm and no wider than 7.0 mm[a]
IA2	Maximum depth of invasion of stroma greater than 3 mm and no greater than 5 mm taken from base of epithelium, either surface or glandular, from which it originates; horizontal invasion not more than 7 mm
IB	Clinical lesions confined to the cervix or preclinical lesions greater than Stage IA
IB1	Clinical lesion no longer than 4.0 cm in size
IB2	Clinical lesion greater than 4.0 cm in size
Stage II	Extension beyond cervix but not to pelvic wall. Involves vagina, but not the lower-third
IIA	Involves vagina, but not lower-third. No obvious extension to parametria
IIB	Involves vagina, but not lower-third. Obvious parametrial involvement
Stage III	Extension to pelvic wall. On rectal exam, no cancer-free space between tumor and pelvic wall. Involves lower-third of vagina
IIIA	No extension to pelvic side wall
IIIB	Extension to pelvic side wall
Stage IV	Extension beyond true pelvis or involvement of bladder or rectal mucosa. Bullous edema does not permit a case to be assigned to Stage IV

FIGO, International Federation of Gynecology and Obstetrics.
[a]Definition of microinvasion by the SGO includes these criteria plus absence of capillary-lymphatic space invasion.

Table 13.11 *Stage-specific frequency, mean age and outcome of cervical carcinoma*[313]

Stage	(%)	Mean age	5-year survival (%)
IA1	(4.4)	44.5	99
IA2	(3.2)	44.6	97
IB	(39)	48.6	80
IIA	(6.9)	55.5	66
IIB	(2.2)	53.7	64
IIIA	(1.5)	63.0	33
IIIB	(19.8)	56.4	39
IVA	(2.5)	60.1	17
IVB	(1.7)	58.1	9

(or suspicious for carcinoma), with 12 out of the 13 showing a tumor diathesis characterized by cellular debris and blood. However, they noted a reduced cellularity in many and suggested that the diathesis and inflammatory cells may block filter coverage by epithelial cells.[222] Einhorn et al. performed a meta-analysis of five studies encompassing 61 cases with both conventional and liquid-based cytology. A diagnosis of cancer was made in 88.5% and 85.2% of the liquid-based and conventional smears, respectively. Cases not diagnosed as cancer were classified as abnormal, ranging from atypical glandular cells of undetermined significance to high-grade squamous intraepithelial lesions.[217]

Tumor diathesis is traditionally associated with invasive squamous cell carcinoma of the cervix but is not invariably present. Rushing and Cibas examined 28 smears from 19 patients with squamous carcinoma and reported diathesis in 54%, with diathesis correlating with depth of invasion. They concluded that the distinction between an intraepithelial lesion and a shallow invasive cancer may not always be possible on cervicovaginal smears.[223]

Cytologic alterations most commonly associated with 'missed' invasive carcinomas

The following changes are uncommonly associated with cancer, but in experience based principally on medical legal consultations, the five major pitfalls in recognizing invasive squamous or glandular carcinomas and their precursors include the misclassification (or under-appreciation) of the following (Fig. 13.29):

1 *Keratinizing lesions*: Abnormal keratinizing cells must be approached with caution (Fig. 13.29a) and the diagnosis of LSIL to describe such lesions without some qualification is not recommended.

2 *Immature squamous cells with a metaplastic cell phenotype* (Fig. 13.29b): Atypical immature squamous cells with a metaplastic phenotype are among the more difficult to identify and appreciate. With the higher index of suspicion seen in current practice, the over-diagnosis of innocuous immature metaplasia is also likely, particularly on liquid-based preparations.

3 *Hyperchromatic clumped groups (HCGs) of cells* (Fig. 13.29c): Invasive squamous or adenocarcinomas may present with sheets of cells with variable degrees of nuclear atypia. Typically, these cell aggregates overlap, exhibit nuclear enlargement and prominent nucleoli. They may be misinterpreted as endometrial, lower

uterine segment and endocervical cells. These are discussed in greater detail in Chapter 14.

4 *HSIL or carcinoma associated with 'classic' koilocytosis (rare)*: It is estimated that approximately 0.1% of LSIL smears will be followed by a diagnosis of squamous cell carcinoma. The authors have encountered two cases of this type, one of which contained in addition cells raising the possibility of a higher-grade SIL in addition to LSIL (Fig. 13.29d,e).

5 *'Reactive appearing' but atypical endocervical cells*. Adenocarcinomas of the cervix may occasionally present with small clusters of cells closely resembling reactive changes.

Clinical detection of invasion

When a mass lesion is present, the diagnosis of invasion is not difficult (Fig 13.30). However, the colposcopist can expect to miss a significant proportion of early invasive squamous cell carcinomas of the cervix. In one study, the sensitivity of colposcopy for microinvasion was 50%, but specificity was 91%. In one-third of cases, neither the colposcopic examination nor the Papanicolaou smear identified invasion.[224] Atypical vessels were found in only one-third of cases in the study by Liu et al.[225]

The principal characteristics of invasion by colposcopy are the following.[226]

Percent of HSILs associated with (micro)invasion

The proportion of biopsy-proven HSILs associated with early invasion varies from less than 1%, to 7%.[221] In a recent clinical trial of 125 women with documented HSIL who were followed for 6 months, one (0.8%) was found to have invasion on cone biopsy.[221]

Risk of invasion following treatment for HSIL

Soutter et al. observed over 2000 women with over 44000 woman-years of follow-up. A total of 33 developed invasive cancer: 14 microinvasive with a cumulative rate of invasion 8 years after treatment of 5.8 per 1000 women and 85 per 100000 woman-years.[227] The risk of developing cancer did not change throughout the follow-up period and the authors concluded that conservative outpatient therapy reduced the risk of invasive cancer by 95% during the first 8 years after treatment. However, even with careful, long-term follow-up, the risk of invasive cervical cancer among these women is about five-fold the general population of women. The authors recommended continued follow-up for at least 10 years after conservative treatment of CIN.[228]

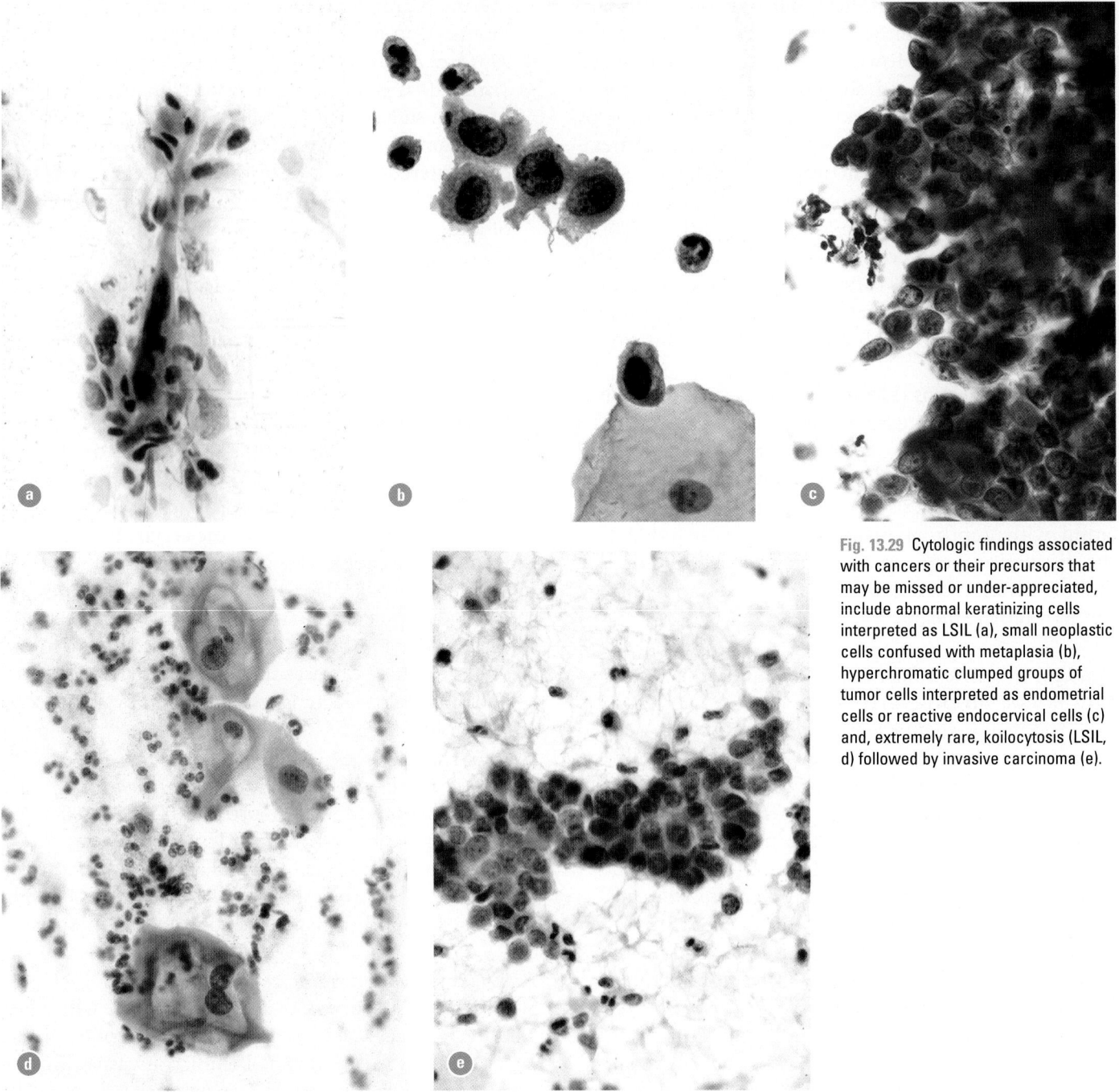

Fig. 13.29 Cytologic findings associated with cancers or their precursors that may be missed or under-appreciated, include abnormal keratinizing cells interpreted as LSIL (a), small neoplastic cells confused with metaplasia (b), hyperchromatic clumped groups of tumor cells interpreted as endometrial cells or reactive endocervical cells (c) and, extremely rare, koilocytosis (LSIL, d) followed by invasive carcinoma (e).

Features of HSIL portending stromal invasion

In general, there is no method that will predict which high-grade SIL will progress to invasion. However, some authors have identified features more commonly seen in HSILs associated with invasive carcinoma. These include: (1) extensive involvement of surface epithelium and deep endocervical crypts by expansile CIN III, (2) luminal necrosis and (3) intraepithelial squamous maturation (Fig. 13.31a,b). Other features of concern include disorganized epithelial growth in which the epithelium contains discrete independent units of proliferating cells (Fig. 13.31c,d), papillary architecture (Fig. 13.31e) and, possibly, the presence of other forms of differentiation in the form of conspicuous mucin production (Fig. 13.31f).[229] Tidbury et al. found that the extent of HSIL was seven-fold higher in cases with invasion.[230] Unusual fibrous proliferations in the stroma should also alert the pathologist to the possible presence

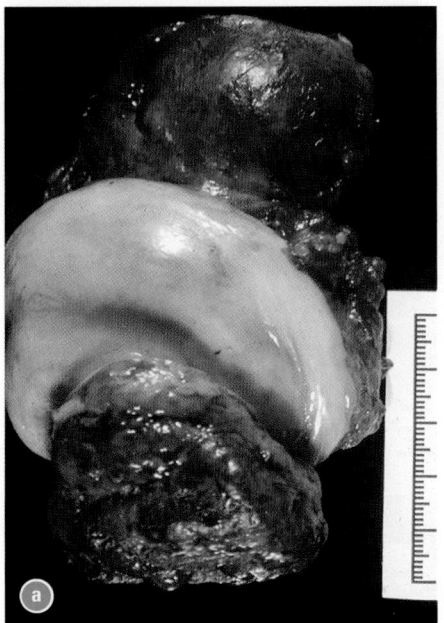 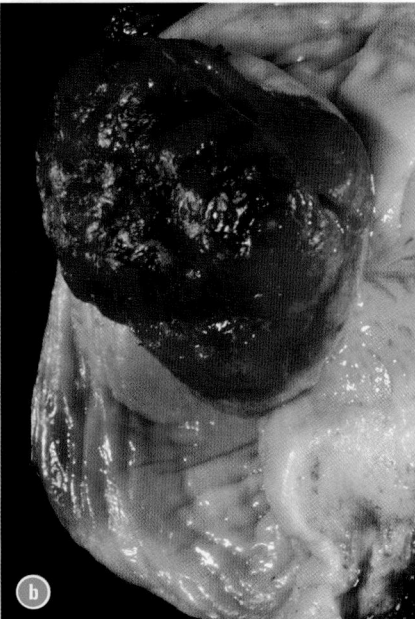 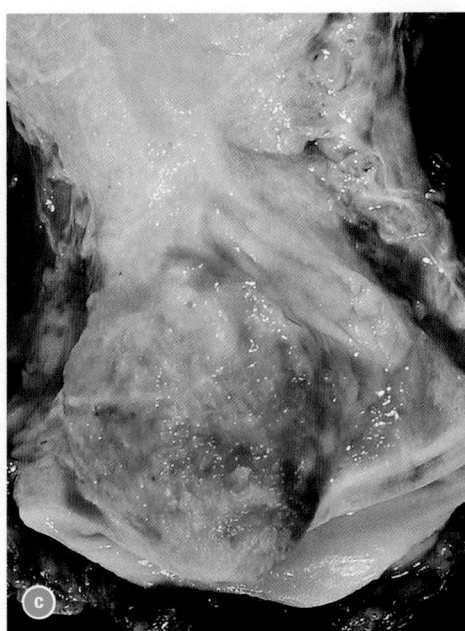

Fig. 13.30 Gross appearance of invasive squamous cell carcinoma (a) seen as a fungating mass at the os in the opened cervix (b). A smaller carcinoma is situated at the squamo-columnar junction (c).

of invasion, although the same may be produced by biopsy artifacts. Under certain circumstances, a diagnosis of invasion may be suspected in the evaluation of an endocervical curettage based on the above criteria.

DIAGNOSIS OF INVASION

Introduction

Before classifying a cervical tissue sample as invasive carcinoma, the pathologist must clear four diagnostic hurdles, which comprise determining if invasion is present, excluding mimics, applying the criteria for microinvasion and advising the clinician with the use of appropriate reporting.

As mentioned above, abnormal differentiation, increased epithelial thickness, loss of polarity, altered differentiation and mucin production may herald a greater risk of invasion.[229,230] The latter is often associated with adenocarcinoma *in situ* and we have observed a high rate of early invasion when this variable is present. However, ultimately, the diagnosis rests on criteria specific for stromal invasion.

How does one approach 'borderline microinvasion'? Although it is not an accepted category, borderline microinvasion (less than 1 mm) was defined by Wilkinson and Komorowski and its risk assessed.[231] The authors noted that 4.8% and 27% of CIS and

microinvasive lesions were reclassified as 'borderline invasion'. They found no metastases in the 29 cases followed. The implication is that a diagnosis of suspicious for, or diagnostic of, very early stromal invasion (or that which is suspicious for invasion) can be managed conservatively.

Criteria for invasive squamous cell carcinoma

The most commonly used criteria for invasion include the following: (1) a desmoplastic response in the adjacent stroma (Fig. 13.32a); (2) focal conspicuous maturation of the neoplastic epithelium with prominent nucleoli (Fig. 13.32a,b); (3) blurring of the epithelial-stromal interface; and (4) loss of polarity of the nuclei at the epithelial-stromal border with absence of the palisaded pattern characteristic of CIN (Fig. 13.32b). Three additional features include: (5) scalloping of the margins at the epithelial-stromal interface (Fig. 13.32c) – scalloping refers to fine irregularities, which are not typically seen with gland (crypt) involvement or tangential sectioning through gland involvement;[232] (6) the appearance of 'pseudo-crypt involvement' (Fig. 13.32d,e); and (7) the apparent 'folding or duplication' of the neoplastic epithelium (Fig. 13.32f). Duplication of epithelium refers to the presence of vascular structures within a sheet of neoplastic epithelial cells, producing an image of incompletely formed

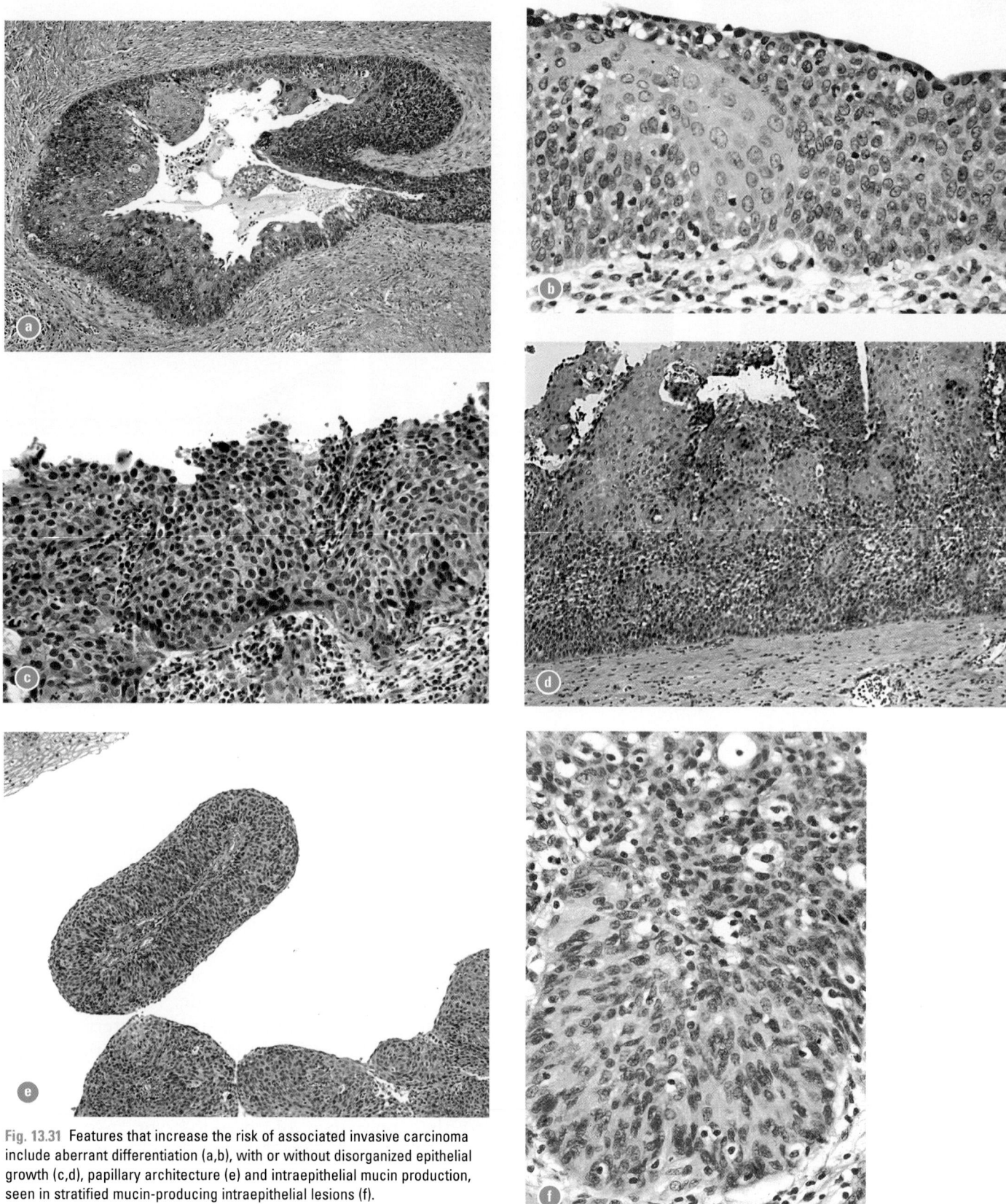

Fig. 13.31 Features that increase the risk of associated invasive carcinoma include aberrant differentiation (a,b), with or without disorganized epithelial growth (c,d), papillary architecture (e) and intraepithelial mucin production, seen in stratified mucin-producing intraepithelial lesions (f).

papillae. These features aid in recognizing invasion in the presence of an intense inflammatory response, which may obscure desmoplasia on the one hand and blur the epithelial-stromal interface on the other.[6] Pseudo-crypt involvement is defined as discrete circumscribed nests of invasive carcinoma, usually with central necrosis, that may mimic crypt involvement. In contrast to crypts, this form of invasive carcinoma does not exhibit glandular epithelium, is often composed of multiple circumscribed nests, often contains central necrosis, and may display a loss of polarity.[229]

Differential diagnosis of invasion (Fig. 13.33a–f)

A previous review of 265 cases of presumed microinvasion sent to the Gynecologic Oncology Group determined that approximately one-third were over-

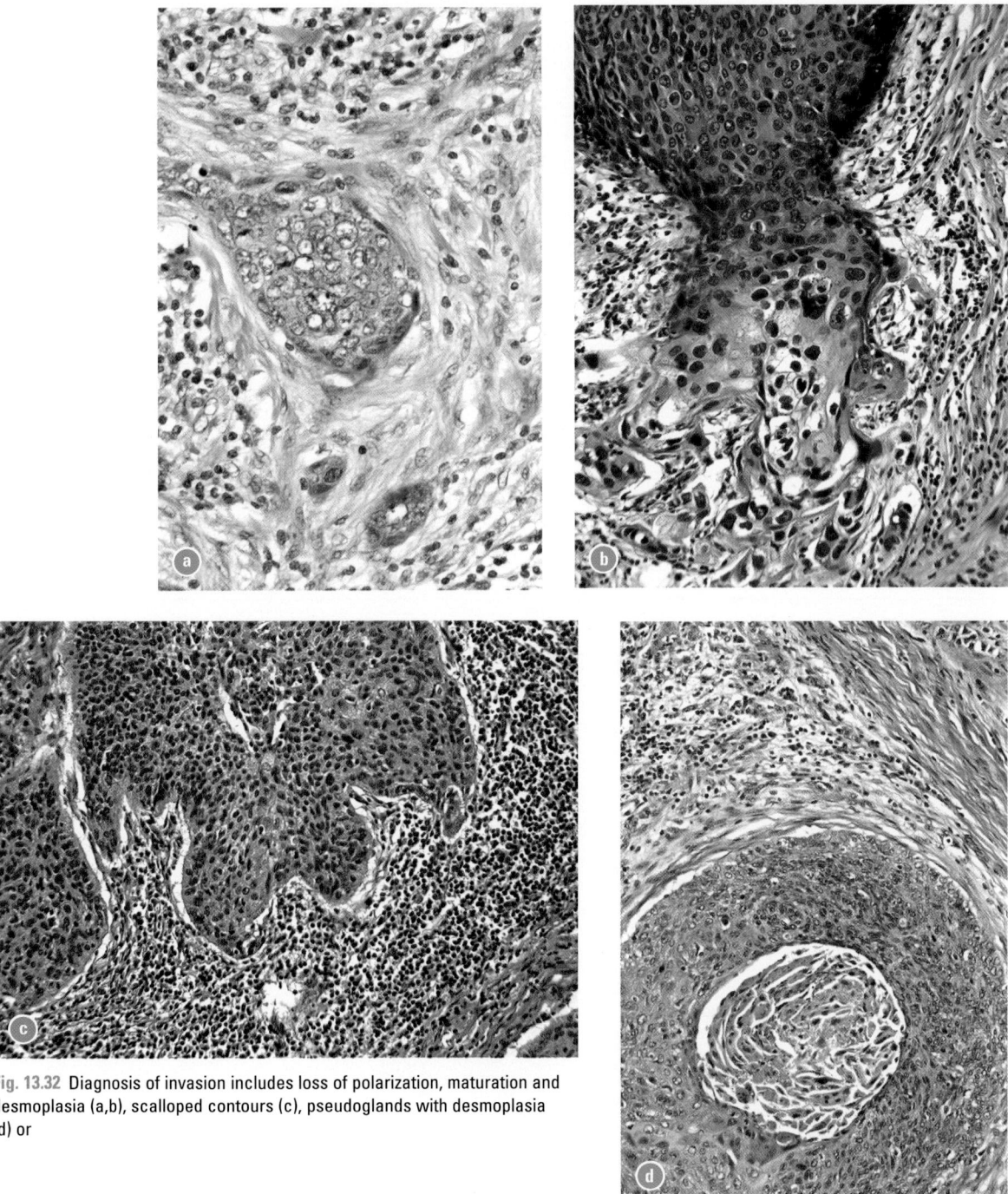

Fig. 13.32 Diagnosis of invasion includes loss of polarization, maturation and desmoplasia (a,b), scalloped contours (c), pseudoglands with desmoplasia (d) or

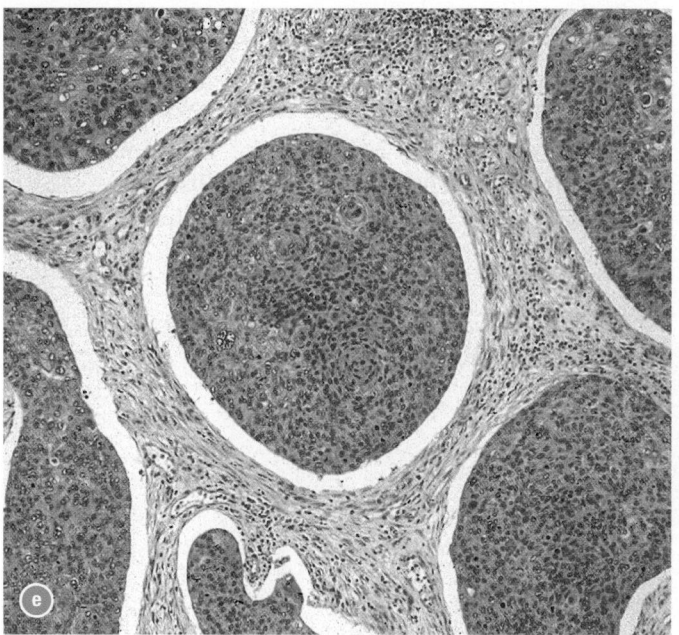

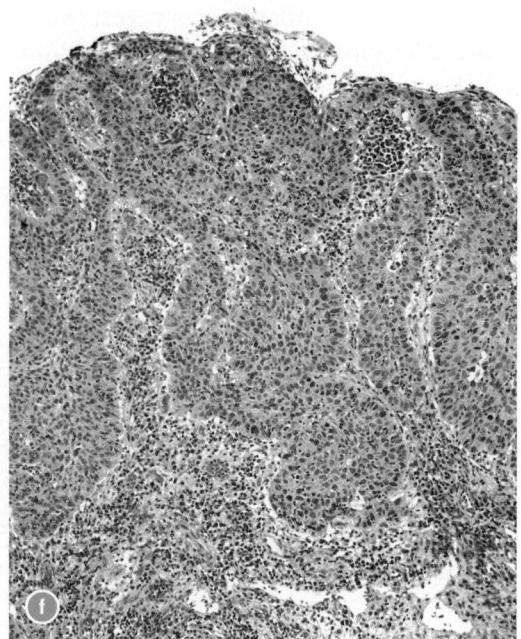

Fig. 13.32 **Cont'd** retraction artifacts (e); and complex interlacing growth patterns ('epithelial duplication', f).

diagnosed intraepithelial lesions, underscoring the potential problems in lesion interpretation.[233] The most important mimics of microinvasion include:

1 Tangentially sectioned epithelium, benign or neoplastic (Fig. 13.33a)
2 Prior biopsy sites (Fig. 13.33b)
3 Inflammatory or reparative changes in CIN, including pseudoepitheliomatous changes (Fig. 13.33c)
4 Obscuring of the epithelial-stromal interface by inflammation or other artifacts (Fig. 13.33d)
5 Crypt (gland) involvement that is inflamed or tangentially sectioned (Fig. 13.33e,f)

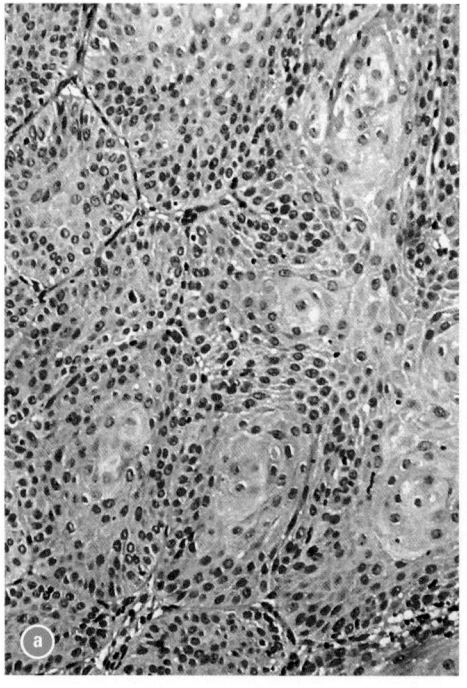

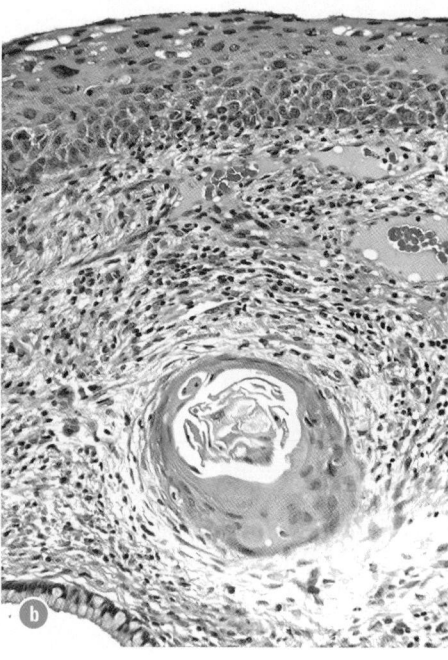

Fig. 13.33 Mimics of invasion include tangential section of metaplasia (a), displaced benign epithelium from a biopsy artifact (b),

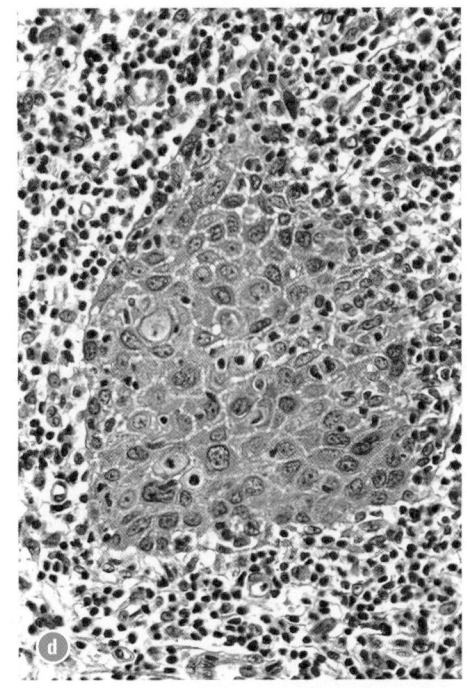

Fig. 13.33 Cont'd
pseudoepitheliomatous hyperplasia in a SIL (due to underlying submucosal leiomyoma) (c), disrupted benign mucosa with inflammation (d) and extensive crypt involvement with inflammation (e). The latter is distinguished form invasive carcinoma by the retention of superficial columnar cells on the lumenal surface (f, lower right).

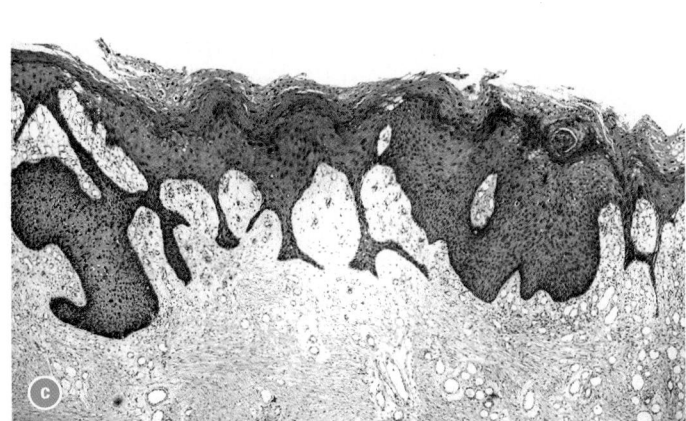

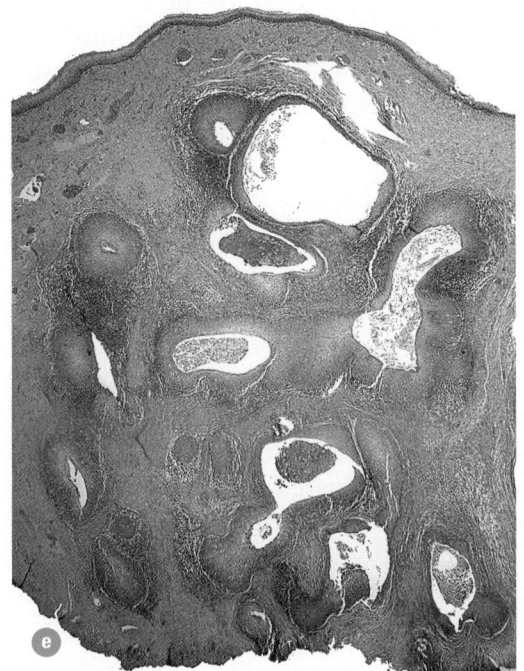

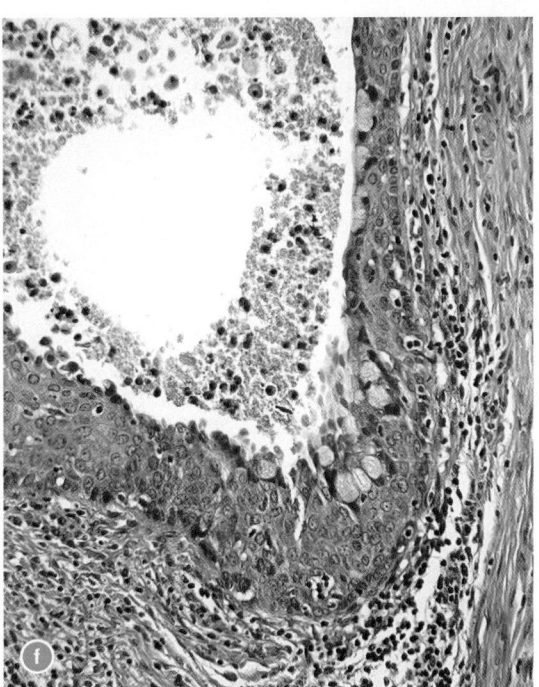

6   Cautery or crush artifact
7   Misinterpretation of cancer in the ECC, including implantation site and floaters from other sites.

Crypt involvement is characterized by preservation of epithelial polarity, a smooth epithelial-stromal interface and, in contrast to the parameter of duplication, each nest of epithelium is discrete and separate from the adjacent one. Artifacts are usually produced by prior biopsy, in which a stromal response may be present. They should not be associated with the other parameters of invasion. Cautery or crush artifact should be recognized and reported if it hinders diagnosis. Inflammatory changes are responsible for the greatest diagnostic difficulty, as these alterations may blur the epithelial-stromal interface or, in combination with prior trauma, be associated with small nests of epithelium in the inflammatory cell infiltrates. The laboratory management of these findings is to obtain levels to determine if additional features of invasive carcinoma are present and obtain consultation if there is a question of invasion in a cone specimen. Factors influencing management include whether the areas in question are in continuity with, or within 1 mm of, the surface epithelium, are limited to one or two foci, are not associated with other parameters of invasion, including capillary-lymphatic space invasion, and are associated with clear margins. Intraepithelial lesions associated with underlying inflammation, either from secondary infection or previous biopsy, must be evaluated carefully to avoid the over-diagnosis of invasion when the epithelial-stromal interface is disrupted by the inflammatory process. Another mimic of invasion is placental implantation site, which was discussed above.

DEFINING MICROINVASIVE SQUAMOUS CELL CARCINOMA

In recent years, the proportion of invasive cervical carcinoma diagnosed at an early stage (less than 5 mm in depth) has increased over 10-fold and currently is approximately 21%. Staging systems for early invasive cervical cancer are designed to integrate biologic behavior and clinical management (Tables 13.10, 13.11). Squamous carcinoma of the cervix was previously staged under two systems endorsed by the Society of Gynecologic Oncologists (SGO) and FIGO (International Federation of Gynecology and Obstetrics), respectively. The principal difference between the two systems was in the staging of early invasion. The SGO endorsed system defined Stage IA as equal to or less than 3.0 mm in depth by 7.0 mm in length without capillary lymphatic space invasion. This cut-off distinguished cases amenable to conservative (excision-only) therapy from those requiring lymph node dissection. The FIGO system originally subdivided Stage I into 'minimal invasion' (less than 1 mm) and invasion less than 5.0 mm in depth, making no recommendation as to management. The two systems have since come into near agreement, using the SGO definition to identify Stage IA squamous cell carcinoma of the cervix (see Appendix).[234]

When cone biopsy should be considered

If either superficial invasion or a growth pattern characterizing invasion (confluent neoplastic growth or papillary carcinoma) is identified in a biopsy specimen, cone biopsy is necessary if:

1 the lesion does not appear grossly invasive clinically or colposcopically and
2 it is not clearly deeper than 3 mm in the original biopsy and does not exhibit capillary-lymphatic space invasion or
3 the amount of tissue in the sample is very small.

Measurement of invasion

Once the cone biopsy is performed, the measurement of depth of invasion should be made from the most superficial epithelial-stromal interface of the adjacent intraepithelial process (Fig. 13.34a). This is not always possible if the tissue is distorted or the epithelium absent, in which case the thickness of the tumor should be measured (Fig. 13.34b,c). This is best accomplished using an ocular micrometer or a method of measurement that makes it possible to identify with certainty if the lesion has invaded to a depth of over 3 mm. If the microscope stage has a micrometer scale, the epithelial-stromal interface or top of the lesion can be placed at the upper edge of the field. Taking note of the scale, the stage can be moved until the top of the field reaches the lower limits of invasion. The distance traveled can be determined by examining the scale (Fig. 13.34c).

Parameters of importance

Issues requiring attention when considering microinvasion are:

Tumor type. This discussion is limited to squamous carcinomas. However, certain subsets of squamous carcinoma, such as papillary squamous carcinomas, may not be as easily evaluated without complete excision. Neuroendocrine carcinomas and adenocarcinomas naturally will be evaluated using different criteria.

Tumor dimension (depth and length). The risk of pelvic lymph node metastases increases significantly between 1 and 5 mm of invasion and is estimated as high as 4.3% for lesions invading between 3.1 and 5.0 mm (Table 13.11).[235–238] In a recent review by Ostor et al., the frequency of nodal involvement increased only slightly (from <1% to 2%) as tumor depth increased from 1 to 5 mm. Ostor et al. questioned the premise that microinvasive carcinoma be defined by a 3 mm cut-off.[238] However, a diagnosis of microinvasion (as defined by the therapeutic alternative of simple hysterectomy) in the USA requires that the carcinoma invade less than 3.0 mm into the stroma, based on recommendations of the SGO.[239] Burghardt et al. proposed that tumor volume be taken into account as a more precise predictor of recurrence and metas-

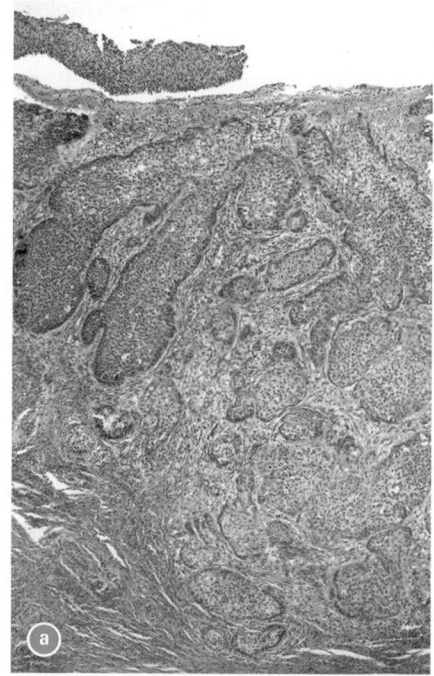

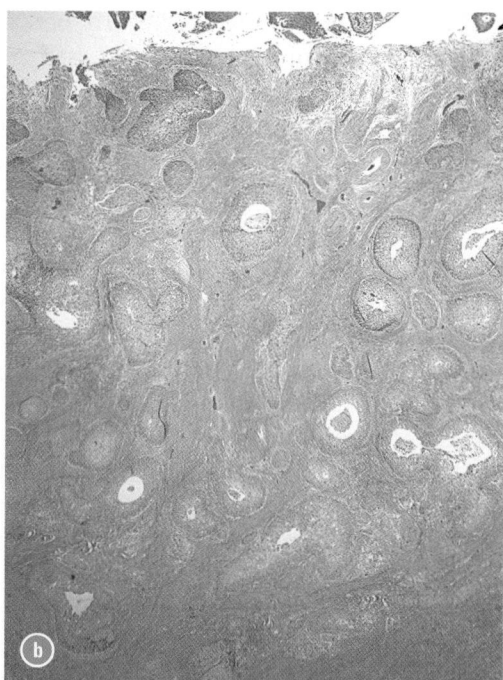

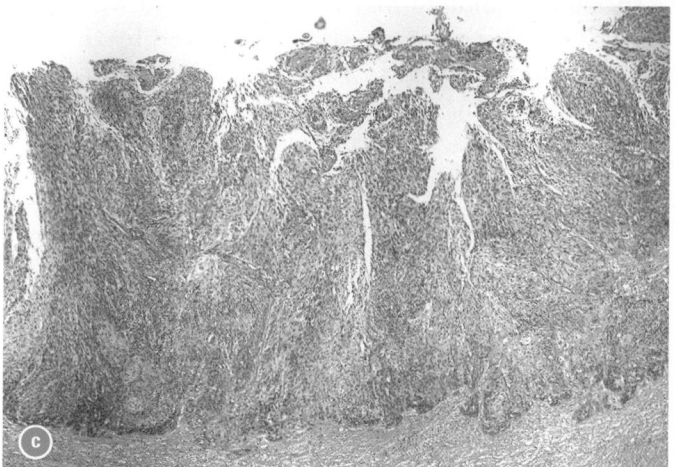

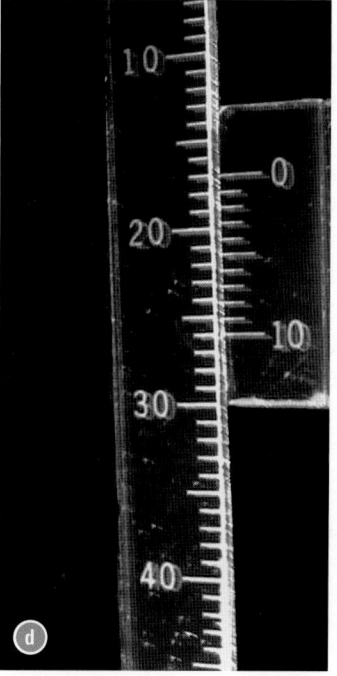

Fig. 13.34 Low-power views of different patterns of stromal invasion. Conventional infiltration is measured from the highest epithelial-stromal interface, seen here as a cleavage plane where the epithelium has lifted from the stroma (a). Invasive patterns mimicking gland involvement are best measured from the surface (b). When the distinction of intraepithelial and invasive components cannot be made, a measure of thickness is most appropriate (c). Microscope stage scale can be used to determine distance in millimeters from one point in the slide to another (d), measuring the distance traveled across a single reference point (microscopic field edge).

tases.[240] Lesions less than 420 mm² rarely recur. A more simplified approach places the cutoff at 7 mm in length.[239]

Confluence of growth pattern

Confluence has been defined as anastomosing tongues of epithelium with pushing borders, or a lesion front of greater than 1 mm.[241] Despite a report emphasizing the prognostic importance of confluent patterns of invasion, others have not found that confluence is an independent factor, once depth of invasion is controlled for.[242–244] In his review, Ostor noted an adverse outcome in less than 3% of cases with this feature.[245]

Capillary-lymphatic space invasion

The frequency of capillary-lymphatic space invasion (CLSI) has varied widely but increases as a function of depth. Van Nagel et al. and Ostor and Rome reported CLSI in 24% of superficially invasive carcinomas based on Ulex Europaeus Agglutin I (UEAI) stains.[245] They noted that 6 of 12 (50%) tumors with lymph node metastases were associated with CLSI notwithstanding the fact that 19% of cases with negative lymph nodes had CLSI. Similarly, 50% of invasive recurrences were associated with CLSI in the original tumor versus 14% of patients with no recurrence.[245] CLSI has been associated with an adverse prognosis in carcinomas exceeding 3 mm in depth in most, if not all, reports.[247,248] The implication from these multiple studies is that the vast majority of cases with CLSI do not present with histologically positive lymph nodes, but CLSI is associated more commonly with an adverse outcome.

In a recent review, Benedet and Anderson computed a 10-fold increased risk (8.3% vs 0.8%) of nodal metastases in Stage IA1 (less than 3.0 mm invasion) tumors with CLSI, conferring a risk of metastases of over 8% and recurrence of 15% (Tables 13.12 and 13.13).[249] Thus, there is sufficient evidence of increased risk to warrant careful counseling of patients whose tumors contain CLSI and serious consideration of lymph node dissection, while recognizing that over 85% of Stage IA1 tumors with CLSI will not have nodal metastases. It is important to emphasize that not all risk can be eliminated by lymph node dissection. One study found a relationship between CLSI and extrapelvic recurrences, while another found that a worse prognosis associated with CLSI was not influenced by lymph node dissection.[48,52] Nevertheless, because an appreciable number of patients with positive pelvic lymph nodes are salvaged, prudence dictates that the nodes be removed or sampled if capillary-lymphatic space invasion is unequivocal.

Table 13.12 *Follow-up of Stage IA cervical cancer*[313]

Stage	Definition	Positive nodes (%)	Recurrences	Deaths
1A1	<1.0 mm	0.07	0.38	0.07
	1–2.9 mm	1.9	1.5	0.5
1A2	3–5 mm	7.8	4.5	2.4

Table 13.13 *Frequency of CLSI, nodal involvement and recurrence risk*[249]

Capillary-lymphatic space invasion (CLSI)	Depth of invasion		
	<1.0 mm	1–2.9 mm	3–5 mm
Frequency	4.4%	16.4%	19.7%
Recurrence risk	Present	3.1%	15.7%
	Absent	0.6%	1.7%
Nodal involvement	Present	8.2%	7.5%
	Absent	0.8%	8.3%

In practice, oncologists request that the presence of CLSI be reported, and will usually opt for radical hysterectomy and pelvic lymphadenectomy if it is seen in a lesion less than 3.0 mm in depth. For these reasons, over- and under-interpretation of CLSI must be avoided.

CLSI typically exhibits the following features: (1) rounded nests of tumor cells, (2) enclosed within a sharply defined space, (3) with molding of the tumor nests to the vascular space and (4) an absence of a surrounding stromal response (Fig. 13.35a,b).

Conditions mimicking vascular space invasion

1 Retraction artifacts may produce confusion in the interpretation of CLSI. To avoid this pitfall, it is best to evaluate CLSI at the periphery of the lesion and to avoid the diagnosis of CLSI in the proximity of desmoplasia (Figs 13.35a, 13.36a,b).

2 Neoplastic epithelium displaced into vascular spaces during injection of anesthetic or during specimen handling may also be confused with CLSI.[250] This condition is characterized by the following features: (a) prominent vascular dilatation in the area due to the injection; (b) intravascular neoplastic epithelium that closely resembles CIN; (c) variable contouring of the epithelium; (d) evidence of trauma, including surface disruption due to the needle tract (Fig. 13.36c–e). A diagnosis of CLSI should be made with caution when invasion is not seen. Conversely, if the characteristic features of CLSI are present, a compulsive search for invasion should be made. In discohesive tumors with abundant neoplastic epithelium, transfer of tumor into larger vascular spaces may occur by the process of 'buttering' wherein sectioning spreads the cells into available spaces. Such artifacts should be obvious by the presence of loose aggregates elsewhere in the specimen and the absence of the characteristic rounded clusters of tumor cells.

3 Other forms of pseudovascular space invasion include menstrual endometrium within small vessels (Fig. 13.36f). Recognition of this pitfall requires attention to the nature of the cells within the vessels.

Reporting microinvasion

We do not use the term 'microinvasive' carcinoma, preferring to report such tumors as 'superficially invasive squamous cell carcinomas' and providing appropriate information that will allow the clinician to come

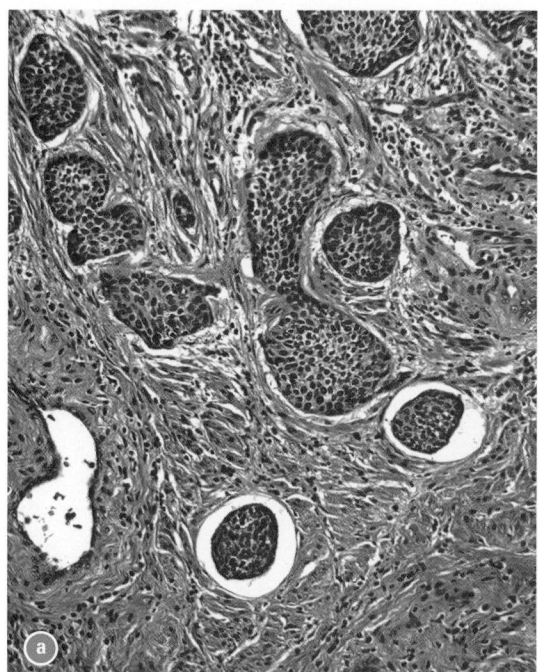
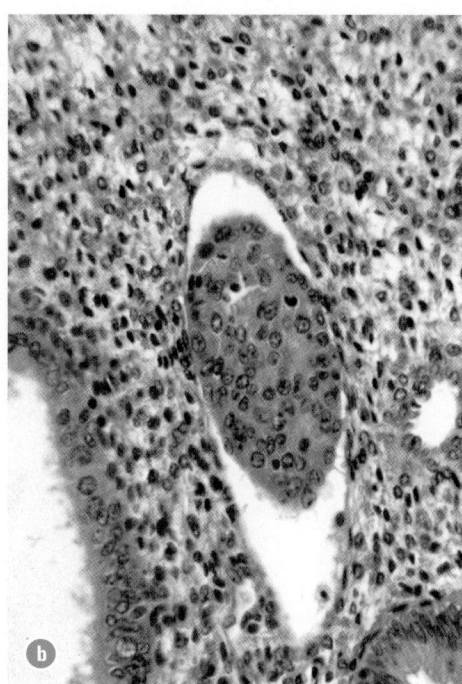

Fig. 13.35 Capillary-lymphatic space invasion (CLSI) is best evaluated at the periphery of the invasive tumor, and should be devoid of tissue reaction (desmoplasia) (a). CLSI is characterized typically by nests of differentiated neoplastic epithelium within discrete spaces (b). Endothelial cells may or may not be conspicuous.

to a conclusion regarding therapy. The purpose of this strategy is two-fold. First, clinicians should not assume that a diagnosis of microinvasion identifies a reproducibly defined entity. Determining which patients are amenable to cone biopsy versus requiring lymph node dissection is a subjective process and clinicians should be discouraged from presuming that a report showing 'microinvasion' does not require further review, both to avoid over- and under-estimation of invasion. As a rule, all cases falling into the range of those defined as microinvasion should prompt a dialogue between the pathologist and clinician and, ideally, be reviewed by two or more pathologists. Secondly, the criteria for microinvasion may vary slightly depending on locale. When reviewing the biopsy, we report the largest dimensions of the lesion to aid the clinician in deciding the next step in management (i.e. cone biopsy *vs* radical hysterectomy), particularly if there is no visible mass on clinical examination. In cone biopsies, the following should be reported: (a) depth; (b) length of the entire lesion; (c) if length constitutes continuous tumor or is composed of multiple small foci; (d) the presence or absence of CLSI; (e) status of endocervical, ectocervical and deep margins and, if negative, distance (in mm) from invasive tumor to these margins; (f) intraepithelial disease and its relationship to the margins and (g) glandular differentiation if present. The latter generally precludes management of

the lesion as microinvasive if there is clear evidence of invasive adenocarcinoma.

Common dilemmas and their management

Multifocal lesions, none of which exceed the criteria for microinvasion. These should be described in detail. It is not uncommon to identify several small foci of early invasion in multiple areas of different sections. These foci may be technically greater than 7.0 mm in aggregate distance from one another. This finding should be reported in a narrative. In the authors' experience, it is unusual to encounter multiple foci, each of which measures less than 3.0 mm by less than 7.0 mm in dimension. The latter circumstances would be more likely to mandate lymph node dissection than the finding of small foci of early stromal invasion.

Invasion originating from an endocervical crypt. This occasionally occurs and will elicit the favorite question of many pathologists who manage this disease, which is, whether to measure the depth from the surface or the crypt (Fig. 13.37). The most important distinction to make when faced with this problem is to ensure that the 'crypts' are not actually cohesive nests of invasive carcinoma (Figs 13.32d,e and 13.34b). If they are, it is likely that the criteria for microinvasion have been exceeded. If not, the appropriate practice is to measure the depth from the epithelial-stromal interface of the crypt. Nevertheless, these findings should

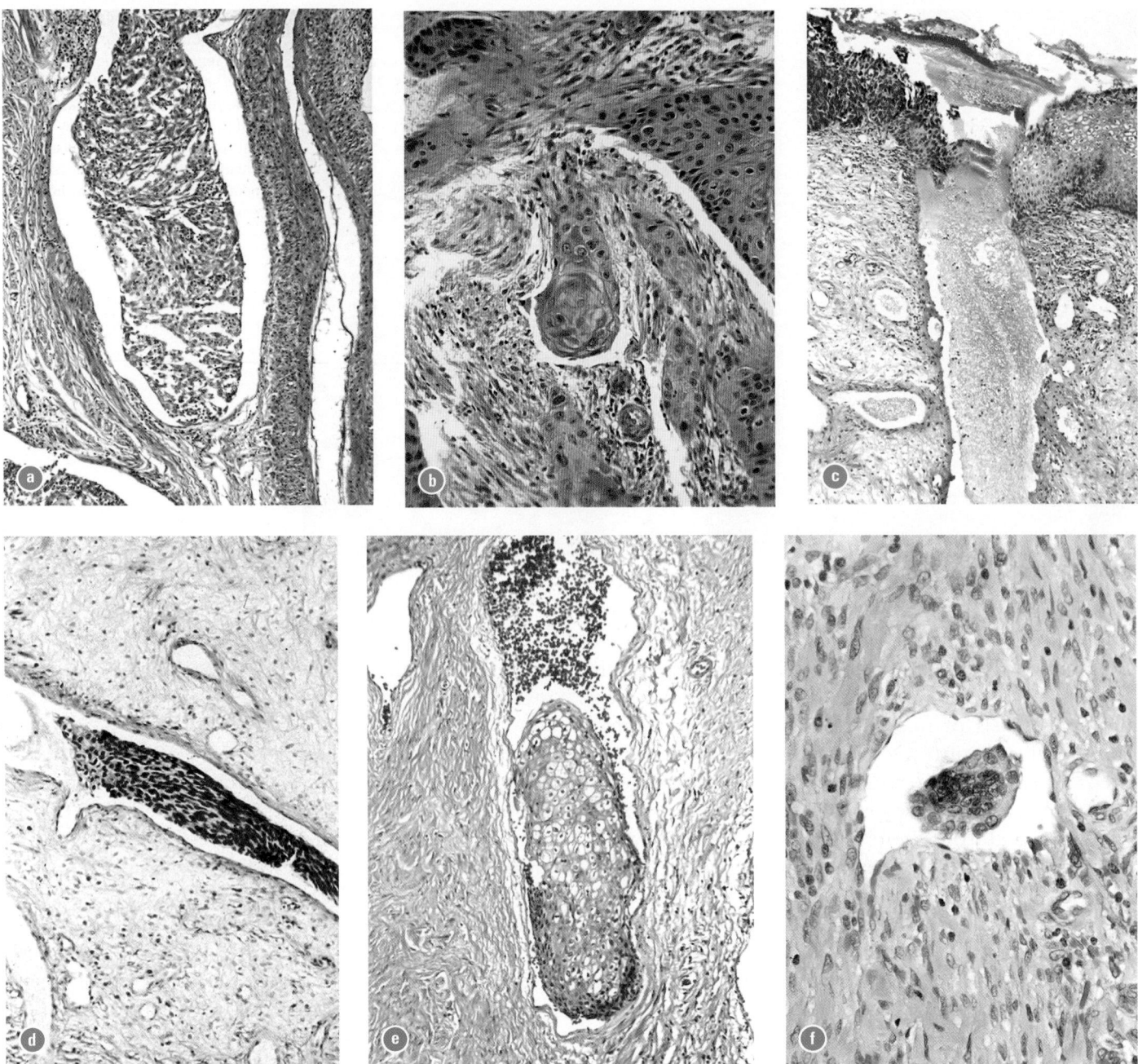

Fig. 13.36 Differential diagnosis of capillary-lymphatic space invasion includes retraction artifacts (a,b); anesthetic needle tracts (c); and displacing neoplastic epithelium into vascular spaces (d,e). This phenomenon is often accompanied by generalized submucosal vascular dilatation. Menstrual endometrium may occasionally be present in vessels, and may confuse the unwary (f).

be detailed in a narrative on the report and taken into account when planning therapy.

Suspicion of CLSI in a single space that is not confirmed on levels. The diagnosis of capillary-lymphatic space invasion – and with it the almost certain decision to perform lymph node dissection – should be based on more than a single focus in a single tissue section. If a single focus is seen or suspected, multiple tissue sections should be reviewed. If one suspicious focus cannot be confirmed on additional sections, it should be reported in a narrative.

Papillary lesions without stromal invasion (Fig. 13.31e). The authors classify these as papillary squamous cell carcinomas based on architecture, but specify that depth of

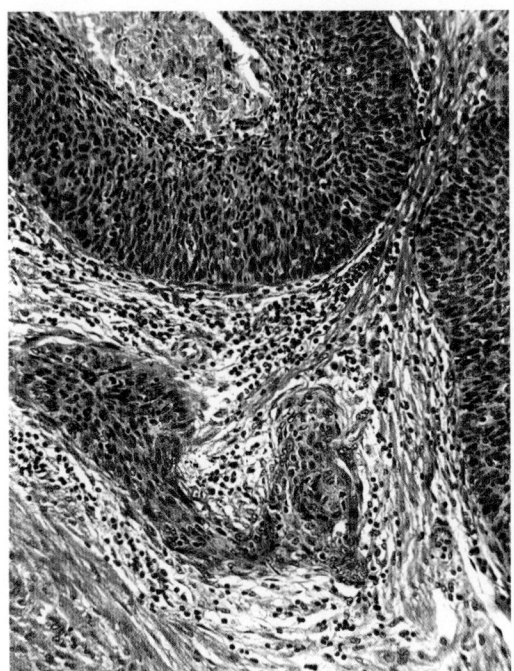

Fig. 13.37 Invasion from a crypt. When present as an isolated focus, the tumor can be measured from the epithelial-stromal interface of the crypt.

invasion cannot be assessed. Further diagnostic strategies (cone biopsy) may be required before deciding whether a radical hysterectomy is indicated (see below).

Capillary-lymphatic space involvement in association with SIL only (see above). When capillary-lymphatic space invasion is present, two causes must be excluded, both of which we have encountered in practice. The first is artifactual introduction of neoplastic epithelium into the vascular space, usually during the injection of local anesthestic prior to the surgical procedure.[250] The second is that an underlying invasive carcinoma is present but has not been sampled. The latter is confirmed by additional sectioning or further tissue biopsies.

MANAGEMENT OF SUPERFICIALLY INVASIVE SQUAMOUS CELL CARCINOMA

Cone biopsy is an acceptable option if the lesion fulfills the criteria for microinvasion and ample margins are identified. Studies of cone biopsy versus hysterectomy have not shown a significantly increased risk of metastatic spread. Hysterectomy is the preferred approach for women who do not desire to maintain their fertility. Modified radical hysterectomy and lymph node dissection is the standard for lesions exceeding the criteria for microinvasion, i.e. extending deeper than 3.0 mm into the cervical stroma and/or exceeding 7.0 mm in length and/or showing unequivocal capillary-lymphatic space invasion. Cases with multifocal disease that collectively span more than 7.0 mm, or cohesive lesions with a blunt epithelial-stromal interface, may be treated on a case-by-case basis.

Radical trachelectomy, combining cervical amputation with lymph node dissection, has been employed by several groups as a fertility-sparing alternative to hysterectomy and pelvic lymph node dissection for the management of Stage IA2 and selected stage IB1 carcinomas. The procedure involves amputation of the cervix and upper vagina combined with lymph node dissection, resulting in a vaginal-lower uterine segment junction. Preliminary studies indicate that the procedure is equal to modified radical hysterectomy; however, the differences in failure between Stage IA1 and IA2 are usually sufficiently small that large numbers will be needed to ascertain the precise degree of risk taken when opting for this procedure versus conventional therapy. Table 13.14 summarizes four studies, each of which reported rare recurrences. A significant minority of patients successfully conceive, but a proportion fail to

Table 13.14 Outcome following radical trachelectomy

Parameter	Main Author			
	Covens[282,314]	Dargent[315]	Roy[316]	Shepherd[317]
Number	81	82	44	30
Stage		IB+	IB–IIA	
Follow-up (mean)		52	25	2
Recurrences	1	3	1	
Deaths	1	1	1	
Attempted conception	37	29	13	13
Pregnancies	22	47	19	14
Live births	18	13+	7+	9

Table 13.15 *Categories of squamous carcinoma*

Squamous cell carcinoma
    Large cell keratinizing (well-differentiated)
    Large cell non-keratinizing (moderately-differentiated)
    Small cell non-keratinizing (poorly-differentiated

Lymphoepithelial-like carcinoma

Spindle cell (sarcomatoid) carcinoma

Verrucopapillary carcinomas
    Papillary (squamo-transitional) carcinoma
    Verrucous carcinoma
    Condylomatous carcinoma
    Giant condyloma (rare)

Basaloid carcinomas[a]

[a]May be associated with adenoid basal and adenoid cystic carcinomas, and carcinosarcomas.

achieve a term pregnancy. Despite these potential limitations, radical trachelectomy is gaining increasing popularity as it the only procedure for more extensive disease that allows the potential for future childbearing.

PATHOLOGY OF INVASIVE SQUAMOUS CARCINOMA

Grading

Grading of squamous cell carcinoma (Table 13.15) has relatively little prognostic significance. There are three classically described categories of differentiation, comprising predominantly keratinizing tumors (Grade 1) that are mainly differentiated with conspicuous keratin pearls (Fig. 13.38a). Large cell non-keratinizing carcinomas (Grade 2) with greater nuclear pleomorphism, infiltrative borders and inflammation (Fig. 13.38b) and small cell non-keratinizing carcinomas (Grade 3) with a predominately high nuclear/ cytoplasmic ratio (Fig. 13.38c).[251]

Four variants of large cell keratinizing and non-keratinizing carcinomas are:

1 Lymphoepithelial-like carcinomas, which consist of poorly-defined aggregates of non-keratinized tumors cells, often with indistinct cytoplasmic borders, intermixed with abundant lymphoid cells, similar to their morphologic counterparts in the pharynx. The term is an adaptation of that used to define similar tumors of the nasopharynx. The differential diagnosis includes lymphoid hyperplasia and lymphoma, both of which can be easily distinguished with stains for epithelial cells (keratin, epithelial membrane antigen) or squamous cells (p63) (Fig. 13.39a–c).[252]

2 Spindle cell squamous cell carcinoma, also termed sarcomatoid squamous cell carcinoma, has been described in the vulva and cervix and consists of a expansile tumor mass with a spindled cell

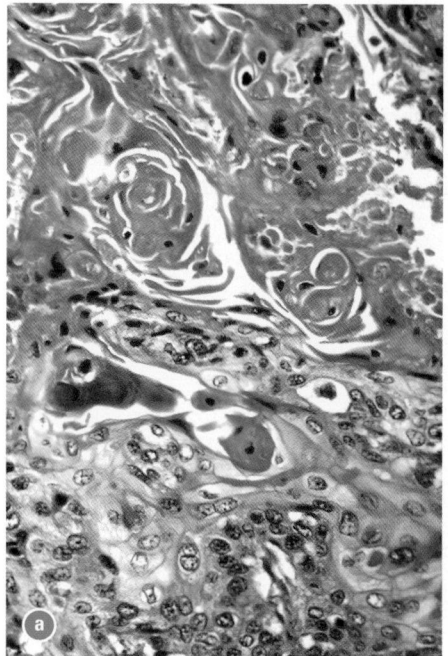
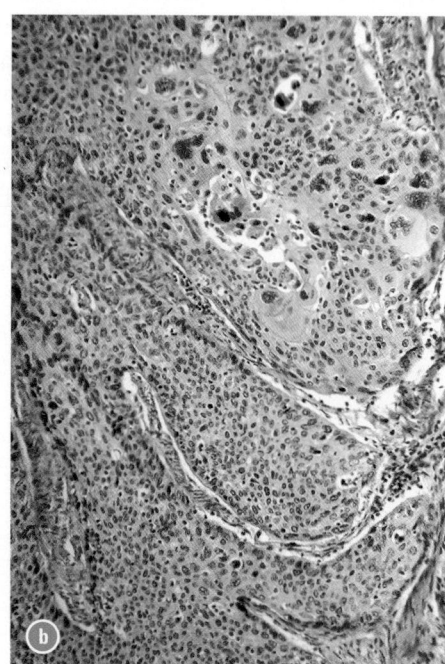
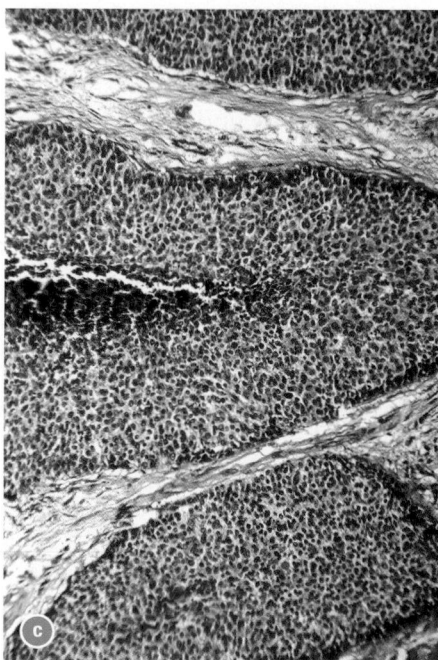

Fig. 13.38 Three common patterns of squamous cell carcinoma of the cervix are large cell keratinizing (well-differentiated) (a), large cell non-keratinizing (moderately-differentiated) (b) and small cell non-keratinizing (poorly-differentiated) (c). Differentiation has minimal influence on prognosis for squamous carcinoma.

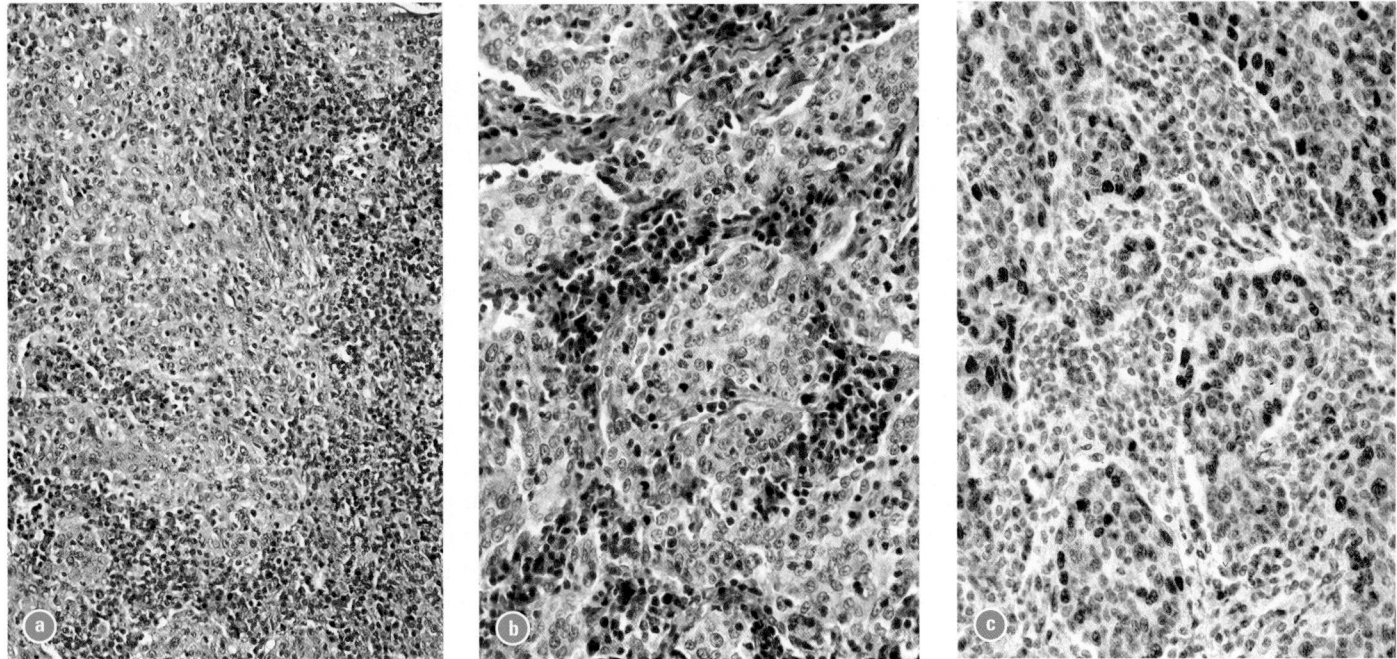

Fig. 13.39 Lymphoepithelial-like carcinoma of the cervix exhibits an indistinct blending of a monomorphic non-keratinizing tumor with a prominent lymphoid infiltrate (a,b). Strong positivity for p63 is consistent with a squamous origin (c).

component.[253,254] The 'sarcoma' is typically not differentiated but tumors with osteoclast giant cells have been reported.[255] The tumors frequently contain both squamous carcinoma and spindle cell components, either separate or subtly blending (Fig. 13.40a–c). Ultrastructural and immunohistochemical studies indicate that these tumors are derived from squamous cell carcinoma and several features will aid in the correct diagnosis of these tumors: (a) True carcinosarcomas of the cervix almost always arise in association with basaloid neoplasms. Thus, if the pathologist

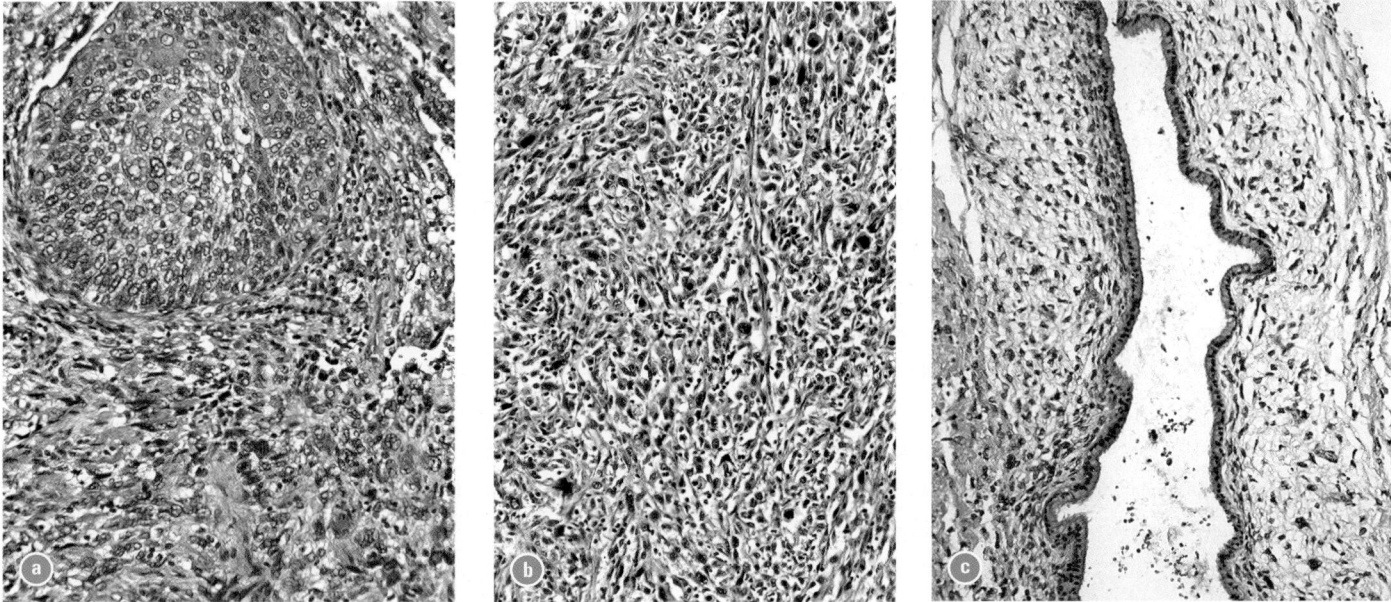

Fig. 13.40 Spindle cell squamous carcinoma displaying the interface between epithelioid (upper) and sarcomatoid (lower) elements (a). Spindle cell component (b). Rare cuffing of normal glands (adenosarcoma-like pattern) by a spindle cell squamous carcinoma (c).

encounters a spindle cell neoplasm of the cervix not associated with a basaloid squamous tumor, the differential diagnosis narrows to a pure sarcoma versus a spindle cell carcinoma. (b) If an epithelial component is appreciated, it will be a typical large cell non-keratinizing squamous cell carcinoma. (c) A spindle cell squamous carcinoma is also likely if a precursor lesion (CIN) is also present. In some cases, a transition from CIN or squamous carcinoma (superficial) to spindle cell morphology (deep) is present. (d) Special stains for keratins will usually be positive and may vary in intensity. An aggressive clinical course has been observed in one study of four cases.[254]

3 Verrucopapillary neoplasms of the cervix include both benign and malignant tumors and will be addressed as a group for clarity (Table 13.16). They include the following (Fig. 13.41a–f): (a) Actual giant condylomata (so-called Buschke–Löwenstein tumors) of the cervix are exceedingly rare, and are more commonly reported in the anogenital mucosa, particularly in men (see Ch. 10). The authors have seen one case in which the histologic features were indistinguishable from condyloma, which scored positive for HPV 11, yet had extended from the cervix into the parametrium. (b) Verrucous carcinomas are extremely uncommon and consist of broad-based exophytic tumors with a uniform epithelial-stromal interface, and minimal atypia (Fig. 13.41d,e). The diagnosis should be made with strict criteria.[256,257] Risk of lymph node metastases is considered negligible; however, these tumors are considered radiation resistant. Reports of association with HPV vary. (c) Papillary squamous neoplasms with conventional invasion comprise a unique subset of tumors in which the papillary component fails to fulfill the criteria for carcinoma but is associated with frankly infiltrative squamous carcinoma (Fig. 13.41a,b). The authors have seen rare examples of this entity. In both, the invasive component was either focal or unrecognized prior to hysterectomy.[258] (d) Papillary squamo-transitional carcinomas of the uterine cervix are characterized by filiform papillae lined by neoplastic cells identical to high-grade CIN and may have features resembling transitional cell carcinoma of urothelial origin (Fig. 13.42a–c).[259] The term 'transitional' is based principally on the light microscopic appearance, inasmuch as special stains for squamous (CK 7) are typically positive and transitional cell differentiation (CK 20) is present in less than 10% of cases. Because these tumors are predominately papillary, invasion may not be confirmed and may require wedge biopsy or LEEP cone.[260,261] However, the majority (90%) will demonstrate invasion with sufficient sampling.[258] Some authors have subdivided papillary carcinomas into (i) predominantly squamous, (ii) mixed squamous and transitional and (iii) predominantly transitional.[258] The value of histologic sub-classification is unclear. (e) More poorly-differentiated papillary carcinomas comprise a rare subset of tumors that score positive for CK 7 but do not score positive for squamous cell markers and are lined by undifferentiated epithelial cells (see Ch. 15).[252,262] These tumors may be associated with glandular neoplasia and presumably are derived from de-differentiated epithelial cells derived from the latter. Such lesions may be associated with both squamous and glandular carcinomas.[252,262] (f) Condylomatous carcinomas consist of well-differentiated exophytic squamous cell carcinomas with conspicuous superficial and basal cell atypia (Fig. 13.41c). The most compelling reason for sub-classifying these tumors is to

Table 13.16 Differential diagnosis of papillary cervical neoplasia

Tumor	Differentiation	Koilocytosis	Basal atypia	Infiltration
Condyloma	Mature	Yes	No	None
Immature condyloma	Immature squamous	Minimal	No	None
Papillary squamo-transitional CA	Immature squamous	No	Yes	Variable
Condylomatous carcinoma	Mature squamous	Variable	Yes	Present
Verrucous carcinoma	Mature squamous	No	Minimal	Blunt
Papillary undifferentiated carcinoma	None	No	Yes	Present

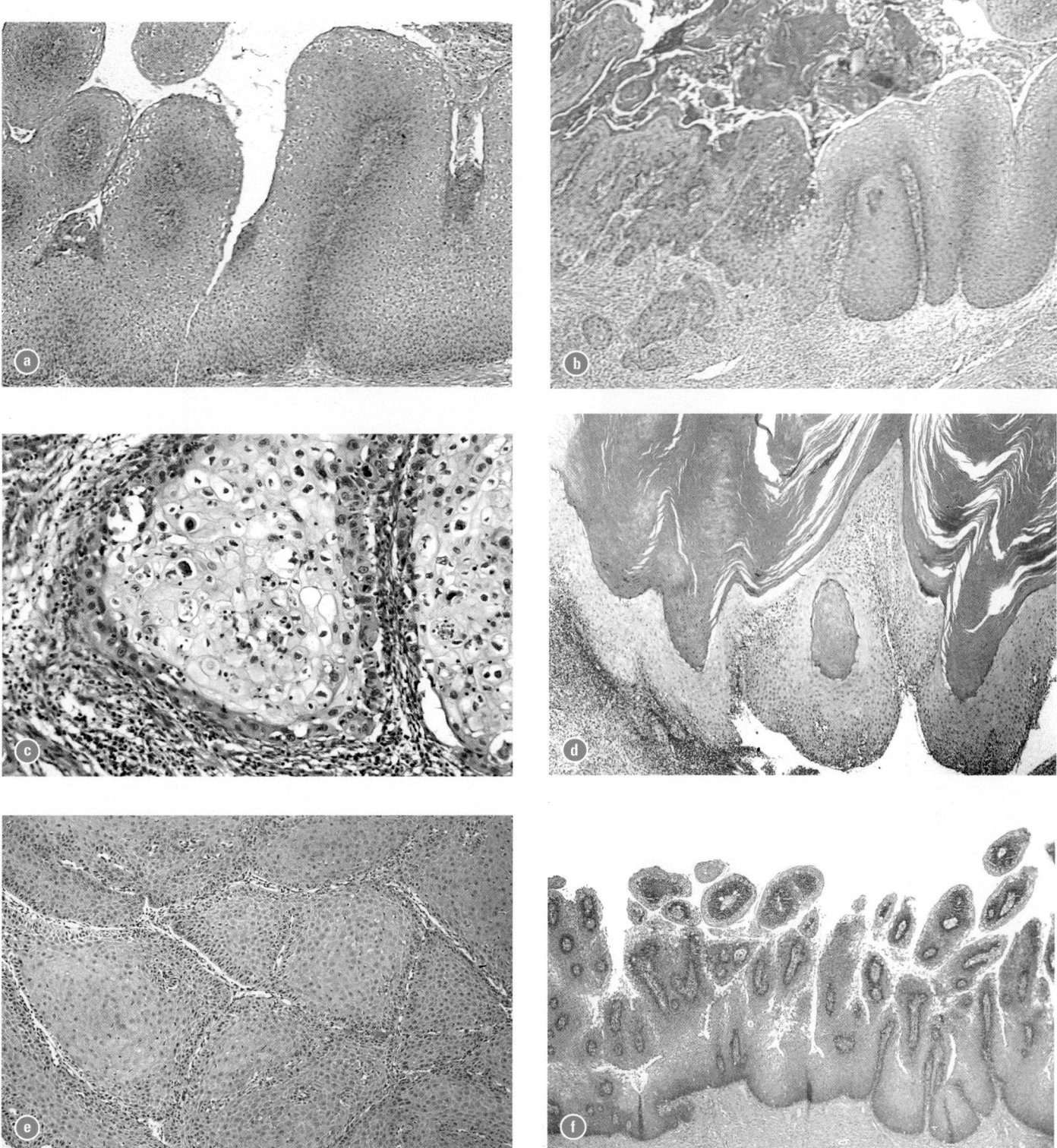

Fig. 13.41 Verrucopapillary neoplasia of the cervix. A well-differentiated papillary neoplasm (a) merges with a carcinoma (b). Condylomatous carcinoma (c) with marked nuclear atypia and 'pseudokoilocytosis'. Verrucous carcinoma (d) with an extremely well-differentiated epithelium devoid of atypia (e). A rare lesion closely resembling a transitional papilloma does not meet criteria for condyloma, immature condyloma, conventional papillary carcinoma, or verrucous carcinoma (f).

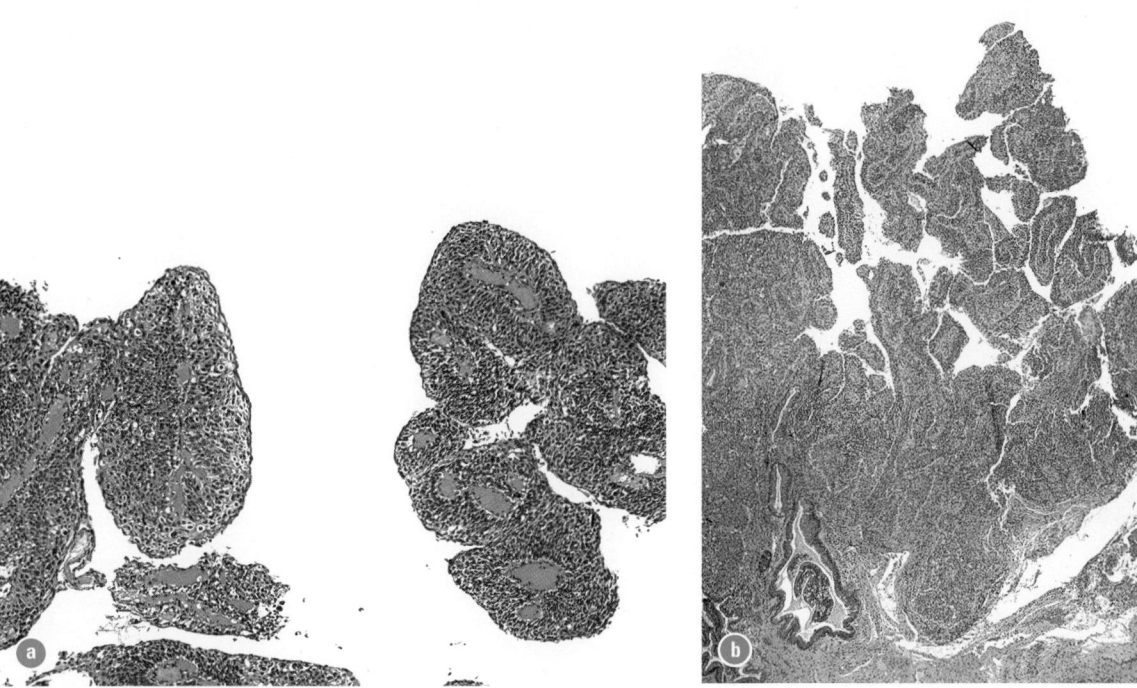

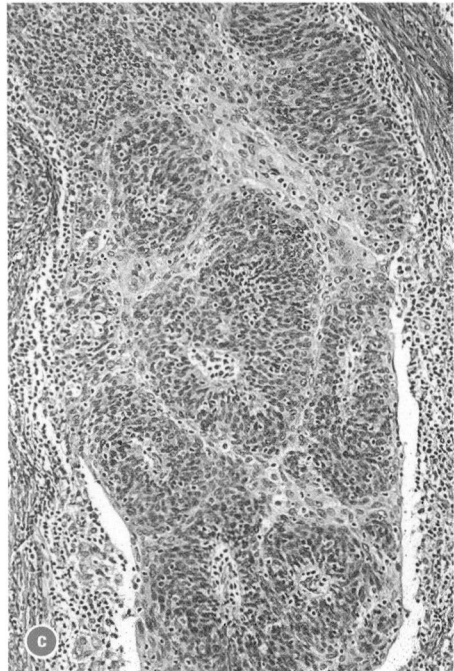

Fig. 13.42 Papillary 'squamo-transitional' carcinoma may show minimal invasion in limited samples (a, b). Confluence of epithelial growth with endoduplication (c) characterizes these tumors.

distinguish them from verrucous carcinomas and condylomata.[263] Benign verrucopapillary lesions include: (g) Condyloma, which as discussed previously, are usually easily distinguished by the presence of koilocytosis and an absence of parabasal atypia. In rare instances, these lesions may be extensive. (h) Immature condyloma (papillary immature metaplasia), may resemble papillary carcinomas and may be identical to tumors classified as 'transitional papilloma'. They are immature in appearance, but are composed of uniform nuclei with nucleoli, a low mitotic index, and minimal nuclear overlap. In contrast to papillary carcinomas, these tumors exhibit a relatively low Ki-67 index.[162,165]

4 Basaloid squamous carcinomas are extremely rare variants of cervical neoplasia that exhibit a mixture of basaloid and variable mature squamous

differentiation (Fig. 13.43a–c). These tumors are technically squamous, but some have been associated with adenoid basal carcinomas and may actually arise from these tumors early in their evolution. They may also be associated with a sarcomatous element.

Significance of columnar cell differentiation

A significant proportion of cervical squamous carcinomas are associated with columnar cell differentiation. The prognostic significance of columnar differentiation is not clear. In one study, 27% of randomly selected squamous carcinomas contained some degree of mucin positivity. Approximately 5% contained sufficient mucin to warrant reclassification as adenosquamous carcinomas, suggesting that mucin stains may in some cases aid in classification.[264]

In a second study, 87 Stage I cervical carcinomas treated by radical hysterectomy were studied. A total of 39% were mucin-positive and this group (and pure adenocarcinomas) was significantly associated with a higher risk of lymph node metastases.[265]

Markers used to distinguish squamous carcinomas from other tumors, including neuroendocrine carcinomas, are discussed in Chapter 16.

Reporting squamous carcinomas

Histologic reporting should include the following:
1 Grade (well-, moderately- or poorly-differentiated)
2 Cell type
3 Depth of invasion or thickness
4 Extent of tumor: the extent of invasion into extra-cervical tissues and metastases to both pelvic and extrapelvic organs should be recorded
5 Angiolymphatic vascular space invasion: the presence of tumor within blood vessels and/or lymphatic vessels should be noted and an attempt made to distinguish, when possible, between them
6 Status of lymph nodes: report the presence or absence of metastases in each submitted group of lymph nodes, recording the total number of involved lymph nodes in relation to the total number of lymph nodes identified
7 Status of resection margins: the adequacy of local excision should be assessed by careful examination of resection margins, the latter preferably marked by the use of ink. The distance from the deepest point of stromal invasion to the closest (inked) margin of resection may be noted in the report.

TREATMENT AND OUTCOME OF SQUAMOUS CARCINOMA

Clinical factors influencing outcome/presentation

Presenting signs/symptoms. Pretorius et al. evaluated a cohort of 81 women with cervical cancer and correlated presentation with outcome.[266] Abnormal vaginal bleeding and an abnormal Papanicolaou smear were the dominant presenting findings (56% and 28%). Other symptoms, such as pain and discharge, were seen in

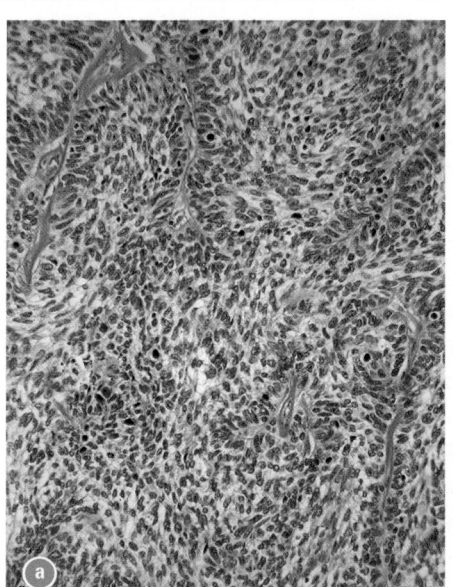 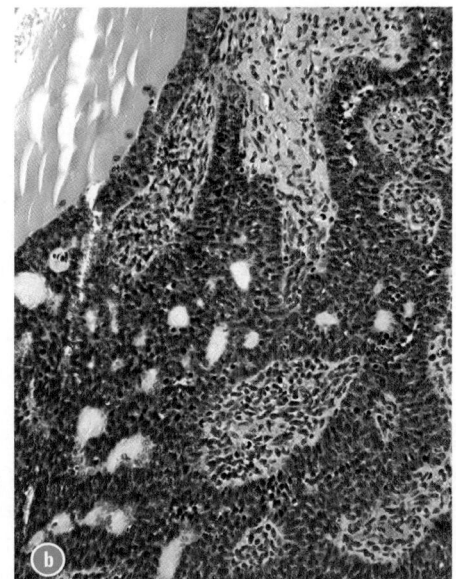 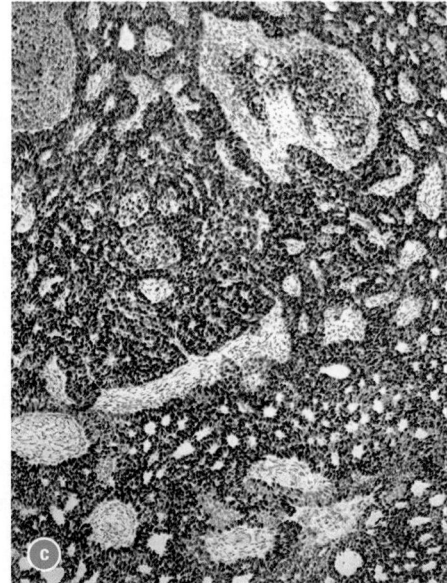

Fig. 13.43 Carcinomas with basaloid phenotype may present as solid (a) or interlacing cord-like (b) growth patterns. Strong staining for p63 confirms the basal (versus columnar) pattern of differentiation (c).

less than 10%. An abnormal Papanicolaou smear was associated with Stage I disease and a significantly longer disease-free survival (96%) than vaginal bleeding (51%). Both exceeded the disease-free survival of those presenting with pain (29%). Thus, early detection (by cytology) is associated with a significantly higher disease-free survival and significantly smaller tumor volume.[266]

Age of presentation. Patients aged under 35 years comprise slightly more than 10% of women with cervical cancer and a disproportionate number of those who have previously been screened. Whether the under-35 age group is at greater risk of an adverse outcome is doubtful. Jennings et al. performed a retrospective cohort study comparing women under and over 35 years of age.[267] They found no significant difference in the incidence of non-squamous tumors, tumor grade, lymph node involvement, HPV status, tumor recurrence or survival between the two groups. Young patients appeared to enter the study at significantly earlier stages of the disease, and a greater proportion of them underwent surgical treatment.[267] Yang et al. studied Stage IB–IIA cervical cancers among women 35 years of age or younger and older and reported a similar overall survival (71.2% *vs* 72.4%) for both groups. Non-squamous carcinomas, including adenocarcinoma and small cell carcinoma, were both associated with HPV 18 and the younger patients and conferred a slightly higher but not significant risk of recurrence/persistence; however, these differences were not significant and 71% of the recurrences were squamous cell carcinomas.[268]

Early studies of HPV prevalence in cervical cancer suggested the existence of an HPV-negative older population, possibly with a worse prognosis. Notwithstanding occasional tumors in older women, such as minimal deviation adenocarcinoma and verrucous carcinoma, that may not be associated with HPV, a relationship between age and HPV prevalence has not been substantiated in cervical cancer. Baay et al. found no statistically significant difference in either the prevalence of HPV DNA or distribution of genotypes between women with cervical cancer who were younger or older than 65 years of age.[269]

Presentation during pregnancy. Carcinoma of the cervix during pregnancy is rare and is diagnosed in approximately 1 per 3000 to 10 000 pregnant patients.[270,271] Conversely, approximately 3% of all cancer patients are pregnant at the time of diagnosis. The two important clinical issues are influence of pregnancy on outcome and the risk of delaying delivery until fetal maturity permits viability, and the potential negative impact of cone biopsy on the pregnancy.

Influence of pregnancy on outcome. Several studies of cervical cancer during pregnancy noted no significant worsening of outcome.[270,272,273] One study noted an increase in blood loss in the pregnant group.[274] Adverse outcome was directly related to tumor extent.

Safety of delays in treatment. In general, management of pregnant patients with cervical cancer is as follows: (1) Patients under gestational age of 20 weeks undergo immediate surgery with fetal loss. (2) Patients at gestational age of 20 weeks or older with low-stage disease may be treated with observation of up to 4 months.[271–276] (3) Conization can be performed safely for cases of early (microinvasive) carcinoma.[271,277] The safety of longer follow-up intervals is unclear based on relatively little data. Sorosky followed seven Stage IB pregnant patients who desired pregnancy retention from 21 to 207 days (median 109 days), with no adverse outcomes and no apparent worsening of clinical stage.[275]

Viral factors and outcome. HPV type 16 predominates in squamous neoplasia in contrast to type 18, which is seen more frequently in glandular and neuroendocrine neoplasms.[278,279] Nevertheless, two studies indicate that HPV type may influence outcome. Lombard et al. studied 197 patients for which HPV typing was available (83%), with a median follow-up of 38 months.[280] Although they reported no significant relationship between virologic data and tumor stage/node status, the 5-year disease-free survival (DFS) rate was 100% for patients with intermediate-risk HPV-associated tumors, 58% for patients with HPV16-positive tumors, and 38% for patients with HPV18-positive tumors ($p = 0.02$). In multivariate analysis, the relative risk (RR) of death conferred by HPV 18 was 2.4 times that of HPV 16, and 4.4 times that for patients with a viral type different from HPV 16/18.[280] Schwartz et al. similarly found the risk of tumor-related mortality to be 2.2-fold higher in HPV 18 *vs* HPV 16-positive tumors with the associations strongest for those with FIGO Stage IB/IIA disease. The HPV-18 associations were strongest for patients with FIGO Stage IB or IIA disease. The increased risk was also seen in the subset of patients with squamous carcinomas, with HPV 18 conferring increased risk, particularly in earlier-stage disease.[281]

Management of squamous cell carcinoma

Improvements in prognosis in the past 30 years

Covens et al. summarized their experience in a large practice and noted a consistent reduction in comorbidity (blood loss, length of stay, transfusion, infections, etc.) associated with cervical cancer therapy over a 16-year period.[282] However, parameters linked to early detection and prognosis (age, tumor size, capillary-lymphatic space invasion and pelvic lymph node involvement) did not change. They also noted a significant increase in the proportion of adenocarcinomas (28%) and a decrease in the proportion of grade 3 tumors (28%). They concluded that most of the progress made was in the realm of operative management than survival.[282]

Standard treatment options

Stage IB: Standard treatment is radical hysterectomy or radiation therapy. Radical hysterectomy is the preferred option for smaller tumors and carries a nearly 100% disease-specific survival rate for tumors under 2 cm.[283–285] For more deeply invasive tumors, tumors exceeding 4 cm and including those with capillary-lymphatic space invasion, adjunctive radiation therapy is preferred.[286] In a randomized prospective trial by the Gynecologic Oncology Group reported by Sedlis et al., patients with intermediate-risk factors following radical hysterectomy who received adjuvant radiation had a decreased risk of recurrence (15% *vs* 28%).[287] Further follow-up will be needed to determine the effect of adjuvant radiation on survival.

The ideal treatment of Stage IB2 cervical cancer remains controversial, as a limited amount of randomized prospective data is available. In view of these poor results, a variety of treatment options for this group of patients has been utilized, including: radical hysterectomy followed by radiation or chemoradiation, radiation or chemoradiation followed by routine or selective hysterectomy, neoadjuvant chemotherapy followed by surgery with or without postoperative radiation or chemoradiation alone. It may be helpful to remember that for Stage IB2 tumors two or more modalities for treatment will usually be necessary for effective treatment.

Stage IIA: For tumors that extend to the vagina but are limited to the upper two-thirds, without involvement of the parametria, both radical hysterectomy and radiation therapy have been utilized. Radical surgery would be suggested for a younger patient if an adequate margin can be obtained and adjuvant radiation can be avoided. However, if radiation is likely to be required, primary radiation alone with both external and intracavitary is usually preferable.

Stage IIB: For tumors that extend into the parametria (Stage IIB) the standard treatment in the USA has been radiation therapy. In contrast, radical hysterectomy and lymphadenectomy followed by adjuvant radiation therapy has been preferred by many European and Japanese gynecologic oncologists. More recently, the introduction of chemotherapy into a multimodality treatment for localized cervical cancer has been extensively studied. Treatment schemas have utilized chemotherapy administered before radical surgery or radiation and concurrently with radiation. Since tumor size is an important predictor of response to radiation therapy and eventual survival, the use of chemotherapy to reduce tumor size prior to definitive radiation therapy is attractive. However, despite significant responses to neoadjuvant chemotherapy, randomized trials have failed to demonstrate improvement in survival, possibly due to the development of cross resistance or tumor re-population. In contrast, the concurrent administration of cisplatin-based chemotherapy has produced reproducible benefit in randomized trials of cervical cancer patients with a variety of stages and indications for radiation therapy.[288–292] These trials demonstrated improvements in disease-free and overall survival of 30–50% with concurrent chemotherapy. While the chemotherapy regimens varied, the unifying theme was that all were cisplatin-based. Based on the favorable results of five large randomized trials in cervical cancer, the NCI issued a clinical announcement advocating the concurrent use of cisplatin-based chemotherapy with radiation for cervical cancer patients who required radiation therapy.

Neoadjuvant chemotherapy followed by radical surgery has also been studied. While chemotherapy may induce radiation resistance, this resistance may be overcome by surgical extirpation. Numerous randomized trials have recently been conducted.[293] The results of two completed trials suggest a benefit to this approach. Sardi and colleagues studied neoadjuvant chemotherapy (cisplatin, vincristine, bleomycin) for three courses followed by radical hysterectomy if technically possible followed by radiation therapy.[294] Resection was possible in 100% of the neoadjuvant patients versus 85% of the control group and after 9 years of follow-up the overall survival was improved in the neoadjuvant group at 80% compared with 61%. In another recent randomized trial, Benedetti-Panici and his Italian colleagues compared neoadjuvant cisplatin-based chemotherapy followed by radical hysterectomy versus radiation therapy.[295] In this study, radiation therapy was only given to patients with positive surgical margins or positive nodes. These authors also found a significant improvement in disease-free and overall survival (69% *vs* 51%, *p* = 0.01) with neoadjuvant chemotherapy and surgery compared with radiation therapy alone. However, this study has been criticized because of the low dose of radiation (70 Gy), which is well below what is accepted in the USA.[295] Whether neoadjuvant chemotherapy and radical surgery is superior to radiation therapy with concurrent cisplatin-based chemotherapy is being evaluated by an ongoing randomized trial by the European Organization for Research and Treatment of Cancer (EORTC).

Recurrent cervical cancer represents a particularly difficult problem, with few long-term survivors. The majority of patients with recurrent disease present initially with locally advanced disease and, as demonstrated in recent randomized trials, their disease-free and overall survival curves are almost identical. For patients who have a localized central recurrence following hysterectomy, radiation therapy can be utilized. More commonly, localized recurrences may follow radiation and radical surgery (usually exenteration) is required, with survivals of 25–50%, depending on patient selection criteria. Recent surgical advances, including continent urinary diversion, anal preservation and vaginal reconstruction, can significantly improve the patient's quality of life. Patients with metastatic disease who receive chemotherapy generally fare poorly, with median survivals of 6–8 months.

Both surgery and radiation therapy can be utilized for the management of Stage IB cervical cancer with similar-appearing results. However, significant selection bias exists in determining who is selected for surgery or radiation therapy.[296] Radical hysterectomy is the preferred treatment option for smaller tumors and carries a nearly 100% disease-specific survival rate for tumors under 2 cm.[283,284] Because of controversy regarding the appropriate management of early-stage disease, Landoni and colleagues performed a randomized study of radical surgery versus radiotherapy for stage IB–IIA cervical cancer.[297] These authors found no difference in overall or disease-free survival. However, 46 out of 55 (84%) patients with bulky tumors in the surgery group received adjuvant radiation for additional risk factors.

It has long been recognized that, among tumors limited to the cervix, tumor size is predictive of nodal involvement and survival.[298] While opinion over the appropriate treatment has varied widely, the designation by FIGO of Stage IB1 and IB2 in 1994 established criteria differentiating the clinical management of smaller from larger gross cervical tumors limited to the cervix. Finan and colleagues, retrospectively applying the FIGO 1994 definition, reported Stage IB2 cervical cancer patients had a significantly higher incidence of nodal metastasis (21% vs 44%) and poorer survival (73% vs

90%) following radical hysterectomy than patients with Stage IB1, despite the more frequent use of postoperative radiation therapy (38% vs 72%).[299] Similarly, Trattner and colleagues found that Stage IB1 patients had an overall survival of 90% compared with 40% 5-year survival of Stage IB2 patients.[300]

Following radical hysterectomy, patients may be at high or intermediate risk for recurrence based on pathologic findings. Factors associated with the highest risk of recurrence include nodal metastasis, parametrial extension and involved surgical margins. These patients typically have received radiation but this has been more recently replaced with concurrent chemotherapy and radiation. Patients with deeply invasive tumors, tumors exceeding 4 cm and vascular/lymphatic invasion are at intermediate risk for recurrence. Some authors have advocated routine adjuvant radiation therapy for this sub-group.[286]

Stages III and IV: The tumor is either locally advanced or it has metastasized. Radiation therapy is also the preferred therapy. Surgery is occasionally helpful to relieve symptoms. Chemotherapy is often added.

PREVENTION AND THERAPY WITH VACCINES

A series of technical breakthroughs began in 1991 that have dramatically changed the field of human papillomavirus prevention. Zhou et al. revealed that HPV particles ultrastructurally similar to papillomavirus particles could be produced by expressing the HPV-16 viral capsid genes (L1 and L2) of HPV 16 from a vaccinia vector in eukaryotic cells.[301] Shortly thereafter, other groups reported producing similar VLPs in HPV 16 and HPV 11 (Fig. 13.44).[302–307] This work culminated in the recently published Merck-sponsored multi-institutional study by Koutsky and colleagues summarized in Table 13.17.[11] This study is the first to show that women vaccinated with HPV 16 VLPs, do not harbor HPV 16 or develop HPV 16 related precursor lesions and, by inference, are unlikely to develop HPV-related cancer or transmit the HPV in question. Currently, additional trials examining types 6, 11, 16 and 18 are in progress. These studies will answer questions about the duration of the immune response and degree to which VLP immunization with additional HPV constructs prevents infection by other high-risk HPV types.

Although vaccines would theoretically eliminate cervical cancer, several issues remain unresolved. First, the lack of cross-protection would require a vaccine

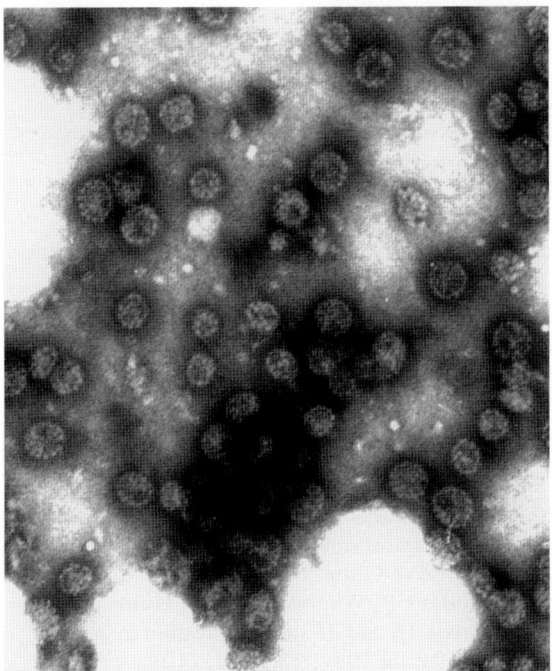

Fig. 13.44 Viral-like particles similar to those currently used in vaccine trials. (VLPs produced by the laboratory of Robert Rose, University of Rochester, Rochester, NY. The micrograph is courtesy of Linda Stannard, University of Cape Town, Cape Town, South Africa.)

Table 13.17 Outcome of vaccination for human papillomavirus

Endpoint	Vaccine (n = 768)	Placebo (n = 765)	Efficacy
Persistent infection	0	41	100.0
Transient infection	6	68	91.2
HPV 16 + CIN	0	9	100.0

From Koutsky et al.[11]

for each type. Nevertheless, types 16, 18, 31, 33, 35 and 45 account for approximately 80% of cervical cancers. Determining whether vaccination should be voluntary or compulsory, delivered to both men and women, instituted in childhood, duration of effect, etc., remains to be resolved. Nevertheless, successes with VLP vaccines are sufficiently compelling to promise a significant reduction in cancer incidence in vaccinated populations. However, this reduction will be gradual and incomplete, unless more efficient and economical methods are devised to provide broad-spectrum oncogenic papillomavirus protection. Issues of vaccine delivery, cost-effectiveness and changes in screening strategies will bear attention and will not be simple or inexpensive in the short run. Nevertheless, a reduc-

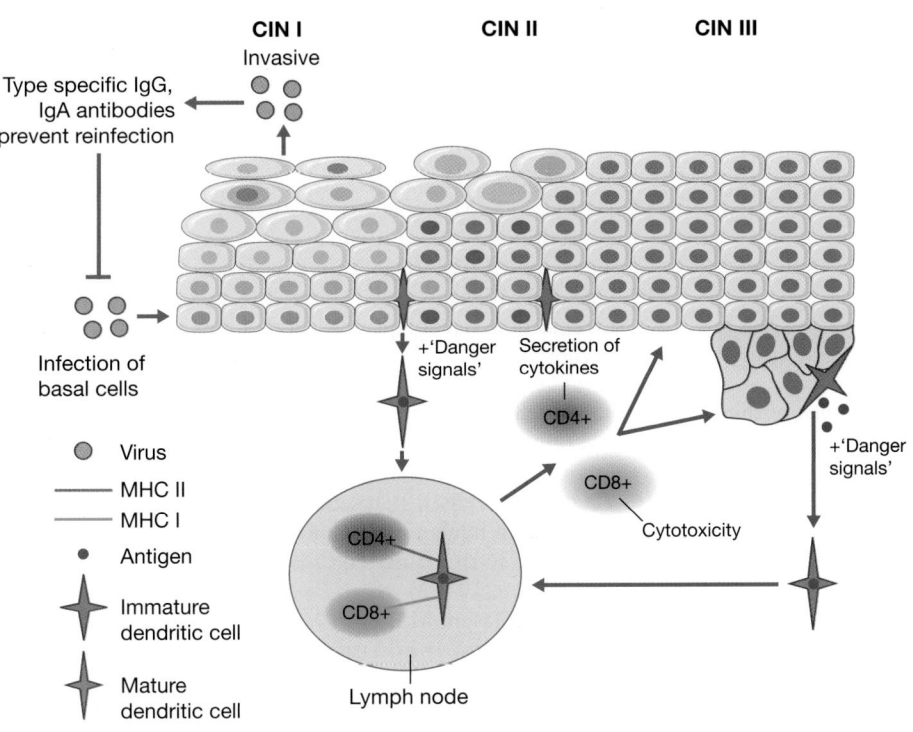

Fig. 13.45 Challenges of inducing antitumor immunity to papillomaviruses include overcoming peripheral tolerance, presenting antigens more effectively than that which occurs during natural infection and stimulating both antigen-presenting cell (dendritic cells) and effector cells pathways. (From Crum and Rivera,[308] copyright 2003, Jones and Bartlett Publishers, with permission.)

tion in the frequency of abnormal Papanicolaou smears and the obligate reduction in colposcopic referrals should be realized in a relatively short period of time even if cytologic screening continues, as it will.

Reversal of cervical cancer and its higher-grade precursors will be much more challenging, as there is no clear-cut example in nature (other than regression of early lesions). Treatment of cancer patients will be complicated by not only difficulties in confirming strong immune responses but also confirming that such responses are indeed efficacious. However, the technology is sufficiently advanced to express tumor antigens *in vivo* and stimulate activated tumor-specific effector cells *in vivo* and *in vitro*, successfully overcoming the obstacles imposed by the natural location of disease problems with antigen presentation and peripheral tolerance that preclude robust T-cell recruitment (Fig. 13.45). The challenge in treating precursor disease will be to bypass difficulties, theoretical or real, that are imposed by the natural location of this disease beyond the reach of cytotoxic lymphocytes. If animal data apply to humans, one possible outcome of vaccinating patients with precursor disease may be to preempt subsequent invasive tumors. This concept bears testing with animal models that include both a precursor and an invasive phase. In the treatment of both cancer and its precursors, a combined approach with high antigen delivery, primed antigen presenting cells and co-administration of cytokines is more attractive for patients with invasive disease. A simpler approach to those with preinvasive disease may be more appropriate for economic reasons. Whether these strategies will be sufficient to overcome the adaptive responses of tumor cells remains to be determined and will represent the next major scientific challenge in treating local and advanced cervical neoplasia.[245]

References

1 Burkett BJ, Peterson CM, Birch LM, et al. The relationship between contraceptives, sexual practices, cervical human papillomavirus infection among a college population. J Clin Epidemiol 1992; 45(11):1295–1302.

2 Kjaer SK, de Villiers EM, Caglayan H, et al. Human papillomavirus, herpes simplex virus and other potential risk factors for cervical cancer in a high-risk area (Greenland) and a low-risk area (Denmark) – a second look. Br J Cancer 1993; 67(4):830–837.

3 Kiviat N. Natural history of cervical neoplasia: overview and update. Am J Obstet Gynecol 1996; 175(4 Pt 2): 1099–1104.

4 O'Hanlan KA, Crum CP. Human papillomavirus-associated cervical intraepithelial neoplasia following lesbian sex. Obstet Gynecol 1996; 88(4 Pt 2):702–703.

5 Rosenfeld WD, Rose E, Vermund SH, Schreiber K, Burk RD. Follow-up evaluation of cervicovaginal human papillomavirus infection in adolescents. J Pediatr 1992; 121(2):307–311.

6 Melkert PW, Hopman E, van den Brule AJ, et al. Prevalence of HPV in cytomorphologically normal cervical smears, as determined by the polymerase chain reaction, is age-dependent. Int J Cancer 1993; 53(6):919–923.

7 Moscicki AB. Genital infections with human papillomavirus (HPV). Pediatr Infect Dis J 1998; 17(7):651–652.

8 Clavel C, Masure M, Bory JP, et al. Human papillomavirus testing in primary screening for the detection of high-grade cervical lesions: a study of 7932 women. Br J Cancer 2001; 84(12):1616–1623.

9 Levert M, Clavel C, Graesslin O, et al. Human papillomavirus typing in routine cervical smears. Results from a series of 3778 patients. Gynecol Obstet Fertil 2000; 28(10):722–728.

10 Stoler MH, Rhodes CR, Whitbeck A, et al. Human papillomavirus type 16 and 18 gene expression in cervical neoplasias. Hum Pathol 1992; 23(2):117–128.

11 Koutsky LA, Ault KA, Wheeler CM, et al. A controlled trial of a human papillomavirus type 16 vaccine. N Engl J Med 2002; 347(21):1645–1651.

12 Lorincz AT, Reid R, Jenson AB, et al. Human papillomavirus infection of the cervix: relative risk associations of 15 common anogenital types. Obstet Gynecol 1992; 79(3):328–337.

13 Munoz N, Bosch FX, de Sanjose S, et al. Epidemiologic classification of human papillomavirus types associated with cervical cancer. N Engl J Med 2003; 348(6):518–527.

14 Koutsky LA, Holmes KK, Critchlow CW, et al. A cohort study of the risk of cervical intraepithelial neoplasia grade 2 or 3 in relation to papillomavirus infection. N Engl J Med 1992; 327(18):1272–1278.

15 Xi LF, Koutsky LA, Galloway DA, et al. Genomic variation of human papillomavirus type 16 and risk for high grade cervical intraepithelial neoplasia. J Natl Cancer Inst 1997; 89(11):796–802.

16 De Marco F, Marcante ML. HPV-16 E6–E7 differential transcription induced in Siha cervical cancer cell line by interferons. J Biol Regul Homeost Agents 1993; 7(1):15–21.

17 Hart KW, Williams OM, Thelwell N, et al. Novel method for detection, typing, quantification of human papillomaviruses in clinical samples. J Clin Microbiol 2001; 39(9):3204–3212.

18 Sun CA, Lai HC, Chang CC, et al. The significance of human papillomavirus viral load in prediction of histologic severity and size of squamous intraepithelial lesions of uterine cervix. Gynecol Oncol 2001; 83(1):95–99.

19 Ylitalo N, Sorensen P, Josefsson AM, et al. Consistent high viral load of human papillomavirus 16 and risk of cervical carcinoma in situ: a nested case-control study. Lancet 2000; 355(9222):2194–2198.

20 Clavel C, Masure M, Levert M, et al. Human papillomavirus detection by the hybrid capture II assay: a reliable test to select women with normal cervical smears at risk for developing cervical lesions. Diagn Mol Pathol 2000; 9(3):145–150.

21 Nagai Y, Maehama T, Asato T, Kanazawa K. Persistence of human papillomavirus infection after therapeutic conization for CIN 3: Is it an alarm for disease recurrence? Gynecol Oncol 2000; 79(2):294–299.

22 Ylitalo N, Josefsson A, Melbye M, et al. A prospective study showing long-term infection with human papillomavirus 16 before the development of cervical carcinoma in situ. Cancer Res 2000; 60(21):6027–6032.

23 Elfgren K, Kalantari M, Moberger B, Hagmar B, Dillner JA. Population-based five-year follow-up study of cervical human papillomavirus infection. Am J Obstet Gynecol 2000; 183(3):561–567.

24 Hopman EH, Rozendaal L, Voorhorst FJ, et al. High-risk human papillomavirus in women with normal cervical cytology prior to the development of abnormal cytology and colposcopy. Br J Obstet Gynaecol 2000; 107(5):600–604.

25 Nobbenhuis MA, Walboomers JM, Helmerhorst TJ, et al. Relation of human papillomavirus status to cervical lesions and consequences for cervical-cancer screening: a prospective study. Lancet 1999; 354(9172):20–25.

26 zur, Hausen H., de Villiers EM. Human papillomaviruses. Annu Rev Microbiol 1994; 48:427–447.

27 Mayrand MH, Coutlee F, Hankins C, et al. Detection of human papillomavirus type 16 DNA in consecutive genital samples does not always represent persistent infection as determined by molecular variant analysis. J Clin Microbiol 2000; 38(9):3388–3393.

28 Xi LF, Demers W, Kiviat NB, et al. Sequence variation in the noncoding region of human papillomavirus type 16 detected by single-strand conformation polymorphism analysis. J Infect Dis 1993; 168(3):610–617.

29 Xi LF, Carter JJ, Galloway DA, et al. Acquisition and natural history of human papillomavirus type 16 variant infection among a cohort of female university students. Cancer Epidemiol Biomarkers Prev 2002; 11(4):343–351.

30 Hu X, Guo Z, Tianyun P, et al. HPV typing and HPV16 E6-sequence variations in synchronous lesions of cervical squamous-cell carcinoma from Swedish patients. Int J Cancer 1999; 83(1):34–37.

31 Nindl I, Rindfleisch K, Lotz B, Schneider A, Durst M. Uniform distribution of HPV 16 E6 and E7 variants in patients with normal histology, cervical intra-epithelial neoplasia and cervical cancer. Int J Cancer 1999; 82(2):203–207.

32 Veress G, Murvai M, Szarka K, et al. Transcriptional activity of human papillomavirus type 16 variants having deletions in the long control region. Eur J Cancer 2001; 37(15):1946–1952.

33 Zehbe I, Tachezy R, Mytilineos J, et al. Human papillomavirus 16 E6 polymorphisms in cervical lesions from different European populations and their correlation with human leukocyte antigen class II haplotypes. Int J Cancer 2001; 94(5):711–716.

34 Odunsi, K, Ganesan T. Motif analysis of HLA class II molecules that determine the HPV associated risk of cervical carcinogenesis. Int J Mol Med 2001; 8(4):405–412.

35 Evans M, Borysiewicz LK, Evans AS, et al. Antigen processing defects in cervical carcinomas limit the presentation of a CTL epitope from human papillomavirus 16 E6. J Immunol 2001; 167(9):5420–5428.

36 McLachlin CM, Tate JE, Zitz JC, Sheets EE, Crum CP. Human papillomavirus type 18 and intraepithelial lesions of the cervix. Am J Pathol 1994; 144(1):141–147.

37 Hecht JL, Kadish AS, Jiang G, Burk RD. Genetic characterization of the human papillomavirus (HPV) 18 E2 gene in clinical specimens suggests the presence of a subtype with decreased oncogenic potential. Int J Cancer 1995; 60(3):369–376.

38 Geraghty DE, Vu Q, Williams L, et al. Mapping HLA for single nucleotide polymorphisms. Rev Immunogenet 1999; 1(2):231–238.

39 Wang SS, Wheeler CM, Hildesheim A, et al. Human leukocyte antigen class I and II alleles and risk of cervical neoplasia: results from a population-based study in Costa Rica. J Infect Dis 2001; 184(10):1310–1314.

40 Herrero R, Hildesheim A, Bratti C, et al. Population-based study of human papillomavirus infection and cervical neoplasia in rural Costa Rica. J Natl Cancer Inst 2000; 92(6):464–474.

41 Brown MR, Noffsinger A, First MR, Penn I, Husseinzadeh N. HPV subtype analysis in lower genital tract neoplasms of female renal transplant recipients. Gynecol Oncol 2000; 79(2):220–224.

42 ter Haar-van Eck SA, Rischen-Vos J, Chadha-Ajwani S, Huikeshoven FJ. The incidence of cervical intraepithelial neoplasia among women with renal transplant in relation to cyclosporine. Br J Obstet Gynaecol 1995; 102(1):58–61.

43 Alloub MI, Barr BB, McLaren KM, et al. Human papillomavirus infection and cervical intraepithelial neoplasia in women with renal allografts. BMJ 1989; 298(6667):153–156.

44 Halpert R, Fruchter RG, Sedlis A, et al. Human papillomavirus and lower genital neoplasia in renal transplant patients. Obstet Gynecol 1986; 68(2):251–258.

45 Wright TC Jr, Sun XW. Anogenital papillomavirus infection and neoplasia in immunodeficient women. Obstet Gynecol Clin North Am 1996; 23(4):861–893.

46 Moscicki AB, Ellenberg JH, Vermund SH, et al. Prevalence of and risks for cervical human papillomavirus infection and squamous intraepithelial lesions in adolescent girls: impact of infection with human immunodeficiency virus. Arch Pediatr Adolesc Med 2000; 154(2):127–134.

47 Ahdieh L, Munoz A, Vlahov D, et al. Cervical neoplasia and repeated positivity of human papillomavirus infection in human immunodeficiency virus-seropositive and -seronegative women. Am J Epidemiol 2000; 151(12): 1148–1157.

48 Cardillo M, Hagan R, Abadi J, Abadi MA. CD4 T-Cell count, viral load, squamous intraepithelial lesions in women infected with the human immunodeficiency virus. Cancer 2001; 93(2):111–114.

49 Heard I, Tassie JM, Schmitz V, et al. Increased risk of cervical disease among human immunodeficiency virus-infected women with severe immunosuppression and high human papillomavirus load (1). Obstet Gynecol 2000; 96(3):403–409.

50 Ellerbrock TV, Chiasson MA, Bush TJ, et al. Incidence of cervical squamous intraepithelial lesions in HIV-infected women. JAMA 2000; 283(8):1031–1037.

51 La Ruche G, You B, Mensah-Ado I, et al. Human papillomavirus and human immunodeficiency virus

infections: relation with cervical dysplasia-neoplasia in African women. Int J Cancer 1998; 76(4):480–486.

52 Parkin DM, Wabinga H, Nambooze S, Wabwire-Mangen F. AIDS-related cancers in Africa: maturation of the epidemic in Uganda. AIDS 1999; 13(18):2563–2570.

53 Franceschi S, Dal Maso L, Arniani S, et al. Risk of cancer other than Kaposi's sarcoma and non-Hodgkin's lymphoma in persons with AIDS in Italy. Cancer and AIDS Registry Linkage Study. Br J Cancer 1998; 78(7):966–970.

54 Chokunonga E, Levy LM, Bassett MT, et al. Aids and cancer in Africa: the evolving epidemic in Zimbabwe. AIDS 1999; 13(18):2583–2588.

55 La Ruche G, Leroy V, Mensah-Ado I, et al. Short-term follow up of cervical squamous intraepithelial lesions associated with HIV and human papillomavirus infections in Africa. Int J STD AIDS 1999; 10(6):363–368.

56 Lomalisa P, Smith T, Guidozzi F. Human immunodeficiency virus infection and invasive cervical cancer in South Africa. Gynecol Oncol 2000; 77(3):460–463.

57 Karlsson R, Jonsson M, Edlund K, et al. Lifetime number of partners as the only independent risk factor for human papillomavirus infection: a population-based study. Sex Transm Dis 1995; 22(2):119–127.

58 Thomas DB, Ray RM, Kuypers J, et al. Human papillomaviruses and cervical cancer in Bangkok. III. The role of husbands and commercial sex workers. Am J Epidemiol 2001; 153(8):740–748.

59 Agarwal SS, Sehgal A, Sardana S, Kumar A, Luthra UK. Role of male behavior in cervical carcinogenesis among women with one lifetime sexual partner. Cancer 1993; 72(5):1666–1669.

60 Kjaer SK, Engholm G, Dahl C, Bock JE. Case-control study of risk factors for cervical squamous cell neoplasia in Denmark. IV: Role of smoking habits. Eur J Cancer Prev 1996; 5(5):359–365.

61 Krebs HB, Helmkamp BF. Treatment failure of genital condylomata acuminata in women: role of the male sexual partner. Am J Obstet Gynecol 1991; 165(2):337–339.

62 Connelly DA, Chan PJ, Patton WC, King A. Human sperm deoxyribonucleic acid fragmentation by specific types of papillomavirus. Am J Obstet Gynecol 2001; 184(6): 1068–1070.

63 Lai YM, Lee JF, Huang HY, et al. The effect of human papillomavirus infection on sperm cell motility. Fertil Steril 1997; 67(6):1152–1155.

64 Kreider JW, Howett MK, Lill NL, et al. In vivo transformation of human skin with human papillomavirus type 11 from condylomata acuminata. J Virol 1986; 59(2):369–376.

65 Elson DA, Riley RR, Lacey A, et al. Sensitivity of the cervical transformation zone to estrogen-induced squamous carcinogenesis. Cancer Res. 2000; 60(5):1267–1275.

66 Salazar EL, Sojo-Aranda I, Lopez R, Salcedo M. The evidence for an etiological relationship between oral contraceptive use and dysplastic change in cervical tissue. Gynecol Endocrinol 2001; 15(1):23–28.

67 Kjellberg L, Hallmans G, Ahren AM, et al. Smoking, diet, pregnancy and oral contraceptive use as risk factors for cervical intra-epithelial neoplasia in relation to human papillomavirus infection. Br J Cancer 2000; 82(7):1332–1338.

68 Coker AL, Sanders LC, Bond SM, Gerasimova T, Pirisi L. Hormonal and barrier methods of contraception, oncogenic human papillomaviruses, cervical squamous intraepithelial lesion development. J Womens Health Gend Based Med 2001; 10(5):441–449.

69 Parazzini F, La Vecchia C, Negri E, et al. Case-control study of oestrogen replacement therapy and risk of cervical cancer. BMJ 1997; 315(7100): 85–88.

70 Lacey JV, Jr, Brinton LA, Barnes WA, et al. Use of hormone replacement therapy and adenocarcinomas and squamous cell carcinomas of the uterine cervix. Gynecol Oncol 2000; 77(1):149–154.

71 Ali S, Astley SB, Sheldon TA, Peel KR, Wells M. Detection and measurement of DNA adducts in the cervix of smokers and non-smokers. Int J Gynecol Cancer 1994; 4(3):188–193.

72 Goodman MT, McDuffie K, Hernandez B, et al. CYP1A1, GSTM1, GSTT1 polymorphisms and the risk of cervical squamous intraepithelial lesions in a multiethnic population. Gynecol Oncol 2001; 81(2):263–269.

73 Lacey JV, Jr, Frisch M, Brinton LA, et al. Associations between smoking and adenocarcinomas and squamous cell carcinomas of the uterine cervix (United States). Cancer Causes Control 2001; 12(2):153–161.

74 Deacon JM, Evans CD, Yule R, et al. Sexual behaviour and smoking as determinants of cervical HPV infection and of CIN3 among those infected: a case-control study nested within the Manchester cohort. Br J Cancer 2000; 83(11):1565–1572.

75 Anttila T, Saikku P, Koskela P, et al. Serotypes of Chlamydia trachomatis and risk for development of cervical squamous cell carcinoma. JAMA 2001; 285(1):47–51.

76 Hildesheim A, Herrero R, Castle PE, et al. HPV co-factors related to the development of cervical cancer: results from a population-based study in Costa Rica. Br J Cancer 2001; 84(9):1219–1226.

77 Reesink-Peters N, Ossewaarde JM, van der Zee AG, et al. No association of anti-Chlamydia trachomatis antibodies and severity of cervical neoplasia. Sex Transm Infect 2001; 77(2):101–102.

78 Marrazzo JM, Stine K, Koutsky LA. Genital human papillomavirus infection in women who have sex with women: a review. Am J Obstet Gynecol 2000; 183(3): 770–774.

79 Fethers K, Marks C, Mindel A, Estcourt CS. Sexually transmitted infections and risk behaviours in women who have sex with women. Sex Transm Infect 2000; 76(5): 345–349.

80 Goldie SJ. Health economics and cervical cancer prevention: a global perspective. Virus Res 2002; 89(2):301–309.

81 Denny L, Kuhn L, Pollack A, Wainwright H, Wright TC Jr. Evaluation of alternative methods of cervical cancer screening for resource-poor settings. Cancer 2000; 89(4):826–833.

82 Wright TC Jr, Denny L, Kuhn L, Pollack A, Lorincz A. HPV DNA testing of self-collected vaginal samples compared with cytologic screening to detect cervical cancer. JAMA 2000; 283(1):81–86.

83 Rosenfeld WD, Vermund SH, Wentz SJ, Burk RD. High prevalence rate of human papillomavirus infection and

association with abnormal Papanicolaou smears in sexually active adolescents. Am J Dis Child 1989; 143(12): 1443–1447.

84 Shen LH, Rushing L, McLachlin CM, Sheets EE, Crum CP. Prevalence and histologic significance of cervical human papillomavirus DNA detected in women at low and high risk for cervical neoplasia. Obstet Gynecol 1995; 86(4 Pt 1): 499–503.

85 Sherman ME, Schiffman M, Cox JT. Effects of age and human papilloma viral load on colposcopy triage: data from the randomized Atypical Squamous Cells of Undetermined Significance/Low-Grade Squamous Intraepithelial Lesion Triage Study (ALTS). J Natl Cancer Inst. 2002; 94(2): 102–107.

86 Levert M, Clavel C, Graesslin O, et al. Human papillomavirus typing in routine cervical smears. Results from a series of 3778 patients. Gynecol Obstet Fertil 2000; 28(10):722–728.

87 Lazcano-Ponce E, Herrero R, Munoz N, et al. Epidemiology of HPV infection among Mexican women with normal cervical cytology. Int J Cancer 2001; 91(3):412–420.

88 Kutza J, Smith E, Levy B, et al. Use of hormone replacement therapy (HRT) and detection of human papillomavirus (HPV) DNA in postmenopausal women. Ann Epidemiol 2000; 10(7):465–466.

89 Ferenczy A, Gelfand MM, Franco E, Mansour N. Human papillomavirus infection in postmenopausal women with and without hormone therapy. Obstet Gynecol 1997; 90(1):7–11.

90 McLachlin CM, Shen LH, Sheets EE, et al. Disparities in mean age and histopathologic grade between human papillomavirus type-specific early cervical neoplasms. Hum Pathol 1997; 28(11):1226–1229.

91 Krane JF, Granter SR, Trask CE, Hogan CL, Lee KR. Papanicolaou smear sensitivity for the detection of adenocarcinoma of the cervix: a study of 49 cases. Cancer 2001; 93(1):8–15.

92 Schwartz PE, Hadjimichael O, Lowell DM, Merino MJ, Janerich D. Rapidly progressive cervical cancer: the Connecticut experience. Am J Obstet Gynecol 1996; 175(4 Pt 2): 1105–1109.

93 Lacey JV Jr, Brinton LA, Abbas FM, et al. Oral contraceptives as risk factors for cervical adenocarcinomas and squamous cell carcinomas. Cancer Epidemiol Biomarkers Prev 1999; 8(12):1079–1085.

94 Linnehan MJ, Groce NE. Counseling and educational interventions for women with genital human papillomavirus infection. AIDS Patient Care STDS 2000; 14(8):439–445.

95 Reitano M. Counseling patients with genital warts. Am J Med 1997; 102(5A): 38–43.

96 Dong SM, Kim HS, Rha SH, Sidransky D. Promoter hypermethylation of multiple genes in carcinoma of the uterine cervix. Clin Cancer Res 2001; 7(7):1982–1986.

97 Conaglen HM, Hughes R, Conaglen JV, Morgan JA Prospective study of the psychological impact on patients of first diagnosis of human papillomavirus. Int J STD AIDS 2001; 12(10):651–658.

98 ALTS Group. Human papillomavirus testing for triage of women with cytologic evidence of low-grade squamous intraepithelial lesions: baseline data from a randomized trial. The Atypical Squamous Cells of Undetermined Significance/Low-Grade Squamous Intraepithelial Lesions Triage Study (ALTS) Group. J Natl Cancer Inst 2000; 92(5):397–402.

99 Wright TC Jr, Schiffman M. Adding a test for human papillomavirus DNA to cervical-cancer screening. N Engl J Med 2003; 348(6):489–490.

100 Dong SM, Kim HS, Rha SH, Sidransky D. Promoter hypermethylation of multiple genes in carcinoma of the uterine cervix. Clin Cancer Res 2001; 7(7):1982–1986.

101 Liao SY, Stanbridge EJ. Expression of MN/CA9 protein in Papanicolaou smears containing atypical glandular cells of undetermined significance is a diagnostic biomarker of cervical dysplasia and neoplasia. Cancer 2000; 88(5): 1108–1121.

102 Keating JT, Cviko A, Riethdorf S, et al. Ki-67, cyclin E, P16INK4 are complimentary surrogate biomarkers for human papilloma virus-related cervical neoplasia. Am J Surg Pathol 2001; 25(7):884–891.

103 Reddy VG, Khanna N, Jain SK, Das BC, Singh N. Telomerase-A molecular marker for cervical cancer screening. Int J Gynecol Cancer 2001; 11(2):100–106.

104 Riethdorf S, Riethdorf L, Schulz G, et al. Relationship between telomerase activation and HPV 16/18 oncogene expression in squamous intraepithelial lesions and squamous cell carcinomas of the uterine cervix. Int J Gynecol Pathol 2001; 20(2):177–185.

105 Koss LG. Diagnostic cytology. Philadelphia: JB Lippincott; 1997.

106 Gray W, McKee G. Diagnostic cytopathology, 2nd edn. Philadelphia, PA: Churchill Livingstone; 2002.

107 Cibas EC, Ducatman BS. Cytology, 2nd edn. Philadelphia, PA: WB Saunders; 2003.

108 Bibbo M. Comprehensive cytopathology. Philadelphia, PA: WB Saunders; 2003.

109 Bryans FE, Boyes DA, Fidler HK. The influence of a cytological screening program upon the incidence of invasive squamous cell carcinoma of the cervix in British Columbia. Am J Obstet Gynecol. 1964; 88:898–906.

110 Miller AB. The (in)efficiency of cervical screening in Europe. Eur J Cancer 2002; 38(3):321–326.

111 Obwegeser JH, Brack S. Does liquid-based technology really improve detection of cervical neoplasia? A prospective, randomized trial comparing the ThinPrep Pap Test with the conventional Pap Test, including follow-up of HSIL cases. Acta Cytol 2001; 45(5):709–714.

112 Lee KR, Ashfaq R, Birdsong GG, et al. Comparison of conventional Papanicolaou smears and a fluid-based, thin-layer system for cervical cancer screening. Obstet Gynecol 1997; 90(2):278–284.

113 Solomon D, Davey D, Kurman R, et al. The 2001 Bethesda System: terminology for reporting results of cervical cytology. JAMA 2002; 287(16):2114–2119.

114 Solomon D, Schiffman M, Tarone R. ASCUS LSIL Triage Study (ALTS) conclusions reaffirmed: response to a November 2001 commentary. Obstet Gynecol 2002; 99(4):671–674.

115 The 1988 Bethesda System for reporting cervical/vaginal cytologic diagnoses. Developed and approved at the National Cancer Institute Workshop, Bethesda, Maryland, USA, 12–13 December, 1988. Acta Cytol 1989; 33(5):567–574.

116 Prasad CJ, Genest DR, Crum CP. Nondiagnostic squamous atypia of the cervix (atypical squamous epithelium of undetermined significance): histologic and molecular correlates. Int J Gynecol Pathol 1994; 13(3):220–227.

117 Sherman ME, Solomon D, Schiffman M. Qualification of ASCUS. A comparison of equivocal LSIL and equivocal HSIL cervical cytology in the ASCUS LSIL Triage Study. Am J Clin Pathol 2001; 116(3):386–394.

118 Melamed MR, Flehinger BJ. Non-diagnostic squamous atypia in cervico-vaginal cytology as a risk factor for early neoplasia. Acta Cytol 1976; 20(2):108–110.

119 Sorosky JI, Kaminski PF, Wheelock JB, Podczaski ES. Clinical significance of hyperkeratosis and parakeratosis in otherwise negative Papanicolaou smears. Gynecol Oncol 1990; 39(2):132–134.

120 Kurman RJ, Henson DE, Herbst AL, Noller KL, Schiffman MH. Interim guidelines for management of abnormal cervical cytology. The 1992 National Cancer Institute Workshop. JAMA 1994; 271(23):1866–1869.

121 Ali S, Niang MA, N'doye I, et al. Secretor polymorphism and human immunodeficiency virus infection in Senegalese women. J Infect Dis 2000; 181(2):737–739.

122 Kiviat NB, Paavonen JA, Brockway J, et al. Cytologic manifestations of cervical and vaginal infections. I. Epithelial and inflammatory cellular changes. JAMA 1985; 253(7): 989–996.

123 Kiviat NB, Peterson M, Kinney-Thomas E, et al. Cytologic manifestations of cervical and vaginal infections. II. Confirmation of Chlamydia trachomatis infection by direct immunofluorescence using monoclonal antibodies. JAMA 1985; 253(7):997–1000.

124 Ward BE, Burkett B, Petersen C, et al. Cytologic correlates of cervical Papillomavirus infection. Int J Gynecol Pathol 1990; 9(4):297–305.

125 De Girolami E. Perinuclear halo versus koilocytotic atypia. Obstet Gynecol 1967; 29(4):479–487.

126 Symmans F, Mechanic L, MacConnell P, et al. Correlation of cervical cytology and human papillomavirus DNA detection in postmenopausal women. Int J Gynecol Pathol 1992; 11(3):204–209.

127 Kaminski PF, Sorosky JI, Wheelock JB, Stevens CW Jr. The significance of atypical cervical cytology in an older population. Obstet Gynecol 1989; 73(1):13–15.

128 Kaminski PF, Stevens CW Jr, Wheelock JB. Squamous atypia on cytology. The influence of age. J Reprod Med 1989; 34(9):617–620.

129 Wilbur DC. False negatives in focused rescreening of Papanicolaou smears: How frequently are 'abnormal' cells detected in retrospective review of smears preceding cancer or high-grade intraepithelial neoplasia? Arch Pathol Lab Med 1997; 121(3):273–276.

130 Crum CP, Genest DR, Krane JF, et al. Subclassifying atypical squamous cells in Thin-Prep cervical Cytology correlates with detection of high-risk human papillomavirus DNA. Am J Clin Pathol 1999; 112(3):384–390.

131 Renshaw AA, Genest DR, Cibas ES. Should atypical squamous cells of undetermined significance (ASCUS) be subcategorized? Accuracy analysis of Papanicolaou smears using receiver operating characteristic curves and implications for the ASCUS/squamous intraepithelial lesion ratio. Am J Clin Pathol 2001; 116(5):692–695.

132 Pitman MB, Cibas ES, Powers CN, Renshaw AA, Frable WJ. Reducing or eliminating use of the category of atypical squamous cells of undetermined significance decreases the diagnostic accuracy of the Papanicolaou smear. Cancer 2002; 96(3):128–134.

133 Wright TC Jr, Cox JT, Massad LS, Twiggs LB, Wilkinson EJ. 2001 Consensus Guidelines for the management of women with cervical cytological abnormalities. JAMA 2002; 287(16):2120–2129.

134 Solomon D, Schiffman M, Tarone R. Comparison of three management strategies for patients with atypical squamous cells of undetermined significance: baseline results from a randomized trial. J Natl Cancer Inst. 2001; 93(4): 293–299.

135 Mitao M, Nagai N, Levine RU, Silverstein SJ, Crum CP. Human papillomavirus type 16 infection: a morphological spectrum with evidence for late gene expression. Int J Gynecol Pathol 1986; 5(4):287–296.

136 Willett GD, Kurman RJ, Reid R, et al. Correlation of the histologic appearance of intraepithelial neoplasia of the cervix with human papillomavirus types. Emphasis on low grade lesions including so-called flat condyloma. Int J Gynecol Pathol 1989; 8(1):18–25.

137 Duensing S, Munger K. Centrosome abnormalities, genomic instability and carcinogenic progression. Biochim Biophys Acta 2001; 1471(2): M81–M88.

138 Munger K. The role of human papillomaviruses in human cancers. Front Biosci 2002; 7:d641–d649.

139 Crum CP, Fu YS, Levine RU, et al. Intraepithelial squamous lesions of the vulva: biologic and histologic criteria for the distinction of condylomas from vulvar intraepithelial neoplasia. Am J Obstet Gynecol 1982; 144(1):77–83.

140 Crum CP, Mitao M, Levine RU, Silverstein S. Cervical papillomaviruses segregate within morphologically distinct precancerous lesions. J Virol 1985; 54(3):675–681.

141 Park J, Sun D, Genest DR, et al. Coexistence of low and high grade squamous intraepithelial lesions of the cervix: morphologic progression or multiple papillomaviruses? Gynecol Oncol 1998; 70(3):386–391.

142 Genest DR, Stein L, Cibas E, et al. A binary (Bethesda) system for classifying cervical cancer precursors: criteria, reproducibility, viral correlates. Hum Pathol 1993; 24(7):730–736.

143 Koss LG. Evolution in cervical pathology and cytology: a historical perspective. Eur J Gynaecol Oncol 2000; 21(6):550–554.

144 Meisels A, Morin C, Casas-Cordero M. Human papillomavirus infection of the uterine cervix. Int J Gynecol Pathol 1982; 1(1):75–94.

145 Prasad CJ, Sheets E, Selig AM, McArthur MC, Crum CP. The binucleate squamous cell: histologic spectrum and relationship to low-grade squamous intraepithelial lesions. Mod Pathol 1993; 6(3):313–317.

146 Mosher RE, Lee KR, Trivijitsilp P, Crum CP. Cytologic correlates of papillary immature metaplasia (immature condyloma) of the cervix. Diagn Cytopathol 1998; 18(6):416–421.

147 Crum CP, Cibas ES, Lee KR. Pathology of early cervical neoplasia. Philadelphia, PA: Churchill Livingstone; 1997.

148 Saito K, Saito A, Fu YS, Smotkin D, Gupta J, Shah K. Topographic study of cervical condyloma and intraepithelial neoplasia. Cancer 1987; 59(12):2064–2070.

149 Lee KR, Minter LJ, Crum CP. Koilocytotic atypia in Papanicolaou smears. Reproducibility and biopsy correlations. Cancer 1997; 81(1):10–15.

150 Hall S, Wu TC, Soudi N, Sherman ME. Low-grade squamous intraepithelial lesions: cytologic predictors of biopsy confirmation. Diagn Cytopathol 1994; 10(1):3–9.

151 Crum CP, Egawa K, Barron B, et al. Human papilloma virus infection (condyloma) of the cervix and cervical intraepithelial neoplasia: a histopathologic and statistical analysis. Gynecol Oncol 1983; 15(1):88–94.

152 Quade BJ, Yang A, Wang Y, et al. Expression of the p53 homologue p63 in early cervical neoplasia. Gynecol Oncol 2001; 80(1):24–29.

153 Richart RM. Cervical intraepithelial neoplasia. Pathol Annu 1973; 8:301–328.

154 Coleman DV. Cytodiagnosis of viral infections. Recent results. Cancer Res 1993; 133:33–44.

155 Laverty CR, Russell P, Black J, Kappagoda N, Booth N. Adenovirus infection of the cervix. Acta Cytol 1977; 21(1):114–117.

156 Geerling S, Nettum JA, Lindner LE, et al. Sensitivity and specificity of the Papanicolaou-Stained cervical smear in the diagnosis of Chlamydia trachomatis infection. Acta Cytol 1985; 29(5):671–675.

157 Freund KM, Buttlar CA, Giampaolo C, et al. The use of cervical cytology to identify women at risk for chlamydial infection. Am J Prev Med 1992; 8(5):292–297.

158 Crum CP, Mitao M, Winkler B, et al. Localizing chlamydial infection in cervical biopsies with the immunoperoxidase technique. Int J Gynecol Pathol 1984; 3(2):191–197.

159 Crum CP. Symposium Part 1: Should the Bethesda System terminology be used in diagnostic surgical pathology? Int J Gynecol Pathol 2003; 22(1):5–12.

160 Anderson MC, Brown CL, Buckley CH, et al. Current views on cervical intraepithelial neoplasia. J Clin Pathol 1991; 44(12):969–978.

161 Albores-Saavedra J, Young RH. Transitional cell neoplasms (carcinomas and inverted papillomas) of the uterine cervix. A report of five cases. Am J Surg Pathol 1995; 19(10):1138–1145.

162 Ward BE, Saleh AM, Williams JV, Zitz JC, Crum CP. Papillary immature metaplasia of the cervix: a distinct subset of exophytic cervical condyloma associated with HPV-6/11 nucleic acids. Mod Pathol 1992; 5(4):391–395.

163 Nuovo GJ, Blanco JS, Leipzig S, Smith D. Human papillomavirus detection in cervical lesions nondiagnostic for cervical intraepithelial neoplasia: correlation with Papanicolaou smear, colposcopy, occurrence of cervical intraepithelial neoplasia. Obstet Gynecol 1990; 75(6):1006–1011.

164 Yang GC, Demopoulos RI, Chan W, Mittal KR. Superficial nuclear enlargement without koilocytosis as an expression of human Papillomavirus infection of the uterine cervix: an in situ hybridization study. Int J Gynecol Pathol 1992; 11(4):283–287.

165 Trivijitsilp P, Mosher R, Sheets EE, Sun D, Crum CP. Papillary immature metaplasia (immature condyloma) of the cervix: a clinicopathologic analysis and comparison with papillary squamous carcinoma. Hum Pathol 1998; 29(6):641–648.

166 Garzetti GG, Ciavattini A, Goteri G, et al. Vaginal micropapillary lesions are not related to human papillomavirus infection: in situ hybridization and polymerase chain reaction detection techniques. Gynecol Obstet Invest 1994; 38(2):134–139.

167 Nuovo GJ, Cottral S, Richart RM. Occult human papillomavirus infection of the uterine cervix in postmenopausal women. Am J Obstet Gynecol 1989; 160(2):340–344.

168 Jovanovic AS, McLachlin CM, Shen L, Welch WR, Crum CP. Postmenopausal squamous atypia: a spectrum including 'pseudo-koilocytosis'. Mod Pathol 1995; 8(4):408–412.

169 Sano T, Oyama T, Kashiwabara K, Fukuda T, Nakajima T. Expression status of p16 protein is associated with human papillomavirus oncogenic potential in cervical and genital lesions. Am J Pathol 1998; 153(6):1741–1748.

170 Klaes R, Benner A, Friedrich T, et al. p16INK4a immunohistochemistry improves interobserver agreement in the diagnosis of cervical intraepithelial neoplasia. Am J Surg Pathol 2002; 26(11):1389–1399.

171 Park JJ, Sun D, Quade BJ, et al. Stratified mucin-producing intraepithelial lesions of the cervix: adenosquamous or columnar cell neoplasia? Am J Surg Pathol 2000; 24(10):1414–1419.

172 Singer G, Kurman RJ, McMaster MT, Shih IeM. HLA-G immunoreactivity is specific for intermediate trophoblast in gestational trophoblastic disease and can serve as a useful marker in differential diagnosis. Am J Surg Pathol 2002; 26:914–920.

173 Huettner PC, Gersell DJ. Placental site nodule: a clinicopathologic study of 38 cases. Int J Gynecol Pathol 1994; 13(3):191–198.

174 Resnick M, Lester S, Tate JE, et al. Viral and histopathologic correlates of MN and MIB-1 expression in cervical intraepithelial neoplasia. Hum Pathol 1996; 27(3):234–239.

175 Mittal K. Utility of proliferation-associated marker MIB-1 in evaluating lesions of the uterine cervix. Adv Anat Pathol 1999; 6(4):177–185.

176 Quade BJ, Park JJ, Crum CP, Sun D, Dutta A. In vivo cyclin E expression as a marker for early cervical neoplasia. Mod Pathol 1998; 11(12):1238–1246.

177 Riethdorf L, Riethdorf S, Lee KR, et al. Human papillomaviruses, expression of p16, early endocervical glandular neoplasia. Hum Pathol 2002; 33(9):899–904.

178 Natarajan E, Saeb M, Crum CP, et al. Co-expression of p16(INK4A) and laminin 5 gamma2 by microinvasive and superficial squamous cell carcinomas in vivo and by migrating wound and senescent keratinocytes in culture. Am J Path 2003; 163(2):477–491.

179 Kobak WH, Roman LD, Felix JC, et al. The role of endocervical curettage at cervical conization for high-grade dysplasia. Obstet Gynecol 1995; 85(2):197–201.

180 Fine BA, Feinstein GI, Sabella V. The pre- and postoperative value of endocervical curettage in the detection of cervical

intraepithelial neoplasia and invasive cervical cancer. Gynecol Oncol 1998; 71(1):46–49.

181 Frost L. Cytobrush in evaluation of cervical dysplasia. Is cervical curettage necessary?. Acta Obstet Gynecol Scand 1990; 69(7–8): 645–647.

182 Andersen W, Frierson H, Barber S, et al. Sensitivity and specificity of endocervical curettage and the endocervical brush for the evaluation of the endocervical canal. Am J Obstet Gynecol 1988; 159(3):702–707.

183 Brown FM, Faquin WC, Sun D, Crum CP, Cibas ES. LSIL biopsies after HSIL smears. Correlation with high-risk HPV and greater risk of HSIL on follow-up. Am J Clin Pathol 1999; 112(6):765–768.

184 Stoler MH, Schiffman M. Interobserver reproducibility of cervical cytologic and histologic interpretations: realistic estimates from the ASCUS-LSIL Triage Study. JAMA 2001; 285(11):1500–1505.

185 Cox JT. Management of atypical squamous cells of undetermined significance and low-grade squamous intra-epithelial lesion by human papillomavirus testing. Best Pract Res Clin Obstet Gynaecol 2001; 15(5):715–741.

186 Turner MJ, Keane DP, Flannelly GM, et al. Cytological screening history of patients with early invasive cervical cancer. Ir Med J 1990; 83(2):61–62.

187 Cooper P, Kirby AJ, Spiegelhalter DJ, Whitehead AL, Patterson A. Management of women with a cervical smear showing a mild degree of dyskaryosis: a review of policy. Cytopathology 1992; 3(6):331–339.

188 Ostor AG. Natural history of cervical intraepithelial neoplasia: a critical review. Int J Gynecol Pathol 1993; 12(2):186–192.

189 Cox JT, Schiffman M, Solomon D; ASCUS-LSIL Triage Study (ALTS) Group. Prospective follow-up suggests similar risk of subsequent cervical intraepithelial neoplasia grade 2 or 3 among women with cervical intraepithelial neoplasia grade 1 or negative colposcopy and directed biopsy. Am J Obstet Gynecol 2003; 188:1406–1412.

190 Pinto AP, Crum CP. Natural history of cervical neoplasia: defining progression and its consequence. Clin Obstet Gynecol 2000; 43:352–362.

191 Robertson JH, Woodend B, Elliott H. Cytological changes preceding cervical cancer. J Clin Pathol 1994; 47(3): 278–279.

192 Vierhout ME, de Planque PM. Concomitant endocervical curettage and cervical conization. Acta Obstet Gynecol Scand 1991; 70(4–5):359–361.

193 Schermerhorn TJ, Hodge J, Saltzman AK, et al. Clinicopathologic variables predictive of residual dysplasia after cervical conization. J Reprod Med 1997; 42:189–192.

194 Lapaquette TK, Dinh TV, Hannigan EV, et al. Management of patients with positive margins after cervical conization. Obstet Gynecol 1993; 82:440–443.

195 Husseinzadeh N, Carter V, Wesseler T. Significance of positive endocervical curettage in predicting endocervical canal involvement in patients with cervical intraepithelial neoplasia. Gynecol Oncol 1989; 35:358–361.

196 Moore BC, Higgins RV, Laurent SL, Marroum MC, Bellitt P. Predictive factors from cold knife conization for residual cervical intraepithelial neoplasia in subsequent hysterectomy. Am J Obstet Gynecol 1995; 173:361–366.

197 Spirtos NM, Schlaerth JB, d'Ablaing G III, Morrow CP. A critical evaluation of the endocervical curettage. Obstet Gynecol 1987; 70:729–733.

198 Weitzman GA, Korhonen MO, Reeves KO, et al. Endocervical brush cytology. An alternative to endocervical curettage?. J Reprod Med 1988; 33:677–683.

199 Zaitoun AM, McKee G, Coppen MJ, Thomas SM, Wilson PO. Completeness of excision and follow up cytology in patients treated with loop excision biopsy. J Clin Pathol 2000; 53:191–196.

200 Phelps JY III, Ward JA, Szigeti J, Bowland CH, Mayer AR. Cervical cone margins as a predictor for residual dysplasia in post-cone hysterectomy specimens. Obstet Gynecol 1994; 84:128–130.

201 Wright TC, Cox JT, Massad LS, et al. 2001 consensus guidelines for the management of women with cervical intraepithelial neoplasia. Am J Obstet Gynecol 2003; 189(1):295–304.

202 Paraskevaidis E, Kitchener H, Adonakis G, Parkin D, Lolis D. Incomplete excision of CIN in conization: further excision or conservative management? Eur J Obstet Gynecol Reprod Biol 1994; 53(1):45–47.

203 Gardeil F, Barry-Walsh C, Prendiville W, Clinch J, Turner MJ. Persistent intraepithelial neoplasia after excision for cervical intraepithelial neoplasia grade III. Obstet Gynecol 1997; 89(3):419–422.

204 McIndoe WA, McLean MR, Jones RW, Mullins PR. The invasive potential of carcinoma in situ of the cervix. Obstet Gynecol 1984; 64(4):451–458.

205 Paterson-Brown S, Chappatte OA, Clark SK, et al. The significance of cone biopsy resection margins. Gynecol Oncol 1992; 46(2): 182–185.

206 Buxton EJ, Luesley DM, Wade-Evans T, Jordan JA. Residual disease after cone biopsy: completeness of excision and follow-up cytology as predictive factors. Obstet Gynecol 1987; 70(4):529–532.

207 Clavel C, Masure M, Bory JP, et al. Hybrid Capture II-based human papillomavirus detection, a sensitive test to detect in routine high-grade cervical lesions: a preliminary study on 1518 women. Br J Cancer 1999; 80(9): 1306–1311.

208 Lin CT, Tseng CJ, Lai CH, et al. Value of human papillomavirus deoxyribonucleic acid testing after conization in the prediction of residual disease in the subsequent hysterectomy specimen. Am J Obstet Gynecol 2001; 184(5):940–945.

209 Jain S, Tseng CJ, Horng SG, Soong YK, Pao CC. Negative predictive value of human papillomavirus test following conization of the cervix uteri. Gynecol Oncol 2001; 82(1):177–180.

210 Chua KL, Hjerpe A. Human papillomavirus analysis as a prognostic marker following conization of the cervix uteri. Gynecol Oncol 1997; 66(1):108–113.

211 Nuovo GJ, Pedemonte BM. Human papillomavirus types and recurrent cervical warts. JAMA 1990; 263(9): 1223–1226.

212 Ferenczy A, Mitao M, Nagai N, Silverstein SJ, Crum CP. Latent papillomavirus and recurring genital warts. N Engl J Med 1985; 313(13):784–788.

213 Strand A, Wilander E, Zehbe I, Rylander E. High-risk HPV persists after treatment of genital papillomavirus infection but not after treatment of cervical intraepithelial neoplasia. Acta Obstet Gynecol Scand 1997; 76(2):140–144.

214 Tate JE, Resnick M, Sheets EE, Crum CP. Absence of papillomavirus DNA in normal tissue adjacent to most cervical intraepithelial neoplasms. Obstet Gynecol 1996; 88(2):257–260.

215 McKee MD, Schechter C, Burton W, Mulvihill M. Predictors of follow-up of atypical and ASCUS Papanicolaou tests in a high-risk population. J Fam Pract 2001; 50(7):609.

216 Benedetti-Panici P, Maneschi F, D'Andrea G, et al. Early cervical carcinoma: the natural history of lymph node involvement redefined on the basis of thorough parametrectomy and giant section study. Cancer 2000; 88(10):2267–2274.

217 Einhorn N. Cancer of the cervix. Trends in the treatment of uterine carcinoma. East Afr Med J 1970; 47(8):410–414.

218 Uyar DS, Eltabbakh GH, Mount SL. Positive predictive value of liquid-based and conventional cervical Papanicolaou smears reported as malignant. Gynecol Oncol 2003; 89:227–232.

219 Johnson SJ, Wadehra V. How predictive is a cervical smear suggesting invasive squamous cell carcinoma? Cytopathology 2001; 12(3):144–150.

220 Nguyen GK, Nguyen-Ho P, Husain M, Husain EM. Cervical squamous cell carcinoma and its precursor lesions: cytodiagnostic criteria and pitfalls. Anat Pathol 1996; 1: 139–164.

221 Crum CP. Dynamics of human papillomavirus infection between diagnosis and therapy: results from the Zyc101A therapeutic trial of high grade cervical intraepithelial neoplasia. N Engl J Med 2003. J Infect Dis 2004; 189:1348–1354.

222 Clark SB, Dawson AE. Invasive squamous-cell carcinoma in thinprep specimens: diagnostic clues in the cellular pattern. Diagn Cytopathol 2002; 26(1):1–4.

223 Rushing, L, Cibas ES. Frequency of tumor diathesis in smears from women with squamous cell carcinoma of the cervix. Acta Cytol 1997; 41(3):781–785.

224 Paraskevaidis E, Kitchener HC, Miller ID, et al. A population-based study of microinvasive disease of the cervix – a colposcopic and cytologic analysis. Gynecol Oncol 1992; 45(1):9–12.

225 Liu WM, Chao KC, Wang KI, Ng HT. Colposcopic assessment in microinvasive carcinoma of the cervix. Zhonghua Yi Xue Za Zhi (Taipei) 1989; 43(3):171–176.

226 Wright VC. When to suspect squamous cancer at colposcopy. Nurse Pract 2001; 26(9):50–61.

227 Soutter WP, Haidopoulos D, Gornall RJ, et al. Is conservative treatment for adenocarcinoma in situ of the cervix safe? Br J Obstet Gynaecol 2001; 108(11):1184–1189.

228 Skehan M, Soutter WP, Lim K, Krausz T, Pryse-Davies J. Reliability of colposcopy and directed punch biopsy. Br J Obstet Gynaecol 1990; 97(9):811–816.

229 Al Nafussi AI, Hughes DE. Histological features of CIN3 and their value in predicting invasive microinvasive squamous carcinoma. J Clin Pathol 1994; 47(9):799–804.

230 Tidbury P, Singer A, Jenkins D. CIN 3: the role of lesion size in invasion. Br J Obstet Gynaecol 1992; 99(7):583–586.

231 Wilkinson EJ, Komorowski RA. Borderline microinvasive carcinoma of the cervix. Obstet Gynecol 1978; 51(4):472–476.

232 Crum CP, Nucci MR Lee KR. The cervix. In: Mills SE, ed. Sternbergs diagnostic surgical pathology, 4th edn. Philadelphia, PA: Lippincott Williams and Wilkins; 2004: 2377–2434.

233 Sedlis A, Sall S, Tsukada Y, et al. Microinvasive carcinoma of the uterine cervix: a clinical-pathologic study. Am J Obstet Gynecol 1979; 133(1):64–74.

234 Kosary CL. FIGO stage, histology, histologic grade, age and race as prognostic factors in determining survival for cancers of the female gynecological system: an analysis of 1973–1987 SEER cases of cancers of the endometrium, cervix, ovary, vulva, vagina. Semin Surg Oncol 1994; 10(1):31–46.

235 Hopkins MP, Morley GW. Microinvasive squamous cell carcinoma of the cervix. J Reprod Med 1994; 39(9): 671–673.

236 Lecuru F, Neji K, Robin F, et al. Microinvasive carcinoma of the cervix. Rationale for conservative treatment in early squamous cell carcinoma. Eur J Gynaecol Oncol 1997; 18(6):465–470.

237 Marana HR, de Andrade JM, Matthes AC, et al. Microinvasive carcinoma of the cervix. Analysis of prognostic factors. Eur J Gynaecol Oncol 2001; 22(1):64–66.

238 Ostor A, Rome R, Quinn M. Microinvasive adenocarcinoma of the cervix: a clinicopathologic study of 77 women. Obstet Gynecol 1997; 89(1):88–93.

239 Creasman WT, Zaino RJ, Major FJ, et al. Early invasive carcinoma of the cervix (3 to 5 mm invasion): risk factors and prognosis. A Gynecologic Oncology Group Study. Am J Obstet Gynecol 1998; 178(1 Pt 1):62–65.

240 Burghardt E, Winter R, Tamussino K, et al. Diagnosis and surgical treatment of cervical cancer. Crit Rev Oncol Hematol 1994; 17(3):181–231.

241 Savage EW. Microinvasive carcinoma of the cervix. Am J Obstet Gynecol 1972; 113(5):708–717.

242 Hasumi K, Sakamoto A, Sugano H. Microinvasive carcinoma of the uterine cervix. Cancer 1980; 45(5):928–931.

243 Benson WL, Norris HJ. A critical review of the frequency of lymph node metastasis and death from microinvasive carcinoma of the cervix. Obstet Gynecol 1977; 49(5):632–638.

244 Roche WD, Norris HJ. Microinvasive carcinoma of the cervix. The significance of lymphatic invasion and confluent patterns of stromal growth. Cancer 1975; 36(1):180–186.

245 Ostor AG, Rome RM. Studies on 200 cases of early squamous cell carcinoma of the cervix. Int J Gynecol Pathol 1993; 12(3):193–207.

246 Buckley SL, Tritz DM, Van Le L, et al. Lymph node metastases and prognosis in patients with stage IA2 cervical cancer. Gynecol Oncol 1996; 63(1):4–9.

247 Delgado G, Bundy BN, Fowler WC, et al. Prospective surgical pathological study of stage I squamous carcinoma of the cervix: a Gynecologic Oncology Group Study. Gynecol Oncol 1989; 35(3):314–320.

248 van Nagell JR, Jr, Greenwell N, Powell DF, et al. Microinvasive carcinoma of the cervix. Am J Obstet Gynecol 1983; 145(8):981–991.

249 Benedet JL, Anderson GH. Stage IA carcinoma of the cervix revisited. Obstet Gynecol 1996; 87:1052–1059.

250 McLachlin CM, Devine P, Muto M, Genest DR. Pseudoinvasion of vascular spaces: report of an artifact caused by cervical lidocaine injection prior to loop diathermy. Hum Pathol 1994; 25(2):208–211.

251 Reagan JW, Fu YS. Histologic types and prognosis of cancers of the uterine cervix. Int J Radiat Oncol Biol Phys 1979; 5(7):1015–1020.

252 Wang TY, Chen BF, Yang YC, et al. Histologic and immunophenotypic classification of cervical carcinomas by expression of the p53 Homologue p63: a study of 250 Cases. Hum Pathol 2001; 32(5):479–486.

253 Raptis S, Haber G, Ferenczy A. Vaginal squamous cell carcinoma with sarcomatoid spindle cell features. Gynecol Oncol 1993; 49(1):100–106.

254 Steeper TA, Piscioli F, Rosai J. Squamous cell carcinoma with sarcoma-like stroma of the female genital tract. Clinicopathologic study of four cases. Cancer 1983; 52(5):890–898.

255 Pang LC. Sarcomatoid squamous cell carcinoma of the uterine cervix with osteoclast-like giant cells: report of two cases. Int J Gynecol Pathol 1998; 17(2):174–177.

256 Robertson DI, Maung R, Duggan MA. Verrucous carcinoma of the genital tract: is it a distinct entity? Can J Surg 1993; 36(2):147–151.

257 Wong WS, Ng CS, Lee CK. Verrucous carcinoma of the cervix. Arch Gynecol Obstet 1990; 247(1):47–51.

258 Koenig C, Turnicky RP, Kankam CF, Tavassoli FA. Papillary squamotransitional cell carcinoma of the cervix: a report of 32 cases. Am J Surg Pathol 1997; 21(8): 915–921.

259 Al Nafussi AI, Al Yusif R. Papillary squamotransitional cell carcinoma of the uterine cervix: an advanced stage disease despite superficial location: report of two cases and review of the literature. Eur J Gynaecol Oncol 1998; 19(5): 455–457.

260 Rose PG, Stoler MH, Abdul-Karim FW. Papillary squamotransitional cell carcinoma of the vagina. Int J Gynecol Pathol 1998; 17(4):372–375.

261 Nakamura E, Shimizu M, Fujiwara K, et al. Papillary squamous cell carcinoma of the uterine cervix: diagnostic pitfalls. APMIS 1998; 106(10):975–978.

262 Robinson CE, Sarode VR, Albores-Saavedra. Mixed papillary transitional cell carcinoma and adenocarcinomas of the uterine cervix: a clinicopathologic study of three cases. Int J Gynecol Pathol 2003; 22:220–225.

263 Mittal KR, Demopoulos RI, Goswami S. Patterns of keratin 19 expression in normal, metaplastic, condylomatous, atrophic, dysplastic, malignant cervical squamous epithelium. Am J Clin Pathol 1992; 98(4):419–423.

264 Husniye, Dilek F, Kucukali T. Mucin production in carcinomas of the uterine cervix. Eur J Obstet Gynecol Reprod Biol 1998; 79(2):149–151.

265 Benda JA. Histopathologic prognostic factors in early stage cervical carcinoma. J Natl Cancer Inst Monogr 1996; (21):27–34.

266 Pretorius R, Semrad N, Watring W, Fotheringham N. Presentation of cervical cancer. Gynecol Oncol 1991; 42(1):48–53.

267 Jennings OG, Soeters RP, Tiltman AJ, et al. The natural history of carcinoma of the cervix in young women. S Afr Med J 1992; 82(5):351–354.

268 Yang YC, Shen J, Tate JE, et al. Cervical cancer in young women in Taiwan: prognosis is independent of papillomavirus or tumor cell type. Gynecol Oncol 1997; 64(1):59–63.

269 Baay MF, Tjalma WA, Weyler J, et al. Prevalence of human papillomavirus in elderly women with cervical cancer. Gynecol Obstet Invest 2001; 52(4):248–251.

270 Duggan B, Muderspach LI, Roman LD, et al. Cervical cancer in pregnancy: reporting on planned delay in therapy. Obstet Gynecol 1993; 82(4 Pt 1):598–602.

271 Allen DG, Planner RS, Tang PT, Scurry JP, Weerasiri T. Invasive cervical cancer in pregnancy. Aust N Z J Obstet Gynaecol 1995; 35(4):408–412.

272 Monk BJ, Montz FJ. Invasive cervical cancer complicating intrauterine pregnancy: treatment with radical hysterectomy. Obstet Gynecol 1992; 80(2):199–203.

273 Sivanesaratnam V, Jayalakshmi P, Loo C. Surgical management of early invasive cancer of the cervix associated with pregnancy. Gynecol Oncol 1993; 48(1):68–75.

274 Sood AK, Sorosky JI, Krogman S, et al. Surgical management of cervical cancer complicating pregnancy: a case-control study. Gynecol Oncol 1996; 63(3):294–298.

275 Sorosky JI, Squatrito R, Ndubisi BU, et al. Stage I squamous cell cervical carcinoma in pregnancy: planned delay in therapy awaiting fetal maturity. Gynecol Oncol 1995; 59(2):207–210.

276 van Vliet W, van Loon AJ, ten Hoor KA, Boonstra H. Cervical carcinoma during pregnancy: outcome of planned delay in treatment. Eur J Obstet Gynecol Reprod Biol 1998; 79(2):153–157.

277 Paraskevaidis E, Koliopoulos G, Malamou-Mitsi V, et al. Large loop excision of the transformation zone for treating cervical intraepithelial neoplasia: a 12-year experience. Anticancer Res 2001; 21(4B):3097–3099.

278 Stoler MH, Mills SE, Gersell DJ, Walker AN. Small-cell neuroendocrine carcinoma of the cervix. A human papillomavirus type 18-associated cancer. Am J Surg Pathol 1991; 15(1):28–32.

279 Pirog EC, Kleter B, Olgac S, et al. Prevalence of human papillomavirus DNA in different histological subtypes of cervical adenocarcinoma. Am J Pathol 2000; 157(4):1055–1062.

280 Lombard I, Vincent-Salomon A, Validire P, et al. Human papillomavirus genotype as a major determinant of the course of cervical cancer. J Clin Oncol 1998; 16(8): 2613–2619.

281 Schwartz SM, Daling JR, Shera KA, et al. Human papillomavirus and prognosis of invasive cervical cancer: a population-based study. J Clin Oncol 2001; 19(7): 1906–1915.

282 Covens A, Rosen B, Murphy J, et al. Changes in the demographics and perioperative care of stage IA(2)/IB (1) cervical cancer over the past 16 years. Gynecol Oncol 2001; 81(2):133–137.

283 Magrina JF, Goodrich MA, Lidner TK, et al. Modified radical hysterectomy in the treatment of early squamous cervical cancer. Gynecol Oncol 1999; 72(2):183–186.

284 Hopkins MP, Morley GW. Radical hysterectomy versus radiation therapy for stage IB squamous cell cancer of the cervix. Cancer 1991; 68(2):272–277.

285 Hopkins MP, Peters WA, III, Andersen W, Morley GW. Invasive cervical cancer treated initially by standard hysterectomy. Gynecol Oncol 1990; 36(1):7–12.

286 Fuller AF Jr, Elliott N, Kosloff C, Hoskins WJ, Lewis JL Jr. Determinants of increased risk for recurrence in patients undergoing radical hysterectomy for stage IB and IIA carcinoma of the cervix. Gynecol Oncol 1989; 33(1):34–39.

287 Sedlis A, Bundy BN, Rotman MZ, et al. A randomized trial of pelvic radiation therapy versus no further therapy in selected patients with stage IB carcinoma of the cervix after radical hysterectomy and pelvic lymphadenectomy: a Gynecologic Oncology Group Study. Gynecol Oncol 1999; 73(2):177–183.

288 Whitney CW, Sause W, Bundy BN, et al. Randomized comparison of fluorouracil plus cisplatin versus hydroxyurea as an adjunct to radiation therapy in stage IIB-IVA carcinoma of the cervix with negative para-aortic lymph nodes: a Gynecologic Oncology Group and Southwest Oncology Group Study. J Clin Oncol 1999; 17(5): 1339–1348.

289 Morris M, Gershenson DM, Burke TW, et al. A phase II study of carboplatin and cisplatin in advanced or recurrent squamous carcinoma of the uterine cervix. Gynecol Oncol 1994; 53(2):234–238.

290 Rose PG, Bundy BN, Watkins EB, et al. Concurrent cisplatin-based radiotherapy and chemotherapy for locally advanced cervical cancer. N Engl J Med 1999; 340(15): 1144–1153.

291 Keys HM, Bundy BN, Stehman FB, et al. Cisplatin, radiation, adjuvant hysterectomy compared with radiation and adjuvant hysterectomy for bulky stage IB cervical carcinoma. N Engl J Med 1999; 340(15):1154–1161.

292 Peters WA III, Liu PY, Barrett RJ, et al. Concurrent chemotherapy and pelvic radiation therapy compared with pelvic radiation therapy alone as adjuvant therapy after radical surgery in high-risk early-stage cancer of the cervix. J Clin Oncol 2000; 18(8):1606–1613.

293 Stewart LA, Parmar MK, Tierney JF. Meta-analyses and large randomized, controlled trials. N Engl J Med 1998; 338(1):61–62.

294 Sardi JE, Giaroli A, Sananes C, et al. Long-term follow-up of the first randomized trial using neoadjuvant chemotherapy in stage Ib squamous carcinoma of the cervix: the final results. Gynecol Oncol 1997; 67(1):61–69.

295 Benedetti-Panici P, Greggi S, Colombo A, et al. Neoadjuvant chemotherapy and radical surgery versus exclusive radiotherapy in locally advanced squamous cell cervical cancer: results from the Italian Multicenter Randomized Study. J Clin Oncol 2002; 20(1):179–188.

296 Zola P, Ferrero A, Fuso L, et al. Different types of hysterectomy in the radio-surgical treatment of early cervical cancer (FIGO Ib-IIa). Eur J Gynaecol Oncol 2002; 23(3):236–242.

297 Landoni F, Maneo A, Colombo A, et al. Randomised study of radical surgery versus radiotherapy for stage Ib-IIa cervical cancer. Lancet 1997; 350(9077): 535–540.

298 Piver MS, Chung WS. Prognostic significance of cervical lesion size and pelvic node metastases in cervical carcinoma. Obstet Gynecol 1975; 46(5):507–510.

299 Finan MA, DeCesare S, Fiorica JV, et al. Radical hysterectomy for stage IB1 vs IB2 carcinoma of the cervix: does the new staging system predict morbidity and survival? Gynecol Oncol 1996; 62(2):139–147.

300 Trattner M, Graf AH, Lax S, et al. Prognostic factors in surgically treated stage Ib–IIb cervical carcinomas with special emphasis on the importance of tumor volume. Gynecol Oncol 2001; 82(1):11–16.

301 Zhou J, Sun XY, Stenzel DJ, Frazer IH. Expression of vaccinia recombinant HPV 16 L1 and L2 ORF proteins in epithelial cells is sufficient for assembly of HPV virion-like particles. Virology 1991; 185(1):251–257.

302 Suzich JA, Ghim SJ, Palmer-Hill FJ, et al. Systemic immunization with papillomavirus L1 protein completely prevents the development of viral mucosal papillomas. Proc Natl Acad Sci USA 1995; 92(25):11553–11557.

303 Rose RC, White WI, Li M, et al. Human papillomavirus type 11 recombinant L1 capsomeres induce virus-neutralizing antibodies. J Virol 1998; 72(7): 6151–6154.

304 Rose RC, Bonnez W, Reichman RC, Garcea RL. Expression of human papillomavirus type 11 L1 protein in insect cells: in vivo and in vitro assembly of viruslike particles. J Virol 1993; 67(4):1936–1944.

305 Schiller JT, Lowy DR. Papillomavirus-like particles and HPV vaccine development. Semin Cancer Biol 1996; 7(6):373–382.

306 Suzich JA, Ghim SJ, Palmer-Hill FJ, et al. Systemic immunization with papillomavirus L1 protein completely prevents the development of viral mucosal papillomas. Proc Natl Acad Sci USA 1995; 92(25):11553–11557.

307 Galloway DA. Is vaccination against human papillomavirus a possibility? Lancet 1998; 351 (Suppl 3):22–24.

308 Crum CP, Rivera MN. Vaccines for cervical cancer. Cancer J 2003; 9:368–376.

309 Hsieh CY, You SL, Kao CL, Chen CJ. Reproductive and infectious risk factors for invasive cervical cancer in Taiwan. Anticancer Res 1999; 19:4495–4500.

310 Hughes SA, Sun D, Gibson C, et al. Managing atypical squamous cells of undetermined significance (ASCUS): human papillomavirus testing, ASCUS subtyping, or follow-up cytology? Am J Obstet Gynecol 2002; 186: 396–403.

311 Cox JT, Schiffman M, Solomon D; ASCUS-LSIL Triage Study (ALTS) Group. Prospective follow-up suggests similar risk of subsequent cervical intraepithelial neoplasia grade 2 or 3 among women with cervical intraepithelial neoplasia grade 1 or negative colposcopy and directed biopsy. Am J Obstet Gynecol 2003; 188:1406–1412.

312 Benedet JL, Bender H, Jones H 3rd, Ngan HY, Pecorelli S. FIGO staging classifications and clinical practice guidelines in the management of gynecologic cancers. FIGO Committee on Gynecologic Oncology. Int J Gynaecol Obstet 2000; 70:209–262.

313 Basil JB, Horowitz IR. Cervical carcinoma: contemporary management. J Reprod Med 2001; 28:727–739.

314 Covens A, Shaw P, Murphy J, et al. Is radical trachelectomy

a safe alternative to radical hysterectomy for patients with stage IA-B carcinoma of the cervix? Cancer 1999; 86:2273–2279.

315 Dargent D, Martin X, Sacchetoni A, Mathevet P. Laparoscopic vaginal radical trachelectomy: a treatment to preserve the fertility of cervical carcinoma patients. Cancer 2000; 88(8):1877–1882.

316 Roy M, Plante M. Radical vaginal trachelectomy for invasive cervical cancer. J Gynecol Obstet Biol Reprod (Paris) 2000; 29(3):279–281.

317 Shepherd JH, Mould T, Oram DH. Radical trachelectomy in early stage carcinoma of the cervix: outcome as judged by recurrence and fertility rates. Br J Obstet Gynaecol 2001; 108:882–885.

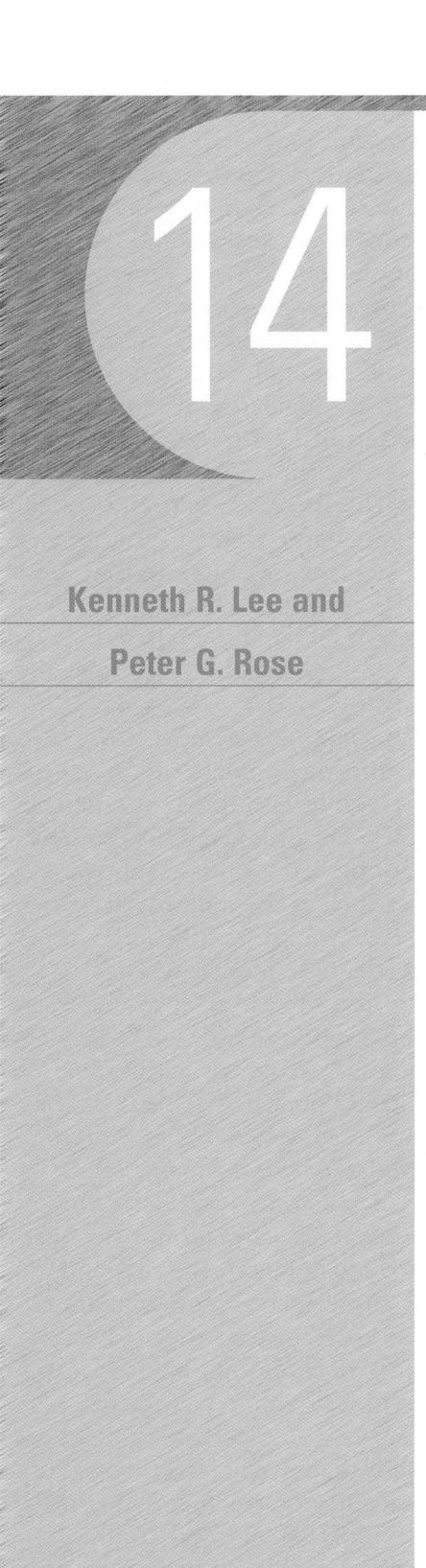

14

Glandular neoplasia of the cervix

Kenneth R. Lee and

Peter G. Rose

Introduction

The precursor-cancer connection
Identifying the woman at risk for
glandular neoplasia

**Principles of cytology in the
diagnosis of glandular neoplasia**

Introduction
Criteria for adenocarcinoma
in situ
Cytologic findings of invasive
adenocarcinoma
False-negative interpretations
False-positive interpretations
Misdiagnosis: HSIL mistaken for
AIS
Atypical glandular cells of
undetermined significance

**Diagnosis and management
of adenocarcinoma *in situ***

Limitations of clinical and
colposcopic detection
Histologic criteria for
adenocarcinoma *in situ*
Glandular atypias that do not
fulfill the criteria for classic
adenocarcinoma *in situ*: the
concept of 'glandular dysplasia'

Differential diagnosis of
adenocarcinoma *in situ*
Treatment of adenocarcinoma
in situ

Early invasive adenocarcinoma

**Diagnosis and management
of adenocarcinoma of the
cervix**

Endocervical (mucinous)
adenocarcinoma
Endometrioid adenocarcinoma
Intestinal adenocarcinoma
Adenosquamous carcinoma
Well-differentiated villoglandular
adenocarcinoma
Clear cell carcinoma
Serous carcinoma
Adenoid basal and adenoid cystic
carcinomas
Mesonephric adenocarcinoma
Adenocarcinoma metastatic to the
cervix
Benign mimics of cervical
adenocarcinoma
Management and prognosis
of adenocarcinomas of the
cervix

Introduction

THE PRECURSOR-CANCER CONNECTION

The concept of adenocarcinoma *in situ* (AIS) was first proposed in 1953 by Friedell and McKay on the basis of two cases of cervical adenocarcinoma that appeared to them to also contain a noninvasive precursor lesion.[1] However, in the ensuing decades, despite remarkable progress in the understanding of the development of cervical squamous carcinoma, AIS remained obscure. It was not until the 1980s that AIS began to receive widespread recognition, highlighted by a detailed description of 72 cases by Jaworski et al. in 1988.[2] AIS is now acknowledged to be the precursor to most invasive adenocarcinomas of the cervix on the basis of the following:

1 The cells of AIS appear neoplastic and AIS is often found adjacent to early invasive adenocarcinomas.[3–6]

2 Human papillomavirus (HPV) is detected in the large majority of AIS cases and with similar frequencies and subtypes (primarily types 16 and 18) in both AIS and adenocarcinoma.[7]

3 Retrospective reviews of biopsies and Papanicolaou (Pap) smears preceding cases of invasive adenocarcinoma have found examples of unrecognized AIS.[8–10]

4 The average age of women with AIS is approximately 38 years, whereas the average age of women with early invasive adenocarcinoma is approximately 43 years (summarized by Lee and Flynn),[5] consistent with AIS being an antecedent to invasion.

5 Markers of aberrant cell cycle regulation, such as p16,[11,12] increased cell turnover, such as Ki-67,[13–16] and alterations of cell membrane adhesion molecules, such as CD44[17,18] and other membrane glycoproteins,[19,20] have regularly been detected in both AIS and adenocarcinoma, but not in normal endocervical cells or benign processes that simulate AIS.

IDENTIFYING THE WOMAN AT RISK FOR GLANDULAR NEOPLASIA

At least 90% of cervical adenocarcinomas contain human papillomavirus (HPV). Types 16, 18 and 45 were identified in approximately 50, 40 and 10% of these tumors in one study.[7] Thus, as with squamous carcinoma, HPV is the most important risk factor for cervical adenocarcinoma.[7,21–23] However, several features distinguish these two cancer types:

1 *Adenocarcinoma of the cervix is increasing in incidence relative to squamous carcinoma.* Since the 1960s, the frequency of cervical adenocarcinoma has been increasing in the USA and other developed countries, where it currently accounts for 20 to 25% of all invasive cervical cancers.[24–32] In a Canadian study, Liu et al. observed that from 1970 to 1996 the incidence of squamous carcinoma declined from 13.4 to 6.6 per 100 000, while the incidence of adenocarcinoma increased from 1.3 to 1.8.[28] This increase has been especially evident among young white women.[32] Although the causes of this increase are not clear, they are likely to include the combined effect of an increased incidence of AIS and the relative ineffectiveness of the Pap smear in detecting early glandular neoplasia.[33–36]

2 *Not all adenocarcinomas are associated with HPV.* There are several different subtypes of adenocarcinoma, possibly with different etiologies and natural histories. For instance, HPV is rarely detected in some of the less common subtypes of adenocarcinoma such as the minimal deviation type.[7] Andersson et al. found that the index of HPV positivity in adenocarcinomas was age-related, decreasing from 89% in women under age 40 to 42% in women over age 60.[37]

3 Contrary to squamous carcinomas, cigarette smoking has not been implicated as a risk factor for adenocarcinomas.[38,39]

4 *The majority of studies support a relationship between adenocarcinoma and its precursors and oral contraceptive use.* This association is stronger than that seen with squamous carcinomas and, depending on the study, increases as a function of length of use and current use.[22,39–45] However, one study of older women did not link cervical adenocarcinoma with estrogen replacement therapy.[46]

The above data suggest that several factors conspire to place a woman at risk for adenocarcinoma. These include young age, exposure to HPV and oral contraceptive use. Unresolved however, is the mechanism by which these events increase the risk of glandular neoplasia relative to squamous neoplasia. One avenue that has not been explored is the relationship between estrogens and the cervical transformation zone. Studies in mice have shown a striking increase in squamous and glandular proliferation with the administration of estrogens, a scenario that is likely played out in the human, following menarche.[47] In humans, a relationship between columnar cell proliferations in the cervix (microglandular change) and hormonal stimuli has been described.[48] Whether the local effects of estrogens include an increase in the index of columnar-derived (or destined) cells that are susceptible to HPV infection remains to be determined, but merits study.[49,50]

Principles of cytology in the diagnosis of glandular neoplasia

INTRODUCTION

A cytologic interpretation of 'atypical endocervical cells', 'adenocarcinoma *in situ*' and 'adenocarcinoma' connote increasingly serious conditions and merit increasingly greater scrutiny. However, because these are often difficult to separate cytologically, the exclusion of glandular neoplasia ultimately requires a colposcopic examination and often a cone biopsy. This is in contrast to the spectrum of squamous abnormalities, the options for which include cytologic follow-up, colposcopy and currently, HPV testing. Thus, because both diagnostic and non-diagnostic glandular atypias require a similar follow-up approach, they merit discussion as a single group and will be addressed together in this segment (Table 14.1).

The key to preventing adenocarcinoma of the cervix is the detection and elimination of its precursor AIS. Unfortunately, Pap smears are not as sensitive for glandular precursors as they are for squamous.[33–36] We calculated a smear sensitivity of 55% to 70% for AIS[34] and of 45% to 76% for invasive adenocarcinoma in our material.[9] This lack of sensitivity is primarily related to

Table 14.1 *The cytologic differential diagnosis of abnormal glandular-appearing cells in Pap smears*

Neoplastic lesions
  Adenocarcinoma *in situ*
  Cervical adenocarcinoma
  High-grade squamous intraepithelial lesion
  Endometrial hyperplasia/carcinoma
  Extrauterine adenocarcinomas
Non-neoplastic lesions
  Tubal metaplasia
  Direct sampling of lower segment endometrium
  Menstrual endometrium
  Reactive endocervical lesions (cervicitis, microglandular hyperplasia, Arias-Stella, radiation effect)
  Atrophy

two factors: (1) Deficient endocervical sampling: this has contributed significantly to low sensitivity in the past. However, the combination of newly designed collection instruments and heightened awareness of the importance of sampling the transformation zone have reduced this component of the problem. (2) Under-appreciation of glandular atypia on smears: we found a screening/interpretive false-negative frequency of 40% to 50% after retrospective review of prior negative Pap smears in women with AIS or invasive adeno-carcinomas.[9,34] Others have reported similar findings.[10] This reflects the difficulties mentioned above that are inherent in distinguishing benign from malignant glandular-appearing cells.

CRITERIA FOR ADENOCARCINOMA *IN SITU*

AIS cells aggregate in hyperchromatic crowded groups. Features of endocervical glandular differentiation in these groups include:

1 strips of columnar cells with crowded, basally oriented nuclei and pale, foamy, or vacuolated cytoplasm;
2 feathering (the perpendicular orientation of the long axis of the cells around the periphery of the group such that the nuclei and small wisps of cytoplasm protrude radially);
3 rosettes (gland-like structures with radially oriented nuclei around a central space).

Neoplastic nuclear features are essential for confirmation. With AIS, there is usually extreme nuclear crowding, often with molding of nuclei around one another. Nuclei are slightly enlarged, ovoid or irregular and hyperchromatic, with diffusely dispersed, slightly to moderately coarse chromatin particles. Nucleoli are usually inconspicuous, but are prominent in some cases. Mitotic figures may be found in about 40% of cases but often only after a diligent search (Figs 14.1–14.7).[51–54]

In thin-layer preparations, AIS groups are smaller and architectural clues, such as columnar cells in strips and rosettes, are not as obvious; the chromatin is finer and nucleoli are more obvious. Importantly however, extreme cell crowding and feathering remain pronounced in thin layers. Also, the chromatin remains coarse relative to that of normal endocervical cells and this can be readily perceived.[55,56]

If definitive features are present, the cytologic interpretation may specify AIS.[57] However, in this setting it is important for clinicians and pathologists to realize that invasion cannot be excluded by cytology and that a cone biopsy is necessary.[58,59]

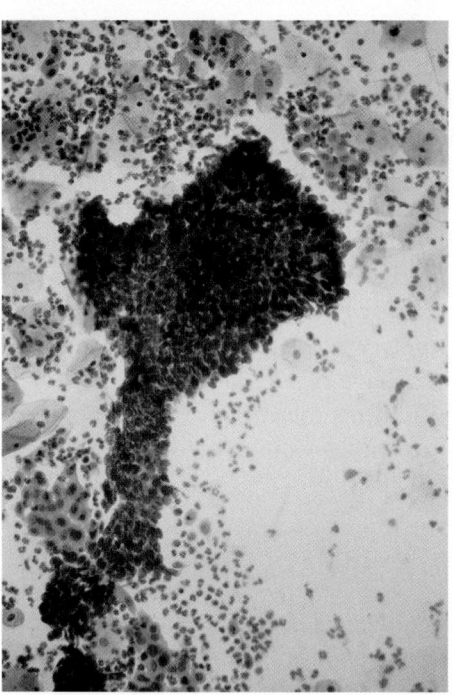

Fig. 14.1
Adenocarcinoma *in situ*. A large crowded group with peripheral feathering is seen.

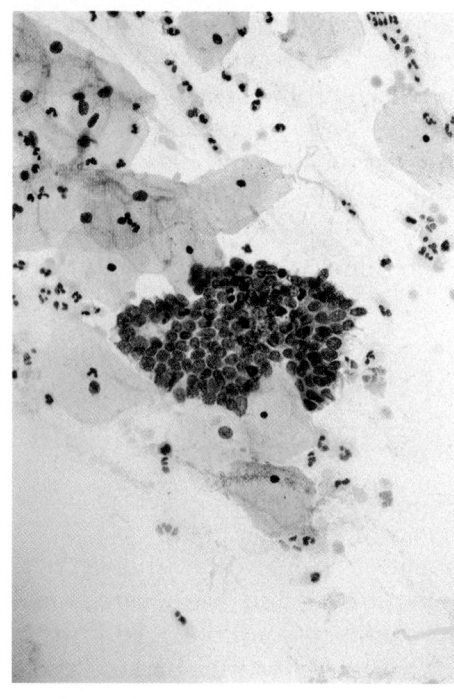

Fig. 14.3
Adenocarcinoma *in situ*. A compact crowded group with feathering and a rosette is seen.

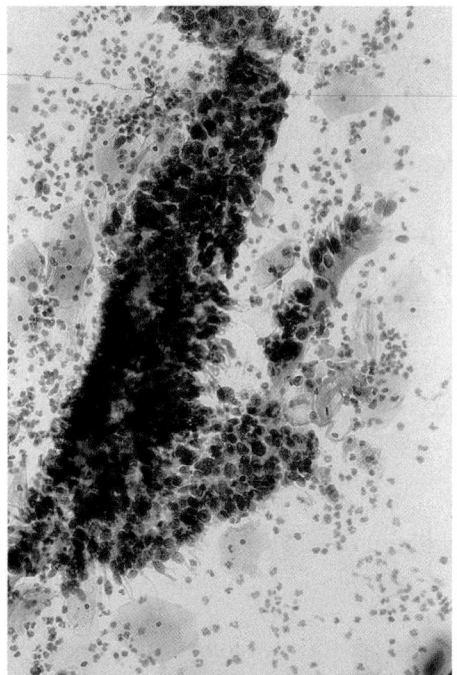

Fig. 14.2
Adenocarcinoma *in situ*. A large crowded group with feathering and a smaller group composed of a strip of columnar cells with polarized nuclei are seen.

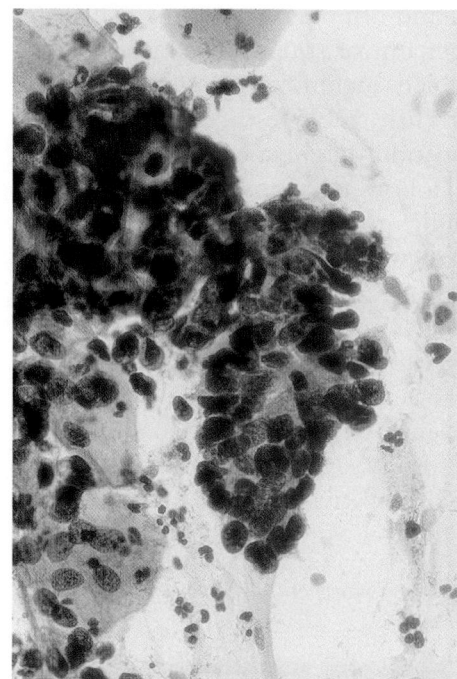

Fig. 14.4
Adenocarcinoma *in situ*. Extreme nuclear crowding with nuclear molding and mild to moderate coarsening of nuclear chromatin is seen. There is a vague rosette in the center.

CYTOLOGIC FINDINGS OF INVASIVE ADENOCARCINOMA

Smear presentation

The smear presentation is more variable than in AIS, being dependent on the cell type and grade of the adenocarcinoma.[60,61] A bloody or necrotic-appearing background is often absent, especially with early adenocarcinoma, and cannot be relied upon to confirm invasion. Conversely, a bloody smear with only a few poorly preserved groups should not be dismissed as unsatisfactory without careful scrutiny, as some advanced adenocarcinomas present with this picture.

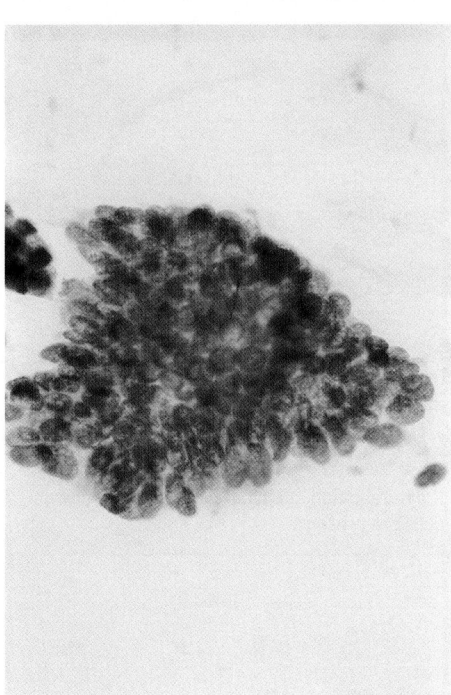

Fig. 14.5
Adenocarcinoma *in situ*. Extreme nuclear crowding with peripheral feathering is seen. Nuclei are only slightly hyperchromatic in this example.

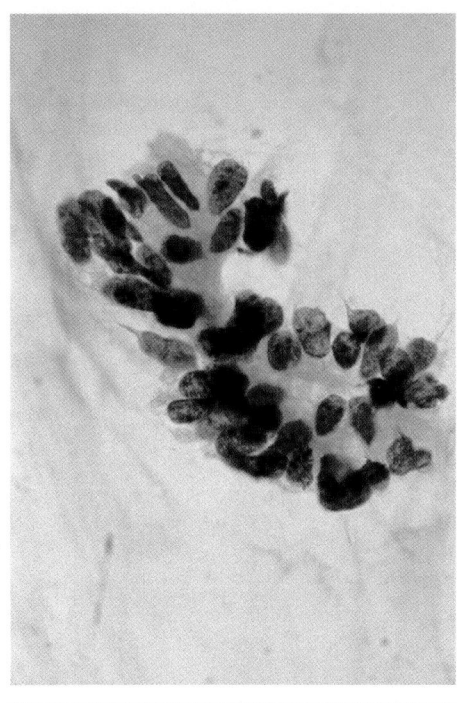

Fig. 14.7
Adenocarcinoma *in situ*. Nuclear irregularity and molding with peripheral feathering and a vague rosette-like structure is seen.

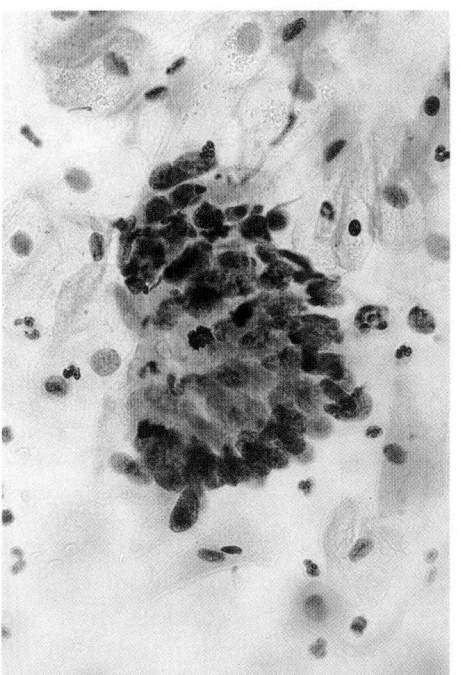

Fig. 14.6
Adenocarcinoma *in situ*. A mitotic figure is present in the center of a group with peripheral feathering and central residual pale to vacuolated cytoplasm.

Features of the cells

These cells are usually larger than those of AIS. The cytoplasm is pale to eosinophilic and is sometimes vacuolated. From case to case, nuclear chromatin ranges from vesicular to coarse, nucleoli vary from absent to prominent and mitotic figures may be frequent or scant (Figs 14.8–14.10).

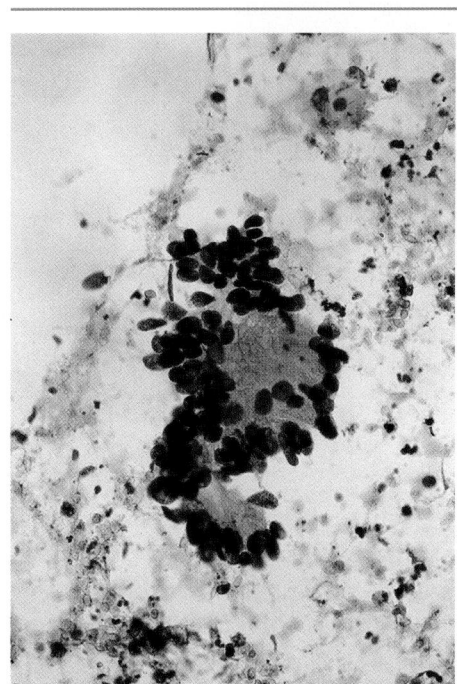

Fig. 14.8 Invasive adenocarcinoma. Degenerated nuclear fragments are present in the background. The group has an AIS-like appearance and would be difficult to distinguish from AIS in the absence of the background diathesis. A diathesis however, cannot be relied on to confirm invasion as it is rarely present in early invasive adenocarcinoma of the cervix.

Cell pattern

Usually the cell groupings in adenocarcinoma are numerous, similar to one another and lack the orderly honeycomb pattern of normal or reactive endocervical cells. Large branching or papillary groups, even if composed of AIS-like cells, suggest invasion. In some cases, single cells and very small groups predominate.

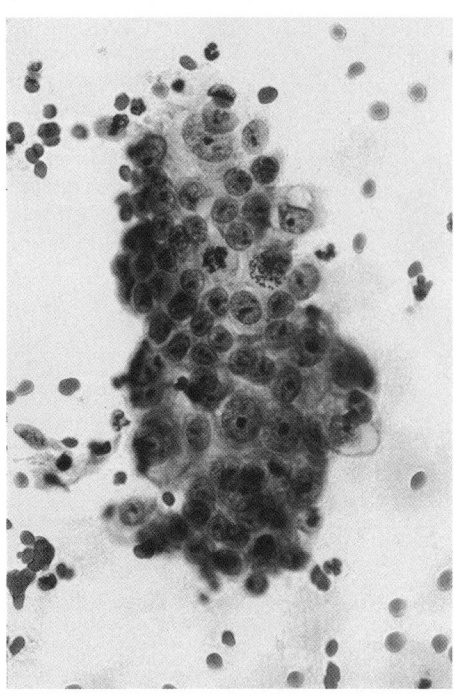

Fig. 14.9 Invasive adenocarcinoma. Crowded enlarged nuclei with prominent nucleoli and mitotic figures. The cytoplasm is foamy and focally vacuolated.

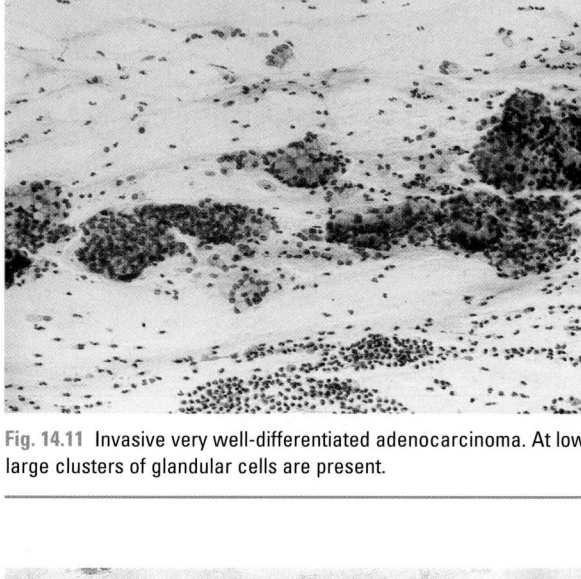

Fig. 14.11 Invasive very well-differentiated adenocarcinoma. At low power, large clusters of glandular cells are present.

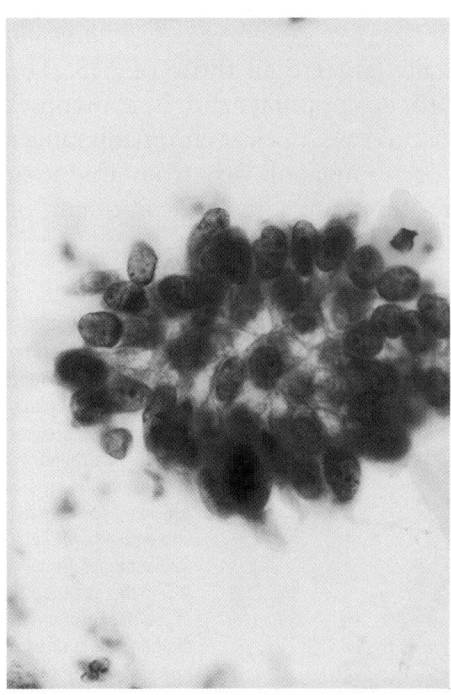

Fig. 14.10 Invasive adenocarcinoma. An AIS-like group with prominent feathering is seen. However, there was deep invasion in the biopsy.

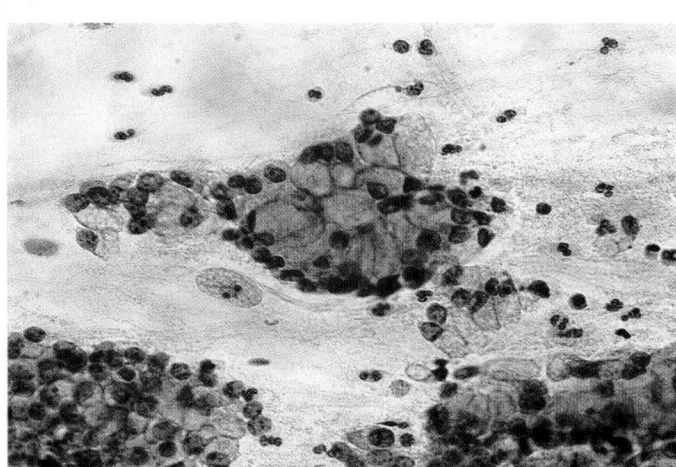

Fig. 14.12 Invasive, very well-differentiated adenocarcinoma. It would be extremely difficult to make the correct diagnosis prospectively in this case. However, the slight nuclear enlargement and monomorphism combined with the voluminous mucin-filled cytoplasm would be unusual in a purely reactive condition.

Similarities with reactive epithelial cells

In some cases of well-differentiated adenocarcinoma, the features that distinguish it from reactive endocervical cells may be very subtle. The finding of numerous groups of similar-appearing, only slightly atypical glandular cells should at least raise the possibility of carcinoma (Figs 14.11, 14.12).

Specific subtypes of adenocarcinoma such as adenoma malignum,[62–64] well-differentiated villoglandular,[65,66] or serous[67] may have characteristic findings. These are important insofar as their recognition invokes the possibility of carcinoma. However, adenocarcinoma subtypes cannot be reliably identified on the basis of their cytologic appearance.

FALSE-NEGATIVE INTERPRETATIONS

The most serious error is mistaking AIS or adenocarcinoma for a benign process. Usually this occurs because the cells are considered to be either endometrial cells or reactive endocervical cells.[9,34,68–71]

AIS mistaken for menstrual or directly sampled endometrial cells

In AIS, as with menstrual endometrium, the cells are extremely crowded, but unlike the latter, the cells in AIS have well-preserved nuclei and at least subtle feathering or small rosettes. The absence of either endometrial stromal fragments, cells in honeycombed sheets, or three-dimensional tubular groups rules against direct sampling of the endometrium (see below) (Fig. 14.13).[69,70,72]

AIS or adenocarcinoma mistaken for reactive endocervical cells

In AIS or adenocarcinoma the abnormal cell population is relatively monomorphous, not a spectrum as is commonly seen with reactive endocervical cells. Neoplastic groups have overlapping or very crowded nuclei that have a range of chromatin coarseness and either small or prominent nucleoli (Figs 14.14–14.16). In some cases this distinction is admittedly very difficult. Smears with only slightly atypical endocervical-appearing cells (Figs 14.11, 14.12) or bloody smears with only a few atypical cells are two patterns of adenocarcinoma that are often underdiagnosed.

FALSE-POSITIVE INTERPRETATIONS

Mistaking benign lesions for AIS or adenocarcinoma is a more common error than false-negative interpretations.

Tubal/tuboendometrial metaplasia

In the most common benign mimic of AIS, tubal metaplasia, the cells, although enlarged and crowded, are usually less so than in AIS.[73,74] Nuclear chromatin is finer than in AIS and feathering and rosettes are absent (Figs 14.17, 14.18). Cytoplasmic cilia are a key finding confirming tubal metaplasia but often are difficult to visualize. One needs to see discrete hair-like cytoplasmic processes, as adherent background debris can mimic cilia. Although very rare, there are ciliated variants of AIS,[75] so, although reassuring, the presence of cilia alone is not sufficient to exclude neoplasia.

Lower segment endometrium, directly sampled

Cells directly scraped from the lower segment of the endometrium are not uncommon. This is especially true in women who have had a cone biopsy.[72,76–78] They appear in fragments that may resemble those of AIS and may include cells with mitotic figures. However, in lower segment endometrium the cells are arranged

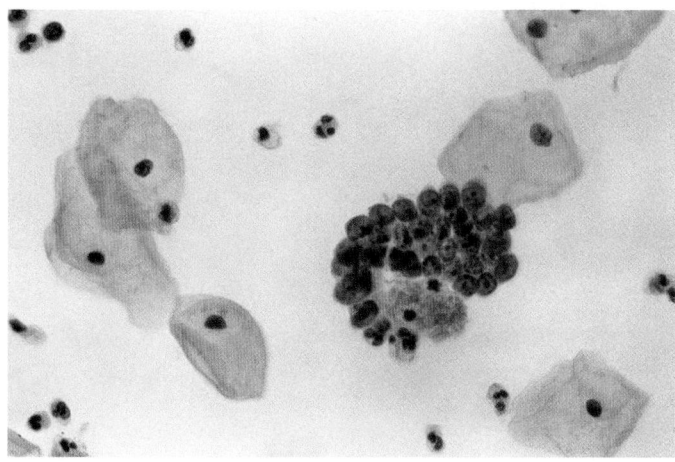

Fig. 14.13 Adenocarcinoma *in situ*. This small group might be confused with menstrual endometrial cells. However, they are well preserved with vague feathering.

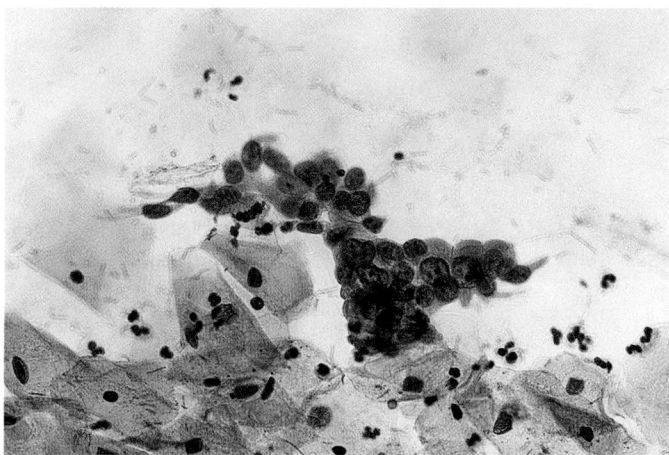

Fig. 14.14 Adenocarcinoma *in situ*. In this example, the cells have a more 'reactive' appearance. However, they are hyperchromatic and quite crowded. Note mitotic figure. Mitotic figures are not specific for neoplasia, as they may be seen with reactive conditions.

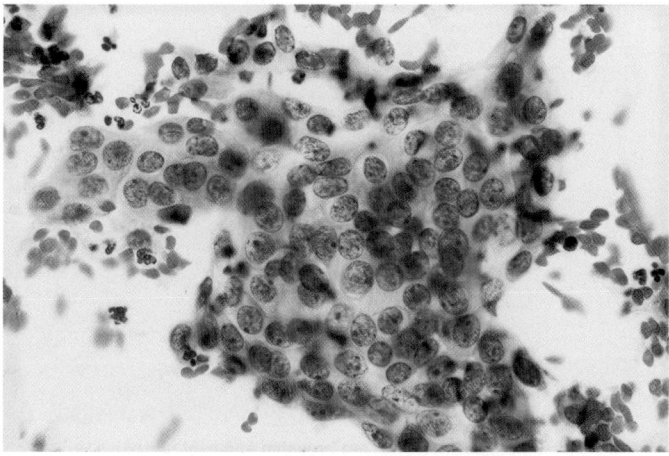

Fig. 14.15 Invasive adenocarcinoma. A sheet of cells with overlapping, similar-appearing nuclei with slightly coarse chromatin and small nucleoli is seen.

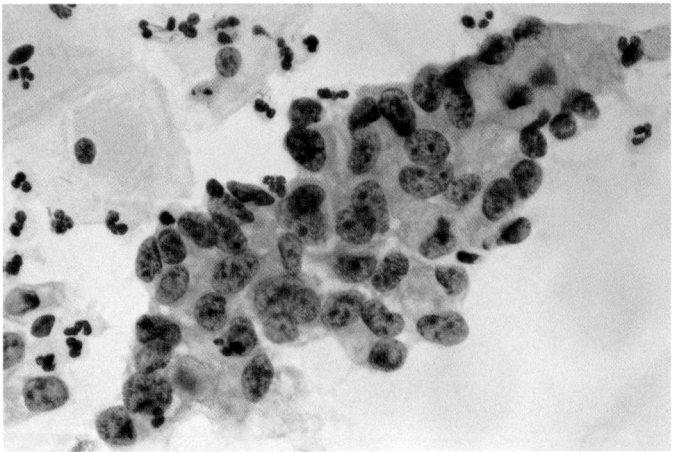

Fig. 14.16 Invasive adenocarcinoma. Nuclei are enlarged and overlapping, chromatin is slightly coarse and nucleoli are prominent.

in flat sheets or three-dimensional tubules that lack feathering or rosettes (Fig. 14.19). Cells are small, uniform and evenly dispersed with either fine or dense (India ink) nuclear chromatin (Fig. 14.20). Groups of endometrial stromal cells (tangles of spindled cells with bland oval nuclei and wispy cytoplasm), either attached to or independent of the epithelial groups, are an important clue (Fig. 14.21).

Menstrual endometrial cells

Perhaps surprisingly, clusters of menstrual endometrial cells may sometimes be difficult to separate from AIS (or HSIL) (Fig. 14.22a). Also, sometimes one encounters large pseudopapillary endometrial fragments that are frightening in their similarity to adenocarcinoma (Fig. 14.22b). In these situations, as in all difficult cytologic

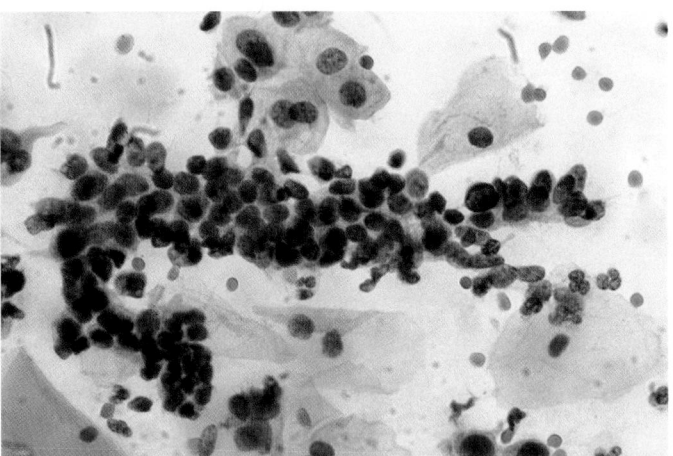

Fig. 14.17 Tubal metaplasia. A dark crowded group simulates the appearance of adenocarcinoma *in situ*. Cilia are present in the columnar cells on the right; however, they are difficult to visualize.

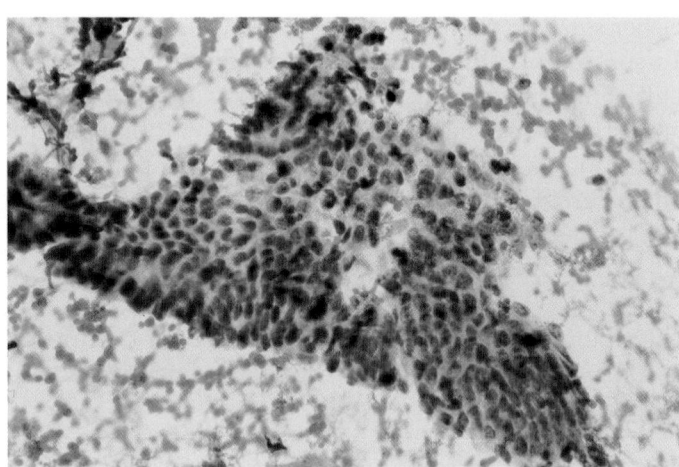

Fig. 14.19 Lower uterine segment, directly sampled. A sheet of cells simulating the appearance of adenocarcinoma *in situ* is present. Nuclei are less crowded than in the usual adenocarcinoma *in situ*.

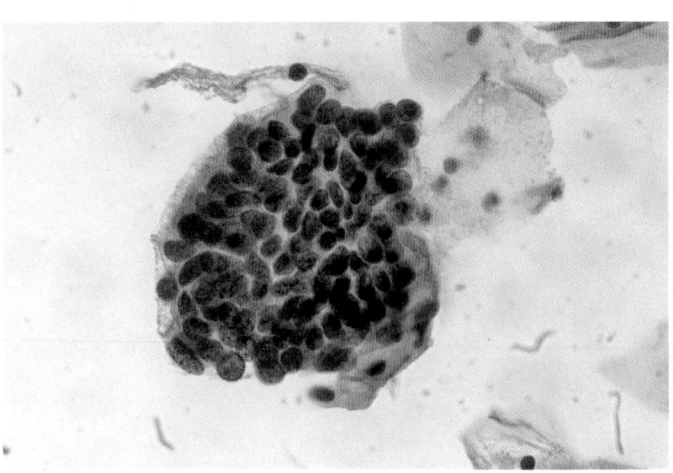

Fig. 14.18 Tubal metaplasia. Nuclei are crowded and hyperchromatic, similar to those of adenocarcinoma *in situ*. Note prominent cilia on left-hand border. Feathering is absent.

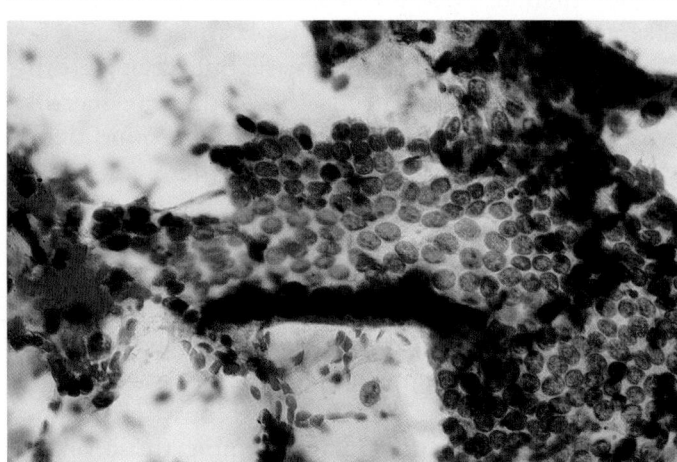

Fig. 14.20 Lower uterine segment, directly sampled. Nuclei are small, uniform, and evenly dispersed; chromatin is bland.

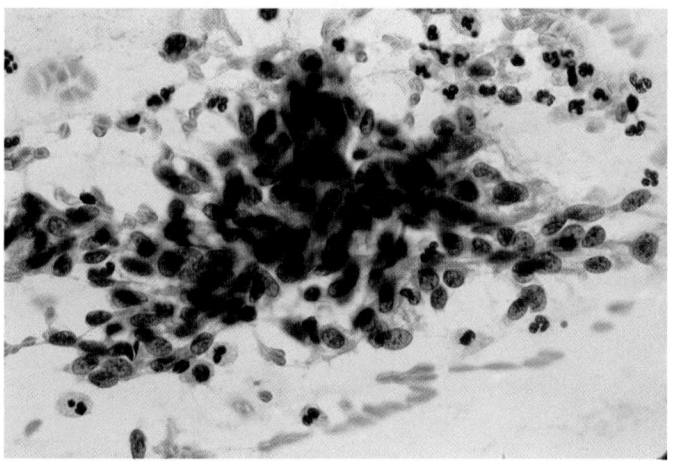

Fig. 14.21 Lower uterine segment, directly sampled. A fragment of spindled endometrial stromal cells with bland chromatin is seen.

interpretations, evaluating the worrisome cells in the context of the entire spectrum of cells on the smear is critical. Most groups of menstrual endometrial cells have very small, molded nuclei with scant or absent cytoplasm and interspersed pyknotic nuclear fragments or are in very tight balls of stromal cells surrounded by larger epithelial cells. Hyperchromasia is present, but is degenerative, with dense, smudged, or beaded chromatin. Feathering, rosettes, or strips of columnar cells, characteristic of AIS, are absent.

Reactive endocervical cells

Reactive endocervical cells, whether from cervicitis or endocervical polyps,[79] microglandular hyperplasia,[80–82] irradiated endocervix,[83] or the Arias-Stella reaction,[84,85] may resemble either AIS or adenocarcinoma. As opposed to neoplasia, in cervicitis or polyps there are sheets of repair-like cells containing evenly distributed nuclei with fine chromatin, sometimes-prominent nucleoli and delicate nuclear membranes. Nuclear size may vary both within and between groups.

Microglandular hyperplasia may yield groups with enlarged, sometimes vacuolated cells that raise the possibility of adenocarcinoma. However, nuclei are variably sized, rather than monomorphic; the chromatin is fine and there may be adherent crowded reserve cells or immature metaplastic cells, some with recognizable intercellular bridges (Fig. 14.23).

With irradiation and the Arias-Stella reaction, there are gigantic cells with voluminous, sometimes vacuolated cytoplasm. Nuclei vary from normal sized to very large, often within the same group and have smudged chromatin and intranuclear vacuoles (Fig. 14.24).

Atrophy

Aside from the well-known problem of benign nuclear atypia in atrophy mimicking squamous dysplasia, atrophic cells may sometimes shed some or all of their cytoplasm and aggregate in pseudoglandular groups that

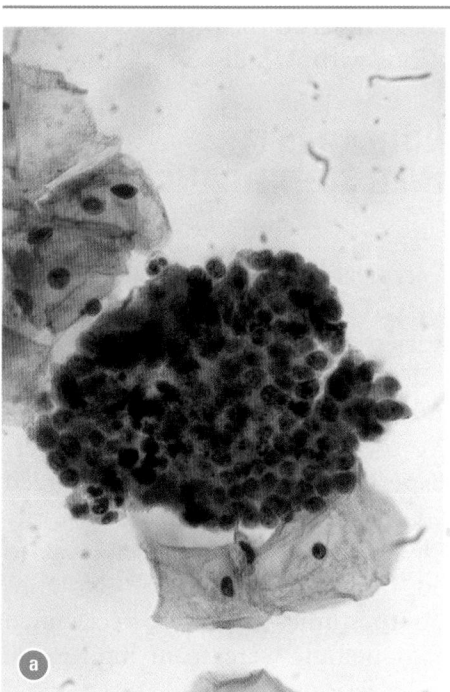

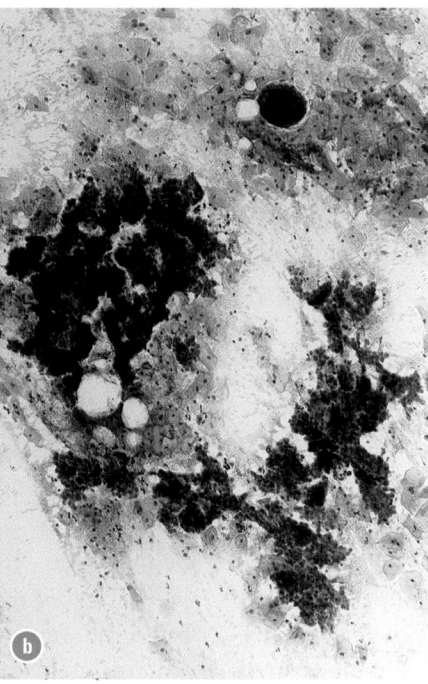

Fig. 14.22 (a) Menstrual endometrial cells. A dark group of extremely crowded, small, degenerated nuclei has a vague suggestion of feathering. (b) Menstrual endometrial cells. Large pseudopapillary groups are present. A stromal ball is seen at the top.

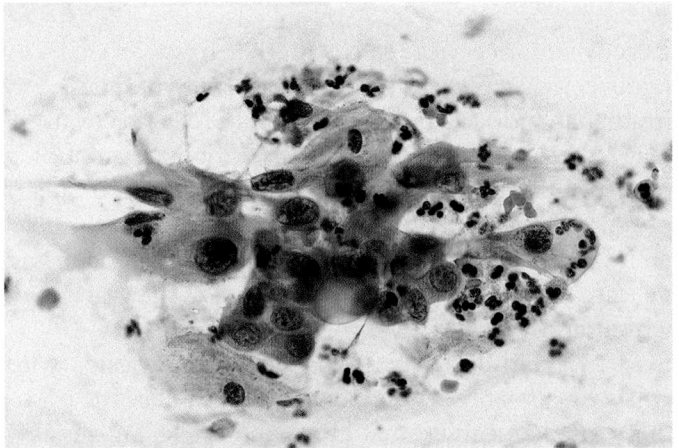

Fig. 14.23 Microglandular hyperplasia. Nuclei are enlarged and slightly hyperchromatic; cytoplasm has an attenuated, pulled-out appearance. Intracytoplasmic leukocytes are present.

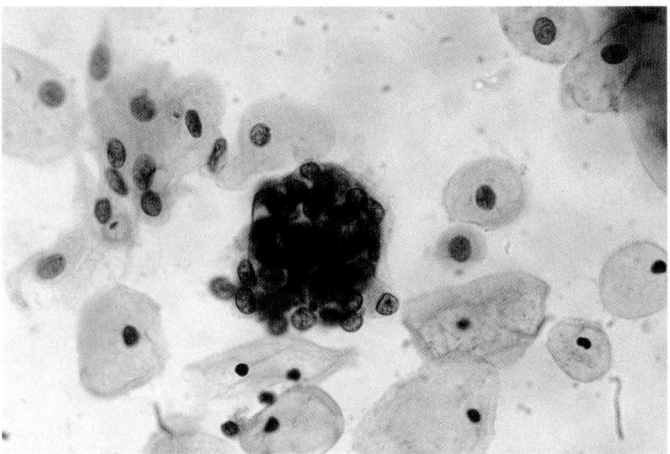

Fig. 14.25 Atrophy. A tightly bound group of nuclei with scant cytoplasm is seen in this smear from a woman with a history of lobular carcinoma of the breast. This pseudoglandular arrangement may be confused with endometrial cells or carcinomas of various types, depending on the history. They are merely atrophic squamous cells without cytoplasm. Note that the individual nuclei are similar to those in the surrounding squamous cells.

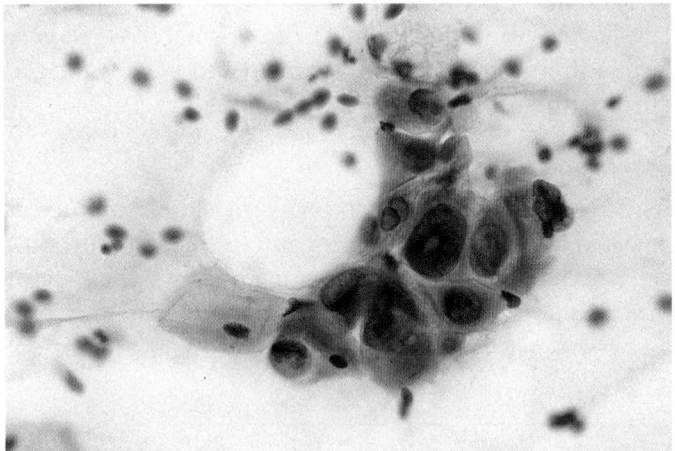

Fig. 14.24 Arias-Stella reaction. Markedly enlarged cells are present in this group. However, there is extreme variability of nuclear size and a smudged or empty appearance to the chromatin.

may be mistaken for endometrial cells, endometrial carcinoma, or even metastatic carcinoma. The atrophic nuclei are small, bland and uniform. Importantly, they are identical to those of the intact cells and cells that have lost only part of their cytoplasm that are present in the background (Fig. 14.25).

MISDIAGNOSIS: HSIL MISTAKEN FOR AIS

High-grade squamous intraepithelial lesion (HSIL) is the most frequent neoplastic mimic of AIS.[86,87] The large majority of biopsies that contain a neoplastic lesion following a report of glandular atypia in Pap smears have HSIL without AIS.[88] In AIS-like HSIL, the abnormal

cells are either in very crowded groups with coarsely hyperchromatic nuclei and scant cytoplasm (Fig. 14.26a) or are loosely arranged with a pale, finely vacuolated cytoplasm (Fig. 14.26b); both appearances mimic glandular differentiation. However, the absence of distinctly columnar shapes, pronounced feathering, or rosettes argues against this. As a general rule, if there is uncertainty whether the cells are HSIL or AIS, they are likely to be the former. As a corollary, gland-like HSIL may be mistaken for reactive rather than neoplastic glandular cells (similar to the problem of falsely negative interpretations with AIS discussed above).

ATYPICAL GLANDULAR CELLS OF UNDETERMINED SIGNIFICANCE

General

The frequencies of atypical glandular cells of undetermined significance (AGUS) reported from individual laboratories have varied from as low as 0.08% to as high as 0.74%.[88] Aside from this wide spectrum of sensitivity, an AGUS interpretation is poorly reproducible. In two retrospective reviews of smears initially interpreted as AGUS, expert reviewers not only disagreed with the initial AGUS interpretation in the majority of cases but also disagreed among themselves as to which cases should remain as AGUS.[88,89] Notably, several cases from both studies that were reclassified by some reviewers as benign were from high-grade squamous or glandular lesions.

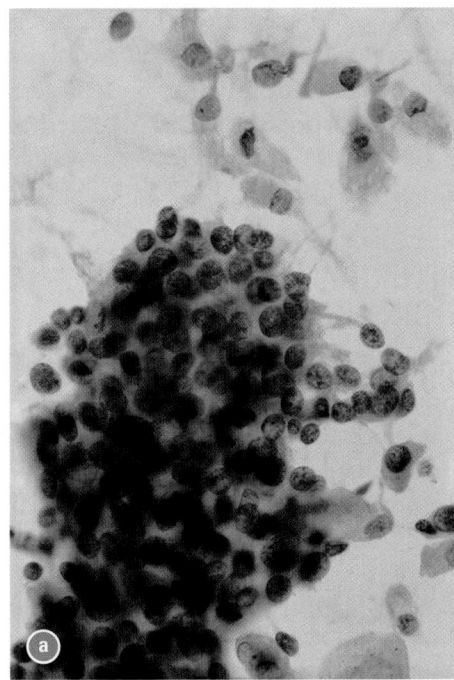 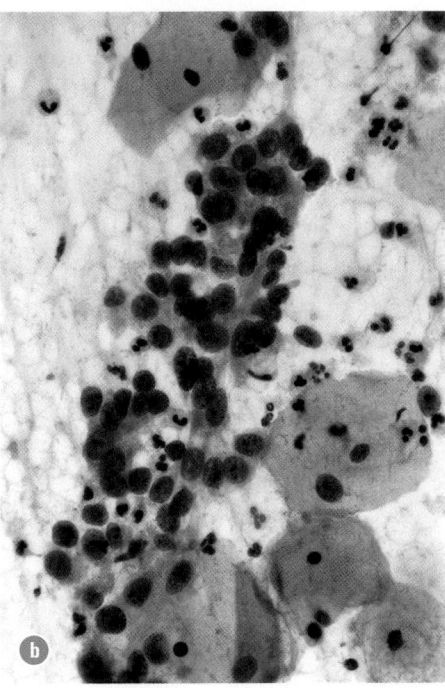

Fig. 14.26 (a) High-grade squamous intraepithelial lesion. A three-dimensional ball-like structure with crowded hyperchromatic nuclei simulates the appearance of AIS. This similarity is accentuated by the presence of benign endocervical cells adherent and adjacent to the group. There is no feathering or rosette formation. In such cases, HSIL is much more likely than AIS. (b) High-grade squamous intraepithelial lesion. In this example, the low density of the cytoplasm and the cell arrangements suggest glandular neoplasia. However, clear-cut feathering or columnar shapes are absent.

However, as noted above, biopsy follow-up after an AGUS interpretation often yields a high-grade squamous rather than a glandular lesion. Thus a smear interpretation of AGUS, although lacking both specificity and reproducibility, carries a significant risk for high-grade neoplasia. In light of this, the 2001 consensus guidelines for Pap smear follow-up recommend colposcopy and biopsy as the initial response to all smears interpreted as 'atypical glandular cells' or 'atypical endocervical cells'.[90]

The Bethesda 2001 terminology for glandular lesions differs from the Bethesda 1991 terminology in that the phrase 'of undetermined significance' has been eliminated from the glandular cell category as has the suffix 'favor reactive' because of concerns that these designations might lead to under-treatment (Table 14.2). In addition, 'endocervical adenocarcinoma *in situ*' is a separate diagnostic category now that enough experience with its cytologic appearance has accrued.

Interpretation of cervical glandular abnormalities with the use of liquid-based preparations

Experience with liquid-based preparations is limited due to the relatively recent introduction of these methods and the infrequency of glandular lesions. In small studies of the ThinPrep (Cytyc, Boxborough, MA) that used patient follow-up to compare its accuracy in detecting abnormal glandular cells with that of conventional smears, use of the ThinPrep was found to be more sensitive and specific in one report,[91] more specific in two reports[92,93] and no different from conventional preparations in one report.[94]

HPV testing following 'atypical glandular cells or atypical endocervical cells'

Data are sparse. Two studies report that the presence of high-risk HPV was highly predictive of high-grade lesions (both glandular and squamous) following AGUS and that false-negative interpretations were infrequent.[95,96] Caveats are that in some cases the atypical glandular cells are from endometrial, tubal, or even ovarian carcinomas that are not HPV related[96] and that a significant minority of cervical adenocarcinomas *in situ* and invasive cervical adenocarcinomas are HPV negative (four cases in 244 patients tested in the two series noted above).[7] Thus, reliance on a negative HPV test

---

Table 14.2 *Bethesda 2001 Pap smear terminology for atypical glandular-appearing cells*

Epithelial cell abnormality
Glandular cell
    Atypical glandular cells (specify endocervical, endometrial, or not otherwise specified)
    Atypical glandular cells, favor neoplastic (specify endocervical or not otherwise specified)
    Endocervical adenocarcinoma *in situ* (AIS)
    Adenocarcinoma, specify as appropriate

result to avoid colposcopy or endometrial biopsy following the reporting of 'atypical endocervical cells' 'or atypical glandular cells' on a smear may lead to under-diagnosis of a serious lesion. Because of this, HPV testing in these situations is not currently recommended.[90] It may, however, be useful in selected clinical situations where a reactive endocervical condition is strongly favored and where biopsy is undesirable, such as during pregnancy.

Diagnosis and management of adenocarcinoma *in situ*

LIMITATIONS OF CLINICAL AND COLPOSCOPIC DETECTION

Unlike squamous lesions of the cervix, the colposcopic criteria for AIS are not defined and colposcopy cannot be relied on to exclude a neoplasm following a cytologic diagnosis of abnormal glandular cells or AIS.[97] However, the majority of women with AIS will, in fact, have a colposcopic abnormality. In one study, 67 (74%) of 90 women with AIS who underwent colposcopy had an abnormal examination. However, a glandular abnormality was suspected prior to colposcopy in only 19 (28%).[98] As discussed above, only a minority of Papanicolaou smears showing AGUS will be confirmed histologically with a glandular abnormality. Upon review of 16 studies with biopsy follow-up after an AGUS, 'favor reactive' or AGUS, 'not specified',[88] only 3.2% of patients had either AIS or invasive endocervical adenocarcinoma, while 3.9% had endometrial carcinoma and 25% had cervical intraepithelial neoplasia (CIN), the majority of the latter being high grade. However, if the AGUS interpretation was qualified as 'favor neoplastic', 62% had either AIS or invasive adenocarcinoma and an additional 18% had CIN.

HISTOLOGIC CRITERIA FOR ADENOCARCINOMA *IN SITU*

Although it may spread widely within the endocervix, AIS almost always involves the transformation zone or the squamocolumnar junction, most likely arising from HPV-infected columnar cells or reserve cells in that location that are committed to glandular differentiation (Fig. 14.27a).[99,100] AIS extends from the surface epithelium into underlying glands, sometimes with an abrupt change to normal within the deeper portion of the affected gland (Fig. 14.27b).[2] It may then extend circumferentially around the cervix and proximally up the canal, sometimes all the way to the endometrium. Rarely AIS initially develops high in the canal or is multifocal.[2,100] About 50% of cases have a concomitant high-grade CIN, the AIS almost always located adjacent and usually proximal to the CIN (Fig. 14.27a).

AIS is recognized by the following:

1 *Epithelial cell crowding*: with stratification or pseudostratification.
2 *Nuclear enlargement*: nuclei are variably enlarged and are oval, elongated, or irregular.
3 *Prominent nuclear hyperchromasia with chromatin coarsening*: nucleoli are usually small or absent, but may be prominent in some cases.

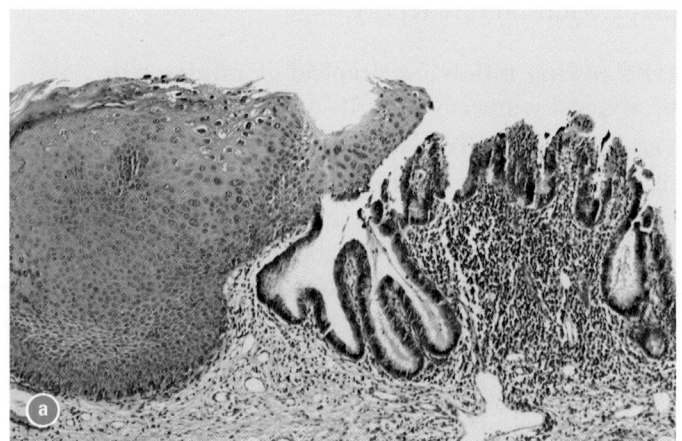
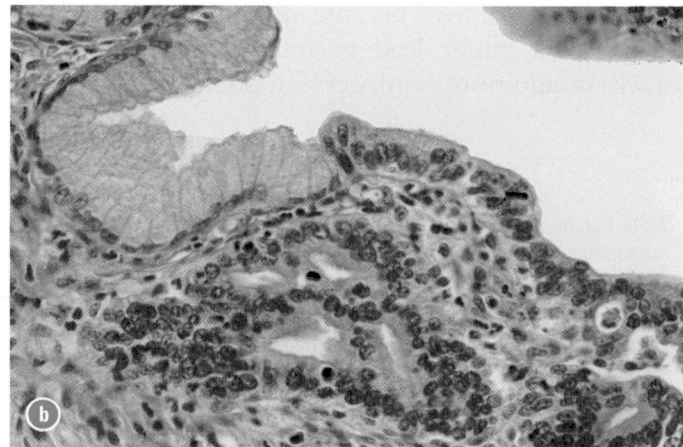

Fig. 14.27 Adenocarcinoma *in situ*. (a) Low-power view of AIS at the transformation zone involving the surface and underlying glands. There is adjacent CIN. (b) ACIS at higher power, showing nuclear hyperchromasia and mitoses. An apoptotic body surrounded by a clear space is seen in the surface epithelium (right).

4 *Mitotic figures*: these are invariably present, often easily visualized at the luminal pole of the cell, but there may be as few as one or two per five high-power fields.[14]

5 *Apoptotic bodies*, located in the basal portion of the gland, are present in about 70% of cases;[101,102] one should require a definitive eosinophilic body containing sharply delineated dark fragments of chromatin so as not to confuse degenerated leukocytes with apoptotic bodies (Fig. 14.27b).

6 *Conspicuous architectural alterations*: sometimes including papillary or cribriform intraglandular growth may be quite florid, suggesting invasive carcinoma. However, the stromal interface of the AIS gland maintains the smooth, well-demarcated appearance of the original benign gland it has replaced (Fig. 14.28). The stroma underlying AIS may contain variable concentrations of acute or chronic inflammatory cells. Their presence alone does not connote invasion.

In addition to the above, there are several AIS subtypes; often these are mixed within the same case.[2] It is important to be aware of these and to be able to identify them all as AIS; however, they have not been shown to differ in their propensity to invade or in the subtype of adenocarcinoma they produce. They include the following:

1 The *endocervical type*, named for its resemblance to endocervical cells. This is the most common. The cells have a columnar cytoplasm that is mucinous-appearing or eosinophilic (Fig. 14.27b).

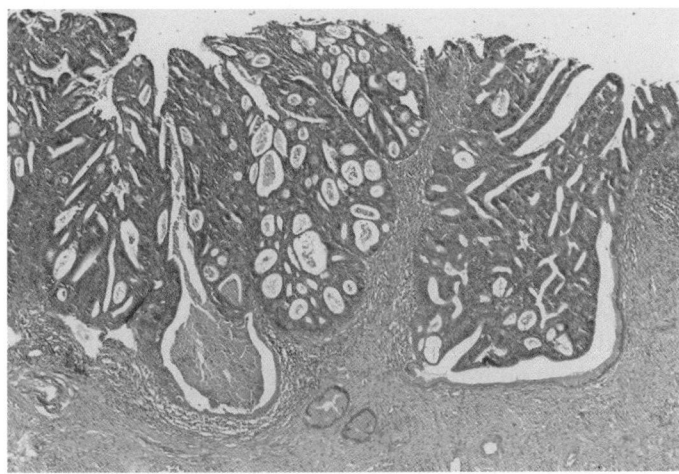

Fig. 14.28 Adenocarcinoma *in situ*. This focus is particularly florid, but is superficial, maintains a uniform epithelial–stromal interface, and merges with normal glandular epithelium (right).

2 The *endometrioid* subtype has more nuclear stratification and less cytoplasm, mimicking neoplastic endometrial glands.

3 The *intestinal* subtype is distinguished by a variable proportion of goblet cells (Fig. 14.29a). There is less nuclear crowding and hyperchromasia in this variant, making confirmation more difficult. However, intestinal differentiation alone is an important clue to AIS, since benign intestinal metaplasia of the cervix is rare.

4 The *tubal* type (Fig. 14.29b).[75] This diagnosis should be made only if there are unequivocal nuclear features of AIS including mitotic figures, since most ciliated lesions are non-neoplastic (see discussion of benign mimics below).

5 The *stratified* type (Fig. 14.29c).[50] At low magnification the lesion appears similar to a squamous intraepithelial lesion, but on close inspection the stratified neoplastic cells contain intracellular mucin. This variant may be a form of adenosquamous carcinoma *in situ*, but more cases with concomitant invasion are needed to confirm this. Currently, we report these as 'AIS, stratified variant'.

True adenosquamous carcinoma *in situ*, containing intimately admixed glandular and squamous differentiation in the same focus, is rarely seen (Fig. 14.29d). Precursor lesions to uncommon subtypes of adenocarcinoma such as adenoma malignum, clear cell carcinoma, or serous carcinoma are not well characterized.

GLANDULAR ATYPIAS THAT DO NOT FULFILL THE CRITERIA FOR CLASSIC ADENOCARCINOMA *IN SITU*: THE CONCEPT OF 'GLANDULAR DYSPLASIA'

Occasionally, there are non-inflammatory glandular atypias with less cellular crowding and stratification than is usually present in AIS. This, along with the long-held theory that preinvasive squamous neoplasia of the cervix evolves through low- and high-grade stages, has attracted some authors to the concept that AIS develops in a similar stepwise manner.[19,103–107] Thus, these lesions have been variously designated as 'glandular dysplasia',[19,106] 'cervical intraepithelial glandular neoplasia' (CIGN),[104,107] or 'atypical hyperplasia'.[108] However, there is currently no proof that lower-grade atypias are precursors to AIS rather than either AIS itself in a less atypical guise (Fig. 14.30a,b) or conversely, non-neoplastic mimics of AIS. Investigations of this question using objective markers such as HPV,[14,104,106,109,110]

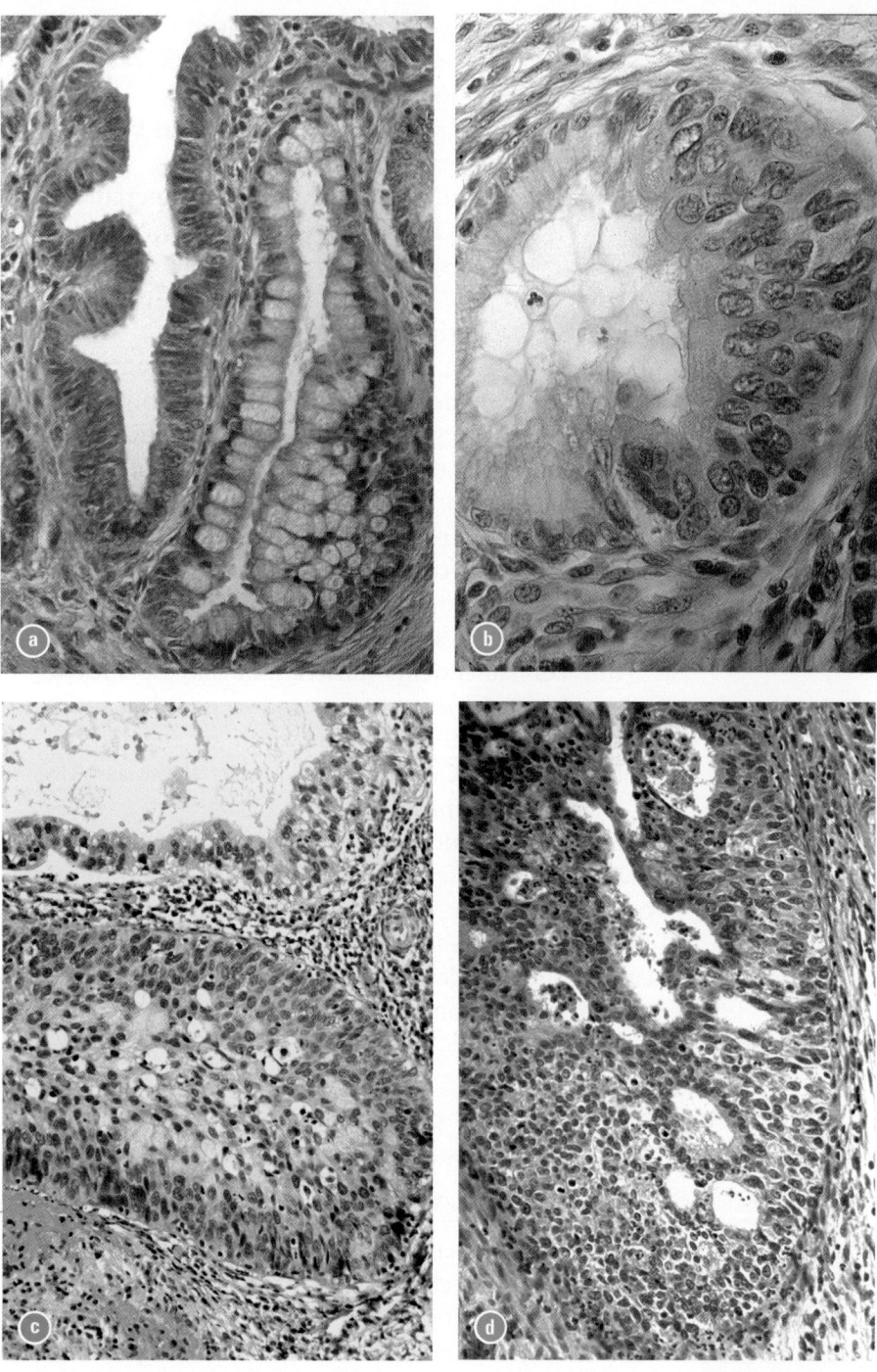

Fig. 14.29 (a) Adenocarcinoma *in situ*, intestinal type. Goblet cells are prominent. Ordinary (endocervical type) AIS is present in an adjacent gland. (b) Adenocarcinoma *in situ*, ciliated type. There is crowding and pronounced nuclear atypia in ciliated cells involving a portion of a gland. (c) Adenocarcinoma *in situ*, stratified type. Cells are stratified; however, there is prominent intracytoplasmic mucin including mucin vacuoles in the cells in all layers. (d) Adenocarcinoma *in situ*, adenosquamous type. There is distinct glandular and squamous differentiation in this *in situ* lesion.

MIB-1/Ki-67,[14] cytoplasmic mucins and lectins[19,20] and p16[11,12] have sometimes reached conflicting conclusions, but most have shown that these less-atypical lesions mark in a manner similar to AIS, especially when present alongside more-diagnostic AIS or high-grade squamous precursor lesions.

Thus, rather than introducing other potentially confusing terms and to avoid the possibility of undertreatment of cancer precursors, we recommend that lesions designated by others as high-grade endocervical 'dysplasia' or 'CIGN' and even some lesions that are considered low-grade endocervical dysplasia by some[19,103,104] be interpreted as AIS in diagnostic reports. In essence, this approach is based on the assumption that some AIS will exhibit a minority of the aforementioned diagnostic criteria. Ciliated atypia is an exception; as noted above, we feel that the diagnosis of the rare tubal variant of AIS requires the presence

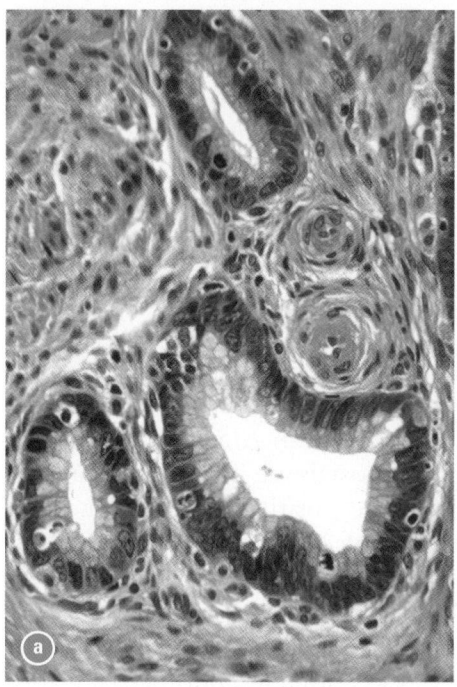
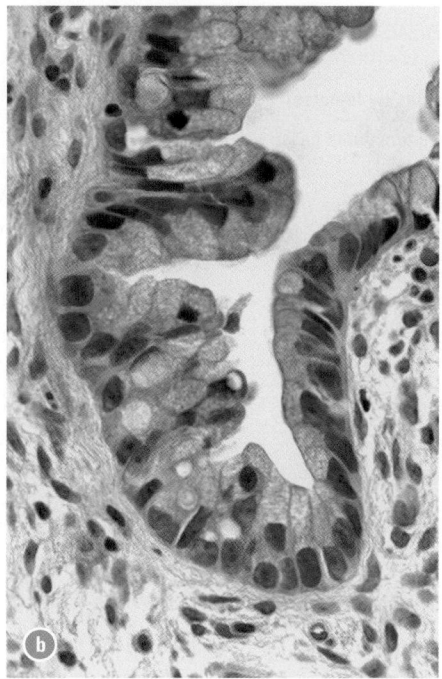

Fig. 14.30 (a) Adenocarcinoma *in situ*. This is a diagnostically borderline lesion. There is less crowding and stratification in this case than in the usual AIS. Note mitotic figures and an apoptotic body in the lower gland. This is an example of a lesion some would call 'glandular dysplasia' (cervical intraepithelial glandular neoplasia). (b) Adenocarcinoma *in situ*. There is less nuclear crowding and hyperchromasia than in the usual AIS. Mitotic figures are not present in this field. This was the highest grade of intraepithelial atypia seen adjacent to an early invasive adenocarcinoma that had a similar cytologic appearance. An isolated *in situ* lesion of this kind is probably not diagnostic of AIS, and might be interpreted as 'glandular dysplasia', perhaps even 'low grade'. In this case, however, it was an immediate precursor to invasive carcinoma.

of features otherwise diagnostic for classic AIS in the absence of cilia in order to distinguish it from atypical tuboendometrial metaplasia.

The uncertainty engendered by the occasional remaining problematic endocervical glandular atypias is best managed with an explanatory comment and, when appropriate, special studies. HPV or p16 positivity, or elevated MIB-1 immunoreactivity may be helpful in selected cases (Fig. 14.31a,b). However, one must keep in mind that even some invasive cervical adenocarcinomas are HPV-negative[7] and that

elevated MIB-1 and p16 reactivity may be present in some benign glandular atypias and absent from some neoplasms.[12,14,111]

DIFFERENTIAL DIAGNOSIS OF ADENOCARCINOMA *IN SITU* (Table 14.3)

Tubal and endometrioid metaplasia

Tubal and endometrioid metaplasias, found in 30% to 100% of completely sectioned cervices, are the most common mimics of AIS.[112,113] In the former, the cells

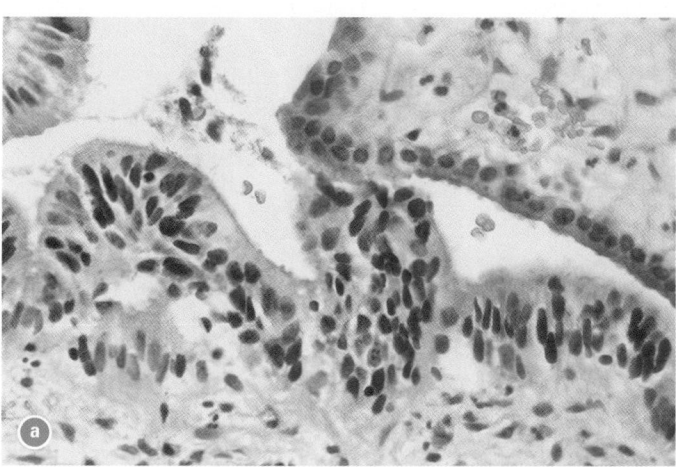
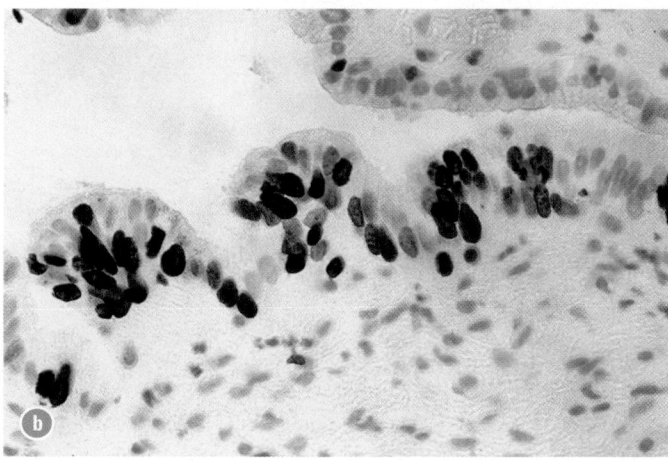

Fig. 14.31 (a) Adenocarcinoma *in situ*. There is a very small focus with nuclear crowding and stratification but without mitotic activity and with suboptimal nuclear preservation. (b) Adenocarcinoma *in situ* stained with MIB-1. The same focus as in Figure 14.31a demonstrates many MIB-1-positive nuclei.

Table 14.3 *Histologic criteria for adenocarcinoma in situ (AIS) and potential pitfalls*

AIS criteria	Benign conditions (helpful exclusionary features)
Cell crowding	Tubal metaplasia, endometriosis (intercalated cells, cilia, less crowding and stratification)
Hyperchromasia	Tubal metaplasia, endometriosis (less coarse, intercalated cells, cilia, less crowding and stratification)
Nuclear enlargement	Reactive endocervical changes: cervicitis, radiation, Arias-Stella, oxyphilic atypia (multinucleation, polymorphism, minimal hyperchromasia, smudged or vacuolated nuclei, low n/c ratio with vacuolated or eosinophilic cytoplasm)
Mitoses	Occasionally seen in mildly stratified endocervix unrelated to Inflammation (other features absent) Endometriosis (endometrial stroma, pseudostratified, uniform nuclei)
Apoptosis	Endometriosis (uncommon)
Goblet cells	Benign intestinal metaplasia (rare, no mitoses)
Complex architecture	Papillary endocervicitis (absence of cytologic atypia) Arias-Stella (smudged, vacuolated nuclei; hobnail cells)

are similar to those lining the fallopian tube; in the latter they resemble those of a proliferative endometrial gland. Frequently, the two blend, warranting the designation 'tuboendometrioid' metaplasia (TEM).

TEM resembles AIS in that the nuclei are larger, darker and more crowded than the usual endocervical gland nuclei. However, nuclear stratification, irregularity and hyperchromasia, although sometimes striking, are less pronounced than in AIS and cilia are usually easily found (Fig. 14.32a). Moreover, mitotic figures or apoptotic bodies are rare or absent in TEM and TEM does not produce the intraglandular papillary and cribriform overgrowth sometimes present in AIS. Also, TEM is usually (but not always) located higher in the canal than AIS, involving deep rather than superficial glands and occupying the entire gland, as opposed to the partial gland involvement often seen in AIS (Fig. 14.32b,c). In difficult cases immunostaining for MIB-1 (absent or infrequent in TEM and positive in 25% or more of the nuclei of most cases of AIS) has been helpful.[13–16]

Cervical endometriosis

Endometriosis may involve the cervix either superficially or deep in the wall.[114] Occasionally, endometrial glands may be entrapped beneath regenerated squamous mucosa following cone biopsy. The diagnostic endometrial stroma may be attenuated, obscured by inflammatory cells or may blend with the cervical stroma, leaving glands lined with crowded and stratified epithelial cells that sometimes have mitotic figures as in proliferative-phase endometrium that may be confused

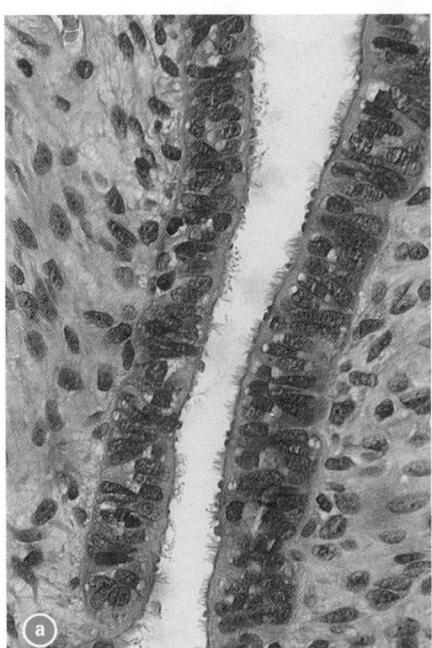
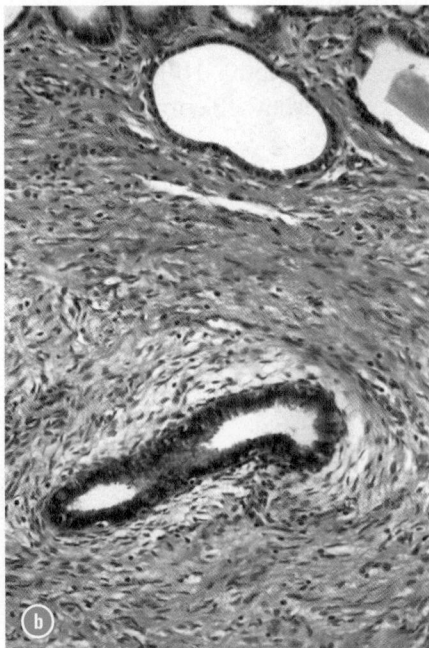
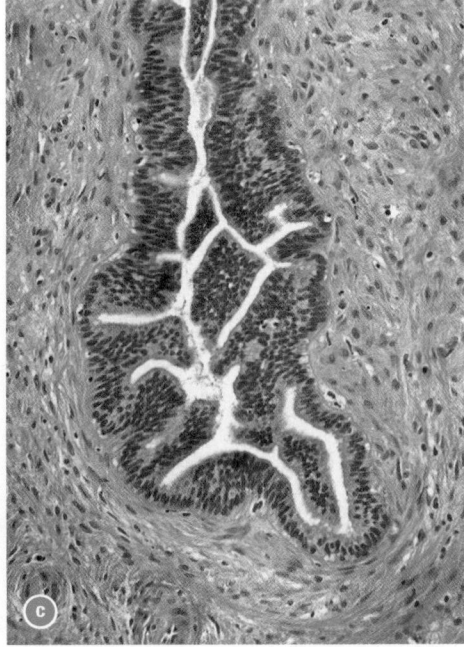

Fig. 14.32 (a) Tubal metaplasia. There is nuclear crowding and enlargement as in AIS. However, nuclei are less hyperchromatic than in the usual AIS, mitotic figures are absent, and many cilia are visible. (b) Tubal metaplasia. The gland is located beneath the normal endocervical glands. There is a periglandular edematous stroma, not to be confused with a stromal reaction to invasion. (c) Tubal metaplasia with some epithelial architectural complexity.

with AIS.[115] Clues to the correct diagnosis include uniform spacing of the glands, occasional ciliated epithelial cells and less pleomorphism and coarse hyperchromasia than in AIS. Surrounding endometrial stromal cells (albeit scant) and evidence of recent or remote stromal hemorrhage are additional clues (Fig. 14.33a–c). Although CD-10 has been a useful marker of endometrial stromal cells, it also marks endocervical periglandular stroma, negating its usefulness in confirming suspected endometriosis.[116] However, a trichrome stain may be useful in distinguishing the stroma of cervical endometriosis (red staining) from the collagen-rich native endocervical stroma (blue staining). This, combined with a reticulin stain outlining the individual endometrial stromal cells, may confirm the diagnosis of endometriosis.[117]

Cervical Arias-Stella reaction and other pregnancy-related epithelial changes

The Arias-Stella reaction is most often recognized in the endometrium, but it also involves the endocervical glands in 10% to 50% of completely examined gravid uteri.[118] It may also be encountered in cervical polyps,[119,120]

a lesion more susceptible to a biopsy during pregnancy. Arias-Stella changes may be confused with either AIS or invasive adenocarcinoma.[120] As opposed to these, Arias-Stella changes are usually focal, involving only a portion of a gland, a single gland, or a small number of glands. The cells are markedly enlarged and may fill the gland space or protrude into it as tufts of cells, filiform papillae, or cells in a hobnail pattern. The cytoplasm is eosinophilic or vacuolated, sometimes with eosinophilic inclusions; nuclei contain smudged, vacuolated, or optically clear chromatin with no or only rare mitotic figures (Fig. 14.34a–c).[120] Knowledge that the patient is pregnant or has recently been pregnant is confirmatory. However, occasionally a similar appearance, usually less pronounced, is seen in non-pregnant patients. Usually they are either receiving hormone therapy or taking oral contraceptives.[120,121]

Another epithelial change sometimes seen in pregnancy is the presence of prominent basal vacuoles. These changes are unlikely to be confused with glandular neoplasia but must be distinguished from intestinal-type AIS (Fig. 14.29a).

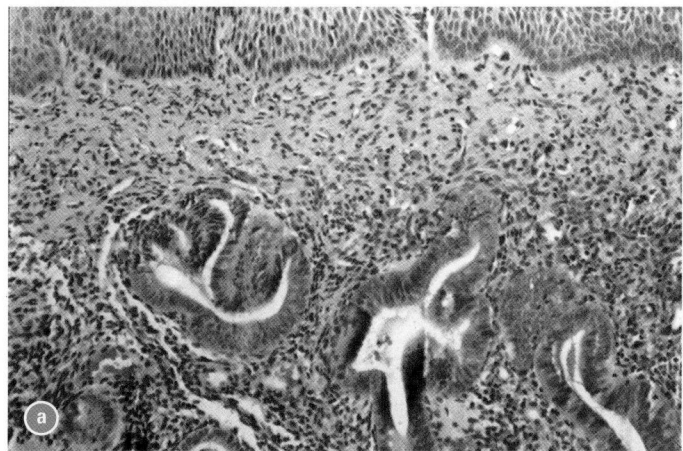

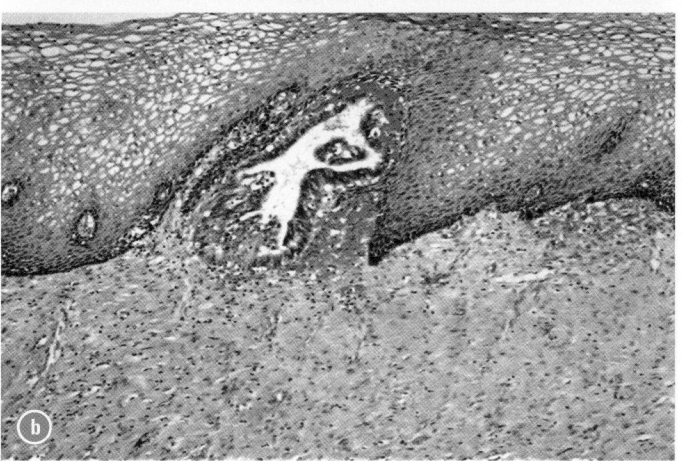

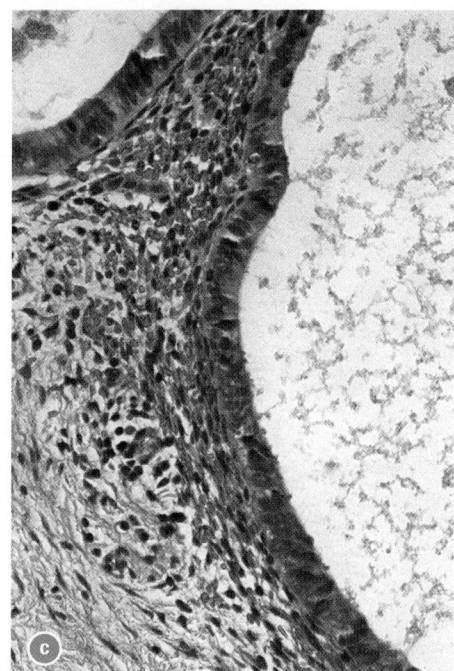

Fig. 14.33 (a) Endometriosis. Irregularly shaped, evenly spaced glands are seen beneath the surface at the squamo-columnar junction. (b) Endometriotic glands entrapped beneath portio epithelium following healing of a cone biopsy site. (c) At higher power the glands are characteristic of endometrial origin. Note the stroma is inconspicuous.

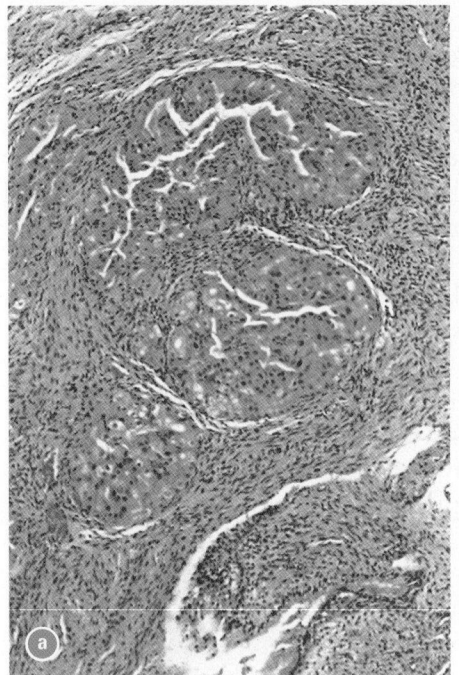

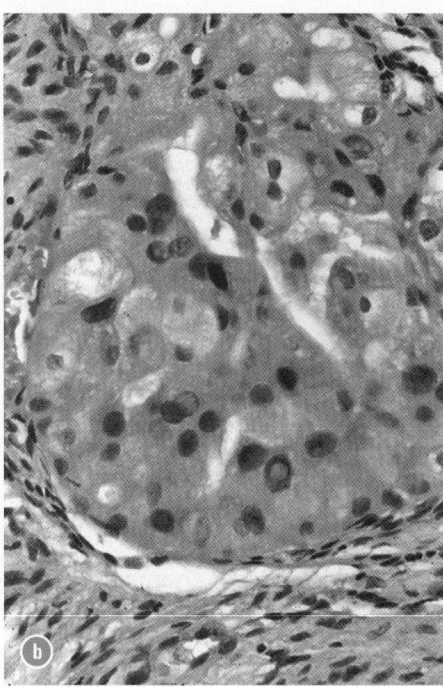

Fig. 14.34 (a) Arias-Stella reaction. Three contiguous glands are occupied by enlarged eosinophilic cells that obliterate the gland lumens. An uninvolved gland is present at bottom. (b) Higher power demonstrates nuclear and cytoplasmic vacuolization, smudged nuclear chromatin, and an absence of mitotic activity. (c) The nuclei have a hobnail appearance.

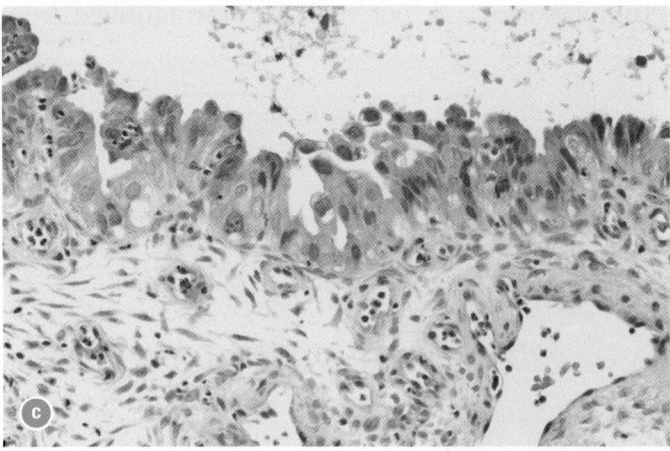

Radiation and cautery effects

Irradiated endocervical cells may become strikingly enlarged, with pleomorphic nuclei (Fig. 14.35a).[122,123] Unlike malignant cells, the nuclear chromatin of irradiated cells is often smudged rather than coarsely hyperchromatic, the nuclei and/or cytoplasm may be vacuolated, the nuclear to cytoplasmic size ratio is not increased and mitotic figures are absent or very rare. The stroma is often hyalinized with ectatic vessels.

Another tissue effect associated with therapy is cautery artifact. This change is more problematic diagnostically when present in squamous epithelium. However, thermal artifacts may also produce nuclear enlargement and distortion of columnar epithelium (Fig. 14.35b).

Cervicitis and reactive epithelial changes

Inflammatory reactions of the endocervix are not often confused with AIS. The reverse error (failure to perceive AIS in the presence of the marked inflammation) is more common. With reactive conditions, the epithelial cells are not as crowded and stratified as in AIS; the chromatin is finer and there is often an enlarged nucleolus (although some AIS cases also feature prominent nucleoli). Although with cervicitis the surface epithelium may be papillary,[124] prominent, stroma-free, intraglandular papillary or cribriform growth is not seen.

Other reactive endocervical cell changes include those associated with repair (Fig. 14.36a), multinucleated

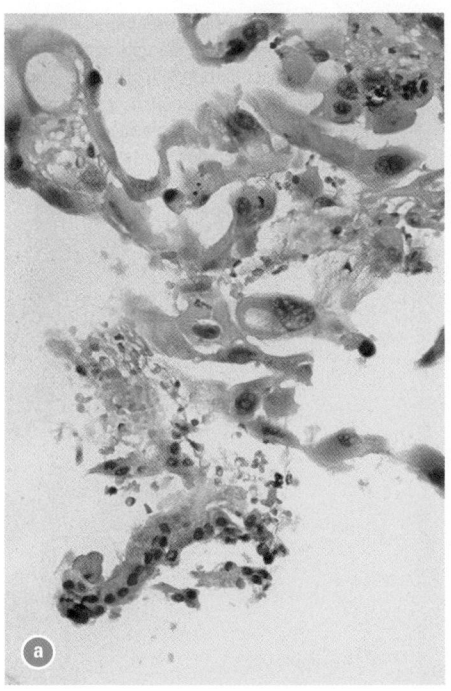

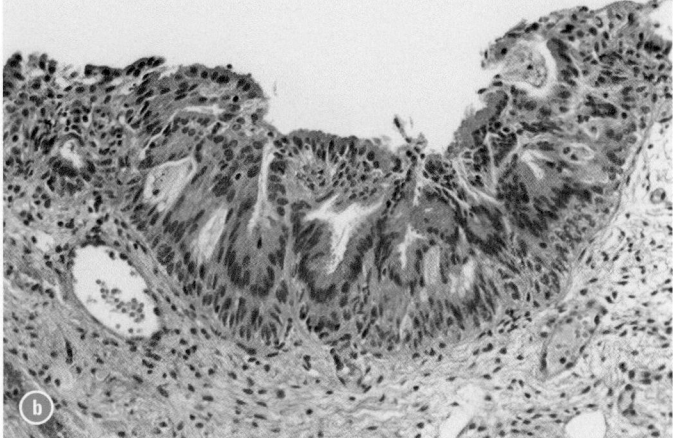

Fig. 14.35 Therapeutic effects on columnar epithelium. (a) Radiation reaction. Markedly enlarged cells with voluminous cytoplasm and irregular nuclei with somewhat smudged, degenerate-appearing chromatin. A strip of normal endocervical cells is seen at lower left. (b) Cautery artifact, producing slightly enlarged hyperchromatic nuclei in endocervical columnar epithelium.

atypias (Fig. 14.36b) and nuclear atypias with prominent eosinophilic cytoplasm (atypical oxyphilic metaplasia) (Fig. 14.36c).[125] The last are usually, but not always, found in women taking hormones or birth control pills.[125] They differ from AIS in that they lack cell crowding and mitotic activity.

Glandular atypia secondary to herpesvirus and cytomegalovirus infections

Although not likely to be confused with AIS, these endocervical reactions are mentioned here for the sake of completeness. Cytomegalovirus (CMV) may infect endocervical epithelial or endothelial cells in either immunosuppressed or normal individuals.[126] The characteristic enlarged cells with large basophilic nuclear inclusions, sometimes with granular cytoplasmic inclusions, are diagnostic (Fig. 14.37). Positive immunohistochemical staining for CMV antigen is confirmatory.

Herpesvirus usually affects the squamous epithelium but also may involve endocervical cells.[127] The infected cells are usually multinucleated with either large nuclear inclusions or with a ground-glass nucleus without inclusions. Multinucleated reactive endocervical cells, a nonspecific finding, may cause confusion. However, these cells lack the characteristic inclusions or ground-glass chromatin. As with CMV, positive immuno-staining for herpesvirus antigen is confirmatory.

TREATMENT OF ADENOCARCINOMA *IN SITU*

Conization is the recommended initial procedure following an AIS diagnosis on a biopsy or a definitive Pap smear. Although most authors recommend 'cold knife' conization, Andersen et al. reported satisfactory results using combination laser conization.[128] The optimal subsequent treatment, if AIS without invasion and with clear margins is confirmed, remains controversial. Hysterectomy eliminates the difficulties encountered in following patients with Pap smears after a cone biopsy.[72,76,77] However, many women with AIS are young and desirous of retaining their fertility. Although several studies have shown that a cone biopsy with clear margins is not fully protective against recurrent AIS or invasive adenocarcinomas,[129–136] others have safely used this approach, emphasizing the necessity of close follow-up.[98,128,137–139]

Early invasive adenocarcinoma

Assessing early invasion in glandular lesions is sometimes difficult because, unlike squamous lesions, preservation of AIS-like gland architecture may accompany invasion. Conversely, AIS itself may be quite complex (Fig. 14.28). Thus, it is generally not advisable to

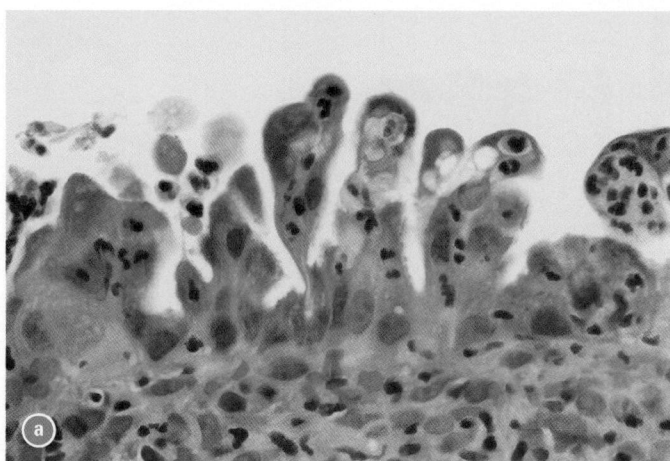

Fig. 14.36 Benign reactive epithelial changes.(a) Reactive changes in columnar epithelium associated with inflammation. (b) Benign multinucleation. (c) Eosinophilic changes (oxyphilic metaplasia). Nuclei are enlarged, irregular, and contain smudged chromatin. A strip of normal endocervical cells is seen at upper left.

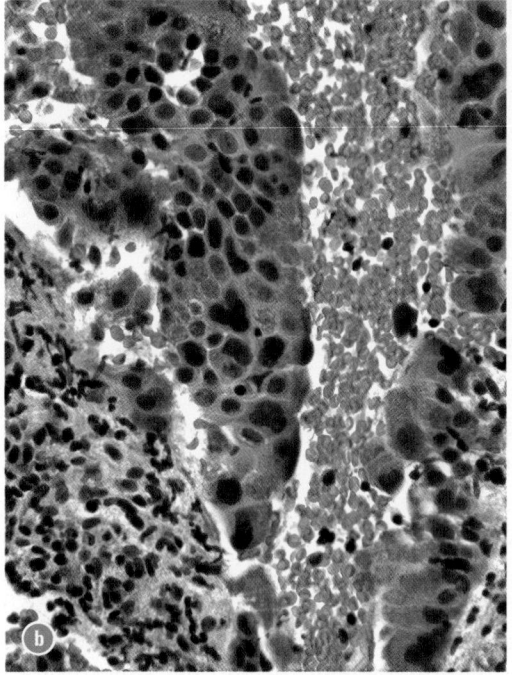

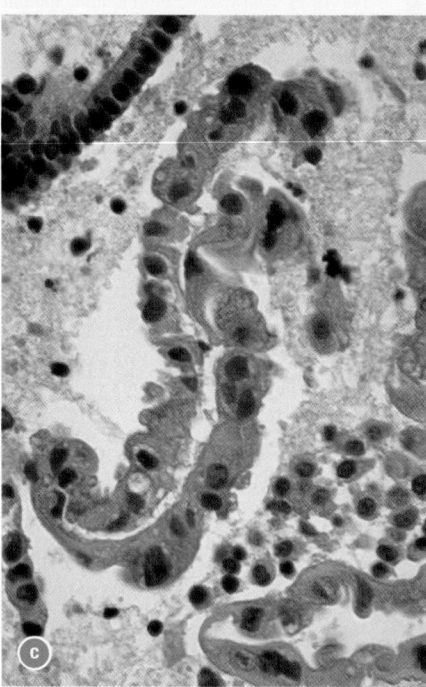

diagnose early invasion from small biopsies. If invasion is suspected in these, one should state this possibility and await a larger specimen or cold-knife cone biopsy for further assessment.

There are three patterns of invasion that typify adenocarcinomas and may be seen in early neoplasms. These comprise infiltrative, expansile and exophytic.[4–6,140,141]

1   *Infiltrative pattern*: the criteria for this pattern are easiest to apply although the infiltration may not be conspicuous. Its earliest manifestation is characterized by small protrusions that appear to bud from AIS glands, extending as separate glands into the stroma, often with an inflammatory response. The cells of the buds and the early invasive glands are often larger than the AIS cells,

with large nuclei, sometimes-prominent nucleoli and an expanded eosinophilic cytoplasm (Fig. 14.38a,b). However, infiltrative invasion is often more subtle, with glands lined by cells similar to those of AIS that permeate the stroma without either an inflammatory or desmoplastic response (Fig. 14.39a,b). In assessing the possibility of invasion in such a case, one must ask whether the arrangement of the glands might possibly be a preexisting benign configuration that has simply been replaced by AIS. The architectural pattern of adjacent benign glands is important for comparison.

2   *Expansile pattern*: the expansile or 'bulky outgrowth'[6] invasive pattern can also be

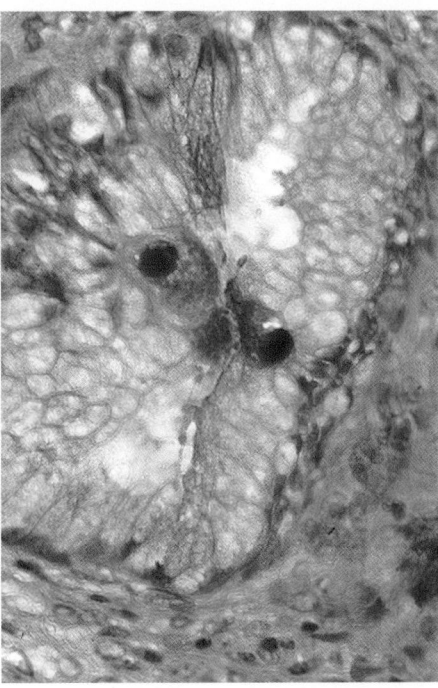

Fig. 14.37
Cytomegalovirus
infection.
An endocervical
gland contains two
cells with huge
intranuclear inclusions
and eosinophilic
granular cytoplasmic
inclusions.

often the problem. Although arbitrary, extension to more than 1 mm below adjacent benign glands generally qualifies.

3 *Exophytic pattern*: this invasive pattern refers to surface polypoid or papillary growth that is more pronounced than the small papillary excrescences that are sometimes present with AIS (Fig. 14.41). Invasion of the underlying stroma may or may not be present. A subset of exophytic adenocarcinomas is the well-differentiated villoglandular adenocarcinoma (see below).

In diagnostic reports the deepest extent of invasion, measured from the overlying surface, is given. The only exceptions are cases of very early invasion where the AIS gland of origin is obvious, in which case the distance from this gland is given (Fig. 14.42). With exophytic tumors, the depth of invasion into the underlying stroma is given, along with the maximum diameter of the exophytic component (Fig. 14.41). The presence or absence of vascular invasion is also reported.

The International Federation of Gynecology and Obstetrics (FIGO, Fr.) system divides early invasive adenocarcinoma into two staging categories.[142] In both there is no grossly visible lesion; in stage IA1, the depth of invasion does not exceed 3 mm and in stage IA2, it is greater than 3 mm but no greater than 5 mm. In both stages, the tumor does not exceed 7 mm in the longest linear extent measured in any one slide. Vascular invasion does not alter the stage. Currently

problematic. Here, well-circumscribed AIS-like glands expand into the stroma as a compact unit rather than as separate infiltrative glands (Fig. 14.40). Often there is no stromal reaction. This pattern, when it extends deeply enough, is recognized intuitively as invasive carcinoma. Defining what constitutes 'deeply enough' is

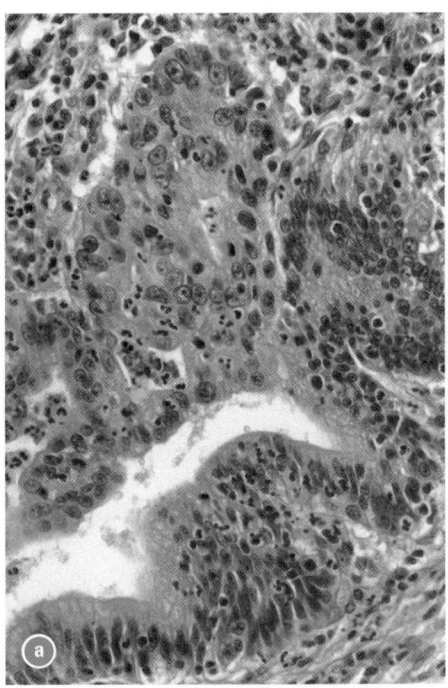

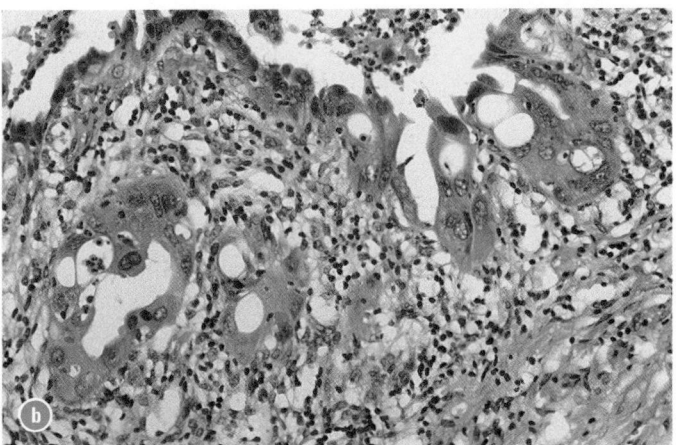

Fig. 14.38 (a) Adenocarcinoma *in situ* with early invasion. In the upper portion of a gland involved by AIS, a bud of enlarged cells with nuclei containing prominent nucleoli protrudes into the underlying inflamed stroma. (b) Early invasive adenocarcinoma. Infiltrative invasion is seen adjacent to an AIS gland containing buds suggesting incipient invasion.

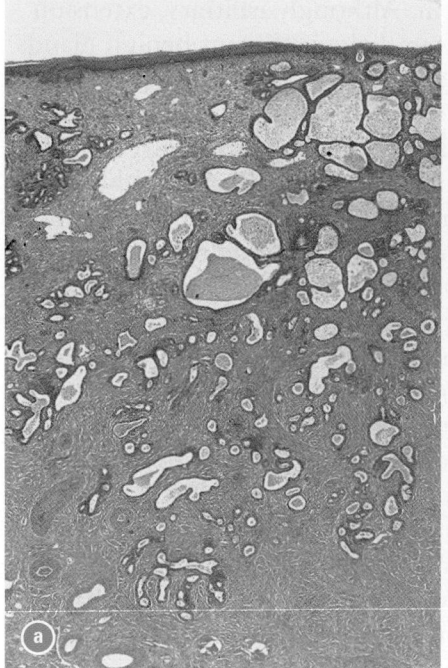 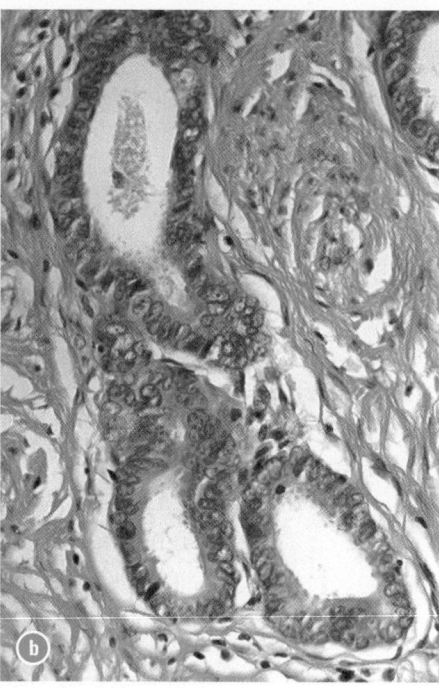

Fig. 14.39 (a) Invasive adenocarcinoma. An infiltrative pattern of glands and cysts extensively infiltrates the underlying stroma. There is no stromal response. (b) Invasive adenocarcinoma. At higher power the deeply invasive glands resemble AIS.

there is no consensus as to the optimal therapy for either stage (cone biopsy alone, simple hysterectomy, or radical hysterectomy with pelvic lymph node dissection), although most cases are treated with the last approach. While staging categories imply a sharp delineation of risk for metastases, in fact some risk exists at all levels of invasion. The risk of pelvic nodal metastases is approximately 1.5% in stage IA1 and only slightly higher in IA2.[3,4,138,143–147] Based on the reported low risk in FIGO stage IA1, a small number of cases have been treated with cone biopsy alone to preserve fertility.[138,148] The additional risk associated with vascular invasion is uncertain because of the small numbers of reported cases; however, of nine patients with early invasion and vascular involvement, none had lymph node metastases.[4,5]

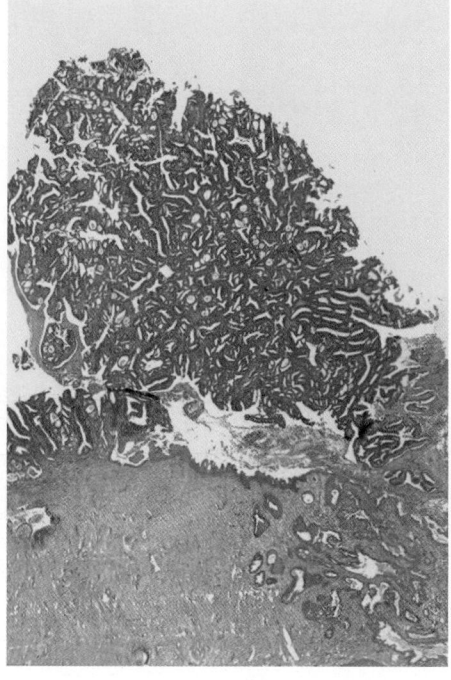

Fig. 14.41 Papillary architecture in a superficial cervical adenocarcinoma.

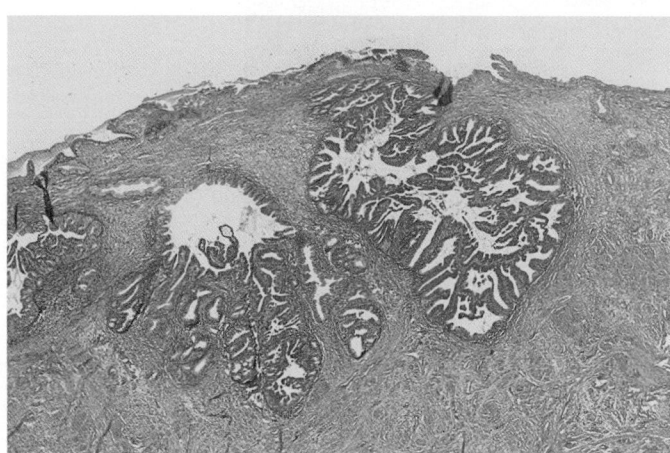

Fig. 14.40 Invasive adenocarcinoma, expansile pattern. Dilated complex glands extend into the underlying stroma in an expansile manner with a sharply circumscribed border. Distinguishing between this pattern and AIS with florid intraglandular growth (Fig. 14.28) may be difficult, sometimes even arbitrary.

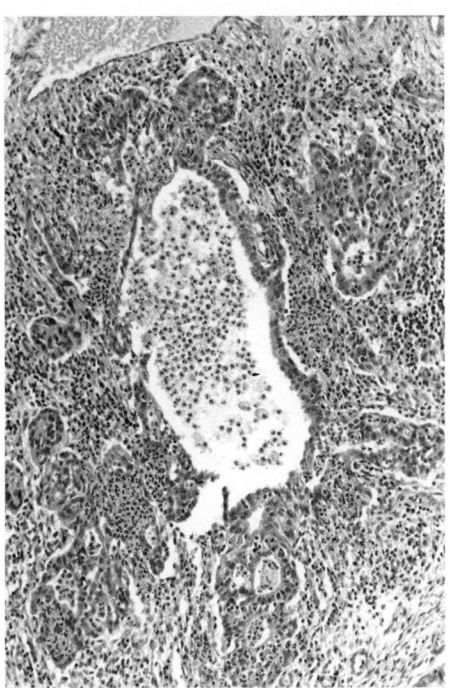

Fig. 14.42 Early invasive adenocarcinoma. An early infiltrative carcinoma emanating from a central gland with AIS is seen in its entirety. In this case, the depth of invasion is measured from the AIS gland to the edge of the furthest invasive gland.

Diagnosis and management of adenocarcinoma of the cervix

Most symptomatic patients with cervical adenocarcinoma have vaginal bleeding and/or pelvic pain or pressure. Less commonly, the presenting sign is a pal-pable pelvic or ovarian mass. Grossly, adenocarcinomas may present as a focus of surface irregularity (Fig. 14.43a), an exophytic mass, an ulcerated plaque, or an indurated, barrel-shaped cervix (Fig. 14.43b).[149,150]

The classification of cervical adenocarcinomas and mixed carcinomas with a glandular component is listed below followed by a description of each subtype (Table 14.4). Adenocarcinomas that contain more than 10% of a second adenocarcinoma subtype are designated mixed-epithelial types and the relative amount of each component is specified. The more common subtypes are graded using a three-tiered system that is based on a combination of architectural and cytologic features keeping in mind that nuclear atypia is an important component of grade and by this criterion most are grade 2 or 3.[151]

ENDOCERVICAL (MUCINOUS) ADENOCARCINOMA

Usual type

The large majority of pure cervical adenocarcinomas are of the endocervical type,[150,151] so named because the epithelial cells simulate, at least to some degree, the appearance of endocervical cells. The cytoplasm may be eosinophilic, mucinous-appearing, or a mixture of these. There are often many mitotic figures and apoptotic bodies (Fig. 14.44a–c).[151] Some classifications separate those tumors in which most of the cells are

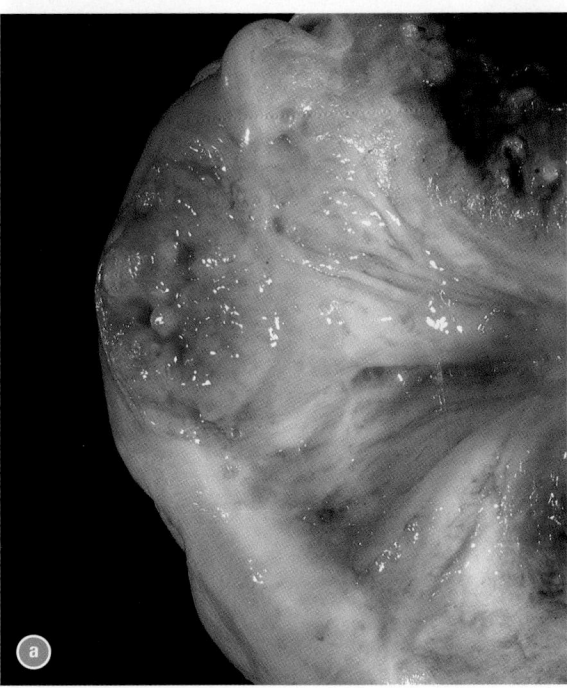

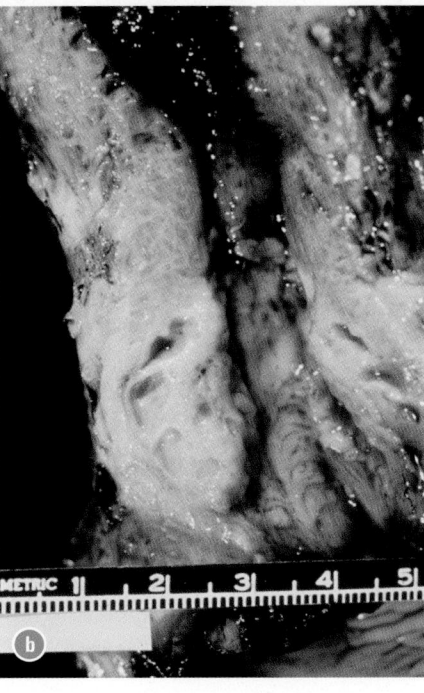

Fig. 14.43 (a) Gross specimen of early adenocarcinoma, presenting as a discoid irregularity in the transformation zone. (b) A more advanced lesion is thickened and indurated circumferentially without an obvious mass.

Table 14.4 *Categories of adenocarcinoma of the cervix*

Endocervical (mucinous)
  Variant:
  Adenoma malignum (minimal deviation type)
Endometrioid
  Variant:
  Minimal deviation endometrioid type
Intestinal
Adenosquamous
  Variants:
  Glassy cell
  Clear cell adenosquamous
Well-differentiated villoglandular
Clear cell
Serous
Adenoid basal
Adenoid cystic
Mesonephric
Metastatic adenocarcinoma

mucinous-appearing into a mucinous type separate from the endocervical category,[151] while others designate the entire endocervical category as the mucinous type with various subtypes.[108,152] These distinctions do not have any known clinical significance, as the prognosis of cervical adenocarcinoma is almost entirely dependent on the tumor stage. In practice, many cases in the endocervical (or mucinous) category are simply designated as 'adenocarcinoma' without specifying a subtype.

Most endocervical-type adenocarcinomas are related to HPV and residual AIS is often present in early invasive lesions. They may have an exophytic papillary growth pattern or invade as irregular glands, cysts, cords, sheets, single cells, or any combination of these. There may or may not be a desmoplastic or inflammatory stromal reaction. Usually the diagnosis of adenocarcinoma is straightforward when specimens are large enough. Two benign lesions that may occasionally cause diagnostic difficulties are microglandular hyperplasia and mesonephric hyperplasia; both are discussed and illustrated below.

Adenoma malignum (minimal-deviation type)

This extremely well-differentiated subtype accounts for 1 to 2% of cervical adenocarcinomas. Because its epithelial cells appear similar to those of the endocervix, it is herein classified as a variant of the endocervical subtype. However, because of its distinctive clinical and pathological features, the terms 'adenoma malignum' or 'minimal-deviation adenocarcinoma' should be specified in diagnostic reports. Approximately 11% of cases have been associated with the Peutz–Jeghers syndrome.[153] In the largest series of 26 cases, the average age of the

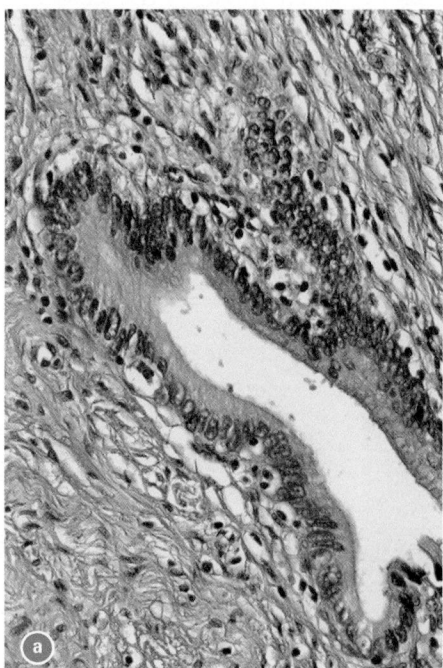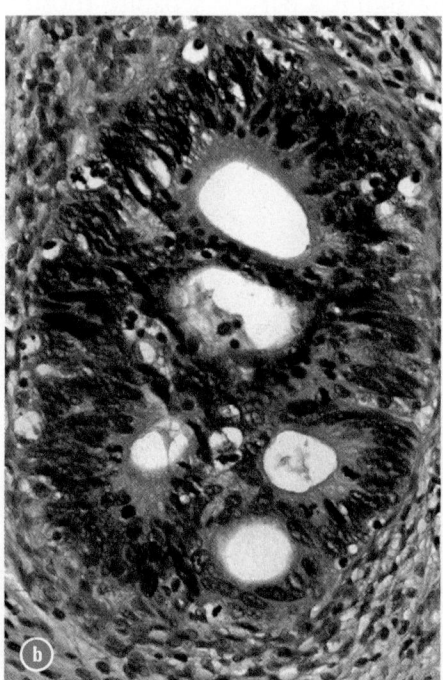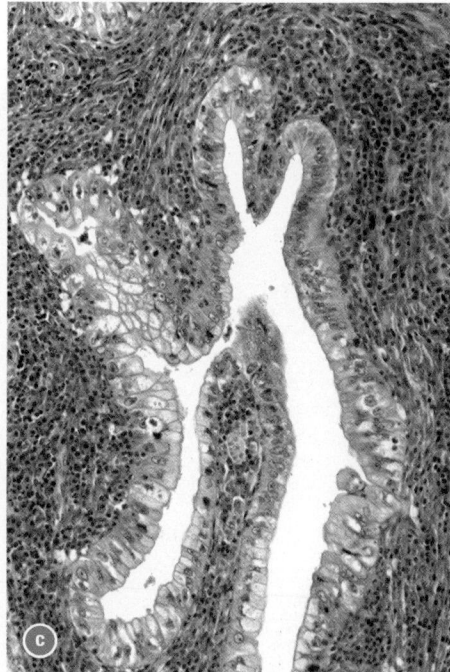

Fig. 14.44 (a) Invasive adenocarcinoma, endocervical type. A malignant gland is lined by columnar cells with eosinophilic cytoplasm. (b) Invasive adenocarcinoma, endocervical type. The cells are columnar with numerous apical mitotic figures and basal apoptotic fragments. (c) Invasive adenocarcinoma, endocervical type. The cells have a pale, mucinous-appearing cytoplasm.

patients was 42 years.[154] In 50% of these 26 cases there was a concomitant mucinous ovarian tumor. Most of these were bilateral and, although some were considered benign primary mucinous tumors of the ovary, it is likely that most (if not all) were actually metastases from the cervical tumor, considering how difficult it is to make this distinction (see section on metastatic tumors to the ovary). The origins of adenoma malignum are obscure; only rare cases are positive for HPV[7,155] and no *in situ* phase has yet been described.

Some patients have a mucinous or watery vaginal discharge, but adenoma malignum often grows insidiously without symptoms, producing an indurated, sometimes barrel-shaped cervix without a discrete mass. It is notorious for escaping notice in small biopsies because of its benign-appearing cells (hence its contradictory appellation). Owing also to the insensitivity of Pap smears,[62–64] adenoma malignum is often discovered in an advanced stage and thus has a worse prognosis than cervical adenocarcinoma in general.[154]

The glands of adenoma malignum are variably sized from small to cystic; many are irregular, with finger-like or bulbous protrusions (Fig. 14.45a). Most of the lining cells are extremely well differentiated, with small, basally located nuclei and pale columnar cytoplasm that are remarkable in their resemblance to normal endocervical cells (Fig. 14.45b). However, on close inspec-

tion, many nuclei are slightly larger than those of normal endocervical cells and they have a small nucleolus (Fig. 14.45c). In rare cases there is a papillary surface component (Fig. 14.46a,b). Most glands elicit no stromal response, but an inflammatory, edematous, or desmoplastic reaction is usually present focally (Fig. 14.47a). Importantly, there is a range of nuclear atypia, with focal enlargement, hyperchromasia and mitotic activity exceeding that of benign endocervical hyperplasias (Fig. 14.47b).

The cytoplasm is positive for carcinoembryonic antigen (CEA) in most cases and negative in most benign mimics.[156,157] However, focal or weak staining should not be interpreted as definitive evidence of cancer; conversely, negative staining, especially in a small biopsy, does not exclude it.[154,158] Adenoma malignum has been shown to be of gastric rather than Müllerian phenotype[159–163] and identification using antibodies to HK1083 for gastric gland mucin, or a positive reaction with the periodic acid–Schiff (PAS) stain at pH 2.5, in addition to CEA staining, has been reported to aid in the diagnosis.[163] It is important to emphasize that most cases can be diagnosed without the use of special stains and that reliance on them may lead to errors unless one is experienced in their use in this rather specialized area.

The differential diagnosis of adenoma malignum includes deep nabothian cysts, florid deep endocervical

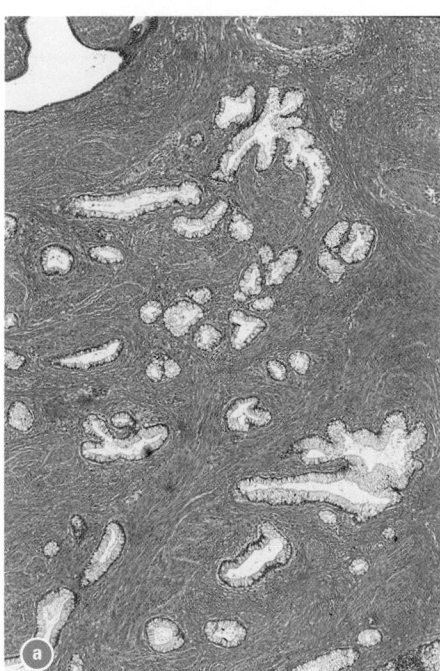 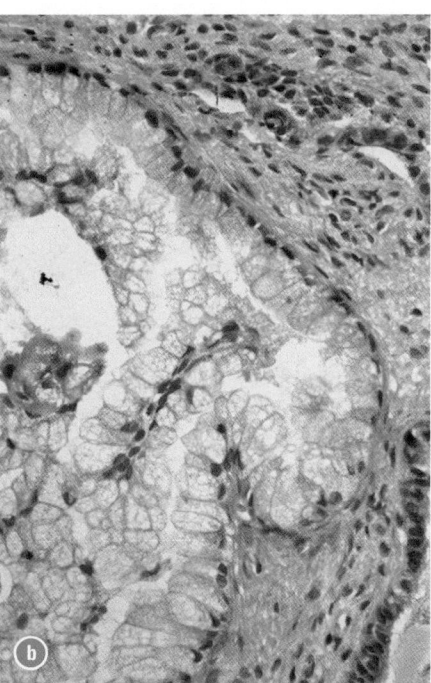 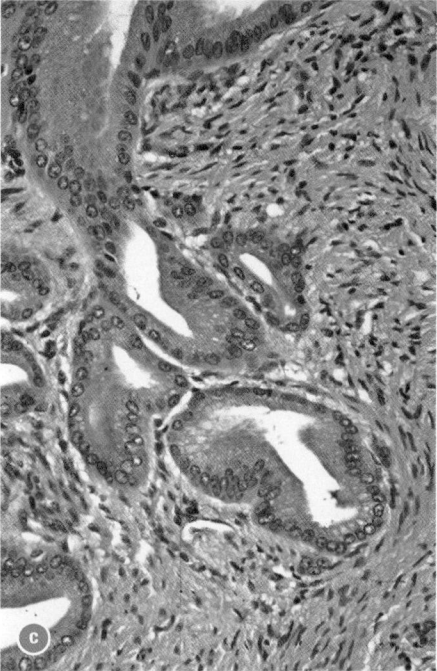

Fig. 14.45 (a) Adenoma malignum. Irregularly shaped glands infiltrate the stroma with no reaction. (b) Adenoma malignum. Malignant glands have abundant mucinous cytoplasm and small benign-appearing nuclei. (c) The cells lining these malignant glands have slightly enlarged nuclei with small nucleoli.

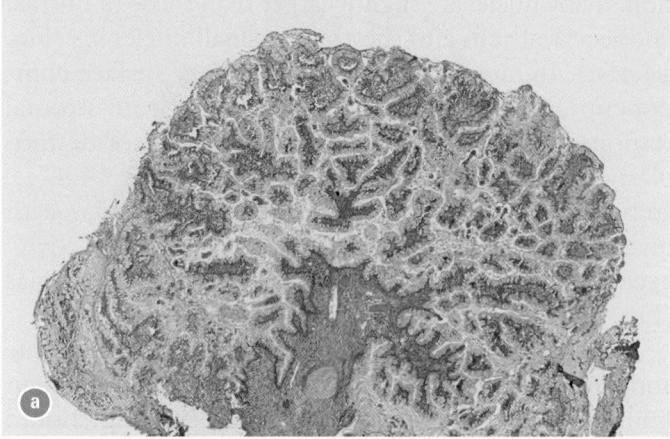

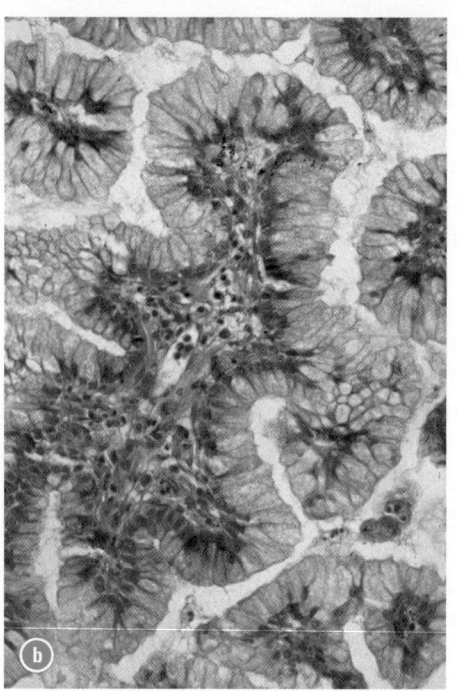

Fig. 14.46 (a) Adenoma malignum. This case was heralded by a small papillary lesion on the ectocervix. (b) The cytologic features are similar to those in Figure 14.45. This case was originally misdiagnosed as a benign papilloma.

glands, tunnel clusters, endocervical gland hyperplasias, adenomyoma of the endocervical type, endocervicosis and mesonephric hyperplasia. These are discussed in detail below. However, all of them lack the infiltrative invasive pattern and focal malignant-appearing nuclei seen in adenoma malignum.

ENDOMETRIOID ADENOCARCINOMA

Usual type

As the name indicates, endometrioid carcinomas appear similar to the usual type of adenocarcinoma of the endometrium, having cells with nonmucinous cytoplasm that are more crowded and stratified than those

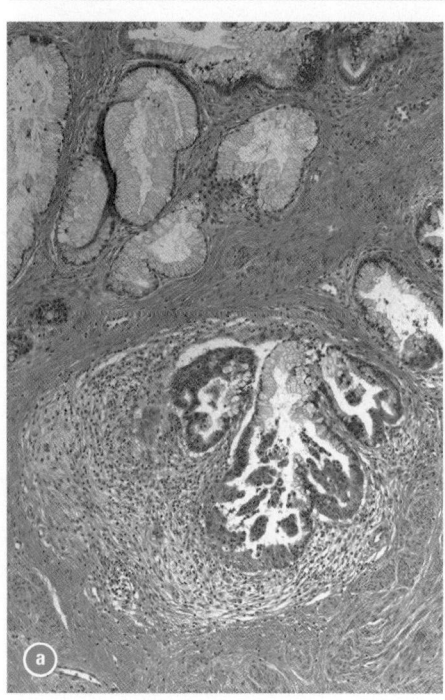

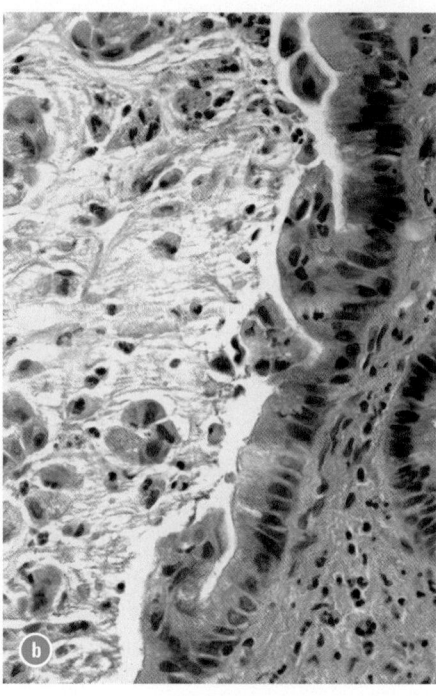

Fig. 14.47 (a) Adenoma malignum. The lower glands have elicited a stromal inflammatory reaction. (b) Adenoma malignum. Here there is focal nuclear enlargement and stratification with sloughing of cells into the lumen of the gland.

of the endocervical type (Fig. 14.48). Some cases may have small areas of bland squamous differentiation (similar to some well-differentiated carcinoma of the endometrium); mixed carcinomas with higher-grade squamous differentiation are classified as adenosquamous carcinomas. Most endometrioid carcinomas are HPV-related and AIS is often present in smaller lesions, indicative of a pathogenesis similar to that of the endocervical type.[5]

The true frequency and the behavior of the endometrioid subtype, as distinct from the endocervical subtype, are not known, since the appearances overlap and the endometrioid designation is often a matter of personal preference. For example, we considered only 4% of 175 consecutive cervical adenocarcinomas as endometrioid,[164] whereas others estimate that the endometrioid subtype accounts for as many as 50% of their cases.[165]

Thus, currently the primary reason for being aware of an endometrioid subtype is to distinguish it from primary carcinoma of the endometrium in curettings and small biopsies. Along with the clinical presentation, the most helpful findings in making this distinction are the presence of AIS, involvement of endocervical-appearing rather than endometrial-appearing stroma and the absence of endometrial hyperplasia. A positive immunohistochemical reaction for CEA and a negative one for vimentin strongly favor an endocervical origin.[165-168] Also, cervical adenocarcinomas are rarely positive for both estrogen-receptor and progesterone-

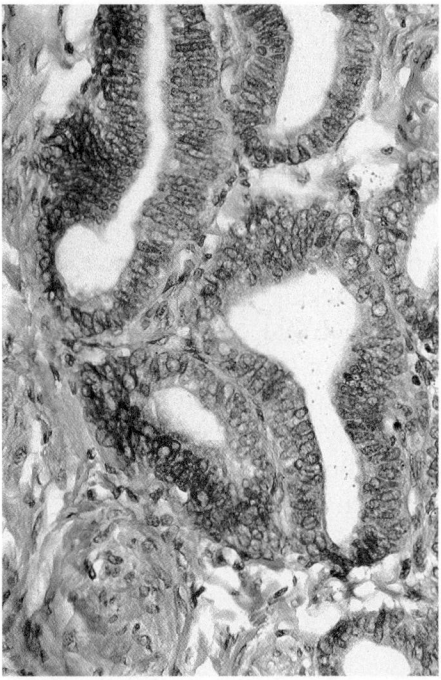

Fig. 14.48 Endometrioid adenocarcinoma. The appearance of the glands is similar to that of a typical carcinoma of the endometrium.

receptor proteins, whereas both are commonly present in endometrial carcinomas.[169] HPV testing by *in situ* hybridization or other means may also be used.[169] However, although immunohistochemical panels may sometimes be useful, results may be equivocal and they are usually not necessary.[168]

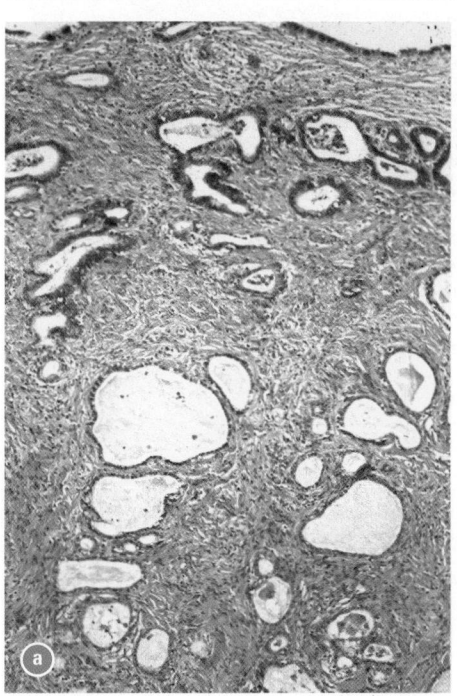

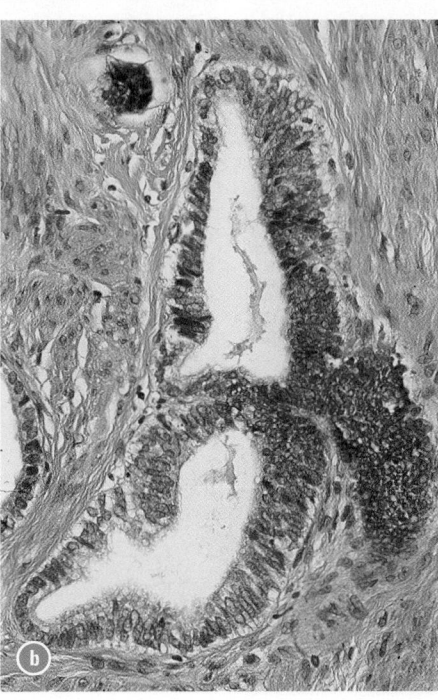

Fig. 14.49 (a) Endometrioid adenocarcinoma, minimal-deviation type. Invasive variably shaped glands with a banal, somewhat attenuated lining epithelium and without any adjacent stromal reaction are present. (b) In this high-power view of an area from the tumor in (a), the glands are similar to those of a proliferative endometrium except for a slight increase in crowding and stratification.

Minimal-deviation adenocarcinoma, endometrioid type

Although the term 'adenoma malignum' is reserved for the endocervical type of minimal deviation adenocarcinoma, rarely an extremely well-differentiated carcinoma will appear endometrioid rather than endocervical.[170–172] In such cases the glands have only mild nuclear atypia and infrequent mitotic figures (Fig. 14.49a). Some cells may even be ciliated or have apical cytoplasmic snouts, mimicking tubal metaplasia.[171] Minimal-deviation endometrioid carcinoma is distinguished from endometriosis or tuboendometrioid metaplasia by its infiltrative architectural pattern (although a stromal reaction is usually absent) and at least focal cytologic atypia (Fig. 14.49b). CEA staining was focally positive in the two cases in which it was studied.[172] In

12 cases with follow-up data, one patient died of her tumor.[170–172]

INTESTINAL ADENOCARCINOMA

Although the endocervical and adenosquamous subtypes may contain foci that appear intestinal, pure intestinal adenocarcinomas of the cervix are rare. Intestinal differentiation is characterized by goblet cells, argentaffin cells and rarely by Paneth's cells.[173–175] Less frequent are cases with extensive extracellular mucin (colloid carcinoma)[176]; rarer still are those composed largely of signet ring cells.[177,178] In all such cases, one should be careful to exclude a primary gastrointestinal carcinoma metastatic to the cervix. Usually this distinction is obvious from

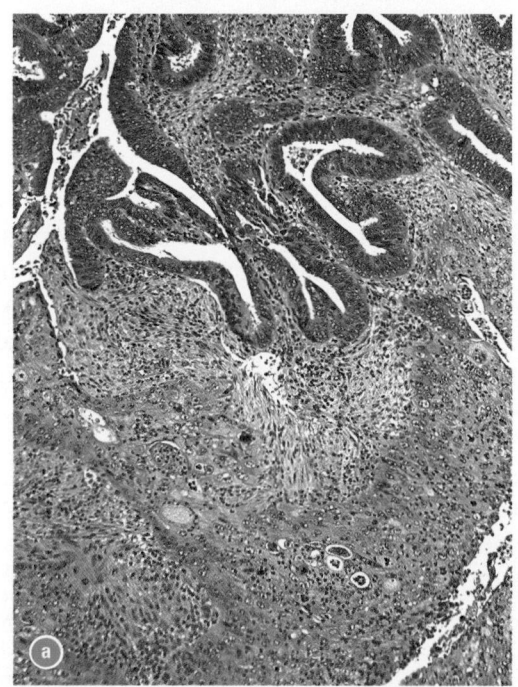

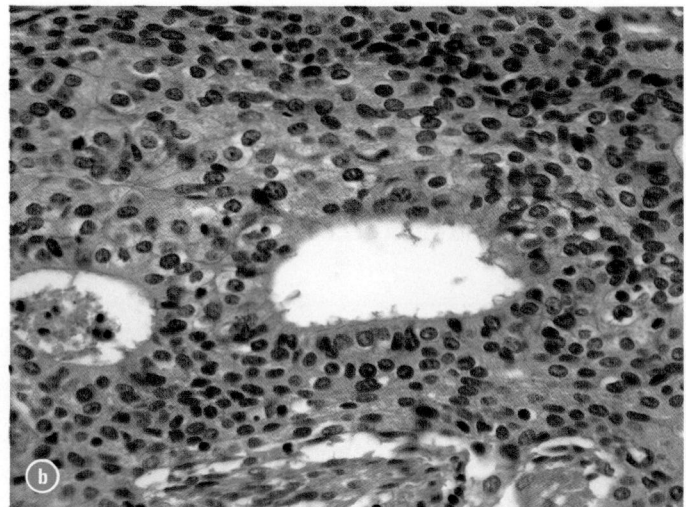

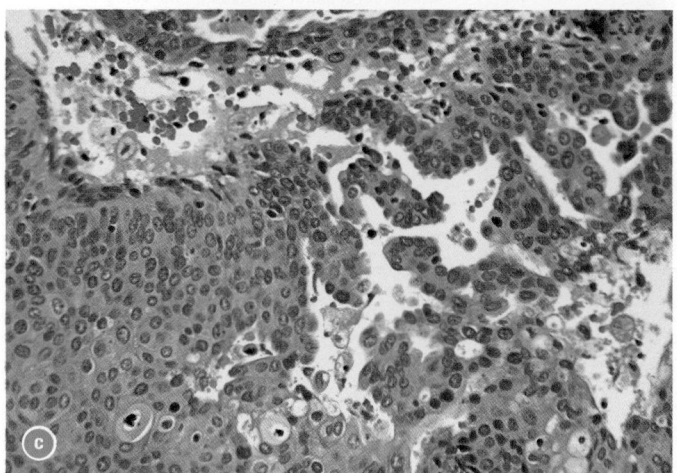

Fig. 14.50 Adenosquamous carcinoma. (a) Juxtaposed distinct glandular and squamous elements. (b) Sheet of squamoid epithelium encloses discrete glandular structures. (c) Blending of squamous with areas of micropapillary glandular differentiation.

the clinical circumstances. Resorting to immunohisto-chemistry may be problematic. Although primary cervical adenocarcinomas of the usual type are characteristically diffusely and strongly CK7-positive[166] while primary intestinal carcinomas are usually either CK 7-negative or only focally positive, CK7 testing of primary cervical adenocarcinomas of the purely intestinal type has not been reported to our knowledge.

ADENOSQUAMOUS CARCINOMA

Usual type

Adenosquamous carcinomas have been reported to constitute from 20% to 50% of all cervical carcinomas that have a glandular component.[108] This wide variation is probably related to different interpretations of what constitutes squamous differentiation. For instance, solid area in poorly-differentiated adenocarcinomas may have eosinophilic cytoplasm that some may interpret as evidence of squamous differentiation, while others may not.[151] Conversely, many pure squamous carcinomas of the cervix have cells that stain positively for mucin.[179] We limit the designation 'adenosquamous' to carcinomas with both squamous and glandular areas that are each clearly recognizable without the use of special stains.[151] Using this definition, we found that adenosquamous carcinomas accounted for 28% of 175 consecutive early-stage adenocarcinomas.[164]

Early adenosquamous carcinomas often contain both residual AIS and CIN, suggesting neoplastic transformation of a stem cell capable of biphasic differentiation.[5] Several patterns may be seen in fully invasive cases, including separate juxtaposed glandular and squamous elements (Fig. 14.50a), sheets of squamoid cells admixed with glands (Fig. 14.50b) and more subtle transitions between squamous and columnar differentiation (Fig. 14.50c). The glandular component in adenosquamous carcinoma may be nonspecific, mucinous (sometimes with signet ring cells), or endometrioid. Adenosquamous carcinomas have been reported to have a worse prognosis than other cervical adenocarcinomas detected at the same stage.[164,180,181] However, some studies found no prognostic difference.[182]

Glassy cell and clear cell adenosquamous carcinomas

If the distinction of squamous from columnar differentiation is based on parameters other than standard hematoxylin and eosin stained sections, the range of lesions in the 'adenosquamous' category expands. Glassy cell carcinoma, first described in 1956, is a rare variant of adenosquamous carcinoma, but its biphasic nature is recognizable only by electron microscopy.[183–185] In glassy cell carcinoma there are solid sheets of large malignant cells with abundant, finely granular (glassy) cytoplasm. Nuclei are large with prominent nucleoli. There is a marked inflammatory infiltrate, often with many eosinophils and plasma cells (Fig. 14.51a,b). In most reports the prognosis has been worse than that for ordinary adenocarcinomas of the cervix, with a tendency for early extra-uterine spread and resistance to radiation.[184–186]

Some authors have pointed out that large cell non-keratinizing squamous carcinomas often have glassy cell-like areas[186] and others note that otherwise typical adenocarcinomas may also have such areas.[151] These cases should not be reported as glassy cell carcinomas, which are quite rare in their pure form.[186]

A rare second category of adenosquamous carcinoma is termed 'clear cell adenosquamous carcinoma'.[187] These carcinomas are strongly associated with HPV 18; they contain recognizable neoplastic glands admixed with sheets of glycogen-rich squamoid cells with a pronounced clear appearance (Fig. 14.51c,d). As with glassy cell carcinomas, clear cell adenosquamous carcinomas have been associated with a poor prognosis.[187]

WELL-DIFFERENTIATED VILLOGLANDULAR ADENOCARCINOMA

This uncommon variant is distinguished by its villous papillary architecture. There may or may not be recognizable underlying stromal invasion (Fig. 14.52a). The average patient age is 33 years.[188,189] Villoglandular adenocarcinoma is HPV-related[190] and adjacent AIS is often present. The finger-like papillae sometimes have a distinctive spindled stroma (Fig. 14.52b) that may contain inflammatory cells. The villi blend with underlying elongated branching glands that push into the stroma over a broad confluent front. The lining cells are either endocervical- or endometrioid-appearing with only mild nuclear atypia and few mitotic figures. Strictly defined, the prognosis for well-differentiated villoglandular adenocarcinoma is excellent. None of the 37 cases in the initial descriptions were reported to have metastasized and the possibility of treatment of selected patients with cone biopsy alone to preserve fertility was suggested.[188,189] However, villoglandular architecture may be superimposed on conventional invasive adenocarcinomas that have the capacity to metastasize to pelvic lymph nodes (Fig. 14.52c).[191,192] Therefore, villous papillary tumors must be composed of cells that are exclusively well-differentiated and must

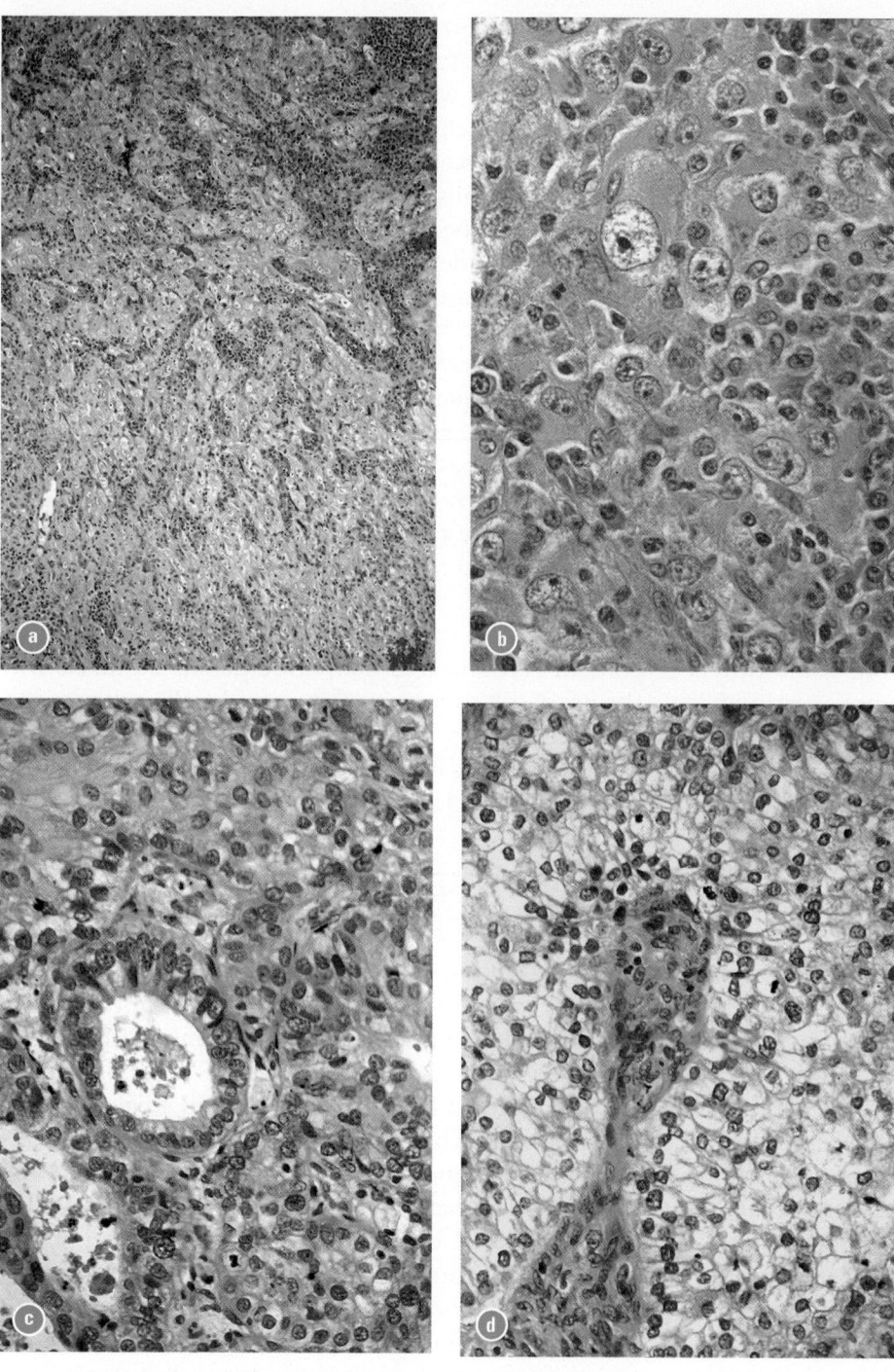

Fig. 14.51 (a) Glassy cell carcinoma. Cells are arranged in sheets (pale clear areas) with a prominent inflammatory reaction. (b) Cells are enlarged and have prominent nuclei and nucleoli; the cytoplasm is granular and eosinophilic (glassy). (c,d) Clear cell adenosquamous carcinoma, characterized by neoplastic glands associated with sheets of glycogen-rich clear squamoid cells.

be removed completely and thoroughly sampled before they are placed in the well-differentiated villoglandular category with its attendant excellent prognosis.[151] Villoglandular carcinomas must also be distinguished from filiform papillary growth patterns that are occasionally present in AIS or in exophytic adenocarcinomas that lack the well-defined villous architecture of well-differentiated villoglandular carcinoma (Fig. 14.41).

CLEAR CELL CARCINOMA

Clear cell carcinoma of the cervix is rare. Its occurrence both in the cervix and vagina of young women has

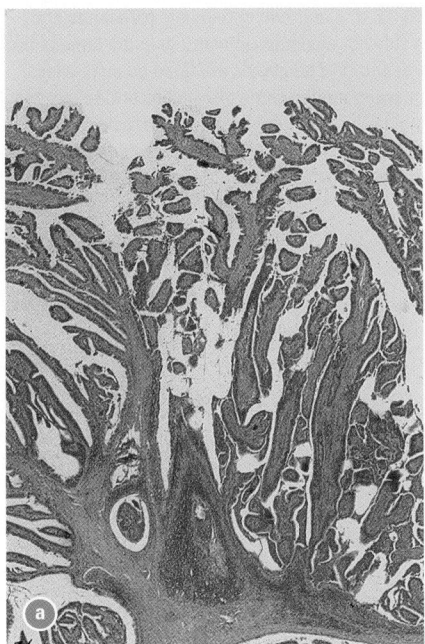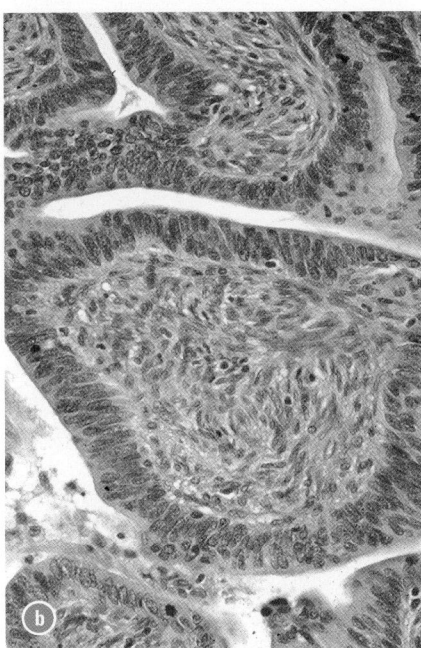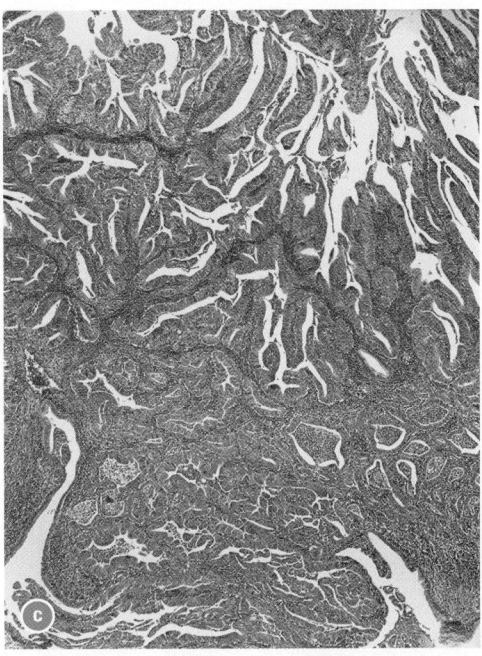

Fig. 14.52 (a) Well-differentiated villoglandular adenocarcinoma. The surface of the tumor contains finger-like villous processes. (b) Well-differentiated villoglandular adenocarcinoma. The villi contain spindle cells and are lined with well-differentiated epithelial cells. (c) Villoglandular architecture (upper) associated with conventional invasion (lower).

been linked to exposure *in utero* to diethylstilbestrol taken by their mothers to avoid miscarriage.[193] Fortunately, the risk for clear cell carcinoma appears to have diminished as this cohort has grown older and currently most cases are sporadic.[194,195] The behavior of sporadic clear cell carcinoma was found to be the same as cervical adenocarcinomas in general in one report,[194] but more aggressive in another.[196]

The histologic appearance is similar to that of the more common clear cell carcinomas of the endometrium and ovary. Tumor cells are arranged in either glandular (Fig. 14.53a), tubulocystic, solid, papillary, or mixed patterns. In the papillary, glandular and tubulocystic areas, the nuclei characteristically protrude into the adjacent space, creating a 'hobnail' appearance (Fig. 14.53b). Papillae often have hyaline stromal cores. The clear cytoplasm, present in most cells, is due to the presence of glycogen, which may be highlighted with a PAS stain. In some cases the cells are focally eosinophilic or mucin-containing rather than clear. The nuclei are usually large, irregular and hyperchromatic with prominent nucleoli but in some cases may be only mildly to moderately atypical (Fig. 14.53c).

The differential diagnosis includes microglandular hyperplasia, mesonephric hyperplasia/carcinoma, the Arias-Stella reaction, glycogen-rich squamous cell carcinoma and other very rare cancers that may contain clear cells, such as yolk sac tumor and alveolar soft part sarcoma, both of which can be primary in the cervix and metastatic renal cell carcinoma. Distinction from the three benign conditions is discussed in detail below. Squamous carcinoma with glycogenated clear cells has other more characteristic, clearly squamous patterns and may have residual CIN. Renal cell carcinoma rarely metastasizes to the cervix but, in a patient with a known renal carcinoma, these may be difficult to distinguish from a primary clear cell carcinoma. Most renal cell carcinomas are CD10 positive while Müllerian-derived clear cell carcinomas are negative.[197] Yolk sac tumor and alveolar soft part sarcoma, both very rare primary tumors of the cervix, have their own characteristic features, which are presented elsewhere in this chapter.

SEROUS CARCINOMA

Serous carcinoma is also rare; it is histologically similar to the much more common serous carcinomas of the ovary and endometrium. The largest series of primary cervical tumors, composed of 17 patients,[198] showed a

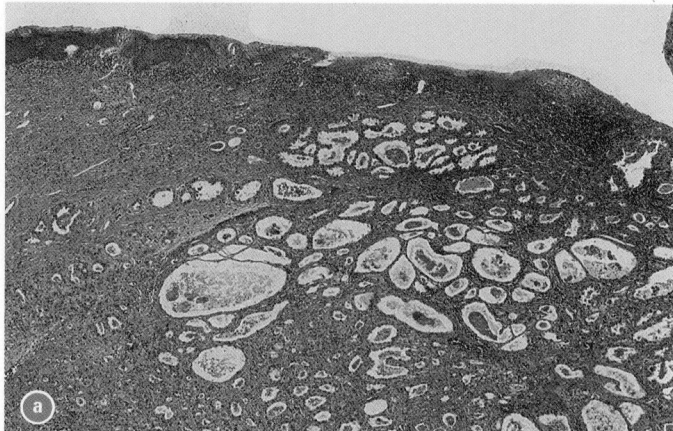

Fig. 14.53 Clear cell carcinoma. (a) Glands and cysts with eosinophilic material in the lumens are present. (b) The glands are lined by cells with enlarged nuclei, some of which protrude into the lumina (hobnail cells). (c) In this example, nuclear atypia is only mild to moderate. Note the prominent cytoplasmic clearing.

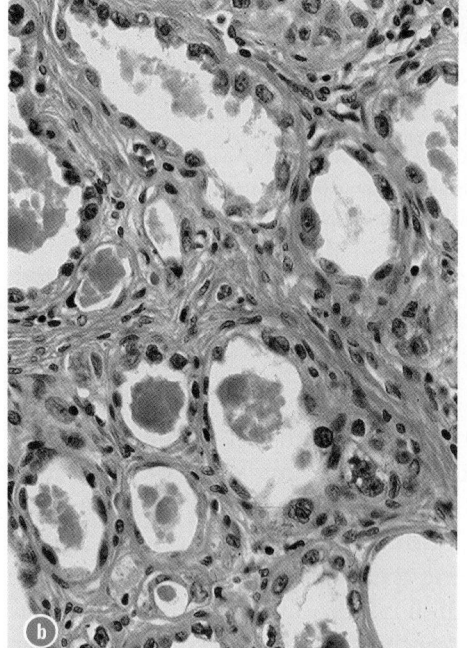

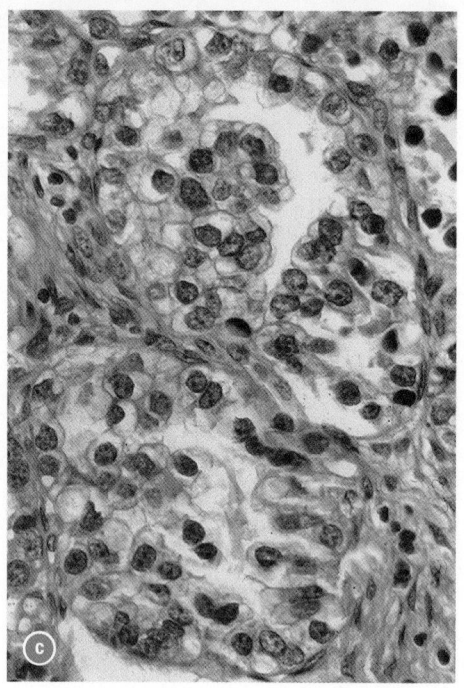

bimodal age distribution, with 10 patients younger than 45 years and four older than 65 years; 14 of the 17 tumors were at stage I at the time of diagnosis, with tumor recurrence in four. All three of the higher-stage tumors were fatal.

The tumor surface contains complex branching papillae, often with inflammatory cells in the stroma (Fig. 14.54a–c). At deeper levels, the tumor may form glands, slit-like spaces, or solid areas. There is nuclear stratification and budding of the epithelial cells into the spaces between papillae. The epithelial cells have large nuclei with prominent nucleoli and conspicuous mitotic figures (Fig. 14.54c). Serous carcinomas are easily distinguished from typical papillary carcinomas of the endo-

cervical type and from well-differentiated villoglandular papillary adenocarcinomas by their complex papillae and high-grade nuclei (Figs 14.41, 14.52a). It is interesting, however, that a well-differentiated villoglandular papillary component was found in five of the 17 reported cases, suggesting a common etiology for these two papillary carcinomas when they occur in the cervix (Fig. 14.54b).[198] Also, unlike endometrial or ovarian serous carcinomas, cervical serous carcinomas in younger women are typically positive for HPV (CP Crum and MR Nucci, pers comm, 2004) and 7 of the 12 cases in the above series that were tested for p53, were negative.[198] Thus, primary cervical serous carcinomas should not be equated with similar-appearing carci-

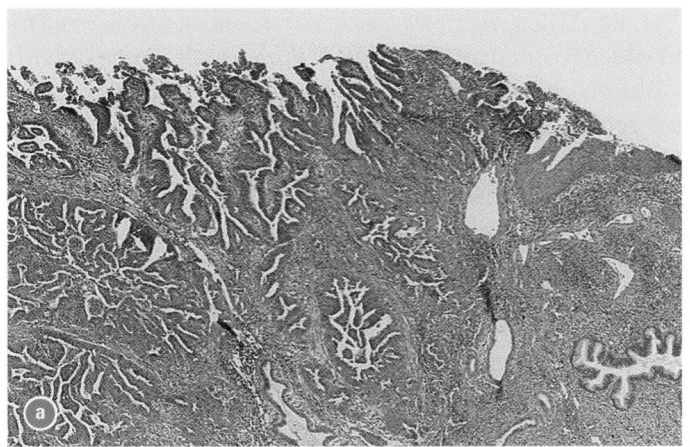

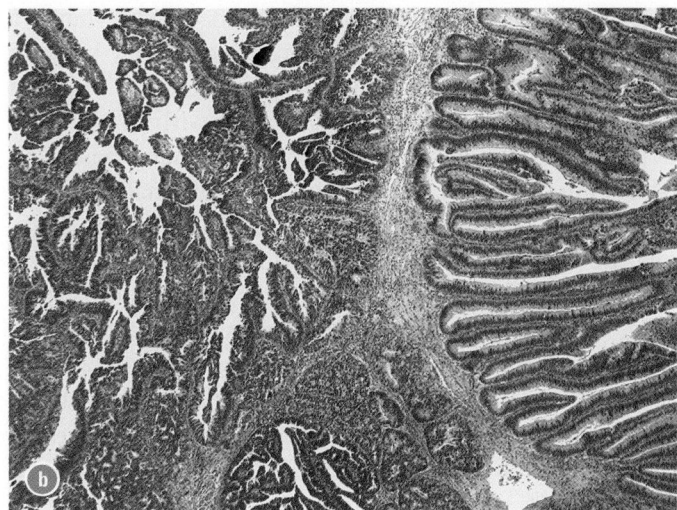

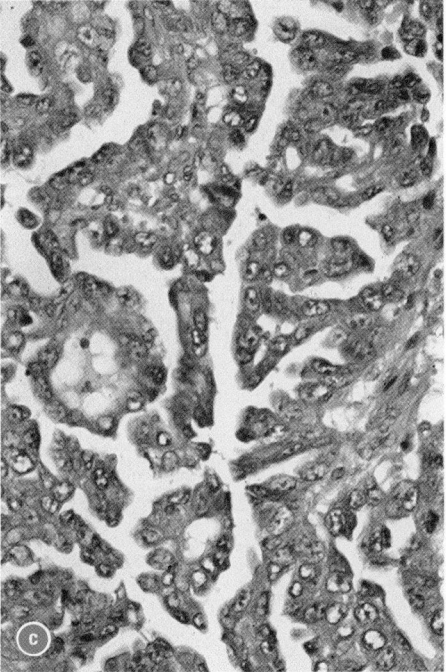

Fig. 14.54 Primary serous carcinoma of the cervix. (a) The surface is papillary. Underlying invasive glands have a fjord-like appearance. (b) Juxtaposed serous (left) and villoglandular architecture (right). (c) At high power, the papillae are complex with buds of epithelial cells with enlarged nuclei and prominent nucleoli.

nomas of the endometrium and ovary. In practice, spread to the cervix from a serous carcinoma of the endometrium or ovary must always be excluded (especially in older women) and if either is present, the cervical lesion is almost certainly metastatic.

ADENOID BASAL AND ADENOID CYSTIC CARCINOMAS

These tumors are discussed together because of certain common features:

1 Both are composed of cells with a basaloid morphology.

2 Both are associated with human papillomavirus.

3 Patients with these tumors are typically postmenopausal.

Adenoid basal and adenoid cystic carcinomas are linked within a spectrum of tumors with basaloid morphology and columnar cell (adenoid) differentiation. Both may be preceded by a squamous intraepithelial lesion that with invasion undergoes a transformation to a basaloid cell proliferation with variable columnar cell differentiation.

Adenoid basal cell carcinomas (ABC) are rare and account for less than 5% of carcinomas of the cervix. ABC is usually an asymptomatic incidental finding in the cervix of postmenopausal women who have a high-grade CIN.[199,200] Three components may be seen underlying the CIN (Fig. 14.55a): these include discrete islands of squamoid cells with a variable degree of atypia and a prominent peripheral basal cell layer (Fig. 14.55b), nests composed of small basaloid cells with scant cytoplasm, sometimes with cystic change and focal columnar differentiation in the form of small acini admixed with the basaloid nests (Fig. 14.55c). There is no stromal reaction (Fig. 14.55a–c). Because there have been no metastases or recurrences among cases fitting this description, some have suggested that they be designated 'adenoid basal epithelioma' to discourage overly radical treatment.[200]

In addition to the above, ABC-like areas are sometimes associated with three other patterns of neoplastic growth: these are basaloid squamous carcinomas, adenoid cystic carcinomas and carcinosarcomas. In pure ABC the peripheral cells of the nests are immunoreactive for CAM 5.2, a helpful feature in excluding a synchronous squamous cell carcinoma in an ABC with severe atypia.[200] The reader is cautioned that sampling may limit an appreciation of more than one pattern in the same patient. Suffice it to say that ABCs do not always signify a predictable biology and may represent one of several pathways of differentiation from a precursor cell.[199,201]

Like ABCs, *adenoid cystic carcinomas (ACC)* occur in older women. Unlike ABCs they usually present with a symptomatic cervical mass and are often complicated by recurrence and metastases.[199] These tumors bear some resemblance to those located more commonly in the salivary glands or respiratory tract. They grow in islands of crowded cells with little cytoplasm in a cribriform arrangement with central hyaline or mucinous material (Fig. 14.56a,b). There may also be a trabecular, solid, or undifferentiated pattern, often with surrounding hyaline material.[202] Focal conspicuous squamous differentiation may be seen.[199] Foci in ACC may mimic ABC (with which these tumors may be associated), but elsewhere ACC has marked nuclear atypia and a stromal response not seen in ABC.[199,201] Like ABCs, ACCs may coexist with mesenchymal elements, forming a carcinosarcoma.

Whether cervical ACCs are derived from myoepithelial cells, as are the more common ACCs found elsewhere, is controversial. One report cited only rare S-100-positive cells of presumed myoepithelial derivation and therefore designated their tumors 'adenoid cystic-like'.[199] Others found S-100 positivity more frequently, as well as staining for type IV collagen and

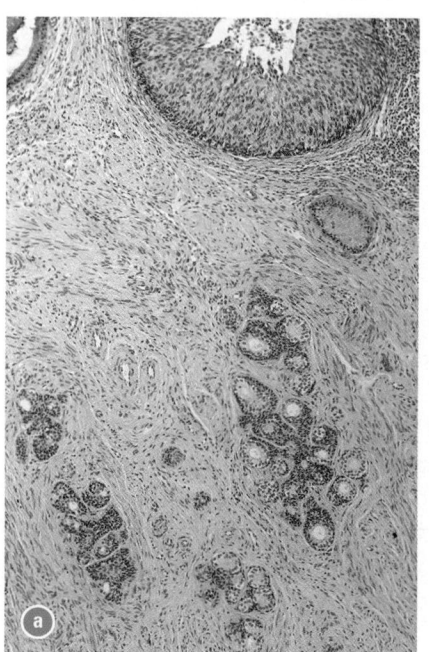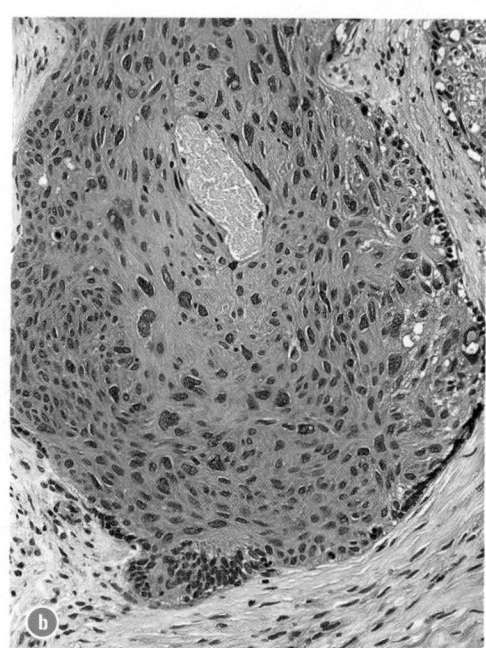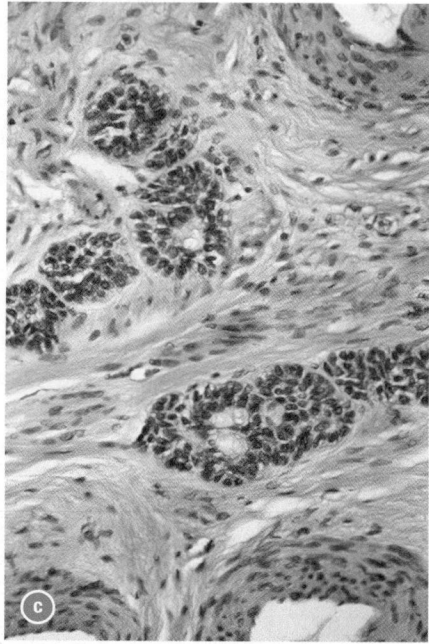

Fig. 14.55 Adenoid basal carcinoma. (a) In this field there is an overlying CIN III. Small 'basaloid' islands are seen in the underlying stroma. (b) Adenoid basal carcinoma with a typical nest of squamoid differentiation with moderate atypia and with prominent basal cells at the epithelial–stromal interface. (c) Higher–power view of infiltrating tumor shows a mix of basal and columnar differentiation.

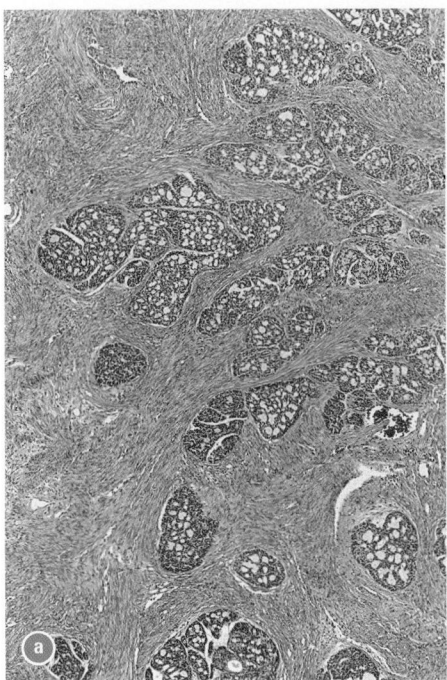
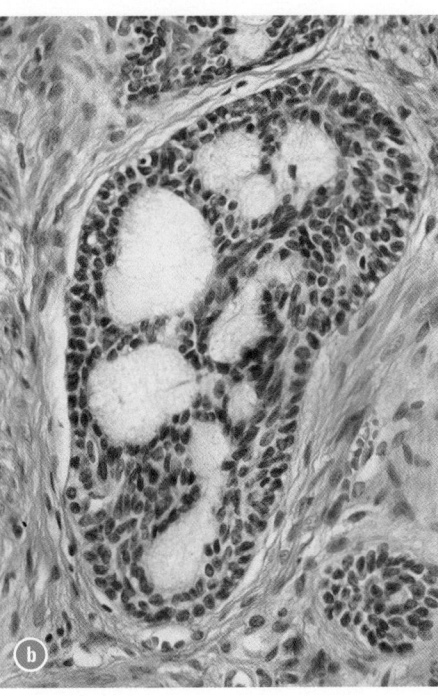

Fig. 14.56 Adenoid cystic carcinoma. (a) A low-power view depicts large complex gland-like aggregates, each having an internal cribriform pattern. (b) The cribriform areas contain dense eosinophilic material. The surrounding nuclei are monomorphous and basaloid but with more atypia than is seen in adenoid basal carcinoma.

laminin in the hyaline material, supporting a basement membrane origin and considered them to be true adenoid cystic carcinomas.[201] Both ABCs and ACCs are usually positive for HPV type 16.[203–205] This finding, combined with the observations that some ACCs have ABC-like areas and that ABCs may be associated with divergent differentiation, suggests further that both may arise from a common precursor.[201]

MESONEPHRIC ADENOCARCINOMA

This rare form of cervical adenocarcinoma is derived from hyperplastic mesonephric remnants usually located in the lateral wall of the cervix. Among 23 reported cases, the mean age of the patients was 53 years.[206–208] The gross findings are sometimes distinct and follow from the origin of this tumor in the cervical wall and its slow growth between the portio and the lower uterine segment, sometimes producing a barrel-shaped cervix (Fig. 14.57).

The histologic patterns are quite variable, including ductal (the most frequent), retiform, papillary, solid, spindle cell and sex-cord-like. Often these are mixed within the same tumor. There is usually no stromal reaction. The nuclei of mesonephric carcinomas are of low to moderate grade and the initial impression is often that of an endometrioid carcinoma or a low-grade mixed epithelial/stromal tumor (Fig. 14.58a–c).

Because of the varied patterns of mesonephric carcinoma, its differential diagnosis ranges widely to include: mesonephric hyperplasia, endometrioid adenocarcinoma, clear cell carcinoma, serous carcinoma, malignant mixed Müllerian tumor (MMMT) and the uterine tumors resembling an ovarian sex-cord tumor (UTROSCT).

The distinction from florid mesonephric hyperplasia may be very difficult since mesonephric hyperplasia often

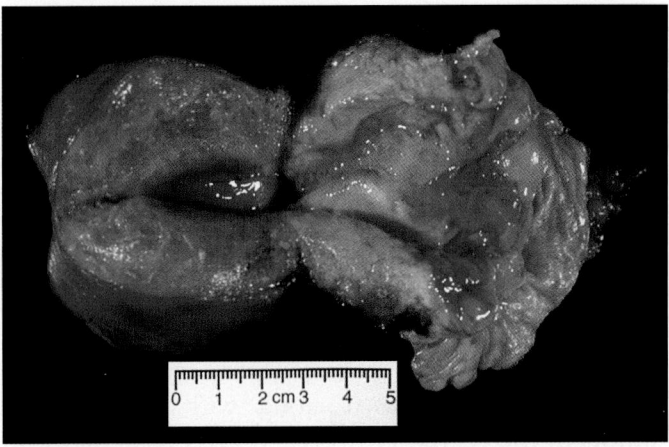

Fig. 14.57 Mesonephric adenocarcinoma, gross specimen. The tumor is present in the wall of the cervix in the right half of the specimen, displacing the overlying unaffected cervical mucosa and producing a barrel-shaped cervix.

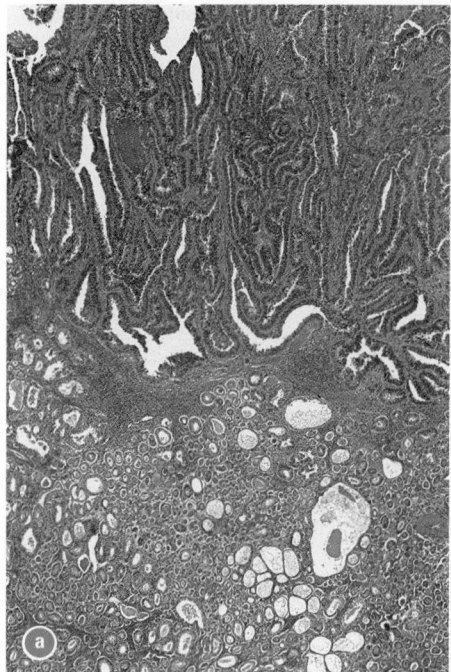 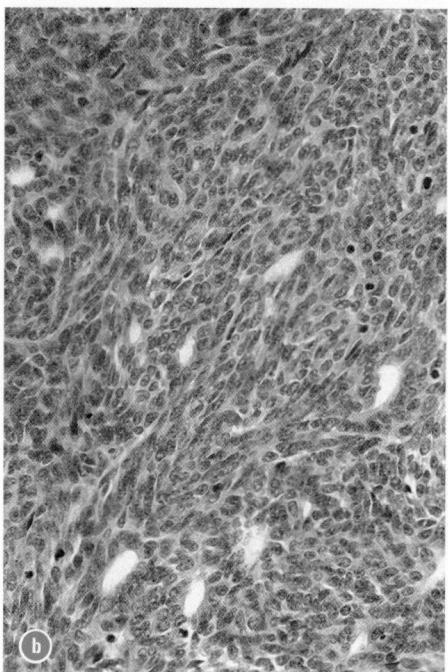 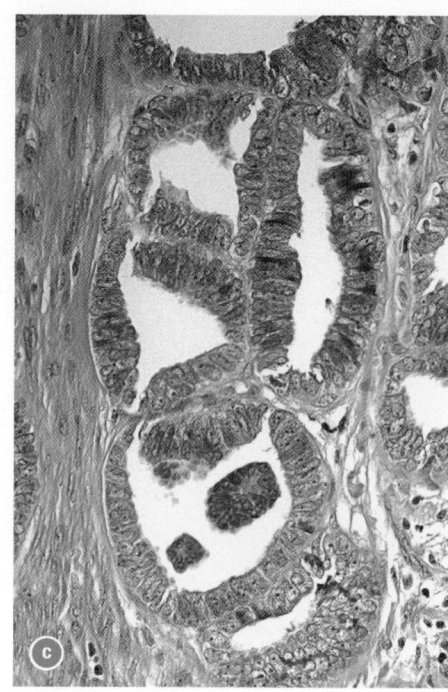

Fig. 14.58 Mesophrenic adenocarcinoma. (a) Two distinctly different patterns are present: papillary and somewhat retiform at the top and tubulocystic at the bottom. (b) A biphasic pattern is seen, with endometrioid-appearing glands separated by spindled cells. (c) In this field, the neoplastic glands have mild to moderate nuclear atypia with endometrioid features.

coexists with and blends with mesonephric carcinoma and both hyperplastic and malignant glands may contain eosinophilic material. Importantly, pure mesonephric hyperplasia is usually an incidental finding and does not form a symptomatic mass, as do most mesonephric carcinomas. Microscopically, the maintenance of a non-infiltrative pattern of evenly spaced, similar-appearing glands, cysts, or tubules is the most important finding distinguishing hyperplasia from carcinoma.

Endometrioid carcinomas are centered on the surface of the cervix, sometimes with residual AIS, whereas mesonephric carcinomas are centered on the deep cervical stroma (although they may extend to the surface). Endometrioid carcinomas usually have higher-grade nuclear atypia than mesonephric adenocarcinomas.

Clear cell and serous carcinomas usually also have higher-grade nuclei than mesonephric carcinomas and exhibit characteristic architectural and cytologic patterns described previously. MMMTs also have higher-grade nuclei than mesonephric carcinomas that have a spindle-cell component (malignant mesonephric mixed tumor).[208] The latter are discussed along with other mixed tumors of the cervix. However, UTROSCTs may also appear biphasic and have less atypia than MMMTs, enhancing their similarity to mesonephric carcinoma with a spindle cell component.

Because of the rarity of mesonephric adenocarcinoma and its wide differential diagnosis, immunohistochemistry is helpful. Most mesonephric carcinomas are positive for cytokeratin (CK) 7, epithelial membrane antigen (EMA), vimentin and calretinin, whereas they are negative for mCEA, CK20 and estrogen and progesterone receptors.[207,208] A report of CD10 staining in benign mesonephric structures as well as in five cervical mesonephric adenocarcinomas suggests that it may also be a useful marker in the distinction from Müllerian-derived tumors.[209] However, UTROSCT is usually also positive for CD10, negating its value in this distinction.[210]

The prognosis for mesonephric adenocarcinoma is uncertain because of the small number of cases reported. However, there is a suggestion that early-stage tumors are more indolent than the usual cervical adenocarcinoma, but that there may be a propensity for recurrence after many years.[207,208]

ADENOCARCINOMA METASTATIC TO THE CERVIX

Most adenocarcinomas metastatic to the cervix come from cancers that arise elsewhere in the genital tract.[211,212] They generally fall into the following types, in order of decreasing frequency (Table 14.5):

Table 14.5 Metastatic versus primary endocervical adenocarcinoma

Pattern or source of metastasis	Histology of metastasis	Helpful biomarkers in metastases
Endometrioid		
Endometrium	Low nuclear grade bland mucinous glands squamous, if present, is low grade	Vimentin (+), ER/PR (+), CEA (−), HPV (−)
Serous		
Endometrium tube, ovary	Complex papillae, high nuclear grade	P53 (++), HPV (−)
Stomach	Signet ring cells diffuse invasion sparing native epithelium	HPV(−)
Breast	Usually lobular subtype sometimes with signet ring forms diffuse invasion sparing native epithelium	HPV(−)
Colon	High-grade nuclei, necrosis, cribriform pattern	CK7 (−), HPV (−), CDX2 (+)
Kidney	Rare, mimics clear cell carcinoma of the cervix	CD10(+), HPV (−)
Lung	Rare, may resemble poorly-differentiated endocervical carcinoma	TTF-1 (+), HPV(−)

1 *Endometrioid adenocarcinomas*: see 'endometrioid adenocarcinoma carcinoma of the cervix' (above) for a detailed discussion of the distinction between carcinoma of the endometrium involving the cervix and primary cervical carcinoma of the endometrioid type. In general, metastatic disease from the endometrium must be considered if (a) an endometrioid tumor has low nuclear grade without AIS (Fig. 14.59a); (b) the squamous component (if present) is well-differentiated; (c) the epithelium is mucinous-appearing and (paradoxically) closely resembles normal endocervix, but is not characteristic of adenoma malignum (Fig. 14.59b) and (d) the patient is in the sixth decade or higher.

2 *Papillary serous carcinomas*: these may originate in the endometrium, fallopian tube or ovary. The most popular theory is spread via 'drop metastases'. This is supported in part by the superficial nature of the metastases in most such cases. Occasionally the primary tumor is not clinically apparent and the initial specimen is obtained from the cervix. Involvement of endocervical crypts in these cases often mimics primary cervical neoplasia (Fig. 14.59c,d). Such tumors exhibit high nuclear grade (Fig. 14.59c), are strongly positive for p53 and are HPV negative. As with endometrioid adenocarcinomas metastatic to the cervix, the patient is usually over age 50.

3 *Other sites*: these include breast (Fig. 14.59e), lung (Fig. 14.59f), kidney and gastrointestinal tract, among others (Table 14.5).[211-213] Often there is widespread disease elsewhere, but occasionally the cervical tumor is the initial finding. Metastases from distant sites usually diffusely infiltrate the stroma of the cervix, sparing the overlying epithelium and endocervical glands (Fig. 14.59e) and tumor emboli may be found in vascular spaces. The morphology is that of the primary tumor and differs in most cases from that of the usual cervical adenocarcinoma.

As discussed in the prior section, human papillomavirus testing is a convenient 'special stain' to establish or exclude a cervical primary adenocarcinoma. Table 14.5 lists helpful distinguishing features and special studies.

BENIGN MIMICS OF CERVICAL ADENOCARCINOMA (Table 14.6)

Deep nabothian cysts, florid deep glands

Endocervical cysts and glands may extend through the entire wall of the cervix grossly and microscopically mimicking adenoma malignum or an adenocarcinoma with a predominantly cystic pattern of invasion (Fig. 14.60).[214,215] Rupture of benign cysts may also invite confusion, since the extravasated mucin may induce reactive changes in the stroma and adjacent glands that suggests invasion.[124] However, adenoma malignum and cystic carcinomas have an infiltrative pattern that is appreciable at low-power magnification (Figs 14.45a, 14.61) and nuclear atypia (albeit sometimes subtle and only focal) exceeds that of benign cysts and glands.

Tunnel clusters

Tunnel clusters, first described by Fluhmann,[216] are clusters of closely packed, interconnected, blind-ended passages or 'tunnels' located in the superficial endocervix. Usually found in parous women, tunnel clusters can be quite florid and can even form a grossly visible mass.[151] In Fluhmann's type A tunnel clusters, the glands are relatively small, whereas in type B, the cystic type, they are dilated, mucin-filled and have an attenuated lining

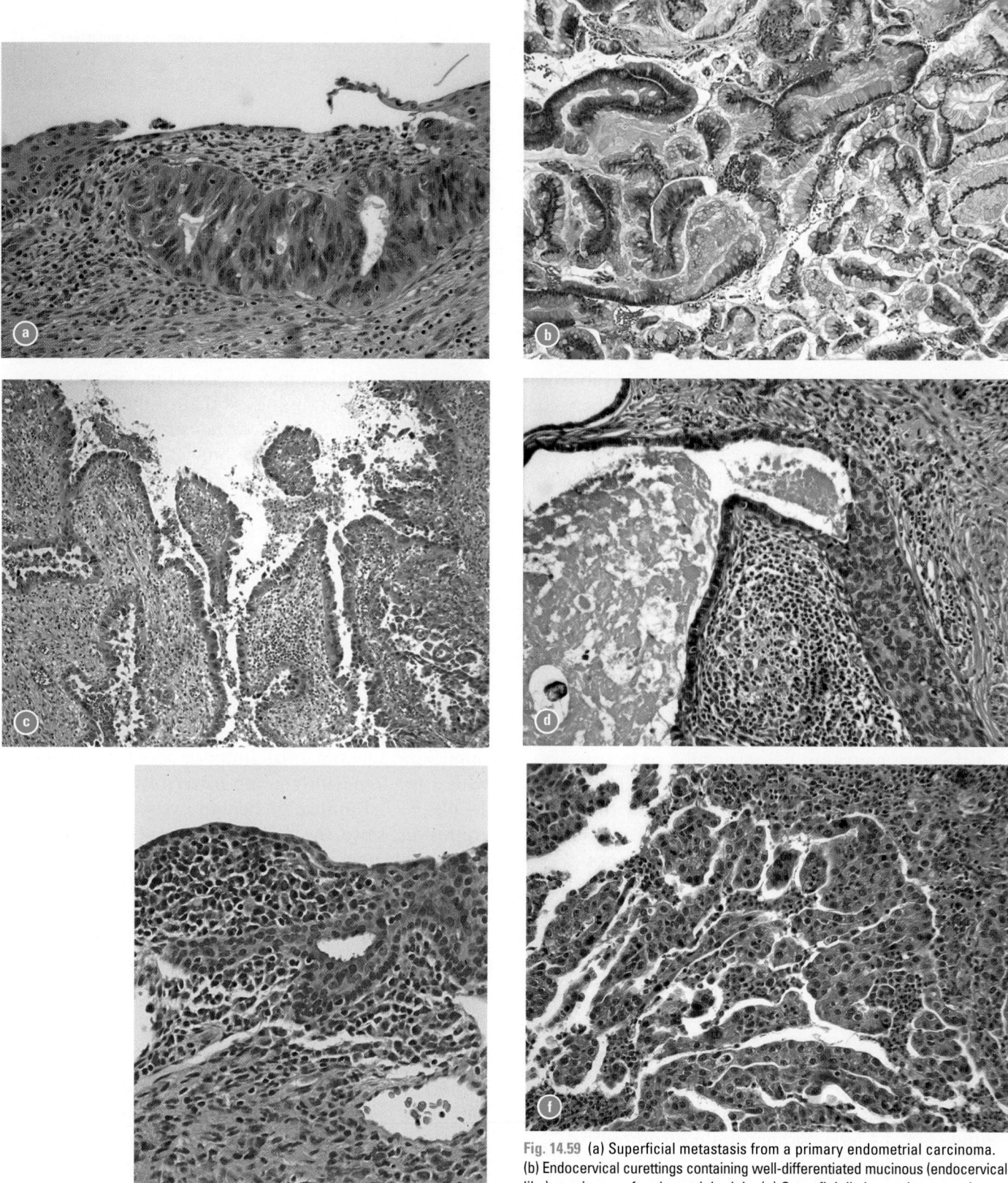

Fig. 14.59 (a) Superficial metastasis from a primary endometrial carcinoma. (b) Endocervical curettings containing well-differentiated mucinous (endocervical-like) carcinoma of endometrial origin. (c) Superficially located metastatic serous carcinoma. (d) Serous carcinoma mimicking intraepithelial neoplasia of the cervix. (e) Metastatic lobular carcinoma of the breast to the cervix. The small malignant cells permeate the superficial stroma without altering the adjacent gland and overlying epithelium. (f) Metastatic lung carcinoma, mimicking serous or poorly differentiated cervical adenocarcinoma.

Table 14.6 *Benign mimics of cervical adenocarcinoma*

1. Deep nabothian cysts, florid deep glands
2. Tunnel clusters
3. Endocervical gland hyperplasias:
   Lobular hyperplasia
   Diffuse laminar hyperplasia
4. Adenomyoma of the endocervical type
5. Endocervicosis, florid cystic endosalpingiosis
6. Müllerian papilloma
7. Microglandular hyperplasia
8. Mesonephric hyperplasia
9. Ectopic prostate
10. Deep tubal metaplasia
11. Villous adenoma

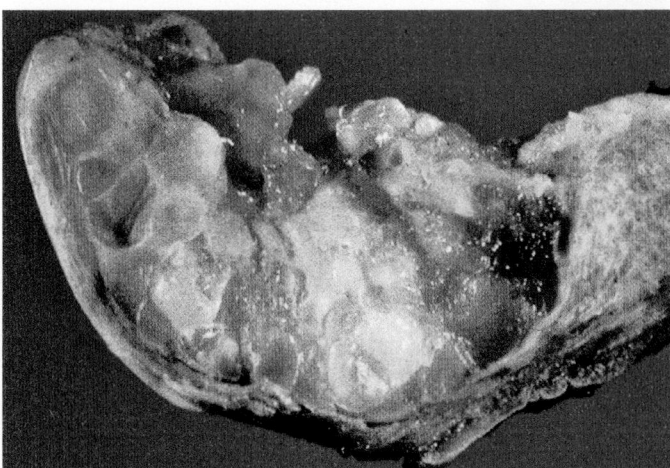

Fig. 14.60 Deep nabothian cysts, gross specimen. A cross-section of the cervix demonstrates mucin-filled cystic glands extending almost entirely through the wall of the cervix, grossly mimicking a cystic mucinous carcinoma (Courtesy, Dr Robert Young, Massachusetts General Hospital).

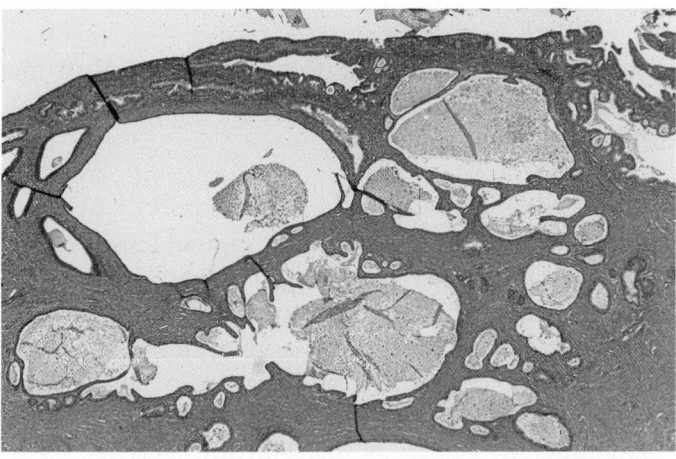

Fig. 14.61 Adenocarcinoma of the cervix, cystic type. Cystic and irregular glands are present in the stroma without a reaction, suggesting the possibility of benign deep cysts. Irregularly shaped glands and intraglandular protrusions are not usually seen in deep nabothian cysts.

(Fig. 14.62a)[217]; often these patterns are mixed (Fig. 14.62b). Tunnel clusters are usually readily distinguished from adenoma malignum or cystic adenocarcinoma by their sharply demarcated periphery, lack of a stromal response and benign-appearing epithelial cells. However, type A tunnel clusters may exhibit nuclear enlargement and slight pleomorphism, sometimes causing them to be mistaken for adenoma malignum (Fig. 14.62c).[218] Awareness of the possibility of nuclear atypia in type A tunnel clusters and observance of a non-infiltrative architectural pattern will help to avoid this error.

Endocervical gland hyperplasias

Idiopathic hyperplasias of the endocervical glands are not known to be precursors to adenocarcinoma. However, they may simulate adenoma malignum. Some endocervical hyperplasias have a non-specific architecture, but two characteristic variants have been described: lobular hyperplasia and diffuse laminar hyperplasia.

1. *Lobular endocervical gland hyperplasia*. This term refers to multiple units of small endocervical glands, often surrounding a central larger gland, arranged in a distinctly lobular pattern.[219] It is usually an incidental finding in the uterus of women of reproductive age, but there may be a grossly apparent abnormality (Fig. 14.63a). Lobular hyperplasia closely mimics adenoma malignum and some cases may have been included as carcinomas in reports published prior to its description. However, it differs from adenoma malignum in that the glands are less irregular, have a noninvasive, distinctly lobular pattern, and lack both a reactive stroma and nuclear atypicality (present at least focally in adenoma malignum) (Fig. 14.63b,c). The epithelial cells are CEA-negative; however, some examples have a gastric pyloric gland phenotype, as does adenoma malignum, negating the usefulness of gastric markers for this distinction.[220]

2. *Diffuse laminar endocervical gland hyperplasia*. In this uncommon hyperplasia evenly spaced round, tubular, or branching endocervical glands extend into the stroma to approximately the same level circumferentially around the cervix.[221] It does not form a mass and is usually an incidental finding in a uterus removed for other reasons. Seen in cross-section, the glands end abruptly in a straight line, usually limited to the inner third of the cervical wall (Fig. 14.64a). Often there is an inflammatory infiltrate, more prominent in the lower levels (Fig. 14.64b). The evenly spaced

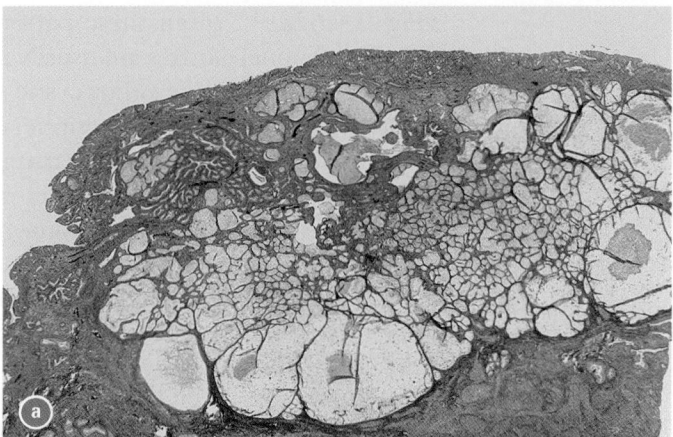

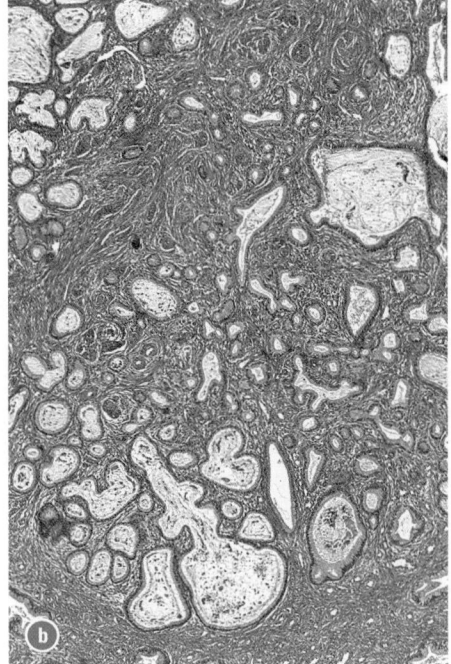

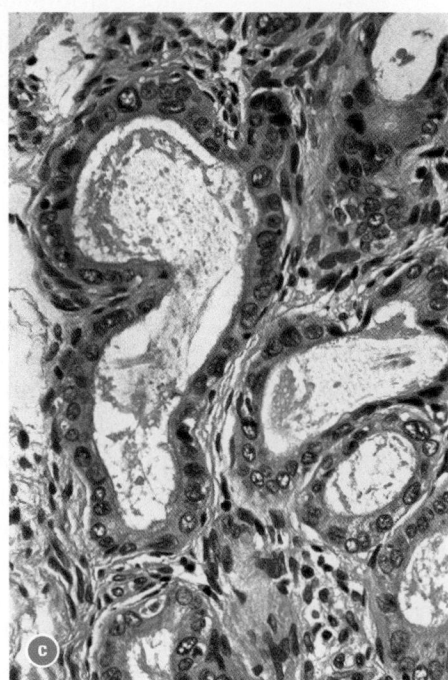

Fig. 14.62 Tunnel clusters. (a) Type B clusters. Note the sharply demarcated border and mucin-filled cysts with attenuated linings. (b) Type B clusters peripherally with type A (smaller) clusters centrally. (c) Type A tunnel clusters with atypia. Note the nuclear enlargement and pleomorphism. In such a case, one needs to judge the overall pattern and possible accompanying type B clusters to avoid overdiagnosis of carcinoma.

glands, abrupt lower border and lack of significant nuclear atypia distinguish this lesion from adenoma malignum.

Endocervicosis, florid cystic endosalpingiosis

Endocervicosis is more commonly encountered in the bladder wall but in rare cases it occurs in the cervix as a grossly recognizable, firm or cystic abnormality in the outer aspect of the anterior wall.[222] Variably sized glands and mucin-filled cysts lined by bland mucinous or flattened epithelium are arranged haphazardly. Cyst rupture may cause mucin extravasation (Fig. 14.65).

In florid cystic endosalpingiosis a deep-seated cystic lesion has tubal rather than endocervical epithelium.[223] As with endocervicosis, the location in the outer wall with an intervening area of uninvolved cervical stroma beneath the surface endocervical glands is an important distinction from cancer.

Müllerian papilloma

This rare papillary ectocervical or vaginal lesion occurs almost exclusively in children, but rarely it is also found in adults.[224,225] The complex branching papillae have broad fibrous cores, sometimes containing inflammatory cells and are lined by a single layer of small, non-ciliated, cuboidal epithelial cells with small nuclei. There is no mitotic activity (Fig. 14.66a,b). It is important to realize that endocervical adenocarcinoma and adenoma malignum can have a papillary surface that may be mistaken for a benign

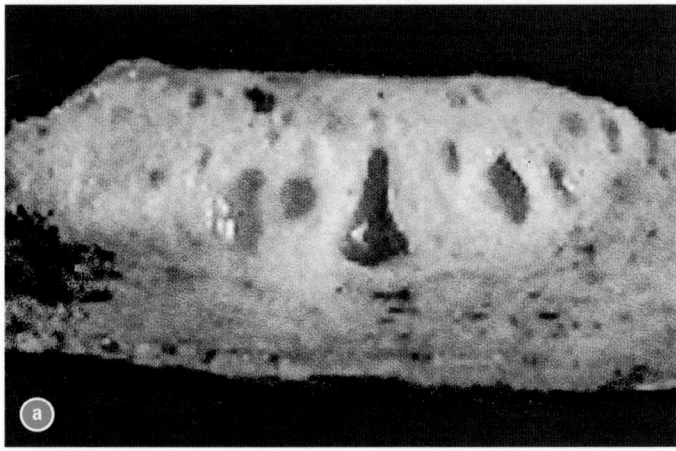

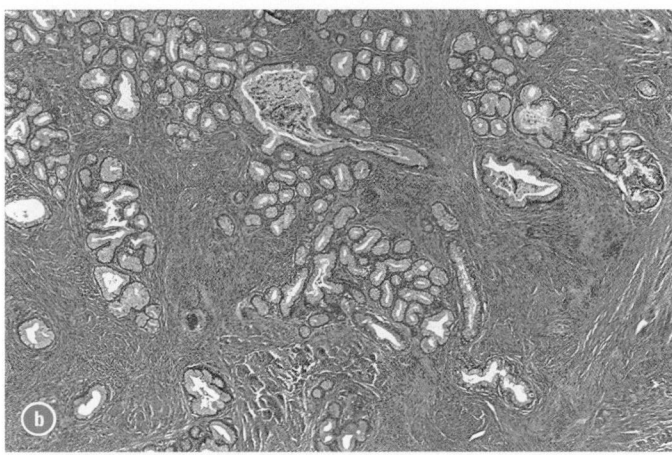

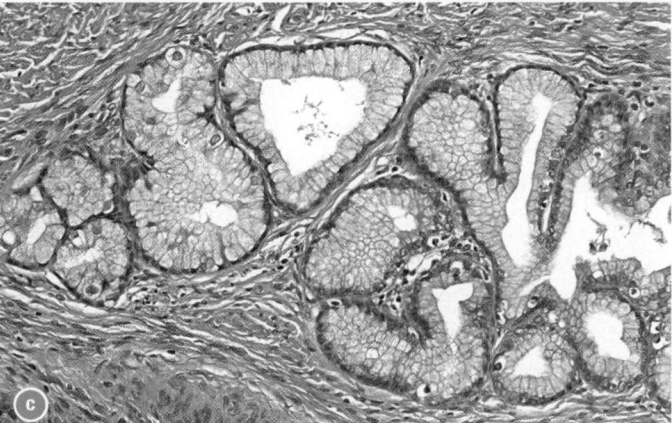

Fig. 14.63 Lobular endocervical gland hyperplasia. (a) Gross specimen. A cross-section of the cervix is seen, with a bulging, partially cystic, sharply circumscribed mass (Courtesy Dr Robert Young, Massachusetts General Hospital). (b) A cystic gland is surrounded by multiple lobules of benign-appearing endocervical glands. There is no stromal reaction. (c) The glands are lined by benign-appearing mucinous cells.

papilloma in a small biopsy (Fig. 14.46a,b). Even slight nuclear atypia in a noninflammatory papillary process involving the cervix should be regarded with suspicion.

Microglandular hyperplasia

Microglandular hyperplasia (MGH) is a common lesion. Usually an incidental microscopic finding, it may form a symptomatic polypoid mass (Fig. 14.67a) or a friable

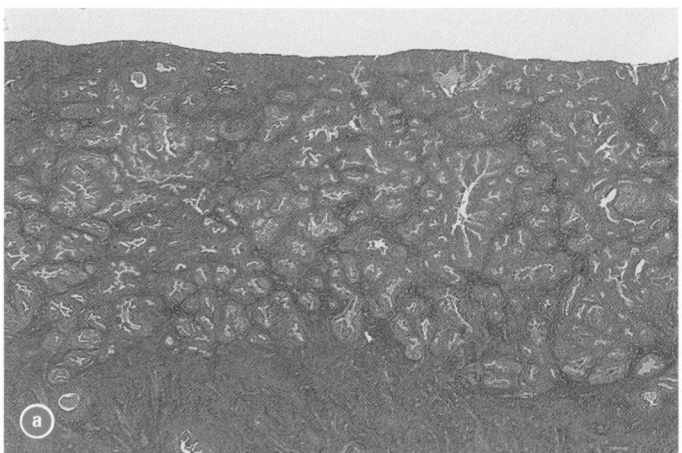

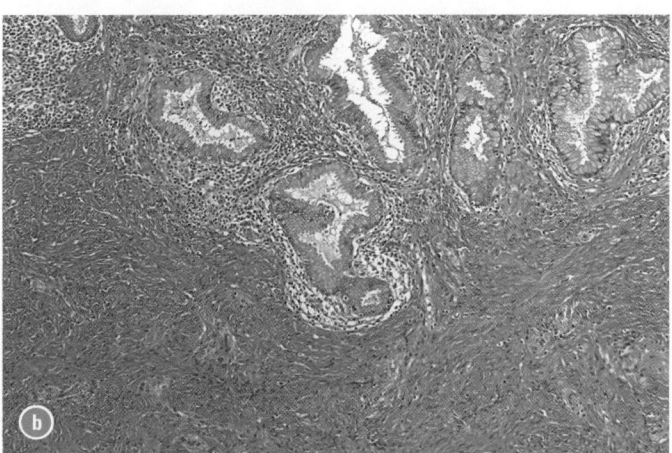

Fig. 14.64 Diffuse laminar endocervical gland hyperplasia. (a) Crowded, evenly spaced benign glands extend into the stroma, terminating in a sharp line. (b) The lower edge of the lesion with benign-appearing glands is surrounded by a prominent inflammatory infiltrate, not to be confused with a reaction to invasion.

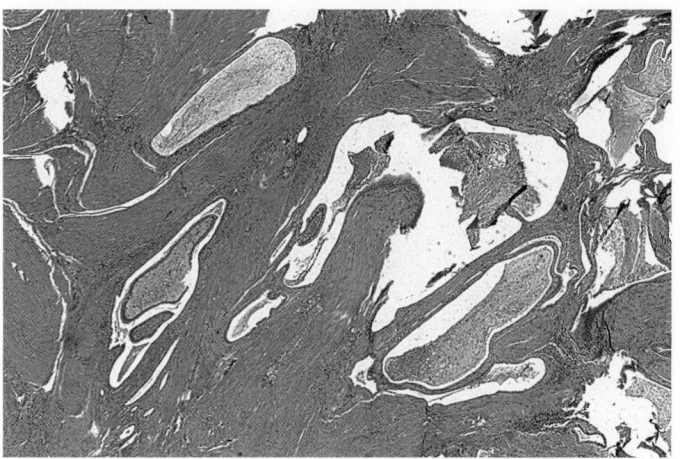

Fig. 14.65 Endocervicosis. Benign-appearing endocervical-like glands are present deep in the wall of the cervix in an edematous stroma containing extravasated mucin. The location in the outer (usually anterior) wall with overlying aglandular stroma is characteristic of this rare benign lesion.

surface 'erosion'. It is usually encountered in young women and has been linked to the use of birth control pills, but it also may occur without their use and in postmenopausal women.[48]

Prior to the first descriptions of MGH in the 1960s,[226,227] some cases were mistaken for carcinoma, principally clear cell carcinoma, because it may produce a striking pattern of crowded glands and cysts that appear to have obliterated the stroma and many of the epithe-

lial cells have a clear or vacuolated cytoplasm (Fig. 14.67b). The vacuoles are usually both sub-nuclear and supra-nuclear and may contain leukocytes, as does the mucin in the gland lumens (Fig. 14.67c). MGH differs from carcinoma in that most of the epithelial cell nuclei have bland chromatin with small or absent nucleoli and mitotic figures are infrequent or absent. Also, unlike carcinoma, the glands are surrounded by a layer of reserve cells or immature squamous metaplastic cells. These may be somewhat inconspicuous (Figs 14.67c, 14.68a), but they may be highlighted by staining for p63, an antigen present in squamous reserve cells and myoepithelial cells. The cytoplasm of MGH is CEA-negative.[156]

Now that MGH is well known, only uncommon variants cause confusion with carcinoma.[228] These may have focal nuclear enlargement and pleomorphism, signet ring cells (Fig. 14.68a), a hobnail pattern (Fig. 14.68b), a solid or trabecular growth pattern, or a myxoid or hyalinized stroma mimicking the hyaline stroma often present in clear cell carcinomas (Fig. 14.68c,d). In all of these, the focal nature of the nuclear and/or architectural changes within the context of more usual MGH is the most important clue to the correct diagnosis.

Pathologists also need to be aware of a variant of endometrial carcinoma that may closely simulate MGH, especially in curettage specimens, because of its muci-

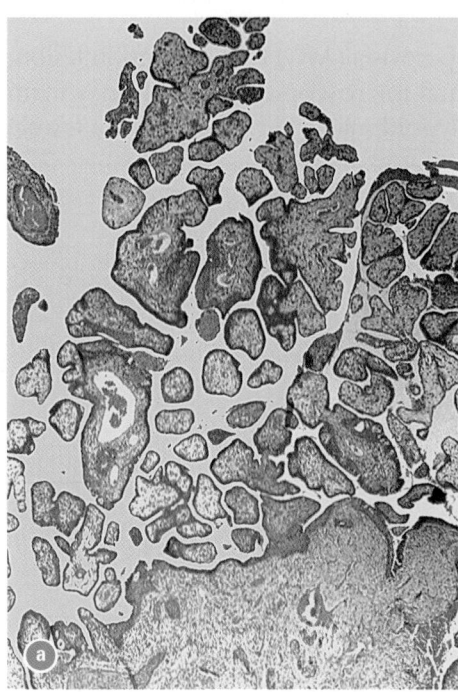
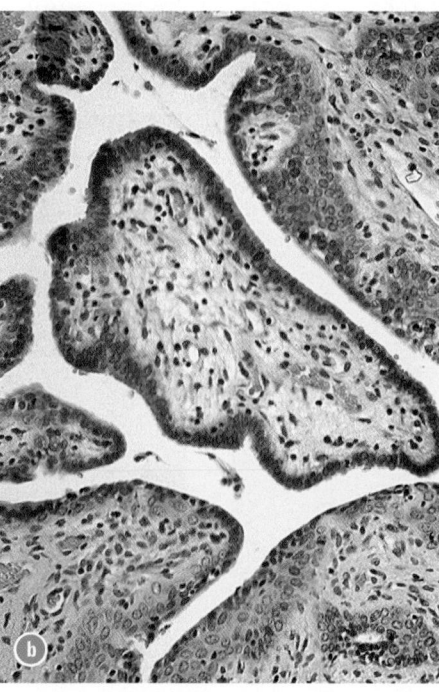

Fig. 14.66 Müllerian papilloma. (a) Broad papillae protrude from the ectocervical surface. (b) The papillae are lined with bland cuboidal cells and squamous cells.

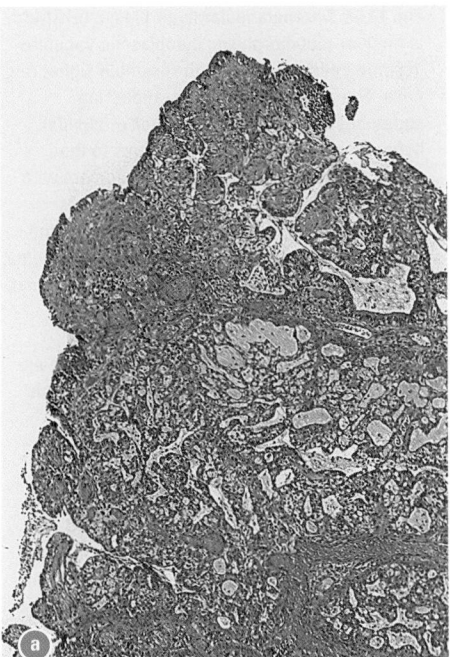 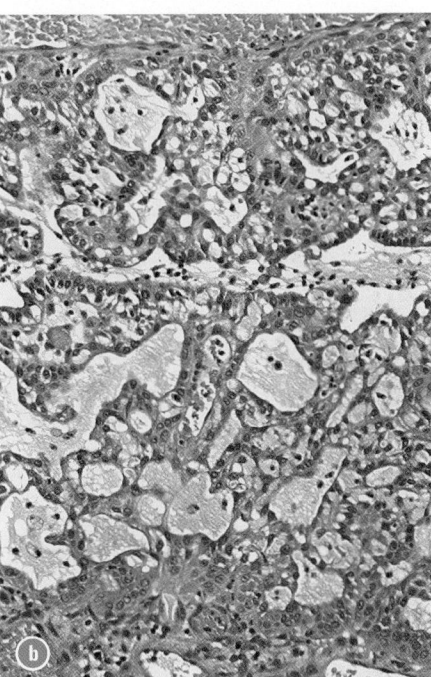 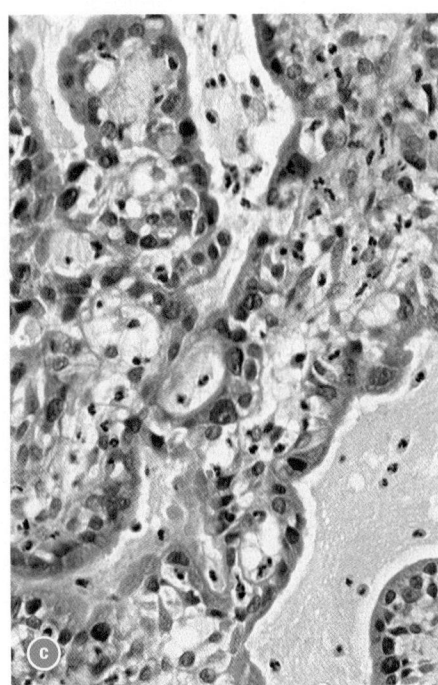

Fig. 14.67 Microglandular hyperplasia. (a) A polypoid cervical mass containing numerous glands is seen. (b) Small and large mucin-filled glands are present. (c) The epithelial cells have a vacuolated cytoplasm and are lined by cuboidal cells with a focal atypia and an attenuated reserve cell lining. Neutrophils are seen in the glandular and intracytoplasmic mucin.

nous epithelium, microglandular pattern, focal squamous differentiation and low nuclear grade (Fig. 14.69).[229,230] MGH-like endometrial carcinomas are associated with endometrial, not endocervical, stroma, often have a cribriform growth pattern, contain cells with slightly hyperchromatic nuclei with scattered mitoses, and do not have the periglandular rim of reserve cells usually seen in MGH (Fig. 14.69).

Mesonephric hyperplasia

Mesonephric remnants were found in 22% of fully sectioned cervices.[231] Usually in the lateral wall, these groups of small glands are reminiscent of thyroid follicles because of their dense eosinophilic luminal material and non-ciliated small cuboidal cells (Fig. 14.70a). Mesonephric remnants may become hyperplastic mimicking endocervical, clear cell, or mesonephric carcinoma. Mesonephric hyperplasia is, however, almost always found incidentally, rarely forming a mass or causing symptoms. Three types of hyperplasia have been described: diffuse, lobular and ductal.[206,232] In the diffuse type (the one most likely to be mistaken for carcinoma), small to cystic glands and tubules are scattered through the endocervical stroma. These may penetrate quite deeply and sometimes also extend to the surface (Fig. 14.70b). The glands are relatively evenly spaced and

thus do not appear infiltrative and do not provoke a stromal response. Nuclei may be slightly larger than those of mesonephric remnants and there may be occasional mitoses (Fig. 14.70c). In the lobular type, the hyperplastic glands are arranged in more or less discrete packets or lobules, sometimes surrounding a central mesonephric duct. In some cases, the duct predominates (ductal hyperplasia), with an intraductal papillary proliferation that may suggest a papillary carcinoma (Fig. 14.70d). Florid examples of mesonephric hyperplasia may merge imperceptibly with mesonephric carcinoma, making this distinction very difficult in some cases. However, mesonephric carcinoma usually forms a cervical mass (Fig. 14.57) and is more obviously invasive than hyperplasia (see discussion above under mesonephric carcinoma of the cervix).

Ectopic prostate

This enigmatic incidental microscopic finding mirrors the histologic appearance of the large prostatic ducts.[233,234] Ectopic prostate is probably a metaplasia, rather than a heterotopia as the name suggests, and it may be more common than its relatively recent description and paucity of reported cases suggest, since it may be dismissed simply as an unusual endocervical gland hyperplasia with squamous metaplasia by those

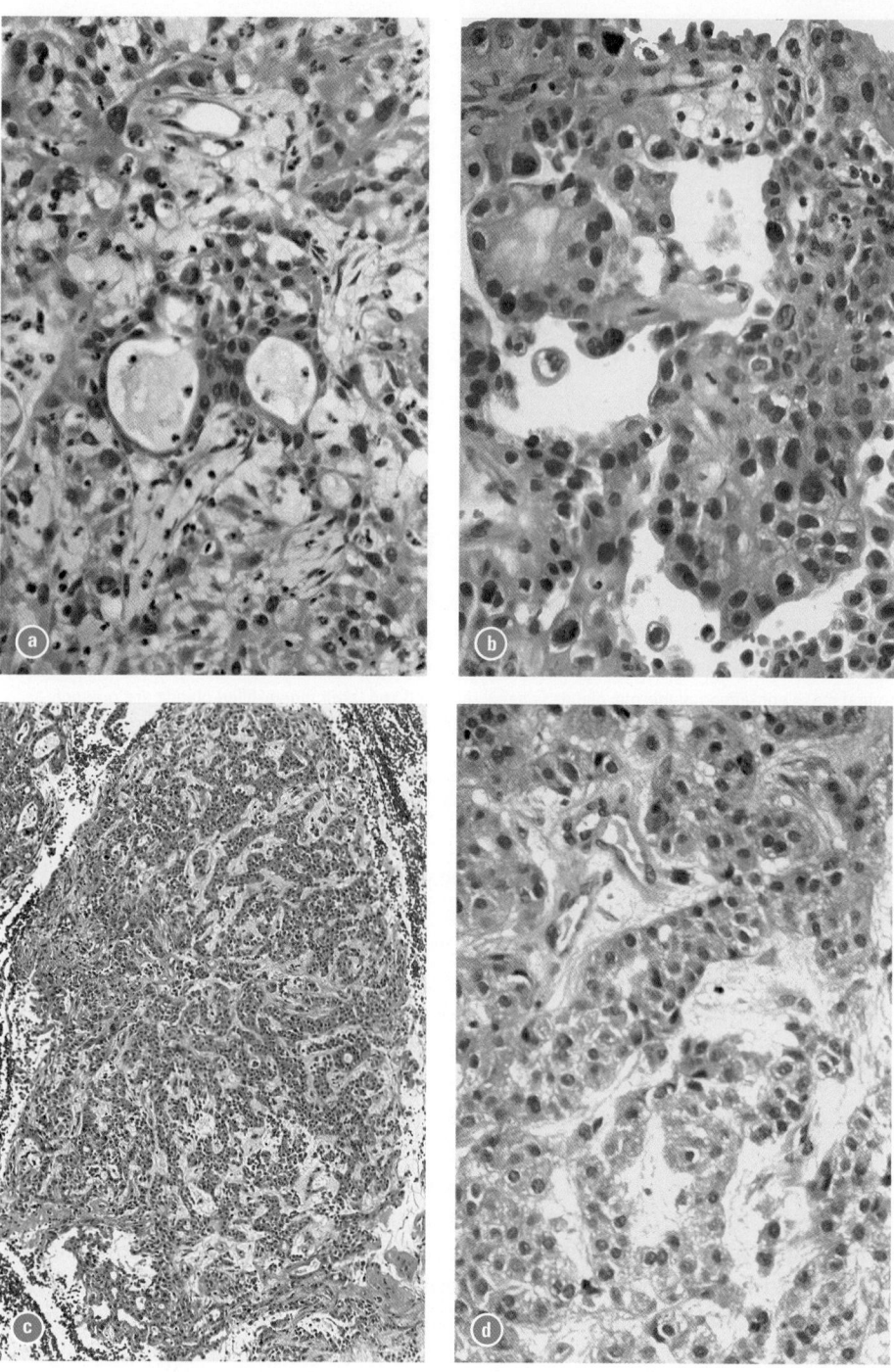

Fig. 14.68 Microglandular hyperplasia. (a) There is nuclear pleomorphism; cytoplasmic vacuoles in some cells cause them to resemble signet ring cells. The central metaplastic-appearing squamous epithelium and the lack of nuclear hyperchromasia are important clues to the correct diagnosis. (b) A papillary fragment with hobnail nuclei is present. (c) The pattern is trabecular rather than microglandular, and the hyaline stroma mimics that of invasive carcinoma. (d) Higher-power magnification of the trabecular pattern and hyaline stroma from (c) is seen. Bland nuclei and the finding of ordinary microglandular hyperplasia seen elsewhere are important clues to the correct diagnosis in this case.

unaware of its existence. Ectopic prostate is composed of variably-sized islands of mixed glandular and squamous epithelium in the wall of the cervix. The peripherally-located glandular epithelium is cuboidal to columnar with mucinous-appearing cytoplasm, small uniform nuclei and a rim of small reserve cells. The central bland squamous cells have abundant clear cytoplasm (Fig. 14.71a–c).

Staining with prostate-specific antigen and/or prostatic acid phosphatase is confirmatory (Fig. 14.71d).

Ectopic prostate is not usually confused with carcinoma. However, adenoid basal carcinoma and possibly very well-differentiated adenosquamous carcinoma might be considered. Adenoid basal carcinomas are more 'basaloid' with more nuclear atypia of the squamous

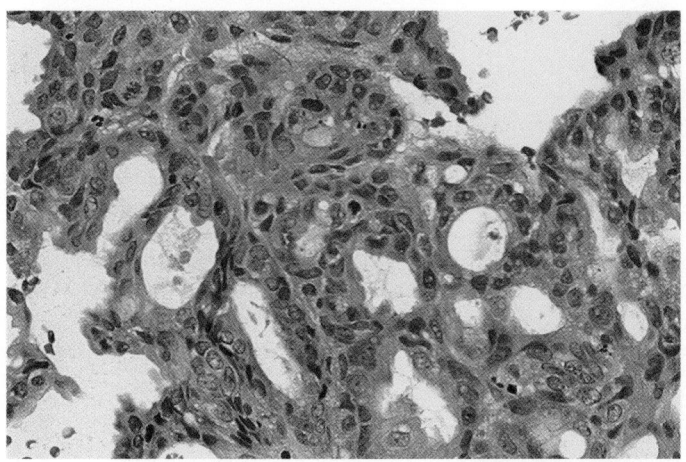

Fig. 14.69 Well-differentiated (microglandular hyperplasia-like) adenocarcinoma of the endometrium. The small glands with somewhat bland nuclei and mucinous material in the gland lumina simulate microglandular hyperplasia. However, the sharp cribriform pattern without a rim of reserve cells and the monomorphic nuclear enlargement with slight atypia serve to distinguish this lesion from microglandular hyperplasia.

cells than is seen in ectopic prostate. They also occur in women who are older than those so far reported to have ectopic prostate. Adenosquamous carcinomas have cytologic atypia and an infiltrative pattern not seen in ectopic prostate.

Deep tuboendometrioid metaplasia

Tuboendometrioid metaplasia of deep endocervical glands that are also crowded, irregular, or cystic may be mistaken for invasive adenocarcinoma of the endometrioid type. Further, a rim of myxoid or edematous stroma may surround these benign glands and be misinterpreted as a reaction to invasion (Fig. 14.32b).[235] However, despite an occasional mitotic figure, the epithelial cells do not have malignant nuclear features and are at least focally ciliated (although some minimal-deviation endometrioid carcinomas may also have ciliated cells). Awareness that slight architectural and cytologic atypia may occur in benign glands of the deep stroma (Fig. 14.32a–c) is essential to prevent a serious diagnostic error.

Villous adenoma

The existence of this entity in the cervix is questionable. Although some state that they have rarely made this diagnosis,[151] we know of only two reported cases.[236,237] Both of these, however, were associated with an underlying well-differentiated adenocarcinoma (one of these of the adenoma malignum type). Therefore these villous adenomas might have been villous papillary components of the carcinoma rather than a separate precursor lesion. As discussed with reference to Müllerian papilloma, any non-inflammatory papillary lesion in the cervix must be regarded with suspicion and an associated invasive adenocarcinoma excluded.

MANAGEMENT AND PROGNOSIS OF ADENOCARCINOMAS OF THE CERVIX

Metastatic spread

Adenocarcinomas have a different pattern of spread than squamous carcinomas. Although most initially spread beyond the cervix by first involving contiguous pelvic structures and pelvic lymph nodes, they are more likely than squamous carcinomas to metastasize to the ovaries, upper abdomen, or distant organs.[238,239] Adenocarcinomas have been reported to have a worse prognosis than squamous carcinomas at similar stages and studies have reported ovarian metastases in approximately 5% of cervical adenocarcinomas, in contrast to 1% of squamous carcinomas.[240–242]

Staging

Adenocarcinoma of the cervix, like its squamous counterpart, is staged according to FIGO guidelines, which is a clinical staging system. However, certain characteristics of adenocarcinoma of the cervix are not as well delineated by FIGO staging as are squamous carcinomas. Squamous carcinoma is largely exophytic, allowing the examiner to better assess the extent of tumor growth on clinical exam. It can be said that with squamous carcinomas 'what you see is what you get'. In contrast, since adenocarcinoma arises from the endocervix, pelvic examination may under-represent the actual extent of the disease. Adenocarcinoma can extensively infiltrate the cervical stroma, resulting in a cervix that may be very firm to palpation. As a result, it is often difficult to be certain that intermediate risk factors, including deep myocervical invasion, large tumor size and vascular/lymphatic invasion, will not be present following radical hysterectomy, even for clinical stage IB1 disease. With more extensive growth, adenocarcinoma of the cervix often results in expansion of the cervix without obvious invasion of the parametria. Since parametrial invasion is required by the staging system to classify disease extent as stage IIB, adenocarcinomas are often classified as barrel-shaped stage IB tumors. Thus, a tumor can be 6 or more centimeters and still be classified as stage I. This has resulted in adenocarcinomas being considered stage for stage as less curable than squamous carcinomas. However, when corrected for tumor size,

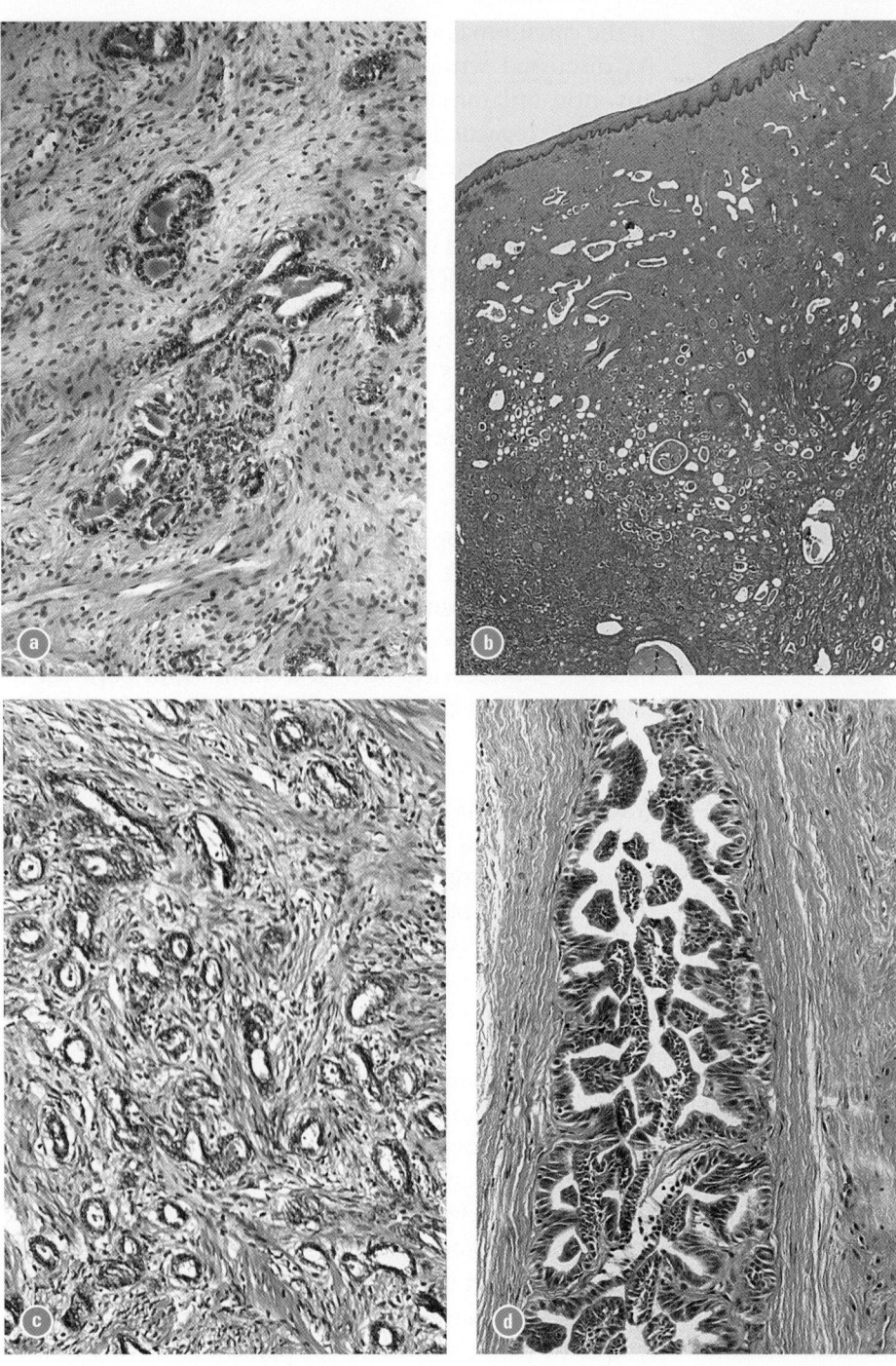

Fig. 14.70 Mesonephric remnants. (a) Small, closely packed glands containing eosinophilic material and lined by benign-appearing cuboidal cells are present in the cervical stroma. (b) Mesonephric hyperplasia, diffuse type. Variably-sized glands permeate the endocervical stroma with an intact overlying surface. (c) Hyperplastic glands are relatively evenly distributed; nuclei are slightly enlarged compared with mesonephric rests.(d) Mesonephric hyperplasia ductal type. A mesonephric duct contains a prominent papillary proliferation.

adenocarcinomas of the cervix can be managed in a similar fashion to their squamous counterpart, with similar outcomes.

Treatment

Stage IB1 adenocarcinoma of the cervix can be effectively treated with radical hysterectomy. In patients with more advanced disease and/or high or intermediate risk factors, adjuvant radiation therapy has been routinely administered. However, the study by Peters et al. comparing concurrent chemotherapy and radiation *vs* radiation alone following radical hysterectomy with high-risk features has established concurrent chemotherapy and radiation as the new standard of care.[243] Interestingly, for patients treated with radiation therapy alone, a significantly poorer outcome was seen for patients with adenocarcinoma than squamous carcinoma. In contrast, the addition of concurrent chemotherapy to radiation

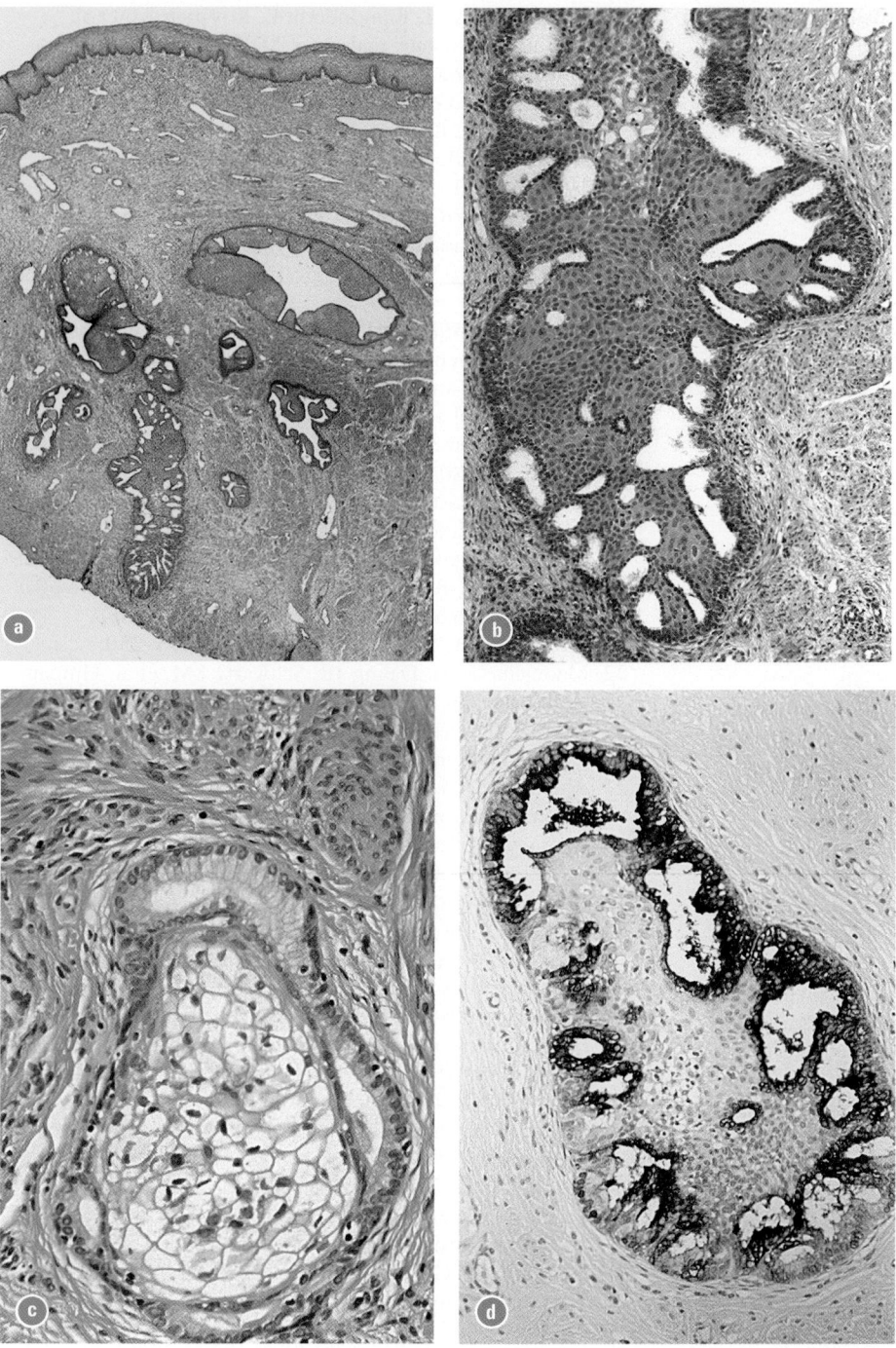

Fig. 14.71 Ectopic prostate. (a) The deep cervical stroma contains variably-sized islands of glandular and squamous epithelium. (b) The glands are arranged peripherally. (c) Glycogenated squamous epithelium and peripheral mucinous glands are seen. (d) Ectopic prostate. An immunoperoxidase stain for prostat-specific antigen is strongly positive.

resulted in an equivalent improved outcome for both glandular and squamous histologies. Although retrospective studies had suggested relative radioresistance for adenocarcinoma, this was the first prospective randomized trial that demonstrated a poorer outcome with radiation therapy alone.

The use of concurrent cisplatin-based chemotherapy during radiation therapy for locally advanced disease (stage IIB to IVA) is a widely accepted practice following the NCI consensus statement. Only approximately 10% of the patients in these cervical cancer trials had adenocarcinoma and, except in the study by Peters et al., their outcome has not been analyzed separately. In advanced and recurrent disease, the treatment principles for squamous and adenocarcinomas are identical. Whereas the Gynecologic Oncology

Group has studied non-squamous tumors separately from squamous tumors, the activity of chemotherapeutic agents is very similar in both histologic groups.

References

1 Friedell GH, McKay DG. Adenocarcinoma *in situ* of the endocervix. Cancer 1953; 6:887–897.

2 Jaworski RC, Pacey NF, Greenberg ML, Osborn RA. The histologic diagnosis of adenocarcinoma *in situ* and related lesions of the cervix uteri. Adenocarcinoma *in situ*. Cancer 1988; 61:1171–1181.

3 Kaku T, Kamura T, Sakai K, et al. Early adenocarcinoma of the uterine cervix. Gynecol Oncol 1997; 65:281–285.

4 Ostor A, Rome R, Quinn M. Microinvasive adenocarcinoma of the cervix: a clinicopathologic study of 77 women. Obstet Gynecol 1997; 89:88–93.

5 Lee KR, Flynn CE. Early invasive adenocarcinoma of the cervix. Cancer 2000; 89:1048–1055.

6 Ostor AG. Early invasive adenocarcinoma of the uterine cervix. Int J Gynecol Pathol 2000; 19:29–38.

7 Pirog EC, Kleter B, Olgac S, et al. Prevalence of human papillomavirus DNA in different histological subtypes of cervical adenocarcinoma. Am J Pathol 2000; 157:1055–1062.

8 Boon ME, Baak JP, Kurver PJ, et al. Adenocarcinoma *in situ* of the cervix: an underdiagnosed lesion. Cancer 1981; 48:768–773.

9 Krane JF, Granter SR, Trask CE, et al. Papanicolaou smear sensitivity for the detection of adenocarcinoma of the cervix: a study of 49 cases. Cancer 2001; 93:8–15.

10 Schoolland M, Allpress S, Sterrett GF. Adenocarcinoma of the cervix: sensitivity of diagnosis by cervical smear and cytologic patterns and pitfalls in 24 cases. Cancer 2002; 96:5–13.

11 Lu X, Shiozawa T, Nakayama K, et al. Abnormal expression of sex steroid receptors and cell cycle-related molecules in adenocarcinoma *in situ* of the uterine cervix. Int J Gynecol Pathol 1999; 18:109–114.

12 Riethdorf L, Riethdorf S, Lee KR, et al. Human papillomaviruses, expression of p16 and early endocervical glandular neoplasia. Hum Pathol 2002; 33:899–904.

13 Cina SJ, Richardson MS, Austin RM, Kurman RJ. Immunohistochemical staining for Ki-67 antigen, carcinoembryonic antigen and p53 in the differential diagnosis of glandular lesions of the cervix. Mod Pathol 1997; 10:176–180.

14 Lee KR, Sun D, Crum CP. Endocervical intraepithelial glandular atypia (dysplasia): a histopathologic, human papillomavirus and MIB-1 analysis of 25 cases. Hum Pathol 2000; 31:656–664.

15 McCluggage WG, Maxwell P, McBride HA, et al. Monoclonal antibodies Ki-67 and MIB1 in the distinction of tuboendometrial metaplasia from endocervical adenocarcinoma and adenocarcinoma *in situ* in formalin-fixed material 1550. Int J Gynecol Pathol 1995; 14:209–216.

16 van Hoeven KH, Ramondetta L, Kovatich AJ, et al. Quantitative image analysis of MIB-1 reactivity in inflammatory, hyperplastic and neoplastic endocervical lesions. Int J Gynecol Pathol 1997; 16:15–21.

17 Ibrahim EM, Blackett AD, Tidy JA, Wells M. CD44 is a marker of endocervical neoplasia. Int J Gynecol Pathol 1999; 18:101–108.

18 Lu D, Tawfik O, Pantazis C, et al. Altered expression of CD44 and variant isoforms in human adenocarcinoma of the endocervix during progression. Gynecol Oncol 1999; 75:84–90.

19 Gloor E, Hurlimann J. Cervical intraepithelial glandular neoplasia (adenocarcinoma *in situ* and glandular dysplasia). A correlative study of 23 cases with histologic grading, histochemical analysis of mucins and immunohistochemical determination of the affinity for four lectins. Cancer 1986; 58:1272–1280.

20 Griffin NR, Wells M. Characterisation of complex carbohydrates in cervical glandular intraepithelial neoplasia and invasive adenocarcinoma. Int J Gynecol Pathol 1994; 13:319–329.

21 Andersson S, Rylander E, Larsson B, et al. The role of human papillomavirus in cervical adenocarcinoma carcinogenesis. Eur J Cancer 2001; 37:246–250.

22 Madeleine MM, Daling JR, Schwartz SM, et al. Human papillomavirus and long-term oral contraceptive use increase the risk of adenocarcinoma *in situ* of the cervix. Cancer Epidemiol Biomarkers Prev 2001; 10:171–177.

23 Altekruse SF, Lacey JV Jr, Brinton LA, et al. Comparison of human papillomavirus genotypes, sexual and reproductive risk factors of cervical adenocarcinoma and squamous cell carcinoma: Northeastern United States. Am J Obstet Gynecol 2003; 188:657–663.

24 Alfsen GC, Thoresen SO, Kristensen GB, et al. Histopathologic subtyping of cervical adenocarcinoma reveals increasing incidence rates of endometrioid tumors in all age groups: a population based study with review of all nonsquamous cervical carcinomas in Norway from 1966 to 1970, 1976 to 1980 and 1986 to 1990. Cancer 2000; 89:1291–1299.

25 Hemminki K, Li X, Mutanen P. Age-incidence relationships and time trends in cervical cancer in Sweden. Eur J Epidemiol 2001; 17:323–328.

26 Hemminki K, Li X, Vaittinen P. Time trends in the incidence of cervical and other genital squamous cell carcinomas and adenocarcinomas in Sweden, 1958–1996. Eur J Obstet Gynecol Reprod Biol 2002; 101:64–69.

27 Herbert A, Singh N, Smith JA. Adenocarcinoma of the uterine cervix compared with squamous cell carcinoma: a 12-year study in Southampton and South-west Hampshire. Cytopathology 2001; 12:26–36.

28 Liu S, Semenciw R, Probert A, Mao Y. Cervical cancer in Canada: changing patterns in incidence and mortality. Int J Gynecol Cancer 2001; 11:24–31.

29 Sasieni P, Adams J. Changing rates of adenocarcinoma and adenosquamous carcinoma of the cervix in England. Lancet 2001; 357:1490–1493.

30 Smith HO, Tiffany MF, Qualls CR, Key CR. The rising incidence of adenocarcinoma relative to squamous cell carcinoma of the uterine cervix in the United States – a 24-year population-based study. Gynecol Oncol 2000; 78:97–105.

31 Vesterinen E, Forss M, Nieminen U. Increase of cervical adenocarcinoma: a report of 520 cases of cervical carcinoma including 112 tumors with glandular elements. Gynecol Oncol 1989; 33:49–53.

32 Zheng T, Holford TR, Ma Z, et al. The continuing increase in adenocarcinoma of the uterine cervix: a birth cohort phenomenon. Int J Epidemiol 1996; 25:252–258.

33 Boon ME, Graaff Guilloud JC, Kok LP, et al. Efficacy of screening for cervical squamous and adenocarcinoma. The Dutch experience. Cancer 1987; 59:862–866.

34 Lee KR, Minter LJ, Granter SR. Papanicolaou smear sensitivity for adenocarcinoma in situ of the cervix. A study of 34 cases. Am J Clin Pathol 1997; 107:30–35.

35 Mitchell H, Medley G, Gordon I, Giles G. Cervical cytology reported as negative and risk of adenocarcinoma of the cervix: no strong evidence of benefit. Br J Cancer 1995; 71:894–897.

36 Nieminen P, Kallio M, Hakama M. The effect of mass screening on incidence and mortality of squamous and adenocarcinoma of cervix uteri. Obstet Gynecol 1995; 85:1017–1021.

37 Andersson S, Rylander E, Larsson B, et al. The role of human papillomavirus in cervical adenocarcinoma carcinogenesis. Eur J Cancer 2001; 37:246–250.

38 Lacey JV Jr, Frisch M, Brinton LA, et al. Associations between smoking and adenocarcinomas and squamous cell carcinomas of the uterine cervix (United States). Cancer Causes Control 2001; 12:153–161.

39 Ursin G, Pike MC, Preston-Martin S, et al. Sexual, reproductive and other risk factors for adenocarcinoma of the cervix: results from a population-based case-control study (California, United States). Cancer Causes Control 1996; 7:391–401.

40 Thomas DB, Ray RM. Oral contraceptives and invasive adenocarcinomas and adenosquamous carcinomas of the uterine cervix. The World Health Organization Collaborative Study of Neoplasia and Steroid Contraceptives. Am J Epidemiol 1996; 144:281–289.

41 Jones MW, Silverberg SG. Cervical adenocarcinoma in young women: possible relationship to microglandular hyperplasia and use of oral contraceptives. Obstet Gynecol 1989; 73:984–989.

42 Lacey JV Jr, Brinton LA, Abbas FM, et al. Oral contraceptives as risk factors for cervical adenocarcinomas and squamous cell carcinomas. Cancer Epidemiol Biomarkers Prev 1999; 8:1079–1085.

43 Ursin G, Peters RK, Henderson BE, et al. Oral contraceptive use and adenocarcinoma of cervix. Lancet 1994; 344:1390–1394.

44 Altekruse SF, Lacey JV Jr., Brinton LA, et al. Comparison of human papillomavirus genotypes, sexual and reproductive risk factors of cervical adenocarcinoma and squamous cell carcinoma: Northeastern United States. Am J Obstet Gynecol 2003; 188:657–663.

45 Lacey JV Jr, Brinton LA, Barnes WA, et al. Use of hormone replacement therapy and adenocarcinomas and squamous cell carcinomas of the uterine cervix. Gynecol Oncol 2000; 77:149–154.

46 Parazzini F, La Vecchia C, Negri E, et al. Case-control study of oestrogen replacement therapy and risk of cervical cancer. Br Med J 1997; 315:85–88.

47 Arbeit JM, Howley PM, Hanahan D. Chronic estrogen-induced cervical and vaginal squamous carcinogenesis in human papillomavirus type 16 transgenic mice. Proc Natl Acad Sci USA 1996; 93:2930–2935.

48 Greeley C, Schroeder S, Silverberg SG. Microglandular hyperplasia of the cervix: a true 'pill' lesion? Int J Gynecol Pathol 1995; 14:50–54.

49 Quade BJ, Yang A, Wang Y, et al. Expression of the p53 homologue p63 in early cervical neoplasia. Gynecol Oncol 2001; 80:24–29.

50 Park JJ, Sun D, Quade BJ, et al. Stratified mucin-producing intraepithelial lesions of the cervix: adenosquamous or columnar cell neoplasia? Am J Surg Pathol 2000; 24:1414–1419.

51 Betsill WL Jr, Clark AH. Early endocervical glandular neoplasia. I. Histomorphology and cytomorphology. Acta Cytol 1986; 30:115–126.

52 Lee KR, Manna EA, Jones MA. Comparative cytologic features of adenocarcinoma in situ of the uterine cervix. Acta Cytol 1991; 35:117–126.

53 Ayer B, Pacey F, Greenberg M, Bousfield L. The cytologic diagnosis of adenocarcinoma in situ of the cervix uteri and related lesions. I. Adenocarcinoma in situ. Acta Cytol 1987; 31:397–411.

54 Biscotti CV, Gero MA, Toddy SM, et al. Endocervical adenocarcinoma in situ: an analysis of cellular features. Diagn Cytopathol 1997; 17:326–332.

55 Roberts JM, Thurloe JK, Bowditch RC, et al. Comparison of ThinPrep and Pap smear in relation to prediction of adenocarcinoma in situ. Acta Cytol 1999; 43:74–80.

56 Wilbur DC, Dubeshter B, Angel C, Atkison KM. Use of thin-layer preparations for gynecologic smears with emphasis on the cytomorphology of high-grade intraepithelial lesions and carcinomas. Diagn Cytopathol 1996; 14:201–211.

57 Solomon D, Frable WJ, Vooijs GP, et al. ASCUS and AGUS criteria. International Academy of Cytology Task Force summary. Diagnostic Cytology Towards the 21st Century: An International Expert Conference and Tutorial. Acta Cytol 1998; 42:16–24.

58 Hayes MM, Matisic JP, Chen CJ, et al. Cytological aspects of uterine cervical adenocarcinoma, adenosquamous carcinoma and combined adenocarcinoma-squamous carcinoma: appraisal of diagnostic criteria for in situ versus invasive lesions. Cytopathology 1997; 8:397–408.

59 Mulvany N, Ostor A. Microinvasive adenocarcinoma of the cervix: a cytohistopathologic study of 40 cases. Diagn Cytopathol 1997; 16:430–436.

60 Kudo R, Sagae S, Hayakawa O, et al. The cytological features and DNA content of cervical adenocarcinoma. Diagn Cytopathol 1987; 3:191–197.

61 Nguyen GK, Daya D. Cervical adenocarcinoma and related lesions. Cytodiagnostic criteria and pitfalls. Pathol Annu 1993; 28 Pt 2:53–75.

62 Granter SR, Lee KR. Cytologic findings in minimal deviation adenocarcinoma (adenoma malignum) of the cervix. A report of seven cases. Am J Clin Pathol 1996; 105:327–333.

63 Ishii K, Katsuyama T, Ota H, et al. Cytologic and cytochemical features of adenoma malignum of the uterine cervix. Cancer 1999; 87:245–253.

64 Szyfelbein WM, Young RH, Scully RE. Adenoma malignum of the cervix. Cytologic findings. Acta Cytol 1984; 28:691–698.

65 Ballo MS, Silverberg SG, Sidawy MK. Cytologic features of well-differentiated villoglandular adenocarcinoma of the cervix. Acta Cytol 1996; 40:536–540.

66 Khunamornpong S, Siriaunkgul S, Suprasert P. Well-differentiated villoglandular adenocarcinoma of the uterine cervix: cytomorphologic observation of five cases. Diagn Cytopathol 2002; 26:10–14.

67 Zhou C, Matisic JP, Clement PB, Hayes MM. Cytologic features of papillary serous adenocarcinoma of the uterine cervix. Cancer 1997; 81:98–104.

68 DiTomasso JP, Ramzy I, Mody DR. Glandular lesions of the cervix. Validity of cytologic criteria used to differentiate reactive changes, glandular intraepithelial lesions and adenocarcinoma. Acta Cytol 1996; 40:1127–1135.

69 Lee KR, Genest DR, Minter LJ, et al. Adenocarcinoma *in situ* in cervical smears with a small cell (endometrioid) pattern: distinction from cells directly sampled from the upper endocervical canal or lower segment of the endometrium. Am J Clin Pathol 1998; 109:738–742.

70 Lee KR. Adenocarcinoma *in situ* with a small cell (endometrioid) pattern in cervical smears: a test of the distinction from benign mimics using specific criteria. Cancer 1999; 87:254–258.

71 Pacey NF. Glandular neoplasms of the uterine cervix. In: Bibbo M, ed. Comprehensive cytopathology. Philadelphia: WB Saunders; 1991:243–255.

72 Ismail SM. Cone biopsy causes cervical endometriosis and tubo-endometrioid metaplasia. Histopathology 1991; 18:107–114.

73 Babkowski RC, Wilbur DC, Rutkowski MA, et al. The effects of endocervical canal topography, tubal metaplasia and high canal sampling on the cytologic presentation of nonneoplastic endocervical cells. Am J Clin Pathol 1996; 105:403–410.

74 Novotny DB, Maygarden SJ, Johnson DE, Frable WJ. Tubal metaplasia. A frequent potential pitfall in the cytologic diagnosis of endocervical glandular dysplasia on cervical smears. Acta Cytol 1992; 36:1–10.

75 Schlesinger C, Silverberg SG. Endocervical adenocarcinoma *in situ* of tubal type and its relation to atypical tubal metaplasia. Int J Gynecol Pathol 1999; 18:1–4.

76 Hong SR, Park JS, Kim HS. Atypical glandular cells of undetermined significance in cervical smears after conization. Cytologic features differentiating them from adenocarcinoma *in situ*. Acta Cytol 2001; 45:163–168.

77 Lee KR. Atypical glandular cells in cervical smears from women who have undergone cone biopsy. A potential diagnostic pitfall. Acta Cytol 1993; 37:705–709.

78 Peralta-Venturino MN, Purslow MJ, Kini SR. Endometrial cells of the 'lower uterine segment' (LUS) in cervical smears obtained by endocervical brushings: a source of potential diagnostic pitfall. Diagn Cytopathol 1995; 12:263–268.

79 Ghorab Z, Hahmood S, Schinella R. Endocervical reactive atypia: a histologic-cytologic study. Diagn Cytopathol 2000; 22:342–346.

80 Selvaggi SM, Heafner HK. Microglandular endocervical hyperplasia and tubal metaplasia: pitfalls in the diagnosis of adenocarcinomas on cervical smears. Diagn Cytopathol 1997; 16(2):168–173.

81 Yahr LJ, Lee KR. Cytologic findings in microglandular hyperplasia of the cervix. Diagn Cytopathol 1991; 7:248–251.

82 Valente PT, Schartz H, Schultz M. Cytologic atypia associated with microglandular hyperplasia. Diagn Cytopathol 1994; 10:326–331.

83 Murad TM, August C. Radiation-induced atypia: a review. Diagn Cytopathol 1985; 1:137–152.

84 Michael CW, Esfahani FM. Pregnancy-related changes: a retrospective review of 278 cervical smears. Diagn Cytopathol 1997; 17:99–107.

85 Pisharodi LR, Jovanoska S. Spectrum of cytologic changes in pregnancy. A review of 100 abnormal cervicovaginal smears, with emphasis on diagnostic pitfalls. Acta Cytol 1995; 39:905–908.

86 Lee KR, Manna EA, St John T. Atypical endocervical glandular cells. Accuracy of cytologic diagnosis. Diagn Cytopathol 1995; 13:202–208.

87 Selvaggi SM. Cytologic features of squamous cell carcinoma *in situ* involving endocervical glands in endocervical cytobrush specimens. Acta Cytol 1994; 38:687–692.

88 Lee KR, Darragh TM, Joste NE, et al. Atypical glandular cells of undetermined significance (AGUS): interobserver reproducibility in cervical smears and corresponding thin-layer preparations. Am J Clin Pathol 2002; 117:96–102.

89 Raab SS, Geisinger KR, Silverman JF, et al. Interobserver variability of a Papanicolaou smear diagnosis of atypical glandular cells of undetermined significance. Am J Clin Pathol 1998; 110:653–659.

90 Wright TC Jr, Cox JT, Massad LS, et al. 2001 Consensus guidelines for the management of women with cervical cytological abnormalities. JAMA 2002; 287:2120–2129.

91 Ashfaq R, Gibbons D, Vela C, et al. ThinPrep Pap Test. Accuracy for glandular disease. Acta Cytol 1999; 43:81–85.

92 Bai H, Sung CJ, Steinhoff MM. ThinPrep Pap Test promotes detection of glandular lesions of the endocervix. Diagn Cytopathol 2000; 23:19–22.

93 Hecht JL, Sheets EE, Lee KR. Atypical glandular cells of undetermined significance in conventional cervical/vaginal smears and thin-layer preparations. Cancer 2002; 96:1–4.

94 Wang N, Emancipator SN, Rose P, et al. Histologic follow-up of atypical endocervical cells. Liquid-based, thin-layer preparation vs. conventional Pap smear. Acta Cytol 2002; 46:453–457.

95 Ronnett BM, Manos MM, Ransley JE, et al. Atypical glandular cells of undetermined significance (AGUS): cytopathologic features, histopathologic results and human papillomavirus DNA detection. Hum Pathol 1999; 30:816–825.

96 Krane J, Lee KR, Sun D, et al. Atypical glandular cells of undetermined significance. Outcome predictions based on human papillomavirus testing. Am J Clin Pathol 2004; 121:87–92.

97 Andersen ES, Arffmann E. Adenocarcinoma *in situ* of the uterine cervix: a clinico-pathologic study of 36 cases. Gynecol Oncol 1989; 35:1–7.

98 Ostor AG, Duncan A, Quinn M, Rome R. Adenocarcinoma *in situ* of the uterine cervix: an experience with 100 cases. Gynecol Oncol 2000; 79:207–210.

99 Crum CP. Contemporary theories of cervical carcinogenesis: the virus, the host and the stem cell. Mod Pathol 2000; 13:243–251.

100 Bertrand M, Lickrish GM, Colgan TJ. The anatomic distribution of cervical adenocarcinoma *in situ*: implications for treatment. Am J Obstet Gynecol 1987; 157:21–25.

101 Biscotti CV, Hart WR. Apoptotic bodies: a consistent morphologic feature of endocervical adenocarcinoma *in situ*. Am J Surg Pathol 1998; 22:434–439.

102 Moritani S, Ioffe OB, Sagae S, et al. Mitotic activity and apoptosis in endocervical glandular lesions. Int J Gynecol Pathol 2002; 21:125–133.

103 Brown LJ, Wells M. Cervical glandular atypia associated with squamous intraepithelial neoplasia: a premalignant lesion? J Clin Pathol 1986; 39:22–28.

104 Higgins GD, Phillips GE, Smith LA, et al. High prevalence of human papillomavirus transcripts in all grades of cervical intraepithelial glandular neoplasia. Cancer 1992; 70:136–146.

105 Kurian K, al Nafussi A. Relation of cervical glandular intraepithelial neoplasia to microinvasive and invasive adenocarcinoma of the uterine cervix: a study of 121 cases. J Clin Pathol 1999; 52:112–117.

106 Tase T, Okagaki T, Clark BA, et al. Human papillomavirus DNA in glandular dysplasia and microglandular hyperplasia: presumed precursors of adenocarcinoma of the uterine cervix. Obstet Gynecol 1989; 73:1005–1008.

107 Jaworski RC. Endocervical glandular dysplasia, adenocarcinoma *in situ* and early invasive (microinvasive) adenocarcinoma of the uterine cervix. Semin Diagn Pathol 1990; 7:190–204.

108 Kurman RJ, Norris HJ, Wilkinson E. Tumors of the cervix. Tumors of the vulva vagina and cervix. Atlas of tumor pathology. Third series fascicle 4: Washington, DC: Armed Forces Institute of Pathology; 1990:78–79.

109 Leary J, Jaworski R, Houghton R. In-situ hybridization using biotinylated DNA probes to human papillomavirus in adenocarcinoma-in-situ and endocervical glandular dysplasia of the uterine cervix. Pathology 1991; 23:85–89.

110 Anciaux D, Lawrence WD, Gregoire L. Glandular lesions of the uterine cervix: prognostic implications of human papillomavirus status. Int J Gynecol Pathol 1997; 16:103–110.

111 Negri G, Egarter-Vigl E, Kasal A, et al. p16INK4a is a useful marker for the diagnosis of adenocarcinoma of the cervix uteri and its precursors: an immunohistochemical study with immunocytochemical correlations. Am J Surg Pathol 2003; 27:187–193.

112 Suh KS, Silverberg SG. Tubal metaplasia of the uterine cervix. Int J Gynecol Pathol 1990; 9:122–128.

113 Jonasson JG, Wang HH, Antonioli DA, Ducatman BS. Tubal metaplasia of the uterine cervix: a prevalence study in patients with gynecologic pathologic findings. Int J Gynecol Pathol 1992; 11:89–95.

114 Clement PB. Pathology of endometriosis. Pathol Annu 1990; 25 Pt 1:245–295.

115 Baker PM, Clement PB, Bell DA, Young RH. Superficial endometriosis of the uterine cervix: a report of 20 cases of a process that may be confused with endocervical glandular dysplasia or adenocarcinoma *in situ*. Int J Gynecol Pathol 1999; 18:198–205.

116 Toki T, Shimizu M, Takagi Y, et al. CD10 is a marker for normal and neoplastic endometrial stromal cells. Int J Gynecol Pathol 2002; 21:41–47.

117 Kim KR. Utility of trichrome and reticulin stains in the diagnosis of superficial endometriosis of the uterine cervix. Int J Gynecol Pathol 2001; 20:173–176.

118 Schneider V. Arias-Stella reaction of the endocervix: frequency and location. Acta Cytol 1981; 25:224–228.

119 Cariani DJ, Guderian AM. Gestational atypia in endocervical polyps – the Arias-Stella reaction. Am J Obstet Gynecol 1966; 95:589–590.

120 Nucci MR, Young RH. Arias-Stella reaction of the endocervix. A report of 18 cases with emphasis on its varied histology and differential diagnosis. Am J Surg Pathol 2004; 28:608–612.

121 Koss LG. The effects of therapeutic procedures and drugs on the epithelium of the female genital tract. In: Koss L, ed. Diagnostic cytology and its histologic bases. Philadelphia: JB Lippincott; 1992:682–683.

122 Lesack D, Wahab I, Gilks CB. Radiation-induced atypia of endocervical epithelium: a histological, immunohistochemical and cytometric study. Int J Gynecol Pathol 1996; 15:242–247.

123 Shield PW, Daunter B, Wright RG. Post-irradiation cytology of cervical cancer patients. Cytopathology 1992; 3:167–182.

124 Young RH, Clement PB. Pseudoneoplastic lesions of the lower female genital tract. Pathol Annu 1989; 24 Pt 2:189–226.

125 Jones MA, Young RH. Atypical oxyphilic metaplasia of the endocervical epithelium: a report of six cases. Int J Gynecol Pathol 1997; 16:99–102.

126 Brown S, Senekjian EK, Montag AG. Cytomegalovirus infection of the uterine cervix in a patient with acquired immunodeficiency syndrome. Obstet Gynecol 1988; 71:489–491.

127 Josey WE, Nahmias AJ, Naib ZM. Viral and virus-like infections of the female genital tract. Clin Obstet Gynecol 1969; 12:161–178.

128 Andersen ES, Nielsen K. Adenocarcinoma *in situ* of the cervix: a prospective study of conization as definitive treatment. Gynecol Oncol 2002; 86:365–369.

129 Im DD, Duska LR, Rosenshein NB. Adequacy of conization margins in adenocarcinoma *in situ* of the cervix as a predictor of residual disease. Gynecol Oncol 1995; 59:179–182.

130 Wolf JK, Levenback C, Malpica A, et al. Adenocarcinoma *in situ* of the cervix: significance of cone biopsy margins. Obstet Gynecol 1996; 88:82–86.

131 Denehy TR, Gregori CA, Breen JL. Endocervical curettage, cone margins and residual adenocarcinoma *in situ* of the cervix. Obstet Gynecol 1997; 90:1–6.

132 Goldstein NS, Mani A. The status and distance of cone biopsy margins as a predictor of excision adequacy for endocervical adenocarcinoma *in situ*. Am J Clin Pathol 1998; 109:727–732.

133 Azodi M, Chambers SK, Rutherford TJ, et al. Adenocarcinoma *in situ* of the cervix: management and outcome. Gynecol Oncol 1999; 73:348–353.

134 Poynor EA, Barakat RR, Hoskins WJ. Management and follow-up of patients with adenocarcinoma *in situ* of the uterine cervix. Gynecol Oncol 1995; 57:158–164.

135 Andersen ES, Nielsen K. Adenocarcinoma *in situ* of the cervix: a prospective study of conization as definitive treatment. Gynecol Oncol 2002; 86:365–369.

136 Kennedy AW, Biscotti CV. Further study of the management of cervical adenocarcinoma *in situ*. Gynecol Oncol 2002; 86:361–364.

137 Shin CH, Schorge JO, Lee KR, Sheets EE. Conservative management of adenocarcinoma *in situ* of the cervix. Gynecol Oncol 2000; 79:6–10.

138 McHale MT, Le TD, Burger RA, et al. Fertility sparing treatment for *in situ* and early invasive adenocarcinoma of the cervix. Obstet Gynecol 2001; 98:726–731.

139 Soutter WP, Haidopoulos D, Gornall RJ, et al. Is conservative treatment for adenocarcinoma *in situ* of the cervix safe? Br J Obstet Gynaecol 2001; 108:1184–1189.

140 Burghardt E. Microinvasive carcinoma in gynaecological pathology. Clin Obstet Gynaecol 1984; 11:239–257.

141 Teshima S, Shimosato Y, Kishi K, et al. Early stage adenocarcinoma of the uterine cervix. Histopathologic analysis with consideration of histogenesis. Cancer 1985; 56:167–172.

142 Creasman WT, DeGeest K, DiSaia PJ, Zaino RJ. Significance of true surgical pathologic staging: a Gynecologic Oncology Group Study. Am J Obstet Gynecol 1999; 181:31–34.

143 Schorge JO, Lee KR, Flynn CE, Goodman A, Sheets EE. Stage IA1 cervical adenocarcinoma: definition and treatment. Obstet Gynecol 1999; 93:219–222.

144 Nicklin JL, Perrin LC, Crandon AJ, Ward BG. Microinvasive adenocarcinoma of the cervix. Aust N Z J Obstet Gynaecol 1999; 39:411–413.

145 Smith HO, Qualls CR, Romero AA, et al. Is there a difference in survival for IA1 and IA2 adenocarcinoma of the uterine cervix? Gynecol Oncol 2002; 85:229–241.

146 Nagarsheth NP, Maxwell GL, Bentley RC, Rodriguez G. Bilateral pelvic lymph node metastases in a case of FIGO stage IA(1) adenocarcinoma of the cervix. Gynecol Oncol 2000; 77:467–470.

147 Berek JS, Hacker NF, Fu YS, et al. Adenocarcinoma of the uterine cervix: histologic variables associated with lymph node metastasis and survival. Obstet Gynecol 1985; 65:46–52.

148 Schorge JO, Lee KR, Sheets EE. Prospective management of stage IA(1) cervical adenocarcinoma by conization alone to preserve fertility: a preliminary report. Gynecol Oncol 2000; 78:217–220.

149 Miller BE, Flax SD, Arheart K, Photopulos G. The presentation of adenocarcinoma of the uterine cervix. Cancer 1993; 72:1281–1285.

150 Young RH, Clement PB. Premalignant and malignant glandular lesions of the uterine cervix. In: Clement PB, Young RH, eds. Tumors and tumor-like lesions of the uterine corpus and cervix. New York: Churchill Livingstone; 1993.

151 Young RH, Clement PB. Endocervical adenocarcinoma and its variants: their morphology and differential diagnosis. Histopathology 2002; 41:185–207.

152 Wells M, Oster AG, Crum CP, et al. Epithelial tumors of the cervix. In: Tavassoli FA, Devilee P, eds. World Health Organization Classification of Tumors. Pathology and genetics of tumors of the breast and female genital organs. Lyon: IARC Press; 2003:272–273.

153 McGowan L, Young RH, Scully RE. Peutz–Jeghers syndrome with 'adenoma malignum' of the cervix. A report of two cases. Gynecol Oncol 1980; 10:125–133.

154 Gilks CB, Young RH, Aguirre P, et al. Adenoma malignum (minimal deviation adenocarcinoma) of the uterine cervix. A clinicopathological and immunohistochemical analysis of 26 cases. Am J Surg Pathol 1989; 13:717–729.

155 Fukushima M, Shimano S, Yamakawa Y, et al. The detection of human papillomavirus (HPV) in a case of minimal deviation adenocarcinoma of the uterine cervix (adenoma malignum) using *in situ* hybridization. Jpn J Clin Oncol 1990; 20:407–412.

156 Speers WC, Picaso LG, Silverberg SG. Immunohistochemical localization of carcinoembryonic antigen in microglandular hyperplasia and adenocarcinoma of the endocervix. Am J Clin Pathol 1983; 79:105–107.

157 Steeper TA, Wick MR. Minimal deviation adenocarcinoma of the uterine cervix ('adenoma malignum'). An immunohistochemical comparison with microglandular endocervical hyperplasia and conventional endocervical adenocarcinoma. Cancer 1986; 58:1131–1138.

158 Michael H, Grawe L, Kraus FT. Minimal deviation endocervical adenocarcinoma: clinical and histologic features, immunohistochemical staining for carcinoembryonic antigen and differentiation from confusing benign lesions. Int J Gynecol Pathol 1984; 3:261–276.

159 Ishii K, Hidaka E, Katsuyama T, et al. Ultrastructural features of adenoma malignum of the uterine cervix: demonstration of gastric phenotypes. Ultrastruct Pathol 1999; 23:375–381.

160 Toki T, Shiozawa T, Hosaka N, et al. Minimal deviation adenocarcinoma of the uterine cervix has abnormal expression of sex steroid receptors, CA125 and gastric mucin. Int J Gynecol Pathol 1997; 16:111–116.

161 Utsugi K, Hirai Y, Takeshima N, et al. Utility of the monoclonal antibody HIK1083 in the diagnosis of adenoma malignum of the uterine cervix. Gynecol Oncol 1999; 75:345–348.

162 Hayashi I, Tsuda H, Shimoda T. Reappraisal of orthodox histochemistry for the diagnosis of minimal deviation adenocarcinoma of the cervix. Am J Surg Pathol 2000; 24:559–562.

163 Ichimura T, Koizumi T, Tateiwa H, et al. Immunohistochemical expression of gastric mucin and p53 in minimal deviation adenocarcinoma of the uterine cervix. Int J Gynecol Pathol 2001; 20:220–226.

164 Schorge JO, Lee KR, Lee SJ, et al. Early cervical adenocarcinoma: selection criteria for radical surgery. Obstet Gynecol 1999; 94:386–390.

165 Zaino RJ. The fruits of our labors: distinguishing endometrial from endocervical adenocarcinoma. Int J Gynecol Pathol 2002; 21:1–3.

166 Castrillon DH, Lee KR, Nucci MR. Distinction between endometrial and endocervical adenocarcinoma: an immunohistochemical study. Int J Gynecol Pathol 2002; 21:4–10.

167 McCluggage WG, Sumathi VP, McBride HA, Patterson A. A panel of immunohistochemical stains, including carcinoembryonic antigen, vimentin and estrogen receptor, aids the distinction between primary endometrial and endocervical adenocarcinomas. Int J Gynecol Pathol 2002; 21:11–15.

168 Kamoi S, AlJuboury MI, Akin MR, Silverberg SG. Immunohistochemical staining in the distinction between primary endometrial and endocervical adenocarcinomas: another viewpoint. Int J Gynecol Pathol 2002; 21:217–223.

169 Staebler A, Sherman ME, Zaino RJ, Ronnett BM. Hormone receptor immunohistochemistry and human papillomavirus in situ hybridization are useful for distinguishing endocervical and endometrial adenocarcinomas. Am J Surg Pathol 2002; 26:998–1006.

170 Kaminski PF, Norris HJ. Minimal deviation carcinoma (adenoma malignum) of the cervix. Int J Gynecol Pathol 1983; 2:141–152.

171 Young RH, Scully RE. Minimal-deviation endometrioid adenocarcinoma of the uterine cervix. A report of five cases of a distinctive neoplasm that may be misinterpreted as benign. Am J Surg Pathol 1993; 17:660–665.

172 Rahilly MA, Williams AR, al Nafussi A. Minimal deviation endometrioid adenocarcinoma of cervix: a clinicopathological and immunohistochemical study of two cases. Histopathology 1992; 20:351–354.

173 Azzopardi JG, Hou LT. Intestinal metaplasia with argentaffin cells in cervical adenocarcinoma. J Pathol Bacteriol 1965; 90:686–690.

174 Lee KR, Trainer TD. Adenocarcinoma of the uterine cervix of small intestinal type containing numerous Paneth cells. Arch Pathol Lab Med 1990; 114:731–733.

175 Fox H, Wells M, Harris M, McWilliam LJ. Enteric tumours of the lower female genital tract: a report of three cases. Histopathology 1988; 12:167–176.

176 Lewis TL. Colloid (mucus secreting) carcinoma of the cervix. J Obstet Gynaecol Br Commonw 1971; 78:1128–1132.

177 Haswani P, Arseneau J, Ferenczy A. Primary signet ring cell carcinoma of the uterine cervix: a clinicopathologic study of two cases with review of the literature. Int J Gynecol Cancer 1998; 8:374–379.

178 Mayorga M, Garcia-Valtuille A, Fernandez F, et al. Adenocarcinoma of the uterine cervix with massive signet-ring cell differentiation. Int J Surg Pathol 1997; 5:95–100.

179 Benda JA, Platz CE, Buchsbaum H, Lifshitz S. Mucin production in defining mixed carcinoma of the uterine cervix: a clinicopathologic study. Int J Gynecol Pathol 1985; 4:314–327.

180 Costa MJ, McIlnay KR, Trelford J. Cervical carcinoma with glandular differentiation: histological evaluation predicts disease recurrence in clinical stage I or II patients. Hum Pathol 1995; 26:829–837.

181 Look KY, Brunetto VL, Clarke-Pearson DL, et al. An analysis of cell type in patients with surgically staged stage IB carcinoma of the cervix: a Gynecologic Oncology Group study. Gynecol Oncol 1996; 63:304–311.

182 Alfsen GC, Kristensen GB, Skovlund E, et al. Histologic subtype has minor importance for overall survival in patients with adenocarcinoma of the uterine cervix: a population-based study of prognostic factors in 505 patients with nonsquamous cell carcinomas of the cervix. Cancer 2001; 92:2471–2483.

183 Glücksmann A, Cherry CC. Incidence, histology and response to radiation of mixed carcinomas (adenoacanthomas) of the uterine cervix. Cancer 1956; 9:971–979.

184 Ulbright TM, Gersell DJ. Glassy cell carcinoma of the uterine cervix. A light and electron microscopic study of five cases. Cancer 1983; 51:2255–2263.

185 Littman P, Clement PB, Henriksen B, et al. Glassy cell carcinoma of the cervix. Cancer 1976; 37:2238–2246.

186 Costa MJ, Kenny MB, Hewan-Lowe K, Judd R. Glassy cell features in adenosquamous carcinoma of the uterine cervix. Histologic, ultrastructural, immunohistochemical and clinical findings. Am J Clin Pathol 1991; 96:520–528.

187 Fujiwara H, Mitchell MF, Arseneau J, et al. Clear cell adenosquamous carcinoma of the cervix. An aggressive tumor associated with human papillomavirus-18. Cancer 1995; 76:1591–600.

188 Young RH, Scully RE. Villoglandular papillary adenocarcinoma of the uterine cervix. A clinicopathologic analysis of 13 cases. Cancer 1989; 63:1773–1779.

189 Jones MW, Silverberg SG, Kurman RJ. Well-differentiated villoglandular adenocarcinoma of the uterine cervix: a clinicopathological study of 24 cases. Int J Gynecol Pathol 1993; 12:1–7.

190 Jones MW, Kounelis S, Papadaki H, et al. Well-differentiated villoglandular adenocarcinoma of the uterine cervix: oncogene/tumor suppressor gene alterations and human papillomavirus genotyping. Int J Gynecol Pathol 2000; 19:110–117.

191 Khunamornpong S, Maleemonkol S, Siriaunkgul S, Pantusart A. Well-differentiated villoglandular adenocarcinoma of the uterine cervix: a report of 15 cases including two with lymph node metastasis. J Med Assoc Thai 2001; 84:882–888.

192 Kaku T, Kamura T, Shigematsu T, et al. Adenocarcinoma of the uterine cervix with predominantly villoglandular papillary growth pattern. Gynecol Oncol 1997; 64:147–152.

193 Herbst AL, Cole P, Colton T, et al. Age-incidence and risk of diethylstilbestrol-related clear cell adenocarcinoma of the vagina and cervix. Am J Obstet Gynecol 1977; 128:43–50.

194 Nordqvist SR, Fidler WJ Jr, Woodruff JM, Lewis JL Jr. Clear cell adenocarcinoma of the cervix and vagina. A clinicopathologic study of 21 cases with and without a history of maternal ingestion of estrogens. Cancer 1976; 37:858–871.

195 Reich O, Tamussino K, Lahousen M, et al. Clear cell carcinoma of the uterine cervix: pathology and prognosis in surgically treated stage IB-IIB disease in women not exposed in utero to diethylstilbestrol. Gynecol Oncol 2000; 76:331–335.

196 Grisaru D, Covens A, Chapman B, et al. Does histology influence prognosis in patients with early-stage cervical carcinoma? Cancer 2001; 92:2999–3004.

197 Ordi T, Cleofe R, Tavassoli F, et al. CD10 expression in epithelial tissues and tumors of the gynecologic tract. A useful marker in the diagnosis of mesonephric, trophoblastic and clear cell tumors. Am J Surg Pathol 2003; 27:178–186.

198 Zhou C, Gilks CB, Hayes M, Clement PB. Papillary serous carcinoma of the uterine cervix: a clinicopathologic study of 17 cases. Am J Surg Pathol 1998; 22:113–120.

199 Ferry JA, Scully RE. 'Adenoid cystic' carcinoma and adenoid basal carcinoma of the uterine cervix. A study of 28 cases. Am J Surg Pathol 1988; 12:134–144.

200 Brainard JA, Hart WR. Adenoid basal epitheliomas of the uterine cervix: a reevaluation of distinctive cervical basaloid lesions currently classified as adenoid basal carcinoma and adenoid basal hyperplasia. Am J Surg Pathol 1998; 22:965–975.

201 Grayson W, Taylor LF, Cooper K. Adenoid cystic and adenoid basal carcinoma of the uterine cervix: comparative morphologic, mucin and immunohistochemical profile of two rare neoplasms of putative 'reserve cell' origin. Am J Surg Pathol 1999; 23:448–458.

202 Albores-Saavedra J, Manivel C, Mora A, et al. The solid variant of adenoid cystic carcinoma of the cervix. Int J Gynecol Pathol 1992; 11:2–10.

203 Cviko A, Briem B, Granter SR, et al. Adenoid basal carcinomas of the cervix: a unique morphological evolution with cell cycle correlates. Hum Pathol 2000; 31:740–744.

204 Grayson W, Taylor L, Cooper K. Detection of integrated high risk human papillomavirus in adenoid cystic carcinoma of the uterine cervix. J Clin Pathol 1996; 49:805–809.

205 Grayson W, Taylor LF, Cooper K. Adenoid basal carcinoma of the uterine cervix: detection of integrated human papillomavirus in a rare tumor of putative 'reserve cell' origin. Int J Gynecol Pathol 1997; 16:307–312.

206 Ferry JA, Scully RE. Mesonephric remnants, hyperplasia and neoplasia in the uterine cervix. A study of 49 cases. Am J Surg Pathol 1990; 14:1100–1111.

207 Silver SA, Devouassoux-Shisheboran M, Mezzetti TP, Tavassoli FA. Mesonephric adenocarcinomas of the uterine cervix: a study of 11 cases with immunohistochemical findings. Am J Surg Pathol 2001; 25:379–387.

208 Clement PB, Young RH, Keh P, et al. Malignant mesonephric neoplasms of the uterine cervix. A report of eight cases, including four with a malignant spindle cell component. Am J Surg Pathol 1995; 19:1158–1171.

209 Ordi J, Romagosa C, Tavassoli FA, et al. CD10 expression in epithelial tissues and tumors of the gynecologic tract. A useful marker in the diagnosis of mesonephric, trophoblastic and clear cell tumors. Am J Surg Pathol 2003; 27:178–186.

210 Oliva E, Young RH, Amin MB, Clement PB. An immunohistochemical analysis of endometrial stromal and smooth muscle tumors of the uterus: a study of 54 cases emphasizing the importance of using a panel because of overlap in immunoreactivity for individual antibodies. Am J Surg Pathol 2002; 26:403–412.

211 Mazur MT, Hsueh S, Gersell DJ. Metastases to the female genital tract. Analysis of 325 cases. Cancer 1984; 53:1978–1984.

212 Mulvany NJ, Nirenberg A, Oster AG. Non-primary cervical adenocarcinomas. Pathology 1996; 28:293–297.

213 Imachi M, Tsukamoto N, Amagase H, et al. Metastatic adenocarcinoma to the uterine cervix from gastric cancer. A clinicopathologic analysis of 16 cases. Cancer 1993; 71:3472–3477.

214 Clement PB, Young RH. Deep nabothian cysts of the uterine cervix. A possible source of confusion with minimal-deviation adenocarcinoma (adenoma malignum). Int J Gynecol Pathol 1989; 8:340–348.

215 Tambouret R, Bell DA, Young RH. Microcystic endocervical adenocarcinomas: a report of eight cases. Am J Surg Pathol 2000; 24:369–374.

216 Fluhmann CF. Focal hyperplasia (tunnel clusters) of the cervix uteri. Obstet Gynecol 1961; 17:206–214.

217 Segal GH, Hart WR. Cystic endocervical tunnel clusters. A clinicopathologic study of 29 cases of so-called adenomatous hyperplasia. Am J Surg Pathol 1990; 14:895–903.

218 Jones MA, Young RH. Endocervical type A (noncystic) tunnel clusters with cytologic atypia. A report of 14 cases. Am J Surg Pathol 1996; 20:1312–1318.

219 Nucci MR, Clement PB, Young RH. Lobular endocervical glandular hyperplasia, not otherwise specified: a clinicopathologic analysis of thirteen cases of a distinctive pseudoneoplastic lesion and comparison with fourteen cases of adenoma malignum. Am J Surg Pathol 1999; 23:886–891.

220 Mikami Y, Manabe T. Lobular endocervical glandular hyperplasia represents pyloric gland metaplasia? Am J Surg Pathol 2000; 24:323–324.

221 Jones MA, Young RH, Scully RE. Diffuse laminar endocervical glandular hyperplasia. A benign lesion often confused with adenoma malignum (minimal deviation adenocarcinoma). Am J Surg Pathol 1991; 15:1123–1129.

222 Young RH, Clement PB. Endocervicosis involving the uterine cervix: a report of four cases of a benign process that may be confused with deeply invasive endocervical adenocarcinoma. Int J Gynecol Pathol 2000; 19:322–328.

223 Clement PB, Young RH. Florid cystic endosalpingiosis with tumor-like manifestations: a report of four cases including the first reported cases of transmural endosalpingiosis of the uterus. Am J Surg Pathol 1999; 23:166–175.

224 Young RH, Scully RE. Invasive adenocarcinoma and related tumors of the uterine cervix. Semin Diagn Pathol 1990; 7:205–227.

225 Smith YR, Quint EH, Hinton EL. Recurrent benign mullerian papilloma of the cervix. J Pediatr Adolesc Gynecol 1998; 11:29–31.

226 Kyriakos M, Kempson RL, Konikov NF. A clinical and pathologic study of endocervical lesions associated with oral contraceptives. Cancer 1968; 22:99–110.

227 Taylor HB, Irey NS, Norris HJ. Atypical endocervical hyperplasia in women taking oral contraceptives. JAMA 1967; 202:185–187.

228 Young RH, Scully RE. Atypical forms of microglandular hyperplasia of the cervix simulating carcinoma. A report of five cases and review of the literature. Am J Surg Pathol 1989; 13:50–56.

229 Young RH, Scully RE. Uterine carcinomas simulating microglandular hyperplasia. A report of six cases. Am J Surg Pathol 1992; 16:1092–1097.

230 Zaloudek C, Hayashi GM, Ryan IP, et al. Microglandular adenocarcinoma of the endometrium: a form of mucinous adenocarcinoma that may be confused with microglandular hyperplasia of the cervix. Int J Gynecol Pathol 1997; 16:52–59.

231 Sherrick JC, Vega JG. Congenital intramural cysts of the uterus. Obstet Gynecol 1962; 19:486–493.

232 Seidman JD, Tavassoli FA. Mesonephric hyperplasia of the uterine cervix: a clinicopathologic study of 51 cases. Int J Gynecol Pathol 1995; 14:293–299.

233 Larraza-Hernandez O, Molberg KH, Lindberg G, Albores-Saavedra J. Ectopic prostatic tissue in the uterine cervix. Int J Gynecol Pathol 1997; 16:291–293.

234 Nucci MA, Ferry JA, Young RH. Ectopic prostate tissue in the uterine cervix. A report of four cases and review of ectopic prostate tissue. Am J Sur Pathol 2000; 24:1224–1230.

235 Oliva E, Clement PB, Young RH. Tubal and tubo-endometrioid metaplasia of the uterine cervix. Unemphasized features that may cause problems in differential diagnosis: a report of 25 cases. Am J Clin Pathol 1995; 103:618–623.

236 Michael H, Sutton G, Hull MT, Roth LM. Villous adenoma of the uterine cervix associated with invasive adenocarcinoma: a histologic, ultrastructural and immunohistochemical study. Int J Gynecol Pathol 1986; 5:163–169.

237 Alvaro T, Nogales F. Villous adenoma and invasive adenocarcinoma of the cervix. Int J Gynecol Pathol 1988; 7:96–97.

238 Lea JS, Sheets EE, Wenham RM, et al. Stage IIB-IVB cervical adenocarcinoma: prognostic factors and survival. Gynecol Oncol 2002; 84:115–119.

239 Natsume N, Aoki Y, Kase H, et al. Ovarian metastasis in stage IB and II cervical adenocarcinoma. Gynecol Oncol 1999; 74:255–258.

240 Nakanishi T, Wakai K, Ishikawa H, et al. A comparison of ovarian metastasis between squamous cell carcinoma and adenocarcinoma of the uterine cervix. Gynecol Oncol 2001; 82:504–509.

241 Nakanishi T, Ishikawa H, Suzuki Y, et al. A comparison of prognoses of pathologic stage Ib adenocarcinoma and squamous cell carcinoma of the uterine cervix. Gynecol Oncol 2000; 79:289–293.

242 Davy ML, Dodd TJ, Luke CG, Roder DM. Cervical cancer: effect of glandular cell type on prognosis, treatment and survival. Obstet Gynecol 2003; 101:38–45.

243 Peters WA, III, Liu PY, Barrett RJ, et al. Concurrent chemotherapy and pelvic radiation therapy compared with pelvic radiation therapy alone as adjuvant therapy after radical surgery in high-risk early-stage cancer of the cervix. J Clin Oncol 2000; 18:1606–1613.

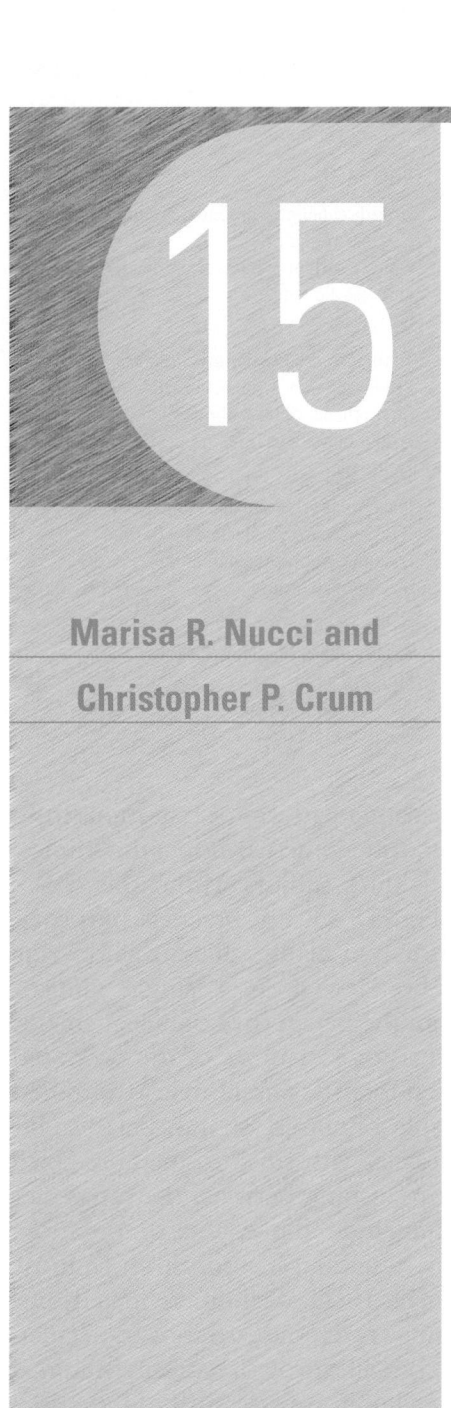

15

Marisa R. Nucci and

Christopher P. Crum

Neuroendocrine carcinoma, mixed epithelial/mesenchymal and mesenchymal tumors and miscellaneous lesions of the cervix

Neuroendocrine carcinoma

Definition
The patient at risk
Cytologic diagnosis
Classification and diagnosis
Differential diagnosis
Management and outcome

Undifferentiated carcinoma

Mixed epithelial/mesenchymal neoplasms

Endocervical polyp
Adenomyoma and polypoid
   adenomyoma of the
   endocervical type
Cervical adenosarcoma
Carcinosarcoma

Mesenchymal neoplasms

Endometrial stromal sarcoma
Alveolar soft-part sarcoma

Smooth muscle tumors
Schwannoma
Peripheral neuroectodermal
   tumor/Ewings sarcoma

Melanocytic lesions

Hematopoietic lesions

Lymphoma
Granulocytic sarcoma

Other conditions

Deciduosis
Ectopic tissues/metaplasias
   (gliosis, cartilage, bone)
Vascular tumors
Amyloidosis
Ligneous cervicitis
Malakoplakia
Trophoblastic lesions
Atypical stromal cells
Gland-poor endometriosis
   (stromatosis)

Neuroendocrine carcinoma

DEFINITION

Neuroendocrine carcinoma of the cervix is an uncommon epithelial malignancy that can usually be distinguished from squamous cell carcinoma and adenocarcinoma by certain morphologic features that correlate strongly with a neuroendocrine immunophenotype. The presence of HPV type 18 is also highly correlative.[1-4]

THE PATIENT AT RISK

Identifying patients at risk for cervical neuroendocrine carcinoma is difficult since it is a rare tumor type. Neuroendocrine differentiation is present in less than 5% of cervical carcinomas.[4] Thus, of the estimated 12 000 cervical cancers each year in the USA, well under 1000 will fall into this diagnostic category. Neuroendocrine carcinoma may coexist with both cervical glandular (more common) and squamous carcinoma, however, it has no defined precursor lesion. Up to 90% of neuroendocrine carcinomas have been associated with HPV type 18 and the age distribution is similar to adenocarcinoma, with most patients being between 25 and 40 years of age.[1-3]

CYTOLOGIC DIAGNOSIS

The diagnosis of neuroendocrine carcinoma is difficult by cytology alone. Small cell clusters with a high nuclear/cytoplasmic ratio and nuclear molding typify this tumor, but these features may be misinterpreted as a high-grade squamous intraepithelial lesion, adenocarcinoma or lymphoma.[5] Furthermore, in liquid-based samples, nuclear molding may not be conspicuous.[6] Moreover, primary neuroendocrine tumors of the cervix and endometrium cannot be distinguished.[7]

CLASSIFICATION AND DIAGNOSIS

Neuroendocrine carcinoma has been classified previously under a wide range of diagnostic terms, ranging from carcinoid to oat cell carcinoma. To promote a more precise classification of these tumors, a consensus workshop convened and subdivided them into four categories: (1) carcinoid, (2) atypical carcinoid, (3) large cell neuroendocrine carcinoma and (4) small cell (oat cell) carcinomas (Table 15.1).[8-10] The reader is advised that this is a morphologic classification only, since the diagnostic reproducibility of these categories is unknown

Table 15.1 Classification of neuroendocrine tumor of the cervix

Type	Criteria
Carcinoid	Orderly tubular to organoid growth pattern Nuclear regularity Finely distributed nuclear chromatin Low mitotic index No necrosis
Atypical carcinoid	Tubular to organoid growth pattern Preservation of cytoplasmic definition Coarsely distributed chromatin Frequent mitoses Necrosis
Large cell	Infrequent organoid growth pattern High nuclear/cytoplasmic (N/C) ratio Loss of cytoplasmic definition Crowding, overlap
Small cell	Same as above Small cells with high N/C ratio Fracture lines Absence of polarity Nuclear molding

and there may be coexisting patterns or transitions from one to another over time. Furthermore, the clinical significance of subdividing tumors within this classification is unclear (Fig. 15.1). For practical purposes, until more information is available, all neuroendocrine neoplasms should be viewed as a single clinicopathologic entity from the perspective of management.

Features common to one or more of the proposed categories of neuroendocrine carcinoma, as outlined above, include variable organoid or trabecular architecture and uniform cells with small to medium-sized nuclei. Features distinguishing between the categories may be subtle and include the extent of organoid architectural pattern, nuclear pleomorphism, mitotic activity and necrosis (Fig. 15.1). Well-differentiated neuroendocrine carcinoma (carcinoid) exhibits trabecular, organoid, nested or cord-like growth patterns, minimal or no necrosis and small uniform cells with round nuclei and finely granular chromatin (Fig. 15.2). Moderately-differentiated neuroendocrine carcinoma (atypical carcinoid) exhibits the above features with increased mitotic activity (usually 5–10 mitoses per 10 high power fields), a greater degree of nuclear atypia and/or conspicuous necrosis (Fig. 15.3). Poorly-differentiated neuroendocrine carcinoma, including large and small cell neuroendocrine carcinoma, exhibits necrosis, abundant mitoses (usually >10 mitoses per 10 high power fields) and progressive loss of organoid architecture (Figs 15.4–15.7).[8-10] In some neuroendocrine carcinomas, an insular/trabecular pattern of growth and/or discohesive architecture may be inconspicuous and may not

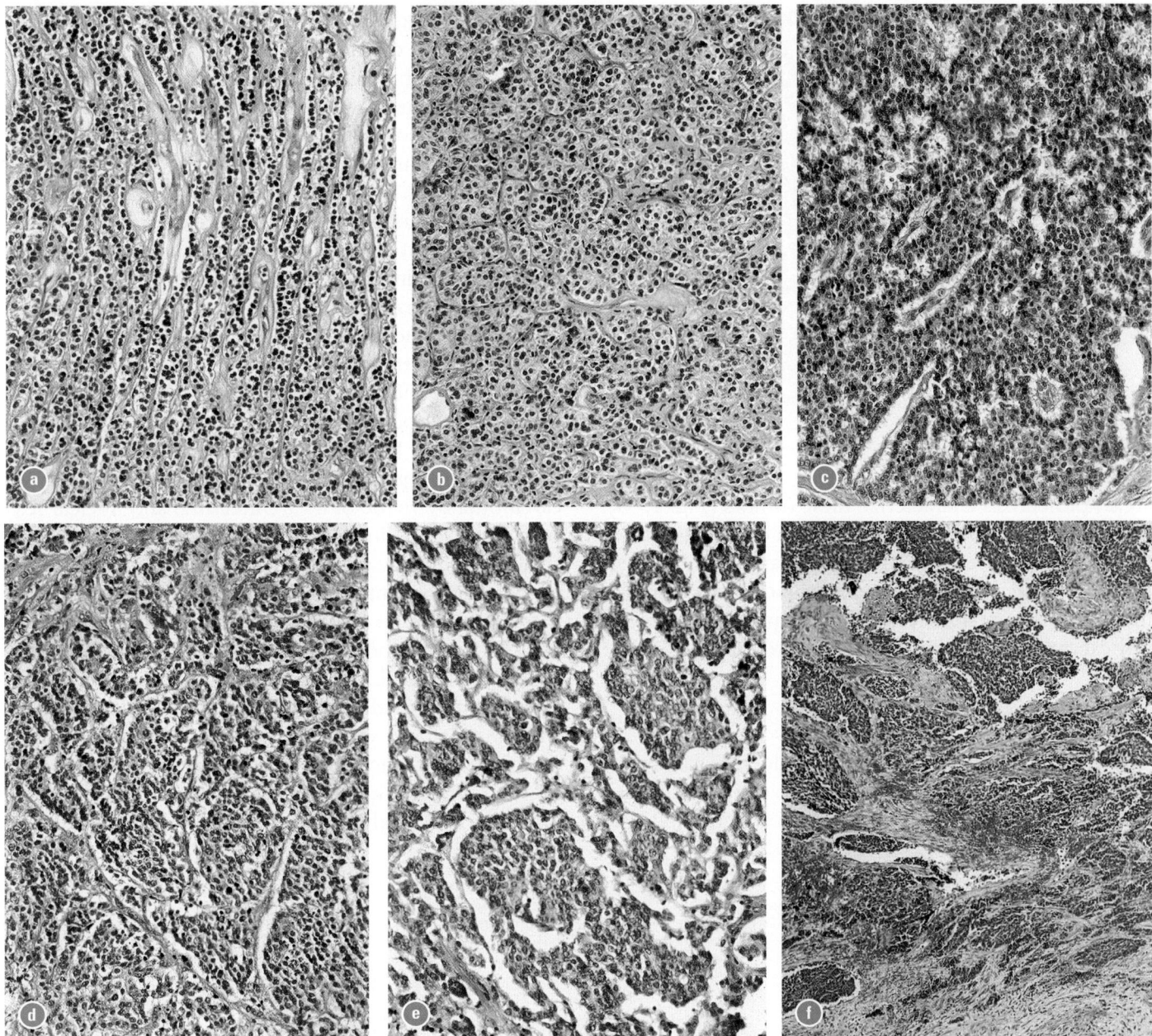

Fig. 15.1 Spectrum of neuroendocrine carcinomas of the cervix, beginning with (a) well-differentiated and terminating in (f) poorly-differentiated morphology.

prompt a consideration of neuroendocrine carcinoma (Fig. 15.7).[11] If the observer is unsure of the distinction, staining with neuroendocrine markers (chromogranin A, synaptophysin, neuron-specific enolase) is advised.

Small cell neuroendocrine carcinoma is morphologically similar to the classic oat cell carcinoma of the lung and demonstrates many of the following features: (1) uniform cell population, (2) hyperchromatic nuclei, (3) a high nuclear-to-cytoplasmic ratio (Fig. 15.4), (4) tumor cells arranged in irregular aggregates, often with little cohesion and (5) occasional rosettes or poorly defined acini. In addition, the nuclei contain coarse to opaque chromatin and, because there is little cytoplasm, they often appear to 'mold' with adjacent nuclei. These tumors may also extensively infiltrate the underlying cervical stroma.[12] Additional histologic features more commonly identified in poorly-differentiated neuroendocrine carcinoma versus squamous cell carcinoma include (1) vascular invasion (Fig. 15.5), observed in up to 90% of cases by Van Nagell et al. and in 78% of early stage lesions by Boruta et al., and (2) conspicuous lack of coexisting inflammation, in contrast to most cases of conventional squamous cell carcinoma.[4,13] Furthermore, by virtue of their rapid growth, broad zones (geographic

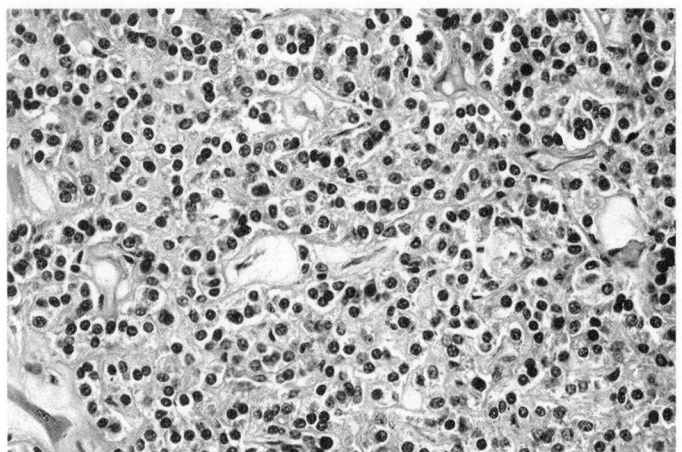

Fig. 15.2 Carcinoid. Organoid arrangement of cells with uniform nuclei, minimal hyperchromasia and low mitotic index.

areas) of necrosis characterize these tumors (Fig. 15.6). Large cell neuroendocrine carcinoma exhibits a similar picture, with a pseudo-trabecular arrangement of cells that have more abundant cytoplasm, large nuclei (similar in nuclear size to small cell non-keratinizing squamous cell carcinoma) and prominent nucleoli (Fig. 15.7).

DIFFERENTIAL DIAGNOSIS

The differential diagnosis of neuroendocrine carcinoma depends on its diagnostic subcategory. Carcinoid tumor must be distinguished from primary or metastatic ade-

nocarcinoma with microacinar architecture (Fig. 15.8a,b). Small and large cell neuroendocrine carcinoma are most easily confused with small cell non-keratinizing squamous cell carcinoma (Fig. 15.9), undifferentiated carcinoma, solid adenocarcinoma, peripheral neuroectodermal tumor, lymphoma or granulocytic sarcoma and melanoma (see below and Table 15.2). The absolute distinction of neuroendocrine carcinoma from some poorly-differentiated cervical carcinomas may be nearly impossible at times, owing to several factors: (1) many neuroendocrine carcinomas arise in association with squamous cell carcinoma or adenocarcinoma (Fig. 15.10a,b); (2) some growth patterns defy the distinction between glandular and neuroendocrine origin (Fig. 15.11); and (3) neuroendocrine carcinoma and other epithelial tumors cannot be distinguished by HPV type.[1–3,11,14]

The pathologist usually recognizes neuroendocrine carcinoma by virtue of its architectural and nuclear features. However, in difficult cases, immunoperoxidase studies to identify neuroendocrine differentiation may be helpful. The majority of neuroendocrine carcinomas in this group will be positive for chromogranin, synaptophysin or both (Fig. 15.12). However, no marker is absolutely reliable. One study compared seven neuroendocrine (small cell undifferentiated) carcinomas with 13 small cell squamous cell carcinomas and found that no single parameter would distinguish between the two, including chromogranin staining and testing for HPV-18.[2] Highly malignant behavior was found to

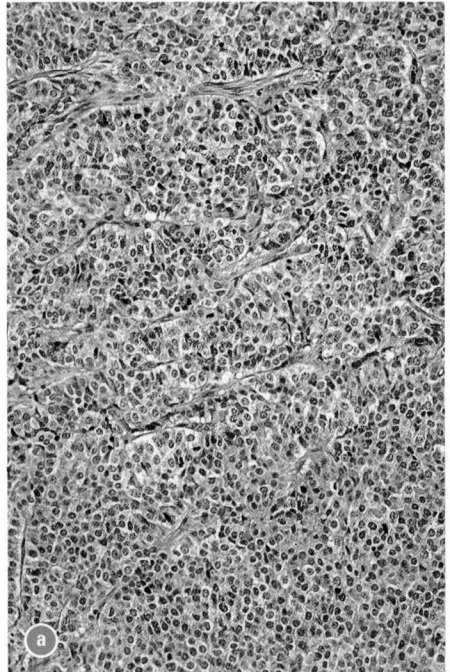

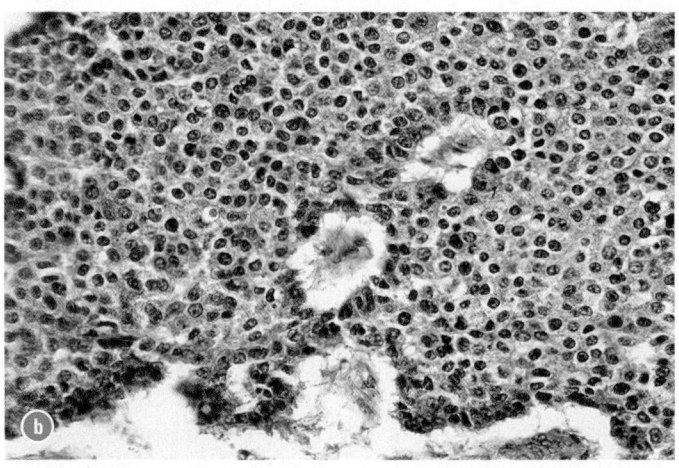

Fig. 15.3 Atypical carcinoid. (a) Greater degree of cellular crowding and increased mitotic index. (b) Nuclear hyperchromasia with variable chromatin coarseness.

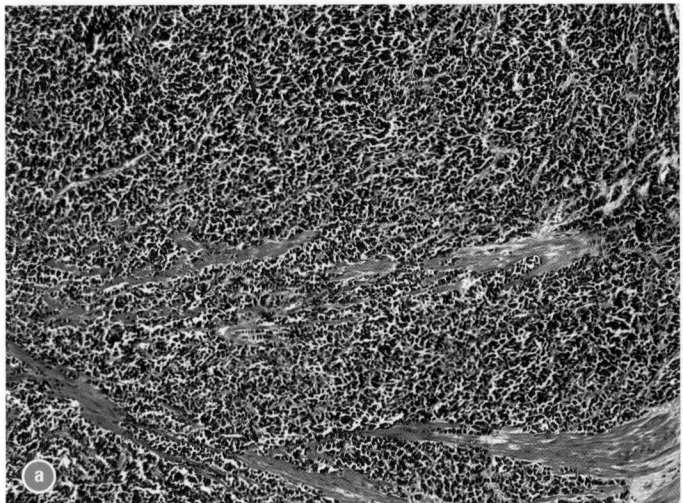
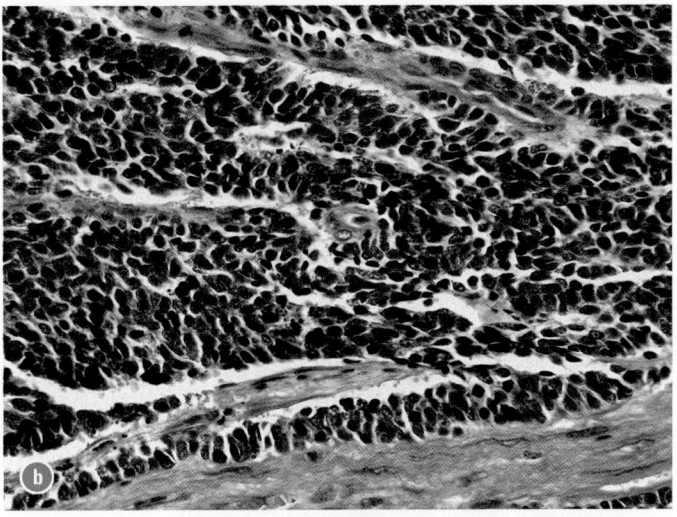
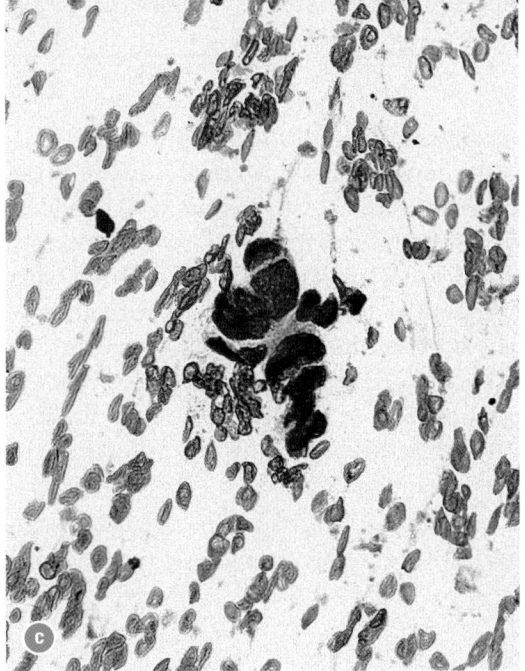

Fig. 15.4 (a) Small cell neuroendocrine carcinoma. The characteristic blue appearance reflects the high nuclear/cytoplasmic ratio and nuclear packing. (b) At higher power, streams of loosely aggregated tumor cells invade the stroma with minimal inflammatory response. (c) Tumor cells in a Papanicolaou smear exhibit the characteristic nuclear molding.

correlate most closely with the histologic pattern (neuroendocrine carcinoma versus small cell squamous) of the tumor. The presence of squamous intraepithelial neoplasia favors small cell squamous carcinoma, but may be associated with neuroendocrine carcinoma.[2,15]

Another study examined the utility of the p53 homolog p63 as a biomarker discriminating squamous from other forms of differentiation in cervical cancers. Some 97% of squamous, 0% of glandular and 0% of neuroendocrine tumors showed strong (>75% positivity) for p63. Transitions from squamous to columnar or undifferentiated morphology coincided with loss of p63 expression. Thus p63 may be useful for differentiating neuroendocrine carcinoma from squamous cell carcinoma, although it will not distinguish neuroendocrine carcinoma from glandular neoplasia. In most cases, these distinctions will be based on histologic features (Fig. 15.13).[3]

As a result of peptide hormone production, neuroendocrine carcinomas have the ability to induce certain clinical syndromes. The best known of these is the carcinoid syndrome, caused by the production of serotonin, but neoplasms of the cervix, like their counterparts elsewhere, may also produce adrenocorticotropic hormone (ACTH), insulin, parathyroid hormone and other substances.[16,17]

The origin of neuroendocrine carcinoma is unclear. As previously mentioned, large and small cell neuroen-

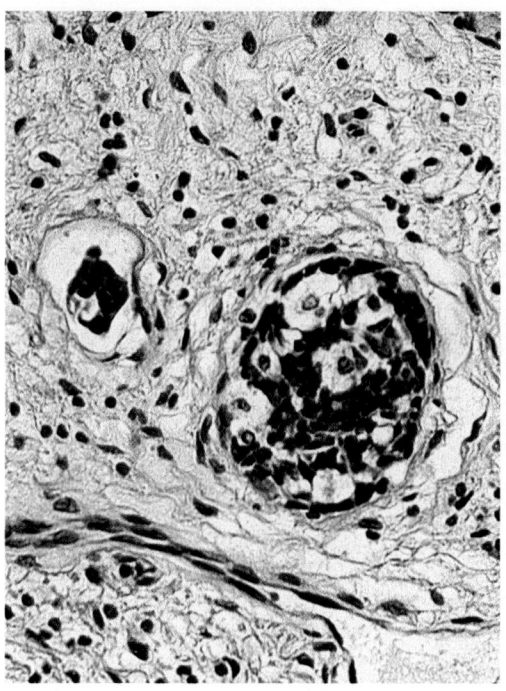

Fig. 15.5 Vascular invasion in neuroendocrine carcinoma. Note the minimal associated inflammation.

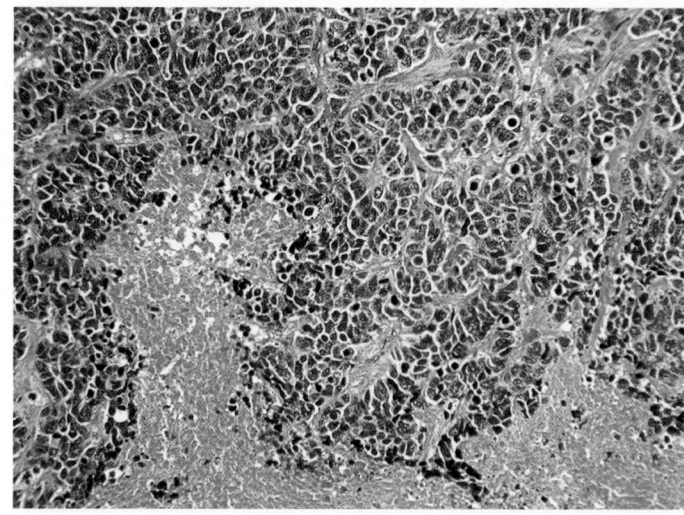

Fig. 15.6 Geographic necrosis in a poorly-differentiated neuroendocrine carcinoma.

docrine carcinomas of the cervix are often observed in association with conventional neoplasms, including adenocarcinoma in situ, invasive adenocarcinoma, cervical intraepithelial neoplasia and conventional squamous cell carcinoma.[2,3,15] Rare reports of neuroendocrine hyperplasias associated with these carcinomas suggest that neuroendocrine differentiation may have preceded cancer; however, in most instances the neuroendocrine phenotype emerges concurrent with or following invasion.[18] Recently, studies of archival tissue have revealed small cell undifferentiated carcinomas to be strongly associated with HPV-18 nucleic acids. Combined with the relatively higher association of HPV-18 with adenocarcinoma of the cervix, this information suggests that this type of HPV may have a propensity to infect a pluripotential population of basal/reserve cells susceptible to shifts in differentiation following infection.[1–3]

Fig. 15.7 Large cell neuroendocrine carcinoma.

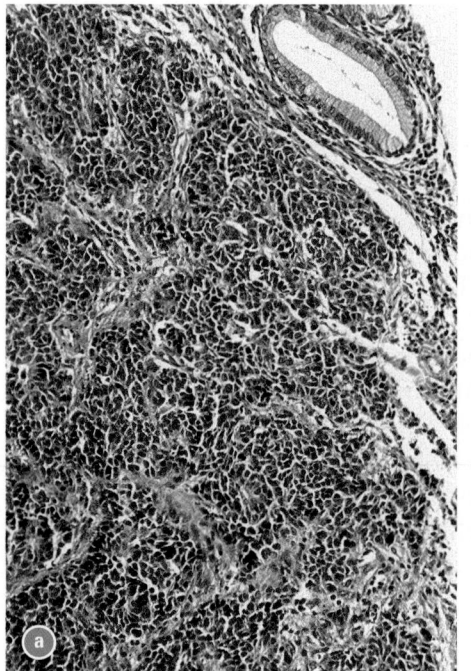

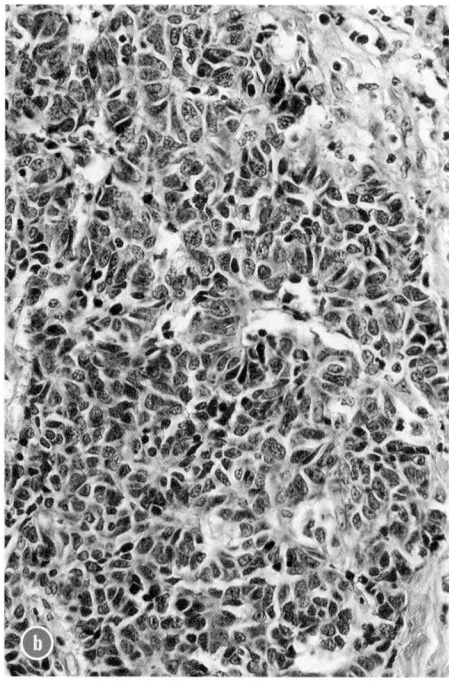

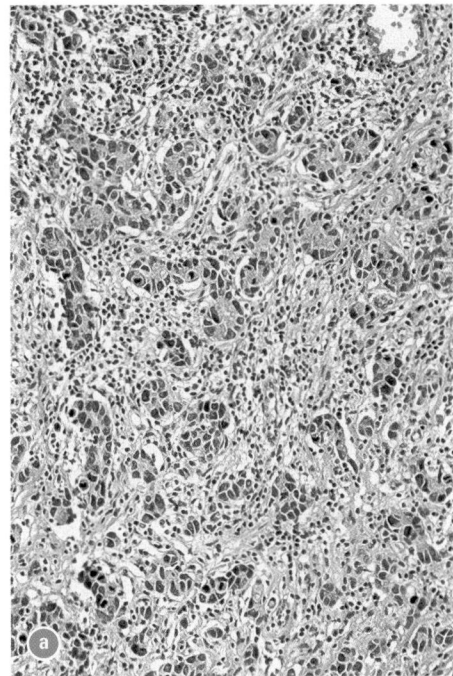
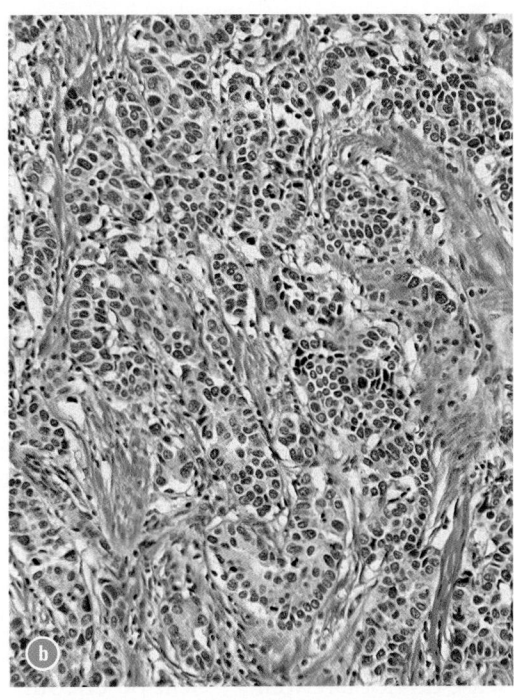

Fig. 15.8 (a) Small tubules in a metastatic adenocarcinoma mimic neuroendocrine carcinoma. (b) A primary adenocarcinoma forming small tubules with uniform nuclei.

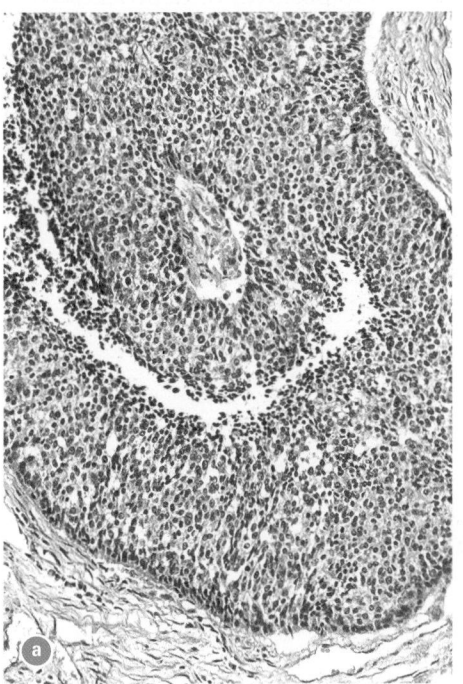
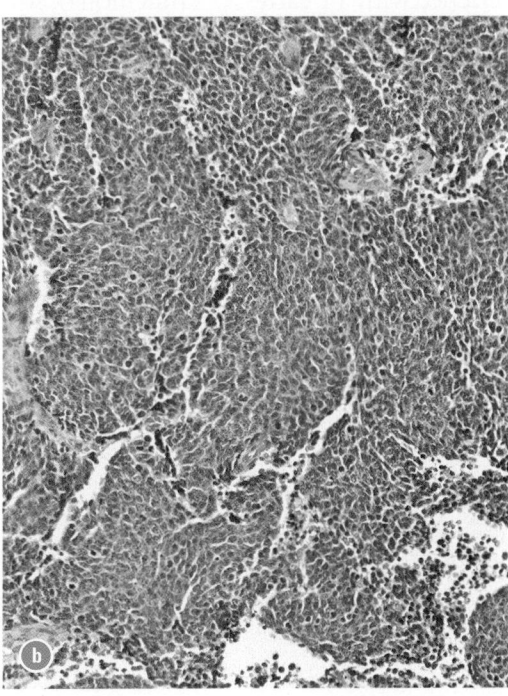

Fig. 15.9 Neuroendocrine carcinoma versus small cell squamous carcinoma. (a) Small cell squamous carcinoma with discrete nesting pattern and preserved polarity. (b) Neuroendocrine carcinoma with more haphazard nesting pattern, showing numerous randomly arranged fracture lines due to poor cohesion and disorganized growth.

MANAGEMENT AND OUTCOME

Neuroendocrine carcinomas have a poor prognosis, although each study contains a few exceptions (Table 15.3).[13,19,20] Over half are stage II or higher when diagnosed, irrespective of the degree of differentiation.[19,21,22] Distant metastases are most frequently to the liver, lung and brain.[19] Current management is similar to that of neuroendocrine carcinoma of the lung, using radiation with a combination of one or more chemotherapeutic agents.[21] Despite aggressive therapy, outcome of patients with neuroendocrine carcinoma is still poor. Delaloge et al. followed 10 patients who were variously treated with surgery, radiation and chemotherapy; eight relapsed within 16 months and one was alive without disease over 4 years later.[20] Weed et al. reviewed 15 patients, of whom 13 died with a median survival of 22 months

Table 15.2 *Histochemical distinction of small cell or undifferentiated tumors of the cervix*

Diagnosis	Immunohistochemistry
Neuroendocrine carcinoma	p63+/−, chromogranin (+), synaptophysin (+)
Small cell non-keratinizing squamous CA	p63 (++), chromogranin (−)
Basaloid carcinoma	p63 (++), chromogranin (−)
Peripheral neuroectodermal tumor	O13 (p30/32MIC2) (+)
Lymphoma	LCA, cd20(L26), cd3 (+)
Granulocytic sarcoma (AML)	Lysozyme, chloracetate esterase (+)
Melanoma	HMB-45, S-100 (+)
Embryonal rhabdomyosarcoma	Myoglobin, myf-4 (+)

and one was alive at nearly 8 years. Other case reports describe long-term survivors treated aggressively with radiation and chemotherapy.[21,23]

Even patients with early stage disease do not fare well. Boruta et al. summarized their experience with 11 early-stage (IB-IIA) neuroendocrine carcinomas and performed a meta-analysis of 23 similar staged cases in the literature.[13] They reported a 2-year survival of 38%. In their study, lymph node metastases (present in 78% of patients) were significantly associated with poor outcome and chemotherapy (VAC or PE) was significantly associated with improved outcome.[13] More

well-differentiated variants, such as carcinoid, have a similarly poor outcome, although the numbers are too small to provide a precise comparison with other neuroendocrine carcinomas.[19,24–26]

Undifferentiated carcinoma

Undifferentiated carcinoma includes both those that can be histochemically linked to a specific line of differentiation and those that are unclassifiable, even by histochemical methods. Lymphoepithelial-like (squamous), glassy cell (columnar) and spindle cell squamous carcinomas are examples of poorly-differentiated tumors whose origins can be confirmed histochemically. Other poorly-differentiated tumors (e.g. transitional carcinoma) are difficult to link to a specific line of differentiation, but are placed in the squamous group by default. Occasionally, both intraepithelial and invasive neoplasms will be encountered that do not exhibit columnar cell (mucinous), squamous (p63 positive) or neuroendocrine (chromogranin-positive) differentiation (Fig. 15.14). The cases that we have seen in this group have typically been associated with mixed precursor lesions, including stratified mucin-producing intraepithelial lesions (SMILE) and may form discrete nests with loosely arranged tumors cells or papillary structures lined by undifferentiated carcinoma.[3,27]

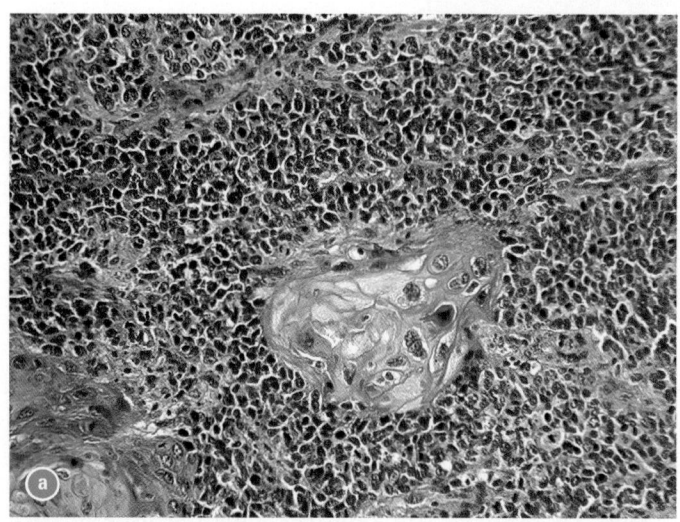

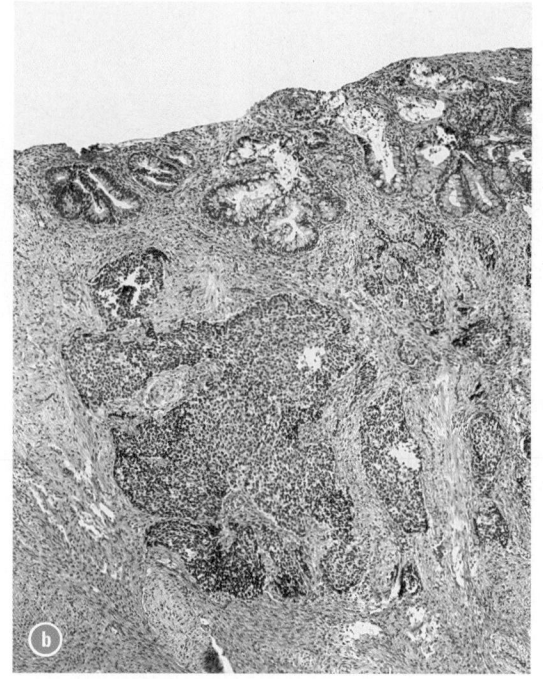

Fig. 15.10 (a) Squamous differentiation in the center of a poorly-differentiated neuroendocrine carcinoma. (b) Adenocarcinoma in situ (upper) merging with neuroendocrine carcinoma (lower).

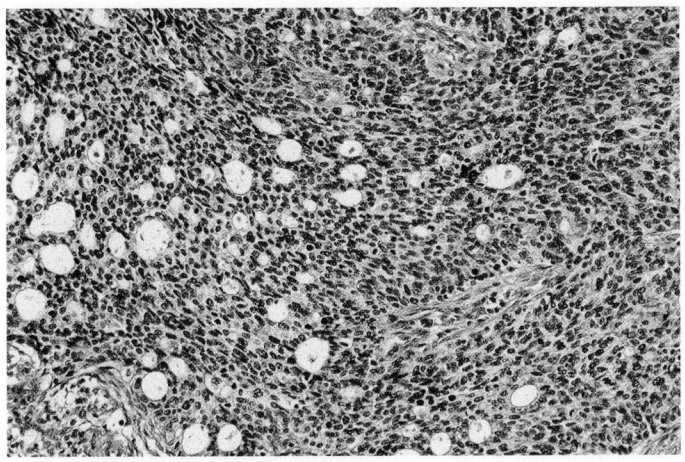

Fig. 15.11 Poorly-differentiated carcinoma with features of both adenocarcinoma and neuroendocrine carcinoma.

Mixed epithelial/mesenchymal neoplasms

ENDOCERVICAL POLYP

Clinical presentation

Endocervical polyps are common and occur over a wide age range, with a mean in the fifth decade (Table 15.4).[28,29] The polyps typically arise within or above the cervical os and range from a few mm to 4 cm in size (with an average of 1 cm). Some polyps occur at the endocervical–lower uterine segment junction and harbor both endometrioid (or tubal) and endocervical epithelium. These are variously termed lower uterine segment polyps or mixed endocervical/endometrial polyps.

Endocervical polyps are clinically relevant because approximately 40% are symptomatic and often present with bleeding.[29] Given the high frequency of association with menopause, symptomatic polyps require an additional endometrial sampling to exclude an endometrial origin or coincident endometrial pathology.[29–33] However, in one large study of over 300 patients, Golan et al. identified malignancy in less than 1% and only in the group that presented with symptoms.[29] Some authors have speculated that unopposed estrogen associated with menopause is responsible for endocervical polyps, but there is no conclusive evidence to support this theory.[29]

Histopathology

The majority of endocervical polyps identified clinically are confirmed histologically (Table 15.4). Endocervical polyps exhibit a wide range of morphologic features reflecting the mixture of glands and stroma with variable predominance of either, including: (1) polypoid microglandular hyperplasia in which the epithelium is the predominant component (Fig. 15.15a); (2) typical epithelial/stromal polyps (Fig. 15.15b); (3) predominately stromal polyps, sometimes with atypical stromal cells, similar to those seen more commonly in the vagina (Fig. 15.15c,d); and (4) polyps with atypical features, defined as hypercellular stroma and irregular gland architecture, but not fulfilling the criteria for adenosarcoma (Fig. 15.16). Rare reports of hamartomatous polyps containing benign cartilage have also been described.[34]

Differential diagnosis

The clinical differential diagnosis on gross examination of a cervical polypoid growth includes prolapsed

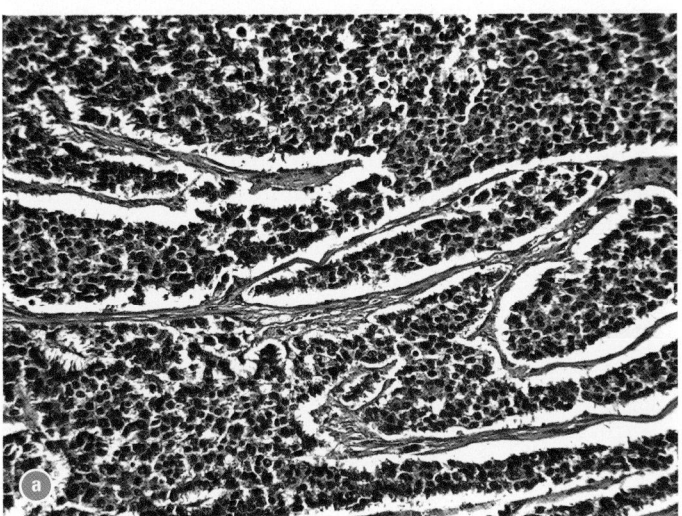

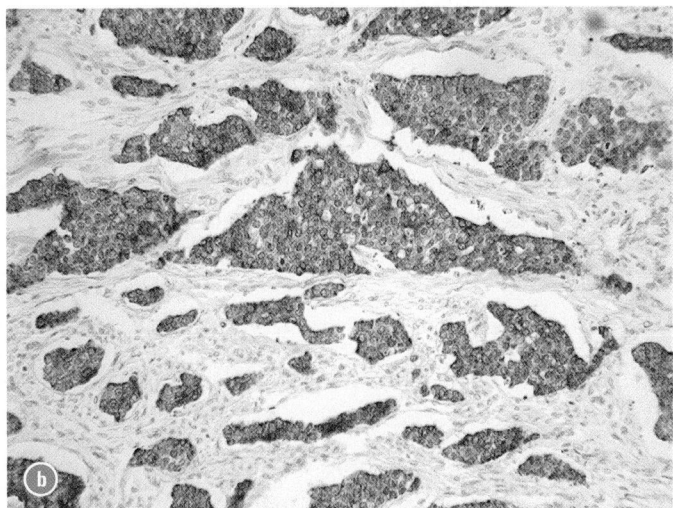

Fig. 15.12 (a) Moderately-differentiated neuroendocrine carcinoma. (b) Chromogranin positivity.

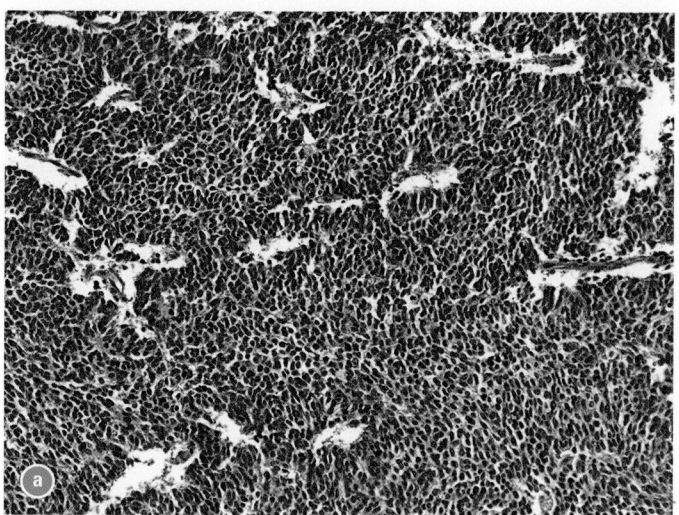 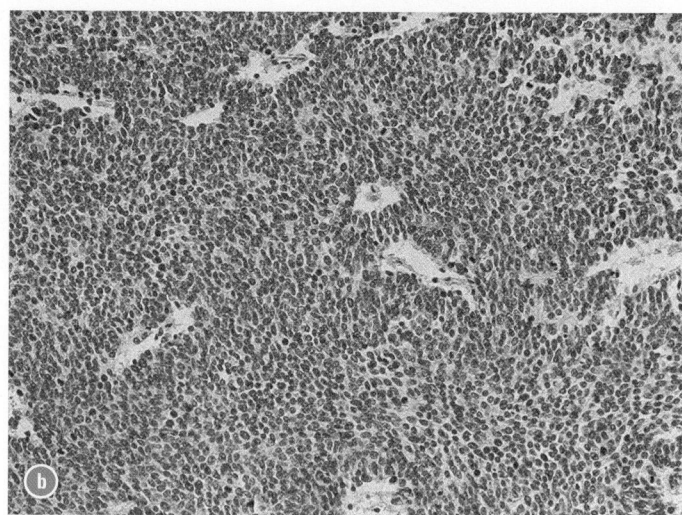

Fig. 15.13 (a) Poorly-differentiated neuroendocrine carcinoma. (b) These tumors are typically negative or weakly positive for p63, as in this case.

endometrial or endocervical submucosal leiomyoma, adenomyoma, adenosarcoma and other malignancies (Table 15.5). Adenosarcoma should be suspected if polyps recur following removal (Figs 15.15,15.16). However, 10–20% of benign polyps will also recur.[34] Very large polyps invariably raise the suspicion of malignancy (sarcoma, adenosarcoma, etc.); however, in a literature survey of extremely large polyps (10–17 cm in diameter), none were malignant.[35] Moreover, reports of adenosarcoma initially misdiagnosed as a benign polyp have not recorded large size as a presenting feature (see below).[36] In general, with the exception of a subtle adenosarcoma, most other polypoid lesions can be distinguished from benign endocervical polyps.

Management

Management of endocervical polyps consists of removal. In patients who are symptomatic (most commonly abnormal bleeding), concurrent endometrial sampling should be performed to exclude concomitant endometrial polyps or other pathology.[29,32] There is no universal agreement that polyps found incidentally require any action other than outpatient (if possible) removal.[29]

ADENOMYOMA AND POLYPOID ADENOMYOMA OF THE ENDOCERVICAL TYPE

Adenomyomas and polypoid adenomyomas are much more common in the uterine corpus, but reports have characterized cases originating in the cervix.[37–40] In

one study of 10 cases, the patients had a mean age of 40 years and the tumors were either polypoid or mural-based cervical masses; one in the latter category was 23 cm wide.[37] The stroma of cervical adenomyoma is predominantly composed of smooth muscle. The admixed glands, which are lined by benign-appearing endocervical cells, are cystic or irregularly shaped, exhibit a somewhat lobular growth pattern and are devoid of stromal reaction (Fig. 15.17a,b). When cervical adenomyoma presents as a mural-based mass, the principal differential diagnosis is with minimal deviation adenocarcinoma (adenoma malignum), because both tumors may exhibit similarly shaped irregular glands lined by bland mucinous epithelium. Distinction between the two is made on the well-circumscribed nature of the former. In addition, lack of a desmoplastic stromal reaction and atypical cytologic features, which is seen at least focally in all cases of adenoma malignum, help differentiate between the two entities. In curettage specimens, the well-circumscribed nature of cervical adenomyoma may not be appreciated and the combination of glands and smooth muscle stroma may suggest invasion if one is not alert to the possibility of adenomyoma.[37–40]

Table 15.3 Presenting stage and survival of neuroendocrine carcinoma

Author	n	I	II	III	IV	Comment
Boruta[13]	34	IB or IIA				38% 2-year survival
Weed[19]	15	5	3	1	6	13/15 died, 1 alive at 80 months
Delaloge[20]	10	6	1	1	2	8/10 relapsed 16 months

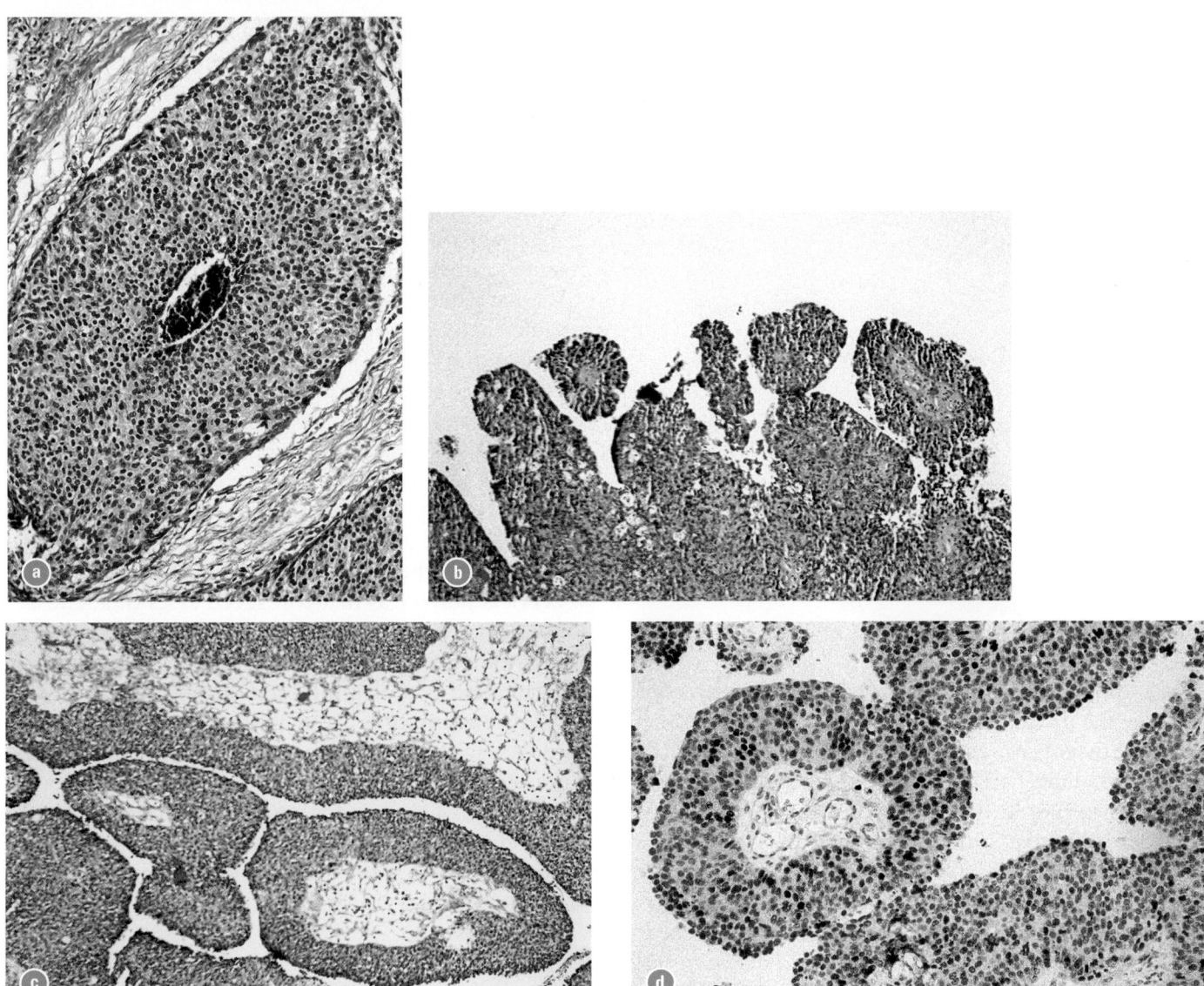

Fig. 15.14 Poorly-differentiated non-neuroendocrine carcinomas. (a) Nests of p63-negative poorly-differentiated carcinoma associated with an adenosquamous carcinoma in situ. (b) Undifferentiated papillary carcinoma associated with an adenocarcinoma. (c) Undifferentiated papillary carcinoma of the cervix (HPV-18 positive). (d) Note the variable p63 staining.

CERVICAL ADENOSARCOMA

Background and clinical presentation

Adenosarcoma is a biphasic tumor composed of a malignant stromal component and a benign epithelial component. Primary cervical adenosarcoma is extremely rare, accounting for a minority (2%) of those that occur in the genital tract (uterine > ovarian/pelvic > cervix) and with fewer than three dozen reports in the English literature.[41-48] The largest series of primary cervical adenosarcomas was published by Jones and Lefkowitz.[48] In their study of 12 cases and a review of an additional 12 from the literature, the average age was 31 years (range 11–65 years) with one-third under age 15 and tumor size varied from 1.0 to 4.5 cm. The majority of the cases personally reviewed (58%) presented with abnormal vaginal bleeding. A polypoid or papillary lesion, often clinically simulating a benign cervical polyp protruding through the cervical os, is one of the more typical clinical presentations.

Histopathology

Cervical adenosarcoma is characterized by the following features: (1) irregularly shaped glands with prominent branching often likened to the pattern seen in cystosarcoma phyllodes of the breast (Fig. 15.18a,b), (2) a

Table 15.4 Clinicopathologic features of endocervical polyps (from Golan et al.[29])

Peak incidence	Fifth decade
Clinical presentation (%)	
Symptomatic	40
Postmenopausal bleeding	30
Postcoital bleeding	12.5
Vaginal discharge	17.5
Size (diameter, mm)	
Range	3–40
Mean	10
Histologic outcome (%)	
Polyp confirmed	84.7
Nabothian cyst	4.3
Leiomyoma	1.2
Endometrial polyp	0.3
Endometrial findings (%)	
Cyclic/atrophic	58.2
Anovulatory	12.4
Endometrial polyp	4.4
Atypical hyperplasia	1.9
Adenocarcinoma	0.8
Other (insufficient findings, etc.)	22.3

periglandular cellular stroma that is discrete and conforms to the gland lining (Fig. 15.18a,b), (3) stromal mitotic activity, (4) variable stromal cell atypia and (5) lining epithelium that often, but not invariably, shows altered differentiation most often as ciliated or endometrioid-type epithelium (Fig. 15.18c). A range of stromal cell atypia and mitotic activity may be seen; at least two mitotic figures are usually stated to be present, although in most cases the mitotic index exceeds 4 per 10 high power fields (Fig. 15.18d). Heterologous elements, including cartilage and striated muscle differentiation, may also be present.[36,44,48]

Differential diagnosis

The differential diagnosis includes (1) adenosarcoma arising in endometriosis or in the endometrium, with secondary involvement of the cervix,[47] (2) atypical endocervical polyp, (3) adenomyoma of the cervix, (4) prolapsed fibroid with reactive stromal changes and (5) rare spindle cell carcinomas that exhibit periglandular condensation. Adenosarcoma of the uterus must always be excluded and the process of exclusion entails hysterectomy or carefully executed fractional curettage. Atypical polyps are the most difficult group because they may contain unusual stroma and irregular gland outlines. Careful attention to stromal atypia and mitoses is critical in distinguishing these lesions from adenosarcoma. Adenomyomas should not be confused with adenosarcoma due to its well-defined myomatous stroma.

Occasionally, endometrial submucosal leiomyomata may prolapse through the cervical os with surface ulceration leading to increased stromal cellularity and vascularity. These histologic features may mimic adenosarcoma or endometrial stromal sarcoma;[49] attention to this possibility as well as immunostains for h-caldesmon, desmin and CD10 will help in distinguishing the origin of these lesions as myomatous (caldesmon and desmin positive) rather than a stromal (CD10 positive) origin.

We have encountered rare examples of spindle cell squamous carcinomas of the cervix that were distributed in an unusual periglandular growth pattern, giving the impression of an adenosarcoma. However, the periglandular 'stroma' was strongly cytokeratin- and p63-positive and was associated with a conventional squamous cell carcinoma (Fig. 15.19).

Adenosarcoma of either endometrial or endocervical origin may present as cervical polyps (Figs 15.18, 15.20). Kerner and Lichtig reported that an initial diagnosis of cervical polyp was made in seven cases of adenosarcoma prior to histologic evaluation.[36] In contrast to benign endocervical polyps, adenosarcoma exhibits the characteristic irregular, infolded or slit-like glands with stromal condensation. In small samples, however, these features may not be conspicuous. The confusion of endocervical polyp with adenosarcoma (and vice versa) is almost a rite of passage for young pathologists, because the latter may be both subtle and/or partially sampled. Suffice it to say that any endocervical polyp with cellular stroma or irregular glands should prompt a re-evaluation.

Management and outcome

Most adenosarcomas are managed with hysterectomy and close clinical follow-up, but are occasionally highly malignant.[50,51] Jones and Lefkowitz reported two deaths and two persistent/recurrent tumors in 23 women with follow-up;[48] outcome was linked to depth of invasion into the uterine wall.[50,51] The wisdom of local excision is unclear given the small number of cases and the need to exclude myometrial invasion. However, this approach may be appropriate if the tumor originates from a narrow stalk and the site of excision can be sampled and monitored to exclude residual disease. Salpingo-oophorectomy is generally recommended; however, there is insufficient evidence to support or discourage ovarian conservation.[50]

CARCINOSARCOMA

Background and clinical presentation

Carcinosarcomas of the cervix are rare, with less than 50 cases reported in the world literature. A significant

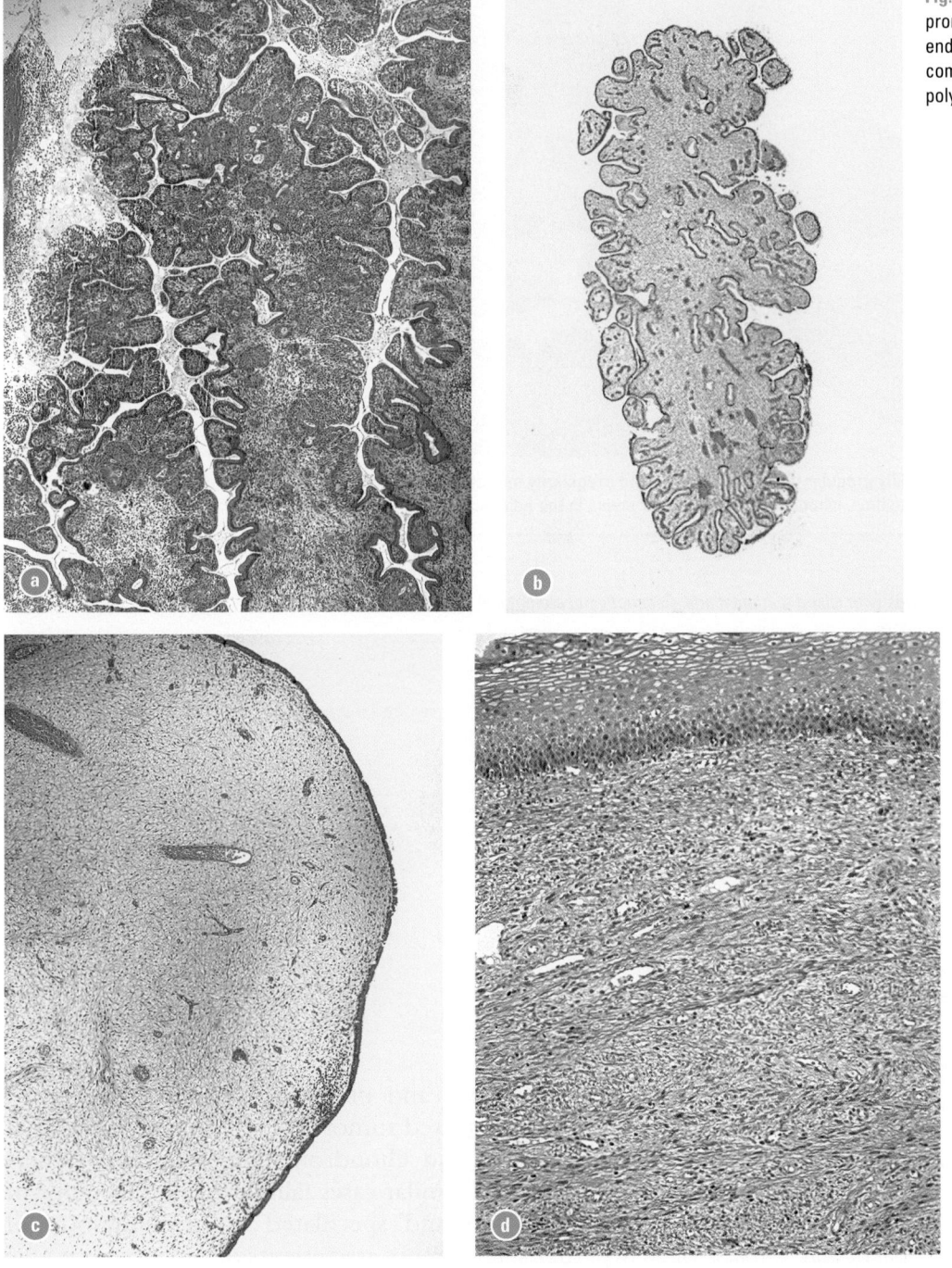

Fig. 15.15 (a) Endocervical polyp with prominent microglandular changes. (b) Typical endocervical polyp. (c) Endocervical polyp composed principally of stroma (stromal polyp). (d) Mild stromal atypia.

subset of these tumors shares distinctive characteristics with adenoid basal carcinoma: (1) they are often associated with human papillomaviruses, (2) they predominate in older women (mean age seventh decade) and (3) both frequently share basaloid epithelial components. There is little data on ethnicity; however, in one study, seven of eight patients were black.[52–57] For other less common forms of carcinosarcoma, including those containing endometrioid and mesonephric histology, the HPV status is doubtful or unknown.[58–62]

Histopathology

Cervical tumors exhibiting mixed epithelial and mesenchymal features fall into at least four categories (Table 15.5). (1) Spindle cell (sarcomatoid) squamous cell carcinomas, discussed previously (Fig. 15.21) are

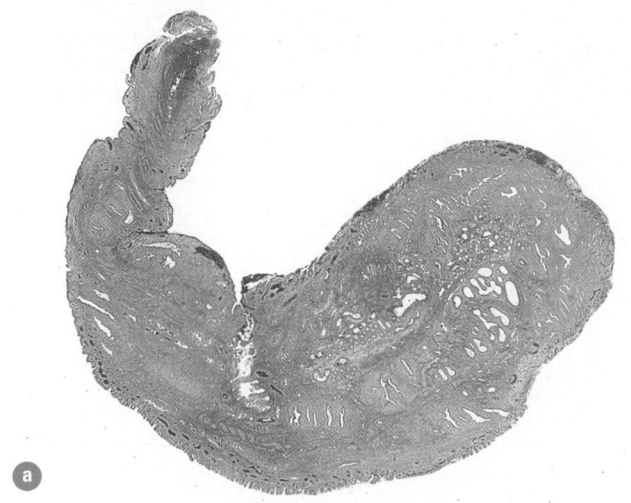
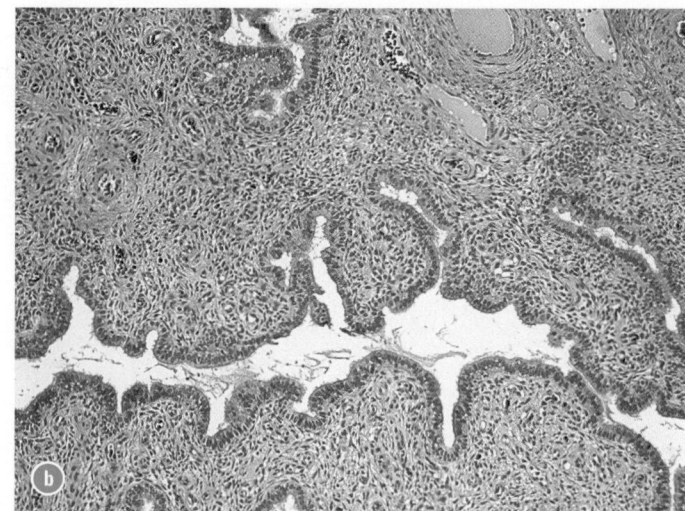

Fig. 15.16 (a) Atypical endocervical polyp with mildly irregular glands. (b) Slight gland irregularity may suggest adenosarcoma. The distinction from the latter requires attention to periglandular stromal accentuation, mitotic index and nuclear atypia in the adjacent stroma.

Table 15.5 *Classification of cervical malignancies with mixed epithelial and mesenchymal phenotype*

Diagnosis	Precursor	Epithelium	Mesenchymal diff.	HPV
Spindle cell SCC	HSIL	LCNK	Spindle cell carcinoma	Positive
Carcinosarcoma				
Cervix specific	HSIL/ACIS, Adenoid basal*	Basaloid/adenoid cyst	Stromal sarcoma	Positive
MMMT	None known	Endometrioid	Variable	UK
Mesonephric carcinoma	Hyperplasia	Mesonephric	Spindle, other	Negative
Wilm's tumor	None known	Tubular	Blastema, cartilage	UK

LCNK, large cell non-keratinizing squamous carcinoma; HSIL, high-grade squamous intraepithelial lesion; ACIS, adenocarcinoma in situ; MMMT, malignant mixed Müllerian tumor; SSC, squamous cell carcinoma
*Rare carcinosarcomas, specifically those associated with basaloid morphology, are associated with or preceded by adenoid basal carcinomas. UK, unknown.

tumors that are not classified as carcinosarcomas but are likely to be confused with the latter and are included for the purpose of comparison. (2) Tumors with basaloid, adenoid basal and adenoid cystic features associated with a sarcoma, usually a nondescript spindle cell sarcomatous component (Fig. 15.22) are a particular subset of carcinosarcoma that has been best characterized as a distinct entity and is closely associated with HPV.[52–57] (3) Conventional carcinosarcoma with endometrioid glandular morphology and a more diverse pattern of stromal differentiation, including rhabdomyosarcomatous and chondroid elements (Fig. 15.23)[53] may be indistinguishable from their endometrial counterpart. (4) Mesonephric tumors with spindle cell or other forms of mesenchymal differentiation (Fig. 15.24a): concerning this latter group, Clement et al. identified four mesonephric carcinomas with a malignant spindle cell component and proposed the term 'malignant mesonephric mixed tumor'.[58] Included were one each with osteoid and chondroid differentiation. Others have reported similar cases falling within this range of differentiation and speculated on the question of whether such tumors are variants of carcinoma or true carcinosarcomas, without resolving this issue.[59–62] In either case, these patterns can be particularly confusing if the characteristic well-differentiated mesonephric remnants are not identified.[58] (5) Variants of Wilms' tumor, which have been reported in both the cervix and endometrium. Whether these tumors can be distinguished from the above is questionable. However, they are mentioned because variants of these tumors have been specifically reported and some have responded to Wilms' specific chemotherapy (Fig. 15.24b).[63–65]

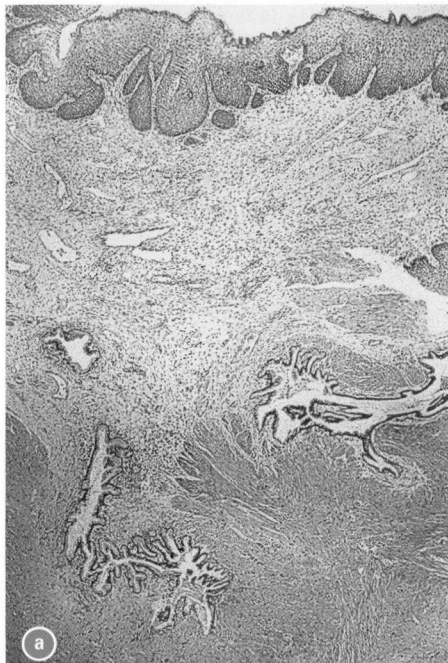
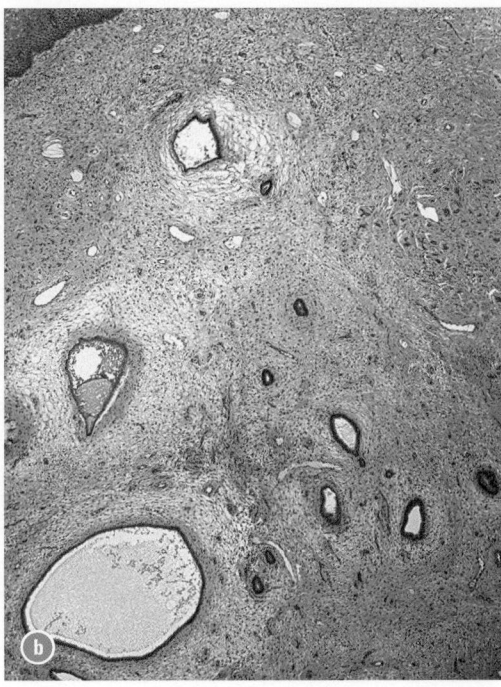

Fig. 15.17 (a,b) Adenomyomas, containing irregular admixture of glands and myomatous stroma.

Differential diagnosis

The distinction of the above entities is outlined in Table 15.5. Other tumors most likely to be confused with carcinosarcoma include: (1) spindle cell carcinomas, which are devoid of glandular and basaloid morphology and show a transition from conventional squamous to a spindle cell component, unusual for a carcinosarcoma as defined above; (2) adenosarcomas, which exhibit a mixture of benign appearing glands and a neoplastic stromal component, but are easily separated by virtue of their benign glandular features; and (3) carcinosarcoma metastatic from the corpus or ovary, which is the most likely mimic of a primary cervical carcinosarcoma. The latter must always be excluded in cases of cervical carcinosarcomas that contain classic endometrioid glandular morphology.

Management and outcome

The majority of patients with carcinosarcoma reviewed by Clement et al. (14 of 16) were stage IB. Of 22 patients (staged and unstaged), with some follow-up in their series, 12 either died of or were alive with disease. The majority are treated with surgery, with or without adjunctive radiotherapy. The value of supplemental chemotherapy is unknown.

Mesenchymal neoplasms

The tumors in this section comprise the bulk of sarcoma categories reported in the literature. The following discussion omits embryonal rhabdomyosarcoma, which is addressed in Chapters 1 and 9. However, rhabdomyosarcoma is discussed in the differential diagnosis of mesenchymal lesions of the cervix (Table 15.6).

ENDOMETRIAL STROMAL SARCOMA

The cervix is frequently the site of endometriosis, most commonly consisting of a variable mixture of endometrial-type glands and stroma (see Ch. 14). However, stromal sarcomas are rarely reported in this site.[66] The diagnosis is based on the cardinal features of any stromal sarcoma, including a uniform population of spindled tumor cells, limited fascicular organization and the characteristic uniformly distributed network of small vessels. Immunostaining with antibodies to CD-10 is a useful adjunct, albeit of questionable specificity. When stromal sarcoma is suspected, benign gland-poor endometriosis (stromatosis, see below), leiomyosarcoma and reactive stromal changes must be excluded (Fig. 15.25).

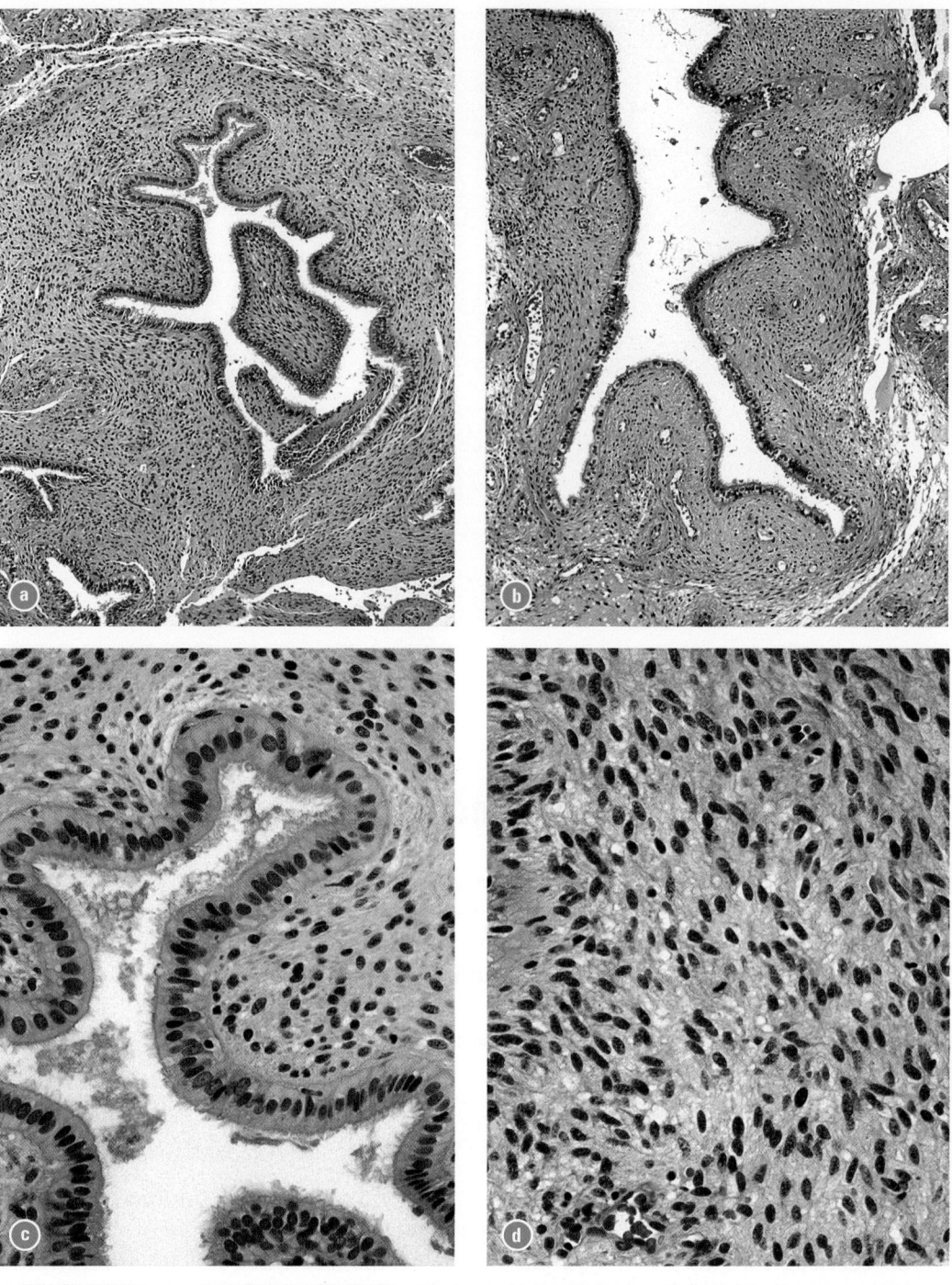

Fig. 15.18 Adenosarcoma of the endocervix. (a,b) Irregular branching glands with stromal cuffing. (c) Tubal metaplasia of the lining epithelium is common. (d) Stromal mitoses (center) confirm the diagnosis in the presence of the above findings.

ALVEOLAR SOFT-PART SARCOMA

Alveolar soft-part sarcoma is a rare tumor of uncertain histogenesis that usually involves the extremities, trunk and the head and neck region. A small number of cases have been described in the reproductive tract, including cervix.[67–73] In the study by Nielsen et al., the age distribution is typically in the reproductive years, ranging from 14–38 years (mean 29).[69]

Histologically, the tumor is composed of sheets of cells with abundant granular eosinophilic cytoplasm arranged in solid nests with well-defined delicate fibrovascular septa. Alternatively, the tumor cells within the nests may be less cohesive and line the septa in an alveolar pattern, hence the name. The tumor cells contain characteristic PAS-positive diastase resistant granules, which correspond to dense

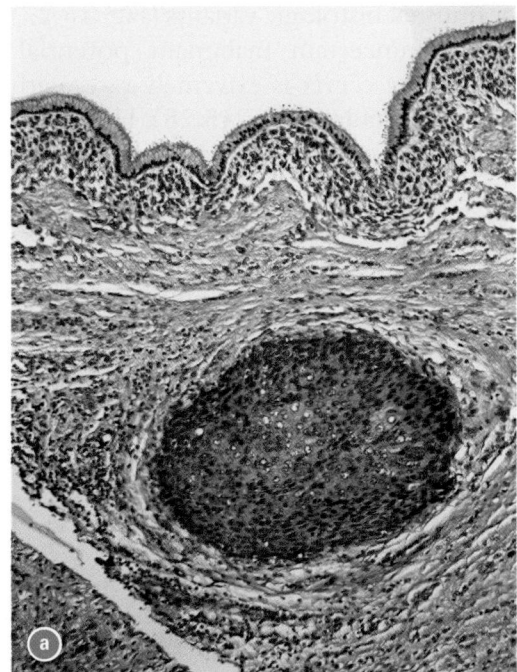 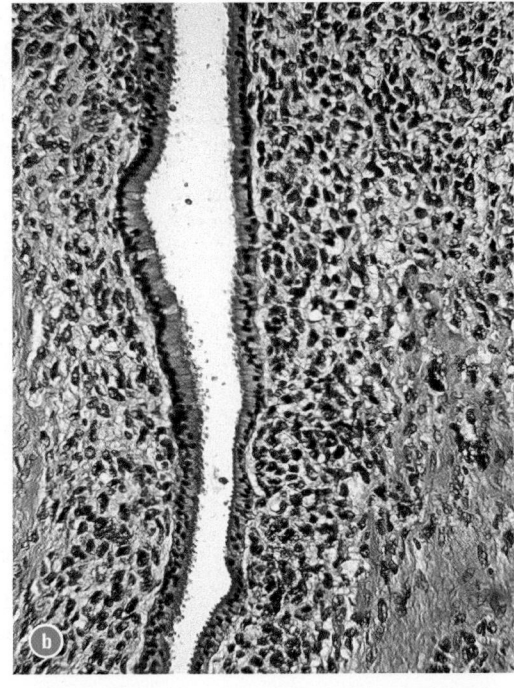

Fig. 15.19 (a) Unusual presentation of spindle cell squamous carcinoma with periglandular (reserve-cell-like) distribution (upper) associated with conventional squamous differentiation (lower). (b) At higher magnification, the periglandular cuffing mimics adenosarcoma.

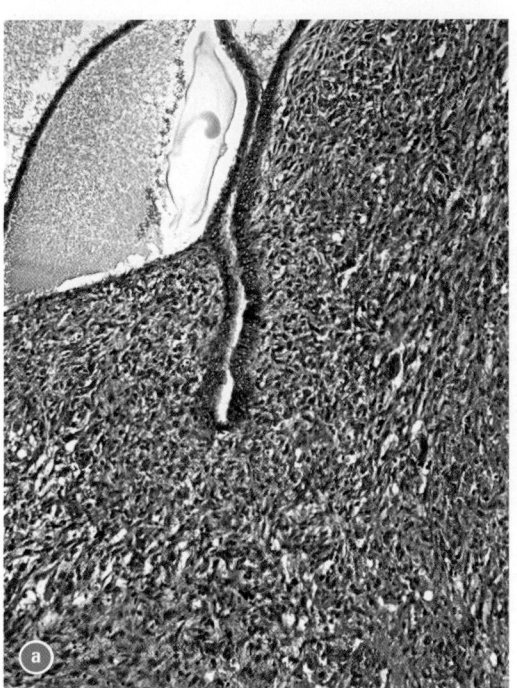 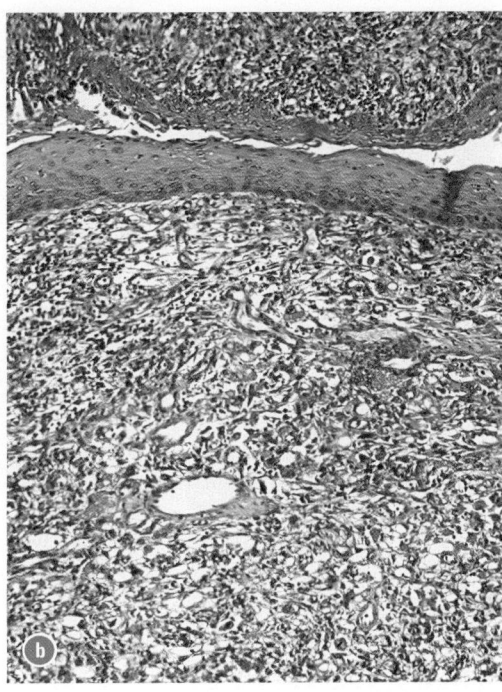

Fig. 15.20 (a,b) Higher-grade adenosarcoma beneath columnar and squamous epithelium.

membrane-bound granules on ultrastructural analysis (Fig. 15.26).[67–73]

The prognosis in genital tract alveolar soft-part sarcoma is good relative to other sites, where 2, 5 and 10-year survivals are 77, 60 and 38%, respectively.[68,69,74] In the series by Nielsen et al.,[69] eight of nine patients were alive over an average follow-up of 5.2 years.[69] However, late recurrences beyond the 5- and 10-year follow-up interval are not uncommon and long-term expectations in individual cases must take this into account.[74]

SMOOTH MUSCLE TUMORS

Leiomyomas are relatively common in the cervix and are usually easily recognized. Three problematic scenarios include: (1) ulceration with superficial necrosis, (2) cel-

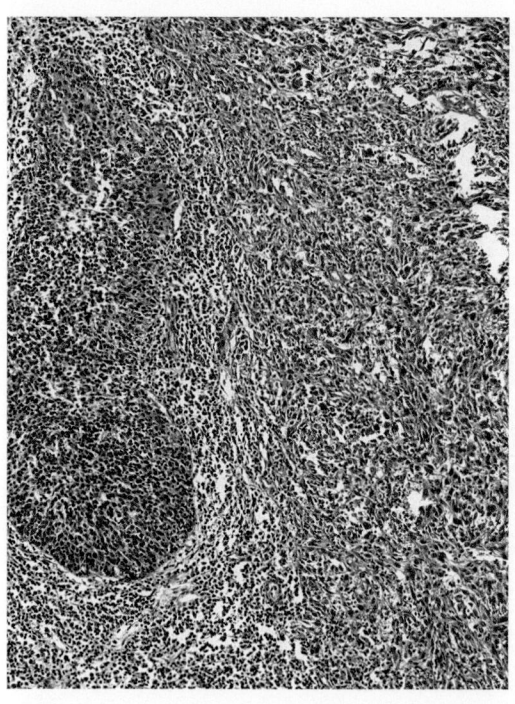

Fig. 15.21 Spindle cell carcinoma, juxtaposing conventional large cell non-keratinizing (left) carcinoma and spindle cell morphology.

lular, atypical or unusual histologic variants (Fig. 15.27) and (3) tumors of uncertain malignant potential. Leiomyosarcoma of the cervix is extremely rare, with some cases reported in children (Fig. 15.28). Histologic variants include myxoid, epithelioid, clear cell and xanthomatous types.[75–83] The characteristic morphology is similar to that of leiomyosarcoma of the myometrium, consisting of a fascicular organization, discrete tumor cell necrosis, variable nuclear atypia and mitotic activity (see criteria for uterine leiomyosarcoma in Ch. 22). Smooth muscle origin can be established by immunostaining for desmin and caldesmon (if necessary). Prognosis is based on tumor stage, similar to that of the uterus.[84]

SCHWANNOMA

Benign schwannomas are exceedingly rare, but have been reported in the cervix.[85,86] Malignant schwanno-

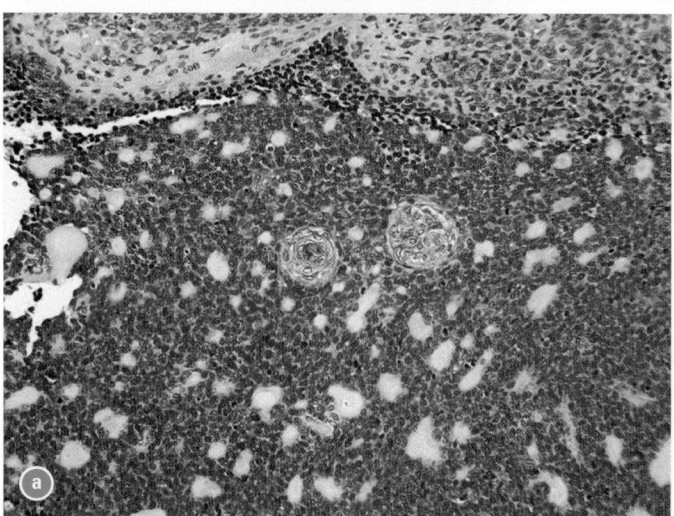

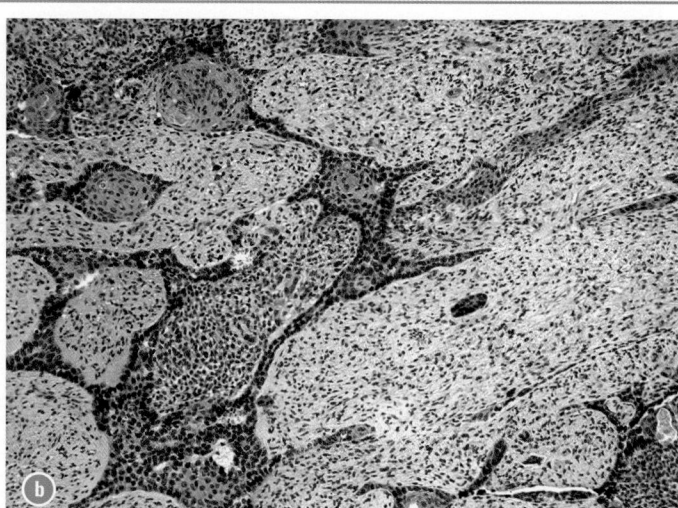

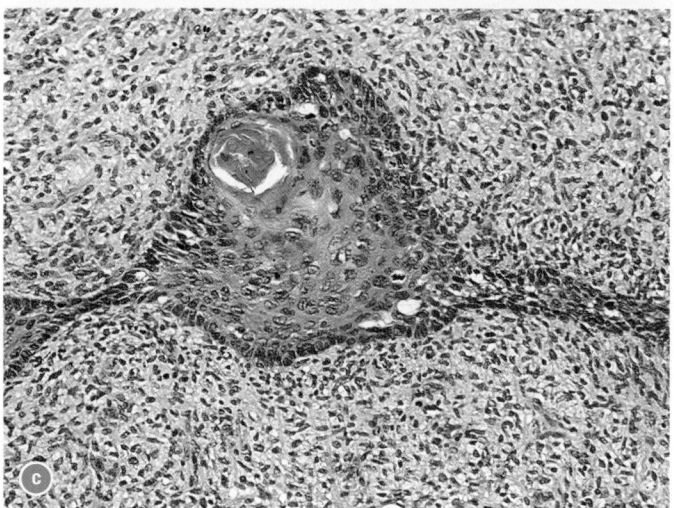

Fig. 15.22 Typical carcinosarcoma of the cervix, combining (a) basaloid (or adenoid basal) squamous neoplasia with (b) sarcoma. (c) Some foci may show prominent keratin formation.

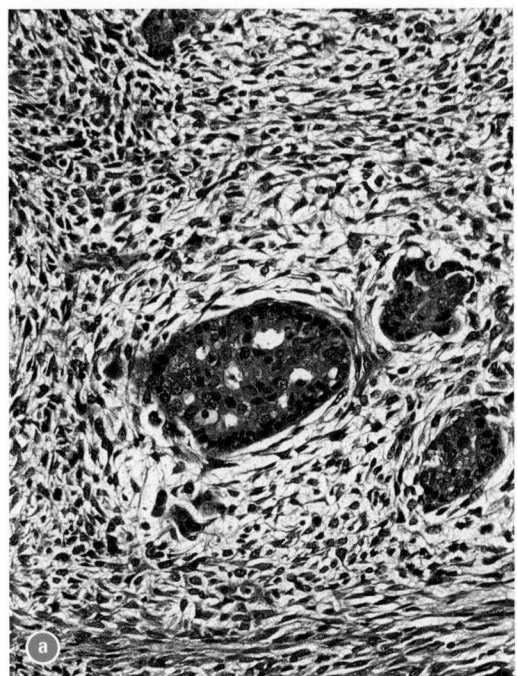
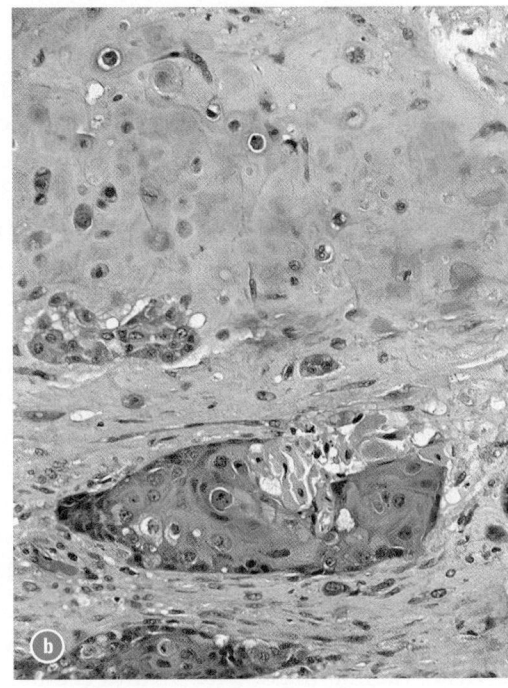

Fig. 15.23 (a) Carcinosarcoma of endometrial origin typically contains glandular and mesenchymal components, in contrast to cervical tumors. (b) Focal squamous differentiation in a carcinosarcoma of the endometrium may mimic cervical carcinoma; however, the squamous differentiation is typically haphazard. Coexisting cartilage (above) is rare in the cervix.

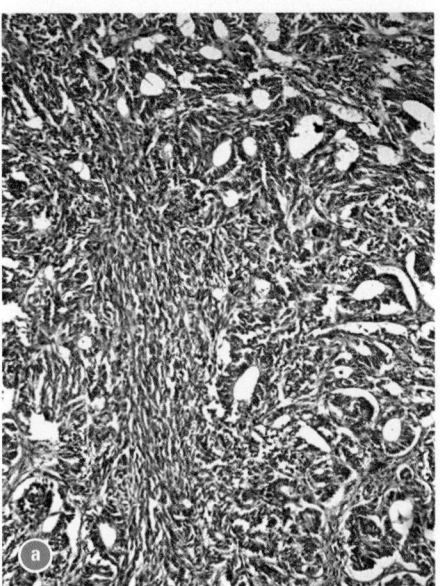
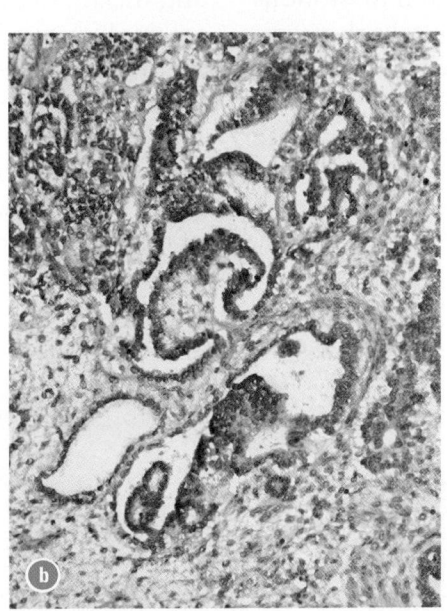
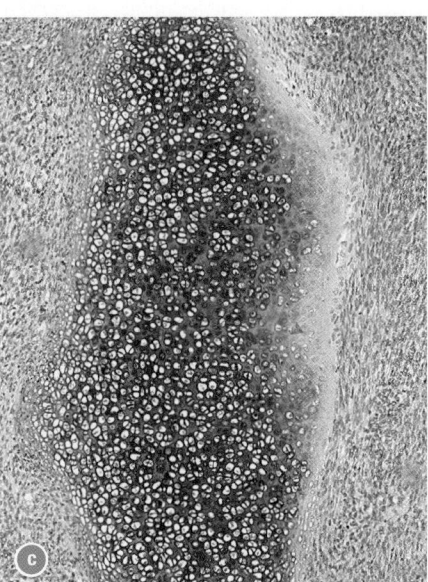

Fig. 15.24 (a) Mesonephric carcinoma with spindle cell (sarcomatoid) differentiation. (b) Mesonephric carcinoma of the uterus resembling Wilms' tumor, with chondroid differentiation (c).

mas (malignant peripheral nerve sheath tumors) of the cervix are also rare and limited principally to case reports.[87,88] The only multi-case report on malignant schwannomas is by Keel et al.[89] They described three cases in adult women with predominantly spindle cells with eosinophilic cytoplasm admixed with hypocellular fibrous/myxoid areas. The tumors were S-100 protein and vimentin-positive and HMB-45- and desmin-negative. The outcome was variable and appeared related to tumor extent. Because of the potential for confusion with other sarcomas, immunostaining was critical to the proper classification.

PERIPHERAL NEUROECTODERMAL TUMOR/EWING'S SARCOMA

These are extremely rare tumors of which only a few have been reported in the cervix and vagina.[90–92] Most

Table 15.6 Differential diagnosis of mesenchymal proliferations of the cervix

Tumor	Distinguishing feature(s)	Immunophenotype (+)
Stromal sarcoma	Non-fascicular, perivascular growth	CD10
Stromatosis	Superficial, stromal breakdown	CD10
Leiomyosarcoma	Interlacing fascicles	Desmin, caldesmon
MPNST	Alternating cellularity, perivascular bundles, slender nuclei	S-100
Embryonal rhabdomyosarcoma	Cambium layer (botryoides)	Myoglobin
Alveolar soft part sarcoma	PAS-positive granules	–

MPNST, malignant peripheral nerve sheath tumor.

patients are in their fourth or fifth decade and present with bleeding or a painless cervical/vaginal mass. The characteristic histologic features are a monotonous population of cohesive small round blue cells that typically lack the morphologic heterogeneity or molding of neuroendocrine carcinoma (Fig. 15.29). However, extensive necrosis may be present, impeding accurate diagnosis.

Peripheral neuroectodermal tumor/Ewing's sarcoma is characterized by a specific cytogenetic abnormality consisting of a 22q12 rearrangement, which can be detected by fluorescent in-situ hybridization (FISH) with appropriate genomic probes. In addition, the rearrangement results in a fusion transcript (EWS/ERG) that can be detected by polymerase chain reaction analysis.[90,93] In addition, expression of the highly restricted surface antigen p30/32MIC2 in membranous pattern is characteristic (Fig. 15.29).[90,93]

The data on outcome for peripheral neuroectodermal tumor of the uterus is limited and, in general, the outcome has been poor, particularly if patients were followed for more than a few months.[94] However, several reports have observed a short to intermediate survival (months to 4.5 years) following chemotherapy and radiation.[92,93,95,96]

Melanocytic lesions

Melanocytic neoplasms of the cervix are exceedingly rare and are basically limited to two categories: blue nevus and melanoma. Blue nevi are typically encountered in routine hysterectomies from middle-aged to elderly women and identified as darkly pigmented foci involving the endocervix.[97] Uehara et al. carefully examined 189 uteri removed for benign conditions, serially sectioned the cervix and identified stromal melanocytic foci (microscopic blue nevi; defined as small highly pigmented groups of melanocytes) in 28.6%, peaking at 40% in women in the sixth decade.[98] They proposed that the origin of these

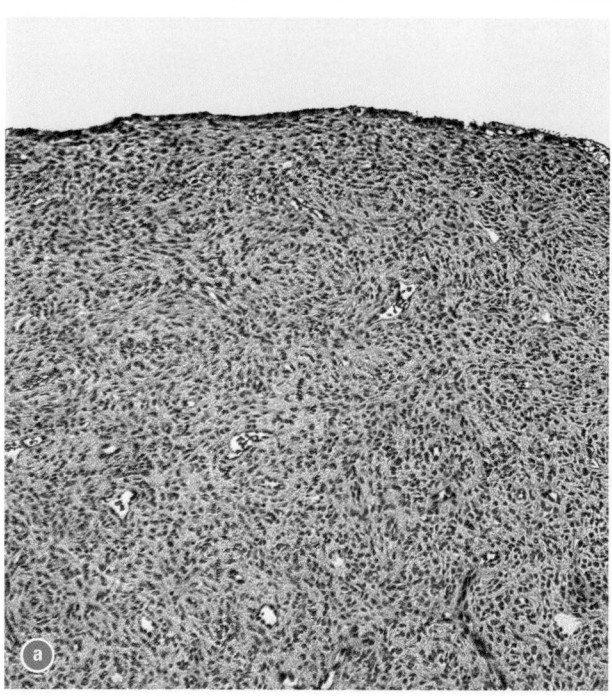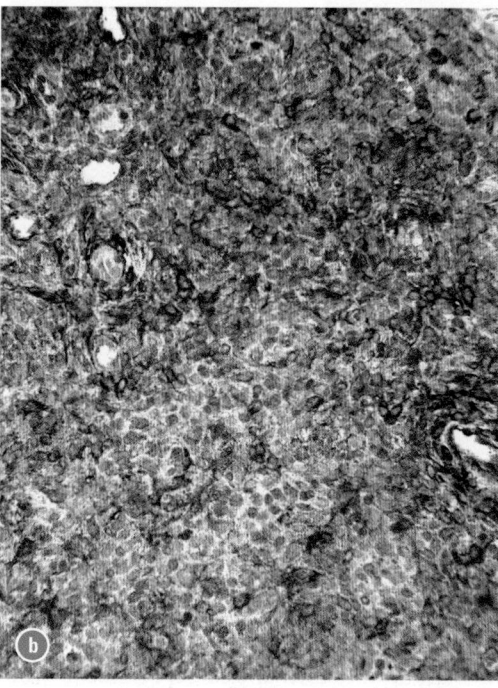

Fig. 15.25 (a) Endometrial stromal sarcoma, (b) following immunostaining for CD10.

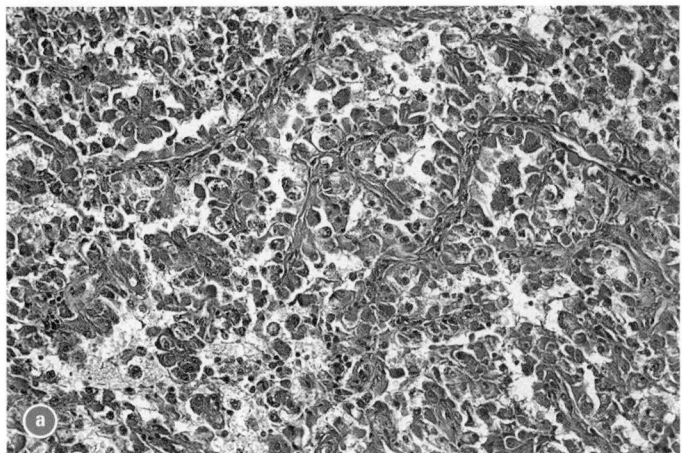
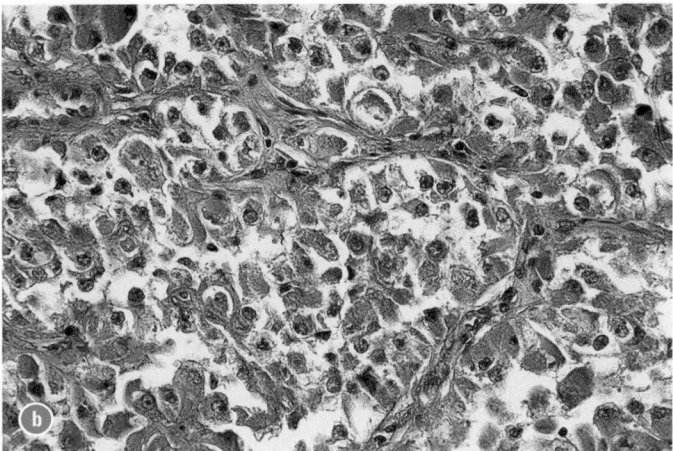

Fig. 15.26 (a,b) Alveolar soft-part sarcoma. These tumors exhibit uniform solid or alveolar-like nests of tumor cells within fibrous septa.

cells was from the stroma with a nerve sheath origin suggested based on S-100 studies.[97,98] The predominately stromal distribution of the melanocytes was proposed by the authors to explain the lack of epithelial involvement in the majority of cervical melanomas (see below).

Melanomas of the cervix are extremely rare. Clark et al. reviewed the world literature, identifying 43 cases of primary melanoma. However, less than one-third contained evidence of intraepithelial neoplastic melanocytes.[99] Like tumors elsewhere, cervical melanomas may be mistaken for sarcomas and poorly-differentiated carcinomas.[100]

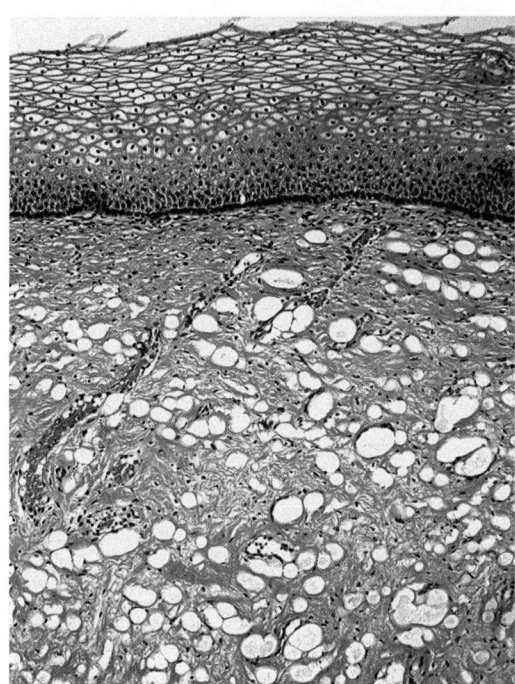

Fig. 15.27 Lipoleiomyoma of the cervix.

Hematopoietic lesions

LYMPHOMA

Lymphomas of the cervix are rare. The largest series of uterine lymphomas by Vang et al. reviewed 26 cases (Fig. 15.30).[101,102] Ten were presumed to arise in the uterus (I or IIE) and nine involved the cervix, with a mean age of 55 years. Five of six patients were still alive at 5 years, in contrast to only two of seven in which the uterine involvement was considered secondary. The dominant pattern is diffuse large B-cell lymphoma.[102] These tumors are usually easily distinguished from the prominent lymphoid follicles seen in follicular cervicitis. However, occasionally, lymphoid infiltrates occur in the cervix and may be confused with lymphoma and require marker studies.

GRANULOCYTIC SARCOMA

Acute myelocytic leukemia rarely presents initially as a cervical neoplasm and, even more rarely, this presentation will precede overt leukemia by more than a few weeks or months.[103–105] Friedman reviewed 28 cases in the female genital tract, including those with or without a history of acute leukemia. The age range is wide, in accordance with the disease itself. The tumors typically presented with abnormal bleeding, variously interpreted as menometrorrhagia, postcoital or postmenopausal bleeding. The tumors typically were situated under an attenuated or ulcerated surface mucosa (Fig. 15.31). The characteristic histology consisted of abnormal mononuclear cells with a high nuclear-to-cytoplasmic ratio, irregular nuclear shapes (ovoid, cleaved and reniform), with delicate chromatin and a moderate-to-high mitotic

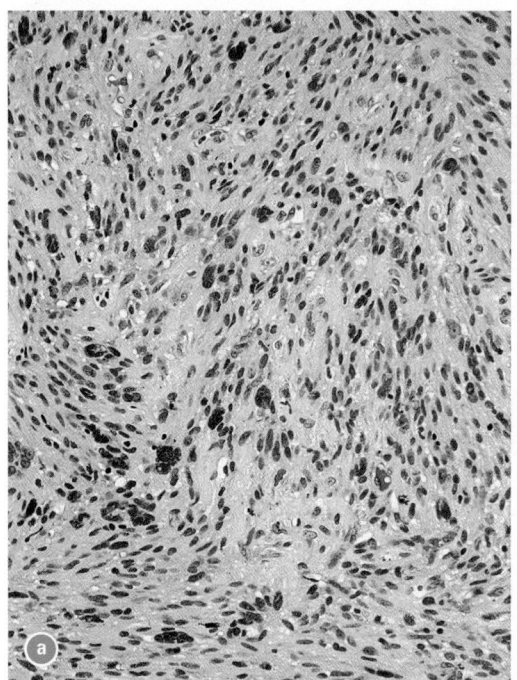

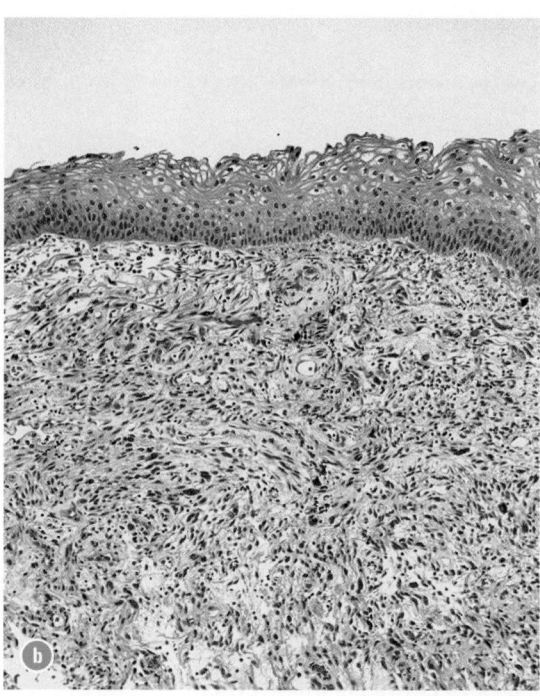

Fig. 15.28 (a,b) Leiomyosarcoma. The tumor abuts the squamous mucosa. The differential diagnosis includes leiomyoma or reactive stromal changes in a cervical polyp (see Fig. 15.15d).

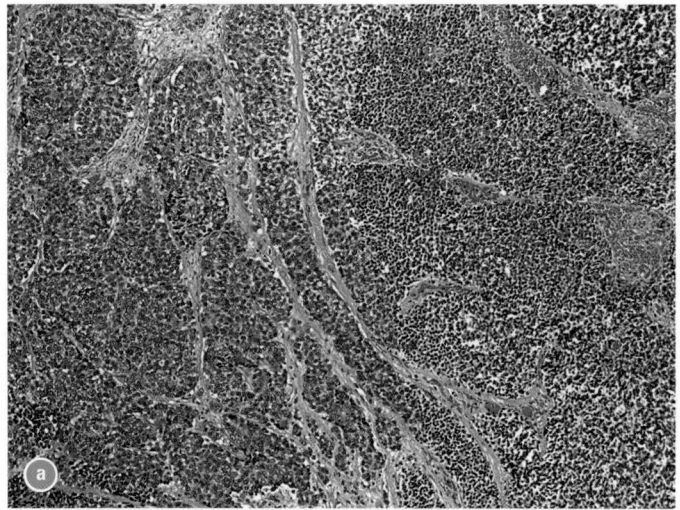

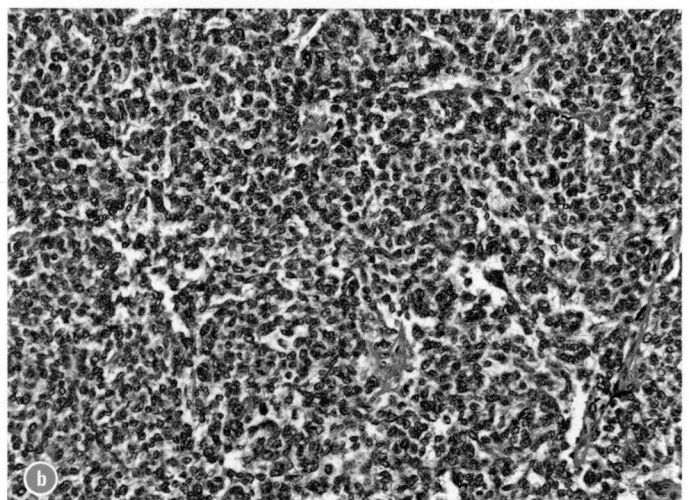

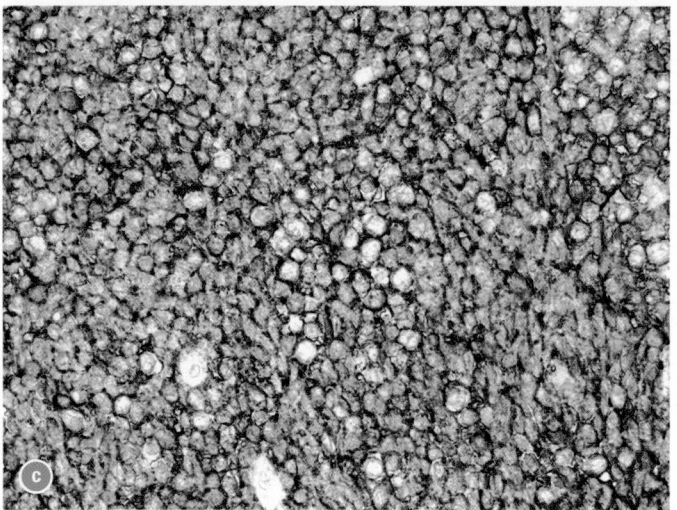

Fig. 15.29 PNET/Ewing's sarcoma. (a) Poorly-differentiated small round blue cell tumor with geographic necrosis (right). (b) Solid growth of uniform cells with a defined vascular network differs from neuroendocrine carcinoma. (c) Immunostaining with O13 shows the characteristic membranous staining pattern.

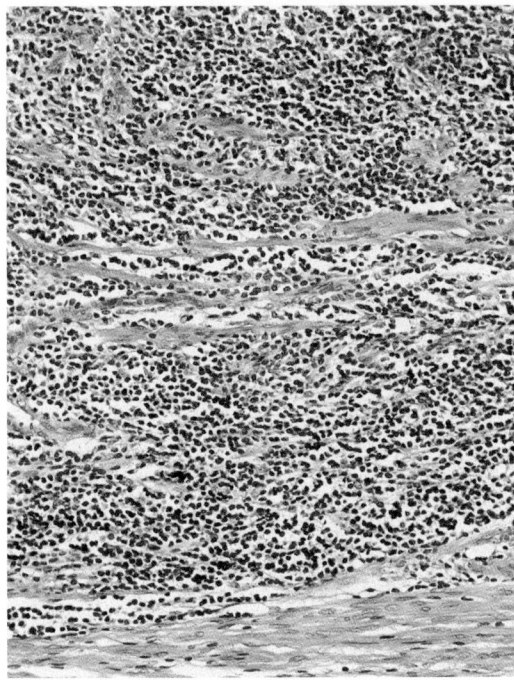

Fig. 15.30 Lymphoma of the cervix, containing diffuse infiltrate of mononuclear cells.

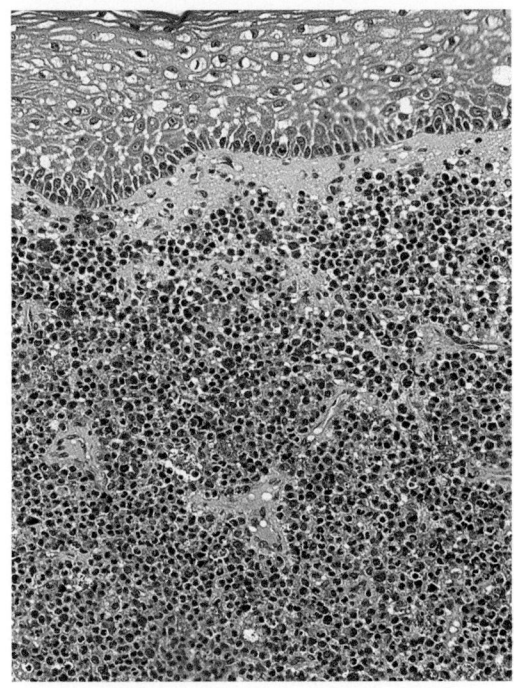

Fig. 15.31 Subepithelial deposit of acute myelocytic leukemia (chloroma, granulocytic sarcoma), seen in this case in the skin.

index (Fig. 15.32a). Positive stains for leukocyte common antigen, anti-lysozyme and naphthol AS-D chloroacetate esterase established the diagnosis (Fig. 15.32b). Lysozyme immunostaining may be necessary to establish the cell of origin when esterase staining may be negative, as in cases with monocytic differentiation. The mortality exceeds 80%, irrespective of the timing of the systemic disease.

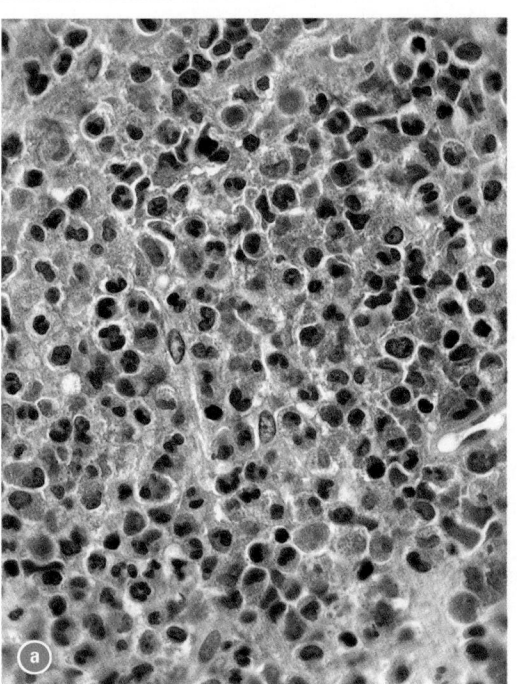

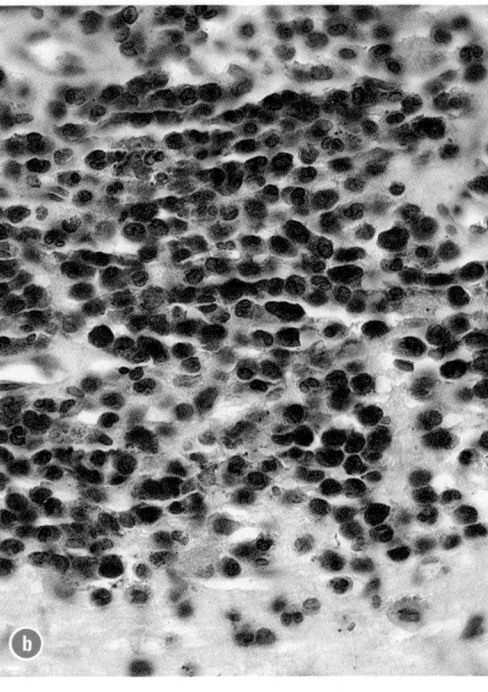

Fig. 15.32 (a) Higher magnification of granulocytic sarcoma depicts a spectrum of myeloid precursor cells. (b) Following staining with chloroacetate esterase.

Other conditions

DECIDUOSIS

Ectopic decidua is common in the cervix in pregnancy.[106] It may present as a polyp, as plaque-like deposits on the surface or within endometriosis. The important points of recognition pertain to the association of a coexisting pregnancy and distinction from mesenchymal neoplasia (Fig. 15.33).

ECTOPIC TISSUES/METAPLASIAS (GLIOSIS, CARTILAGE, BONE)

Glial tissue, cartilage and bone have all been identified in the cervix. As in the uterus, there may be a relationship to pre-existing pregnancy (Fig. 15.34).[107,108] Other mechanisms include hamartomatous origins or metaplasia of endocervical mesenchyme.[109]

VASCULAR TUMORS

Vascular lesions of the cervix are extremely rare and include capillary hemangioma and cavernous hemangioma.[110] Lymphangiomas of the cervix have not been described, but have been observed on the vulva following radiation therapy.[111,112] Some of these can be extensive, requiring hysterectomy.[113]

AMYLOIDOSIS

Amyloidosis has been reported in the cervix in individuals with multiple myeloma.[114] An example is shown in Chapter 21. Localized amyloidosis has typically been associated with squamous cell carcinoma and may be

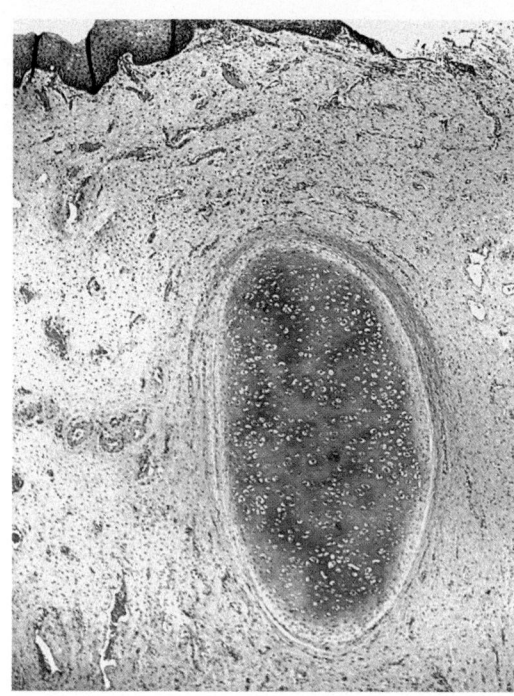

Fig. 15.34 Ectopic cartilage in the cervix. This may be associated with pre-existing pregnancy.

associated with systemic amyloidosis in these patients.[115–117] Rare instances of primary amyloidosis without an associated tumor have been reported.[117]

LIGNEOUS CERVICITIS

Ligneous mucositis is a rare, chronic, recurrent and sometimes spontaneously resolving condition associated with pseudomembrane formation that may involve mucous membranes in the mouth, nasopharynx or trachea.[118] Ligneous changes of the female genital tract typically involve the cervix or vagina. The pathologic hallmark is the deposition of amorphous fibrinoid material (not amyloid) containing immunoglobulins A and G with a sparse inflammatory infiltrate (see Ch. 10). Involvement of the upper genital tract has also been reported, possibly explaining the link between this disorder and infertility.[119] The pathogenesis is unknown and a proportion of cases involving the conjunctiva have been reported to resolve.[120]

MALAKOPLAKIA

Malakoplakia is a granulomatous disease of uncertain etiology characterized by a histiocytic infiltrate (von Hansemann cells) with calcified structures called Michaelis–Gutmann bodies. These can be seen both intra- and extracellularly. One of the more popular theories of pathogenesis is an abnormal response to an infection mediated by defective lysosomes and abnormal micro-

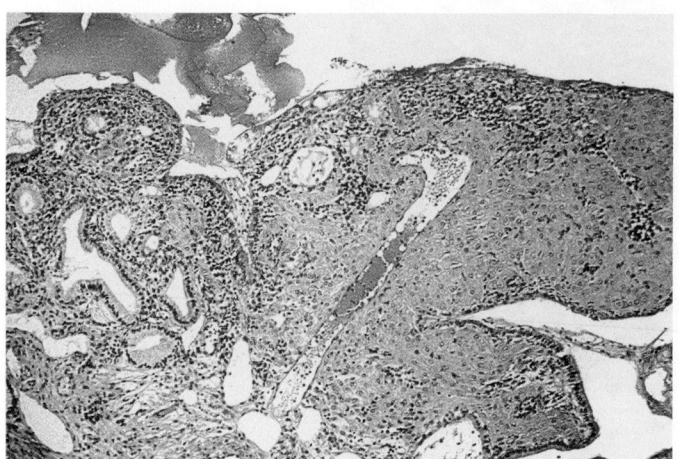

Fig. 15.33 Ectopic decidua in the cervix (right), commonly seen during pregnancy.

tubule assembly.[121,122] The disease is typically described in the urinary tract but can be seen in other organs. The most common site of genital tract involvement is the vagina, with the cervix rarely involved. The morphologic features of malakoplakia include epithelial ulceration and a histiocytic infiltrate with the characteristic PAS-positive Michaelis–Gutmann bodies.[123]

TROPHOBLASTIC LESIONS

Three principal forms of trophoblastic cell growth may be seen in the cervix.

The first, placental site nodule, which is described in Chapter 32, is distinctive in appearance, but to the uninitiated may be confused with an epithelial or mesenchymal lesion (Fig. 15.35). Cervical placental site nodule may be present for years following pregnancy. The second is placental site trophoblastic tumor arising in intermediate trophoblast that implanted in the cervix. A subset of these, with an epithelial appearance, is termed epithelioid trophoblastic tumor (Fig. 15.36).[124,125] The third is metastatic placental site trophoblastic tumor, which occurs as a nodular lesion in the vagina or cervix (see Ch. 9). The last two entities may not be immediately recognized as a placental site trophoblastic tumor and may be confused with other epithelial or mesenchymal lesions.[126] An important clue is the young age of the patient. A recent history of pregnancy may or may not be recorded. Inasmuch as the pregnancy may have gone unnoticed. A serum B-HCG should be performed (see Chapter 32). Helpful immunohistochemical stains include HPL, HCG and Mel-CAM.

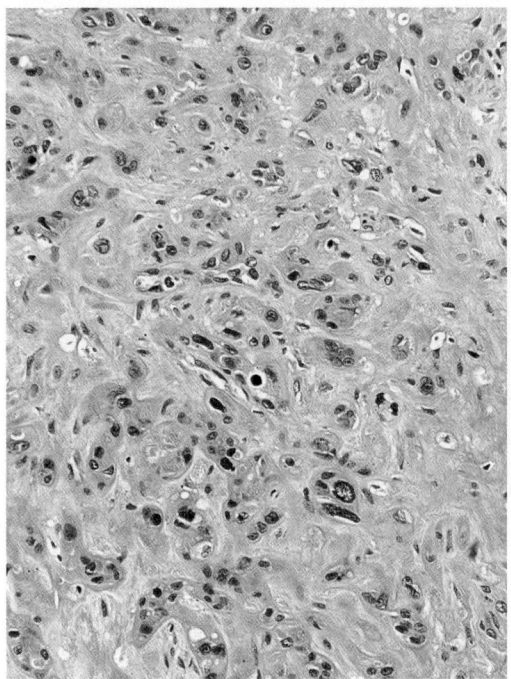

Fig. 15.36 Epithelioid placental site trophoblastic tumor.

ATYPICAL STROMAL CELLS

Large atypical stromal cells may be seen in fibroepithelial stromal polyps of the cervix (Fig. 15.37). Their importance lies in their potential confusion with other mesenchymal neoplasms (see Chapter 9).

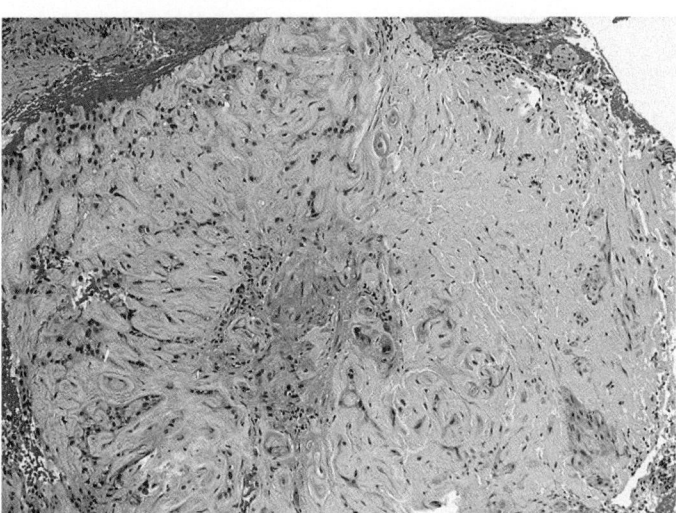

Fig. 15.35 Implantation site nodule, containing intermediate trophoblast in a keratin-rich background.

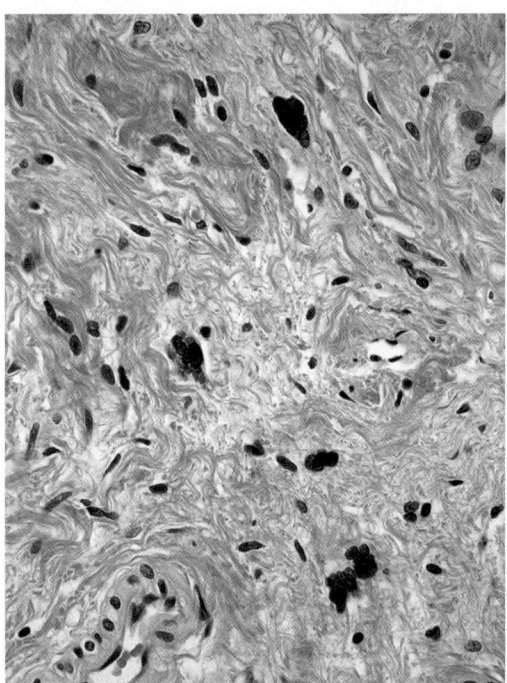

Fig. 15.37 Atypical stromal cells, often seen alone or in association with fibroepithelial polyps.

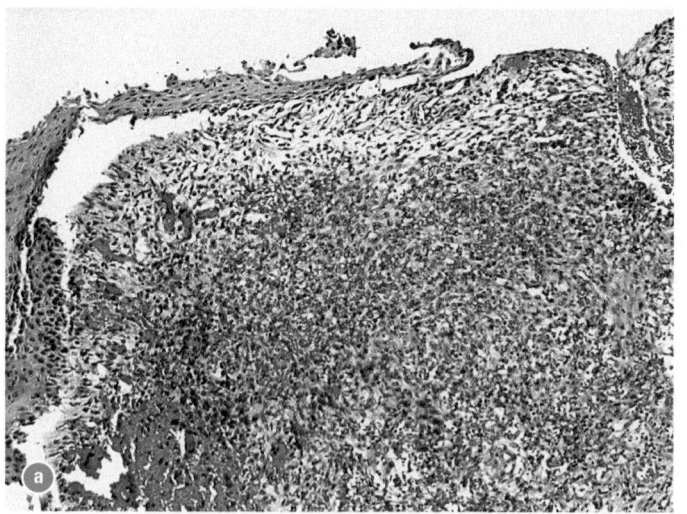
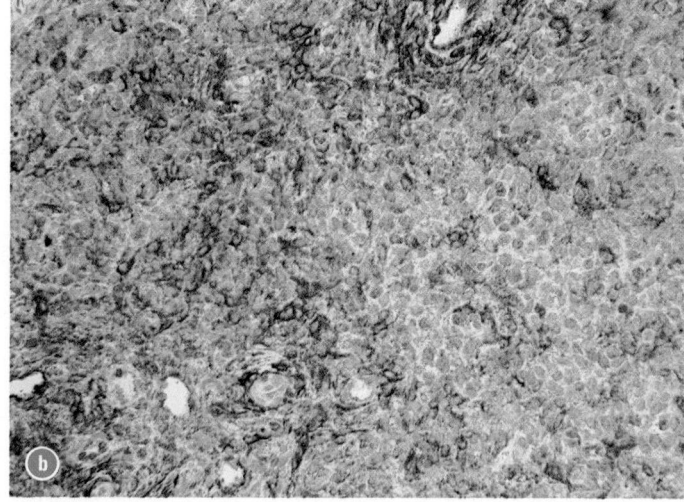

Fig. 15.38 (a) Endometrial stromatosis of the cervix, (b) positive staining with CD10.

GLAND-POOR ENDOMETRIOSIS (STROMATOSIS)

Gland-poor endometriosis (stromatosis) can occur at any site and when present may be misclassified as a mesenchymal neoplasm. The differential diagnosis includes endometrial stromal sarcoma, stromal components of adenosarcoma, other mesenchymal lesions and, conceivably, reactive stromal changes in the cervix (Fig. 15.38).[127] Helpful features include a superficial location, absence of a mass lesion, presence of stromal breakdown and/or evidence of old hemorrhage with hemosiderin.

References

1 Stoler MH, Mills SE, Gersell DJ, Walker AN. Small-cell neuroendocrine carcinoma of the cervix. A human papillomavirus type 18-associated cancer. Am J Surg Pathol 1991; 15:28–32.

2 Ambros RA, Park JS, Shah KV, Kurman RJ. Evaluation of histologic, morphometric and immunohistochemical criteria in the differential diagnosis of small cell carcinomas of the cervix with particular reference to human papillomavirus types 16 and 18. Mod Pathol 1991; 4:586–593.

3 Wang TY, Chen BF, Yang YC, et al. Histologic and immunophenotypic classification of cervical carcinomas by expression of the p53 homologue p63: a study of 250 cases. Hum Pathol 2001; 32:479–486.

4 Nagell J van Jr, Powell DE, Gallion HH, et al. Small cell carcinoma of the uterine cervix. Cancer 1988; 62:1586–1593.

5 Ciesla MC, Guidos BJ, Selvaggi SM. Cytomorphology of small-cell (neuroendocrine) carcinoma on ThinPrep cytology as compared to conventional smears. Diagn Cytopathol 2001; 24:46–52.

6 Hoerl HD, Schink J, Hartenbach E, et al. Exfoliative cytology of primary poorly differentiated (small-cell) neuroendocrine carcinoma of the uterine cervix in ThinPrep material: a case report. Diagn Cytopathol 2000; 23:14–18.

7 Proca D, Keyhani-Rofagha S, Copeland LJ, Hameed A. Exfoliative cytology of neuroendocrine small cell carcinoma of the endometrium. A report of two cases. Acta Cytol 1998; 42:978–982.

8 Albores-Saavedra J, Larraza O, Poucell S, Rodriguez Martinez HA. Carcinoid of the cervix uteri. Additional observations on a new neoplastic entity. Gac Med Mex 1976; 111:397–410.

9 Albores-Saavedra J, Rodriguez-Martinez HA, Larraza-Hernandez O. Carcinoid tumors of the cervix. Pathol Annu 1979; 14:273–291.

10 Albores-Saavedra J, Gersell D, Gilks CB, et al. Terminology of endocrine tumors of the uterine cervix: results of a workshop sponsored by the College of American Pathologists and the National Cancer Institute. Arch Pathol Lab Med 1997; 121:34–39.

11 Gilks CB, Young RH, Gersell DJ, Clement PB. Large cell neuroendocrine carcinoma of the uterine cervix: a clinicopathologic study of 12 cases. Am J Surg Pathol 1997; 21:905–914.

12 Walker AN, Mills SE. Unusual variants of uterine cervical carcinoma. Pathol Annu 1987; 22:277–310.

13 Boruta DM 2nd, Schorge JO, Duska LA, et al. Multimodality therapy in early-stage neuroendocrine carcinoma of the uterine cervix. Gynecol Oncol 2001; 81(1):82–87.

14 Pirog EC, Kleter B, Olgac S, et al. Prevalence of human papillomavirus DNA in different histological subtypes of cervical adenocarcinoma. Am J Pathol 2000; 157:1055–1062.

15 Stassart J, Crum CP, Yordan EL, et al. Argyrophilic carcinoma of the cervix: a report of a case with coexisting cervical intraepithelial neoplasia. Gynecol Oncol 1982; 13(2):247–251.

16 Akiba Y, Mikami M, Komuro Y, et al. A case of neuroendocrine carcinoma of uterine cervix with the elevated plasma level of serotonin. Nippon Sanka Fujinka Gakkai Zasshi 1996; 48:897–900.

17 Koch CA, Azumi N, Furlong MA, et al. Carcinoid syndrome caused by an atypical carcinoid of the uterine cervix 1. J Clin Endocrinol Metab 1999; 84:4209–4213.

18 Chan JK, Tsui WM, Tung SY, Ching RC. Endocrine cell hyperplasia of the uterine cervix. A precursor of neuroendocrine carcinoma of the cervix? Am J Clin Pathol 1989; 92:825–830.

19 Weed JC Jr, Graff AT, Shoup B, Tawfik O. Small cell undifferentiated (neuroendocrine) carcinoma of the uterine cervix. J Am Coll Surg 2003; 197(1):44–51.

20 Delaloge S, Pautier P, Kerbrat P, et al. Neuroendocrine small cell carcinoma of the uterine cervix: what disease? What treatment? Report of ten cases and a review of the literature. Clin Oncol (R Coll Radiol) 2000; 12(6):357–362.

21 Abulafia O, Sherer DM. Adjuvant chemotherapy in stage IB neuroendocrine small cell carcinoma of the cervix. Acta Obstet Gynecol Scand 1995; 74:740–744.

22 Louka MH, Danoff B, Brodovsky HS, Jahshan AE. Carcinoid tumors of the uterine cervix: response to combination chemotherapy and radiotherapy. Am J Clin Oncol 1982; 5(5):487–493.

23 Balderston KD, Tewari K, Gregory WT, et al. Neuroendocrine small cell uterine cervix cancer in pregnancy: long-term survival following combined therapy. Gynecol Oncol 1998; 71(1):128–132.

24 Hariri J, Rasmussen EA, Hage E. Carcinoid tumor of the uterine cervix. Acta Obstet Gynecol Scand 1983; 62(5):539–540.

25 Groben P, Reddick R, Askin F. The pathologic spectrum of small cell carcinoma of the cervix. Int J Gynecol Pathol 1985; 4(1):42–57.

26 Seidel R Jr, Steinfeld A. Carcinoid of the cervix: natural history and implications for therapy. Gynecol Oncol 1988; 30(1):114–119.

27 Park JJ, Sun D, Quade BJ, et al. Stratified mucin-producing intraepithelial lesions of the cervix: adenosquamous or columnar cell neoplasia? Am J Surg Pathol 2000; 24(10):1414–1419.

28 Caroti S, Siliotti F. Cervical polyps: a colpo-cyto-histological study. Clin Exp Obstet Gynecol 1988; 15(3):108–115.

29 Golan A, Ber A, Wolman I, David MP. Cervical polyp: evaluation of current treatment. Gynecol Obstet Invest 1994; 37(1):56–58.

30 Lee WH, Tan KH, Lee YW. The aetiology of postmenopausal bleeding – a study of 163 consecutive cases in Singapore. Singapore Med J 1995; 36(2):164–168.

31 Spiewankiewicz B, Stelmachow J, Sawicki W, et al. Hysteroscopy in cases of cervical polyps. Eur J Gynaecol Oncol 2003; 24(1):67–69.

32 Vilodre LC, Bertat R, Petters R, Reis FM. Cervical polyp as risk factor for hysteroscopically diagnosed endometrial polyps. Gynecol Obstet Invest 1997; 44(3):191–195.

33 Neri A, Kaplan B, Rabinerson D, et al. Cervical polyp in the menopause and the need for fractional dilatation and curettage. Eur J Obstet Gynecol Reprod Biol 1995; 62(1):53–55.

34 Ilhan R, Yavuz E, Iplikci A, Tuzlali S. Hamartomatous endocervical polyp with heterologous mesenchymal tissue. Pathol Int 2001; 51(4):305–307.

35 Khalil AM, Azar GB, Kaspar HG, et al. Giant cervical polyp. A case report. J Reprod Med 1996; 41(8):619–621.

36 Kerner H, Lichtig C. Müllerian adenosarcoma presenting as cervical polyps: a report of seven cases and review of the literature. Obstet Gynecol 1993; 81:655–659.

37 Gilks CB, Young RH, Clement PB, et al. Adenomyomas of the uterine cervix of endocervical type: a report of ten cases of a benign cervical tumor that may be confused with adenoma malignum. Mod Pathol 1996; 9:220–224.

38 Silverberg SG. Adenomyomatosis of endometrium and endocervix – a hamartoma. Am J Clin Pathol 1975; 64:192–199.

39 Mikami Y, Maehata K, Fujiwara K, Manabe T. Endocervical adenomyoma. A case report with histochemical and immunohistochemical studies. APMIS 2001; 109:546–550.

40 Kuwabara H, Ohno M, Moriwaki S. Uterine adenomyoma of endocervical type. Pathol Int 1999; 49:1019–1021.

41 Clement PB, Scully RE. Müllerian adenosarcoma of the uterus: a clinicopathologic analysis of 100 cases with a review of the literature. Hum Pathol 1990; 21(4):363–381.

42 Kaku T, Silverberg SG, Major FJ, et al. Adenosarcoma of the uterus: a Gynecologic Oncology Group clinicopathologic study of 31 cases. Int J Gynecol Pathol 1992; 11(2):75–88.

43 Zaloudek CJ, Norris HJ. Adenofibroma and adenosarcoma of the uterus: a clinicopathologic study of 35 cases. Cancer 1981; 48(2):354–366.

44 Ramos P, Ruiz A, Carabias E, et al. Müllerian adenosarcoma of the cervix with heterologous elements: report of a case and review of the literature. Gynecol Oncol 2002; 84:161–166.

45 Bhandare D, Madiwale C, Kothari K, et al. Müllerian adenosarcoma of the uterine cervix. Indian J Pathol Microbiol 2001; 44:371–372.

46 Verschraegen CF, Vasuratna A, Edwards C, et al. Clinicopathologic analysis of müllerian adenosarcoma: the M.D. Anderson Cancer Center experience. Oncol Rep 1998; 5:939–944.

47 Toral JA. Extraendometrial müllerian adenosarcoma. Philipp J Obstet Gynecol 1998; 22:87–97.

48 Jones MW, Lefkowitz M. Adenosarcoma of the uterine cervix: a clinicopathological study of 12 cases. Int J Gynecol Pathol 1995; 14:223–229.

49 McCluggage WG, Alderdice JM, Walsh MY. Polypoid uterine lesions mimicking endometrial stromal sarcoma. J Clin Pathol 1999; 52:543–546.

50 Michener CM, Simon NL. Ovarian conservation in a woman of reproductive age with müllerian adenosarcoma. Gynecol Oncol 2001; 83(2):424–427.

51 Gal D, Kerner H, Beck D, et al. Müllerian adenosarcoma of the uterine cervix. Gynecol Oncol 1988; 31(3):445–453.

52 Abell MR, Ramirez JA. Sarcomas and carcinosarcomas of the uterine cervix. Cancer 1973; 31:1176–1192.

53 Clement PB, Zubovits JT, Young RH, Scully RE. Malignant müllerian mixed tumors of the uterine cervix: a report of nine cases of a neoplasm with morphology often different from its counterpart in the corpus. Int J Gynecol Pathol 1998; 17:211–222.

54 Grayson W, Taylor LF, Cooper K. Carcinosarcoma of the uterine cervix: a report of eight cases with immunohistochemical analysis and evaluation of human papillomavirus status. Am J Surg Pathol 2001; 25:338–347.

55 Hall-Craggs M, Toker C, Nedwich A. Carcinosarcoma of the uterine cervix: a light and electron microscopic study. Cancer 1981; 48:161–169.

56 Manhoff DT, Schiffman R, Haupt HM. Adenoid cystic carcinoma of the uterine cervix with malignant stroma. An unusual variant of carcinosarcoma? Am J Surg Pathol 1995; 19:229–233.

57 Yannacou N, Gerolymatos A, Parissi-Mathiou P, et al. Carcinosarcoma of the uterine cervix composed of an adenoid cystic carcinoma and an homologous stromal sarcoma. A case report. Eur J Gynaecol Oncol 2000; 21:292–294.

58 Clement PB, Young RH, Keh P, et al. Malignant mesonephric neoplasms of the uterine cervix. A report of eight cases, including four with a malignant spindle cell component. Am J Surg Pathol 1995; 19:1158–1171.

59 Bloch T, Roth LM, Stehman FB, et al. Osteosarcoma of the uterine cervix associated with hyperplastic and atypical mesonephric rests. Cancer 1988; 62:1594–1600.

60 Yamamoto Y, Akagi A, Izumi K, Kishi Y. Carcinosarcoma of the uterine body of mesonephric origin. Pathol Int 1995; 45:303–309.

61 Bague S, Rodriguez IM, Prat J. Malignant mesonephric tumors of the female genital tract: a clinicopathologic study of 9 cases. Am J Surg Pathol 2004; 28(5):601–607.

62 Silver SA, Devouassoux-Shisheboran M, Mezzetti TP, Tavassoli FA. Mesonephric adenocarcinomas of the uterine cervix: a study of 11 cases with immunohistochemical findings. Am J Surg Pathol 2001; 25(3):379–387.

63 Roberts DJ, Haber D, Sklar J, Crum CP. Extrarenal Wilms' tumors. A study of their relationship with classical renal Wilms' tumor using expression of WT1 as a molecular marker. Lab Invest 1993; 68(5):528–536.

64 Muc RS, Grayson W, Grobbelaar JJ. Adult extrarenal Wilms tumor occurring in the uterus. Arch Pathol Lab Med 2001; 125(8):1081–1083.

65 Babin EA, Davis JR, Hatch KD, Hallum AV 3rd. Wilms' tumor of the cervix: a case report and review of the literature. Gynecol Oncol 2000; 76(1):107–111.

66 Boardman CH, Webb MJ, Jefferies JA. Low-grade endometrial stromal sarcoma of the ectocervix after therapy for breast cancer. Gynecol Oncol 2000; 79(1):120–123.

67 Abeler V, Nesland JM. Alveolar soft-part sarcoma in the uterine cervix. Arch Pathol Lab Med 1989; 113:1179–1183.

68 Emerich J, Senkus E, Konefka T. Alveolar rhabdomyosarcoma of the uterine cervix. Gynecol Oncol 1996; 63:398–403.

69 Nielsen GP, Oliva E, Young RH, et al. Alveolar soft-part sarcoma of the female genital tract: a report of nine cases and review of the literature. Int J Gynecol Pathol 1995; 14(4):283–292.

70 Flint A, Gikas PW, Roberts JA. Alveolar soft part sarcoma of the uterine cervix. Gynecol Oncol 1985; 22:263–267.

71 Kopolovic J, Weiss DB, Dolberg L, et al. Alveolar soft-part sarcoma of the female genital tract. Case report with ultrastructural findings. Arch Gynecol 1987; 240:125–129.

72 Morimitsu Y, Tanaka H, Iwanaga S, Kojiro M. Alveolar soft part sarcoma of the uterine cervix. Acta Pathol Jpn 1993; 43:204–208.

73 Sahin AA, Silva EG, Ordonez NG. Alveolar soft part sarcoma of the uterine cervix. Mod Pathol 1989; 2:676–680.

74 Lieberman PH, Foote FW Jr, Stewart FW, Berg JW. Alveolar soft-part sarcoma. JAMA 1966; 198:1047–1051.

75 Abdul-Karim FW, Bazi TM, Sorensen K, Nasr MF. Sarcoma of the uterine cervix: clinicopathologic findings in three cases. Gynecol Oncol 1987; 26:103–111.

76 Colombat M, Sevestre H, Gontier MF. Epithelioid leiomyosarcoma of the uterine cervix. Report of a case. Ann Pathol 2001; 21:48–50.

77 Fraga M, Prieto O, Garcia-Caballero T, et al. Myxoid leiomyosarcoma of the uterine cervix. Histopathology 1994; 25:381–384.

78 Fujiwaki R, Yoshida M, Iida K, et al. Epithelioid leiomyosarcoma of the uterine cervix. Acta Obstet Gynecol Scand 1998; 77:246–248.

79 Gotoh T, Kikuchi Y, Takano M, et al. Epithelioid leiomyosarcoma of the uterine cervix. Gynecol Oncol 2001; 82:400–405.

80 Grayson W, Fourie J, Tiltman AJ. Xanthomatous leiomyosarcoma of the uterine cervix. Int J Gynecol Pathol 1998; 17:89–90.

81 Kasamatsu T, Shiromizu K, Takahashi M, et al. Leiomyosarcoma of the uterine cervix. Gynecol Oncol 1998; 69:169–171.

82 Silva EG, Tornos C, Ordonez NG, Morris M. Uterine leiomyosarcoma with clear cell areas. Int J Gynecol Pathol 1995; 14:174–178.

83 Lack EE. Leiomyosarcomas in childhood: a clinical and pathologic study of 10 cases. Pediatr Pathol 1986; 6:181–197.

84 Irvin W, Presley A, Andersen W, et al. Leiomyosarcoma of the cervix. Gynecol Oncol 2003; 91(3):636–642.

85 LeMaire WJ, Kreiss C, Commodore A, Barker EA. Neurilemmoma: an unusual benign tumor of the cervix. Alaska Med 2002; 44(3):63–65.

86 Gwavava NJ, Traub AI. A neurilemmoma of the cervix. Br J Obstet Gynaecol 1980; 87(5):444–446.

87 Lallas TA, Mehaffey PC, Lager DJ, et al. Malignant cervical schwannoma: an unusual pelvic tumor. Gynecol Oncol 1999; 72(2):238–242.

88 Bernstein HB, Broman JH, Apicelli A, Kredentser DC. Primary malignant schwannoma of the uterine cervix: a case report and literature review. Gynecol Oncol 1999; 74(2):288–292.

89 Keel SB, Clement PB, Prat J, Young RH. Malignant schwannoma of the uterine cervix: a study of three cases. Int J Gynecol Pathol 1998; 17:223–230.

90 Pauwels P, Ambros P, Hattinger C, et al. Peripheral primitive neuroectodermal tumour of the cervix. Virchows Arch 2000; 436:68–73.

91 Sato S, Yajima A, Kimura N, et al. Peripheral neuroepithelioma (peripheral primitive neuroectodermal tumor) of the uterine cervix. Tohoku J Exp Med 1996; 180:187–195.

92 Tsao AS, Roth LM, Sandler A, Hurteau JA. Cervical primitive neuroectodermal tumor. Gynecol Oncol 2001; 83:138–142.

93 Cenacchi G, Pasquinelli G, Montanaro L, et al. Primary endocervical extraosseous Ewing's sarcoma/PNET. Int J Gynecol Pathol 1998; 17:83–88.

94 Rose PG, O'Toole RV, Keyhani-Rofagha S, et al. Malignant peripheral primitive neuroectodermal tumor of the uterus. J Surg Oncol 1987; 35(3):165–169.

95 Malpica A, Moran CA. Primitive neuroectodermal tumor of the cervix: a clinicopathologic and immunohistochemical study of two cases. Ann Diagn Pathol 2002; 6(5):281–287.

96 Horn LC, Fischer U, Bilek K. Primitive neuroectodermal tumor of the cervix uteri. A case report. Gen Diagn Pathol 1997; 142(3/4):227–230.

97 Patel DS, Bhagavan BS. Blue nevus of the uterine cervix. Hum Pathol 1985; 16(1):79–86.

98 Uehara T, Izumo T, Kishi K, et al. Stromal melanocytic foci ('blue nevus') in step sections of the uterine cervix. Acta Pathol Jpn 1991; 41(10):751–756.

99 Clark KC, Butz WR, Hapke MR. Primary malignant melanoma of the uterine cervix: case report with world literature review. Int J Gynecol Pathol 1999; 18:265–273.

100 Ishikura H, Kojo T, Ichimura H, Yoshiki T. Desmoplastic malignant melanoma of the uterine cervix: a rare primary malignancy in the uterus mimicking a sarcoma. Histopathology 1998; 33:93–94.

101 Omari-Alaoui H, Kebdani T, Benjaafar N, et al. Non-Hodgkin's lymphoma of the uterus: apropos of 4 cases and review of the literature. Cancer Radiother 2002; 6:39–45.

102 Vang R, Medeiros LJ, Ha CS, Deavers M. Non-Hodgkin's lymphomas involving the uterus: a clinicopathologic analysis of 26 cases. Mod Pathol 2000; 13:19–28.

103 Friedman HD, Adelson MD, Elder RC, Lemke SM. Granulocytic sarcoma of the uterine cervix – literature review of granulocytic sarcoma of the female genital tract. Gynecol Oncol 1992; 46:128–137.

104 Kapadia SB, Krause JR, Kanbour AI, Hartsock RJ. Granulocytic sarcoma of the uterus. Cancer 1978; 41:687–691.

105 Seo IS, Hull MT, Pak HY. Granulocytic sarcoma of the cervix as a primary manifestation: case without overt leukemic features for 26 months. Cancer 1977; 40:3030–3037.

106 Schneider V, Barnes LA. Ectopic decidual reaction of the uterine cervix: frequency and cytologic presentation. Acta Cytol 1981; 25(6):616–622.

107 Roca AN, Guajardo M, Estrada WJ. Glial polyp of the cervix and endometrium. Report of a case and review of the literature. Am J Clin Pathol 1980; 73(5):718–720.

108 Gronroos M, Meurman L, Kahra K. Proliferating glia and other heterotopic tissues in the uterus: fetal homografts? Obstet Gynecol 1983; 61(2):261–266.

109 Ilhan R, Yavuz E, Iplikci A, Tuzlali S. Hamartomatous endocervical polyp with heterologous mesenchymal tissue. Pathol Int 2001; 51(4):305–307.

110 Kondi-Pafiti A, Kairi-Vassilatou E, Spanidou-Carvouni H, et al. Vascular tumors of the female genital tract: a clinicopathological study of nine cases. Eur J Gynaecol Oncol 2003; 24(1):48–50.

111 Jappe U, Zimmermann T, Kahle B, Petzoldt D. Lymphangioma circumscriptum of the vulva following surgical and radiological therapy of cervical cancer. Sex Transm Dis 2002; 29(9):533–535.

112 Schwab RA, McCollough ML. Acquired vulvar lymphangiomas: a sequela of radiation therapy. Cutis 2001; 67(3):239–240.

113 Weerasinghe DS, Walton SM, Bilous AM. Haemangioma of the uterine cervix – case report. Aust N Z J Obstet Gynaecol 1980; 20(1):60–61.

114 Taylor E, Gilks B, Lanvin D. Amyloidosis of the uterine cervix presenting as postmenopausal bleeding. Obstet Gynecol 2001; 98(5):966–968.

115 Gibbons D, Lindberg GM, Ashfaq R, Saboorian MH. Localized amyloidosis of the uterine cervix. Int J Gynecol Pathol 1998; 17(4):368–371.

116 Tsang WY, Chan JK. Amyloid-producing squamous cell carcinoma of the uterine cervix. Arch Pathol Lab Med 1993; 117(2):199–201.

117 Sakemi T, Nakamura K, Baba N, Watanabe T. Rapidly progressive renal amyloidosis associated with uterine cervical cancer. Clin Nephrol 1992; 38(3):173–174.

118 Shimabukuro M, Iwasaki N, Nagae Y, et al. Ligneous conjunctivitis: a case report. Jpn J Ophthalmol 2001; 45(4):375–377.

119 Scurry J, Planner R, Fortune DW, et al. Ligneous (pseudomembranous) inflammation of the female genital tract. A report of two cases. J Reprod Med 1993; 38(5):407–412.

120 Hidayat AA, Riddle PJ. Ligneous conjunctivitis. A clinicopathologic study of 17 cases. Ophthalmology 1987; 94(8):949–959.

121 Dasgupta P, Womack C, Turner AG. Blackford HN. Malacoplakia: von Hansemann's disease. BJU Int 1999; 84:464–469.

122 Agnarsdóttir M, Hahn L, Sellgren U, Willen R. Malacoplakia of the cervix uteri and vulva. Acta Obstet Gynecol Scand 83(2):214–216.

123 Chen KTK, Hendricks EJ. Malakoplakia of the female genital tract. Obstet Gynecol 1985; 65:84S–87S.

124 Shih IM, Kurman RJ. The pathology of intermediate trophoblastic tumors and tumor-like lesions. Int J Gynecol Pathol 2001; 20(1):31–47.

125 Shih IM, Kurman RJ. Epithelioid trophoblastic tumor: a neoplasm distinct from choriocarcinoma and placental site trophoblastic tumor simulating carcinoma. Am J Surg Pathol 1998; 22(11):1393–1403.

126 Baergen RN, Rutgers J, Young RH. Extrauterine lesions of intermediate trophoblast. Int J Gynecol Pathol 2003; 22(4):362–367.

127 Clement PB, Young RH, Scully RE. Stromal endometriosis of the uterine cervix. A variant of endometriosis that may simulate a sarcoma. Am J Surg Pathol 1990; 14(5):449–455.

16

Evaluation of cyclic endometrium and benign endometrial disorders

Christopher P. Crum,

Mark D. Hornstein and

Elizabeth A. Stewart

Introduction

Cycling endometrium (third and fourth decade)

Introduction
Menstrual phase
Early proliferative phase with
    residual stromal breakdown
    (late menstrual/early
    proliferative endometrium)
Proliferative phase endometrium
16-day endometrium (POD 2)
Vacuole phase of secretory
    endometrium (17–19 days;
    POD 4–6)
Exhaustive phase of secretory
    endometrium (20–22 days;
    POD 6–8)
Predecidual phase of secretory
    endometrium (23–28 days;
    POD 9–14)

Disorders of secretory maturation that are the focus of infertility management

Luteal phase defect
Ovulation induction and defects in
    secretory maturation

The role of biomarkers in
    endometrial evaluation

Abnormal uterine bleeding

Introduction
Dysfunctional uterine
    bleeding
Menorrhagia
Causes of abnormal uterine
    bleeding as a function of age
    group
Clinical work-up

Endometrial pathology

Patterns commonly associated
    with abnormal (and
    dysfunctional) bleeding
Postmenopausal endometrium
Current or post-pregnancy/ post-
    partum endometrium
Benign atypias/artifacts
    encountered in routine
    evaluation of endometrium

Management of endometrial bleeding

Introduction

Pathologists routinely evaluate endometrial biopsies, which account for at least 20% of gynecologic specimens requiring pathology consultation. The majority of endometrial biopsies are performed for abnormal uterine bleeding and questions that are posed in each situation requiring biopsy and the clinical information required vary for each individual case (Table 16.1). For adolescent women, abnormal uterine bleeding will most likely be transient, but can at times be severe, often due to the presence of underlying bleeding disorders. For women in the third and fourth decades, a range of disorders must be excluded.[1] Bleeding on contraceptives, if transient, may not require sampling. However, persistent bleeding or situations in which the status of the endometrium must be evaluated such as during fertility evaluations or to rule out hyperplasia in the setting of polycystic ovarian disease, or disturbances in luteal phase warrant sampling. The fifth decade witnesses the approach of menopause when abnormal bleeding heralds the cessation of ovulation. In the six and seventh decades, the questions shift to causes of bleeding in the patient on hormonal replacement therapy, or if the patient is not on hormones, other causes of unexpected bleeding, particularly the possibility of a neoplastic process. In all age groups, the clinical and laboratory management of abnormal bleeding is designed to determine whether the bleeding is a function of a structural (histologically abnormal) disturbance such as endometrial polyps, submucosal leiomyomata, inflammatory/infectious or unopposed estrogen effect) disturbance or a functional disorder devoid of a structural or histologic anomaly (dysfunctional bleeding). Superimposed on this test matrix of ultrasound, hysteroscopy, biopsy and histologic evaluation is the not-infrequent urgency imposed by unusually heavy (menorrhagia) or both heavy and frequent (menometrorrhagia) bleeding (Table 16.2).

Although not specified as a cause of abnormal bleeding, concurrent pregnancy, including ectopic gestations, may be reported as 'abnormal bleeding' in unsuspecting women of reproductive age or interpreted as such by the caregiver. Thus, where appropriate, pregnancy must be excluded.

Several books, chapters and reviews are available on the interpretation of benign endometrium and have clarified, or introduced improvements, in the original scheme put forth by Noyes et al.[2–9] Nevertheless, the wide range of alterations seen in the endometrium during reproductive and menopausal years poses a challenge to many practitioners. This chapter addresses a framework on which to superimpose the histologic images that are encountered when reviewing the endometrial biopsy. The goal of this chapter is to integrate a range of overlapping templates, including age and disturbances that are peculiar to age with morphology and differential diagnosis and ultimately, the clinical scenarios of presentation on one end and management on the other.

Table 16.1 Causes of abnormal uterine bleeding

Age (years)	Causes (in order of decreasing frequency)
Prepubertal	Precocious puberty (hypothalamic, pituitary, ovarian)
Adolescence	Disorders in the hypothalamic–pituitary axis (transient) Disorders in folliculogenesis (transient) Sexually transmitted infections, undiscovered pregnancy Hematologic disorders (von Willebrand's, factors VII, XI)
Third and fourth decade	Oral contraceptive related Post-pregnancy Dysfunctional uterine bleeding Organic lesions (polyps, leiomyomata, endometritis) Anovulatory cycle
Fifth decade	Anovulatory or altered cycle Organic lesions (polyps, leiomyomata, endometritis, IUDª) Neoplasia
Sixth decade	Hormone replacement therapyª Benign organic lesions (polyps, leiomyomata, endometritis) Atrophy Neoplasia

ªFrequency of hormone replacement therapy (HRT) and intrauterine device (IUD) usage will vary according to population.

Cycling endometrium (third and fourth decade)

INTRODUCTION

The endometrial cycle (Table 16.3) entails the interplay of four participants: the hypothalamus, pituitary, ovarian cortex and endometrium. These regulators of menstrual cycle interact to direct the two major phases, termed follicular and luteal phases, based on ovarian function or their synonyms, proliferative- and secretory-based endometrial morphology (Fig.

Table 16.2 Definitions of abnormal uterine bleeding

Abnormal uterine bleeding	Unscheduled or unexpected uterine bleeding
Dysfunctional uterine bleeding	Unscheduled bleeding that is presumed to be a consequence of a hormonal/functional (usually anovulatory) abnormality. Thus it can only be applied in the strict sense after all structural causes have been excluded
Oligomenorrhea	Intervals greater than 35 days
Polymenorrhea	Intervals less than 24 days
Menorrhagia (hypermenorrhea)	Excessive bleeding with normal intervals
Metrorrhagia	Excessive flow and duration at irregular intervals
Menometrorrhagia	Irregular menses
Withdrawal bleeding	Bleeding following the withdrawal of hormones

16.1).[10] Gonadotropin-releasing hormone (GNRH) is released in pulsatile fashion from the arcuate nuclei of the hypothalamus and orchestrates the release of follicle-stimulating hormone (FSH) and luteinizing hormone (LH) from the pituitary. Regulation of these hormones is dependent (positively) on the GNRH and (negatively) on the production of estrogens and progesterone by the follicle and corpus luteum, respectively, that feedback on the pituitary.

FSH increases prior to menstruation and initiates the process of recruitment of several follicles during stromal breakdown and regeneration. Subsequently, a dominant follicle emerges and is self-sustaining at the expense of its neighbors, converting androgen to estrogen with the aid of LH, maximizing its response

Table 16.3 Classification of cyclic endometrium

Category	Patterns (corresponding figures)
ME	Secretory exhausted glands, predecidua, diffuse breakdown Acute inflammatory exudates (Fig. 16.2a,b)
Late ME	Tubular glands, surface breakdown, blue aggregates of stroma Lack of surface epithelial/stromal cohesion (Fig. 16.4a–c)
PE	Tubular glands, mitoses (Fig. 16.5a–d)
16-day EM	Tubular glands, mitoses, scattered sub-nuclear vacuoles (Fig. 16.6b)
SE	Vacuoles[18–20] (Fig. 16.7a–d) Exhausted glands[21–29] (Figs 16.8–16.11) Stromal edema[22–23] (Fig. 16.8c) Predecidua[24–29] (Fig. 16.9a–e) Mononuclear cells[27–29] (Fig. 16.9e)

ME, menstrual (ovulatory) endometrium; PE, proliferative endometrium; EM, endometrium; SE, secretory endometrium.

to FSH by the production of activins while suppressing FSH by inhibins and the estrogen feedback loop. Ultimately this process confers the dominant follicle selective advantage over the now regressing surrounding follicles. Estradiol production by this follicle maintains proliferation and growth of the endometrium in the first 2 weeks of the cycle.

The mid-cycle LH surge coincides with the peak of estradiol levels, resulting in follicle rupture and release of the ovum. The LH surge is followed by increase in progesterone production by the now luteinized granulosa cells. The latter marks the transition from follicle to corpus luteum and initiates the vacuole phase of early secretory endometrium. Progesterone levels rise rapidly and remain elevated for approximately 14 days, terminating endometrial gland proliferation and promoting secretory conversion and predecidual changes in the latter half of the luteal phase. Estrogen secretion continues during this phase of the cycle, albeit at lower levels.

The onset of menstruation occurs if fertilization does not take place. The corpus luteum begins to regress and the highly vascular predecidualized endometrium with its complex secretory gland architecture rapidly disintegrates over an average of 5 days. This process of dissolution levels off at the basalis and the onset of the next cycle is characterized by restoration of an intact surface epithelium by migration from the gland crypts and resumption of the integrity of the endometrial stroma. The cycle begins anew.[8]

Less than 15% of all women have a 'prototypical' menstrual cycle lasting 28 days. Most fall between 24 and 35 days and 20% of women will at some time experience an irregular cycle. Durations of flow may range from 2–7 days, although most are within 4–6 days. Blood loss should be less than 30 ml. Thus, cycles with durations of flow of less than 2 or greater than 7 days with blood loss exceeding 80 ml are abnormal. Anovulatory cycles are most common before 20 and after age 40.[7]

Cyclic endometrium can be subdivided into seven phases based on morphologic appearance; these are summarized in Table 16.3. These include: (1) menstrual phase composed of scheduled (ovulatory) breakdown, (2) early proliferative phase with residual stromal breakdown leftover from the prior menstrual cycle which was just completed, (3) mid to late proliferative phase, (4) 16-day endometrium, (5) the vacuolar phase of early secretory endometrium, (6) the secretory exhausted phase and (7) the predecidua phase. Cycle phase assignment is often described in terms of an idealized 28-day cycle in which day 1 corresponds to

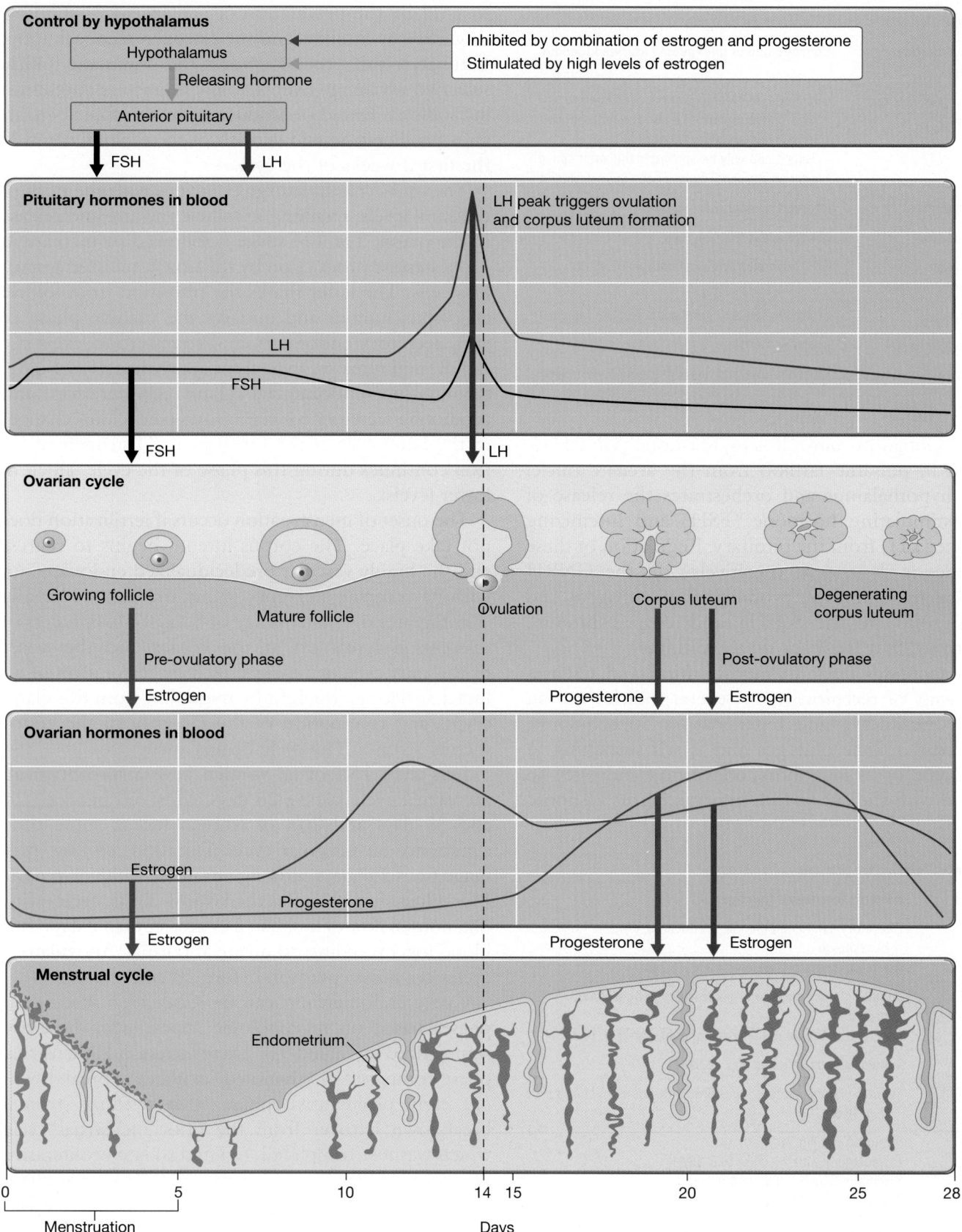

Fig. 16.1 Schematic of the menstrual cycle. Interplay of the hypothalamic, pituitary, ovarian and endometrial components and a schematic of events related to the menstrual cycle. (Adapted from Starr and McMillan.[10])

the first day of clinical menses. Women whose regular cycle length differs from this 28-day model typically have variations in length of the pre-ovulatory interval. Post-ovulatory phases (post-ovulatory days (POD) 17–28 in an idealized cycle) however, are quite consistent in duration even amongst women with differing overall cycle lengths.

There are five reasons for assigning a precise date to an endometrial biopsy.

1 The need to establish that ovulation has or has not taken place.

2 To determine if the assigned date falls within the expected range based on the patient's last menstrual period. This requires cooperation of both the clinician and the pathologist in determining whether a disturbance in the luteal phase has occurred.

3 To determine if a morphologically visible maturation disturbance exists, such as dyssynchronous maturation of endometrial glands in relation to the stroma.

4 To become accustomed to small differences in morphology of benign endometrial changes. An appreciation of such nuances may facilitate the recognition of subtle neoplastic processes.

5 To determine if sufficient endometrial luteal maturation has occurred in a preparatory cycle for potential recipients of egg donation or frozen embryo.

MENSTRUAL PHASE

Menstrual phase is morphologically defined by collapse of the stroma and shedding of the functionalis.[11] Lytic enzymes are confined within lysosomes in the early part of the luteal phase, maintained by progesterone. Release of matrix metalloproteinases (collagenases, gelatinases, stomolysins, etc.) occurs with the drop in progestin and is accompanied by activation of clotting followed by fibrinolysis.[11] The earliest feature of this process is condensation of predecidual cells into discrete aggregates or cord-like arrangements admixed with blood and inflammatory cells (Fig. 16.2a). Subsequently, a pattern of 'scheduled breakdown' ensues, with coordinate collapse of the functionalis, sheets of neutrophils and the characteristic plump aggregates of necrotic predecidua. Included in this detritus of ovulation are exhausted secretory glands that range from large, irregularly shaped glands with slightly stratified nuclei (a consequence of epithelial collapse and nuclear condensation) to single-cell layered epithelium

with a thin or delicate appearance (Fig. 16.2b). The presence of predecidual stromal aggregates and/or exhausted glands typifies ovulatory breakdown and, when encountered, this pattern of scheduled (diffuse) breakdown with acute inflammatory debris most commonly signifies that ovulation has occurred.[1] At day 3 of the menses, the diagnosis of ovulation can still be made provided sufficient secretory exhausted glands are still present (Fig. 16.2c). Following this, the remainder of the breakdown occurs in the lower functionalis and the diagnosis of ovulation cannot be confirmed on histologic grounds.

The diagnosis rendered for these changes is: *Menstrual (ovulatory) endometrium.*

Two variations in menstrual endometrium have been reported in the past. The first is irregular shedding. In this pattern, fragments of intact predecidualized endometrium coexist with early proliferative-pattern endometrium. The explanation for this picture is persistent corpus luteum, leading to a greater range of findings in which features of early breakdown (predecidualized fragments) coexist with later regenerative (tubular glands) components (Fig. 16.2d,e). The second variation is 'membranous dysmenorrhea', consisting of cohesive sheets of predecidualized endometrium with scarce glands, alternating with conventional disaggregated endometrium (Fig. 16.2f). This pattern was anecdotally associated with dysmenorrhea in some instances, hence the term.

Certain diagnostic pitfalls may be encountered in association with real or perceived menstrual endometrium. The first is the misdiagnosis of menstrual endometrium as endometrial adenocarcinoma, which may be simulated by the collapse of glands and the associated necrotic predecidua (Fig. 16.3a). The second pitfall is the reverse. Small disaggregated fragments of adenocarcinoma that may simulate stromal breakdown (Fig. 16.3b). Less serious pitfalls are other patterns of breakdown that may be associated with a variety of disturbances that do not signify ovulation. These are summarized in Table 16.4 and illustrated elsewhere in this chapter.

EARLY PROLIFERATIVE PHASE WITH RESIDUAL STROMAL BREAKDOWN (LATE MENSTRUAL/EARLY PROLIFERATIVE ENDOMETRIUM)

The process of scheduled (ovulatory) stromal breakdown involves both shedding of the overlying secretory functionalis and, later in menses, continued breakdown

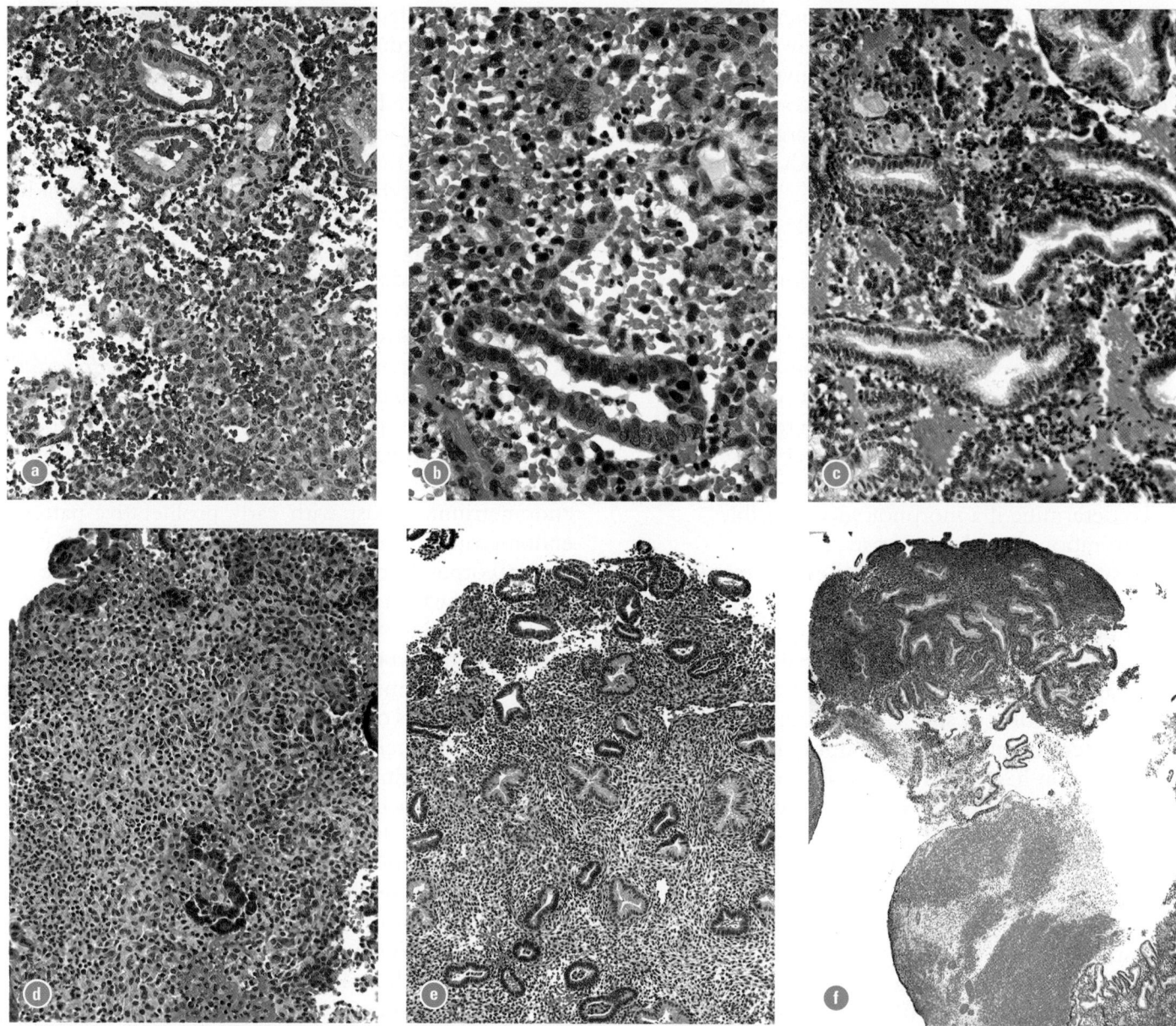

Fig. 16.2 (a) Menstrual endometrium exhibits a diffuse pattern of stromal breakdown. (b) At higher power the exhausted glands contain delicate single-layered epithelium and cord-like aggregates of necrotic predecidualized stroma. (c) At day 3 of menses the features of ovulation can still be appreciated. (d,e) Irregular shedding, characterized by early breakdown of predecidualized endometrium (d) combined with an early proliferative pattern with star-shaped glands (e). (f) 'Membranous dysmenorrhea', with intact sheets of necrotic predecidua (lower).

of the lower functionalis. The cessation of bleeding is in part aided by vasoconstriction and rising estrogen levels, which reduce the production of proteinases and prompt 'healing'.[7] The end of the menses is characterized by the re-epithelialization of the basalis. Three features characterize this phase: (1) basal tubular glands with slightly stratified nuclei, variable sub-nuclear vacuoles and occasional mitoses; (2) residual breakdown (shedding) of lower functionalis stroma; and (3)

variable detachment of the surface epithelium (Fig. 16.4a). The latter phenomenon occurs in association with the process of re-epithelialization (as the endometrium attempts to stem the bleeding, repair itself and proliferate), leading to a combination of increasingly rare stromal clumps representing residual stromal breakdown or shedding (so-called 'blue balls') and epithelial resurfacing (Fig. 16.4b).[4] The latter may be quite tenuous at first, leading to the appearance of poor

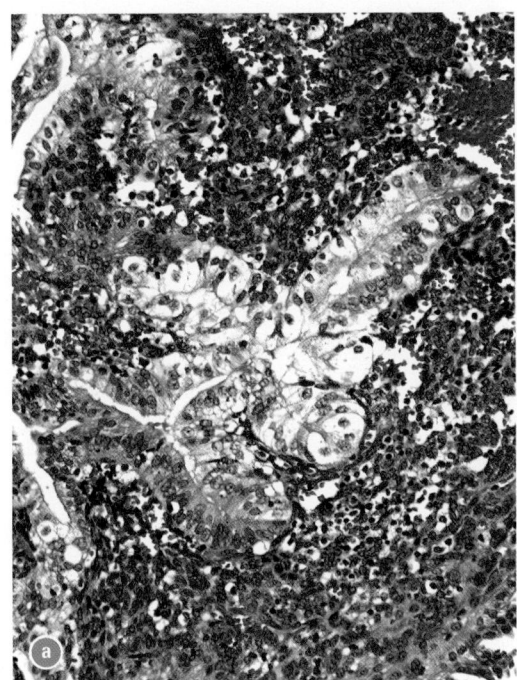

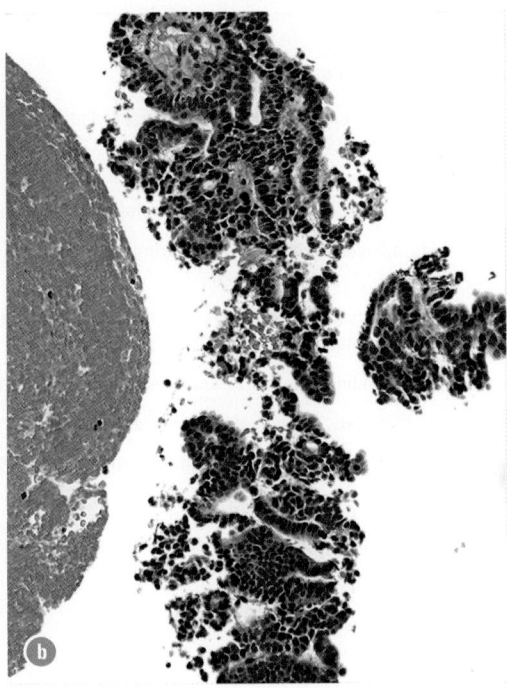

Fig. 16.3 (a) Crowded endometrial glands with breakdown simulating endometrial carcinoma. (b) Small fragments of endometrial carcinoma simulating menstrual endometrium.

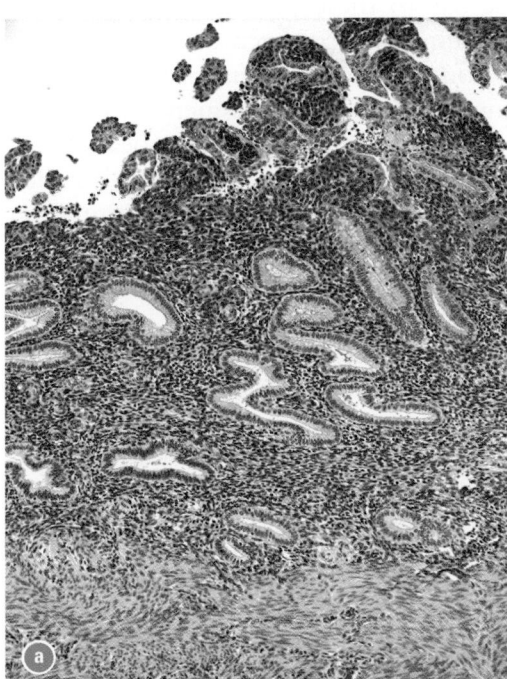

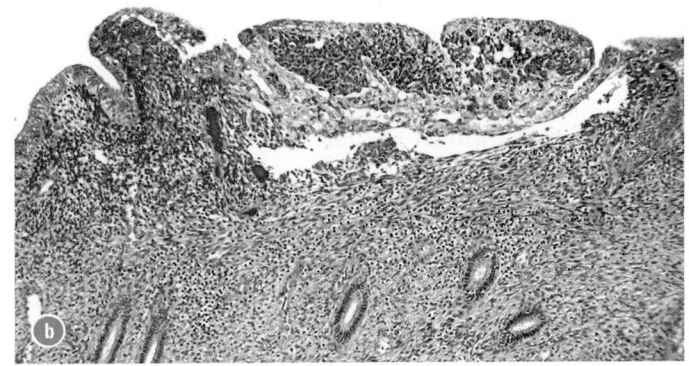

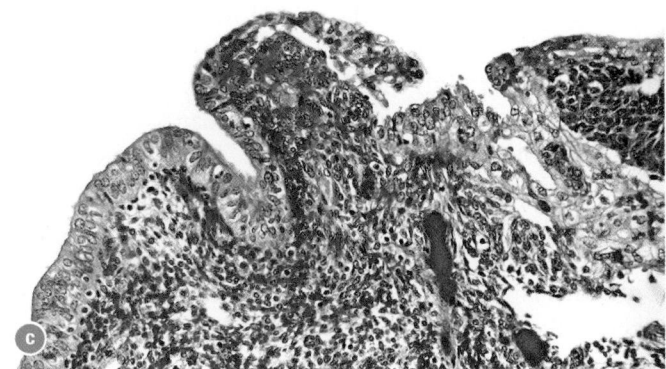

Fig. 16.4 (a) Late menstrual endometrium with surface breakdown. (b) Clusters of necrotic surface stroma. (c) Detachment of surface epithelium overlying stromal breakdown.

Table 16.4 Differential diagnosis of stromal breakdown

Cause	Pattern (corresponding figure)
Ovulatory	Exhausted glands, diffuse breakdown, necrotic predecidua, acute inflammation (Fig. 16.2a,b)
Late menstrual	Tubular glands, variable vacuoles, rare mitoses, surface breakdown, poor surface epithelial-stromal cohesion (Fig. 16.4a–c)
Replacement therapy	Tubular glands, spindled stroma, variable stromal cohesion (Fig. 16.37a)
Anovulation (persistent follicle)	Patchy breakdown, cystic, irregular glands, fibrin thrombi, blue stromal aggregates, gland karyorrhexis (Fig. 16.15c)
Dysfunctional[a]	Intact functionalis, tubular glands, diffuse breakdown (Fig. 16.16c)
Unknown[b]	Stromal breakdown only, minimal glands, similar to late menstrual
Chronic endometritis	Lymphoplasmacytic infiltrates, intra-glandular exudates (Fig. 16.21c)
Endometrial polyp	Surface breakdown
Post pregnancy	Similar to late menstrual, necrotic decidua (decidual cast)
Post progestin therapy	Similar to post pregnancy

[a]A diagnosis of dysfunctional uterine bleeding is permitted once any pathology has been excluded.
[b]In the absence of glandular tissue ovulation, anovulation and dysfunctional causes can neither be excluded nor confirmed.

cohesion with, or detachment from, the underlying stroma (Fig. 16.4c). Because all morphologic signs of ovulation (such as predecidualized stroma, secretory exhausted glands) are no longer present, ovulation cannot be confirmed. The diagnosis rendered for this phase of the cycle is as follows: 'Early proliferative endometrium with residual stromal breakdown. It is not possible to confirm ovulation in the late stage of endometrial shedding'.

PROLIFERATIVE PHASE ENDOMETRIUM

Proliferative phase endometrium reflects the influence of estrogenic hormones from the developing ovarian follicle, which stimulate gland proliferation and produce the classic tubular gland with pseudostratified epithelium and increased mitotic activity. At low power, the glands appear blue or dark due to the pseudostratified basophilic nuclei (Fig. 16.5a). The pathologist who examines these glands at high magnification may be initially concerned by the coarse-appearing nuclear chromatin and high mitotic index (Fig. 16.5b). The critical features which aids in the recognition that these glands are benign are the orderly arrangement of the nuclei in an architecturally normal, i.e. round to minimally irregular, gland. As the cycle progresses some edema may be seen followed by increased gland tortuosity prior to ovulation. Subclassification or assign-

ment of a cycle day to these nuances of proliferative phase endometrium is not required inasmuch as they have no bearing on diagnosis and management. There are three diagnostic pitfalls in assessment of the proliferative phase. The first is the variable appearance of the stroma, which may include a prominent spindled appearance. The novice may sometimes misinterpret this feature as predecidua or progestin effect (Fig. 16.5c); however, the lack of prominent spiral arterioles and the presence of abundant mitoses are inconsistent with progestin effect. The second pitfall is intraluminal material misinterpreted as secretions. 'Secretions' can be found in the lumen of any endometrial gland irrespective of cycle day and should not be used to assign a cycle date. A third pitfall is a technical one where gland tracts are susceptible to intussusception, also termed 'telescoping' or 'gland in gland' artifact (Fig. 16.5d). This may be misinterpreted as hyperplasia; however, this pattern has been sufficiently well described that it should not be confused with neoplasia. The diagnosis we render for this phase of the cycle is simply: Proliferative endometrium.

16-DAY ENDOMETRIUM (POD 2)

Ovulation as defined occurs on day 14 of the cycle. Both 15- and 16-day endometrium are technically synonymous with the first and second days following

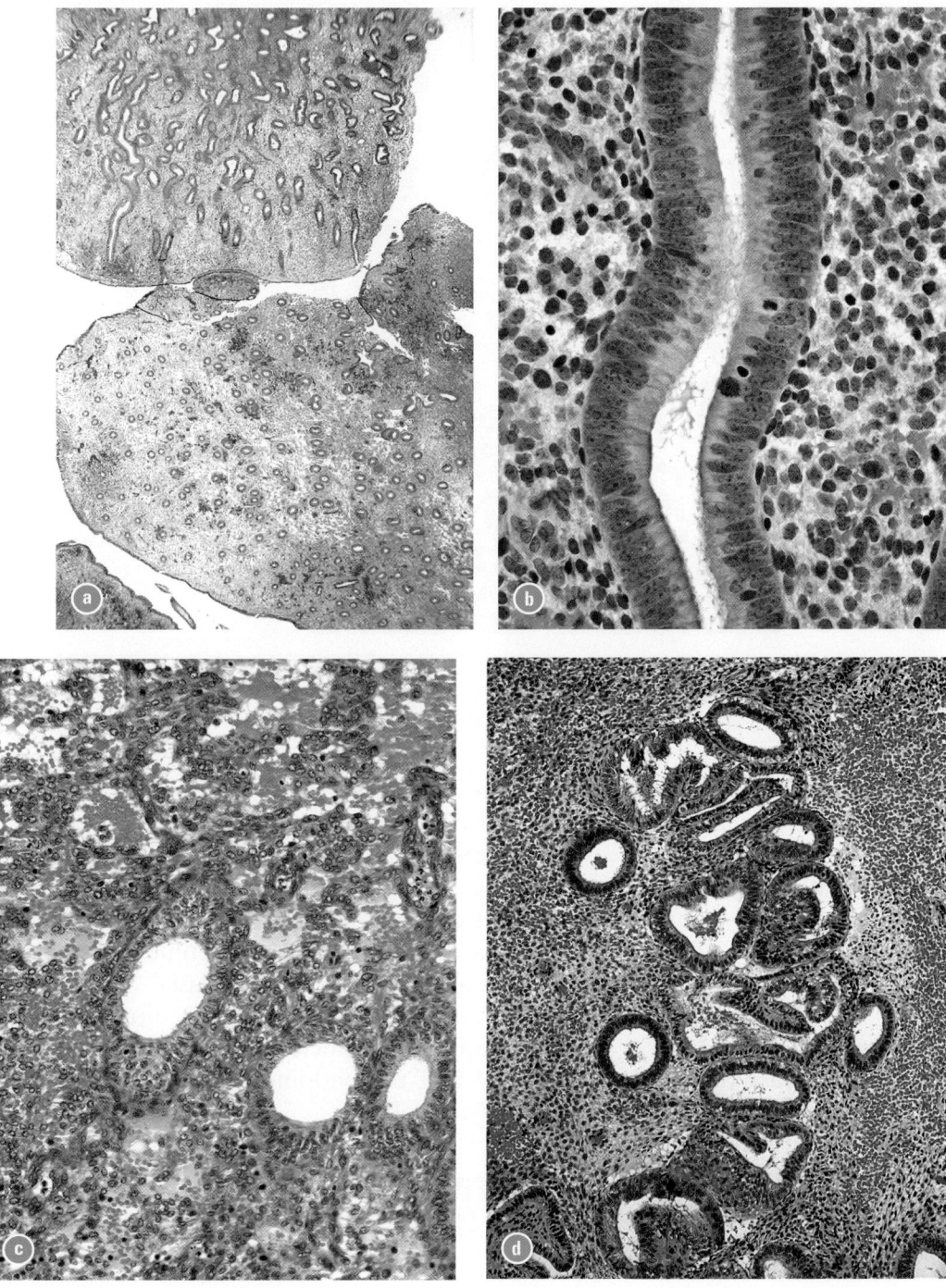

Fig. 16.5 (a) Low-power microphotograph of proliferative endometrium illustrating abundant tubular glands. (b) At higher power the pseudostratified epithelium contains prominent nuclei with mitoses. (c) Pseudo-predecidual changes in a proliferative endometrium. (d) Gland in gland (telescoping) artifact.

ovulation. Both may be characterized by the presence of sub-nuclear vacuoles in an endometrium that has the glandular architecture (and mitotic activity) of proliferative endometrium. These findings are subtle in day 15 and conspicuous in 16-day endometrium (Fig. 16.6a,b).[1] The endometrial glands will appear slightly larger and slightly less basophilic at low power due to the interruption of the pseudostratified epithe-

lium by vacuoles. Mitoses must be present, but will be less conspicuous. The transition to a pattern that is diagnostic of ovulation (day 17 secretory phase) occurs when a discrete group of glands with no mitoses and uniform sub-nuclear vacuoles is identified. The reader is reminded that sub-nuclear vacuoles alone are not sufficient for a diagnosis of ovulation if mitoses are present. Thus, the diagnosis rendered for this pattern

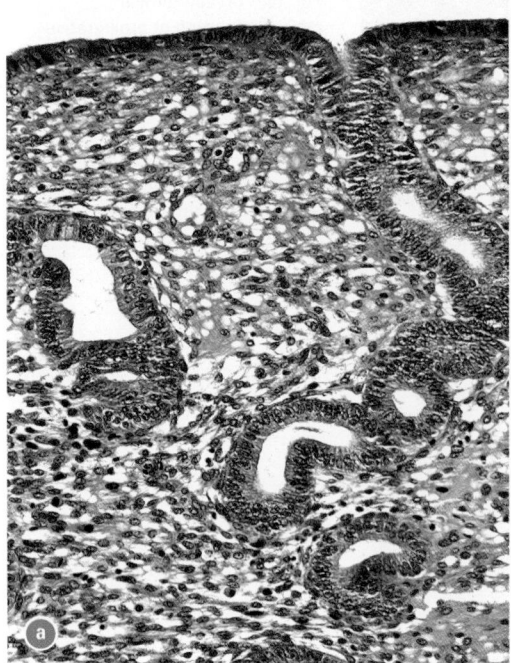
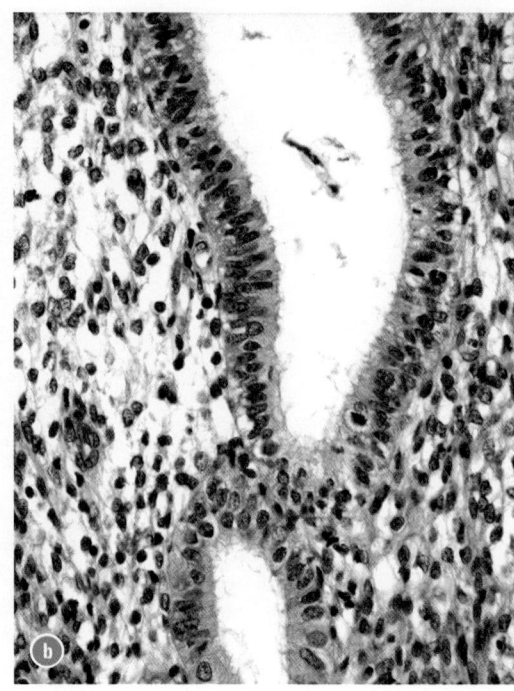

Fig. 16.6 (a) A 15-day endometrium contains rare vacuoles. (b) A 16-day endometrium contains sub-nuclear vacuoles and regular mitoses. This pattern may be associated with ovulation, but is not specific.

is: 16-day endometrium. This pattern may be associated with ovulation; however it is not specific for ovulation and may be seen with estrogen alone. Clinical correlation is advised.

VACUOLE PHASE OF SECRETORY ENDOMETRIUM (17–19 DAYS; POD 4–6)

The vacuole phase of secretory endometrium (SE) signifies the first phase of the post-ovulatory period. The low-power appearance of the endometrium contains glands that are larger and slightly undulating and which appear more eosinophilic due to the absence of pseudostratified nuclei combined with vacuoles and intracellular secretions (Fig. 16.7a). As described above, 17-day SE is characterized by uniform sub-nuclear vacuoles and virtually no mitotic activity (see Fig. 16.7a inset). In 18-day secretory endometrium, the vacuoles are staggered toward the lumen and are accompanied by supranuclear discharge, seen as a ragged surface change (Fig. 16.7b). The vacuoles may or may not be conspicuous; however, the nuclei are prominently situated in the center of each cell, forming a uniform monolayer amidst eosinophilic cytoplasm. In day 19 secretory endometrium, the nuclei have nearly migrated back to the base and are accompanied by scattered residual sub-nuclear vacuoles and the appearance of

early secretory exhaustion; mitotic activity typically is not present (Fig. 16.7c).

One diagnostic pitfall commonly encountered in the vacuole phase of the endometrial cycle is an irregular random pattern of gland enlargement leading to foci of gland crowding. This is sometimes erroneously interpreted as a 'secretory hyperplasia' (Fig. 16.7d). In contrast to hyperplasia, there is no appreciable cellular stratification, nuclear changes in comparison with the rest of the endometrium or other features seen in early neoplasia.

EXHAUSTIVE PHASE OF SECRETORY ENDOMETRIUM (20–22 DAYS; POD 6–8)

Conclusion of the vacuole phase is characterized by secretory exhaustion. This pattern persists for the remainder of the cycle, with the exception of occasional hypersecretory changes that might accompany the late secretory phase. The early phases of this latter portion of the cycle are relatively indistinct. SE day 20 demonstrates peak intraluminal secretions accompanied by occasional residual sub-nuclear vacuoles combined with slight gland enlargement and a compact subsurface stroma (Fig. 16.8a). The presence of this subsurface change may be misinterpreted as stroma exhibiting predecidual change, leading to

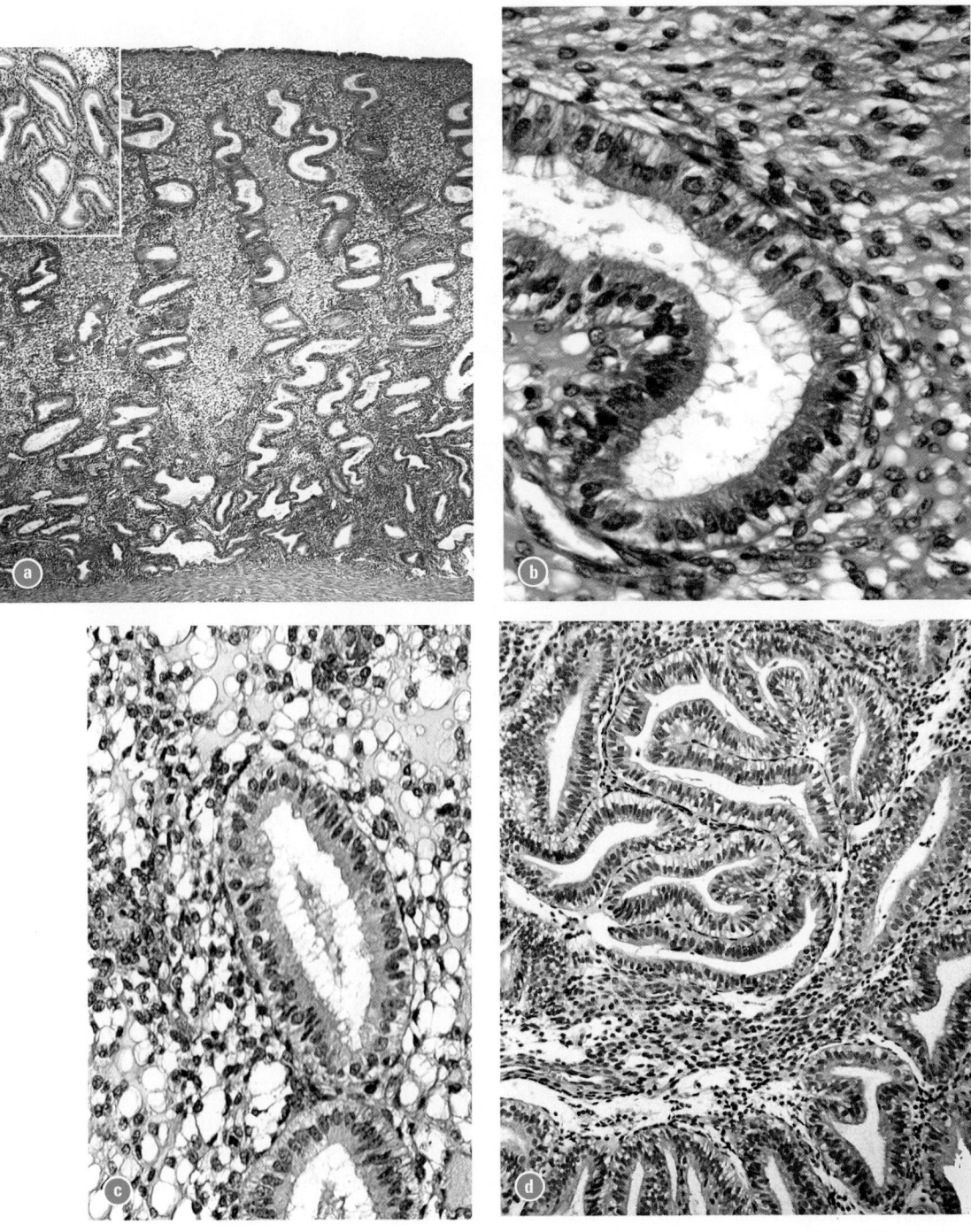

Fig. 16.7 (a) Low power of 17-day secretory endometrium (compare with Fig. 16.5a). Inset illustrates prominent sub-nuclear vacuoles. (b) Secretory day 18. (c) Secretory endometrium day 19. (d) Artifactual crowding of glands in early secretory endometrium may simulate hyperplasia.

misinterpretation of the cycle day as day 25. However, the former does not display prominent perivascular cuffing and, unlike predecidua, the stromal cells still exhibit dark nuclei and scant cytoplasm. Secretory endometrium day 21 exhibits an increase in stromal edema, highlighting the spiral arterioles (Fig. 16.8b). SE day 22 is characterized by a peak in stromal edema and exhibits the first hint of perivascular cuff-

ing but conspicuous predecidual changes are lacking (Fig. 16.8c).

PREDECIDUAL PHASE OF SECRETORY ENDOMETRIUM (23–28 DAYS; POD 9–14)

This phase is initiated by the condensation of predecidua around spiral arterioles. Predecidua is not

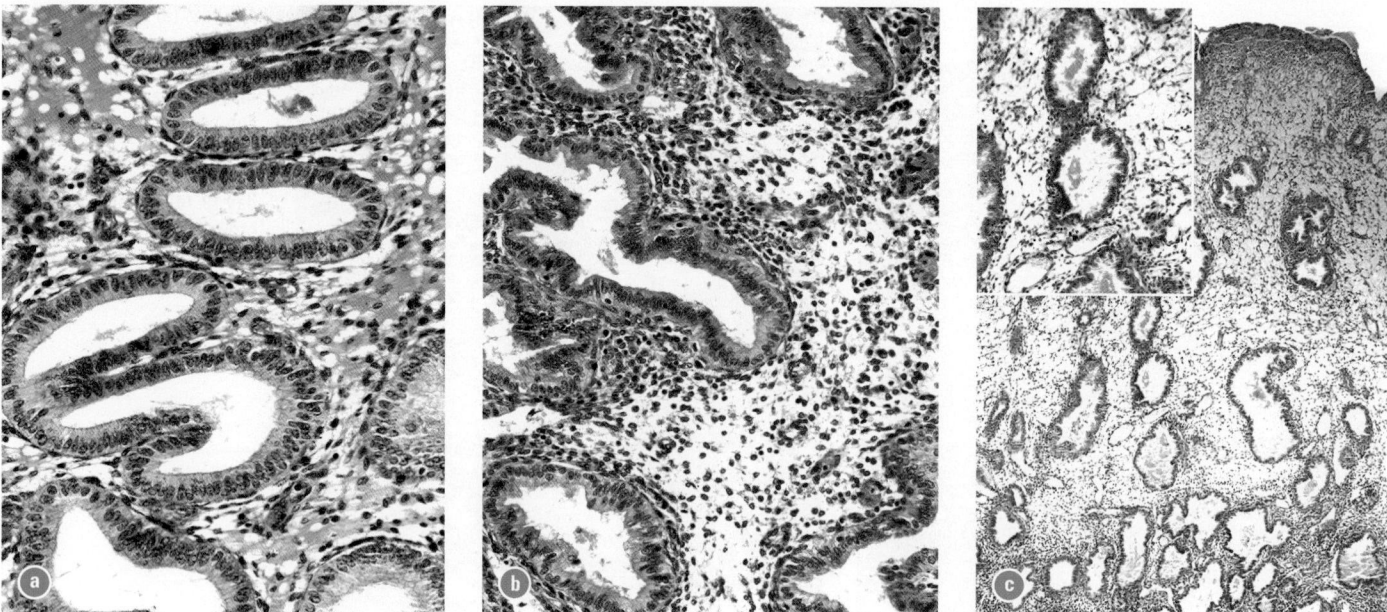

Fig. 16.8 (a) Secretory endometrium day 20, (b) day 21, (c) day 22, with prominent edema and secretory exhausted glands (inset).

actually decidua because it is not the result of pregnancy; nevertheless, the term predecidua is used because the cells bear some morphologic resemblance to pregnancy-related decidual change. Predecidua has three characteristics. The first is spiral aggregates of spindled cells around vessels (Fig. 16.9a). A potential pitfall is the interpretation of larger arteries as spiral arterioles and confusing the two to three layers of investing adventitia around these larger arteries as predecidua. However, predecidua exhibits two additional distinctions, being the acquisition of slightly basophilic (as opposed to eosinophilic) cytoplasm, often with distinct cell borders and nuclear changes that are characterized by a reduction in basophilia with finer chromatin texture. This combination of abundant darker cytoplasm mixed with paler nuclei reduces the nuclear/cytoplasmic contrast, making the cells less distinct and lending a slightly 'smudged' or 'out of focus' appearance to the aggregates. This relative 'softness' amidst the higher contrast of the lower functionalis distinguishes predecidua from its mimics (Fig. 16.9b). As a rule of thumb, perivascular aggregates involving single vessels signifies day 23, aggregates bridging multiple vessels are day 24 (Fig. 16.9a), subsurface aggregates are present in day 25, linear sheets beneath the surface signify day 26 (Fig. 16.9c) and continuous subsurface with expansion downward between the folds of the functionalis are assigned day 27 (Fig. 16.9d,e). In mid to late secretory phase

endometrium, adjacent glands may display a transition from dilated glands with a simple contour to those having a 'saw-toothed' configuration (Fig. 16.10a), but in the late phase the glands may be variably dilated or tubular (similar to the changes seen with progestin effect (Fig. 16.10b)). The prominent saw-toothed glands may be confused with pregnancy but are not diagnostic in the absence of the nuclear features characterizing Arias-Stella change.

Scattered endometrial stromal granulocytes may be seen by secretory day 24–25 but are conspicuous by day 26 (Fig. 16.9d). One potential diagnostic pitfall is edematous predecidua, which may be confused with day 21, particularly by the inexperienced (Fig. 16.11a,b). Closer examination of the edematous areas will confirm the presence of cells with the characteristic basophilic cytoplasm and other features of individual predecidual cells as described above. In general, the spaces between the stromal cell nuclei in late secretory phase are occupied by cytoplasm in contrast to earlier in the phase when the nuclei are separated by fluid (Fig. 16.11b). A second diagnostic pitfall is interpretation of stromal granulocytes as inflammation or chronic endometritis. However, in contrast to the latter, no plasma cells are present and the setting of late secretory endometrium is inconsistent with chronic endometritis. The diagnosis for secretory endometria is simply: 'Secretory endometrium (day specified)'.

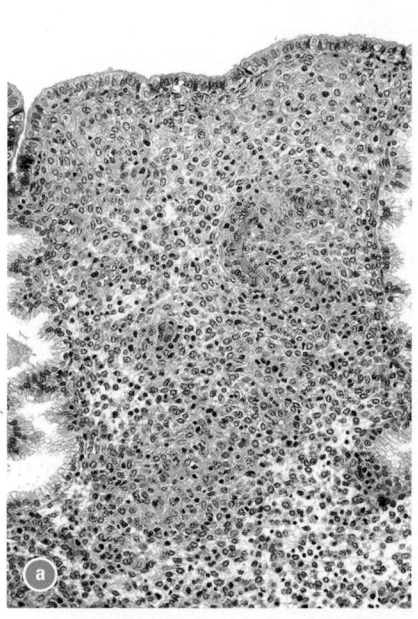
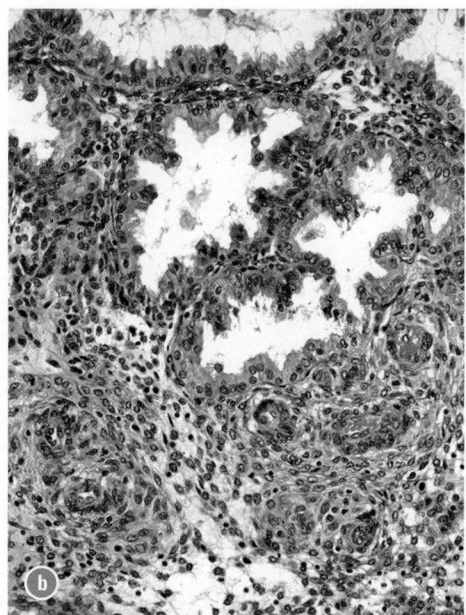
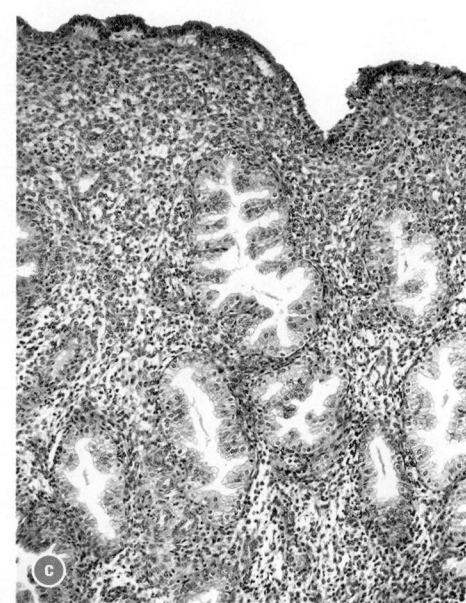
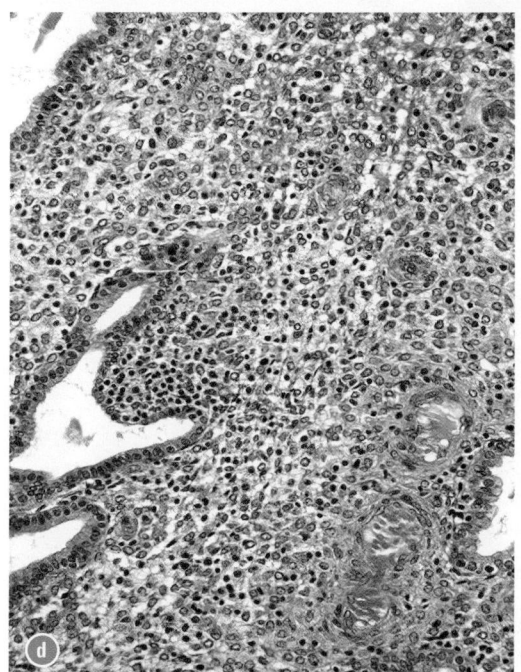
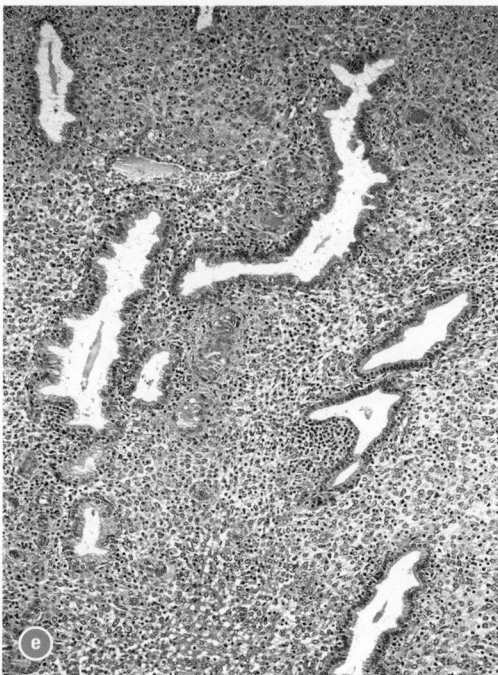

Fig. 16.9 (a) Predecidua cuffing around spiral arterioles begins at day 23. (b) Cytoplasmic basophilia and nuclear hypochromasia produce a loss of cell contrast. (c) Predecidua distributed on the surface by day 25/26. (d) Extension of predecidua between glands occurs by day 27. (e) Endometrial granulocytes emerge around day 26.

Disorders of secretory maturation that are the focus of infertility management

LUTEAL PHASE DEFECT

Luteal phase defect (LPD, or inadequate luteal phase) is not defined as a specific alteration of the endometrium, but as secretory maturation that is morphologically at least 2 days earlier than expected relative to the expected post-ovulatory day on two endometrial samplings. LPD was first described by Jones and encompasses a range of conditions, including disorders in folliculogenesis, defective corpus luteum function and abnormal luteal rescue by the early pregnancy.[12] Certain conditions known to cause ovulatory dysfunction, such as hyperprolactinemia, hyperandrogenic states, weight loss, stress and athletic training, may also contribute to LPD in ovulating women.[13]

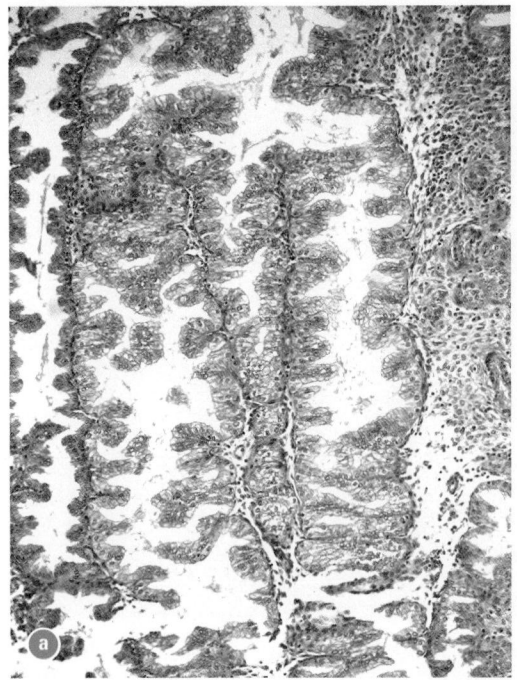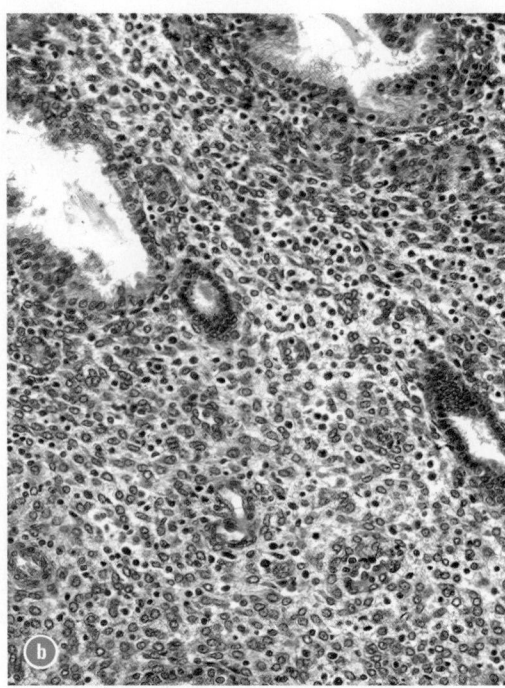

Fig. 16.10 (a) Saw-toothed glandular configuration seen in late secretory endometrium. (b) Small tubular glands may be present, simulating exogenous hormonal effect.

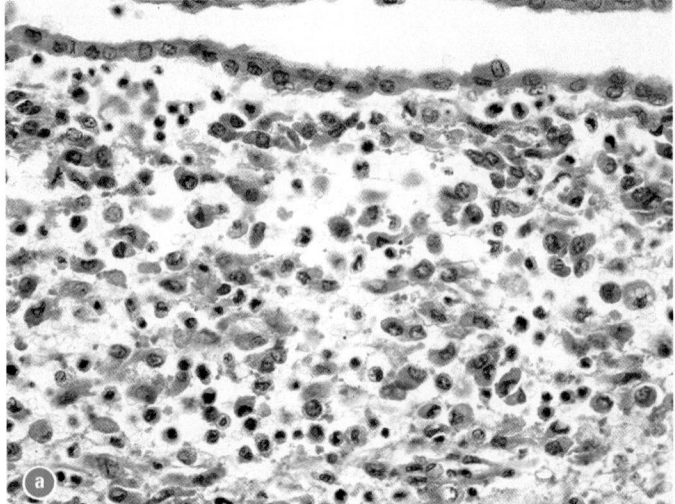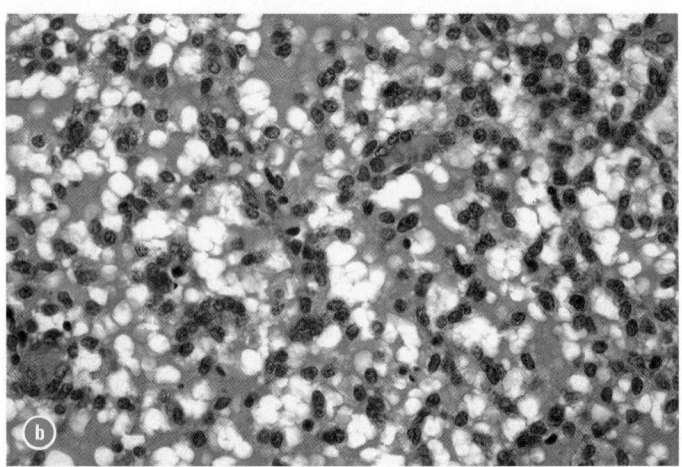

Fig. 16.11 (a) Edematous predecidua. (b) Stromal changes in a 21-day secretory endometrium may mimic predecidua.

The endometrial biopsy has been termed the 'gold standard' in LPD diagnosis while at the same time raising questions about the extent to which LPD can be considered a clinical entity. Central to this discussion has been (1) whether progesterone levels or endometrial biopsies are more reliable indicators of ovarian function, (2) whether either alone is sufficient to define LPD and whether (3) these tests are reproducible. One study concluded that the most reliable test was a single serum progesterone level from the mid-luteal phase, or three random progesterone measurements.[14] Endometrial biopsy was not considered as reliable. Another attributed the disparity between endometrial response and (normal) progesterone levels to an insufficient response of the endometrium to progesterone. The conclusion was that histologic examination was indicated irrespective of the progesterone level.[15] However, others have observed delayed endometrial development in nearly one-fourth of cases in which biochemical parameters and follicle development were observed.[16]

Review of the available literature supports the above, that endometrial biopsy (1) frequently underestimates the cycle day, (2) shows a lag in secretory maturation at similar frequencies in both cases and controls, (3) is not consistent from cycle to cycle and (4) cannot be estimated with sufficient inter-observer reliability to be an accurate barometer of LPD. For example, Davis et al. examined 39 biopsies in five women with regular cycles. Using a 2-day or greater lag in endometrial maturity to define LPD, the incidence of single and sequential out-of-phase endometrial biopsies was 51.4% and 26.7%, respectively. Using a 3-day or greater lag to define an LPD, the incidence of single and sequential out-of-phase EMBs was 31.4% and 6.6%, respectively. Because the frequency of discrepancies in these normal women approached that seen in those with infertility, the authors questioned the traditional definition and prevalence of LPD.[17]

In one study, five observers twice analyzed split endometrial biopsies from 25 women. A total of 65 and 27% of discrepancies, respectively, were explained by inter- and intra-observer variation.[18] Duggan et al. showed that considerable variation existed between observers although 77% fell within 2 days.[19] Murray et al. recently correlated observer endometrial dating, inter-observer reproducibility and relationship to cycle day by hormonal measurements. They found that traditional dating criteria were not as precise as originally assumed and subject to observer variability. They concluded that histologic dating of the endometrium was an inadequate measure for evaluating luteal phase deficiency.[20] In a study which evaluated 774 endometrial biopsies performed for infertility, Davidson et al. concluded that, although endometrial biopsies are relatively safe, the diagnostic and therapeutic consequences are limited and endometrial biopsies may be useful only if performed in cases of habitual abortion or ovulation induction with clomiphene citrate.[21]

OVULATION INDUCTION AND DEFECTS IN SECRETORY MATURATION

Although controversial for fertility, LPD is a generally accepted cause of recurrent pregnancy loss. Studies of assisted reproduction (donor insemination) have correlated failure to conceive with insufficient endometrial response to progesterone.[22] It is generally held that a normal corpus luteum will result in a normal transi-

tion to and progression through secretory maturation. Conversely, a deficiency in corpus luteum development results in dyssynchrony of the endometrium, which may be corrected by the administration of progesterone.[23] Paradoxically, therapy with synthetic gestagens depresses glandular secretion, induces glandular atrophy and pseudodecidualization of the stroma and the magnitude of the change depends on the dosage and type of drug.[3] Clomiphene depresses normal secretion by its anti-estrogenic effect, which causes deficient estrogen priming. On the other hand, clomiphene counteracts excessive estrogen and will normalize its secretion in a deficient luteal phase that was preceded by follicular persistence. A luteal phase defect is associated with gonadotropin-releasing hormone analogue/human menopausal gonadotropin-stimulated cycles used in assisted reproduction. Potential mechanisms include the effects of Lupron on the endometrium and loss of granulose cells during egg retrieval. This can be counteracted by the administration of progesterone either by suppository or i.m. injections. The goal is to increase the progestogen bioavailability of the endometrium.[24] In an artificial cycle, depending upon the state of endogenous hormonal stimulation, the patients will benefit either from clomiphene or gonadotropin to maintain or normalize their secretory endometrium.[25]

The pathologist usually has a peripheral role in *in vitro* fertilization, where much of the strategy is based on hormonal parameters. However, prepcycles designed to prepare the endometrium for a donor-fertilized ovum often rely on an assessment of endometrial maturation. These hormonal regimens typically do not precisely recapitulate the normal luteal phase, but the pathologist will be asked to estimate the degree of predecidual changes, the development of which are considered germane to a successful trial. The findings in such instances may range from well-developed mid secretory phase endometrium (Fig. 16.12a,b) to one with a wide range of maturation (Fig. 16.13). The pathologist may encounter evidence of anovulation or other disturbances signifying either an unreceptive environment or worse hyperplasia.

THE ROLE OF BIOMARKERS IN ENDOMETRIAL EVALUATION

Citing the lack of inter-observer reproducibility and consistency in recognizing cycle defects, several groups have examined a range of biomarkers in providing an objective assessment of endometrial receptivity to implantation (see summary by Dubowy et al.[26]). Recently,

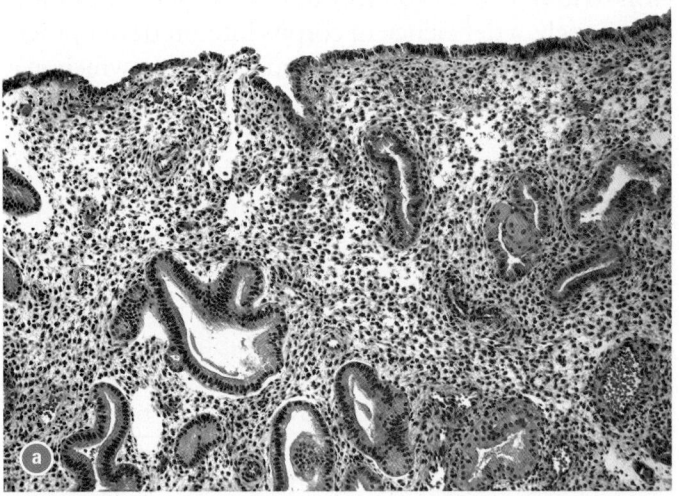 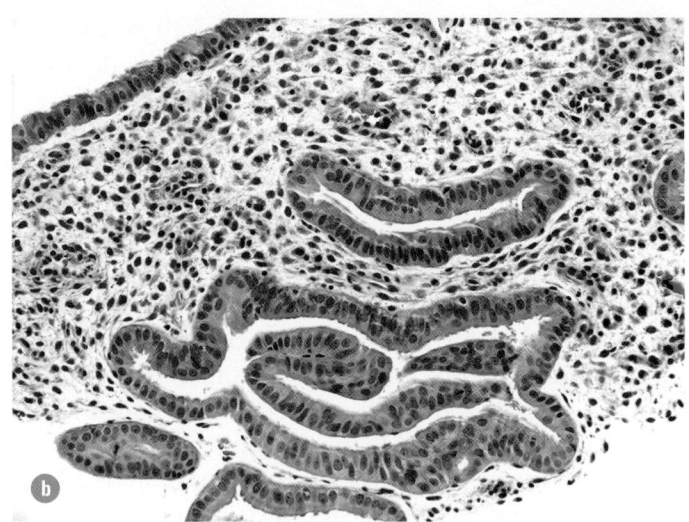

Fig. 16.12 (a) Typical endometrial prep cycle. The glands exhibit some delay in secretory maturation. (b) At higher power, predecidual changes can be recognized, albeit subtle.

Dubowy et al. observed preferential expression of cyclin E and p27 in the proliferative and luteal phases of the cycle, respectively.[26] With their eye towards an 'endometrial function test', the authors noted that continued nuclear expression of cyclin E in glands in the luteal phase correlated with infertility and may signify decreased endometrial receptivity. Presumably, this extended expression of cyclin E has its correlate in dyssynchronous glands that are functionally delayed. Although their findings will require validation by additional studies, such studies endeavor to categorize the mor-

Fig. 16.13 Another prep cycle sample shows a wide disparity in response, with both lag in secretory maturation (tubular glands) and a dominant early secretory pattern with sub-nuclear vacuoles.

phologic disturbances that typify dyssynchronous endometrium with more objective means.

Abnormal uterine bleeding

INTRODUCTION

Abnormal uterine bleeding has been estimated to occur in 20 per 1000 women-years in a family practice and comprises up to 30% and 75% of gynecologic visits in pre- and postmenopausal women, respectively.[27,28] Abnormal bleeding is categorized according to the underlying cause and morphology (Tables 16.1, 16.4). In women in the second to fourth decades, contraceptive-related bleeding (28%) is the most common abnormality. For women in the fifth decade, bleeding is most often associated with anovulation (perimenopausal bleeding). Additional disorders that may produce abnormal bleeding include chronic endometritis, endometrial polyps and submucosal leiomyomata. In women over age 55, bleeding is often associated with hormonal replacement therapy. However, the risk of endometrial carcinoma increases in this population and, depending on the proportion of patients on hormones, may comprise a considerable proportion of patients with abnormal bleeding. In one study, it was 29%.[29]

Cyclic (menstrual) bleeding takes place in the upper two-thirds of the endometrium, is initiated by the release of proteolytic enzymes of endometrial and leukocyte origin, and is characterized by tissue necrosis, loss of vascular integrity, inflammatory cell infiltrates and thrombi in small vessels. Moreover, cyclic bleeding occurs in a diffuse (programmed) manner. Abnormal bleeding tends to localize to the upper-third of the functionalis, where it may be focal or diffuse. The breakdown is mediated by inflammatory (endometritis) or vascular (fragility) phenomena, which may accompany chronic endometritis, polyps, submucosal leiomyomata, atrophy and other organic causes. Similarly, alterations in vasculature that predispose to bleeding may be found in altered hormonal environments, including anovulation and progestational hormonal therapy. In the absence of a morphologic abnormality, impaired vasoconstriction and fibrinolysis are presumed to be the mechanisms.[11]

DYSFUNCTIONAL UTERINE BLEEDING

Depending on the woman's age, a significant proportion of cases of uterine bleeding, and up to 50% of those with menorrhagia, occur in the absence of an organic cause. This is referred to as dysfunctional uterine bleeding (DUB). As strictly defined, DUB is bleeding in the absence of *both* ovulation and an organic cause; however, some authors attribute a proportion of DUB (30%) to causes other than ovulation.[30] Thus, a diagnosis of DUB cannot be made until histologic examination excludes an organic lesion. In clinical practice, DUB is frequently listed on the pathology requisition *prior to* the pathology diagnosis. In this setting DUB is not specific and is essentially synonymous with abnormal bleeding. In either setting the pathologist is not required to make the diagnosis; rather he or she must exclude organic causes and be aware of patterns that may signify DUB.

Three general patterns may be included under dysfunctional uterine bleeding. The first is a visible change (cystic) in the endometrial glands for which a presumptive diagnosis of anovulation can be made. In a study of 1282 cases of dysfunctional bleeding, 77% were attributed to anovulation and, of these, 89% to persistent follicle or other glandular disturbance ('hyperplasia').[30] This pattern may be classified as 'estrogen breakthrough bleeding'. Over half of patients with DUB are menopausal. The second is a proliferative-pattern endometrium with subnormal proliferation, which could signify subnormal estrogen stimulation and/or a disturbance in folliculogenesis. This group comprised approximately 11% in the study by Vakiani et al. and may be loosely termed 'estrogen withdrawal bleeding'. Other patterns attributed to DUB include the finding of ovulatory endometrium with disturbances in the follicular (prolonged) or luteal phase or in premenopausal patients, impaired vasoconstriction and coagulation disturbances.[11,30,31]

MENORRHAGIA

An important subset of abnormal bleeding is menorrhagia. Menorrhagia is defined subjectively as a heavy and/or prolonged menstrual bleeding and objectively measured as menstrual blood loss of greater than 80 ml.[31] Menorrhagia is common, seen in approximately 30% of women and is one of the most common reasons for patient-initiated visits to gynecologists. Moreover, nearly two-thirds of these patients become candidates for hysterectomy or endometrial destructive surgery. Approximately 50% are idiopathic (dysfunctional bleeding) and abnormalities in prostaglandin metabolism have been implicated.[31] Long-term treatment of idiopathic menorrhagia includes intrauterine progestogens, antifibrinolytic agents (tranexamic acid) and nonsteroidal anti-inflammatory agents (mefenamic acid). Since the early 1990s, there has been increasing use of endometrial destructive techniques (endometrial ablation) as an alternative to hysterectomy. These are discussed at the conclusion of this chapter. Their further refinement and the advent of fibroid embolization has increased the options available to women.[31]

Inherited bleeding disorders may play a prominent role in abnormal bleeding and those fulfilling strict criteria (by a pictorial bleeding assessment chart or PBAC) comprised 17% of women presenting with menorrhagia in one study.[32] Some 60–74% of women with von Willebrand's disease (vWD) and factors XI and VII deficiency present with menorrhagia.[32,33]

CAUSES OF ABNORMAL UTERINE BLEEDING AS A FUNCTION OF AGE GROUP

Adolescence

The conditions that may produce abnormal bleeding after menarche can be subdivided into four categories:

1 Disorders of the hypothalamic–pituitary axis are common in the first 5 years of the menstrual cycle, leading to periodic anovulation.[9] Reindollar and McDonough found that 55–82% of the cycles were anovulatory in the first 2 years; by the 4th and 5th years only 20% of cycles were anovulatory.[34] Anovulatory bleeding was the cause in 50–74% of patients who were admitted for inpatient stay because of severe bleeding.[35]

2 Anovulation due to disorders in the follicular phase, leading to unopposed estrogen effect and eventual breakdown.[36–38]

3 Unrecognized pregnancy and sexually transmitted diseases, which may cause irregular bleeding.

4 Unexplained menorrhagia. This latter category is emphasized due to the fact that a substantial minority of these patients (8–25%) may have unrecognized coagulation disorders.[33,37,38] Menorrhagia with onset at the menarche was predictive of an inherited bleeding disorder in 65% of von Willebrand's disease and 67% of factor XI (FXI)-deficient patients.[32]

Bleeding during third and fourth decades

In this age group, a common cause of bleeding is oral contraceptive therapy.[39] Other causes that must be considered include recent pregnancy, dysfunctional causes and, occasionally, anovulatory cycles. Organic lesions are less common causes of bleeding during this time.

Fifth decade

In the fifth decade, organic lesions (submucosal leiomyomata, polyps, chronic endometritis, neoplasia) predominate as defined causes of abnormal bleeding. Dysfunctional (persistent follicle and abnormal folliculogenesis) is also common early in this decade.

Sixth decade and older

Early in menopause, the most common causes of bleeding in this age group are hormonal replacement therapy, benign organic lesions and involutional changes. The risk of neoplasia increases progressively with age. Hormone replacement therapy (HRT) is a common cause of bleeding. In most instances, no pathology is found, other than the characteristic histopathologic findings related to the hormonal regimen. In one study, intrauterine pathology was found in 16 (18.6%) of 99 women with AUB. This frequency of pathology was four-fold higher in those patients who had first become amenorrheic *vs* those early in their course of HRT and in those with persistent bleeding over more than 6 months.[40] In another study of women on HRT, the frequency of normal findings, atrophy, polyps and suspicious lesions on hysteroscopy was 48, 20, 27 and 4%, respectively. Overall, in one study, biopsies of women on HRT showed normal findings (76%), inadequate sample (19%), hyperplasia (2.6%) and adenocarcinoma (1.2%), respectively.[41]

CLINICAL WORK-UP

The evaluation of abnormal uterine bleeding requires exclusion of structural abnormalities by a combination of physical examination, endometrial sampling and uterine imaging, with sonographic techniques and/or hysteroscopy[42] and exclusion of coagulation defects, especially in younger women. In recent years, hysteroscopy has emerged as the gold standard for evaluating abnormal bleeding associated with anatomic causes, supplanting the blind endometrial biopsy.[27] It should be emphasized that hysteroscopy will not replace sampling for excluding endometrial neoplasia. Visualization of the endometrial cavity by hysteroscopy has been reported to uncover a visible cause in up to 50% of cases of abnormal bleeding.[27,43] This approach is most sensitive to identify endometrial polyps, submucosal leiomyomata, congenital malformations and Asherman's syndrome (Fig. 16.14a).[27] It is not useful for excluding endometritis.[44]

The present indications for hysteroscopy include abnormal uterine bleeding, diagnosis and possible removal of submucosal leiomyomas or endometrial polyps, location and removal of lost intrauterine devices (IUDs), evaluation of infertile patients with abnormal hysterosalpingograms, diagnosis and treatment of uterine adhesions and division of small uterine septa. Hysteroscopy is contraindicated during pregnancy and in the setting of infection, profuse uterine bleeding and cervical malignancy. With proper technique and patient selection few complications arise, but uterine perforation, infection and bleeding are possible. Other complications related to the uterine distending medium or to operative hysteroscopy may occur.[45]

Transvaginal ultrasound is also used as a screening tool for postmenopausal women with vaginal bleeding. It is painless, complication-free and more sensitive for detecting neoplasia than blind biopsy. However, it is not specific. While a thin endometrial stripe is unlikely to produce pathology, the converse, a thick stripe, may or may not signify significant pathology (Fig. 16.14b,c). Nevertheless, some consider transvaginal sonography combined with Pipelle endometrial biopsy and outpatient hysteroscopy to be as effective as inpatient hysteroscopy and curettage. Currently, transvaginal ultrasound (TVU) is considered a viable first-line management tool combined with both biopsy and hysteroscopy when indicated.[45] Equivalent techniques are sonohysterogram or saline infusion sonograms for premenopausal women. In general, sonohysterogram is superior to ultrasound alone for excluding endometrial pathology.

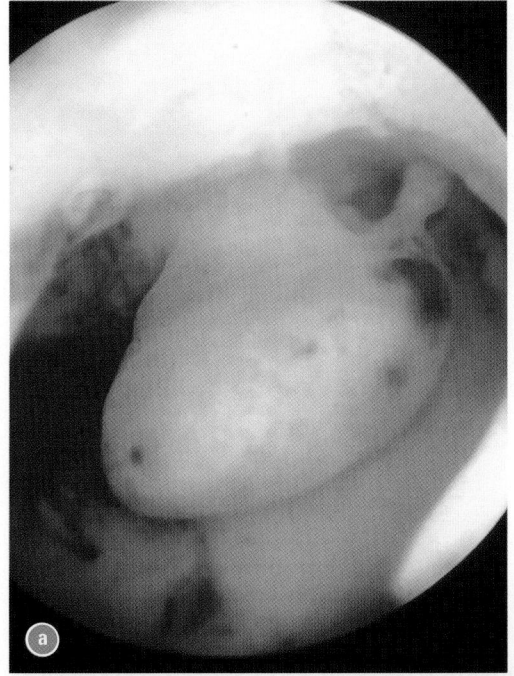

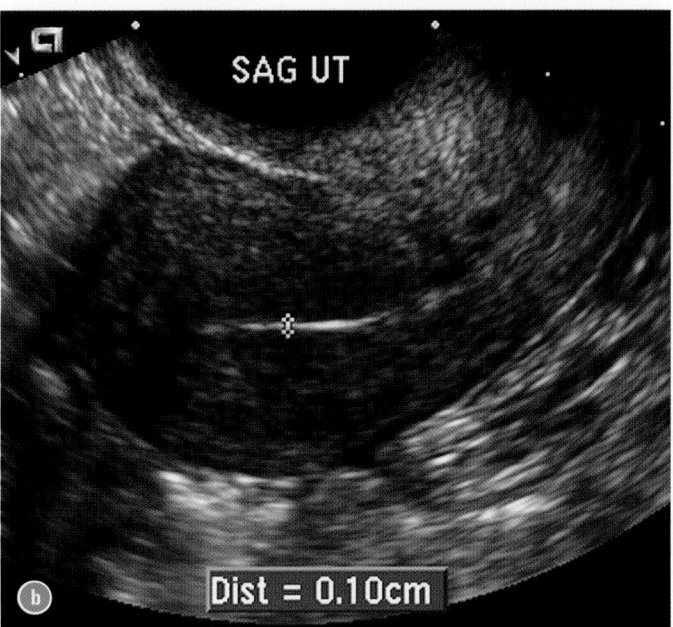

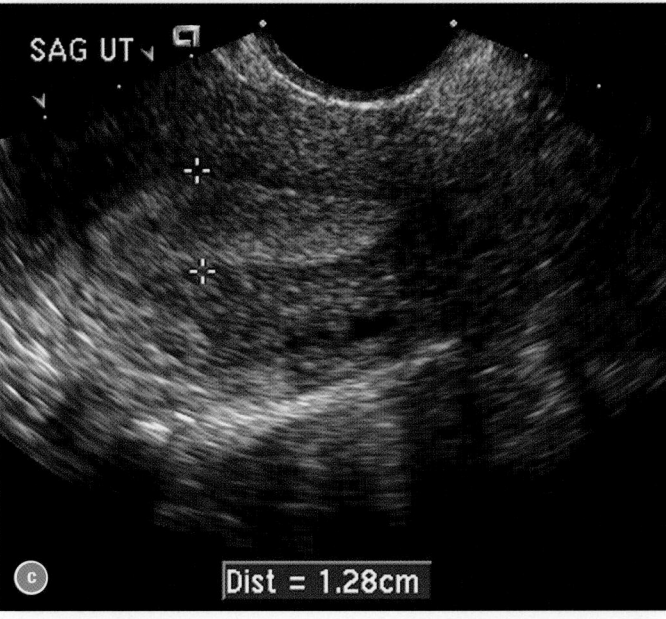

Fig. 16.14 (a) Hysteroscopic image of a lesion pathologically confirmed as an endometrial polyp. The tenuous attachment to the uterine wall suggests that this is an endometrial lesion and not a submucosal leiomyoma. Ultrasonogram of normal (b) and (c) abnormal endometrial stripes, both framed by the asterisks. (Courtesy of P. Doubilet, Brigham and Women's Hospital.)

Endometrial pathology

PATTERNS COMMONLY ASSOCIATED WITH ABNORMAL (AND DYSFUNCTIONAL) BLEEDING

The majority of endometrial samples received for evaluation come from women in the third to sixth decade. In this age range, the dominant group is the fifth. The following is a list of pathologic abnormalities that may be recognized by light microscopic examination (Table 16.5). The frequency of each category varies as a function of the age group. In general, most patients with abnormal bleeding who require endometrial sampling are being evaluated for infertility (third and fourth decade), are experiencing menorrhagia (any age), or bleeding of any form in the fifth decade or older.

Table 16.5 *Causes of abnormal uterine bleeding in the fourth and fifth decades*

Cause	Differential diagnosis
Anovulation (Fig. 16.15a–d)	Endometrial polyp (Fig. 16.17) Basalis (Fig. 16.20b)
Endometrial polyp (Fig. 16.17)	Basalis/lower uterine segment (Fig. 16.20b) Tangentially sectioned functionalis Atypical polypoid adenomyoma (Fig. 16.18d) Adenomyomatous polyp (Fig. 16.18a,b) Intraendometrial leiomyoma (Fig. 16.18c) Adenosarcoma (Fig. 16.19a)
Chronic endometritis (Fig. 16.21)	Late menstrual endometrium (Fig. 16.4a–c) Post-partum/post-abortal endometrium (Fig. 16.43e) Cervical tissue (plasma cells) Menstrual endometrium (Fig. 16.2a,b) Lymphoproliferative disorder (Fig. 16.28a,b)
Submucosal myoma	Progestin/tamoxifen therapy (Figs 16.32a, 16.38a,b) Endometrial polyp (Fig. 16.17) Stromal neoplasm (Fig. 16.32b,c)

Anovulation

Anovulatory cycles are one of the most common causes of dysfunctional uterine bleeding. Vakiani et al. studied 1282 cases of out-of-phase endometria and noted anovulatory cycle in 77%, which could be divided between anovulatory changes and hyperplasia. Of the latter, less than 2% demonstrated atypical hyperplasia, testifying to the predominance of anovulatory changes. Most of the patients were menopausal.[30]

Anovulatory changes may manifest as several histologic patterns in the endometrium depending on whether the anovulatory cycle was accompanied by persistent estrogen production. The continued stimulus of estrogen results in conformational changes in the endometrial glandular epithelium, the most prominent being cystic glandular dilatation and regularly irregular gland distribution (Fig. 16.15a,b). Stromal breakdown, when present, is patchy, resulting from focal fibrin thrombi (Fig. 16.15c,d). If anovulation is not accompanied by persistent estrogen production, the cystic glandular changes may not be evident. However, other features in keeping with an anovulatory cycle, including gland cell karyorrhexis, patchy breakdown with fibrin thrombi, surface repair and tubal metaplasia, are often present. In the presence of these findings, a diagnosis of anovulation is appropriate (Table 16.4).

Published literature suggests that many anovulatory endometria have previously been interpreted as simple non-atypical hyperplasias, particularly if the latter diagnosis does not require gland crowding.[2,4,46] Another common term is disordered proliferative endometrium.[2]

The risk of endometrial cancer is estimated to be less than 2% in this group.[2,4] In the absence of gland crowding or other features of early neoplasia, the following diagnosis is made: Proliferative endometrium with alterations in gland architecture (or other features) consistent with anovulation, with stromal breakdown (if present). The term 'cystic glandular dilatation' is generally avoided, inasmuch as such terms have previously connotated hyperplasia.

Alterations signifying breakdown in the absence of persistent follicle

This group comprises endometria with stromal breakdown and gland karyorrhexis, in the absence of cystic glandular dilatation (Fig. 16.16a–c). By virtue of the normalcy of the endometrium, this qualifies for a diagnosis of 'dysfunctional uterine bleeding'.[30] Depending on the timing of sampling, the pattern may be indistinguishable from a late menstrual pattern (Fig. 16.16a). Alternatively, the picture may be that of uniformly arranged tubular glands associated with diffuse stromal breakdown (Fig. 16.16c). This pattern is consistent with either breakdown occurring in the middle of the proliferative phase or initiated by a defect in either follicle growth or transition to corpus luteum. As previously described in the section on the menstrual phase, this pattern is distinguished from ovulatory breakdown by the absence of secretory stromal or epithelial changes. However, it is not readily distinguished from hormonal replacement therapy, which may be associated with tubular glands and diffuse breakdown when the hormone is withdrawn. The

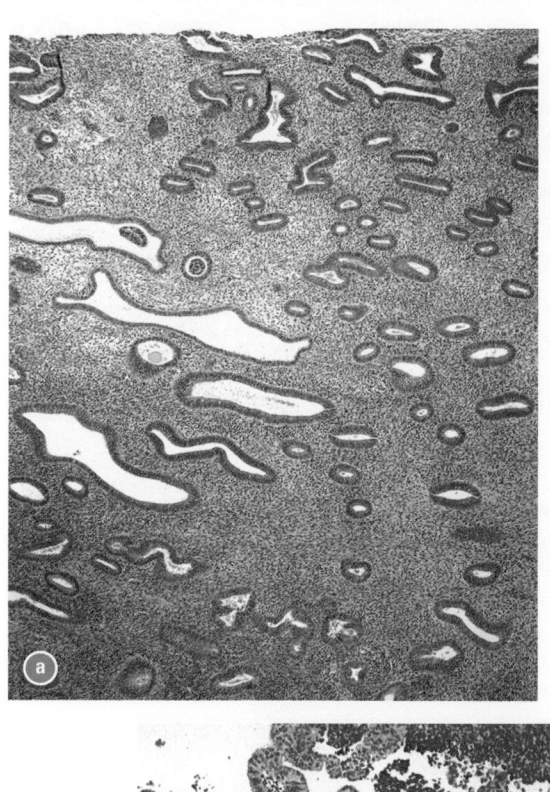
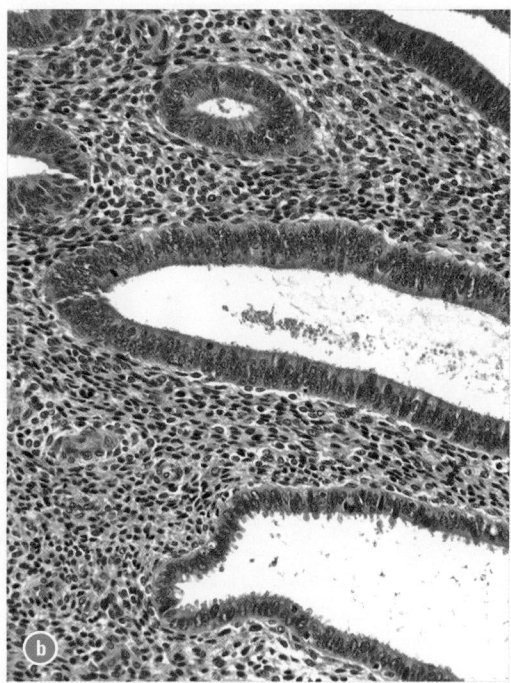
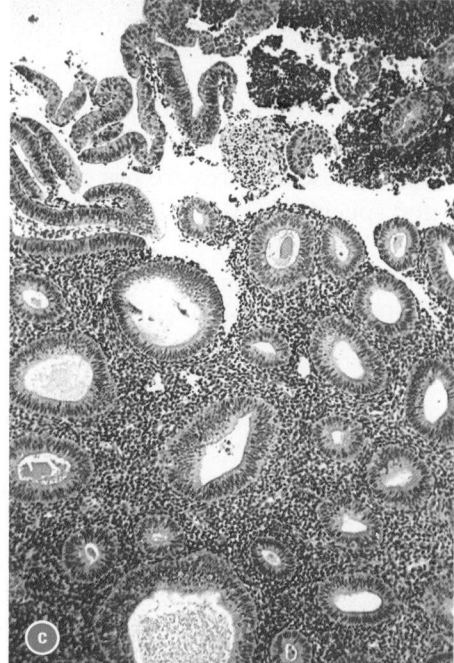
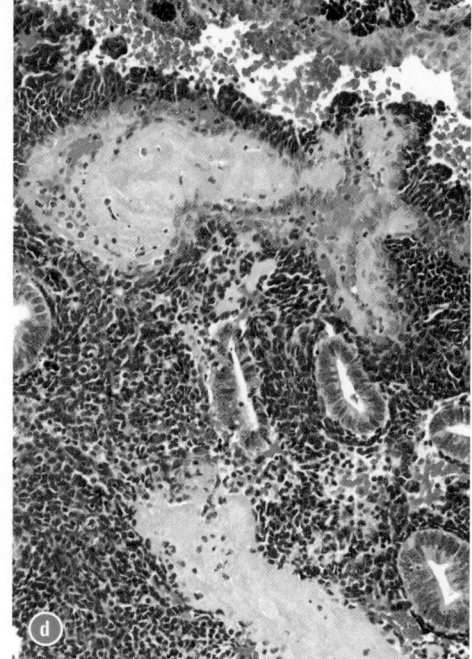

Fig. 16.15 (a) Anovulation with persistent follicle. (b) Higher-power view of cystic glands including focal tubal metaplasia, (c) with stromal breakdown, (d) fibrin thrombi.

diagnosis in such cases may be 'Benign endometrium with stromal breakdown. The differential diagnosis includes hormonal therapy or altered cycle'.

Endometrial polyp

A second and one of the most common causes of abnormal uterine bleeding is endometrial polyp (EMP).[47] This benign tumor is defined as a mono-

clonal neoplastic proliferation of stromal cells incorporating a non-neoplastic glandular component. The stromal lesion has been associated with defined cytogenetic abnormalities, most commonly alterations in chromosome 6p that have been attributed to mutations in the HMGIC gene locus.[48,49]

Hypertension, obesity and late menopause are associated with endometrial polyps. Postmenopausal bleed-

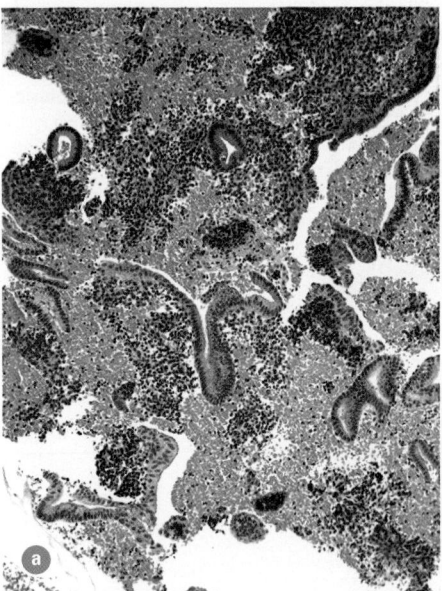 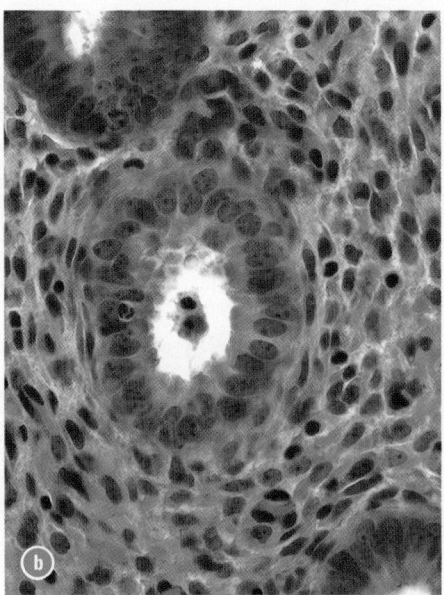 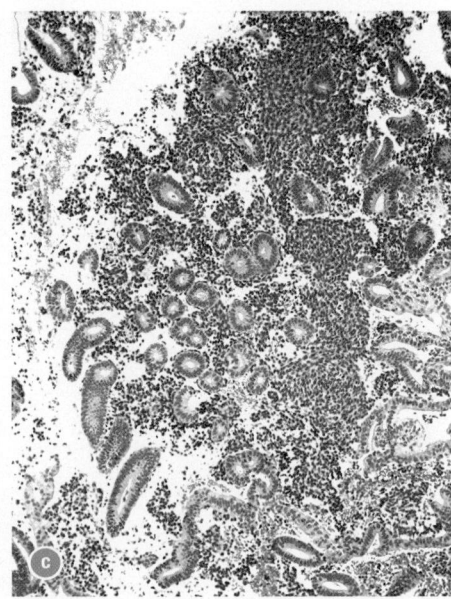

Fig. 16.16 (a) Breakdown without glandular dilatation. The differential diagnosis is typically late menstrual versus unscheduled (dysfunctional) bleeding. The distinction is made based on menstrual history; (b) gland karyorrhexis, (c) cohesive groups of tubular glands with diffuse breakdown. This could represent spontaneous breakdown due to hormonal or coagulation disturbances. A 'failed follicle' could also produce rapid disintegration and loss of proliferative activity.

ing (44%) and abnormal bleeding (82%) in premenopausal women are common presenting symptoms. Multiple lesions have been reported in 15–26% of women.[50] In one study, approximately 24% of symptomatic woman were found to have endometrial polyps with the highest frequency in the fifth decade. More than half experienced metrorrhagia.[51] Endometrial polyps increase in frequency as a function of age and are common findings in tamoxifen-treated patients.[52] They may occur at any age, but are more likely to be associated with abnormal bleeding in older patients.[53] Endometrial polyps may regress, but larger lesions tend to persist.[54] Overall, the risk of malignancy in endometrial polyps is low (less than 2%) and confined principally to women who are postmenopausal.[55] Endometrial polyps have also been strongly associated with endometriosis, being reported in nearly 50%.[56]

Transvaginal ultrasonography supplemented by sonohysterography in cases with abnormal ultrasonographic findings has become the preferred approach, with ultrasound increasing the diagnosis by five-fold and hysteroscopy by three-fold compared with standard ultrasound.[47,57] Diagnosis by ultrasound increased five-fold (3.6 vs 16.8%) and operative hysteroscopy increased three-fold (6.4 vs 19.7).[47]

Several characteristic histologic features are often used to describe these benign mesenchymal tumors with secondary inclusion of benign glands, including central vessels and the presence of a connecting stalk (Fig. 16.17a,b). Some of these tumors may be sessile (Fig. 16.17c). These features are not always evident in a fragmented specimen. We require that at least two of the following three features be present within a region of endometrial functionalis for a diagnosis of EMP: (1) thick-walled vessels, (2) altered stroma, usually fibrous or collagenous, or (3) irregular gland architecture (Fig. 16.17d,e). Although intact polyps sectioned in their entirety will be surfaced on several sides by epithelium, the majority is removed piecemeal. The number of tissue surfaces covered by epithelium is thus an inconsistent feature of polyps. Furthermore, irregularly shaped sheets of normal functionalis removed by curettage may be cut tangentially to yield apparent circumferential coverage by surface epithelium. In a practical sense, small fragments without surface epithelium pose a less compelling argument for polyp. In contrast, larger fragments with two or more of the above-mentioned features support the diagnosis of polyp. Aside from identification of surface to exclude a basal location, the geometry of surface coverage is of little utility in the differential diagnosis of endometrial polyps. Glands may be irregularly spaced and focally slightly crowded in EMPs but if unaccompanied by complex architecture or altered cytology, do not fulfill a diagnosis of endometrial intraepithelial neoplasia.[46] Following menopause, endometrial polyps may become atrophic.

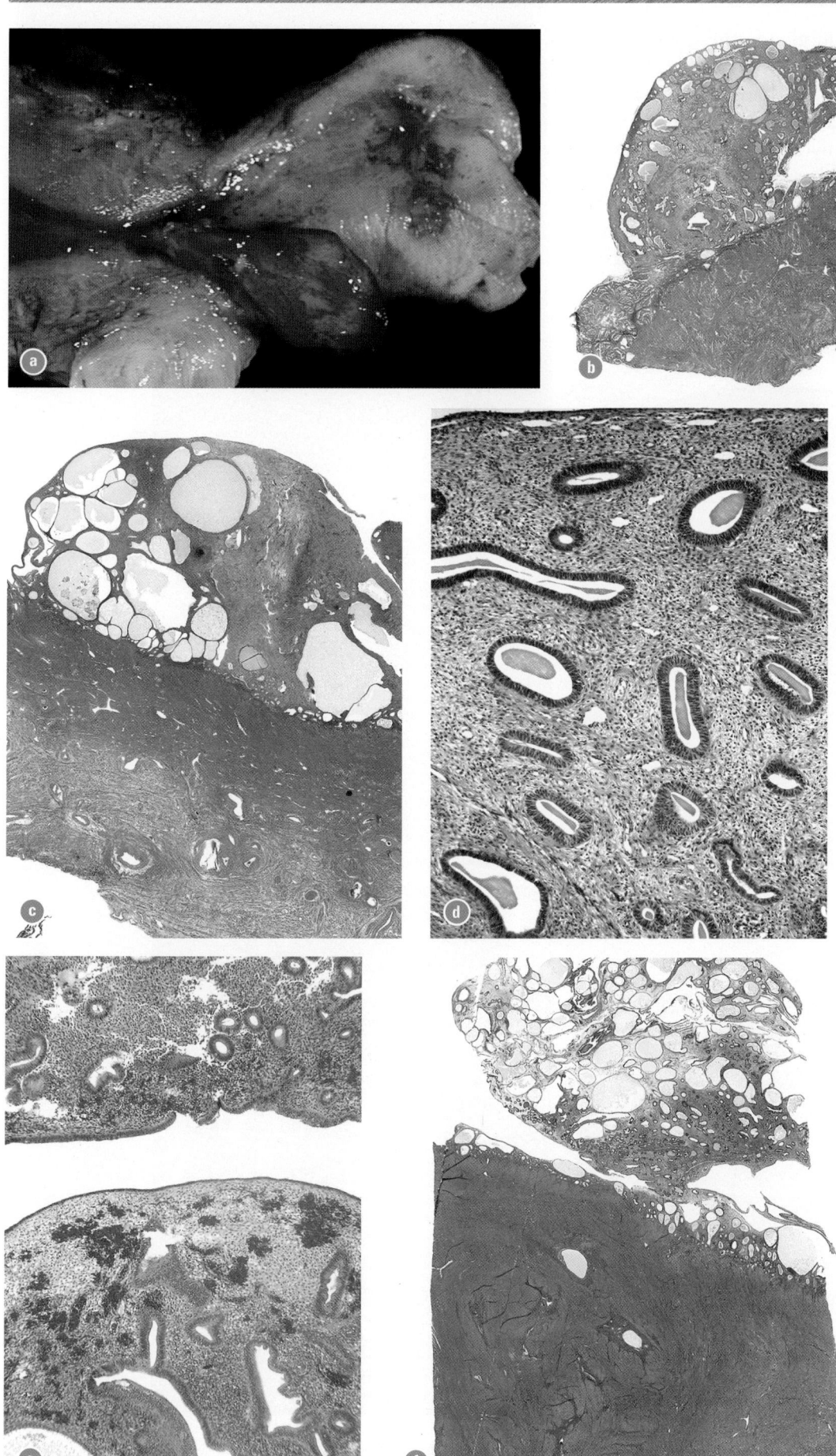

Fig. 16.17 (a) Gross appearance of endometrial polyp. (b,c) Low-power photomicrographs of pedunculated and sessile polyps, respectively. (d) Higher-power view illustrates altered glands and stroma with surface epithelium. (e) Contrast between functionalis (upper) and polyp stroma (lower). (f) Cystic atrophic (senile) polyp.

When accompanied by cystic glands these lesions are referred to as cystic atrophic (senile) polyps (Fig. 16.17f).

The differential diagnosis of EMP includes (a) adenomyomatous polyp, (b) intraendometrial leiomyomas, (c) atypical polypoid adenomyomas and (d) low-grade or subtle adenosarcomas and basalis. Adenomyomatous polyps have a uniform admixture of myomatous stroma and glands (Fig. 16.18a,b). Intraendometrial leiomyomas are similar to adenomyomatous polyps with the excep-

tion that the smooth muscle forms a discrete nodular lesion in the endometrium (Fig. 16.18c). Atypical polypoid adenomyomas have, in addition to a myomatous stroma, irregular gland architecture typically accompanied by squamous morules (Fig. 16.18d). These neoplasms are discussed under preinvasive endometrial lesions.

The distinction with potentially the most important consequences is between endometrial polyp and adenosarcoma (Fig. 16.19a–c). The great majority of adeno-

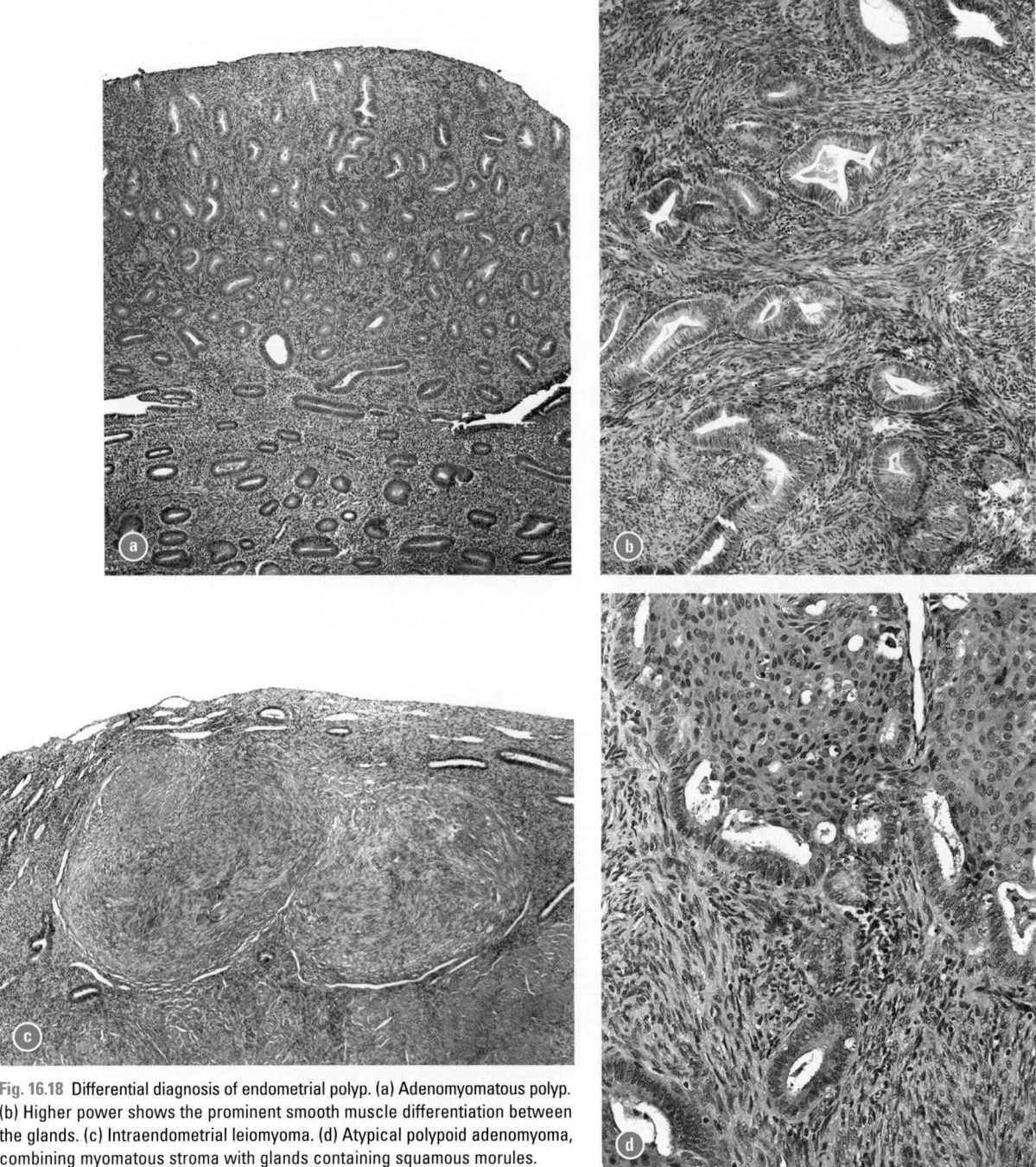

Fig. 16.18 Differential diagnosis of endometrial polyp. (a) Adenomyomatous polyp. (b) Higher power shows the prominent smooth muscle differentiation between the glands. (c) Intraendometrial leiomyoma. (d) Atypical polypoid adenomyoma, combining myomatous stroma with glands containing squamous morules.

sarcomas exhibit conspicuous altered gland architecture accompanied by periglandular stromal condensation, stromal cellular atypia and increased mitotic activity (Fig. 16.19a).[58] Nevertheless, a proportion of endometrial polyps may exhibit altered gland architecture and variable stromal cellularity (Fig. 16.19b,c). Hattab et al. noted that mild increases in mitotic index and prominent stromal changes were common in large polyps, but did not increase the risk of recurrence.[59]

Another variant of polyp contains atypical stromal changes (Fig. 16.19d).[60] The most prudent approach to these lesions is to carefully monitor them with a follow-up endometrial sample. These are discussed in more detail in Chapter 20. EMP must be distinguished from lower uterine segment and basalis (Fig. 16.20). The former often exhibits a pale eosinophilic stroma with focally cystic glands (Fig. 16.20a). Basalis lacks the thick-walled vessels and surface epithelium (Fig. 16.20b).

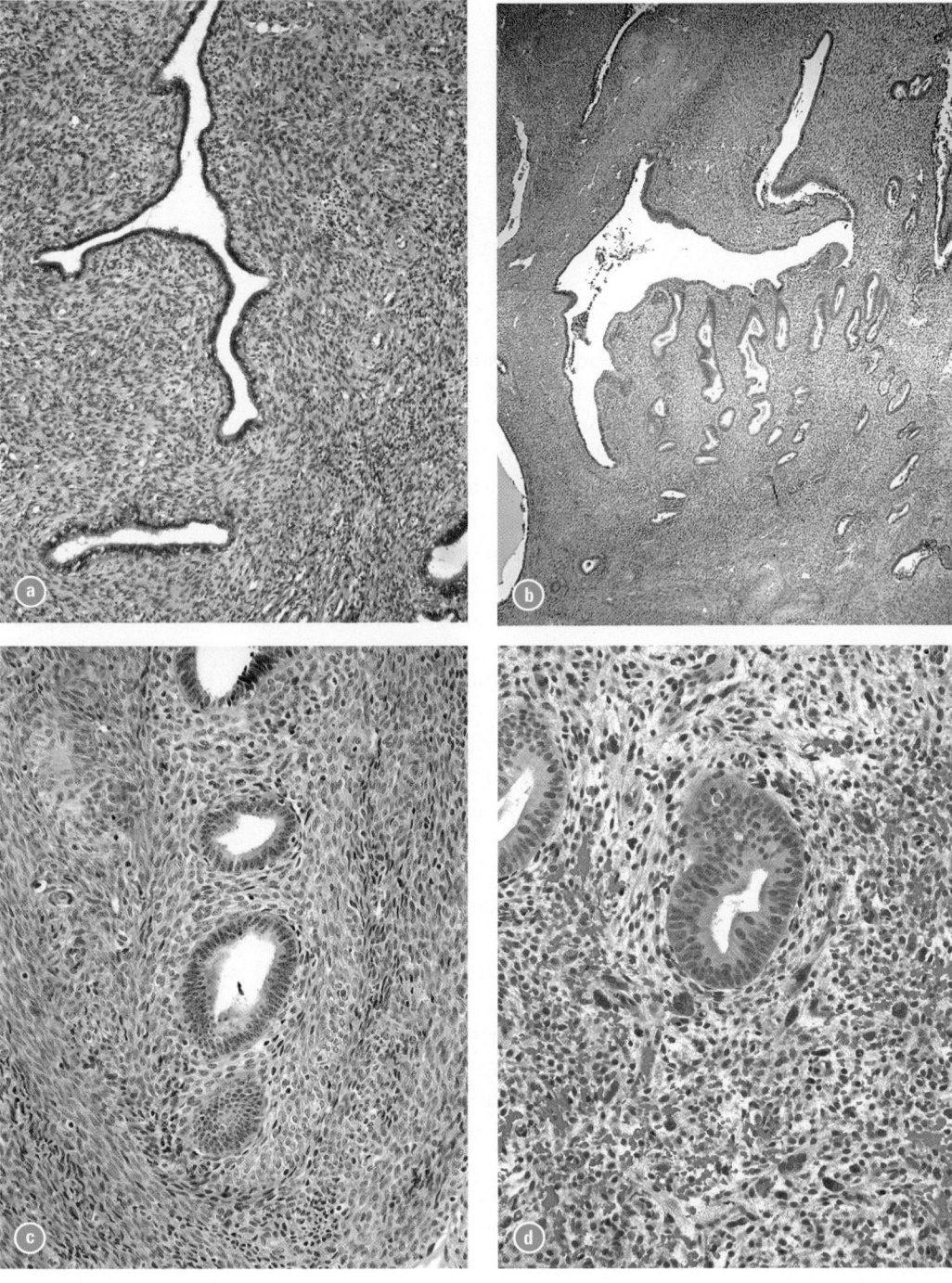

Fig. 16.19 Atypical polyp versus adenosarcoma. (a) Adenosarcoma. (b,c) Atypical polyp, with endometrial stroma. (d) Focal stromal atypia in polyp.

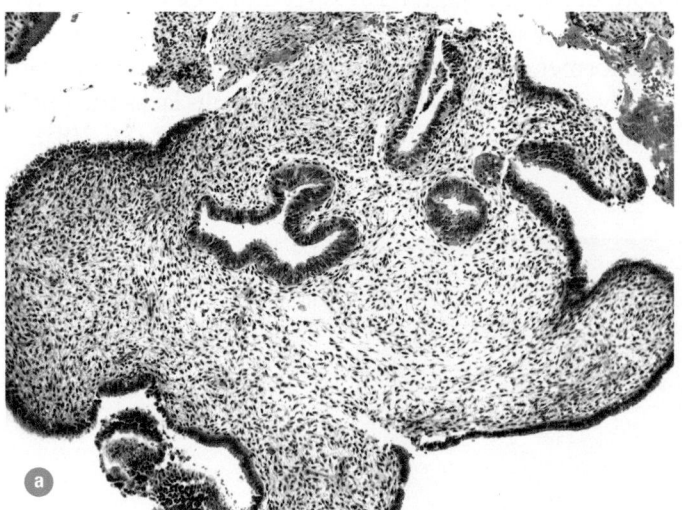

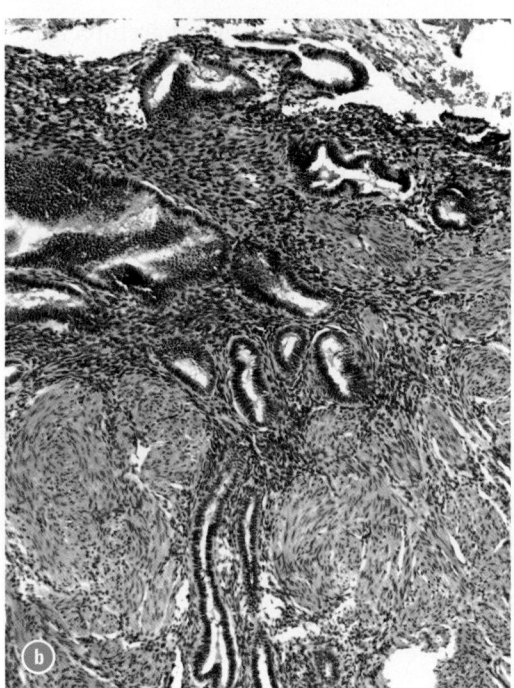

Fig. 16.20
(a) Lower uterine segment.
(b) Basalis.

Endometritis

Endometritis is defined as endometrial inflammation and includes a number of entities summarized in Table 16.6. Excepting purpural sepsis, granulomatous endometritis, actinomycosis (IUD) exotic causes (such as schistosomiasis) and inflammation associated with structural abnormalities (polyps or submucosal leiomyomata), the term is synonymous with chronic (plasmacytic) endometritis (CPE).[61,62] CPE is considered an infectious process until proven otherwise and is a component of pelvic inflammatory disease (PID). CPE is strongly associated with acute salpingitis, being present in over half of cases.[62] In a population of 152 women suspected of PID, Eckert et al. noted 43 women had neither endometritis nor salpingitis; 26 women had endometritis alone without salpingitis and 83 women had salpingitis. They noted a relationship between endometritis alone and both chlamydia and gonorrhea and fewer generalized symptoms in this group.[63] Hillier et al. examined 178 patients with PID and identified endometritis in 65%. A total of 23% of those with acute salpingitis did not have coexisting endometritis. The odds ratios for gonorrhea, chlamydia and anaerobic Gram-negative rods (bacterial vaginosis) for CPE were 5.7, 4.8 and 2.6, respectively, arguing for a role of these organisms in its pathogenesis.[64] Paavonen et al. noted that in a group of women with cervicitis, endometritis was associated with a history of intermenstrual vaginal bleeding, the presence of *Chlamydia trachomatis*, *Neisseria gonorrhoeae*, or *Streptococcus agalactiae* in the cervix and serum antibodies to *C. trachomatis* or to *Mycoplasma hominis*.[65] Others have associated *mycoplasma* with both endometritis and salpingitis.[66] Based on these studies, it is clear that CPE is a component of the syndrome of pelvic inflammatory disease, although not necessarily a concurrent disorder with, or predictor of, the latter. The work-up requires attention to the above pathogens.

The above studies specifically targeted women who were the most likely to manifest with CPE and for whom the significance of this disorder was easily deduced. In

Table 16.6 Endometritis

Category	Pathogen
Purpural sepsis	Staphylococcus, clostridia
Chronic (or acute and chronic) plasmacytic endometritis	Chlamydia, gonorrhea, enteric organisms
Granulomatous endometritis	TB, HSV, CMV, idiopathic
Xanthogranulomatous endometritis	
Lymphocytic endometritis	Unknown
Reactive endometritis	
Endometrial polyp	
Submucosal leiomyoma	
Intrauterine device	
Ablation-related	

TB, tuberculosis; HSV, herpes simplex virus infection; CMV, cytomegalovirus infection.

practice, the pathologist may encounter CPE under a variety of circumstances and these will vary according to the age of the patient, which, in general, will determine the most likely underlying causes. Table 16.7 summarizes 200 consecutive diagnoses of CPE at Brigham and Women's Hospital and breaks them down according to age group. In women under 40, over two-thirds of cases will be identified in women who have either been recently pregnant (post-partum or post-abortal endometritis) or have presented with unexplained uterine bleeding. In women between 41 and 50 the majority either present with unexplained bleeding or a history of intrauterine device. In women over 50, the more common findings include unexplained bleeding, associated with structural (prolapse, polyps, etc.) and obstructive (pyometra) conditions. Importantly, nearly one-third of patients with chronic endometritis will not manifest with structural abnormalities or concurrent conditions other than unexplained bleeding. Moreover, chronic endometritis is not recognizable by hysteroscopic examination.[67] The bleeding presumably reflects a functional disturbance in the endometrium imposed by the inflammatory infiltrate and its influence on the stroma and epithelium.[11]

The features that signify CPE include the following: (1) the appearance of increased stromal densities associated with mononuclear cells, (2) intraluminal acute inflammatory exudate, (3) lymphoid follicles and (4) alterations in proliferative or secretory phase pattern, (5) stromal breakdown and not infrequently, (6) focal squamous metaplasia on the surface (Fig. 16.21a–e). The most common pattern seen is proliferative. Whether this signifies an increased susceptibility of proliferative phase to infection, or a relationship between CPE and anovulatory states, is unclear. When searching for plasma cells, the pathologist should focus on the stroma just beneath the surface epithelium (particularly in areas where there is focal stromal breakdown) and at the periphery of the lymphoid aggregates.

Although the presence of plasma cells *and* lymphoid follicles is pathognomonic of CPE, follicles are not sufficient for the diagnosis without plasma cells. Rare plasma cells in the absence of the other stigmata of CPE may be seen in late menstrual phase, associated with submucosal leiomyomata, or in endometrial polyps (Fig. 16.22). In these settings their presence should be noted but with the caveat that a diagnosis of CPE cannot be confirmed.[2] Similarly, the association of plasma cells and inflammation with other organic lesions, such as squamous morules, is interpreted as secondary. In contrast, foci of squamous metaplasia on the endometrial surface is a recognized feature in CPE (Fig. 16.21e).

In younger women, CPE is often seen in post-partum or post-abortal endometria (Fig. 16.21a). In these instances, the diagnosis of CPE should be made and management will depend on the setting and symptoms. Plasma cells may also be seen in the decidua underlying the implantation site in placental specimens, a condition referred to as 'plasmacytic deciduitis'. However, the significance of plasma cells in decidua (and in fallopian tube mucosa) during pregnancy is unclear and not always assumed to be infectious in origin (Fig. 16.23) (see Chapter 33).

Another variant of endometritis is pyometra, typically seen postmenopause and often preceded by signs of obstruction.[68] The curetting typically exhibits abundant acute inflammatory exudate, necrotic tissue and fragments of superficial endometrium with inflammation and repair. Pyometrium carries a significant risk of associated endometrial carcinoma, which should be excluded by repeat curettage if there are clinical concerns (Fig. 16.24a,b). It may also develop following other obstructive conditions, including cervical carcinoma.[68–70]

Granulomatous endometritis is associated with tuberculosis (Fig. 16.25a,b), endometrial ablation (Fig. 16.25c), coccidioidomycosis, schistosomiasis and cytomegalovirus and, rarely, herpetic infections.[71–76] It may also be seen with non-infectious causes, such as sarcoid. Cytomegalovirus (CMV) endometritis is often linked to immunosuppression. Although granulomatous endometritis is not invariably associated with tuberculosis, a skin test and special stains for acid-fast bacilli (AFB) are necessary to exclude that possibility.

Table 16.7 *Chronic endometritis at Brigham and Women's Hospital*[a]

Age range (years)	PP	IUCD	AUB	Organic	Pyometra	Other[b]
18–30	40	10	31	5	2	12
31–40	28	9	35	9		19
41–50	6	13	29	11	1	41
51–60	0	25	37	12	7	19
60+	0	3	16	17	17	47

PP, post-partum; IUCD, intrauterine contraceptive device; AUB, abnormal uterine bleeding. Organic, organic (structural) cause identified.

[a]Listed as a percentage of cases of chronic endometritis containing an organic lesion or in which the above information was available from the pathology requisition.

[b]No clinical information was provided on the pathology requisition.

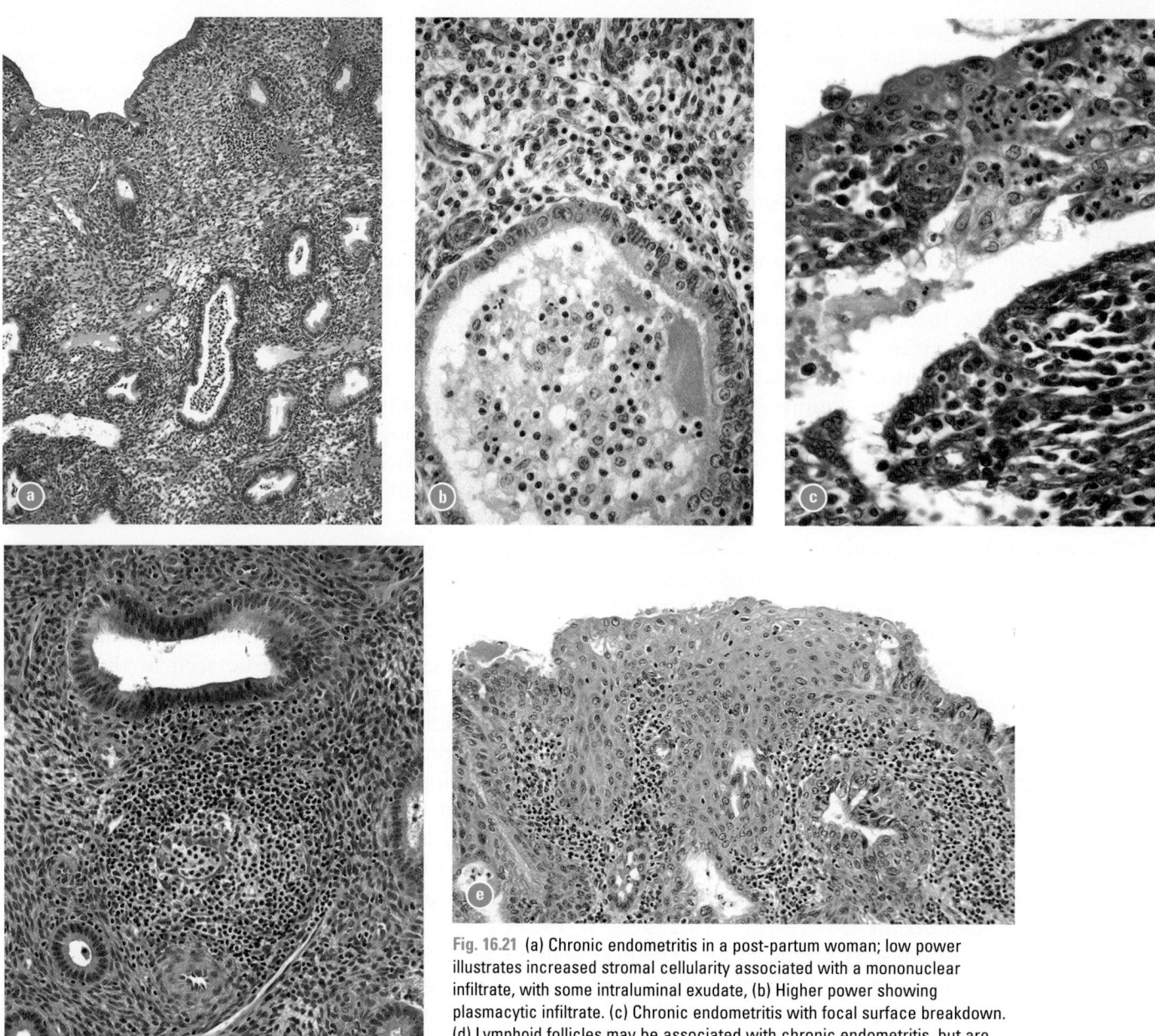

Fig. 16.21 (a) Chronic endometritis in a post-partum woman; low power illustrates increased stromal cellularity associated with a mononuclear infiltrate, with some intraluminal exudate, (b) Higher power showing plasmacytic infiltrate. (c) Chronic endometritis with focal surface breakdown. (d) Lymphoid follicles may be associated with chronic endometritis, but are not specific in the absence of plasma cells. (e) Focal squamous metaplasia of the surface epithelium.

The differential diagnosis of chronic endometritis includes conditions in which inflammatory cells are present in the absence of plasma cells. Additional inflammatory lesions of the endometrium may be caused by non-specific alterations such as prolapse (Fig. 16.26). An uncommon inflammatory lesion consists of dense clusters of activated lymphocytes in the absence of plasma cells (lymphocytic endometritis), presumably signifying an immune response (Fig. 16.27a–c). Late menstrual, post-abortal and post-partum endometria without plasma cells may mimic chronic endometritis by virtue of the lymphocytic infiltrates. Rarely, a primary lymphoma will manifest in the endometrium and may mimic chronic endometritis (Fig. 16.28a,b).

Intrauterine contraceptive devices

Intrauterine contraceptive devices (IUDs) have been in use since the early 1960s. Complications arising

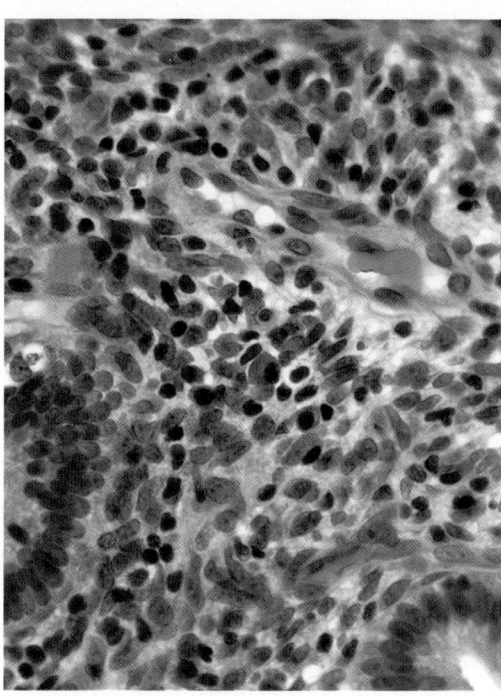

Fig. 16.22 Plasma cell in an endometrial polyp (center).

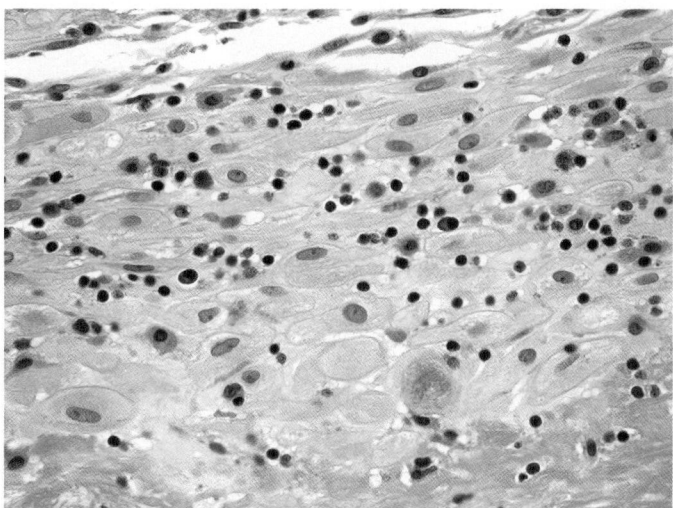

Fig. 16.23 Plasmacytic deciduitis.

from the Dalcon Shield in the early 1970s resulted in changes in design, leading to several generations of devices with increasing efficiency of contraception and reduced complications.[77] Nevertheless, the frequency of use in the USA dropped from approximately 20% of reproductive-age women in the 1970s to less than 1% in 2000.[77] Rates of usage are higher in Europe and South American and highest in Asia, where the proportion of women is as high as 49% (in Korea).[78]

At least three mechanisms explain the contraceptive effect of IUDs. The first is induction of a localized inflammatory response in the endometrium that is spermatocidal. The second is an influence on ovum transport rate and/or a direct ovicidal effect (copper-containing devices). The third, seen with progesterone-coated devices such as the Levonorgestrel-20 IUDs, is

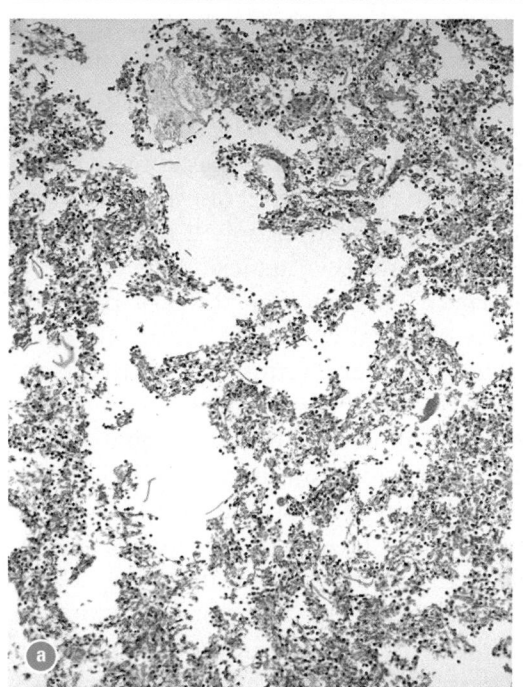

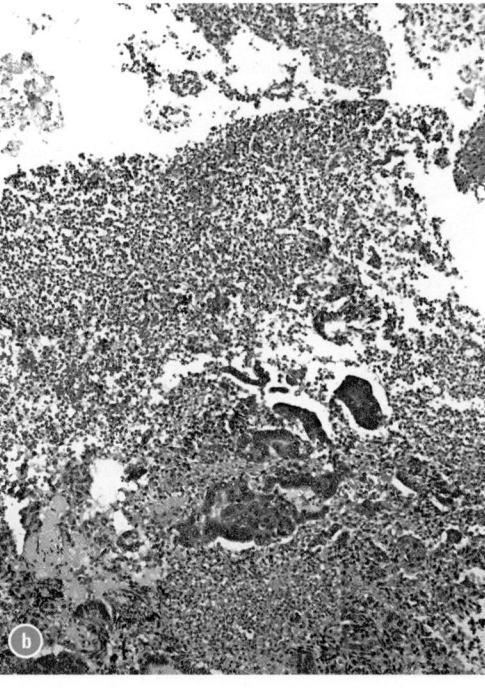

Fig. 16.24 (a) Pyometra, with prominent acute inflammatory exudates and cellular debris, (b) with associated adenocarcinoma (lower center).

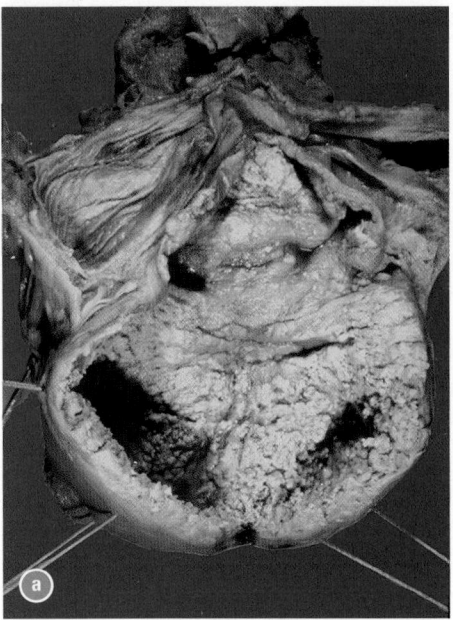 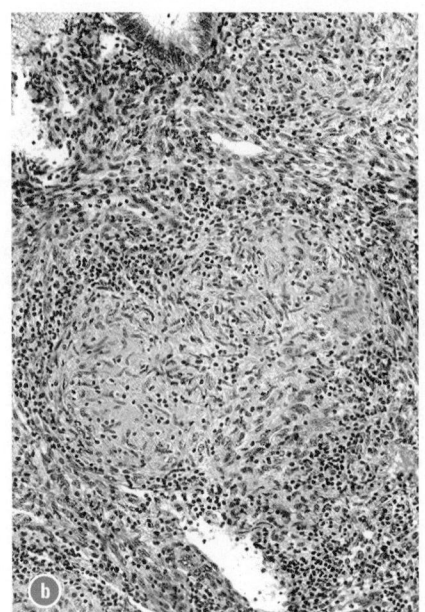 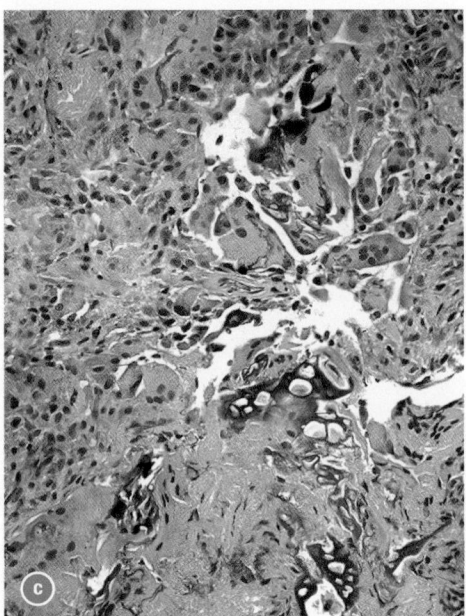

Fig. 16.25 (a) Gross pathology of endometrial tuberculosis. The endometrial cavity has been opened, showing striking caseous necrosis. (b) Microphotograph of granuloma. (c) Giant cell reaction associated with recent endometrial ablation.

a suppression of both endometrial and tubal mucosa by the direct effects of the hormone itself. This is assumed to directly suppress implantation.[79]

The pregnancy rates for copper devices have been estimated at slightly less than 1 per 100 years of usage.

Fig. 16.26 Non-specific inflammation with a lymphoid aggregate, associated with prolapse.

The progesterone-coated devices have a significantly lower rate of approximately 0.1 per 100 years of usage. In both groups, a disproportionate percentage (up to 25%) of these pregnancies are ectopic in nature.[78]

The risk of bacterial infection following the insertion of an IUD is low and not a contraindication for its use. Studies have shown that IUDs do not increase the risk of sexually transmitted disease, although insertion of copper IUDs is not encouraged in women who are prone to infection, such as HIV-infected individuals.[80,81] The most publicized complication of IUDs is actinomycosis (*Actinomyces israelii*). However, the relationship of IUDs to actinomycosis is controversial. What is known is the following: (1) Despite over 30 million women years of use, only a few hundred cases of pelvic actinomycosis associated with IUDs have been reported. (2) Less than 0.5% of removed IUDs have histologically visible actinomycotic granules. (3) *Actinomyces* are frequently cultured from the female genital tract and are considered indigenous flora. (4) Less than 1 in over 120 000 hospital admissions are related to pelvic actinomycosis. (5) The risk of actinomycosis, even when associated with an IUD, is extremely low.[77,82] (6) However, despite the above, cases of pelvic actinomycosis associated with IUDs have been reported to follow a prolonged period in which *Actinomyces* were detected in the Papanicolaou smear.[83] Thus, despite arguments to the contrary, it is

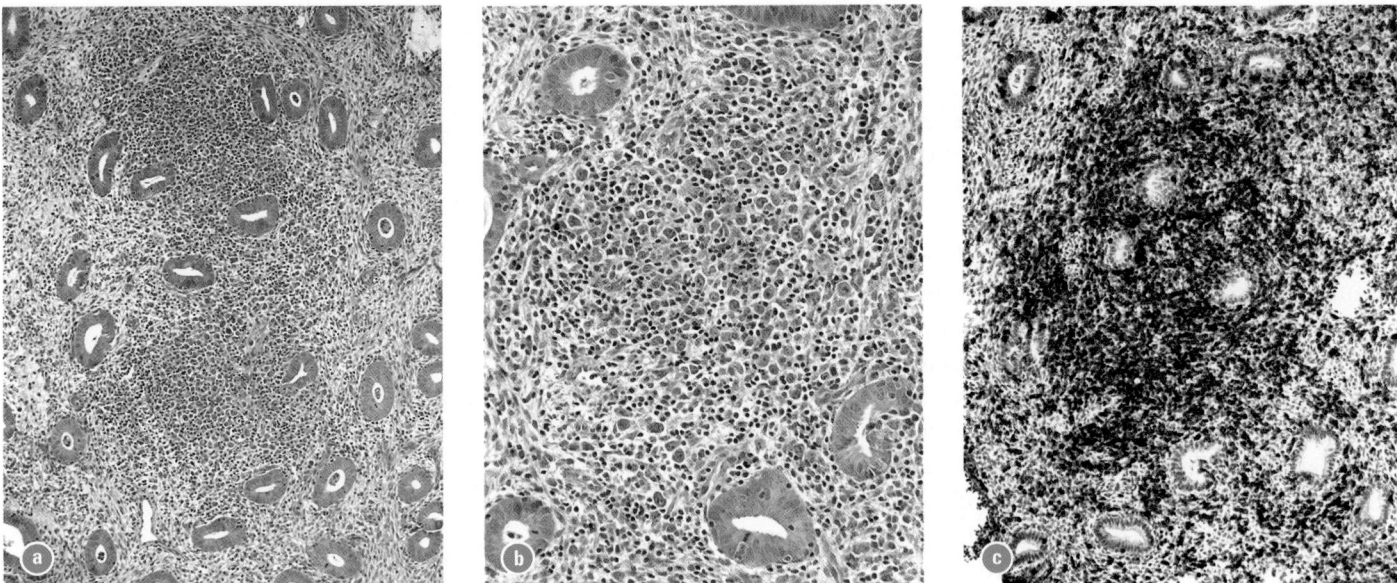

Fig. 16.27 (a,b) Prominent lymphoid infiltrates in the endometrium of a woman who recently underwent cone biopsy. There are no plasma cells present. (c) A stain for cd3 (polyclonal) is strongly positive.

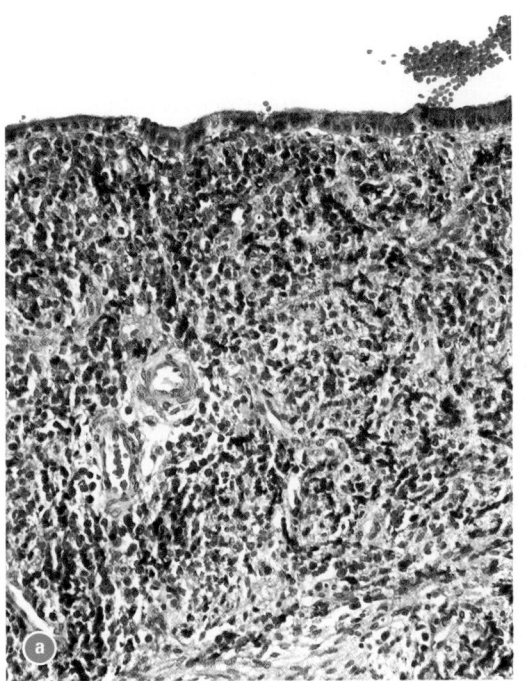

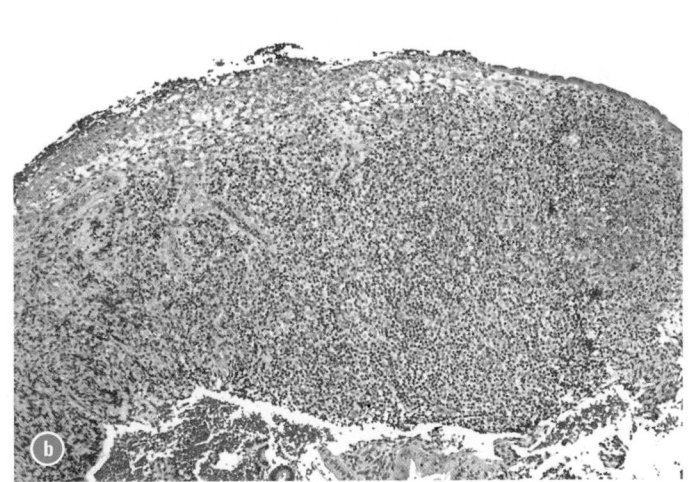

Fig. 16.28 (a) Endometrial lymphoma, consisting of a homogeneous infiltrate of lymphoid cells. (b) Dense infiltrate of plasma cells and lymphoid cells in chronic endometritis.

assumed that the focal accumulation of abundant organisms in the presence of an IUCD does increase the risk, albeit small, to a proportion of users.

Management options for patients with an IUD and documented *Actinomyces* include follow-up alone, treatment with antibiotics without removing the IUD and removal of the IUD with or without treatment and replacing the IUD after the colonization with *Actinomyces* has cleared. Treatment of patients with the IUD *in situ* has been successful in 67% of cases in contrast to 100% when the device was removed.[83] Overall, despite arguments to the contrary, the weight of opinion is to remove the device if *Actinomyces* are identified.[77,83,84] One caveat is the potential misclassification of mimics of sulfur granules (pseudoactinomycotic radiate granules or PAMRAGs) that are associated with IUDs. The presence of these artifacts may needlessly prompt the removal of an IUD with no other indications.[85]

Intrauterine devices are associated with a wide range of inflammatory alterations, including the following: (1) spindle stroma due to inflammatory change or focal progestin effect (Fig. 16.29a), (2) squamous metaplasia (Fig. 16.29b), (3) surface atypia of repair (Fig. 16.29c) and, (4) in rare instances, marked inflammation with granulation tissue infiltrates (Fig. 16.29d).[86] Plasma cells may also be present. The most important pathogen is *Actinomyces* (Fig. 16.30a,b), which must be distinguished from PAMRAGs (Fig. 16.30c).

Submucosal leiomyoma/fibroid

Submucosal leiomyomas (SMF) are a common finding in patients with abnormal uterine bleeding.[1] Although endometrial sampling may not detect SMF, the presence of surface functionalis with few or no glands (aglandular functionalis) should raise suspicion of this lesion (Fig. 16.31a,b). If we identify two or more strips of aglandular functionalis at least 2 mm in length the following diagnosis is made: Strips of aglandular functionalis suggestive of submucosal leiomyoma (clinical correlation advised).

The practitioner is cautioned that not all aglandular functionalis signifies a submucosal leiomyoma, and its presence may be confused with other conditions, including atrophy, hormone replacement therapy (Fig. 16.32a), polyps and rarely endometrial stromal neoplasms (stromal nodule, stromal sarcoma and adenosarcoma) (Fig. 16.32b,c) or even lymphoma (Fig. 16.28). Concerning the latter, any hypercellular aglandular stromal process should be investigated with further sampling.

Hormonal therapy

Hormonal therapy (Table 16.8) encompasses a wide range of regimens prescribed for the purposes of continuous contraception,[86,87] temporary (emergency) contraception,[88] control of dysfunctional uterine bleeding,[89] therapy of endometriosis,[90] hormone replacement therapy at menopause,[91] reducing the risk of ovarian (oral contraceptives) and breast (tamoxifen) cancer,[87,92] reducing the size of leiomyomata (Lupron)[93] and as first-line management of early endometrial neoplasia.[94] The morphologic effects of hormonal therapy

Table 16.8 Mixed pattern endometrium

Cause	Pattern
Hormonal therapy	
Oral contraceptives (Fig. 16.33)	Small (tiny) tubular glands
	Secretory exhaustion
	Spindled stroma
Provera (Fig. 16.34)	Variable glands
	Pseudodecidualized stroma
Megestrol (Fig. 16.35)	Small, slit-like glands
	Exaggerated pseudodecidual response
	Arias-Stella effect (rarely)
Sequential (HRT) (Fig. 16.37)	Tubular glands
	Spindled stroma
	Variable secretory changes
Tamoxifen (Fig. 16.38)	Similar to HRT
	Polyps
Anovulation + progestin effect	
Plus ovulation (Fig. 16.39c)	Cystic glands
	Secretory exhaustion
Plus progestin therapy (Fig. 16.39a)	Cystic glands
	Variable secretory change
	Pseudodecidua
Altered secretory maturation	
Due to deficient CL development (Fig. 16.40)	Inadequate secretory conversion
Tubular, secretory exhausted glands	
Due to clonal alterations (Fig. 16.41)	Sharply demarcated
	Pseudostratified glands
	Secretory maturation

can be subdivided into at least five different categories, comprising oral contraceptives, short-term progesterone to manage abnormal bleeding, short- or long-term treatment with powerful progestins such as megestrol, hormonal replacement therapy at menopause and other compounds such as tamoxifen.

Oral contraceptives

At least four generations of oral contraceptives (OCPs) have been developed since their inception in the 1960s.[87] Early preparations were associated with higher complications of vascular accidents and myocardial infarction (because of higher dose) and increased risk of endometrial carcinoma (sequential preparations).[87,95] Current preparations employ continuous combined estrogen and progesterone. Currently, 10 million women in the USA and over 100 million women worldwide use oral contraceptives. Risk of pregnancy is approximately 5 users per 100 and 1 per 100 women-years in use. Benefits of OCPs include a reduction in risk of ovarian and endometrial cancer and possibly colorectal cancer. Risks of OCPs are principally

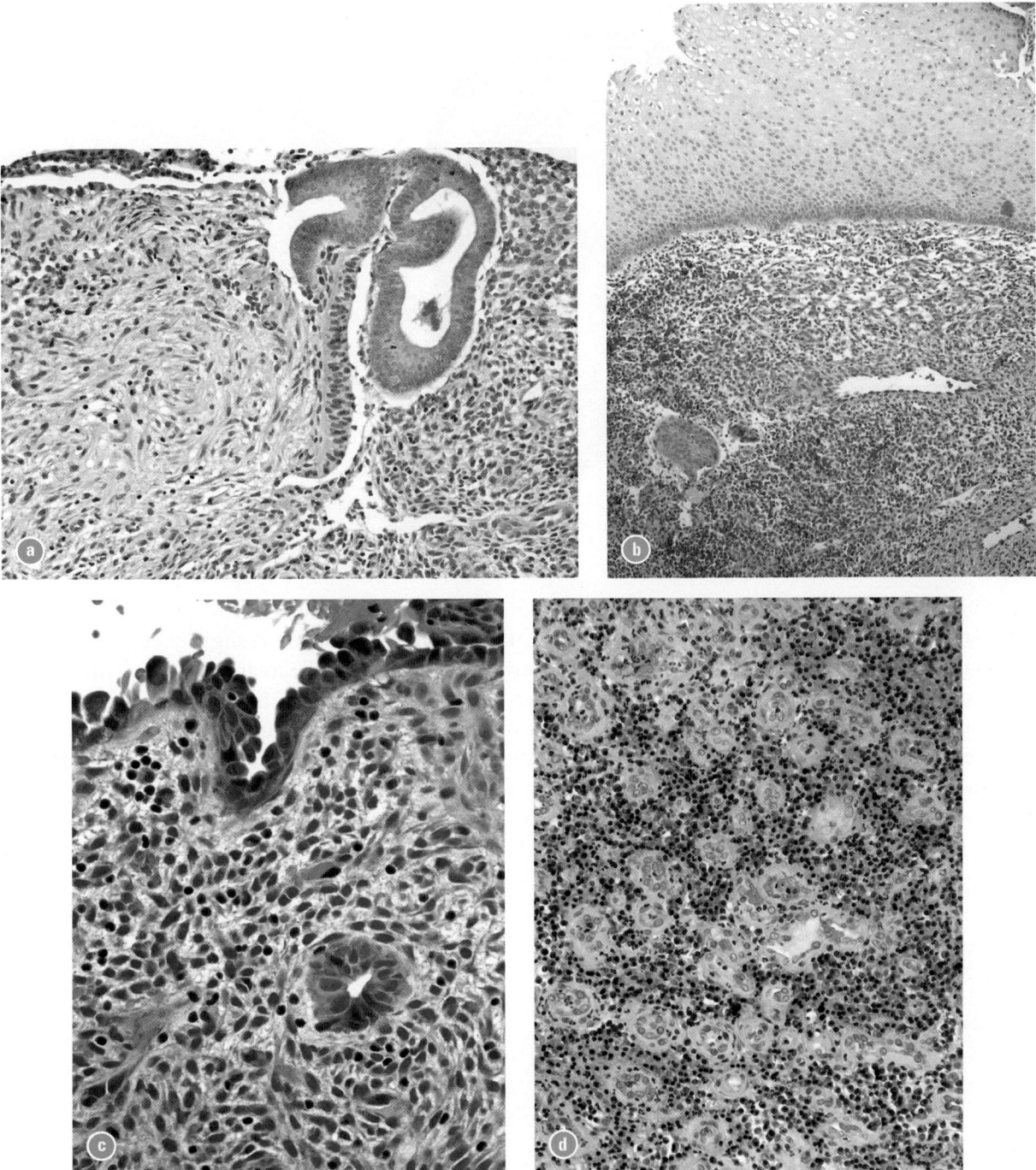

Fig. 16.29 Endometrial changes associated with intrauterine device. (a) Altered stroma (pseudodecidual changes, left) associated with a progestin-coated device. (b) Squamous metaplasia. (c) Surface reactive changes with atypia. (d) Granulation tissue associated with a long-standing IUD that became imbedded in the myometrium.

cardiovascular, in the form of myocardial infarction, venous thrombosis and ischemic stroke. All of the latter risks are magnified significantly in women who smoke.[87,96]

Emergency contraception is administered within 5 days of unprotected sexual intercourse and includes either combined estradiol–levonorgestrel (Yuzpe regimen) and levonorgestrel-only therapy, given in two (Yuzpe regimen) or as a double dose.[97]

Bleeding is common in women on oral contraceptives, particularly in the first 3 months of use.[98] It is

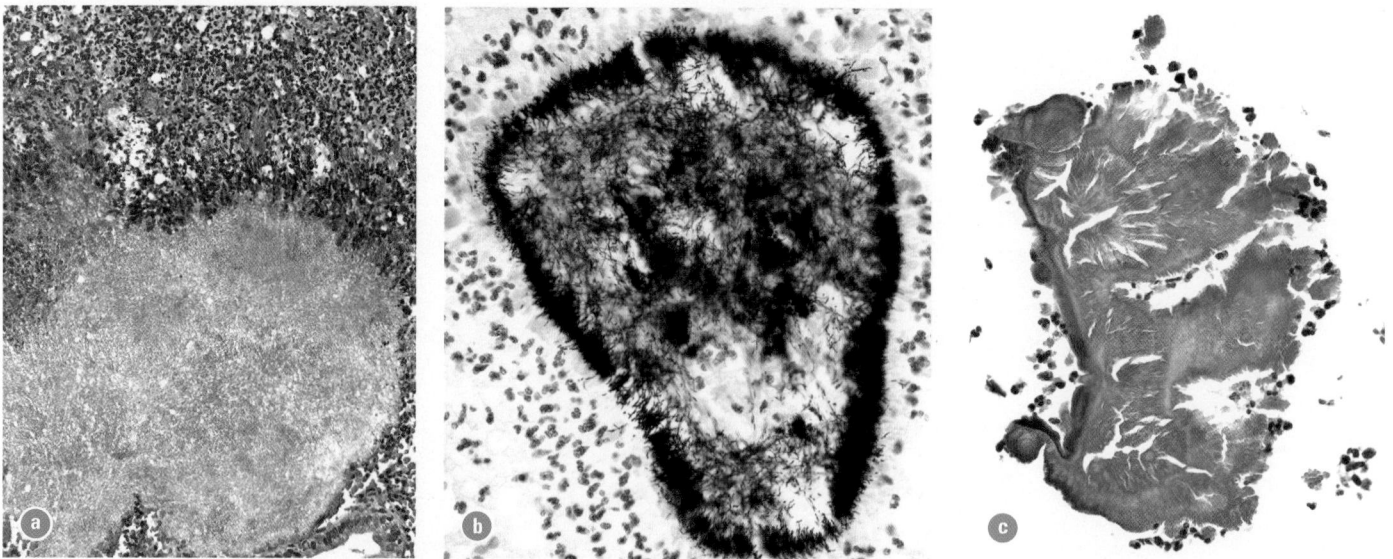

Fig. 16.30 Actinomycotic granules. (b) Following Gram stain, illustrating hyphae. (c) Pseudoactinomycotic radiate granules (PAMRAGs).

rarely threatening, but if continuous merits an evaluation with endometrial sampling to exclude an organic cause. First-line management usually consists of assessing patient compliance (most common factor) and adjusting the hormonal regimen as needed.[98]

The pathologist generally encounters biopsies from patients on OCPs when abnormal bleeding has occurred. The morphologic hallmark of OCP effect is progressively smaller glands (tiny tubular glands) lined by cuboidal epithelium and small or absent vacuoles (Fig. 16.33a,b). The stroma is slightly edematous and the stromal cells are spindle in appearance. This pattern is the expected sequela to the continuous administration of combined estrogen and progestin. It is distinguished from late menstrual endometrium by the absence of larger glands, pseudostratification and the characteristic stroma. It is distinguished from atrophy by the stromal changes, the uniformly small glands

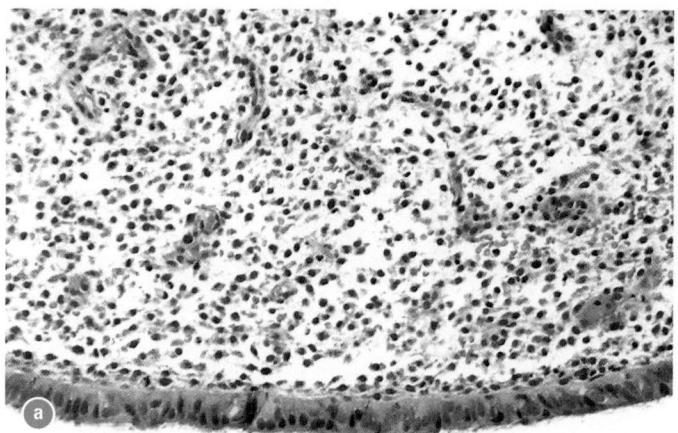

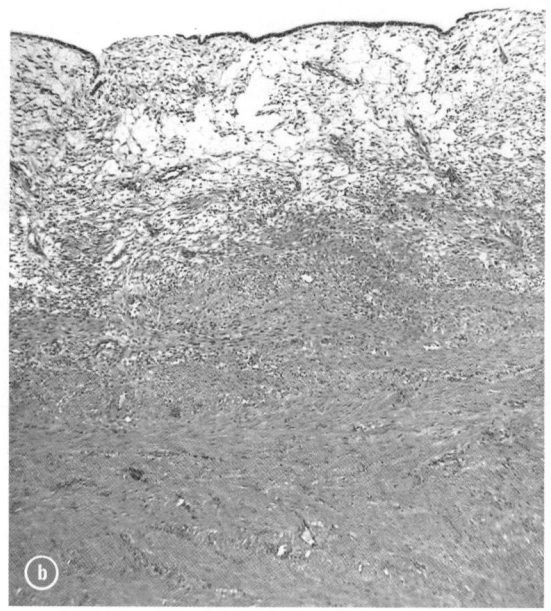

Fig. 16.31 (a) Aglandular functionalis associated with submucosal leiomyoma. (b) Compression atrophy produced by submucosal leiomyoma, shown in a hysterectomy.

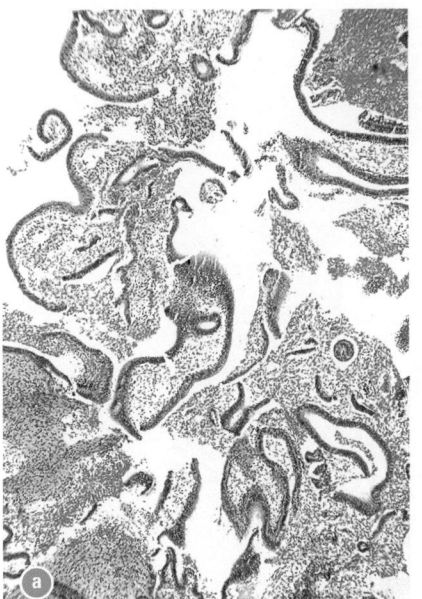
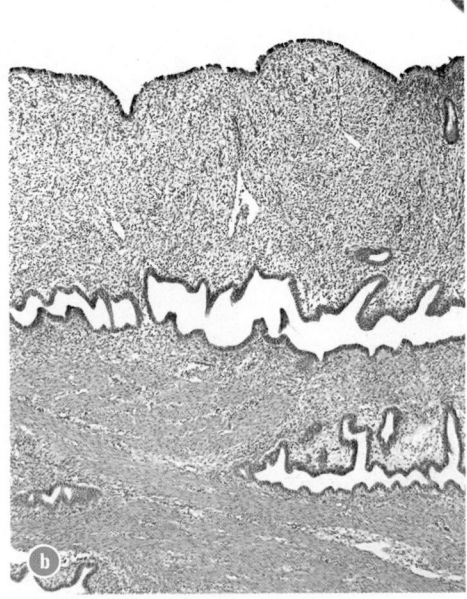
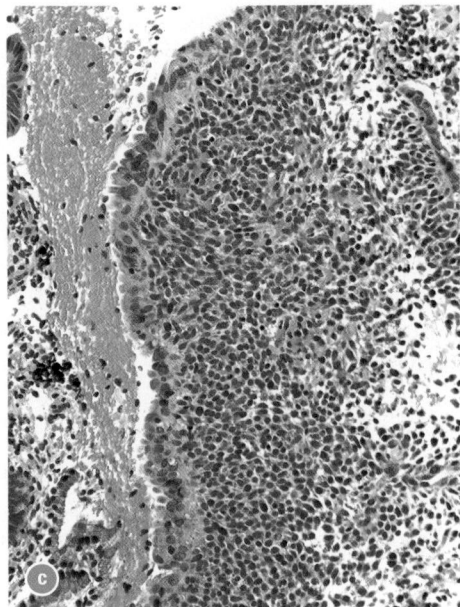

Fig. 16.32 (a) Hormone replacement therapy, with attenuated superficial functionalis, may mimic the effect of submucosal leiomyoma. (b) Endometrial adenosarcoma, with aglandular surface. (c) Strips of highly cellular sarcomatous stroma from an adenosarcoma.

and the patient's age. Another contraceptive currently used is Depo-Provera. The findings are similar to that of progestin therapy outlined below.

Progesterone administration

Exogenous progestogen (Provera) therapy is often administered cyclically to women with anovulation, abnormal bleeding or a diagnosis of endometrial hyperplasia.[99] In contrast to oral contraceptives, the effect is limited to progesterone and produces a more conspicuous pseudodecidual stromal response accompanied by a range of glandular changes (Fig. 16.34). The latter typically present a mixture of tubular inactive appearing glands and glands that show secretory

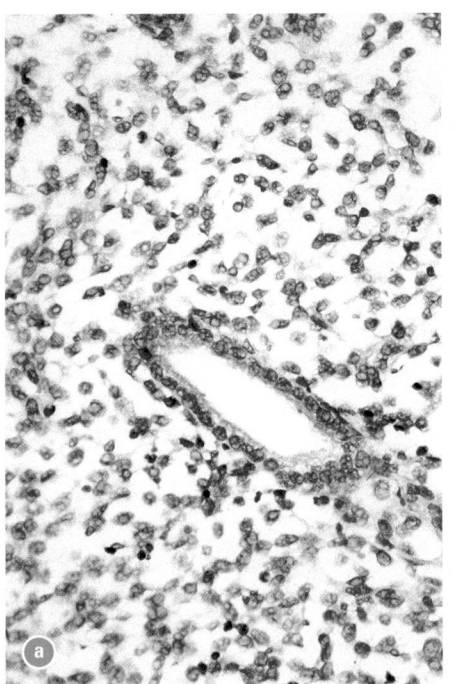
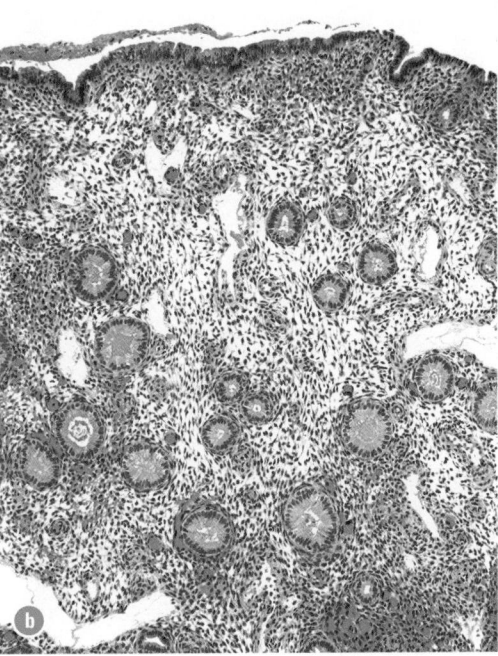

Fig. 16.33 (a,b) Oral contraceptive effect with tubular glands and a range of secretory exhaustion.

effect. Early on, there is a subtle reduction in gland epithelial cell stratification, with a corresponding reduction in nuclear size and mitotic activity. With prolonged administration, the glands closely resemble those of oral contraceptive effect; however, the changes in the stroma are much more striking. The glandular morphology may vary considerably, particularly when polyps are present. Variable cystic glandular change may also be seen and, in the presence of progestins, cannot necessarily be construed as resulting from prior anovulation.

Strong progestins

Powerful progestins such as megestrol (Megace) are administered in response to severe menorrhagia or atypical hyperplasia.[100–102] This hormone produces even more pronounced stromal changes, including marked pseudodecidual effect with a pavement-like arrangement of polyhedral stromal cells. Glands may be small and tubular, cystic and slit-like with high-dose therapy (Fig. 16.35a,b). Stretches of aglandular functionalis may be seen and must not be confused with the effects of submucosal leiomyoma.

A confusing variant of prolonged progestin therapy is the presence of sheets of amorphous functionalis in the curetting. This is caused by withdrawal of the hormonal stimulus, leading to wholesale shedding of intact necrotic pseudodecidua (pseudodecidual cast) (Fig. 16.36). The differential diagnosis is an altered menstrual endometrium (membranous dysmenorrhea) (Fig. 16.2c),[103] necrotic gestational endometrium, necrotic smooth muscle, fibrin and necrotic polyp. The principal exclusion is concurrent pregnancy, which can usually be ruled out by history.

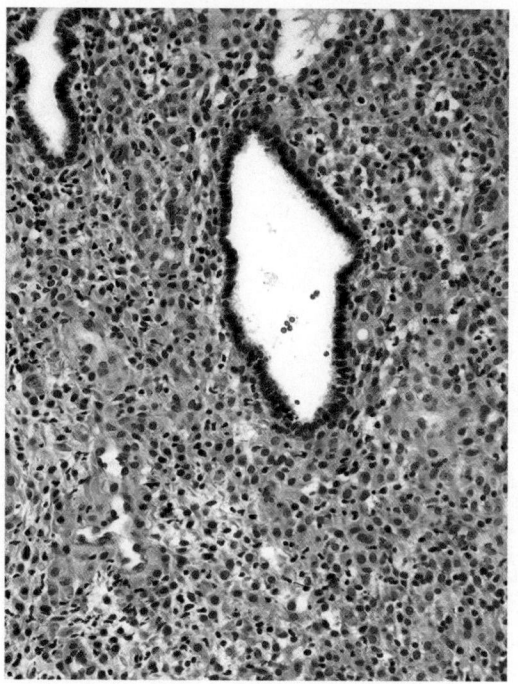

Fig. 16.34 Progestin (Provera) effect with attenuated exhausted glands and pseudodecidua.

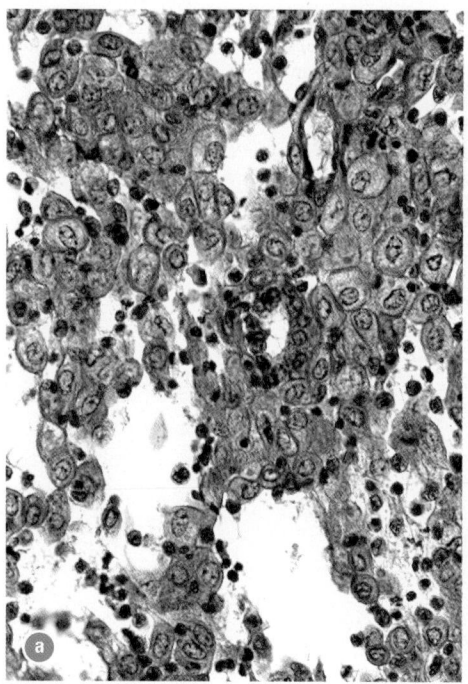
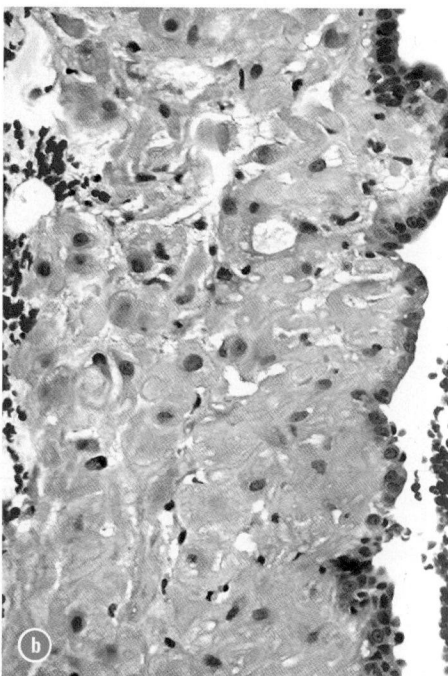

Fig. 16.35 Megestrol effect with (a) tiny tubular glands and prominent polyhedral pseudodecidual cells, (b) pronounced pseudodecidual change creating a zone of aglandular functionalis.

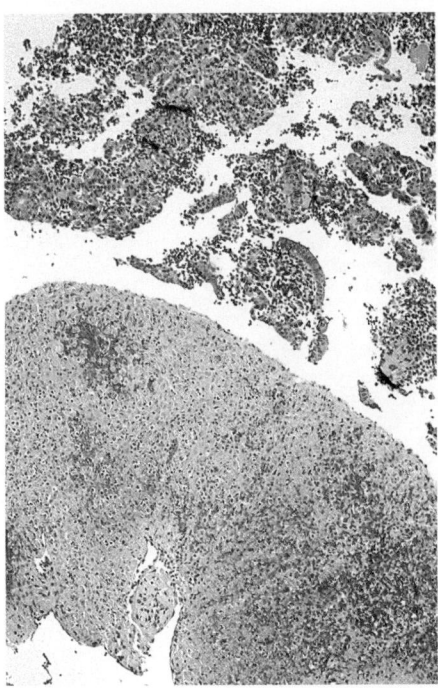

Fig. 16.36 Degenerating pseudodecidual cast produced by intense hormonal effect followed by withdrawal. Note the adjacent regenerating basalis with residual stromal breakdown (upper).

Hormonal replacement therapy

Hormone replacement therapy (HRT) typically employs sequential estrogen-progestogen administration.[104] The typical findings on biopsy are a combination of several elements, including tubular but quiescent appearing glands in a nondescript stroma (Fig. 16.37a) and variable stromal disaggregation (Fig. 16.37b). Additional findings typically include tubal metaplasia, or its variant eosinophilic metaplasia and variable syncytial epithelial groups characteristic of repair (Fig. 16.37c). In essence, HRT produces an attenuated inactive endometrium with scant tubular glands and principally surface epithelium, with minimal mitotic activity. Spindled stroma and marked gland shrinkage seen in OCPs is generally absent.

Diagnosis: Benign endometrial fragments with gland and stromal changes consistent with hormone replacement therapy.

Patients on HRT may either request estrogen-only preparations or not take the progestins, or be highly sensitive to the estrogen component. In such instances, findings consistent with unopposed estrogen effect may be encountered (Fig. 16.37d). At such times, a comment should be made to the effect that excessive estrogen effect is present, to alert the clinician of the possible need to alter the dose.[105]

Diagnosis: Fragments of benign endometrium with changes consistent with unopposed or poorly opposed estrogen effect.

Tamoxifen

Tamoxifen is currently recommended in the prevention and treatment of breast cancer.[106,107] The histologic findings in patients on tamoxifen therapy are essentially an inactive endometrium similar to hormone replacement therapy (Fig. 16.38a). Tamoxifen is also associated with endometrial polyps (which may be multiple) (Fig. 16.38b) and a variety of endometrial neoplasms, such as adenosarcoma and malignant mixed Müllerian tumor.[107–110]

Clomiphene therapy

Clomiphene is best known for the production of marked secretory changes with prominent sub-nuclear vacuoles (Fig. 16.38c).

Mixed pattern endometria (Table 16.8)

Mixed patterns are most commonly produced by hormonal therapy, but can usually be appreciated by attention to the aforementioned categories combined with clinical information. The entities discussed in this segment are those showing gland dyssynchrony. Endometritis may be associated with endometrial dyssynchrony and is not considered in this category. The definition of 'mixed pattern' endometrium is the presence of alterations comprising both a proliferative and secretory pattern. With uncommon exceptions, a mixed pattern does not imply mitotic activity in secretory glands.

Apart from hormonal therapy and assisted reproduction, mixed pattern endometria can be subdivided into three groups: (a) sporadic ovulation, (b) intrinsic disturbances in folliculogenesis and (c) clonal events leading to distinctly different gland patterns or in the endometrium *per se.*

Anovulation followed by hormonal therapy or ovulation

This pattern exhibits a combination of tubular glands with cystic glandular dilatation and variable stromal changes. The presence of prominent pseudodecidual change indicates progestin therapy (Fig. 16.39a). The reader is reminded that intense progestin therapy alone will also generate cystic glandular changes (Fig. 16.39b).

If anovulation is followed by ovulation (Fig. 16.39c), the endometrium will exhibit glands of irregular size containing secretory features accompanied by edematous stroma typical of secretory phase. Alternatively, prominent vacuoles may be seen, although it is uncertain whether this finding is pathognomonic of ovulation (Fig. 16.39d). Mitotic activity may be absent yet some of the glands may contain tubal metaplasia. This is characteristic of anovulatory pattern with superimposed ovulation.

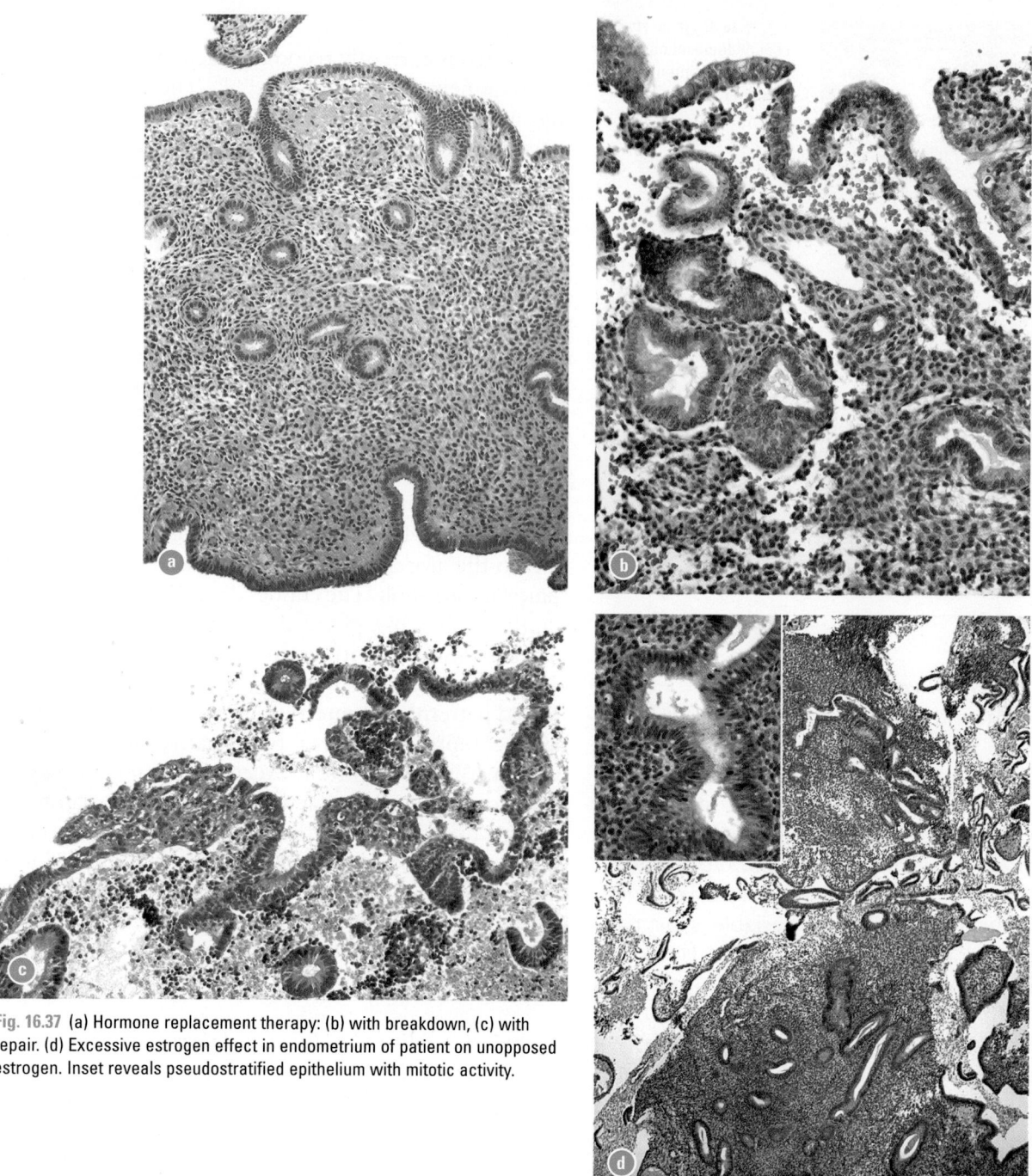

Fig. 16.37 (a) Hormone replacement therapy: (b) with breakdown, (c) with repair. (d) Excessive estrogen effect in endometrium of patient on unopposed estrogen. Inset reveals pseudostratified epithelium with mitotic activity.

Diagnostic terms for the above include: Altered endometrium with a mixed secretory and proliferative pattern. This pattern may be associated with anovulation and superimposed ovulation or hormonal (progestin) therapy.

Intrinsic disturbances in secretory maturation

Intrinsic disturbances in secretory maturation may be mediated by either a deficient signal from the ovary that is reflected in the entire specimen or a localized phenomenon in the target tissue. In the first, there may be evidence of deficient secretory maturation characterized by minimal pseudostratification with or without sub-nuclear vacuoles or more advanced stromal changes characterizing mid-secretory phase (Fig. 16.40). The persistence of tubular glands into what should be day 19 or higher, indicates either suboptimal follicle maturation, absent corpus luteum

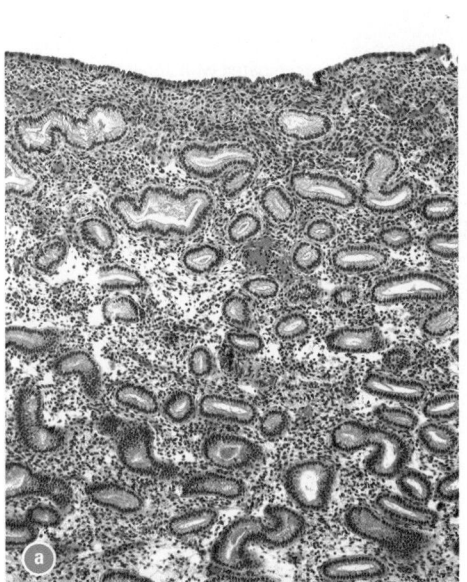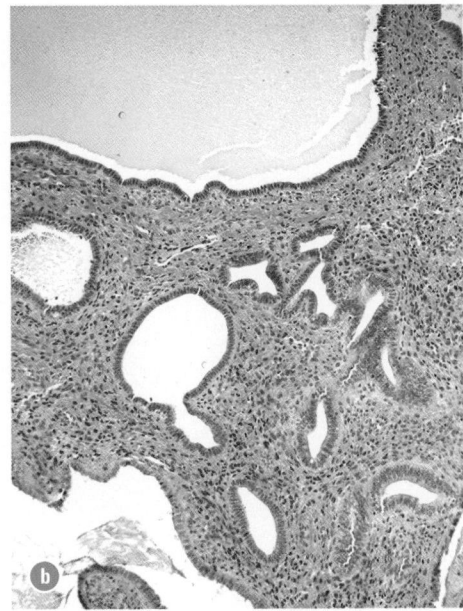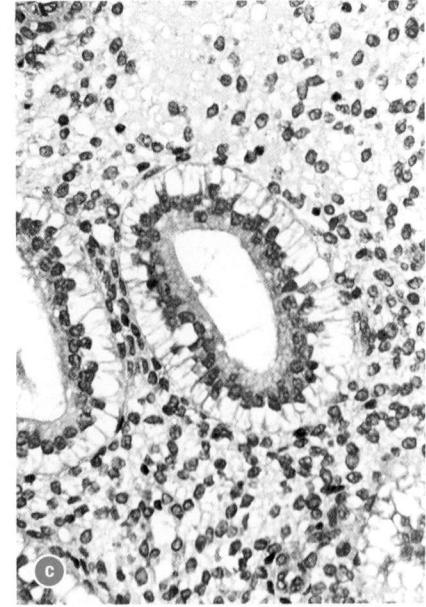

Fig. 16.38 (a) Tamoxifen, resembling replacement therapy. (b) Tamoxifen-associated polyp. (c) The effects of clomiphene therapy, shown as prominent columnar sub-nuclear vacuoles ('sky-scraper vacuoles').

development or a defect in endometrial response. In essence, there is a defect in secretory conversion. Altered secretory maturation is more typically seen near menopause, as is the end result of this process in which diffuse stromal breakdown ensues as the follicle degenerates in the absence of a corpus luteum. This pattern closely resembles hormone replacement therapy, the latter characterized by mitotically quiet tubular glands and nondescript stromal changes.

Diagnostic terms for the above include: Altered endometrium with delayed secretory maturation. This pattern could be caused by hormonal therapy or altered cycle (clinical correlation is advised).

Clonal events leading to mixed gland phenotypes
In a third scenario, clonal events lead to mixed gland phenotypes (Fig. 16.41a,b). This is the least common mixed pattern in which discrete pseudostratified glands, sometimes accompanied by mitotic activity, are ensconced within an otherwise normal-appearing secretory phase endometrium. By all appearances, this pattern is a juxtaposition of two physiologic groups of endometrial glands, one progressing normally through the secretory phase and the other lagging due to a molecular event that has targeted a discrete gland tract. The most plausible explanation is a clonal event resulting in loss of a gene required for this

transition, such as that encoding the progesterone receptor. Indeed, progesterone receptors may be lost in such instances. The impact of this phenomenon on fertility would seem negligible given the focal nature of these changes and the otherwise normal-appearing secretory phase endometrium. As a lesson in what molecular perturbations may be in store for most endometria during reproductive life, this finding is intriguing.[111]

POSTMENOPAUSAL ENDOMETRIUM

Following age 50, a surprisingly small number of endometrial samples will exhibit a classic proliferative or secretory endometrium or changes secondary to a persistent follicle. Rather, the patterns fall into one of several groups with decreasing frequency.

Inactive

The term 'inactive' is more descriptive than a functional term, inasmuch as an inactive-appearing pattern may be encountered at the end of ovulatory shedding, following oral contraceptive or replacement therapy and during the transition from a cycling to atrophic endometrium at menopause. In essence, it is defined as sparse tubular glands in the absence of mitotic activity. The difference between an inactive

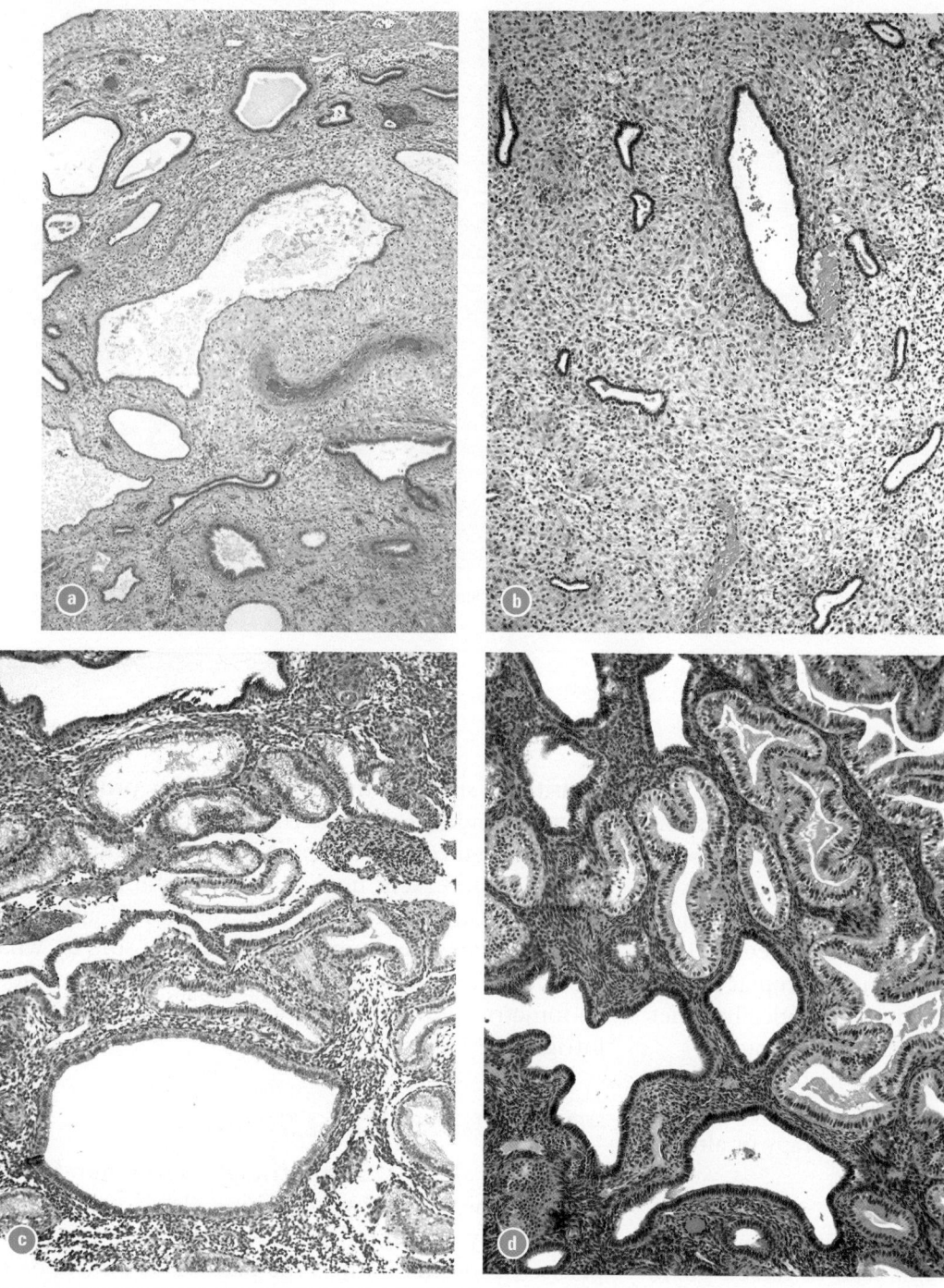

Fig. 16.39 (a) Anovulation followed by progestin. (b) Marked progestin effect may simulate cystic changes associated with anovulation. (c) Anovulation followed by ovulation. (d) Mixed pattern with prominent sub-nuclear vacuoles. This suggests recent ovulation or altered hormonal condition.

and atrophic pattern is simply one of degree. In practice, the diagnosis of inactive should be made sparingly and only after transient phenomena, such as hormonal therapy or a late menstrual pattern have been excluded. Otherwise, the diagnosis should reflect the conditions (such as hormonal effect, late menstrual, etc.).

Atrophy

This natural pattern in the postmenopausal patient may be increasingly observed if hormone replacement therapy falls into disfavor. Endometrium from a postmenopausal woman who is not on replacement therapy typically consists of attenuated scant strips of surface epithelium with minimal underlying stroma (Fig. 16.42).

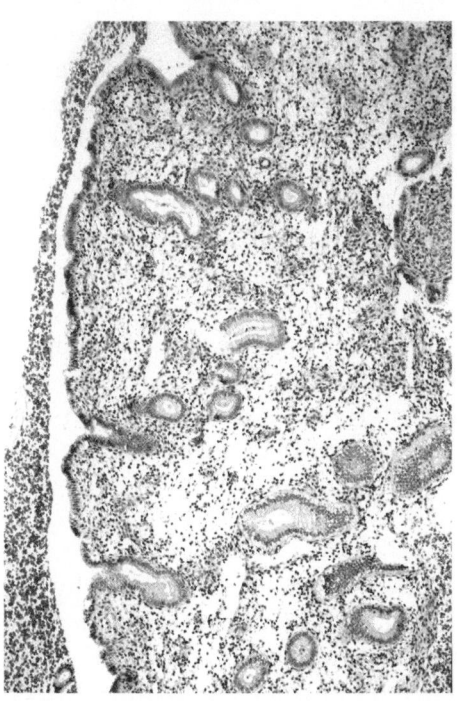

Fig. 16.40 Altered cycle with dyssynchronous pattern. This pattern is indistinguishable from recent hormonal therapy.

resembles combined therapy and can be achieved by appropriately low levels of estrogen replacement. The second is a characteristic proliferative endometrium, which by definition increases the risk of endometrial cancer by several-fold. It would not be an over-estimation to say that excess estrogen effect in post-menopausal woman carries a higher risk of cancer than the persistent estrogen of ovulation in a perimenopausal patient. The third pattern is distinctly uncommon, consisting of proliferative endometrium with glandular dilation analogous to anovulation (Fig. 16.37d). Either of the last two patterns could be seen with either estrogen therapy or endogenous estrogen effect (obesity, cortical stromal hyperplasia).

When excess estrogen effect is encountered, the following diagnosis is rendered: Proliferative (with our without cystic glands) endometrium consistent with unopposed or poorly opposed estrogen effect. The physician should be notified and advised of this condition and the increased risk it entails for subsequent endometrial neoplasia.

This pattern is at the extreme end of a spectrum of benign changes in postmenopausal women with conspicuous estrogen effect at the other end of this spectrum.

Excess estrogen effect

Women on continuous estrogen may present with a range of endometrial findings. The first closely

CURRENT OR POST-PREGNANCY/POST-PARTUM ENDOMETRIUM

The most important issues faced in management of patients who are recently pregnant include exclusion of ectopic pregnancy, confirming or excluding retained products of conception, excluding trophoblastic neo-

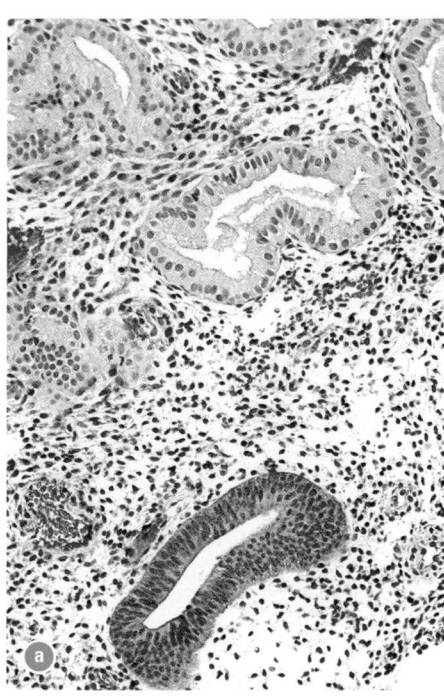

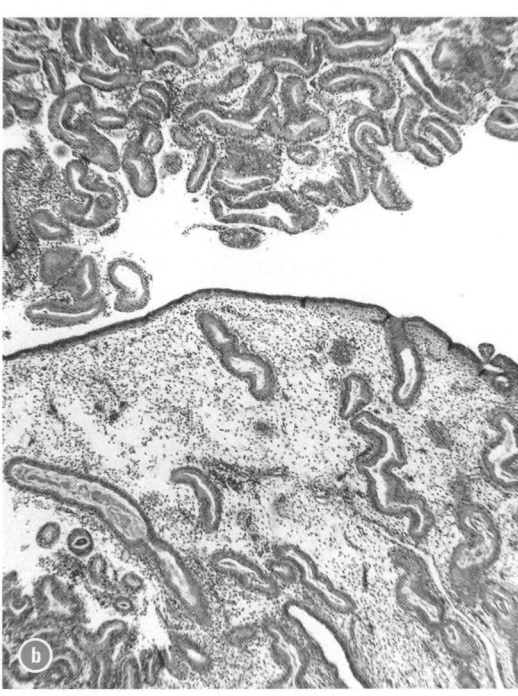

Fig. 16.41 (a) Mixed pattern due to clonal population of progestin-unresponsive glands. The latter appears to have a defect in the progestin receptor pathway. (b) Juxtaposition of proliferative endometrium (lower) and a clonal population of slightly more crowded, uniform glands (above). The latter do not fulfill the criteria for endometrial intraepithelial neoplasia.

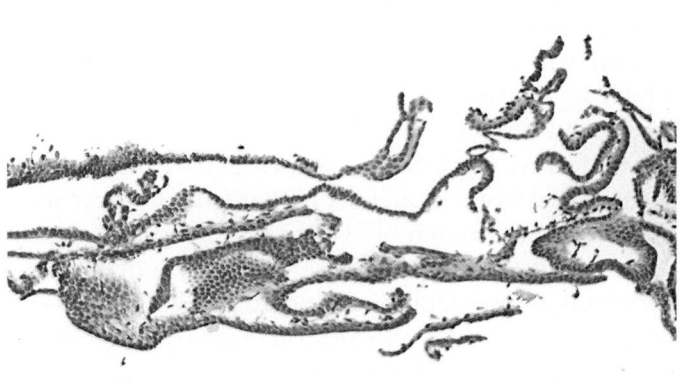

Fig. 16.42 Atrophic endometrium with strips of attenuated surface epithelium.

plasia and other conditions, such as endometritis. The first three are covered under disorders of early pregnancy in the chapter on placenta and the fourth is addressed previously under endometritis. This discussion will be limited to simply reviewing patterns that may be encountered in suspected or unsuspected pregnancy. This topic will be discussed in detail in Chapter 32.

Decidua

The full term is *decidua vera* and corresponds to uterine lining of a pregnant woman under the influence of the corpus luteum. Decidua must be distinguished from *predecidua,* which signifies the luteal phase and is not diagnostic of pregnancy, and *pseudodecidua,* which, as described previously, is morphologically similar except it is caused by something other than pregnancy, including stromal changes induced by exogenous progestin. Gestational stromal changes seen in sites other than the uterine lining, including cervix (decidual polyp) and upper genital tract (tube, ovarian cortex and peritoneum) fall into the category of *ectopic decidua.*

Decidua is characterized by small rounded nuclei with ample cytoplasm and inconspicuous spiral arterioles. Variable amounts of inflammation may be present (Fig. 16.43a). When the goal is to exclude ectopic pregnancy, the pathologist may be compelled to make the distinction between inflamed decidua and decidua with implantation site. The latter is distinguished by enlarged hyperchromatic nuclei with a higher nuclear/cytoplasmic ratio (Fig. 16.7b).

Implantation site

Recent implantation site is associated with decidua, does not form a discrete nodule and is invariably asso-

ciated with Nitabuch's fibrin (Fig. 16.43b). Mimics include the following. The first is old implantation site, characterized by uniform nodular aggregates of intermediate trophoblast with abundant cytoplasm (Fig. 16.43d). We have seen an old implantation site in samples of decidua from patients with concurrent ectopics; thus, the age of the implantation site may be critical to the decision of whether ectopic pregnancy can be excluded. The second is the presence of hyaline degeneration seen in cervix or endometrium secondary to injury or infarction, which to the unaware may be misinterpreted, as implantation site; the lack of associated trophoblast helps exclude this possibility.

Arias-Stella effect

Arias-Stella effect (ASE) is characterized by hypersecretory glands lined by cells that typically have abundant vacuolated cytoplasm and enlarged often hyperchromatic polyploid nuclei (sometimes 16N). The effected cells often project into the lumen of the gland, imparting a hobnail appearance (Fig. 16.43c). When these features are present in a secretory endometrium a diagnosis of pregnancy can be made. However, the location of the pregnancy (intra- versus extra-uterine) cannot be ascertained. Historically, the main diagnostic pitfall of ASE was misinterpretation as clear cell adenocarcinoma (CCA) of the endometrium. CCA characteristically will have readily identifiable mitotic figures that may include atypical forms as well as prominent nucleoli and a more diffuse degree of cytologic atypia involving the gland tract. In contrast, ASE typically does not have mitotic activity and exhibits a spectrum of nuclear atypia with an admixture of normal-appearing cells with enlarged affected cells. Another, perhaps less well-known, diagnostic pitfall is the misclassification of ASE as implantation site, particularly when an involved gland is tangentially sectioned (Fig. 16.43c, see below).

BENIGN ATYPIAS/ARTIFACTS ENCOUNTERED IN ROUTINE EVALUATION OF ENDOMETRIUM (FIG. 16.37)

A list of these entities is given in Table 16.9, some of which have been addressed previously. Additional ones to be aware of include the following:

Exfoliation (fixation) artifacts

We are witnessing an increasingly common phenomenon termed 'exfoliation artifact'. This is characterized by

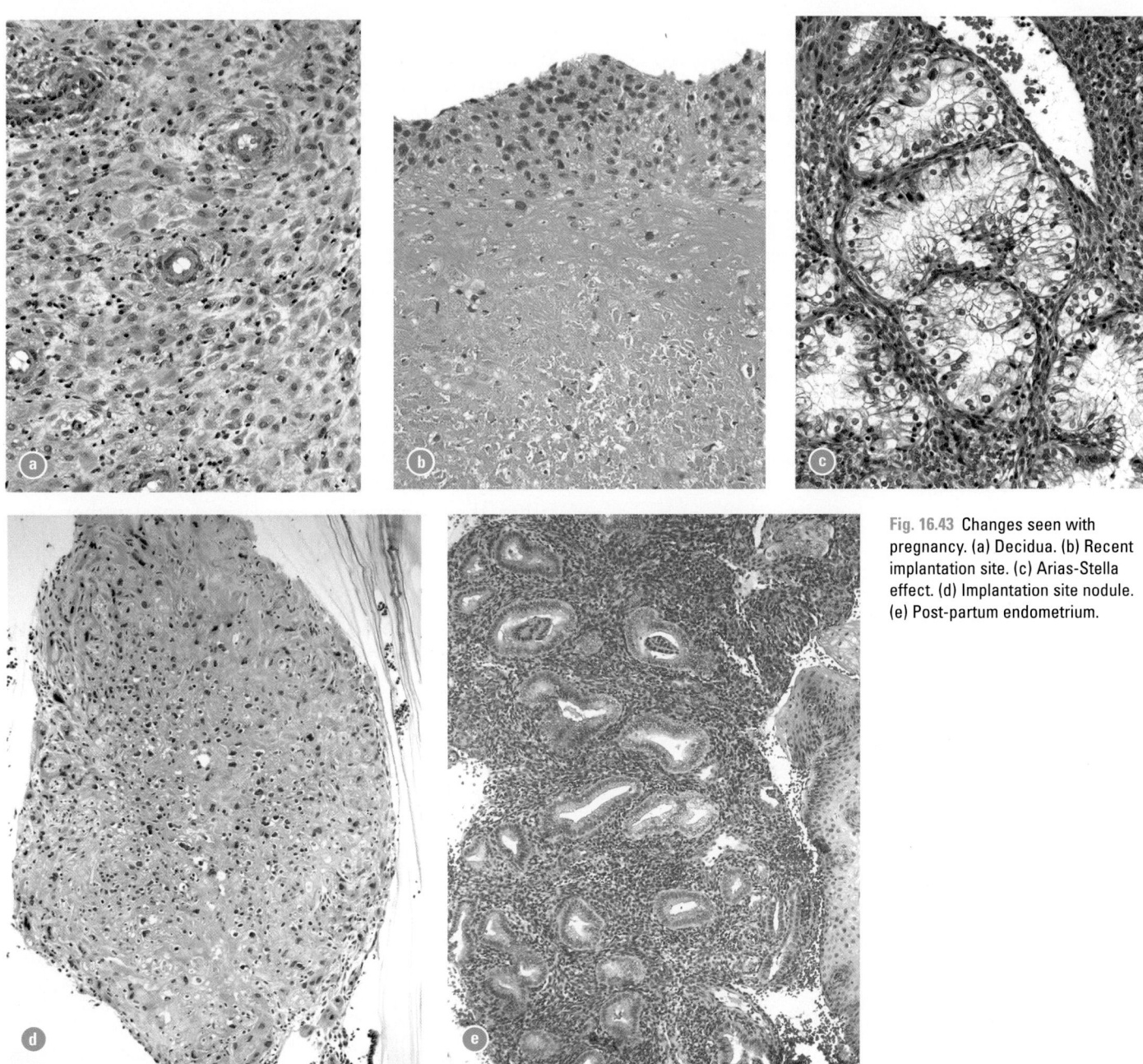

Fig. 16.43 Changes seen with pregnancy. (a) Decidua. (b) Recent implantation site. (c) Arias-Stella effect. (d) Implantation site nodule. (e) Post-partum endometrium.

disaggregation of the luminal cells of proliferative and secretory endometrium giving rise to a pseudo-micropapillary appearance to the endometrial lining or, in extreme cases, occlusion of the lumen (Fig. 16.44a,b). The differential diagnosis includes a papillary serous carcinoma. However, the following features will usually distinguish this artifact: (1) absence of nuclear atypia, (2) a relatively low nuclear/cytoplasmic ratio, (3) areas in which the artifact blends with normal-appearing endometrium and (4) subtle but discernible stromal changes adjacent to the altered glands, in the form of poor preservation. The cause of this artifact is not clear, but most likely relates to the instillation of fluids during hysteroscopy.[112]

Table 16.9 *Categories of benign endometrial epithelial atypia. Atypias are principally cellular with minimal architectural irregularity*

Radiation	Reactive/reparative (endometritis, repair) (Fig. 16.46a)
	Arias-Stella effect (pregnancy, post-partum) (Figs 16.43c, 16.45a)
	Arias-Stella effect-like (hormones, idiopathic) (Fig. 16.45d)
	Viral (CMV)
Artifacts	Neoplastic (serous carcinoma) (Fig. 16.46b,c)
	Pseudocarcinoma (menstrual) (Fig. 16.3a)
	Telescoping artifact (Figs 16.5d, 16.7d)
	Exfoliation artifact (Fig. 16.44a,b)
	Inspissated material (Fig. 16.44c)
Pitfalls	Small cell undifferentiated carcinoma masquerading as breakdown
	Fragments of adenocarcinoma masquerading as breakdown (Fig. 16.3b)
	Stromal neoplasms appearing as breakdown or aglandular functionalis (Fig. 16.32b,c)
	Surface serous carcinomas appearing to be surface reactive atypia (Fig. 16.46b,c)

CMV, cytomegalovirus infection.

Inspissated gland artifacts

These are also likely to be due to mechanical means and are characterized by amorphous debris packed into the superficial glands of the functionalis. The debris does not contain a dominant inflammatory cell component and must be distinguished from intraluminal inflammation (Fig. 16.44c).

Arias-Stella-like patterns

We have encountered these under four circumstances. The first is exaggerated ASE in gestational endometrium (Fig. 16.45a). The second is ASE in regenerating endometria following pregnancy or associated with ectopic gestation. This is uncommon, but is characterized by the unique juxtaposition of proliferating glands and prominent nuclear atypia (Fig. 16.45b). The third is ASE confined to the surface epithelium and adjacent glands. This pattern may mimic implantation site (Fig. 16.45c). The fourth is ASE-like changes in association with hormone replacement therapy (Fig. 16.45d).[113] These are easily recognized by the presence of a prominent pseudodecidual response. In the latter settings, it is important to exclude clear cell carcinoma. Invariably, the former exhibit preserved nuclear/cytoplasmic ratio, a tendency for intermittent rather than continuous atypia and focal rather than diffuse strong staining for p53.

Altered surface epithelial changes, including repair

These may take several forms and are associated with post-partum or post-abortal endometria, intrauterine devices, degenerative changes in endometrial polyps or endometrium adjacent to submucosal leiomyomata and bleeding post menopause. They are typically focal, at times syncytial in appearance, may be associated with stromal breakdown and generally are a 'sporadic' rather than diffuse atypia (Fig. 16.46a). The princi-

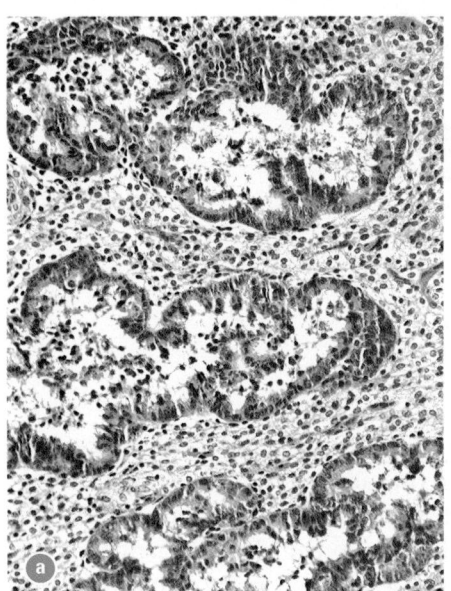 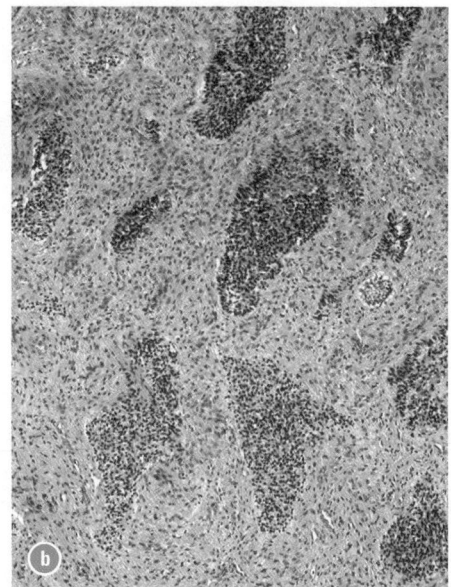 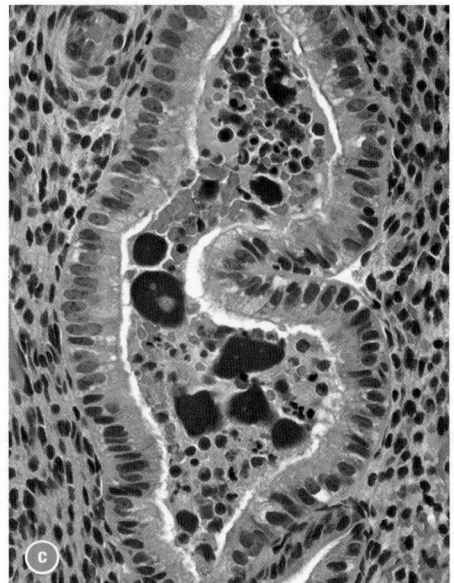

Fig. 16.44 (a) Exfoliation artifact mimicking serous neoplasia or hypersecretory endometrium. (b) Exfoliation of cells fills the glandular lumens in this polyp. (c) Inspissated amorphous material in surface gland lumina, presumably introduced during procedure (hysteroscopy).

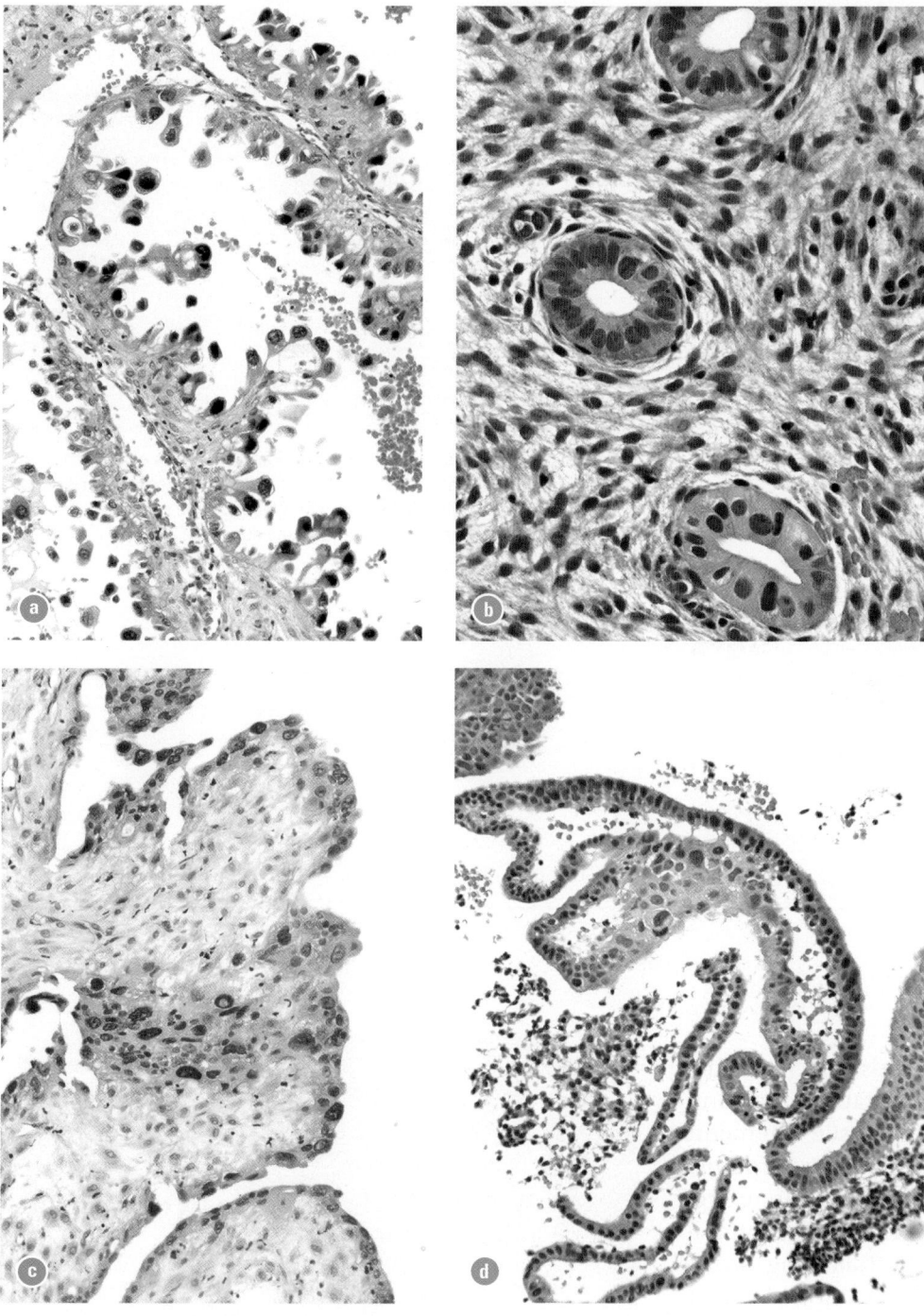

Fig. 16.45 (a) Exaggerated Arias-Stella effect in gestational endometrium. (b) Arias-Stella effect associated with regenerating endometrium. (c) Atypical Arias-Stella effect, mimicking implantation site. (d) Arias-Stella-like changes in progestin therapy. There is focal nuclear enlargement (center).

pal distinction is between a benign process and a small or early uterine papillary serous carcinoma (intra-epithelial carcinoma). The reader is reminded that vigilance is important in postmenopausal women and that a p53 stain may be prudent if any index of suspicion exists for the latter. In our experience, non-neoplastic epithelial changes will stain positive with antibodies to p53, but typically in a weak to moderate and heterogeneous manner. Diffuse intense stain-

ing typifies serous carcinoma (Fig. 16.46b,c). Repair is discussed in greater detail under metaplasias (Ch. 18).

Ablation

Ablation produces tissue necrosis, hyaline change and prominent foreign body giant cell reaction (Fig. 16.25c). The differential diagnosis includes necrotic polyps or submucosal leiomyomata.

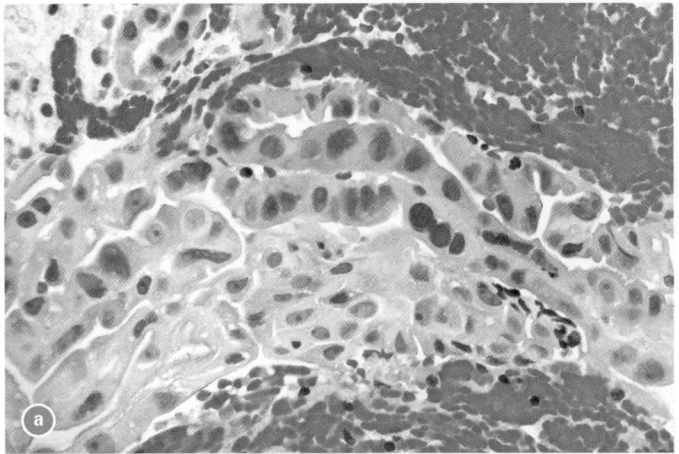

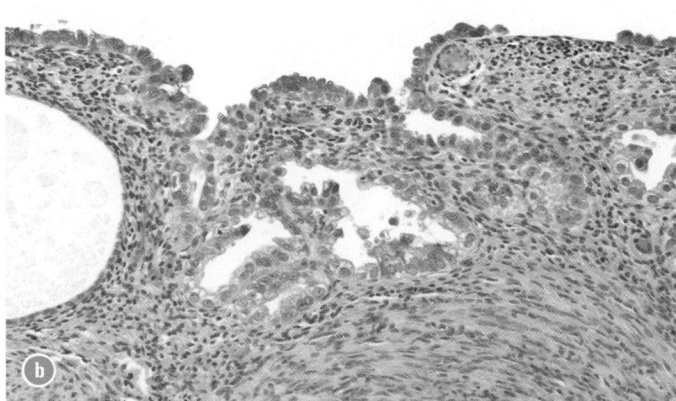

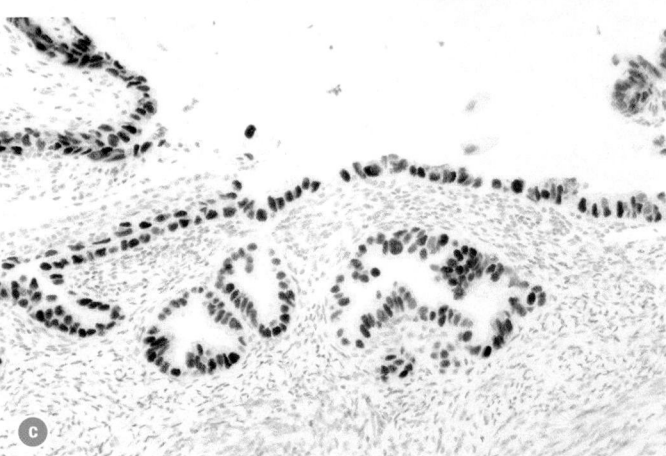

Fig. 16.46 (a) Surface reactive changes. (b) Papillary serous carcinoma, confined to the endometrial surface. When focal it may be misinterpreted as a reactive surface epithelial change. (c) Confirmation of (b) with immunostaining showing uniform and intense nuclear accumulation of p53.

Contamination from other samples

This may occur under three scenarios: (1) introduction of tissue during specimen preparation and sampling (Fig. 16.47), (2) transport of tissue fragments during processing and (3) transfer during embedding. Some contaminants are obvious and others are extremely subtlc. The laboratory management of contaminants is to review procedures in the following order: (1) Other cases accessioned and/or sectioned at the same bench on the same day should be reviewed for similar pathology. (2) If there is no relationship found, other specimens in the laboratory should be evaluated. (3) If the question is a critical one (i.e. excluding cancer), analysis of the tissue in question and tissue of known source from the patient can be evaluated by molecular means to prove or exclude a common patient source.

Introduction of tissues via perforation

These typically consist of adipose tissue from the mesentery or other peritoneal surfaces. However, bowel,

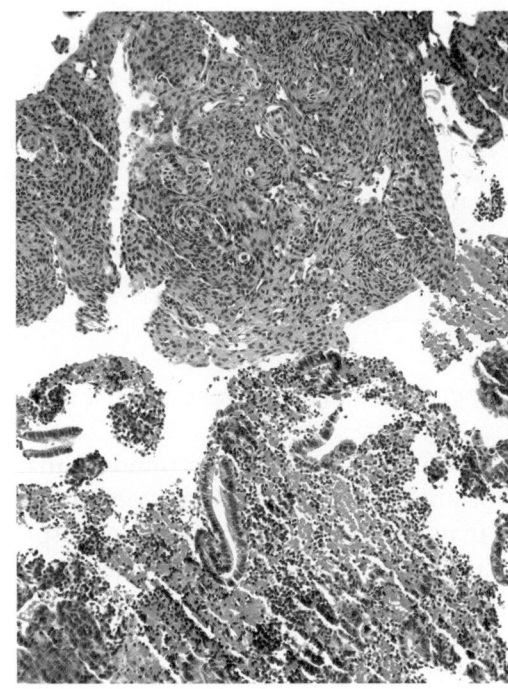

Fig. 16.47 Fragments of meningioma (upper) admixed with normal endometrium (lower). Both samples were processed at the same bench.

bladder and other tissues may be present (Fig. 16.48a). The clinician should be notified immediately in such instances to ensure close follow-up and further therapy, if required. A mimic of perforation is a 'swiss cheese' artifact in blood clot (Fig. 16.48b). Careful examination will exclude adipose tissue.

Focal necrotic polyps, hyaline changes, macrophage responses

These encompass surface injuries accompanied by degenerative stromal changes and reactive macrophage/epithelial responses (Fig. 16.49a,b). Sheets of cohesive macrophages may occasionally be mistaken for neoplasia (Fig. 16.49b). Repair and reactive changes are discussed in greater detail in the context of endometrial metaplasia (see Ch. 18).

Management of endometrial bleeding

Management of abnormal uterine bleeding varies according to the underlying disorder, which will in turn determine whether pathologic examination is required. Bleeding associated with precocious puberty will initiate a search for a hormonally active lesion. Similarly, sporadic or irregular bleeding in early adoles-

cence and bleeding in the first few months of oral contraceptive therapy will usually not necessitate endometrial sampling unless heavy. Heavy menstrual bleeding can cause considerable discomfort depending on the individual, and perceptions will be highly subjective.[114]

Management of abnormal bleeding depends on the cause and degree of discomfort and extent, if any, of anemia. Although not initially suspected in most cases of abnormal bleeding, bleeding secondary to coagulation disturbances may be managed with correction of the coagulopathy with tranexamic acid, desmopressin spray and oral contraceptives. A coagulation abnormality must always be considered if prolonged bleeding complicates diagnostic procedures, particularly in the setting of easy bruising, gum bleeding or abnormal bleeding following other surgical procedures.[32]

Three methods that are used most frequently are the administration of progestogens, including oral contraceptives, endometrial ablation and hormone-releasing intrauterine devices. One study summarized five trials with 311 patients managed surgically and 314 by hormone-releasing intrauterine systems. Ablation was superior to progestin delivery systems in controlling bleeding at 1 year, although the advantage was less after 2 to 3 years. Predictably, hysterectomy stopped all bleeding but caused serious complications

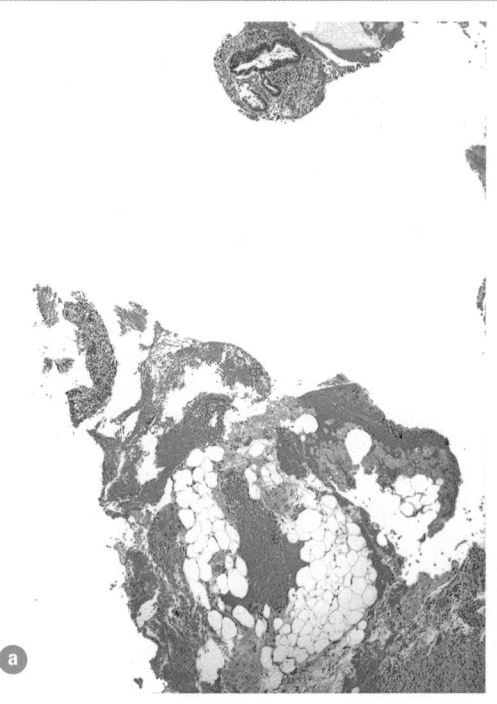
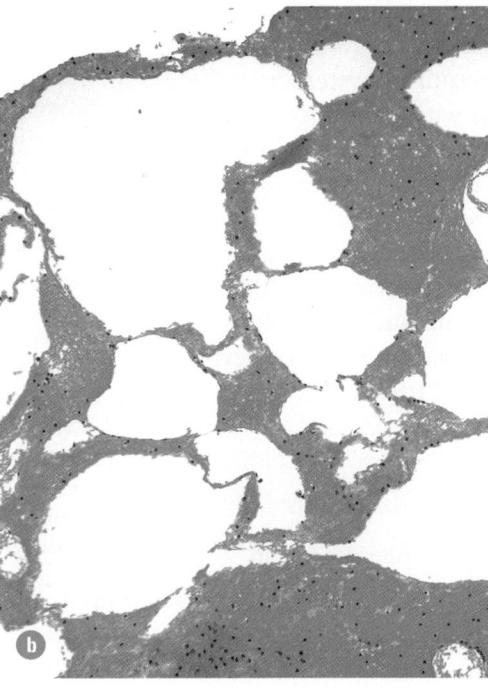

Fig. 16.48 (a) Adipose tissue (lower) admixed with benign endometrial glands (upper) from an endometrial sampling that perforated the uterine wall. (b) Swiss cheese artifact in blood clot may mimic adipose tissue.

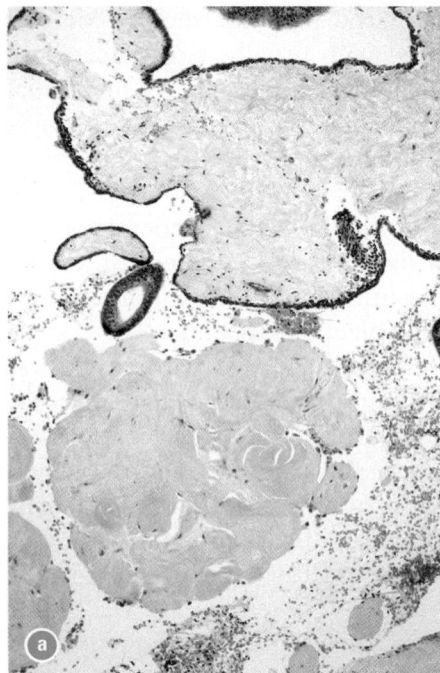
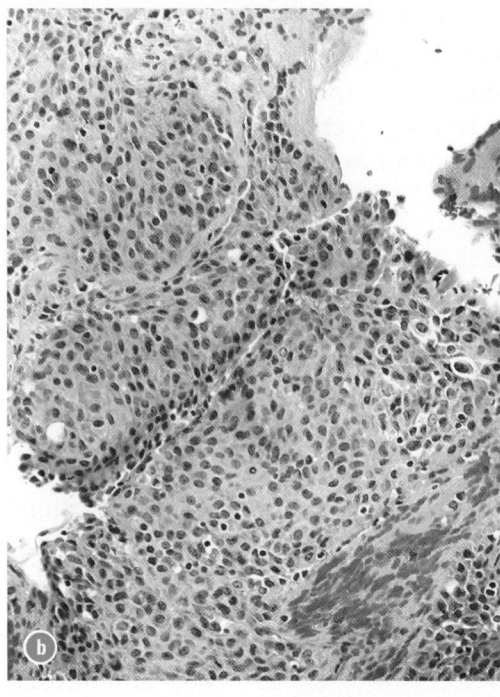

Fig. 16.49 (a) Hyaline degenerative change in an endometrial polyp. (b) Accumulation of macrophages, in the form of pseudoepithelioid sheets, may be associated with IUDs, surface disturbances associated with infarcted polyps or submucosal leiomyomas, or for unknown reasons.

for some women. The implication from this analysis is that oral therapy is less likely to produce the desired effect in cases of significant bleeding and one or more conservative options (LNG-IUS or ablation) are preferable for long-term control.[114]

Hysteroscopic surgery is the method of choice for structural lesions, principally polyps and submucosal leiomyomata, whereas ablation may be required for dysfunctional bleeding. In one study of 395 patients with all of these disorders, bleeding was controlled in 75%, with failure in 18%. Some 10% required a repeat procedure and 50 eventually required hysterectomy.[115] In a second study, 568 patients with benign conditions were treated by laser or electrosurgery. A total of 58% had cessation of bleeding, 34% had continued lesser bleeding and 8% did not improve.[116]

Based on these studies and others, it is generally concluded that hysteroscopic removal yields the best results for anatomic lesions such as polyps or fibroids, whereas endometrial ablation is the preferred approach to intractable abnormal uterine bleeding.

References

1 Strickland JL, Wall JW. Abnormal uterine bleeding in adolescents. Obstet Gynecol Clin North Am 2003; 30(2):321–335.

2 Noyes FW, Hertig AT, Rock J. Dating the endometrial biopsy. Fertil Steril 1950; 1:3–25.

3 Hendrickson MR, Longacre TA, Kempson RL. The uterine corpus. In: Sternberg SS, ed. Diagnostic surgical pathology, Philadelphia, PA: Lippincott; 1999:2203–2224.

4 Dallenbach-Hellweg G. Histopathology of the endometrium, 3rd edn. New York: Springer; 1981.

5 Sherman ME, Mazur MT, Kurman RJ. Benign diseases of the endometrium, St Louis, MO: Mosby; 1996: 422–454.

6 Anderson MC, Robboy SJ, Russell P, Morse A. The normal endometrium. In: Robboy SJ Anderson MC, Russell P, eds. Pathology of the female reproductive tract. London: Churchill Livingstone; 2002:241–265.

7 Fox H, Wells M. Haines and Taylor obstetrical and gynaecological pathology, 5th edn. London: Churchill Livingstone; 2002.

8 Speroff L, Blass RH, Kase NG. Clinical gynecologic endocrinology and infertility. Baltimore: Lippincott, Williams and Wilkins; 1999:575–579.

9 Mutter GL, Ferenczy A. Anatomy and histology of the uterine corpus. In: Kurman RJ, ed. Blaustein's pathology of the female genital tract, 5th edn. New York: Springer Verlag; 2001:383–419.

10 Starr C, McMillan B. Human biology. Belmont, CA: Wadsworth Publishing Co; 1997.

11 Ferenczy A. Pathophysiology of endometrial bleeding. Maturitas 2003; 45(1):1–14.

12 Jones GS. Luteal phase defect: a review of pathophysiology. Curr Opin Obstet Gynecol 1991; 3(5):641–648.

13 Ginsburg KA. Luteal phase defect. Etiology, diagnosis and management. Endocrinol Metab Clin North Am 1992; 21:85–104.

14 Jordan J, Craig K, Clifton DK, Soules MR. Luteal phase defect: the sensitivity and specificity of diagnostic methods in common clinical use. Fertil Steril 1994; 62:54–62.

15 Kusuhara K. Clinical importance of endometrial histology and progesterone level assessment in luteal-phase defect. Horm Res 1992; 37:53–58.

16 Grunfeld L, Sandler B, Fox J, et al. Luteal phase deficiency after completely normal follicular and periovulatory phases. Fertil Steril 1989; 52:919–923.

17 Davis OK, Berkeley AS, Naus GJ, et al. The incidence of luteal phase defect in normal, fertile women, determined by serial endometrial biopsies Fertil Steril 1990; 53:189–190.

18 Gibson M, Badger GJ, Byrn F, et al. Error in histologic dating of secretory endometrium: variance component analysis. Fertil Steril 1991; 56(2):242–247.

19 Duggan MA, Brashert P, Ostor A, et al. The accuracy and interobserver reproducibility of endometrial dating. Pathology 2001; 33(3):292–297.

20 Murray MJ, Meyer WR, Zaino RJ, et al. A critical analysis of the accuracy, reproducibility, and clinical utility of histologic endometrial dating in fertile women. Fertil Steril 2004; 81:1333–1343.

21 Davidson BJ, Thrasher TV, Seraj IM. An analysis of endometrial biopsies performed for infertility. Fertil Steril 1987; 48:770–774.

22 Li TC, Klentzeris L, Barratt C, et al. A study of endometrial morphology in women who failed to conceive in a donor insemination programme. Br J Obstet Gynaecol 1993; 100(10):935–938.

23 Dallenbach-Hellweg G. The endometrium in natural and artificial luteal phases. Hum Reprod 1988; 3:165–168.

24 Bourgain C, Smitz J, Camus M, et al. Human endometrial maturation is markedly improved after luteal supplementation of gonadotrophin-releasing hormone analogue/human menopausal gonadotrophin stimulated cycles. Hum Reprod 1994; 9(1):32–40.

25 Ben-Nun I, Jaffe R, Fejgin MD, Beyth Y. Therapeutic maturation of endometrium in *in vitro* fertilization and embryo transfer. Fertil Steril 1992; 57(5):953–962.

26 Dubowy RC, Feinberg RF, Keefe DL, et al. Improved endometrial assessment using cyclin E and p27. Fertil Steril 2003; 80:146–156.

27 Wieser F, Tempfer C, Kurz C, Nagele F. Hysteroscopy in 2001: a comprehensive review. Acta Obstet Gynecol Scand 2001; 80(9):773–783.

28 Mencaglia L, Perino A, Hamou J. Hysteroscopy in perimenopausal and postmenopausal women with abnormal uterine bleeding. J Reprod Med 1987; 32(8):577–582.

29 Schneider LG. Causes of abnormal vaginal bleeding in a Family Practice Center. J Fam Pract 1983; 16:281–283.

30 Vakiani M, Vavilis D, Agorastos T, et al. Histopathological findings of the endometrium in patients with dysfunctional uterine bleeding. Clin Exp Obstet Gynecol 1996; 23(4): 236–239.

31 Oehler MK, Rees MC. Menorrhagia: an update. Acta Obstet Gynecol Scand 2003; 82(5):405–422.

32 Lee CA. Women and inherited bleeding disorders: menstrual issues. Semin Hematol 1999; 36(3 Suppl. 4): 21–27.

33 Oral E, Cagdas A, Gezer A, et al. Hematological abnormalities in adolescent menorrhagia. Arch Gynecol Obstet 2002; 266(2):72–74.

34 Reindollar RH, McDonough PG. Adolescent menstrual disorders. Clin Obstet Gynecol 1983; 26(3):690–701.

35 Claessens EA, Cowell CA. Acute adolescent menorrhagia. Am J Obstet Gynecol 1981; 139(3):277–280.

36 Hillard PJA. Menstruation in young girls: a clinical perspective. Obstet Gynecol 2002; 99(4):655–662.

37 Quint EH, Smith YR. Abnormal uterine bleeding in adolescents. J Midwifery Womens Health 2003; 48(3):186–191.

38 Falcone T, Desjardins C, Bourque J, et al. Dysfunctional uterine bleeding in adolescents. J Reprod Med 1994; 39(10):761–764.

39 Schrager S. Abnormal uterine bleeding associated with hormonal contraception. Am Fam Physician 2002; 15(10):2073–2080.

40 Leung PL, Tam WH, Kong WS, Yuen PM. Intrauterine pathology in women with abnormal uterine bleeding taking hormone replacement therapy. J Am Assoc Gynecol Laparosc 2003; 10(2):260–262.

41 Munro MG. Dysfunctional uterine bleeding: advances in diagnosis and treatment. Curr Opin Obstet Gynecol 2001; 13(5):475–489.

42 Nagele F, O'Connor H, Davies A, et al. 2500 outpatient diagnostic hysteroscopies. Obstet Gynecol 1996; 88(1):87–92.

43 Polisseni F, Bambirra EA, Camargos AF. Detection of chronic endometritis by diagnostic hysteroscopy in asymptomatic infertile patients. Gynecol Obstet Invest 2003; 55(4):205–210.

44 Valle RF. Hysteroscopy. Curr Opin Obstet Gynecol 1991; 3(3):422–426.

45 Davidson KG, Dubinsky TJ. Ultrasonographic evaluation of the endometrium in postmenopausal vaginal bleeding. Radiol Clin North Am 2003; 41(4):769–780.

46 Mutter GL. Diagnosis of premalignant endometrial disease. J Clin Pathol 2002; 55:326–331.

47 Biron-Shental T, Tepper R, Fishman A, et al. Recurrent endometrial polyps in postmenopausal breast cancer patients on tamoxifen. Gynecol Oncol 2003; 90(2):382–386.

48 Fletcher JA, Pinkus JL, Lage JM, et al. Clonal 6p21 rearrangement is restricted to the mesenchymal component of an endometrial polyp. Genes Chromosomes Cancer 1992; 5(3):260–263.

49 Dal Cin P, Wanschura S, Kazmierczak B, et al. Amplification and expression of the HMGIC gene in a benign endometrial polyp. Genes Chromosomes Cancer 1998; 22(2):95–99.

50 Reslova T, Tosner J, Resl M, et al. Endometrial polyps. A clinical study of 245 cases. Arch Gynecol Obstet 1999; 262(3–4):133–139.

51 Van Bogaert LJ. Clinicopathologic findings in endometrial polyps. Obstet Gynecol 1988; 71(5):771–773.

52 Hachisuga T, Miyakawa T, Tsujioka H, et al. K-ras mutation in tamoxifen-related endometrial polyps. Cancer 2003; 98:1890–1897.

53 Goldstein SR, Monteagudo A, Popiolek D, et al. Evaluation of endometrial polyps. Am J Obstet Gynecol 2002; 186(4):669–674.

54 DeWaay DJ, Syrop CH, Nygaard IE, et al. Natural history of uterine polyps and leiomyomata. Obstet Gynecol 2002; 100(1):3–7.

55 Anastasiadis PG, Koutlaki NG, Skaphida PG, et al. Endometrial polyps: prevalence, detection and malignant potential in women with abnormal uterine bleeding. Eur J Gynaecol Oncol 2000; 21(2):180–183.

56 Kim MR, Kim YA, Jo MY, et al. High frequency of endometrial polyps in endometriosis. J Am Assoc Gynecol Laparosc 2003; 10(1):46–48.

57 Chavez NF, Garner EO, Khan W, et al. Does the introduction of new technology change population demographics? Minimally invasive technologies and endometrial polyps. Gynecol Obstet Invest 2002; 54(4):217–220.

58 Clement PB, Scully RE. Müllerian adenosarcoma of the uterus: a clinicopathologic analysis of 100 cases with a review of the literature. Hum Pathol 1990; 21(4): 363–381.

59 Hattab EM, Allam-Nandyala P, Rhatigan RM. The stromal component of large endometrial polyps. Int J Gynecol Pathol 1999; 18(4):332–337.

60 Sington JD, Manek S. Cytological atypia in endometrial polyps and immunostaining for p16, p53 and Ki67. Histopathology 2002; 41(1):86–88.

61 Kaminski PF, Podczaski ES. Benign conditions of the uterus. In: Hernandez E, Atkinson BF, eds. Clinical gynecologic pathology. Philadelphia, PA: WB Saunders; 1996:256.

62 Wasserheit JN, Bell TA, Kiviat NB, et al. Microbial causes of proven pelvic inflammatory disease and efficacy of clindamycin and tobramycin. Ann Intern Med 1986; 104(2):187–193.

63 Eckert LO, Hawes SE, Wolner-Hanssen PK, et al. Endometritis: the clinical-pathologic syndrome. Am J Obstet Gynecol 2002; 186(4):690–695.

64 Hillier SL, Kiviat NB, Hawes SE, et al. Role of bacterial vaginosis-associated microorganisms in endometritis. Am J Obstet Gynecol 1996; 175(2):435–441.

65 Paavonen J, Teisala K, Heinonen PK, et al. Microbiological and histopathological findings in acute pelvic inflammatory disease. Br J Obstet Gynaecol 1987; 94(5):454–460.

66 Taylor-Robinson D. Mycoplasma genitalium – an up-date. Int J STD AIDS 2002; 13(3):145–151.

67 Mitettinen A. Mycoplasma hominis in patients with pelvic inflammatory disease. Isr J Med Sci 1987; 23:713–716.

68 Scott WW Jr, Rosenshein NB, Siegelman SS, Sanders RC. The obstructed uterus. Radiology 1981; 141:767–770.

69 Zidi YS, Bouraoui S, Atallah K, et al. Primary in situ squamous cell carcinoma of the endometrium, with extensive squamous metaplasia and dysplasia. Gynecol Oncol 2003; 88:444–446.

70 Babarinsa IA, Campbell OB, Adewole IF. Pyometra complicating cancer of the cervix. Int J Gynaecol Obstet 1999; 64:75–76.

71 Smart PJ, Hetherington JF. Postoperative uterine granulomata following endometrial resection. Pathology 1995; 27:209–211.

72 Frank TS, Himebaugh KS, Wilson MD. Granulomatous endometritis associated with histologically occult cytomegalovirus in a healthy patient. Am J Surg Pathol 1992; 16:716–720.

73 Bylund DJ, Nanfro JJ, Marsh WL Jr. Coccidioidomycosis of the female genital tract. Arch Pathol Lab Med 1986; 110:232–235.

74 Namavar Jahromi B, Parsanezhad ME, Ghane-Shirazi R. Female genital tuberculosis and infertility. Int J Gynaecol Obstet 2001; 75:269–272.

75 El Maraghy MA, Elyan A, El-Leithy AG, et al. Bilharziasis of the female genital tract; new concepts. J Egypt Soc Parasitol 1982; 12:179–186.

76 Schneider V, Behm FG, Mumaw VR. Ascending herpetic endometritis. Obstet Gynecol 1982; 59:259–262.

77 International Planned Parenthood Federation, IPPF. International Medical Advisory Panel IMAP. The Dalkon Shield IUD. IPPF Med Bull 1980; 14:3.

78 Thonneau P, Goulard H, Goyaux N. Risk factors for intrauterine device failure: a review. Contraception 2001; 64:33–37.

79 Stanford JB, Mikolajczyk RT. Mechanisms of action of intrauterine devices: update and estimation of postfertilization effects. Am J Obstet Gynecol 2002; 187:1699–1708.

80 Rivera R, Best K. Current opinion. Consensus statement on intrauterine contraception. Contraception 2002; 65:385–388.

81 World Health Organization. Improving access to quality care in family planning: medical eligibility criteria for contraceptive use, 2nd edn. Geneva: World Health Organization; 2000:1.

82 Lippes J. Pelvic actinomycosis: a review and preliminary look at the evidence. Am J Obstet Gynecol 1999; 180:265–269.

83 Arend SM, Oosterhof H, van Dissel JT. Actinomyces and the intrauterine device. Arch Int Med 1998; 158:1270.

84 Bonacho I, Pita S, Gomez-Besteiro MI. The importance of removal of the intrauterine device in genital colonization by actinomyces. Gynecol Obstet Invest 2001; 52:119–123.

85 O'Brien PK, Roth-Mayo LA, Davis BA. Pseudo-sulfur granules associated with intra-uterine contraceptive devices. Am J Clin Pathol 1981; 75:822–825.

86 Budden GC, Walford NQ, Hawkins DF. Intra-uterine granulation tissue with an intra-uterine contraceptive device in situ for 16 years. J Obstet Gynecol 1985; 5:190–191.

87 Petitti DB. Clinical practice: combination estrogen-progestin oral contraceptives. N Engl J Med 2003; 349:1443–1450.

88 Dunn S, Guilbert E, Lefebvre G, et al. Clinical practice gynaecology and social sexual issues committees, Society of Obstetricians and Gynaecologists of Canada (SOGC). Emergency contraception. J Obstet Gynaecol Can 2003; 25:673–687.

89 Apgar BS, Greenberg G. Using progestins in clinical practice. Am Fam Physician 2000; 62:1839–1846, 1849–1850.

90 Olive DL, Pritts EA. Treatment of endometriosis. N Engl J Med 2001; 345(4):266–275.

91 Manson JE, Martin KA. Clinical practice. Postmenopausal hormone-replacement therapy. N Engl J Med 2001; 345:34–40.

92 Jones KL, Buzdar AU. A review of adjuvant hormonal therapy in breast cancer. Endocr Relat Cancer 2004; 11:391–406.

93 Deligdisch L. Hormonal pathology of the endometrium. Mod Pathol 2000; 13:285–294.

94 Figueroa-Casas PR, Ettinger B, Delgado E, et al. Reversal by medical treatment of endometrial hyperplasia caused by estrogen replacement therapy. Menopause 2001; 8:420–423.

95 Silverberg SG, Makowski EL. Endometrial carcinoma in young women taking oral contraceptive agents. Obstet Gynecol 1975; 46:503–506.

96 Wentz AC. Cigarette smoking and infertility. Fertil Contracept 1986; 46:365–367.

97 Yuzpe AA. Postcoital contraception. Int J Gynaecol Obstet 1978–1979; 16:497–501.

98 Endrikat J, Gerlinger C, Plettig K, et al. A meta-analysis on the correlation between ovarian activity and the incidence of intermenstrual bleeding during low-dose oral contraceptive use. Gynecol Endocrinol 2003; 17:107–114.

99 Albers JR, Hull SK, Wesley RM. Abnormal uterine bleeding. Am Fam Physician 2004; 69:1915–1926.

100 Guven M, Dikmen Y, Terek MC, et al. Metabolic effects associated with high-dose continuous megestrol acetate administration in the treatment of endometrial pathology. Arch Gynecol Obstet 2001; 265(4):183–186.

101 Schacter L, Rozencweig M, Canetta R, et al. Megestrol acetate: clinical experience. Cancer Treat Rev 1989; 16(1):49–63.

102 Gal D. Hormonal therapy for lesions of the endometrium. Semin Oncol 1986; 13(Suppl 4):33–36.

103 Rabinerson D, Kaplan B, Fisch B, et al. Membranous dysmenorrhea: the forgotten entity. Obstet Gynecol 1995; 85(5 Part 2):891–892.

104 Kocjan T, Prelevic GM. Hormone replacement therapy update: who should we be prescribing this to now? Curr Opin Obstet Gynecol 2003; 15(6):459–464.

105 Smith RE. A review of selective estrogen receptor modulators and national surgical adjuvant breast and bowel project clinical trials. Semin Oncol 2003; 30(5 Suppl 16):4–13.

106 Brown K. Breast cancer chemoprevention: risk-benefit effects of the antioestrogen tamoxifen. Expert Opin Drug Saf 2002; 1(3):253–267.

107 Biron-Shental T, Tepper R, Fishman A, et al. Recurrent endometrial polyps in postmenopausal breast cancer patients on tamoxifen. Gynecol Oncol 2003; 90(2):382–386.

108 Clement PB, Oliva E, Young RH. Mullerian adenosarcoma of the uterine corpus associated with tamoxifen therapy: a report of six cases and a review of tamoxifen-associated endometrial lesions. Int J Gynecol Pathol 1996; 15(3):222–229.

109 Bouchardy C, Verkooijen HM, Fioretta G, et al. Increased risk of malignant mullerian tumor of the uterus among women with breast cancer treated by tamoxifen. J Clin Oncol 2002; 20(21):4403.

110 Deligdisch L, Kalir T, Cohen CJ, et al. Endometrial histopathology in 700 patients treated with tamoxifen for breast cancer. Gynecol Oncol 2000; 78(2):181–186.

111 Elvin JA, Peerwani Z, Crum CP, Mutter GL. The 'mixed-pattern secretory' endometrium: is it clonal rather than hormonal? Mod Pathol 2005; 18:182A.

112 Elvin JA, Crum CP. Exfoliation artifact in endometrial samples. A unique mimic of uterine papillary serous carcinoma (UPSC) associated with hysteroscopy. Mod Pathol 2005; 18:182A.

113 Huettner PC, Gersell DJ. Arias-Stella reaction in nonpregnant women: a clinicopathologic study of nine cases. Int J Gynecol Pathol 1994; 13(3):241–247.

114 Marjoribanks J, Lethaby A, Farquhar C. Surgery versus medical therapy for heavy menstrual bleeding. Cochrane Database Syst Rev 2003; 2:CD003855.

115 Cravello L, D'Ercole C, Roge P, Boubli L, Blanc B. Hysteroscopic management of menstrual disorders: a review of 395 patients. Eur J Obstet Gynecol Reprod Biol 1996; 67(2):163–167.

116 Baggish MS, Sze EH. Endometrial ablation: a series of 568 patients treated over an 11-year period. Am J Obstet Gynecol 1996; 174(3):908–913.

17 Endometrial intraepithelial neoplasia

George L. Mutter,

Linda R. Duska and

Christopher P. Crum

Introduction

Definition of EIN
Historical background
Discordance of WHO
   hyperplasias with EIN

The patient at risk

Endocrine factors
Genetic risk factors
Epidemiologic risk factors
Medication risk factors

Screening and detection

Hysteroscopy and sonography
Endometrial sampling

Pathology of EIN

Rationale
Biomarkers
A combined molecular and
   histopathologic model for EIN
Diagnostic criteria of EIN

Differential diagnosis

Common benign patterns that
   may be misclassified as EIN
Interpretative problems in EIN
   diagnosis
Exclusion of carcinoma

Management of EIN

Introduction

DEFINITION OF EIN

Endometrial intraepithelial neoplasia (EIN) is a clonal proliferation of architecturally and cytologically altered premalignant endometrial glands which are prone to malignant transformation to endometrioid (Type I) endometrial adenocarcinoma. EIN lesions are non-invasive genetically altered neoplasms that arise focally and may convert to malignant phenotype upon acquisition of additional genetic damage. Diagnostic criteria for EIN have been developed by histopathologic correlation with clinical outcomes, molecular changes and objective computerized histomorphometry. EIN is conceptually similar to complex atypical hyperplasia (CAH) of the endometrium and the majority of EINs overlap with CAH. However, as defined, EIN is not exclusive to CAH and not all CAH are EIN lesions. This is due to both differences in classification criteria and inconsistent application of hyperplasia diagnostic by pathologists, as will be discussed below.

EIN should not be confused with unrelated serous intraepithelial carcinoma (serous EIC), which is an early phase of (Type II) papillary serous adenocarcinomas of the endometrium.

HISTORICAL BACKGROUND

In 1949 Arthur T. Hertig, a pathologist at Harvard Medical School and the Boston Hospital for Women, described 'adenomatous hyperplasia' and 'anaplasia' of the endometrium as precancerous lesions that may antedate appearance of endometrial adenocarcinoma by 1–5 years.[1–3] At that time estrogens were recognized as participants in promotion of endometrial carcinoma, but there were inadequate tools to resolve field effects due to systemic hormonal exposures from neoplastic proliferation caused by somatic mutation. This remained a major source of confusion and contention for the next 50 years, during which the pace of nomenclature proposals by far outstripped actual advances in the understanding of this disease.[4]

A 1985 landmark paper showed that subjective cytologic 'atypia' within a lesion increased cancer risk 14-fold, the single variable conferring the largest incremental endometrial cancer risk discovered up to that time.[5] In 1994, the World Health Organization sanctioned a classification system whereby four classes of hyperplasia were divided by architecture (complex/simple) and cytology (non-atypical/atypical).[6] Atypical endometrial

hyperplasias, whether of simple or complex architecture, were widely construed as premalignant lesions requiring therapeutic ablation. The dominance of cytology in risk assessment has since been tempered by the realization that pathologists are unable to reproducibly classify individual lesions as atypical vs non-atypical,[7–10] and recognition that architectural features have a predictive value at least as important as cytology.[11,12]

A parallel effort to use computers to classify low vs high cancer risk endometrial lesions played out against this backdrop of pathologist-derived classification systems. Availability of software and hardware for computerized tissue morphometry in the late 1970s enabled a greater degree of objectivity in histopathologic description of premalignant endometrial lesions than previously possible.[13–16] When statistically modeled against clinical outcomes of interest, individual cytologic[17,18] and architectural[19] predictive variables measured in an H&E (hematoxylin and eosin) stained slide could be discovered and validated. This reached its pinnacle in the D-Score, a morphometric scoring system with superb cancer predictive performance exceeding anything seen previously. Implementation into practice, however, required placing the morphometry results into a context that is both understandable and accessible to pathologists. Primarily in Europe, this has taken the form of reference laboratories where morphometry can be centrally performed in appropriately equipped facilities.[20] Most recently, the architectural variable of volume percentage stroma, a measure of gland crowding central to the D-Score, has been incorporated as a key EIN criterion as described here.

Microdissection of targeted small lesions in paraffin-embedded tissues enabled precise correlation between molecular genetic and histopathologic features of endometrial precancers. Molecular studies showing a clonal growth pattern[21–23] for endometrial precancers established their focality of origin and subsequent centripetal expansion as geometric properties of evolving lesions. By the time that such clones can be seen under the microscope, there are evident changes in both cytology and architecture that offset them from the background.[24] Lesion size and contrast of localizing lesion cytology and architecture to that of the background endometrium are characteristics that must be assessed during routine diagnosis and have been incorporated into EIN diagnostic criteria.[25]

A formal proposal[26] for the EIN diagnostic schema emerged from realization that those histologic changes seen in genetically altered monoclonal endometrial precancers were identical to those previously defined by computerized morphometry of H&E stained sections as increasing the likelihood of carcinoma.[12] A high degree of clinical relevance was immediately justified by a series of pre-existing clinical outcome studies, all of which[11,19,27–29] validated the cancer predictive value of the original D-Score based diagnostic algorithm. Just as diverse and independent methods of discovery were integrated to define the group of lesions we now know as EIN, this is an entity that may be diagnosed in several ways. For those with access to the commercially available QProdit software and morphometry workstation (Leica, Cambridge, UK), EIN lesions are those with a D-Score less than a threshold of 1. EIN identified by morphometry as a lesion with D-Score<1 identifies lesions with a 27% chance of concurrent,[28] or 46-fold increased risk for future endometrial carcinoma (Fig. 17.1).[28,30] Practical implementation of subjective criteria for EIN diagnosis by pathologists working at a standard microscope with routine H&E slides[25,31] is the subject of the remainder of this chapter.

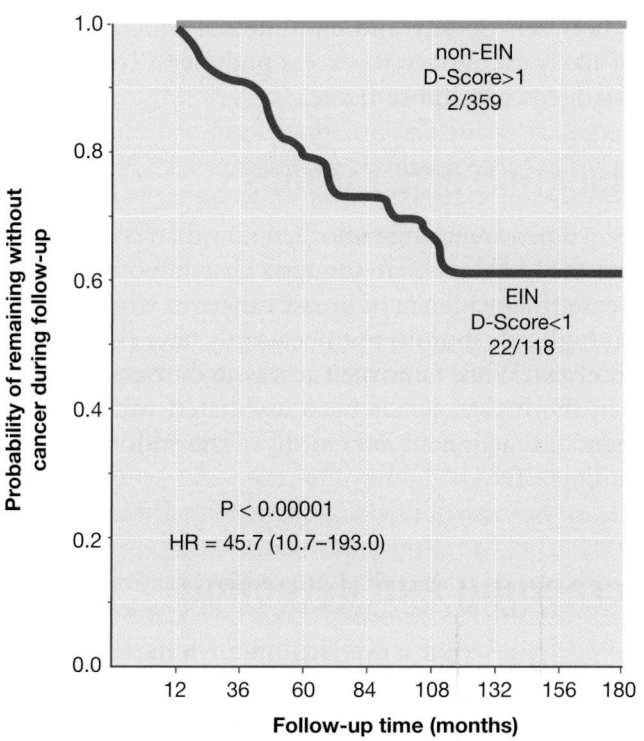

Fig. 17.1 Prospective cancer risk of an endometrial intraepithelial neoplasia (EIN) diagnosis. Long-term cancer-free survival of 477 endometrial 'hyperplasias' stratified by morphometry into high-risk EIN (D-Score <1) and low-risk benign (D-Score >1) subgroups. A total of 27% of women with EIN will have a concurrent adenocarcinoma diagnosed within 1 year of EIN diagnosis;[28] these were excluded as instances of 'concurrent' carcinoma. The resulting plot shows long-term cancer occurrences evolving from an EIN lesion, an event which is 46-fold more likely in EIN-bearing compared with non-EIN-bearing women. (Data from Baak et al., with permission.)[30]

DISCORDANCE OF WHO HYPERPLASIAS WITH EIN

EIN diagnostic criteria are sufficiently different from those used previously in the WHO hyperplasia schema that there is no fixed correlation. Cytology assessment as atypical or non-atypical on an absolute scale has been replaced by a relative (internal background comparison) standard for cytology interpretation in EIN in which classic 'atypia' need not be present, but rather a change from the background cytology takes place. Most, but not all, EIN lesions are culled from the previous atypical category. Introduction of size criteria and the concept of localizing clonal origin in EIN enables diagnosis of high-risk lesions that previously were overlooked. In practice, assignment of hyperplasia diagnoses has always varied between individual pathologists. 'Complex non-atypical hyperplasia', for example, can either be a very common or rarely invoked diagnosis. This has a substantial impact on how your prior practice patterns will relate to more standardized EIN groups. Figure 17.2[32] is based upon combined experience of multiple European and American groups.

The patient at risk

ENDOCRINE FACTORS

Endocrine risk factors for endometrial precancers are essentially identical to those for endometrioid endometrial adenocarcinoma, with estrogens acting as promoters and progestins as protectors.[33] In the Postmenopausal Estrogen/Progestin Interventions (PEPI) trial, 12% of women receiving unopposed estrogens developed atypical hyperplasia over the 3-year surveillance period compared with 0% of placebo controls.[34] Estrogen risks are obviated by addition of progestins such as medroxyprogesterone acetate, which protects against development of endometrial hyperplasia,[34,35] and when administered in a combined low-dose oral contraceptive formulation may reduce endometrial cancer risk below that of the population background.[36,37]

GENETIC RISK FACTORS

Sporadic EIN lesions are precursors to that subset of endometrial carcinomas characterized by endometrioid differentiation, PTEN gene inactivation and microsatellite instability. Although there are few studies reporting precancer histology seen in women with hereditary

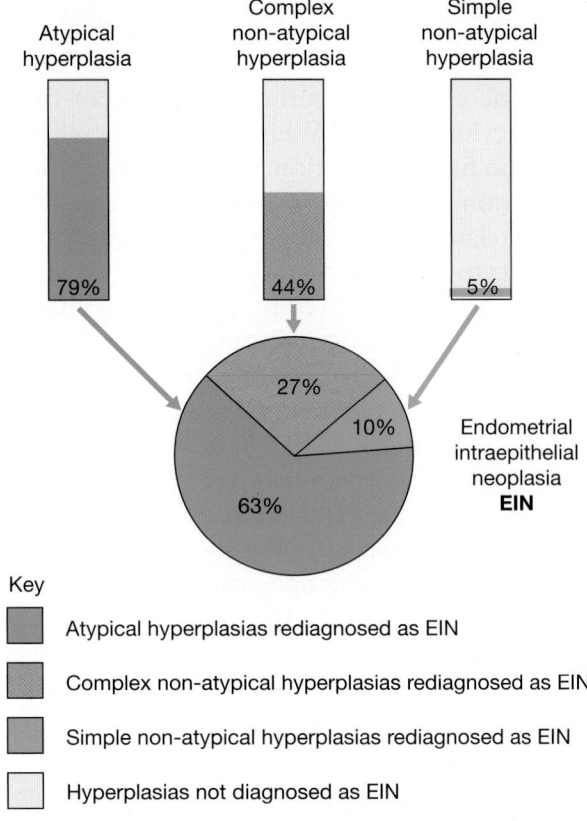

Atypical hyperplasia
Complex non-atypical hyperplasia
Simple non-atypical hyperplasia

79%   44%   5%

27%

10%

63%

Endometrial intraepithelial neoplasia
EIN

Key

■ Atypical hyperplasias rediagnosed as EIN

▦ Complex non-atypical hyperplasias rediagnosed as EIN

▨ Simple non-atypical hyperplasias rediagnosed as EIN

□ Hyperplasias not diagnosed as EIN

Fig. 17.2 WHO hyperplasias rediagnosed by EIN criteria. EIN lesions are diagnosed using different criteria than WHO hyperplasias, so the correlation is not fixed. Colored portions of bar graphs show approximate percentages of each WHO hyperplasia class that will be diagnosed as EIN. Remaining WHO hyperplasias not diagnostic of EIN (gray) will be allocated to unopposed estrogen (anovulatory), polyp and other benign categories. The pie chart shows relative contributions of each hyperplasia type to the EIN diagnostic category in a biopsy series of sequential endometrial hyperplasias seen in a busy hospital practice.[32]

endometrial cancer risk, it is reasonable to assume that familial endometrial cancers with these characteristics may transit a comparable premalignant phase of EIN. Hereditary non-polyposis colon cancer (HNPCC), caused by abnormalities of factors involved in DNA mismatch repair, is an autosomal dominant condition conferring a 60% lifetime risk for endometrial cancer, generally of the endometrioid type, with >75% showing microsatellite instability,[38–40] and 68% having loss of PTEN tumor suppressor function.[41] These tumors occur on average about 30 years earlier than their sporadic counterparts, leading to a current management recommendation to begin annual or semiannual endometrial biopsies by age 30–35.[42] A second heritable cancer syndrome characterized by an elevated risk for that type of endometrial cancer with a premalignant EIN phase is Cowden's syndrome, caused by germline transmission of a mutant PTEN allele.[43]

Early detection and treatment of premalignant endometrial disease is a mainstay of endometrial cancer therapy. Lifetime risk for endometrial cancer is 2.4% in the USA,[44] primarily a sporadic disease driven by complex interactions between somatically acquired genetic lesions and ambient hormonal selection factors. The majority of endometrial cancers are discovered when the patient develops symptomatic bleeding, followed by a diagnostic endometrial biopsy. Under these circumstances, 21% of endometrial adenocarcinomas at the time of initial diagnosis have already extended beyond the subjacent myometrium, having extended to the cervix (Stage 2, 5.8%), regional nodes or extrauterine tissues (Stage 3, 7.7%) or distant sites (Stage 4, 8.3%).[45] If detected earlier, many of these patients could achieve surgical cure by hysterectomy alone.

EPIDEMIOLOGIC RISK FACTORS

EIN has risk factors similar to those of endometrioid endometrial cancer. Specifically, women who are obese are at increased risk to develop EIN.[46] This relationship between obesity and endometrial proliferation is most likely secondary to excess peripheral conversion of estrogens in adipose tissue.

MEDICATION RISK FACTORS

More women are taking tamoxifen now than ever before, in the face of data that suggests that tamoxifen may decrease the incidence of breast cancer in women who are at high risk (but do not necessarily have the disease themselves). While tamoxifen acts as an estrogen antagonist in the breast, it has been associated with various benign and malignant alterations of the endometrium, including EIN.[47,48]

Screening and detection

HYSTEROSCOPY AND SONOGRAPHY

Endometrial visualization by hysteroscopy or vaginal ultrasonography can be a useful adjunct to biopsy, but practice in this regard is not standardized. Hysteroscopically guided endometrial biopsies are increasingly performed in clinical settings where practitioners are comfortable with this technology.[49–52] A smooth regular lining by hysteroscopy can reassure the clinician that an occult carcinoma was not missed and direct visual guidance can improve access to remote regions of an irregularly shaped cavity. Transvaginal ultrasound is an insensitive and nonspecific screen for endometrial cancer and there is little data on ability to detect physically small EIN lesions. Cancer detection sensitivity for transvaginal ultrasound with a threshold endometrial thickness of 6 mm is only 17%; and 33% for a threshold value of 5 mm. Specificity is very low, making this an expensive (during follow-up of numerous false positives) as well as insensitive test.[53] Ultrasound will, however, identify conformational abnormalities of the uterine cavity that may complicate access for sampling.

ENDOMETRIAL SAMPLING

Endometrial biopsy and curettage remain the primary diagnostic modality to evaluate potential endometrial disease. These are invasive procedures that can cause cramping and bleeding and carry minimal risks of uterine perforation or contamination of the cavity by pathogens. For these reasons, endometrial sampling cannot be considered a screening test, but rather a procedure undertaken in response to specific symptoms or cancer risk factors. The most common setting in which an EIN-yielding endometrial biopsy is performed is work-up of menstrual irregularity in a perimenopausal woman, or symptomatic bleeding in a postmenopausal patient. Introduction of the Pipelle biopsy apparatus, which unlike curettage does not necessitate cervical dilatation and anesthesia, greatly reduced the cost and morbidity of endometrial sampling. Outpatient office-based Pipelle biopsies are now the most commonly performed endometrial sampling procedure.

Sampling devices

Transcervical endometrial sampling is the mainstay of endometrial diagnosis. Sampling adequacy is of particular concern with localizing EIN lesions that are not uniformly represented in all fragments. Coverage is affected by the device used, guidance by hysteroscopy or ultrasound, operator performance and uterine anatomy. Short of hysterectomy, no sampling strategy is foolproof. If there is any clinical or pathologic concern that the available sample is inadequate or non-representative, the diagnostic process is incomplete and resampling should be undertaken.[54] It is incumbent upon the pathologist to have a clear understanding of sources of sampling and interpretative errors, of how these influence options for follow-up diagnostic procedures and to communicate clearly to the clinician.

Curettage by a rigid sharp device is the most established method, but has the drawback of requiring cervical dilatation and attendant anesthesia. For those lesions whose distribution or site of origin is particularly relevant to management, separate acquisition of endometrial and endocervical curettage fractions ('fractional curettage') may facilitate physical resolution of the sites of involvement. Curettage is not without its limitations, however, sampling less than half of the uterine cavity in about 60% of cases.[55]

The Pipelle biopsy instrument, a 3.2 mm diameter flexible cannula that aspirates an approximately 1.5–2 mm 'core' of tissue (Fig. 17.3) as it is sweeps across the endometrial surface, is sufficiently small that cervical dilation is unnecessary. Because no anesthesia is needed, it may be used readily in a private office setting and is more comfortable to patients than a sharp curettage[56] or Vabra aspiration biopsy.[57] These clinical benefits have led to widespread use of the Pipelle instrument in many outpatient contexts.

There are now many studies comparing the endometrial sampling adequacy of Pipelle biopsy to curettage. In aggregate, tissue adequacy[58] and diagnostic accuracy weigh in favor of the Pipelle with a few notable caveats. Physical mass lesions which impinge upon the uterine cavity, such as polyps or uterine leiomyomata, may deflect the flexible Pipelle device and lead to blind spots.[59] Insight regarding these underlying conditions may be gained by ultrasonographic studies or physical exam and sampling errors reduced by use of a rigid sampling device or hysteroscopic guidance.[52] Overall sensitivity/specificity of endometrial precancer (atypical hyperplasia) diagnosis is 82–100% for Pipelle, 67–99.8% for Vabra aspiration. Detection of endometrial carcinoma, generally bulky lesions, is even more sensitive, at 99.6% for Pipelle and 97.1% for Vabra aspiration.[60]

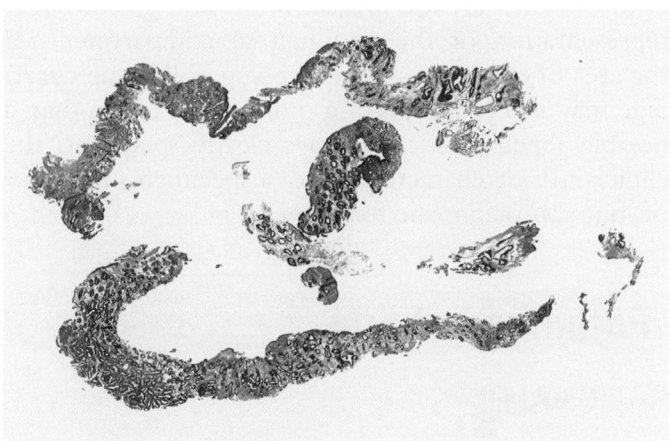

Fig. 17.3 Macroscopic view of endometrial fragment configuration of a specimen obtained by Pipelle device.

Hysteroscopic biopsies are the scantiest tissue biopsy format, relying upon accurate target selection rather than coverage extent to minimize sampling error. In the case of physically small grossly inapparent EIN lesions, a larger random sample may be advantageous. Small, often crushed, tissue fragments yielded by tiny jaws of the hysteroscopic biopsy device present a diagnostic challenge to the pathologist. Not only is interpretation usually compromised by artifact but also the background context necessary to recognize a localizing EIN lesion may be missing or poorly represented.

Specimen adequacy

Tissue fragment size, quality of technical processing and presence or absence of potentially confounding factors will determine the degree of confidence that an EIN lesion can be recognized or excluded within an individual sample. It is common to receive a rather scanty specimen from the postmenopausal woman whose endometrium is atrophic or inactive. Most of these will simply be scanty specimens in which there are no findings suggestive of an EIN or adenocarcinoma. A simple diagnosis describing what is actually present, annotated by a comment regarding abundance, is usually sufficient in these cases. A special case is when the stated endometrial curettage contains no endometrial tissue at all, but perhaps only material from an endocervical or vaginal source. A specific comment that no endometrial tissue was identified will alert the clinician to a significant sampling problem.

Specific recommendations for dealing with small, sub-diagnostic or hormonally treated lesions are provided in Table 17.3. Some inadequate specimens should be followed by resampling. Interpretative problems in a crushed tiny hysteroscopic biopsy might be subsequently resolved by Pipelle or curettage sampling, both of which are less artifact prone and give broader representation of the endometrial compartment. If the area of concern is within a polyp, follow-up curettage may succeed in getting more of the lesion than a flexible Pipelle device. Always clearly specify to the clinician those characteristics of a specimen suggestive of, but sub-diagnostic for, EIN.

Pathology of EIN

RATIONALE

Much as the German pathologist Koch developed a series of postulates that must be fulfilled in order to scientifically prove pathogenesis of disease by a specific infectious organism, similar postulates may be formulated for premalignant disease. We here list predictions to be met for a clinically relevant and biologically distinctive category of endometrial precancers, all of which have been fulfilled in the case of EIN.

Criterion 1: EIN differs from normal tissues

EIN are bona fide neoplasms, comprising a monoclonal outgrowth of a single transformed cell[22,23] from a polyclonal source field. These benign expansile clones have only a marginal advantage beyond normal endometrial tissues and in the absence of additional genetic damage lack the ability to invade or metastasize. Lesions with microsatellite instability have marker genotypes different than normal source tissues.[61]

Criterion 2: EIN shares some, but not all features with carcinoma

Cells in the early stages of endometrial carcinogenesis should have some features which distinguish them from normal tissues and whose retention during progression establishes them as the physical progenitors of carcinoma. Both EIN and endometrial carcinoma are monoclonal lesions and those markers characteristic of monoclonality (nonrandom inactivation of a particular X chromosome copy, presence of a particular altered microsatellite) are conserved between the EIN and carcinoma lesions of individual patients.[12,21–23,61,62] Genetic alteration of specific genes implicated in endometrial carcinogenesis has been shown to be conserved between EIN and carcinomas which occur in individual patients. This is true for inactivation of the PTEN tumor suppressor gene,[63–65] mutation of the K-ras oncogene[66–68] and epigenetic inactivation of the DNA repair gene MLH1:[69] 63% of EIN lesions, for example, have lost the ability to express the tumor suppressor protein from the PTEN gene, a phenotype shared with over 80% of endometrial cancers.[24,65]

Criterion 3: EIN can be diagnosed

Diagnostic criteria applicable to a routine pathology practice are presented below.[25,26,31] Additionally, there is an objective reference standard for EIN diagnosis in computerized morphometry of H&E-stained slides.[12] Cytologic and architectural characteristics of H&E-stained tissues are measured to calculate a D-Score which indicates EIN when less than a threshold of 1.0.[11,12]

Criterion 4: EIN increases risk for carcinoma

Available clinical outcome studies have applied image analysis of pathologic endometria to identify subsets of women with EIN and correlated this diagnosis with future or concurrent carcinoma.[11,27–29] Some 26% of women diagnosed with EIN already have cancer at the time of diagnosis and the remainder have a 46-fold elevated cancer risk in the ensuing years (Fig. 17.1).[28,30]

Criterion 5: Genetic and hormonal mechanisms of carcinogenesis converge in EIN

Endometrial expression of the tumor suppressor gene PTEN normally increases in an estrogenic environment.[70] This functional requirement for increased tumor suppression activity of PTEN under estrogen-rich conditions cannot be met in PTEN-defective EIN lesions. Thus, most EIN lesions (those 63% with lost PTEN protein) will have a defective tumor suppressor response to estrogens. Correspondingly, if the mitogenic effects of estrogens are mitigated by progestins, PTEN mutant endometrial glands undergo selective involution relative to PTEN-intact glands.[71]

Criterion 6: Introducing EIN genotype into an animal produces premalignant lesions and heightened cancer risk

Some 63% of EIN lesions comprise cells which are defective in production of the PTEN tumor suppressor gene product.[24] Heterozygote PTEN mutant mice uniformly (100%) develop endometrial 'hyperplasia,' and 21% of these progress to carcinoma.[72]

BIOMARKERS

Anti-PTEN antibodies are the first commercially available 'special stain' for neoplastic endometrioid (Type I) endometrial disease. Paraffin tissue immunohistochemistry with anti-PTEN antibody 6H2.1 (Cascade Biosciences, Winchester, MA)[65,73] shows that over half of endometrioid endometrial adenocarcinomas and their precursor EIN lesions have lost PTEN protein due to genomic mutational or deletional inactivation.[24,65] Many commercial anti-PTEN antibodies do not work on paraffin-embedded tissues. A working protocol for successful use of antibody 6H2.1 is available online at www.endometrium.org. The most common problems are inadequate antigen retrieval, failure to incubate primary antibody overnight at 4°C, too low an antibody titration (use 1:100 for older blocks), use of old sections (must be cut and used within days), lack of adequate controls to recognize when it is working and use of dark obscuring counterstains.

Caution is advised in using PTEN immunohistochemistry to make diagnoses of individual patients. It is an insensitive (half of EIN lesions have normal PTEN expression) and nonspecific (over a third of normal proliferative and anovulatory endometria contain PTEN-null glands) marker for EIN. PTEN expression is greatly affected by the endocrine and clinical context in which it is applied. Normal endometrial PTEN expression is greatly reduced or lost in secretory and atrophic glands.[70] Absence of expression in these circumstances cannot be equated with loss of function. Correspondingly, an estrogenic environment increases endometrial stromal and normal gland PTEN expression, improving contrast with a localizing PTEN-mutant clone.

PTEN immunohistochemistry can, however, be a useful educational tool for pathologists to delineate the extent and configuration of mutant clones and relate these features to routinely stained slides. Figure 17.4 shows an H&E-stained EIN lesion with matching PTEN immunohistochemistry images to delimit clonal precancerous lesions with single cell resolution. This educational objective can be segregated from the diagnostic process by setting aside interesting cases and undertaking a batch staining after they have already been signed out. This provides the benefit of comparison of multiple examples without compromising patient care. PTEN immunohistochemistry is not a routine or requisite part of EIN diagnosis.

There are actually quite a few genes whose inactivation in endometrial carcinogenesis occurs during the premalignant phase and may be detected in EIN lesions, but none have diagnostic value at present and most are inaccessible without specialized facilities. Microsatellite instability caused by epigenetic inactivation of the MLH1 gene[74] accompanies 17–23% of sporadic endometrial carcinomas,[40,61,75–77] and may be seen in premalignant lesions.[22,69,76] Direct DNA analysis is needed for microsatellite instability detection, although MLH1 immunohistochemistry shows loss of protein in most of these cases.[78] K-ras mutation occurs in 16–20% of premalignant endometrial lesions,[67,68] but this prevalence is too low to be diagnostically pathognomonic and its detection requires direct sequencing rather than immunohistochemistry. p53, a tumor suppressor commonly inactivated in papillary serous endometrial carcinomas, is only rarely inactivated in endometrioid carcinomas and EIN lesions.[79,80]

A COMBINED MOLECULAR AND HISTOPATHOLOGIC MODEL FOR EIN

Latent, premalignant and malignant phases of EIN-mediated endometrial carcinogenesis are diagrammed

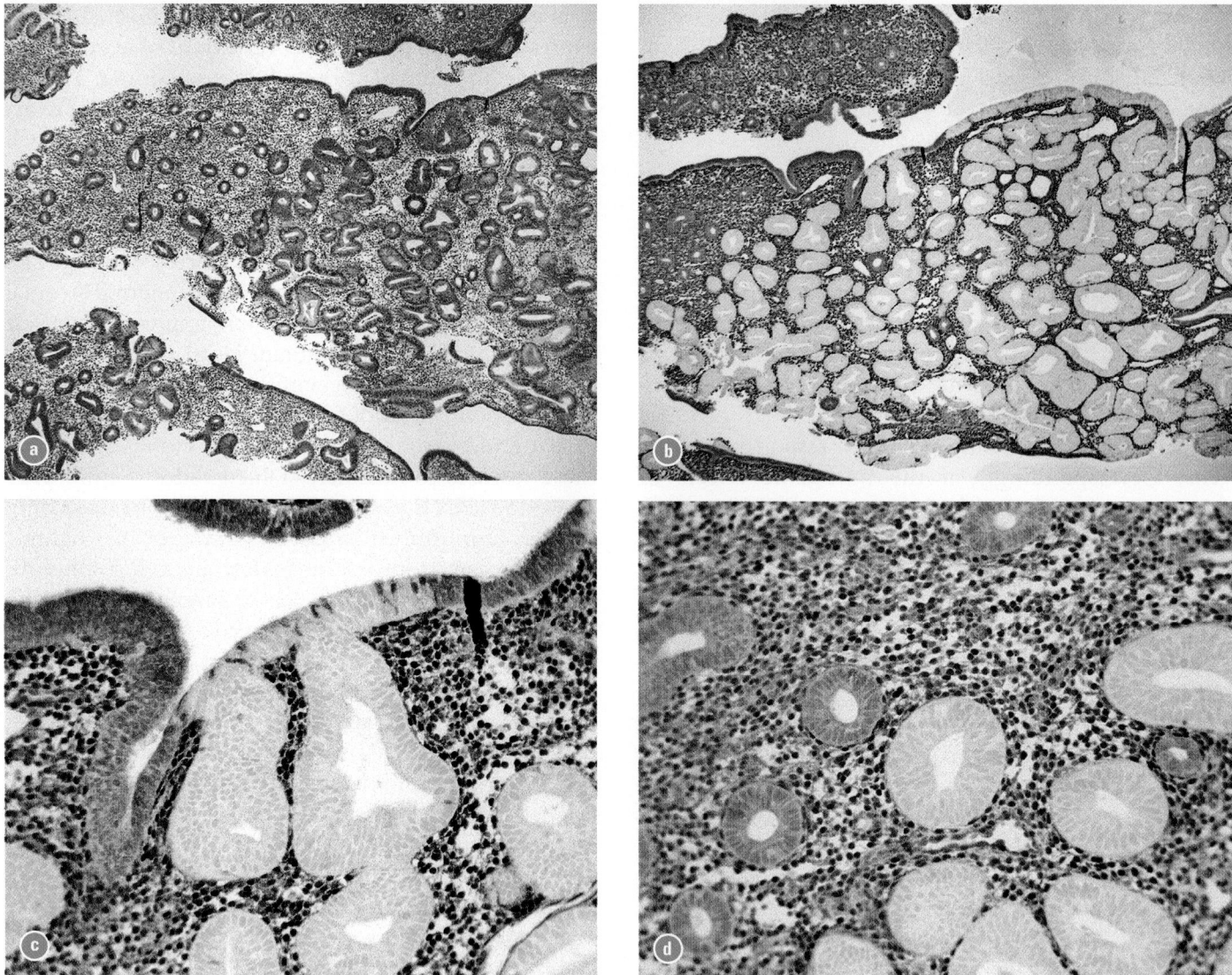

Fig. 17.4 Loss of PTEN function in EIN. A localizing EIN lesion occupying the right half of the large tissue fragment (a) has clonally inactivated the PTEN tumor suppressor gene (b–d). Immunohistochemistry with anti-PTEN antibody 6H2.1. Note the higher density and epithelial thickening in the EIN glands (pale, devoid of PTEN signal) compared with background glands.

in Figure 17.5. In almost half of apparently normal women, histologically unremarkable proliferative endometria contain a small fraction of (PTEN tumor suppressor gene) mutant endometrial glands. This phase may be construed as 'latent' because not only do the mutated glands look completely normal under the microscope but they also progress to EIN and cancer at very low efficiency. This latent phase may persist for years, with continued presence of scattered and interspersed mutant glands after many menstrual cycles.[24] Mutant glands are probably represented in the reserve population of cells that regenerate a new functionalis each month. Endocrine factors act upon these 'latent precancers' to modulate involution, or progression to EIN.

Transition to EIN requires accumulation of additional genetic damage in at least one 'latent precancer' cell, which then clonally expands from its point of origin (indicated by expanding arrows) to form a contiguous grouping of a tightly packed and cytologically altered glands recognizable as EIN. The monoclonal precancer (EIN) develops internal heterogeneity through mutation and advantageous events selected by local conditions result in hierarchical subclones (left to right) of varying success. EIN lesions have only marginal increases in growth potential and retain susceptibility to further growth modulation by hormonal factors. Some involute. Others, through additional mutation and selection, reach a stage where hormonal support is no

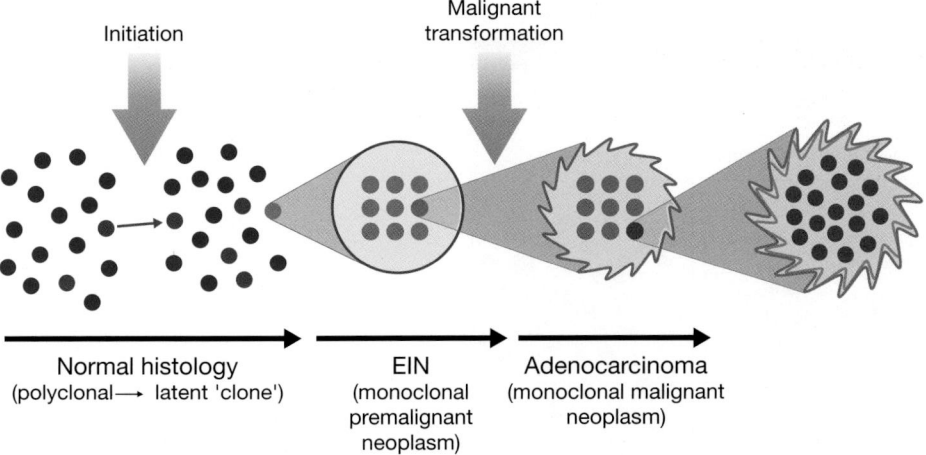

Initiation

Malignant
transformation

Normal histology
(polyclonal → latent 'clone')

EIN
(monoclonal
premalignant
neoplasm)

Adenocarcinoma
(monoclonal malignant
neoplasm)

Fig. 17.5 Clonal origin of EIN. The first genetic changes (such as PTEN inactivation) which initiate endometrial carcinogenesis are unaccompanied by any phenotypic alterations at the light microscopic level. This 'latent' phase of cytologically and architecturally normal but genetically altered cell may persist for years in a normally menstruating woman. Low cancer risk, combined with lack of a rational therapeutic response, are reasons that systematic screening and treatment of these 'latent' phase lesions is unwarranted at present. As additional genetic damage accumulates, higher-risk morphologically altered mutant clones declare themselves by demonstrating those architectural and cytologic alterations that distinguish EIN. Malignant transformation of EIN lesions, which occurs at least 46-times more frequently than non-EIN tissues (Fig. 17.1), warrants careful diagnosis and treatment. Endocrine modifiers of endometrial cancer risk act upon the latent and EIN phases of this sequence by tipping the balance of clonal expansion *vs* involution.

longer required for survival. Malignant transformation to cancer is defined by accumulation of sufficient genetic damage to permit invasion of adjacent stromal tissues.

DIAGNOSTIC CRITERIA OF EIN

A framework for EIN diagnosis is shown in Table 17.1. Notable is the clear separation of endometrial changes caused by unopposed estrogens and carcinoma, from EIN.

Topography of EIN

The distribution of a lesion is useful in distinguishing between the diffuse, field-wide effects, of an abnormal

hormonal environment (anovulation, or persistent estrogen effect), surface changes secondary to stromal breakdown and more focal EIN (Fig. 17.6). Clonal origin from a single cell requires EIN lesions to begin as local processes within the endometrial compartment. Early EIN lesions are easily diagnosed by their contrast in architecture and cytology with the background from which they have emerged. Over time, EIN lesions may completely overrun the background endometrium, thereby removing the convenient lesion-to-background contrast in morphology which assists in EIN diagnosis. For this reason, or because of fragmentation, many EIN lesions must be diagnosed without the benefit of comparison with companion benign tissues. Exclusion of artifact and careful evaluation of the architectural and cytologic features of EIN usually permit accurate diagnosis in these instances.

EIN diagnostic criteria

All of the diagnostic criteria of Table 17.2,[31] and listed below, must be met in order to make an EIN diagnosis. The entire slide should first be scrutinized under low magnification for localizing lesions and, if found, these areas examined under higher power to assess possible changes in cytology within the architecturally distinct focus. Widespread EIN lesions that have replaced the entire endometrial compartment tend to have a suffi-

Table 17.1 EIN diagnostic schema

EIN nomenclature	Topography	Functional category	Treatment
Benign architectural changes of unopposed estrogen	Diffuse	Estrogen effect	Hormonal therapy
EIN: endometrial intraepithelial neoplasia	Focal progressing to diffuse	Precancer	Hormonal or surgical
Carcinoma	Focal progressing to diffuse	Cancer	Surgical stage-based

Benign	Premalignant	Malignant

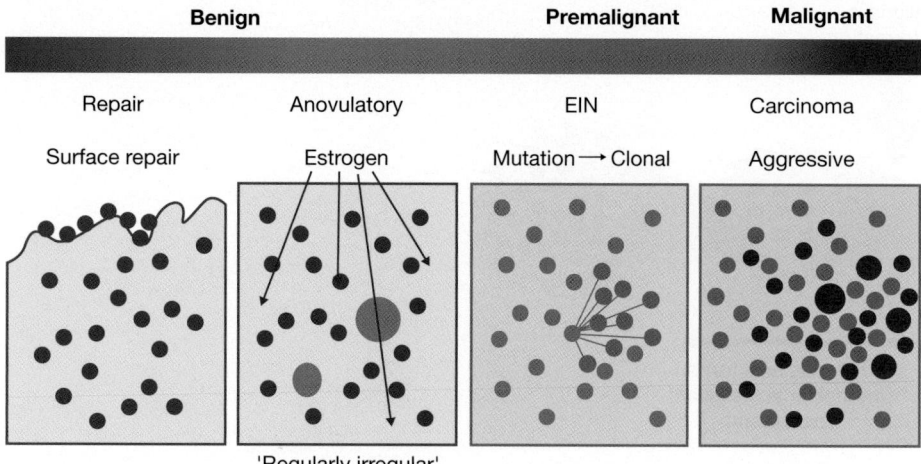

Repair   Anovulatory   EIN   Carcinoma

Surface repair   Estrogen   Mutation → Clonal   Aggressive

'Regularly irregular'

Fig. 17.6 Schematic topography of EIN. Benign, premalignant and malignant endometrial processes have differing large-scale architectures and distribution within the endometrial compartment. Reparative or degenerative changes lead to epithelial piling up and loss of polarity in regions of stromal breakdown or offending stimulus. Benign systemic effects (such as unopposed estrogens) tend to induce changes throughout the endometrial field, with responsive individual glands randomly scattered throughout. In contrast, EIN lesions begin at a single point in space, growing outwards as a compact mass of individual glands with altered cytology. Initially they have the appearance of a physical 'patch' or geographic domain composed of glands with altered cytology and architecture, eventually overtaking the entire endometrial compartment. Malignant transformation is accompanied by loss of the single-layered individual glands of EIN. The epithelium may become stratified, cribriform or solid, and arranges itself in folded sheets or complex villoglandular structures. Myoinvasion is rarely seen in biopsies, because of sampling limitations.

ciently atypical cytology that background normal endometrium is no longer required as a reference point for accurate diagnosis.

Size, architecture and cytology features are easy EIN diagnostic criteria. Much more difficult are exclusion of benign mimics and adenocarcinoma from the differential diagnosis. There are no simple rules for benign mimic exclusion. The broad universe of competing entities can only be recognized on sight by one who has the easy familiarity that comes with experience. Consistent demarcation of the EIN–adenocarcinoma threshold remains important clinically because it provides a basis for the clinician to evaluate the risks of electing hormonal rather than surgical therapy in younger patients who wish to retain fertility.

Special diagnostic challenges, such as recognition of EIN within polyps, interpretation of subdiagnostically small or fragmented lesions and interpretation of lesions with non-endometrioid differentiation have specific caveats presented below that should be carefully studied.

Architecture

Gland area exceeds stromal area: A cardinal architectural feature of endometrial precancers is glandular crowding, with a threshold quantitative cutoff for EIN lesions of less than half of the tissue area occupied by stroma (volume percentage stroma or VPS). Areas with large dominant cysts should always be avoided in making this assessment. Although EIN is an epithelial disease, visual assessment of the glands themselves is complicated by frequent artifactual displacement from associated stroma, pale staining of most epithelia and visual 'shimmering' between gland epithelia and lumens. These may all be avoided by focusing on the stromal compartment, which has the significant advantages of a more uniform composition throughout the specimen and superior staining qualities. By focusing on the

Table 17.2 *EIN diagnostic criteria*

EIN criterion	Comments
Architecture	Area of glands greater than stroma
Cytology	Cytology differs between architecturally crowded focus and background, or clearly abnormal
Size >1 mm	Maximum linear dimension exceeds 1 mm
Exclude mimics	Benign conditions with overlapping criteria: basalis, secretory, polyps, repair, etc.
Exclude cancer	Carcinoma if mazelike glands, solid areas, polygonal 'mosaic-like' glands, myoinvasion or significant cribriforming

Modified from Silverberg et al. 2003.[31]

stroma itself, only intact fragments in which stroma has not been avulsed from glands will be evaluated.

Careful review of graphic (Fig. 17.7)[11,12,28,29] and histologic examples of varying stromal densities will assist in training your eye to classify patient material as above or below the diagnostic threshold. EIN lesions tend to cluster with a median volume percentage stroma of about 40% and non-EIN (benign) lesions cluster at a median of approximately 75%. These differences are sufficiently great that visual assessment by a trained eye can be informative.

Cytology

Cytology of architecturally crowded area is different than background, or clearly abnormal: There is no absolute standard for cytologic features of EIN lesions, but the cytology of EIN is usually clearly demarcated as divergent from that of coexisting benign endometrial tissues in the same patient (Fig. 17.8). The manner of cytologic change in EIN varies considerably from patient to patient

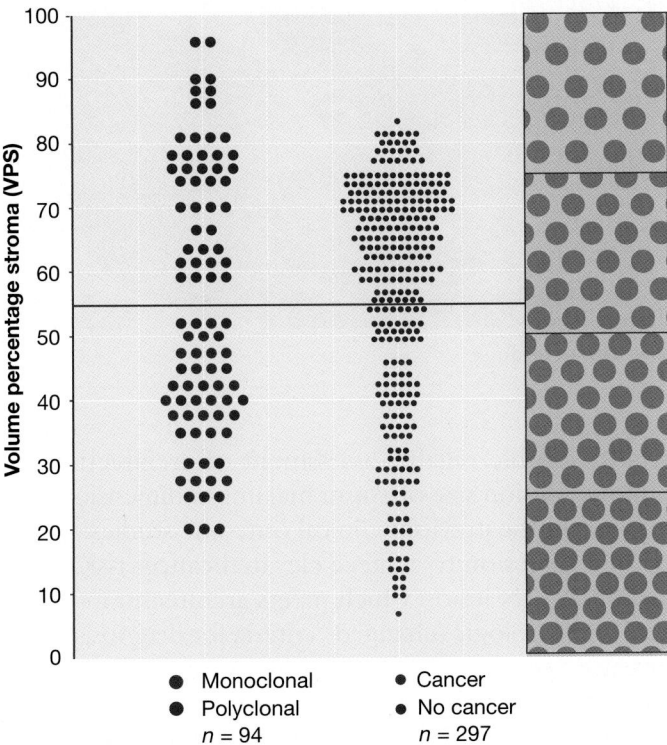

Fig. 17.7 Gland crowding (volume percentage stroma, VPS) correlates with clonal precancers and clinical cancer outcome. Correlation of architectural feature of volume percentage stroma with molecular benchmarks of premalignant disease (monoclonal growth, red symbols in left scattergram) and clinical cancer outcome (red symbols, right scattergram). Note the threshold of 55% for both, approximately where the area of glands is that of stroma (VPS 55%). Tiles on the right show the stromal compartment in dark gray for a range of gland packing densities. Data compiled from Mutter and Baak.[11,12,28,29]

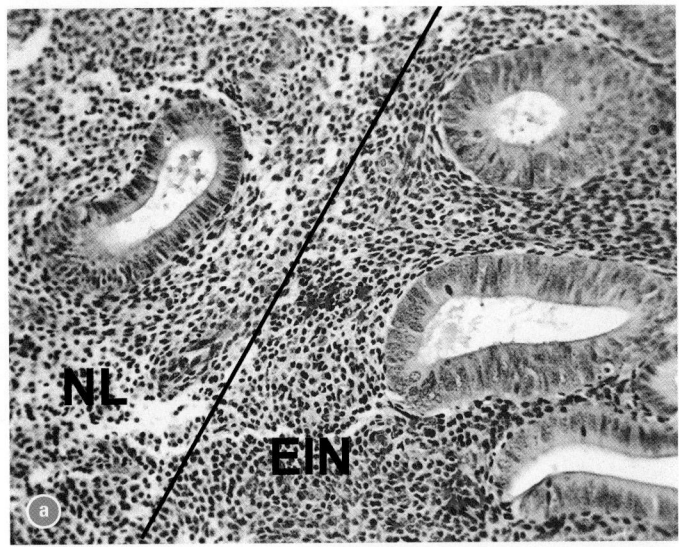
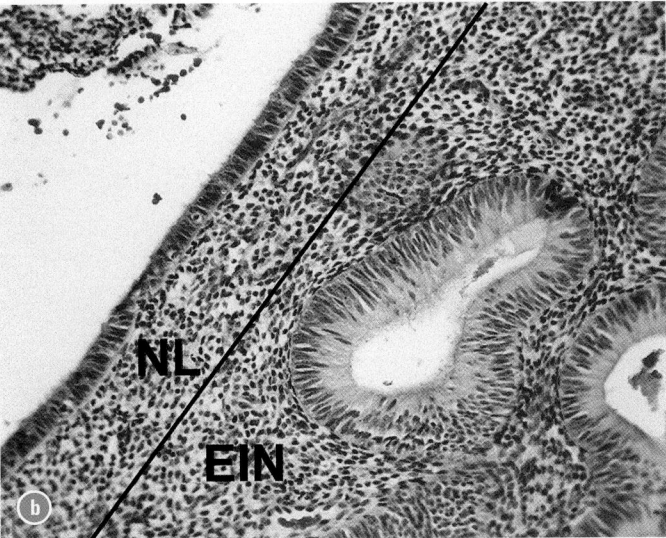

Fig. 17.8 Cytologic demarcation at the EIN perimeter. (a,b) Two different examples of the perimeter of EIN lesions. EIN glands are in the lower right, normal background glands are upper left.

and can include, but is not be limited to, increased variation in nuclear size and contour, clumped or granular chromatin texture, change in nucleoli, change in nuclear/cytoplasmic ratio and altered cytoplasmic differentiation (Fig. 17.9). Stereotypical static descriptions of cytologic atypia, such as nuclear rounding and appearance of nucleoli are met in many but not all EIN lesions. In this sense, a fixed presentation of cytologic atypia is not a prerequisite for EIN. Attempts to define an absolute standard are confounded by the extreme morphologic plasticity of endometrial glandular cells under changing hormonal, repair and differentiation conditions.

Cytologic changes in some EIN lesions are manifest as a change in differentiation state to a tubal (Fig. 17.10),[12] mucinous (Fig. 17.11),[12] micropapillary (Fig. 17.12)[12]

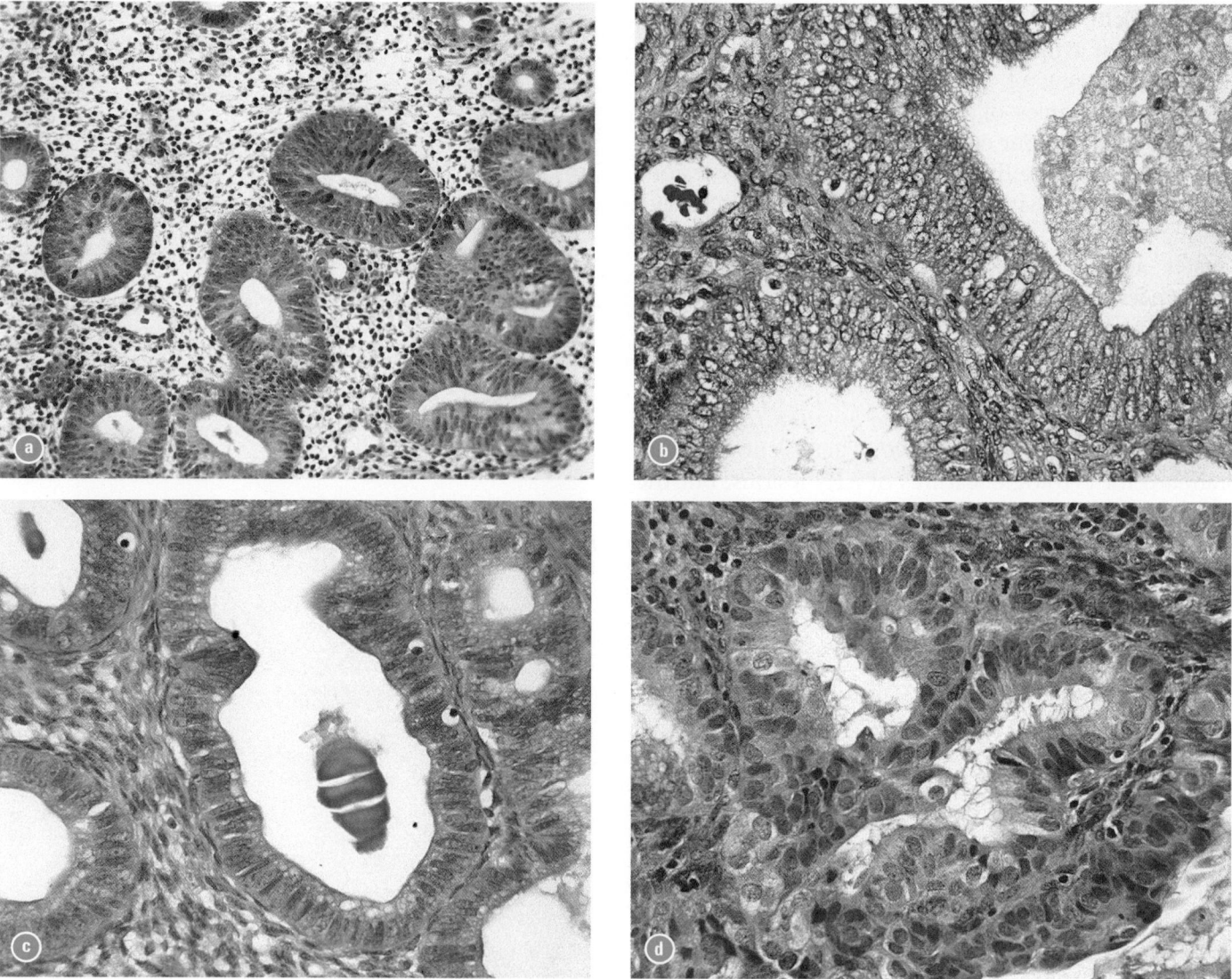

Fig. 17.9 Endometrioid cytology in EIN. Nuclear cytomorphology can vary greatly between patients (a–d).

or eosinophilic (Fig. 17.13)[12] phenotype. These must be distinguished from the scattered random pattern of hormonally, or surface-located repair-induced 'metaplasias'. Further details of how to interpret nonendometrioid EIN lesions are presented in the Pitfalls section below.

In those cases with no normal glands for internal reference, it is necessary to assess the freestanding cytology of relevant fragments in the context of their architectural features. Some EIN lesions occupy the entire tissue sample and should not be underdiagnosed for lack of a convenient benign gland in the area.

Size

>1 mm in maximum dimension: Accurate EIN diagnosis requires a contiguous field of glands sufficiently large to enable reliable assessment of architecture. A minimum lesion size of 1 mm maximum dimension was required in the previous clinical outcome studies[11,27,28,30] for an EIN lesion to achieve elevated cancer risk. That area of an EIN lesion which meets architectural (gland area) and cytologic (changed) criteria for diagnosis must measure a minimum of 1 mm in maximum dimension, a scale which usually encompasses more than 5–10 glands (Fig. 17.14). Most biopsy formats produce tissue fragments in excess of 1.5–2 mm. The size requirement must be met in a single tissue fragment, not added amongst multiple fragments. There is no formal evidence that once beyond the minimum 1 mm, EIN lesions should be stratified by size, but if a lesion is discretely focal, it may be of interest to the clinician to know what fraction of the available curettings contain lesion.

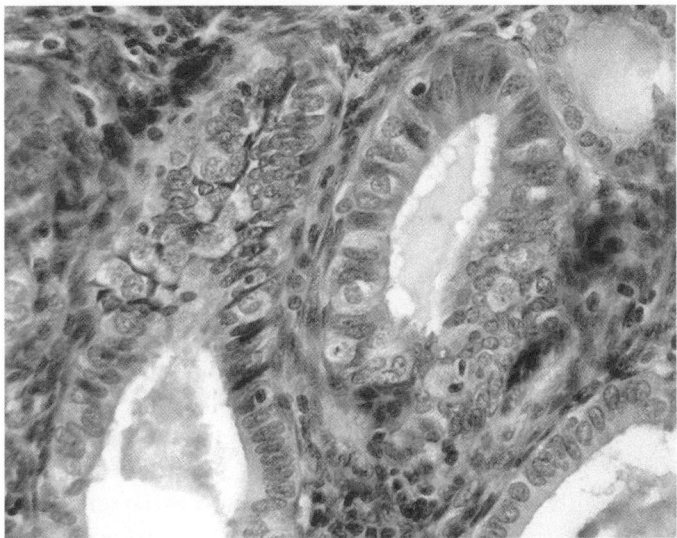

Fig. 17.10 EIN with tubal differentiation. This lesion evolved into a Type I (endometrioid class) adenocarcinoma, shown by conservation of genetic changes between this EIN and subsequent carcinoma.[12]

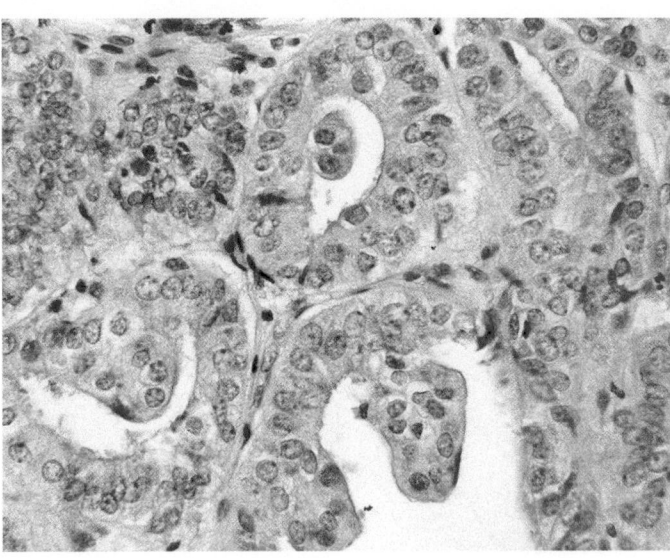

Fig. 17.12 EIN with micropapillary differentiation. This lesion evolved into a Type I (endometrioid class) adenocarcinoma, shown by conservation of genetic changes between this EIN and subsequent carcinoma.[12]

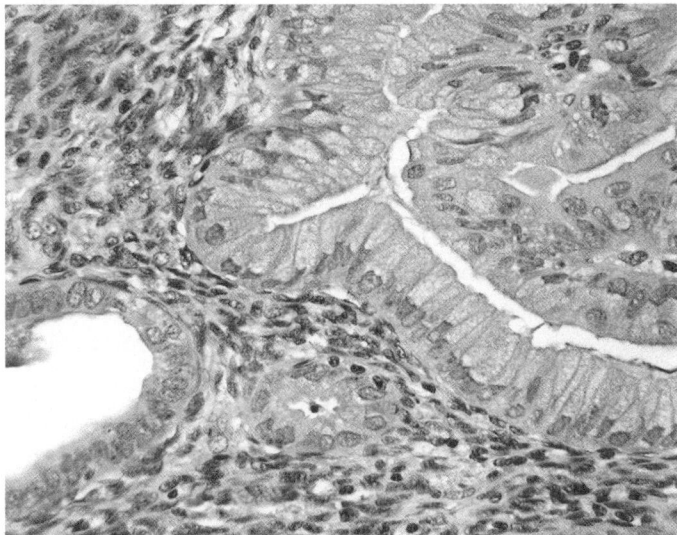

Fig. 17.11 EIN with mucinous differentiation. This lesion evolved into a Type I (endometrioid class) adenocarcinoma, shown by conservation of genetic changes between this EIN and subsequent carcinoma.[12]

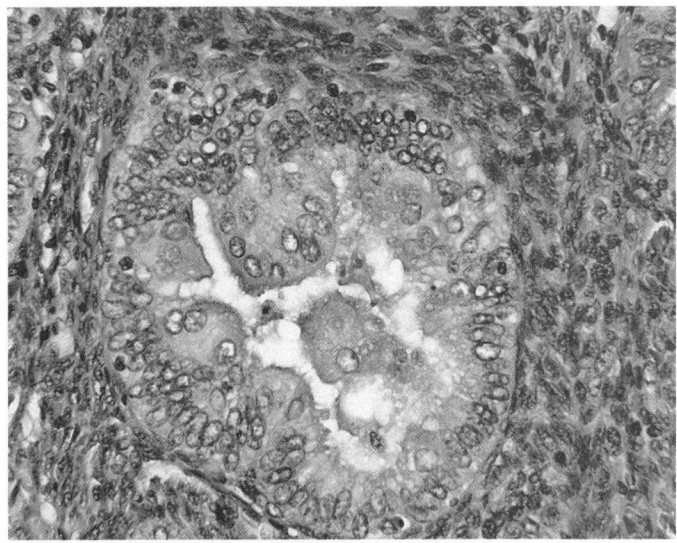

Fig. 17.13 EIN with eosinophilic differentiation. This lesion evolved into a Type I (endometrioid class) adenocarcinoma, shown by conservation of genetic changes between this EIN and subsequent carcinoma.[12]

Individual or small clusters of cytologically altered glands have an undefined natural history and are best diagnosed descriptively (see Pitfalls section, below).

Exclusion of benign mimics and adenocarcinoma

Features of EIN overlap with benign and malignant conditions, which must be carefully discriminated from EIN itself. These are described in detail in the section that follows.

Differential diagnosis

The differential diagnosis of EIN can be subdivided into several categories. The first consists of common patterns encountered in practice. The second consists of unique situations wherein interpretation is influenced by other factors, such as polyp, progestin therapy, metaplasia, etc. The third consists of malignancies that may be confused with EIN

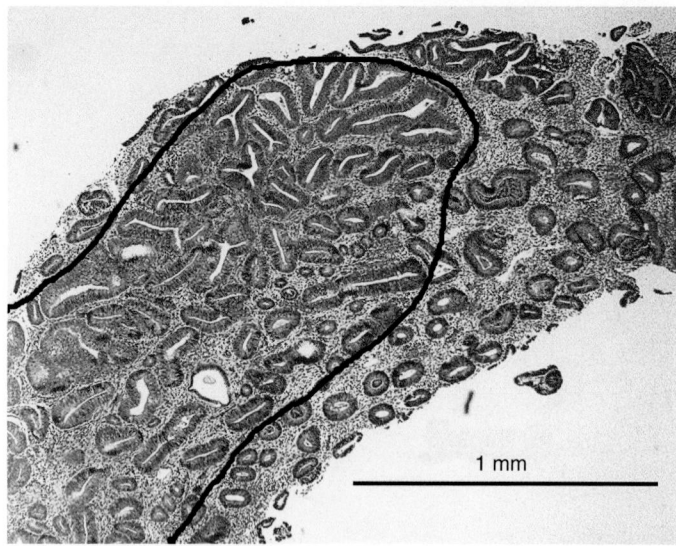

Fig. 17.14 EIN size criteria. EIN distributed in a localizing pattern with the perimeter marked. Lesion size is in excess of 1 mm maximum dimension, as required for EIN diagnosis. This patient got endometrial adenocarcinoma 4 years following this biopsy.

COMMON BENIGN PATTERNS THAT MAY BE MISCLASSIFIED AS EIN

Patients with one of the conditions listed below may still have an EIN, but this diagnosis should be made with careful consideration into how the coexisting factor(s) may modify the criteria for EIN diagnosis. If a specimen is refractory to confident diagnosis, a comment as to the nature of the problem may be useful in directing management.

Reactive changes

Reactive changes are caused by infection, physical disruption, recent pregnancy or recent instrumentation. These can cause piling up of the epithelium and loss of nuclear polarity (Fig. 17.15).

Artifactual gland displacement

Beware diagnosing an EIN lesion if the cytology is identical between areas with crowded compared with uncrowded glands. Many of these are artifactual disruptions where the stroma is sheared and glands pushed in apposition (Fig. 17.16).

Persistent estrogen effect

Randomly scattered cysts of protracted estrogen exposure and occasional branching glands are commonly encountered in anovulatory or estrogen-exposed endometria. Gland density is uniformly irregular throughout the endometrial compartment, with occasional clusters of glands having a cytology identical to the uncrowded areas (Fig. 17.17). These can be diagnosed as 'proliferative endometrium with architectural changes of unopposed estrogens'. With increasing duration, microthrombi form and scattered stromal breakdown may be associated with epithelial piling along the collapsed stromal surfaces.

Mid to late secretory endometrium

Mid to late secretory endometrium displays loss of nuclear polarity, nuclear enlargement and variation in nuclear size which, if measured objectively by computerized

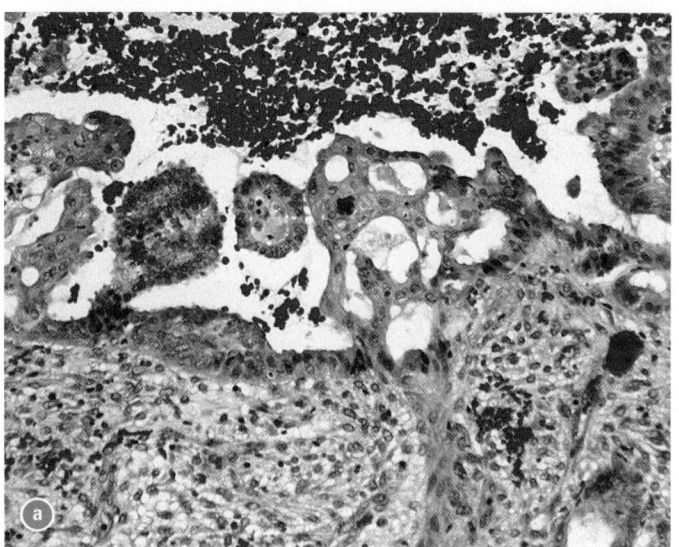

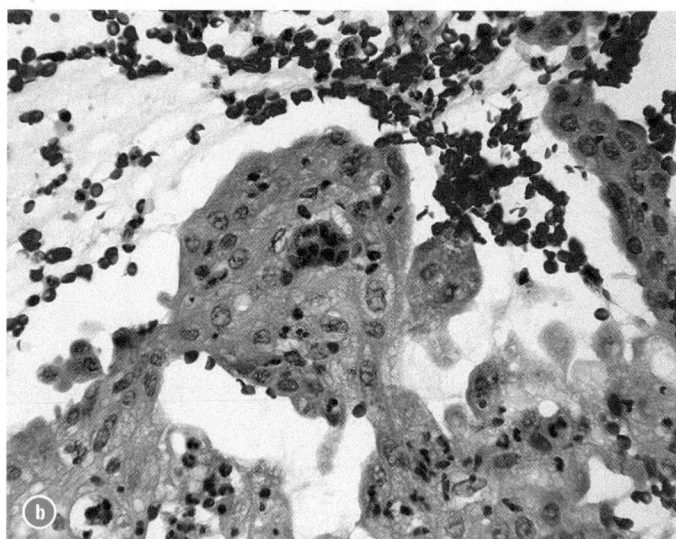

Fig. 17.15 Benign mimics of EIN: reactive surface changes. Piling of surface epithelium caused by recent breakdown. Note the stromal aggregate embedded in a papillary area of surface epithelium.

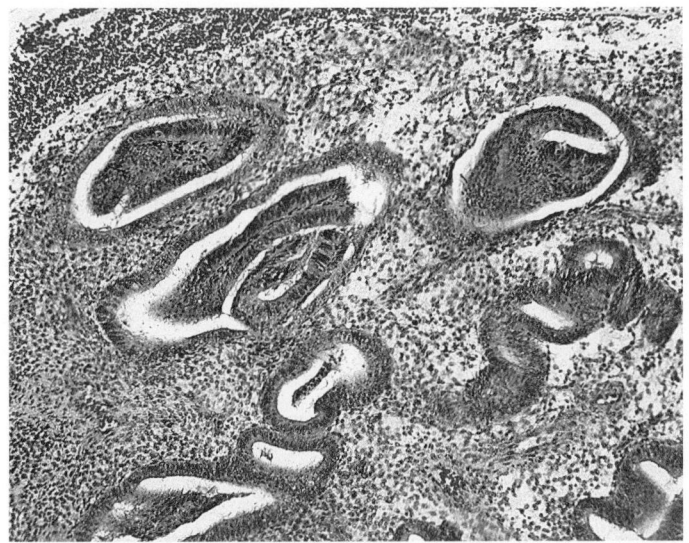

Fig. 17.16 Benign mimics of EIN: artifactual gland displacement. Telescoping artifact, which in some cases may be associated with lateral gland displacement, pushing glands into proximity at high density.

morphometry, overlaps substantially with EIN lesions. Stromal responsiveness to progesterone is not homogeneous at all endometrial depths. Lack of stromal pre-decidualization in the deeper functionalis and superficial basalis makes glands appear crowded and these same glands may display a worrisome cytology and complicated saw-toothed luminal profiles (Fig. 17.18).

Endometrial polyps

Endometrial polyps contain irregularly spaced glands in which scattered glands may differ from native endometrium due to their tendency to have reduced hormonal responsiveness. Benign polyps may also have low VPS caused by cysts (senile polyps) or random aggregations of glands (Fig. 17.19). Approximately 10% of EIN lesions, however, will present within an endometrial polyp and these must be diagnosed as described below in the Pitfalls section.

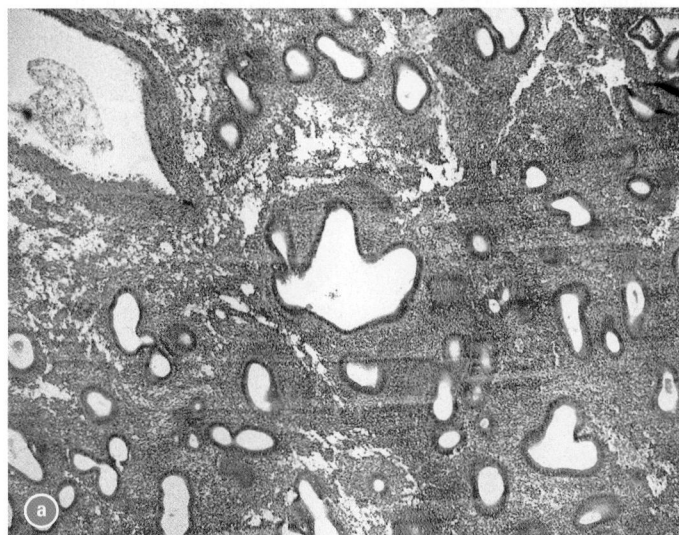

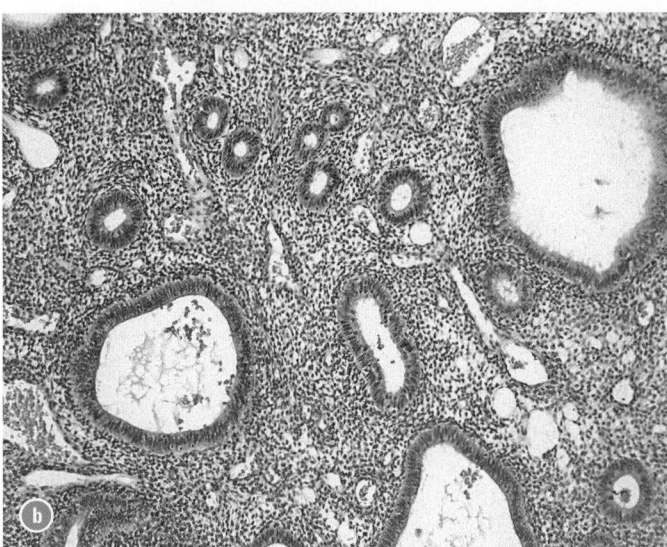

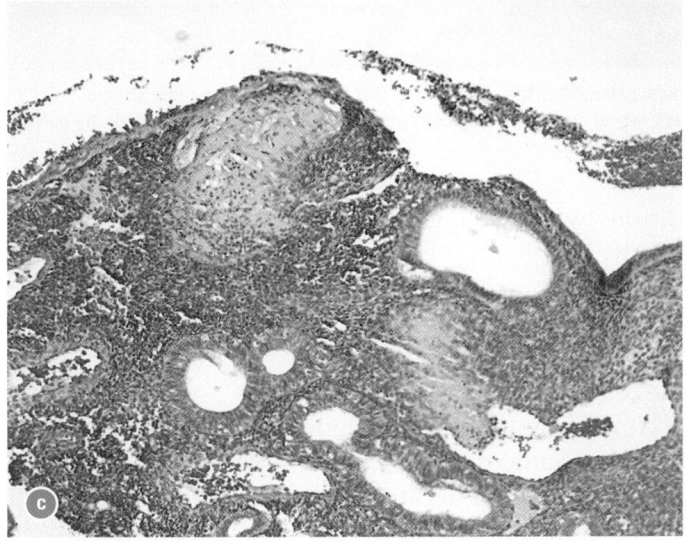

Fig. 17.17 Benign mimics of EIN: anovulatory endometrium. A scattered distribution 'regularly irregular' (a,b) of cystically dilated proliferative glands is caused by excess estrogen exposure. There are some non-discrete clusters of glands but this will not be confused with EIN because they do not have a change in cytology relative to the background and do not have sufficient gland density and perimeter size. Fibrin thrombi (c) cause microinfarcts with stromal breakdown and secondary adjacent epithelial collapse. Tubal metaplasia occurs frequently, but like the cysts, is distributed in scattered fashion.

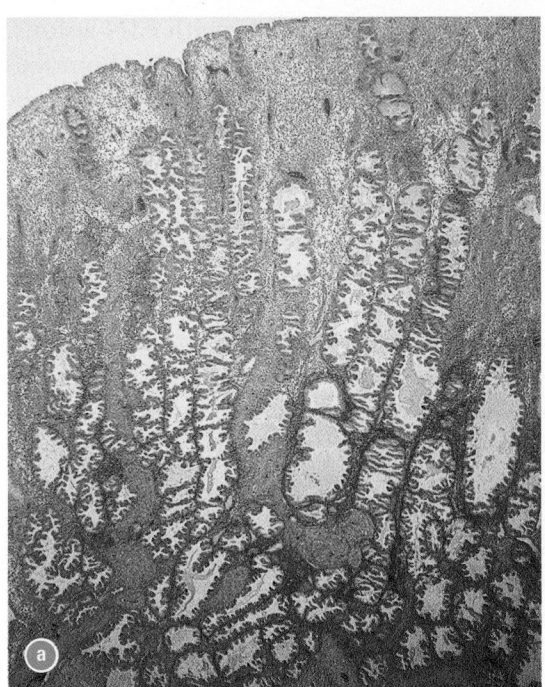

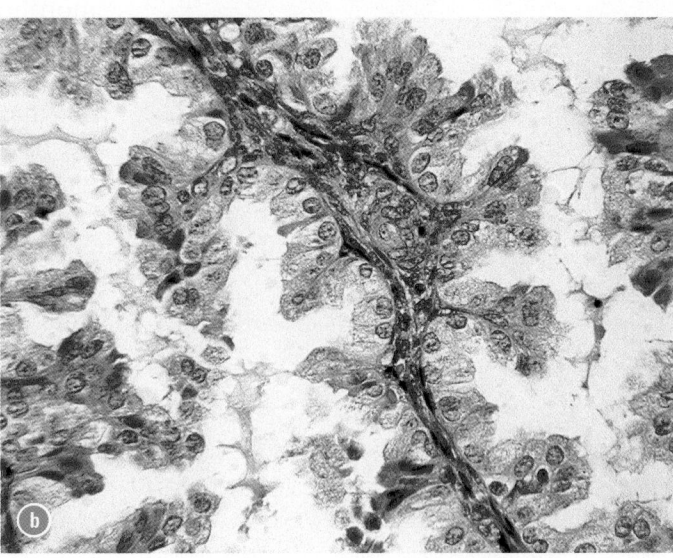

Fig. 17.18 Benign mimics of EIN: secretory endometrium. Glands are distributed at high density deep in the functionalis and basalis where there is little predecidual change. In those areas, the lumens are redundant and lined by larger round-to-oval nuclei.

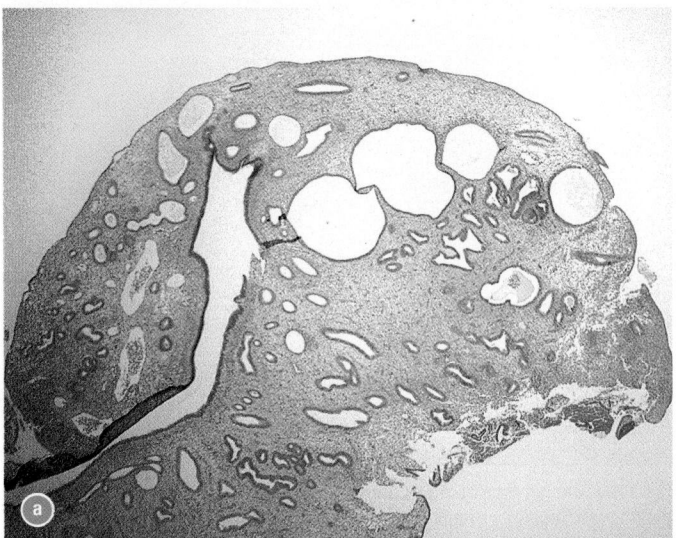

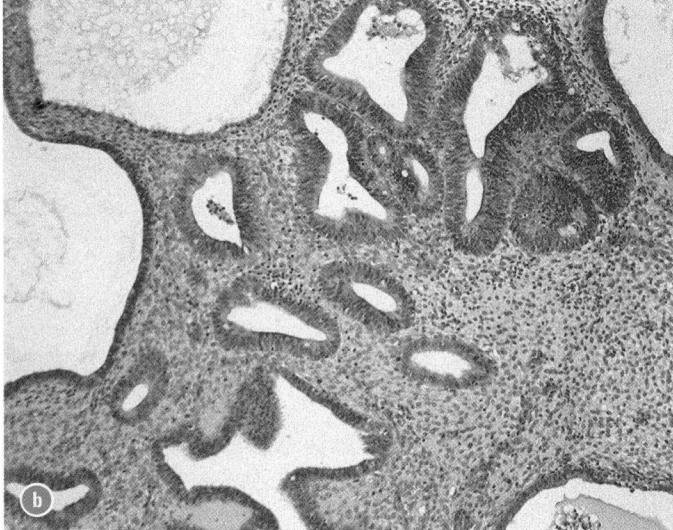

Fig. 17.19 Benign mimics of EIN: endometrial polyps. Dominant cysts should always be avoided when diagnosing EIN. This benign polyp has a low stromal percentage because of cysts. Other regions have random aggregation of benign glands, which are not cytologically altered relative to the remainder of the polyp.

Endometrial breakdown

Endometrial breakdown is one of the most common settings for overdiagnosis of a benign endometrium as a precancer or cancer. Breakdown may follow an ovulatory or anovulatory cycle and persist into the transitional period between late menses and early proliferative endometrium. Altered cytology is due to piling up of epithelial cells unsupported by stroma and associated nuclear changes such as loss of polarity (Fig. 17.20) which may be accentuated under certain fixation con-

ditions which exaggerate chromatin texture (Bouin's fixative).

INTERPRETATIVE PROBLEMS IN EIN DIAGNOSIS

If confounding factors preclude a definitive classification of the specimen at hand, make a descriptive diagnosis and clearly communicate the character of the unresolved differential and specific reason for diagnostic uncer-

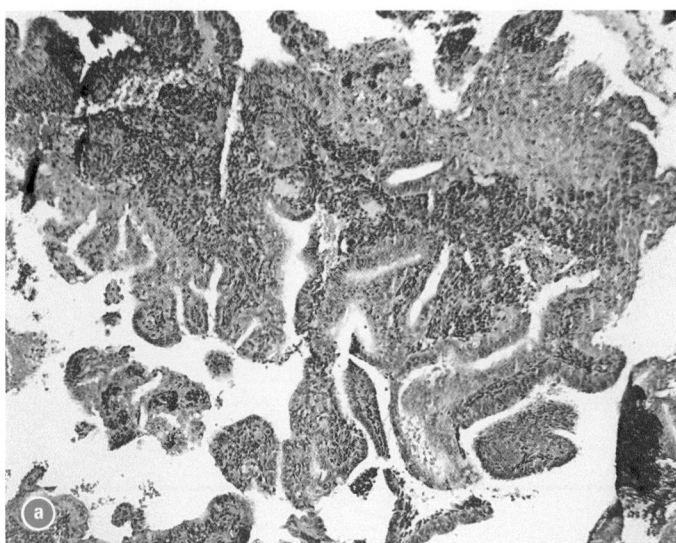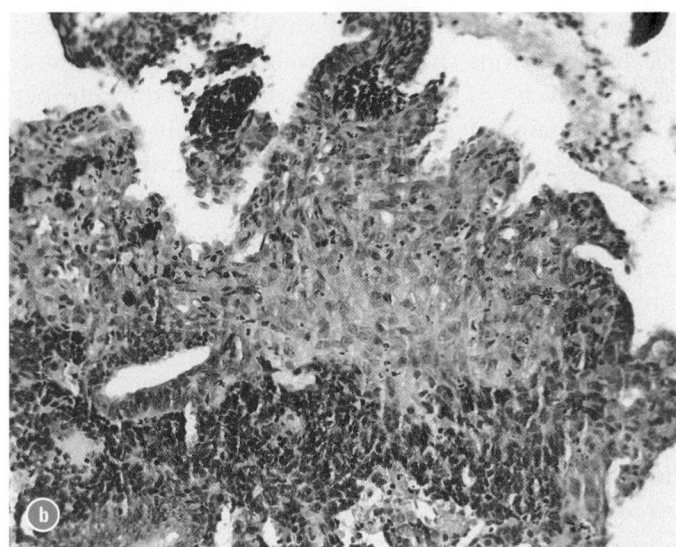

Fig. 17.20 Benign mimics of EIN: menstrual endometrium. Extensive stromal breakdown in this endometrium has caused surface epithelial piling up.

tainty (Table 17.3). Pathologists vary in their attitudes towards making clinical recommendations for follow-up within the pathology report. We do this routinely, especially if the sampling instrument or strategy needs

Table 17.3 Pitfalls in EIN diagnosis

Problem	Response
Fragmented or distorted	Get levels and ask for a rebiopsy soon (within 3 months) if still worried
Suspicious for EIN but <1 mm	Section deeper and evaluate context: 1 If extends to edge of fragment <1 mm, likely sampling error: recommend rebiopsy soon (within 3 months) 2 If small area in larger fragment, likely a sub-diagnostic 'pre-EIN': make descriptive diagnosis and recommend follow-up biopsy in 6 months
Suspicious for EIN but >50% VPS	Descriptive diagnosis and follow-up in 6 months
EIN in polyp	Apply usual EIN criteria, using polyp itself as the background for cytologic comparison. EIN in polyps are usually discrete
Non-endometrioid differentiation	If glandular, can use EIN criteria but must rule out specific cancer
Squamous morules	Make diagnosis based upon gland component, mentally subtracting morules. Do not consider cribriform if morule separates peripheral lumens
Progestin effect	Diagnose EIN if criteria met. Descriptive diagnosis of any other suspicious localizing lesions. Suggest withdrawal of hormones and rebiopsy 2–4 weeks after cessation of withdrawal bleed in cases where interpretation is confounded by hormonal therapy

to be changed in the next diagnostic procedure, or the clinician must discontinue progestins to improve diagnostic accuracy. Whatever the venue for communication, the pathologist is often well equipped to contribute a constructive plan for resolution of the diagnostic problem. For example, the patient who is biopsied while on exogenous progestins may be easier to evaluate after withdrawal of hormones. Confusing histologies such as those obscured by extensive altered cellular differentiation ('metaplasias') should be described clearly. Other specimens may be compromised by sampling errors, or superimposed regenerative epithelial changes. All should be clarified by additional studies, deeper levels or immediate resampling to detect the presence of diagnostic areas elsewhere, or follow-up with re-biopsy. If the patient is symptomatic, some clinicians will elect to treat with a trial of high-dose progestins followed by a post-withdrawal biopsy. Recommendations for interpretation of some commonly encountered diagnostic problems are listed below and in Table 17.3.

Sub-diagnostic EIN-like lesion

Lesions suspicious for but sub-diagnostic for EIN deserve clear description and, if clinically appropriate, resampling. Obvious localizing lesions characterized by a changed cytology sometimes do not meet either the minimal 1 mm size or 50% VPS EIN requirements. This is a heterogeneous group composed of examples of poorly sampled EIN lesions, very early precursors of EIN that have not yet reached the diagnostic threshold and subtle benign mimics.

The fragment context of small or loosely packed localizing lesions should be evaluated after obtaining deeper levels. If the affected fragments in deeper levels remain <1 mm in size, with densely packed lesional glands extending from edge to edge, there is a high likelihood that tissue disruption of a larger lesion is the problem (Fig. 17.21). These may be diagnosed as 'fragments of crowded glands with altered cytology consistent with, but not diagnostic of, EIN' with a recommendation to resample within 3 months.

If the fragment is large, but the focus of clustered cytologically altered glands remains <1 mm, or has insufficient gland density for EIN (Fig. 17.22), then sampling error is unlikely. This is a small category of cases, comprising roughly one-fifth or one-quarter of the frequency of easily diagnosed EIN lesions. These rare lesions are probably pre-EIN precursors with a lower cancer risk than bona fide EIN. They should be diagnosed descriptively (microscopic cluster of cytologically altered glands) with a recommendation for follow-up biopsy in 6 months.

Every effort should be made to avoid overdiagnosis of small groups of contrasting glands as EIN. Patients with unopposed estrogens may randomly have a few tubal glands in proximity, polyps can contain irregular distributions of glands and the patient with endometritis or repair can have local effects, which polarize the endometrium. Examination of the background context is most helpful in these circumstances.

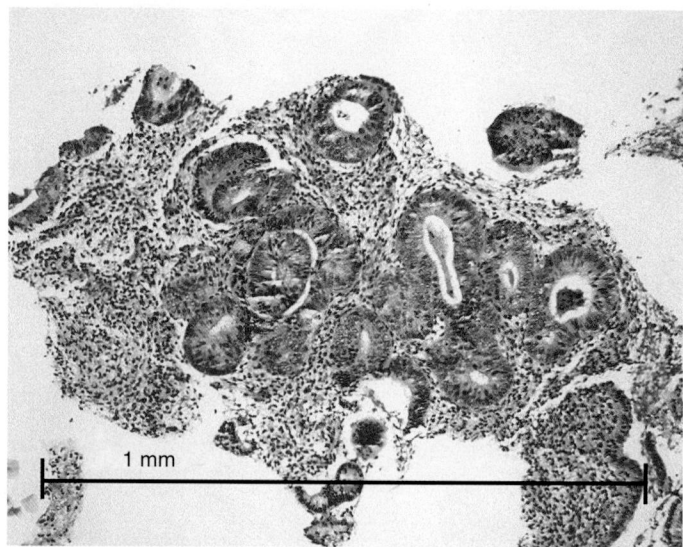

Fig. 17.21 Localizing clonal processes subdiagnostic for EIN: size <1 mm. This cytologically altered lesion with very crowded glands extending from the top to bottom fragment edges is probably an EIN in which the small fragment size prevents meeting the 1 mm minimum size. Deeper levels should be examined to see if better diagnostic areas are present elsewhere. If not, a diagnosis is made of 'fragments of crowded glands with altered cytology consistent with, but not diagnostic of, EIN', with a recommendation for clinical correlation and resampling within 3 months.

EIN within an endometrial polyp

In general, all criteria for EIN diagnosis apply to EIN arising within a polyp, but the reference point for interpretation of EIN cytology and architecture is the background polyp itself, not the normal endometrial functionalis (Fig. 17.23). EIN within polyps are best

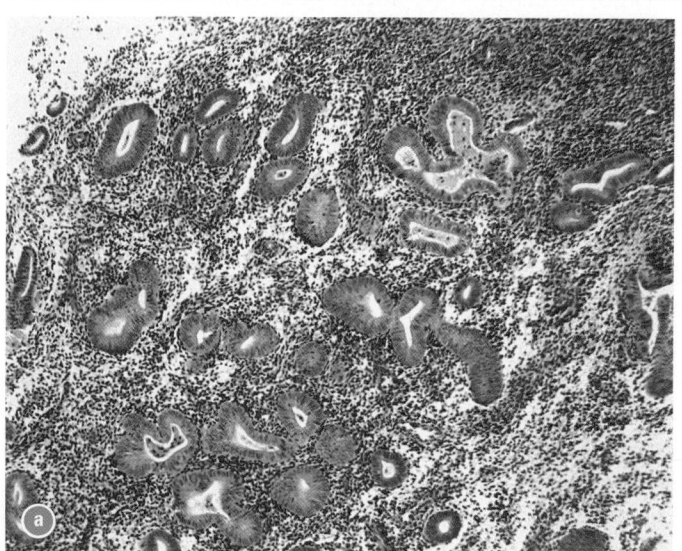

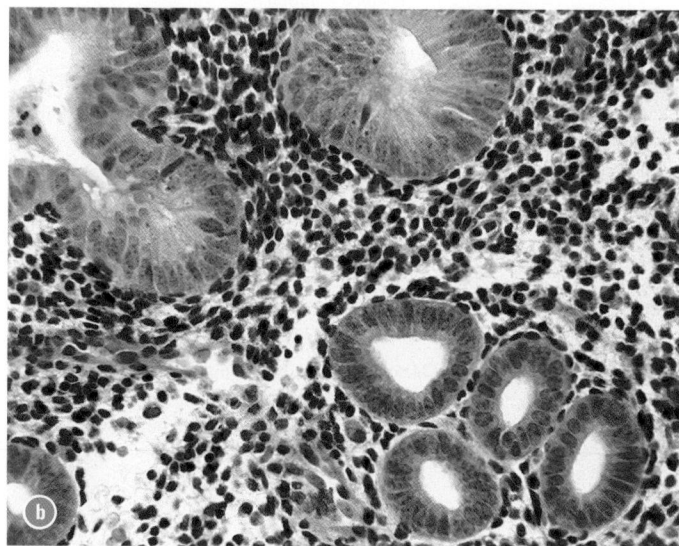

Fig. 17.22 Localizing clonal processes sub-diagnostic for EIN: gland area less than stroma. There is a distinct loose cluster of cytologically altered glands in a large tissue fragment. The focus did not become more cohesive on deeper sectioning, so it was judged not to meet the architectural requirement of gland area in excess of that for stroma. A descriptive diagnosis and recommendation for follow-up sampling in 6 months is advisable for these lesions with an uncertain natural history.

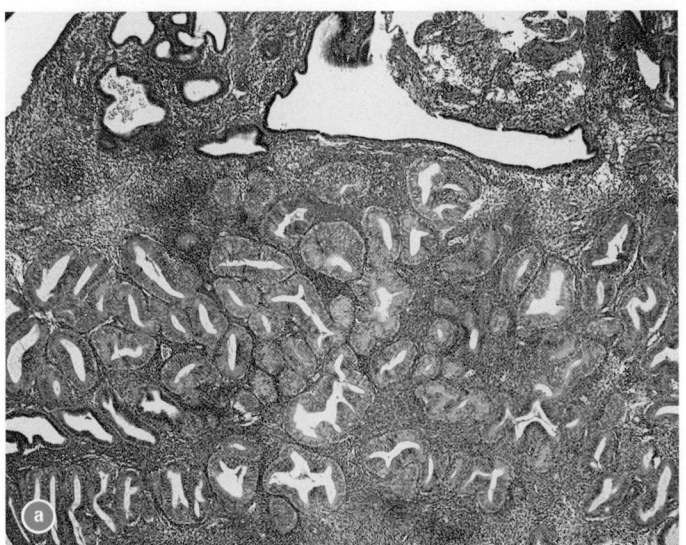
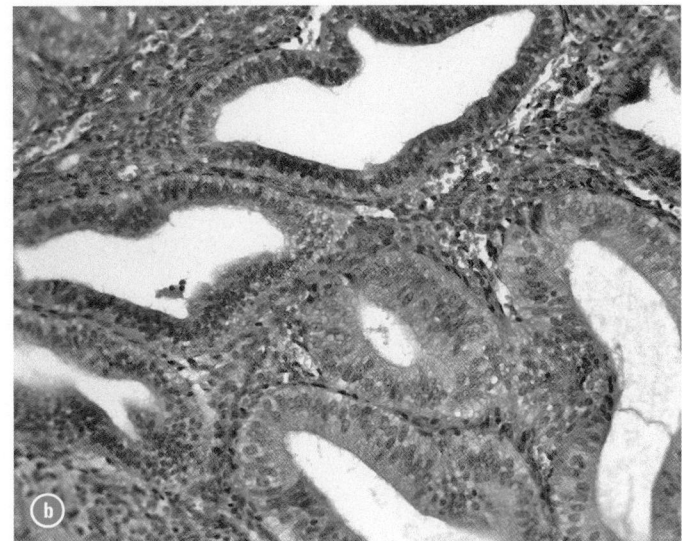

Fig. 17.23 EIN arising in endometrial polyp. Comparison of the discrete EIN area with the polyp background shows a clonal pattern of cytologic change against this setting.

recognized as geographic regions of contiguous glands with an architecture and cytology readily distinguished from that of the background polyp. Avoid overreaction to bland dominant cysts lined by atrophic epithelium, as these are a common component of benign senile polyps or mixed endocervical-endometrial polyps.

The benign polyp will have a regularly irregular distribution of glands. Cytologic variation will not appear in geographic clusters of glands, but rather interspersed or splayed on the periphery with loose boundaries. Random apposition of glands in proximity can be recognized by a cytology identical to that of more dispersed glands elsewhere in the polyp.

On those occasions when EIN is diagnosed within a polyp, the polyp setting should be clearly mentioned in the report. If completely excised, a polypectomy may be curative. If incompletely excised, the physical bulk of a polyp can prevent adequate follow-up sampling by flexible devices (Pipelle).

Non-endometrioid EIN *vs* 'metaplasia'

EIN lesions with non-endometrioid cytology must be distinguished from benign 'metaplasias'. A shift in cytodifferentiation may be the cytologic change which characterizes some EIN examples, which also meet other size, architecture and exclusion criteria (Figs 17.10–17.13). In most instances they are localizing lesions with a classic EIN geography composed of mucinous, tubal or eosinophilic glands. A special case are those glandular lesions containing round intraluminal expan-

sile squamous morules. These morules may be quite abundant, creating distortion of the volumetric relationships between gland and stromal compartments. Since it is the glandular not morular component of these lesions which has premalignant behavior, the bulk contributed by morules should be mentally excluded when assessing the size of the glandular *vs* stromal compartments. If possible, search for morule poor areas with glands that meet EIN criteria (Fig. 17.24).

The differential diagnosis between EIN and carcinoma may have special considerations in non-endometrioid lesions. Solid morules surrounded by a peripheral garland of lumen-containing glands resemble a cribriform pattern that may easily be over-interpreted as adenocarcinomas (Fig. 17.25). True cribriforming involves glandular epithelium only and should not be diagnosed when the cells separating individual lumens are squamous. Criteria for diagnosis of mucinous and squamous adenocarcinomas are different than those for endometrioid adenocarcinomas. The distinction between EIN and carcinoma in these cases must be made using differentiation-state appropriate criteria.

Confounding progestin exposure

Progestins, whether endogenous or pharmacologic, alter endometrial gland cytology and variably expand the stromal compartment to modify gland–stromal relationships. EIN lesions exposed to progestins tend to display nuclear shrinkage and homogenization of coarse chromatin (Fig. 17.26), with pseudodecidual change respon-

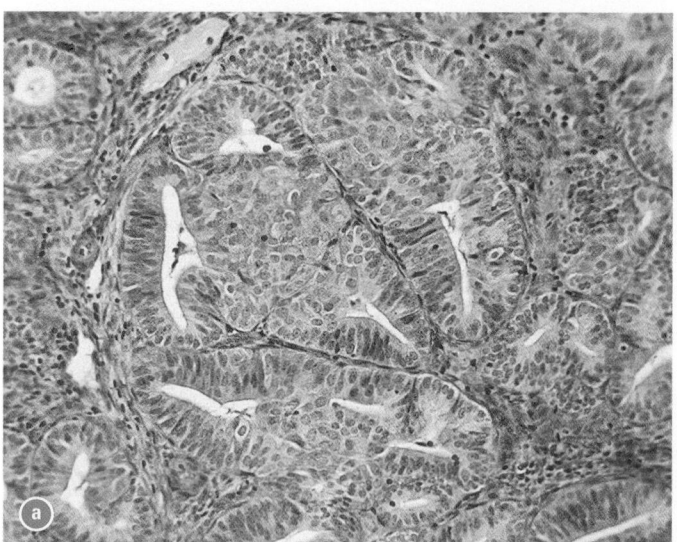 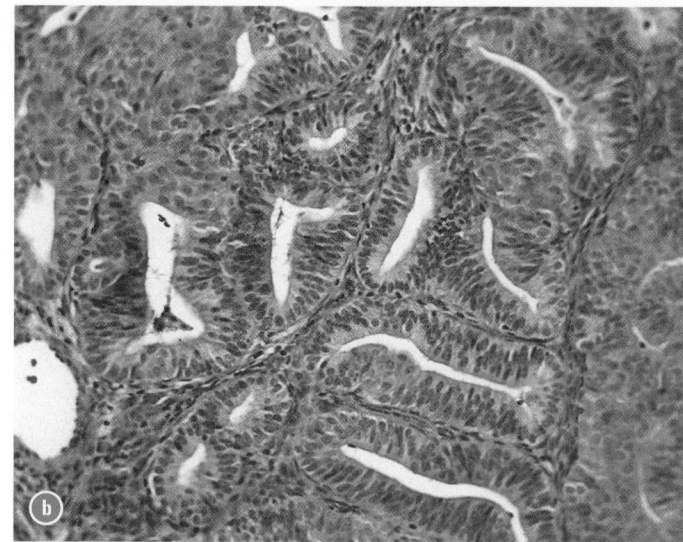

Fig. 17.24 Non-endometrioid EIN: squamous differentiation (morules). (a) Abundant squamous morules vary in density between illustrated areas. Closer examination shows a morule-poor region (b) where architectural criteria for EIN are met.

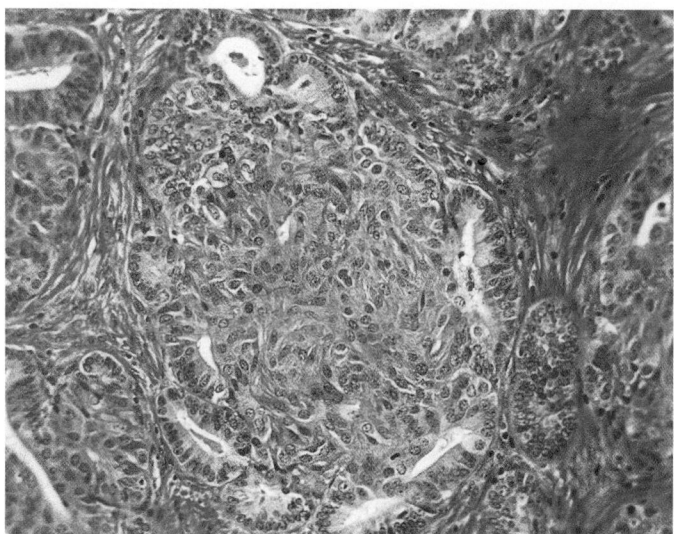

Fig. 17.25 Pseudo-cribriform pattern caused by squamous morule. A large intraluminal morule separates hemi glands on the periphery. This should not be confused with adenocarcinoma.

sible for separation of glands making them appear less crowded. In contrast, nuclei of glands in normal secretory endometrium greatly enlarge and the proportion of glands to stroma varies by height within the functionalis. The paradoxical result is that in the presence of progestins, EIN lesions become more bland and normal endometrium more worrisome. In its most extreme form, pregnant patients with Arias-Stella phenomenon have dramatic epithelial atypia caused by polyploidy and these areas typically demonstrate minimal stromal decidualization, resulting in very crowded gland architecture.

The schedule of progestin therapy for EIN may be continuous or non-continuous and this will influence the hormonal background against which follow-up surveillance biopsies must be interpreted. Protracted, essentially indefinite, progestin therapy is preferred by some clinicians, whereas others employ an interrupted regimen with intermittent endometrial shedding. There is no consensus in recommending one approach over the other, an issue that must be resolved by future clinical trials and the unique considerations of individual patients. Withdrawal of progestins in an interrupted regimen may induce massive apoptosis and endometrial shedding which contribute to clearance of neoplastic tissue.[81] On the other hand, continuous progestin therapy, such as that provided by a progestin-impregnated intrauterine device, has been reported to be effective in treating some endometrial cancers.[82]

For those patients on interrupted progestin regimens, or who have completed a trial of progestins, surveillance biopsies should be performed several weeks after a post-progestin withdrawal bleed. This avoids the interpretative difficulties of confounding stromal and glandular changes caused by progestins and the usual EIN diagnostic criteria apply.

Diagnosis of the endometrium biopsied under the influence of progestins presents the pathologist with interpretative and semantic difficulties. None of the endometrial precancer histopathologic diagnostic schemas, including WHO hyperplasia and EIN diagnostic criteria, were intended to be applied in the setting of active progestin therapy. Nonetheless, when diag-

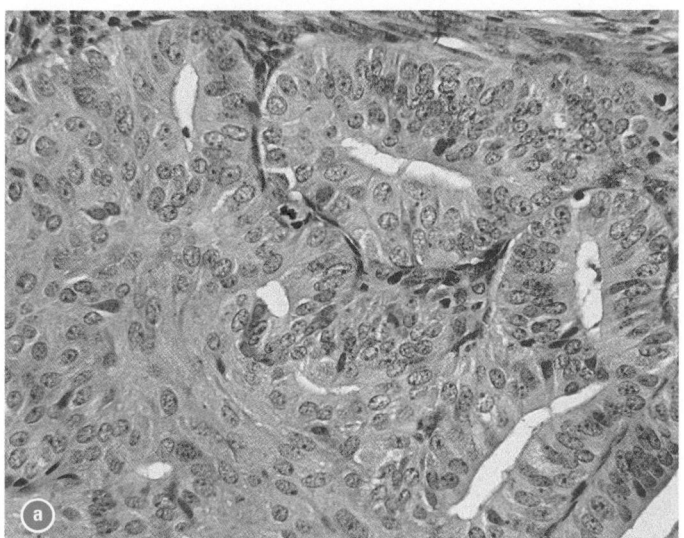
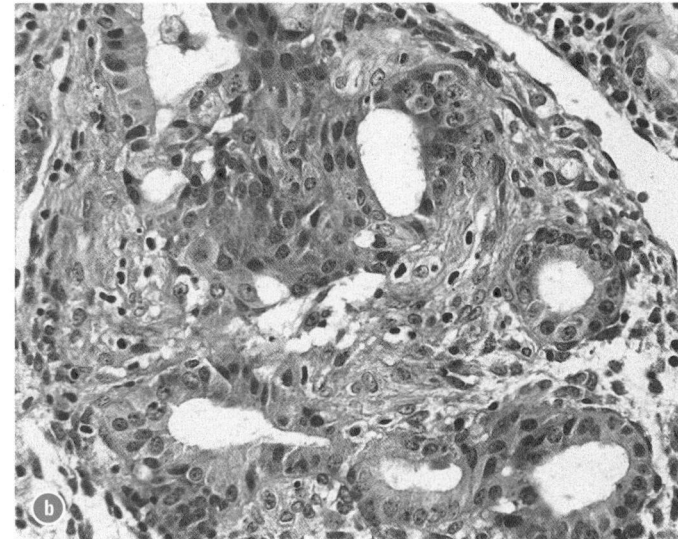

Fig. 17.26 Effects of progestin therapy on EIN. An EIN lesion with squamous morules (a) was rebiopsied after a 4-month trial of progestin Megac (b). Persistence of the morules allows precise identification of the lesion location. Note the dramatic shrinkage of nuclei after treatment. Both photomicrographs taken at identical magnification.

nostic features are present, EIN lesions can and should be diagnosed through a progestin effect. Many EIN lesions rebiopsied in the midst of a course of therapeutic progestins will, however, no longer be diagnostic because of changes in cytology and architecture. These may persist as localizing lesions which should be diagnosed descriptively with a recommendation for rebiopsy, preferably after progestin withdrawal. The pathologist should clearly communicate these progestin-induced diagnostic difficulties to the clinician, so that they may understand the potential benefits of interrupting therapy in order to obtain a more definitive endpoint.

EXCLUSION OF CARCINOMA

Malignancy must always be excluded during the evaluation of EIN and falls into two categories: endometrioid adenocarcinomas and other carcinomas arising in the endometrium or elsewhere.

Endometrioid adenocarcinomas

Cancer may coexist with EIN in an individual patient, but should be always be separately diagnosed because current management of carcinoma differs from that for EIN. Keep in mind that absence of carcinoma in a tissue biopsy does not exclude the possibility that the patient has a cancer which was unsampled during the biopsy procedure. An opinion should always be rendered based upon available material and should be clearly stated.

EIN is composed of individual glands lined by an epithelium one cell layer thick. The epithelium may be pseudostratified or occasionally micropapillary (Fig. 17.12), but should not be cribriform or composed of solid areas of epithelial cells. Presence of any of the following features involving neoplastic glands is inconsistent with EIN and a diagnosis of carcinoma should be entertained:
- Meandering or 'mazelike' lumens (Fig. 17.27).
- Solid epithelium (Fig. 17.28).

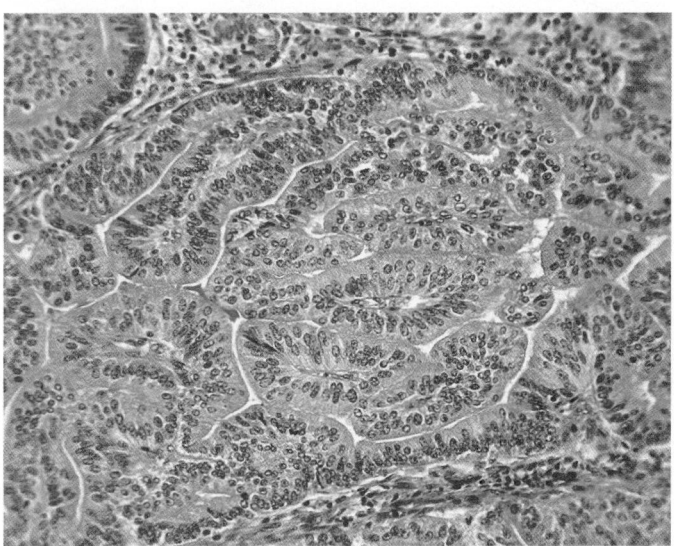

Fig. 17.27 Patterns distinguishing endometrial carcinoma from EIN: meandering lumens in adenocarcinoma. Mazelike luminal connections characteristic of folded epithelial sheets are inconsistent with an EIN. This is a well-differentiated adenocarcinoma.

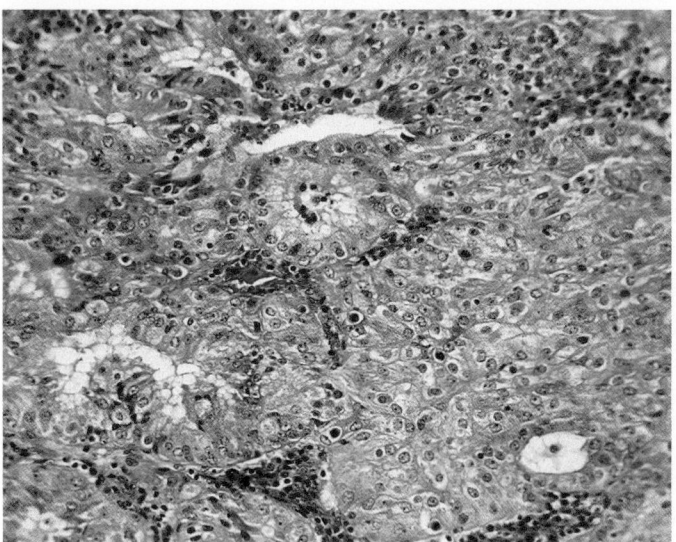

Fig. 17.28 Patterns distinguishing endometrial carcinoma from EIN: solid epithelium in adenocarcinoma. EIN glands have a simple non-stratified lining without solid areas.

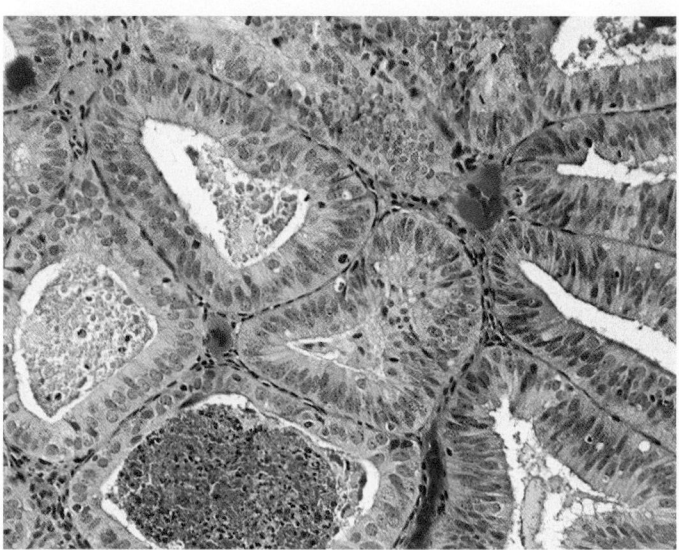

Fig. 17.30 Patterns distinguishing endometrial carcinoma from EIN: 'mosaic' gland pattern. Threadlike dividing stroma between polygonally distorted endometrial glands is unusual for EIN, which in most cases maintains each gland as a separate unit. This has crossed the boundary to well-differentiated carcinoma.

- Cribriform architecture (Fig. 17.29).
- 'Mosaic' gland pattern of distorted polygonal glands with threadlike intervening stroma (Fig. 17.30).
- Myoinvasion. Unfortunately, myometrium is rarely available for evaluation in a biopsy or curettage specimen.

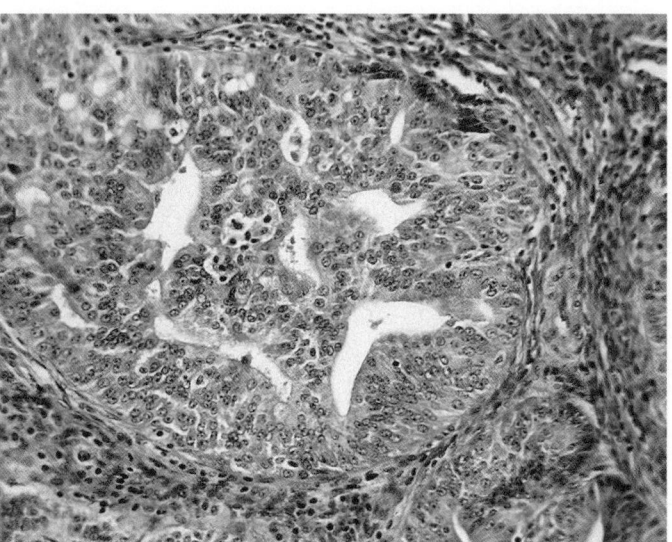

Fig. 17.29 Patterns distinguishing endometrial carcinoma from EIN: cribriform architecture in adenocarcinoma. True cribriform architecture does not appear in EIN, but as shown here may be seen in adenocarcinoma. Caution must be exercised in identification of cribriform architecture, as degenerative areas, tangential sectioning and intraluminal squamous morules can mimic this pattern.

Other carcinomas that may mimic EIN

These include the following:

- Uterine papillary serous carcinomas (UPSCs) extending into endometrial glands. The majority of UPSCs are sufficiently extensive that confusion with EIN will not occur. However, in limited samples, UPSC may appear as uniform enlarged glands with stratified hyperchromatic nuclei. If an intraluminal micropapillary or hobnail pattern is not conspicuous, or if discretely enlarged individual nuclei are not seen, the lesion may be misinterpreted as EIN (Fig. 17.31a). The practitioner should be suspicious of UPSC if the nuclear features of the glands exceed that normally associated with EIN. An immunostain for p53 may be helpful (Fig. 17.31b)
- Endocervical adenocarcinomas. The diagnostic pitfalls introduced by endocervical adenocarcinomas or adenocarcinomas in situ are 2-fold. First, uniform fragments of endocervical adenocarcinoma in an endometrial sample may mimic EIN. EIN is usually excluded by the characteristic nuclear hyperchromasia, luminal eosinophilia, apical mitoses and compact architecture of cervical neoplasia (Fig. 17.32a). Secondly, direct extension of endocervical adenocarcinoma into the endometrial lining epithelium closely mimics EIN. The presence of the above features in addition to a conspicuous neoplasm in the endocervix should be

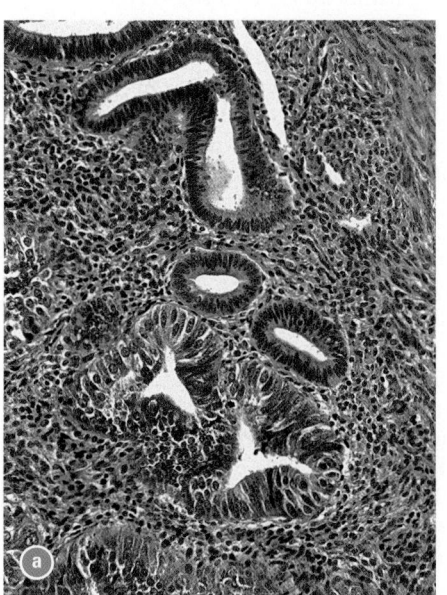
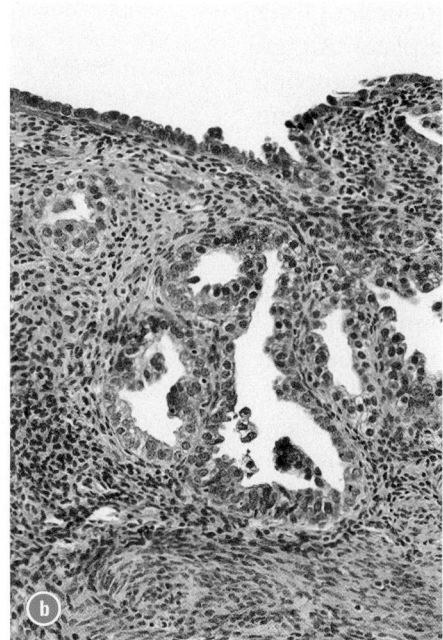
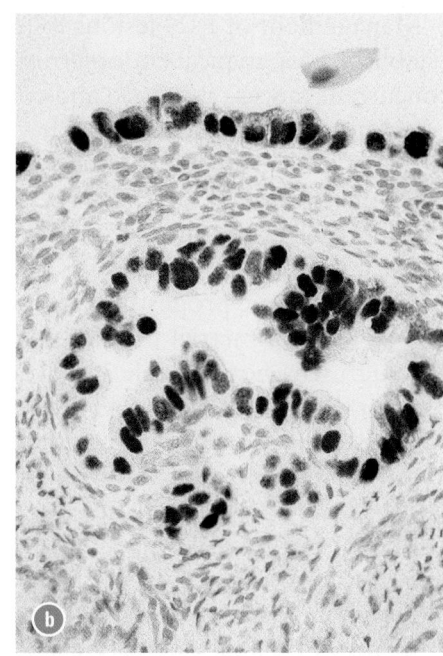

Fig. 17.31 Uterine papillary serous carcinoma (UPSC) involving endometrial glands. (a) Endometrioid growth cellular growth pattern in a UPSC may mimic EIN. (b) Hyperchromatic epithelial cells with a slight 'hobnail' pattern, associated with uniformly contoured glands. (c) A p53 immunostain is strongly positive.

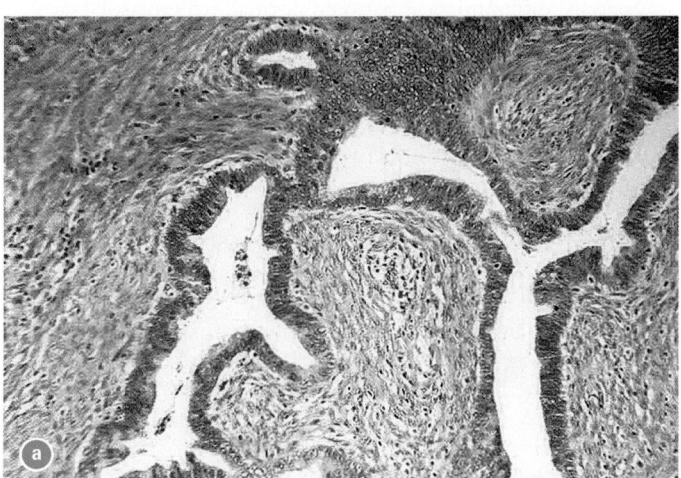
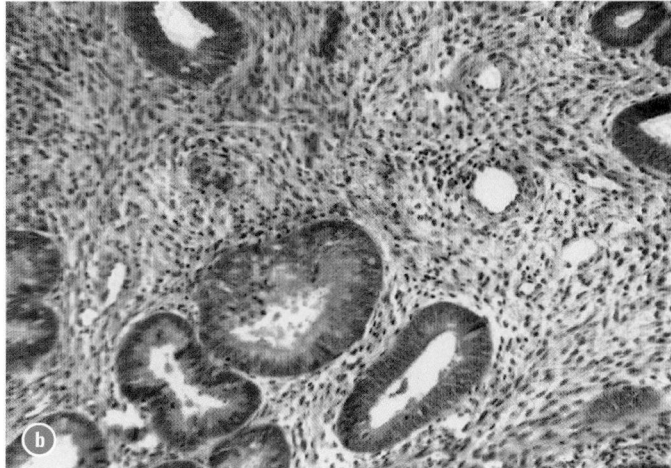

Fig. 17.32 Endocervical adenocarcinoma mimicking EIN. (a) A curetting contains fragments of endocervical adenocarcinoma with villoglandular architecture. (b) The same adenocarcinoma extended cephalad into the functionalis.

sufficient, but endocervical involvement can be subtle (Fig. 17.32b).

Management of EIN

Unopposed estrogen exposure and constitutive genetic risk factors for endometrial carcinoma are managed quite differently than a premalignant EIN lesion. This is a nontrivial point, as in the past pathologists have lumped endocrine effects (anovulatory-type changes of unopposed estrogens) and premalignant disease (EIN) into an assumed disease continuum of hyperplasia subsets stratified by architecture and cytology. Assignment amongst these various categories is poorly reproducible and the implied broad continuum belies a clinical need for assignment into dichotomous treatment groups of patients managed either by endometrial surveillance or lesion ablation. The types and number of EIN diagnostic categories correspond well with therapeutic options, facilitating ready acceptance by clinicians.

Management of EIN lesions follows guidelines long established for atypical endometrial hyperplasia. A high concurrent cancer rate (26%) and concern that sampling errors may miss an occult tumor have led to a prevailing view that immediate hysterectomy is justified by its combined diagnostic and therapeutic benefits. Young patients wishing to preserve fertility and women who are poor surgical risks are candidates for hormonal (progestin) therapy. Systemic progestins can successfully ablate up to 90% of endometrial precancers in young women,[83] although it is not possible in advance to predict that fraction which will respond. A decision to treat hormonally must thus be made between the clinician and patient in full light of the risks and with the precondition that regular follow-up surveillance can be performed.

There is interest in improving efficacy and reducing side effects of progestin-based hormonal therapies. Hormone-impregnated intrauterine devices may deliver high local doses capable of treating endometrial neoplasia while reducing systemic exposures.[82,84,85] Alternatively, there is now basic experimental evidence suggesting interrupted systemic delivery may be more efficient in destroying neoplastic cells than a continuous regimen.[81] Controlled clinical studies will need to be performed to define these options.

Acknowledgments

Some of the text and many of the figures have been used, with permission, from the website www.endometrium.org.[86]

References

1 Hertig A, Sommers S. Genesis of endometrial carcinoma. I. Study of prior biopsies. Cancer 1949; 2:946–956.

2 Hertig A, Sommers S, Bengloff H. Genesis of endometrial carcinoma. III. Carcinoma in situ. Cancer 1949; 2:964–971.

3 Sommers S, Hertig A, Bengloff H. Genesis of endometrial carcinoma. II. Cases 19 to 35 years old. Cancer 1949; 2:957–963.

4 Winkler B, Alvarez S, Richart R, Crum C. Pitfalls in the diagnosis of endometrial neoplasia. Obstet Gynecol 1984; 64:185–194.

5 Kurman R, Kaminski P, Norris H. The behavior of endometrial hyperplasia: a long term study of 'untreated' hyperplasia in 170 patients. Cancer 1985; 56:403–412.

6 Scully RE, Bonfiglio TA, Kurman RJ, et al. Uterine corpus. Histological typing of female genital tract tumors. New York: Springer; 1994:13–31.

7 Bergeron C, Nogales F, Masseroli M, et al. A multicentric European study testing the reproducibility of the WHO Classification of endometrial hyperplasia with a proposal of a simplified working classification for biopsy and curettage specimens. Am J Surg Pathol 1999; 23:1102–1108.

8 Kendall BS, Ronnett BM, Isacson C, et al. Reproducibility of the diagnosis of endometrial hyperplasia, atypical hyperplasia and well-differentiated carcinoma. Am J Surg Pathol 1998; 22:1012–1019.

9 Zaino RJ. Endometrial hyperplasia: is it time for a quantum leap to a new classification? Int J Gynecol Pathol 2000; 19(4):314–321.

10 Zaino R, Trimble C, Silverberg S, et al. Reproducibility of the diagnosis of atypical endometrial hyperplasia (AEH): a Gynecologic Oncology Group (GOG) study [Abstract]. Lab Invest 2004; 84:218A.

11 Baak JPA, Nauta J, Wisse-Brekelmans E, Bezemer P. Architectural and nuclear morphometrical features together are more important prognosticators in endometrial hyperplasias than nuclear morphometrical features alone. J Pathol 1988; 154:335–341.

12 Mutter GL, Baak JPA, Crum CP, et al. Endometrial precancer diagnosis by histopathology, clonal analysis and computerized morphometry. J Pathol 2000; 190:462–469.

13 Bezemer PD, Baak JP, With C de. Discriminant analysis, exemplified with quantitative features of endometrium. Eur J Obstet Gynecol Reprod Biol 1977; 7:209–214.

14 Diegenbach PC, Baak JP. Quantitative nuclear image analysis: differentiation between normal, hyperplastic and malignant appearing uterine glands in a paraffin section. II. Computer assisted recognition by discriminant analysis. Eur J Obstet Gynecol Reprod Biol 1977; 7:389–394.

15 Diegenbach PC, Baak JP. Quantitative nuclear image analysis: differentiation between normal, hyperplastic and malignant appearing uterine glands in a paraffin section. III. The use of texture features for differentiation. Eur J Obstet Gynecol Reprod Biol 1978; 8:109–116.

16 Diegenbach PC, Baak JP. Quantitative nuclear image analysis: differentiation between normal, hyperplastic and malignant appearing uterine glands in a paraffin section. IV. The use of Markov chain texture features in discriminant analysis. Eur J Obstet Gynecol Reprod Biol 1978; 8:157–162.

17 Ausems EW, Kamp JK van der, Baak JP. Nuclear morphometry in the determination of the prognosis of marked atypical endometrial hyperplasia. Int J Gynecol Pathol 1985; 4:180–185.

18 Colgan TJ, Norris HJ, Foster W, et al. Predicting the outcome of endometrial hyperplasia by quantitative analysis of nuclear features using a linear discriminant function. Int J Gynecol Pathol 1983; 1:347–352.

19 Baak JP, Wisse-Brekelmans EC, Fleege JC, et al. Assessment of the risk on endometrial cancer in hyperplasia, by means of morphological and morphometrical features. Pathol Res Pr 1992; 188:856–859.

20 Baak JPA. The role of computerized morphometric and cytometric feature analysis in endometrial hyperplasia and cancer prognosis. J Cell Biochem 1995; 59 (Suppl 23):137–146.

21 Esteller M, Garcia A, Martinez-Palones JM, et al. Detection of clonality and genetic alterations in endometrial Pipelle biopsy and its surgical specimen counterpart. Lab Invest 1997; 76:109–116.

22 Jovanovic AS, Boynton KA, Mutter GL. Uteri of women with endometrial carcinoma contain a histopathologic spectrum of monoclonal putative precancers, some with microsatellite instability. Cancer Res 1996; 56:1917–1921.

23 Mutter GL, Chaponot M, Fletcher J. A PCR assay for non-random X chromosome inactivation identifies monoclonal endometrial cancers and precancers. Am J Pathol 1995; 146:501–508.

24 Mutter GL, Ince TA, Baak JPA, et al. Molecular identification of latent precancers in histologically normal endometrium. Cancer Res 2001; 61:4311–4314.

25 Mutter GL. Diagnosis of premalignant endometrial disease. J Clin Pathol 2002; 55(5):326–331.

26 Mutter GL. The Endometrial Collaborative Group. Endometrial intraepithelial neoplasia (EIN): Will it bring order to chaos? Gynecol Oncol 2000; 76:287–290.

27 Baak JP, Orbo A, Diest PJ van, et al. Prospective multicenter evaluation of the morphometric D-score for prediction of the outcome of endometrial hyperplasias. Am J Surg Pathol 2001; 25(7):930–935.

28 Dunton C, Baak J, Palazzo J, et al. Use of computerized morphometric analyses of endometrial hyperplasias in the prediction of coexistent cancer. Am J Obstet Gynecol 1996; 174:1518–1521.

29 Orbo A, Baak JP, Kleivan I, et al. Computerised morphometrical analysis in endometrial hyperplasia for the prediction of cancer development. A long-term retrospective study from northern Norway. J Clin Pathol 2000; 53(9):697–703.

30 Baak JPA, Mutter GL, Robboy S, et al. The molecular genetics and morphometry-based Endometrial Intraepithelial Neoplasia (EIN) classification scheme predicts the risk of progression to cancer more effectively than the WHO94 'Endometrial hyperplasia' system. Cancer 2005; 103(11): in press.

31 Silverberg SG, Mutter GL, Kurman RJ, et al. Tumors of the uterine corpus: epithelial tumors and related lesions. In: Tavassoli FA, Stratton MR, eds. WHO Classification of Tumors: Pathology and Genetics of Tumors of the Breast and Female Genital Organs. Lyon, France: IARC Press; 2003:221–232.

32 Hecht JL, Ince TA, Baker HE, Mutter GL. Concordance of WHO hyperplasia and EIN classification of endometrial precancers. Mod Path 2005; 18:324–330.

33 Parazzini F, Vecchia C La, Bocciolone L, Franceschi S. The epidemiology of endometrial cancer. Gynecol Oncol 1991; 41:1–16.

34 Writing Group for the PEPI Trial. Effects of hormone replacement therapy on endometrial histology in postmenopausal women. The postmenopausal estrogen/progestin interventions (PEPI) Trial. JAMA 1996; 275:370–375.

35 Woodruff JD, Pickar JH. Incidence of endometrial hyperplasia in postmenopausal women taking conjugated estrogens (Premarin) with medroxyprogesterone acetate or conjugated estrogens alone. Am J Obstet Gynecol 1994; 170:1213–1223.

36 Stanford JL, Brinton LA, Berman ML, et al. Oral contraceptives and endometrial cancer: Do other risk factors modify the association? Int J Cancer 1993; 54:243–248.

37 Weiderpass E, Adami HO, Baron JA, et al. Use of oral contraceptives and endometrial cancer risk (Sweden). Cancer Causes Control 1999; 10(4):277–284.

38 Aaltonen LA, Peltomaki P, Mecklin JP, et al. Replication errors in benign and malignant tumors from hereditary nonpolyposis colorectal cancer patients. Cancer Res 1994; 54:1645–1648.

39 Millar AL, Pal T, Madlensky L, et al. Mismatch repair gene defects contribute to the genetic basis of double primary cancers of the colorectum and endometrium. Hum Mol Genet 1999; 8(5):823–829.

40 Risinger JI, Berchuck A, Kohler MF, et al. Genetic instability of microsatellites in endometrial carcinoma. Cancer Res 1993; 53:5100–5103.

41 Zhou XP, Kuismanen S, Nystrom-Lahti M, et al. Distinct PTEN mutational spectra in hereditary non-polyposis colon cancer syndrome-related endometrial carcinomas compared to sporadic microsatellite unstable tumors. Hum Mol Genet 2002; 11(4):445–450.

42 Powell MA, Mutch DG. Identifying and treating hereditary colon and endometrial cancer. Cont Ob Gyn 2001:85–90.

43 Mutter GL. PTEN, a protean tumor suppressor. Am J Pathol 2001; 158:1895–1898.

44 Curry S, Kelly S. Cancer of the female genital tract: Overview. In: Osteen R, ed. Cancer manual. Boston, MA: American Cancer Society; 1990:253–257.

45 Wolfson AH, Sightler SE, Markoe AM, et al. The prognostic significance of surgical staging for carcinoma of the endometrium. Gynecol Oncol 1992; 45(2):142–146.

46 Anastasiadis PG, Skaphida PG, Koutlaki NG, et al. Descriptive epidemiology of endometrial hyperplasia in patients with abnormal uterine bleeding. Eur J Gynaecol Oncol 2000; 21(2):131–134.

47 Cheng WF, Lin HH, Torng PL, Huang SC. Comparison of endometrial changes among symptomatic tamoxifen-treated and nontreated premenopausal and postmenopausal breast cancer patients. Gynecol Oncol 1997; 66(2):233–237.

48 Cohen I, Perel E, Flex D, et al. Endometrial pathology in postmenopausal tamoxifen treatment: comparison between gynaecologically symptomatic and asymptomatic breast cancer patients. J Clin Pathol 1999; 52(4):278–282.

49 Cooper JM, Erickson ML. Endometrial sampling techniques in the diagnosis of abnormal uterine bleeding. Obstet Gynecol Clin North Am 2000; 27(2):235–244.

50 Epstein E. Management of postmenopausal bleeding in Sweden: a need for increased use of hydrosonography and hysteroscopy. Acta Obstet Gynecol Scand 2004; 83(1):89–95.

51 Loverro G, Bettocchi S, Cormio G, et al. Diagnostic accuracy of hysteroscopy in endometrial hyperplasia. Maturitas 1996; 25(3):187–191.

52 Tahir MM, Bigrigg MA, Browning JJ, et al. A randomised controlled trial comparing transvaginal ultrasound, outpatient hysteroscopy and endometrial biopsy with inpatient hysteroscopy and curettage. Br J Obstet Gynaecol 1999; 106(12):1259–1264.

53 Fleischer AC, Wheeler JE, Lindsay I, et al. An assessment of the value of ultrasonographic screening for endometrial disease in postmenopausal women without symptoms. Am J Obstet Gynecol 2001; 184(2):70–75.

54 Farrell T, Jones N, Owen P, Baird A. The significance of an 'insufficient' Pipelle sample in the investigation of post-menopausal bleeding. Acta Obstet Gynecol Scand 1999; 78(9):810–812.

55 Stock RJ, Kanbour A. Prehysterectomy curettage. Obstet Gynecol 1975; 45(5):537–541.

56 Stovall TG, Ling FW, Morgan PL. A prospective, randomized comparison of the Pipelle endometrial sampling device with the Novak curette. Am J Obstet Gynecol 1991; 165(5):1287–1290.

57 Kaunitz AM, Masciello A, Ostrowski M, Rovira EZ. Comparison of endometrial biopsy with the endometrial Pipelle and Vabra aspirator. J Reprod Med 1988; 33(5):427–431.

58 Ben Baruch G, Seidman DS, Schiff E, et al. Outpatient endometrial sampling with the Pipelle curette. Gynecol Obstet Invest 1994; 37(4):260–262.

59 Guido RS, Kanbour-Shakir A, Rulin MC, Christopherson WA. Pipelle endometrial sampling. Sensitivity in the detection of endometrial cancer. J Reprod Med 1995; 40(8):553–555.

60 Dijkhuizen FP, Mol BW, Brolmann HA, Heintz AP. The accuracy of endometrial sampling in the diagnosis of patients with endometrial carcinoma and hyperplasia: a meta-analysis. Cancer 2000; 89(8):1765–1772.

61 Mutter GL, Boynton KA, Faquin WC, et al. Allelotype mapping of unstable microsatellites establishes direct lineage continuity between endometrial precancers and cancer. Cancer Res 1996; 56:4483–4486.

62 Faquin WC, Fitzgerald JT, Boynton KA, Mutter GL. Intratumoral genetic heterogeneity and progression of endometrioid type endometrial adenocarcinomas. Gynecol Oncol 2000; 78:152–157.

63 Levine RL, Cargile CB, Blazes MS, et al. PTEN mutations and microsatellite instability in complex atypical hyperplasia, a precursor lesion to uterine endometrioid carcinoma. Cancer Res 1998; 58:3254–3258.

64 Maxwell G, Risinger J, Gumbs C, et al. Mutation of the PTEN tumor suppressor gene in endometrial hyperplasias. Cancer Res 1998; 58:2500–2503.

65 Mutter GL, Lin MC, Fitzgerald JT, et al. Altered PTEN expression as a diagnostic marker for the earliest endometrial precancers. J Natl Cancer Inst 2000; 92:924–930.

66 Duggan BD, Felix JC, Muderspach LI, et al. Early mutational activation of the c-Ki-ras oncogene in endometrial carcinoma. Cancer Res 1994; 54:1604–1607.

67 Mutter GL, Wada H, Faquin W, Enomoto T. K-ras mutations appear in the premalignant phase of both microsatellite stable and unstable endometrial carcinogenesis. Mol Pathol 1999; 52:257–262.

68 Sasaki H, Nishii H, Takahashi H, et al. Mutation of the Ki-ras protooncogene in human endometrial hyperplasia and carcinoma. Cancer Res 1993; 53:1906–1910.

69 Esteller M, Catasus L, Matias-Guiu X, et al. hMLH1 Promoter hypermethylation is an early event in human endometrial tumorigenesis. Am J Pathol 1999; 155(5):1767–1772.

70 Mutter GL, Lin MC, Fitzgerald JT, et al. Changes in endometrial PTEN expression throughout the human menstrual cycle. J Clin Endocrinol Metab 2000; 85:2334–2338.

71 Zheng W, Baker HE, Mutter GL. Involution of PTEN-null endometrial glands with progestin therapy. Gynecol Oncol 2004; 92:1008–1013.

72 Stambolic V, Tsao MS, Macpherson D, et al. High incidence of breast and endometrial neoplasia resembling human Cowden syndrome in PTEN mice. Cancer Res 2000; 60(13):3605–3611.

73 Perren A, Weng L, Boag A, et al. Immunocytochemical evidence of loss of PTEN expression in primary ductal adenocarcinomas of the breast. Am J Pathol 1999; 155:1253–1260.

74 Esteller M, Levine R, Baylin SB, Ellenson LH, Herman JG. MLH1 promoter hypermethylation is associated with the microsatellite instability phenotype in sporadic endometrial carcinomas. Oncogene 1998; 17:2413–2417.

75 Burks RT, Kessis TD, Cho KR, Hedrick L. Microsatellite instability in endometrial carcinoma. Oncogene 1994; 9:1163–1166.

76 Duggan BD, Felix JC, Muderspach LI, et al. Microsatellite instability in sporadic endometrial carcinoma. J Natl Cancer Inst 1994; 86:1216–1221.

77 Faquin WC, Fitzgerald JT, Lin MC, et al. Sporadic microsatellite instability is specific to neoplastic and preneoplastic endometrial tissues. Am J Clin Pathol 2000; 113(4):576–582.

78 Simpkins SB, Bocker T, Swisher EM, et al. MLH1 promoter methylation and gene silencing is the primary cause of microsatellite instability in sporadic endometrial cancers. Hum Mol Genet 1999; 8(4):661–666.

79 Lax SF, Kendall B, Tashiro H, et al. The frequency of p53, K-ras mutations and microsatellite instability differs in uterine endometrioid and serous carcinoma: evidence of distinct molecular genetic pathways. Cancer 2000; 88(4):814–824.

80 Sherman ME, Bur ME, Kurman RJ. p53 in endometrial cancer and its putative precursors: evidence for diverse pathways of tumorigenesis. Hum Pathol 1995; 26:1268–1274.

81 Wang S, Pudney J, Song J, et al. Mechanisms involved in the evolution of progestin resistance in human endometrial hyperplasia – precursor of endometrial cancer. Gynecol Oncol 2003; 88:108–117.

82 Montz FJ, Bristow RE, Bovicelli A, et al. Intrauterine progesterone treatment of early endometrial cancer. Am J Obstet Gynecol 2002; 186(4):651–657.

83 Randall TC, Kurman RJ. Progestin treatment of atypical hyperplasia and well-differentiated carcinoma of the endometrium in women under age 40. Obstet Gynecol 1997; 90(3):434–440.

84 Perino A, Quartararo P, Catinella E, et al. Treatment of endometrial hyperplasia with levonorgestrel releasing intrauterine devices. Acta Eur Fertil 1987; 18(2):137–140.

85 Sturridge F, Guillebaud J. A risk-benefit assessment of the levonorgestrel-releasing intrauterine system. Drug Saf 1996; 15(6):430–440.

86 Mutter GL. A focus on premalignant lesions of the endometrium. www.endometrium.org; 2003.

18

Altered endometrial differentiation (metaplasia)

Christopher P. Crum,

Marisa R. Nucci and

George L. Mutter

Introduction

Origins of metaplasia

The patient at risk

Classification and outcome

Squamous metaplasia
Surface epithelial changes
(the repair–metaplasia sequence)

Mucinous metaplasia
Tubal metaplasia
Eosinophilic metaplasia
Other epithelial (oxyphilic)
 metaplasias
An algorithm for assessing
 metaplasia
Non-epithelial metaplasias/
 heterotopias of the
 endometrium

Introduction

Endometrial metaplasia is defined as epithelial differentiation that differs from the conventional endometrioid epithelium. Altered differentiation is a preferred term to avoid implying that the distinction between metaplasia and neoplasia can always be made. However, for simplicity, the term metaplasia will be used in this chapter.

In a sense, metaplastic changes are the 'pathologist's disease'. They are not recognized clinical disorders and the clinician does not routinely record 'rule out metaplasia' on the pathology requisition. Rather, metaplastic changes are a spectrum of processes that may be benign, or signal the presence of a neoplastic process. When the pathologist encounters altered differentiation during the examination of endometrial biopsies or curettings, he or she must determine the risk of neoplasia and advise the clinical caregiver to pursue the most appropriate course of action.

Metaplasia in the endometrium may occur in benign conditions, arise in association with endometrial intraepithelial neoplasia (EIN) or be associated with endometrial carcinomas. Because of the wide range of entities associated with metaplasia, these changes can be viewed as a 'parallel universe' composed of altered differentiation that interdigitates with and mirrors the biology of, the endometrial surface and glandular epithelium (Table 18.1). Not unexpectedly, the precise distinction of an endometrial metaplastic phenomenon from a neoplastic lesion may at times be difficult and the practitioner will be tempted to use certain descriptive terms, such as 'atypical metaplasia' or 'complex metaplasia' to convey the diagnostic uncertainty that these changes evoke. The purpose of this chapter is to review the spectrum of altered differentiation of the endometrium, identify those changes that carry the greatest risk of cancer and distinguish them from those that pose a lesser risk.

Table 18.1 Location of endometrial metaplasia

Metaplasia	Location
Papillary syncytial	Surface epithelium
Squamous	
Reactive	Surface epithelium
Morular	Glands
Ichthyosis	Surface and glands
Ciliated	Glands, surface epithelium
Mucinous	Glands, surface epithelium
Eosinophilic	Glands, surface epithelium
Hobnail	Glands, surface epithelium

Origins of metaplasia

The prototype metaplasia in the uterus is inherently related to the transition from columnar to squamous epithelium. This transition is essentially a redirection of cell fate and begins in the lower genital tract during fetal life, when Müllerian epithelium undergoes transformation to a squamous phenotype via the development of reserve cells (Fig. 18.1).[1,2] This process occurs via the induction of p63, which is induced in the basal cells of these primitive epithelia and mediates a redirection of cell differentiation to squamous (and urothelial) (Figs 18.1, 18.2).[1,2] A second consequence of this process is the appearance of reserve cells in the cervix (Figs 18.2a, 18.3a). These cells are best known for their capacity to undergo squamous (and possibly columnar) metaplasia in the cervix during adult life.[3]

Basal cells of the prostate and myoepithelial cells of the breast have a similar origin as reserve cells, but are uniformly and permanently distributed beneath the columnar epithelium of their respective sites. In contrast, reserve cells of the cervix vary in distribution and number and may appear *de novo* at any time during the reproductive years. A commonly encountered scenario which supports the latter concept is the proliferation of columnar epithelium in the form of microglandular change, which is common in reproductive life, although its relationship with specific hormonally active conditions (contraceptives or pregnancy) remains unclear.[4] Immunohistochemical studies have shown that this proliferation is characterized by the gradual transition from an immature columnar to a reserve cell and ultimately to a squamous phenotype (Fig. 18.3b–d).[5,6] In this setting the reserve cells, like the other basal or squamous epithelia generated during fetal life, are produced from proliferating Müllerian columnar epithelium.

Although reserve cells are traditionally associated with the cervix, cells with a similar appearance can be identified in the endometrium.[7] p63-positive columnar cells are conspicuous by immunostaining in the uterus during fetal life, presumably due to stromal–epithelial interactions that occur under the influence of hormones (Fig. 18.2b).[8] These cells essentially disappear after birth in both the lower uterine segment and endometrium but remain in the cervix. In, proliferative phase endometrium, occasional p63-positive cells may be seen; these cells are sporadically distributed in the glands, are not basal in orientation and range from 1–3 nuclei per gland. Whether these cells represent endometrial reserve cells is unlikely. In premenopausal women,

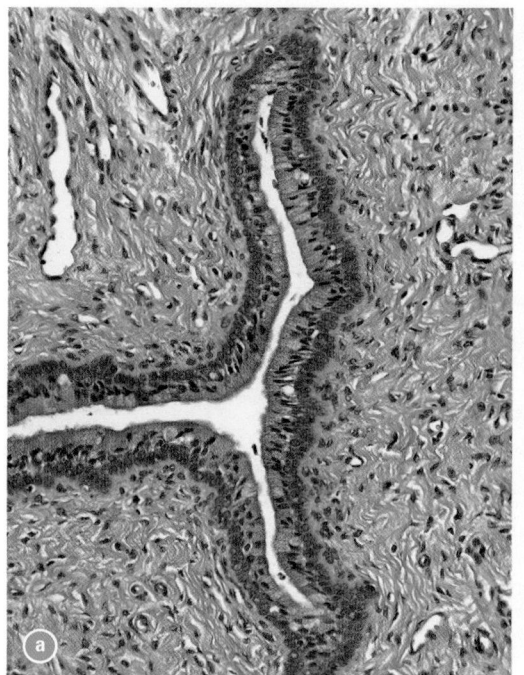 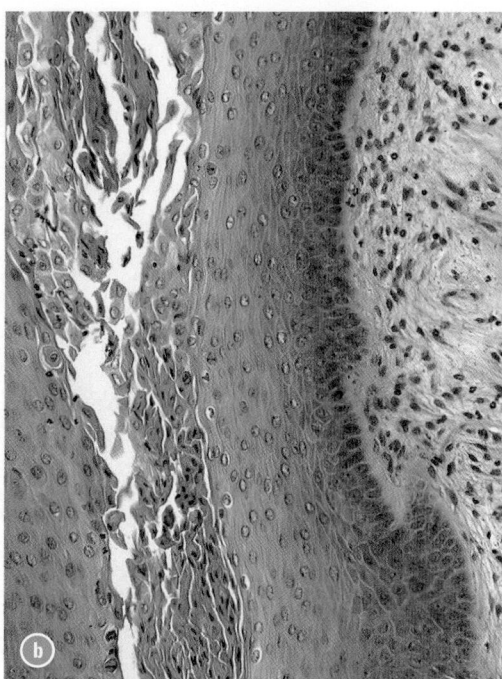

Fig. 18.1 Origins of squamous epithelium in the lower genital tract. (a) In the newborn mouse, reserve cells are induced at the epithelial–stromal interface in the vagina, resulting in a bilayered epithelium at birth. (b) Following estrogenic stimulation, these cells undergo squamous differentiation with shedding of the overlying columnar epithelium. In the human, the process of squamous differentiation occurs prior to birth.

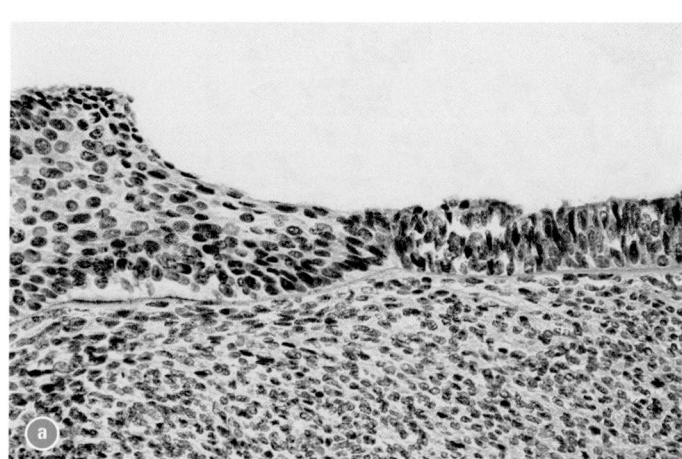 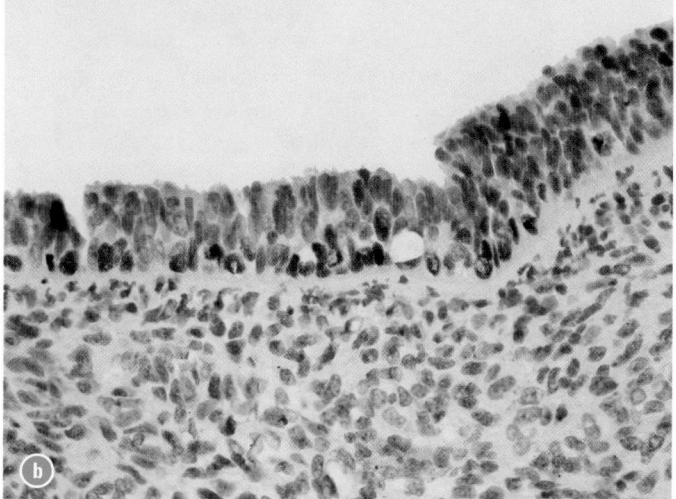

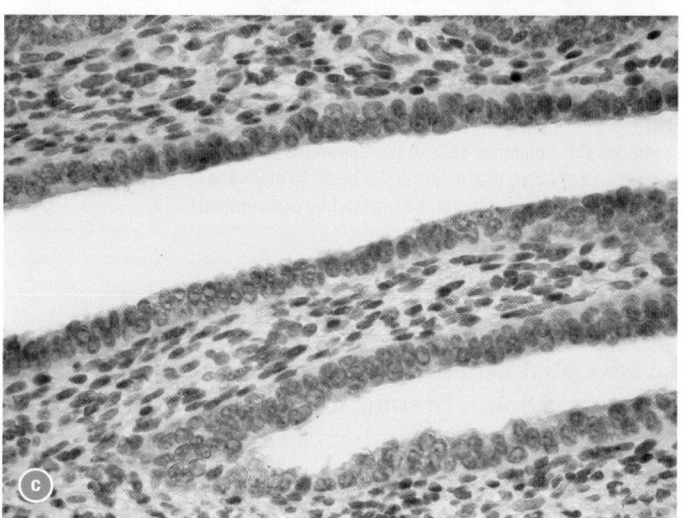

Fig. 18.2 p63 expression in the epithelial cells of the cervix and uterus prior to birth. (a) The squamous epithelium stains strongly for p63 (left), merging with Müllerian epithelium (right) with basal p63 staining. (b) Focal basal cells are highlighted in the uterine fundus, but (c) the fallopian tubes are devoid of staining. This underscores the importance of the epithelial–stromal relationships in the cervix and uterus.

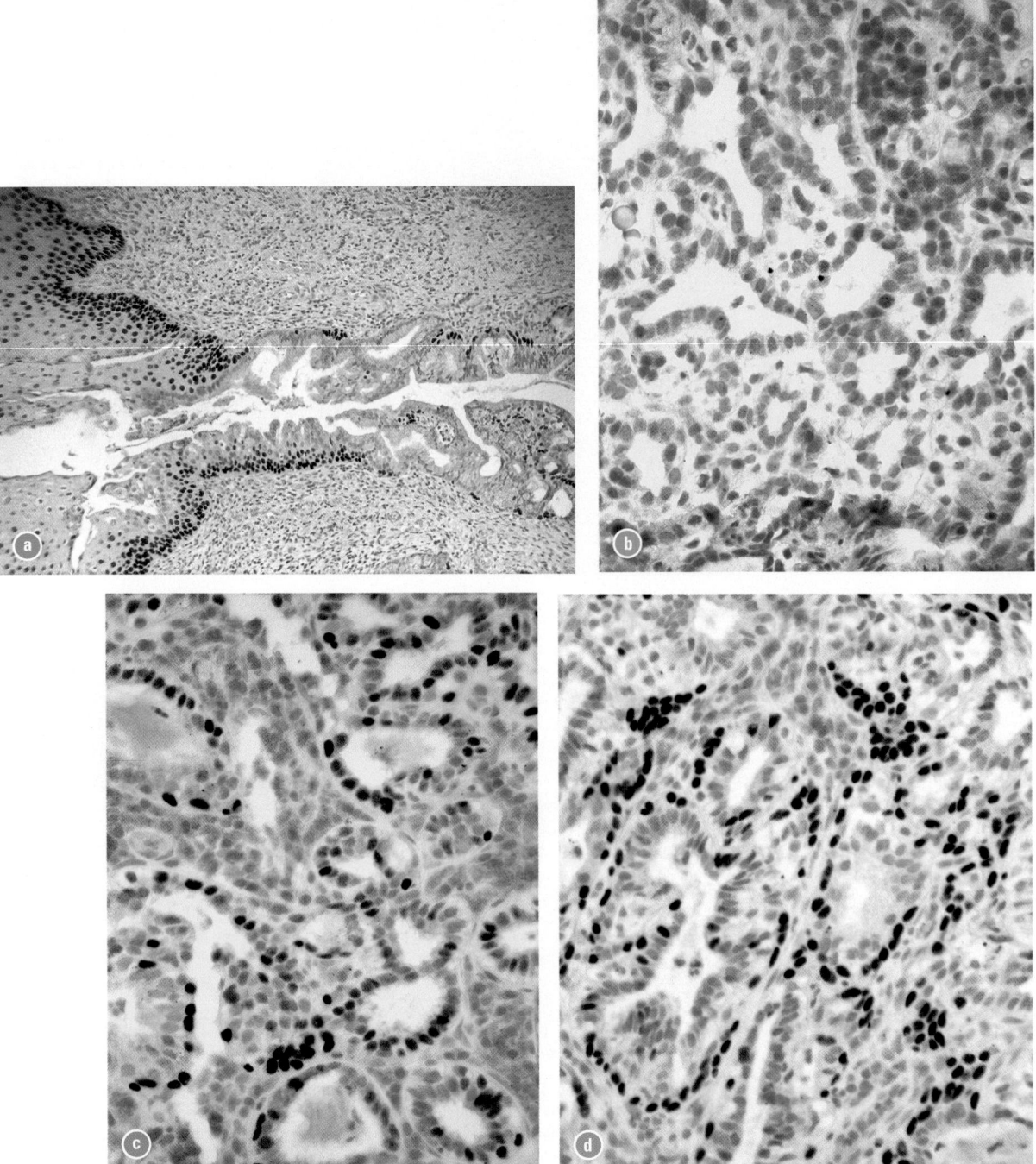

Fig. 18.3 (a) p63 expression in cervix typically diminishes cephalad (right) to involve scattered sub-columnar cells in the upper endocervix. (b) In microglandular change, p63 expression is weakly present in early glandular proliferation. (c) Later, glandular nuclei begin to stain and still later (d) distinct populations of reserve cells emerge. (d) This conforms to a model in which reserve cells can be created by proliferation of surface columnar cells. (From reference 5, with permission).

regenerating endometrium following menstrual or anovulatory breakdown, a situation in which one might expect to find these cells, does not typically demonstrate p63 positive basal or reserve cells. However, postmenopausal endometria, particularly polyps, may be associated with foci of p63-positive basal or 'reserve' cells (Fig. 18.4a). In some instances, the basal/reserve cells are not conspicuous but can be highlighted by p63 immunostaining (Fig. 18.4b,c). Squamous (including morular) metaplasia is strongly p63 positive and may

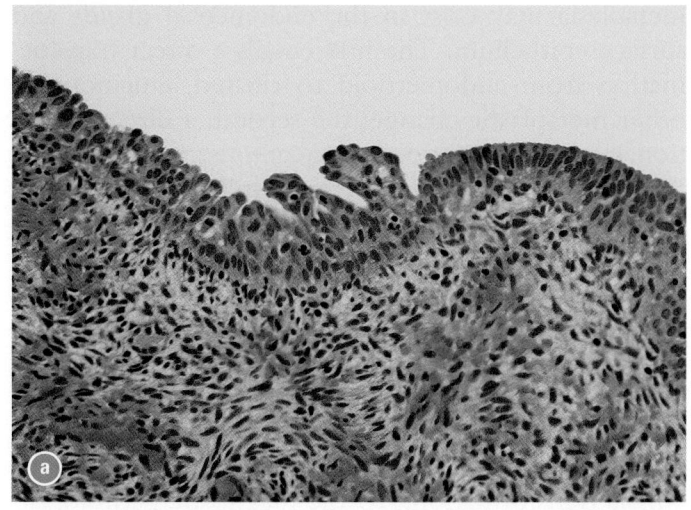

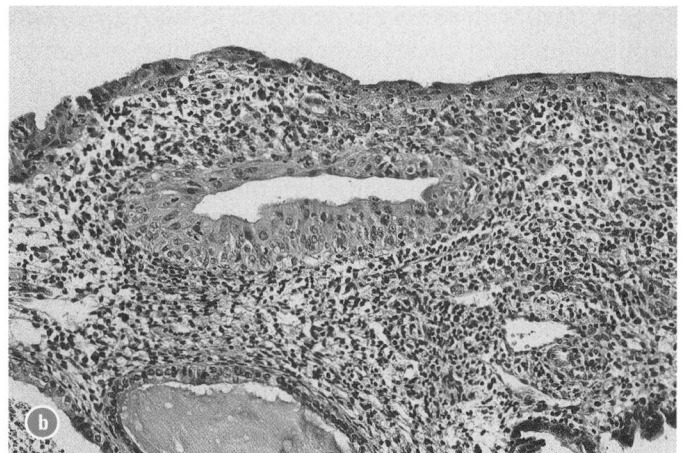

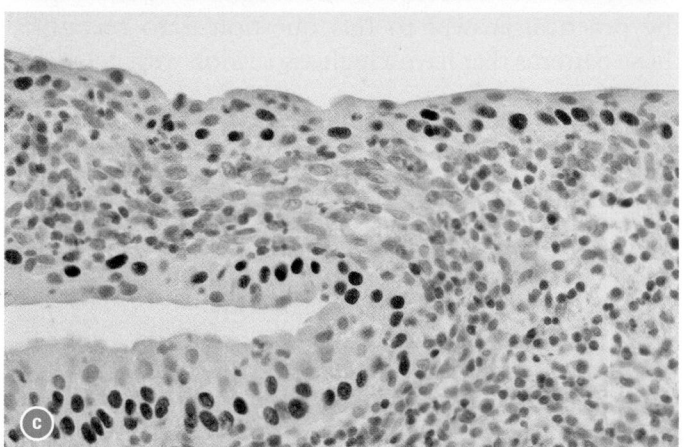

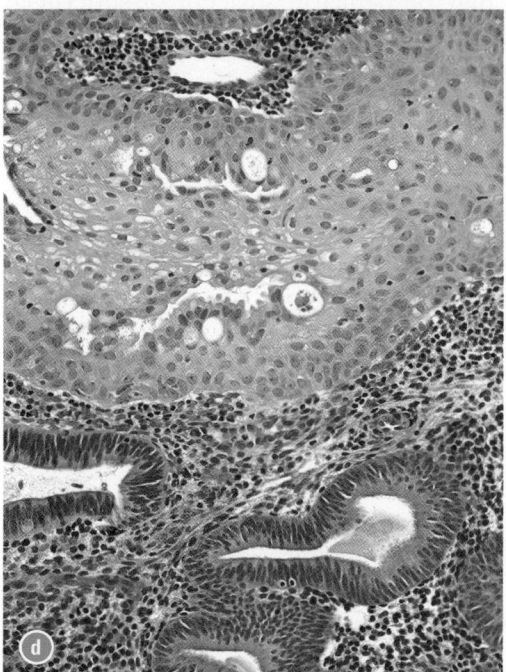

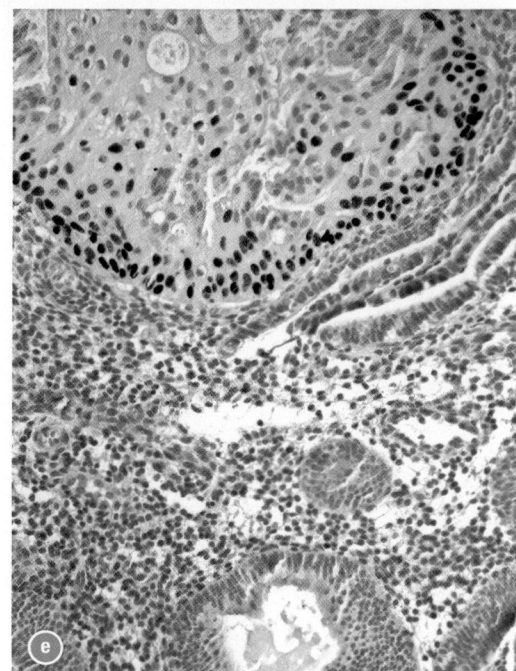

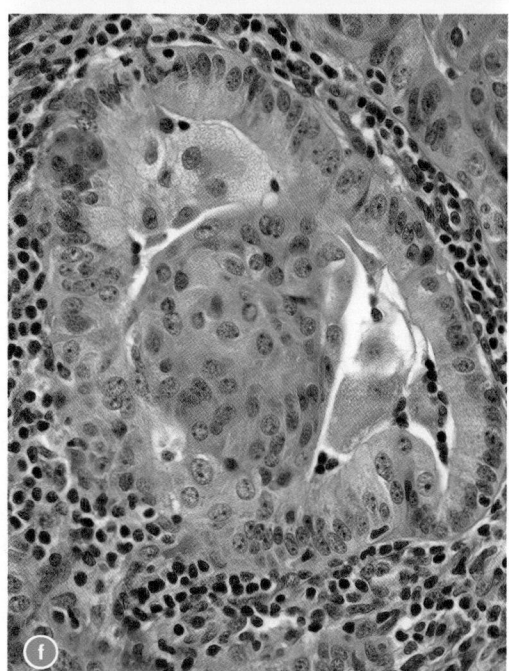

Fig. 18.4 Possible origins of basal or reserve cells in the uterus in a postmenopausal woman. (a) Reserve cells underly a micropapillary proliferation of surface epithelium (center). (b) Otherwise inconspicuous basal cells in this postmenopausal uterus are highlighted by p63 staining (c). Squamous metaplasia (d, upper) is admixed with and distinguished from, columnar epithelium by the presence of p63-positive cells (e). (f) Squamous metaplasia is often present on the luminal surface in the glandular epithelium (center).

be associated with reserve-type cells (Fig. 18.4d,e).[7] The implication from these associations is that columnar epithelial cells of the uterus are capable, under certain conditions, of forming reserve-type cells. Although the cause is unknown, the alterations in hormonal status that characterize menopause coupled with epithelial–stromal breakdown and repair may set the stage for these changes to occur.[8]

Because mucinous and tubal metaplasias occur in both the endocervix and endometrium in the absence of reserve cells, their development does not appear dependent on transition through a reserve cell phase. Moreover, squamous metaplasia (morules) in the endometrium may be beneath, adjacent or superficial to the columnar epithelium, suggesting an origin directly from either the columnar cells or subcolumnar reserve cells (Fig. 18.4e,f). Thus, at least three pathways to

metaplasia may exist in the endometrial glands and surface epithelium. The first entails a direct transformation from endometrioid to ciliated/mucinous or other metaplastic change; the second, a direct transition from endometrioid to squamous; and the third, the creation of a reserve cell population that subsequently undergoes squamous (or perhaps other forms of) metaplasia. Conceivably, more than one pathway is initiated in the same epithelium or one pathway may lead to different alterations in differentiation, explaining the not infrequent coexistence of mucinous, tubal and/or squamous elements in the same lesion (Fig. 18.4d). What is not clear is when and to what degree metaplastic changes in the endometrium signify *neoplastic* transformation. To the diagnostic pathologist, the practical answer to this question is to recognize those patterns that have a high association with neoplasia.

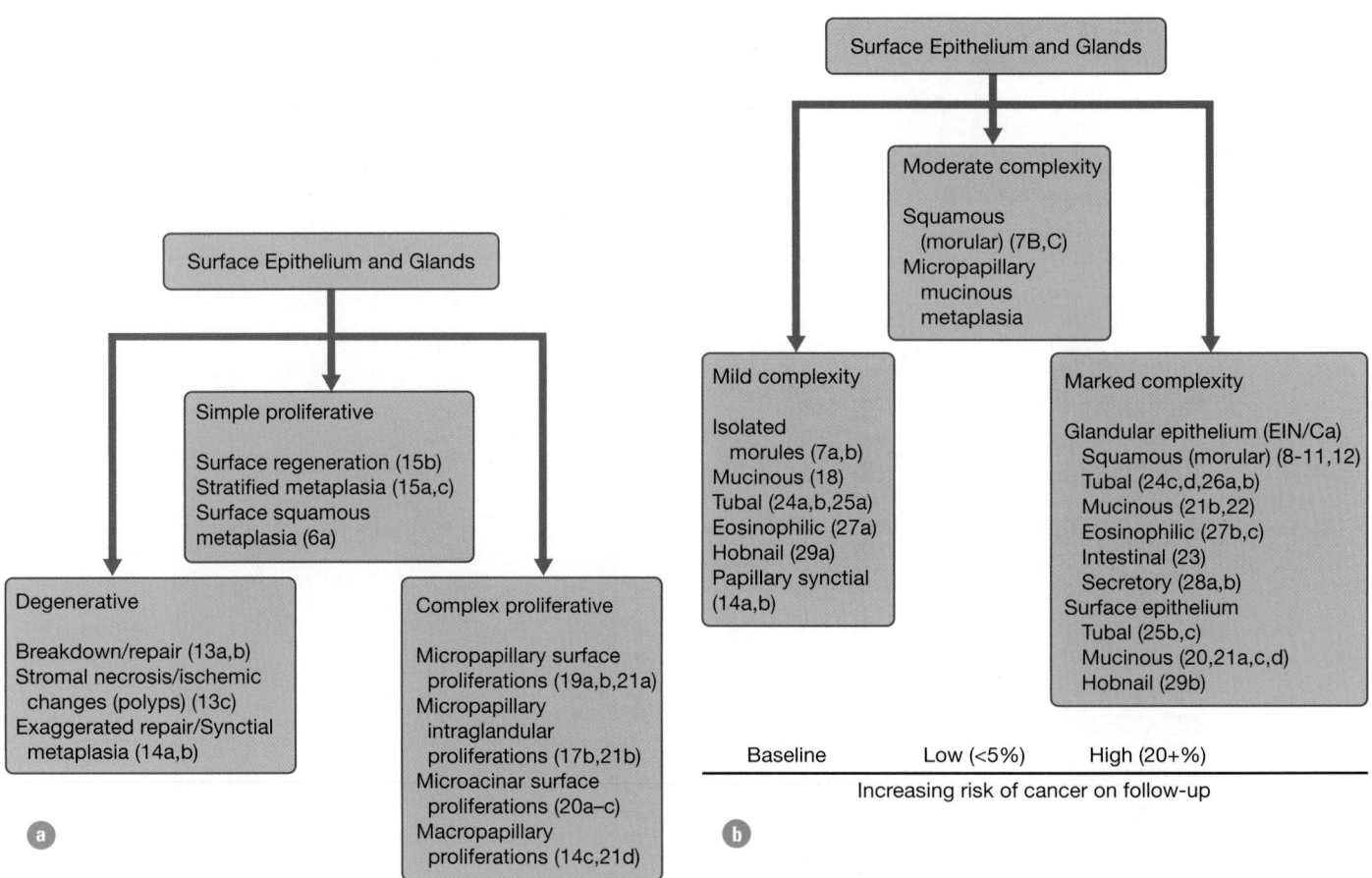

Fig. 18.5 Two parallel schematics for epithelial proliferations of the endometrium. (a) Range of generic epithelial alterations in the surface epithelium and within glands. (b) Range of metaplastic alterations. In both, risk of coexisting or subsequent cancer increases as a function of epithelial complexity. Corresponding figures are in parentheses.

The patient at risk

Metaplasia may be encountered in curettings from both pre- and postmenopausal women. Squamous metaplasia (morules) are most common in women who are menopausal or undergoing evaluation for infertility, but can emerge spontaneously in association with normal cycling endometrium.[9,10] Other metaplasias, specifically tubal, mucinous, syncytial and other variants, are most common in association with menopause, including hormone replacement therapy.[9] All of these forms of metaplasia exhibit a range of architectural complexity, from non-complex simple strips of surface or glandular epithelia, to glands with architectural complexity synonymous with endometrial intraepithelial neoplasia, to frank adenocarcinoma (Fig. 18.5a,b).[11–13] The following is a breakdown of their categories and morphologic patterns.

Classification and outcome of endometrial metaplasia

Each of the following categories illustrates a range of epithelial changes that depict a spectrum from benign to malignant. Lesions in the latter category are addressed in Chapters 17 and 19. The portrayed range of epithelial atypias does not necessarily imply that each is part of a biologic progression or continuum. Rather, each is shown to assist the reader in identifying patterns and identifying those that deserve careful follow-up. The reader is advised that the morphologic distinction between syncytial, mucinous, ciliated (tubal), eosinophilic and even squamous metaplasia may not always be clear-cut, inasmuch as many of these patterns may be present in the same specimen or intermingled within the same gland or focus. Moreover, certain 'metaplasias' cannot be classified into a certain subtype, consisting only of cells with pale or eosinophilic cytoplasm and no specific form of differentiation.

Metaplasias vary in their presentation. Squamous metaplasia is viewed as a process that most frequently involves the gland unit or the interglandular space (morular metaplasia). Syncytial metaplasia characteristically predominates in the surface epithelium in areas of stromal breakdown and mucinous and tubal metaplasias can arise from either surface epithelium or underlying glands. In this discussion, two perspectives of metaplasia will be addressed. The first is the catego-rization of metaplasias *per se* by cell differentiation, each with its own range of complexity. The second is the attention to two parameters that may signal increased risk of endometrial cancer: (1) coexisting endometrioid glandular complexity and (2) epithelial complexity within the metaplastic epithelium *per se*. The latter is subdivided into three components, comprising stratified, papillary and microglandular architecture. Thus, when confronted with a metaplastic change, the pathologist must assess: (1) the degree of complexity in the associated endometrial glandular epithelium, (2) the extent of stratification and atypia in surface epithelial changes and (3) the extent of complex architecture produced by the metaplastic process, including microglandular and papillary features. These parameters must be addressed repeatedly by the pathologist and comprise an algorithm of exclusions applied to every endometrial sample.

SQUAMOUS METAPLASIA

Squamous metaplasia manifests as a range of changes from benign reactive processes to squamous differen-tiation in carcinomas. Benign changes include those associated with chronic endometritis, intrauterine devices and trauma (Fig. 18.6a).[14,15] Typically, reactive metaplasia is present as scattered surface foci. A poorly under-stood variant of squamous metaplasia is *ichthyosis uteri* (Fig. 18.6b).[16] Although such lesions have been classi-fied as exaggerated metaplasias of the endometrium, they may be extensive, forming cyst-like spaces in the myometrium and on occasion, may be associated with squamous neoplasia.[17] Extensive squamous prolifera-tions, even if morphologically benign, deserve careful scrutiny.

The second and more common pattern of squa-mous differentiation is *morular metaplasia*, depicted as small, round, cohesive and regular 'granuloma-like' aggregates of immature squamous cells located within the gland tract (Fig. 18.7a–d). The central location of the morule suggests replacement of the gland tract by squamous metaplasia, with a secondary proliferation of columnar epithelium, not unlike cervical microglan-dular metaplasia (Fig. 18.7b). The squamous morule may be centrally placed (luminal) or between glands, often exhibits central necrosis and may merge with more mature squamous differentiation (Fig. 18.7d). Isolated morular metaplasia – with minimal or no glandular proliferation – is not uncommon in reproductive age women (Fig. 18.7a). However, morular metaplasia is frequently associated with some degree of gland crowd-

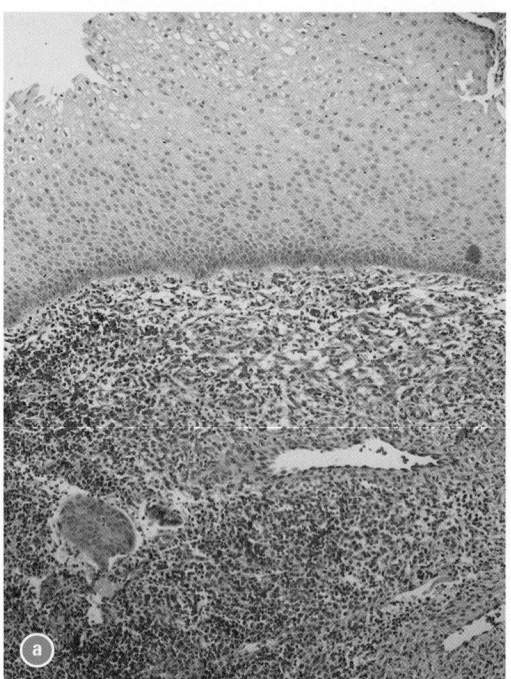
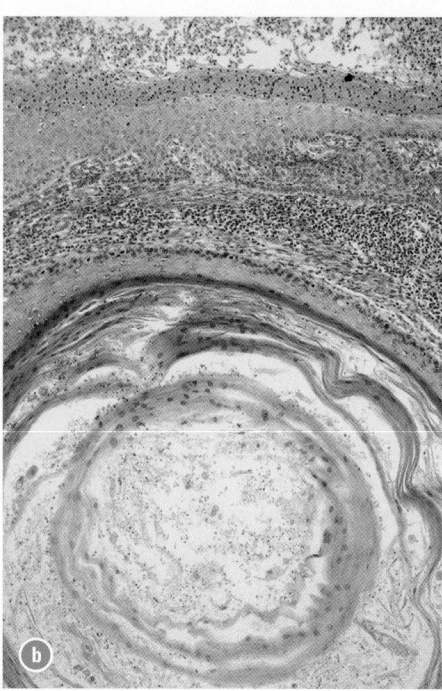

Fig. 18.6 Reactive changes. (a) Associated with IUD. (b) Ichthyosis uteri, with extensive squamous differentiation.

ing, which makes its interpretation more challenging. (Fig. 18.7b).[9,10]

The classification of these minor gland proliferations associated with morular metaplasia is problematic, inasmuch as the degree of gland crowding and/or altered epithelial appearance required to justify a diagnosis of EIN may not be present. When these benign-appearing changes are more extensive, they may raise a concern for EIN or cancer (Fig. 18.7c). The transition from squamous morules (or morular metaplasia) to EIN with squamous differentiation requires the presence of both glandular crowding and altered cytologic features within the glandular epithelium as compared to the surrounding normal endometrial glands (Fig. 18.8). Nevertheless, as discussed below, gland crowding alone without cytologic changes may be a risk factor for subsequent endometrial carcinoma irrespective of its degree of stratification and atypia.

Squamous morules are cytologically and architecturally uniform in EIN as wells as lesions that cannot be classified as EIN. In contrast, squamous differentiation associated with endometrial adenocarcinomas is more variable. In some lesions, discrete morules are present and the diagnosis of cancer is based strictly on the glandular architecture (Fig. 18.9). In others, there is aberrant differentiation or keratinization (Fig. 18.10). As discussed in Chapter 19, the terms 'adenoacanthoma' and 'adenosquamous carcinoma' have been abandoned in lieu of 'adenocarcinoma with squamous differentiation'.[18] In some instances, the carcinomatous/glandular component may be very subtle. More poorly-differentiated neoplasms include squamous carcinoma (which will be discussed in Chapter 19), as well as rare well-differentiated squamous neoplasms, including condylomata of the endometrial cavity and atypical polypoid adenomyomas.[19–22]

Most morular metaplasias have a benign outcome.[9,10,23,24] In a recent follow-up study of morular metaplasia at the Brigham and Women's Hospital, we found that less than 5% of endometrial biopsies or curettings classified as uncomplicated (i.e. without hyperplasia) morular metaplasia were followed by a histologically proven endometrial adenocarcinoma (Table 18.2).[24] In contrast, morular metaplasias described in association with either gland proliferation/crowding or EIN were followed by adenocarcinoma in 14% of cases.[23,24] Rarely, ovarian neoplasms have developed concurrently or subsequent to a diagnosis of endometrial morular metaplasia.[25] Because in occasional cases morules re-emerge after an interval of normal biopsies, periodic follow-up is warranted. Unfortunately, morular metaplasia is often encountered in reproductive aged women and the chances of a successful pregnancy following treatment are considered low, which may be a reflection of the altered hormonal state (estrogenic) presumed asso-

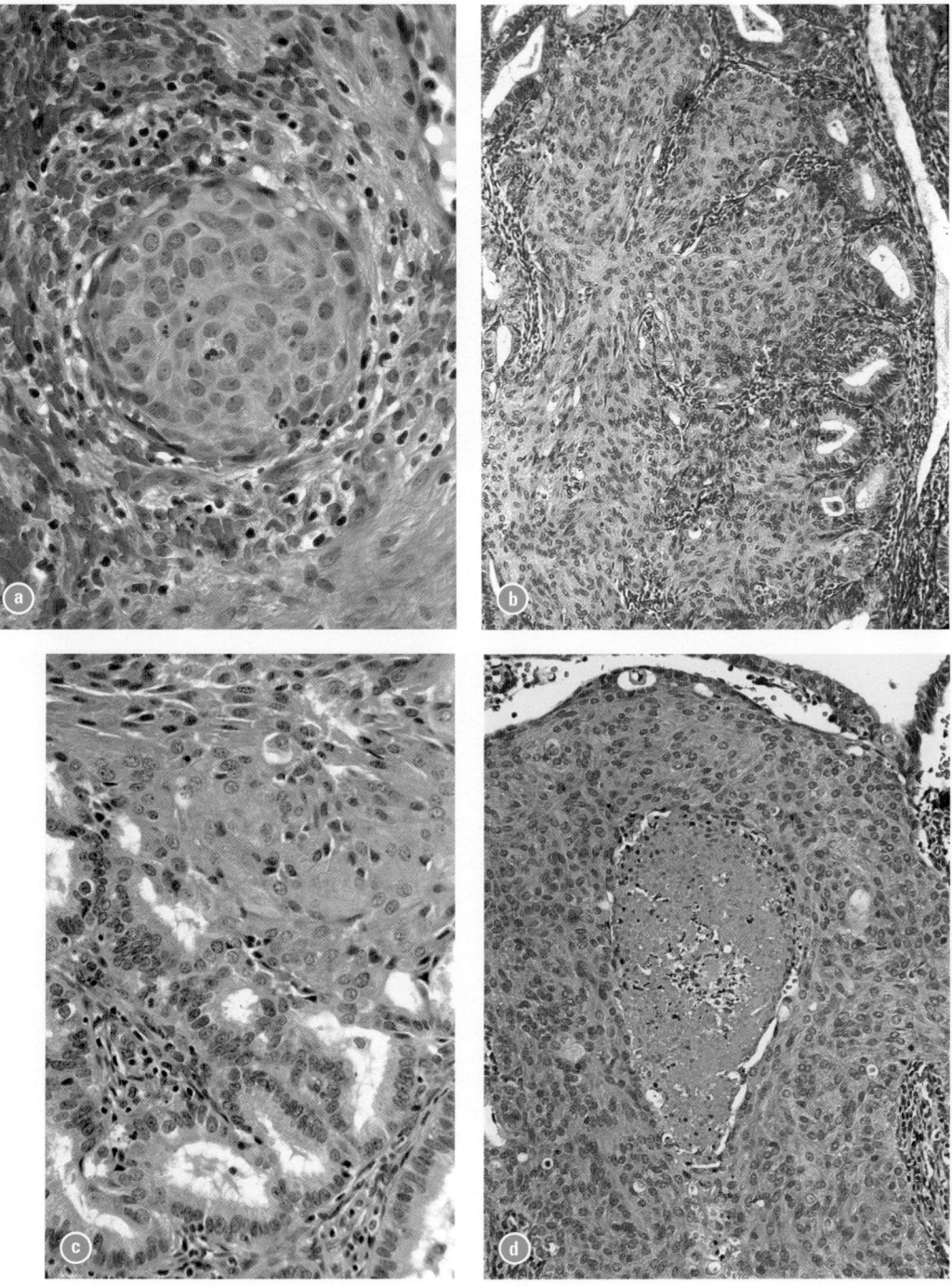

Fig. 18.7 (a) Isolated squamous morules with no coexisting glandular proliferation. This carries a low risk of subsequent adenocarcinoma. (b) Squamous morules associated with a collar of non-crowded glands. (c) Morular metaplasia with gland crowding and minimal atypia. (d) Central necrosis is common in morules.

Table 18.2 *Follow-up of cases diagnosed with morular metaplasia*[24]

Pattern	N	Morphology	Follow-up (%) (mean 25 months)		
			Normal	Hyperplasia	Cancer
Grade 1	29	Isolated/no gland crowding	89.7	6.7	3.4
Grade 2	28	Gland crowding	57.1	28.6	14.3
Grade 3	19	Crowding/cytologic change (EIN)	42.1	42.1	15.7

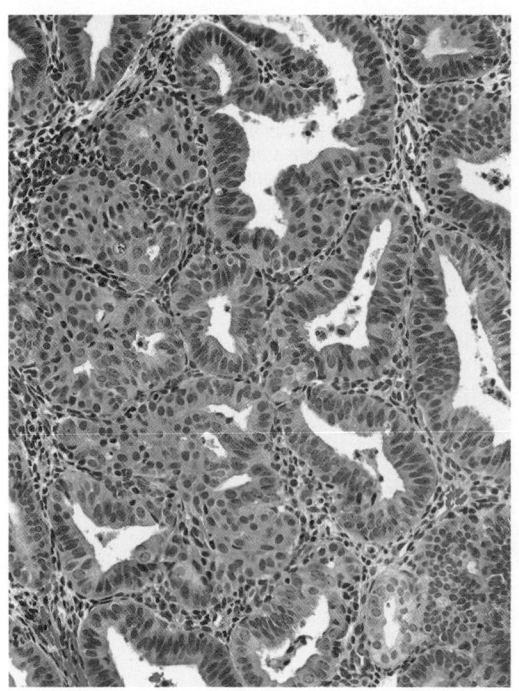

Fig. 18.8 Squamous morules with gland crowding and atypia, justifying a diagnosis of endometrial intraepithelial neoplasia.

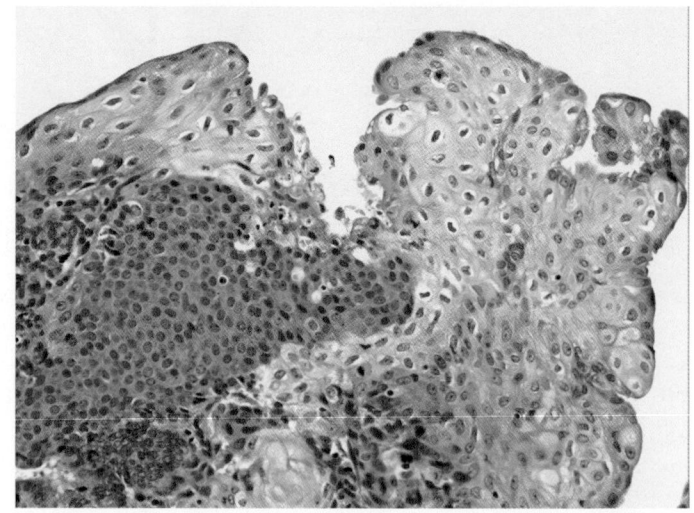

Fig. 18.10 Disorganized squamous differentiation associated with endometrial adenocarcinoma.

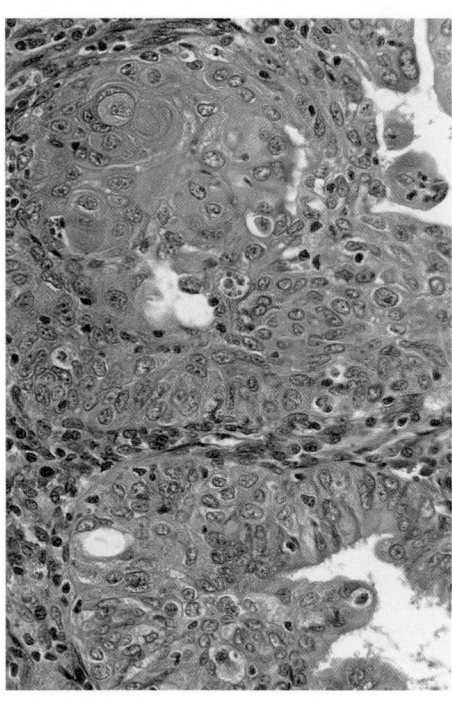

Fig. 18.9 Endometrial adenocarcinoma with discrete nests of squamous differentiation (top center).

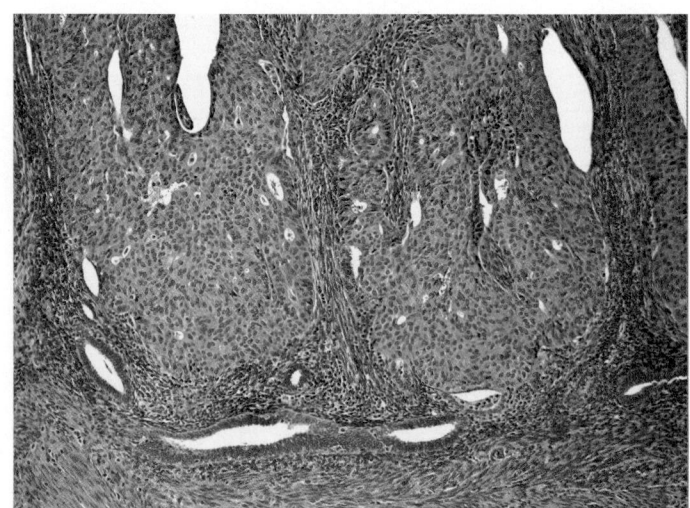

Fig. 18.11 Sheets of cohesive morular metaplasia with focal glandular differentiation.

ciated with the formation of morules as well as possibly a cause for infertility.

Pitfalls in the diagnosis of squamous metaplasia of the endometrium include both the over- and under-diagnosis of endometrial cancer. Sheets of endometrial squamous metaplasia may be difficult to distinguish from malignancy (Fig. 18.11). Alternatively, foci of apparently benign squamous epithelium may be present in the endometrium associated with more advanced disease, including squamous carcinoma (Fig. 18.12).[26] A similar pitfall is the misinterpretation of metastatic carcinoma to the cervix as native squamous metaplasia. These are discussed in greater detail in the chapter on endometrial cancer. Lastly, atypical polypoid adenomyomas, which combine morular metaplasia with atypical glands in a myomatous stroma, may be confused with either conventional morular metaplasia in

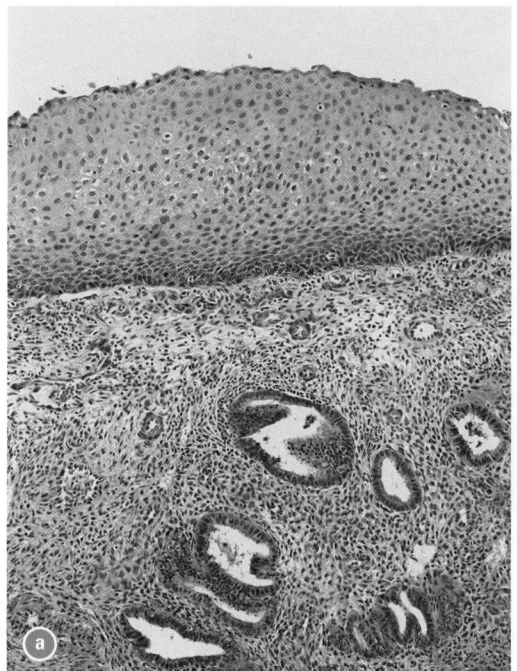 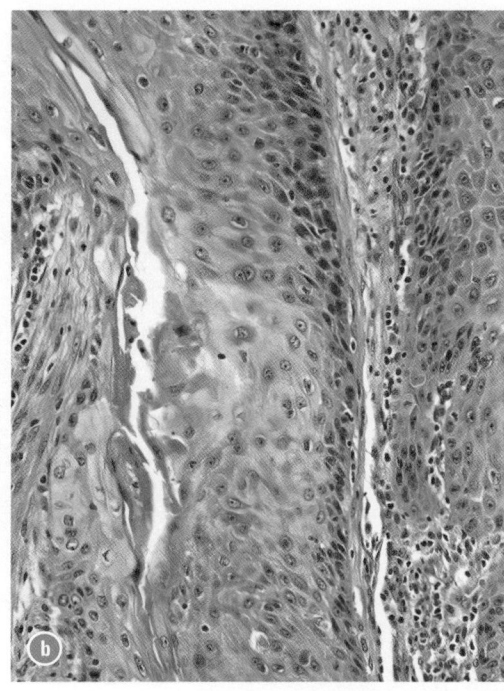

Fig. 18.12 (a) Benign-appearing squamous differentiation on the endometrial surface. (b) Squamous carcinoma of the endometrium from the same case.

polyps or adenocarcinoma. These are discussed in greater detail in Chapter 19.

SURFACE EPITHELIAL CHANGES (THE REPAIR-METAPLASIA SEQUENCE)

As previously discussed, metaplasias can occur both in the glands and on the endometrial surface. Origins for the latter include (1) *de novo* transformation of the surface epithelium and (2) extension of glandular lesions to the surface. Irrespective of the origin of surface metaplasias, they may morphologically imperceptibly merge with a range of surface proliferations that include repair (and breakdown) on one end to complex lesions including cancer on the other. Whether or not there is a direct relationship between repair and metaplasia, the practitioner often confronts altered surface epithelial changes and must determine whether they signify a risk for neoplasia. The term 'repair' may be a misnomer, as the epithelial changes are degenerative in some settings but proliferative in others.[27] Similarly, the changes, while designated as metaplasias, may be difficult to classify.

Degenerative surface epithelial changes (repair) are typically seen in unscheduled breakdown during menopause, or in association with hormonal replacement therapy (Fig. 18.13a). Characteristically, degenerative repair exhibits layered, unpolarized epithelial cell aggregates overlying stromal breakdown; in addition, some stratification (Fig. 18.13b), apoptosis and scant inflammatory cells may be present. The most likely cause of the epithelial changes is the underlying degenerative process in the stroma with loss of vascular supply. A second pattern is seen with necrotic polyps. In this scenario, the underlying stimulus is not breakdown but stromal ischemia and necrosis (Fig. 18.13c). In contrast to the syncytial clusters of epithelial cells seen in breakdown, the epithelium often exhibits mild papillary change, which in this setting is presumed to represent a benign degenerative phenomenon.

Stratified syncytial epithelial changes with breakdown exhibit a range of morphologies that quantitatively and qualitatively exceed degenerative repair. In this process, there is exaggerated epithelial growth with a disorganized exfoliative pseudopapillary arrangement of epithelial cells, which is characterized by syncytial, haphazardly arranged, aggregates of epithelial cells with ample cytoplasm and occasional mucin droplets. Characteristically, there is a conspicuous lack of epithelial organization (Fig. 18.14a,b). Although stromal breakdown is often present adjacent to the process or elsewhere in the specimen, in some cases it may be absent. Small, loosely arranged epithelial clusters may project away from the stroma, but are devoid of epithelial architecture. This latter change has been termed papillary syncytial metaplasia.[10]

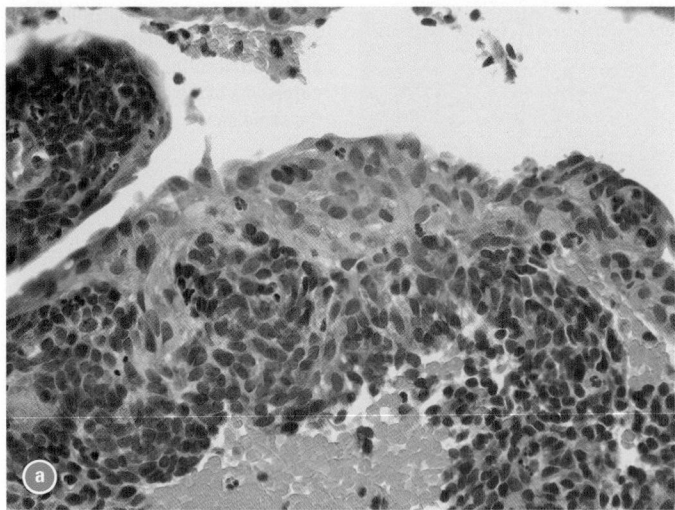

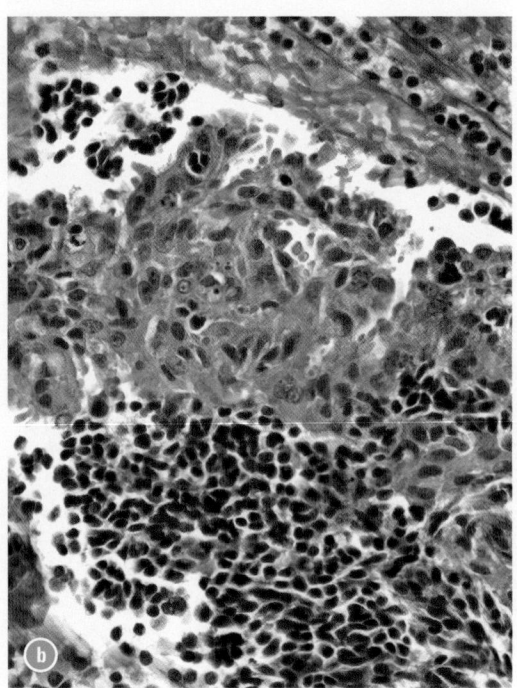

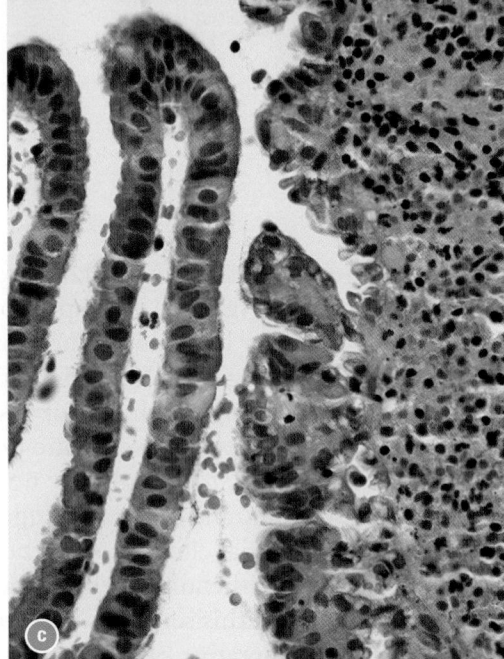

Fig. 18.13 Degenerative repair. (a) Associated with breakdown and (b) with mild stratified appearance. (c) Stratified degenerative epithelial changes associated with necrotic polyp (center right).

Because papillary syncytial metaplasia has an exfoliative papillary appearance, it must be distinguished from neoplasia. In particular, the absence of breakdown combined with defined papillary architecture with stromal cores should raise this concern (Fig. 18.14c).

Stratified or pseudo-stratified surface epithelial changes comprise the third category. These epithelia exhibit one or more layers and occur in the absence of breakdown.[7] These changes in cell appearance present as one to three layers of discrete cuboidal to columnar eosinophilic cells which lack the characteristic disorganized syncytial groupings of

degenerative or syncytial repair (Fig. 18.15a,b). These cells may also contain eosinophilic, mucinous, or tubal differentiation and will be discussed further under the subsequent headings. Alternatively, the cells may not display a characteristic pathway of differentiation, being composed of stratified groups of cells with round nuclei and pale to eosinophilic cytoplasm (Fig. 18.15c).

As defined, the above changes are considered benign. However, the reader should be aware that, in some instances, both endometrial intraepithelial neoplasia (atypical hyperplasia) and endometrial cancer might arise in or be associated with endometria undergoing

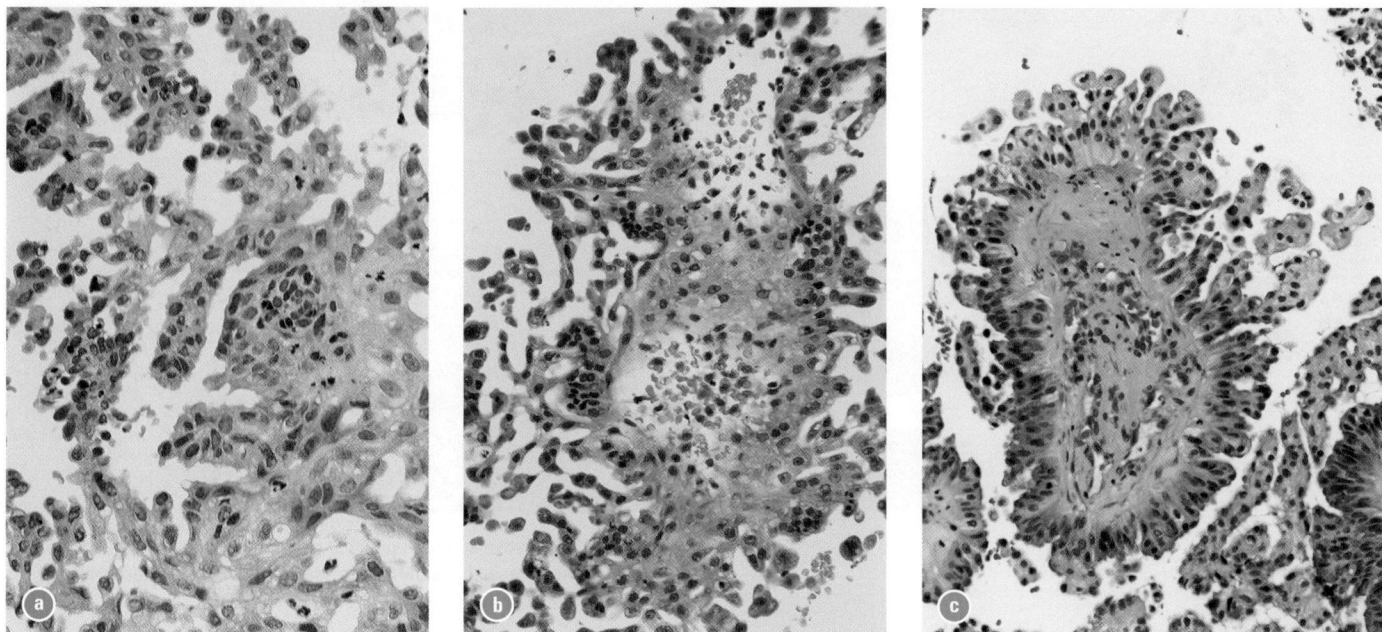

Fig. 18.14 (a,b) Exaggerated repair (papillary syncytial metaplasia) associated with breakdown. Despite the designation as papillary, important features seen in both panels is a lack of architectural organization with a 'pseudopapillary' architecture (stromal cores are absent) and low nuclear cytoplasmic ratio. (c) Papillary structures in an endometrial adenocarcinoma. Note the well-defined fibrotic stromal core.

breakdown. Typically, the changes will be more complex and the cells will exhibit a greater degree of cytologic atypia than that typically seen in metaplasias associated with benign processes (Figs 18.16a,b, 18.17a). Stratified epithelia with combinations of tubal and mucinous metaplasia forming multiple layers on the endometrial surface and occurring in the absence of conspicuous breakdown must be approached with care (see below). The possibility of neoplasia must be considered if the following are present: (1) evidence of glandular (or microglandular) organization, (2) defined papillae with stromal cores or an organized epithelial lining and (3) coexisting glands with disturbed intraglandular architecture (Fig. 18.17b). These alterations may be subtle and the reader is cautioned that with small specimens the pathologist may require a repeat sample.

MUCINOUS METAPLASIA

Like squamous differentiation, mucinous metaplasia ranges from simple cuboidal or columnar mucinous epithelium to complex proliferations associated with adenocarcinoma. A rare variant termed *intestinal metaplasia* is detailed below. Mucinous metaplasia may accompany tubal or squamous metaplasia, either in glands or on the surface,[9] and this combination of changes is typically seen in endometria from patients on hormonal replacement therapy.

The extent of mucinous metaplasia determines the level of concern by the pathologist.[28–32] Nucci et al. described three (types A–C): the first (type A) consisted of cuboidal endocervical-type epithelium involving the endometrial surface, or present within polyps or glands (Fig. 18.18a).[28] This pattern most commonly occurs in samples from perimenopausal women and presumably signifies epithelial transitions related to hormonal effects.[30] Type B metaplasias exhibit mild architectural complexity and slight papillary architecture (Fig. 18.18b). The papillary features are typically not as striking as those described by others as 'papillary hyperplasia' that are discussed below (Fig. 18.19).[33] In our experience, when papillary architecture is subtle or focal, there is a low risk of coexistent endometrial neoplasia. Nevertheless, periodic sampling should be considered if defined micropapillae are present lined by mucinous epithelial cells (Table 18.3). The third (type C) consists of either cribriform arrangements of mucinous epithelium within glands (Fig. 18.20a) or free-floating mucinous epithelium

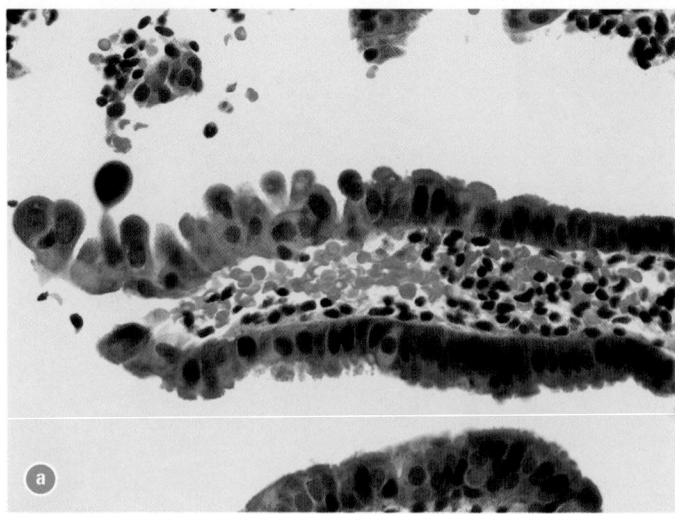

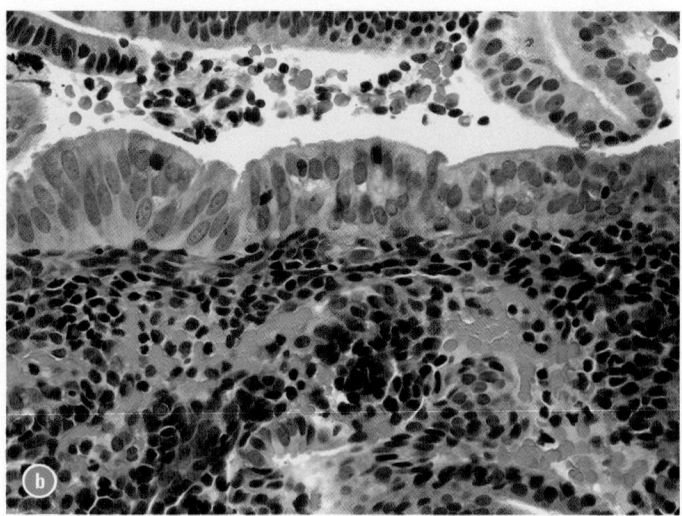

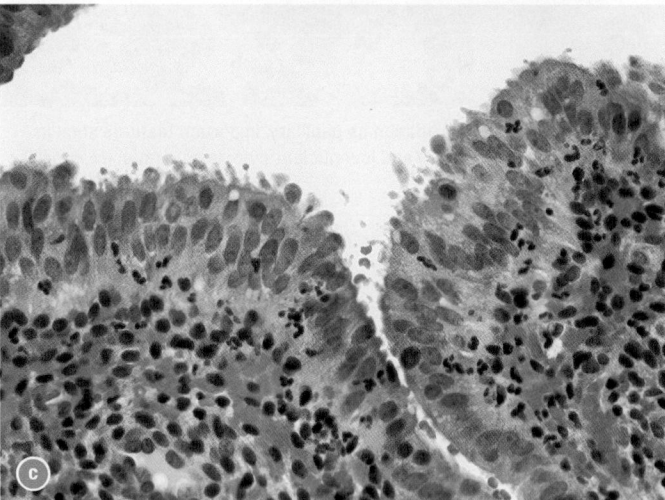

Fig. 18.15 Proliferative surface epithelial changes associated with breakdown. (a) Mild changes resemble tubal metaplasia. (b) Pseudostratified epithelial changes. (c) Multilayered epithelium.

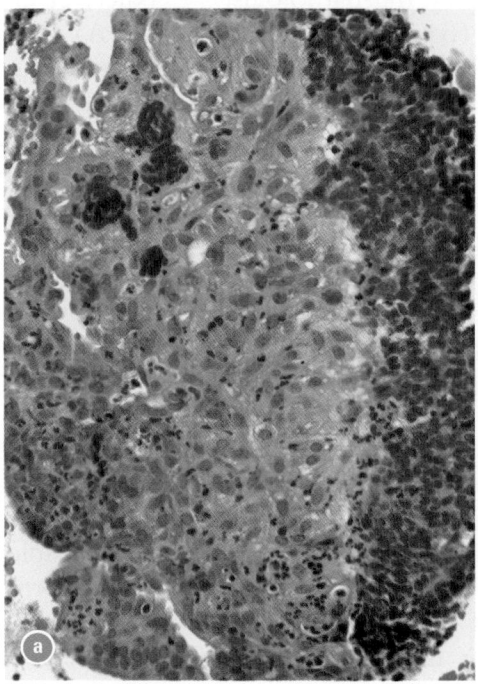

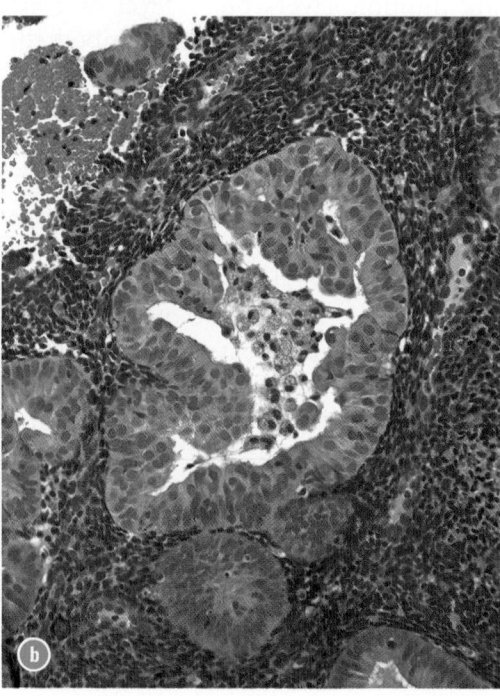

Fig. 18.16 (a) Exuberant surface changes associated with an endometrial intraepithelial neoplasia. This should be distinguished from repair, syncytial metaplasia and lesser forms of surface metaplasia. (b) Similar changes within a gland in an area of breakdown, associated with EIN.

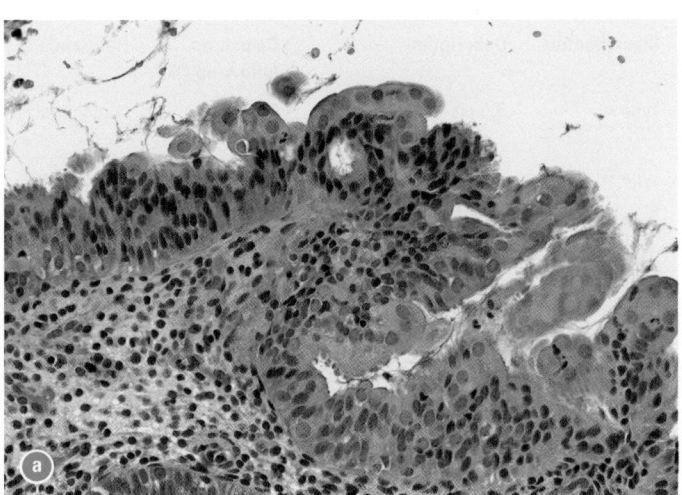

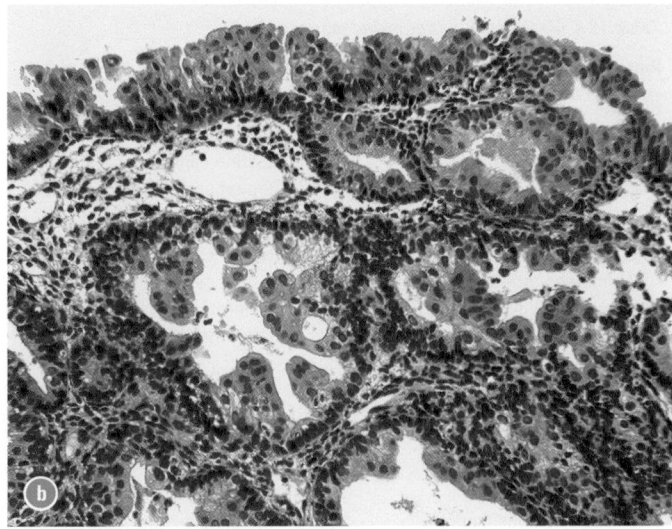

Fig. 18.17 (a) Surface 'metaplasia' with stratified appearance and gland-like structures associated with endometrial adenocarcinoma. (b) Papillary growth within endometrial glands. The complex growth pattern should be classified as EIN irrespective of form of differentiation.

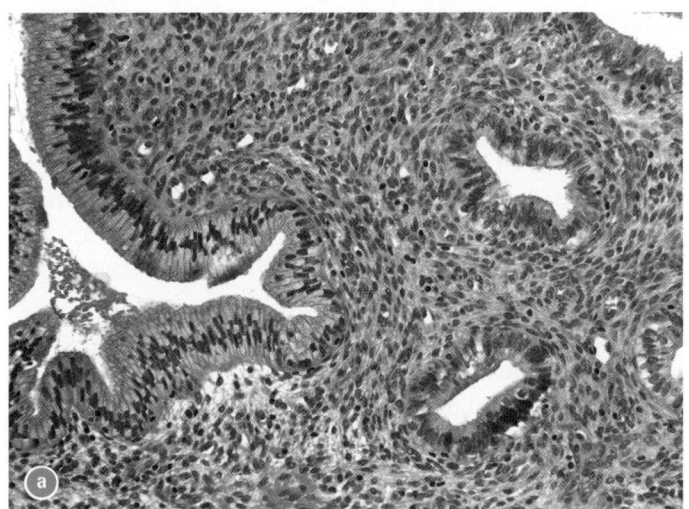

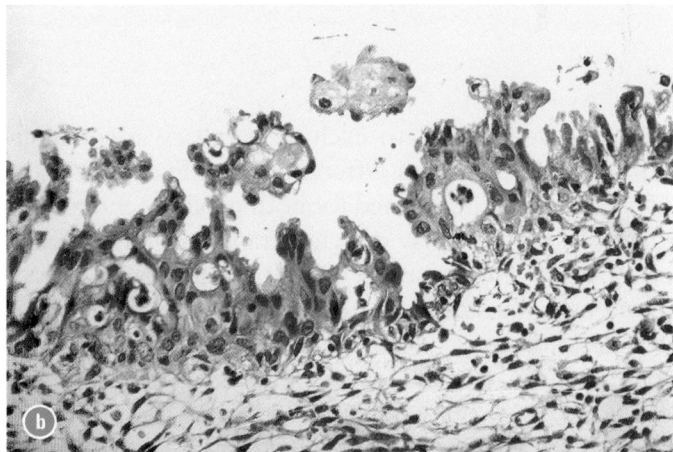

Fig. 18.18 (a) Minor mucinous metaplasia present as a cuboidal epithelium (type A by Nucci et al.). (b) Small papillary excrescences with mucinous metaplasia (type B).

exhibiting a microglandular or villous architecture (Fig. 18.20b–d).[26] These carry a significant risk (75%) of adenocarcinoma on subsequent samplings or hysterectomy, although most do not demonstrate myoinvasion (Table 18.4).[26,31] Another worrisome pattern consists of conspicuous papillary architecture and/or endometrial glands with papillary mucinous, ciliated or combined muco-ciliated epithelium (Fig. 18.21a,b). A small series of papillary lesions was not associated with cancer and may signify a subset with limited neoplastic potential.[31,32] However, similar changes within glands or polyps may be associated with neoplasia and should be managed with the intent to exclude EIN

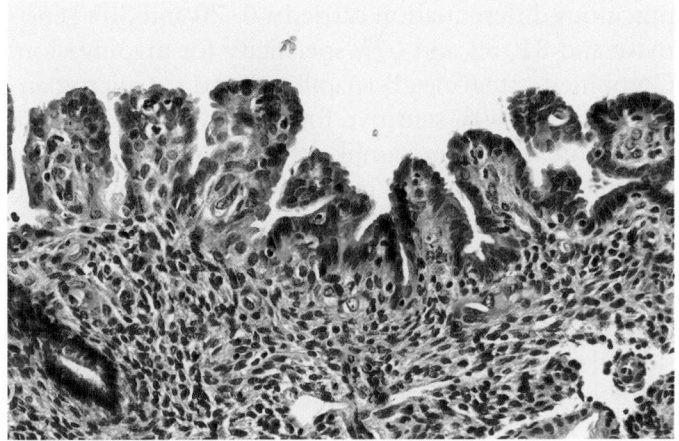

Fig. 18.19 Papillary hyperplasia of the endometrial surface.

Table 18.3 Metaplastic patterns and management

Pattern(s)	Management
Surface	
Repair	Routine clinical
Papillary syncytial	Routine clinical
Atypical (stratified) repair	Repeat sample in 3–6 months
Squamous	
Isolated morule	Repeat sample in 6 months
Morule and proliferation	Repeat sample in 6 months
Morule and EIN	EIN protocol
Morule and cancer	Cancer protocol
Ciliated	
Simple tubal metaplasia	Routine clinical
Complex tubal metaplasia	EIN protocol (See Ch. 17)
EIN with tubal metaplasia	EIN protocol
Mucinous	
Simple mucinous metaplasia	Routine clinical
Papillary mucinous proliferation	EIN protocol
Microglandular mucinous proliferation	EIN protocol
Eosinophilic	
Eosinophilic metaplasia	Routine clinical
Eosinophilic EIN	EIN protocol

EIN, endometrial intraepithelial neoplasia.

Table 18.4 Follow-up of mucinous metaplasia[28,33]

Classification	Description	Cancer on follow-up (%)	Reference
Type A	Simple or focal papillary	0	Nucci et al.[26]
Type B	Complex microglands	64[a]	Nucci et al.[26]
Type C	Type B + atypia	100	Nucci et al.[26]

[a]The majority were noninvasive or invasive through less than one-third of the myometrial thickness.

and followed closely to exclude papillary adenocarcinomas with mucinous differentiation (Fig. 18.21c,d). Hysterectomies performed for both papillary and microglandular patterns may not yield frankly invasive adenocarcinomas. However, they merit classification as neoplasia and warrant close follow-up if hysterectomy is not desired.

Recently, Vang and Tavassoli examined the criteria of Nucci et al. and compared them with published criteria for endometrioid proliferations.[30] The sensitivity and specificity of classic endometrioid criteria (diagnostic of neoplasia) for myoinvasion were 20.0% and 71.4%, respectively. In contrast, type A, B and C categories of mucinous differentiation carried a 0, 70 and 30% sensitivity and 81, 52 and 67% specificity for myoinvasion. Combined categories B (papillary) and C (microglandular) were 100% sensitive for myoinvasion with 19% specificity. This is not unlike the findings of Nucci et al., who noted that the majority of cancers associated with groups C lesions were not myoinvasive.[26,30]

The natural history of mucinous metaplasias is not well defined. In general, those metaplasias that are not accompanied by architectural complexity are not considered at risk. In our practice, mucinous lesions with any epithelial complexity are recommended for a follow-up sample in 6 months (Tables 18.3, 18.4). Microglandular or papillary lesions require at the least a dilatation

and curettage and, if persistent, hysterectomy.[26,33–35] These lesions, even with a bland cytology, may be aggressive. Approximately 75% of lesions with microacinar architecture will be followed by a diagnosis of endometrial adenocarcinomas, which may demonstrate either mucinous or endometrioid differentiation.

The primary distinction that the pathologist must make when confronted with mucinous differentiation in an endometrial curetting is between microglandular changes of cervical origin and abnormal mucinous epithelium of uterine origin. Qiu and Mittal compared these two entities and found the following features to favor an endometrial origin: (1) absence of prominent sub-nuclear vacuoles, (2) luminal squamous metaplasia, (3) stromal foam cells, (4) high mitotic index (over 3 per 10 HPF) and (5) absence of vimentin staining (Fig. 18.22a–c, Table 18.5).[36] The presence of reserve-like subsurface epithelial populations in the areas flanking the microglandular pattern suggest a cervical origin.

A rare variant of mucinous metaplasia is *intestinal metaplasia* of the endometrium. Recently, McCluggage et al. showed that 17% of mucin-positive endometrioid adenocarcinomas contain mucin intracytoplasmic O-acetylated sialomucins, which they concluded to signify

Table 18.5 Differential diagnosis of microglandular mucinous epithelia[36]

Parameter	MGC	Endometrial carcinoma
Foamy stromal cells	Absent	Present
MIB-1 staining	Low	High
Sub-nuclear vacuoles	Present	Absent
Sub-columnar squamous metaplasia	Present	Rare
Luminal squamous metaplasia	Absent	Present
Vimentin	Negative	Positive

MGC, microglandular change.

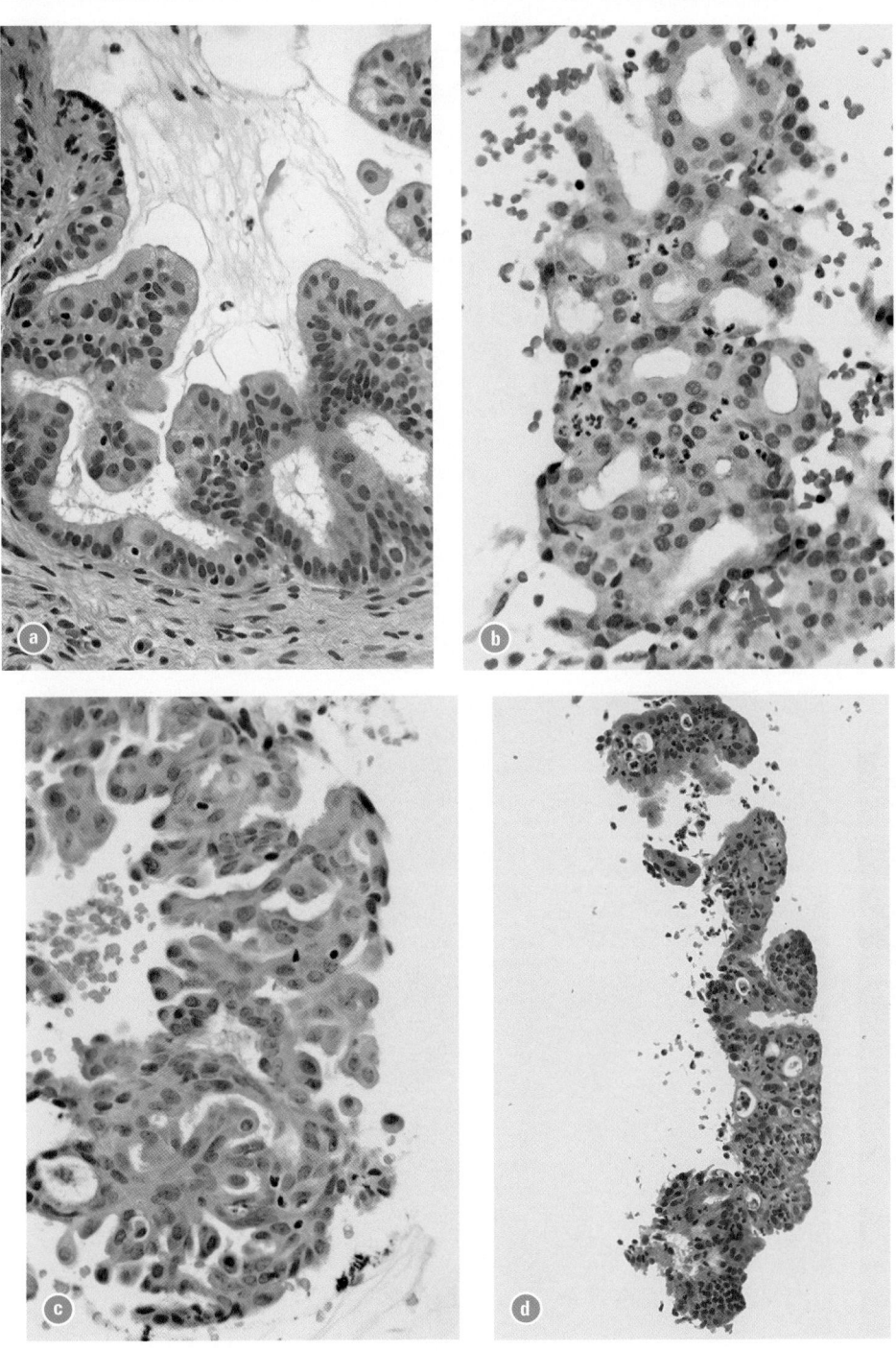

Fig. 18.20 Mucinous metaplasia with complex (micro-acinar) architecture (type B). (a) In an endometrial gland. (b–d) As detached fragments in a curetting. All of these samples were associated with endometrial adenocarcinoma.

intestinal differentiation.[37] In this setting, the morphologic features of intestinal differentiation were not appreciated. However, others have shown conspicuous intestinal and/or gastric differentiation, either in uterine polyps or on the endometrial surface (Fig. 18.23).[26,38] The implication of these studies is that Müllerian epithelium is capable of undergoing intestinal differentiation.

In the absence of neoplasia, the prospective risk of intestinal metaplasia is unknown.

TUBAL METAPLASIA

Cilia are common in the cervix and lower uterine segment and endometrial lining epithelium during the

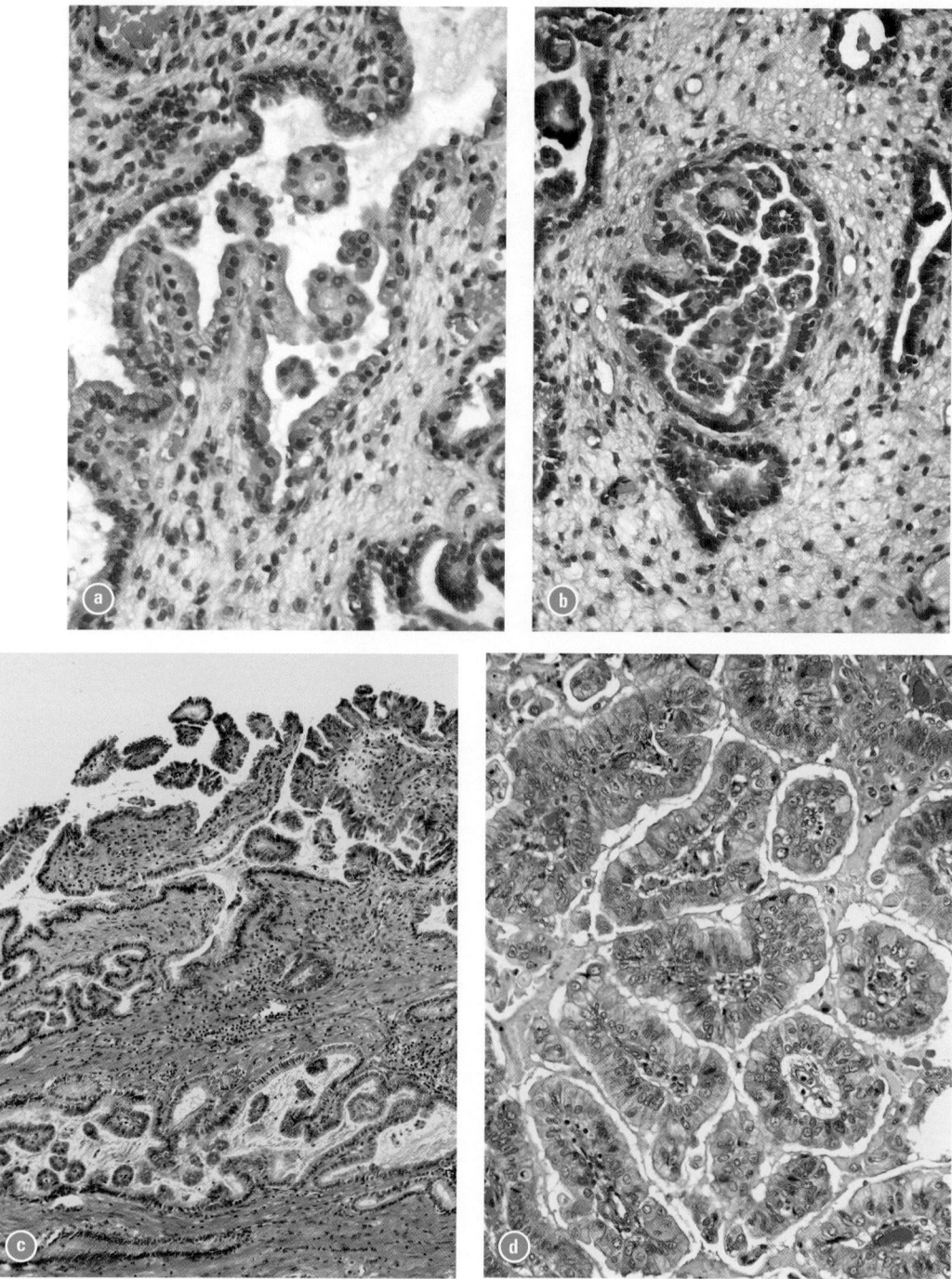

Fig. 18.21 Papillary architecture. (a,b) Papillary architecture on the surface and within a gland respectively. (c) Surface muco-papillary architecture in a polyp associated with a well-differentiated (ciliated) adenocarcinoma. (d) Complex papillary architecture with atypia in a well-differentiated adenocarcinoma.

endometrial cycle, being most conspicuous in the follicular phase and do not merit mention on the pathology report.[39] Extensive tubal metaplasia is most commonly encountered at menopause, associated with anovulatory states (persistent follicle), endometrial polyps and in endometria that are either responding to hormonal replacement therapy or undergoing evolution to a postmenopausal (inactive or atrophic) pattern. These associations suggest a relationship to excess estrogen.

The histologic features of tubal metaplasia include conspicuous cilia, clear round cells similar to those seen in the fallopian tube and eosinophilic luminal borders (Fig. 18.24a,b). Like the other forms of metaplasia, tubal metaplasia may be seen in glands (Fig. 18.24a–d) or as

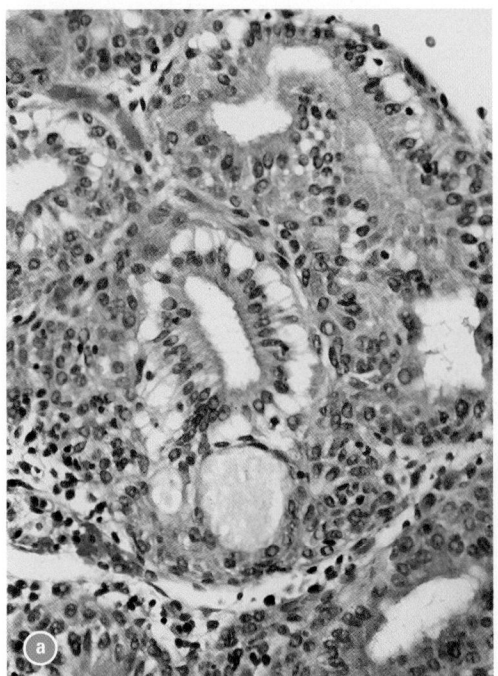

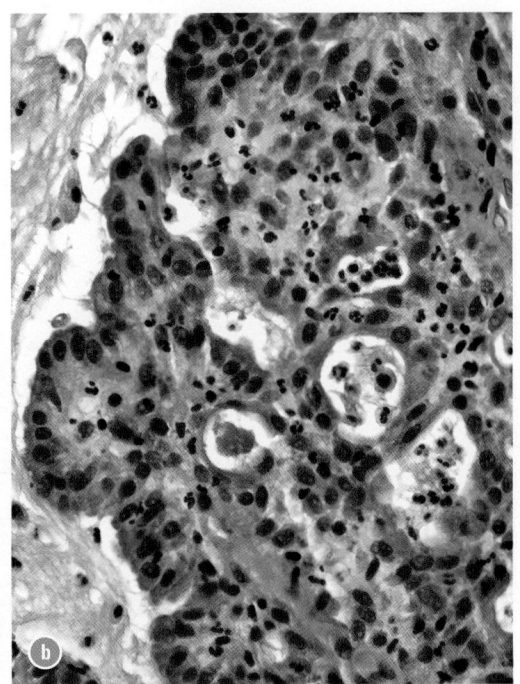

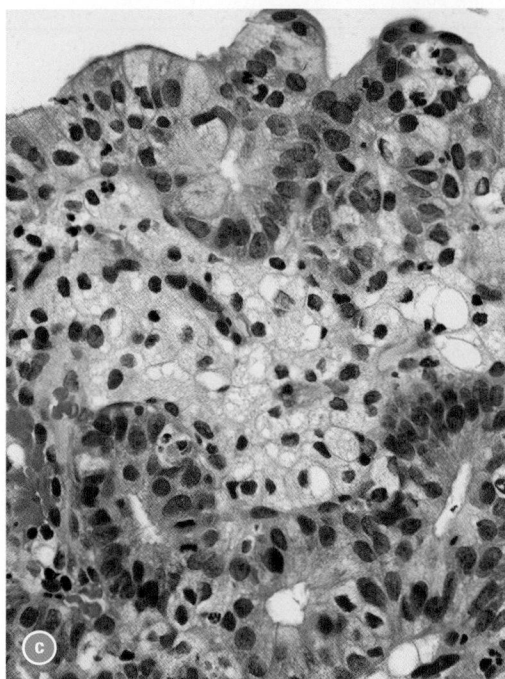

Fig. 18.22 Microglandular change versus endometrial adenocarcinoma. (a) Prominent vacuoles and sub-columnar squamous metaplasia in microglandular change from the cervix, (b) MGH-like changes in adenocarcinoma. (c) Foamy stromal cells beneath bland-appearing glands in adenocarcinoma. Mitoses are also present.

detached fragments of epithelium (Fig. 18.25a–c). It may be simple (Figs 18.24a, 18.25a), associated with mild epithelial complexity (Fig. 18.24b,c), or associated with frank neoplasia (Figs 18.24d, 18.25b,c). The latter includes three entities. EIN with tubal differentiation exhibits the characteristic gland crowding and altered epithelial architecture with focal epithelial tufting and stratification (Fig. 18.24d). Rarely, microglandular patterns akin to those seen in mucinous metaplasia may be encountered and carry the same significance (Fig. 18.25b,c). Finally, frank adenocarcinomas can exhibit prominent tubal differentiation (Fig. 18.26). Like the other forms of altered differentiation, management should be tailored to the degree of complexity of both the metaplasia and coexisting glands (Table 18.3).[40]

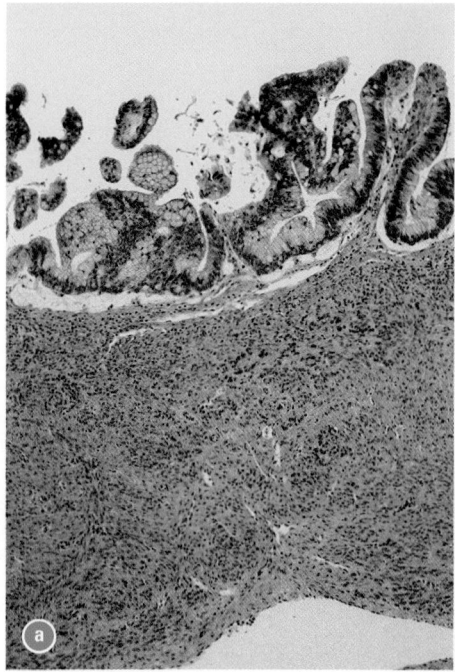
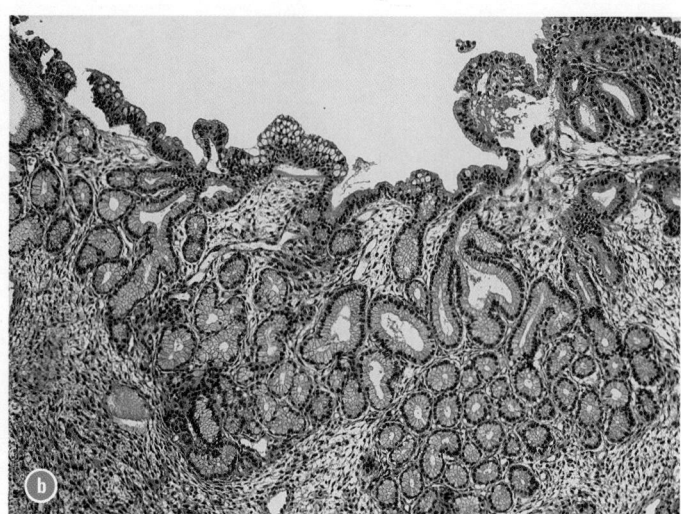

Fig. 18.23 (a) Intestinal metaplasia in the surface epithelium of the endometrium. (b) Gastric differentiation in a polyp.

EOSINOPHILIC (OXYPHILIC) METAPLASIA

Eosinophilic metaplasia is an uncommon form of differentiation characterized by an oxyphilic appearance to the individual cells. Eosinophilic metaplasia bears some resemblance to tubal metaplasia, but is devoid of cilia. Because its distinguishing feature is eosinophilic cytoplasm, eosinophilic metaplasia is basically a descriptive entity.[9] The epithelium is typically arranged in a single layer of cuboidal cells with uniform round nuclei (Fig. 18.27a). Similar to tubal and mucinous metaplasias, classification of eosinophilic metaplasia is linked to degree of complexity. Eosinophilic changes are occasionally seen in EIN and in endometrial carcinoma (Fig. 18.27b,c).[41–43]

OTHER EPITHELIAL METAPLASIAS

Other forms of altered differentiation include *secretory* and *hobnail* metaplasia. Secretory changes may be seen in EIN (Fig. 18.28a,b). Hobnail metaplasia likely comprises a range of changes, including surface alterations linked to underlying necrosis, exfoliation artifacts, pseudo-Arias-Stella changes and changes in polyps (Fig. 18.29a).[9,31] We have even witnessed hobnail meta-

Table 18.6 *Pitfalls in the diagnosis of metaplasia*

Differentiation (Fig.)	Exclusion (Fig.)
Papillary syncytial (14a,b)	Papillary carcinoma (14c) Coexistent EIN (16a,b, 17b) Coexistent adenocarcinoma (17a)
Squamous (morular)(7a–c)	Adenocarcinoma with sq. diff. (9, 10) EIN with morular metaplasia (8) Squamous carcinoma Atypical polypoid adenomyoma
Mucinous (18,19,22c)	Microglandular change (cx) (22a,b) Adenocarcinoma (20a–d)
Eosinophilic (27a)	EIN (27b,c)
Hobnail (29a)	Uterine papillary serous CA (29c,d) Clear cell CA (29b)
Growth pattern	**Consider**
Cribriform architecture	Pseudo cribriform (repair) (13b) Papillary syncytial metaplasia (14a) Intraglandular (EIN) (20a) Microglandular change (cervix)(22a) Adenocarcinoma (20a–d)
Papillary architecture	Papillary syncytial metaplasia (14b). Pseudo-papillary reactive change (13b,13c). Intraglandular (EIN) (21b) Surface changes assoc. with EIN (16a, 17b) Adenocarcinoma (17a, 21c,d)

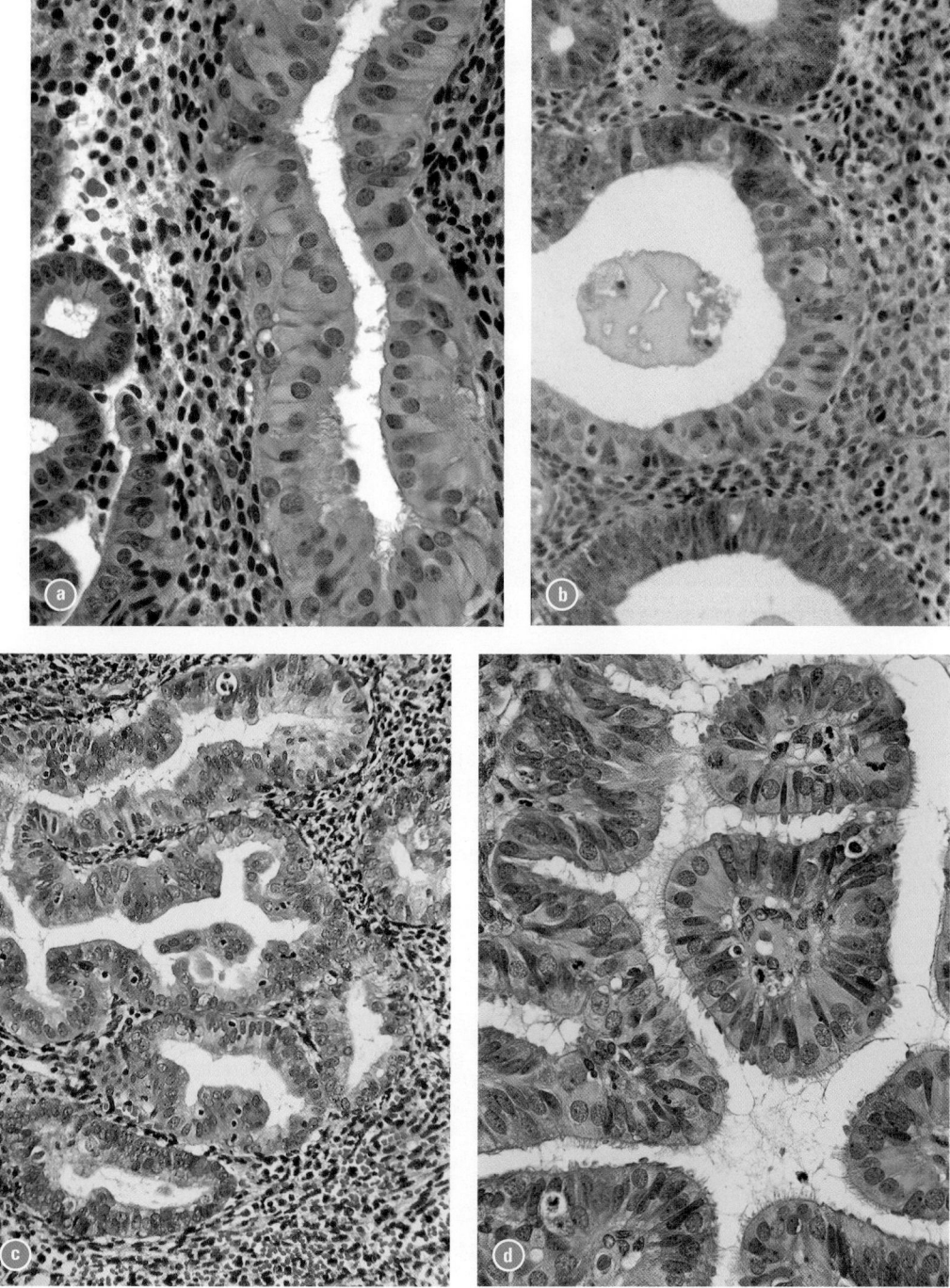

Fig. 18.24 Tubal metaplasia in glands. (a) Simple, (b) mildly complex, (c) EIN, with intraglandular complexity, (d) EIN, with papillary architecture.

plasia associated with clear cell carcinomas, likely signifying degenerative changes in these tumors (Fig. 18.29b). Hobnail metaplasia may be confused with uterine papillary serous carcinoma. Special stains for p53 may be helpful in distinguishing the two, inasmuch as serous neoplasms are strongly positive (Fig. 18.29c,d).[44]

AN ALGORITHM FOR ASSESSING METAPLASIA

The management of metaplasias entails both excluding clinically important mimics (Table 18.6) and using an established strategy to ensure consistent management.

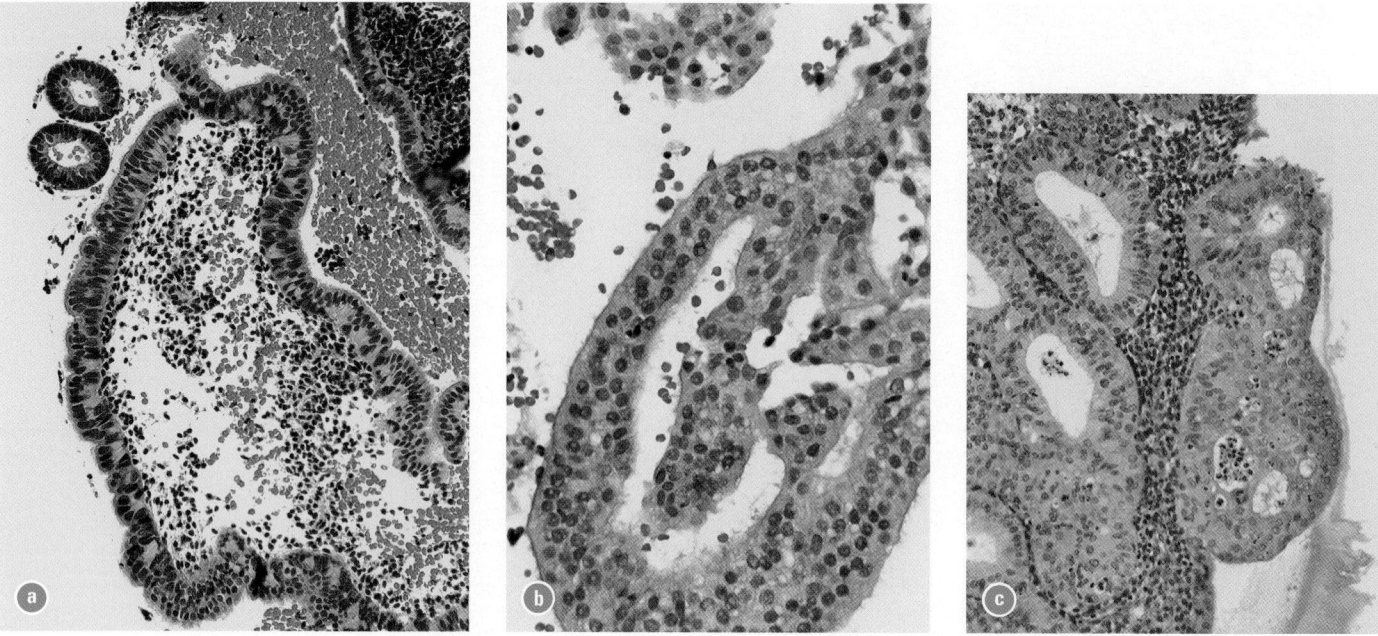

Fig. 18.25 Tubal metaplasia on the surface. (a) Simple, (b,c) complex with microacinar change. The underlying glands are also atypical in (c). (b,c) Associated with endometrial carcinoma.

The reader can appreciate from this discussion that metaplasia is a descriptive entity that parallels the classification of endometrial glandular lesions. The degree of architectural complexity determines the risk of a coexisting or subsequent adenocarcinoma Table 18.3 outlines an approach to metaplastic processes. In brief, the approach is as follows.

1 *Squamous metaplasia*: the classification parallels the degree of gland complexity and cytologic change.

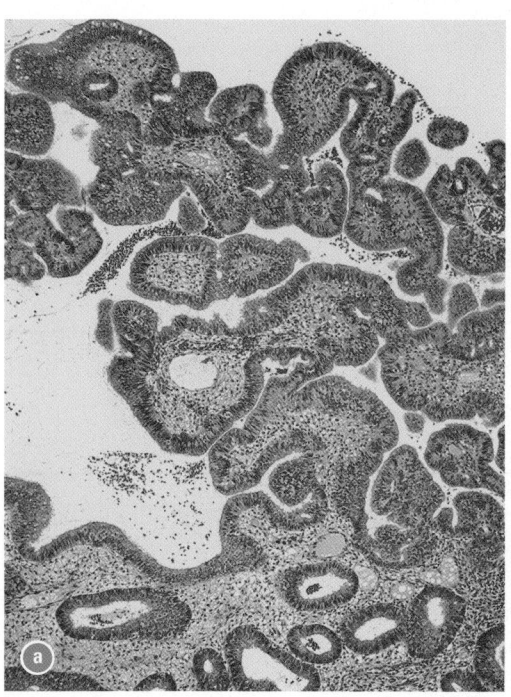
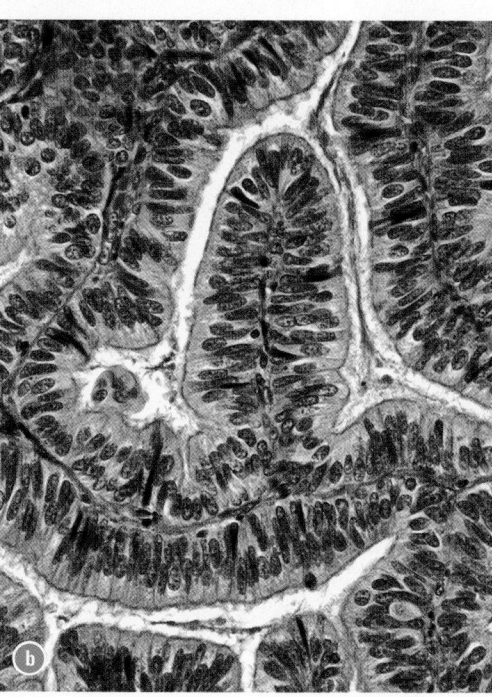

Fig. 18.26 (a) Endometrial adenocarcinoma with tubal differentiation (ciliated adenocarcinoma). (b) Higher-power illustrates the prominent cilia.

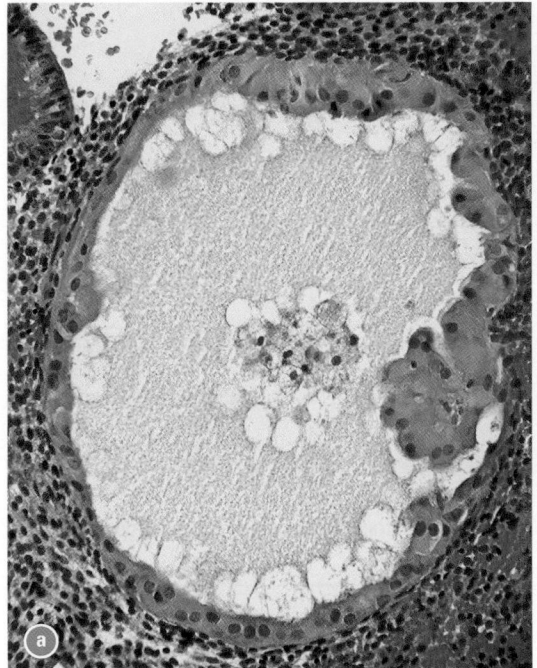

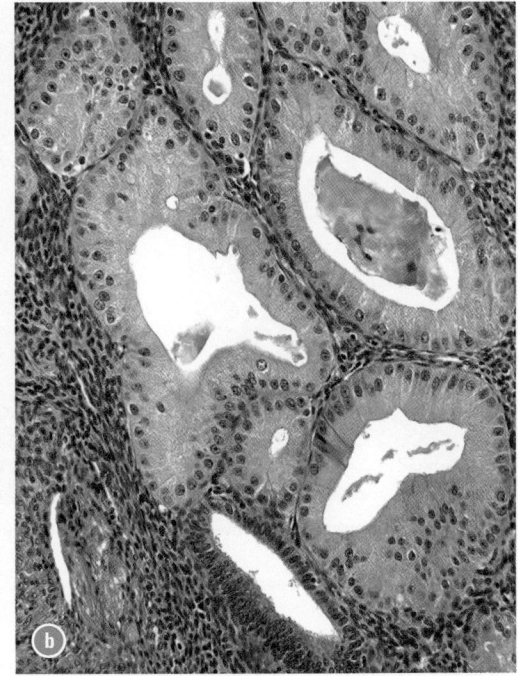

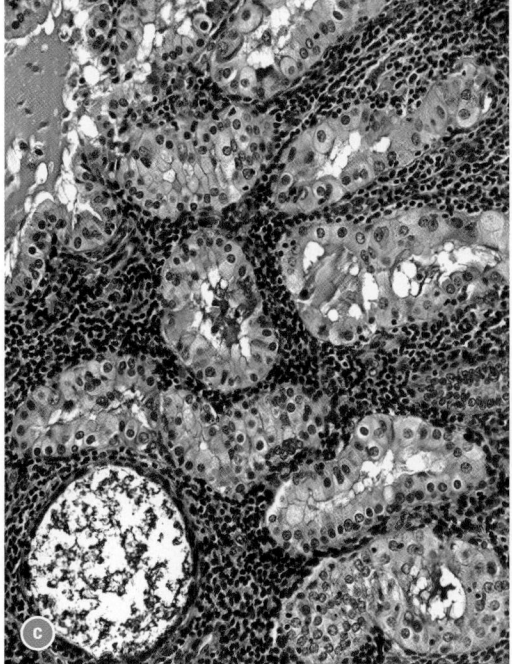

Fig. 18.27 (a) Eosinophilic metaplasia. (b,c) Eosinophilic change in EIN.

2 *Mucinous and ciliated metaplasia*: when confined to glands, the degree of stratification and disturbance in the glandular lining dictates the diagnosis with complex intraglandular metaplasias classified as EIN. Because the changes may be subtle and/or limited in amount, metaplastic changes present on the surface or in detached or exfoliated groups may be difficult to classify.

These lesions are best classified according to the degree of microglandular change or complexity. In those cases where a limited amount of lesion is present, or a diagnosis of a precancerous or cancerous change cannot be made, a repeat sample should be advised. If enough lesional tissue is present and it has a complex microglandular architecture then it is classified as a well-

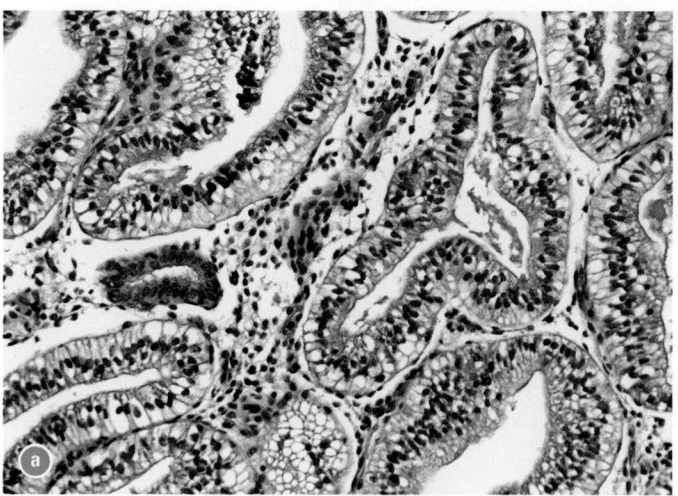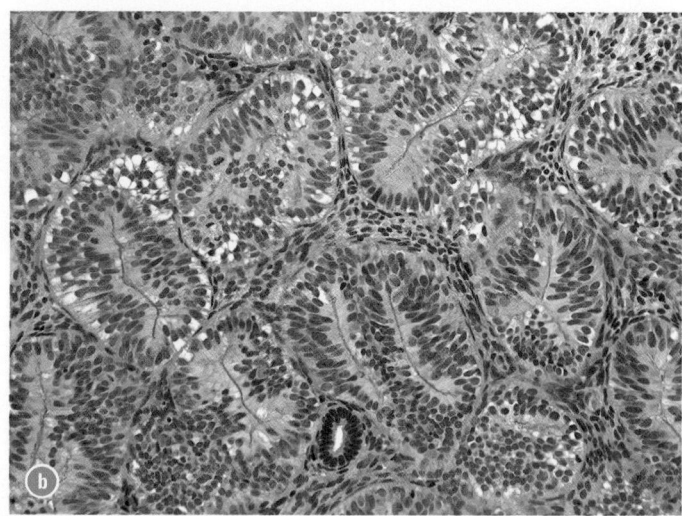

Fig. 18.28 (a,b) Secretory differentiation in EIN. In both there is gland crowding and stratified epithelium. Note the contrast to normal inactive gland (lower center) in (b).

differentiated adenocarcinoma. In those cases with suboptimal material a diagnosis of atypical (mucinous or ciliated) metaplasia is permitted, with the comment that well-differentiated adenocarcinoma cannot be excluded. Obviously, the distinction of a complex metaplasia from a well-differentiated adenocarcinoma is dictated by the degree of atypia and the practitioner's experience. The important issue is identifying the process and initiating careful follow-up.

3 *Papillary lesions*: slight micropapillary changes, or pseudo-papillary surface changes associated with stromal breakdown, carry a low index of concern. Well-differentiated papillary architecture within glands should be classified as EIN. Other 'extra-glandular' well-differentiated papillary changes should be classified as EIN (papillary) and further sampling recommended.

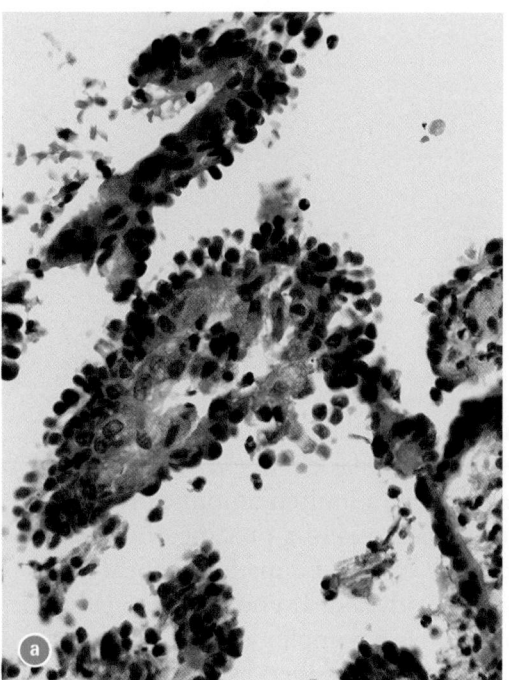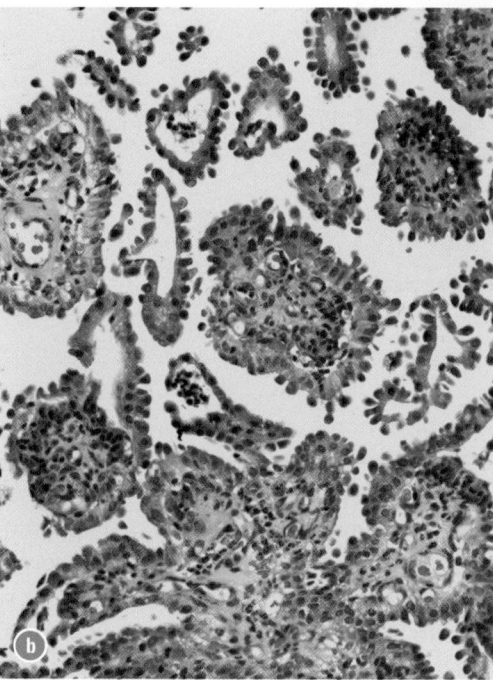

Fig. 18.29 Hobnail metaplasia. (a) Benign, associated with a polyp. (b) Associated with a clear cell carcinoma. In the latter there are numerous discrete papillary structures.

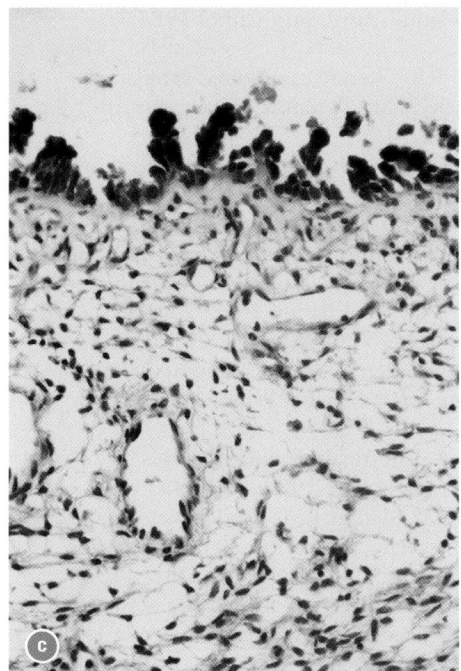 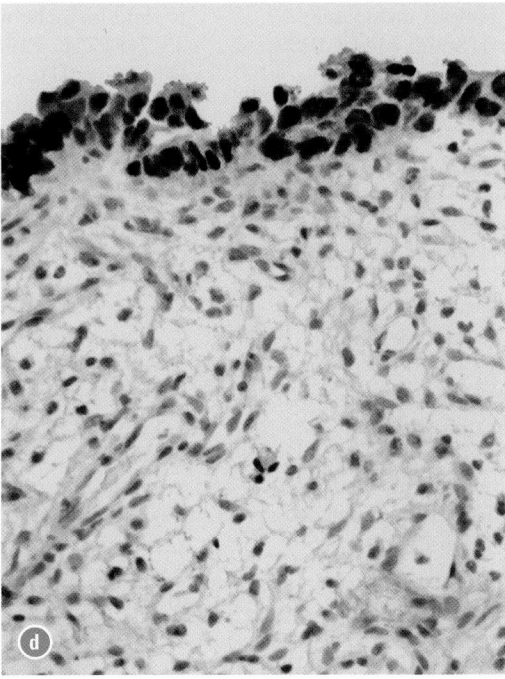

Fig. 18.29 Cont'd (c) Uterine papillary serous carcinoma may present with a subtle surface change resembling hobnail metaplasia. (d) Intense immunostaining for p53 distinguishes serous carcinoma from benign metaplasias.

NON-EPITHELIAL METAPLASIAS/HETEROTOPIAS OF THE ENDOMETRIUM

Several reports in the literature have described mature glia, bone and cartilage in the endometrium, in some instances following pregnancy.[45–50] In one report, mature glia was found in curettings on successive samplings.[51] Presumably, these structures are derived from fetal tissue remaining following a prior evacuation.[50,52] However, this hypothesis has not been tested by genetic analysis.

References

1 Kurita T, Cunha GR. Roles of p63 in differentiation of Müllerian duct epithelial cells. Ann NY Acad Sci 2001; 948:9–12.

2 Ince TA, Cviko AP, Quade BJ, et al. p63 Coordinates anogenital modeling and epithelial cell differentiation in the developing female urogenital tract. Am J Pathol 2002; 161(4):1111–1117.

3 Quade BJ, Yang A, Wang Y, et al. Expression of the p53 homologue p63 in early cervical neoplasia. Gynecol Oncol 2001; 80(1):24–29.

4 Greeley C, Schroeder S, Silverberg SG. Microglandular hyperplasia of the cervix: a true 'pill' lesion? Int J Gynecol Pathol 1995; 14(1):50–54.

5 Witkiewicz AK, Hecht JL, Cviko A, et al. Microglandular hyperplasia: a model for the denovo emergence and evolution of endocervical reserve cells. Human Pathol 2005; 36:154–161.

6 Elson DA, Riley RR, Lacey A, et al. Sensitivity of the cervical transformation zone to estrogen-induced squamous carcinogenesis. Cancer Res 2000; 60(5):1267–1275.

7 O'Connell JT, Mutter GL, Cviko A, et al. Identification of a basal/reserve cell immunophenotype in benign and neoplastic endometrium: a study with the p53 homologue p63. Gynecol Oncol 2001; 80(1):30–36.

8 Kurita T, Cooke PS, Cunha GR. Epithelial-stromal tissue interaction in paramesonephric (Müllerian) epithelial differentiation. Dev Biol 2001; 240(1):194–211.

9 Hendrickson MR, Kempson RL. Endometrial epithelial metaplasias: proliferations frequently misdiagnosed as adenocarcinoma. Report of 89 cases and proposed classification. Am J Surg Pathol 1980; 4(6):525–542.

10 Crum CP, Richart RM, Fenoglio CM. Adenoacanthosis of endometrium: a clinicopathologic study in premenopausal women. Am J Surg Pathol 1981; 5(1):15–20.

11 Kaku T, Silverberg SG, Tsukamoto N, et al. Association of endometrial epithelial metaplasias with endometrial carcinoma and hyperplasia in Japanese and American women. Int J Gynecol Pathol 1993; 12(4):297–300.

12 Kaku T, Tsukamoto N, Tsuruchi N, et al. Endometrial metaplasia associated with endometrial carcinoma. Obstet Gynecol 1992; 80(5):812–816.

13 Andersen WA, Taylor PT Jr, Fechner RE, Pinkerton JA. Endometrial metaplasia associated with endometrial adenocarcinoma. Am J Obstet Gynecol 1987; 157(3):597–604.

14 Risse EK, Beerthuizen RJ, Vooijs GP. Cytologic and histologic findings in women using an IUD. Obstet Gynecol 1981; 58(5):569–573.

15 Hameed M, Heller DS, Murphy G. Squamous metaplasia of endometrium after uterine artery embolization for symptomatic leiomyomata. J Am Assoc Gynecol Laparosc 2002; 9(1):70–72.

16 Brown D Jr, Spjut HJ. Extensive squamous metaplasia of the endometrium (ichthyosis uteri). South Med J 1982; 75(5):593–595.

17 Kucukali T, Ertoy D, Ayhan A. Ichthyosis uteri associated with a uterine squamous papilloma. Eur J Gynaecol Oncol 1996; 17(1):37–41.

18 Clement PB, Young RH. Endometrioid carcinoma of the uterine corpus: a review of its pathology with emphasis on recent advances and problematic aspects. Adv Anat Pathol 2002; 9(3):145–184.

19 Stastny JF, Ben-Ezra J, Stewart JA, et al. Condyloma and cervical intraepithelial neoplasia of the endometrium. Gynecol Obstet Invest 1995; 39(4):277–280.

20 Sherwood JB, Carlson JA, Gold MA, et al. Squamous metaplasia of the endometrium associated with HPV 6 and 11. Gynecol Oncol 1997; 66(1):141–145.

21 Fujita M, Shroyer KR, Markham NE, et al. Association of human papillomavirus with malignant and premalignant lesions of the uterine endometrium. Hum Pathol 1995; 26(6):650–658.

22 Mazur MT. Atypical polypoid adenomyomas of the endometrium. Am J Surg Pathol 1981; 5(5):473–482.

23 Hendrickson MR, Kempson RL. Surgical pathology of the uterine corpus. Major Probl Pathol 1979; 12:1–580.

24 Crum CP, Lomo L, Lin MC, et al. Morular metaplasia of the endometrium revisited: a follow-up study. Abstract, USCAP meeting, Vancouver, 2004.

25 Zidi YS, Bouraoui S, Atallah K, et al. Primary in situ squamous cell carcinoma of the endometrium, with extensive squamous metaplasia and dysplasia Gynecol Oncol 2003; 88(3):444–446.

26 Nucci MR, Prasad CJ, Crum CP, Mutter GL. Mucinous endometrial epithelial proliferations: a morphologic spectrum of changes with diverse clinical significance. Mod Pathol 1999; 12(12):1137–1142.

27 Mount SL. Mucinous metaplasias of the endometrium: biologically meaningful subsets for the practicing surgical pathologist. Adv Anat Pathol 2000; 7(4):197–200.

28 Deligdisch L. Hormonal pathology of the endometrium. Mod Pathol 2000; 13(3):285–294.

29 Dallenbach-Hellweg G. Histopathology of functional and neoplastic changes in cervix and endometrium. Verh Dtsch Ges Pathol 1997; 81:240–244.

30 Vang R, Tavassoli FA. Proliferative mucinous lesions of the endometrium: analysis of existing criteria for diagnosing carcinoma in biopsies and curettings. Int J Surg Pathol 2003; 11(4):261–270.

31 Lehman MB, Hart WR. Simple and complex hyperplastic papillary proliferations of the endometrium: a clinicopathologic study of nine cases of apparently localized papillary lesions with fibrovascular stromal cores and epithelial metaplasia. Am J Surg Pathol 2001; 25(11):1347–1354.

32 Rorat E, Wallach RC. Papillary metaplasia of the endometrium: clinical and histopathologic considerations. Obstet Gynecol 1984; 64(3):90S–92S.

33 Ross JC, Eifel PJ, Cox RS, et al. Primary mucinous adenocarcinoma of the endometrium. A clinicopathologic and histochemical study. Am J Surg Pathol 1983; 7(8):715–729.

34 Young RH, Scully RE. Uterine carcinomas simulating microglandular hyperplasia. A report of six cases. Am J Surg Pathol 1992; 16:1092–1097.

35 McCluggage WG, Perenyei M. Microglandular adenocarcinoma of the endometrium. Histopathology 2000; 37(3):285–287.

36 Qiu W, Mittal K. Comparison of morphologic and immunohistochemical features of cervical microglandular hyperplasia with low-grade mucinous adenocarcinoma of the endometrium. Int J Gynecol Pathol 2003; 22(3):261–265.

37 McCluggage WG, Roberts N, Bharucha H. Enteric differentiation in endometrial adenocarcinomas: a mucin histochemical study. Int J Gynecol Pathol 1995; 14(3):250–254.

38 Wells M, Tiltman A. Intestinal metaplasia of the endometrium. Histopathology 1989; 15(4):431–433.

39 Husami N, Crum CP, Richart RM, Vande Wiele R. Ciliated endocervical cells: a cyclic 'pseudo-protozoal infestation' of the endocervix. Fertil Steril 1981; 36(1):116–118.

40 Hendrickson MR, Kempson RL. Ciliated carcinoma – a variant of endometrial adenocarcinoma: a report of 10 cases. Int J Gynecol Pathol 1983; 2(1):1–12.

41 Zamecnik M. Atypical oxyphilic metaplasia of the uterine cervix. Report of a case. Cesk Patol 2000; 36(2):60–64.

42 Fukuoka K, Hirokawa M, Shimizu M, et al. Oxyphilic cell variant of endometrioid adenocarcinoma. Pathol Int 1998; 48(9):754–756.

43 Pitman MB, Young RH, Clement PB, et al. Endometrioid carcinoma of the ovary and endometrium, oxyphilic cell type: a report of nine cases. Int J Gynecol Pathol 1994; 13(4):290–301.

44 Quddus MR, Sung CJ, Zheng W, Lauchlan SC. p53 immunoreactivity in endometrial metaplasia with dysfunctional uterine bleeding. Histopathology 1999; 35(1):44–49.

45 Bahceci M, Demirel LC. Osseous metaplasia of the endometrium: a rare cause of infertility and its hysteroscopic management. Hum Reprod 1996; 11(11):2537–2539.

46 Basu M, Mammen C, Owen E. Bony fragments in the uterus: an association with secondary subfertility. Ultrasound Obstet Gynecol 2003; 22(4):402–406.

47 Zettergren L. Glial tissue in the uterus. Am J Pathol 1973; 71(3):419–426.

48 Roca AN, Guajardo M, Estrada WJ. Glial polyp of the cervix and endometrium. Report of a case and review of the literature. Am J Clin Pathol 1980; 73(5):718–720.

49 Aabye R. Cartilage in the endometrium. Acta Obstet Gynecol Scand 1955; 34(1):105–110.

50 Al-Shawaf T, Brown J, Keegan C. Retention of fetal bones 8 years following termination of pregnancy. Ultrasound Obstet Gynecol 1992; 2(1):61–63.

51 Russell P, Costa C de, Yeoh G. Fetal glial allograft in the endometrium: case report of a recurrent pseudo-tumor. Pathology 1993; 25(3):247–249.

52 Newton CW 3rd, Abell MR. Iatrogenic fetal implants. Obstet Gynecol 1972; 40(5):686–691.

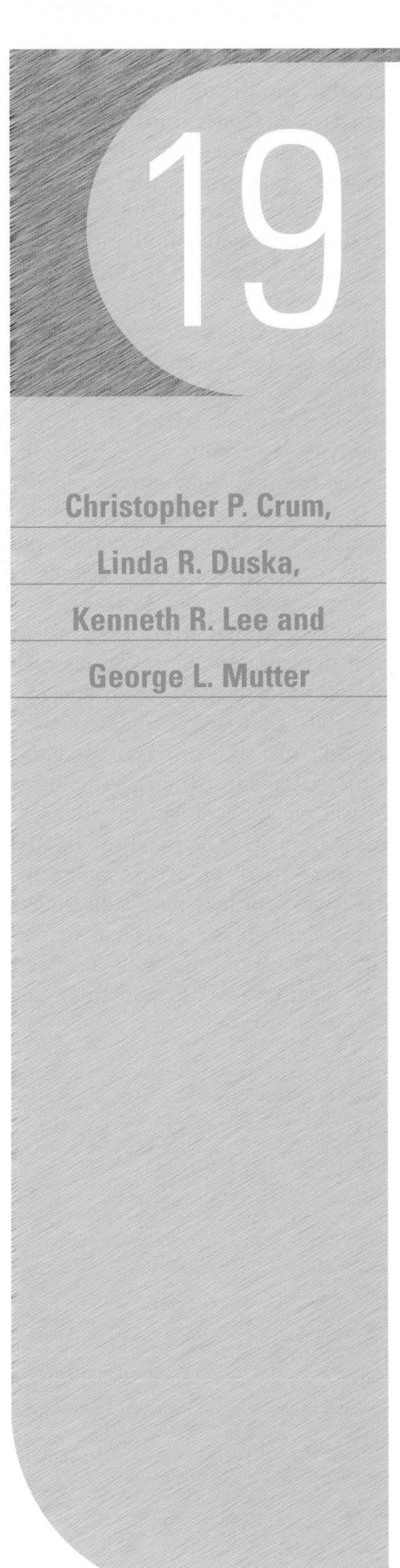

19

Adenocarcinoma, carcinosarcoma and other epithelial tumors of the endometrium

Christopher P. Crum,

Linda R. Duska,

Kenneth R. Lee and

George L. Mutter

Introduction

Endometrial adenocarcinoma

The patient at risk
Clinical parameters for assessing
    risk
Histopathology of endometrial
    adenocarcinoma
Differential diagnosis of
    endometrial adenocarcinoma
Components of laboratory
    management
Biomarkers and other parameters
    associated with outcome
Management and outcome

Carcinosarcomas

Introduction and definition
Pathogenesis

The patient at risk
Clinical presentation
Pathology
Staging, management and
    outcome

**Other epithelial neoplasms
arising in the endometrium**

Atypical polypoid adenomyoma
Condylomata
Squamous cell carcinomas
Poorly-differentiated papillary
    (transitional cell) tumors
Small cell undifferentiated tumors
Other undifferentiated tumors
Metastatic epithelial tumors to the
    endometrium

Introduction

This chapter will address endometrial carcinomas, including those with mesenchymal differentiation (carcinosarcomas). Primary endometrial carcinomas comprise a range of morphologies including carcinomas closely resembling pre-existing endometrial epithelium (endometrioid), clear cell carcinomas, uterine papillary serous carcinomas (UPSCs), carcinomas sharing one or more of these features, undifferentiated carcinomas and tumors with mixed epithelial-mesenchymal differentiation (carcinosarcomas). They can also be divided according to pathogenesis, including (1) excess estrogen effect via obesity, hormonal replacement, or abnormal estrogen production by ovarian lesions, (2) the absence of hyperestrogenism (3) tamoxifen therapy and (4) prior radiation therapy.

The issues most critical to proper diagnosis and management are (1) identifying the patient at risk for these neoplasms, (2) the appropriate methods for identifying or excluding endometrial adenocarcinoma, (3) an appreciation of the different forms of endometrial carcinomas that have prognostic significance and (4) the assessment of variables that impact on outcome and influence therapy.

Endometrial adenocarcinoma

THE PATIENT AT RISK

Demographics

Endometrial carcinoma is the most common invasive cancer of the female genital tract in the USA (cervical cancer remains the most common worldwide) and accounts for 7% of all invasive cancers in women, excluding skin cancer. Previously, it was far less common than cancer of the cervix, but earlier detection and effective treatment of cervical intraepithelial neoplasia (CIN) and an increase in endometrial carcinomas in younger age groups have reversed this ratio. In the USA, there are now 34 000 new endometrial cancers per year, compared with less than 12 000 new cervical cancers. Endometrial cancers usually arise in postmenopausal women and over 80% present with abnormal (postmenopausal) bleeding, which often permits detection and cure at an early stage.[1]

From 2% to 14% of endometrial carcinomas occur in women younger than 40 years of age. The peak incidence is in the 55–65-year-old age group with a median age of 63.[2,3] Two general patient groups emerge from demographic and histopathologic studies (Table 19.1).[4] The first is endometrioid adenocarcinomas and their variants, which are often termed Type I endometrial carcinomas. As a group, these account for about 90% of endometrial cancers and arise in a background of chronic estrogen stimulation. The source of estrogen may be from ovarian dysfunction (either polycystic ovarian disease or cortical stromal hyperplasia (stromal thecosis)), estrogen-secreting tumors (rare), and unopposed estrogen in the form of continuous estrogen therapy. Obesity, which encourages conversion of androstenedione to estrone in adipose tissue via aromatase activity, is strongly associated with this subset of endometrial tumors. Nulliparity is another risk factor. Because ovarian dysfunction and obesity are associated with adult-onset diabetes mellitus, the latter is also a risk factor.[2] However, the reader is cautioned that not every woman with a Type I tumor will share these risk factors, and that attention to these variables alone will not determine which women with postmenopausal bleeding merit diagnostic studies.[5,6]

Endometrial carcinomas that are associated with unopposed estrogen tend to be well-differentiated and mimic normal endometrial glands (hence the term 'endometrioid') in histologic appearance and are associated with a favorable prognosis. The presumed pathway to endometrial cancer involves excess estrogen, development of anovulatory endometrium, subsequent endometrial intraepithelial neoplasia (atypical hyperplasia) and, ultimately, adenocarcinoma. This has been discussed in detail in Chapter 17. Predictably, this

Table 19.1 Pathogenetic subsets of endometrial carcinoma[1,2,4,21]

Parameter	Type 1	Type 2
Age	50s–60s	60s–70s
Obesity	Common	Uncommon
Estrogenic stimuli	Common	Uncommon
Endometrium	Anovulatory	Atrophic
Precursor	EIN	Unknown
Transition	Slow	Rapid
Type	Endometrioid	Papillary serous or mixed
Molecular genetics	MSI, PTEN mutation	p53 mutation, 1p deletions
Familial	HNPCC	
Spread	Lymph nodes	Peritoneum
Concurrent ovarian	Common	Uncommon
Prognosis	Good	Poor

subset of tumors affects women in their mid- to late-50s but encompasses most of adenocarcinomas seen in the younger age groups.[4,7]

The second and much less common group of endometrial carcinomas (Type II) is more commonly seen in the seventh and eighth decades, does not arise in association with hyperestrogenism, obesity or diabetes, and has a distinctly different morphologic growth pattern. In this group, tumors are generally more poorly-differentiated, and include both clear cell and papillary serous carcinoma.[8] These tumors overall have a poorer prognosis than endometrioid tumors, and the factors predisposing to their development are less well defined.[9] A small proportion of these tumors arise in association with endometrioid carcinomas, indicating either independent processes, or more likely, a single tumor which has evolved to develop heterogeneity through multiple pathogenetic pathways. These pathways are illustrated in the schematic in Figure 19.1.

A third mechanism of carcinogenesis is radiation related. In one study of 23 women who developed endometrial cancer following radiation therapy, the average duration from radiation exposure to cancer development was 14 years. Some 69% were in unfavorable histologic categories, including carcinosarcomas.[10]

Ethnicity

Studies have shown that endometrial carcinoma is less common in African-American women, but that this group nonetheless has a higher mortality.[11,12] Blacks have a cancer incidence of 13 per 100 000, compared with 23 for whites and 14 for white Hispanics. However, blacks have a four-fold higher risk of dying from endometrial cancer. The excess mortality in this group has been attributed to one or more variables, including later stage at diagnosis, unfavorable tumor type or stage, socio-demographic factors, treatment and comorbidities.[11] Tumor histologic type probably accounts for the bulk of this effect, as blacks have significantly higher incidence rates of poor prognostic cell types of serous/clear cell carcinoma, carcinosarcoma and sarcoma. Rare aggressive tumor types accounted for

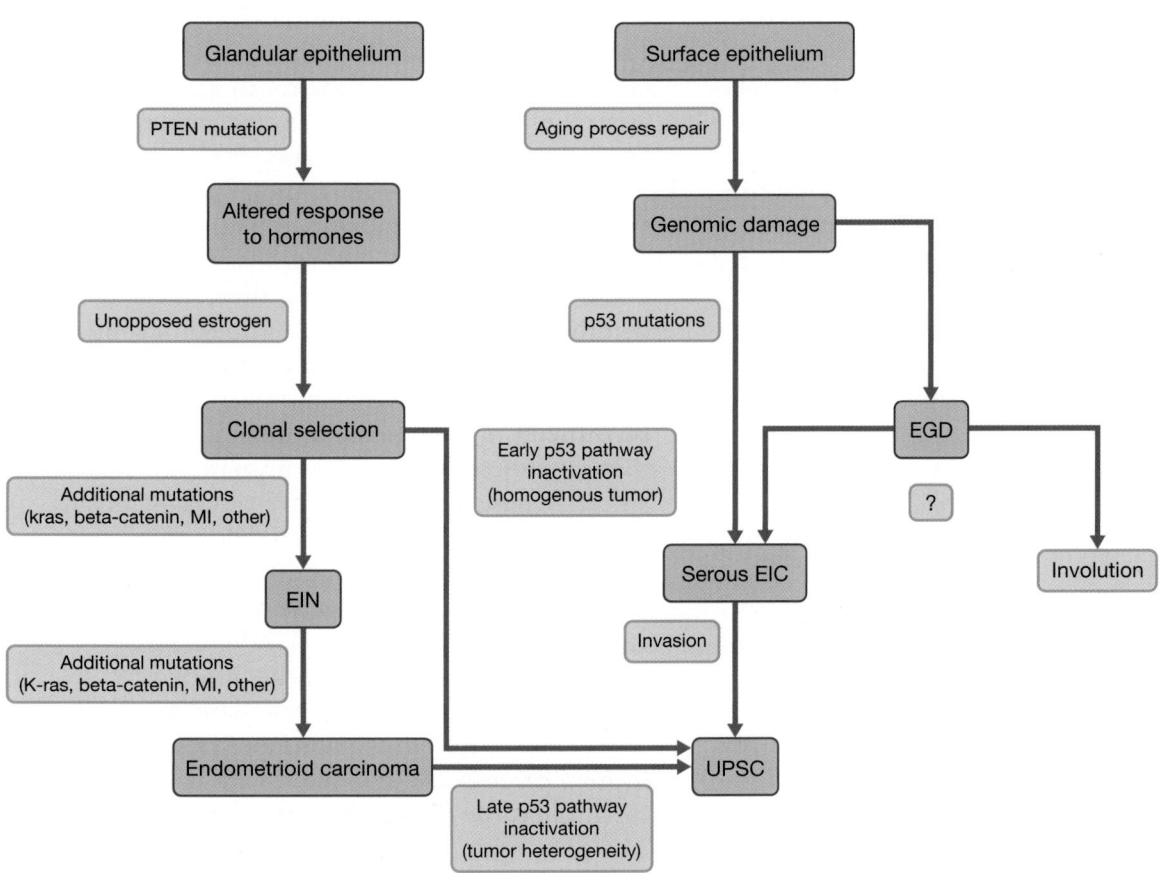

Fig. 19.1 Schematic of pathways to endometrial adenocarcinoma. The dominant routes are via PTEN/MSI and p53 mutations, which define the endometrioid and serous phenotypes. Other pathways play a lesser role.

53% of mortality among blacks, compared with 36% among whites in one study.[12] However, survival is poorer for blacks than for whites even when controlled for in histopathologic category, stage, grade and age.[12]

Hormone replacement/suppressive therapy

Estrogens

Continuous (unopposed) estrogen exposure is associated with an increased risk of endometrial adenocarcinoma, with a risk of approximately six-fold higher than controls (Table 19.2).[2] Shorter intervals of estrogen followed by progesterone, such as encountered in use of sequential contraceptives and sequential replacement therapy, have a normal or marginal increase in risk. Screening of the latter population with endometrial sampling has not proven to be cost-effective. In two studies combined, only one malignancy was discovered in 1398 patients on replacement therapy who were screened by biopsy.[13,14]

Tamoxifen

Tamoxifen is a non-steroidal antiestrogen used chiefly for prophylaxis for, and as a maintenance drug for, breast carcinoma.[15] The dominant histologic pattern seen with tamoxifen use is an atrophic or inactive endometrium. However, in the mid-1990s studies emerged linking more prolonged use with endometrial polyps and a range of endometrial neoplasms, including endometrioid, serous and mixed epithelial and mesenchymal tumors.[16] The risk of these conditions, which includes an increased endometrial stripe on ultrasound, increases as a function of dose and duration of therapy. A total of 18% of 317 treated patients developed some form of pathology in one study and 5 (1.6%) developed malignancy after 3 years of exposure.[17] The malignancy rate was 0.5% (5) in another of 1010 women followed an average of 51 months. The computed standard incidence ratio was 4.0–4.8.[18]

Some authors have linked tamoxifen to more aggressive subtypes of endometrial cancers;[19] others have not demonstrated an increased risk of poor outcome.[15] Some of the observed differences may be due to selection bias of consultation material-based studies compared with more inclusive studies of exposed populations.

Familial syndromes and risk factors for other cancers

Endometrial cancer is overwhelmingly (>98% of occurrences) a sporadic disease, but rarely may be a manifestation of hereditary cancer syndromes that also include ovarian, colonic and other neoplasms. What is known can be summarized in the following points:

1 Endometrial carcinoma is the most common gynecologic cancer associated with hereditary non-polyposis colonic cancer syndrome (HNPCC or Lynch II syndrome); the two cancers are linked by the replication error phenotype (RER+) attributed to defects in mismatch repair genes.[2,20,21] From 40–70% of women with HNPCC develop endometrial cancer and the mean age is approximately 10–20 years younger than non-familial occurrences (46 years).[2,20–22]

2 The risk of synchronous or metachronous ovarian tumors is increased in women with endometrial cancer, ranging from 10% to 23%.[23] Like isolated endometrial adenocarcinoma, these occur most commonly in a sporadic, non-familial setting. Especially when a histologically similar tumor is seen in both endometrial and ovarian sites, it may be difficult or impossible to distinguish whether these represent independent primaries or metastatic spread. These alternatives have repercussions in interpretation of a heightened field effect (hereditary) versus late-stage sporadic disease. Some of the familial risk of endometrial cancer appears independent of the HNPCC link.[24] This strong relationship appears limited to endometrioid tumors only. Standard incidence (risk) ratios (SIRs) for synchronous or metachronous ovarian carcinomas in women with endometrioid carcinomas (or the reverse) range as high as 140.[25] The SIRs of endometrial cancer and endometrioid ovarian cancer in a daughter whose mother had endometrial cancer are similar (3.4 and 3.2).[25]

Table 19.2 Risk factors for endometrial cancer[25,26,33]

Factor		Relative risk
Overweight	(20–50 lb)	3.0
	(50+ lb)	10.0
Nulliparous	(vs 1 child)	2.0
	(vs 5 children)	5.0
Late menopause (>52 vs 49)		2.4
Diabetes mellitus		2.7
Unopposed estrogen therapy		6.0
Tamoxifen therapy		2.0
Sequential oral contraceptives		7.0
Combination oral contraceptives		0.5
Cowden's syndrome (PTEN mutation)		3–5-fold increased risk
HNPCC		40–60% lifetime risk
Family member with endometrial cancer		3.4

If a sister was affected by colorectal cancer the SIR increased to 31.4, and the mean age predictably decreased.[24] There is a mildly elevated endometrial cancer risk in familial kindreds with Cowden's syndrome, caused by constitutive inactivation of the PTEN tumor suppressor gene.[26] The low magnitude of increased risk (probably only 3–5-fold) may be due to lack of those non-genetic hormonal factors which interact with mutations to define lifetime cancer risk.

3 Patients who present with familial endometrial cancer have a high frequency of genetic mutations in those mismatch repair genes inactivated in HNPCC families. Most commonly, these are structural genomic defects in the DNA mismatch repair genes MLH1, MSH2 and MSH6, and a genetic instability phenotype can be observed in histologically normal, as well as neoplastic, tissues. Sporadic, non-familial endometrial cancers also have a high incidence (17–23%) of microsatellite instability caused by inactivation of the MLH1 gene.[27–31] The mechanism of MLH1 inactivation in these sporadic cases is, however, epigenetic rather than mutational, and the genetic instability phenotype is seen only in transformed neoplastic tissues.[27] The accumulated data thus support a relationship between inactivation of mismatch repair genes and endometrioid tumors of the female genital tract. When the mismatch repair system is constitutively inactivated through a heritable mechanism, affected individuals are younger at time of cancer presentation and have a shared risk for other neoplasms, most notably colorectal cancer.

Molecular genetics

Serous and endometrioid endometrial cancer subtypes have a divergent pathogenesis. Mutations in the PTEN gene and the replication error (RER) phenotype with microsatellite instability (MSI) are strongly associated with the endometrioid subgroup (Table 19.1).[32,33] Mutations of the PTEN tumour suppressor gene – active in cell cycle control and apoptosis – have been identified in up to 80% of endometrioid carcinomas and are also commonly detected in isolated glands of histologically normal proliferative endometrium and EIN (see Ch. 17) (Figs 19.1, 19.2a,b). The pathogenesis of endometrial carcinoma and its transition from normal to neoplastic also involves a wide range of other molecular disturbances, including K-ras mutation, beta-catenin inactivation, and loss of cyclin-dependent kinase activity.[34,35]

In contrast to the endometrioid carcinomas, serous tumors are rarely associated with PTEN inactivation or MSI. Rather, over 80% of these tumors possess mutations in the p53 tumor suppressor gene. Mutations in p53 are found in the earliest identifiable manifestations of these tumors (Figs 19.1, 19.2c,d). Until recently, no studies have identified a *bona-fide* precursor to UPSC (see below).[36,37]

Despite the above, the pathogenesis of endometrial adenocarcinoma is complex. Endometrioid and serous carcinomas may coexist, p53 mutations can associated with 'endometrioid' carcinomas as well as a proportion of epithelial tumors contain mesenchymal differentiation.[36,37] These differences will be addressed in the discussion of morphologic patterns, biomarker identification and outcomes.

Precursor lesions

Preinvasive endometrial glandular neoplasia has been discussed in detail in Chapters 17 and 18. It is generally assumed that the common (endometrioid) forms of endometrial adenocarcinoma have their beginnings as endometrial intraepithelial neoplasms (EIN).[38] This is supported by temporal, genetic and morphologic continuity between EIN and endometrioid endometrial adenocarcinoma as well as the increased risk of endometrial cancer clinical outcomes associated with EIN.[39–41]

The lag period between premalignant lesions and development of endometrial cancers and the precise percentage of endometrial cancers which transit a diagnosable premalignant phase is unclear, both due to previous imprecision in precancer diagnosis under the old 'hyperplasia' system and difficulties in obtaining longitudinal tissue samples on individual patients. Koss screened asymptomatic women and found a prevalence rate of endometrial cancer of 6.96 per 1000 women-years, with an incidence of 1.71 per 1000 women-years.[5] In spite of an active search for endometrial hyperplasias, the rate of these lesions was nearly identical to the prevalence and incidence rates for carcinoma – a striking contrast to the disparity in prevalence rates for invasive and preinvasive squamous neoplasms of the cervix. A systematic search for residual EIN in women having hysterectomies for endometrial adenocarcinoma shows that approximately 40% of women with endometrioid types of carcinoma retain persistent premalignant lesions at the time of definitive therapy. Those cancers that transit a premalignant phase are most likely to show inactivation of the PTEN gene, a genetic change noted in two-thirds of EIN

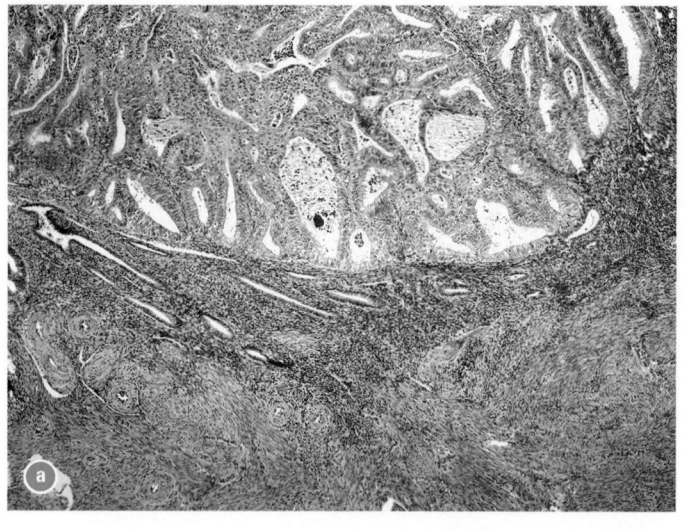
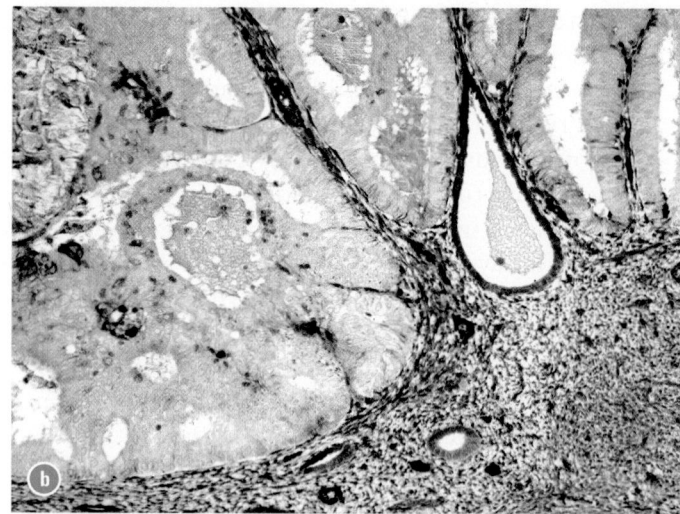
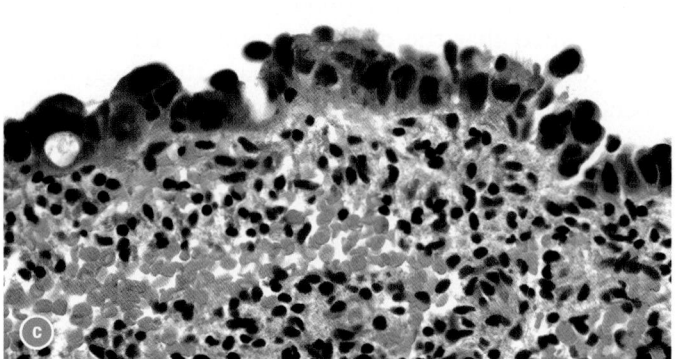
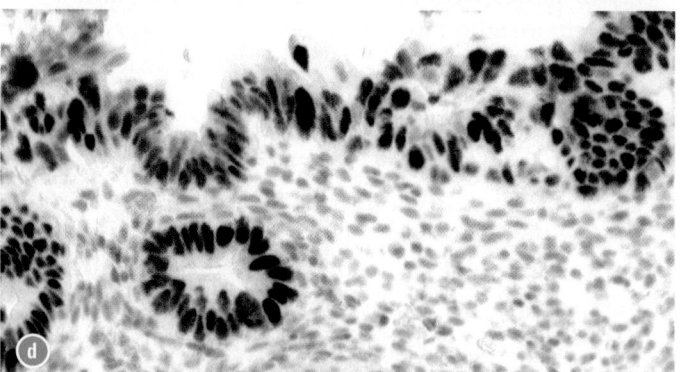

Fig. 19.2 (a) Endometrioid adenocarcinoma, (b) absence of PTEN (note positive normal gland at right), (c) uterine papillary serous carcinoma, (d) expression and retention of mutant p53.

lesions.[42] This is strong evidence that not only is the endometrioid subtype of carcinoma most strongly associated with premalignant EIN lesions but also that this progression scenario is functionally defined by accumulation of genetic defects within affected tissues over a period of years. The tempo of progression was first estimated by Hertig and Sommers, who found an average progression interval of 3–5 years from 'endometrial anaplasia' to adenocarcinoma.[43] This timeframe was confirmed in a follow-up study of 'atypical endometrial hyperplasia', which showed a median progression interval to adenocarcinoma of 4.1 years.[44]

In contrast to endometrioid carcinomas, uterine papillary serous carcinomas are not associated with an unequivocal precursor lesion that can be distinguished morphologically and genetically. p53 mutant atypical cells deployed on the endometrial surface, 'serous endometrial intraepithelial carcinoma' (serous EIC) have been proposed as a precursor lesion, but the majority of these occur in association with coexisting carcinoma and are likely an early manifestation of the carcinoma, rather than a premalignant lesion. UPSC either develops quickly or emerges from morphologically normal endometrial surface epithelium as a full-blown carcinoma, making detection of an intervening premalignant phase difficult.[30] A small percentage emerge as a secondarily mutated subclone from a pre-existing endometrioid adenocarcinoma, in which case the malignant endometrioid tumor might be viewed as a 'precursor.'

Zheng et al. have recently described a lesion, termed 'endometrial glandular dysplasia', which may be a precursor to UPSC (Fig. 19.3). This is based upon a histologic appearance and genotype which is intermediate between that of normal epithelium and papillary serous

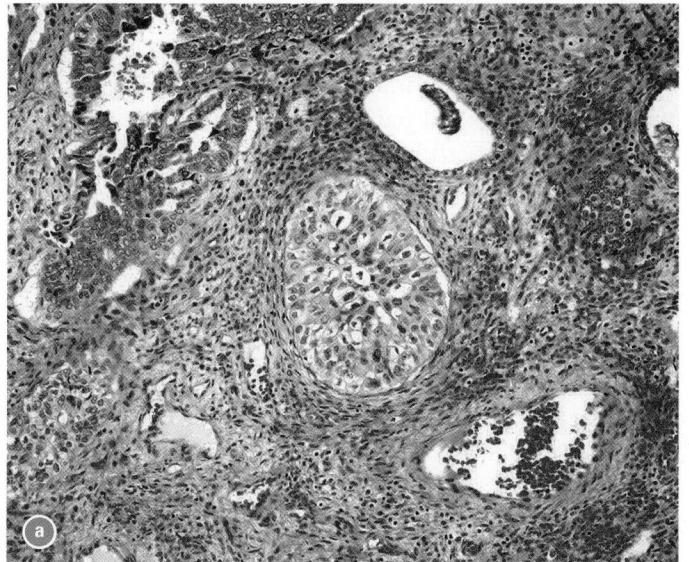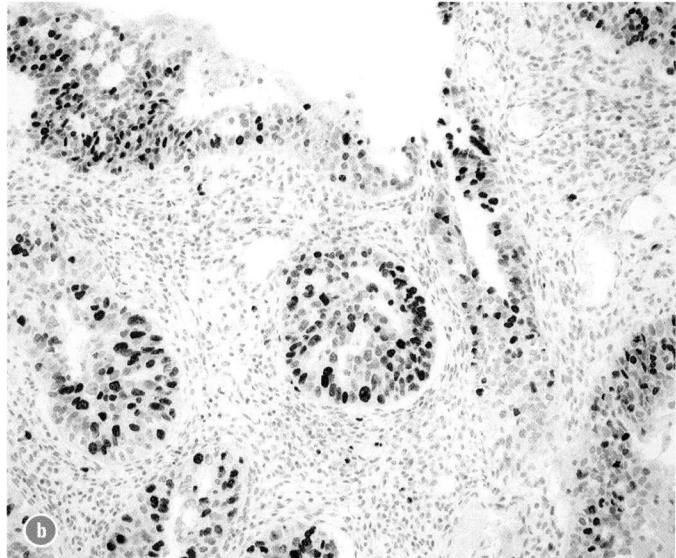

Fig. 19.3 (a) Endometrial glandular dysplasia, a possible precursor to early uterine papillary serous carcinoma. (b) p53 immunostaining (Courtesy of Wenxin Zheng, MD).

carcinoma.[45] It remains be determined whether this rare lesion is a common precursor to UPSC or one of several phenotypes (including endometrioid adenocarcinomas) that predate this tumor. Nevertheless, as will be revealed below, the diagnostic pathologist who routinely reviews the histology of endometrial carcinomas will experience an increasing appreciation for the more subtle variants of uterine papillary serous carcinoma.

CLINICAL PARAMETERS FOR ASSESSING RISK

Postmenopausal bleeding

Postmenopausal bleeding confers a 64-fold increase in risk of endometrial carcinoma and the risk is maximized by recurrent bleeding.[46] In one study, 91% of patients presented with postmenopausal or irregular bleeding. More ominous but less frequent symptoms were abdominal pain or other symptoms (9.4%).[47] Important variables that influence the significance of bleeding include the following.

Age (menopausal status)

The risk of cancer is a function of the age when bleeding occurs, increasing from 9% in the sixth to 60% in the ninth decade.[2,48] Overall, the risk in postmenopausal women with bleeding is approximately 8–11%. In the majority, atrophic (83%) and other benign non-atrophic

(6%) patterns are present.[49,50] However, any abnormal bleeding should be investigated, including intermenstrual bleeding and oligomenorrhea (particularly in the setting of ovarian dysfunction).

Setting

Hormone replacement therapy (HRT) is associated with a lower risk of carcinoma in the setting of bleeding. Elliott et al. examined 299 postmenopausal women and 204 women on HRT. The incidence of endometrial carcinoma was significantly higher in older women and those who were not on HRT (RR >10).[51] Gemer and Segal observed a rate of only 0.08% for women under 50 *vs* 3.7% for women over age 50.[52]

Persistent bleeding

Twu and Chen studied 77 patients with postmenopausal bleeding whose initial tissue diagnosis was benign. A total of 16 subsequently were diagnosed with carcinoma or hyperplasia, and the risk was particularly high for those over 65 years of age (44.8%).[53] The authors concluded that repeated bleeding in a postmenopausal patient may justify hysterectomy.

The recurrence rate of uterine bleeding was highest in carcinoma of the endometrium but not exclusive to this group. However, another study of 40 hysterectomies for persistent postmenopausal bleeding but with normal prior endometrial sampling found no cancers and four (10%) hyperplasias, suggesting that persistent postmenopausal bleeding with non-malignant pathology on endometrial sampling is not necessarily an indication for hysterectomy.[54]

Transvaginal ultrasound

Transvaginal ultrasound (TVU) has increased in popularity, principally as a device to screen women on tamoxifen therapy and identify women at low risk for endometrial cancer. The parameter of importance is endometrial thickness. The following are important variables when using TVU:

1 As a rule, the mean endometrial thickness increases as a function of the pathology, averaging 3.4, 9.7 and 18.2 mm for atrophic, hyperplastic and malignant endometrium.[55]

2 The cut-off level varies between studies but generally ranges between 5 mm (for the general population) and 8 mm (for women on tamoxifen). Predictably, the lower the threshold the higher the sensitivity and the lower the positive predictive value. In a screening population, nearly 100% of cancers can be excluded with the value set at 5 mm.[56] However, the positive predictive value is poor, being 9% in one screening study.[57] In a meta-analysis of four studies of women with postmenopausal bleeding, Gupta et al. noted a positive predictive value of 31.3% for a positive test (>5 mm); however, 2.5% of negatives were confirmed to have cancer on histologic examination.[58] Other literature reviews and reports using a 5 or 6 mm cut-off have found similar results and, despite some showing a 100% sensitivity, the consensus is that symptomatic women should undergo endometrial sampling.[59,60]

3 In many institutions, TVU is most popular in the follow-up of women on replacement therapy or tamoxifen. The cut-off is usually 8 mm and the test is limited by lack of specificity. Endometrial thickness increases as a function of duration of treatment and will exceed 8 mm in half after prolonged use.[61] Moreover, there is little relationship between thickness and cancer. The cause of the endometrial thickness in most women on tamoxifen is sub-endometrial thickening.[62]

Hysteroscopy

It is generally accepted that hysteroscopy is a useful adjunct to evaluating the endometrium but is not sufficient without histologic examination. One meta-analysis based on 208 articles found established a pretest probability of endometrial cancer at 3.9%; a positive and negative hysteroscopy yielded a cancer diagnosis in 71.8 and 0.6%, respectively.[63] Others concur that while few cancers are identified in setting of normal or atrophic findings, all patients must undergo biopsy.[64]

One concern with hysteroscopy is that it will increase the risk of a positive peritoneal washing at the time of hysterectomy, effectively upstaging the tumor to a FIGO IIIA. However, it does not influence overall prognosis.[65]

HISTOPATHOLOGY OF ENDOMETRIAL ADENOCARCINOMA

Introduction

The pathologist may be involved in four phases of endometrial carcinoma management, including (1) detection of the tumor on Papanicolaou smear, (2) interpretation of a biopsy or curetting which may be prompted by the cytology, but much more frequently by abnormal bleeding, (3) intraoperative assessment of the uterus to facilitate staging and (4) postoperative evaluation of the hysterectomy specimen to determine the risk of recurrence and to guide therapy. Each of these components of laboratory management has its priorities, limitations and diagnostic pitfalls and will be discussed subsequently. However, addressing each requires first a comprehensive understanding of the histologic classification and grading of endometrial neoplasia.

Tumor types

Endometrial adenocarcinomas can be subdivided into the following categories: (1) endometrioid adenocarcinomas, including those associated with related but 'non-endometrioid' forms of differentiation; (2) papillary serous carcinoma; (3) clear cell carcinomas; (4) carcinomas with features intermediate between endometrioid and papillary serous; (5) poorly-differentiated or undifferentiated carcinomas without clear-cut endometrioid or serous features; (6) mixed carcinomas; and (7) rare carcinomas such as pure squamous carcinomas or small cell neuroendocrine types (Table 19.3).[66] Carcinosarcomas will be discussed separately.

Endometrioid adenocarcinomas

Introduction Endometrioid adenocarcinomas, including those with non-endometrioid forms of differentiation, account for nearly 90% of endometrial adenocarcinomas. Most endometrioid carcinomas are characterized histologically by well-defined glands lined by cytologically malignant columnar epithelial cells. However, they are

Table 19.3 *Classification of endometrial epithelial neoplasia*[66]

Precursors
  Type I pathway: endometrial intraepithelial neoplasia (EIN)
  Type II pathway: serous EIC/endometrial glandular dysplasia

Common types
  Endometrioid adenocarcinoma
    Pure endometrioid carcinoma
    With squamous differentiation
    With mucinous differentiation
    With ciliated (tubal) differentiation
    With secretory differentiation
    With squamo-transitional differentiation
    Villoglandular carcinoma
  Uterine papillary serous carcinoma
    Confined to mucosal surface (endometrial intraepithelial carcinoma)
    Invasive
    Mixed endometrioid and serous carcinoma
  Clear cell carcinoma
  Carcinosarcoma

Rare variants
  Condyloma
  Squamous carcinoma (incl. verrucous carcinoma)
  Small cell carcinoma
  Giant cell carcinoma
  Non-gestational choriocarcinoma

Metastatic tumors
  Cervix carcinoma
  Breast carcinoma
  Gastrointestinal carcinoma

subdivided into several morphologic subsets, each of which may vary in the degree of differentiation. Three important parameters to keep in mind when evaluating tumors in this category are: (1) glandular pattern, (2) degree of nuclear atypia and (3) non-endometrioid cellular differentiation (or metaplasia). The grading systems are detailed below.[66]

Morphologic patterns Patterns of endometrioid differentiation fall into the following categories: (1) conventional endometrioid carcinoma and other patterns accounting for a small or large percentage of the tumor, including (2) squamous, (3) mucinous, (4) tubal, (5) secretory, (6) villoglandular and (7) other forms of differentiation. These additional cell patterns are often classified in separate 'non-endometrioid' categories because they differ in appearance from normal endometrium.[7,67] This is technically correct. However, the separation of endometrioid from these other patterns is superfluous, inasmuch as these variant patterns are characteristically associated with endometrioid carcinomas in contrast to serous or clear cell carcinomas and do not alter outcome. For this reason, they will be discussed with the endometrioid tumors.

Endometrioid gland patterns Endometrioid adenocarcinomas are those in which the malignant glands resemble those of the normal proliferative phase endometrium. They are distinguished from normal endometrium and preinvasive disease (EIN) by the presence of some or all of the following in addition to malignant cytologic features: (a) confluent cribriform growth; (b) loss of individual gland integrity with 'rambling' glands with minimal or no intervening stroma; (c) villoglandular architecture and (d) nuclear atypia in excess of that associated with EIN (see Ch. 17) (Fig. 19.4). They are typically graded as well-differentiated (grade 1), with easily recognizable glandular patterns (Fig. 19.5a); moderately-differentiated (grade 2)(Fig. 19.5b), showing well-formed glands mixed with solid sheets of malignant cells; or poorly-differentiated (grade 3) (Fig. 19.5c), characterized by solid sheets of cells with barely recognizable glands, often with greater nuclear atypia and mitotic activity.[68] Most endometrioid carcinomas are grades 1 or 2.

Because they resemble normal endometrium, endometrioid carcinomas usually display nuclear uniformity with preservation of polarity (Fig. 19.6a). The neoplastic glands are larger and typically more irregular than those of the normal endometrium. When conspicuous atypia is present, it will influence grading (Fig. 19.6b). Rarely, some exhibit a uniform tubular pattern similar to Sertoli cell tumors of the ovary (Fig. 19.7).[69] Another characteristic feature of some endometrioid tumors is the presence of compact clusters of foamy histiocytes in the stroma adjacent to the neoplastic glands (Fig. 19.8a). In curettage specimens, foamy cells should be distinguished from smaller sheets of macrophages that are commonly seen in benign endometria (Fig. 19.8b). Foamy stromal histiocytes do not invariably signify cancer, but their presence in association with a uterine carcinoma signifies an endometrial rather than a cervical origin.

Squamous differentiation Squamous differentiation accompanies approximately 25% of endometrioid carcinomas and includes a range of atypia that parallels the degree of glandular atypia. This range includes the following: (a) Discrete nests (morules) or uniformly demarcated sheets of uniform non-keratinizing squamous cells, as commonly seen in EIN and metaplasias, typically accompany well-differentiated tumors and those lesions straddling the interface between EIN and well-differentiated adenocarcinoma (Fig. 19.9a). (b) More irregular or bizarre squamous differentiation, with prominent keratinization and nuclear atypia, is

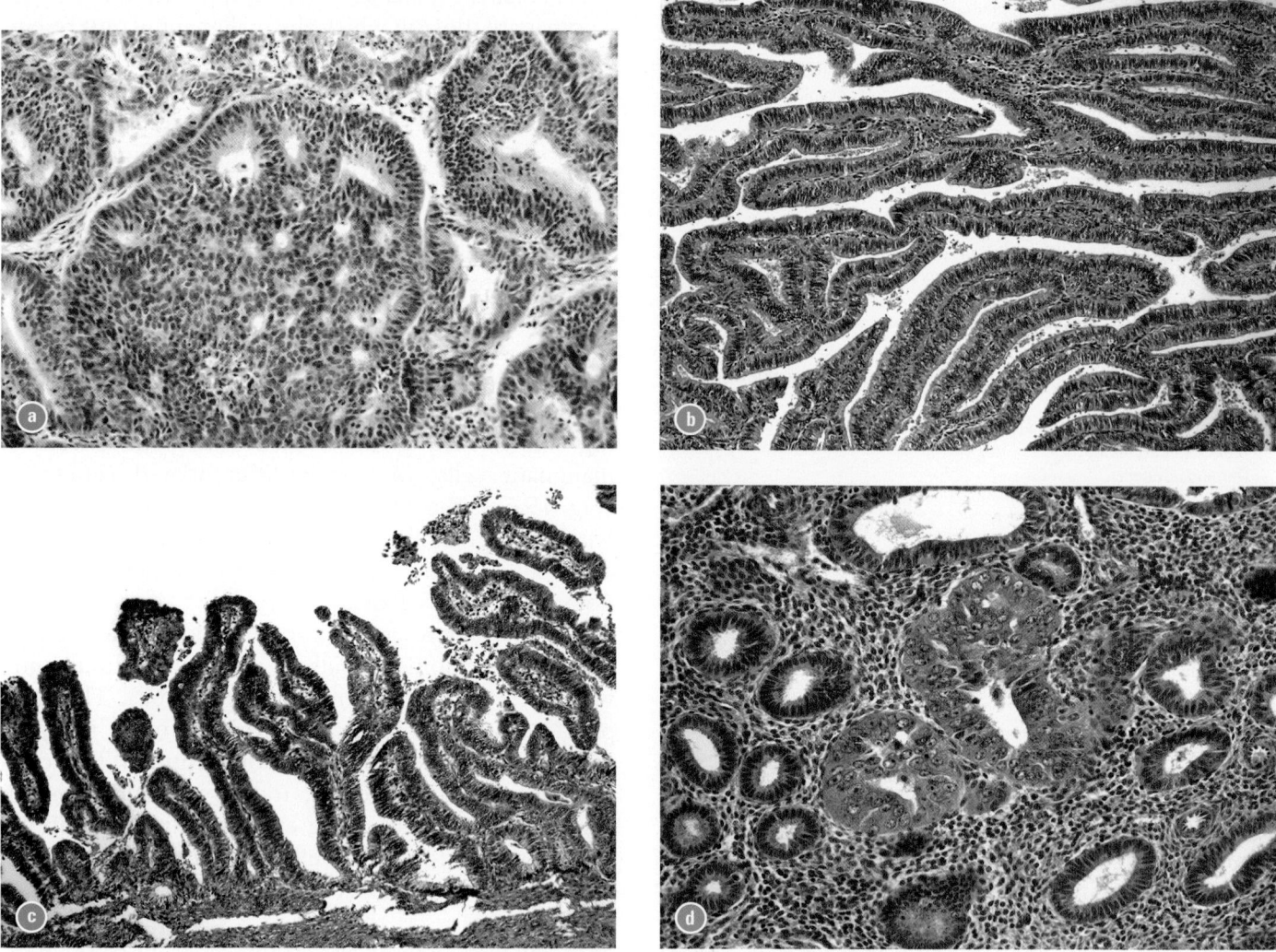

Fig. 19.4 Diagnosis of endometrial cancer: (a) confluent cribriform growth, (b) rambling gland, (c) villoglandular architecture, (d) conspicuous nuclear atypia.

usually associated with higher-grade tumors (Fig. 19.9b). (c) Conspicuous nuclear atypia or less well-defined squamous differentiation with focal keratinization and higher nuclear grade may be indistinguishable from squamous carcinoma; this pattern accompanies high-grade endometrioid adenocarcinomas (Fig. 19.9c).

The clinical significance of squamous differentiation in endometrioid carcinomas has been debated in the past, with disagreement over whether squamous differentiation *per se* influences outcome. Traditionally, adenocarcinomas with squamous differentiation were assigned unique diagnostic categories, such as adenoacanthoma or adenosquamous carcinoma, on the assumption that they portended better and worse outcomes, respectively.[70] Although this was generally correct, experts ultimately decided that the degree of glandular differentiation primarily governed the prognosis of these tumors. Consequently, nomenclatures replaced the above terms with 'adenocarcinoma (of specific type and grade) with squamous differentiation'.[71] Because the range of squamous differentiation varies in endometrioid carcinomas and because the transitions between squamous and glandular components can be subtle, the pathologist may not always be able to determine whether the tumor in question is a poorly-differentiated endometrioid carcinoma or a high-grade carcinoma with mixed differentiation. However, in high-grade tumors this distinction is not critical, as the tumor will be assigned a high-risk histology. In some tumors, the non-glandular component may appear transitional or squamo-transitional (see below), reflecting further the plasticity of these tumors in terms of differentiation pathway (Fig. 19.10).[72,73]

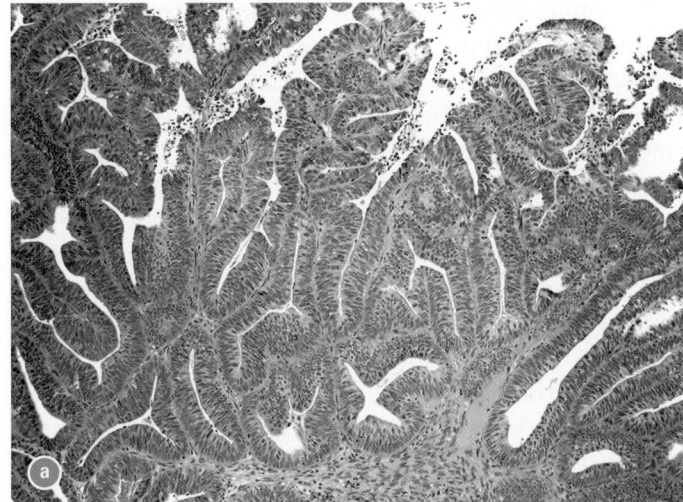

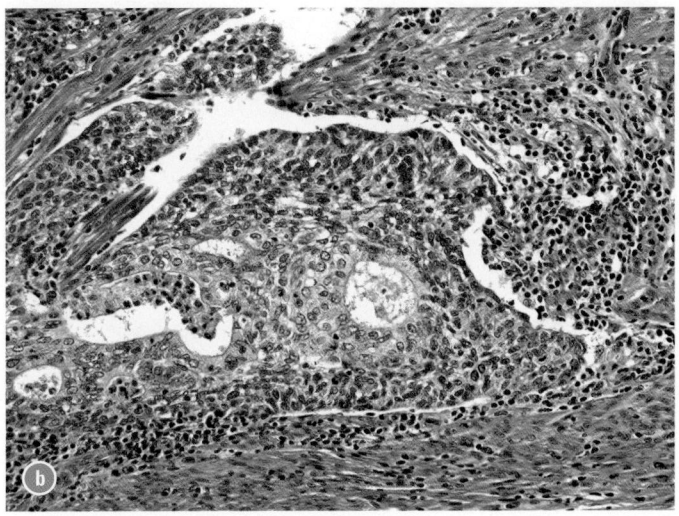

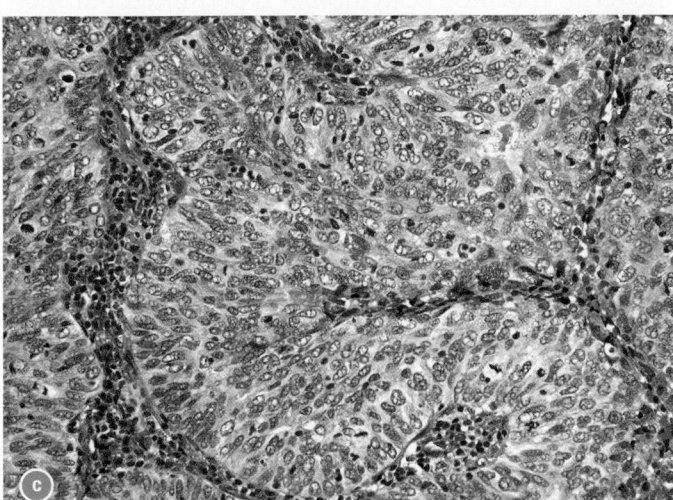

Fig. 19.5 Endometrial adenocarcinoma: (a) grade 1, (b) grade 2, (c) grade 3.

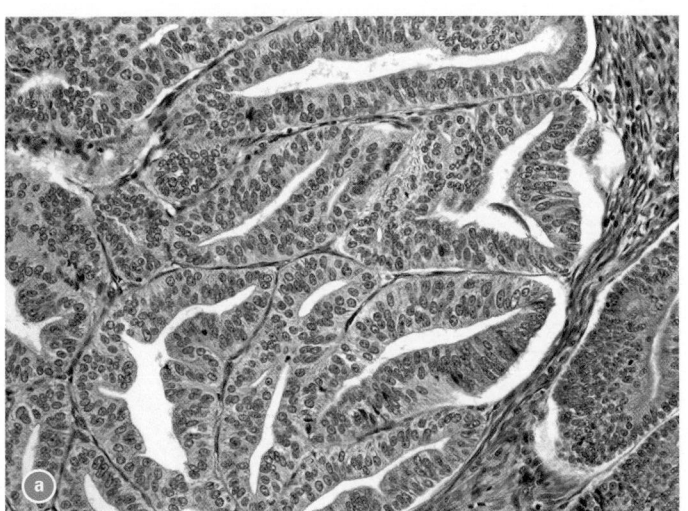

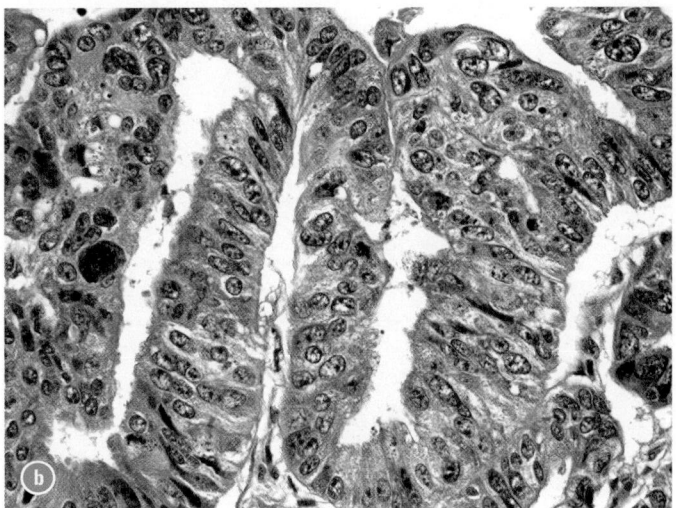

Fig. 19.6 Most endometrioid adenocarcinomas contain pseudostratified epithelial cells with uniform (low- grade) nuclei (a). Others contain foci of conspicuous nuclear enlargement and hyperchromasia (b). The latter justifies a one-step increase in grade.

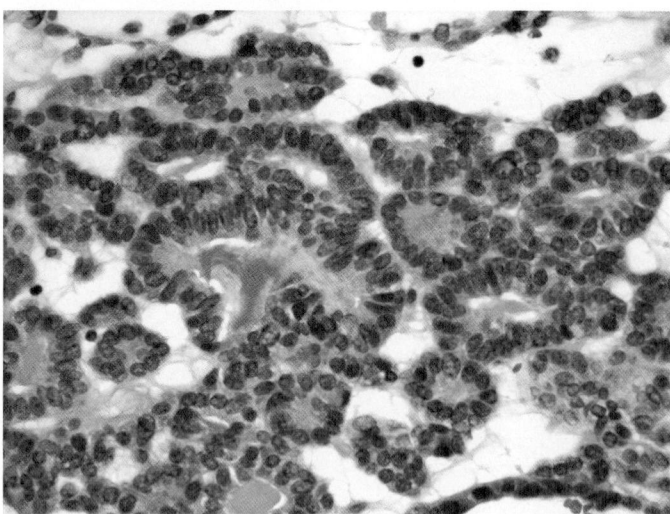

Fig. 19.7 Sertoli-like patterns occasionally occur in endometrial carcinomas.

The diagnostic pitfalls associated with squamous differentiation include both under- and over-grading of the tumor. Squamous sheets lacking keratinization may be misclassified as a grade 2 or 3 endometrioid carcinoma (Fig. 19.11a). Eosinophilic degenerative changes in glandular areas may be misclassified as squamous differentiation, but this error is not clinically significant (Fig. 19.11b). In rare cases, bland squamous areas of under-sampled carcinoma may be dismissed as benign cervical epithelium (Fig. 19.11c). This latter circumstance could delay the diagnosis of cancer.

Mucinous differentiation Mucinous differentiation is frequently present as a minor component in endometrioid adenocarcinomas and is defined by the presence of prominent intracellular mucin. As has been emphasized previously in Chapter 18, bland-appearing mucinous glands, while resembling endocervix, are much more commonly seen in endometrial than endocervical carcinomas, from which they must be distinguished.

A minority of endometrial carcinomas are purely mucinous and, in rare cases, marked mucin production will be visible on gross examination. In most, mucinous differentiation occurs in an otherwise well-differentiated endometrioid neoplasm, prompting the diagnosis of 'endometrioid adenocarcinoma (grade specified) with mucinous differentiation'. If nearly pure, the term 'mucinous carcinoma' is permitted but there is no clinical significance to this distinction. The range of atypia, however, may be, in terms of influencing the diagnosis and prompt recognition of these tumors.[74-76]

Histologically, tumors with mucinous differentiation range from banal to obviously malignant. The most subtle variants exhibit either cribriform or papillary glandular architecture lined by uniform cuboidal to low-stratified cells with round, slightly enlarged nuclei and conspicuous mucin (Figs 19.12, 19.13). Those with microacinar architecture may closely resemble microglandular change of the cervix. Those with micropapillary architecture must be distinguished from benign surface metaplasias. (These are discussed in Chapter 17 and under differential diagnosis, below.)

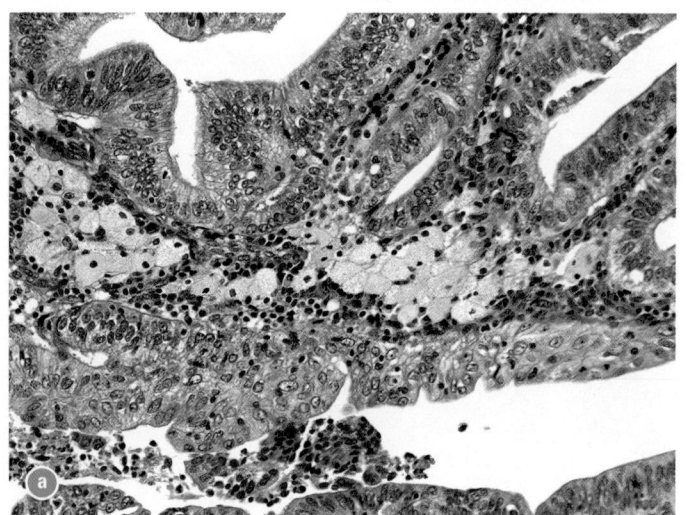
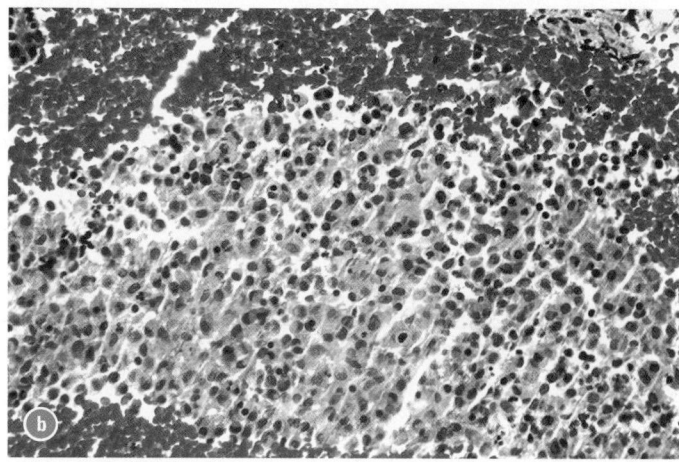

Fig. 19.8 (a) Foamy histiocytes are frequently associated with endometrial cancer (center). (b) Macrophages are not specific and are more commonly seen with benign conditions.

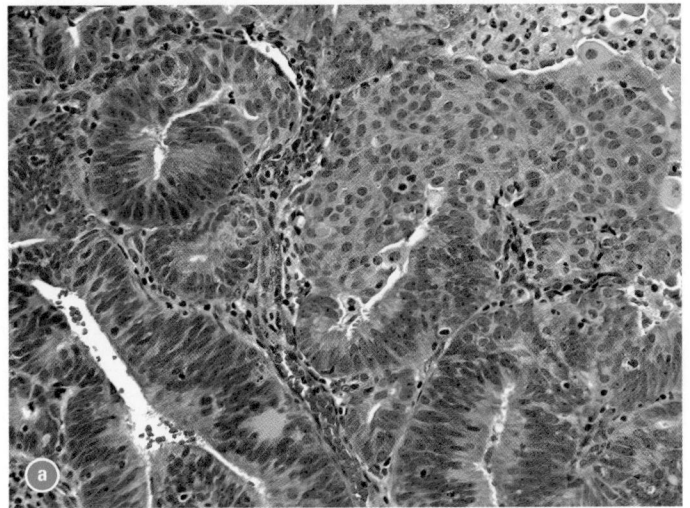

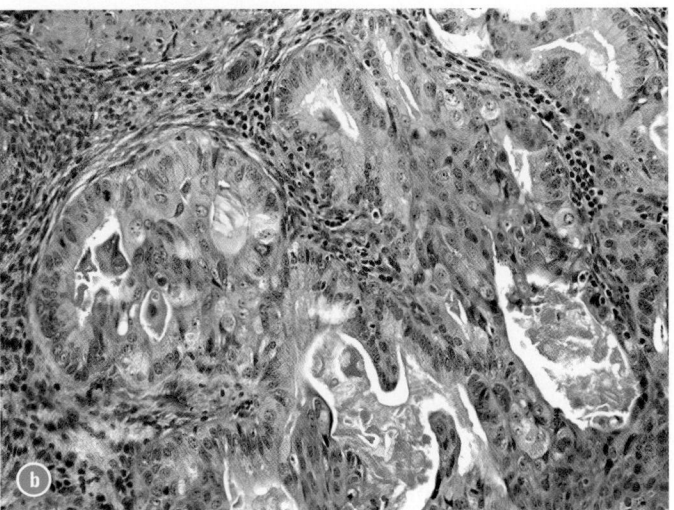

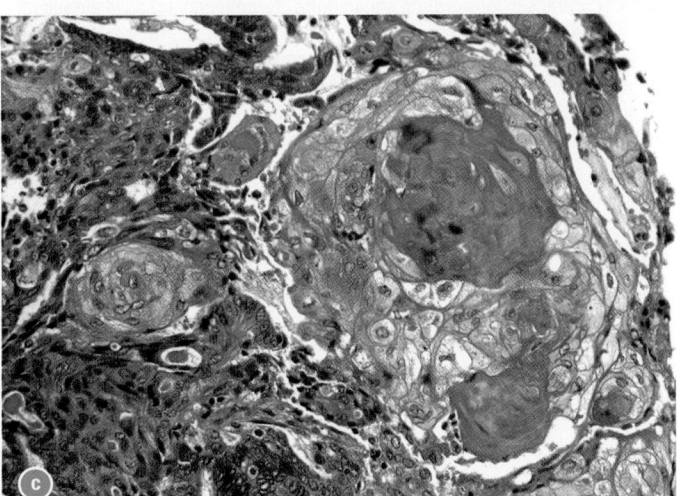

Fig. 19.9 The spectrum of squamous differentiation in endometrial cancer includes (a) morules, (b) aberrant differentiation and (c) solid sheets of squamous differentiation.

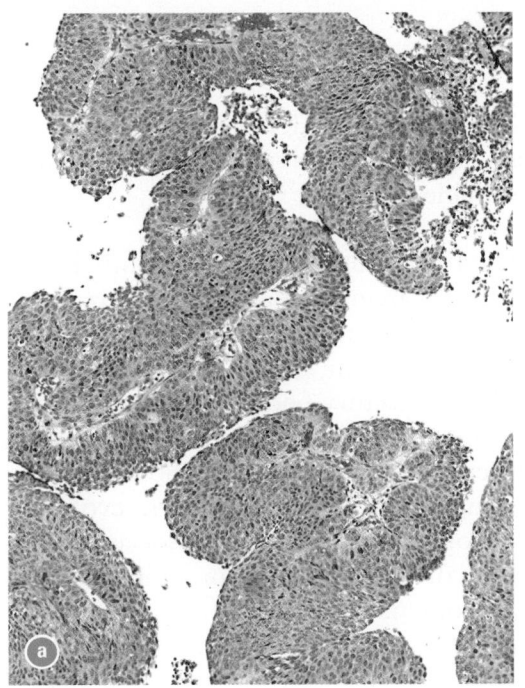

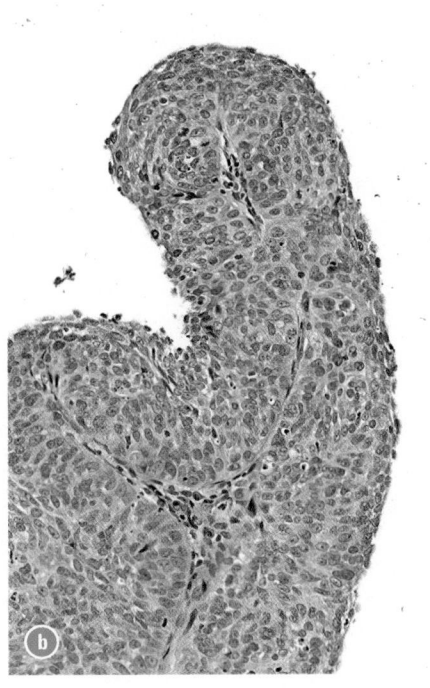

Fig. 19.10 Poorly-differentiated squamo-transitional differentiation in an endometrial carcinoma. Note the loosely arranged papillae (a) lined by uniform cells with preserved polarity (b).

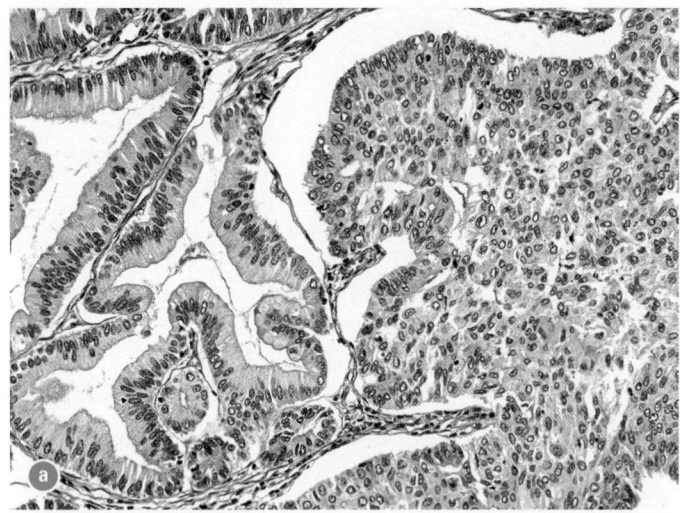

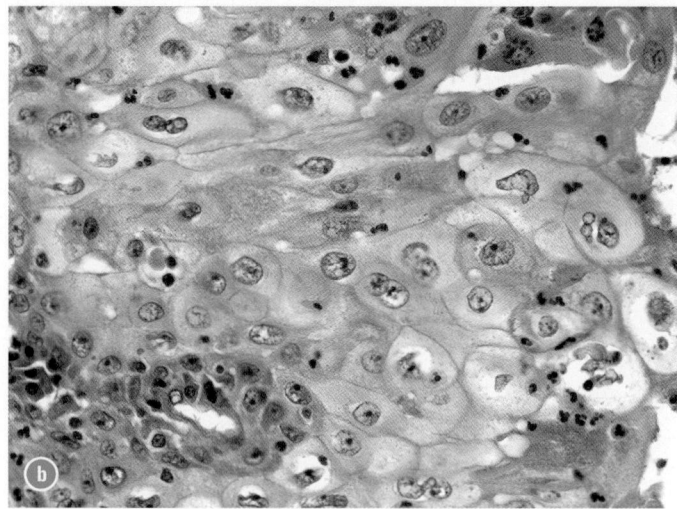

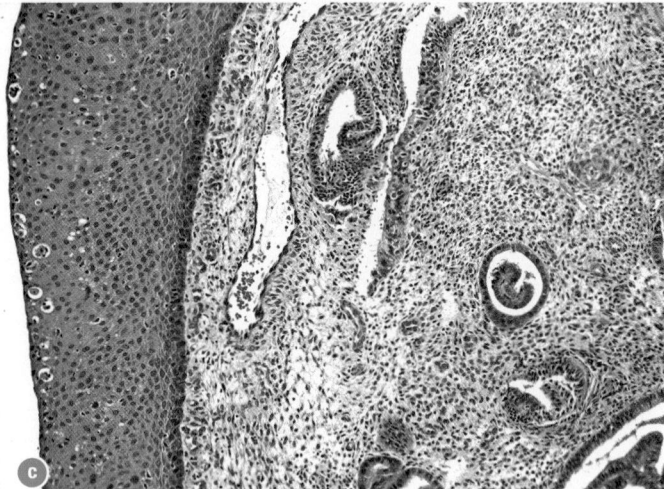

Fig. 19.11 Pitfalls in interpreting squamous differentiation: (a) solid sheets of squamous differentiation (right) may be misinterpreted as grade 2 adenocarcinoma, (b) eosinophilic areas in conventional adenocarcinomas may mimic squamous differentiation, (c) squamous differentiation associated with an endometrial carcinoma lining the surface of the lower uterine segment and mimicking cervical epithelium.

Others contain more irregular architecture and conspicuous nuclear atypia and are unmistakably malignant (Fig. 19.14). Rare variants of mucin-producing endometrial carcinomas include those with gastric or intestinal differentiation (Fig. 19.15a,b).[77] In general, lesions with mild atypia will be minimally invasive. However, there have been cases in which the mucinous component was superficial and focal, with a subjacent higher-grade adenocarcinoma or, rarely, a carcinosarcoma.

Tubal (ciliated cell) differentiation Tubal differentiation is common in both benign and neoplastic endometrium. When the tumor has widespread ciliated cells, the term 'ciliated carcinoma' has been used.[78] By definition, these tumors are well-differentiated (Fig. 19.16). They have uniform but confluent glands composed of stratified cells with round nuclei, focal cytoplasmic clearing, prominent eosinophilic cytoplasm with terminal bars and well-defined cilia projecting into the lumen above a portion of the cells. They portend a favourable outcome.[78]

Secretory differentiation A small number of endometrioid adenocarcinomas are characterized by basal or supranuclear vacuoles akin to those seen in early secretory endometrium.[7,79] The glands are similar in contour to early secretory endometrium but differ by their size (larger), back-to-back orientation and prominent differential epithelial stratification with luminal scalloping. Although the pattern evokes a connection to progestins and may be associated with hormonal therapy or ovulatory endometrium in some premenopausal women, the majority of patients are postmenopausal (Fig. 19.17a). The most important

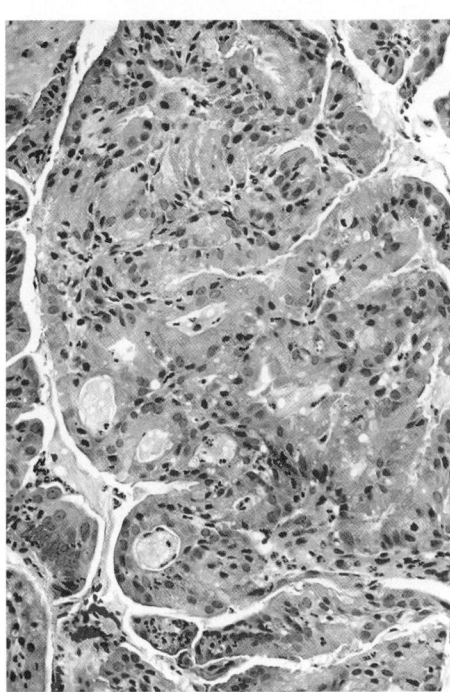

Fig. 19.12 Bland-appearing mucinous changes in a well-differentiated adenocarcinoma with microglandular architecture.

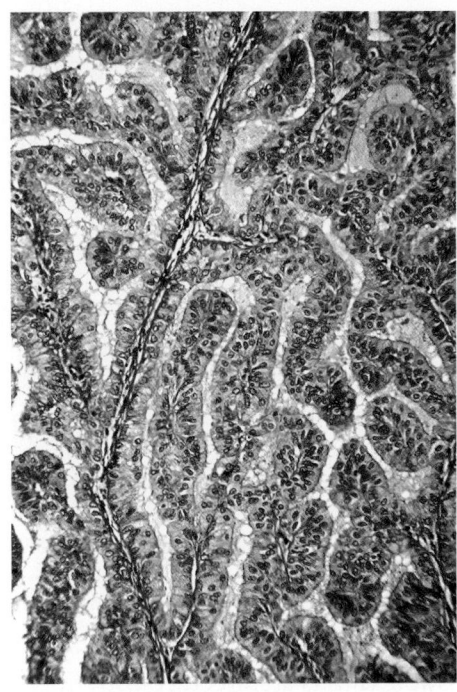

Fig. 19.14 Mucinous adenocarcinoma of the endometrium composed of larger glands.

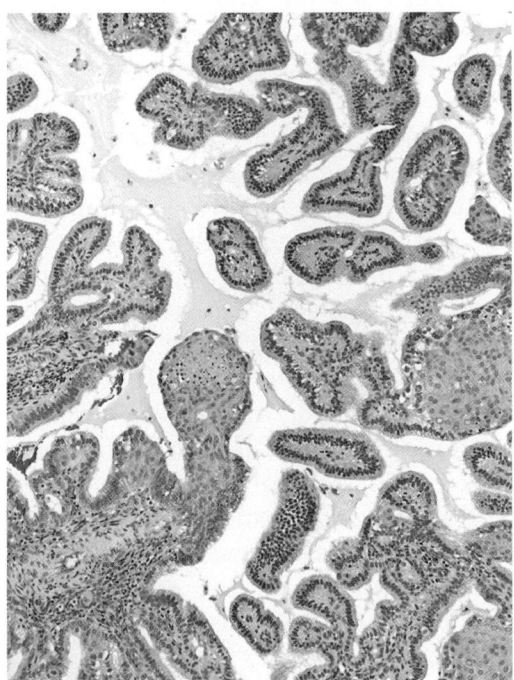

Fig. 19.13 Micropapillary architecture in an adenocarcinoma with mucinous differentiation. Note the coexisting squamous differentiation.

exclusions are secretory endometrium with artifactual crowding (Fig. 19.17b) and EIN with secretory change (see Ch. 17). In addition, two other forms of endometrial carcinoma will exhibit clear cytoplasm.

The first is clear cell carcinoma, in which the lining cells are cuboidal and minimally stratified, with more prominent nuclear atypia than is present in secretory carcinomas (Fig. 19.17c). The second is more subtle and consists of glands with higher nuclear/cytoplasmic ratio and small discrete vacuoles in the glandular epithelium, or sheets of cells with cytoplasmic vacuolation lacking gland architecture. These features characterize more poorly-differentiated adenocarcinomas, including the epithelial components of carcinosarcomas (see below)(Fig. 19.17d).

Villoglandular carcinoma Villoglandular endometrioid adenocarcinomas exhibit a predominately tree-like branching architecture with discrete fibrovascular cores lined by defined pseudostratified endometrioid-type epithelium (Fig. 19.18). Some degree of villoglandular architecture has been described in up to 30% of endometrioid adenocarcinomas.[7] However, this pattern is seen to dominate in less than 5% of endometrioid carcinomas. The prognostic importance of this pattern varies depending on the study. One associated the villoglandular pattern with other aggressive histologic features.[80] A larger study did not detect a difference in outcome between villoglandular carcinomas and conventional endometrioid adenocarcinomas.[81]

A variety of other endometrial lesions, some benign (papillary metaplasia) and others malignant (uterine papillary serous, clear cell, mucinous, and transitional

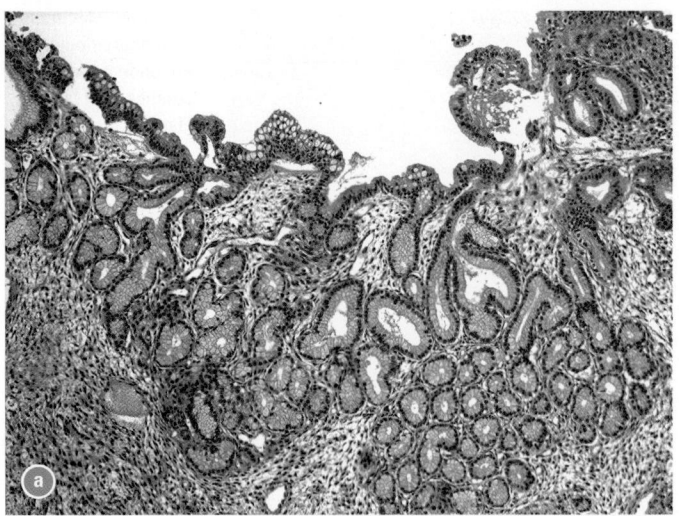
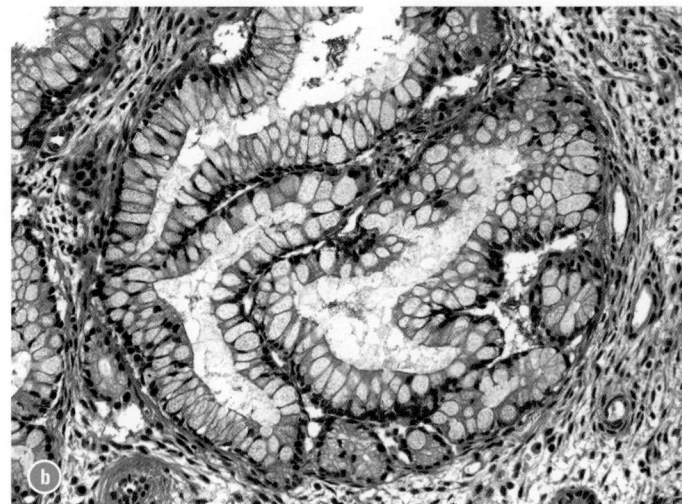

Fig. 19.15 Endometrial adenocarcinoma with (a) gastric and (b) intestinal differentiation.

carcinoma), may exhibit villous architecture with fibro-vascular cores. These will be discussed below under differential diagnosis.[81,82]

Uterine papillary serous carcinomas

Introduction Although classification as a poorly-differentiated endometrioid adenocarcinoma typically requires a loss of glandular differentiation and the presence of solid growth, two histologic patterns behave as if poorly-differentiated, regardless of their degree of architectural differentiation: uterine papillary serous carcinomas (UPSCs) and clear cell carcinomas. Neither of these types is associated with a morphologically definable non-cancerous precursor lesion, although

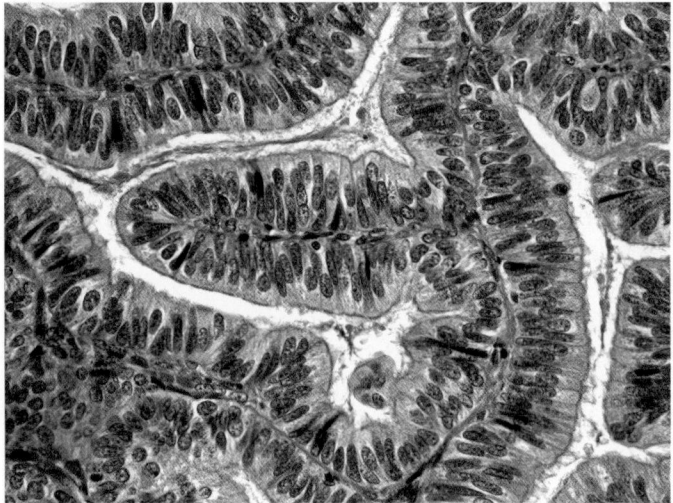

Fig. 19.16 Endometrial adenocarcinoma with tubal (ciliated) differentiation.

non-invasive forms of serous carcinoma (so-called 'serous endometrial intraepithelial carcinoma') exist. UPSCs are derived via mutations in the p53 tumor suppressor gene and (from a morphologic perspective) appear to develop abruptly in atrophic endometrium, within endometrial polyps and, occasionally, within pre-existing endometrioid carcinomas.

UPSCs have been recognized as a distinct entity for over 20 years.[83] Their place as a highly aggressive form of uterine cancer was solidified in 1982.[8,84] Additional studies have essentially confirmed the integrity of this entity while expanding its spectrum to include three non-exclusive patterns: (1) mixed serous and endometrioid carcinomas; (2) serous carcinomas arising in endometrial polyps; and (3) serous carcinomas confined to the endometrial surface or endometrial glandular mucosa (so-called intraepithelial carcinomas). All three can be deceptive and are identified more efficiently as the practitioner gains experience. Despite the absence of invasion and the small amount of neoplastic epithelium in some of these UPSCs, they have a strong tendency to spread to peritoneal surfaces, possibly by retrograde expulsion through the fallopian tubes. The discrete nature of these neoplasms underscores the abrupt transformation from benign to malignant seen in serous endometrial carcinomas and supports the concept that even the earliest, non-invasive forms are capable of metastasizing and killing the patient.

Pure serous carcinomas comprise as few as 1.1% of endometrial carcinomas in one study and as many as 10% in others.[67,85] The actual frequency is elusive,

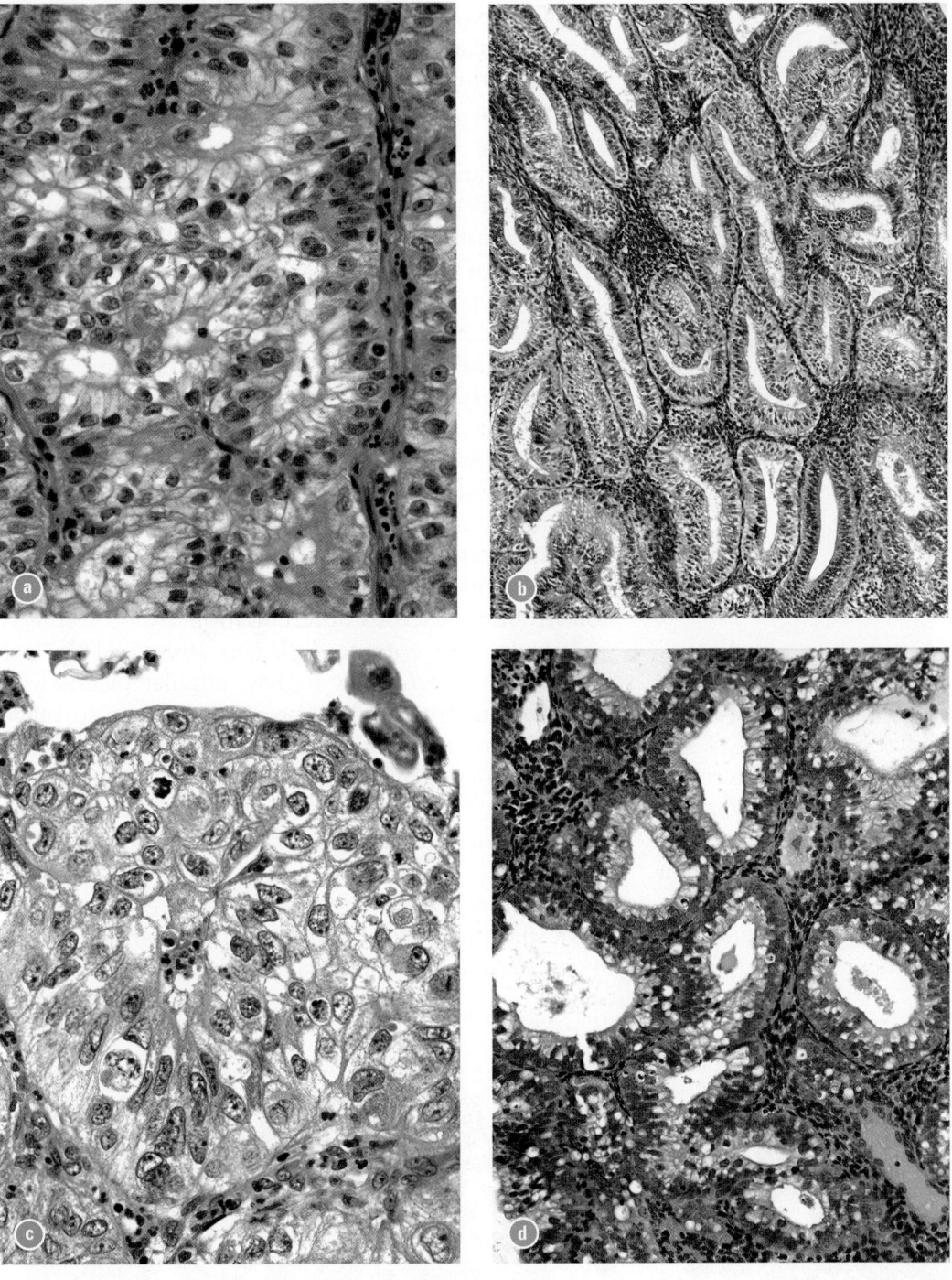

Fig. 19.17 Secretory differentiation in an endometrial carcinoma (a). Mimics of secretory differentiation include secretory endometrium with gland crowding (b), clear cell carcinoma (c) and stratified vacuoles in a primitive epithelium associated with more poorly-differentiated carcinomas and carcinosarcomas (d).

subject to both the vagaries of misclassification (such as in the misinterpretation of villoglandular endometrioid tumors as serous or the under-appreciation of mixed endometrioid and serous patterns) and the variable emphasis assigned to certain histologic and immunohistochemical (p53) parameters in making the diagnosis of a serous tumor.

Growth patterns All serous tumors, including those arising in combination with endometrioid tumors, have features in common, which are high-grade nuclear atypia, a cuboidal to low stratified epithelium and macronuclei and prominent nucleoli in at least a portion of the lesion. The architectural patterns encountered vary from those that are obviously papillary to

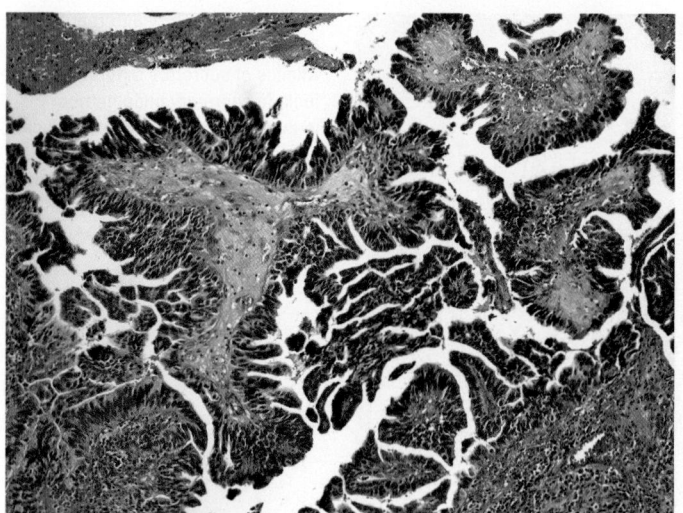

Fig. 19.18 Villoglandular adenocarcinoma. These tumors contain well-defined papillae lined by pseudostratified endometrioid epithelium. The degree of nuclear atypia is mild to moderate with exfoliation of cohesive cell clusters rather than individual lining cells.

those that exhibit characteristic glandular features. Many of these patterns can be encountered in a single tumor. The patterns are as follows.

Papillary glandular architecture. The pattern of papillary growth in UPSC has three components. The first consists of large, broad, irregular papillae lined by cuboidal to irregularly stratified tumor cells with a high nuclear/cytoplasmic ratio and macro nuclei (Fig. 19.19a). The second is associated with the first and consists of cells exfoliated from these papillae (micro-

papillary growth) (Fig. 19.19a). The third consists of intraglandular micropapillae. All three are commonly present in the same tumor (Fig. 19.19b).

Disturbed glandular architecture with slit-forming glands (Fig. 19.20a). This is a common pattern seen in both ovarian and endometrial serous carcinomas. As the papillae become less well defined, especially as they invade the uterine wall, the epithelium is often separated by narrow linear spaces, producing small slits between the epithelial cords. This is inconsistent with endometrioid tumors, which maintain either a macroglandular or microglandular architecture.

Poorly-differentiated 'large cell' patterns. These patterns can take the form of architectural confluent or solid growth and papillae with larger cells containing abundant cytoplasm (Fig. 19.20b). This pattern may not be immediately recognized as serous. However, the absence of a recognizable endometrioid growth pattern combined with the marked nuclear atypia is consistent with serous differentiation.

Tumors with organized fibrous stroma. This is a pattern characterized by narrow angular glands with organized interglandular fibrosis, similar to so-called 'carcinofibromas' of the ovary. The interglandular stroma is well defined, similar to villoglandular carcinomas of the cervix. The diagnosis of UPSC is based on the characteristic micropapillary changes and atypia (Fig. 19.20c).

Microcystic patterns. Like the solid pattern, this pattern is not specific. However, this pattern is commonly seen in ovarian serous carcinomas (Fig. 19.20d). The micro-

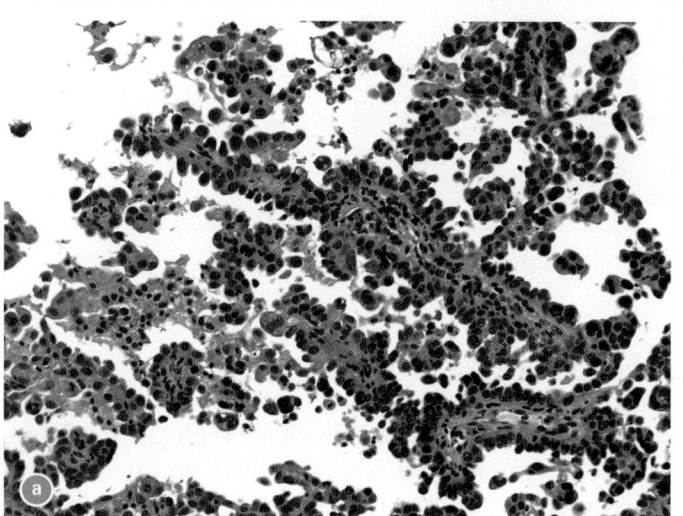

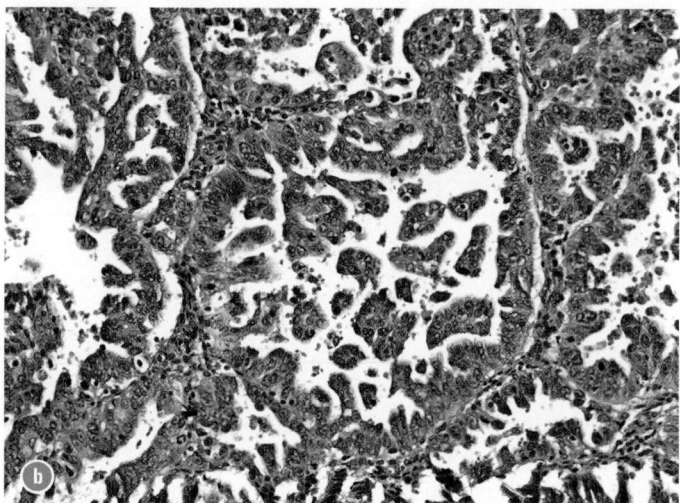

Fig. 19.19 Papillary patterns seen in serous carcinoma include (a) larger irregular papillae and micropapillary growth with exfoliation of tumor cells and (b) intraglandular micropapillary growth.

cystic pattern is distinguished from the microglandular pattern of endometrioid carcinomas (with mucinous differentiation).

Tumors confined to the surface mucosa ('serous endometrial intraepithelial carcinomas') or endometrial polyps. We interpret these as uterine papillary serous carcinomas that are earlier in their natural history but otherwise biologically developed. This pattern may be particularly inconspicuous, either as single neoplastic cells on the surface of an atrophic endometrium (Fig. 19.21a) or an endometrial polyp (Fig. 19.21b). This lesion often extends into the subsurface epithelium, replacing normal glandular lining similar to cervical neoplasms (Fig. 19.21c). However, in contrast to cervix, this pattern is distinctly malignant, capable of widespread intra-abdominal metastases, and mandates complete staging in the manner performed for ovarian carcinomas.[86]

The common association of UPSC with endometrial polyps appears to be more than coincidence.[87] Whether the polyps are predisposed to p53 mutations, or more likely to generate proliferations that take advantage of these mutations, is unknown.

Tumors with features intermediate between serous and endometrioid. These may be better classified with p53 immunostaining and attention to morphologic

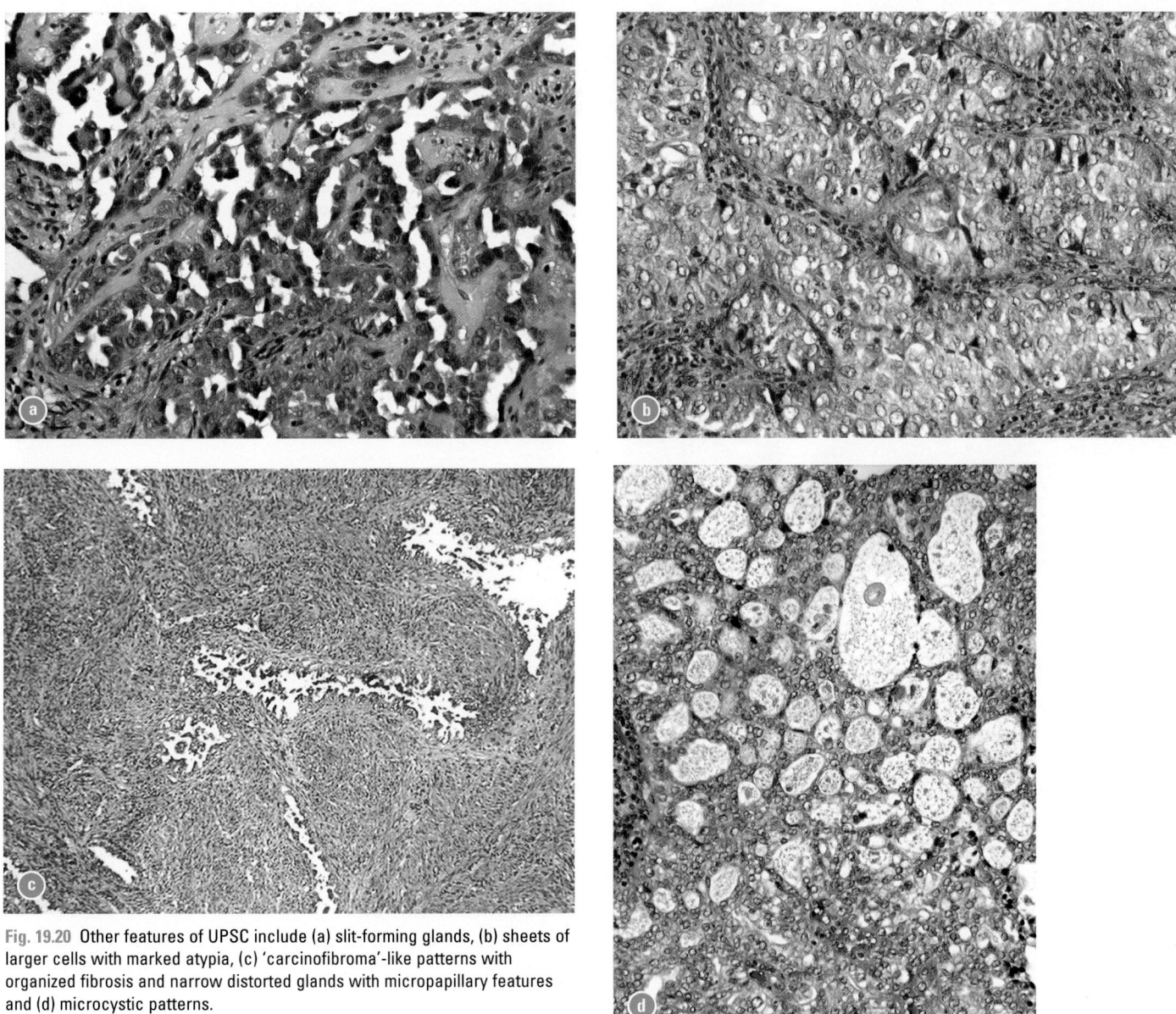

Fig. 19.20 Other features of UPSC include (a) slit-forming glands, (b) sheets of larger cells with marked atypia, (c) 'carcinofibroma'-like patterns with organized fibrosis and narrow distorted glands with micropapillary features and (d) microcystic patterns.

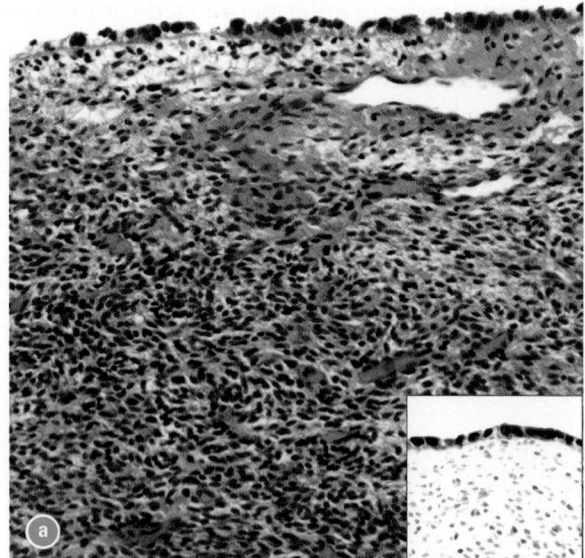

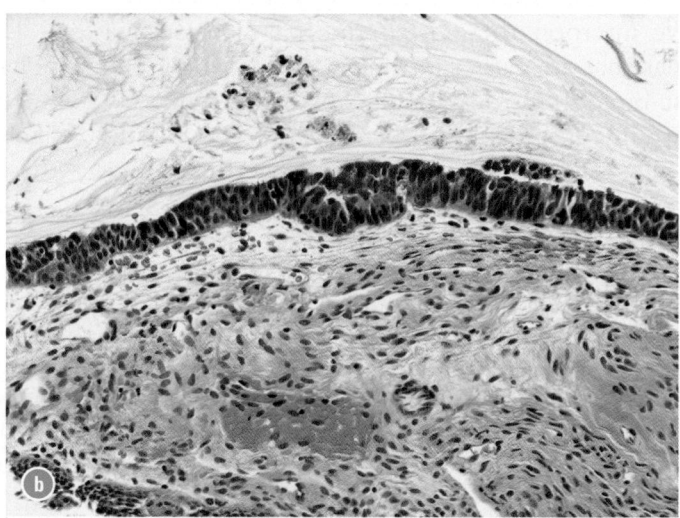

Fig. 19.21 UPSC involving the surface mucosa only (a) – a p53 immunostain (inset) highlights the tumors cells on the surface; involving the surface of an endometrial polyp (b), extending into subsurface glands as non-invasive carcinoma (c).

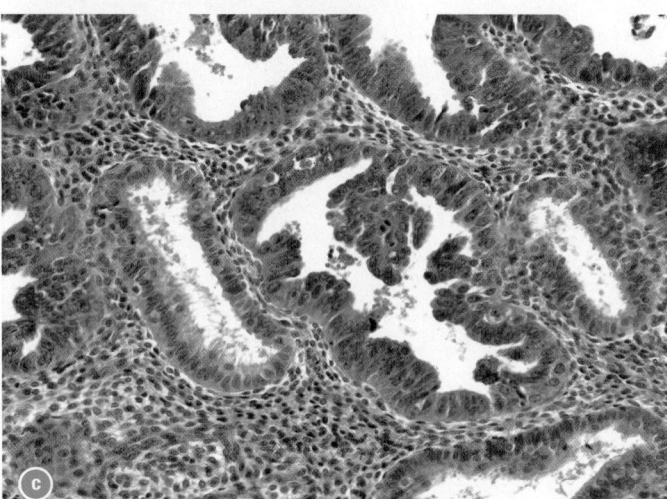

patterns as discussed below. However, pathologists who use p53 as a biomarker must be aware of the multiplicity of staining patterns.

1 Immunostaining for p53. The accumulation of p53 in a high percentage of tumor cells is due to p53 gene mutations in papillary serous cancers, and defects elsewhere in the p53 pathway in rare endometrioid cancers (Figs 19.22–19.25). Reports differ on whether p53 immunostaining is an independent prognostic parameter, primarily because it correlates so closely with nuclear atypia and the serous phenotype. However, p53 staining is a useful biomarker to confirm the presence of a serous

neoplasm and possibly, to identify endometrioid patterns that may be more aggressive.[77,78,88]

The precise cut-off level of staining that defines a p53 mutation varies according to reports.[89] In our laboratory, at least a portion of the tumor must contain 70% or greater strongly positive nuclei. Others use lower cut-off levels between 30 and 70%. In practice, most will score less than 30% or more than 70%.

The most common distribution pattern includes the following: (a) diffuse (>70%) intense nuclear staining (Fig. 19.22a,b), (b) no staining or cytoplasmic staining only (Fig. 19.23a,b) and

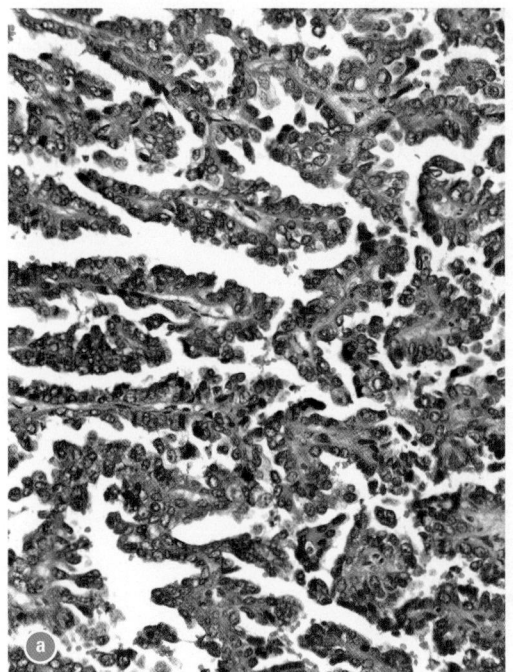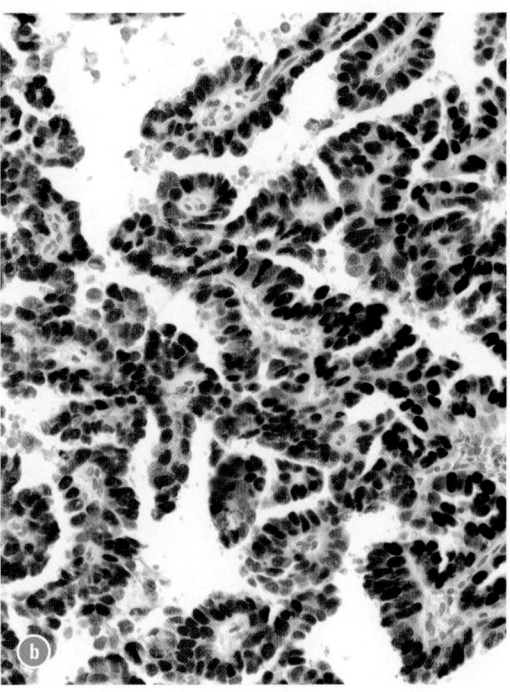

Fig. 19.22 UPSC (a) with diffuse intense staining associated with p53 mutation (b).

(c) focal weak to intense staining of scattered neoplastic cells (less than 30%) (Fig. 19.24a,b). A fourth pattern defines the juxtaposition of two distinct staining (and morphologic) patterns, including an abrupt transition from minimal to marked staining, befitting the dual histologic patterns (Fig. 19.25a–c).

2 Although most serous and endometrioid carcinomas are readily distinguished, a subset of tumors are diagnostically problematic.

  a Villoglandular endometrioid adenocarcinomas are not usually confused with UPSCs but can be distinguished by p53 immunostaining (Fig. 19.26a,b). Micropapillary architecture

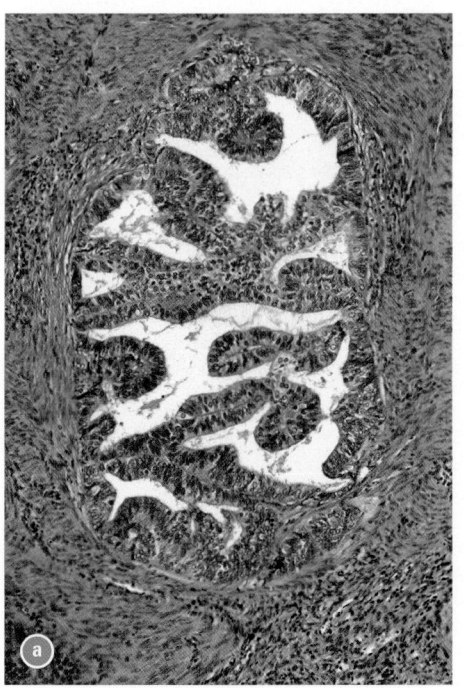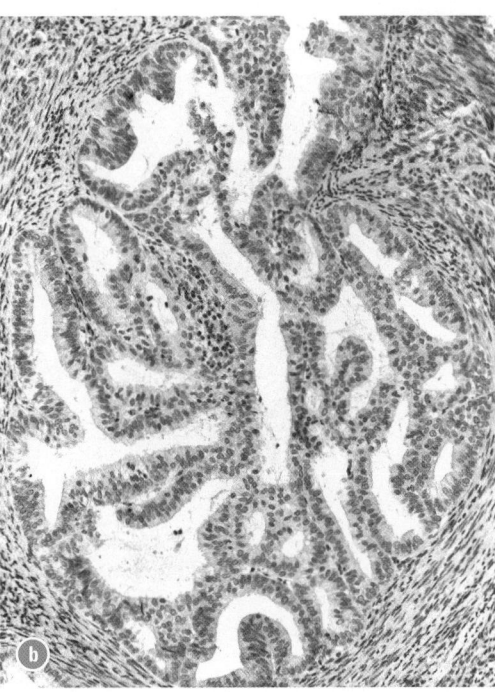

Fig. 19.23 Endometrioid adenocarcinoma (a) with absent staining for p53 (b).

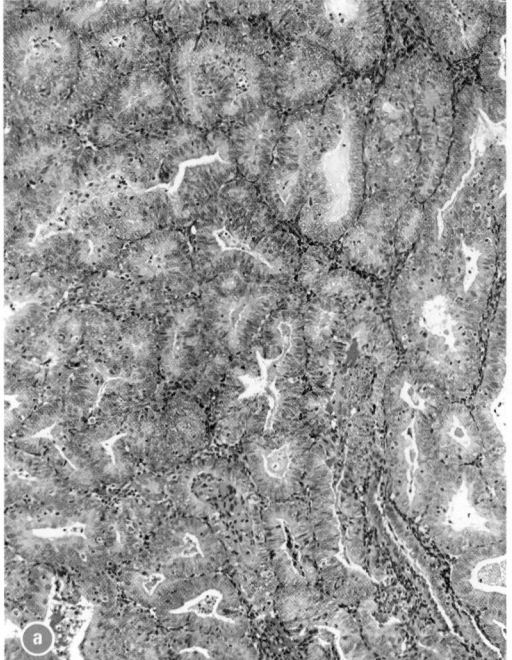 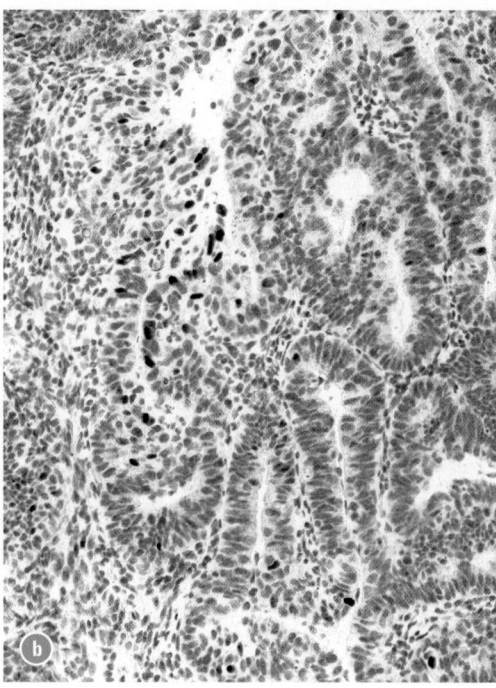

Fig. 19.24 Endometrioid adenocarcinoma (a) exhibiting focal intense staining for p53 (b).

in endometrioid carcinomas can be easily distinguished by the preservation of a higher nuclear/cytoplasmic ratio and minimal atypia relative to UPSC (Fig. 19.23c, compare with Figure 19.19b).

b Tumors with a predominately endometrioid growth pattern accompanied by nuclear atypia of a degree usually seen in serous carcinomas.

The glands are typically well defined with pseudostratified epithelium; however, the epithelial lining usually contains conspicuous nuclear atypia (Fig. 19.27a,b). Further examination may reveal more classic serous patterns.

c Tumors with a distinct biphasic morphology, in which a well-differentiated endometrioid adenocarcinoma merges with a classic serous

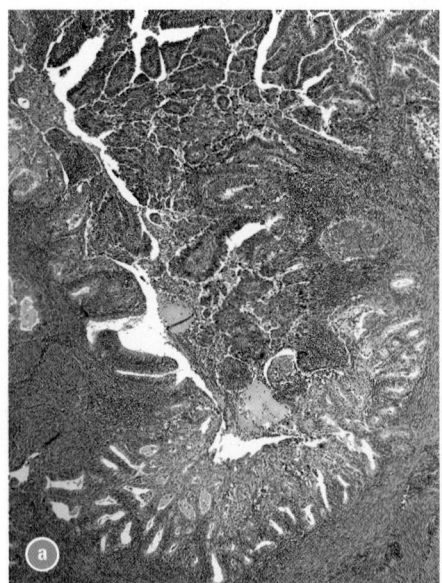 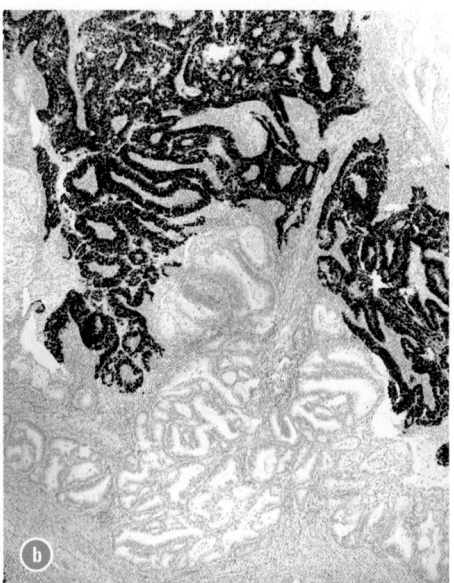 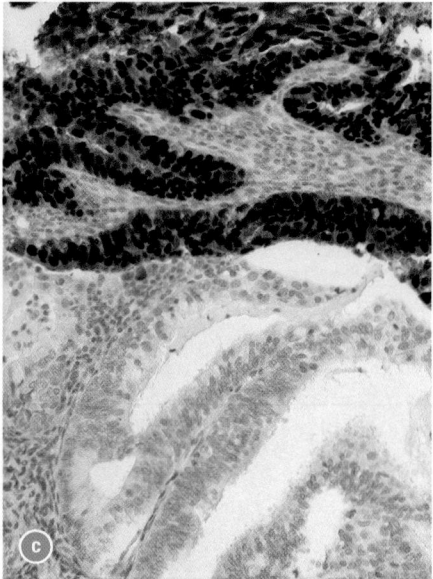

Fig. 19.25 A true combined endometrioid (lower) and serous (upper) carcinoma (a) also exhibits a biphasic p53 staining pattern at (b) low and (c) high power.

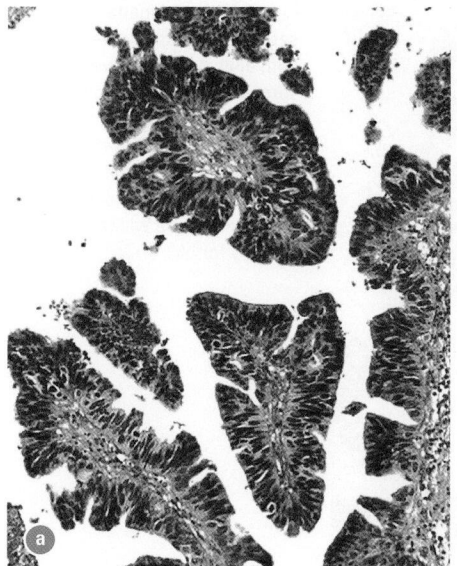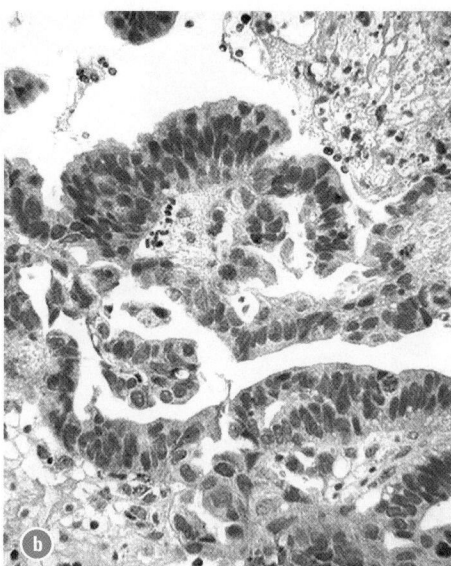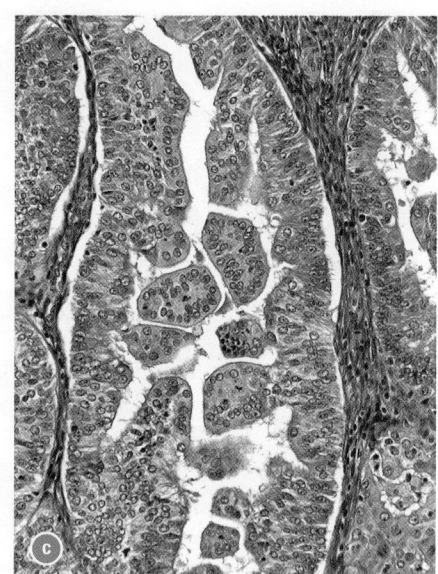

Fig. 19.26 Villoglandular carcinoma (a) and following p53 staining (b). Micropapillary architecture in an endometrioid carcinoma can be distinguished from UPSC on morphologic grounds (c). (Compare with Fig. 19.19b.)

neoplasm. The former may also have mucinous, tubal or squamous differentiation, features inconsistent with serous carcinoma. In some instances the transition is subtle, whereas in others it is abrupt (Fig. 19.25a–c). In some, the endometrioid component is small while in others the reverse is the case. These tumors often exhibit a biphasic pattern of p53 immunostaining as well.[9,37] In rare instances, a conventional endometrioid carcinoma will overlie a deeply invasive serous component (Fig. 19.28a,b).

A serous carcinoma, even one that is admixed with an endometrioid component, confers a poor prognosis (Table 19.4).[81,85,90–94] Carcangiu and Chambers analyzed three parameters associated with serous carcinomas: tumors apparently confined to polyps, tumors associated with endometrioid components and tumors coexisting with ovarian carcinomas of similar morphology.[90] The outcome of all three groups was poor, with an endometrioid component having no beneficial impact on survival. Tumors confined to polyps behaved as aggressively as those of similar stage with myometrial invasion, and tumors associated with ovarian involve-

Table 19.4 Outcome of endometrial carcinoma as a function of cell type

Type	Ref.	Stage I (<2mm) (%)	Stage I (all) (%)	All cases (%)
EM	70, 86[a]	98	91	91
VG	81	–	–	94[b]
ASCA	70, 69	–	64	65
CCA	92, 85	90	43–59	39–42
UND	252	100	79	58
UPSC	86, 95, 98	60–93[c]	75	27–38

EM, endometrioid, including adenoacanthoma; VG, endometrioid villoglandular; ASCA, adenosquamous carcinoma; CCA, clear cell carcinoma; UND, undifferentiated carcinoma; UPSC, uterine papillary serous carcinoma.

[a]Combines recurrences and deaths.
[b]Stage I and II combined 3-year survival.
[c]Survival in this group increases as a function of thorough staging to exclude extrauterine disease.

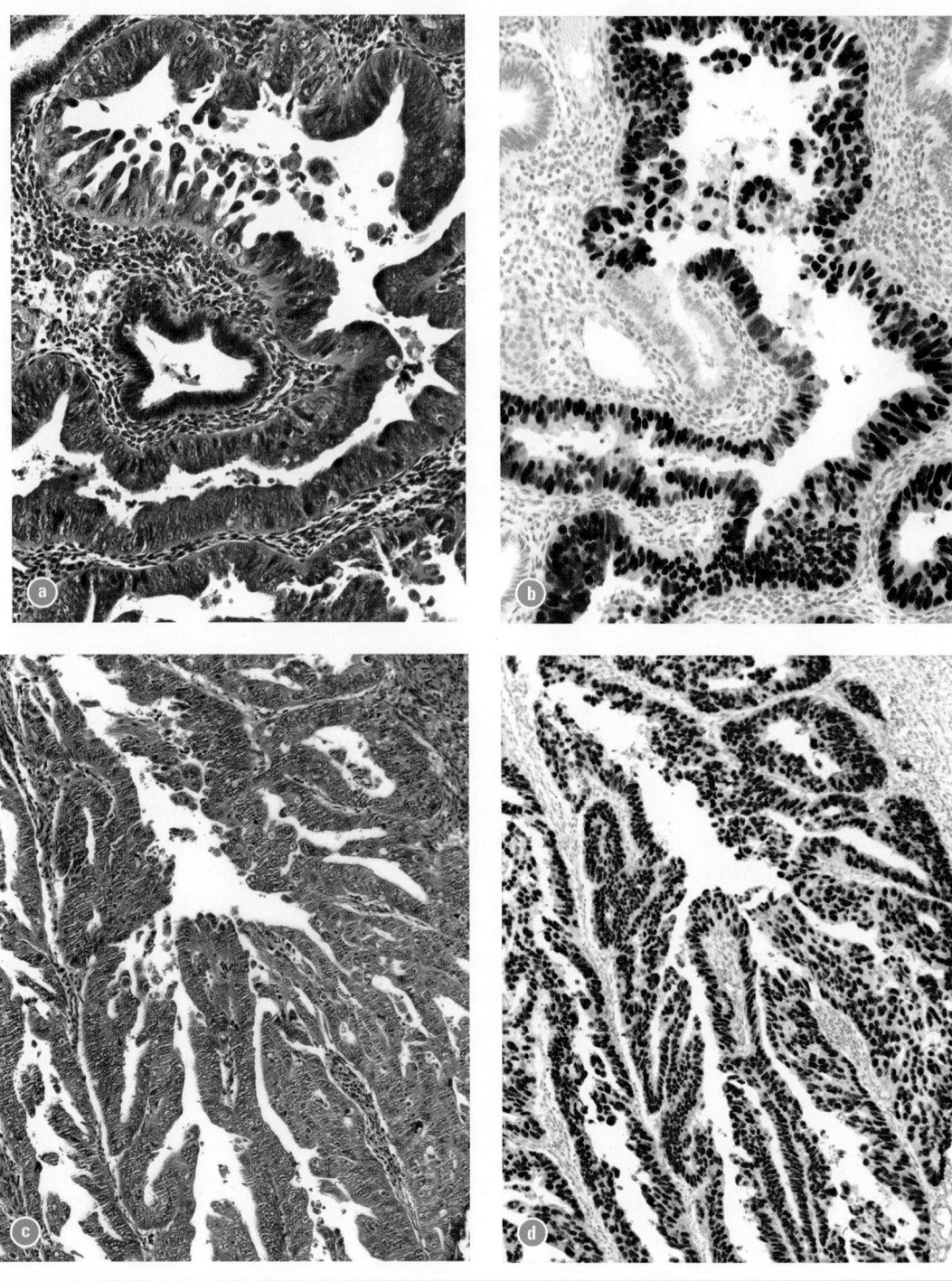

Fig. 19.27 (a) A bipatterned serous carcinoma containing both endometrioid (lower) and serous (upper) differentiation. (b) The entire tumor stained positive for p53. (c) In rare instances, a tumor that is a consensus endometrioid adenocarcinoma will (d) stain strongly for p53.

ment behaved as high-stage carcinomas, observations also shared by others.[87,95] Goff et al. came to similar conclusions with UPSCs involving the surface or underlying glands only, noting that lack of myometrial invasion did not preclude positive peritoneal washings and a poor outcome.[96] However, most have found that if meticulous staging was performed (identical in scope to that for ovarian serous carcinomas), Stage I tumors had a favorable outcome, with relapse rates less than 20%.[97–100]

Clear cell carcinomas

Clear cell carcinomas of the endometrium account for less than 1% of endometrial carcinomas and are recognized by the presence of tumor cells with generally polyhedral shape, clear, glycogen-rich cytoplasm and

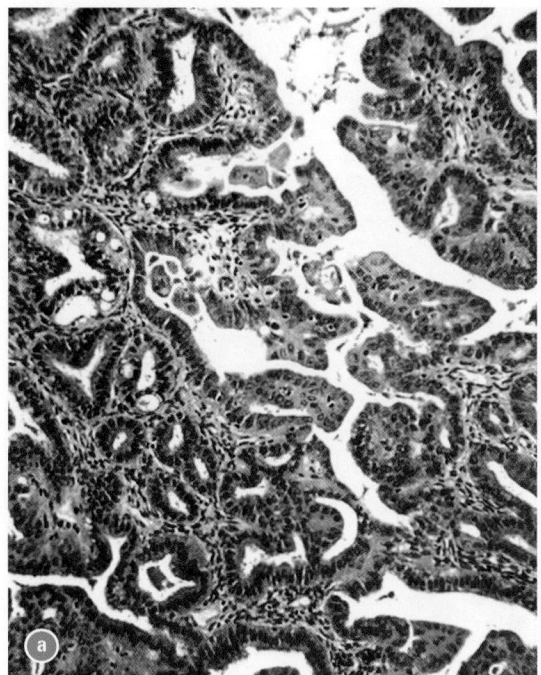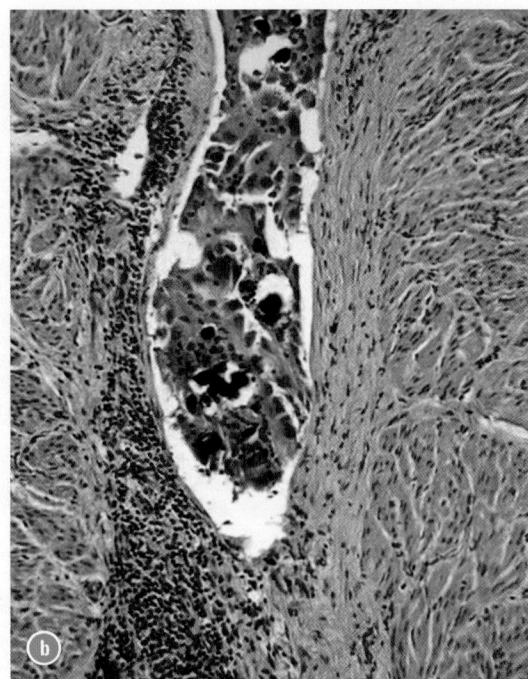

Fig. 19.28 A superficial endometrioid adenocarcinoma (a), beneath which is a serous neoplasm predominating in vascular spaces (b).

high-grade nuclei.[67,101] The tumors grow in tubular, solid and papillary patterns. The tubular variants differ from endometrioid carcinomas by tubular gland architecture, the lack of pseudostratified growth, cuboidal lining cells and an eosinophilic PAS-positive acellular matrix between the glands. Papillary variants differ from serous types in two ways: (1) In clear cell carcinomas glands or papillae are lined by a single layer of polyhedral cells with uniform nuclei and prominent nucleoli (Fig. 19.29a,b). (2) In contrast to serous carcinomas, prominent exfoliation is typically absent. When the tumor cells are arranged in solid sheets, the preservation of distinct cell borders is maintained, although there may be marked nuclear atypia, as in serous carcinomas (Fig. 19.29c). Immunostaining for p53 in clear cell carcinomas has been reported to be less consistent than for UPSC, implying that these tumors are a biologically heterogeneous group (Fig. 19.29d).[102] In our experience, clear cell carcinomas are usually strongly positive.

Aside from UPSC discussed immediately above, the differential diagnosis of clear cell carcinoma includes endometrioid carcinomas with secretory differentiation. Since clear cell carcinomas stain strongly for p53 in many cases, a positive reaction with this biomarker will distinguish them from non-neoplastic reactive changes or Arias-Stella effects. Lastly, some poorly-differentiated endometrioid carcinomas may have focal clear cell features. These usually do not contain the distinct architectural features of a clear cell carcinoma. However, if the diagnosis of clear cell carcinoma is uncertain, the pathologist should classify the lesion as a poorly-differentiated (grade 3) adenocarcinomas with clear cell features.

Clear cell carcinomas of the uterus have a less favorable outcome than endometrioid carcinomas (Table 19.4). However, they do not share the propensity to involve peritoneal surfaces that characterizes UPSC. Abeler and Kjorstad reported crude 5- and 10-year survival rates of 42 and 39%, respectively.[91]

Histologic grading of endometrial carcinomas

Adenocarcinomas of endometrioid type, including those with other forms of differentiation described above are graded according to, and without marked nuclear atypia or other stigmata of serous carcinoma, can be subdivided into the following grades by the FIGO system (Table 19.5) (Fig. 19.5a–c). The distinction of

Table 19.5 *FIGO grading system for endometrioid carcinoma*[a]

Grade 1	Less than 5% solid growth (excludes squamous differentiation)
Grade 2	Solid growth involving 5–50%
Grade 3	Solid growth involving over 50%

[a]Tumor grade is increased by one step if conspicuously enlarged nuclei and prominent nucleoli are present. Lesser atypias do not justify an increase in grade. FIGO, International Federation of Gynecology and Obstetrics.

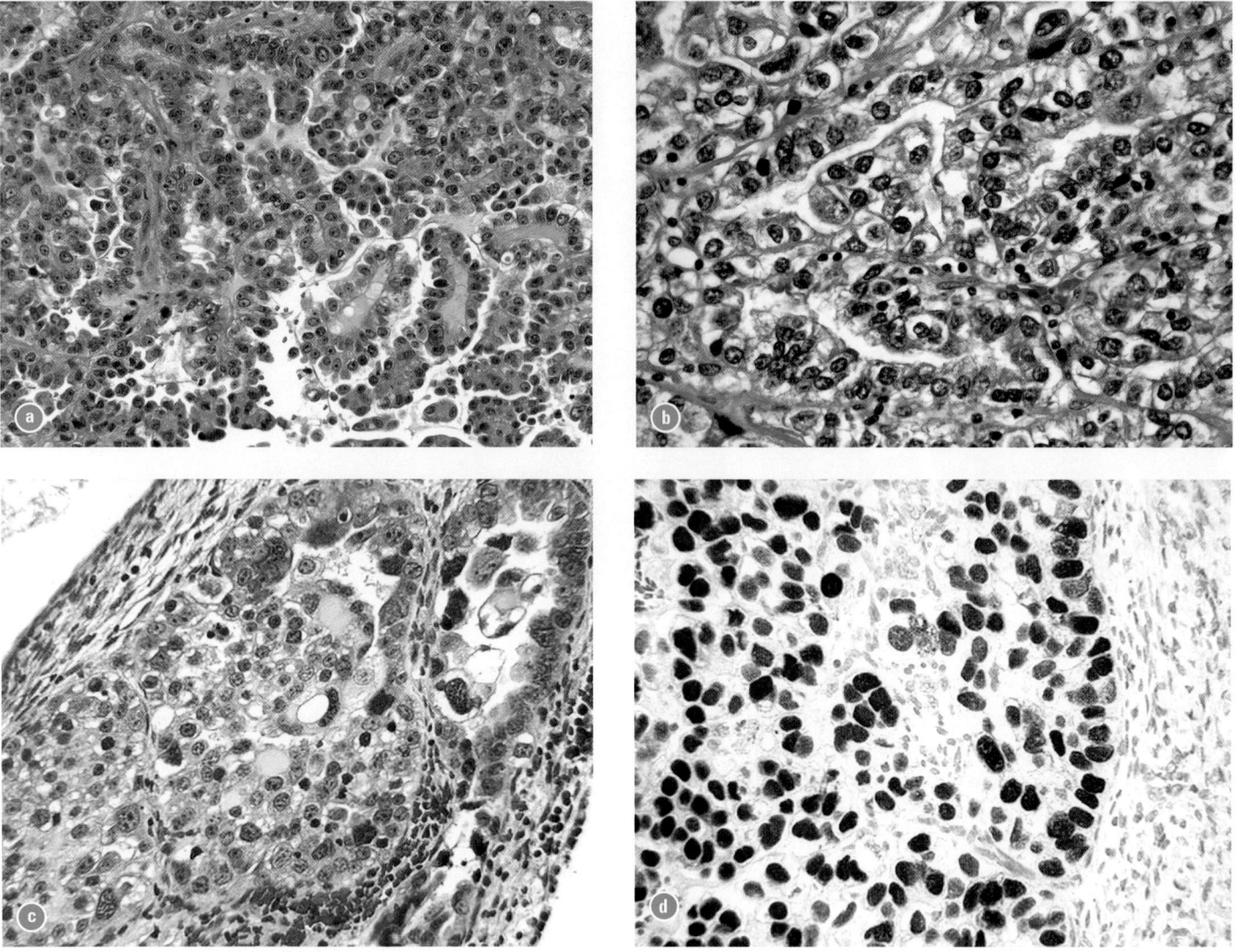

Fig. 19.29 Clear cell carcinomas of the endometrium, including (a) papillary, (b) tubulo-glandular and (c) more solid variants. (d) The latter was strongly positive for p53.

grades 1, 2 and 3 is based on less than 5%, 5–50% and greater than 50% solid growth, respectively.

The pathologist is permitted to increase the grade by one step if severe nuclear atypia is present (Fig. 19.6a,b). Both the architectural and nuclear grading scheme are summarized in Table 19.5.

The cut-off of 5% solid between grades 1 and 2 can be problematic due to the relatively small difference in prognosis between the two grades (92% *vs* 88% 5-year survival) and a cut-off point of 5% solid growth.[103] Other systems have been proposed: Taylor et al. offered a two-tiered system in which grade 2 was assigned to tumors with greater than 20% solid growth. They reported much higher inter-observer reproducibility (κ 0.97 *vs* 0.53 for a three-grade system) and improved

agreement with outcome histology in the hysterectomy (90% *vs* 63%).[104]

In a second study, Lax et al. proposed a binary system in which grade 2 was assigned to tumors with two or more of the following: (1) more than 50% solid growth (squamous and non-squamous were not distinguished); (2) diffusely infiltrative versus expansive myometrial invasion; and (3) tumor cell necrosis.[105] For tumors that were confined to the endometrium, 50% solid growth or greater and tumor necrosis designated high grade. Inter-observer agreement was also high in contrast to the traditional system (κ 0.65 *vs* 0.22). In their analysis, grade 1, Stage IA/IB had a 100% 5-year survival (FYS). Grade 1/Stage IC–IV and grade 2, Stage IB and IC had FYS of 67 and 76%, respectively. However, because the pattern of myometrial infiltration was an important variable, this system is more appropriate to the hysterectomy specimen than the curetting.[105]

Tumors that are classified as papillary serous adenocarcinomas and clear cell carcinomas are exempt from grading, as they are by definition high-risk tumors and will require full surgical staging.

Other important variables in grading

As implied in the prior discussions, the standard grading system for endometrioid carcinomas is a guideline and not an absolute. This is due to three additional variables: (a) not all solid areas of tumor impose a higher grade; (b) assessment of nuclear grade – which can be used to upgrade endometrioid carcinomas – is subjective; and (c) a small proportion of endometrioid tumors are strongly p53 immunopositive. The following rules should be followed:

1 Squamous differentiation (metaplasia or morules). When recognized, squamous differentiation does not factor as solid growth and does not upgrade the tumor. Cytologically bland grade 1 neoplasms with focally solid growth exceeding 5% do not merit upgrading if the solid areas resemble squamous metaplasia (so-called abortive squamous differentiation) and exhibit bland cytologic features (Fig. 19.11a).

2 Some tumors are biphasic, consisting of juxtaposed well- and poorly-differentiated endometrioid tumors without a more gradual shift in grade. If such cases contain less than 50% solid growth, the pathologist should call attention to the biphasic pattern and the fact that a portion of the tumor is essentially a grade 3 (Fig. 19.30).

3 Irrespective of the grading system, the presence of pronounced nuclear atypia warrants upgrading of the tumor. This is defined as the anisokaryosis, macronuclei, nuclear pleomorphism and prominent nucleoli (Fig. 19.6b). As discussed previously, if p53 immunostaining is performed and is diffusely (greater than 70% nuclei) positive, the tumor warrants upgrading. Whether the tumor should be ultimately classified as a high-grade endometrioid carcinoma or serous carcinoma has not been established. At Brigham and Women's Hospital, the findings are reported and the clinician is advised that the presence of p53 immunostaining warrants designation as a high-grade endometrial adenocarcinoma.

DIFFERENTIAL DIAGNOSIS OF ENDOMETRIAL ADENOCARCINOMA (TABLE 19.6)

When a biopsy or curetting from a woman with postmenopausal bleeding is evaluated histologically, proper management hinges on attention to both excluding benign mimics of carcinoma and not misinterpreting carcinoma as benign. This issue is addressed on a daily basis by the pathologist who evaluates cyclic or noncyclic endometrium (Ch. 16) and endometrial intraepithelial neoplasia (Ch. 17), and who must sort out the various metaplastic lesions that occur in the endometrium (Ch. 18). The most important pitfalls encountered in practice are discussed below.

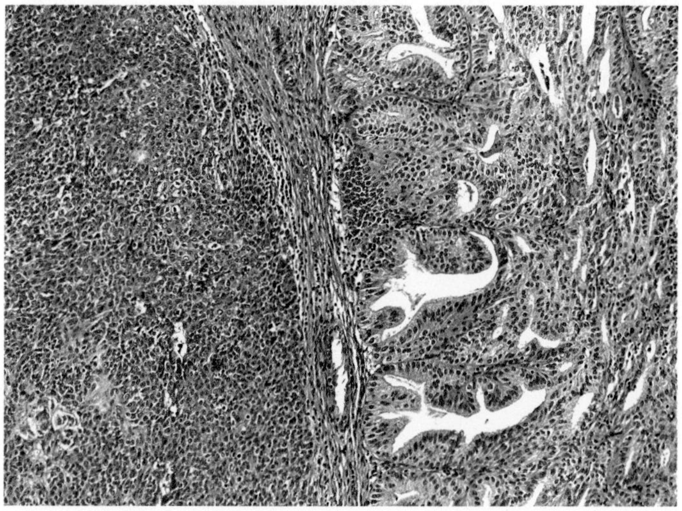

Fig. 19.30 Biphasic carcinoma with well- (right) and poorly- (left) differentiated areas juxtaposed.

Table 19.6 Differential diagnosis of endometrial carcinoma (curettings)

Parameter	Mimicking	Differential diagnosis
Gland architecture	Cancer	Telescoping artifact
		Stromal collapse, breakdown
		Sectioning artifacts
	Benign	Microglandular mucinous carcinoma
		Surface endometrioid carcinoma
Nuclear atypia	Cancer	Surface or glandular repair
		Arias-Stella changes (hormonal therapy)
		Radiation effect
Papillary changes	Cancer	Exfoliation artifact
		Stromal breakdown with papillary changes
		Papillary syncytial change
	Benign	Papillary mucinous carcinoma

Lesions are recognized but are difficult to classify due to inherent problems of applying criteria: for all practical purposes, this is not a serious transgression, inasmuch as the experts in the field are unable to come to consensus when evaluating curettings. The entities of note including morular metaplasia (Ch. 18), EIN (Ch. 17) and atypical polypoid adenomyomas (see below) and may be difficult to distinguish from carcinoma because the squamous differentiation obscures the degree of gland complexity.

Misclassification of patterns that are shared by benign and neoplastic epithelium:

1 Gland crowding that is misinterpreted as neoplasia, including gland crowding in small fragments (Fig. 19.31a), tangential or oblique sectioning of benign glands (Fig. 19.31b) and gland crowding with stromal collapse associated with breakdown (Fig. 19.31c).

2 Gland crowding associated with endometrial carcinoma that may go under-appreciated, including surface gland crowding that may mimic repair (Fig. 19.32a), small microglandular clusters of well-differentiated (microglandular hyperplasia-like) carcinomas that mimic endocervix (Fig. 19.32b) and disaggregated fragments of cancer that could mimic stromal breakdown (Fig. 19.32c).

3 Atypias that may be misdiagnosed as carcinoma include Arias-Stella-like reactions linked to hormonal therapy (Fig. 19.33a) and idiopathic and reactive/ reparative atypias in polyps or surface epithelium (Fig. 19.33b).

4 Subtle atypias that may go unappreciated in a minority of cases include small foci of UPSC or scant strips of clear cell carcinoma in a curetting (Fig. 19.34a,c). These atypias may be less

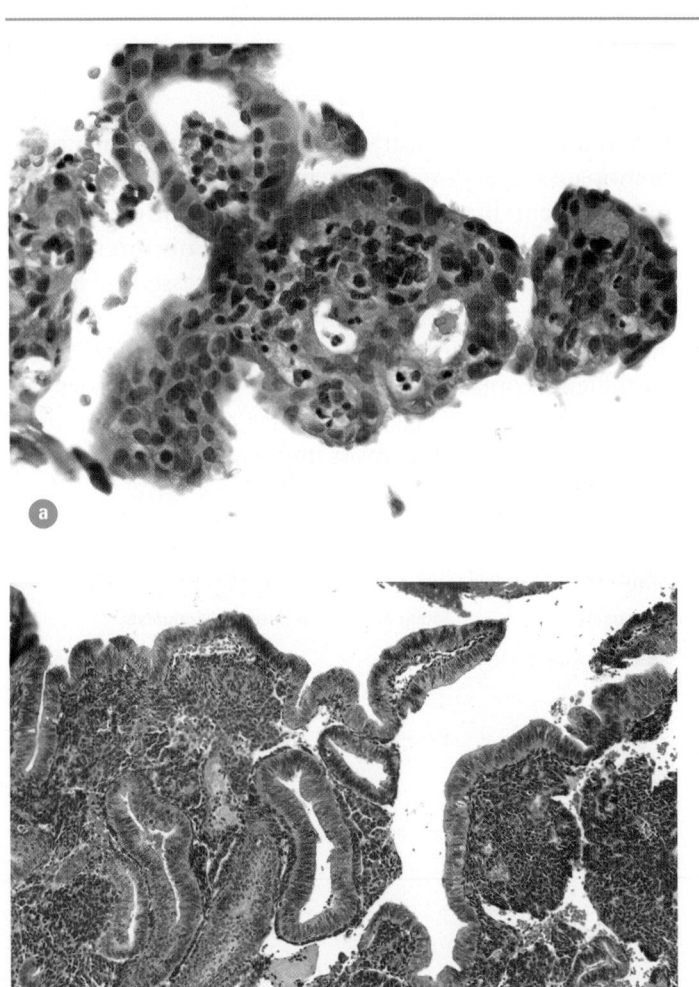

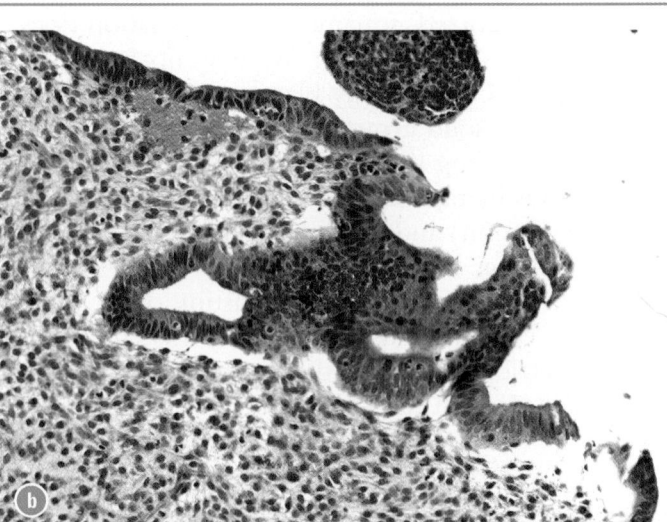

Fig. 19.31 Gland crowding in (a) small fragments, (b) tangential sections and (c) stromal collapse (breakdown) may mimic adenocarcinoma.

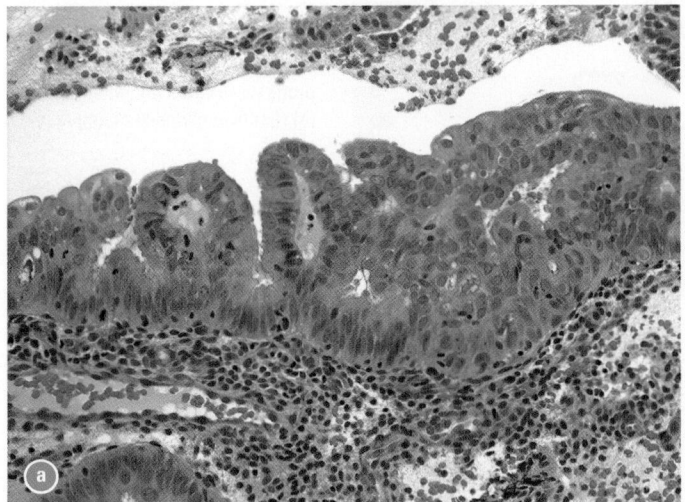

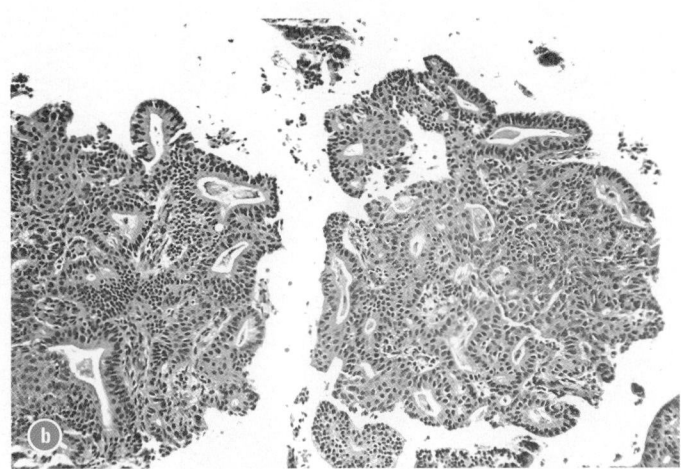

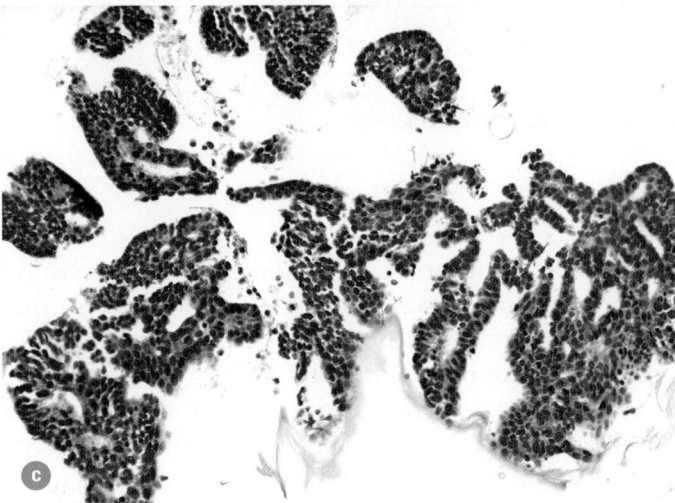

Fig. 19.32 (a) Gland crowding in carcinomas may mimic repair. (b) Microglandular growth patterns of well-differentiated mucinous carcinomas may mimic endocervix. (c) When the glandular organization is not well developed, it may be confused with stromal breakdown.

conspicuous than reactive or Arias-Stella-like epithelial changes, but are highlighted by p53 immunostaining (Fig. 19.34b,d).

5 Papillary architectures are recognized as abnormal but are difficult to classify: many benign and malignant processes exhibit papillary architecture, including villoglandular, mucinous, clear cell and transitional carcinomas. In practice, most of these are easily distinguished by all but the most inexperienced pathologist. The most problematic from the perspective of differential diagnosis are the following:

a Villoglandular endometrioid adenocarcinomas may exhibit considerable complexity and, in some cases, a higher nuclear grade than usual. However, they lack the micropapillary architecture and complex pattern of exfoliation seen in UPSC (Fig. 19.19).

b Peculiar exfoliation artifacts can be seen in curettings that appear to be related to hysteroscopic evaluation (Fig. 19.35a). In these instances, otherwise normal glands display a loss of cohesion of the lining cells with exfoliation into the lumen.

c Foci of necrosis or breakdown may be associated with small clusters of papillary surface change in the overlying epithelium (Fig. 19.35b).

d Papillary changes may be produced by potent progestins (Fig. 19.33a).

e Reactive epithelial changes in surface mucosa associated with ischemia (Fig. 19.33b).

f The presence of micropapillary architecture in conventional adenocarcinomas may reflect degenerative changes. All of these can be excluded by attention to the clinical setting, histologic details and, if needed, p53 immunostaining (see below).

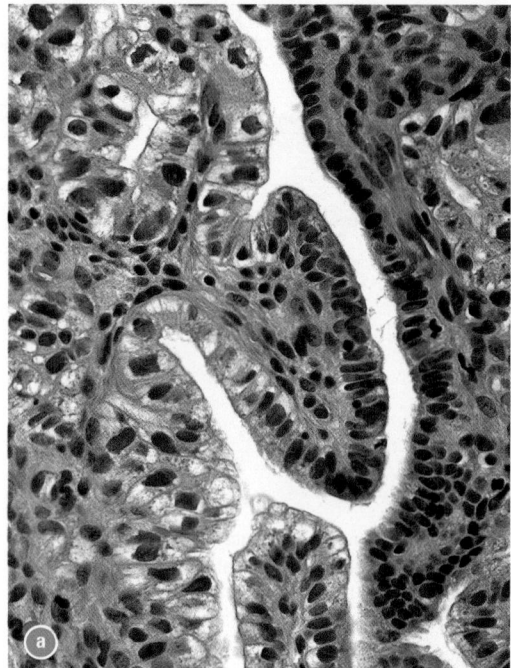
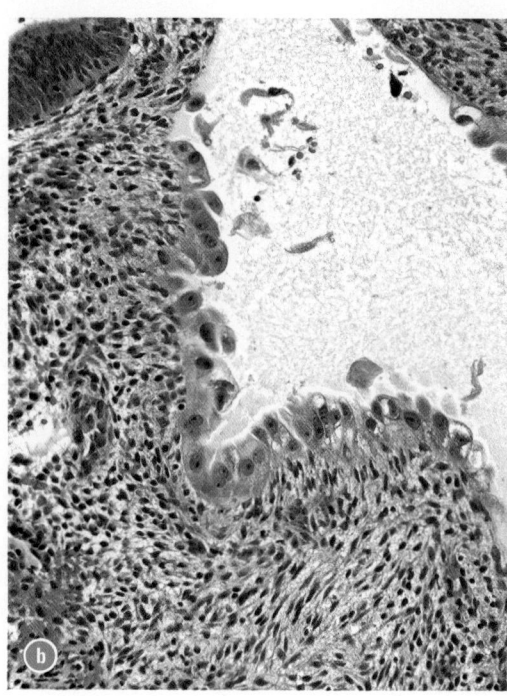

Fig. 19.33 Atypias often over-diagnosed as carcinoma include (a) Arias-Stella-like changes in progestin-treated endometrium and (b) reactive epithelial changes in polyps.

COMPONENTS OF LABORATORY MANAGEMENT (TABLE 19.7)

Cytologic detection

The sensitivity of cervical cytology for detecting endometrial adenocarcinoma has been reported as high as 65% using liquid-based preparations, but may much lower, particularly in women who are not bleeding.[106] Overall, the sensitivity of the cervical smear is not sufficient to warrant Pap cytology as a single test to triage abnormal uterine bleeding. The critical issues in cytologic detection of endometrial cancers include the following:

Significance of atypical glandular cells in general. Atypical glandular cells in a cervical smear are typically associated with an endocervical adenocarcinoma *in situ* or a high-grade squamous intraepithelial lesion. A small percentage are associated with endometrial cancer, but the risk increases in women over 40 years of age, when cervical adenocarcinoma is uncommon.[107,108] Older patients have a 13-fold higher risk of endometrial neoplasia than younger women.[109]

Significance of endometrial histiocytes. Histiocytes alone are not a risk factor for endometrial adenocarcinoma. Nassar et al. evaluated the significance of histiocytes alone in cervical smears. The positive predictive value (PPV) for endometrial cancer was 1.3% overall and 20% if additional Pap smear (endometrial or atypical glandular cells) or clinical (postmenopausal bleeding) findings.[110] These findings indicate that histiocytes alone are a poor indicator of coexisting endometrial pathology. Nguyen et al. found also that histiocytes alone did not increase the odds ratio of coexisting endometrial neoplasia.[111]

Significance of endometrial cells. The significance of endometrial-type cells (ETCs) in a cervical Pap specimen as an indicator of endometrial carcinoma is influenced by several factors: (1) age of the patient, (2) presence or absence of abnormal bleeding and (3) cellular atypia or a diathesis. Although benign-appearing

Table 19.7 Critical variables in management

Cytology	
Positive	Increases risk of cervical involvement (does not alter initial staging)
Biopsy	
Type	Clear cell/UPSC will result in nodal sampling
Grade	Grade 2 or greater increases likelihood of nodes
Cervix	Involvement will prompt preoperative radiation
Intraoperative	
Type	Clear cell/UPSC will result in nodal sampling
Grade	Grade 2 or greater increases likelihood of nodes
Depth	Nodal sampling if depth exceeds 50% for any grade
Hysterectomy	
Cervix	Postoperative radiation to reduce local recurrence
Grade	Grade 3 may receive postoperative radiation
Depth	Greater than 50% will receive post operative radiation
CLSI	Postoperative radiation
Nodes	Involvement = postoperative radiation

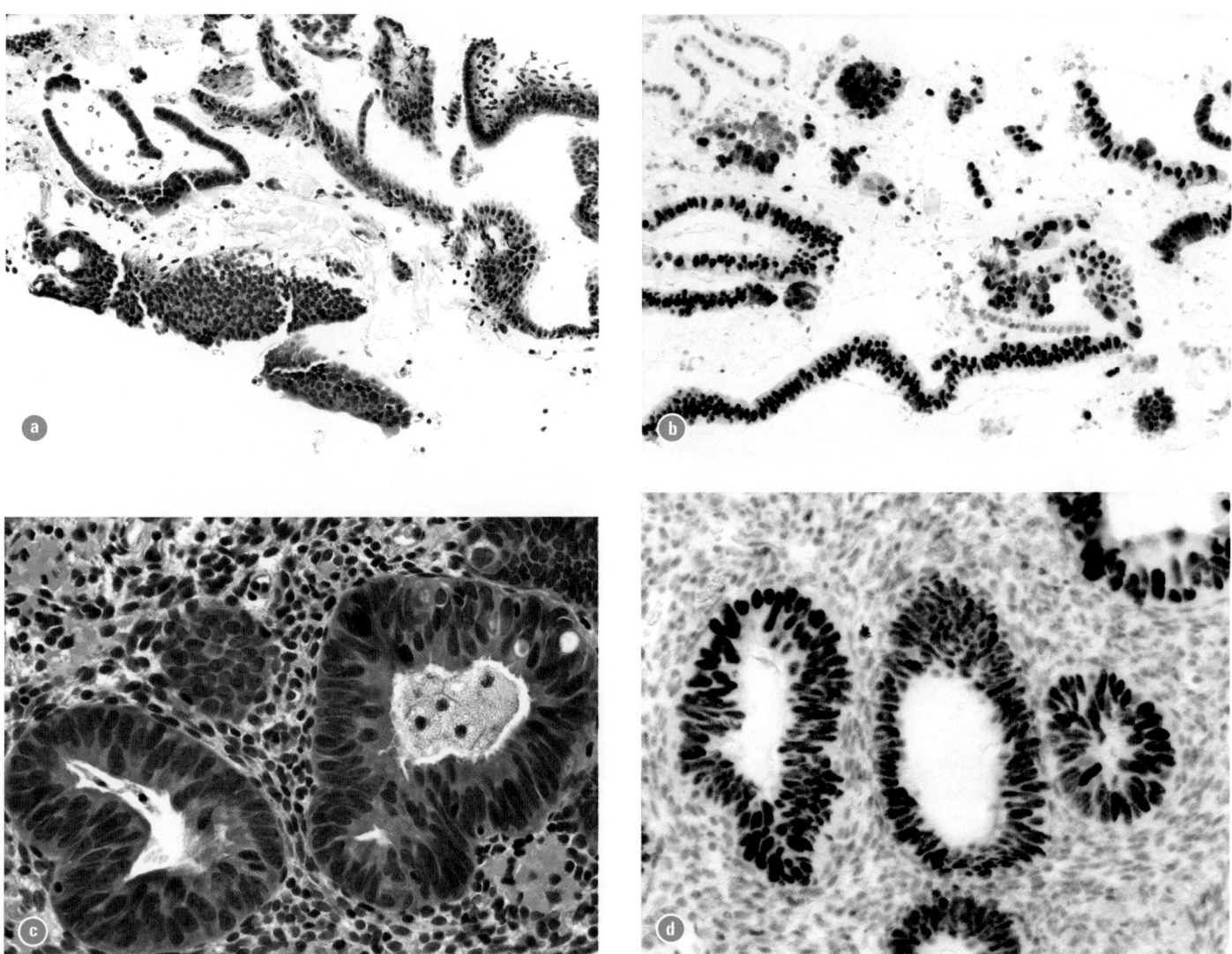

Fig. 19.34 Atypias associated with cancer that may be subtle or overlooked include (a) small fragments in curettings, particularly UPSC. (b) When suspicious, the pathologist should consider a p53 immunostain. (c) Another subtle serous carcinoma in a polyp (akin to what has been termed endometrial 'glandular dysplasia') and (d) following staining for p53.

endometrial cells in Pap smears confer a low risk of concomitant adenocarcinoma, the risk is substantially increased if there is concomitant abnormal bleeding or cytologic atypia. Karim et al. studied 1162 smears from patients 45 years and older with ETCs; adenocarcinoma was found in 4.2% with tissue follow-up.[112] Chang et al. found only one carcinoma in 132 cases with normal ETCs.[113] Van den Bosch et al. recorded a positive predictive value of 13–17% for ETCs. The risk increased to 50% when the cells were atypical.[114]

The positive smear as a predictor of cervical involvement. Several studies indicate that the presence of endometrial cancer in a cervical smear correlates strongly with cervical involvement.[115] Leminen et al.

reported that the accuracy of the Papanicolaou smear was 50%, and that of endocervical curettage 51% for cervical involvement.[116] Nevertheless, other than raising the suspicion of cervical involvement, the cervical smear is not useful for staging and should not prompt preoperative therapy on its own.

Interpretation of the endometrial and endocervical biopsy/curettage

Virtually all patients with endometrial carcinoma undergo a biopsy or curettage, where most of the initial diagnoses are made. The variables addressed in interpretation of the endometrial sampling include the following:

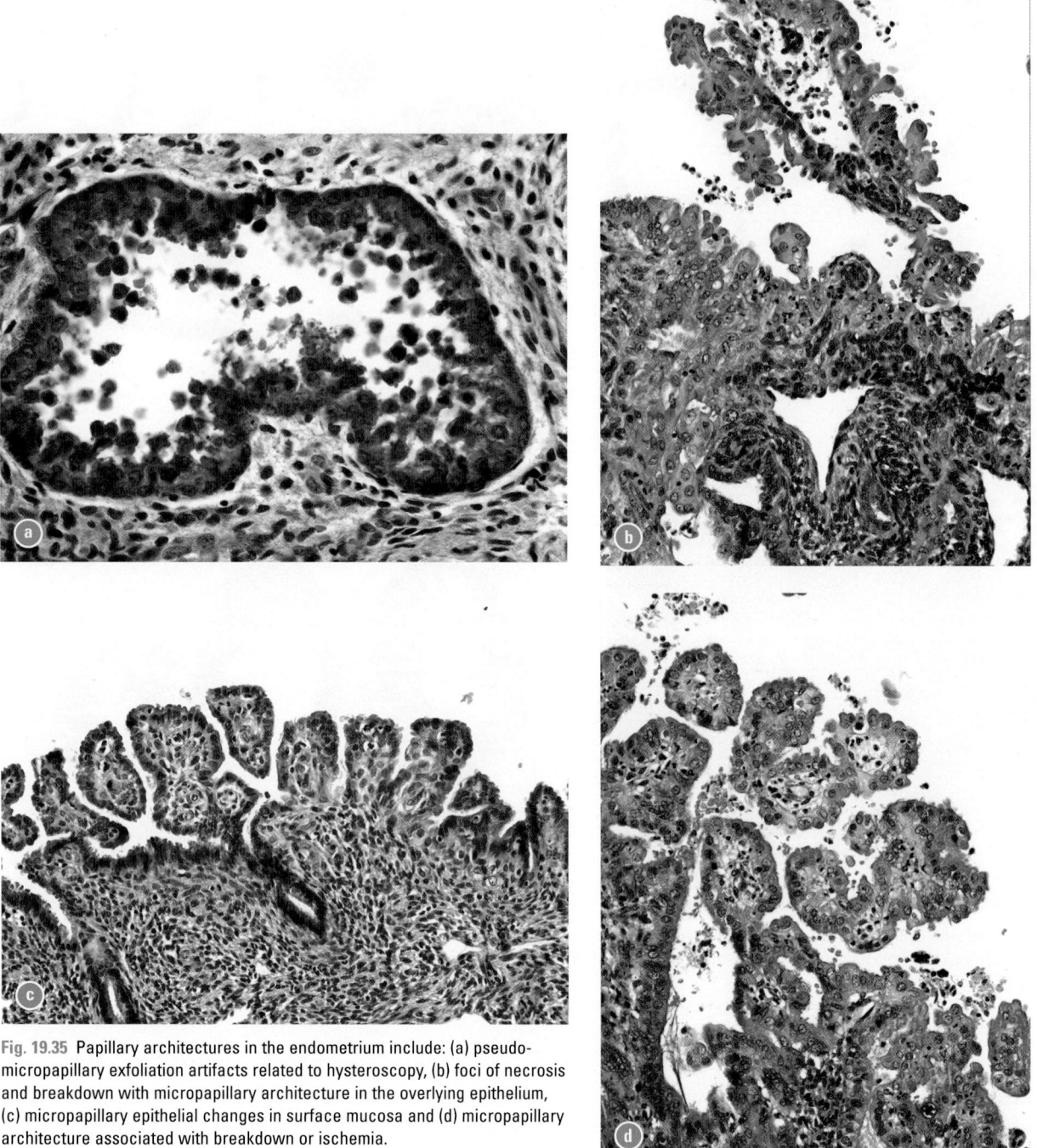

Fig. 19.35 Papillary architectures in the endometrium include: (a) pseudo-micropapillary exfoliation artifacts related to hysteroscopy, (b) foci of necrosis and breakdown with micropapillary architecture in the overlying epithelium, (c) micropapillary epithelial changes in surface mucosa and (d) micropapillary architecture associated with breakdown or ischemia.

Sensitivity and predictive value for cancer on follow-up. The overall reliability of this approach is high. Clark et al. performed a quantitative review of published research encompassing over 1000 cases. A positive (cancer) result in the biopsy/curettage was followed by a diagnosis of cancer in 82% of hysterectomy specimens. Importantly, a negative biopsy did not guarantee the absence of neoplasia, underscoring the importance

of follow-up and attention to persistent symptoms despite a negative result.[117] Other studies report detection rates of 90–100%.[118–121] Suffice it to say that endometrial sampling devices are sensitive but not infallible.

Significance of a preoperative diagnosis of EIN. Prior studies have shown that the risk of cancer (on hysterectomy) following a diagnosis of EIN approaches 25%.[122]

However, in the absence of an outright diagnosis of cancer in the curettings, the chance that the hysterectomy will contain deeply invasive tumor is low.[123] In our prior experience, the average pathologist is more likely to over- than under-diagnose endometrial precancers.[124] However, a recent study by the Gynecologic Oncology Group in which a central expert panel re-reviewed approximately 300 biopsies referred by community pathologists as 'atypical endometrial hyperplasias' reported an inordinately high percentage of these cases, which were reinterpreted as adenocarcinoma on review, with many examples of myoinvasion at immediate hysterectomy.[125,126] This reflects difficulties within the community of discrimination of the precancer-cancer as well as benign-precancer threshold. The EIN schema, which uses more precise definitions to define these boundaries, has great promise in improving upon this performance. The clinician who manages patients with EIN conservatively must ensure close surveillance with repeated sampling and, if contemplating surgery, should approach the patient with the possibility of invasive cancer in mind.[125,126]

Concordance with grade on hysterectomy. Once an unequivocal diagnosis of cancer is made in curettings, concordance with the final hysterectomy is dependent on sampling. Most studies have demonstrated good concordance between biopsy and hysterectomy grade for biopsy grades 2 or 3. However, in view of the fact that only 5% solid component will upgrade a grade 1 tumor, a grade 1 diagnosis is often revised following examination of the entire surgical specimen. Overall, concordance rates range from 56 to 65% and most are due to underestimation of grade.[123,124] In one study, 30%, 46% and 100% of patients presenting with grade 1, 2 and 3 endometrial adenocarcinomas, respectively, ultimately required full surgical staging at the time of their primary surgery.[124]

This issue becomes particularly relevant when a practitioner manages a grade 1 endometrial carcinoma without anticipating the possible need for complete staging.

Cervical involvement. Cervical involvement occurs in 15–30% of cases and cannot always be excluded preoperatively (Fig. 19.31).[127,128] The pathologist must carefully evaluate the endocervical curetting because this variable has traditionally influenced decisions regarding preoperative radiotherapy or choice of a more aggressive surgical approach. The fundamental question concerns the predictive value of a positive endocervical curetting for true endocervical involvement. Pete et al. confirmed cervical involvement in only 30% of their cases with a positive preoperative ECC.[129] Several other studies have shown that the ECC has a high sensitivity and negative predictive value (about 91% and 96%, respectively), but a lower specificity (89%) and positive predictive value (45%).[127,129–131] Some, but not all of this uncertainty can be addressed with attention to endocervical stromal invasion. Rubin et al. distinguished two groups, including 25 (32%) with demonstrable involvement of cervical stroma and 52 (68%) with only detached fragments of carcinoma present in endocervical curettings. They noted a significant association between extent of cervical involvement and outcome.[132] Because *bona-fide* cervical invasion carries a poor prognosis, the pathologist should not report cervical involvement without invasion and should advise the clinician accordingly if a tumor is present but invasion is not within the endocervical curetting.[133]

Intraoperative management

Most endometrial carcinomas are confined to the uterus at the time of diagnosis, but removal of the uterus and surgical staging is required to assess the extent of disease. The purpose of intraoperative evaluation of the uterus is to confirm grade assigned on the biopsy or curetting and assess the depth of invasion, the extent of which might determine whether a lymph node dissection takes place (Fig. 19.36) (Table 19.7). However, the degree to which the intraoperative pathology examination is useful depends on (1) the accuracy with which information can be obtained and (2) the consistency with which the results are interpreted by the gynecologist or gynecologic oncologists. The latter hinges in part on the existence of published recommendations with established criteria for ascertaining risk of lymph node metastases.

The two most important intraoperative determinations are depth of invasion and tumor grade, which in turn determine the need for lymph node dissection. Traditionally, all tumors in which the depth of invasion exceeds 50% of the myometrial thickness and grade 2 or 3 tumors exceeding one-third are candidates for lymph node dissection. However, the reader is advised that some authors support surgical staging in all but the most superficial well-differentiated carcinomas. This philosophy is prompted by a few more recent (and still controversial) studies correlating improved long-term survival with complete surgical staging.[134]

Gross and/or microscopic evaluation of tumor grade and depth of invasion will predict final pathologic outcome in from 85 to 94% of cases.[135–140] Most authors feel that gross examination or, if preferred, frozen

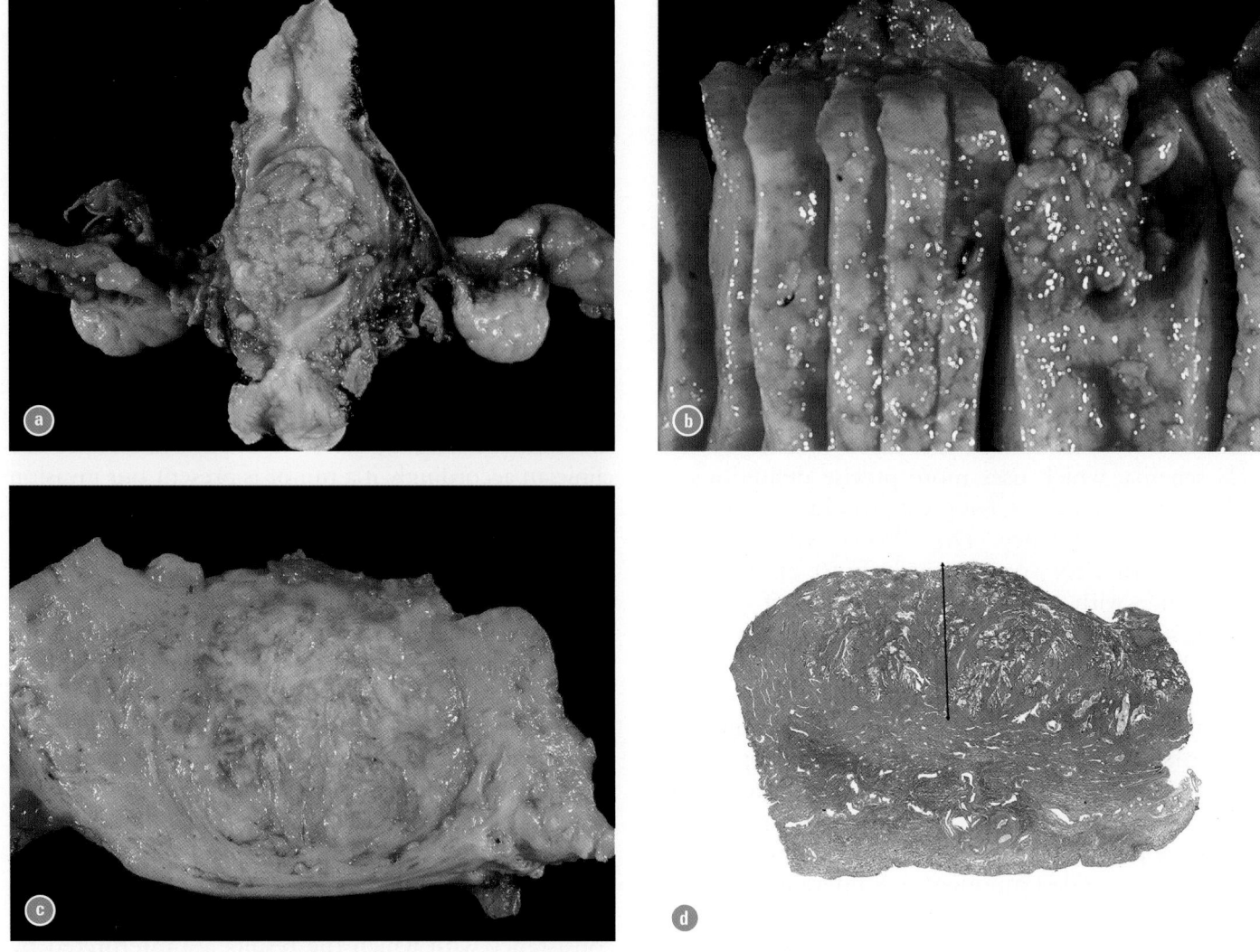

Fig. 19.36 (a) Gross appearance of endometrial carcinoma. (b) Sectioning of endomyometrium. (c) Gross assessment of myometrial invasion. (d) Assessment of depth by microscopy.

section, is a useful approach to ascertain depth and grade, respectively. The most common errors are underestimation of grade or depth, based on sampling error or inability to appreciate invasion. The latter most commonly occurs with diffusely infiltrating carcinomas or poorly-differentiated tumors in lymphatics. Conversely, involvement of adenomyosis may result in an overestimation of myometrial invasion. Predictably, UPSCs and clear cell carcinomas are fully staged with total abdominal hysterectomy, nodal, omental and peritoneal sampling.[141]

The approach to the intraoperative pathologic evaluation is as follows:

1 The uterus is opened by the pathologist in the frozen section room, carefully sectioned with attention to keeping the specimen intact for further evaluation, and at least one transverse section submitted for frozen section (Fig. 19.36).

2 Attention should be paid to gross lesions, but equally important, to subtle changes in color and consistency in the myometrium that may herald subtle or diffuse invasion. Conversely, careful attention to areas of suspected adenomyosis is important.

3 The cervix and vaginal reflections should also be scrutinized and sampled if suspicious areas are found. Evaluation of the section should focus on cell type (endometrioid versus serous or clear cell or other), grade and depth of invasion. The latter is provided as a percentage estimate of the myometrial thickness. At the time of final examination of permanent sections, these

parameters should be compared with those recorded during intraoperative evaluation and any discrepancies addressed and explained. In most cases with a discrepancy it is due to sampling error. In some instances, a subtle diffuse invasion may be missed or a grade under-assigned. If the discrepancies are clinically significant, the clinician should be notified and advised.

4 Communication between the surgeon and pathologist. The pathologist should be aware of the original biopsy diagnosis, if available, and determine if the intraoperative findings are consistent with or at variance to the original endometrial sampling. This information, including the current assessment of depth and grade, should be communicated to the surgeon. Interpretive problems, including those introduced by adenomyosis or other artifacts, should be discussed. The surgeon must ensure that the pathologist has all the clinical information required to complete their assessment. Conversely, the pathologist should query the surgeon to confirm that they have all the information required to proceed with the surgery.

Postoperative pathologic evaluation

Gross pathology

The decision regarding nodal and omental/peritoneal sampling is the critical determinant of intraoperative management. Subsequent evaluation of the uterus involves submission of sufficient endomyometrium to ensure accurate staging and ascertain the need for additional therapy. In all cases, the entire endomyometrium should be sectioned (bread-loafed) at 2–3 mm intervals and carefully inspected. The amount of endomyometrium submitted will vary depending on the circumstances. For example, if a well-differentiated adenocarcinoma was the original diagnosis and nothing is found on gross examination, representative sections may be sufficient. In contrast, if the original diagnosis was uterine papillary serous carcinoma, the entire endometrium will be submitted. In all cases, at least 2–3 sections from each side should be submitted (Fig. 19.36). The entire adnexa (ovaries and tubes) should be processed if any of the following criteria are met: (1) the clinician or pathologist suspect extrauterine disease; (2) there is a history of breast cancer or suspected familial risk for breast or ovarian cancer; (3) peritoneal washing cytology is returned as positive; and (4) the endometrial tumor is a serous carcinoma or contains a serous or high-grade component.[141]

Histopathologic features

Histopathologic examination of the uterus is necessary to final staging. While this process is unlikely to result in a second surgical procedure, it is important in terms of deciding whether adjunctive postoperative therapy is needed. The latter will be considered if certain high-risk parameters are found, inasmuch as they may increase the risk of local recurrence. Some of these include histologic type, depth of invasion, grade, presence of cervical involvement and the presence or absence of capillary-lymphatic space invasion, among others.[142] A complete assessment is therefore integral to the next step in therapeutic triage.

In 1988, FIGO redefined staging for endometrial carcinoma according to final surgical–pathologic evaluation and this has influenced the management of a significant minority of women.[143–146] The staging system for endometrial cancer is summarized in Table 19.8 (see also the Appendix). Combined with the grade, stage predicts the natural history of the disease. The 5-year survival for Stages I–IV is approximately 90+%, 75%, 60% and 15–26%, respectively. A more precise estimate in individual cases can be obtained with attention to the following parameters, which are critical to management.

Table 19.8 FIGO surgical staging for endometrial cancer

Stage I	Tumor confined to the uterine fundus
Stage IA	The tumor is limited to the endometrium
Stage IB	The tumor invades through less than 50% of the myometrial thickness
Stage IC	The tumor invades through greater than 50% of the myometrial thickness
Stage II	The tumor extends to the cervix (the lower part of the uterus)
Stage IIA	Cervical extension is limited to the columnar epithelium of surface and crypts
Stage IIB	Tumor invades the cervical stroma
Stage III	There is regional tumor spread
Stage IIIA	The tumor penetrates the uterine serosa, involves adnexa, or is detected in peritoneal washings
Stage IIIB	Tumor involves vagina
Stage IIIC	The tumor involves regional lymph nodes
Stage IV	Tumor invades contiguous organs or has metastasized to remote organ sites
Stage IVA	Tumor invades the bladder or rectum
Stage IVB	Distant metastases are present

FIGO, International Federation of Gynecology and Obstetrics.

Tumor type or grade Tumor type and grade in the hysterectomy is correlated with the curetting. Table 19.4 and Table 19.9 summarize the relationship between tumor grade and type and outcome – the important histologic variables. Grading (FIGO) is applied to endometrioid adenocarcinomas and outcomes are similar for grade 1 and 2 tumors (92% and 87%) for Stage I, with a more pronounced reduction in survival for grade 3.[146] Nuclear grade is also an important parameter in the grading assignment, and should be carefully evaluated.

As implied in the prior discussion, the highest percentage of recurrences occur in the papillary serous and clear cell categories versus endometrioid carcinomas. In the study of Stage I patients by Cirisano et al. the estimated 5-year survival for UPSC and clear cell carcinoma (CCC) was 56% *vs* 93% for endometrioid carcinoma.[147] The overall 5-year survival for Stage I-II UPSC/CCC is 36–40% *vs* 70–90% for endometrioid carcinoma.[8,90,95] When all stages were considered by Nordstrom et al., 49% with UPSC or CCC died of their cancer compared with 31% of endometrioid tumors.[148]

Depth of invasion Depth of invasion is an important variable in both management and prognosis. In general, the measurement of invasion is made from the nearest normal endomyometrial interface. It is most optimally determined in a full-thickness section (Fig. 19.36). If the myometrium is too thick to manage a single section in a cassette, the section can be inked appropriately and divided horizontally at the center and submitted in two cassettes. Both depth in millimeters and percentage of myometrial thickness involved can be conveyed, although the latter is used for staging purposes.

Invasive patterns Invasion of the myometrium can present in a variety of patterns, including the following:
1 Obvious infiltration with small or large tumor nests, irregular epithelial stromal border with loss of epithelial polarity, altered differentiation, and stromal reaction (Fig. 19.37a)
2 More subtle patterns in which the stromal reaction dominates and the glands are less conspicuous (Fig. 19.37b)
3 Invasion along a broad interface with minimal stromal reaction (Fig. 19.37c)
4 Infiltration by tumor cells in small groups with minimal stromal reaction. This pattern is the most subtle and may be missed, particularly on frozen section (Fig. 19.37d)
5 Invasion of well-differentiated neoplastic glands with virtual absence of stromal reaction (so-called adenoma malignum-type of growth pattern; also referred to as 'diffusely invasive').[149,150]

Distinguishing invasion from involvement of adenomyosis

The pathologist frequently must determine whether the tumor is within adenomyosis or invading the myometrium. This is frequently an important distinction because adenomyosis is often situated more deeply in the myometrium.[150] Involvement of adenomyosis manifests as 'regularly irregular' nests of tumor in the myometrium that are similar in outline to adenomyosis without carcinoma and lack evidence of 'directed' downward growth (Fig. 19.38a). Normal glands should be visible at the epithelial-stromal interface of some of these nests (Fig. 19.38b). In contrast, invasive carcinoma is defined as either multiple small glands penetrating into the myometrium in similar orientation or dense clusters of glands extending as a unit vertically into the myometrium (directed growth). The other features of invasion discussed above may be present, and it is not uncommon for the involvement of adenomyosis to be accompanied by myometrial invasion as well (Fig. 19.39).

Some authors have examined endometrial stroma-specific markers such as CD10 to highlight the endometrial stroma in an attempt to distinguish adenomyotic involvement from myometrial invasion. Unfortunately, this approach has not been successful, because CD10 positivity is seen at the tumor-endometrial stromal

Table 19.9 *Important variables in the evaluation of hysterectomy specimen*

Parameter	Exclusions
Histologic type	Distinguish UPSC/CCC from endometrioid
Histologic grade	Squamous metaplasia *vs* solid adenocarcinoma
Depth of invasion	Adenomyosis, specimen distortion
Capillary-lymphatic space invasion	Transfer artifacts
Cervical involvement	Benign cervical atypias, superficial *vs* invasive
Parametrium	Endometriosis
Serosa	Endometriosis, second primary neoplasms
Tubes and ovaries	Incidental tumor cell transfer, second primaries
Omentum/peritoneum	Endosalpingiosis, second primaries, keratin granulomas
Regional lymph nodes	Müllerian inclusions, macrophages/histiocytes

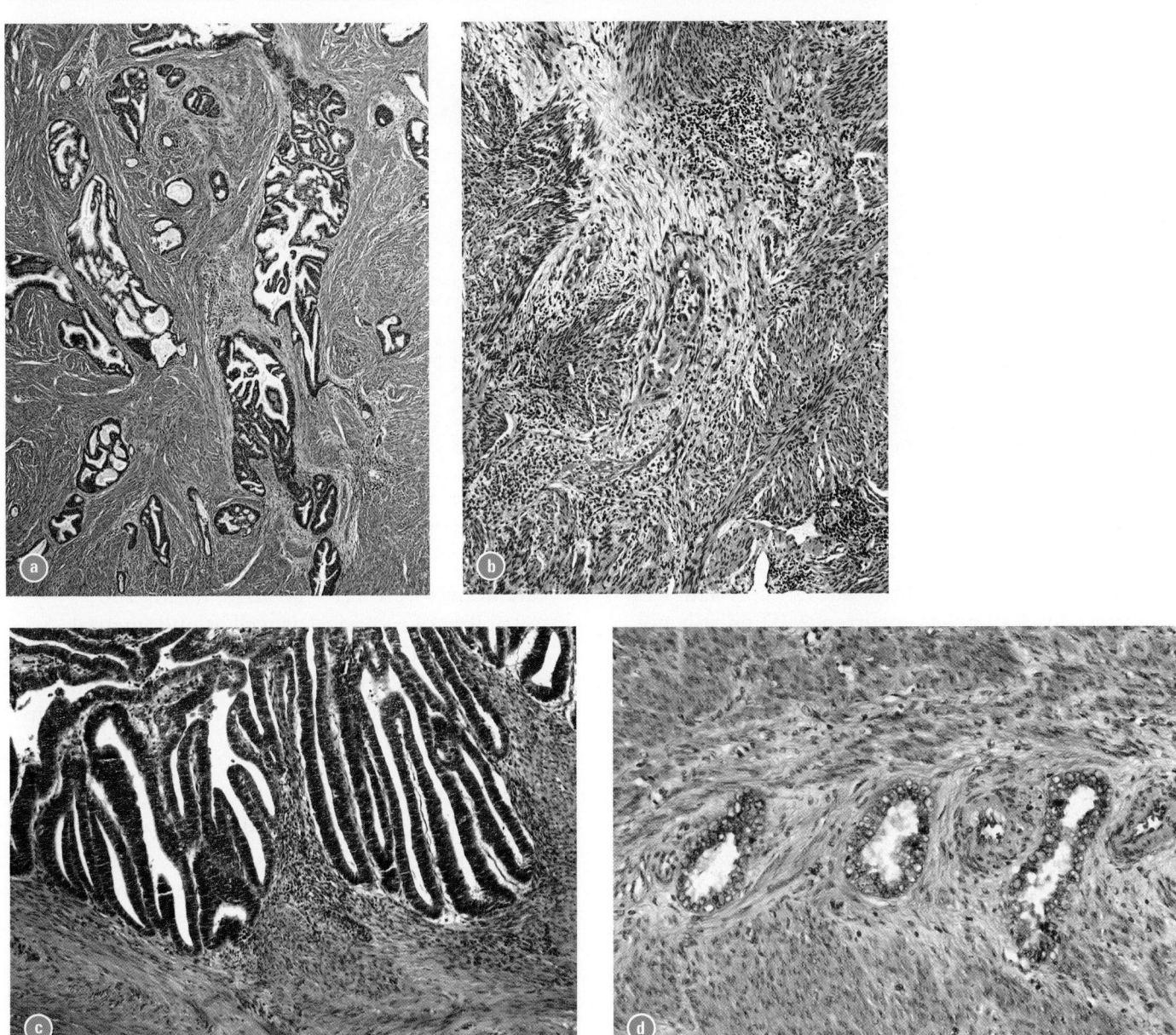

Fig. 19.37 Patterns of invasion in endometrial carcinoma include (a) classic invasion with stromal inflammation or fibrosis, (b) scant invasive epithelium (center) with predominately stromal myxoid change, (c) invasion along a broad interface with little or no stromal reaction and (d) invasion as small glands with negligible stromal reaction.

interface of frankly invasive tumors. Presumably the CD10 is induced by the tumor *per se*.[151,152] Because there is no absolutely reliable method to distinguish all invasive cancer from that within adenomyosis, pathologists can expect to occasionally encounter extensive 'adenomyosis-like' tumor involvement. If it is not accompanied by evidence of adenomyosis in the adjacent non-involved endometrium, the diagnosis of myometrial invasion should be considered.

Lower uterine segment (LUS) involvement

The lower uterine segment (LUS) (Fig. 19.40) is involved in as many as 44% of endometrial carcinomas.[153] Three issues must be addressed in management:
1 *The risk of poor outcome.* Phelan et al. found LUS involvement showed a trend towards a less favorable outcome when it was a component of a conventional corpus carcinoma.[153] However, LUS involvement by itself, in the absence of other

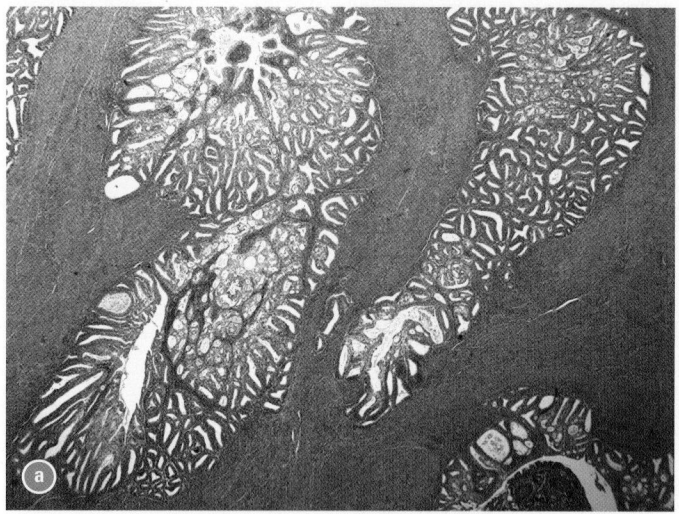 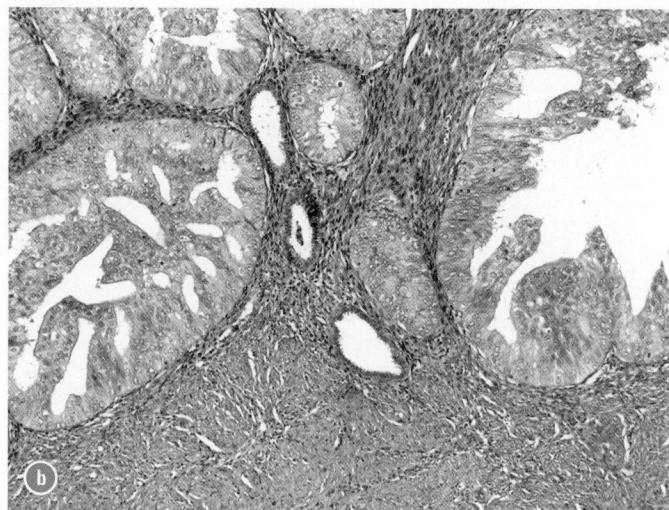

Fig. 19.38 Involvement of adenomyosis by endometrial adenocarcinoma. (a) The diagnosis is based on the absence of 'directed' invasion. (b) Endometrial stroma or glands at the tumor–myometrial interface (center) are not always conspicuous but is helpful in the diagnosis.

adverse pathologic features, did not correlate with increased risk of pelvic recurrence. Thus, it is not an indication for adjuvant radiation therapy.

2 *The significance of LUS carcinomas as a distinct entity.* Hachisuga et al. examined 88 cancers in women under 50 years of age and noted that 16 were confined to the LUS.[154] These tumors were more frequently of higher grade and more deeply invasive than conventional corpus carcinomas.

3 *The possibility of a primary cervical neoplasm.* Hachisuga et al. noted that 20% of LUS carcinomas were HPV positive, raising the possibility of a cervical as well as endometrial origin for these tumors.[155] However, although we do employ HPV testing to resolve this question, in our experience most appear to be derived from the endometrium and are HPV negative.

Cervical involvement

The cervix is involved in 13–29% of cases of endometrial cancer and this increases the risk of both local relapse and nodal involvement and a lower survival

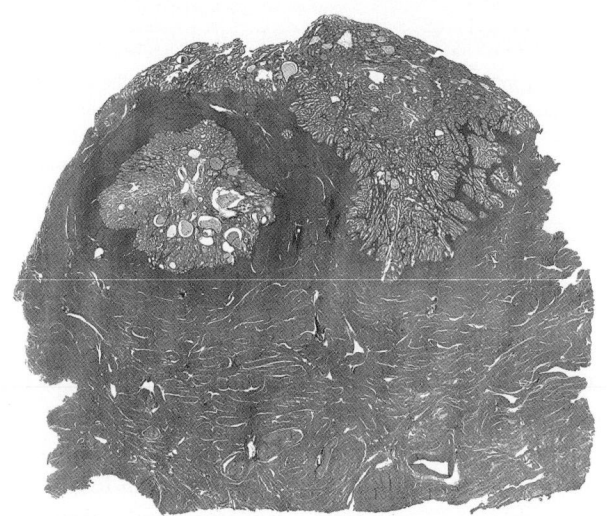

Fig. 19.39 Adenomyosis (left) associated with myometrial invasion in a 'directed' pattern of invasion (right).

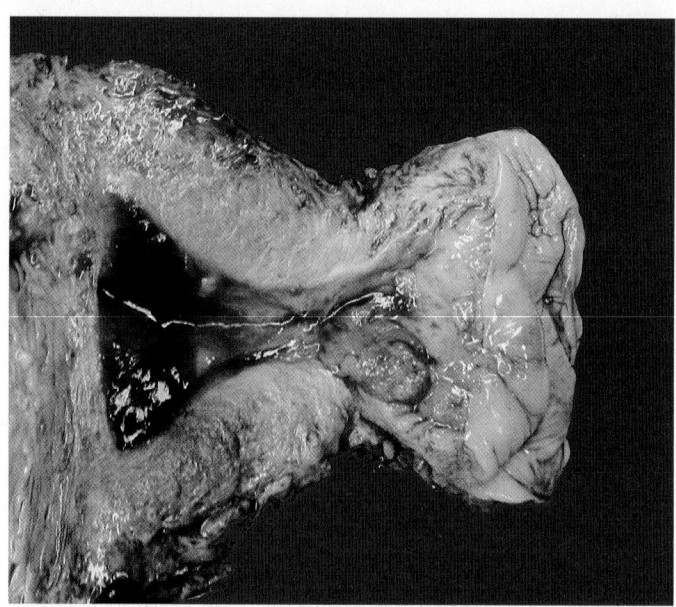

Fig. 19.40 Gross appearance of lower uterine segment adenocarcinoma.

(see Table 19.9).[127,156–158] When cervical involvement coexists with other variables such as extrauterine disease, deep myometrial invasion and papillary serous morphology, the prognosis is particularly poor.[130]

The following aspects of cervical involvement are important to recognize histologically:

Degree of involvement. The precise stage is determined by whether the tumor involves the surface glands only (Stage IIA) (Fig. 19.41a) or invades the cervical stroma (Stage IIB) (Fig. 19.41b). Superficial implants in the cervix with minimal or no stromal invasion occurred in 40% of cases with cervical involvement in one study.[156] Another noted a significantly higher survival for IIA than IIB (86 *vs* 46%).[159] Observers have correctly assumed that the surface involvement seen in Stage IIA tumors is due to implants of tumor settling on the endocervical mucosa following curettage.

Subtle forms of endometrial adenocarcinoma involving cervix may mimic primary cervical cancer. Recently, Tambouret et al. summarized a small number of cases in which endometrial adenocarcinoma deeply invaded the cervix with a deceptively bland histology and minimal stromal response (Fig. 19.42a–c).[160] This pattern may be confused with minimal deviation adenocarcinoma of the cervix, mesonephric lesions and endometriosis.

Excluding endocervical adenocarcinoma. This has been discussed in Chapter 14 and can be summarized by the following statements. (a) It is extremely unlikely that tumors in both the cervix and endometrium will be attributed to two separate primary neoplasms. (b) Carcinomas occurring at any age with extensive endometrial involvement are rarely derived from the cervix. (c) Predominately mucinous, clear cell or papillary serous carcinomas occurring in older women are highly likely to originate from the endometrium. (d) Poorly-differentiated carcinomas extensively involving the cervix in younger women are more likely (but not invariably) to be primary cervical neoplasms, including those that closely resemble serous carcinomas. The two can be distinguished in most cases by HPV testing (cervix) or vimentin, estrogen and progesterone receptors (endometrium).[161,162]

Peritoneal cytology and peritoneal spread

The following must be considered in the evaluation of peritoneal spread:

Cytologic findings. Malignant cells are identified in peritoneal washings in up to 20% of cases and increase in frequency as a function of stage, from 17% in Stage I to 85% in Stage IV (Fig. 19.43a,b).[2] Positive peritoneal washings also correlate with relapse.[163,164] What has been unclear is whether peritoneal cytology is an independent prognostic indicator of poor outcome in endometrial carcinoma.[165] In a gynecologic oncology group study by Creasman et al., positive washings were an independent risk factor for relapse.[166] However, that study included *clinical* Stage I tumors. A subsequent study of *surgical* Stage I tumors (excepting the washings) found no difference in prognosis.[167] Kennedy et al. observed positive washings in 5.2% of tumors limited to the uterus on histologic examination, with a 5-year survival of 67% *vs* 85% for those without

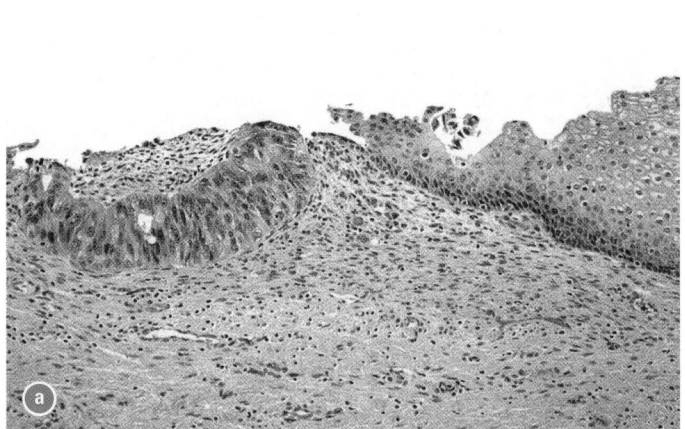
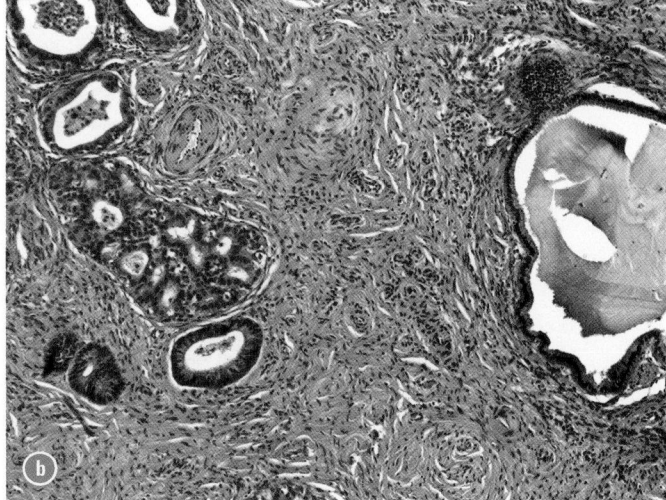

Fig. 19.41 (a) Superficial deposit of endometrial carcinoma in the cervical transformation zone (left). (b) Frank endocervical stromal invasion by an endometrial adenocarcinoma.

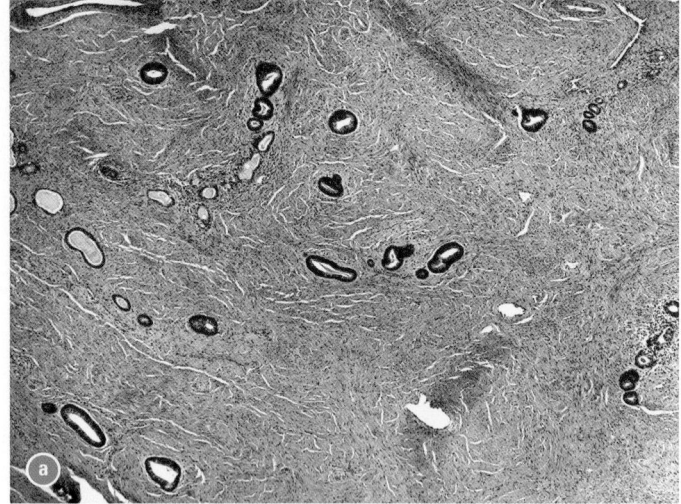

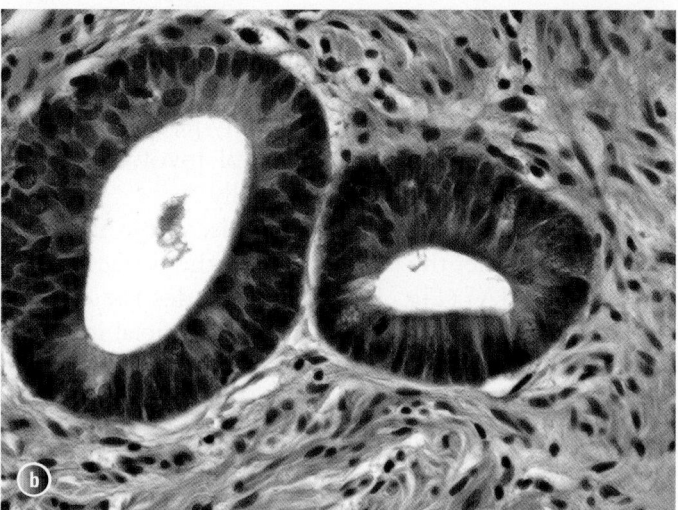

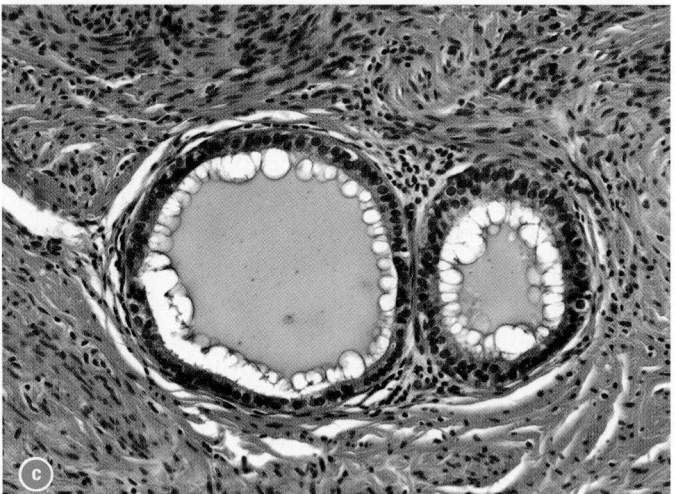

Fig. 19.42 Deceptively bland involvement of the cervix by an endometrial adenocarcinoma. (a) At low power, the neoplastic glands are well spaced and maintain an orderly architecture. (b) At high power, some glands are typical of endometrioid epithelium, whereas others (c) are lined by cuboidal epithelium with minimal atypia, resembling mesonephric or endocervical epithelium.

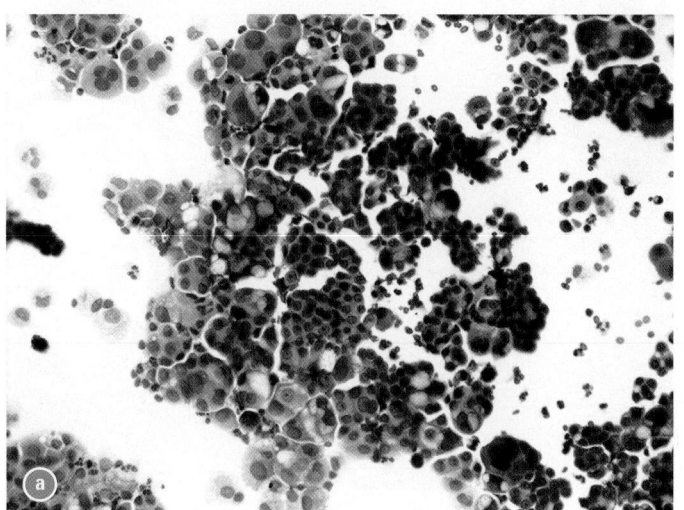

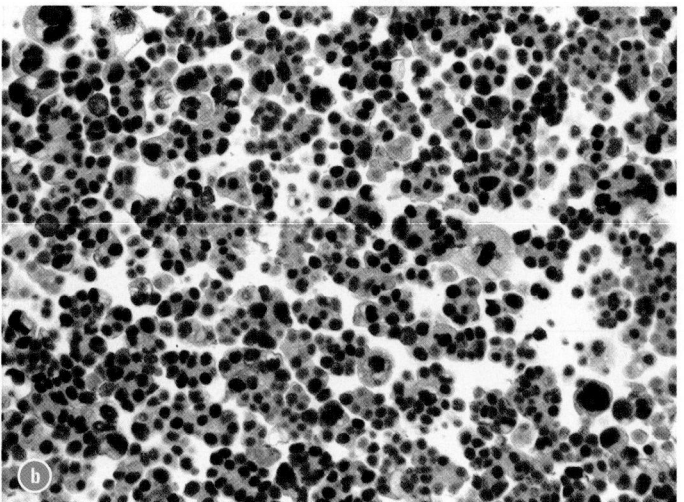

Fig. 19.43 (a) Peritoneal cell block from a uterine papillary serous carcinoma with (b) strongly positive p53 immunostaining.

positive washings. Nevertheless, confounding variables prevented an independent correlation of relapse with positive washings.[168] Another study resampled the peritoneal fluid 1–2 weeks following surgery of washing-positive patients and found no cells, suggesting that they were transient.[169]

Histologic spread to the peritoneum. As mentioned above, most endometrioid and clear cell adenocarcinomas relapse in sites other than the peritoneal surfaces, with serous tumors responsible for the majority. Exceptions include occasional aggressive endometrioid carcinomas and tumors arising in pelvic endometriosis.

Mimics of peritoneal spread. The two entities most likely to be confused with peritoneal spread are atypical endometriosis and keratin granulomas. The latter are presumably a reaction to the keratin accompanying squamous differentiation in the primary tumor transported through the fallopian tubes. However, despite the spread of these cells to the peritoneum, they do not increase the risk of relapse. Notably, malignant glandular or squamous epithelium is not identified (Fig. 19.44).[7]

Coexisting tubo-ovarian involvement

Coexisting involvement of the endometrium or ovary is found in 10% and 5% of women with ovarian and endometrial cancer, respectively. Synchronous endometrioid carcinomas of uterus and ovary are associated with a younger age in general (41–52 years), an association that might delineate a unique group with

a genetic predisposition, as discussed previously.[170–172] Tumors with endometrioid histology in both organs typically fare well. Eifel et al. reported a 100% survival in cases where the concurrent endometrial and ovarian tumors were endometrioid, in keeping with the assumption that these are separate primary tumors.[170] In contrast, those with other histologic types had more extensive myometrial involvement and higher risk of extragenital spread, with a survival of only 55%. Predictably, evidence of spread beyond both the uterus and ovary identifies the more aggressive group. Falkenberry et al. reported a 100% survival in patients with Stage I ovarian and endometrial tumors, respectively.[171] Soliman et al. reported a median survival of 10 years for patients with concordant endometrioid histology.[173]

For the pathologist, sorting out tumor origins in an individual case may be difficult. The presence of coexisting endometrial and ovarian carcinoma can be explained by three scenarios: (1) primary uterine carcinoma metastatic to the ovary, (2) primary ovarian carcinoma metastatic to the endometrium and (3) concurrent endometrial and ovarian primary neoplasms. A few practical guidelines may be helpful:

1 If involvement of either the endometrium or the ovary is due to metastatic disease, extension to other sites beyond either organ is likely to be clinically evident, in which case management will be similar irrespective of primary site.

2 Even if this is not the case, synchronous serous, clear cell, or high-grade endometrioid carcinomas will mandate more aggressive management.

3 Patients with synchronously discovered grade 1 endometrioid carcinomas, without clinically evident spread beyond these organs, can be considered for no further therapy.

With respect to the exercise of distinguishing independent from co-dependent (metastatic) tumors, the following should be considered.

1 Metastatic involvement of the endometrium by an ovarian carcinoma is rare. This is only considered if small, discrete plaques of carcinoma are present in an otherwise normal endometrium.

2 Deeply invasive endometrioid carcinomas, those associated with tubal spread, or with capillary-lymphatic space invasion, are more likely to metastasize to the ovaries. However, there is no reliable evidence that these parameters exclude separate primary endometrioid tumors. In either instance, cases with these adverse findings would likely be managed more aggressively.

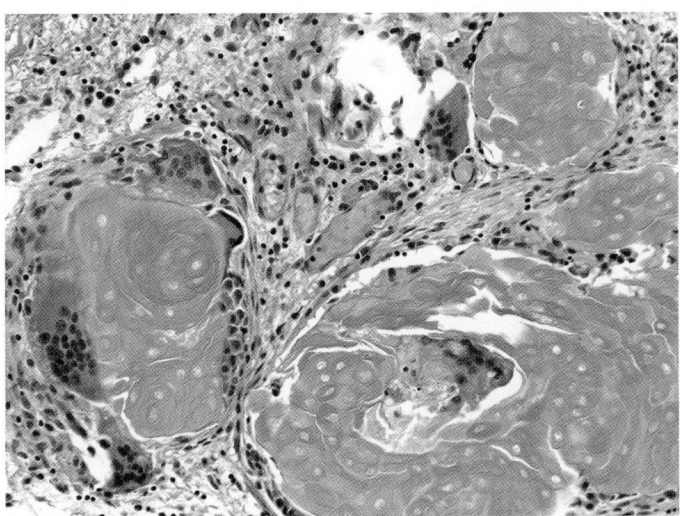

Fig. 19.44 Keratin granulomas in the peritoneum in a patient with an endometrial adenocarcinoma with squamous differentiation. The carcinoma was confined to the uterus.

3 Because synchronous extrauterine primary tumors presumably arise from endometriosis, additional primaries, arising in the retroperitoneum or cul-de-sac, are also possible. Conceivably, some higher-stage tumors (involving uterus, ovary, cul-de-sac, etc.) are in fact multiple independent primary neoplasms.

In summary, for the purposes of management, the most important issue is whether either tumor is non-endometrioid (clear cell or serous) and whether there is disease beyond the ovary and uterus.[172,173]

Although their value is still unclear, molecular assays designed to determine if both ovarian and uterine (endometrioid) tumors share common aberrations in the PTEN gene may refine the assignment of status as a separate primary or metastasis. In one study, the staging of 3 from 10 concurrent uterine/ovarian neoplasms was revised once the tumors were matched by molecular means.[174]

Parametrial spread

Parametrial spread (6%) increases as a function of stage, being associated with 6 and 17% of Stage II and III tumors, respectively. When present, there is a high (38%) rate of recurrence and eventual death in 5 or more years.[175]

Nodal status

The status of the pelvic and para-aortic lymph nodes ultimately governs outcome and most of the other staging parameters are indexed to this risk. Patients with pelvic or para-aortic lymph node involvement (Stage IIIC) have a disease-free survival of 36% at 5 years. Further, if pelvic nodes are involved, the risk of para-aortic involvement is as high as 50% *vs* less than 5% if negative (Fig. 19.45).[176,177] The extent of nodal involvement further influences outcome. In a study of 17 patients with only a single pelvic lymph node involved, the actuarial 5-year disease-free survival was 81%.[178] Other variables adversely influencing outcome in node-positive cases include higher percentage of positive nodes, a desmoplastic response in the lymph node to the tumor and extension of the tumor into the perinodal adipose tissue.[179] Predictably, unresectable macroscopic nodal metastases are associated with a significantly shorter disease-specific survival.[180]

Pathologic examination of the lymph nodes entails a detailed dissection of the nodal tissue, preferably in the fresh state. Larger nodes should be sectioned at 1–2 mm intervals. Microscopically, as with any nodal examination, the pathologist should pay close attention to the subcapsular region to exclude small foci of metastatic tumor (Fig. 19.45a,b). When metastases are detected, the number of nodes involved, and presence or absence of extranodal direct extension should be recorded. Two important pitfalls are the misdiagnosis of Müllerian inclusions (Fig. 19.46) as tumor and of reactive mesothelial cells as metastatic deposits (Fig. 19.47a,b).[181,182] If desired, immunostaining with calretinin (mesothelial cells) or epithelial membrane

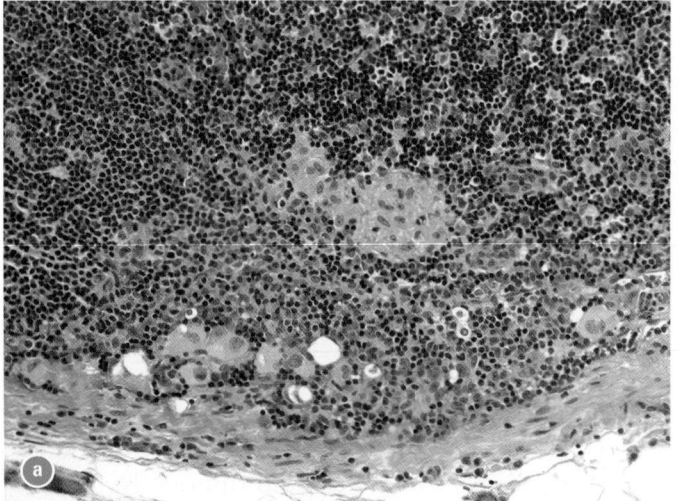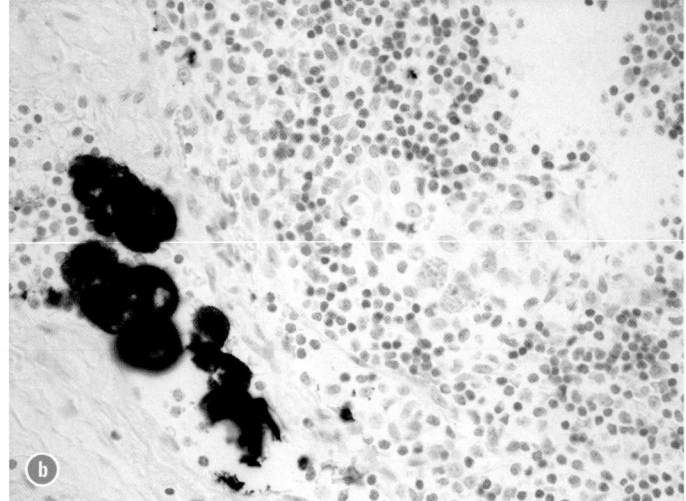

Fig. 19.45 (a) Metastatic endometrial adenocarcinoma involving a pelvic lymph node; (b) keratin staining marks the cells in the periphery, whereas the nest of macrophages in the center are negative.

antigen (carcinoma) will distinguish cancer from mesothelial cells or macrophages (Fig. 19.45b).

Although not yet recommended as standard in the laboratory management of endometrial cancer, immunostaining of pelvic lymph nodes with keratin antibodies has been shown to increase the detection of tumor cells (Fig. 19.45a,b).[183] Yabushita et al. reported no recurrences in 22 Stage I patients with negative nodes *vs* 5 of 15 with cytokeratin-positive nodes.[184] It is important to emphasize that other elements in nodes, including macrophages, mesothelial cells and Müllerian inclusions, may also stain for cytokeratins.

Capillary-lymphatic space invasion

Myometrial capillary-lymphatic space invasion is typically not detected until after the decision regarding lymph node dissection has been made. Nonetheless, the risk of positive pelvic and para-aortic lymph nodes in presumably Stage I patients has been significantly associated with capillary-lymphatic space invasion in the uterus.[185] Studies have shown vascular invasion to be particularly important, exceeding depth of invasion (Stage IA *vs* IB) as a risk factor. When combined with grade, this parameter identified patients with a high relapse potential.[186]

Vascular space invasion is best evaluated at the periphery of the tumor where retraction artifacts will not introduce problems in its assessment. The finding of recognizable endothelial cells surrounding the potentially involved space is important in confirming them as vascular.[187] The tumor nests typically occur in

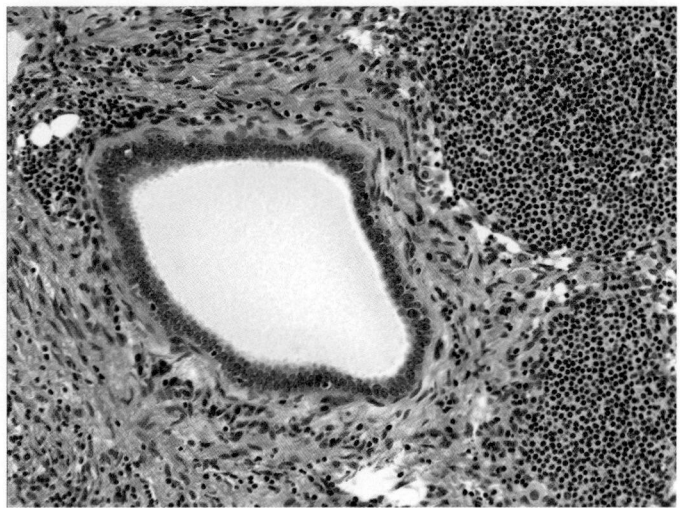

Fig. 19.46 Müllerian inclusions in a pelvic lymph node.

smaller vessels and characteristically take the shape of the vessel. The degree of nuclear atypia may be deceptively bland and be accompanied by a more conspicuous eosinophilic cytoplasm relative to the original carcinoma (Fig. 19.48a).

When considering capillary-lymphatic space invasion, the pathologist should be careful to exclude artifacts that occur due to sectioning the endomyometrium, such as introduction of neoplastic epithelium into vascular spaces. Groups of unaltered tumor cells in large vessels are commonly artifactual and these should be distinguished from vascular invasion (Fig. 19.48b).

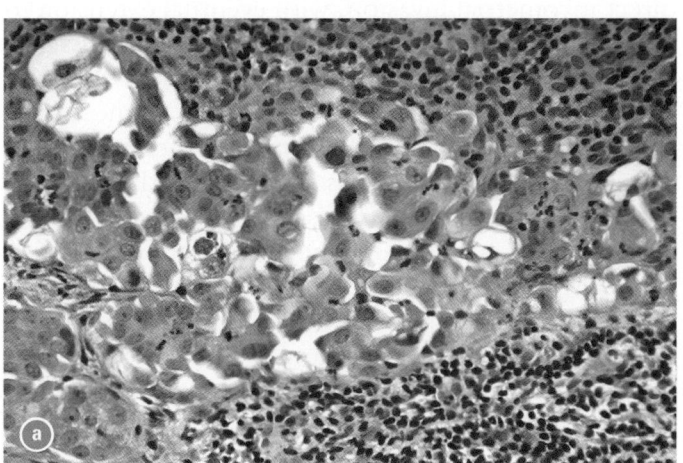
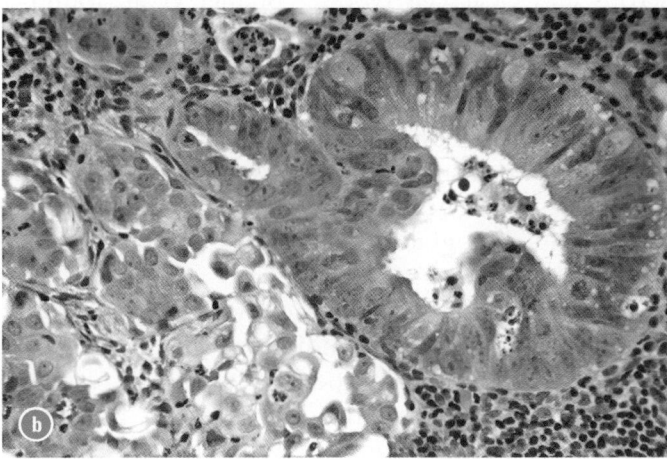

Fig. 19.47 Reactive mesothelial cells in (a) a lymph node and (b) associated with adenocarcinoma.

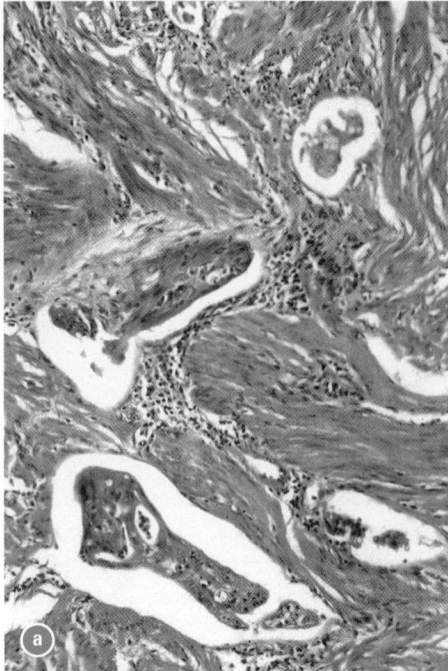 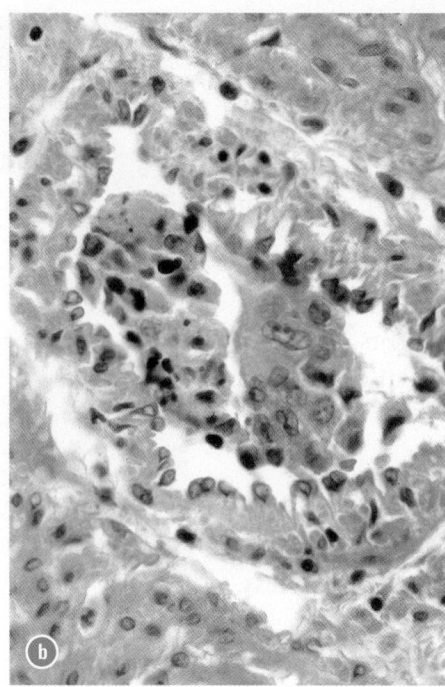

Fig. 19.48 (a) Capillary-lymphatic space invasion. (b) Pseudovascular space invasion due to sectioning artifacts.

BIOMARKERS AND OTHER PARAMETERS ASSOCIATED WITH OUTCOME

A variety of other markers influence outcome; most are of academic interest in current practice. In addition to p53, unfavorable parameters include Ki-67, p21, S-phase fraction (unfavorable) and progesterone receptor (favorable).[188,189] Favorable indicators include estrogen and progesterone receptors.[190]

Ploidy, nuclear grade and morphometric grade have all been linked to unfavorable outcome.[191] In another study, Nordstrom et al. found that nuclear grade explained all of the differences in survival attributed to serous and clear cell types.[192] Steiner et al. found a combination of DNA index (fresh frozen tissue) and the mean values of the shortest nuclear diameter and the SD of the longest diameter (paraffin-embedded tissue) gave the best prognostic information *vis-à-vis* cancer-related death in an all-possible-subsets regression analysis.[193] The above studies validate the importance of nuclear grade in evaluating any endometrial adenocarcinoma.

Molecular profiling is currently permitting study of additional prognostic indicators. Increased DNA methylation, a process associated with many cancers, may inactivate or alter the expression of important tumor-related genes. One study simply examined the state of ribosomal DNA methylation as a surrogate of methylation status in tumors and determined that it was associated with a poorer prognosis.[194] Others are actively profiling genome-wide protein expression patterns in tumors in an attempt to identify so-called 'proteomic signatures', the identification of which may have utility as early detection markers.

MANAGEMENT AND OUTCOME

Overview

Spread of endometrial carcinomas generally occurs via direct myometrial invasion, with eventual extension to contiguous periuterine structures. Eventually, dissemination to regional lymph nodes occurs; in the later stages, tumor may be hematogenously borne to the lungs, liver, bones and other organs. In certain types, specifically papillary serous carcinoma, there is the added risk of peritoneal disease, suggesting spread via peritoneal seeding. A range of prognostic factors, including grade and cell type, depth of myometrial invasion, vascular space invasion, status of peritoneal washings, and age, influence outcome.[148,195] The reader is reminded that a single parameter, such as stage, is not used in isolation, and may be modified in the context of other variables.

The outcome of endometrial cancer is stage-dependent. Overall, 5- and 10-year actuarial survivals for all stages are 83% and 80%, respectively.[195] Life table 5-year survivals for Stages IA, IB, II, III and IV were 89%, 92%, 77%, 27% and 0%, respectively.[146]

The most common pathology-related management scenarios are as follows:

1 Tumor has a favorable histologic type (endometrioid), is grade 1 or 2 and is confined to the endometrium or the inner third of the myometrium. Risk of lymph node involvement is 5% or less.

2 Tumor has deep myometrial invasion, grade 2 or 3 endometrioid, or evidence of vascular space invasion. Recommendations include adjuvant pelvic irradiation.

3 Tumor is an unfavorable histologic type (serous or clear cell) of any stage. Risk of relapse is at least 30% and will usually mandates adjunctive therapy.

4 Tumor is a favorable histologic type with involvement of the inner third (grade 3) or outer two-thirds (grades 1 and 2). This is an intermediate-risk category.

5 Additional parameters influencing outcome are present.

Two studies have established a rationale for reviewing the pathology in questionable cases. In one, one-third of diagnoses were revised; the revised diagnoses altered management in 8% and 12% of the total. Changes included grade, depth of invasion and the presence of cervical involvement.[196,197]

Controversies

Should preoperative irradiation be performed for a positive endocervical curetting? It is the opinion of these authors that the specificity of a positive endocervical curetting is not sufficient to justify preoperative irradiation. In particular, in a younger patient, a radical hysterectomy would be strongly considered. However, if the cervix is grossly involved – which is uncommon – radiation is a viable consideration although most will opt for a surgical route if the cervix is clinically normal.[198–201]

Should lymph nodes be dissected for grade 1 tumors involving the inner one-half of the myometrium? This is an important question because (a) it arises during the intraoperative procedure and (b) it may add significance to the detection of *any* myometrial invasion. From a practical standpoint, this question cannot be answered in the scope of this chapter due to the level of controversy that exists. Suffice it to say that some authors recommend nodal sampling of all patients, whereas others use it sparingly, particularly in Europe.[202,203] Currently, if a tumor invades through less than 50% of the myometrial thickness and is confirmed to be a grade 1 endometrioid, most practitioners will not dissect the lymph nodes. However, as a rule, if the surgeon or pathologist is uncertain about grade or depth in this setting, dissection should be considered.[202,203] One survey of gynecologic oncologists noted that nearly one-half will attempt sampling in all surgical cases.[204]

Does complete lymph node dissection (*vs* limited sampling) improve survival rates? Although some studies have suggested that survival may be improved, others have not and the question remains unanswered.[204] Nevertheless, many investigators feel that whole pelvic radiation therapy can be avoided in such cases and/or replaced with vaginal brachytherapy as needed.[205]

Does adjuvant radiation or chemotherapy prolong life, particularly in low-stage tumors? This question applies in particular to low-stage high-grade tumors. Creasman et al. reported death rates for Stage I serous, clear cell and grade 3 endometrioid of between 19 and 28%. Radiation was associated with a 6–8% improvement in survival but was not significant. There is currently insufficient data to determine if adjunctive chemotherapy will alter the outcome in this group.[206]

Carcinosarcomas

INTRODUCTION AND DEFINITION

Carcinosarcomas, formerly termed malignant mixed Müllerian tumors (MMMTs), account for approximately 10% of endometrial malignancies. The diagnosis requires the combination of epithelial and mesenchymal (sarcomatous) differentiation. It should be emphasized that the latter is presumed to derive from the epithelial component (or concurrent with it from the same progenitor cell) via shifts in differentiation. Accordingly, the sarcomatous portion may score positive with both epithelial- and mesenchymal-specific biomarkers. However, the tumor is defined by the histologic *appearance* of mesenchymal differentiation, which produces a unique clinical and histologic presentation relative to conventional adenocarcinomas.

PATHOGENESIS

Two general theories or pathways might explain carcinosarcomas: the conversion and the collision. In the collision theory, the sarcomatous element evolves from the carcinoma. In the collision theory, the two components presumably develop independently of each other, and occupy distinct areas with no visible transition at the interface of the two. This pattern theoretically could also be produced by a complete subclonal transition to a mesenchymal phenotype with outgrowth of the latter as a separate mass.[207]

Irrespective of pattern, most studies support a common origin of the components of carcinosarcomas and a strong genetic similarity to adenocarcinomas. A microdissection and allelic loss/retention study of 172 carcinomatous or sarcomatous foci from 17 gynecologic carcinosarcomas strongly supported a monoclonal origin for these neoplasms.[208] In another, X-chromosome inactivation pattern, K-ras and p53 mutation analysis linked the two patterns of diffentiation.[209] A third noted that 21 of 25 carcinosarcomas were monoclonal throughout although a few could be explained as polyclonal.[210] Patterns of allelic imbalance have also been attributed to an origin from epithelial rather than mesenchymal cells.[211]

THE PATIENT AT RISK

Prior radiation

Carcinosarcomas occur almost exclusively in postmenopausal patients (most often over the age of 60), some of whom have a history of prior pelvic irradiation.[212–216] Varela-Duran et al. proposed that carcinosarcomas originating in younger women are more likely to be radiation-related.[217]

Tamoxifen therapy

In one small study of six patients diagnosed with carcinosarcoma who had been taking tamoxifen, five had been maintained on the drug for at least 6 years and one for 3 years. However, the risk is not tumor-type specific, given the wide range of endometrial neoplasms associated with tamoxifen.[218]

Race

There is some evidence that African-Americans are more susceptible to these tumors, with one study reporting a rate of 4.3 per 100 000 in blacks in contrast to 1.7 for whites and 0.99 for women of other races. However, a precise assessment of the role of ethnicity will require larger studies in which prior radiation therapy is taken into account.[219]

CLINICAL PRESENTATION

Women with carcinosarcomas are typically postmenopausal, with a median age in the late seventh or early eighth decade. It most commonly presents with postmenopausal bleeding or as a prolapsing, polypoid uterine mass.[220]

PATHOLOGY

Gross examination

Grossly, carcinosarcomas are more fleshy in appearance than adenocarcinomas; they may be bulky and polypoid and sometimes protrude through the cervical os (Fig. 19.49).

Histopathology

By definition, carcinosarcomas consist of adenocarcinoma admixed with the mesenchymal elements. Both components exhibit a wide range of patterns and the pathologist will often immediately suspect a carcinosarcoma by the irregularity of growth patterns. The sarcomatous component may include endometrial stromal, smooth muscle, skeletal muscle, mesonephroid, Wilms' tumor-like and other patterns of differentiation. Accurate sub-classification of the sarcomatous component is a useful exercise, but is not relevant to management. What is important, for both prognostic and staging purposes, is its recognition as a carcinosarcoma. Important aspects of this exercise include the following:

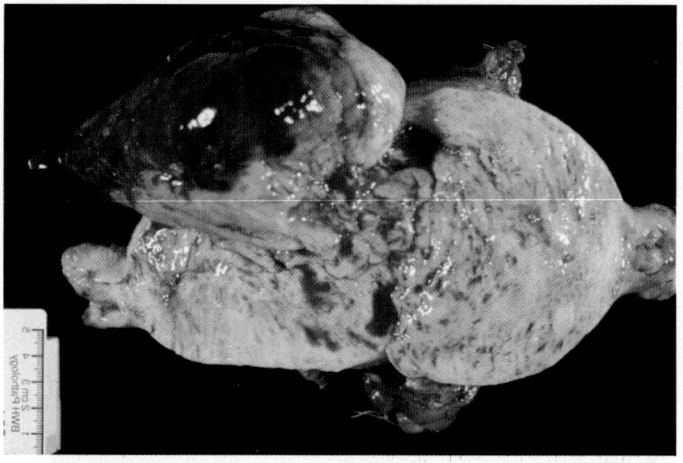

Fig. 19.49 Gross appearance of a carcinosarcoma, seen here as a large, irregular fleshy polypoid mass in the uterine cavity.

Features that are not sarcomatous per se but may signify the presence of a carcinosarcoma. These include: (1) extensive necrosis or a necrotic tumor that is not clearly recognized as epithelial in origin and (2) unusual patterns of epithelial differentiation that are not customarily seen in pure adenocarcinomas. The entire spectrum of epithelial differentiation may be seen in these tumors, ranging from the most well-differentiated endometrioid to poorly-differentiated papillary serous or clear cell types. However, some patterns appear more strongly associated with carcinosarcoma. These include solid components with marked pleomorphism and variable differentiation, bizarre squamous differentiation and more primitive or 'embryonal' glandular growth patterns (Fig. 19.50a). Some patterns consist of lace-like arrangements that are not characteristic of conventional adenocarcinomas (Fig. 19.50b). Other patterns include stratified epithelia with moderate atypia and small 'cascading' cytoplasmic vacuoles that are reminiscent of a more primitive epithelial differentiation (Figs 19.17c, 19.50c). (3) Mesenchymal differentiation patterns that are not readily classified as endometrial stromal sarcoma or leiomyosarcoma, including skeletal muscle, chondroid and unclassifiable mesenchymal differentiation (Fig. 19.51a–c). All of these may be seen with pure heterologous sarcomas, but are much more likely to signify the presence of a carcinosarcoma.

Patterns of carcinosarcoma. Carcinosarcomas are highly variable, with irregular frequencies in both epithelial and mesenchymal differentiation, often in the same tumor, and diverse patterns of transition between the two. Some transitions consist of discrete epithelial and mesenchymal elements and these are

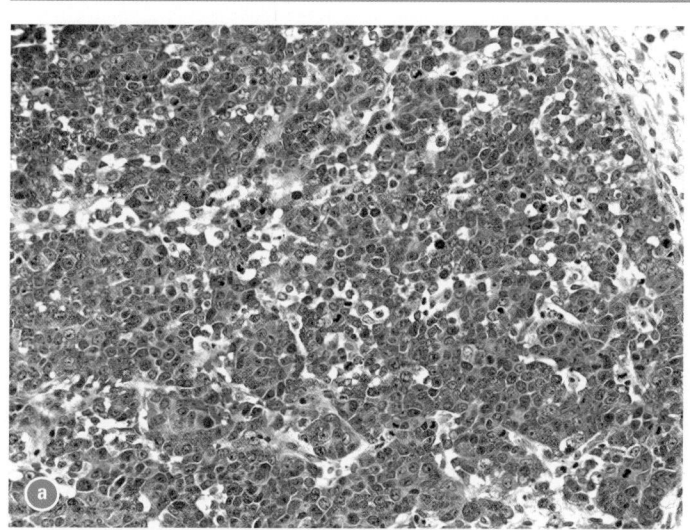

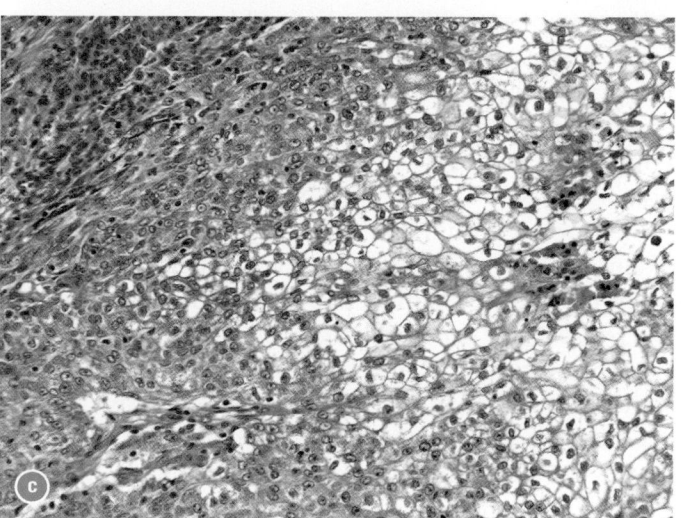

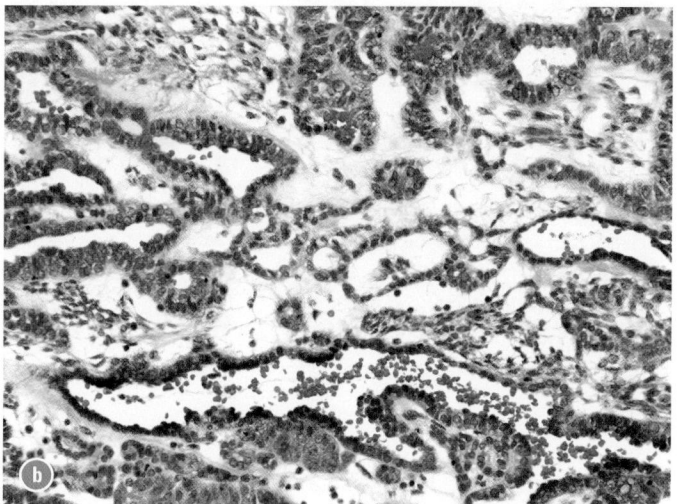

Fig. 19.50 Epithelial patterns that may herald the presence of carcinosarcoma include (a) poorly-differentiated nondescript sheets of tumor cells, (b) irregular lace-like epithelial patterns and (c) sheets of glycogen-rich cells which do not conform to typical mucinous, secretory or clear cell patterns.

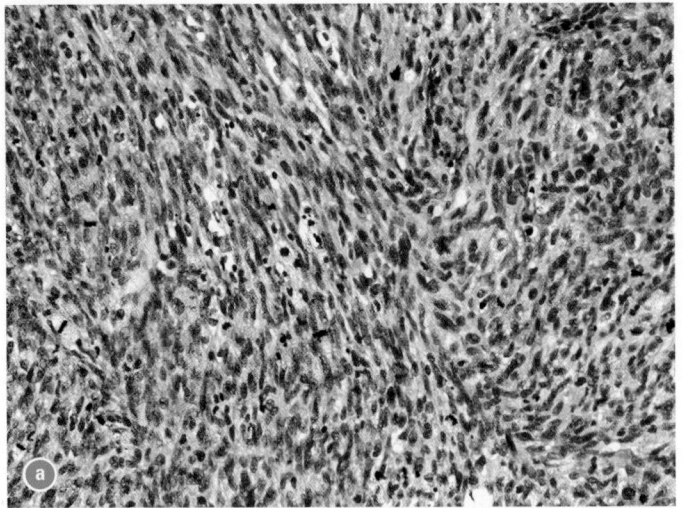

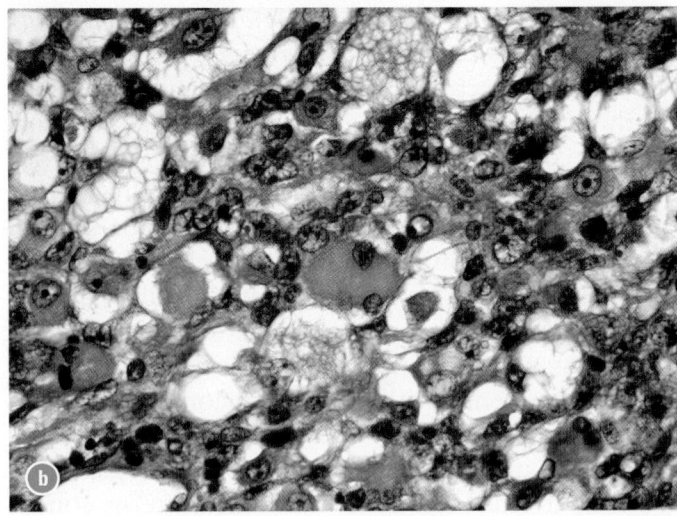

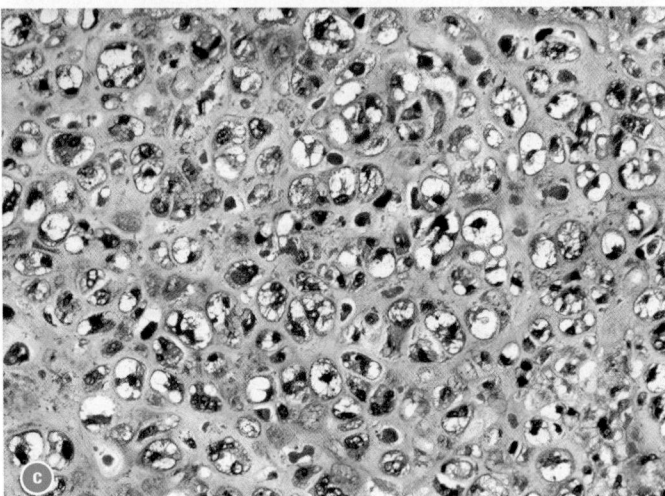

Fig. 19.51 Patterns of stromal differentiation in carcinosarcomas include (a) stromal sarcoma, (b) rhabdomyosarcoma and (c) chondrosarcoma.

easily recognized (Fig. 19.52); others contain a subtle blending of the two (Fig. 19.53). Some tumors are predominantly epithelial, with less conspicuous sarcomatous areas (Fig. 19.54). In predominantly epithelial patterns, the pathologist must distinguish between variations of epithelial differentiation, or a non-neoplastic, desmoplastic stroma when attempting to identify a sarcomatous component. In problematic cases, immunostains (AE1/AE3, keratin) may be helpful in distinguishing between an unusual pattern of carcinoma and sarcomatous differentiation.[207,221]

Some carcinosarcomas are predominantly mesenchymal and in some instances will mimic adenosarcomas. Because any given tumor can exhibit most if not all of these patterns concurrently, the appearance will range from predominantly epithelial to epithelial-mesenchymal to predominantly mesenchymal. A predominantly sarcomatous tumor may resemble an adenosarcoma or stromal sarcoma with preservation of benign glands. This is presumably the consequence of 'overgrowth' of the mesenchymal component. The important distinguishing feature is the presence of malignant epithelium (Fig. 19.55). The reader can take comfort in the fact that the diagnosis of carcinosarcoma is based as much on the diversity of patterns (combined with uncertainty of classifying each) as the exclusion of epithelial or sarcomatous differentiation by immunohistochemistry (Fig. 19.56).

Heterologous vs homologous tumors. Carcinosarcomas were traditionally divided into homologous and heterologous malignant mixed Müllerian tumors according to whether the mesenchymal component expressed differentiation that was intrinsic (stromal or leiomyosarcoma) or extrinsic (rhabdomyosarcoma,

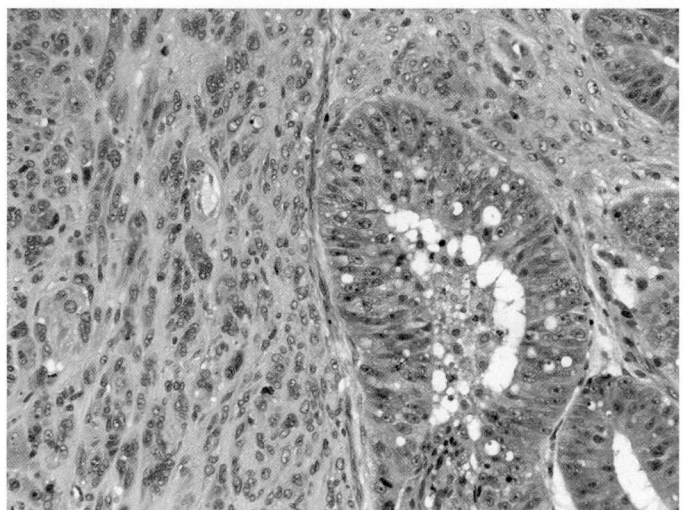

Fig. 19.52 Carcinosarcoma exhibiting a sharp contrast between the epithelial and mesenchymal components.

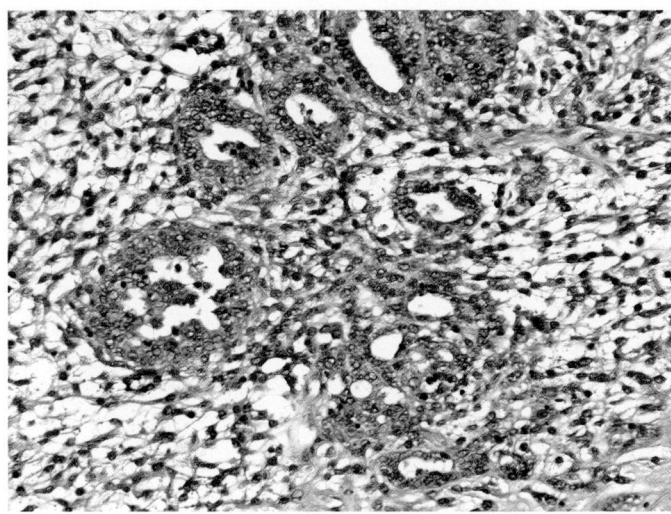

Fig. 19.53 In this carcinosarcoma, the transition between epithelial and mesenchymal components is more subtle.

chondrosarcoma, etc.) to the uterus. This separation was based on reports suggesting a more ominous prognosis for the heterologous tumors.[222] However, the prognosis for both forms is currently considered equally poor and all tumors are now termed 'carcinosarcomas'.[221]

Composition of metastases versus primary tumors. The metastases from carcinosarcomas are highly variable but the majority contain an epithelial component, whether discovered in the lymph nodes, peritoneum or distant sites. One study evaluated the cellular com-

position of 62 metastases, 51 of which were diagnosed at the time of surgery. Carcinoma or carcinosarcoma accounted for over 90% of metastatic tumor, with only a few containing a pure sarcoma.[207] One example of the disparity in appearance between primary and metastatic carcinosarcomas is illustrated in Figure 19.57.

Patterns associated with adverse or favorable prognosis. As mentioned above, the stromal component, including grade, mitotic index and the presence and types of heterologous elements, has not correlated with poor outcome. In contrast, an epithelial compo-

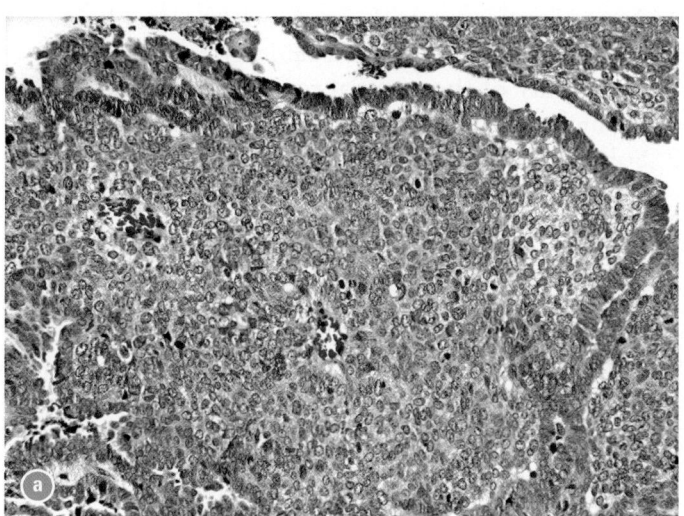

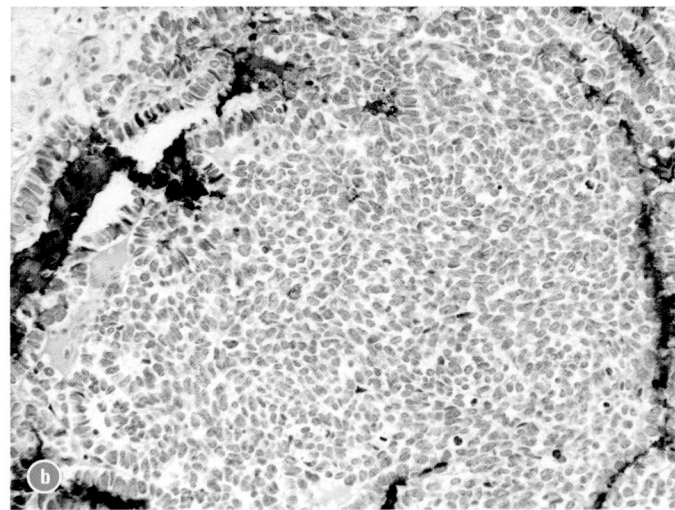

Fig. 19.54 (a) In this carcinosarcoma, the underlying sarcoma has a more epithelioid appearance. (b) However, it is distinctly keratin-negative in contrast to the surface epithelium.

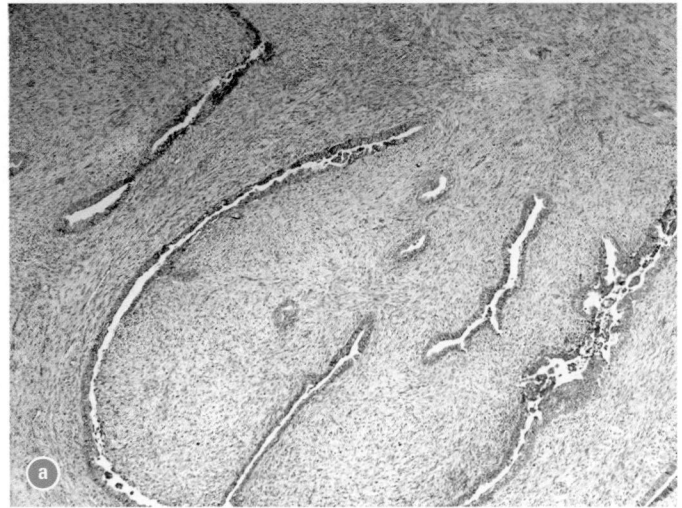

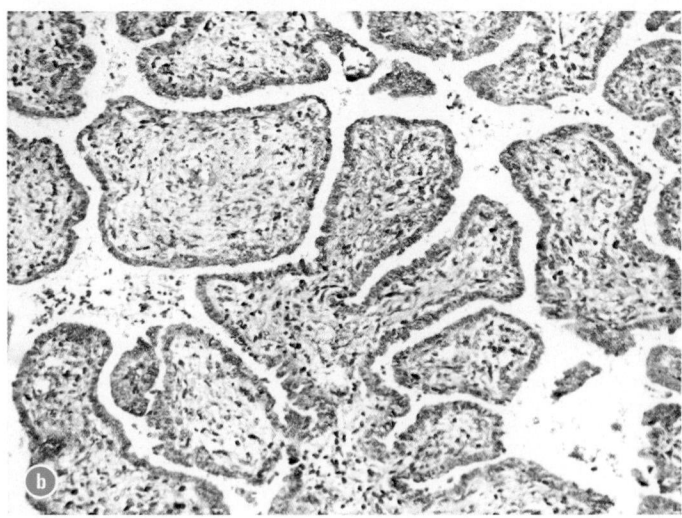

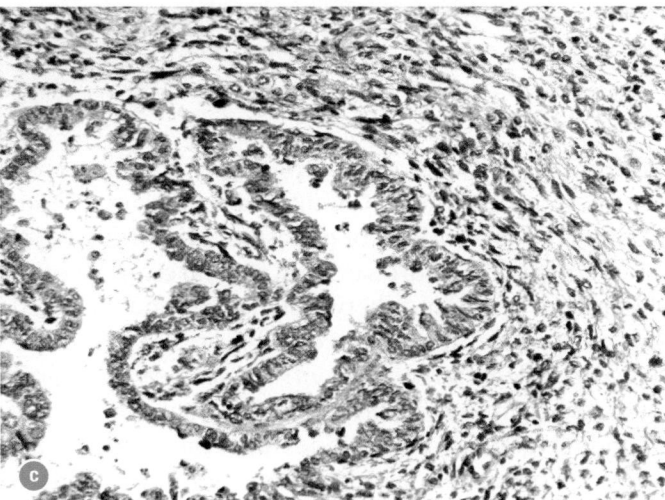

Fig. 19.55 (a) This carcinosarcoma resembles an adenosarcoma at low magnification; (b) including papillary fibromatous growth. (c) However, the epithelial component is malignant.

nent consisting of high-grade, serous and clear cell neoplasia correlates with a higher frequency of metastases. Other features associated with poor outcome in carcinomas, such as deep myometrial invasion, capillary lymphatic-space invasion and cervical involvement, impose a similar adverse prognosis in carcinosarcoma.[221]

In our practice, tumors of mixed epithelial and mesenchymal differentiation are simply classified as carcinosarcomas, with additional comments clarifying the cell type and grade of the epithelial component, and other parameters that are associated with prognosis in epithelial tumors. Rare patterns that may merit other therapeutic approaches, such as Wilms' tumor-like differentiation, are also mentioned, if present.[223]

Differential diagnosis. The differential diagnosis of carcinosarcoma includes the following:

1. Adenocarcinomas with prominent desmoplasia (Fig. 19.58a). These are excluded by the uniformity of the stromal reaction and the lack of nuclear atypia
2. Solid carcinomas or carcinomas with a spindle cell architecture (Fig. 19.58b)
3. Bizarre carcinomas with metaplastic growth
4. Biphasic carcinomas
5. Stromal sarcomas with sex cord-like differentiation (Fig. 19.58c)
6. Adenosarcomas.

STAGING, MANAGEMENT AND OUTCOME

Frequency of surgical upstaging

Treatment of choice consists of total abdominal hysterectomy, bilateral salpingo-oophorectomy and

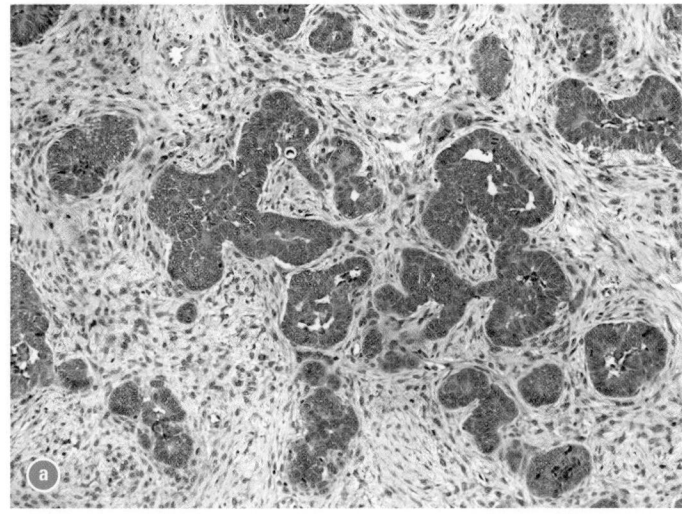

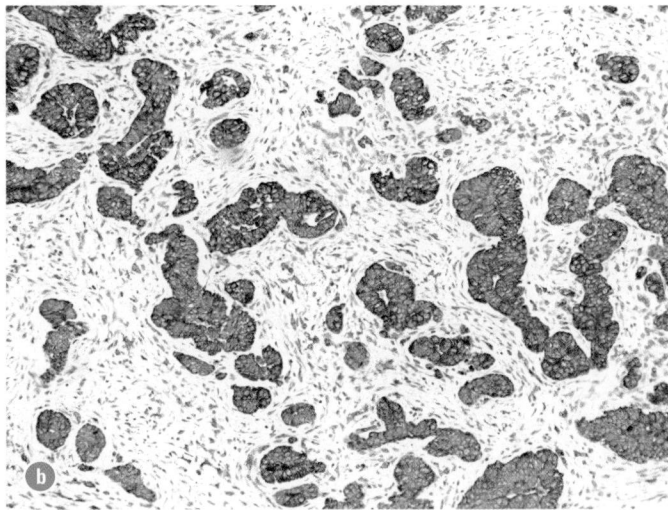

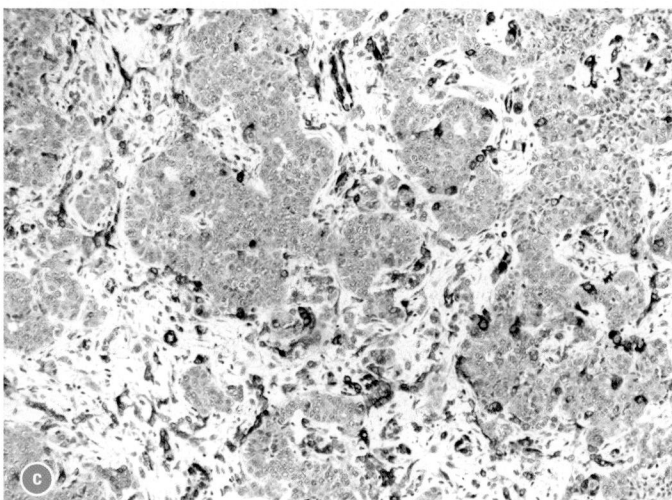

Fig. 19.56 Differentiation between epithelial and mesenchymal components of (a) a carcinosarcoma (b) with keratin and (c) smooth muscle actin.

complete surgical staging. Surgical findings determine further therapy. Le noted 84% to be clinical Stage I; however, the high frequency of lymph node metastases will increase the stage in many cases.[224] Approximately 15% of endometrial adenocarcinomas are upstaged when surgical staging has been completed. In two studies of clinical Stage I carcinosarcomas, 20–30% and 55% were upstaged following surgical staging.[220,225] The most significant prognostic factors were pathologic extent of disease and vascular invasion in the myometrium. There was no difference in outcome between homologous and heterologous tumors. Initial surgery for staging is essential for the adequate evaluation and treatment of these patients. Yamada et al. examined pathologic variables influencing prognosis in 62 patients with carcinosarcoma. Occult metastases were found in 38 (61%) of 62 patients.[226]

Prognosis

Surgical stage at time of surgery is the most important prognostic factor. In stage I–II disease, depth of myometrial invasion and lymphatic/vascular space involvement are significantly related to outcome.[227–229]

In one study, 61% recurred in a median of 10 months, with a median survival of 26 months and a five year survival of 30%.[228] In another study, five year survival was 43%.[227] Survival was highly stage dependent, ranging from 74% for tumors confined to the corpus to 24% with advanced disease.[226]

Impact of therapy on outcome

The two most effective drugs for carcinosarcomas are ifosfamide and cisplatin. Thigpen et al. evaluated 44 women with the frequency of complete, partial, stable disease and progressive diseases seen in 2%, 18%, 23%

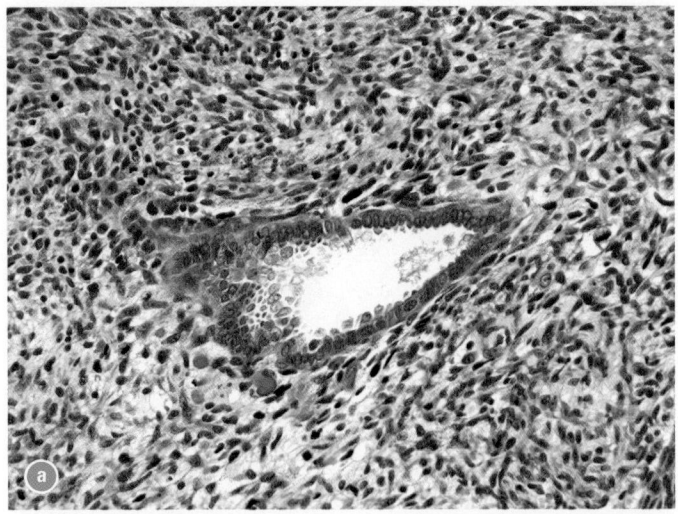

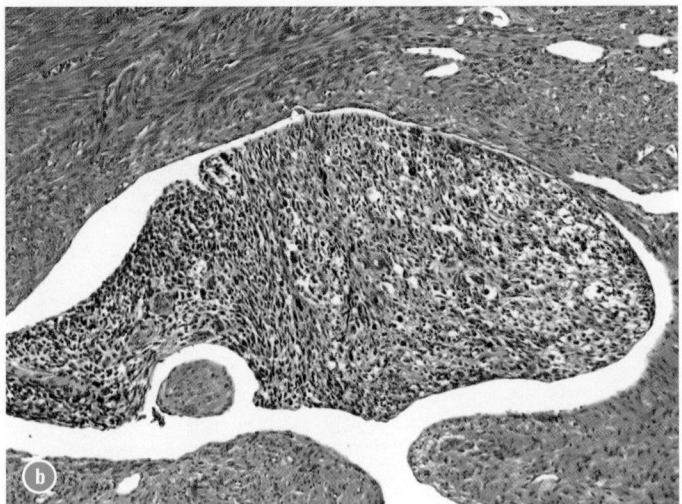

Fig. 19.57 Primary carcinosarcoma composed principally of (a) a stromal component; (b) with capillary-lymphatic space invasion. (c) The regional lymph node contains metastatic adenocarcinoma.

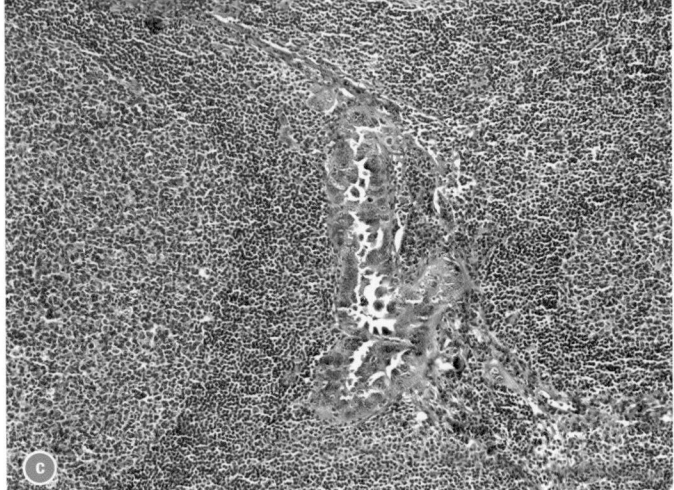

and 57%, with median progression-free and overall survivals of 5.2 and 11.7 months.[230] Sutton et al. examined 194 patients with cisplatin added to ifosfamide. The addition of cisplatin to ifosfamide appears to offer a small improvement in progression-free survival over ifosfamide alone in the management of advanced carcinosarcoma of the uterus; the added toxicity may not justify the use of this combination.[231] Chemotherapy has been limited to advanced or recurrent disease, although its role in the adjuvant setting is currently under investigation. The most active single agents are ifosfamide and cisplatin.[220]

The value of radiotherapy depends on the study. One study reported that the addition of radiotherapy significantly reduced the local recurrence rate from 55% (17 patients) to 3% (one patient). Adjuvant radio-

therapy reduced the risk of distant failure and death in patients with disease confined to the uterus but did not impact distant recurrence or survival in Stage III patients.[232]

Other studies recommend radiotherapy for reducing local failure and have not noted an increase in survival. A total of 32 patients are reported by Le.[224] There is no statistically significant difference in the progression-free or overall survival in the radiated group compared to the expectantly treated group. Sartori et al. found that in Stage I–II patients postoperative radiation did not improve 5-year disease-free survival.[229]

Yamada et al. found that neither adjuvant radio-therapy nor chemotherapy was identified as an independent prognostic variable for recurrence or survival.[226] A number of early-stage patients survive without adju-

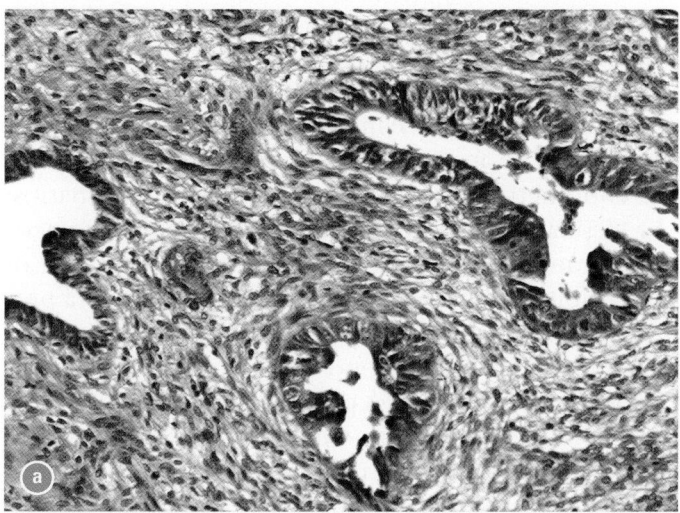

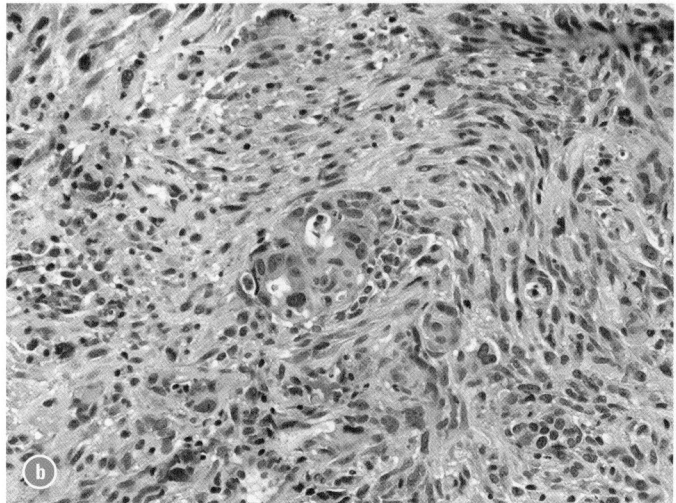

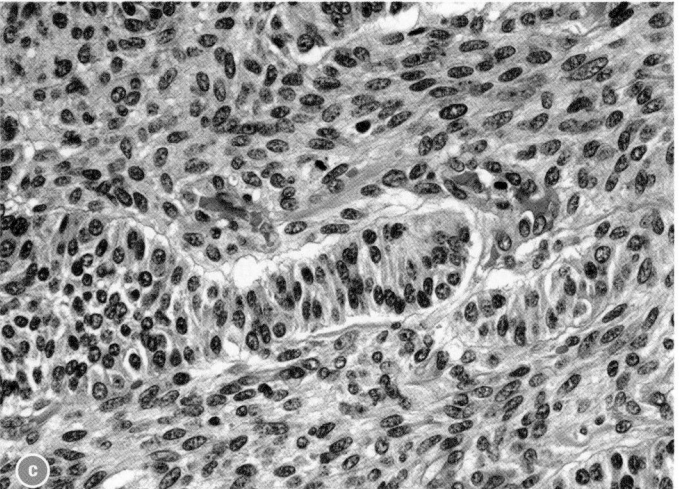

Fig. 19.58 The differential diagnosis of carcinosarcoma includes (a) conventional carcinomas with prominent stromal reaction, (b) adenocarcinomas with a spindle cell architecture and (c) endometrial stromal tumors with epithelioid (sex cord-like) areas.

vant therapy. This argues for extending the International Federation of Gynecology and Obstetrics' endometrial carcinoma surgical staging system to include carcinosarcomas, and also for conducting prospective trials to examine the benefits of adjuvant therapy for patients with early-stage disease.

Sartori et al. followed 118 cases of carcinosarcoma. In Stage I–II patients, postoperative radiation did not improve 5-year disease-free survival.[229]

These are aggressive neoplasms and have a 5-year survival rate of 25–30%, with major adverse prognostic factors being adnexal spread, nodal metastases and the histologic type of carcinoma. Adjunctive therapy may provide local control but is unproven for advanced disease.

Other epithelial neoplasms arising in the endometrium

ATYPICAL POLYPOID ADENOMYOMA

Atypical polypoid adenomyoma (APA) is defined as an adenomyomatous polyp containing an endometrial intraepithelial neoplasm with squamous morules. Unlike endometrial polyps, these tumors are often sessile, with a broader base and, at times, a less well demarcated polyp-myometrial interface (Fig. 19.59). In addition the stroma is distinctly myofibromatous, exhibiting fascicles of stroma and interdigitating sharply demarcated nests of hyperplastic endometrial glands. Squamous morules are conspicuous (Fig. 19.60a,b).

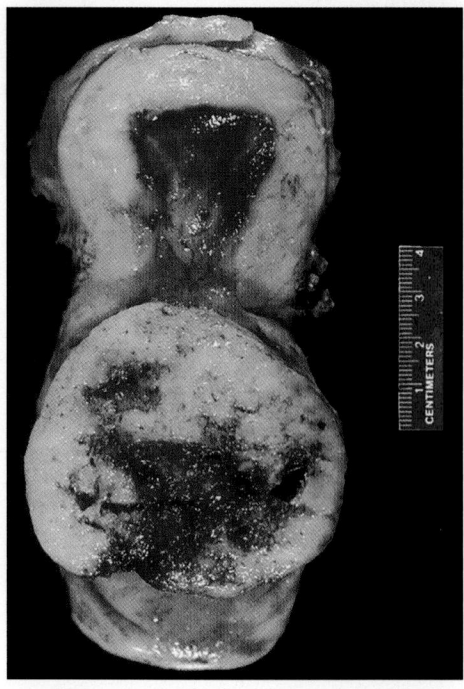

Fig. 19.59 Gross appearance of an atypical polypoid adenomyoma. The tumor presents as a broad-based polypoid mass in the lower uterine segment.

The principal concern generated by these neoplasms is the risk of malignancy, a concern fueled by the appearance of many tumors. In one study nearly one-half had areas of complex glandular architecture that otherwise merited the diagnosis of well-differentiated carcinoma (Fig. 19.60c,d). Half of APAs persist and subsequent myoinvasive carcinoma is most frequent (17% vs 0%) in tumors with a high versus low glandular complexity. Pregnancy has been achieved following conservative management in a minority of patients. Overall, if coexisting cancer is not suspected, conservative management of APAs is an option, provided the tumor can be removed and the patient followed. Otherwise, hysterectomy is the most practical option.[233–236]

CONDYLOMATA

Rare reports of condylomata have been published. We have likewise seen occasional lesions that were indistinguishable from condyloma growing in the uterus. Interestingly, these tumors have been reported in postmenopausal women. Conceivably the older age reflects the atypical presentation with persistence of the lesions and extension into the endometrial cavity. Whether it is a function of direct extension or transformation of reserve cells in the endometrium is unknown.[237] Giant condylomata have also been reported, although it is not clear if these are distinguished from condylomata.

SQUAMOUS CELL CARCINOMAS

Primary squamous carcinomas of the endometrium are rare, with only a handful of reports in the literature.[238–241] The appearance of a squamous carcinoma in the endometrium can be attributed to four scenarios. (1) Cephalad extension of a cervical squamous neoplasm can occur but is rare. (2) HPV infection of susceptible cells in the endometrium, leading to a preinvasive and invasive tumor, can occur, based on occasional reports of HPV-positive carcinomas in the endometrium.[242–246] (3) A primary carcinoma arising in the glandular epithelium with conversion to a squamous tumor would be the most common scenario, but the coexisting adenocarcinoma would not strictly qualify the tumor as a primary squamous carcinoma. (4) A primary squamous carcinoma arises in either rare foci of reserve cells or pre-existing squamous metaplasia. This is supported by the association of squamous carcinoma with pre-existing benign-appearing squamous epithelium, as in chronic pyometra or other inflammatory conditions.

Histologically, squamous tumors of the endometrium vary in degree of differentiation, from tumors resembling verrucous carcinomas to moderate to poorly-differentiated squamous variants (Fig. 19.61). Either can exhibit prominent keratinization, as well as areas which may be appear benign. Similar to endometrial adenocarcinomas, prognosis of squamous carcinomas is a function of stage.[242–248]

POORLY-DIFFERENTIATED PAPILLARY (TRANSITIONAL CELL) TUMORS

A small number of reports have detailed tumors resembling transitional cell carcinomas of the urothelium (Fig. 19.10a,b).[249] Like their counterparts in the ovary, these tumors are strictly Müllerian in their immunophenotype and are typically CK7 positive and CK20 negative. They occasionally score positive for human papillomavirus. They may be pure or occur in association with endometrioid carcinomas. Follow-up data are limited and these tumors should be managed as higher-grade adenocarcinomas.

SMALL CELL UNDIFFERENTIATED TUMORS

Small cell undifferentiated carcinomas have been reported in the endometrium and may be pure or develop concurrently with a conventional endometrioid adenocarcinoma.[250] Most, but not all of these tumors

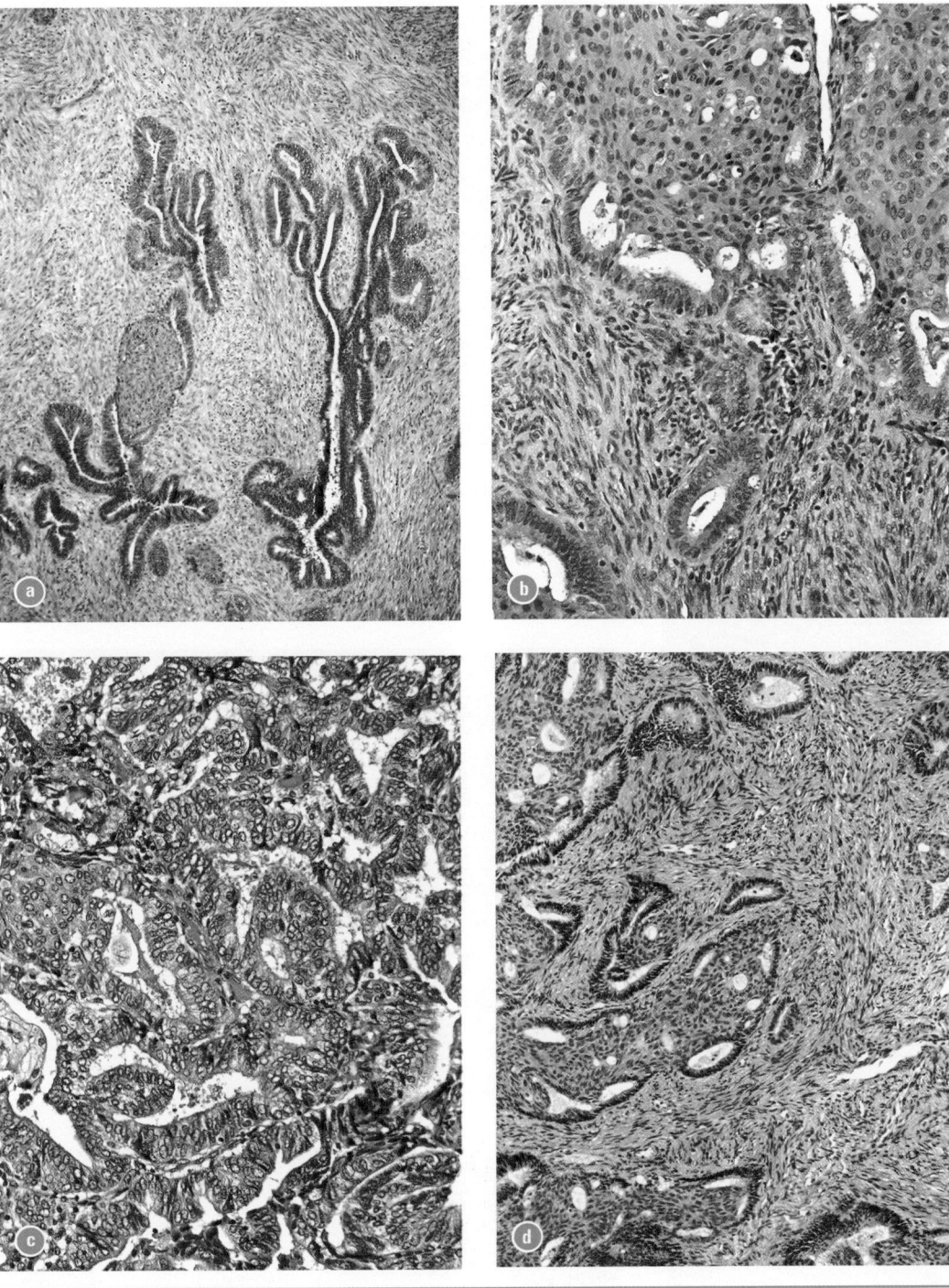

Fig. 19.60 Microscopic appearance of atypical polypoid adenomyoma (APA) containing lower architectural complexity, with prominent squamous morular metaplasia (a, b). A well-differentiated endometrioid adenocarcinoma (c) associated with an APA (d) illustrates the histologic spectrum associated with these tumors. In this case, there was no myometrial invasion.

will score positive with neuroendocrine markers, including chromogranin, synaptophysin and others. The morphology usually resembles neuroendocrine carcinomas of the cervix, with an intermediate cell phenotype, with vascular invasion and loss of tumor cell cohesion prominent (Fig. 19.62).[251]

OTHER UNDIFFERENTIATED TUMORS

These include large cell undifferentiated carcinomas (Fig. 19.63a),[252] lympho-epithelial-like carcinomas,[253] giant (Fig. 19.63b) or pleomorphic (Fig. 19.63c) cells, glassy cell carcinomas (Fig. 19.63d) and tumors

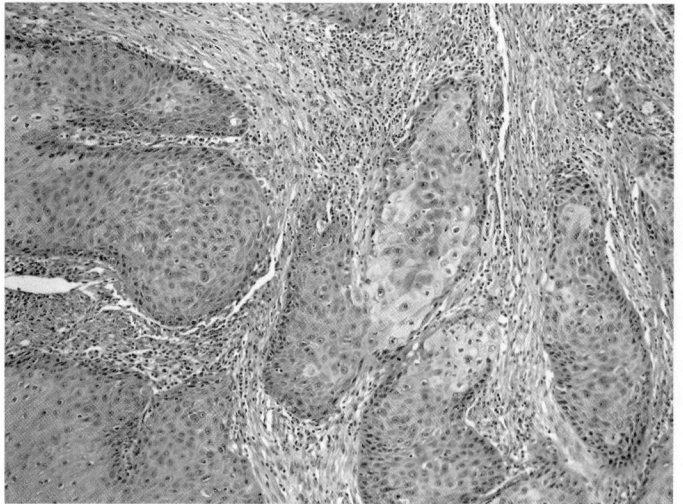

Fig. 19.61 Primary squamous carcinoma of the endometrium.

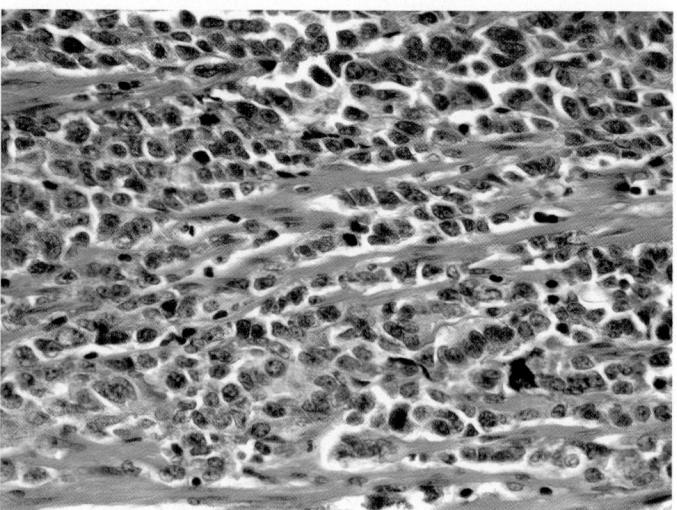

Fig. 19.62 Small cell undifferentiated carcinoma of the endometrium.

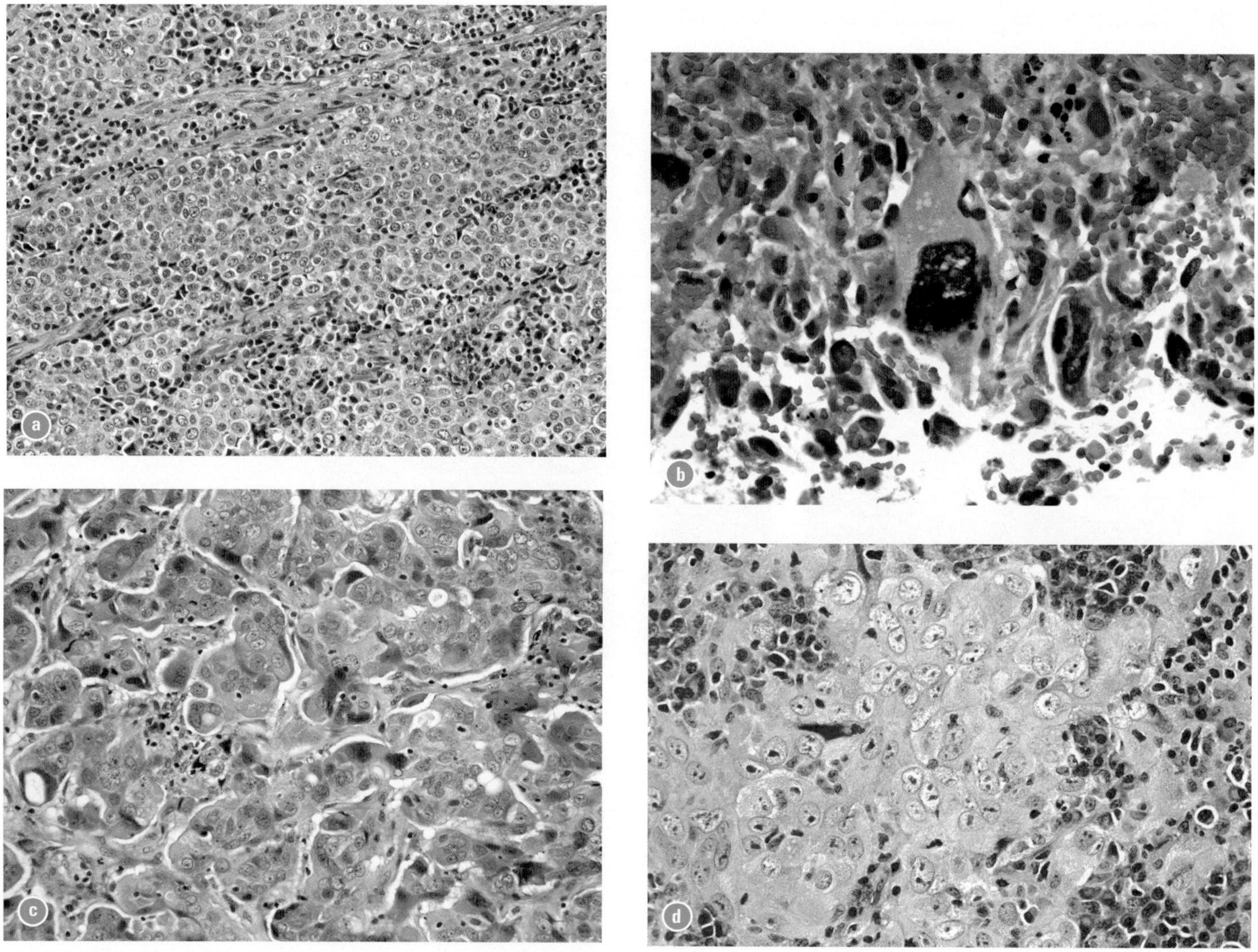

Fig. 19.63 Other patterns seen in the endometrium include (a) large cell undifferentiated patterns, (b) those with giant cells, (c) pleomorphic patterns and (d) glassy cell carcinomas.

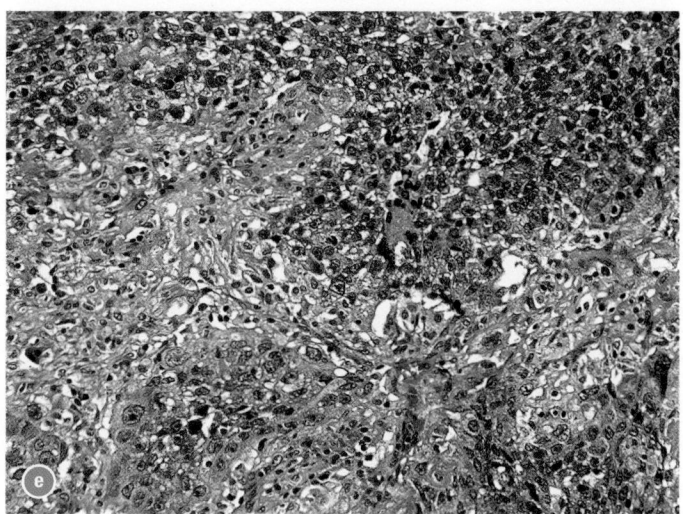

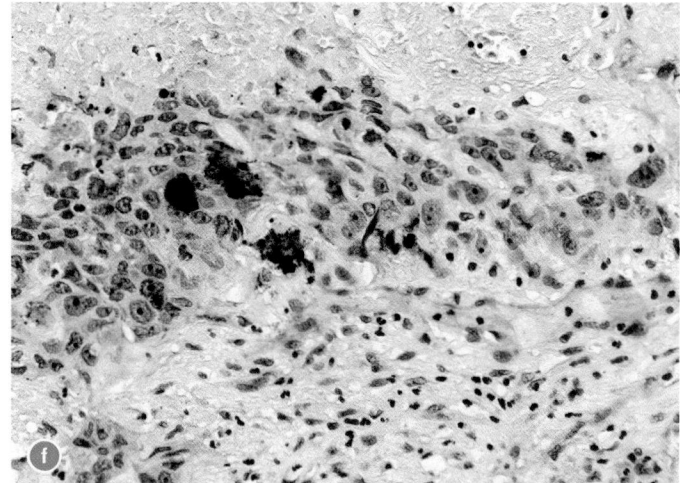

Fig. 19.63 **Cont'd** (e) A tumor with choriocarcinomatous differentiation and (f) following staining for hCG.

with hepatoid trophoblastic differentiation (Fig. 19.63e,f).[67] All of these tumors justify classification as high risk, based on differentiation and nuclear atypia.

METASTATIC EPITHELIAL TUMORS TO THE ENDOMETRIUM

The most common non-primary tumors of the endometrium originate from cervix (adenocarcinoma) (Fig. 19.64a,b), breast (lobular or ductal carcinomas) (Fig. 19.64c) and gastrointestinal tract (including signet ring cell carcinomas) (Fig. 19.64d). As mentioned above, direct implants on the endometrial surface from ovarian carcinomas are rare. Additional sites that must be considered if metastatic tumor is suspected include melanoma, renal cell carcinoma and lung carcinoma. The characteristic features of metastatic carcinoma are a solid architecture, diffusely infiltrative pattern with sparing of individual normal glands and capillary-lymphatic space invasion. This should be expected with gastrointestinal and breast primaries, melanomas and small cell tumors. An exception is

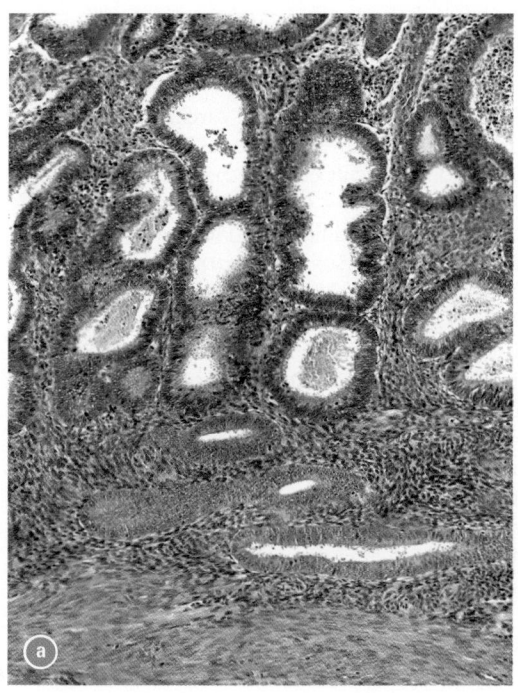

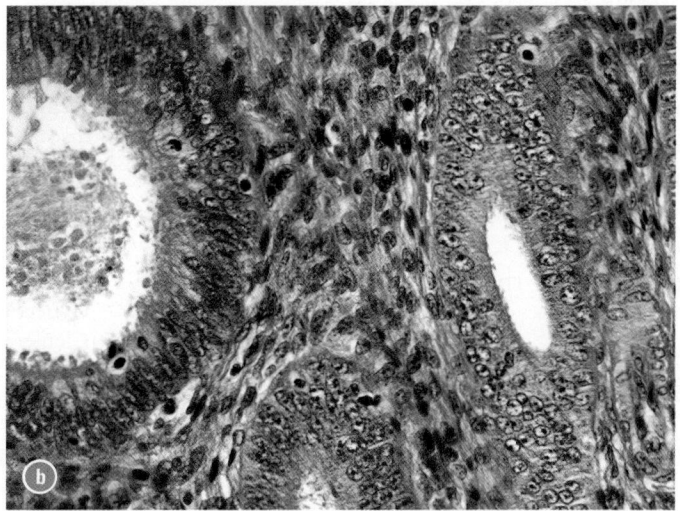

Fig. 19.64 (a) Extension of a cervical adenocarcinoma into the endometrium; (b) at higher power, the subtle difference between endocervical tumor and endometrial glands is seen;

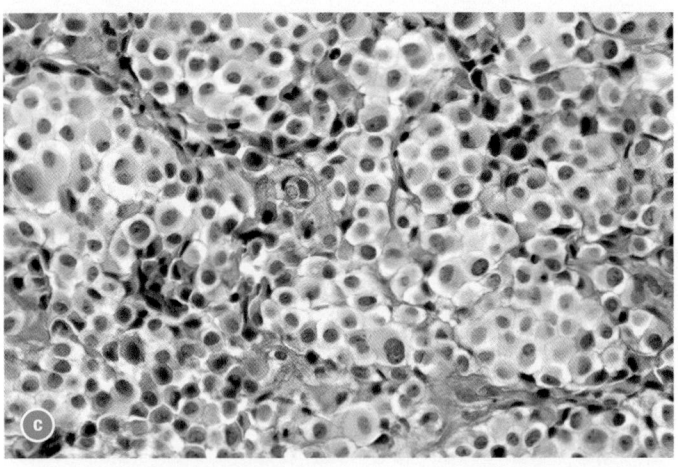

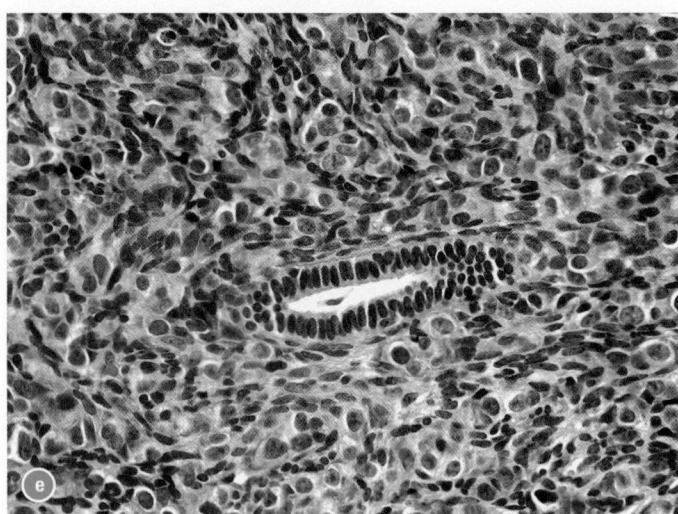

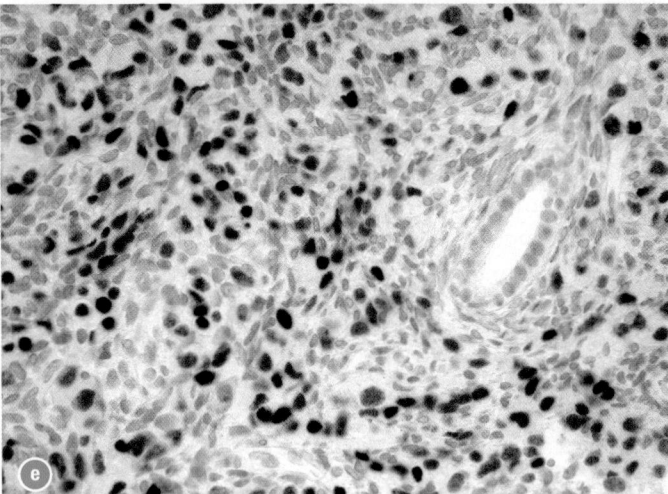

Fig. 19.64 **Cont'd** (c) metastatic breast carcinoma; (d) metastatic gastrointestinal carcinoma; and (e) following staining with CDX.

cervical adenocarcinomas that typically grow superficially and blend with the normal endometrial glands, giving the initial impression of a primary endometrial neoplasm. In the case of obvious metastatic disease, immunophenotyping with CK7/CK20, IDX and other markers will help pinpoint the origin (Fig. 19.64e).

References

1 Curry S, Kelly S. Cancer of the female genital tract: overview. In: Osteen R, ed. Cancer manual. Boston, MA: American Cancer Society; 1990:253.

2 Rose PG. Endometrial carcinoma. N Engl J Med 1996; 335:640–649.

3 Duska LR, Garrett A, Rueda BR, et al. Endometrial cancer in women 40 years old or younger. Gynecol Oncol 2001; 83:388–393.

4 Deligdisch L, Holinka C. Endometrial carcinoma: two diseases? Cancer Detect Prev 1987; 10:237–246.

5 Koss LG. Detection of occult endometrial carcinoma. J Cell Biochem Suppl 1995; 23:165–173.

6 Weber AM, Belinson JL, Bradley LD, Piedmonte MR. Vaginal ultrasonography versus endometrial biopsy in women with postmenopausal bleeding. Am J Obstet Gynecol 1997; 177(4):924–929.

7 Clement PB, Young RH. Endometrioid carcinoma of the uterine corpus: a review of its pathology with emphasis on recent advances and problematic aspects. Adv Anat Pathol 2002; 9(3):145–184.

8 Hendrickson M, Ross J, Eifel P, et al. Uterine papillary serous carcinoma: a highly malignant form of endometrial adenocarcinoma. Am J Surg Pathol 1982; 6:93–108.

9 Sherman ME. Theories of endometrial carcinogenesis: a multidisciplinary approach. Mod Pathol 2000; 13(3):295–308.

10 Pothuri B, Ramondetta L, Martino M, et al. Development of endometrial cancer after radiation treatment for cervical carcinoma. Obstet Gynecol 2003; 101(5 Pt 1):941–945.

11 Hill HA, Eley JW, Harlan LC, et al. Racial differences in endometrial cancer survival: the black/white cancer survival study. Obstet Gynecol 1996; 88(6):919–926.

12 Sherman ME, Devesa SS. Analysis of racial differences in incidence, survival, and mortality for malignant tumors of the uterine corpus. Cancer 2003; 98(1):176–186.

13 Archer DF, McIntyre-Seltman K, Wilborn WW Jr, et al. Endometrial morphology in asymptomatic postmenopausal women. Am J Obstet Gynecol 1991; 165(2):317–320; discussion 320–322.

14 Gronroos M, Salmi TA, Vuento MH, et al. Mass screening for endometrial cancer directed in risk groups of patients with diabetes and patients with hypertension. Cancer 1993; 71(4):1279–1282.

15 Barakat RR. Tamoxifen and endometrial neoplasia. Clin Obstet Gynecol 1996; 39(3):629–640.

16 Fisher B, Costantino JP, Redmond CK, et al. Endometrial cancer in tamoxifen-treated breast cancer patients: findings from the National Surgical Adjuvant Breast and Bowel Project (NSABP) B-14. J Natl Cancer Inst 1994; 86(7):527–537.

17 Voss SC, Lacey CG, Pupkin M, Degefu S. Ultrasound and the pelvic mass. J Reprod Med 1983; 28(12):833–837.

18 Cecchini S, Ciatto S, Bonardi R, et al. Risk of endometrial cancer in breast cancer patients under long-term adjuvant treatment with tamoxifen. Tumor 1998; 84(1):21–23.

19 Magriples U, Naftolin F, Schwartz PE, Carcangiu ML. High-grade endometrial carcinoma in tamoxifen-treated breast cancer patients. J Clin Oncol 1993; 11(3):485–490.

20 Mecklin JP, Jarvinen HJ. Tumor spectrum in cancer family syndrome (hereditary nonpolyposis colorectal cancer). Cancer 1991; 68(5):1109–1112.

21 Watson P, Vasen HFA, Mecklin JP, Järvinen H, Lynch HT. The risk of endometrial cancer in hereditary nonpolyposis colorectal cancer. Am J Med 1994; 96:516–520.

22 Millar AL, Pal T, Madlensky L, et al. Mismatch repair gene defects contribute to the genetic basis of double primary cancers of the colorectum and endometrium. Hum Mol Genet 1999; 8(5):823–829.

23 Maruyama A, Miyamoto S, Saito T, et al. Clinicopathologic and familial characteristics of endometrial carcinoma with multiple primary carcinomas in relation to the loss of protein expression of MSH2 and MLH1. Cancer 2001; 91:2056–2064.

24 Fornasarig M, Viel A, Bidoli E, et al. Familial risk of endometrial cancer after exclusion of families that fulfilled Amsterdam, Japanese or Bethesda criteria for HNPCC. Ann Oncol 2004; 15(4):598–604.

25 Hemminki K, Aaltonen L, Li X. Subsequent primary malignancies after endometrial carcinoma and ovarian carcinoma. Cancer 2003; 97(10):2432–2439.

26 Mutter GL. PTEN, a protean tumor suppressor. Am J Pathol 2001; 158:1895–1898.

27 Esteller M, Levine R, Baylin SB, Ellenson LH, Herman JG. MLH1 promoter hypermethylation is associated with the microsatellite instability phenotype in sporadic endometrial carcinomas. Oncogene 1998; 17:2413–2417.

28 Burks RT, Kessis TD, Cho KR, Hedrick L. Microsatellite instability in endometrial carcinoma. Oncogene 1994; 9:1163–1166.

29 Goodfellow PJ, Buttin BM, Herzog TJ, et al. Prevalence of defective DNA mismatch repair and MSH6 mutation in an unselected series of endometrial cancers. Proc Natl Acad Sci USA 2003; 100(10):5908–5913.

30 Mutter GL, Boynton KA, Faquin WC, Ruiz RE, Jovanovic AS. Allelotype mapping of unstable microsatellites establishes direct lineage continuity between endometrial precancers and cancer. Cancer Res 1996; 56:4483–4486.

31 Risinger JI, Berchuck A, Kohler MF, et al. Genetic instability of microsatellites in endometrial carcinoma. Cancer Res 1993; 53:5100–5103.

32 Charames GS, Millar AL, Pal T, Narod S, Bapat B. Do MSH6 mutations contribute to double primary cancers of the colorectum and endometrium? Hum Genet 2000; 107(6):623–629.

33 Dubeau L. Etiology and detection of gynecologic cancer. In: Morrow CP, Curtin JP, Townsend DE, eds. Synopsis of gynecologic oncology, 4th edn. New York: Churchill Livingstone; 1993:1–22.

34 Enomoto T, Inoue M, Perantoni A, et al. K-ras activation in premalignant and malignant epithelial lesions of the human uterus. Cancer Res 1991; 51:5304–5314.

35 Machin P, Catasus L, Pons C, et al. CTNNB1 mutations and beta-catenin expression in endometrial carcinomas. Hum Pathol 2002; 33(2):206–212.

36 Berchuck A, Boyd J. Molecular basis of endometrial cancer. Cancer 1995; 76(10 Suppl):2034–2040.

37 Sherman ME, Bur ME, Kurman RJ. p53 in endometrial cancer and its putative precursors: evidence for diverse pathways of tumorigenesis. Hum Pathol 1995; 26(11): 1268–1274.

38 Mutter GL, Baak JPA, Crum CP, et al. Endometrial precancer diagnosis by histopathology, clonal analysis, and computerized morphometry. J Pathol 2000; 190:462–469.

39 Hecht JL, Ince TA, Baak JPA, et al. Prediction of endometrial carcinoma by subjective EIN diagnosis. Mod Pathol 2005; 18(3):324–330.

40 Orbo A, Baak JP, Kleivan I, et al. Computerised morphometrical analysis in endometrial hyperplasia for the prediction of cancer development. A long-term retrospective study from northern Norway. J Clin Pathol 2000; 53(9):697–703.

41 Baak JP, Orbo A, van Diest PJ, et al. Prospective multicenter evaluation of the morphometric D-score for prediction of the outcome of endometrial hyperplasias. Am J Surg Pathol 2001; 25(7):930–935.

42 Mutter GL, Lin MC, Fitzgerald JT, et al. Altered PTEN expression as a diagnostic marker for the earliest endometrial precancers. J Natl Cancer Inst 2000; 92:924–930.

43 Hertig A, Sommers S. Genesis of endometrial carcinoma. I. Study of prior biopsies. Cancer 1949; 2:946–956.

44 Kurman RJ, Kaminski PF, Norris HJ. The behavior of endometrial hyperplasia. A long-term study of 'untreated' hyperplasia in 170 patients. Cancer 1985; 56(2): 403–412.

45 Zheng W, Liang SX, Yu H, et al. Endometrial glandular dysplasia: a newly defined precursor lesion of uterine papillary serous carcinoma. Part I: morphologic features. Int J Surg Pathol 2004; 12(3):207–223.

46 Gull B, Karlsson B, Milsom I, Granberg S. Can ultrasound replace dilation and curettage? A longitudinal evaluation of postmenopausal bleeding and transvaginal sonographic measurement of the endometrium as predictors of endometrial cancer. Am J Obstet Gynecol 2003; 188(2):401–408.

47 Krissi H, Chetrit A, Menczer J. Presenting symptoms of patients with endometrial carcinoma. Effect on prognosis. Eur J Gynaecol Oncol 1996; 17(1):25–28.

48 Hawwa ZM, Nahhas WA, Copenhaver EH. Postmenopausal bleeding. Lahey Clin Found Bull 1970; 19:61–70.

49 Gredmark T, Kvint S, Havel G, Mattsson LA. Histopathological findings in women with postmenopausal bleeding. Br J Obstet Gynaecol 1995; 102(2):133–136.

50 Iatrakis G, Diakakis I, Kourounis G, et al. Postmenopausal uterine bleeding. Clin Exp Obstet Gynecol 1997; 24(3):157.

51 Elliott J, Connor ME, Lashen H. The value of outpatient hysteroscopy in diagnosing endometrial pathology in postmenopausal women with and without hormone replacement therapy. Acta Obstet Gynecol Scand 2003; 82(12):1112–1119.

52 Gemer O, Segal S. Endometrial cancer in patients undergoing diagnostic curettage. Arch Gynecol Obstet 1998; 261(2):79–81.

53 Twu NF, Chen SS. Five-year follow-up of patients with recurrent postmenopausal bleeding. Zhonghua Yi Xue Za Zhi (Taipei) 2000; 63(8):628–633.

54 Fung Kee Fung M, Burnett M, Faught W. Does persistent postmenopausal bleeding justify hysterectomy? Eur J Gynaecol Oncol 1997; 18(1):26–28.

55 Granberg S, Wikland M, Karlsson B, Norstrom A, Friberg LG. Endometrial thickness as measured by endovaginal ultrasonography for identifying endometrial abnormality. Am J Obstet Gynecol 1991; 164(1 Pt 1):47–52.

56 Karlsson B, Granberg S, Wikland M, et al. Transvaginal ultrasonography of the endometrium in women with postmenopausal bleeding – a Nordic multicenter study. Am J Obstet Gynecol 1995; 172(5):1488–1494.

57 Langer RD, Pierce JJ, O'Hanlan KA, et al. Transvaginal ultrasonography compared with endometrial biopsy for the detection of endometrial disease. Postmenopausal Estrogen/Progestin Interventions Trial. N Engl J Med 1997; 337(25):1792–1798.

58 Gupta JK, Chien PF, Voit D, Clark TJ, Khan KS. Ultrasonographic endometrial thickness for diagnosing endometrial pathology in women with postmenopausal bleeding: a meta-analysis. Acta Obstet Gynecol Scand 2002; 81(9):799–816.

59 Tabor A, Watt HC, Wald NJ. Endometrial thickness as a test for endometrial cancer in women with postmenopausal vaginal bleeding. Obstet Gynecol 2002; 99(4):663–670.

60 Taipale P, Tarjanne H, Heinonen UM. The diagnostic value of transvaginal sonography in the diagnosis of endometrial malignancy in women with peri- and postmenopausal bleeding. Acta Obstet Gynecol Scand 1994; 73(10): 819–823. Erratum in: Acta Obstet Gynecol Scand 1995; 74(4):324.

61 Hann LE, Kim CM, Gonen M, et al. Sonohysterography compared with endometrial biopsy for evaluation of the endometrium in tamoxifen-treated women. Obstet Gynecol Surv 2004; 59(6):440–441.

62 Symonds I. Ultrasound, hysteroscopy and endometrial biopsy in the investigation of endometrial cancer. Best Pract Res Clin Obstet Gynaecol 2001; 15(3):381–391.

63 Clark TJ. Outpatient hysteroscopy and ultrasonography in the management of endometrial disease. Curr Opin Obstet Gynecol 2004; 16(4):305–311.

64 Lo KW, Yuen PM. The role of outpatient diagnostic hysteroscopy in identifying anatomic pathology and histopathology in the endometrial cavity. J Am Assoc Gynecol Laparosc 2000; 7(3):381–385.

65 Sainz de la Cuesta R, Espinosa JA, Crespo E, Granizo JJ, Rivas F. Does fluid hysteroscopy increase the stage or worsen the prognosis in patients with endometrial cancer? A randomized controlled trial. Eur J Obstet Gynecol Reprod Biol 2004; 115(2):211–215.

66 Silverberg SG, Kurman RJ, Nogales F, et al. Tumors of the uterine corpus: epithelial tumours and related conditions. In: Tavassoli FA, Devilee Pl, eds. Tumors of the breast and gynecologic tract. Lyon: WHO; 2002:218.

67 Clement PB, Young RH. Non-endometrioid carcinomas of the uterine corpus: a review of their pathology with emphasis on recent advances and problematic aspects. Adv Anat Pathol 2004; 11(3):117–142.

68 Zaino RJ, Kurman RJ, Diana KL, Morrow CP. The utility of the revised International Federation of Gynecology and Obstetrics histologic grading of endometrial adenocarcinoma using a defined nuclear grading system. A Gynecologic Oncology Group study. Cancer 1995; 75(1):81–86.

69 Lurain JR, Rice BL, Rademaker AW, et al. Prognostic factors associated with recurrence in stage I adenocarcinoma of the endometrium. Obstet Gynecol 1991; 78:63-69.

70 Abeler VM, Kjorstad KE. Endometrial adenocarcinoma with squamous cell differentiation. Cancer 1992; 69:488–495.

71 Zaino RJ, Kurman RJ. Squamous differentiation in carcinoma of the endometrium: a critical appraisal of adenoacanthoma and adenosquamous carcinoma. Semin Diagn Pathol 1988; 5(2):154–171.

72 Lininger RA, Ashfaq R, Albores-Saavedra J, Tavassoli FA. Transitional cell carcinoma of the endometrium and endometrial carcinoma with transitional cell differentiation. Cancer 1997; 79:1933–1943.

73 O'Connell JT, Mutter GL, Cviko A, et al. Identification of a basal/reserve cell immunophenotype in benign and neoplastic endometrium: a study with the p53 homologue p63. Gynecol Oncol 2001; 80(1):30–36.

74 Ross JC, Eifel PJ, Cox RS, Kempson RL, Hendrickson MR. Primary mucinous adenocarcinoma of the endometrium. A clinicopathologic and histochemical study. Am J Surg Pathol 1983; 7:715–729.

75 Young RH, Scully RE. Uterine carcinomas simulating microglandular hyperplasia: a report of six cases. Am J Surg Pathol 1992; 16:1092–1097.

76 Nucci MR, Prasad CJ, Crum CP, Mutter GL. Mucinous endometrial epithelial proliferations: a morphologic spectrum of changes with diverse clinical significance. Mod Pathol 1999; 12(12):1137–1142.

77 Zheng W, Yang GC, Godwin TA, Caputo TA, Zuna RE. Mucinous adenocarcinoma of the endometrium with intestinal differentiation: a case report. Hum Pathol 1995; 26(12):1385–1388.

78 Hendrickson MR, Kempson RL. Ciliated carcinoma – a variant of endometrial adenocarcinoma: a report of 10 cases. Int J Gynecol Pathol 1983; 2(1):1–12.

79 Silverberg SG. Problems in the differential diagnosis of endometrial hyperplasia and carcinoma. Mod Pathol 2000; 13(3):309–327.

80 Ambros RA, Malfetano JH. Villoglandular adenocarcinoma of the endometrium. Am J Surg Pathol 2000; 24(1):155–156.

81 Zaino RJ, Kurman RJ, Brunetto VL, et al. Villoglandular adenocarcinoma of the endometrium: a clinicopathologic study of 61 cases: a gynecologic oncology group study. Am J Surg Pathol 1998; 22(11):1379–1385.

82 Hendrickson MR, Kempson RL. Endometrial epithelial metaplasias: proliferations frequently misdiagnosed as adenocarcinoma. Report of 89 cases and proposed classification. Am J Surg Pathol 1980; 4(6):525–542.

83 Lauchlan SC. Tubal (serous) carcinoma of the endometrium. Arch Pathol Lab Med 1981; 105(11):615–618.

84 Christopherson WM, Alberhasky RC, Connelly PJ. Carcinoma of the endometrium. II. Papillary adenocarcinoma: a clinical pathological study, 46 cases. Am J Clin Pathol 1982; 77(5):534–540.

85 Abeler VM, Kjorstrad KE. Serous papillary carcinoma of the endometrium: a histopathological study of 22 cases. Gynecol Oncol 1990; 39:266–271.

86 Wheeler DT, Bell KA, Kurman RJ, Sherman ME. Minimal uterine serous carcinoma: diagnosis and clinicopathologic correlation. Am J Surg Pathol 2000; 24(6):797–806.

87 Silva EG, Jenkins R. Serous carcinoma in endometrial polyps. Mod Pathol 1990; 3:120–128.

88 Geisler JP, Geisler HE, Wiemann MC, et al. p53 expression as a prognostic indicator of 5-year survival in endometrial cancer. Gynecol Oncol 1999; 74(3):468–471.

89 Alkushi A, Lim P, Coldman A, et al. Interpretation of p53 immunoreactivity in endometrial carcinoma: establishing a clinically relevant cut-off level. Int J Gynecol Pathol 2004; 23(2):129–137.

90 Carcangiu ML, Chambers JT. Uterine papillary serous carcinoma: a study on 108 cases with emphasis on the prognostic significance of associated endometrioid carcinoma, absence of invasion, and concomitant ovarian carcinoma. Gynecol Oncol 1992; 47:298–305.

91 Abeler VM, Kjorstad KE. Clear cell carcinoma of the endometrium: a histopathological and clinical study of 97 cases. Gynecol Oncol 1991; 40(3):207–217.

92 Murphy KT, Rotmensch J, Yamada SD, Mundt AJ. Outcome and patterns of failure in pathologic stages I–IV clear-cell carcinoma of the endometrium: implications for adjuvant radiation therapy. Int J Radiat Oncol Biol Phys 2003; 55:1272–1276.

93 Nordstrom B, Strang P, Lindgren A, Bergstrom R, Tribukait B. Endometrial carcinoma: the prognostic impact of papillary serous carcinoma (UPSC) in relation to nuclear grade, DNA ploidy and p53 expression. Anticancer Res 1996; 16:899–904.

94 Malpica A, Tornos C, Burke TW, Silva EG. Low-stage clear-cell carcinoma of the endometrium. Am J Surg Pathol 1995; 19:769–774.

95 Cirisano FD, Robboy SJ, Dodge RK, et al. The outcome of stage I-II clinically and surgically staged papillary serous and clear cell endometrial cancers when compared with endometrioid carcinoma. Gynecol Oncol 2000; 77:55–65.

96 Goff BA, Kato D, Schmidt RA, et al. Uterine papillary serous carcinoma: patterns of metastatic spread. Gynecol Oncol 1994; 54(3):264–268.

97 Grice J, Ek M, Greer B et al. Uterine papillary serous carcinoma: evaluation of long-term survival in surgically staged patients. Gynecol Oncol 1998; 69:69–73.

98 Carcangiu ML, Tan LK, Chambers JT. Stage Ia uterine serous carcinoma. A study of 13 cases. Am J Surg Pathol 1997; 21:1507–1514.

99 Nguyen NP, Sallah S, Karlsson U, et al. Prognosis for papillary serous carcinoma of the endometrium after surgical staging. Int J Gynecol Cancer 2001; 11(4):305–311.

100 Grice J, Ek M, Greer B, et al. Uterine papillary serous carcinoma: evaluation of long-term survival in surgically staged patients. Gynecol Oncol 1998; 69(1):69–73.

101 Christopherson WM, Alberhasky RC, Connelly PJ. Carcinoma of the endometrium: I. A clinicopathologic study of clear-cell carcinoma and secretory carcinoma. Cancer 1982; 49(8):1511–1523.

102 Lax SF, Pizer ES, Ronnett BM, Kurman RJ. Clear cell carcinoma of the endometrium is characterized by a distinctive profile of p53, Ki-67, estrogen, and progesterone receptor expression. Hum Pathol 1998; 29(6):551–558.

103 Bilgin T, Ozuysal S, Ozan H. A comparison of three histological grading systems in endometrial cancer. Arch Gynecol Obstet 2005; 272(1):23–25.

104 Taylor RR, Zeller J, Lieberman RW, O'Connor DM. An analysis of two versus three grades for endometrial carcinoma. Gynecol Oncol 1999; 74(1):3–6.

105 Lax SF, Kurman RJ, Pizer ES, Wu L, Ronnett BM. A binary architectural grading system for uterine endometrial endometrioid carcinoma has superior reproducibility compared with FIGO grading and identifies subsets of advance-stage tumors with favorable and unfavorable prognosis. Am J Surg Pathol 2000; 24(9):1201–1208.

106 Schorge JO, Hossein Saboorian M, Hynan L, Ashfaq R. ThinPrep detection of cervical and endometrial adenocarcinoma: a retrospective cohort study. Cancer 2002; 96(6):338–343.

107 Duska LR, Flynn CF, Chen A, Whall-Strojwas D, Goodman A. Clinical evaluation of atypical glandular cells of undetermined significance on cervical cytology. Obstet Gynecol 1998; 91(2):278–282.

108 Parellada CI, Schivartche PL, Pereyra EA, et al. Atypical glandular cells on cervical smears. Int J Gynaecol Obstet 2002; 78(3): 227–234.

109 Koonings PP, Price JH. Evaluation of atypical glandular cells of undetermined significance: is age important? Am J Obstet Gynecol 2001; 184(7):1457–1459.

110 Nassar A, Fleisher SR, Nasuti JF. Value of histiocyte detection in Pap smears for predicting endometrial pathology. An institutional experience. Acta Cytol 2003; 47(5):762–767.

111 Nguyen TN, Bourdeau JL, Ferenczy A, Franco EL. Clinical significance of histiocytes in the detection of endometrial adenocarcinoma and hyperplasia. Diagn Cytopathol 1998; 19(2):89–93.

112 Karim BO, Burroughs FH, Rosenthal DL, Ali SZ. Endometrial-type cells in cervico-vaginal smears: clinical significance and cytopathologic correlates. Diagn Cytopathol 2002; 26(2):123–127.

113 Chang A, Sandweiss L, Bose S. Cytologically benign endometrial cells in the Papanicolaou smears of postmenopausal women. Gynecol Oncol 2001; 80(1):37–43.

114 Van den Bosch T, Vandendael A, Wranz PA, Lombard CJ. Cervical cytology in menopausal women at high risk for endometrial disease. Eur J Cancer Prev 1998; 7(2):149–152.

115 Zuna RE, Erroll M. Utility of the cervical cytologic smear in assessing endocervical involvement by endometrial carcinoma. Acta Cytol 1996; 40:878–884.

116 Leminen A, Forss M, Lehtovirta P. Endometrial adenocarcinoma with clinical evidence of cervical involvement: accuracy of diagnostic procedures, clinical course, and prognostic factors. Acta Obstet Gynecol Scand 1995; 74(1):61–66.

117 Clark TJ, Mann CH, Shah N, et al. Accuracy of outpatient endometrial biopsy in the diagnosis of endometrial cancer: a systematic quantitative review. Br J Obstet Gynaecol 2002; 109(3):313–321.

118 Vorgias G, Lekka J, Katsoulis M, et al. Diagnostic accuracy of prehysterectomy curettage in determining tumor type and grade in patients with endometrial cancer. Med Gen Med 2003; 5(4):7.

119 Machado F, Moreno J, Carazo M, et al. Accuracy of endometrial biopsy with the Cornier pipelle for diagnosis of endometrial cancer and atypical hyperplasia. Eur J Gynaecol Oncol 2003; 24(3–4):279–281.

120 Dijkhuizen FP, Mol BW, Brolmann HA, Heintz AP. The accuracy of endometrial sampling in the diagnosis of patients with endometrial carcinoma and hyperplasia: a meta-analysis. Cancer 2000; 89(8):1765–1772.

121 Wu HH, Casto BD, Elsheikh TM. Endometrial brush biopsy. An accurate outpatient method of detecting endometrial malignancy. J Reprod Med 2003; 48(1):41–45.

122 Dunton C, Baak J, Palazzo J, et al. Use of computerized morphometric analyses of endometrial hyperplasias in the prediction of coexistent cancer. Am J Obstet Gynecol 1996; 174:1518–1521.

123 Mitchard J, Hirschowitz L. Concordance of FIGO grade of endometrial adenocarcinomas in biopsy and hysterectomy specimens. Histopathology 2003; 42(4):372–378.

124 Petersen RW, Quinlivan JA, Casper GR, Nicklin JL. Endometrial adenocarcinoma – presenting pathology is a poor guide to surgical management. Aust NZ J Obstet Gynaecol 2000; 40(2):191–194.

125 Trimble CL, Kauderer J, Silverberg S, et al. Concurrent endometrial carcinoma (ED) in women with biopsy diagnosis of atypical endometrial hyperplasia (AEH): a Gynecologic Oncology Group (GOG) Study. Gynecol Oncol 2004; 92:393–394.

126 Zaino R, Trimble C, Silverberg S, Kauderer J, Curtin J. Reproducibility of the diagnosis of atypical endometrial hyperplasia (AEH): A Gynecologic Oncology Group (GOG) study. Lab Invest 2004; 84(Suppl 1):218A.

127 Jordan LB, Al-Nafussi A. Clinicopathological study of the pattern and significance of cervical involvement in cases of endometrial adenocarcinoma. Int J Gynecol Cancer 2002; 12(1):42–48.

128 Toki T, Oka K, Nakayama K, Oguchi O, Fujii S. A comparative study of pre-operative procedures to assess cervical invasion by endometrial carcinoma. Br J Obstet Gynaecol 1998; 105(5):512–516.

129 Pete I, Godeny M, Toth E, et al. Prediction of cervical infiltration in Stage II endometrial cancer by different preoperative evaluation techniques (D&C, US, CT, MRI). Eur J Gynaecol Oncol 2003; 24(6):517–522.

130 Caron C, Tetu B, Laberge P, Bellemare G, Raymond PE. Endocervical involvement by endometrial carcinoma on fractional curettage: a clinicopathological study of 37 cases. Mod Pathol 1991; 4:644–647.

131 Lampe B, Kurzl R, Dimpfl T, Fawzi H. Accuracy of preoperative histology and macroscopic assessment of cervical involvement in endometrial carcinoma. Eur J Obstet Gynecol Reprod Biol 1997; 74(2):205–209.

132 Rubin SC, Hoskins WJ, Saigo PE, et al. Management of endometrial adenocarcinoma with cervical involvement. Gynecol Oncol 1992; 45(3):294–298.

133 Fanning J, Alvarez PM, Tsukada Y, Piver MS. Prognostic significance of the extent of cervical involvement by endometrial cancer. Gynecol Oncol 1991; 40:46–47.

134 Irvin WP, Rice LW, Berkowitz RS. Advances in the management of endometrial adenocarcinoma. A review. J Reprod Med 2002; 47(3):173–189; discussion 189–190.

135 Larson DM, Connor GP, Broste SK, Krawisz BR, Johnson KK. Prognostic significance of gross myometrial invasion with endometrial cancer. Obstet Gynecol 1996; 88(3):394–398.

136 Altintas A, Cosar E, Vardar MA, Demir C, Tuncer I. Intraoperative assessment of depth of myometrial invasion in endometrial carcinoma. Eur J Gynaecol Oncol 1999; 20(4):329–331.

137 Franchi M, Ghezzi F, Melpignano M, et al. Clinical value of intraoperative gross examination in endometrial cancer. Gynecol Oncol 2000; 76(3):357–361.

138 Quinlivan JA, Petersen RW, Nicklin JL. Accuracy of frozen section for the operative management of endometrial cancer. Br J Obstet Gynaecol 2001; 108(8):798–803.

139 Vorgias G, Hintipas E, Katsoulis M, et al. Intraoperative gross examination of myometrial invasion and cervical infiltration in patients with endometrial cancer: decision-making accuracy. Gynecol Oncol 2002; 85(3):483–486.

140 Noumoff JS, Menzin A, Mikuta J, et al. The ability to evaluate prognostic variables on frozen section in hysterectomies performed for endometrial carcinoma. Gynecol Oncol 1991; 42(3):202–208.

141 Chan JK, Loizzi V, Youssef M, et al. Significance of comprehensive surgical staging in noninvasive papillary serous carcinoma of the endometrium. Gynecol Oncol 2003; 90:181–185.

142 Mutter GM, Crum CP. Endometrial carcinoma. In: Fletcher CDM, ed. Pathology of tumors. London: Churchill Livingstone; 2005: in press.

143 Creasman WT, Morrow CP, Bundy BN, et al. Surgical pathologic spread patterns of endometrial cancer. A Gynecologic Oncology Group Study. Cancer 1987; 60(8 Suppl):2035–2041.

144 Creasman WT, DeGeest K, DiSaia PJ, Zaino RJ. Significance of true surgical pathologic staging: a Gynecologic Oncology Group Study. Am J Obstet Gynecol 1999; 181(1):31–34.

145 Burke C, Hickey K. Does surgical staging of clinical Stage I endometrial carcinoma significantly alter adjuvant management? J Obstet Gynaecol 2004; 24(3):289–291.

146 Zaino RJ, Kurman RJ, Diana KL, Morrow CP. Pathologic models to predict outcome for women with endometrial adenocarcinoma: the importance of the distinction between surgical stage and clinical stage – a Gynecologic Oncology Group study. Cancer 1996; 77(6):1115–1121. Erratum in: Cancer 1997; 79(2):422.

147 Cirisano FD Jr, Robboy SJ, Dodge RK, et al. The outcome of stage I–II clinically and surgically staged papillary serous and clear cell endometrial cancers when compared with endometrioid carcinoma. Gynecol Oncol 2000; 77:55–65.

148 Nordstrom B, Bergstrom R, Strang P. Prognostic index models in stage I and II endometrial carcinoma. Anticancer Res 1998; 18(5B):3717–3724.

149 Longacre TA, Hendrickson MR. Diffusely infiltrative endometrial adenocarcinoma: an adenoma malignum pattern of myoinvasion. Am J Surg Pathol 1999; 23(1):69–78.

150 Lee KR, Vacek PM, Belinson JL. Traditional and nontraditional histopathologic predictors of recurrence in uterine endometrioid adenocarcinoma. Gynecol Oncol 1994; 54:10–18.

151 Nascimento AF, Hirsch MS, Cviko A, Quade BJ, Nucci MR. The role of CD10 staining in distinguishing invasive endometrial adenocarcinoma from adenocarcinoma involving adenomyosis. Mod Pathol 2003; 16(1):22–27.

152 Srodon M, Klein WM, Kurman RJ. CD10 immunostaining does not distinguish endometrial carcinoma invading myometrium from carcinoma involving adenomyosis. Am J Surg Pathol 2003; 27(6):786–789.

153 Phelan C, Montag AG, Rotmensch J, et al. Outcome and management of pathological stage I endometrial carcinoma patients with involvement of the lower uterine segment. Gynecol Oncol 2001; 83(3):513–517.

154 Hachisuga T, Fukuda K, Iwasaka T, et al. Endometrioid adenocarcinomas of the uterine corpus in women younger than 50 years of age can be divided into two distinct clinical and pathologic entities based on anatomic location. Cancer 2001; 92(10):2578–2584.

155 Hachisuga T, Matsuo N, Iwasaka T, Sugimori H, Tsuneyoshi M. Human papilloma virus and P53 overexpression in carcinomas of the uterine cervix, lower uterine segment and endometrium. Pathology 1996; 28(1):28–31.

156 Mariani A, Webb MJ, Keeney GL, Aletti G, Podratz KC. Endometrial cancer: predictors of peritoneal failure. Gynecol Oncol 2003; 89(2):236–242.

157 Mariani A, Webb MJ, Keeney GL, et al. Stage IIIC endometrioid corpus cancer includes distinct subgroups. Gynecol Oncol 2002; 87(1):112–117.

158 Elia G, Garfinkel DA, Goldberg GL, Davidson S, Runowicz CD. Surgical management of patients with endometrial cancer and cervical involvement. Eur J Gynaecol Oncol 1995; 16(3):169–173.

159 Reisinger SA, Staros EB, Feld R, Mohiuddin M, Lewis GC. Preoperative radiation therapy in clinical stage II endometrial carcinoma. Gynecol Oncol 1992; 45(2):174–178.

160 Tambouret R, Clement PB, Young RH. Endometrial endometrioid adenocarcinoma with a deceptive pattern of spread to the uterine cervix: a manifestation of stage IIb endometrial carcinoma liable to be misinterpreted as an independent carcinoma or a benign lesion. Am J Surg Pathol 2003; 27(8):1080–1088.

161 Castrillon DH, Lee KR, Nucci MR. Distinction between endometrial and endocervical adenocarcinoma: an immunohistochemical study. Int J Gynecol Pathol 2002; 21(1):4–10.

162 Ansari-Lari MA, Staebler A, Zaino RJ, Shah KV, Ronnett BM. Distinction of endocervical and endometrial adenocarcinomas: immunohistochemical p16 expression correlated with human papillomavirus (HPV) DNA detection. Am J Surg Pathol 2004; 28(2):160–167.

163 Zuna RE, Behrens A. Peritoneal washing cytology in gynecologic cancers: long-term follow-up of 355 patients. J Natl Cancer Inst 1996; 88(14):980–987.

164 Mulvany NJ, Arnstein MB, Ryan VA. Prognostic significance of fallopian tube cytology: a study of 99 endometrial malignancies. Pathology 2000; 32(1):5–9.

165 Mulvany NJ, Arnstein M, Ostor AG. Fallopian tube cytology: a histocorrelative study of 150 washings. Diagn Cytopathol 1997; 16(6):483–488.

166 Creasman WT, Disaia PJ, Blessing J, et al. Prognostic significance of peritoneal cytology in patients with endometrial cancer and preliminary data concerning therapy with intraperitoneal radiopharmaceuticals. Am J Obstet Gynecol 1981; 141(8): 921–929.

167 McLellan R, Dillon MB, Currie JL, Rosenshein NB. Peritoneal cytology in endometrial cancer: a review. Obstet Gynecol Surv 1989; 44(10):711–719.

168 Kennedy AW, Webster KD, Nunez C, Bauer LJ. Pelvic washings for cytologic analysis in endometrial adenocarcinoma. J Reprod Med 1993; 38(8):637–642.

169 Hirai Y, Fujimoto I, Yamauchi K, et al. Peritoneal fluid cytology and prognosis in patients with endometrial carcinoma. Obstet Gynecol 1989; 73(3 Pt 1):335–338.

170 Eifel P, Hendrickson M, Ross J, et al. Simultaneous presentation of carcinoma involving the ovary and the uterine corpus. Cancer 1982; 50(1):163–170.

171 Falkenberry SS, Steinhoff MM, Gordinier M, et al. Synchronous endometrioid tumors of the ovary and endometrium. A clinicopathologic study of 22 cases. J Reprod Med 1996; 41(10):713–718.

172 Zaino R, Whitney C, Brady MF, et al. Simultaneously detected endometrial and ovarian carcinomas – a prospective clinicopathologic study of 74 cases: a gynecologic oncology group study. Gynecol Oncol 2001; 83(2):355–362.

173 Soliman PT, Slomovitz BM, Broaddus RR, et al. Synchronous primary cancers of the endometrium and ovary: a single institution review of 84 cases. Gynecol Oncol 2004; 94(2):456–462.

174 Ricci R, Komminoth P, Bannwart F, et al. PTEN as a molecular marker to distinguish metastatic from primary synchronous endometrioid carcinomas of the ovary and uterus. Diagn Mol Pathol 2003; 12(2):71–78.

175 Sato R, Jobo T, Kuramoto H. Parametral spread is a prognostic factor in endometrial carcinoma. Eur J Gynaecol Oncol 2003; 24(3–4):241–245.

176 Ozsoy M, Dilek S, Ozsoy D. Pelvic and paraaortic lymph node metastasis in clinical stage I endometrial adenocarcinoma: an analysis of 58 consecutive cases. Eur J Gynaecol Oncol 2003; 24(5):398–400.

177 Mariani A, Keeney GL, Aletti G, et al. Endometrial carcinoma: paraaortic dissemination. Gynecol Oncol 2004; 92(3):833–838.

178 Nelson G, Randall M, Sutton G, et al. FIGO stage IIIC endometrial carcinoma with metastases confined to pelvic lymph nodes: analysis of treatment outcomes, prognostic variables, and failure patterns following adjuvant radiation therapy. Gynecol Oncol 1999; 75(2):211–214.

179 Yasunaga M, Yamasaki F, Tokunaga O, Iwasaka T. Endometrial carcinomas with lymph node involvement: novel histopathologic factors for predicting prognosis. Int J Gynecol Pathol 2003; 22(4):341–346.

180 Bristow RE, Zahurak ML, Alexander CJ, Zellars RC, Montz FJ. FIGO stage IIIC endometrial carcinoma: resection of macroscopic nodal disease and other determinants of survival. Int J Gynecol Cancer 2003; 13(5):664–672.

181 Horn LC, Bilek K. Frequency and histogenesis of pelvic retroperitoneal lymph node inclusions of the female genital tract. An immunohistochemical study of 34 cases. Pathol Res Pract 1995; 191:991–996.

182 Clement PB, Young RH, Oliva E, Sumner HW, Scully RE. Hyperplastic mesothelial cells within abdominal lymph nodes: mimic of metastatic ovarian carcinoma and serous borderline tumor – a report of two cases associated with ovarian neoplasms. Mod Pathol 1996; 9(9):879–886.

183 Gonzalez Bosquet J, Keeney GL, et al. Cytokeratin staining of resected lymph nodes may improve the sensitivity of surgical staging for endometrial cancer. Gynecol Oncol 2003; 91(3):518–525.

184 Yabushita H, Shimazu M, Yamada H, et al. Occult lymph node metastases detected by cytokeratin immunohistochemistry predict recurrence in node-negative endometrial cancer. Gynecol Oncol 2001; 80(2):139–144.

185 Watanabe M, Aoki Y, Kase H, Fujita K, Tanaka K. Low risk endometrial cancer: a study of pelvic lymph node metastasis. Int J Gynecol Cancer 2003; 13(1):38–41.

186 Lindahl B, Einarsdottir M, Iosif C, Ranstam J, Willen R. Endometrial carcinoma: results of primary surgery on FIGO stages Ia–Ic and predictive value of histopathological parameters. Anticancer Res 1997; 17(3C):2297–2302.

187 Lee KR, Vacek PM, Belinson JL. Traditional and nontraditional histopathologic predictors of recurrence in uterine endometrioid adenocarcinoma. Gynecol Oncol 1994; 54(1):10–18.

188 Oreskovic S, Babic D, Kalafatic D, Barisic D, Beketic-Oreskovic L. A significance of immunohistochemical determination of steroid receptors, cell proliferation factor Ki-67 and protein p53 in endometrial carcinoma. Gynecol Oncol 2004; 93(1):34–40.

189 Stendahl U, Strang P, Wagenius G, Bergstrom R, Tribukait B. Prognostic significance of proliferation in endometrial adenocarcinomas: a multivariate analysis of clinical and flow cytometric variables. Int J Gynecol Pathol 1991; 10(3): 271–284.

190 Palmer DC, Muir IM, Alexander AI, et al. The prognostic importance of steroid receptors in endometrial carcinoma. Obstet Gynecol 1988; 72(3 Pt 1):388–393.

191 Zaino RJ, Davis AT, Ohlsson-Wilhelm BM, Brunetto VL. DNA content is an independent prognostic indicator in endometrial adenocarcinoma. A Gynecologic Oncology Group study. Int J Gynecol Pathol 1998; 17:312–319.

192 Nordstrom B, Strang P, Lindgren A, Bergstrom R, Tribukait B. Carcinoma of the endometrium: do the nuclear grade and DNA ploidy provide more prognostic information than do the FIGO and WHO classifications? Int J Gynecol Pathol 1996; 15(3):191–201.

193 Steiner E, Eicher O, Sagemuller J, et al. Multivariate independent prognostic factors in endometrial carcinoma: a clinicopathologic study in 181 patients: 10 years experience at the Department of Obstetrics and Gynecology of the Mainz University. Int J Gynecol Cancer 2003; 13(2):197–203.

194 Powell MA, Mutch DG, Rader JS, et al. Ribosomal DNA methylation in patients with endometrial carcinoma: an independent prognostic marker. Cancer 2002; 94(11):2941–2952.

195 Poulsen MG, Roberts SJ. Prognostic variables in endometrial carcinoma. Int J Radiat Oncol Biol Phys 1987; 13(7): 1043–1052.

196 Chafe S, Honore L, Pearcey R, Capstick V. An analysis of the impact of pathology review in gynecologic cancer. Int J Radiat Oncol Biol Phys 2000; 48(5):1433–1438.

197 Eifel PJ, Hendrickson M. Stage I endometrial carcinoma: the importance of pathologic review in retrospective analyses. Int J Radiat Oncol Biol Phys 1990; 18(5):1271–1273.

198 Mariani A, Webb MJ, Keeney GL, Calori G, Podratz KC. Role of wide/radical hysterectomy and pelvic lymph node dissection in endometrial cancer with cervical involvement. Gynecol Oncol 2001; 83(1):72–80.

199 Calvin DP, Connell PP, Rotmensch J, Waggoner S, Mundt AJ. Surgery and postoperative radiation therapy in stage II endometrial carcinoma. Am J Clin Oncol 1999; 22:338–343.

200 Ng TY, Nicklin JL, Perrin LC, Cheuk R, Crandon AJ. Postoperative vaginal vault brachytherapy for node-negative Stage II (occult) endometrial carcinoma. Gynecol Oncol 2001; 81(2):193–195.

201 Feltmate CM, Duska LR, Chang Y, et al. Predictors of recurrence in surgical stage II endometrial adenocarcinoma. Gynecol Oncol 1999; 73:407–411.

202 Orr JW. Surgical staging of endometrial cancer: does the patient benefit? Gynecol Oncol 1998; 71(3):335–339.

203 Orr JW Jr, Holimon JL, Orr PF. Stage I corpus cancer: is teletherapy necessary? Am J Obstet Gynecol 1997; 176:777–788.

204 Naumann RW, Higgins RV, Hall JB. The use of adjuvant radiation therapy by members of the Society of Gynecologic Oncologists. Gynecol Oncol 1999; 75(1):4–9.

205 Seago DP, Raman A, Lele S. Potential benefit of lymphadenectomy for the treatment of node-negative locally advanced uterine cancers. Gynecol Oncol 2001; 83(2):282–285.

206 Creasman WT, Kohler MF, Odicino F, Maisonneuve P, Boyle P. Prognosis of papillary serous, clear cell, and grade 3 stage I carcinoma of the endometrium. Gynecol Oncol 2004; 95:593–596.

207 Sreenan JJ, Hart WR. Carcinosarcomas of the female genital tract. A pathologic study of 29 metastatic tumors: further evidence for the dominant role of the epithelial component and the conversion theory of histogenesis. Am J Surg Pathol 1995; 19(6):666–674.

208 Fujii H, Yoshida M, Gong ZX, et al. Frequent genetic heterogeneity in the clonal evolution of gynecological carcinosarcoma and its influence on phenotypic diversity. Cancer Res 2000; 60(1):114–120.

209 Watanabe M, Shimizu K, Kato H, et al. Carcinosarcoma of the uterus: immunohistochemical and genetic analysis of clonality of one case. Gynecol Oncol 2001; 82(3):563–567.

210 Wada H, Enomoto T, Fujita M, et al. Molecular evidence that most but not all carcinosarcomas of the uterus are combination tumors. Cancer Res 1997; 57(23):5379–5385.

211 Micci F, Teixeira MR, Haugom L, et al. Genomic aberrations in carcinomas of the uterine corpus. Genes Chromosomes Cancer 2004; 40(3):229–246.

212 Fehr PE, Prem KA. Malignancy of the uterine corpus following irradiation therapy for squamous cell carcinoma of the cervix. Am J Obstet Gynecol 1974; 119(5):685–692.

213 Bird CC, Willis RA. The possible carcinogenic effects of radiations on the uterus. Br J Cancer 1970; 24(4): 759–768.

214 Schaepman-van Geuns EJ. Mixed tumors and carcinosarcomas of the uterus evaluated five years after treatment. Cancer 1970; 25(1):72–77.

215 Thomas WO Jr, Harris HH, Enden JA. Postirradiation malignant neoplasms of the uterine fundus. Am J Obstet Gynecol 1969; 104(2):209–219.

216 Bukowski S, Cicholska A, Meyer J. Combined mesenchymal carcinosarcoma of the uterus in patient after successful radiotherapy of carcinoma of the uterine cervix. Nowotwory 1967; 17(1):53–57.

217 Varela-Duran J, Nochomovitz LE, Prem KA, Dehner LP. Postirradiation mixed mullerian tumors of the uterus: a comparative clinicopathologic study. Cancer 1980; 45(7):1625–1631.

218 Evans MJ, Langlois NE, Kitchener HC, Miller ID. Is there an association between long-term tamoxifen treatment and the development of carcinosarcoma (malignant mixed Müllerian tumor) of the uterus? Int J Gynecol Cancer 1995; 5(4):310–313.

219 Brooks SE, Zhan M, Cote T, Baquet CR. Surveillance, epidemiology, and end results analysis of 2677 cases of uterine sarcoma 1989–1999. Gynecol Oncol 2004; 93(1):204–208.

220 Vaccarello L, Curtin JP. Presentation and management of carcinosarcoma of the uterus. Oncology 1992; 6(5):45–49; discussion 53–54, 59.

221 Silverberg SG, Major FJ, Blessing JA, et al. Carcinosarcoma (malignant mixed mesodermal tumor) of the uterus. A Gynecologic Oncology Group pathologic study of 203 cases. Int J Gynecol Pathol 1990; 9(1):1–19.

222 Barwick KW, LiVolsi VA. Malignant mixed mullerian tumors of the uterus. A clinicopathologic assessment of 34 cases. Am J Surg Pathol 1979; 3(2):125–135.

223 Roberts DJ, Haber D, Sklar J, Crum CP. Extrarenal Wilms' tumors. A study of their relationship with classical renal Wilms' tumor using expression of WT1 as a molecular marker. Lab Invest 1993; 68(5):528–536.

224 Le T. Adjuvant pelvic radiotherapy for uterine carcinosarcoma in a high risk population. Eur J Surg Oncol 2001; 27(3): 282–285.

225 Macasaet MA, Waxman M, Fruchter RG, et al. Prognostic factors in malignant mesodermal (Müllerian) mixed tumors of the uterus. Gynecol Oncol 1985; 20(1):32–42.

226 Yamada SD, Burger RA, Brewster WR, et al. Pathologic variables and adjuvant therapy as predictors of recurrence and survival for patients with surgically evaluated carcinosarcoma of the uterus. Cancer 2000; 88(12):2782–2786.

227 Bodner-Adler B, Bodner K, Obermair A, et al. Prognostic parameters in carcinosarcomas of the uterus: a clinico-pathologic study. Anticancer Res 2001; 21(4B):3069–3074.

228 Jereczek B, Jassem J, Kobierska A. Sarcoma of the uterus. A clinical study of 42 patients. Arch Gynecol Obstet 1996; 258(4):171–180.

229 Sartori E, Bazzurini L, Gadducci A, et al. Carcinosarcoma of the uterus: a clinicopathological multicenter CTF study. Gynecol Oncol 1997; 67(1):70–75.

230 Thigpen JT, Blessing JA, DeGeest K, Look KY, Homesley HD. Cisplatin as initial chemotherapy in ovarian carcinosarcomas: a Gynecologic Oncology Group study. Obstet Gynecol Surv 2004; 59(8):589–590.

231 Sutton G, Brunetto VL, Kilgore L, et al. A phase III trial of ifosfamide with or without cisplatin in carcinosarcoma of the uterus: a Gynecologic Oncology Group study. Gynecol Oncol 2000; 79(2):147–153.

232 Gerszten K, Faul C, Kounelis S, et al. The impact of adjuvant radiotherapy on carcinosarcoma of the uterus. Gynecol Oncol 1998; 68(1):8–13.

233 Mazur MT. Atypical polypoid adenomyomas of the endometrium. Am J Surg Pathol 1981; 5(5):473–482.

234 Lee KR. Atypical polypoid adenomyoma of the endometrium associated with adenomyomatosis and adenocarcinoma. Gynecol Oncol 1993; 51(3):416–418.

235 Longacre TA, Chung MH, Rouse RV, Hendrickson MR. Atypical polypoid adenomyofibromas (atypical polypoid adenomyomas) of the uterus. A clinicopathologic study of 55 cases. Am J Surg Pathol 1996; 20(1):1–20.

236 Sugiyama T, Ohta S, Nishida T, et al. Two cases of endometrial adenocarcinoma arising from atypical polypoid adenomyoma. Gynecol Oncol 1998; 71(1):141–144.

237 Stastny JF, Ben-Ezra J, Stewart JA, et al. Condyloma and cervical intraepithelial neoplasia of the endometrium. Gynecol Obstet Invest 1995; 39(4): 277–280.

238 Zidi YS, Bouraoui S, Atallah K, Kchir N, Haouet S. Primary in situ squamous cell carcinoma of the endometrium, with extensive squamous metaplasia and dysplasia. Gynecol Oncol 2003; 88(3):444–446.

239 Houissa-Vuong S, Catanzano-Laroudie M, Baviera E, et al. Primary squamous cell carcinoma of the endometrium: case history, pathologic findings, and discussion. Diagn Cytopathol 2002; 27(5): 291–293.

240 Rodolakis A, Papaspyrou I, Sotiropoulou M, Markaki S, Michalas S. Primary squamous cell carcinoma of the

endometrium. A report of 3 cases. Eur J Gynaecol Oncol 2001; 22(2):143–146.

241 Shidara Y, Karube A, Watanabe M, et al. A case report: verrucous carcinoma of the endometrium – the difficulty of diagnosis, and a review of the literature. J Obstet Gynaecol Res 2000; 26(3):189–192.

242 Sherwood JB, Carlson JA, Gold MA, et al. Squamous metaplasia of the endometrium associated with HPV 6 and 11. Gynecol Oncol 1997; 66(1):141–145.

243 Kataoka A, Nishida T, Sugiyama T, et al. Squamous cell carcinoma of the endometrium with human papillomavirus type 31 and without tumor suppressor gene p53 mutation. Gynecol Oncol 1997; 65(1):180–184.

244 Kataoka A, Nishida T, Okina H, et al. Squamous cell carcinoma of the endometrium with human papillomavirus type 31. Kurume Med J 1997; 44(1):67–69.

245 Czerwenka K, Lu Y, Heuss F, Manavi M, Kubista E. Human papillomavirus detection of endometrioid carcinoma with squamous differentiation of the uterine corpus. Gynecol Oncol 1996; 61(2):210–214.

246 Goodman A, Zukerberg LR, Rice LW, et al. Squamous cell carcinoma of the endometrium: a report of eight cases and a review of the literature. Gynecol Oncol 1996; 61(1):54–60.

247 Im DD, Shah KV, Rosenshein NB. Report of three new cases of squamous carcinoma of the endometrium with emphasis in the HPV status. Gynecol Oncol 1995; 56(3):464–469.

248 Yamamoto Y, Izumi K, Otsuka H, et al. Primary squamous cell carcinoma of the endometrium: a case report and a suggestion of new histogenesis. Int J Gynecol Pathol 1995; 14(1):75–80.

249 Spiegel GW, Austin RM, Gelven PL. Transitional cell carcinoma of the endometrium. Gynecol Oncol 1996; 60(2):325–330.

250 Shaco-Levy R, Manor E, Piura B, Ariel I. An unusual composite endometrial tumor combining papillary serous carcinoma and small cell carcinoma. Am J Surg Pathol 2004; 28(8):1103–1106.

251 Varras M, Akrivis Ch, Demou A, et al. Primary small-cell carcinoma of the endometrium: clinicopathological study of a case and review of the literature. Eur J Gynaecol Oncol 2002; 23(6):577–581.

252 Abeler VM, Kjorstad KE, Nesland JM. Undifferentiated carcinoma of the endometrium. A histopathologic and clinical study of 31 cases. Cancer 1991; 68:98–105.

253 Vargas MP, Merino MJ. Lymphoepithelioma-like carcinoma: an unusual variant of endometrial cancer. A report of two cases. Int J Gynecol Pathol 1998; 17(3):272–276.

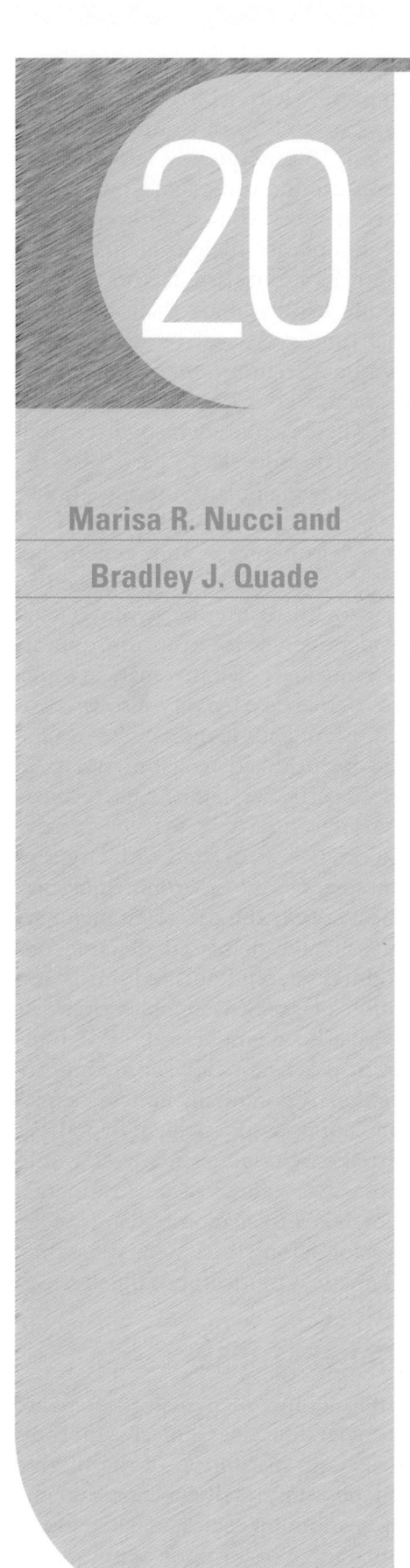

20

Uterine mesenchymal tumors

Marisa R. Nucci and

Bradley J. Quade

Introduction

Definition
Identifying patients at risk for
    mesenchymal neoplasia
General clinical features

Endometrial stromal tumors

Definition and classification
Clinicopathologic features
Molecular genetics
Interpretation of curettings
Management and prognosis
Biomarkers and differential
    diagnosis

Tumors of the myometrium

Definition and classification
Benign leiomyoma
Malignant leiomyosarcoma
Histological variants of leiomyoma

Smooth muscle tumors that are
    difficult to classify
Application of biomarkers to
    smooth muscle neoplasia
Practical approaches to the
    intraoperative examination of
    uterine smooth muscle tumors
Quasi-malignant smooth muscle
    proliferations
Tumors mimicking smooth
    muscle tumors

**Mixed epithelial and
mesenchymal tumors**

Adenosarcoma
Carcinosarcoma (malignant mixed
    Müllerian tumor)

Miscellaneous tumors

Uterine perivascular epithelioid
    cell tumor

Introduction

DEFINITION

Uterine mesenchymal tumors are neoplasms derived from or differentiating towards mesodermally derived tissues. Differentiation is typically towards normal constituents of the uterine corpus – endometrial stromal and myometrial smooth muscle cells; however, differentiation towards heterologous tissues, i.e. mesenchymal tissue not normally present in the uterus (e.g. striated muscle, cartilage or bone) also may be seen.

Mixed epithelial and mesenchymal uterine tumors are composed of either benign or malignant mesenchymal elements combined with benign or malignant epithelium. The classification of such mixed tumors depends upon morphologic assessment of both components.

IDENTIFYING PATIENTS AT RISK FOR MESENCHYMAL NEOPLASIA

The degree of risk for developing mesenchymal tumors is not uniform for all types of uterine mesenchymal neoplasia and assessment of risk is further hindered by the rarity of most of these tumors. In fact, uterine sarcomas account for only 4–9% of uterine malignancy.[1] Moreover, it is estimated that there are only 0.01 to 0.02 cases of uterine sarcoma per 1000 women.[2]

Despite their rarity, there has been recent insight into potential risk factors for certain subtypes of uterine mesenchymal neoplasia. Tamoxifen, an anti-estrogenic drug widely prescribed for women at risk for breast cancer or used to treat women with breast cancer, is known to increase the risk for uterine carcinoma presumably due to its agonistic effect at this site; recently it has become evident that this drug may also increase a women's risk for certain subtypes of uterine mesenchymal neoplasia, particularly adenosarcoma and carcinosarcoma.[3–8] In some cases, there is a long latency period such that long-term follow-up of all patients on tamoxifen is warranted.[9] Follow-up ultrasound evaluation in patients *with* clinical symptoms may be useful in stratifying those women who need to undergo sampling of their endometrium.[10] An abnormal ultrasound finding (i.e. thickened endometrial stripe, polyp or uterine mass) in this group should prompt sampling. The risk for uterine malignancy (both epithelial and mesenchymal types) associated with raloxifene, a drug currently prescribed to prevent osteoporosis and being tested in women with and at risk for breast cancer, is not clear.[11,12]

In contrast to malignant mesenchymal tumors, the frequency of benign uterine leiomyomata is extremely high, with estimates of up to 85% of women of reproductive age and beyond.[13] Consequently, leiomyomata are the most common uterine tumor and one of the most common tumors to affect women. Although their high frequency may complicate their epidemiological analysis, more is known about risk factors for the development of uterine leiomyomata than any other uterine mesenchymal tumor. As will be discussed in greater detail in subsequent sections, there is substantial evidence that genetic factors contribute to the development of leiomyomata. These factors are recognized both at the familial and population levels. In particular, the risk of benign, and possibly malignant, uterine smooth muscle tumors are 2–3-fold higher in black women.[1,14–16]

Non-genetic (i.e. environmental and genetic-by-environmental) factors also have been implicated in the development or growth of uterine leiomyomata. The most frequently identified factor, smoking, appears to reduce the clinical frequency of leiomyomata in some, but not all studies.[17–24] Increased parity also is associated with a reduced risk of leiomyomata.[19,22,24–28] Oral contraceptive use has been linked to leiomyomata in most studies.[19,24,25,29,30] In particular, higher age at menarche and early oral contraceptive use may be protective.[25,28] In contrast, obesity is associated with larger or more symptomatic tumors.[18,23–25,31] Environmental (perineal) exposure to talc increases the risk of leiomyomata by a factor of two.[32] Finally, increased dietary consumption of soy products, alcohol and red meats and decreased consumption of green vegetables or foods rich in ß-carotenes have been implicated.[22,33–35] Individually, these apparent risk factors for leiomyoma are a confusing hodge-podge. A potentially unifying explanation emphasizes the 'unopposed estrogen' hypothesis invoked in endometrial carcinogenesis.[35] Diet would tie into this hypothesis as a source of environmental estrogens. Another potential explanation is that gravidity alters the propensity for leiomyomata by structural, biochemical and epigenetic remodeling of the uterus.[21]

GENERAL CLINICAL FEATURES

In general, most uterine mesenchymal tumors are intramural or intracavitary lesions. Clinical symptoms are related to their size and disruption of the uterine lining, with pelvic pain, pressure and dysfunctional uterine bleeding being the most common clinical manifestations. While size is not a guarantee of a tumor being malignant, in general, most mesenchymal malignancies of the uterine corpus tend to be large (>10 cm) and may have already spread to involve contiguous structures at the time of presentation. Radiographic studies, particularly ultrasound and MRI, may be useful in clinically assessing whether a mass is more likely benign or malignant.[36-43] In addition to spread beyond the uterus, radiographic features suggestive of tumor necrosis may be present. Caveats include central infarction and degeneration of benign tumors such as can be seen in large leiomyomata.

Endometrial stromal tumors

DEFINITION AND CLASSIFICATION

Endometrial stromal tumors are neoplasms composed of cells that morphologically resemble non-neoplastic proliferative phase endometrial stroma. In addition, these tumors also contain numerous small blood vessels, mimicking physiologic spiral arterioles, around which the neoplastic stromal cells typically proliferate in a concentric pattern. Endometrial stromal tumors are separated into benign and malignant categories, termed endometrial stromal nodule and endometrial stromal sarcoma respectively, based upon the presence or absence of an infiltrative border.

Currently, the WHO classifies endometrial stromal tumors into the following categories: (1) endometrial stromal nodule, (2) endometrial stromal sarcoma, low grade and (3) undifferentiated endometrial sarcoma. This classification reflects terminology first proposed in 1966 by Norris and Taylor in their seminal paper on endometrial stromal neoplasms,[44] although current definitions of these categories have changed. The main difference in the current classification centers upon the definition of low-grade endometrial stromal sarcoma and its separation from what was originally termed high-grade endometrial stromal sarcoma. As originally proposed in 1966, separation into low- and high-grade categories was solely based upon mitotic activity; if a tumor which morphologically resembles endometrial stroma had less than 10 mitoses per 10 high power fields, it was considered low- grade, whereas a tumor with greater than 10 mitoses per 10 high power fields was considered high grade. However, since this original publication, the clinical relevance of separating those examples of endometrial stromal sarcoma with morphology similar to normal proliferative phase stroma into low- and high-grade categories based upon mitotic activity has not been confirmed in subsequent studies, most notably by Evans[45] and Chang et al.[46] Moreover,

the category of high-grade endometrial stromal sarcoma had represented a heterogenous group of tumors including those that resembled endometrial stroma and those that were poorly differentiated, being composed of larger cells with a greater degree of nuclear anaplasia akin to the mesenchymal component of carcinosarcoma. Therefore, in the current (2002) WHO classification scheme, there remain two categories of endometrial sarcoma – low grade and undifferentiated, which is based on differences in tumor morphology rather than mitotic activity. A low-grade endometrial stromal sarcoma is a tumor composed of cells that morphologically resemble non-neoplastic proliferative phase endometrial stroma that infiltrates the surrounding myometrium in a characteristic 'finger-like' permeative fashion and typically invades lymphatic or vascular spaces. In contrast, an undifferentiated endometrial sarcoma is a poorly differentiated sarcoma composed of cells that do not resemble proliferative phase endometrial stroma, which usually shows destructive infiltration of the myometrium. Despite this attempt at a neat separation into diagnostic categories, there are examples of endometrial sarcoma that have features of both undifferentiated endometrial sarcoma and low-grade endometrial stromal sarcoma. These tumors show either a combination of low-grade and undifferentiated areas or have the morphologic appearance of an undifferentiated endometrial sarcoma but also exhibit features suggesting differentiation towards endometrial stroma, such as the presence of finger-like infiltrative pattern of the surrounding myometrium or extension into lymphatic or vascular spaces typical of its low-grade counterpart. It is these types of tumors that should perhaps be considered 'high-grade endometrial stromal sarcoma' and that will be discussed under that title in this forum.

CLINICOPATHOLOGIC FEATURES

Endometrial stromal nodule

Endometrial stromal nodules may occur at any age but are typically encountered in women in their fifth and sixth decade.[47-50] They may be located intramurally with no connection to the endometrial surface (raising interesting possibilities concerning histogenesis and shared developmental origin of uterine stroma and smooth muscle), they may be located submucosally at the endomyometrial junction, or they may project into the endometrial cavity as a polypoid mass. On gross examination, they are characteristically well circumscribed and may be mistaken for a leiomyoma; however, endometrial stromal nodules are usually softer in consistency, tend more commonly to be yellow and lack the characteristic whorled, bulging appearance of a typical leiomyoma (Fig. 20.1). Endometrial stromal nodules can vary in size but are usually less than 10.0 cm, although larger tumors have been described.[46,47,49,51]

Histologically, an endometrial stromal nodule is characterized by sharp circumscription between the neoplastic cells and surrounding endometrium or myometrium, with a pushing interface or an interface with minimal extension of the neoplastic cells (<3 mm) into surrounding myometrium (Fig. 20.2).[47] By definition, no lymphatic or vascular invasion is present. The neoplastic

cells of endometrial stromal nodules resemble proliferative phase endometrial stroma, being composed of cells with uniform round to ovoid nuclei that have scant to moderate amounts of eosinophilic to amphophilic cytoplasm (Fig. 20.3). These cells appear to whorl around the prominent vascular component, which resembles the spiral arterioles of non-neoplastic endometrium; foamy stromal cells may be conspicuous (Fig. 20.4). The vessels are typically evenly spaced and uniform in caliber throughout the neoplasm; however, on occasion, larger, thick-walled vessels may be present, although this is usually only a focal finding in a minority of cases.

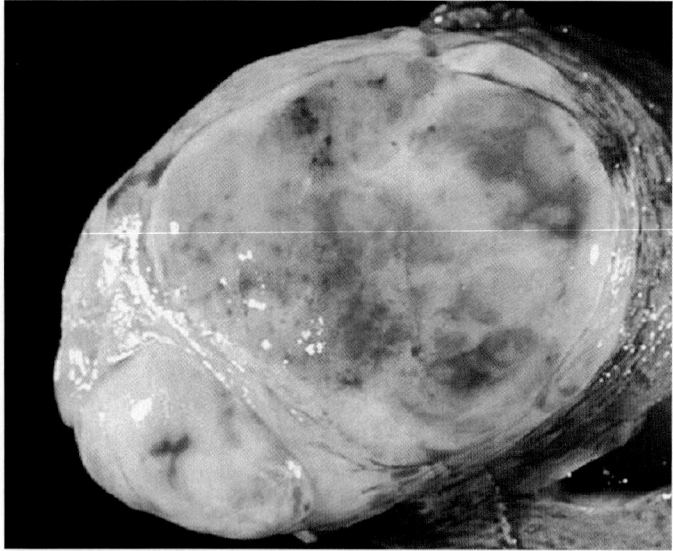

Fig. 20.1 Endometrial stromal nodule. This tumor is bilobate and has areas of smooth muscle differentiation, which are apparent as the tan areas within the distinctive yellow appearance of the neoplastic stroma.

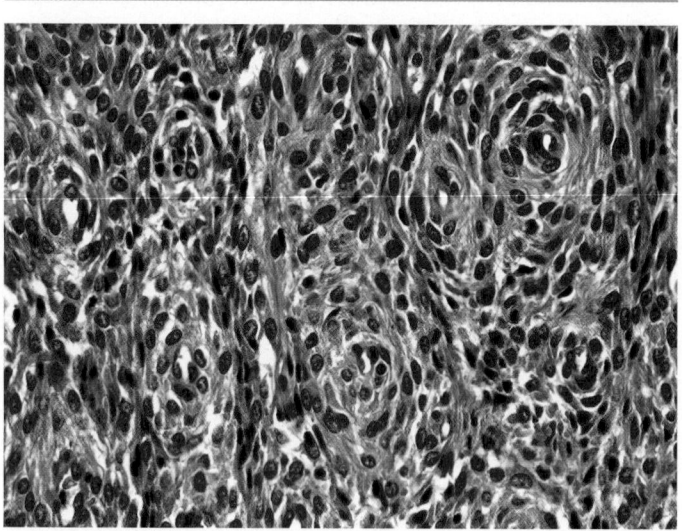

Fig. 20.3 Endometrial stromal nodule. Characteristic cytomorphology and vasculature.

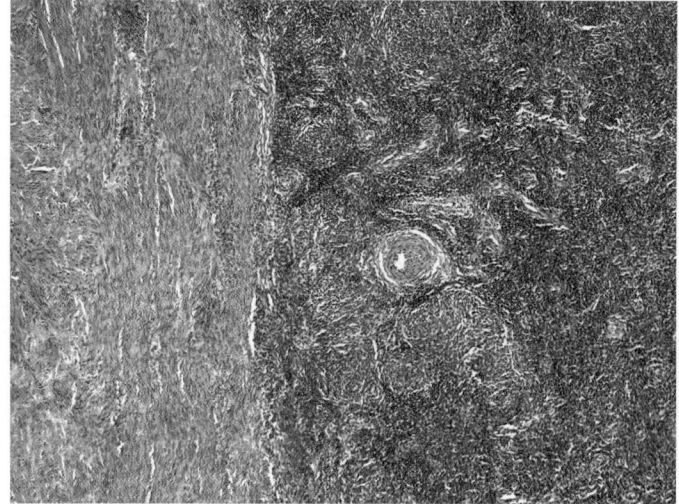

Fig. 20.2 Endometrial stromal nodule. Well-demarcated border with myometrium.

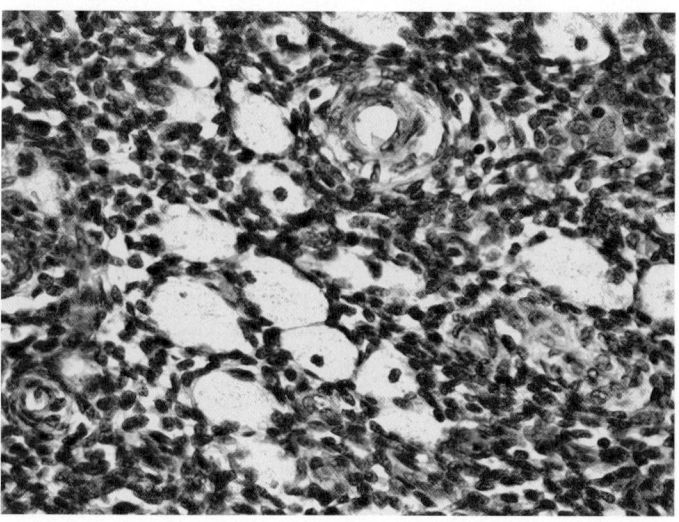

Fig. 20.4 Endometrial stromal nodule. Foamy cells are a characteristic feature.

Low-grade endometrial stromal sarcoma

Women with low-grade endometrial stromal sarcoma tend to be younger than those who present with other types of uterine sarcoma. The gross appearance of low-grade endometrial stromal sarcoma can be variable. Tumors may present as: (1) intramyometrial nodular masses, (2) an intracavitary polypoid mass, (3) diffuse myometrial infiltration with expansion of the uterine wall, or (4) any combination of these patterns (Fig. 20.5). Extension beyond the uterus may be seen and extensive involvement of parametrial vessels may impart a 'worm-like' appearance on gross examination.

Histologically, the neoplastic cells of low-grade endometrial stromal sarcoma are morphologically indistinguishable from those of an endometrial stromal nodule. Diagnosis of sarcoma is based upon the presence of myometrial infiltration (Fig. 20.6) or invasion of lymphatic or vascular spaces (Fig. 20.7). Characteristically, the neoplastic cells invade as rounded to irregularly shaped nests of varying size that has been often likened to a 'finger-like' permeation of the surrounding myometrium.

Endometrial stromal tumors with divergent differentiation

Endometrial stromal tumors can occasionally exhibit a diverse range of differentiation including sex-cord like, epithelial (e.g. endometrioid type glands) and smooth muscle differentiation.[48,52–54]

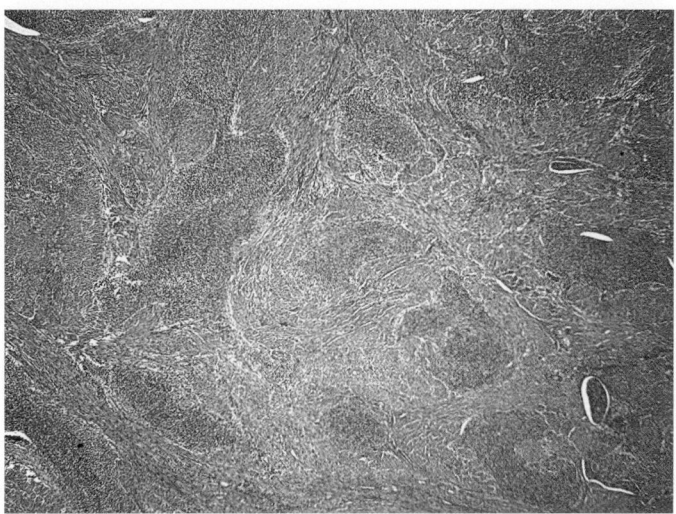

Fig. 20.6 Endometrial stromal sarcoma, low-grade. Tumor permeates myometrium in a finger-like pattern of growth.

Mixed endometrial stromal–smooth muscle tumors

Endometrial stromal neoplasms with smooth muscle differentiation have been the focus of a limited number of studies, partly due to under-recognition of these tumors and their uncommon occurrence.[52,53] If greater than 30% of the tumor comprises smooth muscle then these tumors are designated mixed endometrial stromal–smooth muscle tumors.[53] Histologic features of smooth muscle differentiation include: (1) typical smooth muscle morphology reminiscent of that seen in leiomyomata, (2) nodules with central prominent hyalinization (the so-called 'starburst' pattern; Fig. 20.8) and (3) irregular islands that can be either discrete or merge imperceptibly with the areas characteristic of stro-

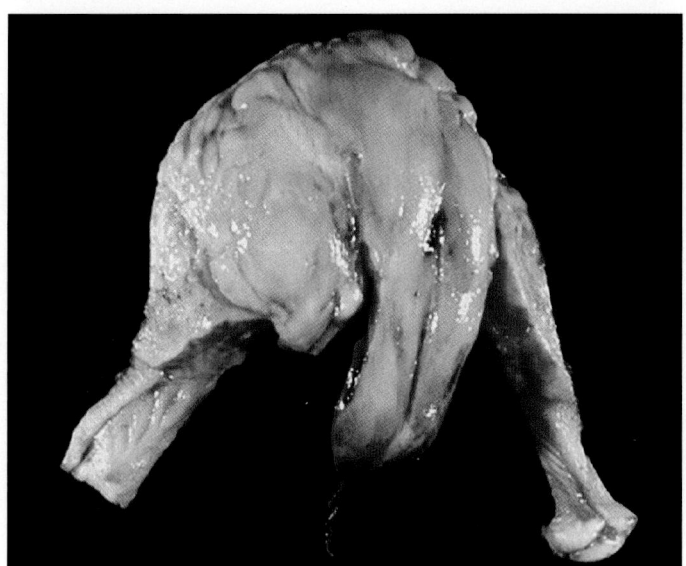

Fig. 20.5 Endometrial stromal sarcoma, low-grade.

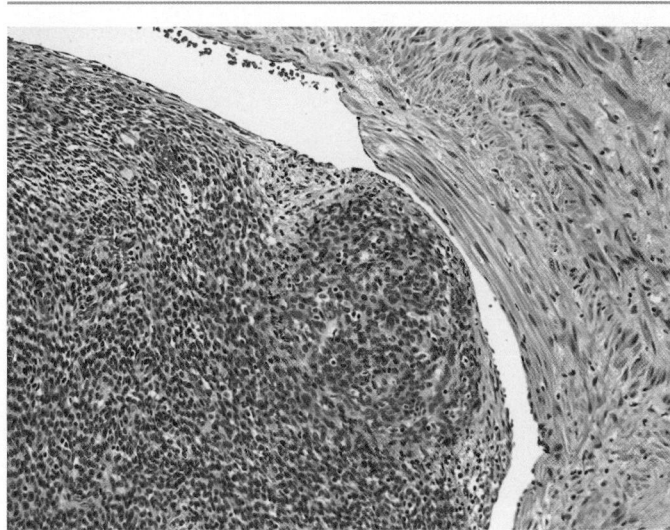

Fig. 20.7 Endometrial stromal sarcoma, low-grade. Vascular invasion.

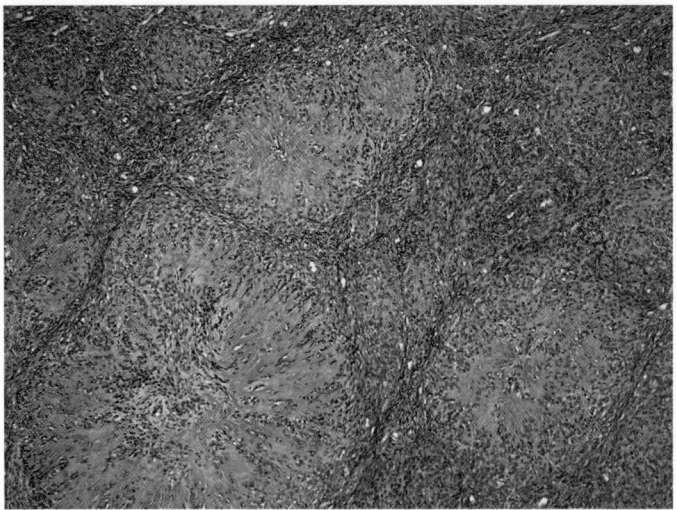

Fig. 20.8 Mixed endometrial stromal–smooth muscle tumor. Nodules of smooth muscle differentiation with central prominent hyalinization ('starburst' pattern).

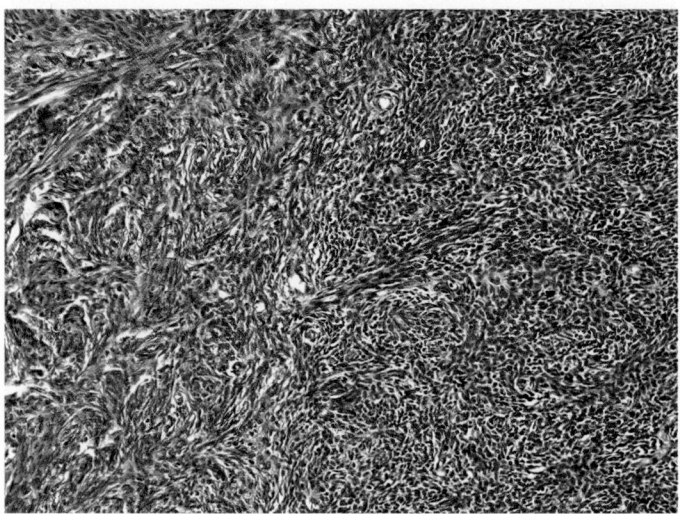

Fig. 20.10 Mixed endometrial stromal–smooth muscle tumor. Imperceptible merging of neoplastic stroma with areas of smooth muscle differentiation.

mal differentiation (Figs 20.9, 20.10). These tumors are of endometrial stromal derivation (see molecular genetics below); therefore, determination of benign *vs* malignant should be made using the criteria for endometrial stromal tumors (e.g. presence/absence of myometrial invasion, lymphatic or vascular invasion).[53]

Endometrial stromal tumor resembling ovarian sex-cord tumor

Endometrial stromal tumors may exhibit morphologic features of ovarian sex-cord-stromal tumors. These elements may be present focally, most often in the form of inter-anastomosing trabeculae (Fig. 20.11), cords and

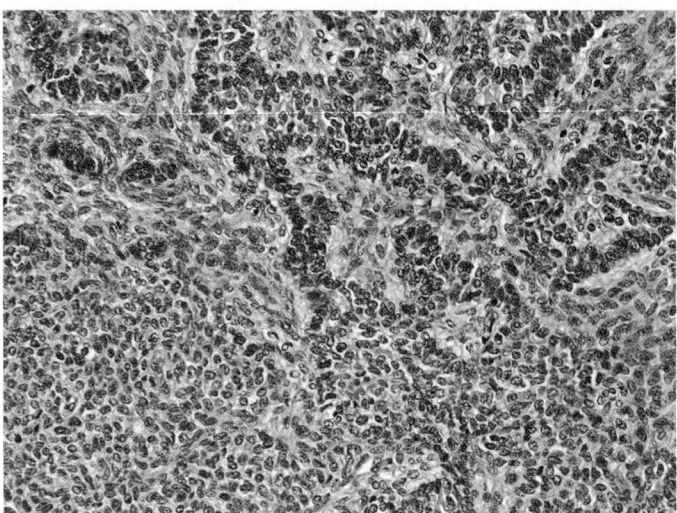

Fig. 20.11 Endometrial stromal sarcoma, low grade. Ovarian sex-cord-like differentiation.

less commonly tubules, or they may be the predominant pattern in which the stromal element is less conspicuous or absent (Fig. 20.12).[55] In the latter case, the term 'uterine tumor resembling ovarian sex cord stromal tumor' has been used. In addition to the morphologic resemblance, these elements also may be positive for markers of sex-cord differentiation, such as inhibin and O-13, suggesting that these foci represent true sex-cord differentiation akin to that seen in the ovary.[56]

Focal sex-cord-like differentiation may be seen in both endometrial stromal nodule and low-grade endometrial stromal sarcoma and does not appear to have an impact on biologic behavior. Histopathologic criteria for the distinction between a stromal nodule and stromal

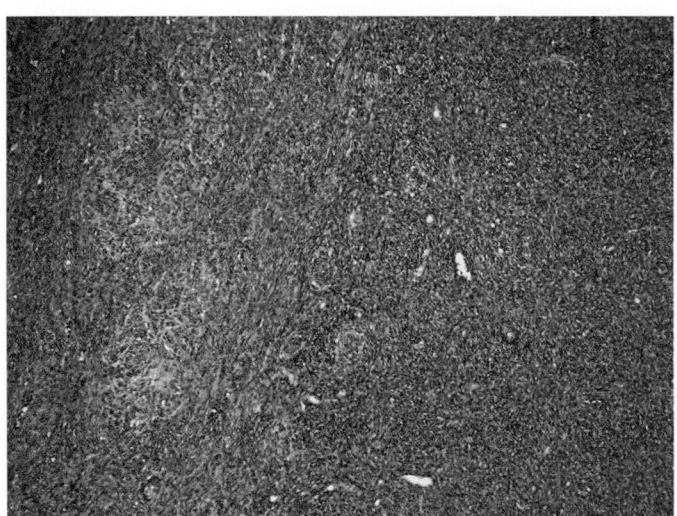

Fig. 20.9 Mixed endometrial stromal–smooth muscle tumor. Area of smooth muscle differentiation on the left.

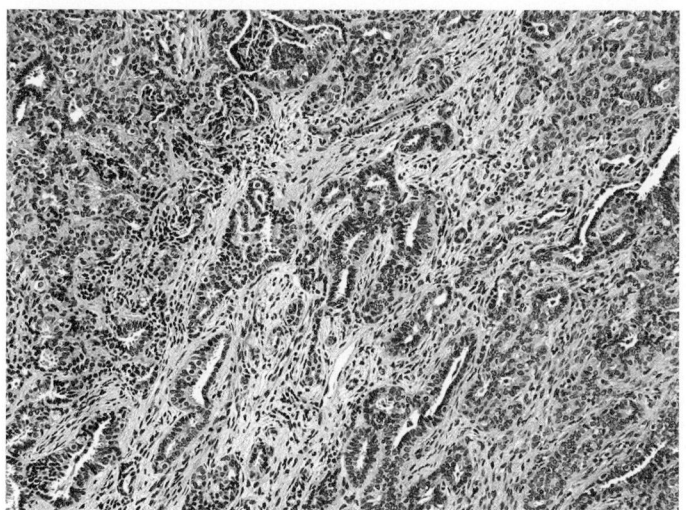

Fig. 20.12 Uterine tumor resembling ovarian sex-cord tumor.

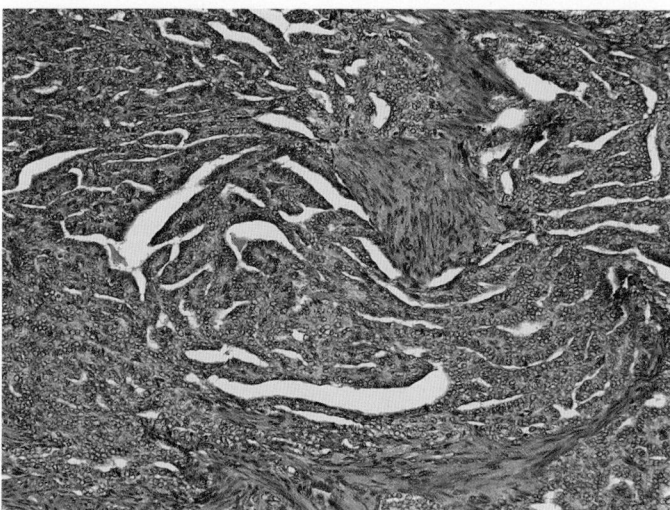

Fig. 20.13 Endometrial stromal sarcoma, low-grade. Prominent endometrioid glandular differentiation.

sarcoma, as outlined previously, are applied regardless of the presence of sex-cord-like elements. Less is known concerning the natural biologic behavior of tumors that show exclusive sex-cord-like differentiation. Although evidence suggests that they are benign – they are generally well-circumscribed, yellow, grey or tan masses and there are no reported incidences of recurrence or metastasis[55] – outcome in patients treated conservatively is not known as all patients typically have undergone hysterectomy.

Endometrial stromal tumor with endometrioid glands

Divergent differentiation down epithelial lines also may be occasionally seen in either endometrial stromal nodule or low-grade endometrial stromal sarcoma, most commonly as well-formed endometrioid glands (Fig. 20.13). While divergent differentiation is the most likely explanation for their presence, some examples may represent entrapped non-neoplastic endometrial glands. In general, this type of differentiation is focal and the main differential diagnosis is the distinction from adenomyosis, particularly adenomyosis with sparse glands. The latter is most commonly encountered as an incidental finding in postmenopausal women and can be distinguished from low-grade endometrial stromal sarcoma primarily based upon the atrophic appearance of the stroma and the lack of grossly identifiable mass.[57]

Undifferentiated endometrial sarcoma (undifferentiated uterine sarcoma)

Usually undifferentiated endometrial sarcoma presents as one or more tan-yellow to gray, fleshy intracavitary

polypoid masses (Fig. 20.14). Hemorrhage and necrosis are common. Histologically, the neoplastic cells show marked cellular atypia and numerous mitoses, including atypical forms, without evidence of differentiation towards endometrial stroma both cytomorphologically (Fig. 20.15) and by pattern of growth within the myometrium. In general, undifferentiated endometrial sarcoma has a diffuse and destructive infiltrative pattern as opposed to the characteristic worm-like pattern and propensity for intravascular extension characteristic of low-grade endometrial stromal sarcoma. Because the tumor cell morphology of undifferentiated endometrial sarcoma is often likened to the mesenchymal component of a carcinosarcoma, exclusion of this latter entity should always be considered. In fact, the diagnosis of undifferentiated endometrial sarcoma should only be considered following exclusion of a poorly differentiated

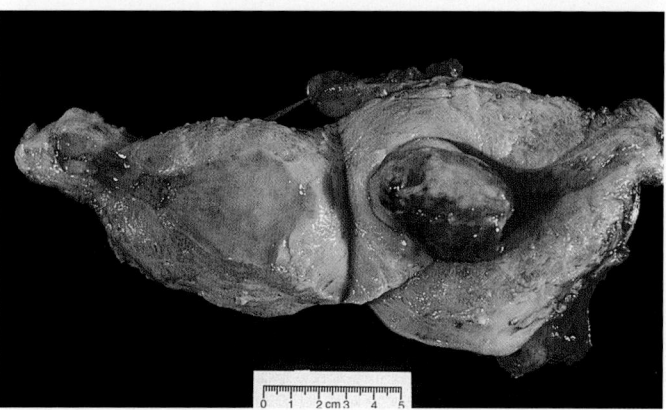

Fig. 20.14 Undifferentiated uterine sarcoma. Polypoid intracavitary mass.

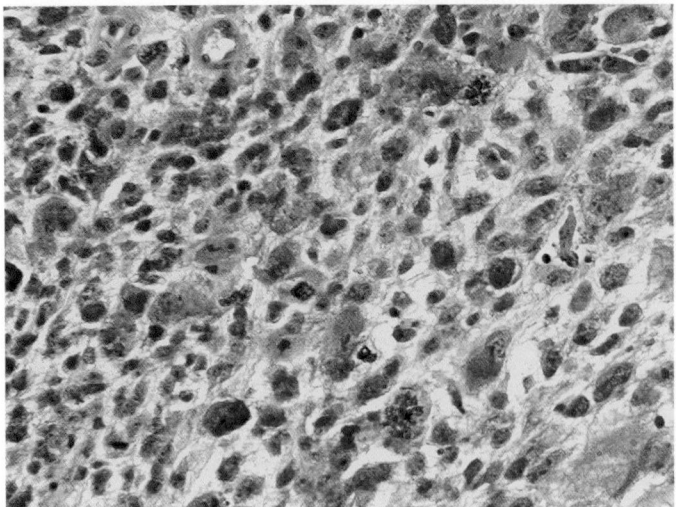

Fig. 20.15 Undifferentiated uterine sarcoma. Pleomorphic sarcoma with numerous, often atypical, mitoses.

carcinoma, leiomyosarcoma and carcinosarcoma, all of which may be morphologically similar in appearance (Fig. 20.16); extensive sampling and immunohisto-chemical staining (e.g. epithelial and smooth muscle markers) may be required.

High-grade endometrial stromal sarcoma

This terminology as applied here does not represent tumors that resemble endometrial stroma that were previously classified as high grade based upon mitotic activity alone, nor does it represent tumors that do not in some fashion exhibit features of endometrial stromal differentiation. Rather this category – and the terminology is controversial (more because of its historical association) – represents those uterine sarcomas that have a greater degree of nuclear atypia but maintain a link to endometrial stromal derivation either by morphology (with a combination of typical low-grade stromal sarcoma morphology merging with areas that exhibit cellular atypia) or growth pattern (namely finger-like myometrial permeation and lymphovascular space protrusion or involvement by tumor cells that have a higher-grade appearance) (Figs 20.17–20.19). In our experience, tumors with these patterns typically present at high stage and the tumors often recur and metastasize. Interestingly, hybrid tumors with both low- and higher-grade areas show loss of staining for CD10, a biomarker for endometrial stromal differentiation, in the higher-grade areas (Fig. 20.20). From these hybrid cases, one could (not surprisingly) argue that a subset of undifferentiated endometrial sarcoma represents undifferentiated endometrial stromal sarcomas.

MOLECULAR GENETICS

Cytogenetic abnormalities have been reported in endometrial stromal tumors, most often as chromosomal rearrangements involving chromosomes 6, 7 and 17.[58] The most common rearrangement is a reciprocal, bal-

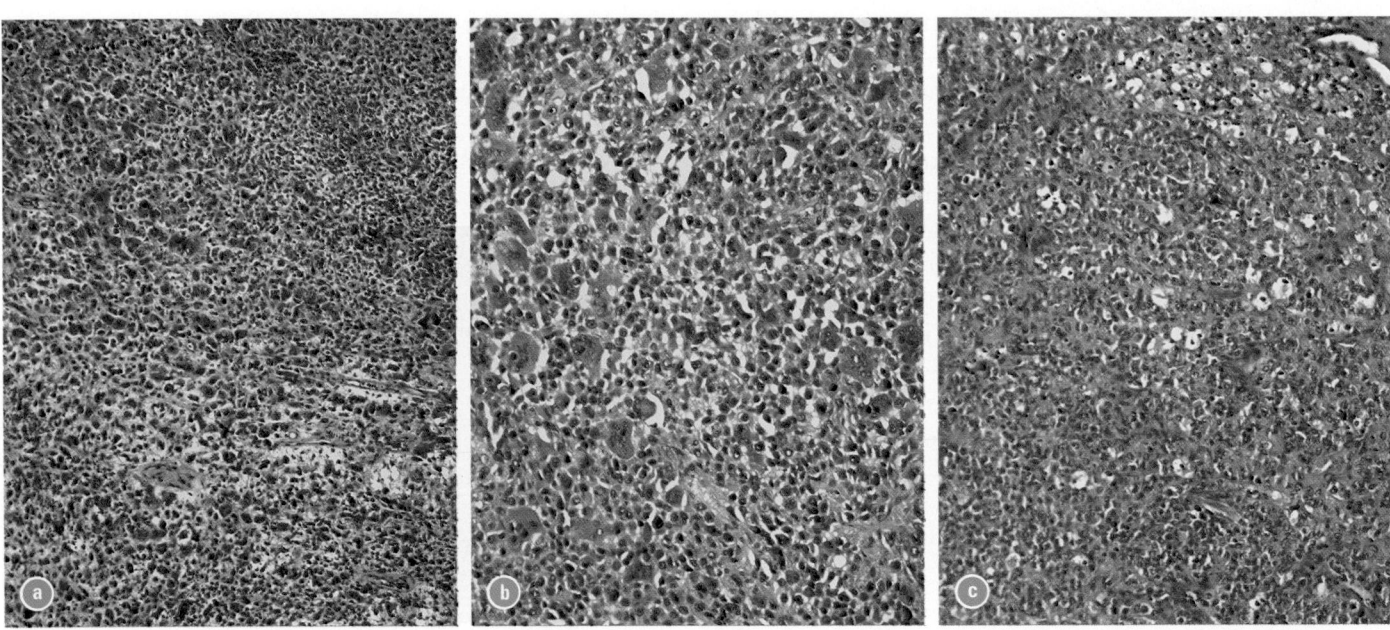

Fig. 20.16 (a) Undifferentiated uterine sarcoma may appear histologically similar to areas of (b) high-grade leiomyosarcoma and (c) poorly-differentiated carcinoma.

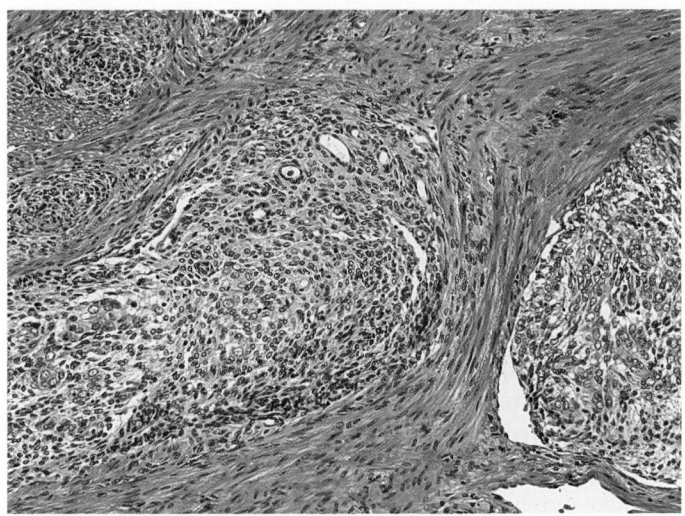

Fig. 20.17 Endometrial stromal sarcoma, low-grade with transition to high-grade areas. Typical growth pattern at low power.

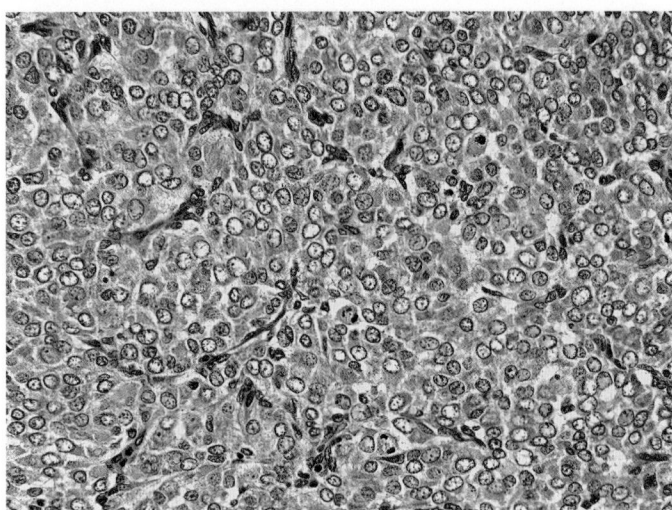

Fig. 20.19 Endometrial stromal sarcoma, high-grade area. Tumor cells appear epithelioid with more abundant cytoplasm. Note the larger, more vesicular nuclei, mitotic activity and karyorrhexis.

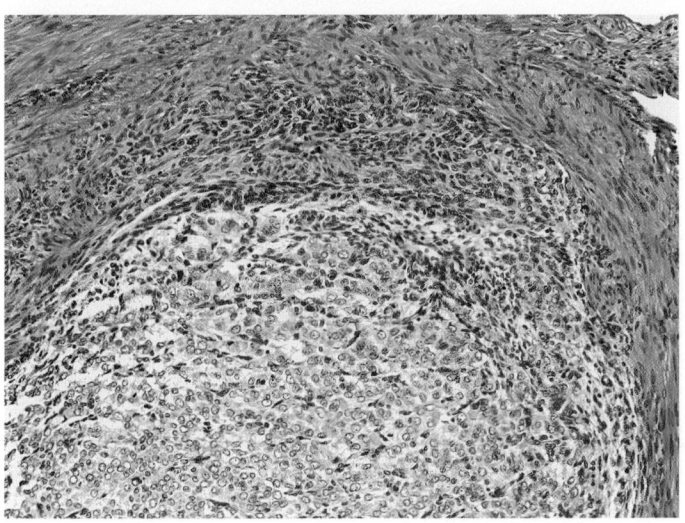

Fig. 20.18 Endometrial stromal sarcoma, low grade, with transition to high-grade areas. Periphery of the tumor nodule shows typical cytomorphology of low-grade stromal sarcoma, whereas the tumor more centrally has a higher-grade appearance with larger, vesicular nuclei and more abundant cytoplasm.

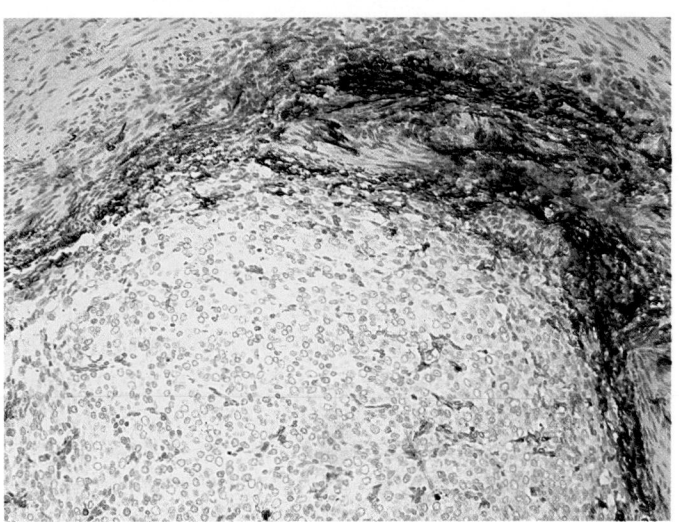

Fig. 20.20 Endometrial stromal sarcoma, low-grade with transition to high-grade areas. Loss of CD10 staining in the high-grade areas.

anced translocation between chromosomes 7 and 17, the t(7;17)(p15;q21).[58] Cytogenetic analysis by karyotyping requires fresh tumor tissue, which may not have been procured at the time of initial examination of the specimen, a scenario not uncommon with endometrial stromal tumors. Recently, two previously unknown genes, termed *JAZF1* and *JJAZ1*, were identified at the chromosomal sites of breakage in 7p15 and 17q21, respectively. In both stromal nodules and low-grade endometrial stromal sarcoma, chimeric *JAZF1-JJAZ1* mRNA transcripts can be detected by reverse transcription PCR in the majority of cases.[59] Moreover, fluo-

rescence *in situ* hybridization analysis can be performed on formalin-fixed, paraffin embedded tissue. In this technique, two fluorescently labeled human genomic probes that flank the chromosome 7 breakpoint in the t(7;17)(p15;q21) are used to test for the presence of the translocation. In a tumor that contains the translocation, the fluorescent-labeled probes are split apart yielding separate red and green signals (Fig. 20.21). A yellow signal is produced by the close apposition of the two probes marking the normal copy of chromosome 7. Endometrial stromal nodules and low-grade endometrial stromal sarcomas may show evidence of the t(7;17)

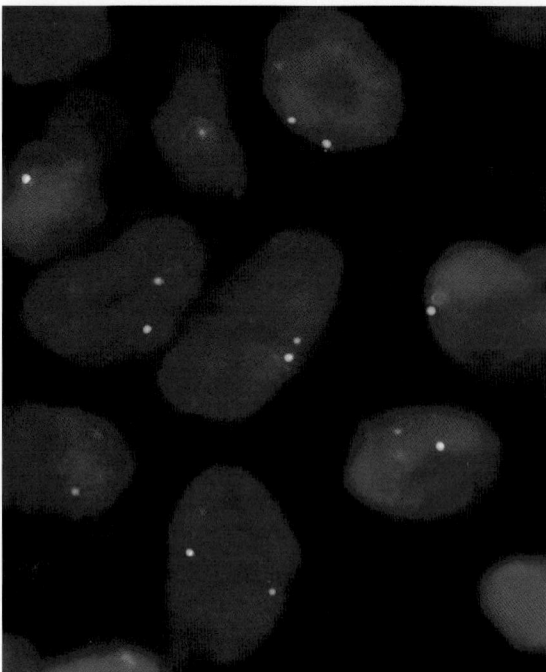

Fig. 20.21 Fluorescence *in situ* hybridization of an endometrial stromal sarcoma. Separation of the red- and green-labeled fluorescent probes that flank the breakpoint on chromosome 7 indicate the presence of the translocation involving the *JAZF1* locus.

translocation by fluorescence *in situ* hybridization, suggesting that the stromal nodule may be a precursor lesion for low-grade endometrial stromal sarcoma and that the t(7;17) is an early genetic abnormality in the development of low-grade endometrial stromal sarcoma. In addition, fluorescence *in situ* hybridization of mixed endometrial stromal–smooth muscle tumors shows evidence for the translocation in both the endometrial stromal and smooth muscle component, supporting the concept that these tumors are of endometrial stromal derivation (M.R.N., unpublished data).

INTERPRETATION OF CURETTINGS

Interpretation of an endometrial stromal neoplasm in biopsy or curettage material first depends upon its recognition as a neoplastic stromal process and its distinction from potential mimics, including endometrial basalis, aglandular functionalis, endometrial polyp and adenosarcoma. Multiple fragments of aglandular cellular stroma containing spiral arteriole-like vessels are characteristic of a stromal neoplasm. Distinction from fragments of basalis is made by virtue of the presence of an orderly component of glands in the latter and lack of the rich vasculature so characteristic of stromal neo-

plasia (Fig. 20.22). Strips of aglandular functionalis, usually associated with submucosal leiomyomata, tend to be less cellular and show features of compression or reactive surface changes (Fig. 20.23). Fragments of stroma-rich endometrial polyps usually exhibit other features of polyp, including large thick-walled vessels and abnormal glandular architecture (Fig. 20.24). Adenosarcoma also may exhibit a cellular stroma but typically have glandular cuffing, albeit sometimes subtle (Fig. 20.25). Appreciation of a more spindled atypical stroma without a rich vascular network helps facilitate this distinction.

Once a stromal neoplasm is suspected based upon histopathologic findings in the endometrial sampling, the next step in interpretation is determination of whether

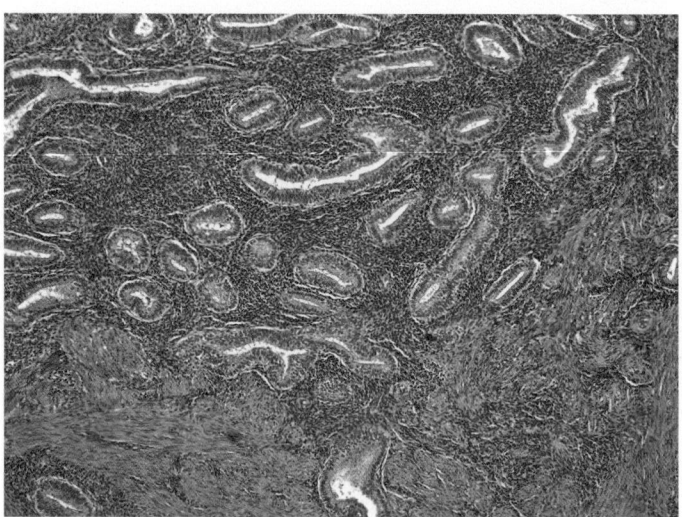

Fig. 20.22 Endometrial basalis. Note the orderly glandular component.

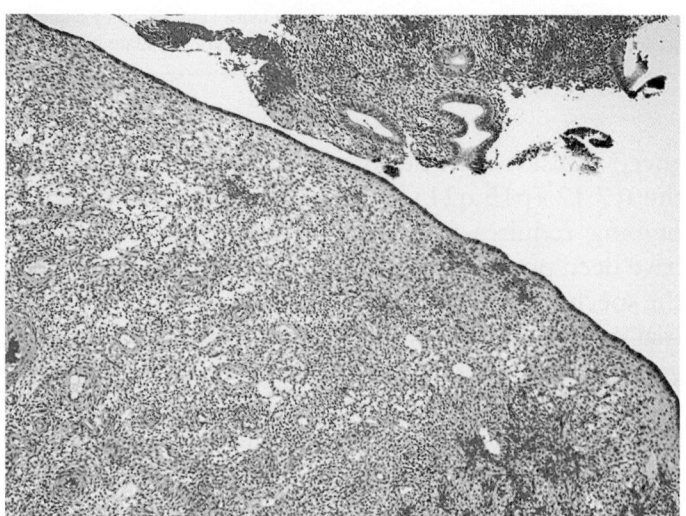

Fig. 20.23 Aglandular functionalis.

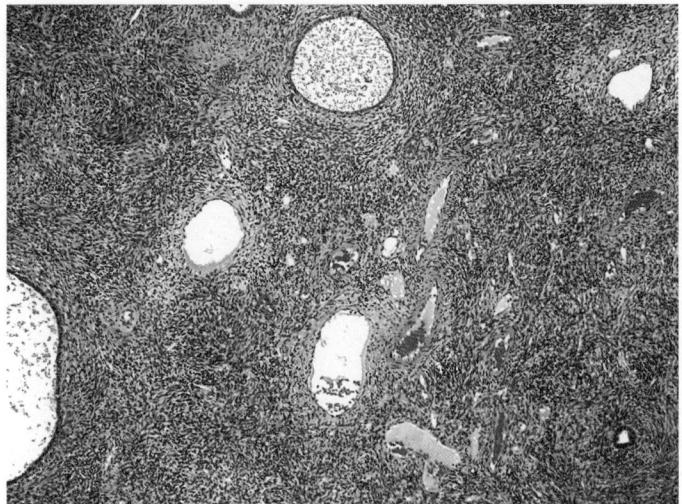

Fig. 20.24 Cellular stroma-rich endometrial polyp. Note the prominent vessels and cystic glands, which are characteristic of polyp.

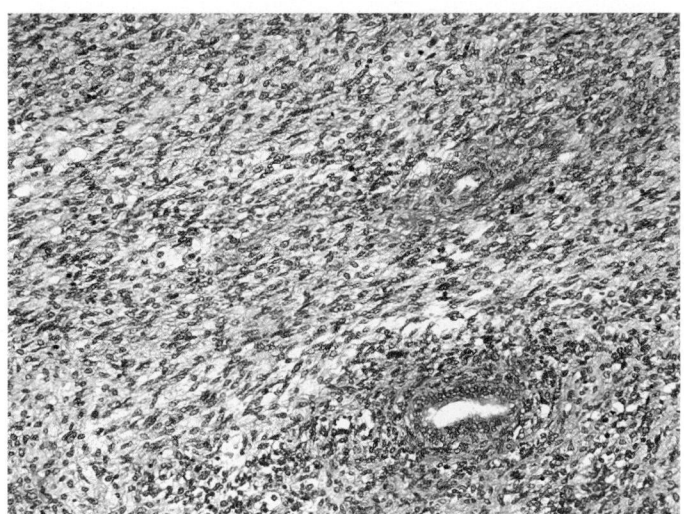

Fig. 20.25 Müllerian adenosarcoma. Periglandular cuffing and atypical stromal cells are characteristic.

or not the tumor is benign or malignant. Unfortunately, this distinction is based upon whether or not there is myometrial or lymphovascular invasion, two criteria that are difficult to interpret in biopsy or curettage material. One could raise the possibility of sarcoma if some fragments of tissue contain myometrium infiltrated by stromal tumor; however, prudent clinicopathologic correlation is critical. In general, diagnosis of an endometrial stromal neoplasm with a comment on one's inability to distinguish between a stromal nodule and sarcoma in the submitted material will be the most likely course of action.

MANAGEMENT AND PROGNOSIS

Endometrial stromal nodule

Endometrial stromal nodules are considered to be benign, non-recurring neoplasms.[47] The vast majority of women with stromal nodules have been treated by hysterectomy, due not only to their incidental discovery in hysterectomy specimens but also to the difficulty in distinguishing between stromal nodules and stromal sarcoma in biopsy or curettage material (see above). In some instances, depending on the location and size of the tumor mass, preservation of fertility may be possible with partial uterine resection, which would include the mass and a rim of myometrium to assess for invasion. Preoperative imaging as to the feasibility of such an approach would be mandatory to assess for circumscription of the mass.

Only a few women with stromal nodules have been treated conservatively (local excision) and none of the tumors have recurred.[47] In a case of an endometrial stromal nodule treated by local excision, an 8-year follow-up has been benign.[50] Occasionally, some endometrial stromal nodules exhibit greater than 3 mm extension into the surrounding myometrium, but lack the typical myometrial permeation seen in endometrial stromal sarcoma. The term 'endometrial stromal nodule with limited infiltration' has been proposed for such tumors.[50] Difficulty in predicting biologic behavior for these tumors is compounded by the fact that very few cases have been described, all have been treated by hysterectomy and long-term follow-up is not known.[50]

Low-grade endometrial stromal sarcoma

Patients with low-grade endometrial stromal sarcoma are treated by hysterectomy and bilateral salpingo-oophorectomy. Patients with tumors confined to the uterus (stage I) have an excellent prognosis, with a 5-year survival rate over 90%.[46] Recurrence is not uncommon, ranging up to 25% in patients with stage I disease.[46,60] Unfortunately, there are no histopathologic parameters to predict which patients with tumors confined to the uterus are at risk for recurrence. Distant metastases, principally involving the lung, may occasionally occur, often close to a decade following initial presentation.[61] Following surgery, treatment options include local radiation therapy (which may reduce local failure). The impact of local radiotherapy on long-term survival, however, is not known.[62] Low-grade endometrial stromal sarcoma typically is positive for progesterone receptor. Therefore hormonal therapy, particularly progestin therapy, is an option often considered in patients who present with advanced-stage disease or have recurrences.[62]

Undifferentiated uterine sarcoma

Most of the studies looking at clinical outcome with different treatment regimens do not clearly distinguish between undifferentiated uterine sarcoma and 'high-grade endometrial stromal sarcoma', with the latter category possibly encompassing tumors that would be classified according to current WHO criteria as low-grade endometrial stromal sarcoma as well as undifferentiated sarcoma. Undifferentiated uterine sarcoma is an aggressive neoplasm and treatment options, in addition to surgery, include consideration of radiation therapy for local control, as well as chemotherapy for systemic control.

BIOMARKERS AND DIFFERENTIAL DIAGNOSIS

Endometrial stromal tumors with smooth muscle differentiation or those that have a more fibrous or myxoid appearance may occasionally be confused with uterine smooth muscle tumors.[53,54,63] Conversely, uterine smooth muscle tumors may mimic endometrial stromal tumors, particularly when the former is markedly cellular (e.g. highly cellular leiomyoma; see later, in Figs 20.73, 20.74) or has prominent vascular invasion (e.g. intravenous leiomyomatosis (see later, in Fig. 20.88) and 'intravenous leiomyosarcomatosis').[51,64–67] In difficult cases, application of a panel of biomarkers may be helpful provided one is aware of potential pitfalls.

Endometrial stromal tumors are usually only focally positive for smooth muscle actin and desmin; however, a subset of morphologically typical cases may show more extensive expression of these markers.[53,63,68–72] In contrast, h-caldesmon is a more specific marker of smooth muscle differentiation than desmin and may be useful in this differential.[68,73] Non-neoplastic and neoplastic endometrial stromal cells are typically negative for this marker, whereas non-neoplastic and neoplastic uterine smooth muscle is positive (Fig. 20.26). h-Caldesmon may, in some cases of highly cellular leiomyoma, only show patchy or focal positivity (see later, in Fig. 20.76).

The role of CD10 as a potential marker of endometrial stromal differentiation was proposed based upon its unexpected expression in endometrial stromal sarcoma.[74–76] Subsequent analyses have shown that CD10 is expressed in endometrial stromal cells of the cycling endometrium (less so in decidua), adenomyosis, endometriosis as well as endometrial stromal tumors,

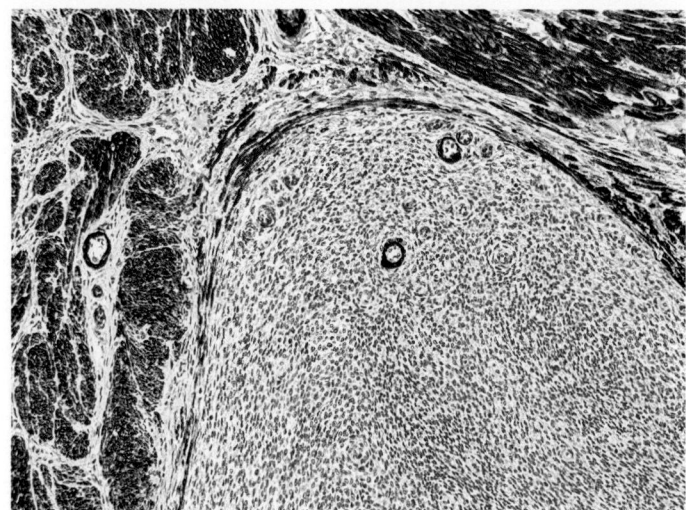

Fig. 20.26 Endometrial stromal sarcoma, low grade. H-caldesmon is diffusely positive in the surrounding myometrium and in the smooth muscle component of the vessels, but negative in the tumor.

both nodules and sarcoma (Fig. 20.27).[76–78] CD10 is typically strongly and diffusely positive in non-neoplastic and neoplastic endometrial stroma; however, some endometrial stromal tumors may be negative for this marker.[79,80] As a further caveat, smooth muscle tumors, particularly highly cellular leiomyomata and leiomyosarcoma, may be positive for CD10 (Fig. 20.28, see later at Fig. 20.77), but usually not to the degree seen in endometrial stromal tumors.

In general, the morphologic appearance of tumor cells and the growth pattern within myometrium can distinguish endometrial stromal sarcoma from

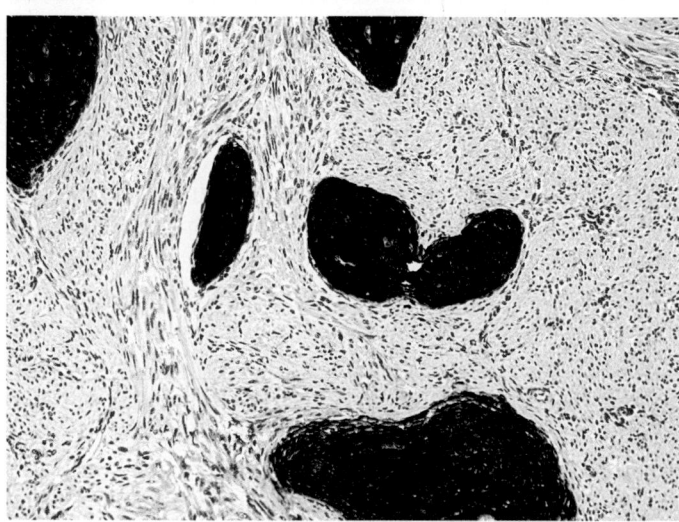

Fig. 20.27 Endometrial stromal sarcoma, low grade. CD10 is typically diffusely positive in endometrial stromal neoplasms.

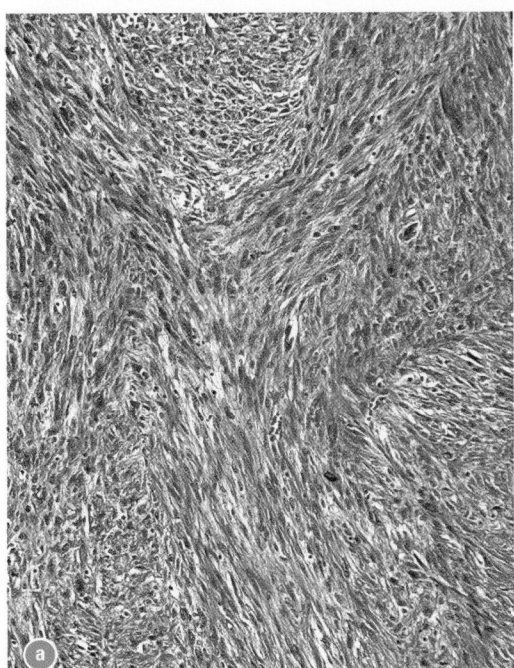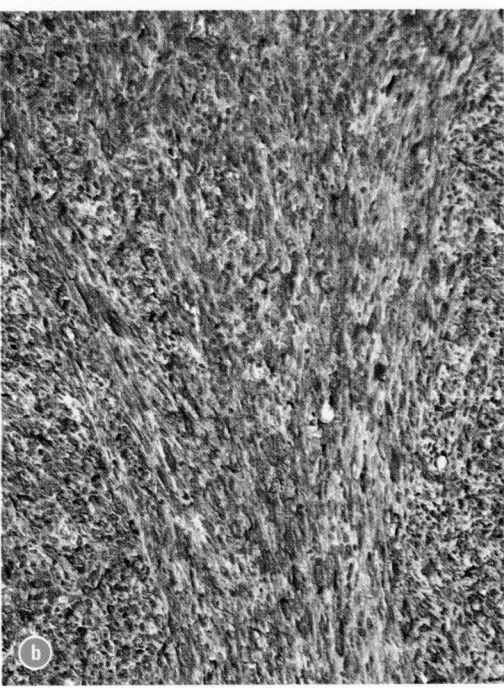

Fig. 20.28 Leiomyosarcoma. (a) Typical histologic appearance (b) with diffuse CD10 positivity.

leiomyosarcoma. In cases in which there is prominent lymphatic or vascular permeation by leiomyosarcoma, endometrial stromal sarcoma may be considered. Although morphologic features such as the presence of a fascicular architecture even in the intravascular component help facilitate its recognition as a malignant smooth muscle tumor, a panel of antibodies including h-caldesmon, desmin and CD10 may be performed in difficult cases. The majority of endometrial stromal sarcomas will be CD10 positive (diffusely)/h-caldesmon negative/desmin variable (but usually focal) and the majority of leiomyosarcoma will be h-caldesmon positive/desmin positive/CD10 variable (often positive).[68,77,79,80] The main pitfalls to consider are that nearly half of leiomyosarcomas can be CD10 positive (sometimes diffusely; Fig. 20.28), some endometrial stromal sarcomas can be diffusely positive for desmin and some endometrial stromal sarcomas can be CD10 negative. Endometrial stromal sarcomas are typically not h-caldesmon positive unless there are areas of smooth muscle differentiation. In the latter situation, interpretation of areas with classic morphology will facilitate the correct diagnosis. In the distinction from leiomyosarcoma, areas of smooth muscle differentiation in endometrial stromal sarcoma tend to be bland and will not exhibit the degree of cellularity and nuclear pleomorphism that can be present in leiomyosarcoma.

Tumors of the myometrium

DEFINITION AND CLASSIFICATION

Benign and malignant uterine smooth muscle tumors occur throughout the female genital tract from the vulva to the broad ligament and ovaries.[81–85] The vast majority of these tumors, however, are located in the uterine corpus, where they are presumed to arise from benign myometrial cells. Their location in the uterus, in combination with their size, largely determines the resulting symptoms. For example, submucosal tumors often present with abnormal bleeding and may be associated with poor reproductive outcome.[86–89] In contrast, subserosal and intramural tumors typically present with pain or impingement on nearby pelvic organs.[90–92] Subserosal leiomyomas are even thought by some to have the capacity to detach from the uterus after development of a new blood supply, earning them the colorful name of 'parasitizing' leiomyoma.[92–95]

In most cases, classification of a smooth muscle neoplasm as benign or malignant is straightforward. Such determination rests entirely on histopathologic features, particularly the presence or absence of atypia, proliferative activity and a particular pattern of necrosis.[96–103] As we shall see, uterine smooth muscle tumors are well-known for their benign variants, which have one of the features of malignancy in isolation.[96,102] Tumors with several features of malignancy (but which do not meet the criteria for the diagnosis of leiomyosarcoma) add further complexity to classification schemes. The prediction of clinical behavior of such morphologic intermediates is difficult at best. Superimposed on this spectrum of smooth muscle neoplasia are a number of morphologically benign smooth muscle proliferations with the biologic features of malignancy, namely dissemination or distant metastasis, vascular invasion, or local infiltration. This morphologic and biologic diversity makes smooth muscle neoplasia a fascinating area of study.

BENIGN LEIOMYOMA

Clinical considerations

Benign tumors of the muscular uterine wall are known variously as leiomyomata, myomas, fibromyomas, fibromas, or fibroids. Leiomyomata are observed in nearly 77% of hysterectomy specimens regardless of the indication for surgery and the average number of independent tumors per uterus has been estimated to be greater than six.[13] Consequently, they are the most common human tumor. Fortunately, only about 25% of women of reproductive age are symptomatic.[91,104]

Women with symptomatic leiomyomata generally present after age 35 years. Symptoms may include abnormal uterine bleeding, pelvic pressure or pain and reproductive dysfunction. Abnormal uterine bleeding due to leiomyomata may be characterized as menorrhagia or hypermenorrhea.[91,105] Leiomyoma-induced menorrhagia may be so severe as to require changing sanitary napkins hourly for more than 5 days; such profound bleeding can result in significant anemia.[91] Leiomyoma-associated bleeding also may become a source of social embarrassment and result in significant lost productivity.[91] Pelvic pain or pressure is typically associated with tumors large enough to distort the uterine corpus. In a testament to the size that uteri with leiomyomata may reach, these 'fibroid uteri' are clinically assessed by comparing them to gravid uteri. Thus, a symptomatic uterus may be as large as a gestational uterus at 16 to 20 weeks. In addition to pain or pressure, large tumors may compress nearby structures and occasionally cause constipation, urinary frequency, or ureteral obstruction.[91,106,107] Although uncommon, the range of reproductive dysfunction associated with leiomyomata includes infertility, spontaneous abortion, premature labor and fetal malpresentation.[108] Pseudo-Meigs' syndrome (ascites and hydrothorax) rarely may be attributed to uterine leiomyoma.[81,85,109–116]

The severity of symptoms associated with leiomyomata is broadly related to tumor size and location.[91] The myometrium can conceptually be divided into three zones: submucosal, intramural and subserosal. Submucosal leiomyomata, as well as larger intramural tumors that distort the endometrial cavity, may cause abnormal uterine bleeding (Fig. 20.29). While all of the pathophysiologic details have yet to be elucidated, attenuation of the endometrium overlying leiomyomata is frequently found. Sampling of these attenuated areas produces strips of aglandular endometrium in curettings, which can be used to suggest the diagnosis of leiomyomata (Fig. 20.23) and a cause for bleeding, provided that no other endometrial pathologies capable of causing bleeding are present. Subserosal or deeper leiomyomata are less likely to cause uterine bleeding, but are more likely to be associated with pelvic pain or pressure.

'Fibroid uterus' is the most common indication for hysterectomy and 2.1 hysterectomies per 1000 women per year are performed for this diagnosis in the USA.[117] Despite the benign nature of leiomyomata, the impact of over 200 000 major surgical procedures per year on public health and medical economics is considerable.[91] Hysterectomies performed for leiomyomata are one of the most plentiful of specimens in the practice of surgical pathology.

'Fibroids' also may be managed expectantly if associated with minimal or no symptoms. Recently, gyne-

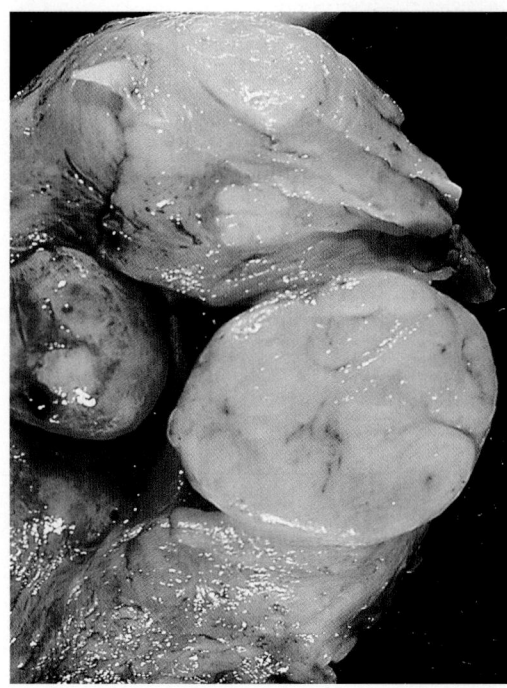

Fig. 20.29 Typical macroscopic appearance of leiomyomata of the usual type. A submucosal leiomyoma protrudes into the endometrial cavity (left). Several intramural leiomyomata have firm, white, incised surfaces that bulge out from the myometrium.

cologists and patients have expressed growing interest in avoiding hysterectomy by developing or selecting less-invasive alternatives to hysterectomy.[118,119] Myomectomy (resection with uterine conservation) is the most widely employed alternative for women who wish to preserve fertility.[120] Myomectomy may be performed using an open abdominal approach or by various closed techniques involving laparoscopy, hysteroscopy or myolysis (which involves *in situ* coagulation using a laparoscopic probe).[91] Tumor size and location play an important role in determining which technique is most appropriate. When compared with hysterectomy, these alternatives are associated with several unique risks: namely, the risks of tumor 'recurrence' and uterine rupture during pregnancy following myomectomy.[91,121–124] The risk of symptomatic recurrence is more likely due to the growth of a second crop of tumors and requires a second operation in 10–26% of cases.[91] More recently, uterine artery embolization with particles of polyvinyl alcohol has been used to treat leiomyoma non-invasively.[21,86,125–140] While uterine artery embolization results in symptomatic improvement for most patients, this technique has been associated with adverse outcomes ranging from post-procedure fevers to amenorrhea, uterine rupture, endomyometritis and fatal sepsis.[127,132,133,141] Uterine artery embolization also has been implicated as a factor delaying the diagnosis of uterine sarcomas.[142,143] The latest non-invasive technique for the treatment of leiomyomata is magnetic resonance imaging-guided focused ultrasound,[144,145] which causes thermolysis of targeted smooth muscle cells (see later, at Figs 20.69, 20.70).

While surgery has been the mainstay of treatment for benign uterine smooth muscle tumors, medical therapy may be helpful in particular circumstances. Androgenic steroids, such as danazol and gestrinone, cause amenorrhea, which may be helpful in treating leiomyoma-associated anemia.[91] Gestrinone also may reduce leiomyoma volume.[146,147] Treatment with gonadotropin releasing hormone agonists, the most widely used medical therapy for leiomyoma, also results in reduction of leiomyoma volume by 35% to 65%[91] by producing a pseudo-menopausal hypoestrogenic state. This therapy places the patient at risk for osteoporosis and other significant complications; consequently, they must be used only for a short-term time (e.g. until definitive surgery can be performed or while waiting for natural menopause to occur).[148,149] Unlike gestrinone, the reduction in tumor volume associated with gonadotropin releasing hormone agonists is rapidly reversible and, in part, may reflect volume shifts in the extracellular matrix of leiomyomata rather than changes in the neoplastic cells.[150] Volume change in treated leiomyomata may be due to changes in apoptosis and IGF-I receptor activity as well.[151,152] Mitigation of the risks associated with hypoestrogenism has been attempted by adding exogenous hormones after an initial period of complete suppression, but these protocols have not been widely adopted.[148,149] Of note to pathologists, there is little or no histologic change in leiomyomata after treatment with gonadotropin releasing hormone agonists.[150,153–155] Lastly, selective estrogen receptor modulators such as raloxifene may inhibit the growth of leiomyomatous smooth muscle cells and reduce leiomyoma volume.[156] Similar to other non-invasive therapies, medical treatment of leiomyomata may delay the diagnosis of leiomyosarcoma.[157]

Pathobiologic features of typical leiomyoma

Hormonal pathophysiology

As their response to gonadotropin releasing hormone agonists illustrate, leiomyomata are hormonally responsive tumors.[158–160] They are very rare before menarche, may grow rapidly during pregnancy or in response to clomiphene administration and often decrease in size after menopause. Moreover, the smooth muscle cells in myometrium and leiomyomata have receptors for both estrogen and progesterone,[161] with some studies suggesting that the abundance of steroid receptors is greater in leiomyoma compared with myometrium.[159,162–167] Mitotic activity in leiomyoma also varies over the course of the menstrual cycle, with the greatest activity in the periphery of the leiomyoma during the secretory (luteal) phase.[168,169] Hormone replacement therapy after menopause stimulates the growth of leiomyomata.[170,171] Finally, the presence of a polymorphism in the estrogen receptor recently has been associated with a increased risk of leiomyomata in some, but not all studies.[172,173]

Clonality

Leiomyomata are independent clonal neoplasms. The unicellular origin of leiomyomata was first established by detecting non-random inactivation of the X chromosome by Linder et al. and Townsend et al.[174,175] In these early studies, the pattern of X chromosome inactivation was established by measuring glucose-6-phosphate dehydrogenase isoforms. All tumor cells expressed only one of the allelic isoforms, indicating that they arose from a single cell in which the other allele had been inactivated by Lyonization, of which X chromosome inactivation by methylation is an important feature. More recently, this strategy has been replicated using a size polymorphism within the androgen receptor locus at Xp12 as a marker of X chromosome inactivation and, by inference, clonality.[176] Within a single uterus, the pattern of allelic inactivation is random as well, indicating that each clonal leiomyoma arose from an independent transformation event. The mechanisms accounting for this high rate of transformation in myometrial smooth muscle cell are unknown.

Genetics

There is substantial evidence of a genetic basis for uterine leiomyomata. One clue to the genetic contribution to leiomyoma tumorigenesis comes from twin studies. It has been observed that the risk for hysterectomy, a surrogate for the diagnosis of leiomyoma, doubles in monozygous (i.e. genetically identical) relative to dizygous (i.e. genetically non-identical) twins.[177,178] In addition, genetic background contributes to the risk of having symptomatic leiomyomata; premenopausal black women have a two- to three-fold increase in symptomatic fibroids compared with other ethnic groups.[14–16] Finally, studies of families also suggest a heritable predisposition to development of leiomyomata.[179,180]

Leiomyomata of the female genital tract are featured in several inherited syndromes. The most prominent of these genetic tumor syndromes is Reed syndrome, also known as multiple cutaneous and uterine leiomyomata (Mendelian Inheritance in Man, No. 150800).[181] This syndrome is characterized by autosomal dominant inheritance of multiple cutaneous leiomyomas (cutaneous leiomyomatosis), which arise from the smooth muscle of erector pili muscles beginning in late adolescence or early adulthood. In addition to cutaneous tumors, affected women in these families frequently have symptomatic uterine leiomyomata at an early age and often undergo hysterectomy before the age of 30 years. Recognition of this syndrome is important because it is also associated with renal cell carcinoma. It has also been suggested that this syndrome is associated with uterine leiomyosarcoma; however, when the uterine pathology was carefully evaluated in one case initially diagnosed as leiomyosarcoma, the tumor was subsequently determined to be an atypical leiomyoma, a histologic variant of leiomyoma described in detail in a latter section. Multiple cutaneous and uterine leiomyomata have been mapped to a locus on chromosome 1 band q42.1.[182–184] Surprisingly, this locus turns out to be fumarate hydratase (fumarase or FH), an enzyme that converts fumarate to malate in the tricarboxylic acid (or citric acid or Kreb's) cycle. The mechanism is not yet understood, but the loss of heterozygosity for the wild-type allele and near complete loss of enzymatic activity suggests that fumarate hydratase behaves like a tumor suppressor gene.[182–184] Of note, mutations in a gene encoding a succinate dehydrogenase subunit, also in the tricarboxylic acid cycle, is associated with familial paraganglioma and this parallel system tends to dispel any residual skepticism that enzymes of intermediary metabolism can act as tumor suppressors.[185–187] Abnormalities of FH, however, are not frequently found in non-syndromic leiomyomata, suggesting that the pathogenetic mechanism causing presumably sporadic leiomyoma is distinct from that causing this familial syndrome.[188,189]

Another genetic syndrome causing smooth muscle proliferation is a variant of Alport syndrome (Mendelian Inheritance in Man, No. 308940).[190] In addition to the well-known kidney manifestations, some affected individuals have esophageal and vulvar leiomyomatosis. The molecular defect in this syndrome is the deletion of the genes for the α5 and 6 chains of type IV (basement membrane) collagen (COL4A5 and COL4A6), which are arranged head-to-head on Xp22.3.[191]

Cytogenetics and molecular genetics About 40% of the typical uterine leiomyomata have at least one clonal cytogenetic aberration.[192–196] In contrast to leiomyosarcoma, the karyotypes of benign smooth muscle tumors are simple. At least six cytogenetic subgroups have been recognized in garden-variety leiomyomata: (1) deletion of 7q, (2) translocation between 12q15 and 14q24, (3) trisomy 12 and (4–6) rearrangements of 6p, 10q22 and 13q.[192–194,196–204] The large number and variety of cytogenetic subtypes suggests that there are multiple pathways to tumorigenesis in uterine smooth muscle. In cases with mosaicism, the cytogenetic abnormalities represent a secondary change acquired after transformation and clonal expansion.[176] Increased tumor size and presence of clonal cytogenetic abnormalities are related, suggesting that chromosomal abnormalities enhance the growth of leiomyomata.[205,206]

The best studied chromosomal aberration in leiomyoma is t(12;14)(q15;q24) (Fig. 20.30). This balanced translocation involves the HMGA2 and RAD51B loci on chromosomes 12 and 14, respectively.[207–216] Interestingly, HMGA2 is associated with a number of other benign mesenchymal tumors, including lipoma, breast fibroadenomas, endometrial polyps, pulmonary chondroid hamartomas, pleomorphic adenomas of the salivary gland and vulvar aggressive angiomyxoma.[207,217–221] HMGA2, also known as high mobility group protein I-C or HMGI-C, is an A-T hook DNA binding protein that contributes to transcriptional regulation. RAD51B,

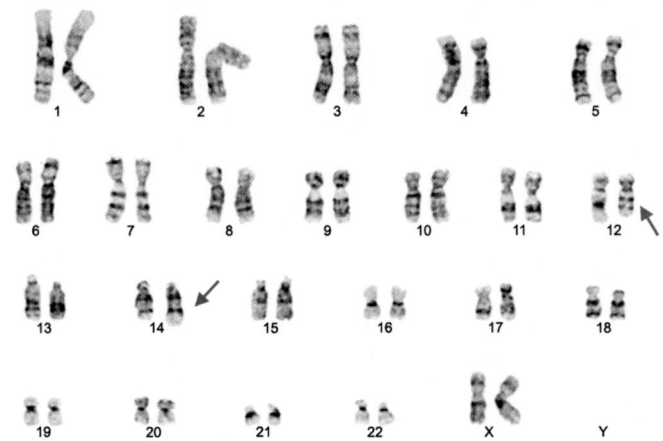

Fig. 20.30 Simple karyotypic abnormalities are found in 40% of leiomyomata. t(12;14)(q15;q24) (red arrows) is a frequent recurrent aberration and results in disruption of the *HMGA2* locus on chromosome 12. (Courtesy of Drs Cynthia Morton and Paola Dal Cin, Brigham and Women's Hospital.)

Histologic examination of typical leiomyoma shows fascicles of bland smooth cells (Fig. 20.31), which often have larger diameters and tend to be arranged with tighter packing as compared with myometrium. Consequently, the small venules are less conspicuous and less random in leiomyoma when compared with myometrium. The neoplastic smooth muscle cells themselves are virtually indistinguishable from their normal counterparts. Specifically, the cells are long and tapered, have abundant pink cytoplasm and contain spindle-shaped nuclei, which have a relatively uniform shape and size (Fig. 20.32). The chromatin is lightly stained, finely textured and uniformly dispersed. Nucleoli may be noted, but should be small and inconspicuous. As we shall see, mitotic figures may be present to varying extents, particularly in the luteal phase.[168,169] Atypical mitotic

or *RAD51-like 1*, is the human homolog of the bacterial DNA repair gene *RecA*. It appears that the critical effect of this rearrangement is inappropriate expression of *HMGA2*, either as a full length or a truncated transcript containing the DNA-binding domains.[209,210,222] This specific rearrangement has been implicated in development of pseudo-Meigs' syndrome.[109] Interestingly, the rearrangement involving 6p in leiomyoma involves the family member of *HMGA2*, namely *HMGA1*, suggesting that the two chromosomal aberrations share a common pathogenetic mechanism.[214,222–224]

Macroscopic and microscopic features of typical leiomyoma

Although the pathologic features of leiomyomata of the usual type are straightforward, a clear understanding of them is required if one is to recognize tumors requiring more scrutiny. In addition, such an understanding is required if we are to forgo sampling every 'fibroid' mass in routine surgical specimens. Fortunately, the features of typical leiomyomata are quite consistent.

The typical leiomyoma is grossly well-circumscribed (Fig. 20.29) and has a firm, rubbery texture. Upon incision, this tumor often bulges out due to increased intratumoral pressure. The cut surfaces are white or slightly pink and the bands of neoplastic smooth muscle are often whorled, giving the impression that the smooth muscle bundles are wrapped around a central core. Lastly, there should be minimal variation in the appearance of the cut surface. Any significant variation or deviation from this appearance must receive additional consideration by the pathologist.

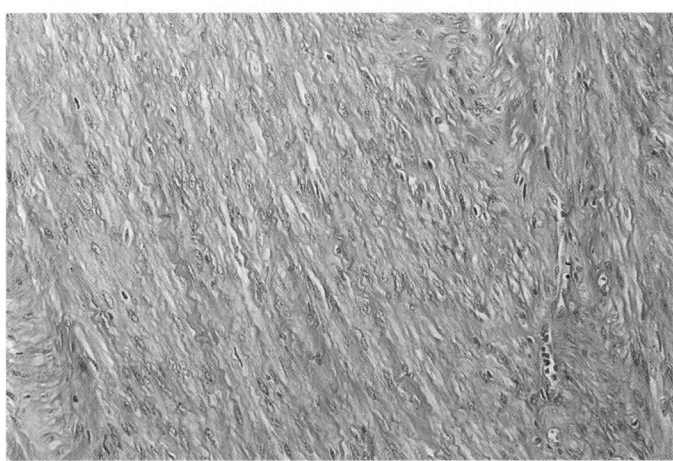

Fig. 20.31 Microscopic appearance of leiomyomata of the usual type.

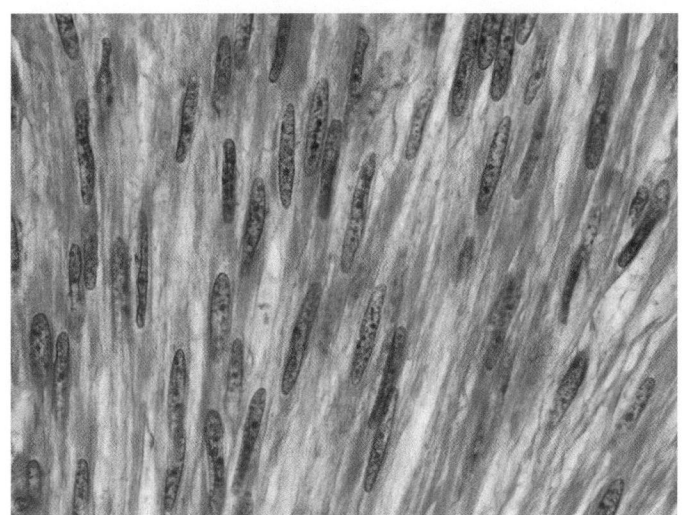

Fig. 20.32 Cytologic features of leiomyomata of the usual type.

figures, however, are worrisome and should prompt further examination and exclusion of malignancy. Interspersed among the benign smooth muscle cells of a leiomyoma, one may see varying numbers of mast cells and occasionally even prominent infiltrates of other chronic inflammatory cells.[225–230] Occasionally, dense lymphocytic infiltrates rarely may simulate lymphoma.[225,228,229] While the pathobiologic basis for the recruitment of inflammatory cells is yet to be elucidated, no specific or worrisome clinical significance has been attached to their presence. One potential exception might be the observation that fewer mast cells are found in leiomyosarcoma, while more are found in cellular and atypical leiomyoma.[227] One also may see a wide variation in the amount of collagenous extracellular matrix within benign leiomyoma. All but the most extremes in the spectrum of cellularity and hyalinization may be readily dismissed without specific comment in routine practice.

Most practitioners will find sampling every 'fibroid' impractical. This, of course, raises the question as to how many fibroids should be sampled. As latter sections will detail, leiomyosarcomas are frequently the largest mass and usually have distinctive gross features. Selective sampling of 'fibroids', therefore, requires a thorough understanding of these distinctive features of malignancy. Minimal deviations from the typical appearance of a benign fibroid merit additional tissue sampling. In typical fibroids, we prefer to sample up to three of the largest tumors in hysterectomies and every fragment in myomectomy specimens.

Alternative patterns of differentiation

From time to time, deviations from the typical spindle cell morphology will be observed. Usually, these alternate patterns of differentiation represents a minor component, but occasionally these unusual patterns may predominate. In most cases, the diagnosis of a benign tumor can be made when the alternative pattern is appreciated as such.

Plexiform and epithelioid leiomyoma

In our practice, the most frequent alternative pattern of differentiation has an epithelioid appearance, which has previously been referred to as being 'plexiform'. In plexiform leiomyoma, small ribbons or islands of rounded smooth muscle cells are present (Fig. 20.33) and it is this non-fascicular component for which the tumors are named. While most attention is focused on the epithelioid appearance of the cells in this pattern, the extracellular matrix plays an important, if not defining, role. Between the ribbons or nests of cells, abundant

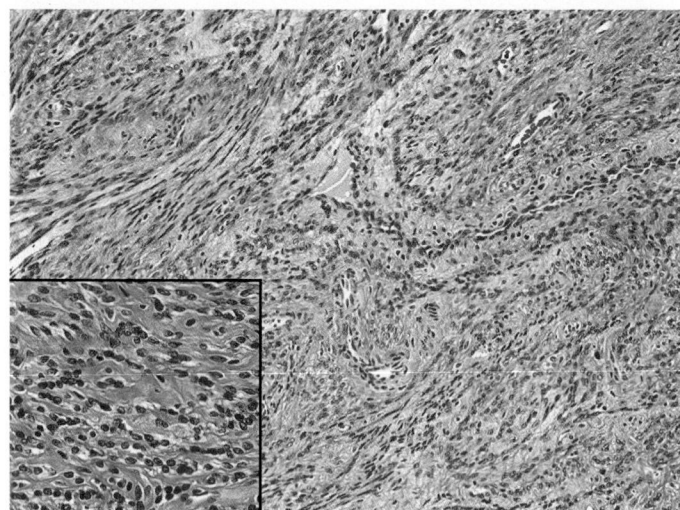

Fig. 20.33 Epithelioid leiomyoma, plexiform subtype.

matrix is present, which acts to entrap these cells and result in loss of the typical spindle shape and gain of an epithelioid appearance. Studies of leiomyoma cells suggest that extracellular matrix constituents are an important part of their repertoire of expressed genes.[231–233] In tumors with plexiform differentiation, it would seem that their capacity to synthesize extracellular matrix is particularly accentuated. In this context, we think it is important to distinguish plexiform leiomyomata (with a pseudo-epithelioid appearance secondary to matrix deposition) from smooth muscle tumors with 'true' epithelioid differentiation (see below). Finally, it has been suggested that the single filing of smooth muscle cells in a plexiform leiomyoma may be confused with metastatic breast cancer.[234] Multiple plexiform tumors also may have an infiltrative pattern and consequently mimic endometrial stromal sarcoma.[235] Thus, this variant of epithelioid leiomyoma deserves recognition as a specific entity in routine practice.

In contrast to plexiform leiomyoma, 'true' epithelioid leiomyoma, also known as leiomyoblastoma (Fig. 20.34) and clear cell leiomyoma (Fig. 20.35), are quite uncommon. Based on immunohistochemical and ultrastructural studies, it has been suggested, perhaps incorrectly, that this tumor mimics fetal myocytes.[236,237] Both epithelioid and clear cell leiomyoma are characterized by rounded or polygonal cells, rather than by spindle cells. Epithelioid leiomyoma (leiomyoblastoma) is composed of rounded cells with abundant eosinophilic cytoplasm (Fig. 20.34), whereas, as its name denotes, the clear cell variant is composed of cells with clear cytoplasm in routinely stained tissue sections (Fig. 20.35).

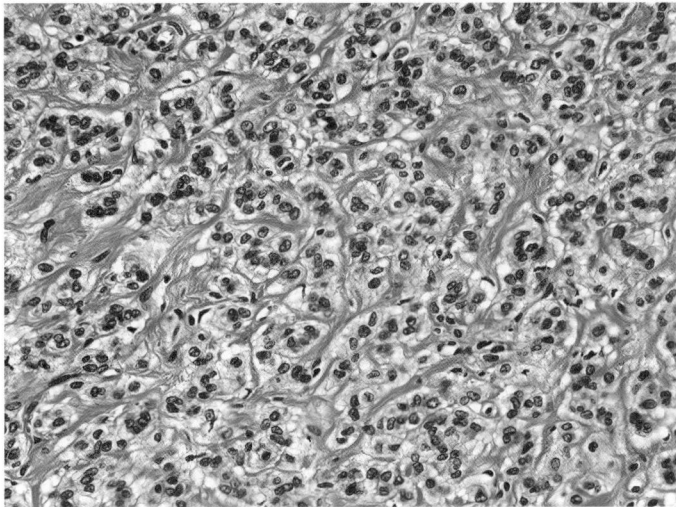

Fig. 20.34 Epithelioid leiomyoma, leiomyoblastoma subtype.

This clear appearance to the cytoplasm is due to vacuolization of mitochondria or lysosomes.[237,238]

Women with epithelioid leiomyomata have clinical characteristics similar to leiomyomata with the typical spindle cell morphology. Specifically, these tumors present in the latter reproductive years, but can occur at any age beginning in the third decade.[239] Epithelioid leiomyomata may have an unusual macroscopic appearance, which would not be specific, but should prompt more histologic sampling. The unusual features noted on inspection of the incised surface might include a softer texture, or a yellow or tan color.

The rarity of this tumor has hindered study of their natural history and, by extension, their prognostication. Their unpredictability has led some to regard epithelioid smooth muscle neoplasms as tumors of low malignant potential.[240] In one of the largest series ($n = 18$) studied to date, Prayson et al. retrospectively correlated pathologic features with clinical outcome.[239] Similar to non-epithelioid smooth muscle tumors, no one histologic feature was predictive of metastatic potential. In general, benign epithelioid smooth muscle tumors were smaller (less than 6 cm), had low mitotic rates (up to three mitoses per 10 high powered fields), lacked severe nuclear atypia and lacked tumor necrosis. In contrast, Atkins et al. have emphasized the strong association of either tumor cell necrosis or mitotic activity in excess of five mitotic figures per 10 high powered fields with poor outcome.[241] Even with these studies, classification and prognostication of epithelioid smooth muscle tumors remains problematic. Recognizing the limited experience with uterine epithelioid smooth muscle tumors, we have adopted a conservative approach to their classification reflecting published criteria,[101,239,241] which is summarized in Table 20.1.

A small number of epithelioid leiomyomata have been analyzed cytogenetically to date. In a series of five tumors, four had simple karyotypic abnormalities similar to those seen in leiomyomata of the usual histologic type.[242] Interestingly, two tumors had del(7)(q21.1q31.2), which includes the critical 7q22 region in typical leiomyoma.[243] This chromosomal deletion, however, was reported to be a secondary change in one instance.[242] Karaiskos et al. also found a balanced translocation between 12q15 and 10q22, which raises the possibility of concurrent rearrangements of the *HMGA2* and *MORF* loci.[242] The similarity between the cytogenetics of typical and epithelioid leiomyomata suggest that they share pathobiologic mechanisms. The greater com-

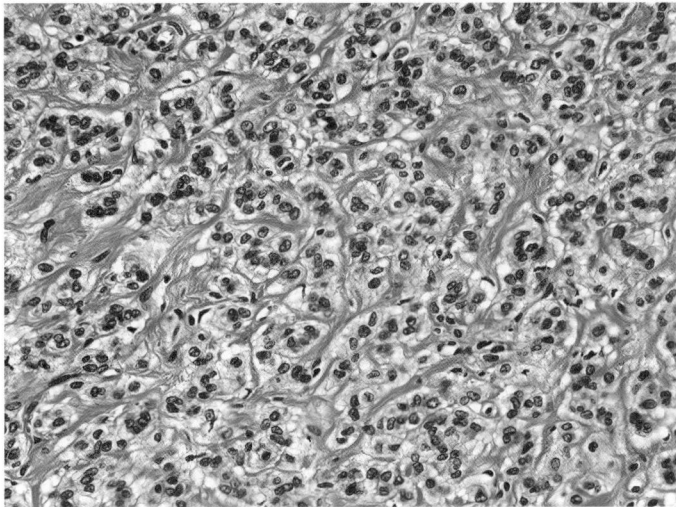

Fig. 20.35 Epithelioid leiomyoma, clear cell subtype.

Table 20.1 Practical classification of smooth muscle tumors with epithelioid differentiation

Diagnosis	Geographic tumor necrosis	Mitotic rate (mitoses per 10 high powered fields)	Atypia
Epithelioid leiomyoma, leiomyoblastoma or cell subtypes	Absent	<5	None or minimal
Epithelioid leiomyosarcoma	Present	Any rate	Present or absent
	Absent	≥5	Present or absent
Epithelioid smooth muscle tumor of uncertain malignancy	Absent		Present

plexity of cytogenetics aberrations and rearrangements involving 17q21 in two epithelioid tumors, however, may distinguish epithelioid and non-epithelioid smooth muscle tumors.[242]

Lipoleiomyoma

Lipoleiomyomata are mixed tumors in which both smooth muscle and adipose cells are present.[244] In general, smooth muscle cells outnumber adipocytes (Fig. 20.36). Rarely, the adipocytes may be so numerous as to replicate a lipoma. The incised surface of a lipoleiomyoma is often bright yellow (Fig. 20.37) and, as the fat content increases, it takes on an increasingly yellow and soft appearance, mimicking the gross appearance of a lipoma

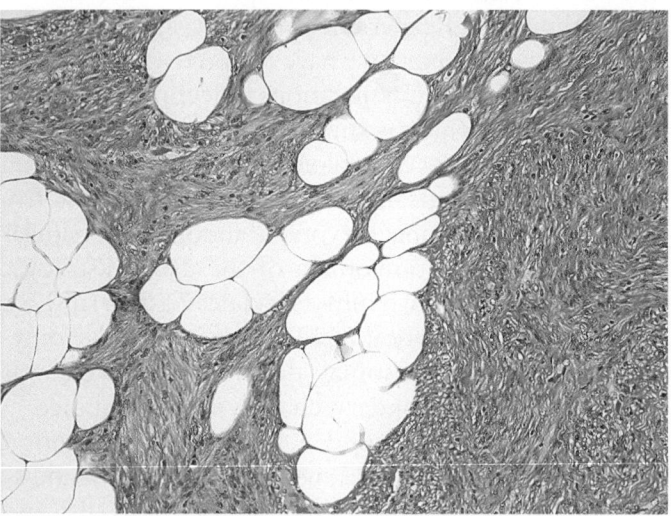

Fig. 20.36 Histologic admixture of adipocytes and smooth muscle cells in lipoleiomyoma.

(Fig. 20.38). Lipoleiomyomata are widely regarded as tumors of older women compared with typical leiomyomata, suggesting that the adipocytic differentiation is degenerative. Cytogenetic analysis of three tumors to date, however, suggests an alternative explanation. Abnormalities of chromosome 5 have been noted in two tumors, raising the possibility of a pathogenetically relevant gene.[245,246] More interestingly, two tumors have rearrangements involving 12q15.[246,247] *HMGA2*, which is located at 12q15, was shown to be aberrantly expressed in one of these tumors.[247] Of note, *HMGA2* is also involved in lipomas, as well as 10% of leiomyomata of the usual type; therefore, aberrant expression of *HMGA2* may account for the occasional adipocytic differentiation in lipoleiomyomata.

Vascular leiomyoma

Vascular leiomyomata or angiomyomata are an uncommon morphologic pattern in leiomyoma.[248] Thick-walled vessels are a characteristic of leiomyoma in general; however, in vascular leiomyomata, this component is particularly prominent (Fig. 20.39). These tumors are benign and their diagnosis carries no particular clinical implication. To date, only one tumor has been analyzed by cytogenetics, revealing the presence of t(X;11)(p11.4;p15) in the mainline and inv(2)(p15q13) and t(5;20)(q13;q13.2) in two stemlines.[249]

Miscellaneous patterns of differentiation

Other patterns of differentiation may rarely be noted and in most cases the alternative differentiation is focal. Some leiomyomas may have patches of cells with nuclear palisading that mimics a schwannoma (Fig. 20.40).[99] In others, sex-cord-like elements or tubules may be seen. Finally, uncommon tumors may harbor impressive

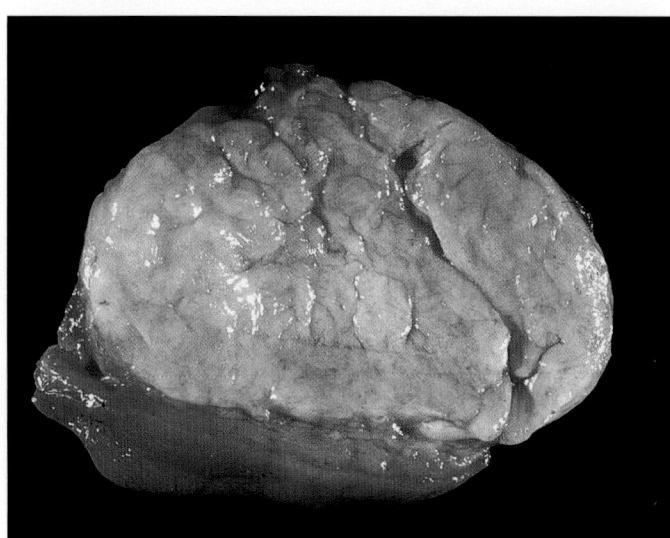

Fig. 20.37 Yellow cut surface of lipoleiomyoma.

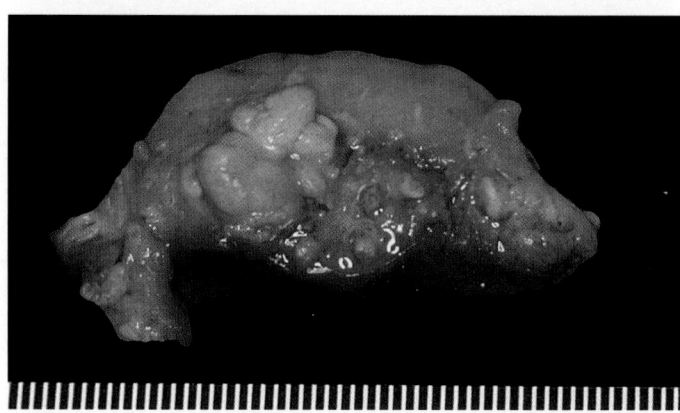

Fig. 20.38 Lipoleiomyoma with prominent adipocytic component (millimeter scale).

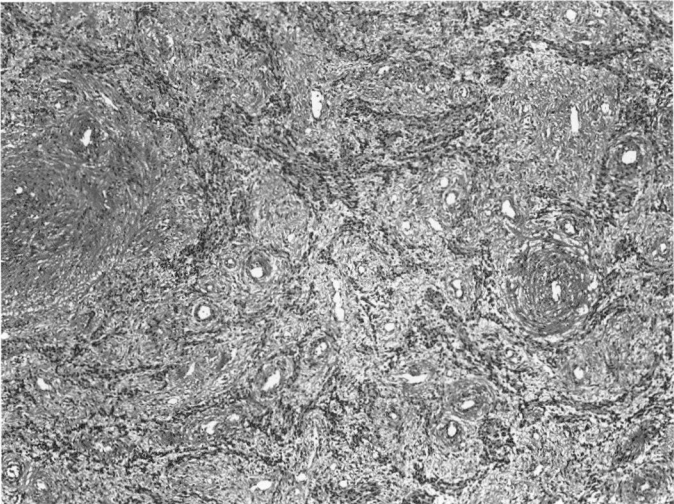

Fig. 20.39 Vascular leiomyoma with plexiform features.

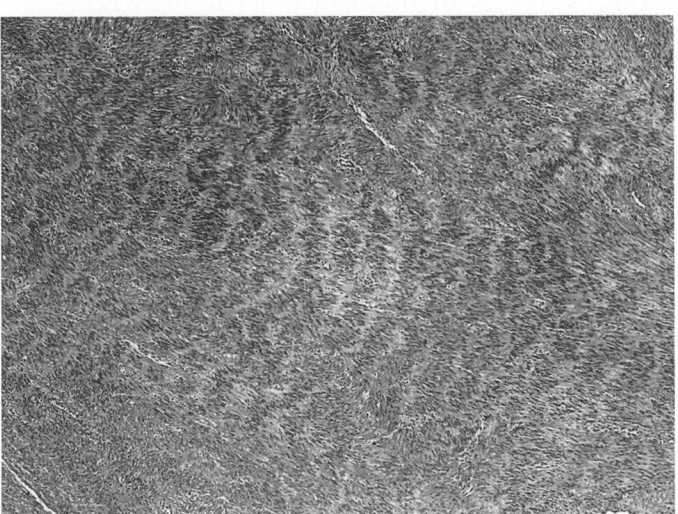

Fig. 20.40 Neurilemmoma-like leiomyoma with nuclear palisading.

numbers of inflammatory or hematopoietic cells.[225–230] While the presence of these admixed cells or aberrant differentiation may pose an interesting scientific puzzle, such tumors behave in benign fashion.

MALIGNANT LEIOMYOSARCOMA

Clinical considerations

In contrast to benign uterine smooth muscle tumors, leiomyosarcomas are fortunately rare, accounting for 1% of all uterine malignancies.[250] Nevertheless, they are the most frequent malignant mesenchymal tumor of the uterus, accounting for 25% of all uterine mesenchymal neoplasms. Their annual incidence has been estimated to be 0.64 cases per 100 000 women.[251] In addition, it has been estimated that the incidence of leiomyosarcoma in women with the preoperative diagnosis of 'fibroid uterus' is between 0.13 and 0.29%.[252] The incidence of leiomyosarcomas may be increased in populations of black women compared with other ethnic backgrounds, but the magnitude of this increase is very modest relative to that noted for benign leiomyomata.[1] In comparison to benign smooth muscle tumors, leiomyosarcomas tend to present later in life, usually around or after menopause. Their incidence rises steadily from 0.2% in the fourth decade to 1.7% in the seventh decade.[252] Consequently, clinical appreciation of a large or rapidly growing 'fibroid' after menopause or during gonadotropin releasing hormone agonist (e.g. leuprolide) therapy is a very worrisome sign.[253–256] Most leiomyosarcomas, however, are unsuspected or presumed to be leiomyomata prior to pathologic examination of a surgical specimen. A small fraction of malignant or suspicious tumors are diagnosed when fragments are obtained by curettage or hysteroscopic myomectomy.

Uterine leiomyosarcomas are highly malignant neoplasms, notable for aggressive growth, local recurrence and frequent distant metastasis.[257–260] Lung and liver are the most frequent sites of metastasis, but unusual sites such as skeletal muscle have been reported.[261–263] Lymph node and ovarian metastasis are uncommon, especially in the absence of extensive extrauterine disease.[264,265]

Pathobiologic features

The cytogenetic changes found in uterine leiomyosarcoma are far more complex than those found in leiomyomata of the usual type.[266–277] These changes include both numerical and structural abnormalities (Fig. 20.41). In addition, specific cytogenetic aberrations may vary from metaphase to metaphase. Such variations suggest that there is a high level of genomic instability in uterine leiomyosarcoma. The high frequency of chromosomal aberrations in leiomyosarcoma correlates with nuclear atypia and accounts for variations from diploidy.[278–280] These changes also hint at the underlying pathobiologic processes that drive malignant smooth muscle neoplasia. Some uterine and extrauterine leiomyosarcomas, however, have been reported to have far simpler karyotypes.[281] The overall complexity of genomic alteration has precluded a positional approach to leiomyosarcoma gene discovery, but tumors with simpler alterations may be targets for positional cloning. With a few exceptions to be noted in subsequent sections, few smooth tumors with features between typical benign and malignant smooth muscle tumors have been characterized by cytogenetic analysis.

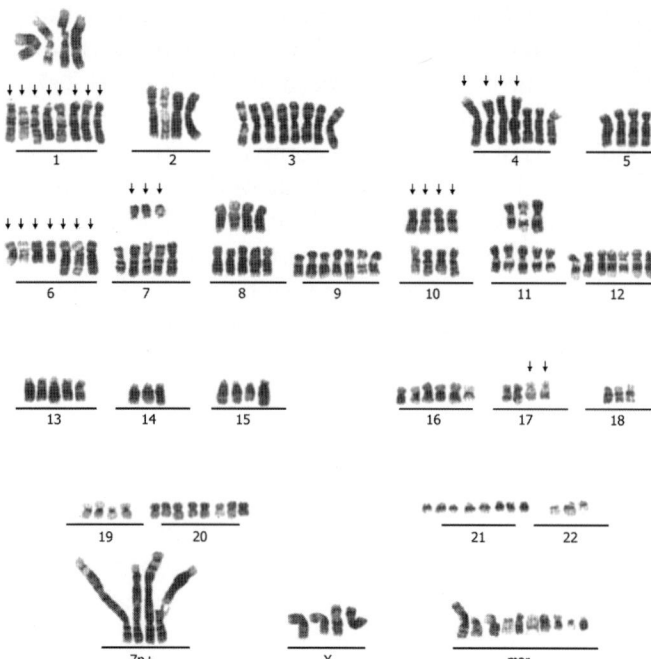

Fig. 20.41 Complex karyotypic abnormalities (including both structural and numerical aberrations) are common in leiomyosarcoma. Marker chromosomes (mar) cannot be classified as to their chromosomal origin. (Courtesy of Dr J. Fletcher, Brigham and Women's Hospital.)

The genomic instability found in leiomyosarcoma by cytogenetic analysis is also reflected by other techniques measuring allelic imbalance. In general, the results of comparative genomic hybridization, a technique for measuring gross chromosomal gains and losses, shows multiple and complex changes in leiomyosarcoma and little, if any, changes in leiomyoma. In particular, loss of heterozygosity for long arms of chromosomes 10 and 13 are found in more than half of leiomyosarcomas, but not in leiomyomata.[246,282] Although not as frequent, gains of 17p, Xp and especially 1q also have been noted.[276,283,284] While these studies have not pointed directly to new diagnostic or therapeutic targets, they reinforce the notion that genomic instability is an important distinction between benign and malignant uterine smooth muscle tumors. Furthermore, the lack of a common pattern of allelic imbalance in uterine smooth muscle tumors suggests that uterine leiomyosarcomas and leiomyomata (at least tumors of the usual type) have different pathogeneses.

Given the complexity of the genomic alteration in leiomyosarcoma, several groups have attempted to understand uterine smooth muscle neoplasia by studying their transcriptional profiles.[233,285–291] As might be expected, the differences in gene expression between myometrium and leiomyomata are small. Larger differences can be

found between the expression profiles of leiomyosarcomas and leiomyomata or myometrium. Down-regulation of gene expression is more frequent in malignant tumors.[233] The distinct clustering of benign and malignant samples provides additional evidence that the pathways to leiomyoma are distinct from the pathway(s) to leiomyosarcoma and are the targets for the development of new clinical biomarkers.

Macroscopic and microscopic features

Most leiomyosarcoma present as large dominant masses, often greater than 10 cm in greatest dimension (Fig. 20.42).[292] Similar to leiomyoma, they may arise throughout the female genital tract. Uterine leiomyosarcomas may be present in the subserosal, intramural and submucosal compartments and they are frequently large enough to span more than one compartment. Most leiomyosarcomas are distinctly different macroscopically from typical leiomyomata (Table 20.2). Their cut surfaces are variegated due to the presence of hemorrhage or necrosis (Figs 20.43–20.45) and the hemorrhagic and necrotic zones are often grossly patchy, involving irregularly shaped areas in an apparently random distribution. The necrotic areas may appear shades of green and yellow while the non-necrotic areas have a prototypical appearance that has been likened to 'fish flesh' by some. Leiomyosarcomas have earned this 'tasteful' description for their grayer color, softer (i.e. non-rubbery) consistency, indistinct bundling and decreased bulging of the cut surface as compared with leiomyomata (Fig. 20.46). Recognition of these gross features cannot be emphasized enough, as they are the trigger for more extensive sampling by the prosector.

Although gross features impact the level of suspicion for malignancy, malignancy is solely determined by histologic examination (Table 20.3). Leiomyosarcomas often have severe nuclear and cytologic atypia,

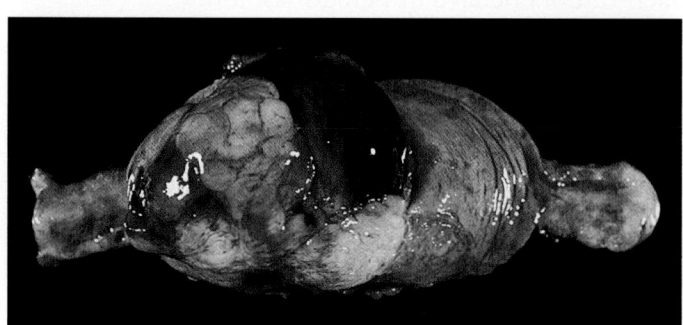

Fig. 20.42 Leiomyosarcoma presenting as a large, intracavitary mass with hemorrhage.

Table 20.2 *Macroscopic pathologic features of leiomyosarcoma compared with leiomyoma*

Pathologic feature	Leiomyosarcoma	Leiomyoma
Multiplicity	Solitary, often dominant mass	Multiple masses
Gross circumscription	Poorly-defined or grossly invasive	Well-defined, usually bulging and compressing adjacent tissues
Variegation of incised surface	Common, often prominent; multifocal hemorrhage or necrosis	Uncommon, often focal or central
Color of incised surface	gray, yellow, or tan	White or tan
Consistency of incised surface	Soft, 'fish-flesh'-like	Firm, whorled

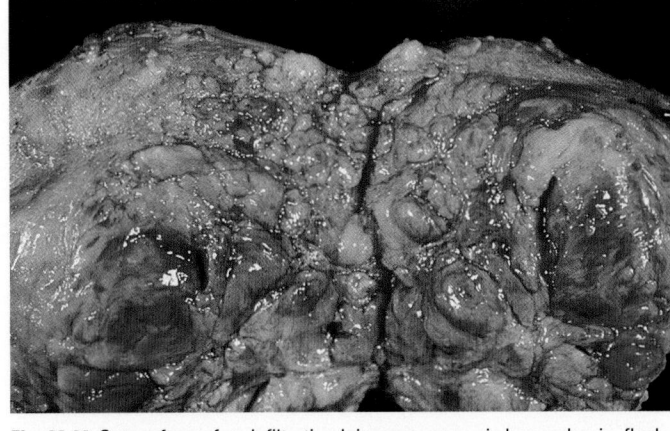

Fig. 20.44 Cut surface of an infiltrating leiomyosarcoma is hemorrhagic, fleshy and partially necrotic (greenish areas). Infiltration into myometrium is seen in the upper left quadrant.

obvious proliferative activity and cellular instability manifested as a particular pattern of necrosis. These three features are the principal factors in the determination of malignancy.[96–101,103] In addition, these tumors may be hypercellular and infiltrate into surrounding myometrium. Diagnosis of malignancy is not difficult when all of these features are present, particularly when florid. Clinical prognostication becomes more difficult when fewer features are present or less pronounced.[96–99,101] It has been long recognized that any

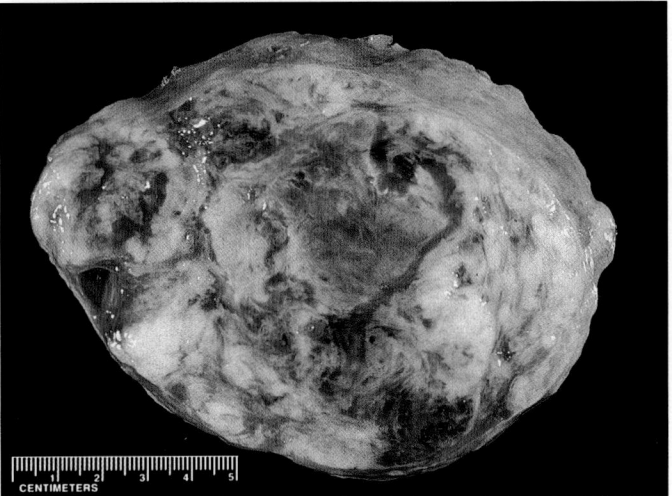

Fig. 20.45 Leiomyosarcoma with hemorrhage and irregular areas of necrosis.

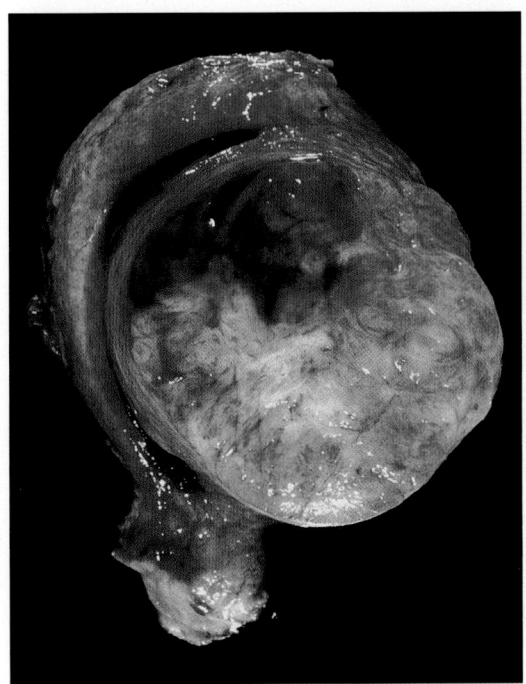

Fig. 20.43 Cut surface of an intracavitary leiomyosarcoma with hemorrhage and variegated color.

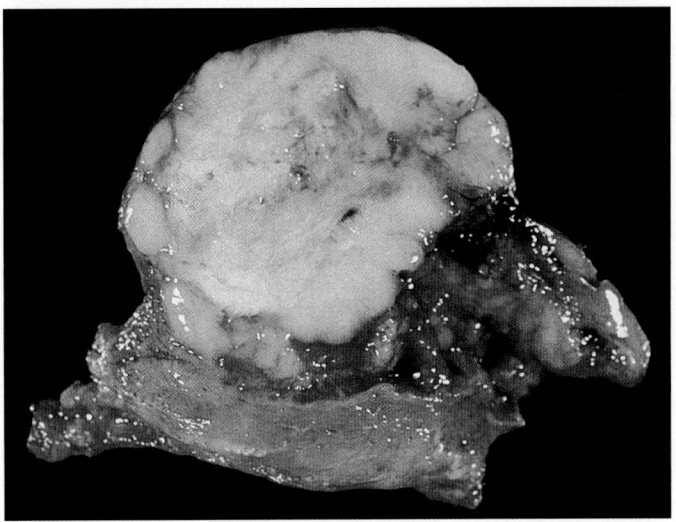

Fig. 20.46 Cut surface of leiomyosarcoma is flat and fleshy, with indistinct non-bulging whorls.

Table 20.3 *Microscopic pathologic features of leiomyosarcoma compared with leiomyoma*

Pathologic feature	Leiomyosarcoma	Leiomyoma
Proliferative activity	Usually elevated, often with abnormal forms	Variable, but usually low
Nuclear and cytologic atypia	Notable at low magnification; may be diffuse or focal; occasionally extreme	Rarely present
Pattern of degeneration	Coagulative, geographic tumor cell necrosis	Infarctive, hyaline, hydropic, or mucinous patterns
Cellularity	Usually hypercellular, sometimes prominent	Variable, but usually only moderately elevated
Microscopic border	Infiltrating adjacent myometrial fascicles	Sharp or interdigitating with adjacent myometrial fascicles

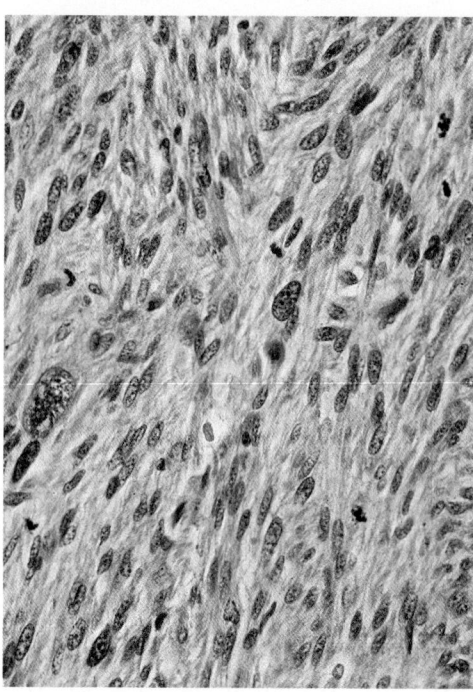

Fig. 20.47 Microscopic appearance of leiomyosarcoma includes frequent mitotic figures, nuclear atypia and hypercellularity.

attempt to classify these tumors must assess several histologic features concurrently.[96,102] Over time and based on a landmark study by Bell et al., the weight of each recognized feature has been evaluated and the classification schema adapted to reflect the relative importance of the various features studied.[101,103] Variants of benign leiomyoma defined by each of these histologic features (see next section) must also be taken into account.[102] Before these conceptual approaches can be applied, however, we must first make careful microscopic observation, guided by thorough gross examination.

Evaluation of mitotic activity

The first feature to be evaluated is proliferative activity (Fig. 20.47).[99] As previously noted, leiomyosarcomas have significant derangements affecting cell cycle control. Mitotic activity may be quite extreme and is amenable to a more quantitative evaluation. Typically, mitotic figures are counted in adjacent high power fields (i.e. with the 40× objective) and averaged over 10 fields. While there is no specific protocol, it is reasonable to count at least 30 and perhaps more fields when calculating this average. It also may be helpful to note the mitotic rate of proliferative 'hot spots' when found.[96] In fact, these counts are probably more clinically meaningful if counting is biased to these areas by starting the count in a proliferative area found at lower magnification. The area to be counted must be selected carefully, as we have seen focal proliferation in benign submucous tumors as they ulcerate into the endometrial or endocervical cavities. A more important caveat is that each potential mitotic figure must be

carefully scrutinized to be sure that it is not a degenerating cell.[96] Such mimics with pyknotic nuclei are common in both benign and malignant tumors and casual counting may drastically overestimate proliferation in a given tumor (Fig. 20.48). It should be recognized that area selection and rigor in counting add a subjective component to an otherwise quantitative parameter.

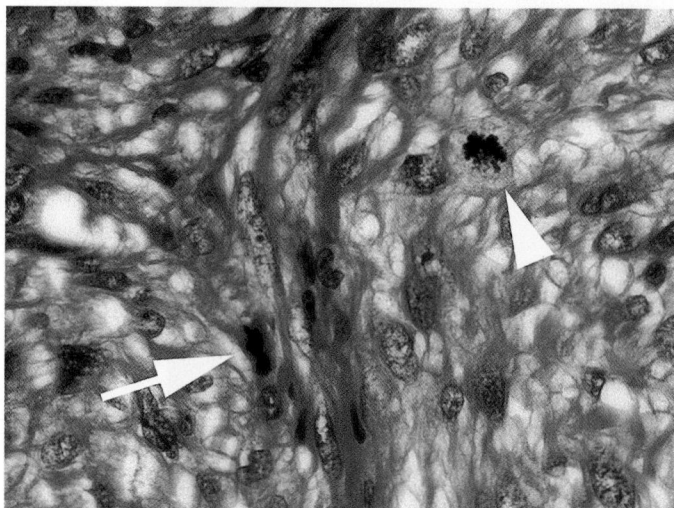

Fig. 20.48 Pyknotic (presumably degenerating) nuclei may mimic mitotic figures in leiomyosarcomas (arrow). Note the eosinophilic cytoplasm of this degenerating cell. An early mitotic figure, with distinct chromosomes visible, is shown for comparison (arrowhead).

Evaluation of atypical mitotic figures

A feature related to mitotic activity is the presence of atypical mitotic figures. Unlike mitotic rate, atypical mitotic figures are not common and consequently not amenable to quantification. Atypical mitotic figures, however, reflect genomic instability, a pathologic feature of leiomyosarcoma and other malignant tumors and may be helpful when found.[103] Declaration of atypia in mitotic figures also has a subjective component. To avoid this pitfall, we look for metaphases with more than one spindle axis (Fig. 20.49) or anaphases in which individual chromosomes lag far behind their companions as they are drawn to the pole of their spindle apparatus (Fig. 20.50). Such aberrations are believed to account for aberrant chromosome segregation or cycles of breakage and fusion, respectively. Mitotic atypia also may be observed in the form of metaphases with far too many chromosomes to be diploid. This criterion may be difficult to apply when subtle and should be used conservatively.

Evaluation of cytologic atypia

Another important feature of malignancy in smooth muscle neoplasia is cytologic atypia (Figs 20.47, 20.51, 20.52). Atypia may be manifested in both the nucleus and cytoplasm of the neoplastic smooth muscle cell. The nuclei of benign smooth muscle cells of myometrium and leiomyoma have a fairly uniform spindle or corkscrew shape and are filled with bland, dispersed chromatin. Nuclear atypia consists of prominent hyperchromasia and coarsening of chromatin texture, nuclear enlargement, multinucleation, multilobation and other varia-

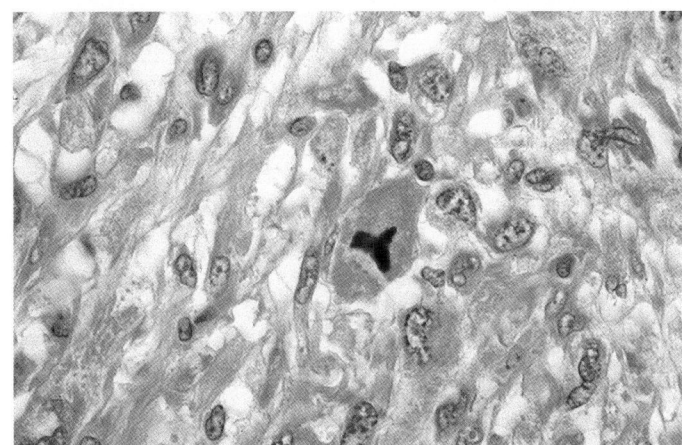

Fig. 20.49 Atypical mitotic figures in leiomyosarcomas include multipolar spindles.

tions in nuclear shape and uniformity. The degree of nuclear atypia found in leiomyosarcomas spans a wide spectrum. In the extreme, it may be evocative of a trophoblastic malignancy (Fig. 20.51). Pleomorphic tumor cells also may resemble inflammatory giant cells (Fig. 20.52). By wide agreement, the atypia should be notable at low (i.e. 10× objective) power for it to warrant classification as significant nuclear atypia. Mild nuclear changes, usually first noticed at higher magnification, do not predict clinical or biologic behavior.[101] Cytologic atypia also may be manifested in leiomyosarcoma by divergent (heterologous) patterns of differentiation, which may include osteosarcomatous, rhabdomyosarcomatous and chondrosarcomatous foci (Fig. 20.53).

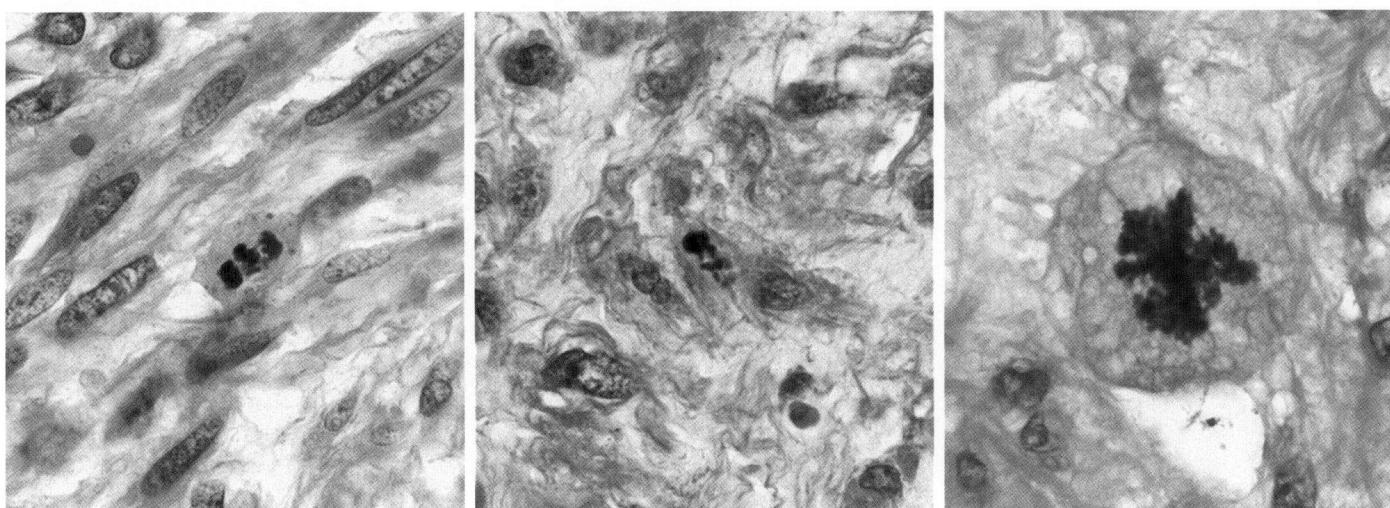

Fig. 20.50 Atypical mitotic figures in leiomyosarcomas include lagging chromosomes (left and middle), as well as extreme aneuploidy (right).

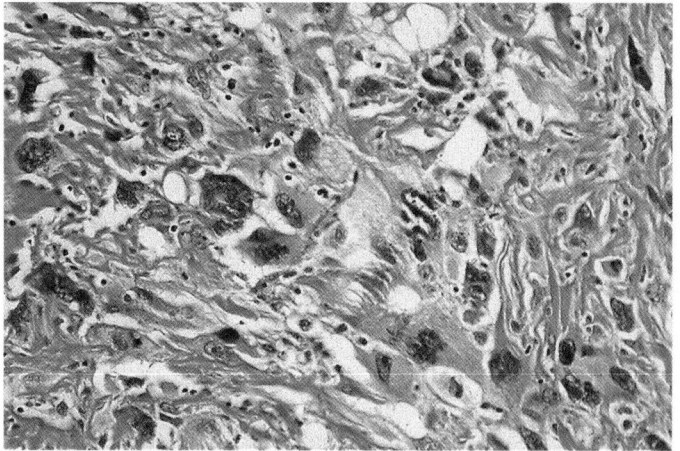

Fig. 20.51 Leiomyosarcoma with extreme nuclear atypia resembling malignant trophoblasts.

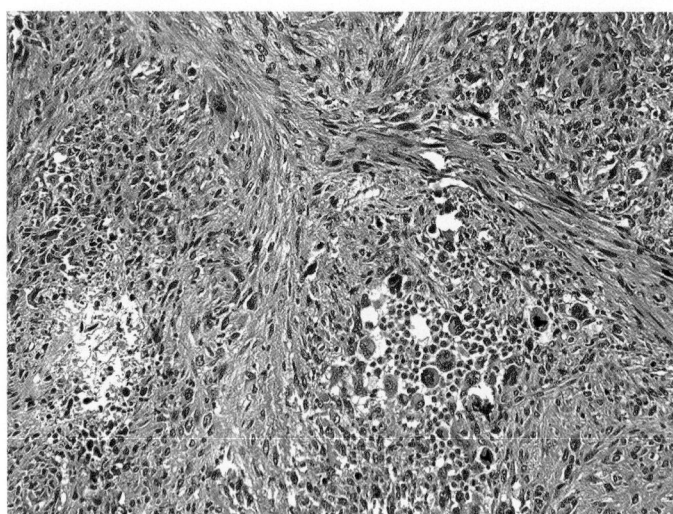

Fig. 20.52 Atypical giant cells in a leiomyosarcoma.

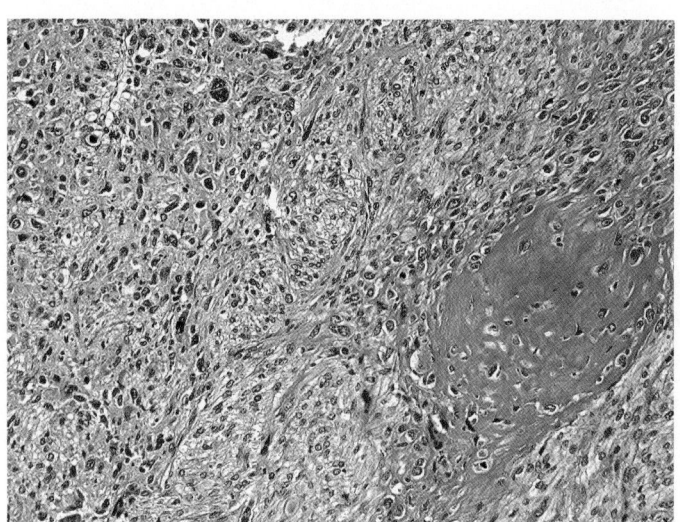

Fig. 20.53 Osteosarcomatous and other heterologous differentiation is another form of atypia in leiomyosarcoma.

Evaluation of tumor cell necrosis

Of the three principal factors, tumor necrosis is considered by some to carry the greatest weight in the determination of malignancy (Figs 20.54–20.56). Malignancy-associated tumor necrosis has to be carefully delineated and distinguished from benign degenerative changes and other therapeutic effects. The elements that should be considered in evaluating non-viable tissue in a uterine smooth muscle tumor are listed in Table 20.4 and compared with degenerating leiomyoma in the later section on leiomyoma variants. Tumor necrosis associated with malignancy is described as being 'geographic' because the contour of the interface with viable tumor

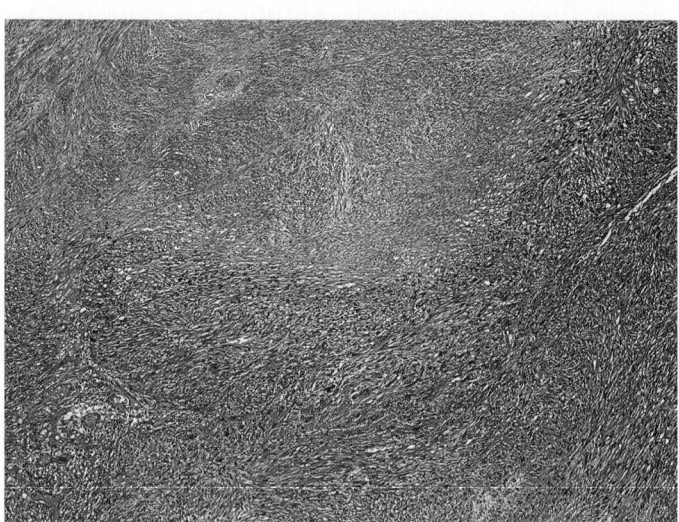

Fig. 20.54 Geographic tumor necrosis in a malignant uterine leiomyosarcoma. Note the sharp border of the island-like zone of tumor cell necrosis.

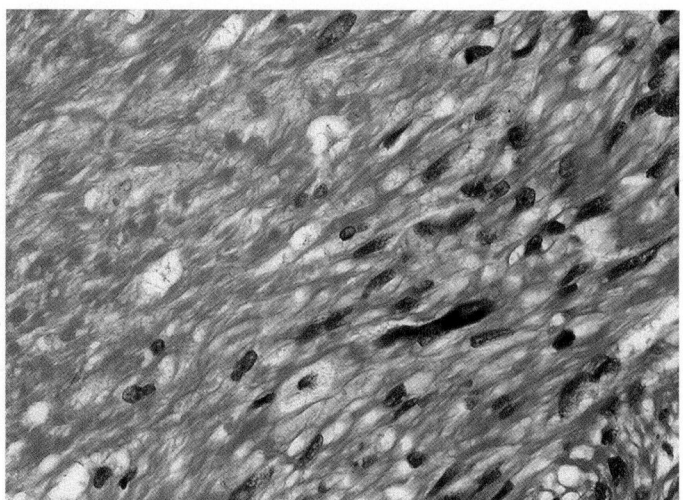

Fig. 20.55 The interface between viable and non-viable cells in geographic tumor necrosis usually spans fewer than five cells.

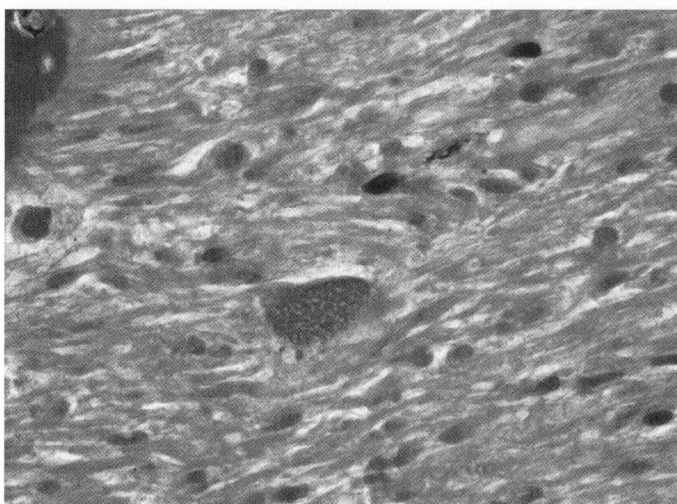

Fig. 20.56 Atypical ghost cell in geographic tumor cell necrosis.

Table 20.5 Practical classification of smooth muscle tumors with typical spindle cell differentiation

Diagnosis	Geographic tumor necrosis	Mitotic rate (mitoses per 10 high powered fields)	Atypia
Leiomyosarcoma	Present Absent	Any rate ≥10	Present or absent Diffuse or multifocal; moderate to severe
Smooth muscle tumor of uncertain malignant potential (STUMP)	Questionable Absent Absent	Any rate >15 Approaching, but less than 10	Present or absent None Diffuse or multifocal; moderate to severe
Atypical leiomyoma	Absent	≤10	Diffuse or multifocal; moderate to severe
Leiomyoma with increased mitotic activity	Absent	≤15	Absent

is often irregular and undulating or angulated, like islands on a map (Fig. 20.54). The transition from viable to necrotic tumor is sharp and on the scale of a few cells (Fig. 20.55). In contrast to benign degeneration due to ischemia, malignant tumor necrosis is not associated with any inflammatory or repair reaction. In addition, atypical 'ghost' cells (necrotic cells in which cell borders and cytologic atypia are still apparent) may be seen in malignant tumor necrosis (Fig. 20.56). Any of these features may herald the diagnosis of malignancy.

Practical diagnostic strategy

The diagnosis of leiomyosarcoma requires the evaluation of multiple individual criteria as described above. The following approach, by integrating the aforementioned microscopic observations, may be helpful in diagnostic deliberations (Table 20.5). The diagnosis of leiomyosarcoma is made when any of the follow

Table 20.4 Distinguishing features of necrosis in malignant and benign uterine smooth muscle tumors

Malignant geographic tumor necrosis	Benign
Multifocal	Single, often central
Irregular, map- or island-like contour	Smooth, rounded contour
Sharp interface	Ill-defined interface
Atypical 'ghost' cells	Bland eosinophilic cells without sharp outlines
Inflammation uncommon	Inflammatory response at the interface
Fibroblastic repair at the interface uncommon	Peripheral fibrosis or central mummifications

conditions are satisfied: (1) geographic tumor necrosis is definitely present; or (2) both proliferative activity greater than or equal to 10 mitotic figures per 10 high powered fields and moderate to severe, diffuse or multifocal atypia are present.

Epithelioid leiomyosarcoma

Epithelioid differentiation in uterine leiomyosarcomas, characterized as rounded, non-spindled tumor cells with abundant eosinophilic cytoplasm, may be focal or uniform (Fig. 20.57). When prominent, specific recognition as an epithelioid leiomyosarcoma is appropriate. These tumors have the other features expected in non-epithelioid leiomyosarcomas. In particular, mitotic activity in excess of five mitotic figures per 10 high powered figures or geographic tumor necrosis are indicative of malignancy (Table 20.1).[241] Other features of malignancy in epithelioid smooth muscle tumors include nuclear atypia, particularly if it is severe, larger tumor size and vascular invasion.[239,241] The prediction of aggressive behavior may be improved if a combination of histologic features is considered.[239] Tumors with a histologic phenotype intermediate between clearly benign and malignant epithelioid smooth muscle tumors or atypical tumors in which the epithelioid phenotype is suspected, but cannot be established with confidence, should be classified as 'tumors of uncertain malignant potential'.

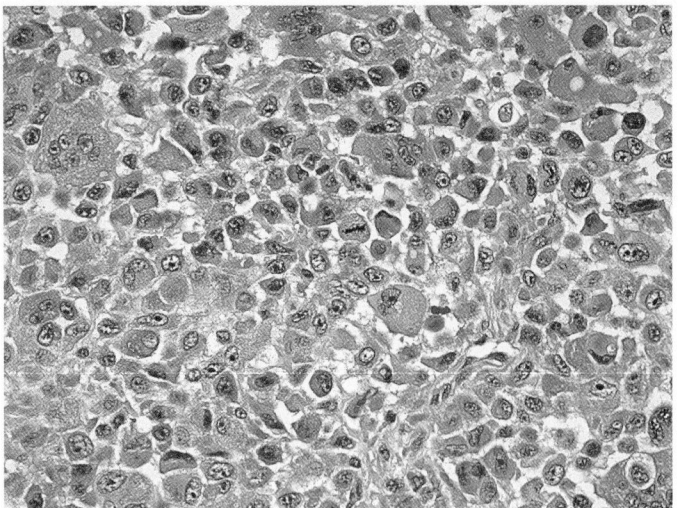

Fig. 20.57 Epithelioid leiomyosarcoma.

Myxoid leiomyosarcoma

Myxoid leiomyosarcoma is a rare variant of uterine leiomyosarcoma.[293-304] Its macroscopic appearance is that of a gelatinous, often large tumor. The criteria for diagnosis of this variant must be adjusted relative to non-myxoid leiomyosarcoma because the increased extracellular matrix reduces cellularity and consequently counts of mitotic activity. Once the myxoid nature of the extracellular matrix is appreciated, a malignancy can be diagnosed by recognizing significant (i.e. moderate to severe) atypia or necrosis in combination with a seemingly low proliferative rate (Fig. 20.58). Atkins et al. have suggested that a rate in excess of two mitotic figures per 10 high powered fields, regardless of the presence or absence of either atypia or necrosis, will separate benign and malignant myxoid tumors.[305] Another important diagnostic feature is infiltration into the adjacent myometrium (Fig. 20.59).[300] For practical purposes, we diagnose myxoid leiomyosarcoma in those cases with any one of the following features: (1) mitoses greater than two per 10 high power fields, (2) significant cytologic atypia (as outlined above), (3) tumor cell necrosis and (4) destructive infiltration of adjacent myometrium. Observation of vascular invasion also may be helpful, but must be distinguished from myxoid intravenous leiomyomatosis.

Prognostic factors and therapeutic decision making

Leiomyosarcoma has a poor prognosis. The 5-year survival has been estimated to be only 30–40%.[250,280,306,307] Even in early-stage (stage I and II) tumors, the recurrence rate for leiomyosarcoma may be as high as 71%.[308] Extrauterine disease (i.e. high stage) at the time of diagnosis is the most potent predictor of survival.[278,307] Five-year survival falls to 8% in stage II–IV patients.[257] The other clinical prognostic factor that has been noted is age.[259,278] Consequently, some feel that the goal of therapy for patients with advanced or recurrent disease should be palliative, although others optimistically note that the outlook for such patients has improved over the last decade.[259,309]

The prognostic importance of mitotic activity

A number of histologic and immunohistochemical features have been investigated as prognostic factors in uterine leiomyosarcoma. Of these, the most important

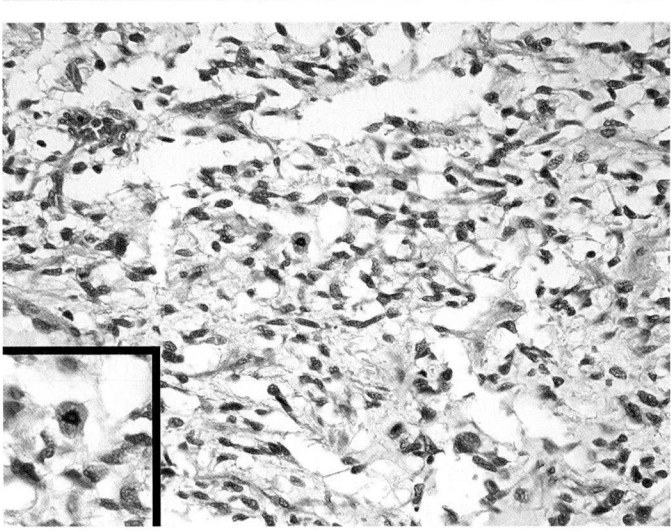

Fig. 20.58 Myxoid leiomyosarcoma. Note the loose collection of atypical cells and an occasional mitotic figure (center and inset) in a rarified stroma.

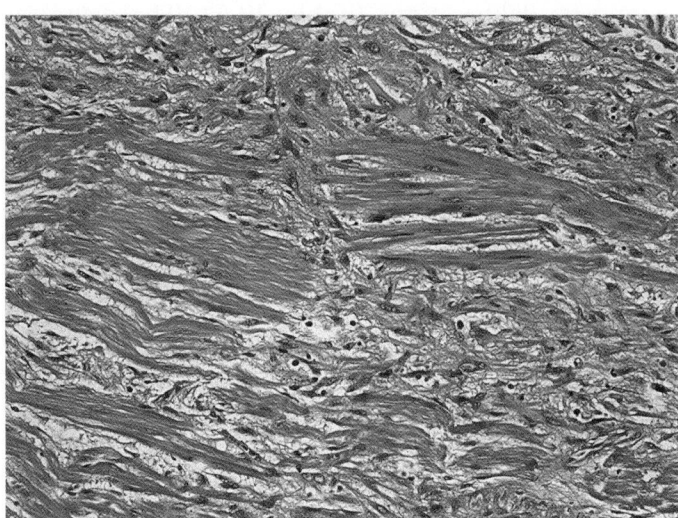

Fig. 20.59 Myxoid leiomyosarcoma. Note the infiltrating tumor cells permeating through myometrial fascicles.

is mitotic count.[259,278,280,308] This can be stated because mitotic count is the prognostic factor identified by the greatest number of studies and it is accessible to all pathologists. Related to mitotic activity, Peters et al. showed that an increasing S phase fraction predicts an adverse outcome.[278] The picture for the Ki-67 antigen, a widely used immunohistochemical surrogate for counting mitotic figures, is far less clear. In one study, Shpitz et al. found that all intermediate or high-grade leiomyosarcomas highly expressed Ki-67 antigen.[310] Despite this observation, Ki-67 expression did not clearly predict outcome in that study. In another study, Layfield et al. found that Ki-67 expression dichotomized the tumors into prognostic groups, but performed no better than histologic diagnosis.[311] Mayerhofer et al. suggested that Ki-67 correlates with vascular space involvement and shorter disease-free survival.[312] Of note, high proliferative rates also may be found in benign leiomyomata (see next section) and Ki-67 immunohistochemistry may play a limited role in the diagnosis of malignancy. In summary, mitotic activity remains the most important histology-based prognostic factor in uterine smooth muscle tumors and should be clearly indicated in pathologic reports diagnosing leiomyosarcoma.

The prognostic importance of histologic grade and size

The significance of histologic grading or tumor necrosis as prognostic factors is somewhat controversial. Some studies show evidence that tumor grading or necrosis is predictive, but most studies do not.[280,308,313,314] Although we include a description of the tumor in our reports, which includes characterization of the atypia and necrosis, we do not routinely grade the histology based on nuclear atypia or necrosis. Tumor size under 5 cm also may be associated with longer survival.[99]

The role of biomarkers in prognostication

The next immunohistochemical marker most commonly considered in uterine smooth muscle neoplasia after Ki-67 is the tumor suppressor p53. p53 is a transcription factor that plays a role in the response to DNA damage and is found mutated or over-expressed in a wide variety of tumors. p53 is not found by immunohistochemistry in myometrium or leiomyoma, but frequently is found in leiomyosarcoma.[315–317] Other studies have reported p53 expression in only about one-half of leiomyosarcomas.[318] In contrast to epitope abundance, p53 transcript level was not significantly altered in leiomyosarcoma compared with leiomyoma or myometrium.[233] Blom et al. suggest that p53 over-expression detected by immunohistochemistry may predict a high risk of recurrence in early-stage uterine leiomyosarcomas.[280] Layfield et al. reported that p53, like Ki-67, divided uterine smooth muscle tumors into prognostic groups, but did not achieve the level of significance achieved by mitotic rate.[311,312] While it is likely that p53 contributes to the pathobiology of leiomyosarcoma, the utility of this prognostic marker has not clearly been established.

A small number of other genes have been investigated as prognostic markers, including c-Kit, CD-34 (a marker of microvessel density), mdm2 (a p53 binding protein), Bcl-2 (an anti-apoptosis factor), estrogen receptor (ESR1), progesterone receptor, vascular endothelial growth factor (VEGF) and telomerase.[280,312,319–324] In our opinion, none of these markers is currently suitable for widespread clinical application.

Clinical management

The treatment of choice for leiomyosarcoma is widely considered to be total abdominal hysterectomy and bilateral salpingo-oophorectomy. The likelihood of nodal disease is low in the absence of more obvious disease, suggesting that lymph node dissection has little prognostic or therapeutic role in the management of leiomyosarcoma.[264,265] Ovarian preservation may be considered in premenopausal patients with early-stage leiomyosarcoma.[250,313] Surgical treatment of isolated pulmonary metastasis may prolong disease-free survival in patients in which adequate local control of the primary tumor has been achieved.[261] Adjuvant chemotherapy or radiotherapy has minimal, if any, effect on survival.[259,260,307,313,325–327] As a result, patients with smooth muscle tumors of uncertain malignant potential are not currently candidates for adjuvant therapies. The advent of a highly efficacious non-surgical therapy for leiomyosarcoma, however, will have a major impact on the pathologic diagnosis of uterine smooth muscle tumors.

HISTOLOGIC VARIANTS OF LEIOMYOMA

Each of the pathologic parameters used in the determination of malignancy in uterine smooth muscle tumors has a benign counterpart. In order to make the diagnosis of a histologic variant, one must be sure that none of the other features of malignancy are present. These variants are discussed in the following sections and listed in Table 20.6. Finally, the approach to tumors with more than one feature of malignancy, yet not satisfying the criteria for malignancy, is considered.

Degeneration

Degeneration in leiomyomata is quite common, but usually easily appreciated (Table 20.4, Figs 20.60, 20.61). In comparison to geographic tumor necrosis associated with malignancy, degeneration is often a homogenous process (Fig. 20.60). The typical gross appearance is that of a bland white, roughly spherical zone centered in the tumor mass. The degeneration also may result in a gelatinous mass or calcification of part or all of the tumor (e.g. the right panel of Fig. 20.60). If hemorrhage or discoloration is present, it also is grossly uniform, resulting in an even pink or frankly red cut surface, which earns it the 'carneous' or 'red' descriptors in older texts (e.g. the lower tumor in the left panel of Fig. 20.60). The interface between the viable and non-viable tissue has a uniform arc with a transition zone comprised of fibroblasts, viable and non-viable smooth muscle cells and scattered inflammatory cells (Fig. 20.61). This granulation tissue-like transition extends over a number of cell lengths and is not easily demarcated. The diffuseness of the border in benign degeneration due to ischemia and other

Table 20.6 Pathologic variants of uterine smooth muscle tumors

Pathologic diagnosis	Defining unusual or quasi-malignant feature
Leiomyoma with increased mitotic activity	5–15 mitotic figures per 10 high powered fields
Atypical (symplastic, bizarre, or pleomorphic) leiomyoma	Pleomorphic or giant tumor cells or cells with prominent nuclear atypia
Cellular leiomyoma	Significantly more cellular than most leiomyomas
Epithelioid leiomyoma	Rounded or polygonal cells resembling epithelial cells
Lipoleiomyoma	Variable, but often high percentage of adipocytes
Vascular leiomyoma	Prominent vascular component
Neurilemmoma-like leiomyoma	Prominent nuclear palisading resembling benign peripheral nerve sheath tumors
Intravascular leiomyomatosis	'Worm-like' venous intrusions of benign-appearing smooth muscle beyond the primary leiomyoma, which may extend into the right heart
Disseminated peritoneal leiomyomatosis	Histologically benign, often numerous smooth muscle tumorlets studding the peritoneum or omentum
Benign metastasizing leiomyoma	Histologically benign smooth muscle mass 'metastatic' to the lung presumably from a benign uterine leiomyoma
Parasitic leiomyoma	Presumably a subserosal uterine leiomyoma that has lost its attachment to the uterine corpus

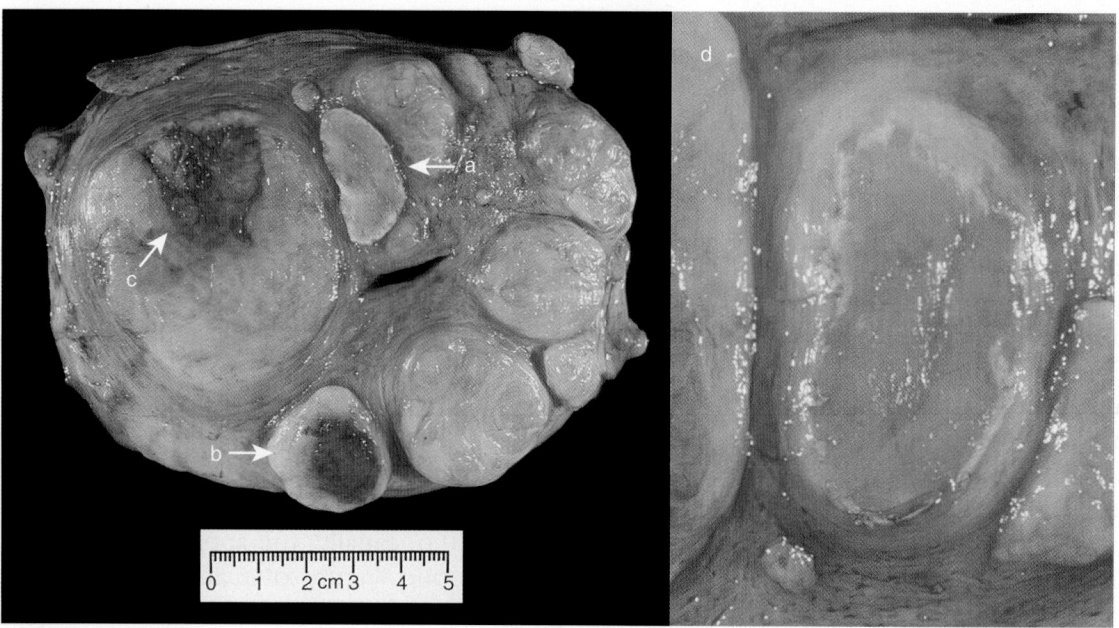

Fig. 20.60 Cross-section of a uterine corpus with multiple leiomyomata displaying several patterns of benign degeneration. (a,d) Uniform gelatinous necrosis with peripheral calcification. (b) Uniform central 'red' necrosis. (c) Wedge-shaped hemorrhagic coagulative necrosis associated with focused ultrasound effect.

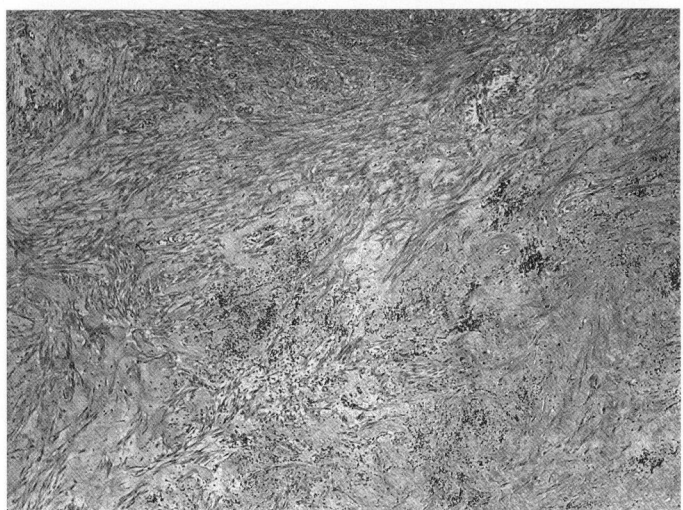

Fig. 20.61 Microscopic appearance of ischemic necrosis in a leiomyoma. Note the poorly demarcated zone between the viable tumor cells and the central degenerative area with hyalinization and hemorrhage. (Compare with Figure 20.62.)

processes is in contrast to the sharply defined border in malignant geographic tumor necrosis (Figs 20.54, 20.55, 20.62). The interface between viable and nonviable in benign smooth muscle tumors occasionally may be as sharp as that seen in malignant tumors, suggesting that the process of necrosis and subsequent repair in benign tumors is evolutionary. The nonviable cells themselves show the eosinophilia (and lack of nuclear staining) of coagulative necrosis. Presence of ghost cells (i.e. necrotic cells with well-defined outline and transparent or eosinophilic contents), with or without atypia (Fig. 20.56), is uncharacteristic

and should prompt a reexamination for other features of malignancy.[103] From time to time, thrombosis may be seen in tumor vessels, suggesting that ischemia is the principal cause of benign coagulative degeneration (Fig. 20.63). Other clinical situations in which rapid degeneration may be noted include pregnancy and other iatrogenic hormonal stimuli (e.g. clomiphene), as well as torsion of a pedunculated subserosal or submucosal tumor.[328] Over time, hyalinization, mummification, or even dystrophic calcification may become prominent.

Upon this typical pattern of degeneration, other appearances may be superimposed. One of the more common alternate tissue reactions is the accumulation of edema fluid. Hydropic foci may be microscopic and patchy. Microscopic foci of hydropic degeneration may be worrisome at lower magnifications because they often have more irregular contours and sharper borders. Careful attention at higher magnifications often resolves this by noting the fluid-filled intercellular spaces and the absence of truly necrotic cells. When more extensive, the wet, slippery cut surface of hydropic degeneration may often be described as 'myxoid' (Fig. 20.64). Such tumors should be histologically examined to exclude a myxoid leiomyosarcoma by recognizing their edematous nature and lack of other malignant features. Like other benign leiomyomata and in distinct contrast to myxoid leiomyosarcomas in the uterus, hydropic leiomyomata do not infiltrate into the fascicles of adjacent myometrium. In rare instances, benign necrosis may cavitate or take on a peculiar multinodular appearance (Figs 20.65, 20.66).[329]

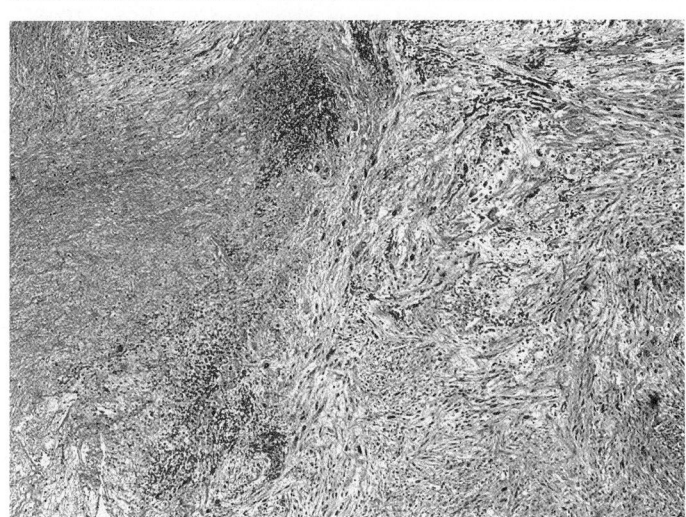

Fig. 20.62 Geographic tumor cell necrosis and hemorrhage in leiomyosarcoma. (Compare with Figure 20.61.)

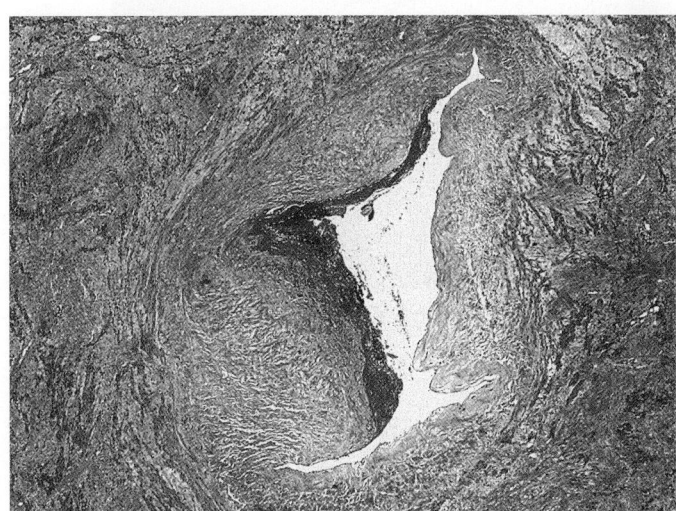

Fig. 20.63 Organizing thrombus associated with necrosis (not shown) in a plexiform leiomyoma.

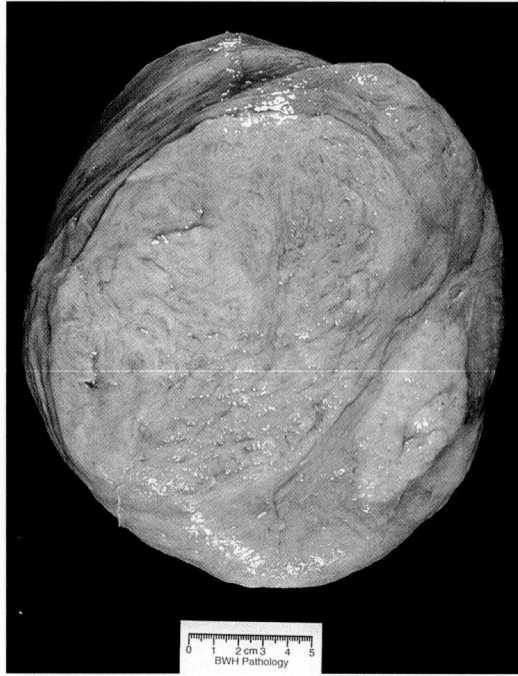

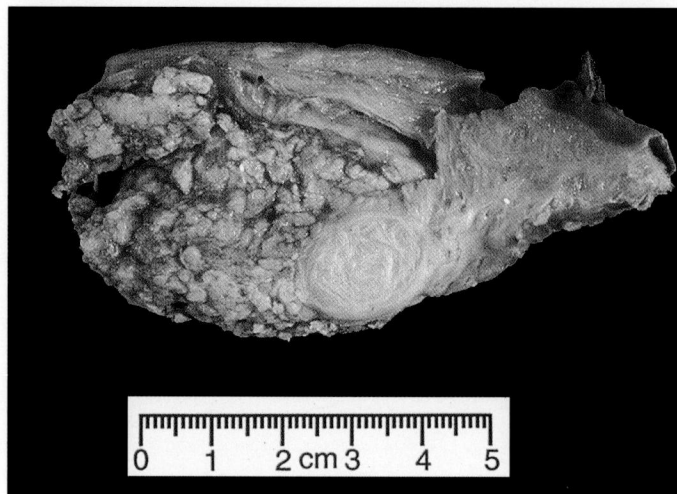

Fig. 20.66 Multinodular appearance of hydropic degeneration in leiomyoma.

Fig. 20.64 Hydropic degeneration in a large leiomyoma.

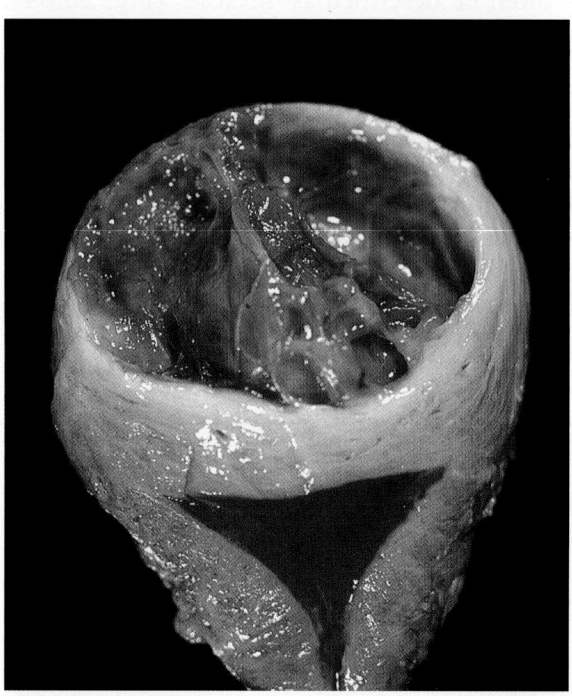

Fig. 20.65 Hydropic degeneration in leiomyoma may cavitate.

In addition to the naturally occurring patterns of degeneration, we now must become accustomed to recognizing iatrogenic necrosis. A number of new therapeutic strategies to non-invasively ablate 'fibroids' have been devised. These new strategies are partly in response to the strong patient preference for uterine conservation. Their clinical utility to date mostly has been limited to the treatment of pre- or perimenopausal women after childbearing.

At the time of this writing, the most widespread of these new procedures is uterine artery embolization, growing to 25 000 case per year since 1996.[21,86,125,126] In this technique, a catheter is threaded into the uterine artery and spheres of synthetic (e.g. polyvinyl alcohol) polymer are injected. As the blood supply to leiomyomata is larger than to the surrounding myometrium, the tumors tend to be more vulnerable to ischemia. Figure 20.67 (upper panel) show an example of yellow ischemic necrosis and calcification in a tumor after an embolization treatment. Of note, spheres of embolization material can easily be seen distending and occluding vessels within and near the tumor (Figs 20.67, 20.68). Of clinical note, this procedure spares the uterus and shortens the recovery interval compared with hysterectomy. Disadvantages of this procedure include costs similar to hysterectomy, the need for special training and equipment, a 10–20% risk of 'recurrence' (or more likely, growth of new tumors) and post-procedure fevers and pain.[91,330] In a few reports, diagnosis and treatment of a uterine sarcoma has been delayed due to the lack of a tissue-based diagnosis prior to this noninvasive therapy.[142,143]

Another new noninvasive treatment for leiomyomata employs magnetic resonance imaging to target thermal ablation by focused application of ultrasound energy. Focused ultrasound treatment is performed by arraying the sonications so as to fill a targeted zone. Of interest to pathologists, the gross appearance of a

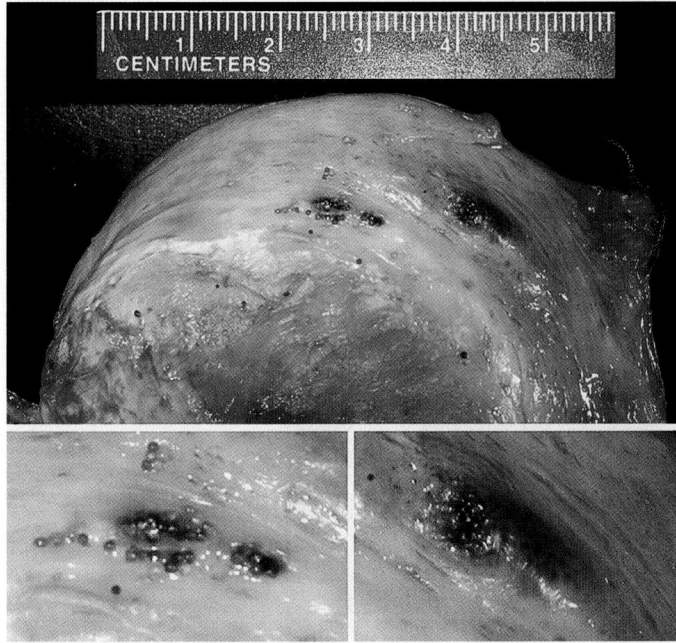

Fig. 20.67 Uterine artery embolization as a treatment of uterine leiomyoma. (Upper panel) Myxoid degeneration and peripheral calcification. (Lower left) Synthetic embolization material distending and spilling out of vessels at the edge of the leiomyoma and in (lower right) adjacent myometrium.

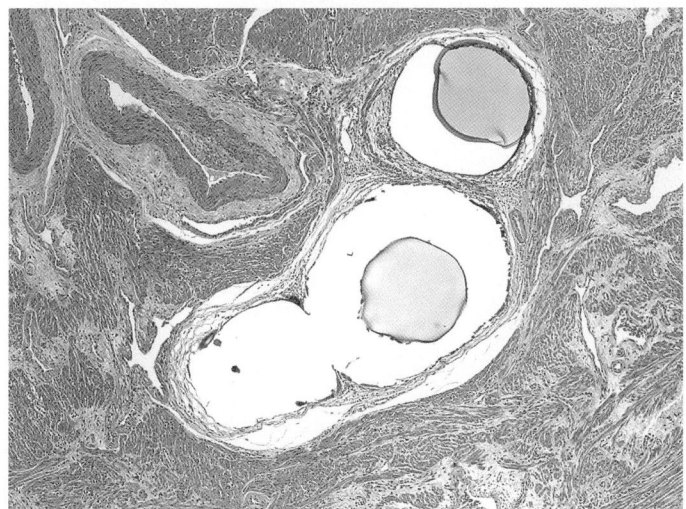

Fig. 20.68 Synthetic embolization material within vessels adjacent to the leiomyoma in Figure 20.67.

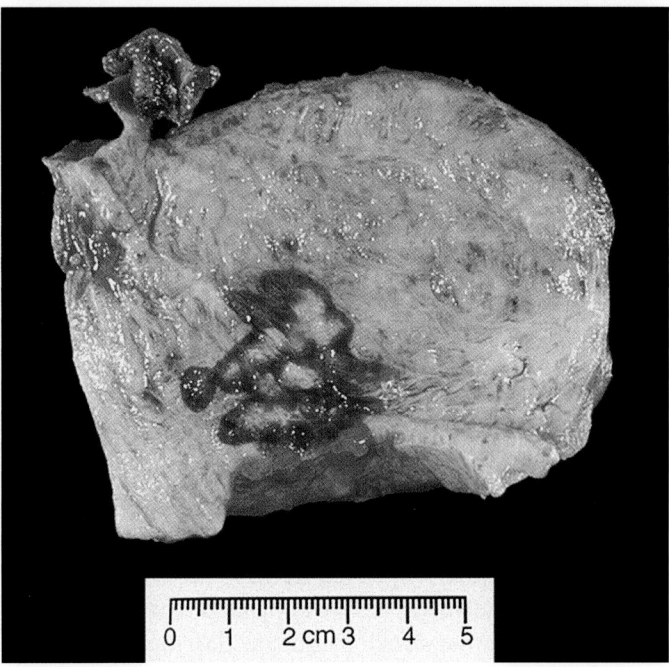

Fig. 20.69 Magnetic resonance guided focused ultrasound application as a treatment of uterine leiomyoma. Note the central blanching and peripheral hemorrhage.

Cellularity

Leiomyomata generally are more cellular than their surrounding myometrium. The exceptions, of course, are those tumors with extensive hyalinization or extracellular matrix deposition (e.g. a plexiform leiomyoma). The term 'cellular leiomyoma' is reserved for notably cellular tumors.[100] While hypercellularity is necessary to

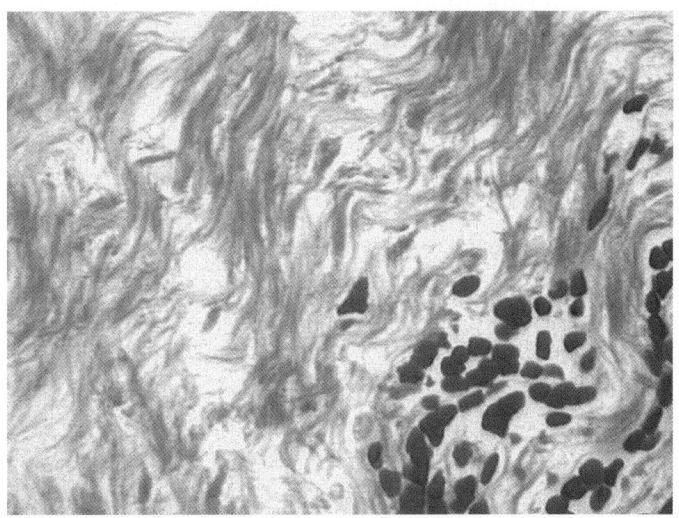

Fig. 20.70 Thermal effect results in bland coagulative necrosis without atypical ghost cells and hemorrhage after magnetic resonance guided focused ultrasound treatment.

leiomyomata early after treatment has many of the features of malignancy (Figs 20.60, 20.69). Specifically, the borders with sonicated and non-sonicated tissues may have complex, map-like, well-defined borders and sonicated tissues may be variegated in color and show extensive hemorrhage. In distinction to geographic tumor necrosis, thermal effect due to focused ultrasound energy transfer is bland coagulative necrosis lacking atypical ghost cells (Fig. 20.70).

classify a tumor as representing this benign variant, it is difficult to quantitate just how cellular a tumor must be before making this diagnosis. It has been suggested by some well-known gynecologic pathologists that only 5% of all leiomyomata should be described as being of the cellular type.[100] This definition may be helpful when considering large numbers of cases, but it is not as useful when a diagnosis must be made on the case at hand.

In practice, cellular leiomyomata must be distinguished from leiomyosarcomas and low-grade endometrial stromal sarcomas. One approach to determining whether an individual tumor merits classification as a cellular leiomyoma is to recognize only those tumors with an extreme or eye-catching degree of cellularity. Another approach would be to reserve this diagnosis for cases in which an endometrial stromal neoplasm was considered in the microscopic differential diagnosis, even if only briefly. By either approach, tumors with an unusual gross appearance might be classified as cellular. Specifically, cellular leiomyomata may have a more gray or pink cut surface with distinct whorls of smooth muscle (Fig. 20.71). The overall gross impression is one of a softer, fleshier tumor. On inspection of tissue sections without the microscope, the heavy hematoxylin staining of a cellular leiomyomata often will stand out, reflecting both the increased number of nuclei and relative lack of extracellular matrix deposition (Fig. 20.72).

Highly cellular leiomyoma is a markedly cellular variant of benign uterine smooth muscle neoplasia that often has an irregular border, which in combination with its marked cellularity particularly may mimic a low-grade endometrial stromal sarcoma (Figs 20.73, 20.74). This variant of leiomyoma can be recognized based upon its characteristic morphologic features,[51] which include (1) the presence of fascicular areas characteristic of smooth muscle neoplasia at least focally in most cases, (2) large thick-walled blood vessels and (3) cleft-like spaces (Figs 20.73, 20.75). In particularly problematic cases, the application of certain immunohistochemical stains may be useful. Highly cellular leiomyomata are positive with markers of smooth muscle differentiation; they are typically diffusely positive for desmin (Fig. 20.75) and are positive for h-caldesmon, although some cases show decreased staining with this marker (Fig. 20.76). This tumor also may be diffusely positive for CD10 (Fig. 20.77); therefore this marker may not be useful in their distinction from endometrial stromal tumors.

Leiomyosarcomas are often markedly hypercellular, but hypercellularity is not a specific diagnostic criterion for the determination of malignancy (Fig. 20.78). More-

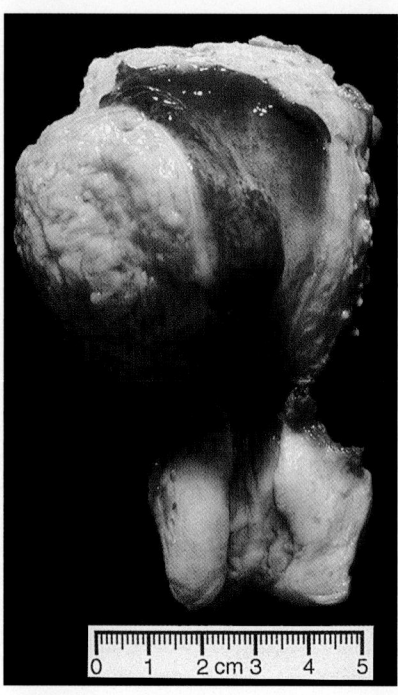

Fig. 20.71 Macroscopic appearance of cellular leiomyoma tends to be softer and more tan than leiomyomata of the usual histologic type.

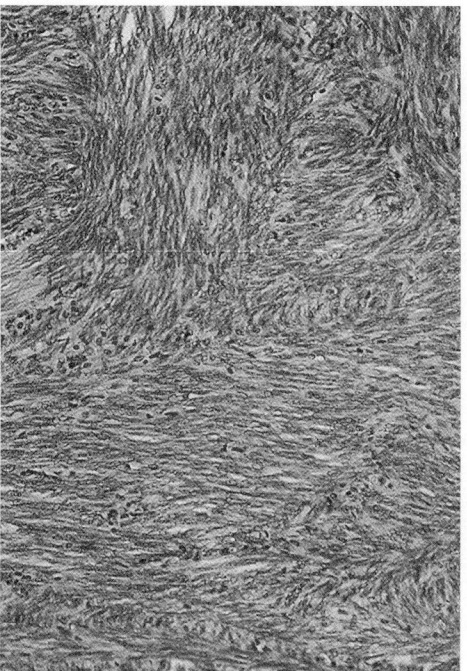

Fig. 20.72 Microscopic appearance of a cellular leiomyoma may mimic an endometrial stromal neoplasm, but is characterized by thick-walled vessels (not shown). Cellular leiomyomata also lack the other key histologic features of leiomyosarcomas.

over, cellular leiomyomas lack the other features of malignant smooth muscle tumors, although they may overlap to some extent with leiomyomata with increased mitotic activity. Cellular leiomyomata are distinguished from endometrial stromal sarcoma based on characteristic histomorphology and immunoprofile. In particular, cellular leiomyomata have large, thick-walled

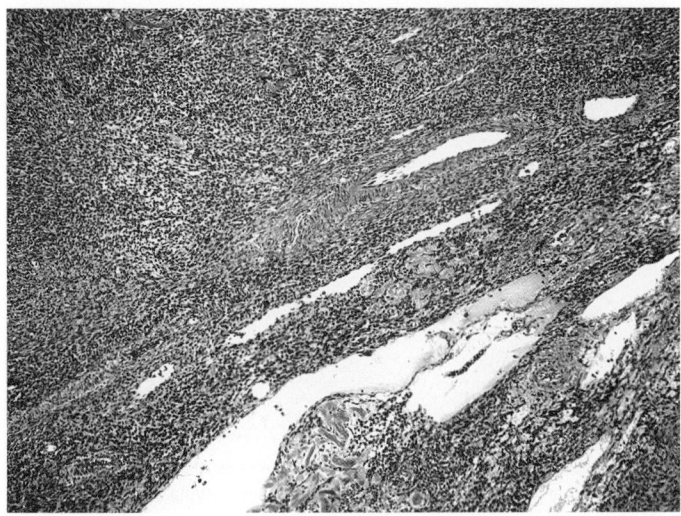

Fig. 20.73 Low-magnification image of a highly cellular leiomyoma. Note the characteristic thick-walled blood vessels and cleft-like spaces.

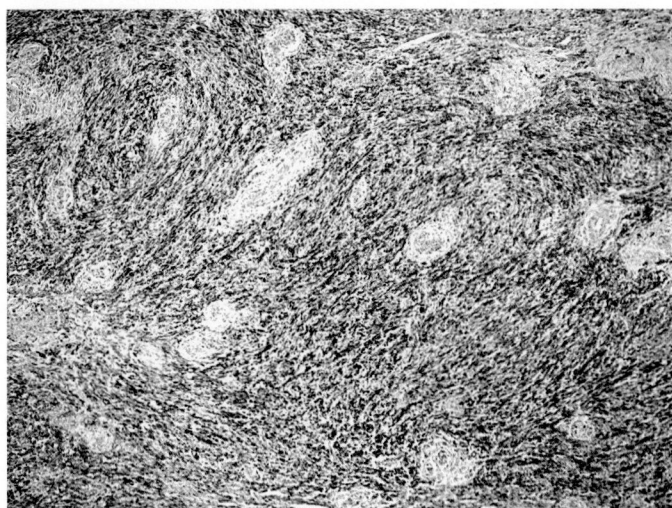

Fig. 20.75 Strong desmin staining in a highly cellular leiomyoma. Note the thick-walled blood vessels.

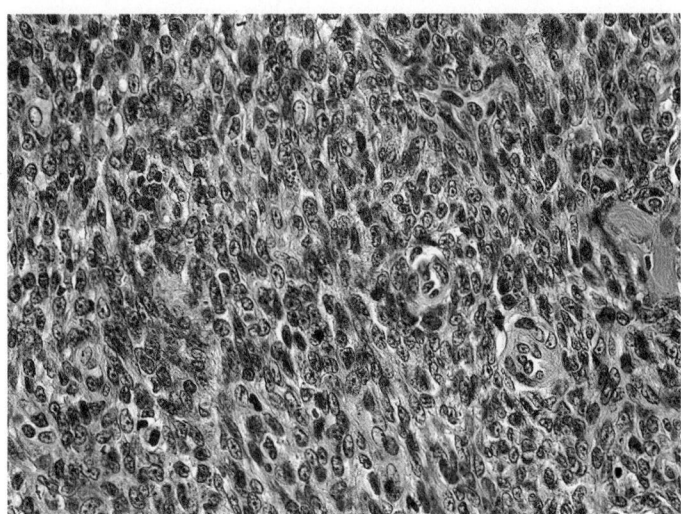

Fig. 20.74 High-magnification image of a highly cellular leiomyoma. Note the resemblance to a low-grade endometrial stromal sarcoma.

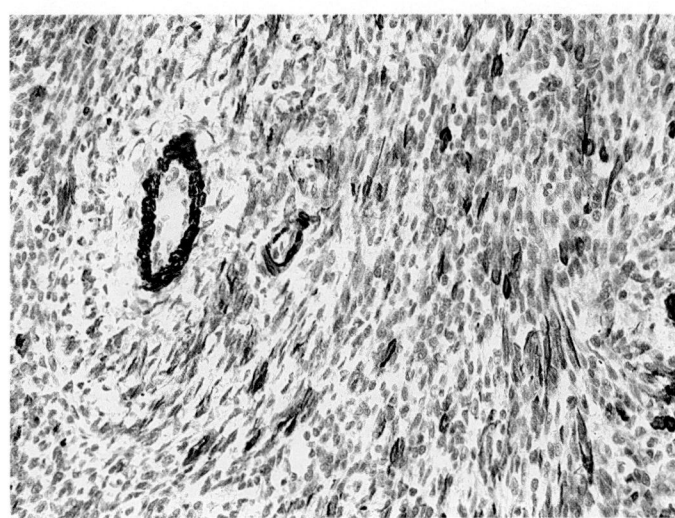

Fig. 20.76 h-Caldesmon staining may be reduced and patchy in highly cellular leiomyomata relative to other leiomyoma.

vessels in comparison to the delicate thin-walled 'spiral arteriole-like' vessels in endometrial stromal sarcoma. In addition, cellular leiomyomata strongly express smooth muscle markers (e.g. h-caldesmon and smooth muscle actin) and generally lack CD10 expression.

Although the diagnosis of a cellular leiomyoma may seem more like our regard for beauty (both are in the eye of the beholder), there is the prospect for a more molecular definition. Recently, disruption of the histone acetyltransferase *MORF* as been associated with rearrangements of 10q22 and the cellular phenotype in a small number of cases.[331] *MORF* also is rearranged in the M4 and M5 subtypes of acute myeloid leukemia. It has been suggested that this rearrangement alters the self-renewal properties in hematopoietic precursor cells. Perhaps a similar molecular mechanism confers the hypercellular phenotype in smooth muscle tumors with rearrangements of *MORF*.

Mitotic activity

Variation in mitotic activity occurring in both myometrial and leiomyomatous smooth muscle cells over the course of the menstrual cycle is a well-established phenomenon. Some investigators have noted that exogenous progesterone increases the mitotic rate in leiomyomata.[168,169] These observations are part of the progesterone stimulation hypothesis of leiomyoma histogenesis.[332] Occasionally, the mitotic rate in benign

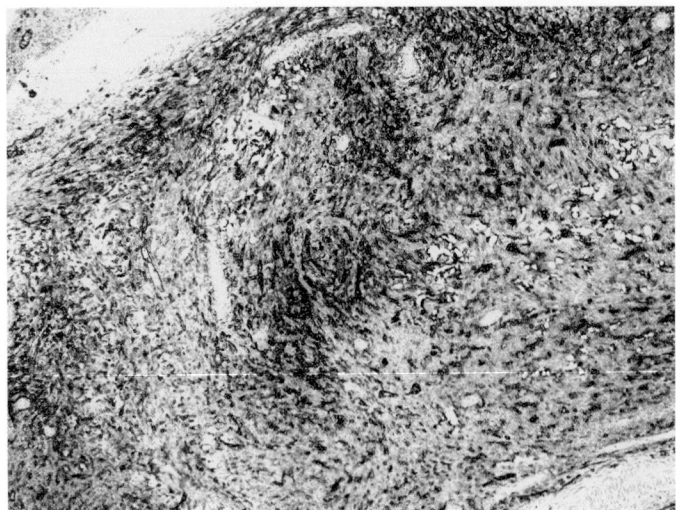

Fig. 20.77 CD10 staining may be diffuse in highly cellular leiomyomata.

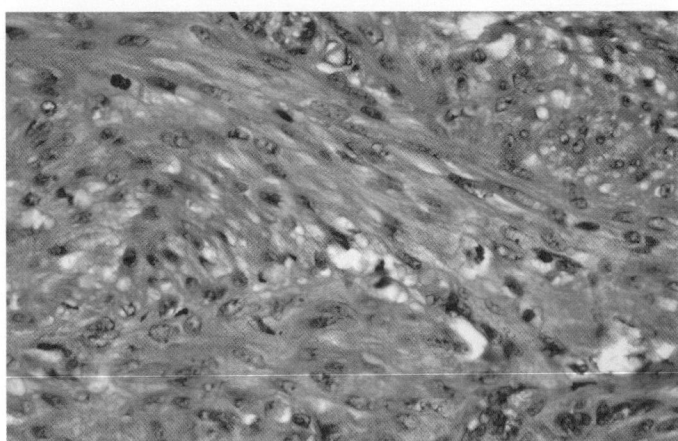

Fig. 20.79 Leiomyomata with increased mitotic activity are characterized by increased proliferative activity. These tumors lack atypia and geographic tumor necrosis.

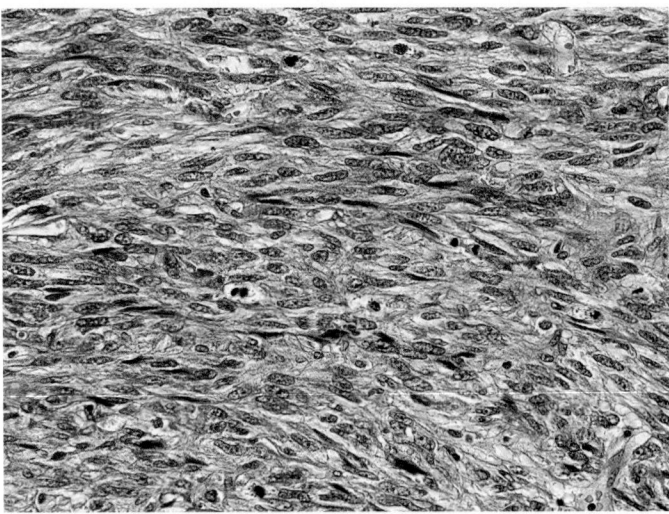

Fig. 20.78 Hypercellularity is a frequent finding in leiomyosarcomas. Several mitotic figures also are present in this field.

tumors may be quite brisk and those with mitotic activity up to 15 mitoses per 10 high power fields are classified as 'leiomyomata with increased mitotic activity' (Fig. 20.79, Table 20.6).[292,333–335] This diagnostic term is useful in denoting the special nature of these tumors, as well as communicating the absence of other worrisome features. Specifically, leiomyomata with increased mitotic activity must not have any significant atypia or geographic tumor necrosis. Presence of any one of these worrisome features warrants additional review.

In practical terms, proliferative activity should be assessed in areas with the highest mitotic rate by visual inspection.[99] Mitotic activity should be reported as an average over 10 high power fields (i.e. using the 40×

objective on most conventionally configured microscopes).[99] Enough fields should be counted to determine a statistically valid average. Generally, 30 high powered fields are sufficient, but occasionally 50 or more fields may be needed. If the mitotic count is highly variable, it may be helpful to report the range. Careful scrutiny of mitotic figures perhaps is as important to the accurate evaluation of proliferative activity as the counting methodology.[96] Pyknotic nuclei are a not infrequent finding in smooth muscle tumors (Fig. 20.48). These apparently degenerating nuclei potentially can be easily mistaken as mitoses by the inexperienced histomorphologist.

Ki-67 antigen, as noted earlier, is a proliferation marker that may have some prognostic value in leiomyosarcoma. It also may be helpful in the diagnosis of leiomyoma with increased mitotic activity and, as we will see, smooth muscle tumors with other features of malignancy. [315,318,336] One way in which Ki-67 immunohistochemistry might be useful is in excluding pyknotic nuclei. We also have found Ki-67 expression useful in understanding intratumoral variation in mitotic activity. In several examples (B.J.Q., unpublished data), proliferative 'hot spot' were discovered in broad zones beneath eroded and attenuated mucosal surfaces of submucosal leiomyoma.

Atypical mitotic figures reflect genomic instability and as such, may be the heralds of a leiomyosarcoma. Detection of atypical mitoses (Figs 20.49, 20.50) in a smooth muscle tumor that would otherwise be classified as a leiomyoma with increased mitotic activity should prompt at least a second look by the pathologist.

Atypia

Leiomyoma with nuclear or cytoplasmic atypia have been known by many names, including pleomorphic leiomyoma, bizarre leiomyoma and symplastic leiomyoma.[100,337] Recently, the term atypical leiomyoma has been adopted as the term to describe this peculiar variant by the World Health Organization and International Agency for Research on Cancer.[101,103] In practice, we often include the older terms as a parenthetical comment, so as to emphasize their benign clinical nature and avoid any extrapolation based on other examples of gynecologic neoplasia (e.g. atypical endometrial hyperplasia and endometrial adenocarcinoma).

This diagnosis should be reserved for those smooth muscle tumors with significant atypia.[101] That is to say, the atypia should be discernible at lower magnifications and evoke the possibility of leiomyosarcoma in the examiner's mind. The atypia may be focal or diffuse (Table 20.5). Nuclear atypia may consist of some combination of nuclear enlargement, multilobation or multinucleation, hyperchromasia, coarsening of the chromatin texture, or prominence of nucleoli (Figs 20.80, 20.81). Cytoplasmic atypia may consist of increases in cytoplasmic volume, particularly by swirls of eosinophilic material suggestive of aberrant cytoskeletal protein accumulation, formation of tumor giant cells and intranuclear invaginations by the cytoplasm (Fig. 20.81).

The distinction between an atypical leiomyoma and leiomyosarcoma is the absolute absence of geographic tumor necrosis and a proliferative rate no higher than ordinary leiomyomata. Bell et al. have suggested that atypical leiomyoma have no more than 10 mitotic

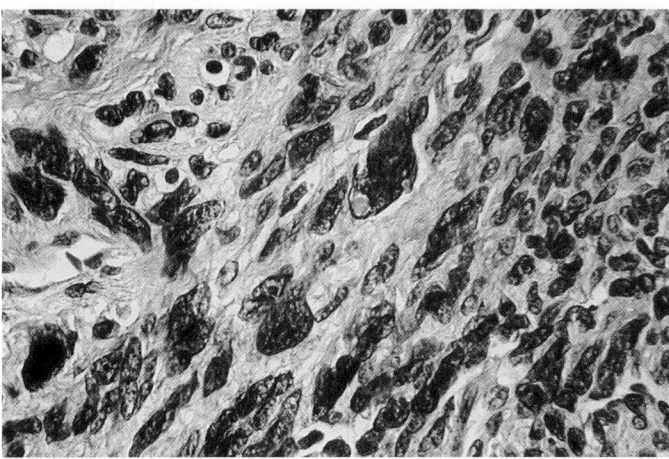

Fig. 20.81 Nuclear and cytoplasmic atypia in an atypical leiomyoma. Note the cytoplasmic inclusion in the enlarged and hyperchromatic nucleus in the center of this image.

figures per 10 high power fields. Obviously, one should be at least a little wary of tumors with counts just under this threshold.

These tumors pose an interesting challenge to pathologists. Their classification as being non-malignant is based on follow-up after hysterectomy. Atypical leiomyoma tumors, however, may not be completely excised with minimally or noninvasive therapies for 'fibroid uteri'. Flow cytometric analysis of atypical leiomyomata shows that some of these tumors are aneuploid.[278,336] Finally, atypical leiomyomata, like leiomyosarcomas, express p53.[162] These pathobiologic observations raise the possibility of a more dynamic natural history for such tumors. Interestingly, we have observed one atypical leiomyoma removed by myomectomy that seemed to recur within a few years. Another group has reported leiomyosarcoma in association with tumors classified as cellular and atypical leiomyomata.[256] Therefore, we encourage careful follow-up or consideration of hysterectomy for an atypical leiomyoma in which there was incomplete exclusion.

Infiltration

While not considered a formal criterion, the invasion of neoplastic smooth muscle cell through adjacent fascicles of myometrial smooth muscle may be a helpful clue as to the malignancy of a tumor (Fig. 20.82). In fact, this feature may be the only evidence of a more aggressive course and is a defining feature of myxoid leiomyosarcomas.[101,296,300] The problem is that infiltration is commonly simulated by benign leiomyoma. This occurs because the fascicles of a leiomyoma and its surrounding myometrium may interdigitate at the tumor's border.

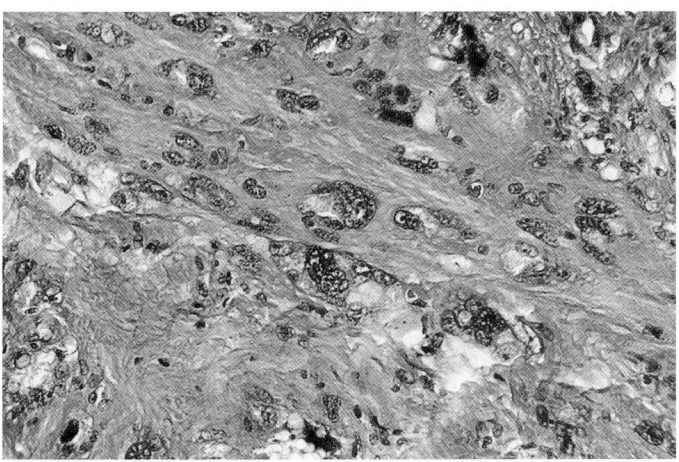

Fig. 20.80 Nuclear atypia in an atypical leiomyoma. Note the absence of other features of malignancy, namely geographic tumor necrosis and increased proliferative activity.

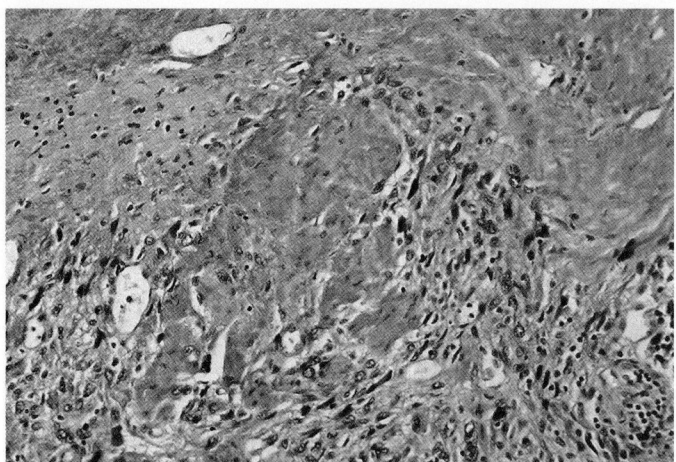

Fig. 20.82 Infiltration by a leiomyosarcoma through adjacent myometrial fascicles.

Such interdigitations may be recognized when the preservation of fascicular bundles in both tissues is appreciated. This feature does not have an established place in the classification of leiomyoma variants and, consequently, we generally do not comment on it in our reports.

SMOOTH MUSCLE TUMORS THAT ARE DIFFICULT TO CLASSIFY

Diagnostic terminology

Under ideal circumstances, the diagnostic categories discussed in the previous sections would encompass all of the uterine smooth muscle tumors encountered in the real world. Unfortunately, they do not. The problem is that an important minority of these tumors have phenotypic features between leiomyomata or the benign variants and the spectrum of tumors we recognize as leiomyosarcomas. To complicate matters further, tumors with intermediate phenotypes are not necessarily benign and may even be as biologically aggressive as high-grade leiomyosarcoma.

When the problem of classifying tumors with intermediate morphologic features was appreciated, a new diagnostic category was introduced: smooth muscle tumor of uncertain malignant potential or STUMP.[97,98,100] Originally, a tumor was so classified if it had either (1) mitotic figures numbering more than 15 per 10 high powered fields, (2) mitotic activity between five and 10 mitotic figures per 10 high powered fields, minimal atypia and increased cellularity, or (3) mitotic activity between two and five mitotic figures per 10 high powered fields and atypia. Any mitotic activity in excess of

these thresholds merited the diagnosis of malignancy. Although this scheme was illustrated with sharp demarcations between benign, uncertain malignant potential and malignant categories, the classification of intermediate tumors with mitotic activity near a threshold remained problematic.

To address these so-called problematic tumors, Bell et al. undertook a comprehensive retrospective analysis of over 200 tumors with intermediate features.[101] A prerequisite for entry of a tumor into the study set was at least five mitotic figures per 10 high powered fields. After gathering information about a number of morphologic features, a recursive partitioning algorithm (viz. classification and regression trees or CART) was used to find the model that predicted the eventual outcome most accurately.

It was this study that placed particular emphasis on the presence of geographic tumor necrosis.[101,103] If geographic tumor necrosis was present, it was not necessary to consider proliferative activity or atypia, although one or the other feature was present in slightly more the 90% of their cases.

If geographic necrosis was not present, it was most efficient to consider atypia next.[101] A tumor could be classified as a benign leiomyoma with increased mitotic activity if there was no atypia (or necrosis). Interestingly, 2 of 89 tumors in this cluster recurred with pulmonary smooth muscle tumors. While these two tumors might be considered examples of the elusive quasi-malignant 'benign metastasizing leiomyoma', there are little data directly relating the pulmonary and uterine smooth muscle neoplasms. In light of the molecular genetic studies on disseminated peritoneal and intravenous leiomyomatosis,[338–340] it could be argued that these two exceptions represent very low-grade leiomyosarcomas.

Of tumors without geographic tumor necrosis but with atypia, the atypia was mostly diffuse in the large series of 'problematic' smooth muscle tumors.[101] It was at this point Bell et al. found that it was appropriate to access the mitotic activity. If the proliferative activity was higher than 10 mitotic figures per 10 high powered fields, tumors were classified as leiomyosarcoma; otherwise, they were classified as 'atypical leiomyoma with a low risk of recurrence'. Only 1 out of 47 tumors in this morphologic group had a poor outcome. Interestingly, only five tumors in their series had focal atypia without necrosis and none was reported to have a poor outcome. Consequently, they also classified these tumors as 'atypical leiomyomata', but appended the disclaimer 'limited experience'.

There are two important points to be made by understanding the evolution in the approach to tumors that are difficult to classify. First, these cases occur in small numbers in all but large referral practices. Consequently, rigorous testing of the performance of these diagnostic approaches in a prospective fashion has yet to be done. Nevertheless, the new emphasis on geographic necrosis and redefinition of atypical leiomyoma has reduced the number of instances in which a tumor would be classified as a 'smooth muscle tumor of uncertain malignant potential', at least in our experience. Secondly, grouping of the remaining difficult cases highlights the ongoing problem areas for gynecologic pathologists (Table 20.7). Situations in which expressing diagnostic uncertainty when using the STUMP term is still appropriate include diagnostic groups in which information about the natural history remains limited.[103] This reservation is particularly true for epithelioid or myxoid smooth muscle tumors that have intermediate atypia or proliferative activity. Another closely related situation might be encountered when presented with a smooth muscle tumor in which one suspects, but cannot be convinced, that epithelioid or myxoid differentiation is present. In our experience, these first two situations represent the minority of cases for which the STUMP term should be used. One of the two more frequent situations arises from the nature of determining whether necrosis is of a benign ischemic or degenerative type or is of a malignant geographic type. Although there are clear criteria (Table 20.4), this determination remains subjective and the inter-observer reproducibility of interpreting necrosis has yet to be determined. It is reasonable, however, to presume greater experience with evaluation of smooth muscle tumors improves the discrimination of benign and malignant patterns. This interpretive skill is further hampered by the fact that necrosis is a dynamic process and early lesions may be hard to classify. Additionally, degenerative processes need not be limited to benign tumors and mixed patterns in a malignant tumor may be confusing. Finally, classification of atypical tumors without necrosis,

but with proliferative rates near the threshold for diagnosis of leiomyosarcoma, remains an area of concern. As noted earlier, consideration of parameters such as the presence of atypical mitoses or the interface with the myometrium may be important in individual cases. In summary, it remains important to recognize that the prediction of prognosis cannot be made safely for all uterine smooth muscle tumors and it is appropriate to convey our uncertainty about the malignant potential in this small number of cases.

Clinical implications

Once the diagnosis of uncertain malignant potential is made, what are the clinical ramifications? First, it depends on the preceding surgical procedure. If a total hysterectomy was performed and the information necessary to stage the patient was obtained, conservative management with periodic follow-up is usually employed. Given the high frequency of pulmonary metastasis of *bona fide* leiomyosarcomas, inclusion of some minimal noninvasive chest imaging in the follow-up regimen can be justified. Perhaps the more important component to post-hysterectomy management of an unusual smooth muscle tumor (and low-stage leiomyosarcoma) is patient awareness and education.

The clinical management of diagnostically challenging smooth muscle tumors is changing in the era of minimally invasive therapy for 'fibroid uteri'. As pointed out for atypical leiomyoma, the potential for 'recurrence' following the diagnosis of an unusual uterine smooth tumor has not been studied in detail. Consequently, we typically advise strong consideration of subsequent hysterectomy when a diagnosis of leiomyoma or a benign variant cannot be made with certainty. Other factors may bear on the clinical decision-making process. The likelihood of complete excision in the original procedure should be considered. In addition, the patient's age, menopausal status and desire to preserve fertility must be taken into account.

APPLICATION OF BIOMARKERS TO SMOOTH MUSCLE NEOPLASIA

Immunoprofiling has made a big impact on the distinction of uterine smooth muscle tumors from other tumor types. Briefly, uterine smooth muscle tumors are characterized by diffuse and strong expression of markers of smooth muscle differentiation. These biomarkers include smooth muscle-specific actin, desmin and h-caldesmon. Uterine smooth muscle tumors may also express CD10, which is frequently expressed in endometrial stromal

---

Table 20.7 *Situations in which diagnosis of Smooth muscle Tumors of Uncertain Malignant Potential (STUMP) may be considered*

1 Tumors in which necrosis is present, but difficult to classify
2 Tumors with significant atypia and mitotic activity near the threshold for malignancy (10 mitotic figures per 10 high powered fields)
3 Epithelioid or myxoid tumors that have atypia or proliferative activity intermediate between their benign and malignant counterparts
4 Worrisome tumors in which one suspects, but cannot be convinced, that epithelioid or myxoid features are present

neoplasms and may be used to distinguish the two tumor types. While the utilization of the markers is detailed in other sections, we simply would remind the reader that the expression of such markers often is reduced in intensity and frequency in malignant tumors, particularly when they are more morphologically deranged.[73,75,80] For example, the transcript level of h-caldesmon is slightly, but consistently reduced by 30–35% in leiomyoma and more dramatically reduced by 85–90% in leiomyosarcoma.[233]

In contrast to the use of biomarkers for tumor classification, utilization of biomarkers has not made as large an impact on the determination of malignancy in uterine smooth muscle neoplasia. Potential markers such as aneuploidy (by flow cytometry), allelic imbalance (by loss of heterozygosity at microsatellites) and genomic instability (by cytogenetics) all reflect aspects of the underlying pathobiology of uterine smooth muscle neoplasia. These techniques, however, require particular expertise and infrastructure and, consequently, are not widely available. Their applicability also is hampered by the limited extent to which unusual smooth muscle tumors (i.e. the benign variants, the quasi-malignant proliferations and the ambiguous tumors) have been characterized.

The three remaining problem areas in difficult uterine smooth muscle tumor include recognition of alternative patterns of differentiation, the type of necrosis and the level of proliferative activity (Table 20.7). The recognition of epithelioid and myxoid tumors remains squarely in the domain of conventional histomorphology. Nor is a marker for worrisome tumor necrosis available. Fortunately, some inroads have been made in applying the use of proliferative markers, primarily Ki-67, to the diagnosis of malignancy in uterine smooth muscle tumors.[315,318,336] As has been emphasized, careful counting of mitotic activity is sufficient in most instances. Furthermore, Ki-67 immunohistochemistry cannot be used to distinguish a mitotically active leiomyoma from leiomyosarcoma, as other morphologic features must be evaluated. Proliferative markers, however, may be useful in distinguishing pyknotic nuclei from dividing cells (Fig. 20.83). This is perhaps most applicable to tumors with atypia and lacking necrosis. High mitotic rates favor malignancy. In this context, immunohistochemistry for Ki-67 may raise or lower the level of concern generated by examination of hematoxylin and eosin stained tissue sections. Although preliminary work has been done, specific definition of a Ki-67-based proliferative index and the criteria upon which to evaluate cases has yet to be firmly established.

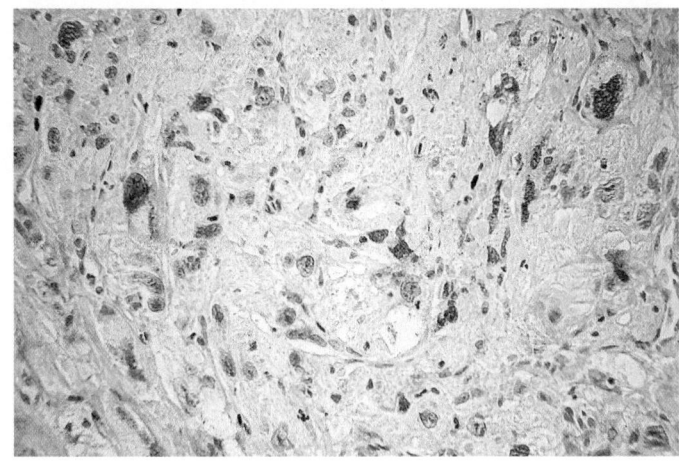

Fig. 20.83 Low Ki-67 staining in atypical leiomyomata.

Investigation into the pathobiology of uterine smooth muscle neoplasia has generated a significant number of other potential biomarkers (e.g. p53, estrogen and progesterone receptors, bcl-2 and VEGF). Undoubtedly, the application of genomics and proteomics to uterine smooth muscle neoplasia will generate additional candidates. The experience with these markers, however, remains limited and their use in wider diagnostic practice cannot be recommended at present.

PRACTICAL APPROACHES TO THE INTRAOPERATIVE EXAMINATION OF UTERINE SMOOTH MUSCLE TUMORS

Clinical considerations will prompt intraoperative consultations of uterine smooth muscle tumors. These considerations include very large fibroids, advanced patient age, peri- or postmenopausal status and rapid 'fibroid' growth, particularly with patients who are postmenopausal or being treated with a gonadotropin releasing agonist. While the final pathologic diagnosis requires thorough sampling of unusual or suspicious tumors, intraoperative evaluation may guide the surgeon in determining what, if any, additional tissues should be sampled to properly stage or cytoreduce the patient. Careful gross examination of the cut surface for hemorrhage, necrosis, or resemblance to fish flesh (viz. tuna steak) can be used to prompt further investigation. Other benign degenerative changes, which are usually more diffuse and centered within the mass, may be used to cautiously reassure the surgeon. In suspicious cases, we take one or two frozen sections to evaluate the level of atypia and presence of microscopic foci of geographic necrosis. High mitotic rates also may be noted, but particular care should be taken to avoid counting pseudomitoses. Perhaps more importantly, a suspicious tumor should provoke consideration of other malignant tumors. Specifically, the differential diagnosis should include endometrial stromal sarcoma, adenosarcoma and carcinosarcoma (malignant mixed Müllerian tumor). Of these, carcinosarcomas are the most frequent.

QUASI-MALIGNANT SMOOTH MUSCLE PROLIFERATIONS

In this section, unusual smooth muscle tumors with quasi-malignant features are described. For the most part, these proliferations are clinically benign, yet have some growth pattern that resembles malignant tumors. Specifically, these features include vascular invasion and growth, disseminated growth within the uterus or abdominal cavity and possibly spread to the lung.

Intravenous leiomyomatosis

This is a peculiar condition in which a tumorous smooth muscle proliferation involves venous spaces.[66,99,338,339,341–352] It affects women in their latter reproductive ages, but has been reported as early as 21 years of age.[65,353] No other specific conditions have been associated with intravenous leiomyomatosis. When the process is limited to the originating tumor, it may be classified as leiomyoma with vascular invasion. There are no long-term studies of intratumoral vascular invasion, but it may be a forerunner of intravenous leiomyomatosis in some cases and the origin of the enigmatic disorder known as benign metastasizing leiomyoma in other cases. With further growth, this smooth muscle proliferation may extend into the uterine wall and a tumorous source may not always be evident (Figs 20.84, 20.85). Worm-like tumor projection may be seen at the parametrial resection margins of hysterectomy specimens with intravenous leiomyomatosis. In more extreme instances, the leiomyomatous tumor may fill the vena cava and even extend into the right cardiac chambers, or involve other tributaries to the inferior vena cava (Fig. 20.86).[338,354] This pattern of intravascular growth also may be seen in renal cell carcinomas, uterine leiomyosarcomas and endometrial stromal sarcoma.[67,355] The first clue that this disorder is clinically benign is provided by examination of the cut surface, which is essentially identical to a uterine leiomyoma (Fig. 20.87). The microscopic appearance in most cases of intravenous leiomyomatosis is that of a typical uterine leiomyoma, but Clement et al. have reported a series of cases in which the histologic features of intravenous leiomy-

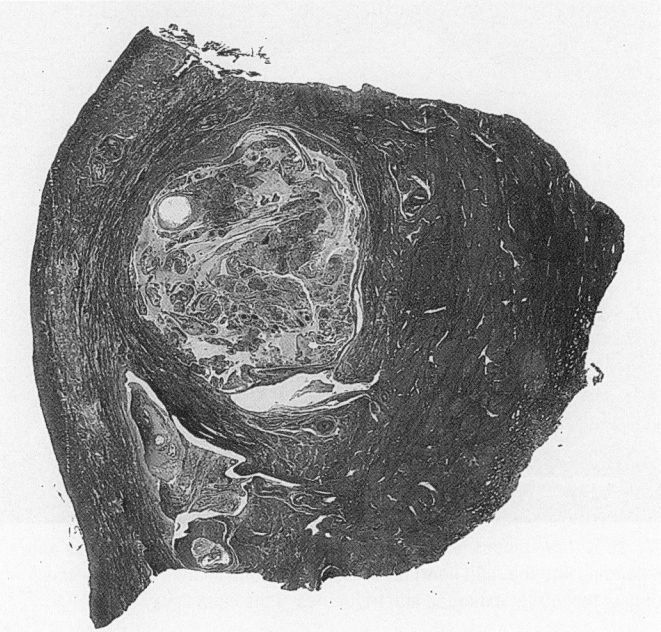

Fig. 20.84 Intravenous leiomyomatosis within the uterine corpus, low magnification.

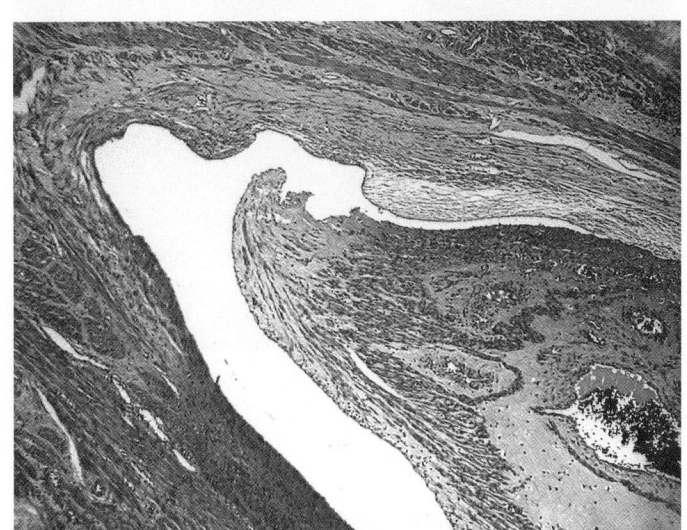

Fig. 20.85 Intravenous leiomyomatosis within the uterine corpus, high magnification.

omatosis exhibited the same spectrum as seen in the benign uterine variants (Fig. 20.88).[64]

The origin of this unusual smooth muscle proliferation is unclear. Some investigators have suggested that intravenous leiomyomatosis arises from vascular smooth muscle, based on microscopic observations in some cases.[341] Similarities between histologic appearances and patient profile, however, suggest that this disorder is related to uterine leiomyomata of the usual type. Kir

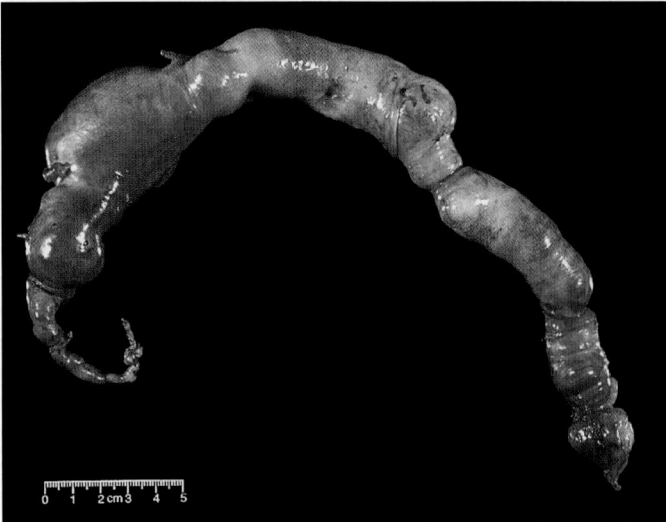

Fig. 20.86 Intravenous leiomyomatosis involving the inferior vena cava and extending into the right heart (at the left side of the image). Note the small tags of tumor that extended into tributaries of the vena cava.

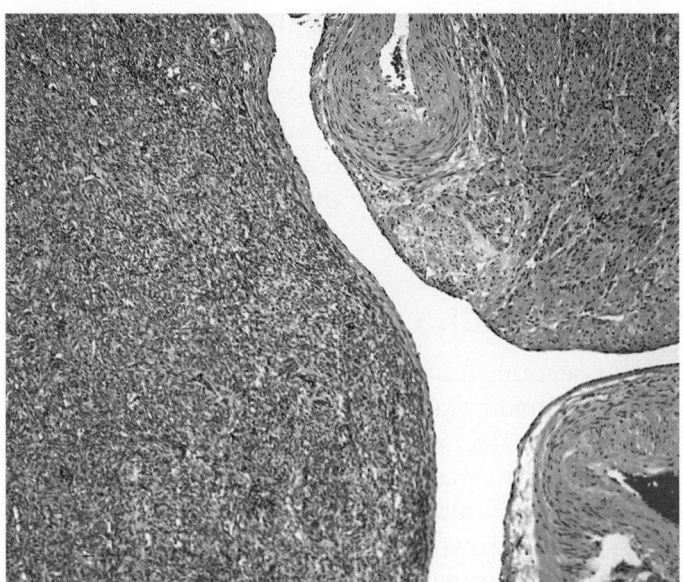

Fig. 20.88 Cellular intravenous leiomyomatosis. The differential diagnosis includes low-grade endometrial stromal sarcoma.

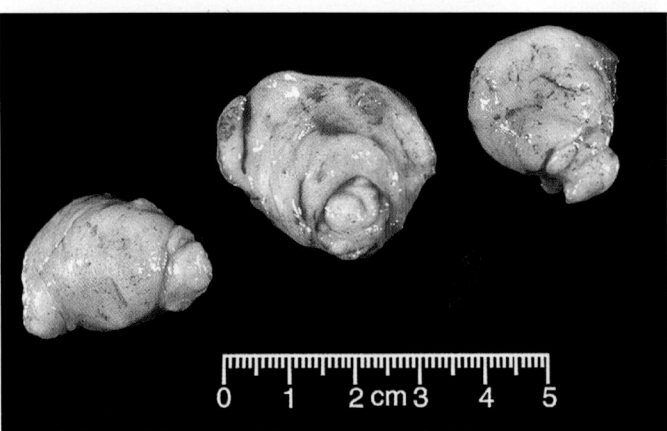

Fig. 20.87 Cut surfaces of intravenous leiomyoma shown in Figure 20.86 resemble a typical uterine leiomyoma.

et al. have pointed out that the immunoprofile of intravenous leiomyomatosis is more like myometrium (and uterine leiomyomata) than subendothelial cells.[353] Cytogenetic analysis also indicates a uterine origin. Karyotypes of two tumors have both shown the presence of a derivative chromosome (*viz.* der(14)t(12;14)(q15;q24)) found frequently in uterine leiomyomata.[338,339] Presumably, the ability to grow within venous spaces reflects some additional genetic alterations.

Intravenous extension might be considered an aggressive biologic property. Despite this malignant appearance, the intravascular growth is usually indolent. The presenting symptoms often depend on the extent of growth. If intravenous leiomyomatosis is associated with a large leiomyoma of the uterus, pelvic pain or bleeding typically predominate. If the extension into the vena cava is significant, symptoms such as syncope and dyspnea may be prominent. In most cases, extirpation to address hemodynamic consequences and hysterectomy to remove associated leiomyomata are sufficient therapy.[354] Expression of estrogen and progesterone receptors has been noted in lesional smooth muscle cells and provides the foundation for gonadotropin releasing hormone agonist (e.g. leuprolide) in the short-term therapy of intravenous leiomyomatosis.[353,356] In rare circumstances, intravenous leiomyomatosis extending into the heart may result in death.[357] Adhesion to the vessel wall and atypical histology may be associated with a more aggressive clinical course.[358] A relationship to benign metastasizing leiomyoma in the lung also has been suggested.[359]

Disseminated peritoneal leiomyomatosis

Disseminated peritoneal leiomyomatosis (leiomyomatosis peritonealis disseminata) is a disorder in which smooth muscle tumorlets are scattered across peritoneal and omental surfaces (Fig. 20.89).[340,360] Although the disorder is quite rare, well over a hundred case have been individually reported, generally in women of reproductive age, but occasionally in postmenopausal women.[361,362] The tumorlets in disseminated peritoneal leiomyomatosis can range in size from microscopic to 10–25 mm and number from a handful to several hundred (Fig. 20.90). The multitude of tumorlets

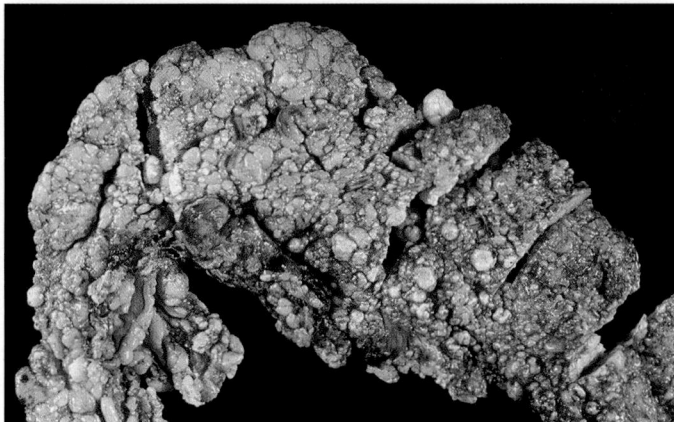

Fig. 20.89 Omentum involved by disseminated peritoneal leiomyomatosis.

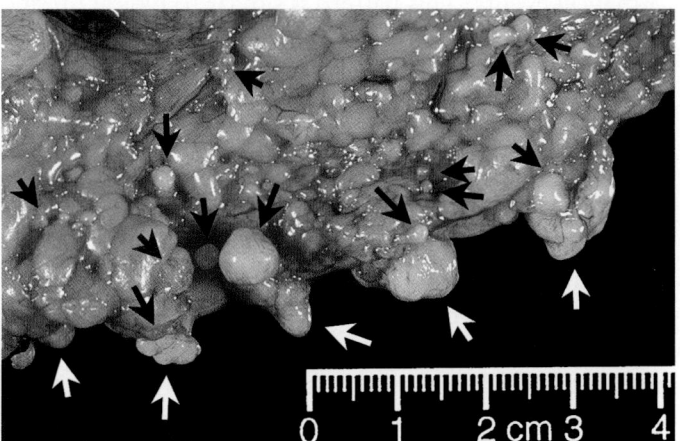

Fig. 20.90 The tumorlets (black and white arrows) of omental disseminated peritoneal leiomyomatosis, which range in size from microscopic up to several cm, are macroscopically identical to small uterine leiomyomata.

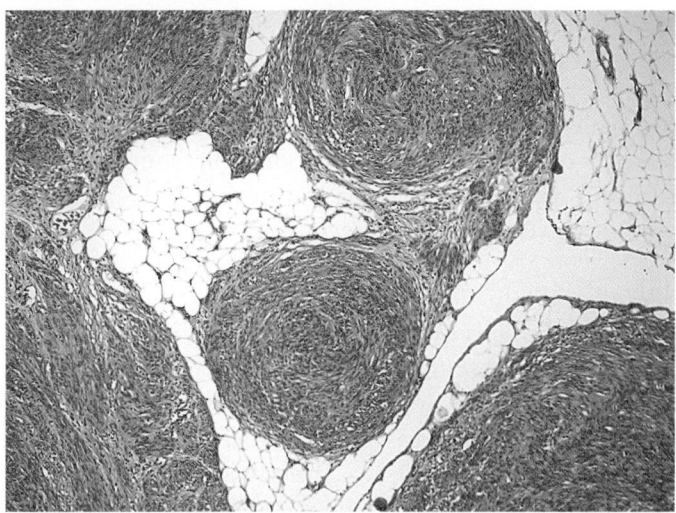

Fig. 20.91 Bland smooth muscle usually comprises the tumorlets of disseminated leiomyomatosis.

studding the peritoneum may initially mimic an aggressive ovarian neoplasm. The correct diagnosis is made by recognizing that each tumorlet is a small leiomyoma. The cut surfaces of the larger tumorlets have the tan, bulging, whorled appearance of their larger uterine counterpart. The microscopic appearances of the tumorlets also are identical to typical uterine leiomyomata (Fig. 20.91). Specifically, the tumorlets are composed of bland smooth cells with low proliferative activity, no significant atypia and no geographic tumor necrosis. Occasionally, the tumorlets may contain foci of endometriosis.[340,363]

Interestingly, disseminated peritoneal leiomyomatosis generally has a benign clinical course. The leiomyomatous nodules may even persist or recur over decades.[340,364] In such cases, the size range of nodules seems to decrease after menopause, pointing the way to one potential therapeutic strategy for perimenopausal women with

peritoneal leiomyomatosis.[365] This proliferation of smooth muscle is often an incidental discovery at the time of Cesarean section or oophorectomy for Brenner tumors, which also suggests that hormonal stimulation plays a role in the pathobiology of this condition.[21,86,366] Experience with these patients by a large number of groups suggests that aggressive therapeutic intervention is unnecessary and potentially harmful. In some circumstances, however, surgical intervention in order to debulk the abdomen or pelvis may be considered when there are signs or symptoms related to mass effect, particularly if there are dominant 'fibroids' among the leiomyomatous lesions.[367] Rarely, malignant transformation has been reported.[368–374]

As noted above, disseminated peritoneal leiomyomatosis is associated with high levels of estrogen. In addition to pregnancy, clomiphene treatment and estrogen-producing ovarian granulosa cell tumors have been reported in association with some, but not all women with disseminated peritoneal leiomyomatosis.[375,376] The tumorlets of this disorder also express progesterone receptor.[366,377] The observation that progesterone can produce ectopic deciduosis in pregnant humans and leiomyoma-like nodules in certain rodent models has led some to conclude that disseminated peritoneal leiomyomatosis is a metaplastic process.[378] If this were to be true, each nodule would be expected to be a polyclonal proliferation, presumably arising from subperitoneal mesenchyme. Clonality analysis of these smooth muscle tumorlets, however, demonstrates that each nodule is clonal.[340] Moreover, these clonality studies indicate that all of the nodules have an identical pattern of X chromosome inactivation, strongly suggesting that all of the nodules arose from a single transformation event. Thus, the disseminated nodules are truly metastatic. The remarkable molecular mechanism(s) permitting intraperitoneal dissemination, yet limiting the proliferation and invasiveness of each nodule have yet to be determined.

Intrauterine leiomyomatosis

Intrauterine leiomyomatosis is a condition in which there are a large number of leiomyomata confined to the uterus. The gross appearance of intrauterine leiomyomatosis is that of an enlarged and usually distorted uterine corpus (Fig. 20.92). Examination of the cut surface may reveal distinct, but confluent tumorous masses, or may reveal a diffuse process without clear delineation of individual masses (Fig. 20.93). This condition is not to be confused with nodular degeneration of myometrium or leiomyomata.[329,379] As one might expect, the associated clinical features often include symptoms referable to mass effect. Similar to disseminated peritoneal leiomyomatosis, intrauterine leiomyomatosis is clinically benign. Clonality studies have shown that each mass within uteri with leiomyomatosis also are clonal.[380] In contrast to peritoneal leiomyomatosis, the intrauterine masses do not necessarily share the same pattern of X chromosome inactivation. This finding suggests that each intrauterine mass arose from independent trans-

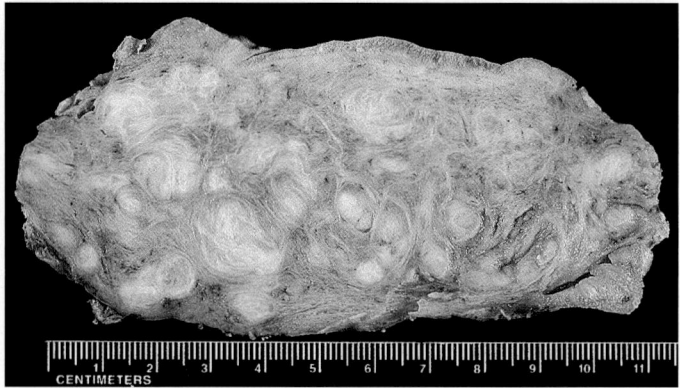

Fig. 20.93 Cut surface of diffuse leiomyomatosis. Note that the numerous masses may have indistinct borders and appear to be confluent.

formation events. This pattern is similar to typical uterine leiomyomata. One possible explanation is that the myometrial smooth muscle cells of some individuals are extremely prone to tumorigenesis. Predisposing genetic or environmental factors in intrauterine leiomyomatosis are unknown at present.

Benign metastasizing leiomyoma

Benign metastasizing leiomyoma is a rare and enigmatic disorder of smooth muscle cell growth.[381,382] The typical clinical scenario is the presentation of one or several small fibroid-like masses in the lung, or occasionally abdominopelvic lymph nodes, in women with a history of hysterectomy (Fig. 20.94). The histologic appear-

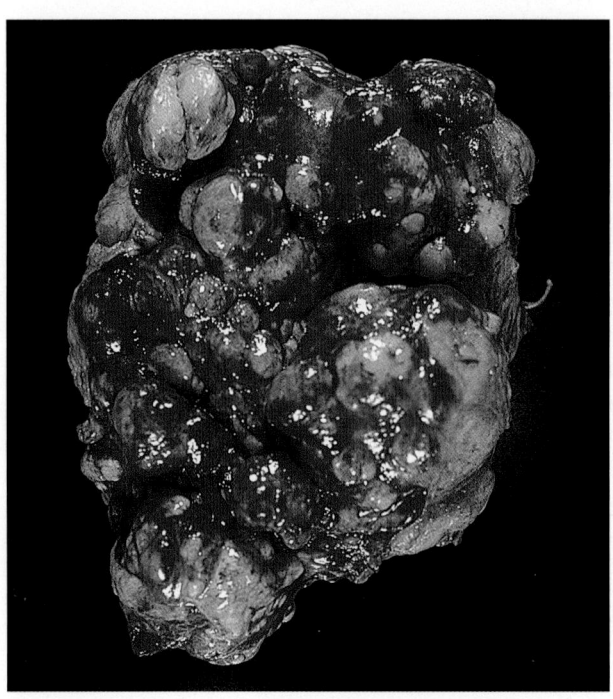

Fig. 20.92 Uterine corpus distorted by diffuse leiomyomatosis.

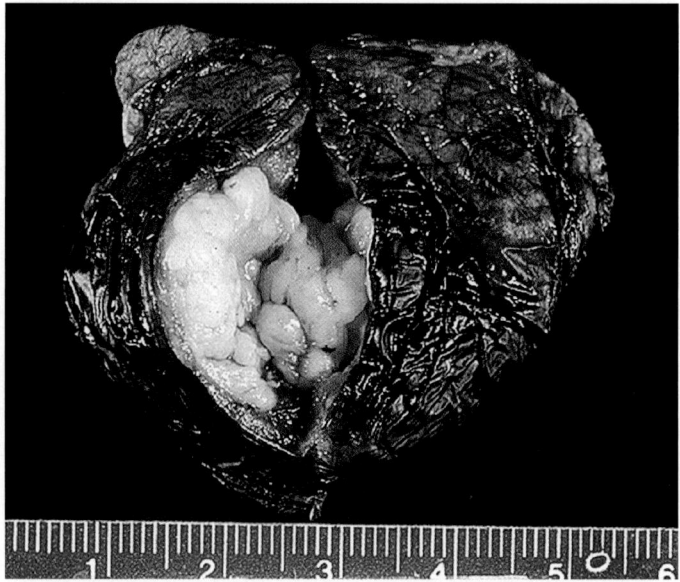

Fig. 20.94 Benign metastasizing leiomyoma is a tumor mass with the macroscopic and microscopic features of a leiomyoma found in the lung (in this case, a pulmonary wedge resection).

ance consists of bland smooth muscle cells. One or more typical leiomyomata are found when the prior hysterectomy specimen, if available, is reviewed. As its name suggests, the clinical course is benign.[382]

Despite its name and the apparent association with prior hysterectomy, there is little evidence establishing a relationship between benign metastasizing leiomyoma and other uterine smooth muscle tumors. The association of benign metastasizing leiomyoma and intravenous leiomyomatosis suggests that the pulmonary lesions may be deported from the intravenous lesions.[359] Analysis of one case by comparative genomic hybridization showed that the pulmonary lesions lacked allelic imbalance, which is more similar to a leiomyoma (or intravenous leiomyomatosis) than a leiomyosarcoma.[383] Furthermore, the multiple lesions had a pattern of X chromosome inactivation compatible with metastasis from a single clone. This observation, however, does not confirm a uterine origin and does not exclude intravenous leiomyomatosis as the source. Cytogenetic analysis of benign metastasizing leiomyoma showed deletions of 19q and 22q, but not other rearrangements found in typical uterine leiomyomata, in all five cases studied.[384] Deletions of 19q and 22q are not commonly found in typical leiomyomata, suggesting that benign metastasizing and typical uterine leiomyomata do not share a common origin.

TUMORS MIMICKING SMOOTH MUSCLE TUMORS

Adenomyosis and adenomyoma

Adenomyosis is defined as the ectopic presence of endometrial glands and stroma within the myometrium, well beyond the normal anatomical interface with the endometrium (Fig. 20.95).[385] In our practice, we require that the glands must be more than the field width of an intermediate magnification (i.e. deeper than the field seen using a 10× objective and 10× ocular lenses in a conventionally configured microscope, or 2–3 mm). Consequently, this is a diagnosis mostly made in well-oriented hysterectomy specimens and essentially never in curetting or hysteroscopic specimens. The imprecision of the diagnostic criteria have led to a wide range (9–30%) in estimating the prevalence of adenomyosis.[386,387] The histologic appearance may vary between foci. The size may range from a single gland with almost no investing stroma to large islands with numerous glands and ample stroma. In most cases, the adenomyotic foci resemble proliferative endometrium, but the ectopic endometrium may undergo secretory differentiation in response to progesterone. This secretory differentiation may lag

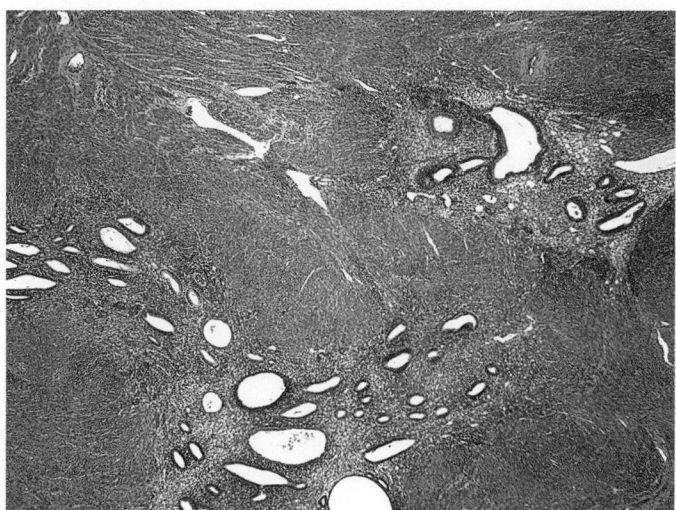

Fig. 20.95 Endometrial glands and stroma well beyond the endomyometrial junction defines adenomyosis.

behind that seen in eutopic endometrium, similar to endometriosis.[388] In some cases, stromal breakdown and subsequent hemorrhage may result in the accumulation of hemosiderin when the adenomyotic foci are deep within the myometrium. The accumulation of blood or its brownish degradation products deep within the myometrium in a seemingly random fashion may provide the first gross clue as to the presence of adenomyosis (Fig. 20.96). Myometrial hypertrophy surrounding adenomyotic foci also may be apparent to the careful observer.

Adenomyosis is a difficult diagnosis to make clinically because it is associated with non-specific signs and symptoms, or it may be asymptomatic. The most frequent

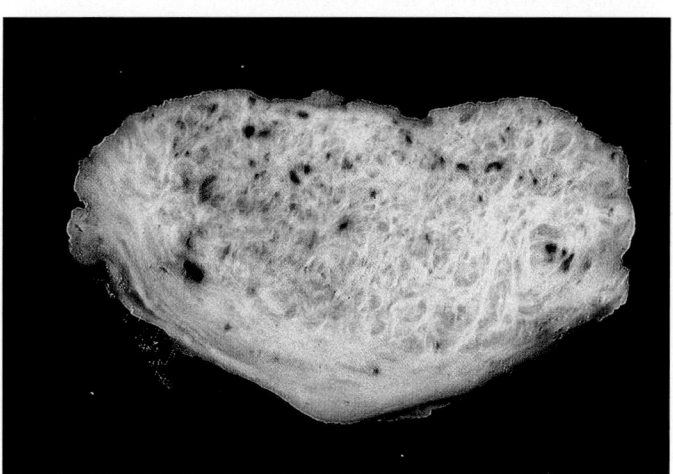

Fig. 20.96 Adenomyosis. Ill-defined smooth muscle hyperplasia and foci of hemosiderin or blood deep within the myometrium are characteristic macroscopic features.

clinical findings include menorrhagia, dysmenorrhea and uterine enlargement, which is presumably due to myometrial hypertrophy. Deeper lesions are more likely to be symptomatic.[389] Hysterectomy, endometrial ablation and hormonal suppression are well-established therapeutic options. Recently, uterine artery ablation has been suggested as an effective minimally invasive alternative.[390]

The origin of adenomyosis is obscure. While it bears a nosological connection to endometriosis, substantive studies to determine the pathobiologic mechanism(s) of adenomyosis are lacking. Hypothetical mechanisms might include instillation of endometrium within the myometrium, *in situ* metaplasia of pluripotent stem cells retained in myometrium, or improper partitioning of the endometrium from the myometrium. Of note, del(7) (q21.2q31.2), a deletion found in typical leiomyoma, also has been found in three cases of adenomyosis, suggesting some pathobiologic overlap between leiomyomata and adenomyosis.[391] Definitive discrimination between these explanations, however, will require further study and new tools.

Adenomyoma is a condition closely related to adenomyosis. The key distinction between the two is the presence of a discernible tumorous mass in adenomyoma (Fig. 20.97). Most often, this mass is grossly identical to a typical leiomyoma. The adenomyomatous mass occasionally may have a softer interface with the surrounding myometrium, but it should still be relatively circumscribed. Like diffuse adenomyosis, the trabeculations seen on the cut surface may be finer than a leiomyoma. In addition, the foci of endometrial glands and stroma may be evident as small (1–2 mm) hemorrhagic spots.

Adenomyomas usually are intramural masses, but occasionally may be submucosal, or even resemble endometrial polyps macroscopically (Fig. 20.97). Of note, adenomyomatous polyps with glandular abnormalities mimicking endometrial hyperplasia with squamous (morular) metaplasia are recognized as a separated entity known as atypical endometrial adenomyoma (APA) or Mazur's polyp (see Ch. 19) (Figs 20.98, 20.99).

Adenomyomas are not usually diagnosed until pathologic examination. Whether adenomyomas are the biologic equivalent of leiomyomata has yet to be studied in detail. Fortunately, they are the clinical equivalent, as they affect the same patient population and can be treated with the same techniques as uterine leiomyomata.

Adenomatoid tumors

Adenomatoid tumors are tumorous masses involving the serosal surfaces of uterus or fallopian tube (Figs 20.100,

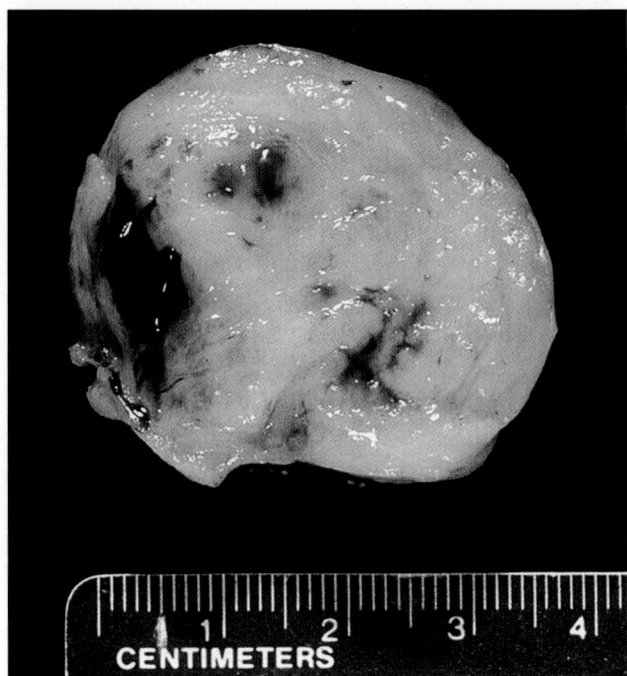

Fig. 20.97 Adenomyoma. Hemosiderin or blood may be seen on the cut surface.

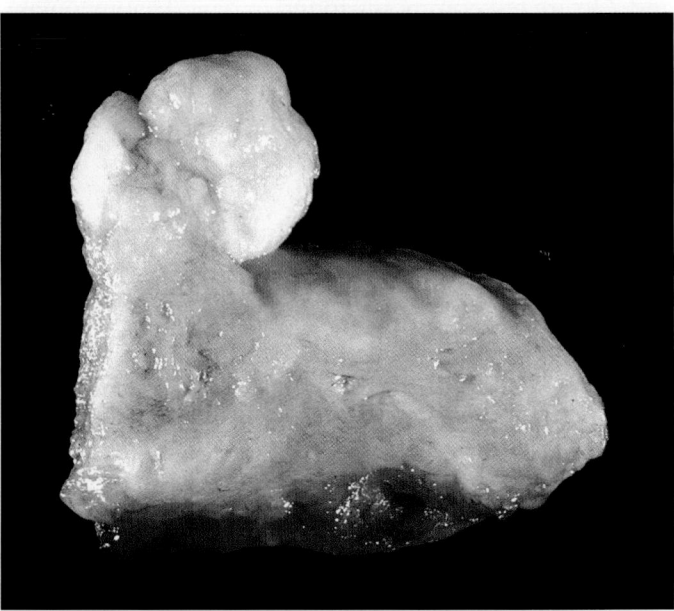

Fig. 20.98 Atypical polypoid adenomyoma. The gross appearance may mimic a usual endometrial polyp.

20.101). Like adenomyomas, these tumors are admixtures of seemingly hyperplastic smooth muscle and another component. In the case of adenomatoid tumors, the second component is derived from the serosal mesothelium. The mesothelial proliferation forms gland-like spaces nestled between smooth muscle fascicles. The

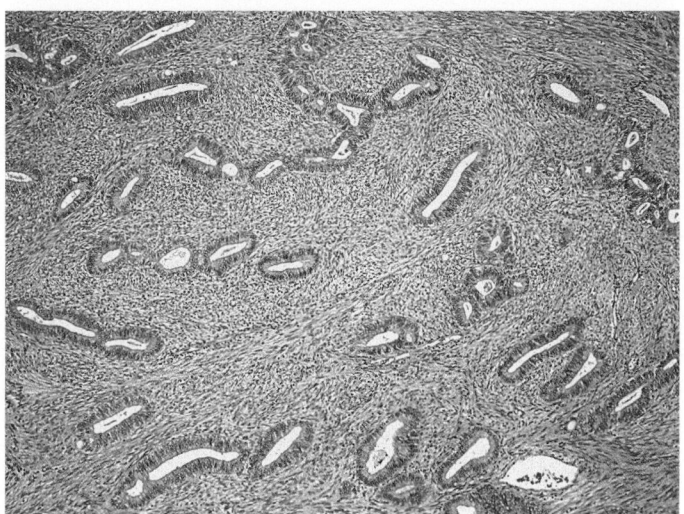

Fig. 20.99 Atypical polypoid adenomyoma. An admixture of fibromyomatous stroma with endometrial-type glands.

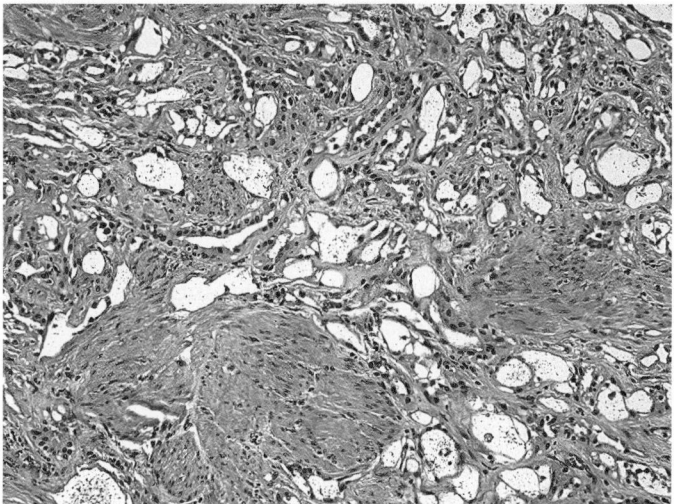

Fig. 20.101 Adenomatoid tumor. A mixed tumor composed of mesothelial cells, which may be inconspicuous, and hyperplastic smooth muscle cells.

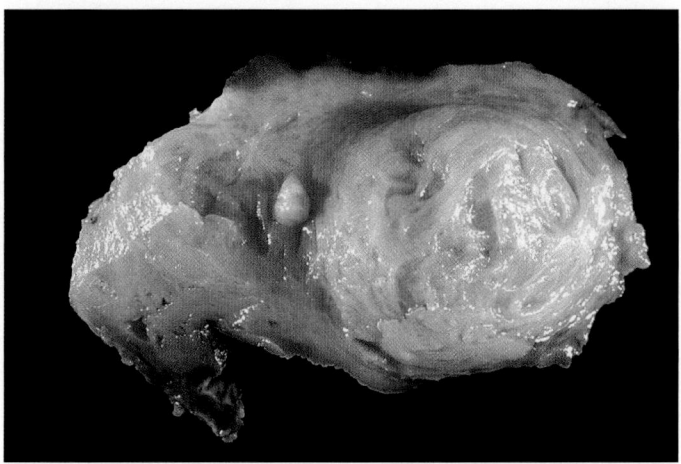

Fig. 20.100 Adenomatoid tumor mimicking a subserosal leiomyoma.

mesothelial origin of these cells can be confirmed by their expression of cytokeratins and calretinin, but not of CD31 or CD34. Presumably, the mesothelial cells are neoplastic and the smooth muscle cells are hyperplastic. This relationship, which remains to be proven, is similar to that between adenomyomas and their companion smooth muscle cells.

In addition to their characteristic location, adenomatoid tumors are firm, rubbery tumors with white or gray cut surfaces. The border with the adjacent myometrium may not bulge out or be as defined as the typical leiomyomata. Microscopically, the mesothelial cells are not infrequently inconspicuous. Consequently, the gland-like spaces may look more like venules, or even adipose or signet ring cells.

As adenomatoid tumors are usually benign, under 2 cm in size and an incidental finding in women in the years before menopause, they have no clinical impact apart from their mimicry of leiomyomata and other tumors.

Mixed epithelial and mesenchymal tumors

Tumors in this category are composed of an admixture of epithelial and mesenchymal elements and classification depends upon whether the epithelial or mesenchymal component is benign or malignant.

ADENOSARCOMA

Definition

Adenosarcoma is composed of a benign epithelial component admixed with a malignant stromal (mesenchymal) component.

Clinical presentation

Uterine Müllerian adenosarcoma can occur over a wide age range, from the second to the tenth decade; however, most occur during the sixth decade in the postmenopausal patient.[392–394] There is no apparent racial predilection.[1] The most common symptoms and clinical findings at presentation include abnormal vaginal bleeding, an enlarged uterus, a pelvic mass or tissue protruding through the os.[392–394] A history of 'recurrent' polyps is not uncommon.[392] Most uterine adenosarcomas are confined to the endometrium; however, myometrial invasion, including deep extension, may occur.[392] The development of adenosarcoma has been linked to tamoxifen therapy in patients being treated with this regimen for breast carcinoma.[3] Prolonged endogenous or exogenous hyperestrinism (as is the case in patients on prolonged tamoxifen therapy) is associated with the development of uterine malignancies, including epithelial and mixed epithelial-mesenchymal tumors.[4–9,395,396]

Histopathologic features

Uterine Müllerian adenosarcomas are typically bulky, soft, polypoid masses that fill the endometrial cavity and may prolapse through the cervical os.[3,392,393,397] They most commonly involve the uterine fundus, but may also occasionally arise in the lower uterine segment or cervix.[392,394,398] Involvement of more than one site in the uterus may be seen less commonly.[392] Histologically, adenosarcoma is characterized by: (1) tubular, dilated or cleft-like glands (as a consequence of intraglandular polypoid projections) lined by benign epithelium which may show a range of appearances from bland cuboidal, to proliferative (similar to proliferative phase endometrium) to epithelium with altered (metaplastic) differentiation (e.g. tubal, mucinous, squamous), (2) periglandular cuffing by hypercellular stroma, (3) stromal mitotic activity (greater than two mitoses per 10 high power fields) and (4) stromal cellular atypia (Figs 20.102, 20.103). Mitotic activity and stromal cellular atypia can be quite variable in this tumor, with some cases exhibiting very little of either, which likely leads to its

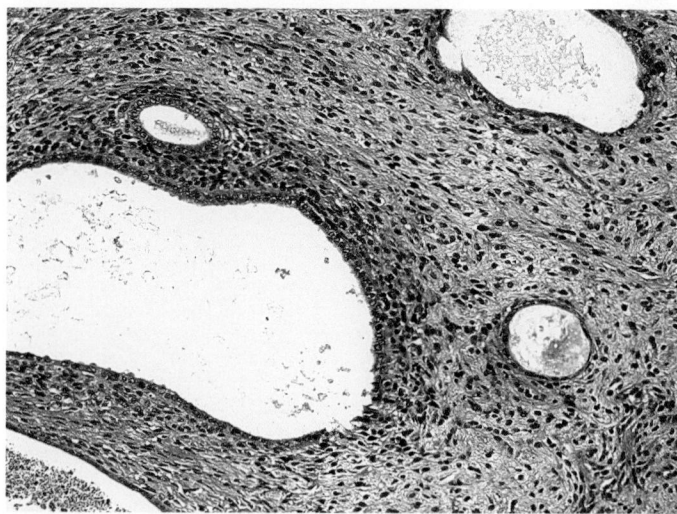
Fig. 20.103 Adenosarcoma. Note the hypercellular stroma cuffing the dilated gland.

under-recognition as well as its over-diagnosis. The mesenchymal component of uterine adenosarcoma is more commonly homologous (with a stromal or fibrous appearance); however, heterologous differentiation, most commonly in the form of rhabdomyosarcoma, also may be seen (Fig. 20.104). Sex-cord-like differentiation may be present as well.[397]

Differential diagnosis

The differential diagnosis of uterine Müllerian adenosarcoma includes: (1) uterine adenofibroma, (2) carcinosarcoma, (3) atypical polypoid adenomyoma, (4) endometrial stromal sarcoma with glandular differentiation and (5) endometrial polyp (Table 20.8). Uterine adenofi-

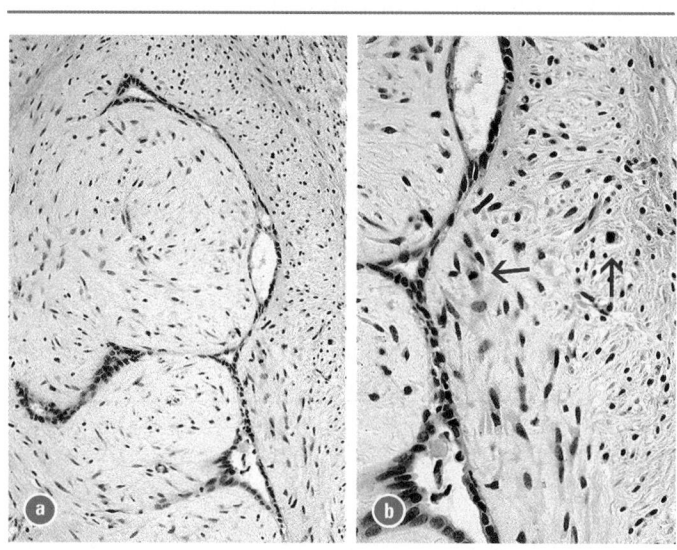
Fig. 20.102 Adenosarcoma. Note the phyllodes-like glands (a) and the mitotically active stromal cells (red arrows in (b)).

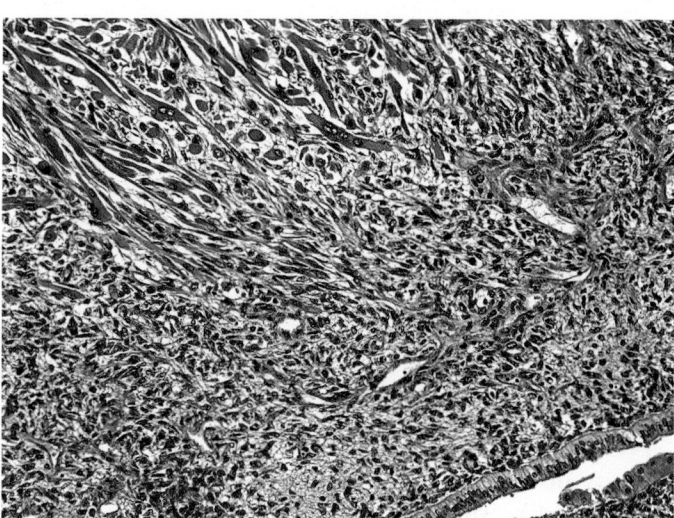
Fig. 20.104 Adenosarcoma. Rhabdomyosarcomatous differentiation.

Table 20.8 *Features of mixed glandular and mesenchymal neoplasia in the uterine corpus*

	Adenosarcoma	Adenofibroma	Atypical polypoid adenomyoma	Low-grade endometrial stromal sarcoma with glandular differentiation	Endometrial polyp
Gland contour	Leaf-like, dilated	Leaf-like, dilated	Tubular, irregular outlines	Tubular	Tubular, dilated
Periglandular cuffing	Yes	Yes	No	No	No
Stromal atypia	Yes	No	No	No	Usually not
Mitotic index	>2/10 hpf[a]	<2/10 hpf[a]	Variable	Variable	Variable
Squamous metaplasia	Rare	Rare	Common	Absent	Occasional; may be associated with endometrial intraepithelial neoplasia
Other epithelial metaplasia	Common	Common	Rare	Rare	Common
Myomatous stroma	No	No	Yes	Occasional	Occasional

[a]high power field.

broma is purportedly a tumor composed of benign epithelial and mesenchymal components similar in appearance to adenosarcoma, except there should not be any stromal atypia and mitoses should not exceed two per 10 high power fields;[399] the diagnosis of adenofibroma should be made with caution and perhaps is best considered as an 'atypical' endometrial polyp (see below). Carcinosarcoma is distinguished from adenosarcoma by its combination of a malignant epithelial as well as mesenchymal component; moreover, the former lacks the typical glandular contours and stromal condensation of the latter. The mesenchymal component of carcinosarcoma also typically has a higher-grade appearance. Atypical polypoid adenomyoma is distinguished adenosarcoma by: (1) fibromyomatous stroma, (2) squamous metaplasia within the glands (which is typically more common and extensive than that seen in adenosarcoma). Occasionally endometrial stromal sarcoma (morphologically 'low-grade') may contain benign-appearing endometrioid glands;[400] usually the glandular elements are focal but they may occasionally be more extensively present (Fig. 20.13). This variant of endometrial stromal sarcoma lacks the periglandular stromal cuffing and the characteristic glandular contours typical of adenosarcoma. Perhaps the most difficult distinction is adenosarcoma from endometrial polyp, particularly benign polyps, which exhibit some but not all features of adenosarcoma. Endometrial polyps with atypical stromal cells may occur similar to stromal polyps seen at other sites in the female genital tract[401] (Fig. 20.105) and occasional cleft-like glands may be seen in otherwise benign polyps. In these instances, a diagnosis of endometrial polyp can be made without further qualification. However, in polyps with glandular

contours and stromal condensation as seen in adenosarcoma, but which lack mitotic activity (or have fewer than two per 10 high power fields) and stromal atypia, it is our opinion that these lesions should be classified as 'endometrial polyp with atypical features' with a comment that although diagnostic features of adenosarcoma are not identified, close clinical follow-up with sampling of any 'recurrent' polyps is recommended.

Prognosis and management

Adenosarcoma is associated with better survival in comparison to other types of uterine sarcoma, particularly carcinosarcoma and leiomyosarcoma;[1] however, recurrence is associated with a poor prognosis.[394] In the largest series of Müllerian adenosarcoma, recurrence

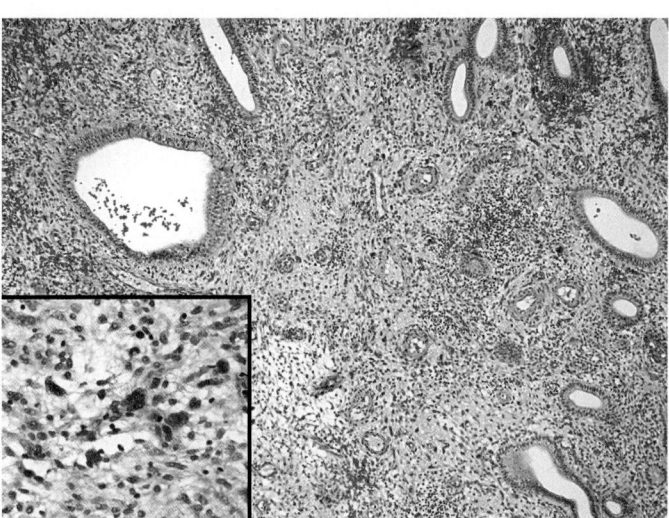

Fig. 20.105 Endometrial polyp with bizarre stromal nuclei. Multinucleated, hyperchromatic stromal cells are present (inset).

occurred in approximately one-fourth of patients, most commonly in the vagina, pelvis or abdomen.[392] Histologic features associated with poor prognosis include the presence of myometrial invasion and sarcomatous overgrowth in the primary tumor.[392–394]

Patients with uterine adenosarcoma are treated by hysterectomy and bilateral salpingo-oophorectomy. Radiotherapy or chemotherapy also may be considered, the latter particularly in patients with inoperable disease.[394] Although the epithelial and stromal component of Müllerian adenosarcoma can be positive for estrogen and progesterone receptor, suggesting tumoral hormonal sensitivity,[402] the impact of bilateral oophorectomy on outcome, particularly in women who wish to maintain their fertility, is not clear.

CARCINOSARCOMA (MALIGNANT MIXED MÜLLERIAN TUMOR)

This tumor type is described in greater detail in the chapter on endometrial carcinoma (Ch. 19). Although this tumor is composed of a malignant epithelial and mesenchymal component, it is now widely accepted (based on morphologic, clinicopathologic and genetic data) that these tumors represent metaplastic carcinomas.

Miscellaneous tumors

UTERINE PERIVASCULAR EPITHELIOID CELL TUMOR

The concept of uterine perivascular epithelioid tumor was introduced because a subset of uterine tumors are composed of cells that are morphologically and immunophenotypically similar to perivascular epithelioid cell-type tumors described at other sites, such as epithelioid angiomyolipoma, clear cell 'sugar' tumor, clear cell myelomelanocytic of the ligamentum teres/falciform ligament, abdominopelvic sarcoma of perivascular epithelioid cells and lymphangioleiomyomatosis (Fig. 20.106).[403] In general, PEComas are composed of epithelioid cells with abundant clear to granular cytoplasm that have a tendency to exhibit a perivascular distribution and which are positive for HMB-45 and desmin (Figs 20.107, 20.108).[403–407] So-called uterine perivascular epithelioid tumors have been described as having two distinctive morphologic subtypes.[403] One subtype closely mimics the growth pattern of low-grade endometrial stromal sarcoma with finger-like permeation of the uterine wall and is composed of cells with abundant eosinophilic,

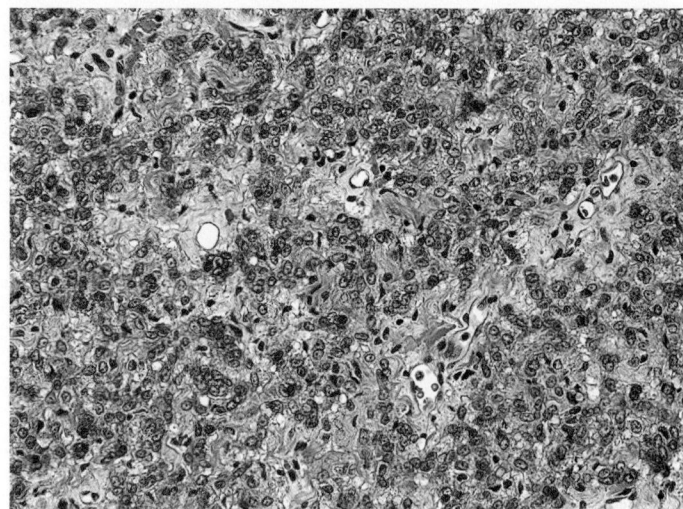

Fig. 20.106 Perivascular epithelioid cell tumor (PEComa).

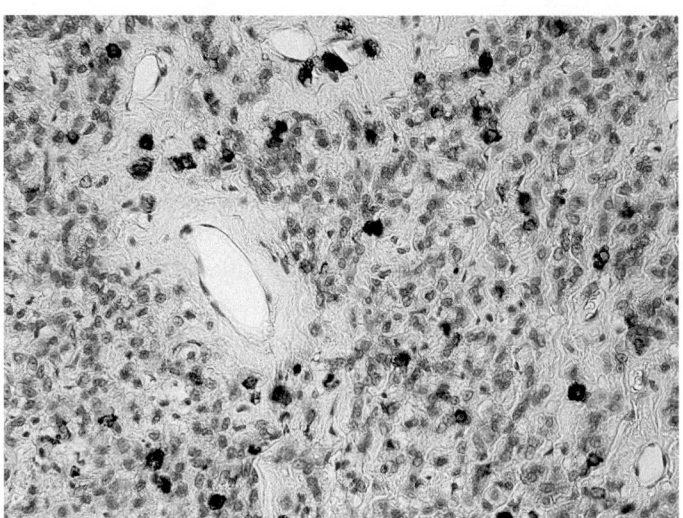

Fig. 20.107 Perivascular epithelioid cell tumor. Focal staining for HMB-45.

clear or granular cytoplasm; these tumors exhibit diffuse HMB-45 expression with only focal muscle marker positivity. The other subtype is composed of epithelioid cells that have less abundant clear cytoplasm, less HMB-45 expression and more extensive muscle marker positivity. The relationship of uterine perivascular epithelioid tumor to epithelioid smooth muscle tumors is unclear; however, it appears that they may be part of a morphologic spectrum.[403,408] Because of this spectrum, use of the term perivascular epithelioid tumor for uterine tumors exhibiting this morphology has been admonished because uterine perivascular epithelioid tumor does not appear yet to be a clinically homogeneous, rigorously defined tumor type.[408] Nevertheless, application of HMB-45 should be considered in all cases of

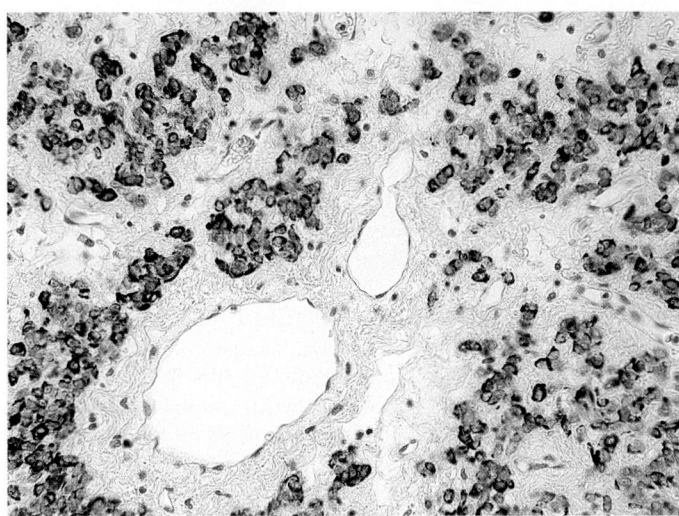

Fig. 20.108 Perivascular epithelioid cell tumor. Diffuse staining for desmin.

uterine mesenchymal tumors with prominent epithelioid cytomorphology not only to further define the concept of uterine perivascular epithelioid tumor but also because some patients with tumors having a uterine perivascular epithelioid tumor-like morphology should be investigated for the possibility of tuberous sclerosis or lymphangioleiomyomatosis.[403,408] Occasionally, low-grade endometrial stromal sarcoma may exhibit an epithelioid cytomorphology,[54] which may raise the possibility of uterine perivascular epithelioid tumor; however, the latter has more prominent thick-walled vessels and lacks the presence of the characteristic spiral arteriole vessels of endometrial stromal sarcoma. Application of HMB-45 will help in this distinction (Fig. 20.107).

References

1 Brooks SE, Zhan M, Cote T, Baquet CR. Surveillance, epidemiology and end results analysis of 2677 cases of uterine sarcoma 1989–1999. Gynecol Oncol 2004; 93:204–208.

2 Nordal RR, Thoresen SO. Uterine sarcomas in Norway 1956–1992: incidence, survival and mortality. Eur J Cancer 1997; 33:907–911.

3 Clement PB, Oliva E, Young RH. Müllerian adenosarcoma of the uterine corpus associated with tamoxifen therapy: a report of six cases and a review of tamoxifen-associated endometrial lesions. Int J Gynecol Pathol 1996; 15:222–229.

4 Fotiou S, Hatjieleftheriou G, Kyrousis G, et al. Long-term tamoxifen treatment: a possible aetiological factor in the development of uterine carcinosarcoma: two case-reports and review of the literature. Anticancer Res 2000; 20:2015–2020.

5 Evans MJ, Langlois NE, Kitchener HC, Miller ID. Is there an association between long-term tamoxifen treatment and the development of carcinosarcoma (malignant mixed Müllerian tumor) of the uterus? Int J Gynecol Cancer 1995; 5:310–313.

6 Moe MM, El Sharkawi S. Is there any association between uterine malignant mixed Müllerian tumour, breast cancer and prolonged tamoxifen treatment? J Obstet Gynaecol 2003; 23:301–303.

7 Curtis RE, Freedman DM, Sherman ME, Fraumeni JF Jr. Risk of malignant mixed Müllerian tumors after tamoxifen therapy for breast cancer. J Natl Cancer Inst 2004; 96:70–74.

8 McCluggage WG, Abdulkader M, Price JH, et al. Uterine carcinosarcomas in patients receiving tamoxifen. A report of 19 cases. Int J Gynecol Cancer 2000; 10:280–284.

9 Kloos I, Delaloge S, Pautier P, et al. Tamoxifen-related uterine carcinosarcomas occur under/after prolonged treatment: report of five cases and review of the literature. Int J Gynecol Cancer 2002; 12:496–500.

10 Bornstein J, Auslender R, Pascal B, et al. Diagnostic pitfalls of ultrasonographic uterine screening in women treated with tamoxifen. J Reprod Med 1994; 39:674–678.

11 Jolly EE, Bjarnason NH, Neven P, et al. Prevention of osteoporosis and uterine effects in postmenopausal women taking raloxifene for 5 years. Menopause 2003; 10:337–344.

12 Goldstein SR. Controversy about uterine effects and safety of SERMs: the saga continues. Menopause 2002; 9:381–384.

13 Cramer SF, Patel A. The frequency of uterine leiomyomas. Am J Clin Pathol 1990; 94:435–438.

14 Marshall LM, Spiegelman D, Barbieri RL, et al. Variation in the incidence of uterine leiomyoma among premenopausal women by age and race. Obstet Gynecol 1997; 90:967–973.

15 Kjerulff KH, Guzinski GM, Langenberg PW, et al. Hysterectomy and race. Obstet Gynecol 1993; 82:757–764.

16 Kjerulff KH, Langenberg P, Seidman JD, et al. Uterine leiomyomas. Racial differences in severity, symptoms and age at diagnosis. J Reprod Med 1996; 41:483–490.

17 Schwartz SM, Marshall LM, Baird DD. Epidemiologic contributions to understanding the etiology of uterine leiomyomata. Environ Health Perspect 2000; 108 (Suppl)(5):821–827.

18 Samadi AR, Lee NC, Flanders WD, et al. Risk factors for self-reported uterine fibroids: a case-control study. Am J Public Health 1996; 86:858–862.

19 Ross RK, Pike MC, Vessey MP, et al. Risk factors for uterine fibroids: reduced risk associated with oral contraceptives. Br Med J (Clin Res Ed) 1986; 293:359–362.

20 Chen CR, Buck GM, Courey NG, et al. Risk factors for uterine fibroids among women undergoing tubal sterilization. Am J Epidemiol 2001; 153:20–26.

21 Baron JA. Beneficial effects of nicotine and cigarette smoking: the real, the possible and the spurious. Br Med Bull 1996; 52:58–73.

22 Wise LA, Palmer JR, Harlow BL, et al. Risk of uterine leiomyomata in relation to tobacco, alcohol and caffeine consumption in the Black Women's Health Study. Hum Reprod 2004; 19(8):1746–1754.

23 Marshall LM, Spiegelman D, Manson JE, et al. Risk of uterine leiomyomata among premenopausal women in relation to body size and cigarette smoking. Epidemiology 1998; 9:511–517.

24 Faerstein E, Szklo M, Rosenshein N. Risk factors for uterine leiomyoma: a practice-based case-control study. I. African-American heritage, reproductive history, body size and smoking. Am J Epidemiol 2001; 153:1–10.

25 Wise LA, Palmer JR, Harlow BL, et al. Reproductive factors, hormonal contraception and risk of uterine leiomyomata in African-American women: a prospective study. Am J Epidemiol 2004; 159:113–123.

26 Parazzini F, Negri E, Vecchia C La, et al. Reproductive factors and risk of uterine fibroids. Epidemiology 1996; 7:440–442.

27 Parazzini F, Vecchia C La, Negri E, Cecchetti G, Fedele L. Epidemiologic characteristics of women with uterine fibroids: a case-control study. Obstet Gynecol 1988; 72:853–857.

28 Marshall LM, Spiegelman D, Goldman MB, et al. A prospective study of reproductive factors and oral contraceptive use in relation to the risk of uterine leiomyomata. Fertil Steril 1998; 70:432–439.

29 Parazzini F, Negri E, Vecchia C La, et al. Oral contraceptive use and risk of uterine fibroids. Obstet Gynecol 1992; 79:430–433.

30 Chiaffarino F, Parazzini F, Vecchia C La, et al. Use of oral contraceptives and uterine fibroids: results from a case-control study. Br J Obstet Gynaecol 1999; 106:857–860.

31 Sato F, Nishi M, Kudo R, Miyake H. Body fat distribution and uterine leiomyomas. J Epidemiol 1998; 8:176–180.

32 Faerstein E, Szklo M, Rosenshein NB. Risk factors for uterine leiomyoma: a practice-based case-control study. II. Atherogenic risk factors and potential sources of uterine irritation. Am J Epidemiol 2001; 153:11–19.

33 Nagata C, Takatsuka N, Kawakami N, Shimizu H. Soy product intake and premenopausal hysterectomy in a follow-up study of Japanese women. Eur J Clin Nutr 2001; 55:773–777.

34 Palan PR, Mikhail M, Romney SL. Decreased beta-carotene tissue levels in uterine leiomyomas and cancers of reproductive and nonreproductive organs. Am J Obstet Gynecol 1989; 161:1649–1652.

35 Chiaffarino F, Parazzini F, Vecchia C La, et al. Diet and uterine myomas. Obstet Gynecol 1999; 94:395–398.

36 Goto A, Takeuchi S, Sugimura K, Maruo T. Usefulness of Gd-DTPA contrast-enhanced dynamic MRI and serum determination of LDH and its isozymes in the differential diagnosis of leiomyosarcoma from degenerated leiomyoma of the uterus. Int J Gynecol Cancer 2002; 12:354–361.

37 Janus C, White M, Dottino P, Brodman M, Goodman H. Uterine leiomyosarcoma–magnetic resonance imaging. Gynecol Oncol 1989; 32:79–81.

38 Kido A, Togashi K, Koyama T, et al. Diffusely enlarged uterus: evaluation with MR imaging. Radiographics 2003; 23:1423–1439.

39 Melia P, Maestro C, Bruneton JN, et al. MRI of uterine leiomyosarcoma. Apropos of 2 cases. J Radiol 1995; 76:69–72.

40 Murase E, Siegelman ES, Outwater EK, Perez-Jaffe LA, Tureck RW. Uterine leiomyomas: histopathologic features, MR imaging findings, differential diagnosis and treatment. Radiographics 1999; 19:1179–1197.

41 Pattani SJ, Kier R, Deal R, Luchansky E. MRI of uterine leiomyosarcoma. Magn Reson Imaging 1995; 13:331–333.

42 Schwartz LB, Zawin M, Carcangiu ML, et al. Does pelvic magnetic resonance imaging differentiate among the histologic subtypes of uterine leiomyomata? Fertil Steril 1998; 70:580–587.

43 Hricak H, Tscholakoff D, Heinrichs L, et al. Uterine leiomyomas: correlation of MR, histopathologic findings and symptoms. Radiology 1986; 158:385–391.

44 Norris HJ, Taylor HB. Mesenchymal tumors of the uterus. I. A clinical and pathological study of 53 endometrial stromal tumors. Cancer 1966; 19:755–766.

45 Evans HL. Endometrial stromal sarcoma and poorly differentiated endometrial sarcoma. Cancer 1982; 50:2170–2182.

46 Chang KL, Crabtree GS, Lim-Tan SK, et al. Primary uterine endometrial stromal neoplasms. A clinicopathologic study of 117 cases. Am J Surg Pathol 1990; 14:415–438.

47 Tavassoli FA, Norris HJ. Mesenchymal tumours of the uterus. VII. A clinicopathological study of 60 endometrial stromal nodules. Histopathology 1981; 5:1–10.

48 Oliva E, Clement PB, Young RH. Endometrial stromal tumors: an update on a group of tumors with a protean phenotype. Adv Anat Pathol 2000; 7:257–281.

49 Fekete PS, Vellios F. The clinical and histologic spectrum of endometrial stromal neoplasms: a report of 41 cases. Int J Gynecol Pathol 1984; 3:198–212.

50 Dionigi A, Oliva E, Clement PB, Young RH. Endometrial stromal nodules and endometrial stromal tumors with limited infiltration: a clinicopathologic study of 50 cases. Am J Surg Pathol 2002; 26:567–581.

51 Oliva E, Young RH, Clement PB, et al. Cellular benign mesenchymal tumors of the uterus. A comparative morphologic and immunohistochemical analysis of 33 highly cellular leiomyomas and six endometrial stromal nodules, two frequently confused tumors. Am J Surg Pathol 1995; 19:757–768.

52 Clement PB. The pathology of uterine smooth muscle tumors and mixed endometrial stromal-smooth muscle tumors: a selective review with emphasis on recent advances. Int J Gynecol Pathol 2000; 19:39–55.

53 Oliva E, Clement PB, Young RH, Scully RE. Mixed endometrial stromal and smooth muscle tumors of the uterus: a clinicopathologic study of 15 cases. Am J Surg Pathol 1998; 22:997–1005.

54 Oliva E, Clement PB, Young RH. Epithelioid endometrial and endometrioid stromal tumors: a report of four cases emphasizing their distinction from epithelioid smooth muscle tumors and other oxyphilic uterine and extrauterine tumors. Int J Gynecol Pathol 2002; 21:48–55.

55 Clement PB, Scully RE. Uterine tumors resembling ovarian sex-cord tumors. A clinicopathologic analysis of fourteen cases. Am J Clin Pathol 1976; 66:512–525.

56 Krishnamurthy S, Jungbluth AA, Busam KJ, Rosai J. Uterine tumors resembling ovarian sex-cord tumors have an immunophenotype consistent with true

sex-cord differentiation. Am J Surg Pathol 1998; 22:1078–1082.

57 Goldblum JR, Clement PB, Hart WR. Adenomyosis with sparse glands. A potential mimic of low-grade endometrial stromal sarcoma. Am J Clin Pathol 1995; 103:218–223.

58 Micci F, Walter CU, Teixeira MR, et al. Cytogenetic and molecular genetic analyses of endometrial stromal sarcoma: nonrandom involvement of chromosome arms 6p and 7p and confirmation of JAZF1/JJAZ1 gene fusion in t(7;17). Cancer Genet Cytogenet 2003; 144:119–124.

59 Koontz JI, Soreng AL, Nucci M, et al. Frequent fusion of the JAZF1 and JJAZ1 genes in endometrial stromal tumors. Proc Natl Acad Sci USA 2001; 98:6348–6353.

60 Gadducci A, Sartori E, Landoni F, et al. Endometrial stromal sarcoma: analysis of treatment failures and survival. Gynecol Oncol 1996; 63:247–253.

61 Aubry MC, Myers JL, Colby TV, et al. Endometrial stromal sarcoma metastatic to the lung: a detailed analysis of 16 patients. Am J Surg Pathol 2002; 26:440–449.

62 Maluf FC, Aghajanian C, Spriggs D. Endometrial stromal sarcoma: etiology, prognosis and treatment options. Am J Cancer 2004; 3:13–23.

63 Oliva E, Young RH, Clement PB, Scully RE. Myxoid and fibrous endometrial stromal tumors of the uterus: a report of 10 cases. Int J Gynecol Pathol 1999; 18:310–319.

64 Clement PB, Young RH, Scully RE. Intravenous leiomyomatosis of the uterus. A clinicopathological analysis of 16 cases with unusual histologic features. Am J Surg Pathol 1988; 12:932–945.

65 Nogales FF, Navarro N, d'Martinez V, et al. Uterine intravascular leiomyomatosis: an update and report of seven cases. Int J Gynecol Pathol 1987; 6:331–339.

66 Mulvany NJ, Slavin JL, Ostor AG, Fortune DW. Intravenous leiomyomatosis of the uterus: a clinicopathologic study of 22 cases. Int J Gynecol Pathol 1994; 13:1–9.

67 Coard KC, Fletcher HM. Leiomyosarcoma of the uterus with a florid intravascular component ('intravenous leiomyosarcomatosis'). Int J Gynecol Pathol 2002; 21:182–185.

68 Nucci MR, O'Connell JT, Huettner PC, et al. h-Caldesmon expression effectively distinguishes endometrial stromal tumors from uterine smooth muscle tumors. Am J Surg Pathol 2001; 25:455–463.

69 Abrams J, Talcott J, Corson JM. Pulmonary metastases in patients with low-grade endometrial stromal sarcoma. Clinicopathologic findings with immunohistochemical characterization. Am J Surg Pathol 1989; 13:133–140.

70 Bonazzi dP, Virtanen I, Lehto VP, et al. Expression of intermediate filaments in ovarian and uterine tumors. Int J Gynecol Pathol 1983; 1:359–366.

71 Franquemont DW, Frierson HF Jr, Mills SE. An immunohistochemical study of normal endometrial stroma and endometrial stromal neoplasms. Evidence for smooth muscle differentiation. Am J Surg Pathol 1991; 15:861–870.

72 McCluggage WG, Date A, Bharucha H, Toner PG. Endometrial stromal sarcoma with sex cord-like areas and focal rhabdoid differentiation. Histopathology 1996; 29:369–374.

73 Rush DS, Tan J, Baergen RN, Soslow RA. h-Caldesmon, a novel smooth muscle-specific antibody, distinguishes between cellular leiomyoma and endometrial stromal sarcoma. Am J Surg Pathol 2001; 25:253–258.

74 Chu P, Arber DA. Paraffin-section detection of CD10 in 505 nonhematopoietic neoplasms. Frequent expression in renal cell carcinoma and endometrial stromal sarcoma. Am J Clin Pathol 2000; 113:374–382.

75 Chu PG, Arber DA, Weiss LM, Chang KL. Utility of CD10 in distinguishing between endometrial stromal sarcoma and uterine smooth muscle tumors: an immunohistochemical comparison of 34 cases. Mod Pathol 2001; 14:465–471.

76 Toki T, Shimizu M, Takagi Y, et al. CD10 is a marker for normal and neoplastic endometrial stromal cells. Int J Gynecol Pathol 2002; 21:41–47.

77 Sumathi VP, McCluggage WG. CD10 is useful in demonstrating endometrial stroma at ectopic sites and in confirming a diagnosis of endometriosis. J Clin Pathol 2002; 55:391–392.

78 Nascimento AF, Hirsch MS, Cviko A, et al. The role of CD 10 staining in distinguishing invasive endometrial adenocarcinoma from adenocarcinoma involving adenomyosis. Mod Pathol 2002; 16(1):22–27.

79 Oliva E, Young RH, Amin MB, Clement PB. An immunohistochemical analysis of endometrial stromal and smooth muscle tumors of the uterus: a study of 54 cases emphasizing the importance of using a panel because of overlap in immunoreactivity for individual antibodies. Am J Surg Pathol 2002; 26:403–412.

80 Hirsch MS, Huettner PC, Cviko A, et al. CD10 (CALLA) positive/h-caldesmon negative immunophenotype effectively distinguishes endometrial stromal tumors from uterine smooth muscle tumors. Mod Pathol 2002; 15:198a.

81 Buckshee K, Dhond AJ, Mittal S, Bose S. Pseudo-Meigs' syndrome secondary to broad ligament leiomyoma: a case report. Asia Oceania J Obstet Gynaecol 1990; 16:201–205.

82 Prayson RA, Hart WR. Primary smooth-muscle tumors of the ovary. A clinicopathologic study of four leiomyomas and two mitotically active leiomyomas. Arch Pathol Lab Med 1992; 116:1068–1071.

83 Neri A, Peled Y, Braslavski D. Vulvar leiomyoma. Acta Obstet Gynecol Scand 1993; 72:221–222.

84 Cheng WF, Lin HH, Chen CK, Chang DY, Huang SC. Leiomyosarcoma of the broad ligament: a case report and literature review. Gynecol Oncol 1995; 56:85–89.

85 Brown RS, Marley JL, Cassoni AM. Pseudo-Meigs' syndrome due to broad ligament leiomyoma: a mimic of metastatic ovarian carcinoma. Clin Oncol (R Coll Radiol) 1998; 10:198–201.

86 Baird DD, Dunson DB. Why is parity protective for uterine fibroids? Epidemiology 2003; 14:247–250.

87 Bajekal N, Li TC. Fibroids, infertility and pregnancy wastage. Hum Reprod Update 2000; 6:614–620.

88 Benson CB, Chow JS, Chang-Lee W, et al. Outcome of pregnancies in women with uterine leiomyomas identified by sonography in the first trimester. J Clin Ultrasound 2001; 29:261–264.

89 Coronado GD, Marshall LM, Schwartz SM. Complications in pregnancy, labor and delivery with uterine leiomyomas: a population-based study. Obstet Gynecol 2000; 95:764–769.

90 Dahan MH, Ahmadi R. Spontaneous subserosal venous rupture overlying a uterine leiomyoma. A case report. J Reprod Med 2002; 47:419–420.

91 Stewart EA. Uterine fibroids. Lancet 2001; 357:293–298.

92 Zaitoon MM. Retroperitoneal parasitic leiomyoma causing unilateral ureteral obstruction. J Urol 1986; 135:130–131.

93 Billings SD, Folpe AL, Weiss SW. Do leiomyomas of deep soft tissue exist? An analysis of highly differentiated smooth muscle tumors of deep soft tissue supporting two distinct subtypes. Am J Surg Pathol 2001; 25:1134–1142.

94 Lurie S, Gorbacz S, Caspi B, Borenstein R. Parasitic leiomyoma: a case report. Clin Exp Obstet Gynecol 1991; 18:7–8.

95 Yeh HC, Kaplan M, Deligdisch L. Parasitic and pedunculated leiomyomas: ultrasonographic features. J Ultrasound Med 1999; 18:789–794.

96 Silverberg SG. Reproducibility of the mitosis count in the histologic diagnosis of smooth muscle tumors of the uterus. Hum Pathol 1976; 7:451–454.

97 Kempson RL, Hendrickson MR. Pure mesenchymal neoplasms of the uterus. In: Fox H, ed. Haines and Taylor obstetrical and gynaecological pathology, 3rd edn. Edinburgh: Churchill Livingstone; 1987:411–456.

98 Kempson RL, Hendrickson MR. Pure mesenchymal neoplasms of the uterine corpus: selected problems. Semin Diagn Pathol 1988; 5:172–198.

99 Evans HL, Chawla SP, Simpson C, Finn KP. Smooth muscle neoplasms of the uterus other than ordinary leiomyoma. A study of 46 cases, with emphasis on diagnostic criteria and prognostic factors. Cancer 1988; 62:2239–2247.

100 Silverberg SG, Kurman RJ. Smooth muscle and other mesenchymal tumors. Tumors of the uterine corpus and gestational trophoblastic disease. In: Rosei J, ed. Atlas of tumor pathology, 3rd Series (Fascicle 3). Bethesda: Armed Forces Institute of Pathology; 1992:113–151.

101 Bell SW, Kempson RL, Hendrickson MR. Problematic uterine smooth muscle neoplasms. A clinicopathologic study of 213 cases. Am J Surg Pathol 1994; 18:535–558.

102 Prayson RA, Hart WR. Pathologic considerations of uterine smooth muscle tumors. Obstet Gynecol Clin North Am 1995; 22:637–657.

103 Hendrickson MR, Tavassoli FA, Kempson RL, et al. Mesenchymal tumours and related lesions. In: Tavassoli FA, Devilee P, eds. Pathology and genetics of tumours of the breast and female genital organs. Lyon: IARC Press; 2003:233–244.

104 Buttram VC. Jr. Uterine leiomyomata – aetiology, symptomatology and management. Prog Clin Biol Res 1986; 225:275–296.

105 Stewart EA, Nowak RA. Leiomyoma-related bleeding: a classic hypothesis updated for the molecular era. Hum Reprod Update 1996; 2:295–306.

106 Jacobs LB, Bhagavan BS. Intraluminal obstruction of distal ileum caused by a uterine leiomyoma. Mod Pathol 1993; 6:229–231.

107 Stanko CM, Severson MA, Molpus KL. Deep venous thrombosis associated with large leiomyomata uteri. A case report. J Reprod Med 2001; 46:405–407.

108 Stovall DW, Parrish SB, Voorhis BJ Van, et al. Uterine leiomyomas reduce the efficacy of assisted reproduction cycles: results of a matched follow-up study. Hum Reprod 1998; 13:192–197.

109 Amant F, Debiec-Rychter M, Schoenmakers EF, et al. Cumulative dosage effect of a RAD51L1/HMGA2 fusion and RAD51L1 loss in a case of pseudo-Meigs' syndrome. Genes Chromosomes Cancer 2001; 32:324–329.

110 Weise M, Westphalen S, Fayyazi A, et al. Pseudo-Meigs syndrome: uterine leiomyoma with bladder attachment associated with ascites and hydrothorax – a rare case of a rare syndrome. Onkologie 2002; 25:443–446.

111 Amant F, Gabriel C, Timmerman D, Vergote I. Pseudo-Meigs' syndrome caused by a hydropic degenerating uterine leiomyoma with elevated CA 125. Gynecol Oncol 2001; 83:153–157.

112 Dunn JS Jr, Anderson CD, Method MW, Brost BC. Hydropic degenerating leiomyoma presenting as pseudo-Meigs syndrome with elevated CA 125. Obstet Gynecol 1998; 92:648–649.

113 Migishima F, Jobo T, Hata H, et al. Uterine leiomyoma causing massive ascites and left pleural effusion with elevated CA 125: a case report. J Obstet Gynaecol Res 2000; 26:283–287.

114 Ollendorff AT, Keh P, Hoff F, et al. Leiomyoma causing massive ascites, right pleural effusion and respiratory distress. A case report. J Reprod Med 1997; 42:609–612.

115 Sinawat S, Seejorn K. Pseudo-Meigs' syndrome secondary to subserous myoma uteri: a case report. J Med Assoc Thai 2002; 85:1240–1243.

116 Terada S, Suzuki N, Uchide K, Akasofu K. Uterine leiomyoma associated with ascites and hydrothorax. Gynecol Obstet Invest 1992; 33:54–58.

117 Keshavarz H, Hillis SD, Kieke BA, Marchbanks PA. Hysterectomy surveillance – United States, 1994–1999. MMWR 2002; 51:1–8.

118 Ingersoll FM, Malone LJ. Myomectomy: an alternative to hysterectomy. Arch Surg 1970; 100:557–561.

119 Verkauf BS. Changing trends in treatment of leiomyomata uteri. Curr Opin Obstet Gynecol 1993; 5:301–310.

120 Acien P, Quereda F. Abdominal myomectomy: results of a simple operative technique. Fertil Steril 1996; 65:41–51.

121 Myomectomy MLJ. Recurrence after removal of solitary and multiple myomas. Obstet Gynecol 1969; 34:200–203.

122 Fedele L, Parazzini F, Luchini L, et al. Recurrence of fibroids after myomectomy: a transvaginal ultrasonographic study. Hum Reprod 1995; 10:1795–1796.

123 Arcangeli S, Pasquarette MM. Gravid uterine rupture after myolysis. Obstet Gynecol 1997; 89:857.

124 Stewart EA, Faur AV, Wise LA, et al. Predictors of subsequent surgery for uterine leiomyomata after abdominal myomectomy. Obstet Gynecol 2002; 99:426–432.

125 McLucas B, Adler L, Perrella R. Uterine fibroid embolization: nonsurgical treatment for symptomatic fibroids. J Am Coll Surg 2001; 192:95–105.

126 McLucas B, Reed RA, Goodwin S, et al. Outcomes following unilateral uterine artery embolisation. Br J Radiol 2002; 75:122–126.

127 Al Fozan H, Dufort J, Kaplow M, et al. Cost analysis of myomectomy, hysterectomy and uterine artery

embolization. Am J Obstet Gynecol 2002; 187:1401–1404.

128 Andersen PE, Lund N, Justesen P, et al. Uterine artery embolization of symptomatic uterine fibroid. Initial success and short-term results. Acta Radiol 2001; 42:234–238.

129 Badawy SZ, Etman A, Singh M, et al. Uterine artery embolization: the role in obstetrics and gynecology. Clin Imaging 2001; 25:288–295.

130 Brunereau L, Herbreteau D, Gallas S, et al. Uterine artery embolization in the primary treatment of uterine leiomyomas: technical features and prospective follow-up with clinical and sonographic examinations in 58 patients. Am J Roentgenol 2000; 175:1267–1272.

131 Burn P, McCall J, Chinn R, Healy J. Embolization of uterine fibroids. Br J Radiol 1999; 72:159–161.

132 Colgan TJ, Pron G, Mocarski EJ, et al. Pathologic features of uteri and leiomyomas following uterine artery embolization for leiomyomas. Am J Surg Pathol 2003; 27:167–177.

133 Blok S de, Vries C de, Prinssen HM, et al. Fatal sepsis after uterine artery embolization with microspheres. J Vasc Interv Radiol 2003; 14:779–783.

134 Goodwin SC, McLucas B, Lee M, et al. Uterine artery embolization for the treatment of uterine leiomyomata midterm results. J Vasc Interv Radiol 1999; 10:1159–1165.

135 Pron G, Bennett J, Common A, et al. The Ontario Uterine Fibroid Embolization Trial. Part 2. Uterine fibroid reduction and symptom relief after uterine artery embolization for fibroids. Fertil Steril 2003; 79:120–127.

136 Pron G, Cohen M, Soucie J, et al. The Ontario Uterine Fibroid Embolization Trial. Part 1. Baseline patient characteristics, fibroid burden and impact on life. Fertil Steril 2003; 79:112–119.

137 Ravina JH, Herbreteau D, Ciraru-Vigneron N, et al. Arterial embolisation to treat uterine myomata. Lancet 1995; 346:671–672.

138 Shashoua AR, Stringer NH, Pearlman JB, et al. Ischemic uterine rupture and hysterectomy 3 months after uterine artery embolization. J Am Assoc Gynecol Laparosc 2002; 9:217–220.

139 Spies JB, Ascher SA, Roth AR, et al. Uterine artery embolization for leiomyomata. Obstet Gynecol 2001; 98:29–34.

140 Zupi E, Pocek M, Dauri M, et al. Selective uterine artery embolization in the management of uterine myomas. Fertil Steril 2003; 79:107–111.

141 Vashisht A, Studd J, Carey A, Burn P. Fatal septicaemia after fibroid embolisation. Lancet 1999; 354:307–308.

142 Dover RW, Ferrier AJ, Torode HW. Sarcomas and the conservative management of uterine fibroids: a cause for concern? Aust N Z J Obstet Gynaecol 2000; 40:308–312.

143 Al Badr A, Faught W. Uterine artery embolization in an undiagnosed uterine sarcoma. Obstet Gynecol 2001; 97:836–837.

144 Stewart EA, Gedroyc WM, Tempany CM, et al. Focused ultrasound treatment of uterine fibroid tumors: safety and feasibility of a noninvasive thermoablative technique. Am J Obstet Gynecol 2003; 189:48–54.

145 Tempany CM, Stewart EA, McDannold N, et al. MR imaging-guided focused ultrasound surgery of uterine leiomyomas: a feasibility study. Radiology 2003; 226:897–905.

146 Coutinho EM, Boulanger GA, Goncalves MT. Regression of uterine leiomyomas after treatment with gestrinone, an antiestrogen, antiprogesterone. Am J Obstet Gynecol 1986; 155:761–767.

147 Coutinho EM, Goncalves MT. Long-term treatment of leiomyomas with gestrinone. Fertil Steril 1989; 51:939–946.

148 Friedman AJ, Daly M, Juneau-Norcross M, et al. Long-term medical therapy for leiomyomata uteri: a prospective, randomized study of leuprolide acetate depot plus either oestrogen-progestin or progestin 'add-back' for 2 years. Hum Reprod 1994; 9:1618–1625.

149 Friedman AJ, Daly M, Juneau-Norcross M, et al. A prospective, randomized trial of gonadotropin-releasing hormone agonist plus estrogen-progestin or progestin 'add-back' regimens for women with leiomyomata uteri. J Clin Endocrinol Metab 1993; 76:1439–1445.

150 Rein MS, Barbieri RL, Welch W, et al. The concentrations of collagen-associated amino acids are higher in GnRH agonist-treated uterine myomas. Obstet Gynecol 1993; 82:901–905.

151 Di Lieto A, Iannotti F, Falco M De, et al. Immunohistochemical detection of insulin-like growth factor type I receptor and uterine volume changes in gonadotropin-releasing hormone analog-treated uterine leiomyomas. Am J Obstet Gynecol 2003; 188:702–706.

152 Bifulco G, Miele C, Pellicano M, et al. Molecular mechanisms involved in GnRH analogue-related apoptosis for uterine leiomyomas. Mol Hum Reprod 2004; 10:43–48.

153 Demopoulos RI, Jones KY, Mittal KR, Vamvakas EC. Histology of leiomyomata in patients treated with leuprolide acetate. Int J Gynecol Pathol 1997; 16:131–137.

154 Gutmann JN, Thornton KL, Diamond MP, Carcangiu ML. Evaluation of leuprolide acetate treatment on histopathology of uterine myomata. Fertil Steril 1994; 61:622–626.

155 Sreenan JJ, Prayson RA, Biscotti CV, et al. Histopathologic findings in 107 uterine leiomyomas treated with leuprolide acetate compared with 126 controls. Am J Surg Pathol 1996; 20:427–432.

156 Walker CL, Burroughs KD, Davis B, et al. Preclinical evidence for therapeutic efficacy of selective estrogen receptor modulators for uterine leiomyoma. J Soc Gynecol Investig 2000; 7:249–256.

157 Meyer WR, Mayer AR, Diamond MP, et al. Unsuspected leiomyosarcoma: treatment with a gonadotropin-releasing hormone analogue. Obstet Gynecol 1990; 75:529–532.

158 Vu K, Greenspan DL, Wu TC, et al. Cellular proliferation, estrogen receptor, progesterone receptor and bcl-2 expression in GnRH agonist-treated uterine leiomyomas. Hum Pathol 1998; 29:359–363.

159 van de Ven J, Sprong M, Donker GH, et al. Levels of estrogen and progesterone receptors in the myometrium and leiomyoma tissue after suppression of estrogens with gonadotropin releasing hormone analogs. Gynecol Endocrinol 2001; 15(Suppl 6):61–68.

160 Maruo T, Ohara N, Wang J, Matsuo H. Sex steroidal regulation of uterine leiomyoma growth and apoptosis. Hum Reprod Update 2004; 10:207–220.

161 Andersen J. Growth factors and cytokines in uterine leiomyomas. Semin Reprod Endocrinol 1996; 14:269–282.

162 Zhai YL, Kobayashi Y, Mori A, et al. Expression of steroid receptors, Ki-67 and p53 in uterine leiomyosarcomas. Int J Gynecol Pathol 1999; 18:20–28.

163 Marugo M, Centonze M, Bernasconi D, et al. Estrogen and progesterone receptors in uterine leiomyomas. Acta Obstet Gynecol Scand 1989; 68:731–735.

164 Chrapusta S, Sieinski W, Konopka B, et al. Estrogen and progestin receptor levels in uterine leiomyomata: relation to the tumour histology and the phase of menstrual cycle. Eur J Gynaecol Oncol 1990; 11:381–387.

165 Chrapusta S, Konopka B, Paszko Z, et al. Immunoreactive and estrogen-binding estrogen receptors and progestin receptor levels in uterine leiomyomata and their parental myometrium. Eur J Gynaecol Oncol 1990; 11:275–281.

166 Brandon DD, Erickson TE, Keenan EJ, et al. Estrogen receptor gene expression in human uterine leiomyomata. J Clin Endocrinol Metab 1995; 80:1876–1881.

167 Andersen J, DyReyes VM, Barbieri RL, et al. Leiomyoma primary cultures have elevated transcriptional response to estrogen compared with autologous myometrial cultures. J Soc Gynecol Investig 1995; 2:542–551.

168 Bourlev V, Pavlovitch S, Stygar D, et al. Different proliferative and apoptotic activity in peripheral versus central parts of human uterine leiomyomas. Gynecol Obstet Invest 2003; 55:199–204.

169 Kawaguchi K, Fujii S, Konishi I, et al. Mitotic activity in uterine leiomyomas during the menstrual cycle. Am J Obstet Gynecol 1989; 160:637–641.

170 Palomba S, Sena T, Morelli M, et al. Effect of different doses of progestin on uterine leiomyomas in postmenopausal women. Eur J Obstet Gynecol Reprod Biol 2002; 102:199–201.

171 Reed SD, Cushing-Haugen KL, Daling JR, et al. Postmenopausal estrogen and progestogen therapy and the risk of uterine leiomyomas. Menopause 2004; 11:214–222.

172 Massart F, Becherini L, Gennari L, et al. Genotype distribution of estrogen receptor-alpha gene polymorphisms in Italian women with surgical uterine leiomyomas. Fertil Steril 2001; 75:567–570.

173 Hsieh YY, Chang CC, Tsai FJ, et al. Estrogen receptor thymine-adenine dinucleotide repeat polymorphism is associated with susceptibility to leiomyoma. Fertil Steril 2003; 79:96–99.

174 Linder D, Gartler SM. Glucose-6-phosphate dehydrogenase mosaicism: utilization as a cell marker in the study of leiomyomas. Science 1965; 150:67–69.

175 Townsend DE, Sparkes RS, Baluda MC, McClelland G. Unicellular histogenesis of uterine leiomyomas as determined by electrophoresis by glucose-6-phosphate dehydrogenase. Am J Obstet Gynecol 1970; 107:1168–1173.

176 Mashal RD, Fejzo ML, Friedman AJ, et al. Analysis of androgen receptor DNA reveals the independent clonal origins of uterine leiomyomata and the secondary nature of cytogenetic aberrations in the development of leiomyomata. Genes Chromosomes Cancer 1994; 11:1–6.

177 Treloar SA, Martin NG, Dennerstein L, et al. Pathways to hysterectomy: insights from longitudinal twin research. Am J Obstet Gynecol 1992; 167:82–88.

178 Luoto R, Kaprio J, Rutanen EM, et al. Heritability and risk factors of uterine fibroids – the Finnish Twin Cohort study. Maturitas 2000; 37:15–26.

179 Voorhis BJ Van, Romitti PA, Jones MP. Family history as a risk factor for development of uterine leiomyomas. Results of a pilot study. J Reprod Med 2002; 47:663–669.

180 Vikhlyaeva EM, Khodzhaeva ZS, Fantschenko ND. Familial predisposition to uterine leiomyomas. Int J Gynaecol Obstet 1995; 51:127–131.

181 McKusik V. Mendelian inheritance in man. Online: Johns Hopkins University and National Center for Biotechnology; http://www.ncbi.nlm.nih.gov/entrez/dispomim.cgi?id=15 0800. 2-28-2002.

182 Alam NA, Bevan S, Churchman M, et al. Localization of a gene (MCUL1) for multiple cutaneous leiomyomata and uterine fibroids to chromosome 1q42.3-q43. Am J Hum Genet 2001; 68:1264–1269.

183 Tomlinson IP, Alam NA, Rowan AJ, et al. Germline mutations in FH predispose to dominantly inherited uterine fibroids, skin leiomyomata and papillary renal cell cancer. Nat Genet 2002; 30:406–410.

184 Toro JR, Nickerson ML, Wei MH, et al. Mutations in the fumarate hydratase gene cause hereditary leiomyomatosis and renal cell cancer in families in North America. Am J Hum Genet 2003; 73:95–106.

185 Pollard PJ, Wortham NC, Tomlinson IP. The TCA cycle and tumorigenesis: the examples of fumarate hydratase and succinate dehydrogenase. Ann Med 2003; 35:632–639.

186 Eng C, Kiuru M, Fernandez MJ, Aaltonen LA. A role for mitochondrial enzymes in inherited neoplasia and beyond. Nat Rev Cancer 2003; 3:193–202.

187 Baysal BE. On the association of succinate dehydrogenase mutations with hereditary paraganglioma. Trends Endocrinol Metab 2003; 14:453–459.

188 Dal Cin P, Morton CC. 1q42 approximately q44 is rarely cytogenetically involved in sporadic uterine leiomyomata. Cancer Genet Cytogenet 2002; 138:92–93.

189 Barker KT, Bevan S, Wang R, et al. Low frequency of somatic mutations in the FH/multiple cutaneous leiomyomatosis gene in sporadic leiomyosarcomas and uterine leiomyomas. Br J Cancer 2002; 87:446–448.

190 McKusik V. Mendelian inheritance in man. Online: Johns Hopkins University and National Center for Biotechnology; http://www.ncbi.nlm.nih.gov/entrez/dispomim.cgi?id=30 8940. 12-29-2003.

191 Zhou J, Mochizuki T, Smeets H, et al. Deletion of the paired alpha 5(IV) and alpha 6(IV) collagen genes in inherited smooth muscle tumors. Science 1993; 261:1167–1169.

192 Mark J, Havel G, Grepp C, et al. Chromosomal patterns in human benign uterine leiomyomas. Cancer Genet Cytogenet 1990; 44:1–13.

193 Meloni AM, Surti U, Contento AM, et al. Uterine leiomyomas: cytogenetic and histologic profile. Obstet Gynecol 1992; 80:209–217.

194 Nilbert M, Heim S, Mandahl N, et al. Karyotypic rearrangements in 20 uterine leiomyomas. Cytogenet Cell Genet 1988; 49:300–304.

195 Pandis N, Heim S, Bardi G, et al. Chromosome analysis of 96 uterine leiomyomas. Cancer Genet Cytogenet 1991; 55:11–18.

196 Rein MS, Friedman AJ, Barbieri RL, et al. Cytogenetic abnormalities in uterine leiomyomata. Obstet Gynecol 1991; 77:923–926.

197 Heim S, Mandahl N, Kristoffersson U, et al. Structural chromosome aberrations in a case of angioleiomyoma. Cancer Genet Cytogenet 1986; 20:325–330.

198 Nilbert M, Heim S, Mandahl N, et al. Ring formation and structural rearrangements of chromosome 1 as secondary changes in uterine leiomyomas with t(12;14)(q14-15;q23-24). Cancer Genet Cytogenet 1988; 36:183–190.

199 Nilbert M, Heim S, Mandahl N, et al. Characteristic chromosome abnormalities, including rearrangements of 6p, del(7q), +12 and t(12;14), in 44 uterine leiomyomas. Hum Genet 1990; 85:605–611.

200 Nilbert M, Heim S, Mandahl N, et al. Trisomy 12 in uterine leiomyomas. A new cytogenetic subgroup. Cancer Genet Cytogenet 1990; 45:63–66.

201 Ozisik YY, Meloni AM, Powell M, et al. Chromosome 7 biclonality in uterine leiomyoma. Cancer Genet Cytogenet 1993; 67:59–64.

202 Ozisik YY, Meloni AM, Surti U, Sandberg AA. Involvement of 10q22 in leiomyoma. Cancer Genet Cytogenet 1993; 69:132–135.

203 Ozisik YY, Meloni AM, Surti U, Sandberg AA. Deletion 7q22 in uterine leiomyoma. A cytogenetic review. Cancer Genet Cytogenet 1993; 71:1–6.

204 Ozisik YY, Meloni AM, Altungoz O, et al. Translocation (6;10)(p21;q22) in uterine leiomyomas. Cancer Genet Cytogenet 1995; 79:136–138.

205 Rein MS, Powell WL, Walters FC, et al. Cytogenetic abnormalities in uterine myomas are associated with myoma size. Mol Hum Reprod 1998; 4:83–86.

206 Hennig Y, Deichert U, Bonk U, et al. Chromosomal translocations affecting 12q14-15 but not deletions of the long arm of chromosome 7 associated with a growth advantage of uterine smooth muscle cells. Mol Hum Reprod 1999; 5:1150–1154.

207 Schoenmakers EF, Wanschura S, Mols R, et al. Recurrent rearrangements in the high mobility group protein gene, HMGI-C, in benign mesenchymal tumours. Nat Genet 1995; 10:436–444.

208 Gattas GJ, Quade BJ, Nowak RA, Morton CC. HMGIC expression in human adult and fetal tissues and in uterine leiomyomata. Genes Chromosomes Cancer 1999; 25:316–322.

209 Quade BJ, Weremowicz S, Neskey DM, et al. Fusion transcripts involving HMGA2 are not a common molecular mechanism in uterine leiomyomata with rearrangements in 12q15. Cancer Res 2003; 63:1351–1358.

210 Schoenberg FM, Ashar HR, Krauter KS, et al. Translocation breakpoints upstream of the HMGIC gene in uterine leiomyomata suggest dysregulation of this gene by a mechanism different from that in lipomas. Genes Chromosomes Cancer 1996; 17:1–6.

211 Schoenmakers EF, Geurts JM, Kools PF, et al. A 6-Mb yeast artificial chromosome contig and long-range physical map encompassing the region on chromosome 12q15 frequently rearranged in a variety of benign solid tumors. Genomics 1995; 29:665–678.

212 Schoenmakers EF, Huysmans C, Ven WJ Van De. Allelic knockout of novel splice variants of human recombination repair gene RAD51B in t(12;14) uterine leiomyomas. Cancer Res 1999; 59:19–23.

213 Schoenmakers EF, Mols R, Wanschura S, et al. Identification, molecular cloning and characterization of the chromosome 12 breakpoint cluster region of uterine leiomyomas. Genes Chromosomes Cancer 1994; 11:106–118.

214 Sornberger KS, Weremowicz S, Williams AJ, et al. Expression of HMGIY in three uterine leiomyomata with complex rearrangements of chromosome 6. Cancer Genet Cytogenet 1999; 114:9–16.

215 Wanschura S, Hennig Y, Deichert U, et al. Molecular-cytogenetic refinement of the 12q14–>q15 breakpoint region affected in uterine leiomyomas. Cytogenet Cell Genet 1995; 71:131–135.

216 Wanschura S, Kazmierczak B, Schoenmakers E, et al. Regional fine mapping of the multiple-aberration region involved in uterine leiomyoma, lipoma and pleomorphic adenoma of the salivary gland to 12q15. Genes Chromosomes Cancer 1995; 14:68–70.

217 Tallini G, Dal Cin P. HMGI(Y) and HMGI-C dysregulation: a common occurrence in human tumors. Adv Anat Pathol 1999; 6:237–246.

218 Kazmierczak B, Rosigkeit J, Wanschura S, et al. HMGI-C rearrangements as the molecular basis for the majority of pulmonary chondroid hamartomas: a survey of 30 tumors. Oncogene 1996; 12:515–521.

219 Nucci MR, Weremowicz S, Neskey DM, et al. Chromosomal translocation t(8;12) induces aberrant HMGIC expression in aggressive angiomyxoma of the vulva. Genes Chromosomes Cancer 2001; 32:172–176.

220 Staats B, Bonk U, Wanschura S, et al. A fibroadenoma with a t(4;12) (q27;q15) affecting the HMGI-C gene, a member of the high mobility group protein gene family. Breast Cancer Res Treat 1996; 38:299–303.

221 Wanschura S, Belge G, Stenman G, et al. Mapping of the translocation breakpoints of primary pleomorphic adenomas and lipomas within a common region of chromosome 12. Cancer Genet Cytogenet 1996; 86:39–45.

222 Klotzbucher M, Wasserfall A, Fuhrmann U. Misexpression of wild-type and truncated isoforms of the high-mobility group I proteins HMGI-C and HMGI(Y) in uterine leiomyomas. Am J Pathol 1999; 155:1535–1542.

223 Kazmierczak B, Bol S, Wanschura S, et al. PAC clone containing the HMGI(Y) gene spans the breakpoint of a 6p21 translocation in a uterine leiomyoma cell line. Genes Chromosomes Cancer 1996; 17:191–193.

224 Kazmierczak B, Dal Cin P, Wanschura S, et al. HMGIY is the target of 6p21.3 rearrangements in various benign mesenchymal tumors. Genes Chromosomes Cancer 1998; 23:279–285.

225 Ferry JA, Harris NL, Scully RE. Uterine leiomyomas with lymphoid infiltration simulating lymphoma. A report of seven cases. Int J Gynecol Pathol 1989; 8:263–270.

226 Maluf HM, Gersell DJ. Uterine leiomyomas with high content of mast cells. Arch Pathol Lab Med 1994; 118:712–714.

227 Orii A, Mori A, Zhai YL, et al. Mast cells in smooth muscle tumors of the uterus. Int J Gynecol Pathol 1998; 17:336–342.

228 Chuang SS, Lin CN, Li CY, Wu CH. Uterine leiomyoma with massive lymphocytic infiltration simulating malignant lymphoma. A case report with immunohistochemical study showing that the infiltrating lymphocytes are cytotoxic T cells. Pathol Res Pr 2001; 197:135–138.

229 Paik SS, Oh YH, Jang KS, et al. Uterine leiomyoma with massive lymphoid infiltration: case report and review of the literature. Pathol Int 2004; 54:343–348.

230 Vang R, Medeiros LJ, Samoszuk M, Deavers MT. Uterine leiomyomas with eosinophils: a clinicopathologic study of 3 cases. Int J Gynecol Pathol 2001; 20:239–243.

231 Stewart EA, Friedman AJ, Peck K, Nowak RA. Relative overexpression of collagen type I and collagen type III messenger ribonucleic acids by uterine leiomyomas during the proliferative phase of the menstrual cycle. J Clin Endocrinol Metab 1994; 79:900–906.

232 Stewart EA, Rhoades AR, Nowak RA. Leuprolide acetate-treated leiomyomas retain their relative overexpression of collagen type I and collagen type III messenger ribonucleic acid. J Soc Gynecol Investig 1998; 5:44–47.

233 Quade BJ, Wang TY, Sornberger K, et al. Molecular pathogenesis of uterine smooth muscle tumors from transcriptional profiling. Genes Chromosomes Cancer 2004; 40:97–108.

234 Nagel H, Brinck U, Luthje D, Fuzesi L. Plexiform leiomyoma of the uterus in a patient with breast carcinoma: case report and review of the literature. Pathology 1999; 31:292–294.

235 Seidman JD, Thomas RM. Multiple plexiform tumorlets of the uterus. Arch Pathol Lab Med 1993; 117:1255–1256.

236 Watanabe K, Ogura G, Suzuki T. Leiomyoblastoma of the uterus: an immunohistochemical and electron microscopic study of distinctive tumours with immature smooth muscle cell differentiation mimicking fetal uterine myocytes. Histopathology 2003; 42:379–386.

237 Mazur MT, Priest JB. Clear cell leiomyoma (leiomyoblastoma) of the uterus: ultrastructural observations. Ultrastruct Pathol 1986; 10:249–255.

238 Hyde KE, Geisinger KR, Marshall RB, Jones TL. The clear-cell variant of uterine epithelioid leiomyoma. An immunohistologic and ultrastructural study. Arch Pathol Lab Med 1989; 113:551–553.

239 Prayson RA, Goldblum JR, Hart WR. Epithelioid smooth-muscle tumors of the uterus: a clinicopathologic study of 18 patients. Am J Surg Pathol 1997; 21:383–391.

240 Kyriazis AP, Kyriazis AA. Uterine leiomyoblastoma (epithelioid leiomyoma) neoplasm of low-grade malignancy. A histopathologic study. Arch Pathol Lab Med 1992; 116:1189–1191.

241 Atkins K, Bell S, Kempson RL, Hendrickson MR. Epithelioid smooth muscle tumors of the uterus. Mod Pathol 2002; 14(1):132A.

242 Karaiskos C, Pandis N, Bardi G, et al. Cytogenetic findings in uterine epithelioid leiomyomas. Cancer Genet Cytogenet 1995; 80:103–106.

243 Sargent MS, Weremowicz S, Rein MS, Morton CC. Translocations in 7q22 define a critical region in uterine leiomyomata. Cancer Genet Cytogenet 1994; 77:65–68.

244 Shintaku M. Lipoleiomyomatous tumors of the uterus: a heterogeneous group? Histopathological study of five cases. Pathol Int 1996; 46:498–502.

245 Havel G, Wedell B, Dahlenfors R, Mark J. Cytogenetic relationship between uterine lipoleiomyomas and typical leiomyomas. Virchows Arch B Cell Pathol Incl Mol Pathol 1989; 57:77–79.

246 Hu J, Surti U, Tobon H. Cytogenetic analysis of a uterine lipoleiomyoma. Cancer Genet Cytogenet 1992; 62:200–202.

247 Pedeutour F, Quade BJ, Sornberger K, et al. Dysregulation of HMGIC in a uterine lipoleiomyoma with a complex rearrangement including chromosomes 7, 12 and 14. Genes Chromosomes Cancer 2000; 27:209–215.

248 Hsieh CH, Lui CC, Huang SC, Ou YC et al. Multiple uterine angioleiomyomas in a woman presenting with severe menorrhagia. Gynecol Oncol 2003; 90:348–352.

249 Hennig Y, Caselitz J, Stern C, et al. Karyotype evolution in a case of uterine angioleiomyoma. Cancer Genet Cytogenet 1999; 108:79–80.

250 Friedrich M, Villena-Heinsen C, Mink D, et al. Leiomyosarcomas of the female genital tract: a clinical and histopathological study. Eur J Gynaecol Oncol 1998; 19:470–475.

251 Harlow BL, Weiss NS, Lofton S. The epidemiology of sarcomas of the uterus. J Natl Cancer Inst 1986; 76:399–402.

252 Leibsohn S, d'Ablaing G, Mishell DR Jr., Schlaerth JB. Leiomyosarcoma in a series of hysterectomies performed for presumed uterine leiomyomas. Am J Obstet Gynecol 1990; 162:968–974.

253 Parker WH, Fu YS, Berek JS. Uterine sarcoma in patients operated on for presumed leiomyoma and rapidly growing leiomyoma. Obstet Gynecol 1994; 83:414–418.

254 Mesia AF, Williams FS, Yan Z, Mittal K. Aborted leiomyosarcoma after treatment with leuprolide acetate. Obstet Gynecol 1998; 92:664–666.

255 Kawamura N, Iwanaga N, Hada S, et al. Transient shrinkage of a uterine leiomyosarcoma treated with GnRH agonist for a presumed uterine leiomyoma: comparison of magnetic resonance imaging finding before and during GnRH agonist treatment. Oncol Rep 2001; 8:1255–1257.

256 Lee WY, Tzeng CC, Chou CY. Uterine leiomyosarcomas coexistent with cellular and atypical leiomyomata in a young woman during the treatment with luteinizing hormone-releasing hormone agonist. Gynecol Oncol 1994; 52:74–79.

257 Salazar OM, Bonfiglio TA, Patten SF, et al. Uterine sarcomas: natural history, treatment and prognosis. Cancer 1978; 42:1152–1160.

258 Berchuck A, Rubin SC, Hoskins WJ, et al. Treatment of uterine leiomyosarcoma. Obstet Gynecol 1988; 71:845–850.

259 Gadducci A, Landoni F, Sartori E, et al. Uterine leiomyosarcoma: analysis of treatment failures and survival. Gynecol Oncol 1996; 62:25–32.

260 Dinh TA, Oliva EA, Fuller AF Jr, et al. The treatment of uterine leiomyosarcoma: results from a 10-year experience (1990–1999) at the Massachusetts General Hospital. Obstet Gynecol Surv 2004; 59:346–347.

261 Anraku M, Yokoi K, Nakagawa K, et al. Pulmonary metastases from uterine malignancies: results of surgical resection in 133 patients. J Thorac Cardiovasc Surg 2004; 127:1107–1112.

262 Funada T, Ohno N, Noguchi T, et al. Pulmonary metastasis of uterine leiomyosarcoma 8 years after hysterectomy; report of a case. Kyobu Geka 2004; 57:509–512.

263 O'Brien JM, Brennan DD, Taylor DH, et al. Skeletal muscle metastasis from uterine leiomyosarcoma. Skeletal Radiol 2004; 33:655–659.

264 Goff BA, Rice LW, Fleischhacker D, et al. Uterine leiomyosarcoma and endometrial stromal sarcoma: lymph node metastases and sites of recurrence. Gynecol Oncol 1993; 50:105–109.

265 Leitao MM, Sonoda Y, Brennan MF, et al. Incidence of lymph node and ovarian metastases in leiomyosarcoma of the uterus. Gynecol Oncol 2003; 91:209–212.

266 Nilbert M, Mandahl N, Heim S, et al. Chromosome abnormalities in leiomyosarcomas. Cancer Genet Cytogenet 1988; 34:209–218.

267 Sait SN, Dal Cin P, Sandberg AA. Consistent chromosome changes in leiomyosarcoma. Cancer Genet Cytogenet 1988; 35:47–50.

268 Boghosian L, Dal Cin P, Turc-Carel C, et al. Three possible cytogenetic subgroups of leiomyosarcoma. Cancer Genet Cytogenet 1989; 43:39–49.

269 Fletcher JA, Morton CC, Pavelka K, Lage JM. Chromosome aberrations in uterine smooth muscle tumors: potential diagnostic relevance of cytogenetic instability. Cancer Res 1990; 50:4092–4097.

270 Nilbert M, Mandahl N, Heim S, et al. Complex karyotypic changes, including rearrangements of 12q13 and 14q24, in two leiomyosarcomas. Cancer Genet Cytogenet 1990; 48:217–223.

271 Nilbert M, Jin YS, Heim S, et al. Chromosome rearrangements in two uterine sarcomas. Cancer Genet Cytogenet 1990; 44:27–35.

272 Laxman R, Currie JL, Kurman RJ, et al. Cytogenetic profile of uterine sarcomas. Cancer 1993; 71:1283–1288.

273 Sreekantaiah C, Davis JR, Sandberg AA. Chromosomal abnormalities in leiomyosarcomas. Am J Pathol 1993; 142:293–305.

274 Han K, Lee W, Harris CP, et al. Comparison of chromosome aberrations in leiomyoma and leiomyosarcoma using FISH on archival tissues. Cancer Genet Cytogenet 1994; 74:19–24.

275 Iliszko M, Mandahl N, Mrozek K, et al. Cytogenetics of uterine sarcomas: presentation of eight new cases and review of the literature. Gynecol Oncol 1998; 71:172–176.

276 Levy B, Mukherjee T, Hirschhorn K. Molecular cytogenetic analysis of uterine leiomyoma and leiomyosarcoma by comparative genomic hybridization. Cancer Genet Cytogenet 2000; 121:1–8.

277 Mandahl N, Fletcher CD, Dal Cin P, et al. Comparative cytogenetic study of spindle cell and pleomorphic leiomyosarcomas of soft tissues: a report from the CHAMP Study Group. Cancer Genet Cytogenet 2000; 116:66–73.

278 Peters WA III, Howard DR, Andersen WA, Figge DC. Deoxyribonucleic acid analysis by flow cytometry of uterine leiomyosarcomas and smooth muscle tumors of uncertain malignant potential. Am J Obstet Gynecol 1992; 166:1646–1653.

279 Peters WA III, Howard DR, Andersen WA, Figge DC. Uterine smooth-muscle tumors of uncertain malignant potential. Obstet Gynecol 1994; 83:1015–1020.

280 Blom R, Guerrieri C, Stal O, et al. Leiomyosarcoma of the uterus: a clinicopathologic, DNA flow cytometric, p53 and mdm-2 analysis of 49 cases. Gynecol Oncol 1998; 68:54–61.

281 Dal Cin P, Boghosian L, Crickard K, Sandberg AA. t(10;17) as the sole chromosome change in a uterine leiomyosarcoma. Cancer Genet Cytogenet 1988; 32:263–266.

282 Quade BJ, Pinto AP, Howard DR, et al. Frequent loss of heterozygosity for chromosome 10 in uterine leiomyosarcoma in contrast to leiomyoma. Am J Pathol 1999; 154:945–950.

283 Packenham JP, du MS, Schrock E, et al. Analysis of genetic alterations in uterine leiomyomas and leiomyosarcomas by comparative genomic hybridization. Mol Carcinog 1997; 19:273–279.

284 Hu J, Khanna V, Jones M, Surti U. Genomic alterations in uterine leiomyosarcomas: potential markers for clinical diagnosis and prognosis. Genes Chromosomes Cancer 2001; 31:117–124.

285 Tsibris JC, Segars J, Coppola D, et al. Insights from gene arrays on the development and growth regulation of uterine leiomyomata. Fertil Steril 2002; 78:114–121.

286 Tsibris JC, Segars J, Enkemann S, et al. New and old regulators of uterine leiomyoma growth from screening with DNA arrays. Fertil Steril 2003; 80:279–281.

287 Tsibris JC, Maas S, Segars JH, et al. New potential regulators of uterine leiomyomata from DNA arrays: the ionotropic glutamate receptor GluR2. Biochem Biophys Res Commun 2003; 312:249–254.

288 Skubitz KM, Skubitz AP. Differential gene expression in leiomyosarcoma. Cancer 2003; 98:1029–1038.

289 Skubitz KM, Skubitz AP. Differential gene expression in uterine leiomyoma. J Lab Clin Med 2003; 141:297–308.

290 Catherino WH, Prupas C, Tsibris JC, et al. Strategy for elucidating differentially expressed genes in leiomyomata identified by microarray technology. Fertil Steril 2003; 80:282–290.

291 Catherino W, Salama A, Potlog-Nahari C, et al. Gene expression studies in leiomyomata: new directions for research. Semin Reprod Med 2004; 22:83–90.

292 Perrone T, Dehner LP. Prognostically favorable 'mitotically active' smooth-muscle tumors of the uterus. A clinicopathologic study of ten cases. Am J Surg Pathol 1988; 12:1–8.

293 Chen KT. Myxoid leiomyosarcoma of the uterus. Int J Gynecol Pathol 1984; 3:389–392.

294 Pounder DJ, Iyer PV. Uterine leiomyosarcoma with myxoid stroma. Arch Pathol Lab Med 1985; 109:762–764.

295 Shroff CP, Deodhar KP, Bhagwat AG. Myxoid leiomyosarcoma of the uterus – a case report with light microscopic and ultrastructural appraisal. Tumori 1984; 70:561–566.

296 Salm R, Evans DJ. Myxoid leiomyosarcoma. Histopathology 1985; 9:159–169.

297 Peacock G, Archer S. Myxoid leiomyosarcoma of the uterus: case report and review of the literature. Am J Obstet Gynecol 1989; 160:1515–1518.

298 Chang E, Shim SI. Myxoid leiomyosarcoma of the uterus: a case report and review of the literature. J Korean Med Sci 1998; 13:559–562.

299 Kasahara K, Nishida M, Iijima S, Kaneko M. Uterine myxoid leiomyosarcoma. Obstet Gynecol 2000; 95:1004–1006.

300 Mittal K, Popiolek D, Demopoulos RI. Uterine myxoid leiomyosarcoma within a leiomyoma. Hum Pathol 2000; 31:398–400.

301 Toki N, Kashimura M, Hasegawa T, et al. Myxoid leiomyosarcoma of the uterus. Report of a case with cytologic findings. Acta Cytol 2000; 44:415–419.

302 Kaleli S, Calay Z, Ceydeli N, et al. A huge abdominal mass mimicking ovarian cancer: p53-negative but aneuploid myxoid leiomyosarcoma of the uterus. Eur J Obstet Gynecol Reprod Biol 2001; 100:96–99.

303 Kagami S, Kashimura M, Toki N, Katuhata Y. Myxoid leiomyosarcoma of the uterus with subsequent pregnancy and delivery. Gynecol Oncol 2002; 85:538–542.

304 Malhotra M, Sharma JB, Wadhwa L, Singh S. Disseminating myxoid leiomyosarcoma of the uterus. Arch Gynecol Obstet 2005; 271:166–167.

305 Atkins K, Bell S, Kempson RL, Hendrickson MR. Myxoid smooth muscle tumors of the uterus. Mod Pathol 2002; 14(1):132A.

306 Bokhman JV, Yakovleva IA, Urmanchejeva AF. Treatment of patients with sarcoma of the uterus. Eur J Gynaecol Oncol 1990; 11:225–231.

307 Echt G, Jepson J, Steel J, et al. Treatment of uterine sarcomas. Cancer 1990; 66:35–39.

308 Major FJ, Blessing JA, Silverberg SG, et al. Prognostic factors in early-stage uterine sarcoma. A Gynecologic Oncology Group study. Cancer 1993; 71:1702–1709.

309 Dinh TA, Oliva EA, Fuller AF Jr, et al. The treatment of uterine leiomyosarcoma. Results from a 10-year experience (1990-1999) at the Massachusetts General Hospital. Gynecol Oncol 2004; 92:648–652.

310 Shpitz B, Tiomkin V, Bomstein Y, et al. Evaluation of putative molecular biomarkers in abdominal and retroperitoneal leiomyosarcomas. Eur J Surg Oncol 2001; 27:203–208.

311 Layfield LJ, Liu K, Dodge R, Barsky SH. Uterine smooth muscle tumors: utility of classification by proliferation, ploidy and prognostic markers versus traditional histopathology. Arch Pathol Lab Med 2000; 124:221–227.

312 Mayerhofer K, Lozanov P, Bodner K, et al. Ki-67 and vascular endothelial growth factor expression in uterine leiomyosarcoma. Gynecol Oncol 2004; 92:175–179.

313 Giuntoli RL, Metzinger DS, DiMarco CS, et al. Retrospective review of 208 patients with leiomyosarcoma of the uterus: prognostic indicators, surgical management and adjuvant therapy. Gynecol Oncol 2003; 89:460–469.

314 Hsieh CH, Lin H, Huang CC, et al. Leiomyosarcoma of the uterus: a clinicopathologic study of 21 cases. Acta Obstet Gynecol Scand 2003; 82:74–81.

315 Zhai YL, Kobayashi Y, Mori A, et al. Expression of steroid receptors, Ki-67 and p53 in uterine leiomyosarcomas. Int J Gynecol Pathol 1999; 18:20–28.

316 Wu X, Blanck A, Olovsson M, et al. Apoptosis, cellular proliferation and expression of p53 in human uterine leiomyomas and myometrium during the menstrual cycle and after menopause. Acta Obstet Gynecol Scand 2000; 79:397–404.

317 Hong T, Shimada Y, Uchida S, et al. Expression of angiogenic factors and apoptotic factors in leiomyosarcoma and leiomyoma. Int J Mol Med 2001; 8:141–148.

318 Mittal K, Demopoulos RI. MIB-1 (Ki-67), p53, estrogen receptor and progesterone receptor expression in uterine smooth muscle tumors. Hum Pathol 2001; 32:984–987.

319 Tsujimura A, Kawamura N, Ichimura T, et al. Telomerase activity in needle biopsied uterine myoma-like tumors: differential diagnosis between uterine sarcomas and leiomyomas. Int J Oncol 2002; 20:361–365.

320 Raspollini MR, Amunni G, Villanucci A, et al. Estrogen and progesterone receptors expression in uterine malignant smooth muscle tumors: correlation with clinical outcome. J Chemother 2003; 15:596–602.

321 Raspollini MR, Villanucci A, Amunni G, et al. C-kit expression in uterine leiomyosarcomas: an immunocytochemical study of 29 cases of malignant smooth muscle tumors of the uterus. J Chemother 2003; 15:81–84.

322 Bodner K, Bodner-Adler B, Kimberger O, et al. Bcl-2 receptor expression in patients with uterine smooth muscle tumors: an immunohistochemical analysis comparing leiomyoma, uterine smooth muscle tumor of uncertain malignant potential and leiomyosarcoma. J Soc Gynecol Investig 2004; 11:187–191.

323 Poncelet C, Fauvet R, Feldmann G, et al. Prognostic value of von Willebrand factor, CD34, CD31 and vascular endothelial growth factor expression in women with uterine leiomyosarcomas. J Surg Oncol 2004; 86:84–90.

324 Raspollini MR, Amunni G, Villanucci A, et al. c-Kit expression in patients with uterine leiomyosarcomas: a potential alternative therapeutic treatment. Clin Cancer Res 2004; 10:3500–3503.

325 Sutton G, Blessing JA, Malfetano JH. Ifosfamide and doxorubicin in the treatment of advanced leiomyosarcomas of the uterus: a Gynecologic Oncology Group study. Gynecol Oncol 1996; 62:226–229.

326 Smith HO, Blessing JA, Vaccarello L. Trimetrexate in the treatment of recurrent or advanced leiomyosarcoma of the uterus: a phase II study of the Gynecologic Oncology Group. Gynecol Oncol 2002; 84:140–144.

327 Giuntoli RL, Bristow RE. Uterine leiomyosarcoma: present management. Curr Opin Oncol 2004; 16:324–327.

328 Myles JL, Hart WR. Apoplectic leiomyomas of the uterus. A clinicopathologic study of five distinctive hemorrhagic leiomyomas associated with oral contraceptive usage. Am J Surg Pathol 1985; 9:798–805.

329 Clement PB, Young RH, Scully RE. Diffuse, perinodular and other patterns of hydropic degeneration within and

adjacent to uterine leiomyomas. Problems in differential diagnosis. Am J Surg Pathol 1992; 16:26–32.

330 Marret H, Alonso AM, Cottier JP, et al. Leiomyoma recurrence after uterine artery embolization. J Vasc Interv Radiol 2003; 14:1395–1399.

331 Moore SD, Herrick SR, Ince TA, et al. Uterine leiomyomata with t(10;17) disrupt the histone acetyltransferase MORF. Cancer Res 2004; 64:5570–5577.

332 Rein MS, Barbieri RL. Friedman AJ. Progesterone: a critical role in the pathogenesis of uterine myomas. Am J Obstet Gynecol 1995; 172:14–18.

333 Dgani R, Piura B, Ben-Baruch G, et al. Clinical-pathological study of uterine leiomyomas with high mitotic activity. Acta Obstet Gynecol Scand 1998; 77:74–77.

334 O'Connor DM, Norris HJ. Mitotically active leiomyomas of the uterus. Hum Pathol 1990; 21:223–227.

335 Prayson RA, Hart WR. Mitotically active leiomyomas of the uterus. Am J Clin Pathol 1992; 97:14–20.

336 Amada S, Nakano H, Tsuneyoshi M. Leiomyosarcoma versus bizarre and cellular leiomyomas of the uterus: a comparative study based on the MIB-1 and proliferating cell nuclear antigen indices, p53 expression, DNA flow cytometry and muscle specific actins. Int J Gynecol Pathol 1995; 14:134–142.

337 Downes KA, Hart WR. Bizarre leiomyomas of the uterus: a comprehensive pathologic study of 24 cases with long-term follow-up. Am J Surg Pathol 1997; 21:1261–1270.

338 Quade BJ, Dal Cin P, Neskey DM, et al. Intravenous leiomyomatosis: molecular and cytogenetic analysis of a case. Mod Pathol 2002; 15:351–356.

339 Dal Cin P, Quade BJ, Neskey DM, et al. Intravenous leiomyomatosis is characterized by a der(14)t(12;14)(q15;q24). Genes Chromosomes Cancer 2003; 36:205–206.

340 Quade BJ, McLachlin CM, Soto-Wright V, et al. Disseminated peritoneal leiomyomatosis. Clonality analysis by X chromosome inactivation and cytogenetics of a clinically benign smooth muscle proliferation. Am J Pathol 1997; 150:2153–166.

341 Norris HJ, Parmley T. Mesenchymal tumors of the uterus. V. Intravenous leiomyomatosis. A clinical and pathologic study of 14 cases. Cancer 1975; 36:2164–2178.

342 Evans AT III, Symmonds RE, Gaffey TA. Recurrent pelvic intravenous leiomyomatosis. Obstet Gynecol 1981; 57:260–264.

343 Cooper MM, Guillem J, Dalton J, et al. Recurrent intravenous leiomyomatosis with cardiac extension. Ann Thorac Surg 1992; 53:139–141.

344 Akatsuka N, Tokunaga K, Isshiki T, et al. Intravenous leiomyomatosis of the uterus with continuous extension into the pulmonary artery. Jpn Heart J 1984; 25:651–659.

345 Nakayama Y, Kitamura S, Kawachi K, et al. Intravenous leiomyomatosis extending into the right atrium. Cardiovasc Surg 1994; 2:642–645.

346 Arinami Y, Kodama S, Kase H, et al. Successful one-stage complete removal of an entire intravenous leiomyomatosis in the heart, vena cava and uterus. Gynecol Oncol 1997; 64:547–550.

347 Andrade LA, Torresan RZ, Sales JF Jr, et al. Intravenous leiomyomatosis of the uterus. A report of three cases. Pathol Oncol Res 1998; 4:44–47.

348 Clement PB. Intravenous leiomyomatosis of the uterus. Pathol Annu 1988; 23:153–183.

349 Itani Y, Otsuka Y, Deguchi F, et al. A case report of intravenous leiomyomatosis extending into the heart. Heart Vessels 2000; 15:291–294.

350 Saitoh M, Hayasaka T, Nakahara K, et al. Intravenous leiomyomatosis with cardiac extension. Gynecol Obstet Invest 2004; 58:168–170.

351 Topcuoglu MS, Yaliniz H, Poyrazoglu H, et al. Intravenous leiomyomatosis extending into the right ventricle after subtotal hysterectomy. Ann Thorac Surg 2004; 78:330–332.

352 Uchida H, Hattori Y, Nakada K, Iida T. Successful one-stage radical removal of intravenous leiomyomatosis extending to the right ventricle. Obstet Gynecol 2004; 103:1068–1070.

353 Kir G, Kir M, Gurbuz A, et al. Estrogen and progesterone expression of vessel walls with intravascular leiomyomatosis; discussion of histogenesis. Eur J Gynaecol Oncol 2004; 25:362–366.

354 Stolf NA, Santos GG, Haddad VL, et al. Successful one-stage resection of intravenous leiomyomatosis of the uterus with extension into the heart. Cardiovasc Surg 1999; 7:661–664.

355 Whitlatch SP, Meyer RL. Recurrent endometrial stromal sarcoma resembling intravenous leiomyomatosis. Gynecol Oncol 1987; 28:121–128.

356 Hameleers JA, Zeebregts CJ, Hamerlijnck RP, et al. Combined surgical and medical approach to intravenous leiomyomatosis with cardiac extension. Acta Chir Belg 1999; 99:92–94.

357 Burke M, Opeskin K. Death due to intravenous leiomyomatosis extending to the right pulmonary artery. Pathology 2004; 36:202–203.

358 Lam PM, Lo KW, Yu MM, et al. Intravenous leiomyomatosis with atypical histologic features: a case report. Int J Gynecol Cancer 2003; 13:83–87.

359 Canzonieri V, D'Amore ES, Bartoloni G, et al. Leiomyomatosis with vascular invasion. A unified pathogenesis regarding leiomyoma with vascular microinvasion, benign metastasizing leiomyoma and intravenous leiomyomatosis. Virchows Arch 1994; 425:541–545.

360 Robboy SJ, Bentley RC, Butnor K, Anderson MC. Pathology and pathophysiology of uterine smooth-muscle tumors. Environ Health Perspect 2000; 108(Suppl 5):779–784.

361 Nguyen GK. Disseminated leiomyomatosis peritonealis: report of a case in a postmenopausal woman. Can J Surg 1993; 36:46–48.

362 Strinic T, Kuzmic-Prusac I, Eterovic D, et al. Leiomyomatosis peritonealis disseminata in a postmenopausal woman. Arch Gynecol Obstet 2000; 264:97–98.

363 Gana BM, Byrne J, McCullough J, Weaver JP. Leiomyomatosis peritonealis disseminata (LPD) with associated endometriosis: a case report. J R Coll Surg Edin 1994; 39:258–260.

364 Heinig J, Neff A, Cirkel U, Klockenbusch W. Recurrent leiomyomatosis peritonealis disseminata after hysterectomy and bilateral salpingo-oophorectomy during combined hormone replacement therapy. Eur J Obstet Gynecol Reprod Biol 2003; 111:216–218.

365 Hales HA, Peterson CM, Jones KP, Quinn JD. Leiomyomatosis peritonealis disseminata treated with a gonadotropin-releasing hormone agonist. A case report. Am J Obstet Gynecol 1992; 167:515–516.

366 Butnor KJ, Burchette JL, Robboy SJ. Progesterone receptor activity in leiomyomatosis peritonealis disseminata. Int J Gynecol Pathol 1999; 18:259–264.

367 Ghosh K, Dorigo O, Bristow R, Berek J. A radical debulking of leiomyomatosis peritonealis disseminata from a colonic obstruction: a case report and review of the literature. J Am Coll Surg 2000; 191:212–215.

368 Abulafia O, Angel C, Sherer DM, et al. Computed tomography of leiomyomatosis peritonealis disseminata with malignant transformation. Am J Obstet Gynecol 1993; 169:52–54.

369 Rubin SC, Wheeler JE, Mikuta JJ. Malignant leiomyomatosis peritonealis disseminata. Obstet Gynecol 1986; 68:126–130.

370 Akkersdijk GJ, Flu PK, Giard RW, et al. Malignant leiomyomatosis peritonealis disseminata. Am J Obstet Gynecol 1990; 163:591–593.

371 Raspagliesi F, Quattrone P, Grosso G, et al. Malignant degeneration in leiomyomatosis peritonealis disseminata. Gynecol Oncol 1996; 61:272–274.

372 Fulcher AS, Szucs RA. Leiomyomatosis peritonealis disseminata complicated by sarcomatous transformation and ovarian torsion: presentation of two cases and review of the literature. Abdom Imaging 1998; 23:640–644.

373 Bekkers RL, Willemsen WN, Schijf CP, et al. Leiomyomatosis peritonealis disseminata: does malignant transformation occur? A literature review. Gynecol Oncol 1999; 75:158–163.

374 Alaniz SA, Castaneda DY. Disseminated peritoneal leiomyomatosis with malignant degeneration. A case report. Gynecol Obstet Mex 1994; 62:336–340.

375 Kitazawa S, Shiraishi N, Maeda S. Leiomyomatosis peritonealis disseminata with adipocytic differentiation. Acta Obstet Gynecol Scand 1992; 71:482–484.

376 Lau WY, Leung ML, Chow CH, Li AK. Leiomyomatosis peritonealis disseminata. Aust N Z J Surg 1990; 60:232–234.

377 Due W, Pickartz H. Immunohistologic detection of estrogen and progesterone receptors in disseminated peritoneal leiomyomatosis. Int J Gynecol Pathol 1989; 8:46–53.

378 Silva EG, Ross JL, Gershenson DM, et al. Peritoneal lesions in guinea pigs treated with hormones. Int J Gynecol Pathol 2002; 21:412–415.

379 Jeffers M, Cowan C, Lunan CB. Degenerative changes in myometrium simulating diffuse leiomyomatosis after treatment with gonadotrophin releasing hormone analogue. J Clin Pathol 1995; 48:278–280.

380 Baschinsky DY, Isa A, Niemann TH, et al. Diffuse leiomyomatosis of the uterus: a case report with clonality analysis. Hum Pathol 2000; 31:1429–1432.

381 Esteban JM, Allen WM, Schaerf RH. Benign metastasizing leiomyoma of the uterus: histologic and immunohistochemical characterization of primary and metastatic lesions. Arch Pathol Lab Med 1999; 123:960–962.

382 Kayser K, Zink S, Schneider T, et al. Benign metastasizing leiomyoma of the uterus: documentation of clinical, immunohistochemical and lectin – histochemical data of ten cases. Virchows Arch 2000; 437:284–292.

383 Tietze L, Gunther K, Horbe A, et al. Benign metastasizing leiomyoma: a cytogenetically balanced but clonal disease. Hum Pathol 2000; 31:126–128.

384 Nucci MR, Dal Cin P, Drapkin R, et al. Unique cytogenetic profile in so-called benign metastasizing leiomyomata: evidence of a distinct clinicopathological entity. Mod Pathol 2003; 16(1):202A.

385 Ferenczy A. Pathophysiology of adenomyosis. Hum Reprod Update 1998; 4:312–322.

386 Benson RC, Sneeden VD. Adenomyosis: a reappraisal of symptomatology. Am J Obstet Gynecol 1958; 76:1044–1057.

387 Owolabi TO, Strickler RC. Adenomyosis: a neglected diagnosis. Obstet Gynecol 1977; 50:424–427.

388 Matsumoto Y, Iwasaka T, Yamasaki F, Sugimori H. Apoptosis and Ki-67 expression in adenomyotic lesions and in the corresponding eutopic endometrium. Obstet Gynecol 1999; 94:71–77.

389 Goswami A, Khemani M, Logani KB, Anand R. Adenomyosis: diagnosis by hysteroscopic endomyometrial biopsy, correlation of incidence and severity with menorrhagia. J Obstet Gynaecol Res 1998; 24:281–284.

390 Kim MD, Won JW, Lee DY, Ahn CS. Uterine artery embolization for adenomyosis without fibroids. Clin Radiol 2004; 59:520–526.

391 Pandis N, Karaiskos C, Bardi G, et al. Chromosome analysis of uterine adenomyosis. Detection of the leiomyoma-associated del(7q) in three cases. Cancer Genet Cytogenet 1995; 80:118–120.

392 Clement PB, Scully RE. Müllerian adenosarcoma of the uterus: a clinicopathologic analysis of 100 cases with a review of the literature. Hum Pathol 1990; 21:363–381.

393 Clement PB. Müllerian adenosarcomas of the uterus with sarcomatous overgrowth. A clinicopathological analysis of 10 cases. Am J Surg Pathol 1989; 13:28–38.

394 Verschraegen CF, Vasuratna A, Edwards C, et al. Clinicopathologic analysis of Müllerian adenosarcoma: the M.D. Anderson Cancer Center experience. Oncol Rep 1998; 5:939–944.

395 Mignotte H, Lasset C, Bonadona V, et al. Iatrogenic risks of endometrial carcinoma after treatment for breast cancer in a large French case-control study. Federation Nationale des Centres de Lutte Contre le Cancer (FNCLCC). Int J Cancer 1998; 76:325–330.

396 Pukkala E, Kyyronen P, Sankila R, Holli K. Tamoxifen and toremifene treatment of breast cancer and risk of subsequent endometrial cancer: a population-based case-control study. Int J Cancer 2002; 100:337–341.

397 Clement PB, Scully RE. Müllerian adenosarcomas of the uterus with sex cord-like elements. A clinicopathologic

analysis of eight cases. Am J Clin Pathol 1989; 91:664–672.

398 Jones MW, Lefkowitz M. Adenosarcoma of the uterine cervix: a clinicopathological study of 12 cases. Int J Gynecol Pathol 1995; 14:223–229.

399 Zaloudek CJ, Norris HJ. Adenofibroma and adenosarcoma of the uterus: a clinicopathologic study of 35 cases. Cancer 1981; 48:354–366.

400 Clement PB, Scully RE. Endometrial stromal sarcomas of the uterus with extensive endometrioid glandular differentiation: a report of three cases that caused problems in differential diagnosis. Int J Gynecol Pathol 1992; 11:163–173.

401 Tai LH, Tavassoli FA. Endometrial polyps with atypical (bizarre) stromal cells. Am J Surg Pathol 2002; 26:505–509.

402 Amant F, Schurmans K, Steenkiste E, et al. Immunohistochemical determination of estrogen and progesterone receptor positivity in uterine adenosarcoma. Gynecol Oncol 2004; 93:680–685.

403 Vang R, Kempson RL. Perivascular epithelioid cell tumor ('PEComa') of the uterus: a subset of HMB-45-positive epithelioid mesenchymal neoplasms with an uncertain relationship to pure smooth muscle tumors. Am J Surg Pathol 2002; 26:1–13.

404 Folpe AL, Goodman ZD, Ishak KG, et al. Clear cell myomelanocytic tumor of the falciform ligament/ligamentum teres: a novel member of the perivascular epithelioid clear cell family of tumors with a predilection for children and young adults. Am J Surg Pathol 2000; 24:1239–1246.

405 Bonetti F, Martignoni G, Colato C, et al. Abdominopelvic sarcoma of perivascular epithelioid cells. Report of four cases in young women, one with tuberous sclerosis. Mod Pathol 2001; 14:563–568.

406 Bonetti F, Pea M, Martignoni G, et al. Clear cell ('sugar') tumor of the lung is a lesion strictly related to angiomyolipoma – the concept of a family of lesions characterized by the presence of the perivascular epithelioid cells (PEC). Pathology 1994; 26:230–236.

407 Chan JK, Tsang WY, Pau MY, et al. Lymphangiomyomatosis and angiomyolipoma: closely related entities characterized by hamartomatous proliferation of HMB-45-positive smooth muscle. Histopathology 1993; 22:445–455.

408 Silva EG, Deavers MT, Bodurka DC, Malpica A. Uterine epithelioid leiomyosarcomas with clear cells: reactivity with HMB-45 and the concept of PEComa. Am J Surg Pathol 2004; 28:244–249.

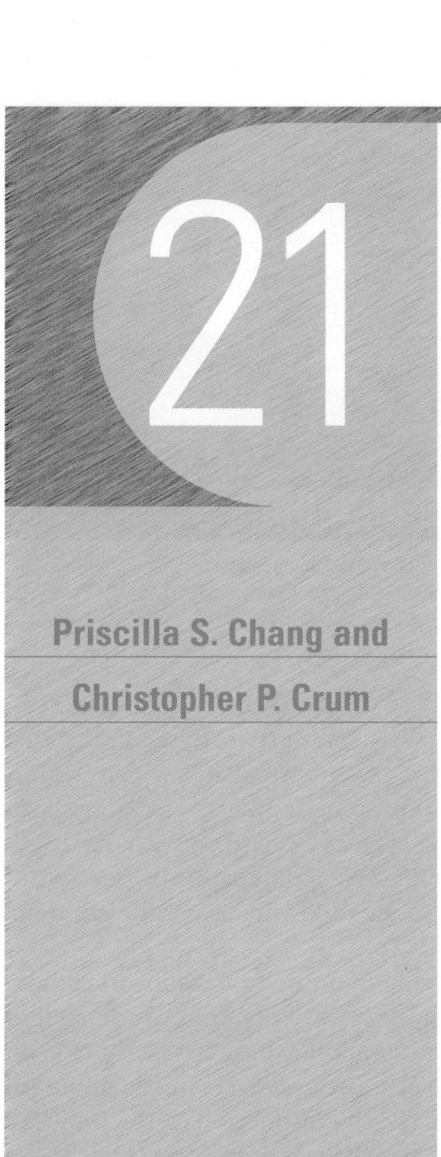

21

The fallopian tube and broad ligament

Priscilla S. Chang and

Christopher P. Crum

Introduction

Tubal anatomy and histology

Approach to commonly received specimens

Tubal ligation
Tubal re-anastomosis
Hysterectomies with attached
    tubes

Infectious disorders

Acute and chronic infectious
    salpingitis
Granulomatous salpingitis

Regional and systemic disorders

Torsion
Vasculitis
Amyloidosis

Ectopic pregnancy

Benign tubal/adnexal masses

Adenomatoid tumor
Serous cystadenoma
Borderline serous tumors
Adenofibromas
Other benign tumors and
    tumor-like lesions

Malignant neoplasms

Introduction
Screening BRCA or familial
    ovarian cancer
Primary carcinoma of the tube
Carcinoma occurring within
    endometriosis
Metastatic neoplasia
Tumors of Wolffian origin
    (FATWO)

Introduction

The fallopian tube comes to the attention of the surgical pathologist under four general scenarios: (1) the tube has been interrupted for sterilization and the pathologist must confirm this; (2) the tube has been removed as a component of the hysterectomy and is examined routinely; (3) the tube is removed for specific reasons, usually tubal pregnancy or rarely, a tubal mass; and (4) the tube becomes an important part of either ovarian cancer screening or staging a Müllerian neoplasm. Each of these scenarios requires from the pathologist a working knowledge of the tubal anatomy and an appreciation of the subtle nature of early tubal cancer.

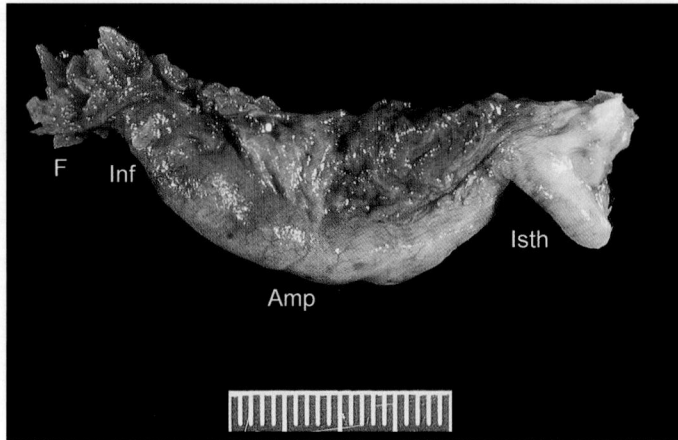

Fig. 21.1 Gross image of the tube with its components including fimbriated end (F), infundibulum (Inf), ampulla (Amp) and isthmus (Isth).

Tubal anatomy and histology

The fallopian tube is formed from the Müllerian (paramesonephric ducts) and lies within the broad ligament located between the ovary and the uterus (see Ch. 1). It is roughly divided into three anatomic regions. The distal portion of the tube (infundibulum) is dilated, opens onto the peritoneal cavity and is ringed by fimbrial projections (Fig. 21.1). The infundibulum merges with the ampulla, gradually narrowing until it nears the isthmus, beyond which it terminates in the intramural region within the uterus. When viewed on cross-sections, the tube displays three distinct layers that are most prominent in the ampulla – the surface mucosa, lamina propria and muscularis (Fig. 21.2). The mucosa consists of a non-stratified epithelial lining composed of three cell types, ciliated, secretory and intercalated cells (Fig. 21.3). The most common are the ciliated cells, followed by secretory cells, which together comprise over 90% of the cell population. The ciliated cells are critical to ovum transport. The secretory cells exhibit fusiform nuclei and apical secretory vacuoles, which often appear blue on hematoxylin and eosin staining. The intercalated cells are presumed to be a variant of the secretory cell and are seen as sporadic elongated nuclei between the ciliated cells. The proportions of these individual cell types vary according to the location in the tube and account for wide variations in the appearance of the tubal epithelium (see below). Scattered lymphocytes are arranged at the epithelial-stromal interface and may signify a form of localized immune system. Beneath this mucosa is the second layer, consisting of the lamina propria with loose connective tissue. In the normal tube, this portion is thrown into redundant slender folds known as plicae. The structural integrity of the plicae is relevant to ovum transport. The third layer consists of the muscularis, which is composed of circular smooth muscle fibers. The outer layer consists of the serosal surface and subserosal loose connective tissue (Fig. 21.2). The isthmus portion of the tube also contains an additional inner longitudinal muscle layer (Fig. 21.2c).[1]

The pathologist will encounter variations in cellular makeup of the tubal mucosa depending on reproductive age, hormonal status and location in the tube. With age, the plicae become progressively more blunt in appearance, owing to both contraction of the lining of the tube and a loss of epithelial complexity (Fig. 21.4). This is analogous to the changes occurring in postmenopausal endometrium. A second variable is the epithelial thickness and composition. Ciliated cells are more prominent in the fimbriated portion of the tube. The number and spacing of the secretory cells varies. In some regions the secretory cells may appear hyperplastic, replacing short stretches of mucosa, or may appear to tuft towards the lumen in small units. Variations in epithelial stratification will be the result. Most are physiologic in nature; however, the pathologist must be familiar with these variations in order to distinguish them from tubal neoplasia. Some authors have reported the presence of both atypical hyperplasias and early intraepithelial carcinomas in tubal mucosa, particularly patients with BRCA mutations. However, precisely which alterations signify early neoplasia is controversial and making this distinction requires a broad understanding of the changes that normally occur.[2–4] Figure 21.5 contrasts some commonly found presumably physiologic patterns with less conspicuous architectural but decidedly

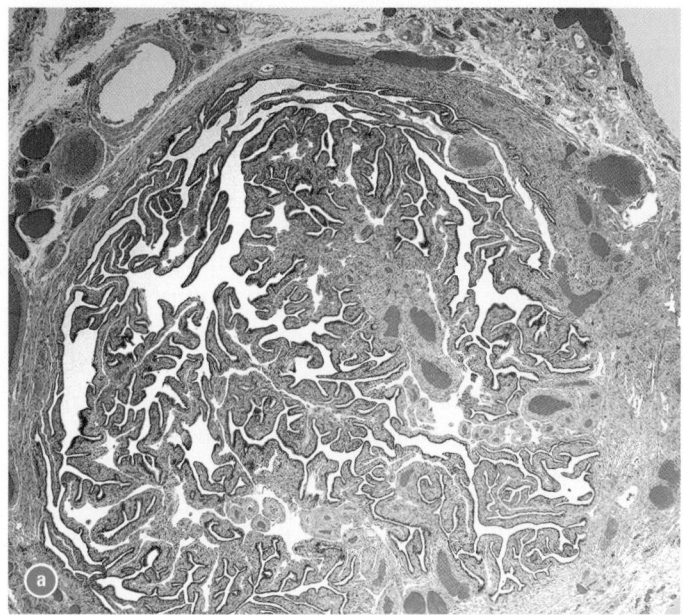

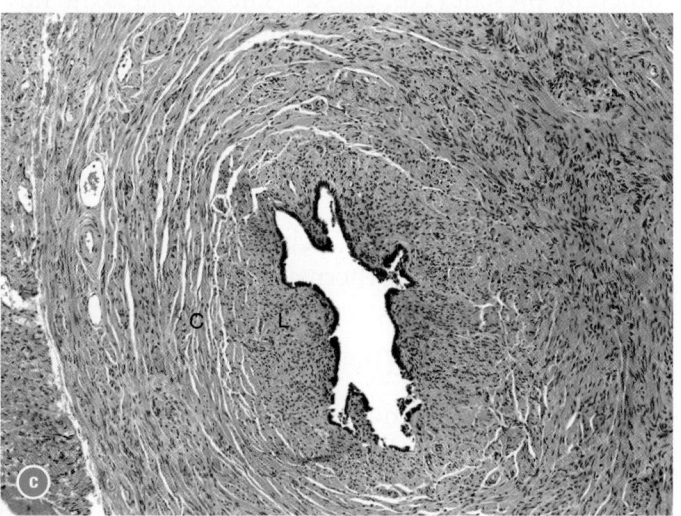

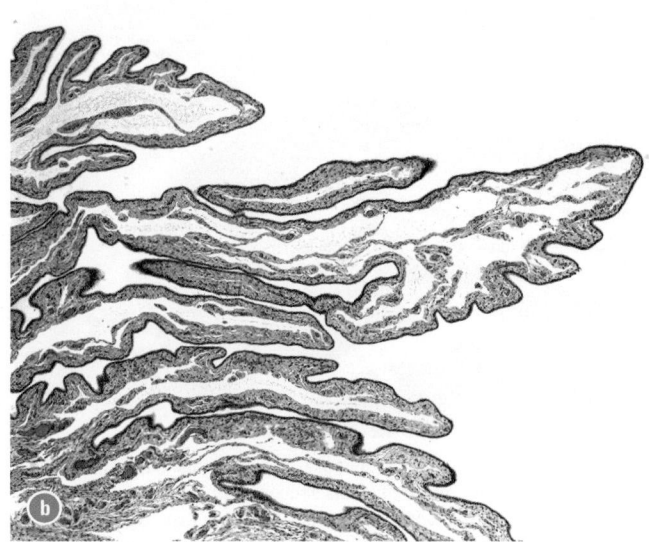

Fig. 21.2 (a) Cross-section of the ampulla displaying the prominent tubal plica. (b) Cross-section at fimbria, where the plica are suspended from the infundibulum in a frond-like appearance. (c) Cross-section at the isthmus, containing both an inner longitudinal (L) and outer circular (C) muscle layer.

malignant epithelium. The obvious importance of these changes lies in their distinction from intraepithelial neoplasia (aka carcinoma *in situ*) of the tube, an exercise that will become more important with the increasingly common use of prophylactic salpingo-oophorectomy. This will be discussed subsequently.

Approach to commonly received specimens

TUBAL LIGATION

The purpose of tubal ligation is to eliminate the risk of subsequent pregnancy. In the USA, nearly one-quarter of reproductive-age women rely on sterilization of either sex to achieve contraception.[5] The success of tubal sterilization is approximately 98%. Significantly, when failures do occur, the risk is greatest at 2–3 years following the procedure; 30% of these will result in ectopic pregnancy. Disadvantages of tubal sterilization include pain, changes in menstruation, dyspareunia, changes in libido and increased risk of gynecologic surgery. Benefits include a reduction in ovarian cancer risk and improved family life.[5–8]

When tubes are transected and ligated, the clinician removes a segment of the tube under laparoscopic guidance and submits it to the pathologist to verify that (a) tube is present and (b) that a complete cross-section is present. The pathologist verifies both and issues a report that a portion of oviduct is present and

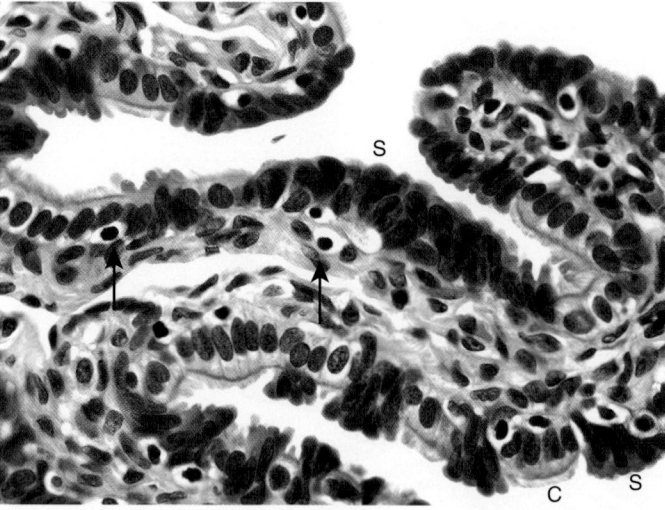

Fig. 21.3 High magnification of tubal mucosa. Darkly-stained elongate nuclei of secretory cells (S) are prominent in this section, with nuclei protruding into the lumen, and are admixed with ciliated cells (C). These two cell types comprise over 90% of the tubal epithelium. Occasional lymphocytes are situated in the basal region, appearing as rounded nuclei (arrows).

consists of a complete cross-section. The pathologist must also report the presence of any tubal abnormalities, although most consist of evidence of old infection (in the form of chronic follicular salpingitis), tubal endometriosis and peritubal adhesions. A common

finding in tubal ligation specimens performed at the time of parturition is focal *ectopic decidual change* of the mucosa (Fig. 21.6a). These changes are occasionally encountered in specimens removed from women undergoing hormonal therapy.[7] Another finding commonly seen in tubes that have been manipulated, either during tubal ligation or routine hysterectomy, is the presence of inflammatory cells that are incidental in nature. These include the margination of neutrophils from submucosal venules, associated with intra-operative manipulation (Fig. 21.6b), or the occasional presence of plasma cells in peripartum tubal ligation specimens. These are frequent and unassociated with other features of salpingitis.

The pathologist faces four potential pitfalls when assessing tubal segments. The first is the diagnosis of tube in the absence of lumen. Because round ligament can mimic tube, the pathologist must require that a lumen be present (Fig. 21.7a). The second is the mis-classification of a paratubal cyst with rudimentary plica as a segment of tube or a hydrosalpinx. Paratubal cysts typically contain a much more attenuated wall with minimal smooth muscle (Fig. 21.7b). The third pitfall is misdiagnosing a segment of ureter as tube. This is unlikely to happen to either the surgeon or an experienced histologist, but is included for completeness. The fourth is mistaking thermal artifacts for neoplasia.[8]

TUBAL RE-ANASTOMOSIS

In some instances, the clinician will attempt a re-anastomosis of the fallopian tube to restore fertility. This is successful in approximately 55% of cases.[9] This procedure typically entails the removal of some segments, which are submitted to the pathologist. The most common findings in these segments are the absence of plica or small foci of hydrosalpinx associated with prior interruption. Other than confirming that no major abnormality (active infection or neoplasia) is present, the pathologist's role is to verify the origin of the tissues.

HYSTERECTOMIES WITH ATTACHED TUBES

In the routine hysterectomy, fallopian tubes are examined with an eye towards excluding concurrent disease. Practically speaking, the following may be seen:

Rests and metaplasias

The most common rests are *Walthard cell rests*, consisting of transitional metaplasia of mesothelial cells (Fig.

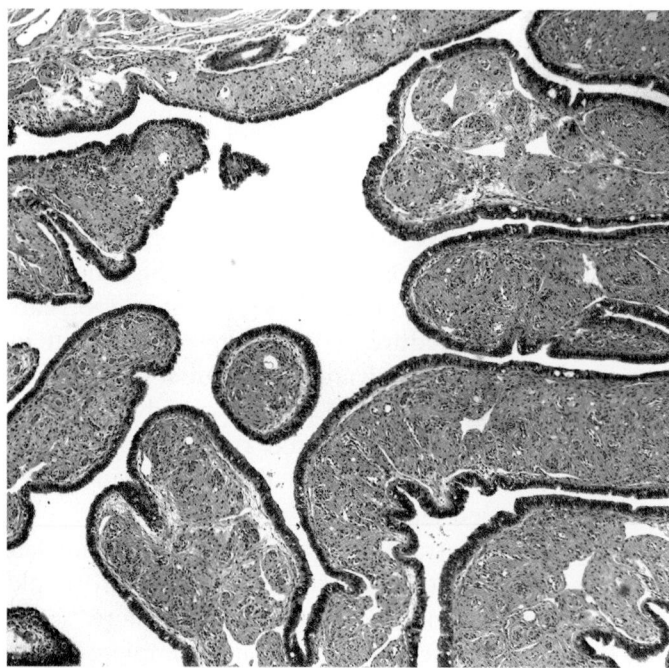

Fig. 21.4 Atrophic tube, with blunt, tubal plicae with collagenized lamina propria (compare with Fig. 21.2a).

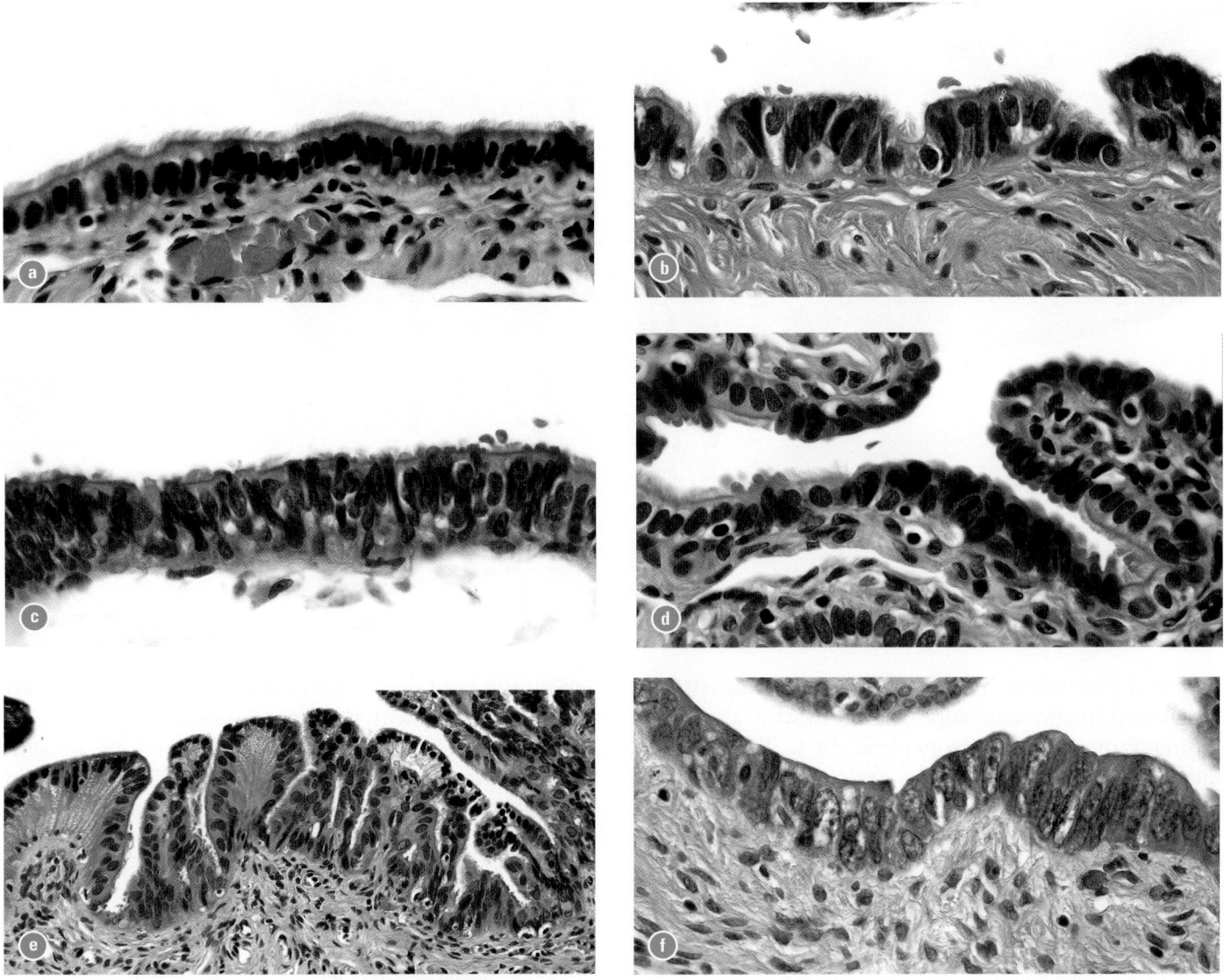

Fig. 21.5 Variations of mucosa in the fallopian tube of adults. (a) Non-stratified predominately ciliated epithelium. (b) Focal irregularities in epithelial thickness produced by mixtures of ciliated and secretory cells. (c) Pseudo-stratified mucosa. (d) Focal concentrations of secretory (and intercalated) cells producing increased cell density. (e) Micropapillary architecture, presumably due to irregularities in epithelial growth. (f) Tubal carcinoma (intraepithelial carcinoma); note the absence of cilia and prominent nuclear atypia.

21.8a). These are most commonly seen adjacent to the fimbria but may be seen on or adjacent to the serosa in any segment of tube. They most likely occur via the development of reserve cells (Fig. 21.8b). This is supported by transitional metaplasia within mesothelial cysts within the mesosalpinx (see below). The lining cells characteristically contain small, uniform fusiform cell nuclei with nuclear grooves (Fig. 21.8c). *Adrenal rests* consist of small discrete microscopic nodules of adrenal cortical cells, typically situated in the connective tissue of the mesosalpinx (Fig. 21.8d). Their presumed origin is from adrenal progenitor cells carried with the mesonephros during development. They are benign but may mimic steroid-producing cells, which occasionally are lipid rich and resemble adrenal cells. However, the latter are situated in the hilus, in contrast to the peritubal connective tissue.

Cysts

Paratubal cysts can be subdivided into the following categories:

Large paratubal Müllerian cysts (hydatids of Morgagni)

These cysts conceivably can arise via three different pathways. The first is Müllerian transformation of the mesothelial surface. The second is detached and

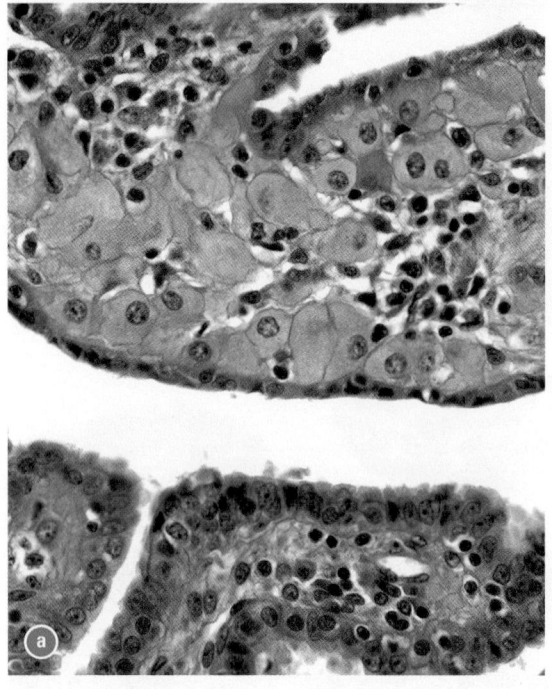

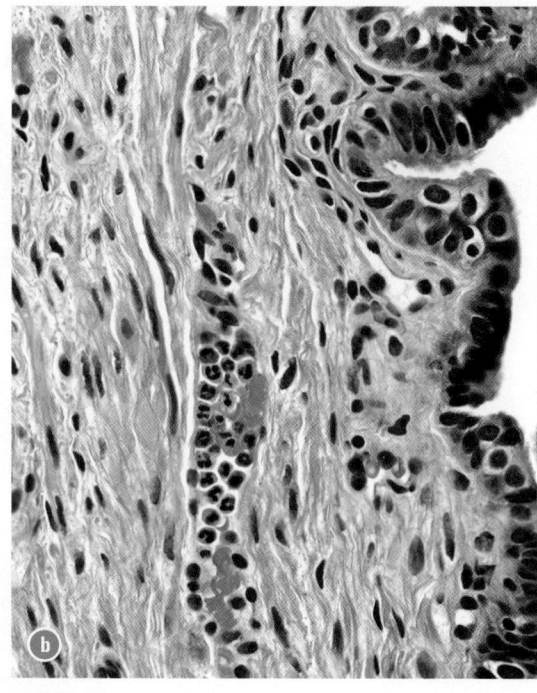

Fig. 21.6 (a) Focal ectopic decidual change in the tubal mucosa, a common feature in peripartum tubal ligation specimens. (b) Marginated neutrophils associated with operative manipulation.

encysted epithelium from the fallopian tube that is ensconced in the mesosalpinx. The third is a vestigial remnant of the paramesonephric duct. The latter is most appealing, as these cysts are characteristically (if not invariably) closely associated with the fallopian tube, typically tethered by a thin band of connective tissue to the tube.[10,11] Paratubal Müllerian cysts charac-

teristically contain an attenuated and translucent cyst wall (Fig. 21.9a) with delicate mesenchyme and variable smooth muscle (Fig. 21.9b). Plicae may be present but are sporadic and the lining epithelium is ciliated (Fig. 21.9c). Paratubal cysts are distinguished from tube (hydrosalpinx) by the absence of a well-developed smooth muscle wall and from serous cystadenomas

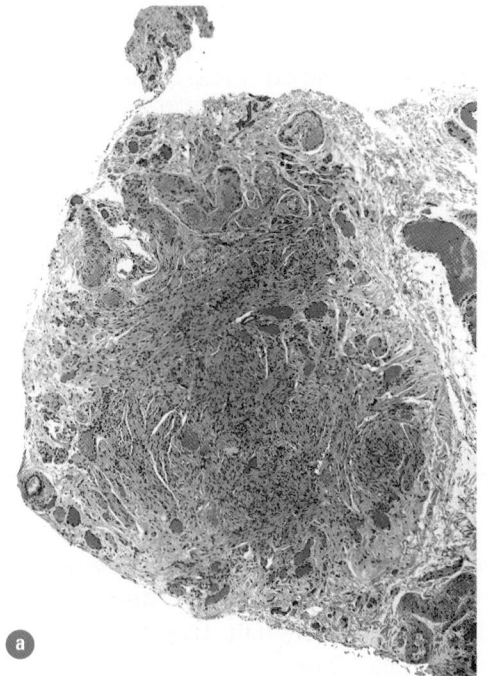

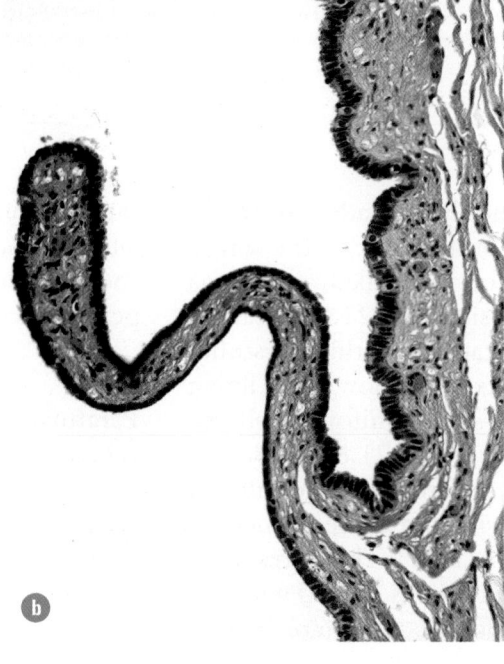

Fig. 21.7 Mimics of normal tube. (a) Round ligament. (b) Paratubal cyst with rudimentary plica can be misclassified as a segment of tube.

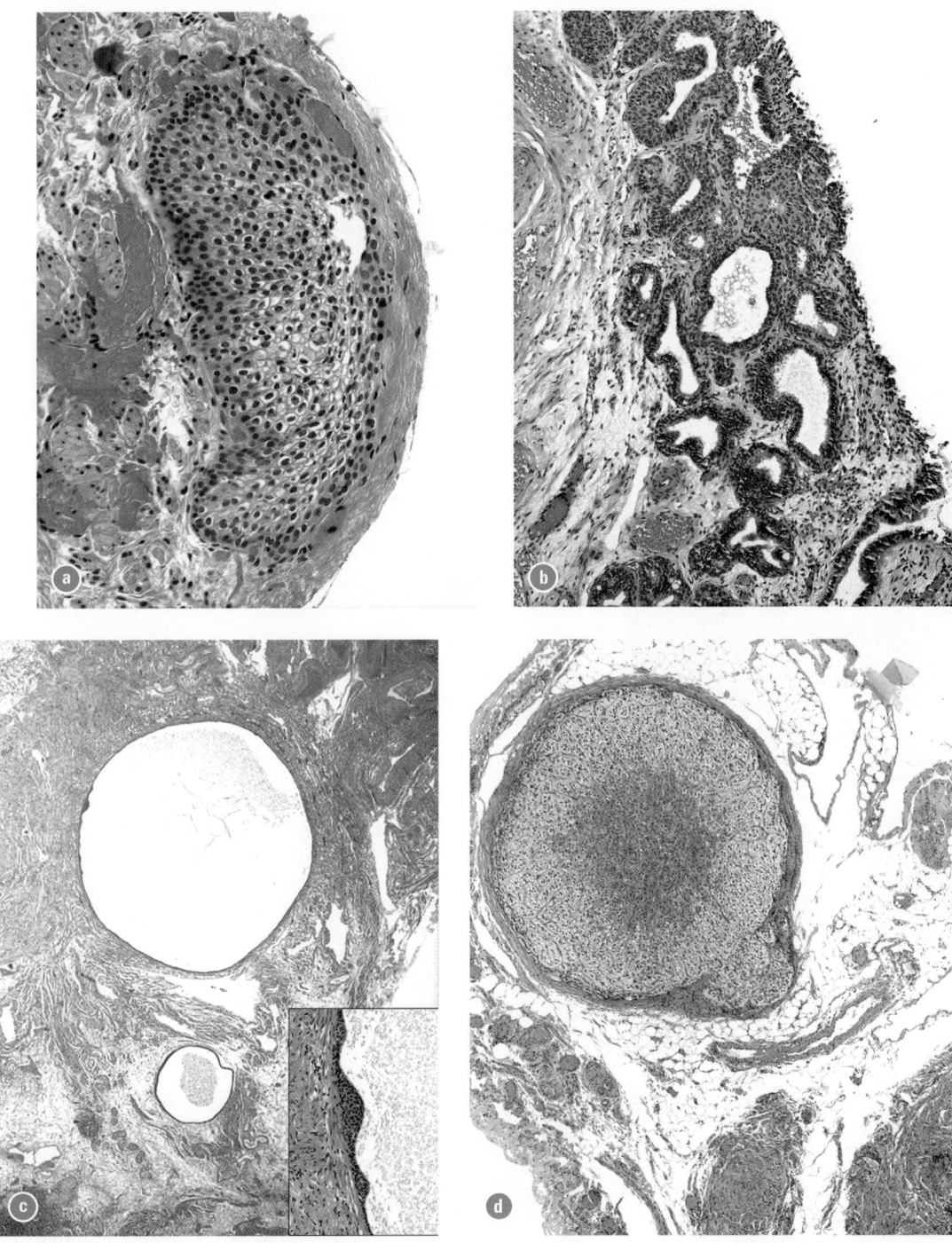

Fig. 21.8 (a) Walthard cell rest. (b) Reserve cells situated beneath the fimbrial columnar cells (lower) expand to give rise to the transitional cells (upper) in this tube. (c) Cystic Walthard cell rest, seen as transitional differentiation within a paratubal cyst (inset, lower right). (d) Ectopic adrenal tissue in the paratubal soft tissue.

by the close similarity to tubal epithelium, occasional rudimentary plica and, specifically, by the absence of a dense collagenized cyst wall that typifies cystomas. Cystadenomas are discussed below.

Endosalpingiosis

These are most likely implants of benign tubal epithelial cells that encyst in the mesosalpinx (Fig. 21.10). Identical epithelial cysts can be seen in the ovarian cortex,

mesentery and lymph nodes, a distribution that precludes origin from paramesonephric (Müllerian) duct remnants. These are distinguished from endometriosis by the well-developed ciliated lining and the absence of endometrial stroma or hemosiderin.

Mesothelial (and simple) cysts

Cysts lined by mesothelium exhibit a range of histologic presentations. The first is *cystic adhesions*, which

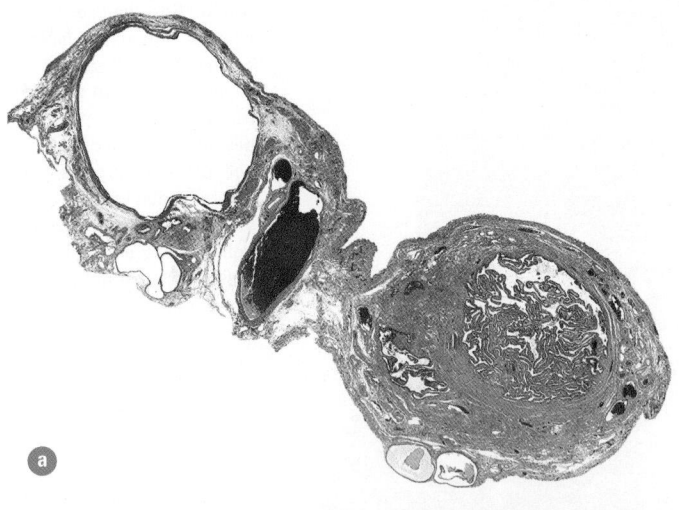

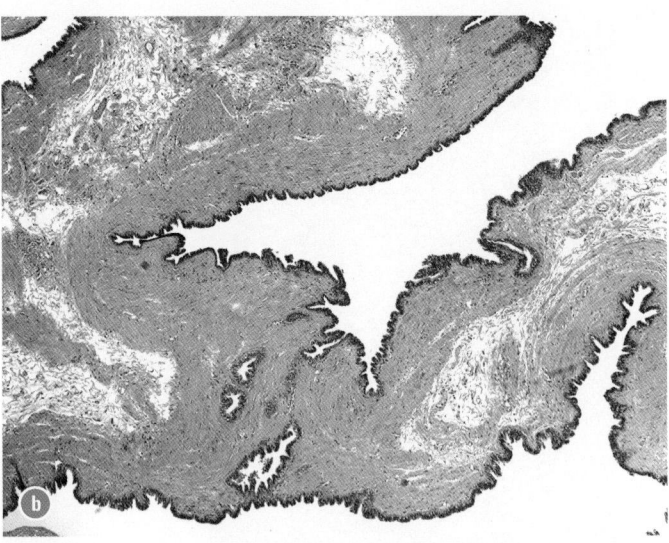

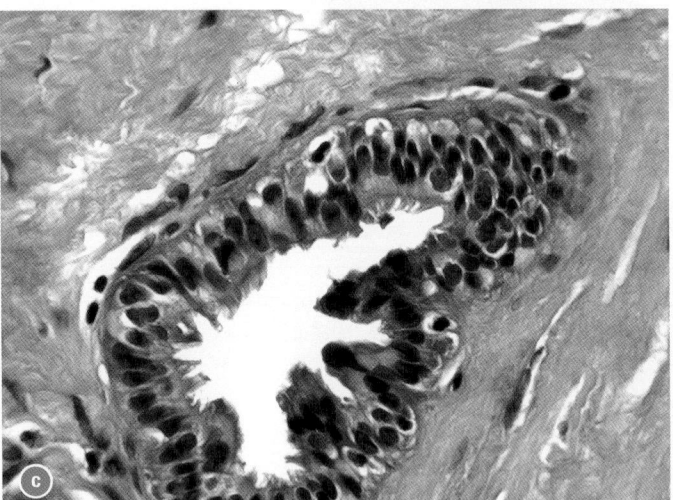

Fig. 21.9 (a) Paratubal Müllerian cyst (hydatid of Morgagni), suspended by a thin soft tissue pedicle. (b) Cyst wall with rudimentary plicae. (c) Ciliated lining epithelium.

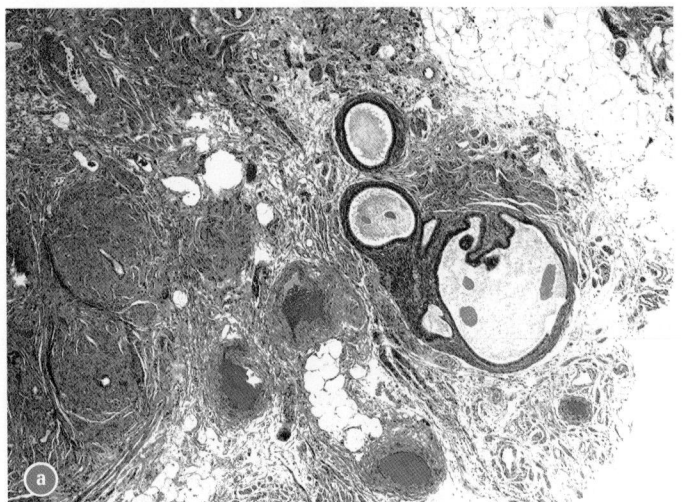

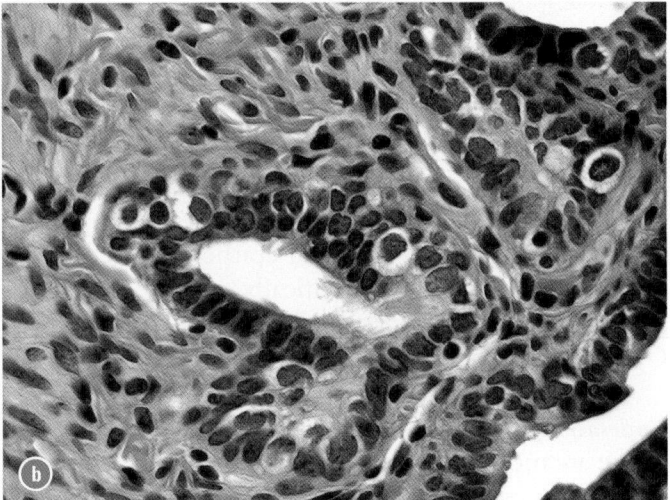

Fig. 21.10 (a) Endosalpingiosis in the broad ligament adjacent to the round ligament. (b) Endosalpingiosis in the round ligament, consisting of ciliated epithelium.

are simply complex adhesions with collections of clear fluid (Fig. 21.11a). A likely related lesion is the *multilocular cyst* with mesothelial proliferation, which is most likely a manifestation of inflammation (Fig. 21.12). These cysts may also exhibit squamoid or transitional metaplasia similar to that seen in Walthard cell rests (Figs. 21.11b, 21.12b). Less commonly, papillary mesothelial hyperplasia is seen (Fig. 21.12c). Another is the solitary cyst lined by cuboidal epithelium with a more collagenized fibrous wall, often termed *simple cyst*. Conceivably, many simple cysts are not mesothelial but epithelial, but in the absence of conspicuous cilia, the pathologist may elect to classify such cysts as simple cysts rather than unilocular cystadenomas (Fig. 21.13).

Endometriosis

Endometriosis is extremely common and is found in approximately 10% of tubal specimens.[11–17] The possible origins of endometriosis are discussed in Chapters 23 and 24 and include transformation of coelomic epithelium and transtubal migration of uterine endometrium during menstruation. In the fallopian tubes, the importance of endometriosis lies in its relationship to infertility in younger women and an increased risk of malignancy with age.

In patients with endometriosis, the principal variable influencing fertility is the condition of the tube, with the rate of successful pregnancy diminishing from over 50% with no abnormality to 0% with bilateral tubal occlusion. In contrast, ovarian and cul-de-sac lesions do not impact on pregnancy rates.[16] History and pelvic examination are of limited predictive value; many lesions are silent and detected by laparoscopy.[17]

Tubal endometriosis has several morphologic presentations. The first is classic endometriosis, characterized by endometrial glands and stroma in the muscularis or more commonly, in the subserosa or mesosalpinx (Fig. 21.14). Younger lesions closely resemble normal endometrium (Fig. 21.14a). Lesions composed of dilated glands surrounded by fibrosis and hemosiderin are more commonly encountered later in the natural history (Fig. 21.14b). In some cases, the process is more subtly present on the serosal surface of the fallopian tube and broad ligament, composed of scant epithelium and hemosiderin-laden macrophages (Fig. 21.14c). A common, albeit nonspecific, feature of endometriosis is the presence of scattered plasma cells (Fig. 21.14d). However, this finding is not considered diagnostic. Similarly, in the absence of stroma or Müllerian epithelium, hemosiderin is not sufficient for a diagnosis of endometriosis.

Of interest and possibly related to endometriosis are inflammatory changes in the fallopian tube lining, including follicular salpingitis. Some authors have proposed a relationship between salpingitis and endometriosis, suggesting that the former is a mechanism for tubal-associated infertility in these patients. This is consistent with the close relationship between tubal adhesions and pregnancy success rates.[16]

Pseudoxanthomatous salpingitis

An uncommon abnormality associated with endometriosis consists of expansion of the tubal plicae by pigmented histiocytes. This is termed 'pseudoxanthomatous salpingitis' and is analogous to the xantho-

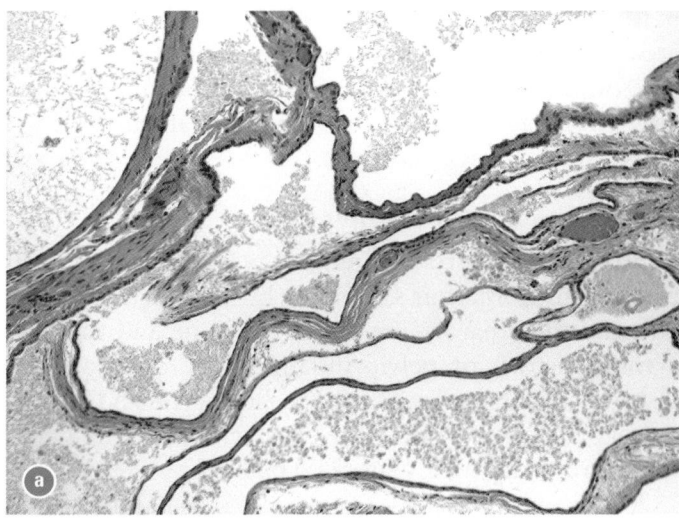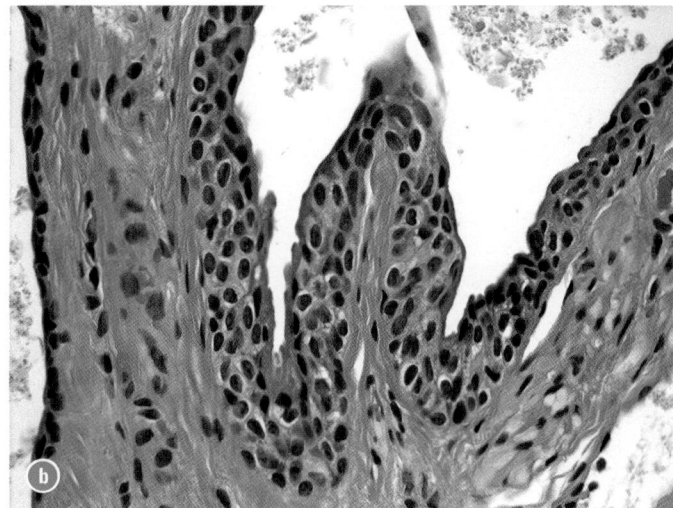

Fig. 21.11 (a) Cystic adhesions. (b) At higher power, there is focal transitional metaplasia.

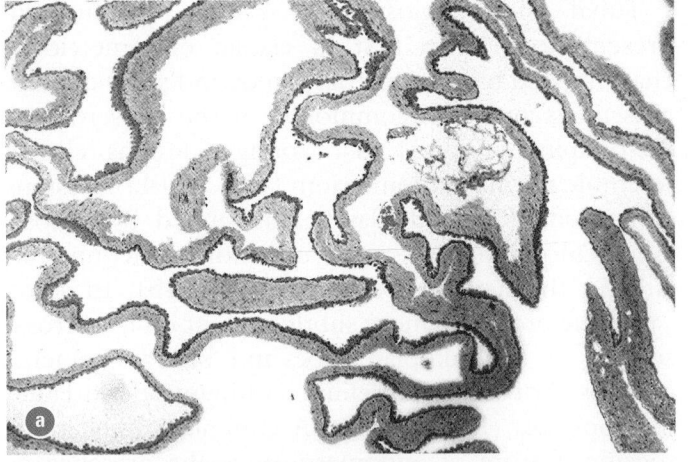

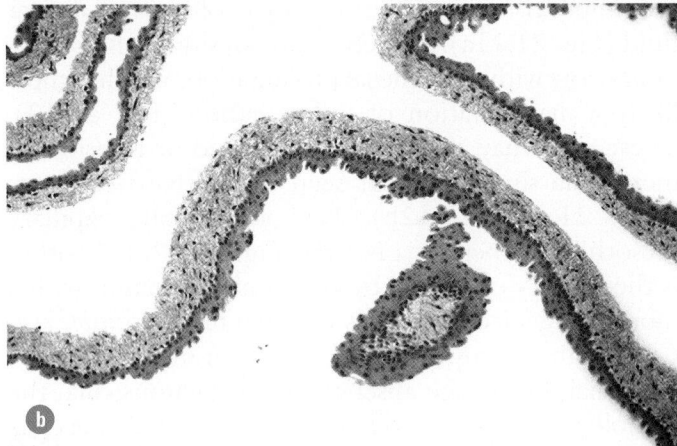

Fig. 21.12 (a) Low power of complex mesothelial cyst. (b) Focal squamoid metaplasia of the lining epithelium. (c) Papillary mesothelial hyperplasia (benign papillary mesothelioma).

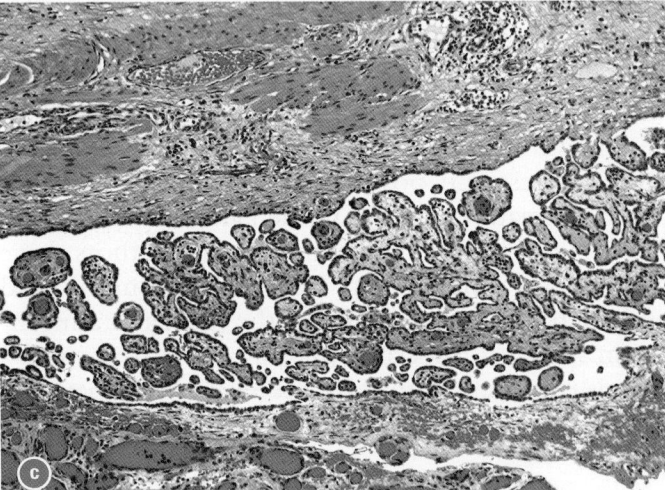

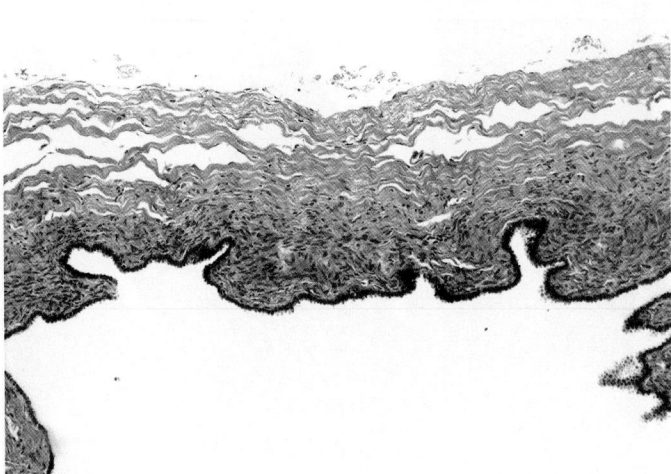

Fig. 21.13 Simple cyst, with collagenized stroma.

matous pseudotumors seen elsewhere in the pelvic area in patients with endometriosis (Fig. 21.15a,b).[18] The origin of this process is not clear, but may be due to hemorrhage directly into the fallopian tube lumen with a macrophage response.

Xanthogranulomatous salpingitis

Xanthogranulomatous salpingitis is distinguished from pseudoxanthomatous salpingitis by its association with a frank inflammatory process of the tube and typically a long history of pelvic inflammatory disease. This disorder is characterized by foamy histiocytes and inflammatory cells in the wall of the tube, with the latter being the more prominent (Fig. 21.16a,b).[19]

A variant of xanthogranulomatous salpingitis is associated with reaction to contrast agents (lipiodol).

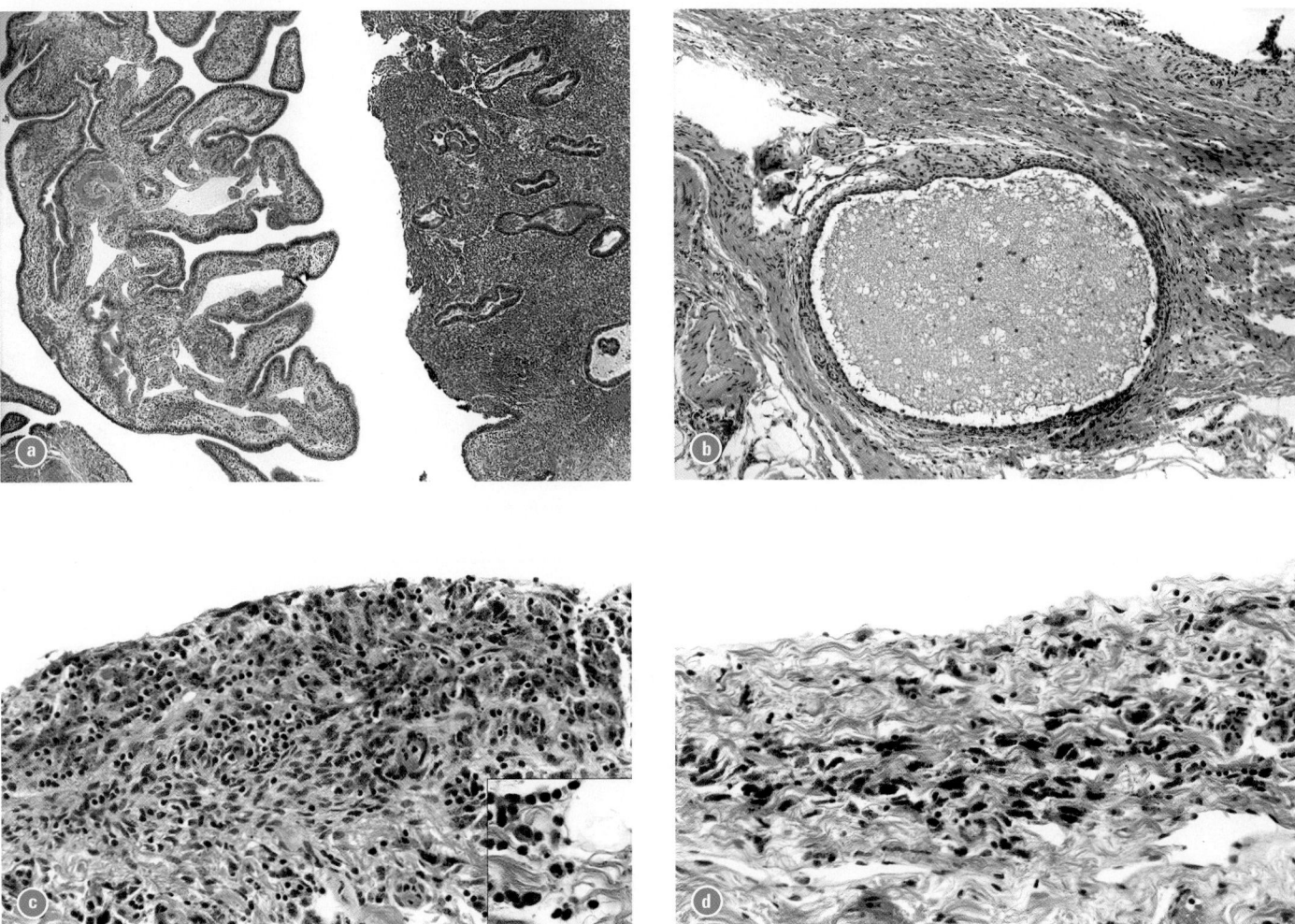

Fig. 21.14 (a) Endometriosis in the tubal wall adjacent to the lumen. (b) Older more subtle lesion with scant hemosiderin in a fibrous matrix. (c) Scant stroma and hemosiderin on the surface of the tube. (d) Plasma cells in endometriosis.

In this condition, the lamina propria contains collections of discrete vacuoles corresponding to the foreign material, with a secondary granulomatous inflammation.[20,21]

Adhesions

Adhesions are common and may follow prior salpingitis, surgery or endometriosis. They may be confined to the tube (paratubal adhesions) (Fig. 21.17a), bridge the tube and ovary (tubo-ovarian adhesions) (Fig. 21.17b) or coalesce and form a cystic mass in which fluid collects (cystic adhesions)(Fig. 21.11a). As discussed above, adhesions are associated with infertility.

Old follicular salpingitis

Chronic (follicular) salpingitis is not uncommon in hysterectomy specimens and reflects prior tubal infec-tion (see below). The characteristic features are plical adhesions forming follicle-like architecture (Fig. 21.18), often accompanied by hydrosalpinx (see below).

Salpingitis isthmica nodosum

Salpingitis isthmica nodosum (SIN) is analogous to 'adenomyosis' of the tube.[22] The prevalence of SIN ranges from 0.6% to 11%, but it is strongly associated with infertility and ectopic pregnancy.[23] SIN consists of a discrete nodular swelling in the more proximal portion of the tube. Histologically this swelling consists of multiple discrete lumina encased in smooth muscle. The assumption is that this process, like adenomyosis of the uterus, develops during the reproductive years (Fig. 21.19).[24] The differential diagnosis is a section at the tubal-uterine junction (cornu) and follicular salpingitis. The former will have evidence of endometrial

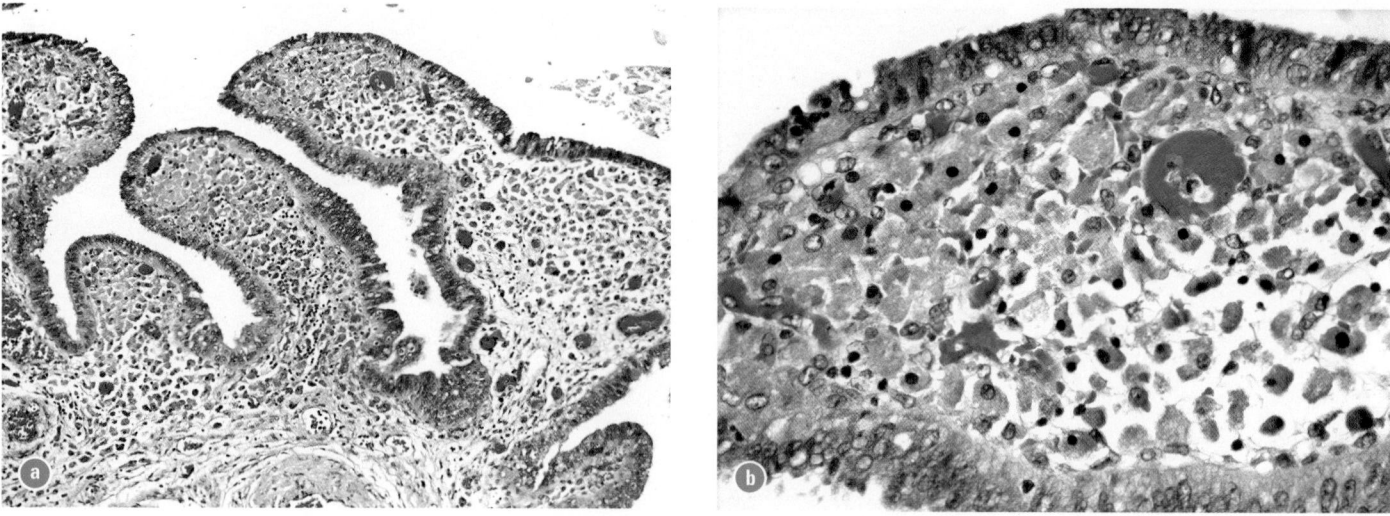

Fig. 21.15 (a) Lower-power image of pseudoxanthomatous salpingitis, with pigmented macrophages in the lamina propria. (b) At higher power the macrophages are associated with minimal inflammatory infiltrate.

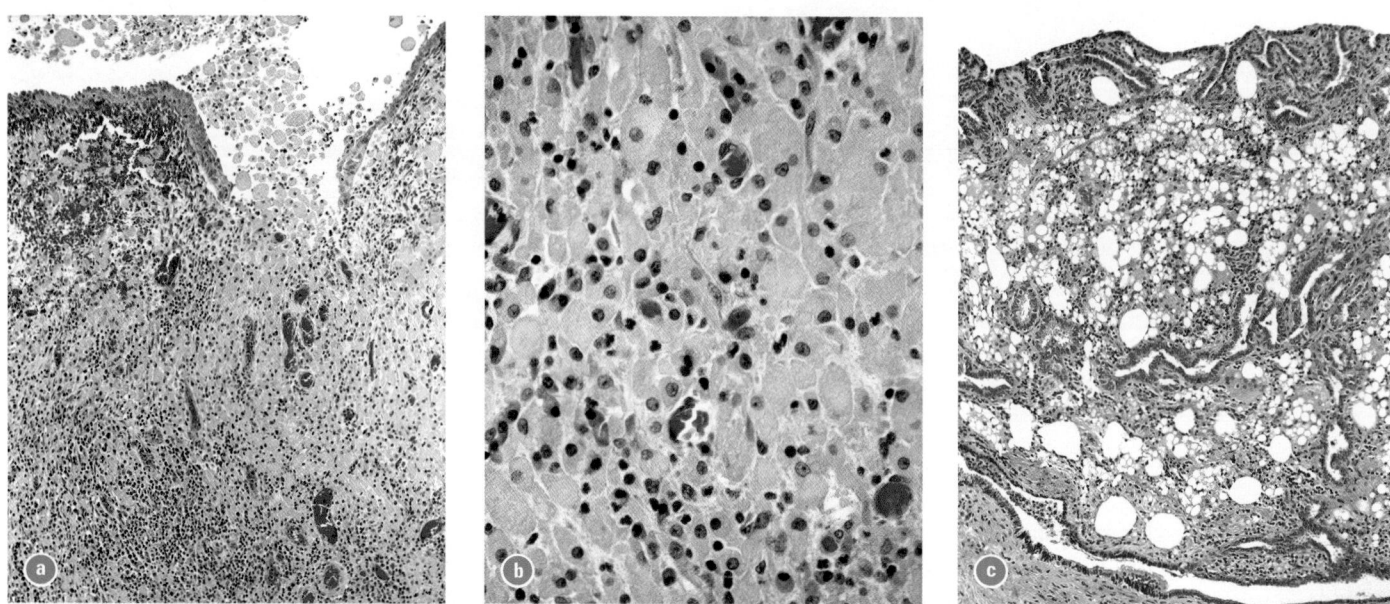

Fig. 21.16 (a) Xanthogranulomatous salpingitis. In this field, the lamina propria is consumed by inflammatory cells; foamy histiocytes are present on the luminal surface (left). (b) At higher magnification the dominant cell population is mononuclear, with scattered foamy histiocytes. (c) Granulomatous salpingitis associated with contrast (lipiodol) material, present here as microscopic spaces, signifying lipid droplets that have dissolved during processing.

stroma and myometrium. In follicular salpingitis, the tissue between the epithelial cysts consists of fibrosis rather than smooth muscle.

The most important clinical sequelae to SIN are infertility and ectopic pregnancy. The prevalence of SIN in fallopian tubes from ectopic pregnancy runs from 10% to 43%, which in some studies amounts to a 50-fold higher rate than controls.[25–27] Some studies have reported SIN to coexist with chronic salpingitis, suggesting a relationship between the two. However, because the focus in such studies is on patients with ectopic pregnancy, the relationship of these two conditions is unclear.[25–27] Others have associated inflammation with SIN, including antibodies to *Chlamydia*.[28] Because of the strong link between SIN and either infertility or ectopic pregnancy, authors recommend microsurgical approaches, which have met with success.[29]

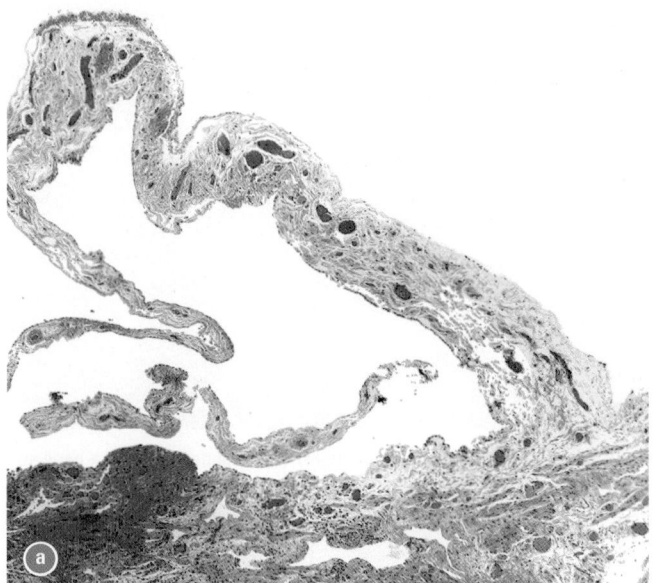

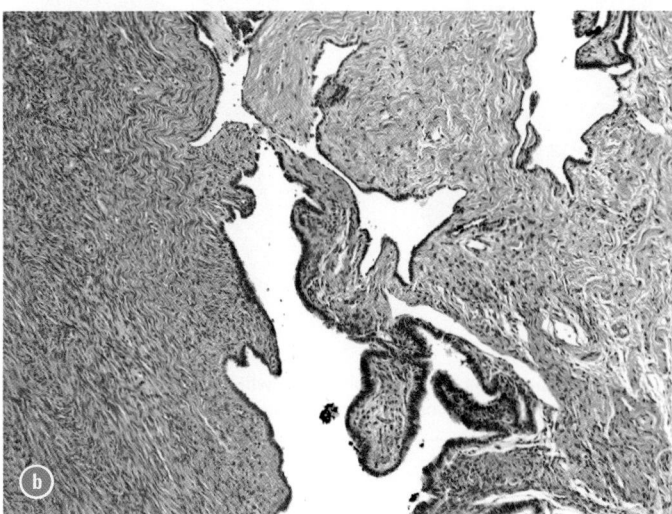

Fig. 21.17 (a) Peritubal adhesions. (b) Tubo-ovarian adhesions. The fimbria (right) are fixed to the ovarian cortex (left).

Benign epithelial proliferations of the fallopian tube

A range of benign morphologic changes can be seen in the mucosal surface of the fallopian tube. These include three distinctive lesions.

1 Papilloma of the tube. Papillomas are uncommon and are characterized by papillary architecture of the mucosa with small discrete detached papillary excrescences in the tubal lumen (Fig. 21.20a,b). These contrast in appearance with plicae, which have a much lower level of architectural complexity. Such lesions may be seen in association with pregnancy or incidental to another procedure. They are benign.[30,31]

2 Mucinous metaplasia of the tubal mucosa. This entity, like mucinous lesions elsewhere in

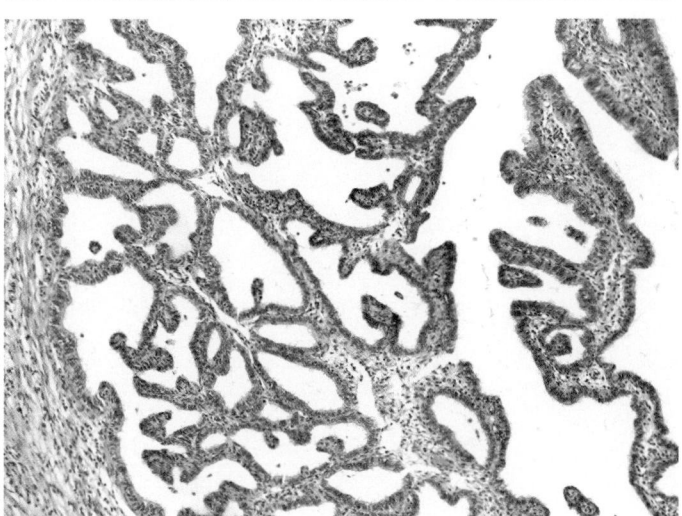

Fig. 21.18 Old follicular salpingitis is characterized by fibrous adhesions of plica with minimal residual inflammation.

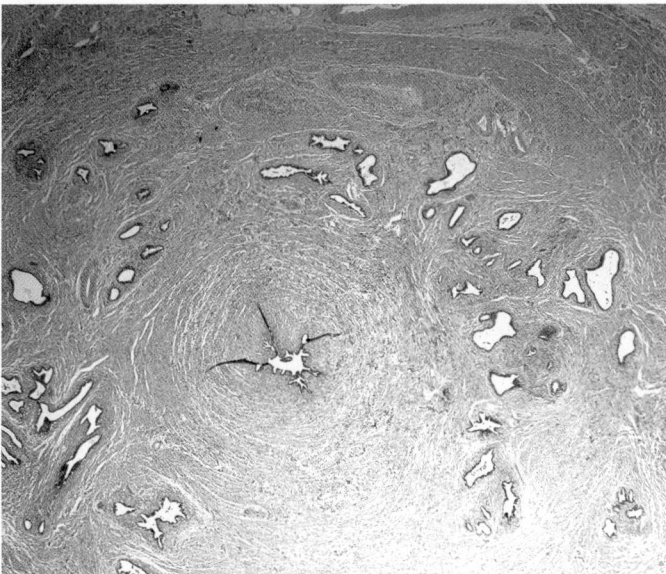

Fig. 21.19 Salpingitis isthmica nodosum. This characteristic lesion is characterized by concentrically arranged lumina in the wall of the fallopian tube, analogous to adenomyosis of the uterus.

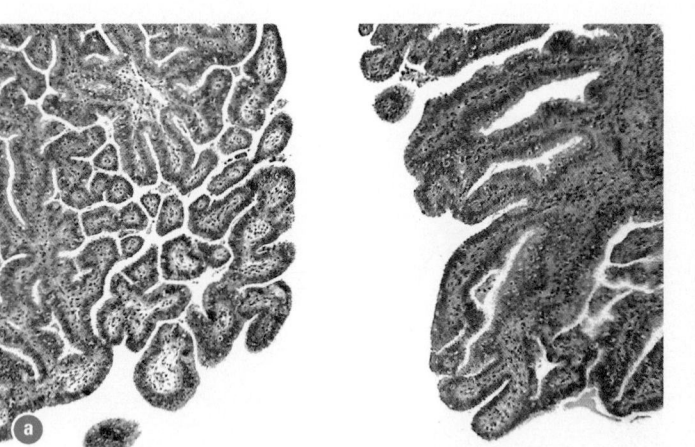
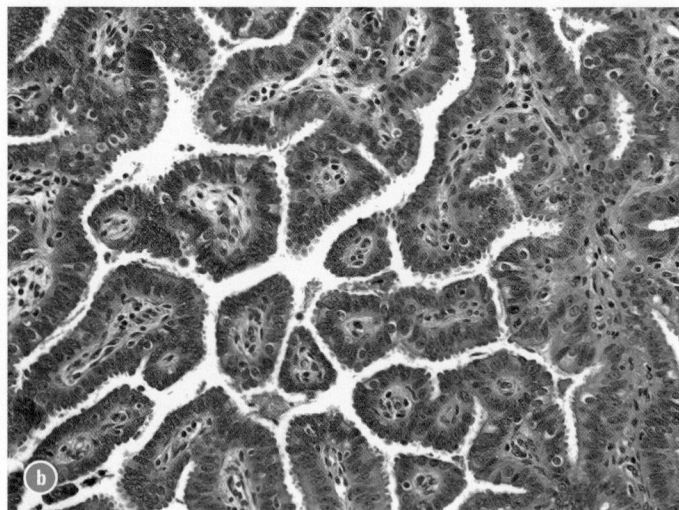

Fig. 21.20 (a) Tubal papilloma (left). The complex growth with individual free-floating papillae contrasts with the tubal plicae (right). (b) At higher power, the papillae are lined by a cuboidal, predominately secretory cells.

the female genital tract, may be associated with Peutz–Jeghers syndrome and mucinous neoplasms of the female genital tract. Some propose that the tubal disease is a manifestation of multifocal mucinous metaplasia. However, the presence of mucinous lesions in the tube should prompt a careful search for similar lesions at other sites, including ovaries (Fig. 21.21a,b).[32] In the latter case, implants from an ovarian neoplasm must be considered if an explanation for multifocal disease (such as Peutz–Jeghers syndrome) is not available.

3 Epithelial pseudoneoplasia associated with salpingitis. Acute salpingitis may be associated with florid epithelial hyperplasia, which can mimic a neoplasm. The disturbance in epithelial architecture gives the appearance of cribriform epithelial growth (Fig. 21.22a). The authors have seen instances in which this process not only disrupted the mucosal–submucosal interface but also delivered epithelium into the submucosal lymphatics with coexisting nodal deposits of benign Müllerian epithelium. However, careful

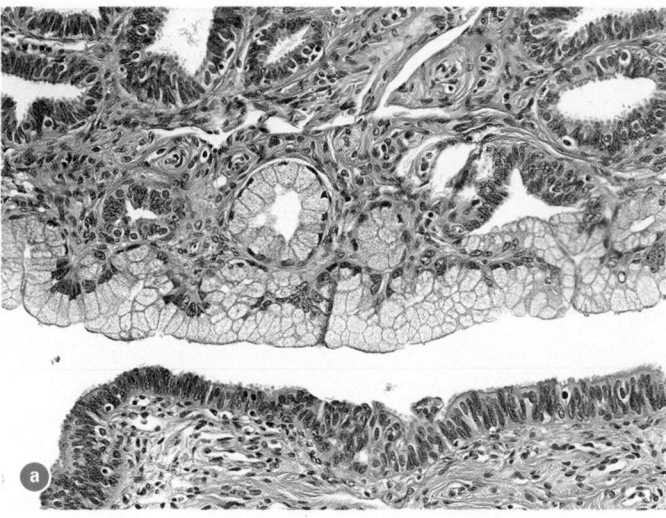
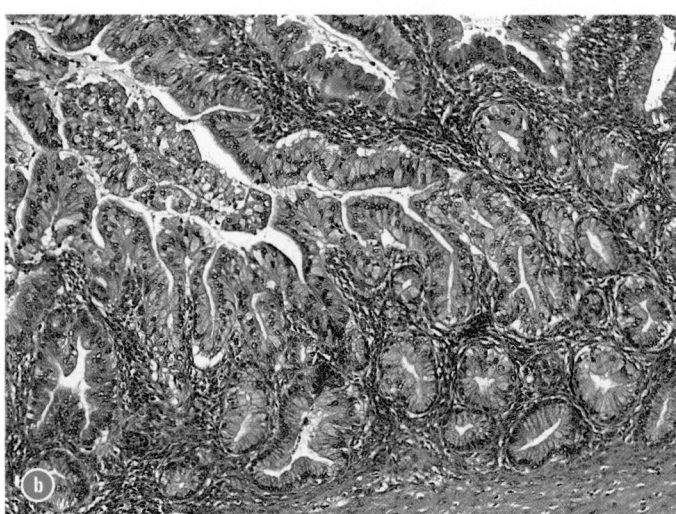

Fig. 21.21 Mucinous epithelium in the mucosa of the fallopian tube. (a) The mucinous epithelium runs in continuity with the tubal mucosa and is cytologically bland. (b) The tubal lesion was associated with an encapsulated well-differentiated mucinous cystadenocarcinoma of the ovary.

scrutiny will reveal the epithelium to be benign, albeit inflamed, in contrast to severe atypia seen with cancer (Fig. 21.22b). The young age of the patient further supports a benign process, Nonetheless, in the study by Cheung et al., some were referred with a diagnosis of carcinoma.[33] The reader is cautioned that less acute inflammatory lesions, including tuberculous salpingitis, may result in dramatic proliferations (Fig. 21.22c). Another source of epithelial complexity, albeit not proliferative, is cautery artifact (Fig. 21.22d).

Calcifications

Calcifications may occur under a variety of conditions, including posttubal ligation or infection, and may be seen as free salpingoliths (Fig. 21.23). Seidman et

al. reviewed a larger series of cases with salpingoliths and linked them to serous borderline tumors, but could not ascertain whether the tubes were the source or recipient of these structures.[34]

Infectious disorders

ACUTE AND CHRONIC INFECTIOUS SALPINGITIS

Introduction

Infectious salpingitis is defined clinically as pelvic inflammatory disease (PID). This discussion will address the form of the disease that is attributed to ascending infection by sexually transmitted pathogens or other

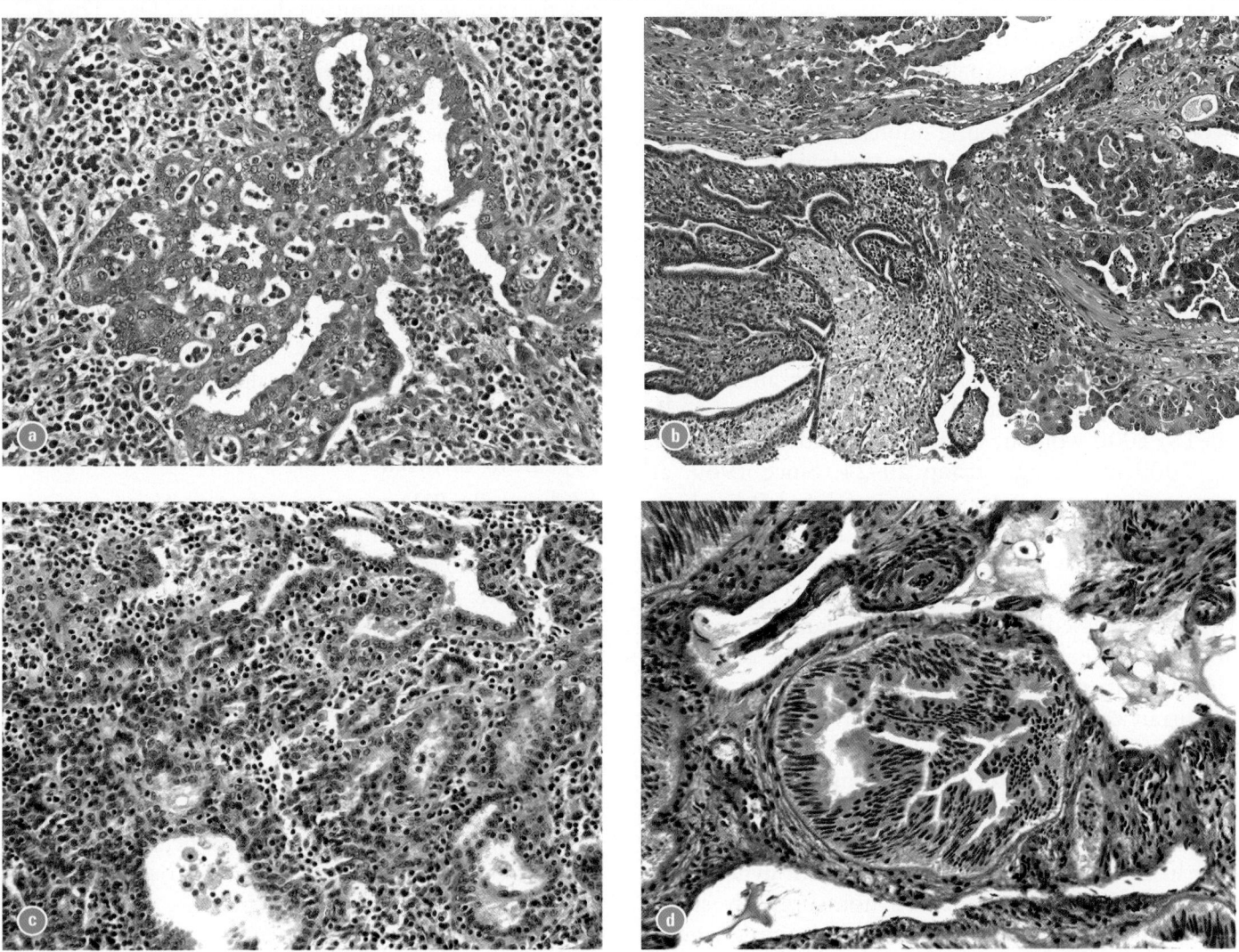

Fig. 21.22 (a) Pseudo carcinomatous change in a fallopian tube associated with acute and chronic salpingitis. (b) Early carcinoma of the fallopian tube (right) associated with salpingitis (left) for comparison. (c) Proliferative epithelial changes in the tube in tuberculosis. (d) Cautery artifact mimicking neoplasia.

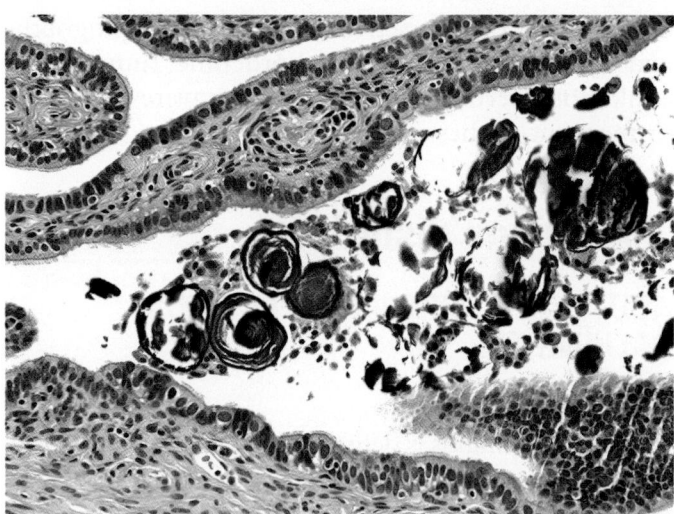

Fig. 21.23 Psammomatous calcifications of the fallopian tube associated with a borderline tumor of the ovary.

microbes harbored in the lower genital tract. The number of visits for sexually transmitted infections has been estimated at 15 million in the USA, with over two-thirds afflicting young adults.[35] Nearly 1 million women each year present with acute salpingitis, imposing a cost of over US$1 billion dollars on the healthcare system. The actual number of women with tubal inflammatory disorders may be considerably higher, due to the fact that many cases are subclinical.[36,37]

The patient at risk

In modern industrialized countries, the annual incidence of PID in women 15–39 years old seems to be 10–13/1000 women, with a peak incidence of about 20/1000 in the age group 20–24. Since 1960, an increase in incidence by a factor of 1.6–1.9 has been observed in women aged 20–29. The prevalence of women who have had PID has increased by a factor of about 1.5 since 1960. Women in this state have a 10-fold increased risk for ectopic pregnancy and 25% of the increase in ectopic pregnancy can be accounted for by the increase in post-PID women.[36]

Curran estimated the reproductive outcome for a cohort of adolescent women reaching reproductive age in 1970. By the turn of the century, there would have been one episode of salpingitis for every two women; 15% will be hospitalized for salpingitis with over half of these women requiring major gynecologic surgery; 10% will be rendered non-surgically sterile and 3% will have experienced an ectopic pregnancy.[38] Adolescent females may be more susceptible to upper genital tract infection than older women due to

possible unique biologic characteristics and sexual behaviors.[39]

At least 80–85% of cases of PID are seen in sexually active women. Risk factors for PID are linked to sexual behavior, including young age, age at first intercourse, multiple sex partners, the presence of bacterial vaginosis, vaginal douching and a history of a sexually transmitted disease.[37] Young, sexually active economically disadvantaged women are considered at greatest risk, and have been the subject of screening efforts.[40]

Two other causes of PID include instrumentation (about 15% of cases) and use of intrauterine devices for contraception (IUD).[41] Approximately 1% of women in the USA use an IUD.[42] Women who use an IUD for contraception are at least 2–4 times more likely to develop PID than non-users. This risk is largely determined by the patient population, with the lowest rates of IUD-associated PID occurring in women at lower risk for sexually transmitted diseases (STDs). The IUD is associated with an increased risk of infection in the first month after insertion. Thus, the practitioner must be certain to insert the device under aseptic conditions and exclude coexisting cervicitis. The value of prophylactic antibiotics at the time of IUD insertion is controversial.[41,43,44] Overall, the risk of infection or ectopic pregnancy (in the post-Dalkon Shield era) attributed to IUDs is considered low and outweighed by the advantages of contraception (Fig. 21.24a).[45,46]

Women who have had PID are twice as likely to develop infection as those who have never had it. Women with one episode of salpingitis run a 25% risk of a subsequent episode.[41]

Organisms involved

Traditionally, PID was been linked to *Neisseria gonorrhoeae*. This organism is sexually transmitted), beginning as an infection of the periurethral glands. Subsequently, the microbe ascends into the lumen of the fallopian tubes and infects the mucosa. Up until the late 1970s, 90% of PID was attributed to *N. gonorrhoeae*. However, by 1989, the pathogenicity of PID had become more diverse, with one-third each attributed to *N. gonorrhoeae* and *Chlamydia trachomatis*, and another third to *Mycoplasma* and *anaerobes*.[47] In particular, *Chlamydia* has attracted attention by its unpredictable symptoms.

Chlamydia is common, infecting nearly one in five under age 20. The most common risk factors for *Chlamydia*, like salpingitis in general, include more than one partner in a year, purulent cervical discharge, failure to use condoms and use of a contraceptive pill. The magnitude of this problem is considered justification for screening for *Chlamydia*, although tailoring the screening to the younger group has a higher cost–benefit ratio.[48]

One of the most problematic aspects of *Chlamydia* infection is the frequent subclinical nature of the disease. A component of this scenario is chronic infection of the fallopian tubes in the form of a 'silent' salpingitis.[49] This is due to the unique nature of *Chlamydia* infection, which includes the following: (1) the organism is intracellular; (2) the initial host inflammatory reaction, mediated by IgA, is brief; (3) chronic or recurrent infection generates a delayed hypersensitivity reaction which is intense and associate with sensitized Th1 lymphocytes; (4) progressive destruction of the mucosa ensues in the presence of few organisms, leading to tubal fibrosis. The irreversibility of this cell-mediated immune attack combined with its asymptomatic nature presents a formidable challenge to treatment and prevention.[50,51]

In recent years *Mycoplasma genitalium* (MG) has been investigated as a third important pathogen in PID. More commonly associated with non-gonococcal urethritis, MG has been associated with bacterial vaginosis, cervical and endometrial infections. Its relationship to salpingitis has been primarily serologic, but it is considered a participant in PID.[52]

Clinical presentation

PID is so difficult to diagnose that 35% of diagnoses are false positives, and perhaps 25% of asymptomatic infertility patients have subclinical *Chlamydia*. Yet the rate of PID seems constant, while STDs multiply. Reported numbers of infertile couples are also higher than ever. Whether this increased infertility is a result of tubal infections with STD organisms is not known.

PID is associated with distinct findings on computed tomography (CT) scan. Early changes include obscuration of the normal pelvic floor fascial planes, thickening of the uterosacral ligaments, and fluid accumulation in the endometrial canal, fallopian tubes and pelvis. Progression is characterized by frank tubo-ovarian or pelvic abscesses. Reactive inflammation of adjacent structures is common and can manifest as small or large bowel ileus or obstruction, hydroureter and hydronephrosis, right upper quadrant inflammation (Fitz-Hugh–Curtis syndrome) or peritonitis. While such changes are not surprising, they underscore the extent of tissue pathology generated when infectious organisms gain entry to the tubal mucosa.[53]

The principal features of PID are bilateral adnexal tenderness and leukorrhea. Other findings of importance include elevated temperature, a palpable adnexal complex, leukocytosis, elevated erythrocyte sedimentation rate and/or C-reactive protein and positive cultures for the associated organisms. Because endometritis is a surrogate for PID in this setting, endometrial biopsy may be useful. Diagnostic laparoscopy is helpful in uncertain cases.[54] Abdominal pain is the most common symptom, although the pain may be mild or even absent in at least 5% of patients with PID verified by laparoscopy.[41]

In patients who have overt PID, it is possible to establish the diagnosis with reasonable certainty by a combination of history, physical examination, Gram stain of cervical secretions, culdocentesis and examination of the sexual partner. Adequate treatment of salpingitis includes an assessment of the severity of the infection, administration of appropriate antibiotics, employment of other health measures, close patient follow-up and treatment of the sexual partner.[43]

Pathology

Gross findings

The gross findings associated with infectious salpingitis vary depending on the severity of the infection and the timing of the examination. The features of salpingitis on display follow a timeline that progresses from mucosal edema to a tube filled with exudate (pyosalpinx) followed by possible tubo-ovarian abscess, and terminating in a damaged distended terminally occluded tube (hydrosalpinx) or tubo-ovarian adhesions. In general, the earliest specimen that the pathologist will encounter is one that has been removed following an interval of disease that was poorly controlled or results in a tubo-ovarian mass. At this point in time, the acute infection has evolved into a tubo-ovarian abscess with adhesions (Fig. 21.24a,b). Older, more common presentations in tubes removed incidentally include hydrosalpinx and tubo-ovarian adhesions (Fig. 21.24c).

Histopathology

In parallel with the natural history of the disease, the histopathology of salpingitis follows a path of acute to chronic inflammation and eventually to adhesions. Typically, early in the course of the disease, the mucosa and lamina propria are involved by an acute inflammatory exudate (Fig. 21.25a). The lumen is filled with pus; hence the term 'pyosalpinx' (Fig. 21.25b). If adhesions partially or completely close the fimbriated end of the tube, the pyosalpinx is resolved and is replaced by clear fluid, termed 'hydrosalpinx'. The histologic correlate is a varied degree of plica loss, producing stretches of a smooth mucosal surface

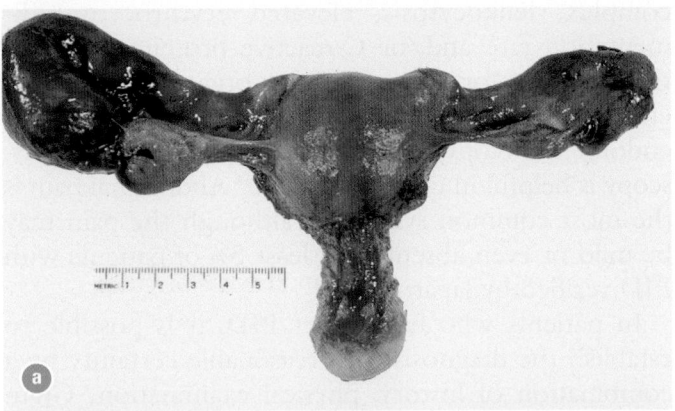

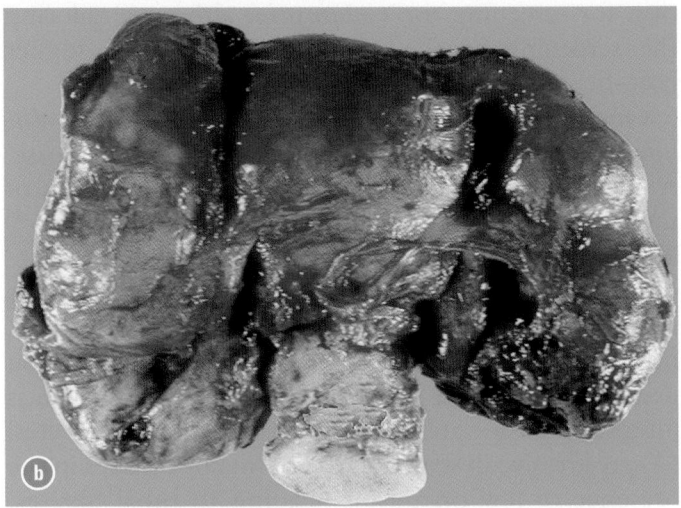

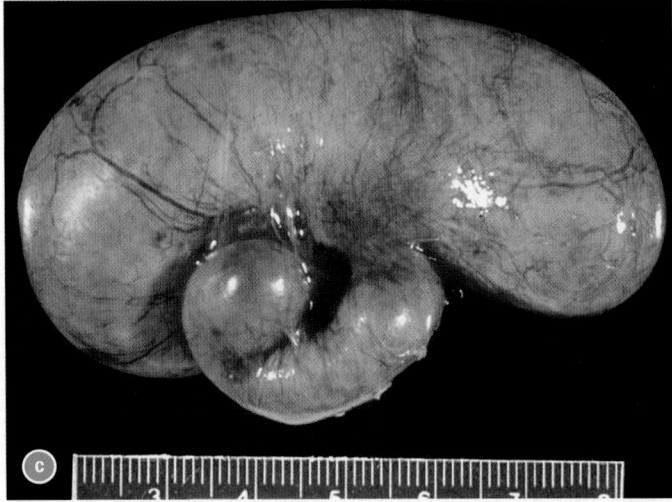

Fig. 21.24 (a) IUD-associated bilateral tubo-ovarian abscesses. (b) Gross image of tubo-ovarian abscess. (c) Hydrosalpinx.

without folds (Fig. 21.25c). A second continuum of morphologic change is formed in the lamina propria. As the infection progresses to a chronic phase and lymphocytes/plasma cells assume a greater proportion of the infiltrate, fusion of the tubal plicae becomes more conspicuous, producing the follicle-like network that is described as 'follicular salpingitis' (Fig. 21.25d).

The third component of salpingitis involves the ovary and mesosalpinx involvement. This may take the form of acute oophoritis, perioophoritis, and perisalpingitis. In the worst case, the oophoritis is suppurative, leading to tubo-ovarian abscess and terminating in extensive tubo-ovarian adhesions and obscured tubal and ovarian anatomy. Less severe infections do not extend past the serosal surfaces, leading to tubo-ovarian adhesions and preserved anatomical relationships.

Pitfalls in diagnosis

Misinterpreting infection as neoplasia: Because acute infection of the tubal mucosa results in a spectrum of destructive, reparative, proliferative and adhesive events, the tubal mucosa may appear complex. The unsuspecting pathologist may misinterpret these changes as neoplastic (Fig. 21.22). This is avoided by attention to the age (usually younger patients), coexisting changes in the tubal mucosa, the architectural regularity of the epithelial proliferation and the lack of the nuclear features of malignancy, including high nuclear/cytoplasmic ratio and coarse chromatin. Chronic infections, such as those seen with *Chlamydia* and tuberculosis, are also likely to produce this picture on occasion.

Misinterpreting neoplasia as infection: The reader is warned that, on occasion, patients with tubal or ovarian carcinoma will present with a picture of acute and chronic salpingitis. In the presence of inflammation, the tumor may not be appreciated grossly and may be missed on frozen section. Suffice it to say that neoplasia should always be included in the differential diagnosis of an elderly patient with salpingo-oophoritis (Fig. 21.22b).

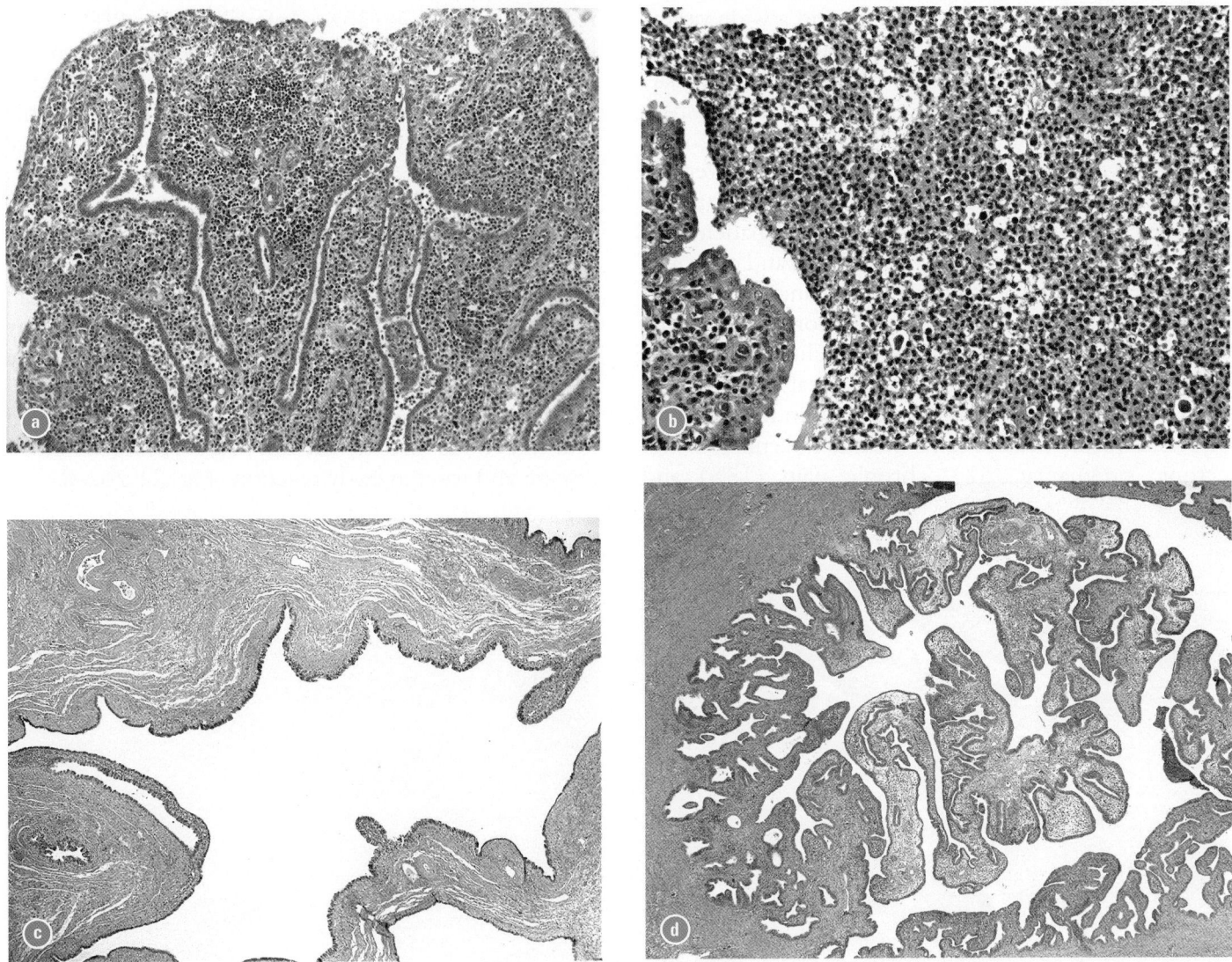

Fig. 21.25 Sequential morphologic changes in ascending infectious salpingitis, including (a) acute salpingitis, (b) pyosalpinx, (c) Hydrosalpinx, following pyosalpinx. (d) Follicular salpingitis.

Management and outcome

The greatest risks associated with acute and chronic salpingitis are infertility and ectopic pregnancy. Infertility will follow approximately one-quarter of cases of acute salpingitis.[55] Westrom correlated outcomes of tubal factor infertility (TFI) by comparing 1309 pregnancy-seeking women 35 years of age and under with laparoscopically verified acute salpingitis with 451 women with normal laparoscopy. The diagnosis of TFI was 12.1% of the patients and 0.9% of the controls, and the first pregnancy was ectopic in 7.8% and 1.3%, respectively. Both infertility and ectopic pregnancy were correlated with number of infections, severity of the infections, age and delayed treatment.[56]

Because the sequelae to infection (once established) are largely unavoidable, the most important management issue is prevention. *Chlamydia* screening programs are considered the mainstay of prevention and employ a range of diagnostic tests, including most recently ligase and polymerase chain reaction analysis of urethral or cervical samples. More recent studies have shown a similar sensitivity with first voided urine specimens, an approach that is more promising if these results are borne out.[55]

Although laparoscopy is helpful for establishing the diagnosis of salpingitis, other less-invasive tests along with selected clinical criteria are recommended. Organisms that cause infection include *N. gonorrhoeae*,

C. trachomatis, genital *Mycoplasma* and a wide variety of facultative and anaerobic bacteria. Prompt recognition and therapy are necessary to reduce the sequelae. Treatment of PID, which is empiric and broad spectrum, is oriented toward polymicrobial PID. Whenever possible, women with PID should be hospitalized for parenteral therapy. The 1989 CDC STD treatment guidelines recommend two regimens for inpatient parenteral therapy: clindamycin/gentamicin and cefoxitin, or equivalent cephalosporin/doxycycline. Outpatient management of PID should be monitored closely; the CDC-recommended regimen includes use of intramuscular cephalosporins and oral doxycycline. Oral penicillins are no longer recommended.[57]

The sequelae to salpingitis include infertility (10%), ectopic pregnancy (5%), chronic pain (15%) and recurrent infection (25%). Infertility after PID ranges between 5.8 and 60%, depending on the severity of the infection, number of infections and age of the woman. The fraction of women rendered infertile due to PID has increased by a factor of about 1.6 since 1960.[36]

GRANULOMATOUS SALPINGITIS

Granulomatous inflammation of the fallopian tube can be caused both by various infectious organisms and by noninfectious processes. Infectious agents include *Mycobacterium tuberculosis*, *Actinomyces*, *Enterobius vermicularis*, *Oxyuris* (pinworm) and *Schistosoma* and non-infectious causes include sarcoidosis, Crohn's disease and foreign body reaction (Fig. 21.26a–d).[58–61]

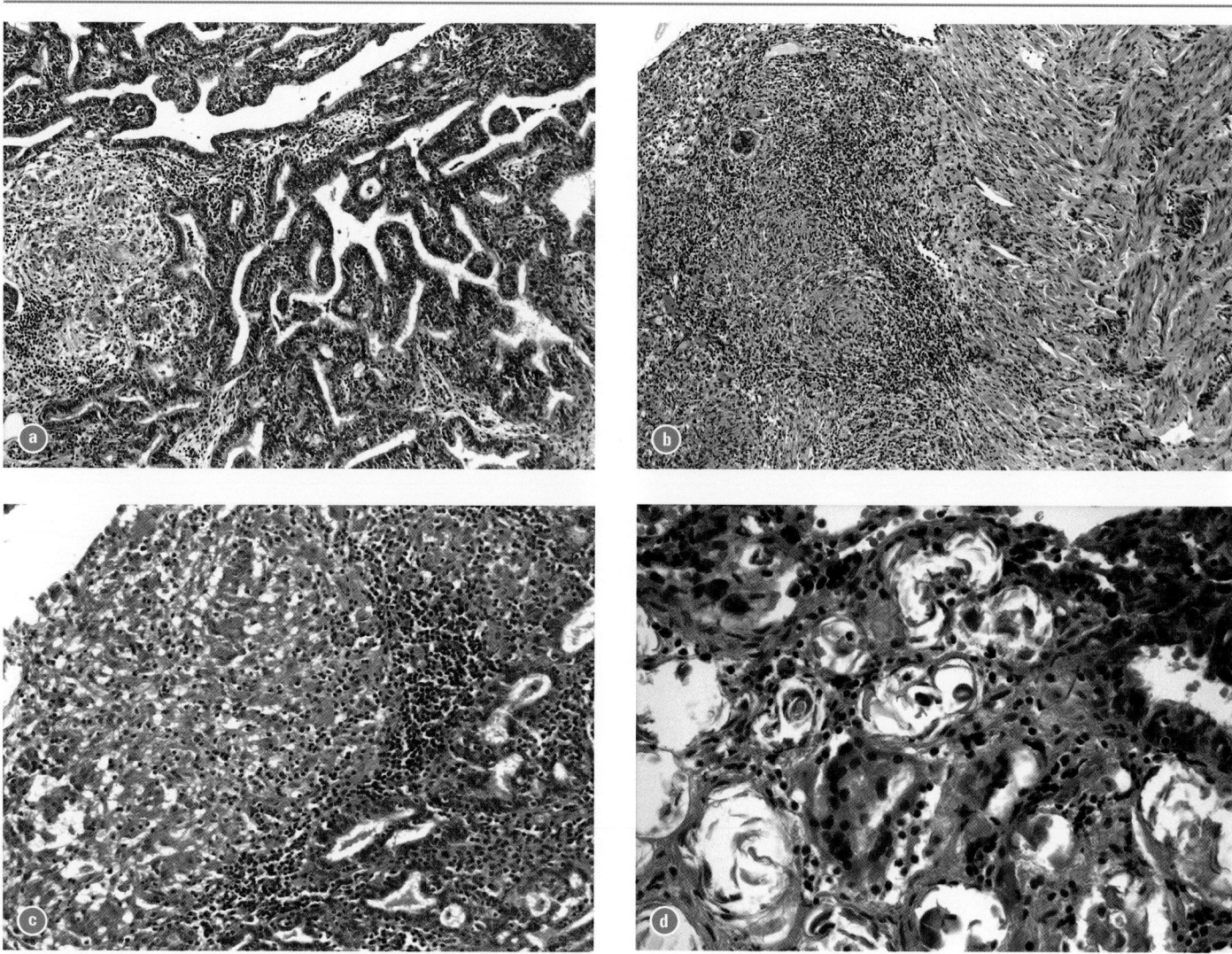

Fig. 21.26 Granulomatous salpingitis. (a, b) Granulomas in the tubal mucosa and round ligament associated with tuberculosis. (c) Granulomatous salpingitis associated with clusters of concentric calcifications (d).

Regional and systemic disorders

TORSION

Torsion of the tube interrupts the venous blood flow with subsequent infarction. Isolated tubal torsion is rare, and is usually associated with pregnancy, hydrosalpinx and ovarian cysts (Fig. 21.27a).[62-65] The characteristic histologic finding of recent torsion is marked congestion of the tubal vasculature and hemorrhagic necrosis. Older lesions will exhibit organized hemorrhage and bland necrosis, with associated serositis. The most important clinical issue is early diagnosis. The pathologist's responsibility is to exclude neoplasia, although torsion is rare in tubal cancer.

VASCULITIS

Vasculitis, in the form of giant cell arteritis (GCA) or necrotizing arteritis resembling periarteritis nodosum (PAN), has been reported in the genital tract, including the vessels in the broad ligament (Fig. 21.27b). Most cases of arteritis are incidental and do not portend a systemic disorder.[66] They occur over a wide age range and approximately half involve a single artery. In the study by Ganesan et al., 10% were associated with either systemic PAN or GCA.[66] Most are asymptomatic.[67] Rarely, vasculitis is associated with systemic disorders or symptoms.[68,69] Others have been attributed to prior surgery or antibiotic treatment.[70]

AMYLOIDOSIS

The abnormal deposition of amyloid protein can involve almost any organ in the body, including the fallopian tubes.[71] The cause of amyloidosis is unknown, but it can be associated with other systemic disease, including diabetes, chronic inflammatory conditions and malignancy, most commonly plasma cell dyscrasias (Fig. 21.28a,b).

Ectopic pregnancy

A discussion of ectopic pregnancy can be found in Chapter 32.

Benign tubal/adnexal masses

ADENOMATOID TUMOR

The most common benign tumor of the fallopian tube is the adenomatoid tumor. These neoplasms are mesothelial in origin, with some authors proposing an endothelial origin in rare tumors (Table 21.1).

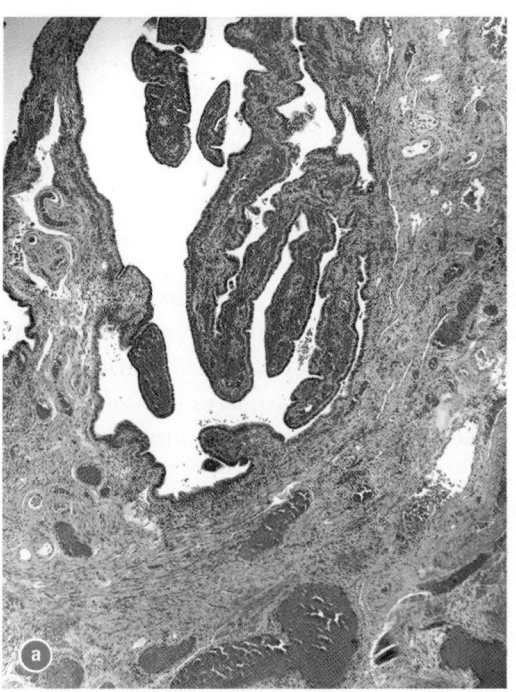
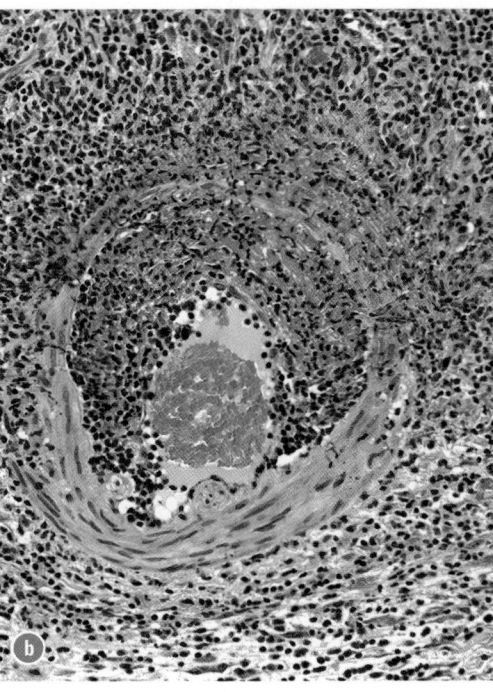

Fig. 21.27 (a) Torsion of the tube, with extensive congestion of tubal vasculature. (b). Isolated necrotizing vasculitis of adnexal artery in an otherwise asymptomatic patient.

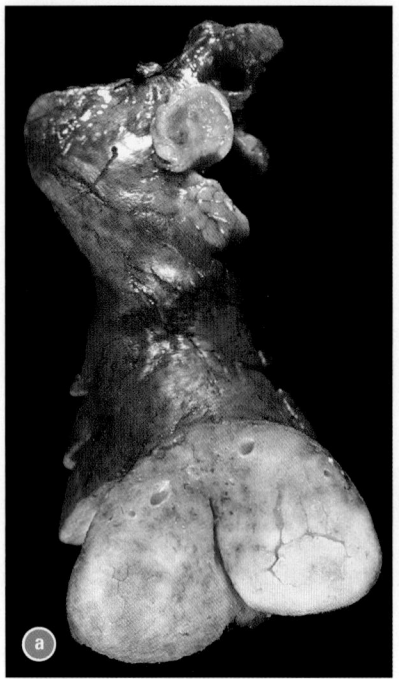
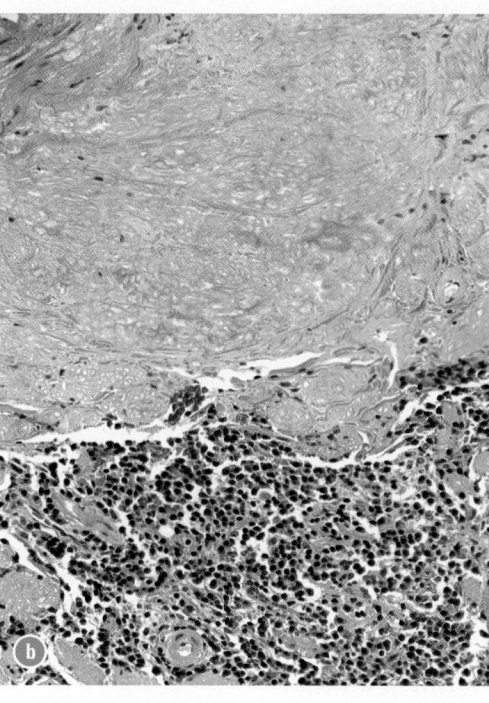

Fig. 21.28 (a) Amyloidosis of the tube, associated with a plasma cell dyscrasia, presenting with an expanded tube with a waxy appearance on sectioning (lower). (b) Histopathology of the tube in (a), revealing a dense infiltrate of plasma cells (lower) beneath amyloid deposits (upper).

The latter has been dispelled by ultrastructural studies, which have confirmed the mesothelial origin by the presence of microvilli and immunohistochemical staining for calretinin and cytokeratin rather than factor VIII.[72]

The gross appearance is that of a small, well-circumscribed nodule, usually located on the serosal surface, with a whitish cut surface. Adenomatoid tumor of the fallopian tube is similar to that of the uterus. These lesions range in size from microscopic to discrete masses in the tubal wall or mesosalpinx.

Histologically, the tumor is composed of small irregular pseudoglandular spaces lined by a single layer of cells, often with intervening smooth muscle or hyalinized stroma (Fig. 21.29). The microscopic appearance can be complex, but few mitoses or pleomorphic cells are present, and should not be mistaken for carcinoma.

The two principal mimics of adenomatoid tumor are signet-ring carcinomas and lipoleiomyoma (Fig. 21.30a,b). The former may be suspected when the tubular architecture is complex and calls to mind signet ring cells. Lipoleiomyoma should be considered if the cystic spaces are larger and resemble adipocytes.

Adenomatoid tumors rarely cause symptoms. A small number of cases undergoing infarction have been reported.[73] They can be multiple, and another was associated with an ectopic pregnancy.[74,75]

SEROUS CYSTADENOMA

Serous cystadenomas are occasionally encountered in the mesosalpinx. They are frequently unilocular and, like their counterparts in the ovary, typically exhibit a dense, collagenized wall and an epithelial lining that varies from essentially flat to focally complex. As mentioned above, these lesions must be distinguished from hydrosalpinx and hydatid of Morgagni (Fig. 21.31a).[76]

BORDERLINE SEROUS TUMORS

Rarely, *borderline serous cystadenomas* have been described in the fallopian tube.[76,77] The criteria for their diagnosis are identical to the ovary (Fig. 21.31b).

ADENOFIBROMAS

Adenofibromas (or an adenofibromatous component of a cystadenoma) consist of a mixture of epithelium with an organized fibrous stroma. These lesions range in size from microscopic foci to larger masses (Fig. 21.31c). The latter are distinctly less common.[78,79]

OTHER BENIGN TUMORS AND TUMOR-LIKE LESIONS

A wide range of extratubal tumors have been described in the broad ligament, which includes both the mesosalpinx, meso-ovarium and round ligament, and include

Table 21.1 *Classification of tumors of the fallopian tube (modified from WHO)[6]*

Benign epithelial
 Endometrioid polyp (Ch. 23)
 Papilloma
 Metaplastic papilloma

Malignant epithelial
 Carcinoma *in situ*
 Serous carcinoma
 Mucinous carcinoma
 Endometrioid carcinoma
 Clear cell carcinoma
 Transitional cell carcinoma
 Squamous carcinoma
 Glassy cell carcinoma
 Mixed carcinoma
 Undifferentiated carcinoma

Mixed epithelial/mesenchymal
 Adenofibroma
 Adenosarcoma
 Carcinosarcoma

Mesothelial
 Solitary mesothelioma (Ch. 23)
 Adenomatoid tumor

Germ cell
 Mature teratoma (incl. monodermal derivatives) (Ch. 29)
 Immature teratoma (Ch. 29)

Trophoblastic neoplasia (Ch. 32)

Metastatic tumors
 Carcinomas of the cervix, endometrium, ovary (Chs 19,27)
 Lymphoma or leukemia (Ch. 31)

Tumor-like lesions
 Atypical hyperplasia
 Endometriosis
 Salpingitis isthmica nodosa
 Tuberculous salpingitis
 Bacterial salpingitis
 Cautery artifact
 Mesothelial hyperplasia
 Ectopic pregnancy (Ch. 32)
 Malakoplakia
 Others

Malignant neoplasms

INTRODUCTION

The most common primary malignant neoplasm of the fallopian tube is adenocarcinoma. Traditionally, pathologists have viewed carcinomas involving the tube as one of three entities. The first category includes neoplasms that arise in the ovary or endometrium and metastasize to the lumen or serosa of the fallopian tube. Second are adenocarcinomas involving endometriosis. Third are primary neoplasms arising in the tubal mucosa, which invade the muscularis and eventually metastasize (Table 21.1). This pathway has traditionally been considered least common, but is being revisited. With the discovery of familial breast-ovarian cancer syndrome and increased attention to the early stage Müllerian carcinomas associated with genetic mutations, investigators have come to conclude that a distinct and possibly significant proportion of Müllerian carcinomas formerly attributed to the ovary or peritoneum originate in the tubal mucosa.[84] Both tubal or ovarian involvement may be seen early in the course of these tumors, and some authors make convincing arguments for the fallopian tube as a critical point of origin, either of the tumor itself, or the cells that give rise to tumors in the ovarian or peritoneal surfaces (Table 21.2; see Ch. 24).[84,85]

Table 21.2 *Evidence supporting the fallopian tube origin for serous carcinoma[84]*

Parameter	Evidence: for = (+); against = (−); neither = (±)
Lining epithelium	Mitotically active, hormone dependent (+)
Ovarian inclusion cysts	Tube is a recognized source (+) Not present prior to menarche (+) More commonly tubal than endometrial (+)
Peritoneal inclusions	Endosalpingiosis (+)
Hysterectomy/ salpingectomy	Reduces ovarian cancer risk (+) High incidence in ovulating hens (+)
Animal models	High frequency of preinvasive disease in the oviduct in hens with ovarian cancer (+)
Precursor lesion in humans	Controversial and yet uncharacterized (±)
Ovarian cancer	Associated with tubal cancer in 8% (±)
Genetic/familial	Associated with both BRCA1 and BRCA2 mutations(+) Associated with family history (+) Early tubal lesions are present in prophylactic salpingectomies (+)

the range of Müllerian tumors from paratubal cysts to carcinomas, as well as *lipomas* (Fig. 21.32a), *leiomyomas*, benign *teratomas*, rare *sex cord stromal tumors* and inflammatory polyps (Fig. 21.32b,c).[11,80,81]

An extremely rare cystic lesion of the fallopian tubes is termed *cystic mesothelioma* (or benign cystic mesothelioma). This is an expansile and often recurrent lesion composed of a prominent stromal component containing multiple variably sized cysts lined by plump mesothelial cells. These features, including the sheer extent of the cystic process, distinguish this entity from multiloculated cystic adhesions or simple cysts (see Ch. 23, Fig. 23.15).[80,82,83]

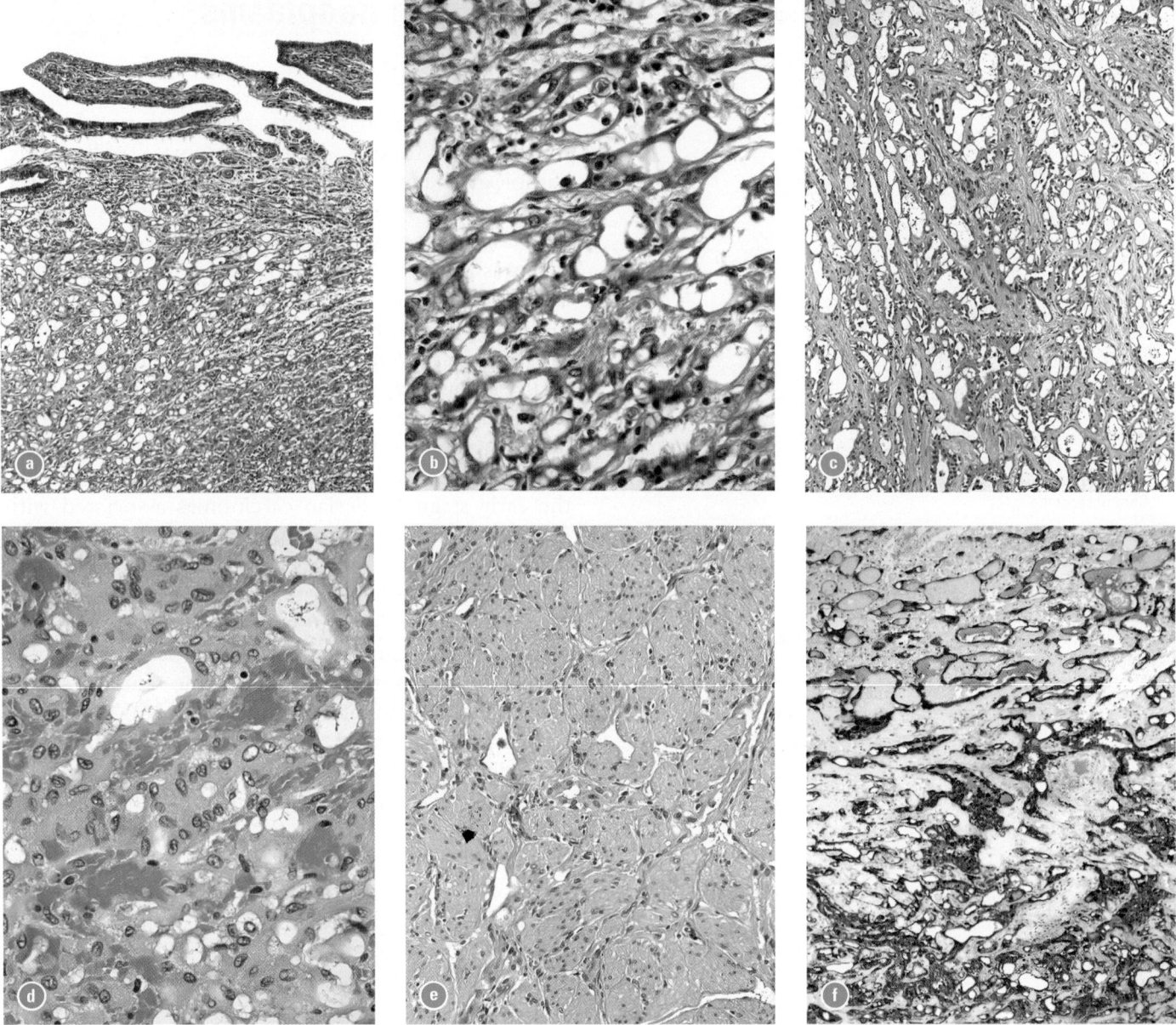

Fig. 21.29 Adenomatoid tumor. (a) At low power, this lesion abuts on the mucosa. (b) Higher power illustrates small endothelial-like spaces lined by flattened mesothelial cells. (c) Adenomatoid tumor with plump-appearing mesothelial cells. (d) Higher power of larger cells (compare with b). (e) Adenomatoid tumor with sparse spaces and predominance of smooth muscle. (f) Staining of an adenomatoid tumor for calretinin.

SCREENING WOMEN WITH BRCA MUTATIONS OR FAMILIAL OVARIAN CANCER

Prophylactic salpingo-oophorectomy is a fundamental component of ovarian cancer prevention in women with BRCA mutations or familial breast/ovarian cancer (see Chs 25 and 27). The standard approach to the prophylactic specimen has been to evaluate the entire ovarian tissue for evidence of occult malignancy.[86] However, in

recent years, a proportion of these tumors have been found in the fallopian tube mucosa, leading investigators to propose a tubal origin in some instances.[84,85] In addition, the frequent location of these early lesions in the fimbriated portion of the tube mandates a thorough examination of this organ. (Fig. 21.33a–d).

In three studies of 180 women undergoing prophylactic salpingo-oophorectomy for familial breast-ovarian cancer, 11 specimens contained occult or early carci-

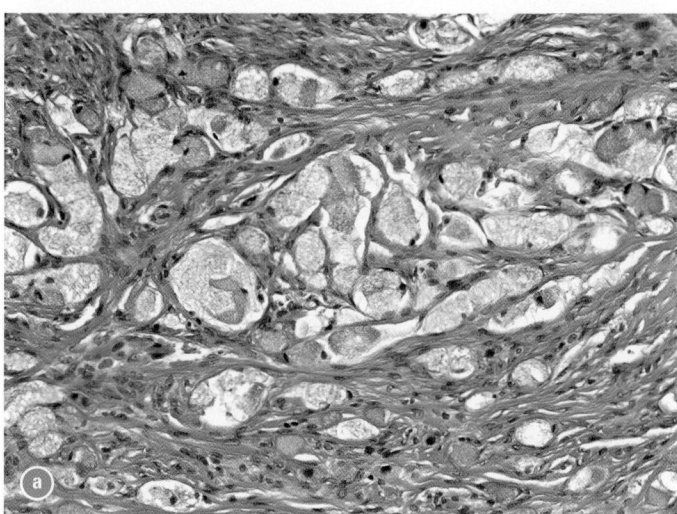

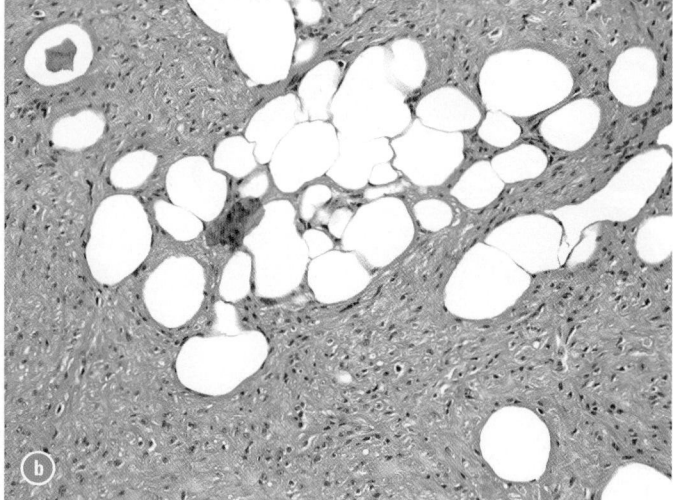

Fig. 21.30 (a) Signet-ring cell carcinoma. The cell nuclei may be inconspicuous but can be distinguished from adenomatoid tumors by the presence of mucin. (b) Lipoleiomyoma. The spaces formed by adipose tissue may be mistaken for adenomatoid tumor but can be distinguished by their characteristic appearance and surrounding smooth muscle.

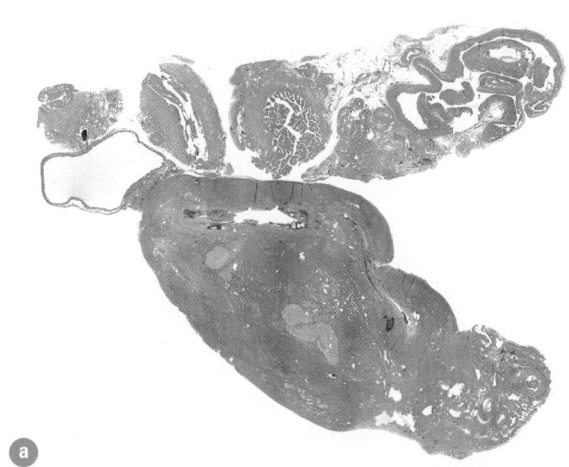

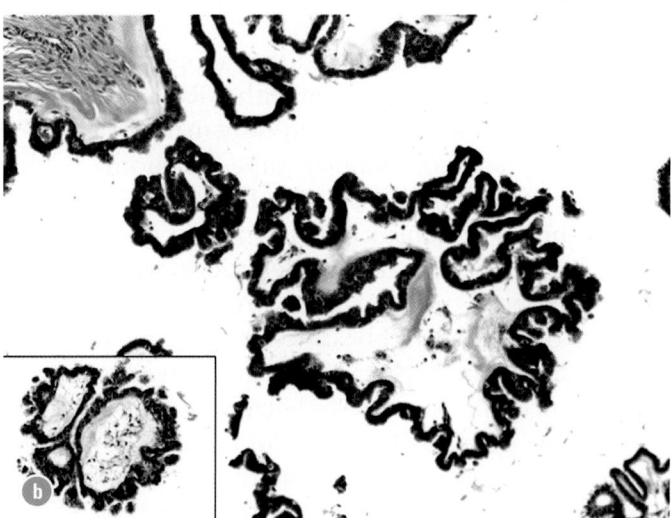

Fig. 21.31 (a) Serous cystadenoma of the paratubal soft tissue at low power. The lesion is at the upper right. A paratubal cyst is adherent to the surface of the ovary (left). (b) Paratubal serous cystadenoma with focal borderline areas (inset left). (c) Intramucosal adenofibroma.

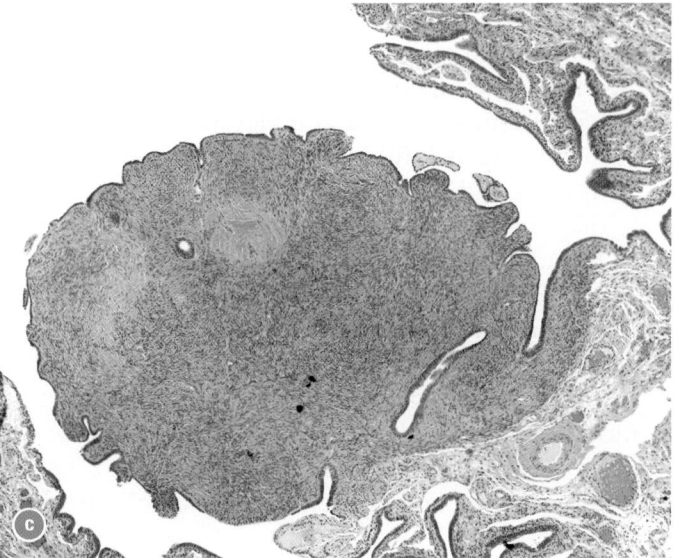

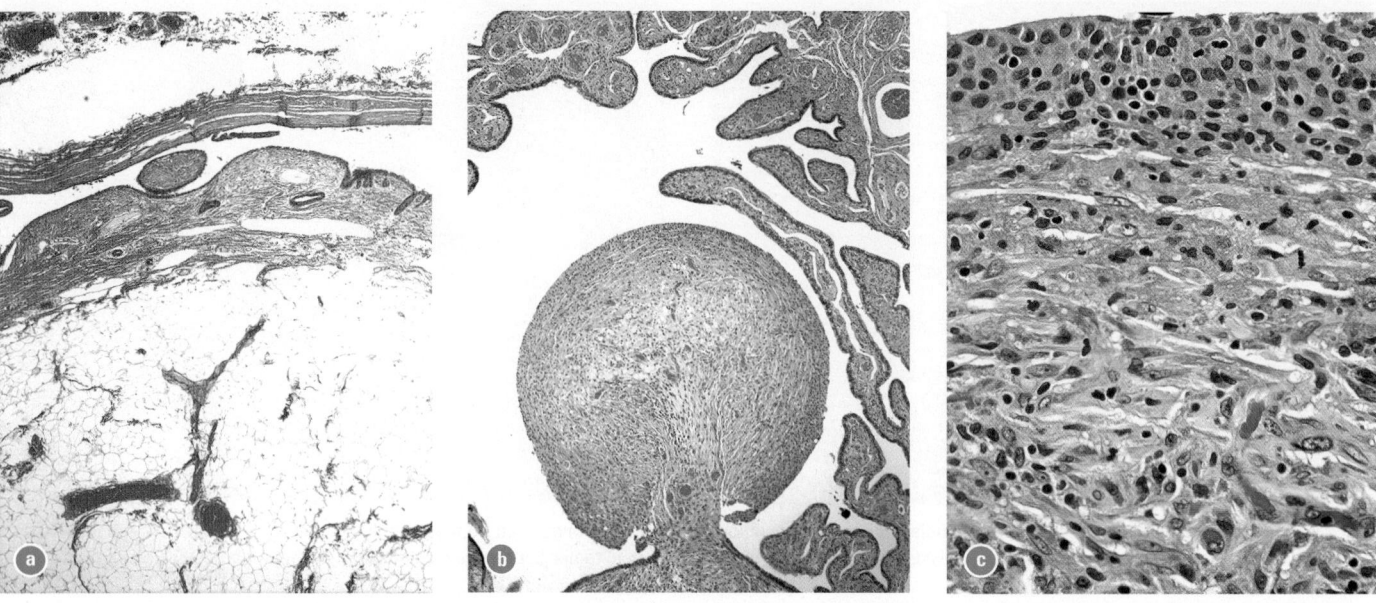

Fig. 21.32 (a) Lipoma of the fallopian tube (left) compressing the mucosa (right). (b) Inflammatory polyp arising in the luminal surface. (c) Higher power showing mixture of foamy histiocytes and young fibroblasts beneath transitional metaplasia of the surface epithelium.

noma, most of which included the fallopian tube. The rate was highest in 30 women with BRCA mutations, of which five (17%) harbored an early malignancy.[85,87,88] Despite the rarity of fallopian tube carcinoma in the general population, BRCA1 and BRCA2 mutation carriers should be considered at increased risk for tubal cancer.[88,89] In one report, 2 of 23 patients with BRCA1 mutations had tubal cancer, providing molecular evidence that fallopian tube cancer may be due to germline mutations in BRCA1. This may have important consequences for the preferred method of prophylactic oophorectomy in BRCA1 mutation carriers.[90] More detailed evaluation of the fallopian tube in these patients has increased the detection rate to as high as 17%.[91] The relatively high rates of occult malignancy in these patients support their designation as a high-risk population for both tubal and ovarian cancer, with the procedures below required following removal of these organs:

1 The fallopian tubes and ovaries should be submitted entirely and be evaluated in serial sections by a pathologist with expertise in gynecologic malignancies. At Brigham and Women's Hospital, the goal is to ensure *se*ctioning and *ex*tensive *ex*amination of the *fim*bria (SEE-FIM protocol), which is as follows:

  • The entire tube is initially fixed for at least 4 hours to minimize loss of epithelium during manipulation.
  • The distal 2 cm of the fimbriated end is transected and opened.
  • The fimbrial mucosa is sectioned longitudinally.

  • The tubal segments combined with the fully sectioned fimbriated end are submitted in toto. Recent studies show increased rates of detection (from less than 2.5 to 17%) with more thorough sectioning.[91] Thus, protocols for examining the fallopian tubes in genetically susceptible patients will continue to evolve.
  • p53 immunostaining is employed in selective cases to assist in identifying potentially abnormal epithelium. However, the diagnosis of early carcinoma must be based on histopathologic parameters. The reader is advised that both extreme caution must be exercised in interpreting epithelial atypia in the fallopian tube, and that at least, a diagnosis of early tubal carcinoma requires the presence of stratified epithelial atypia that otherwise fulfills the criteria for superficial tubal carcinoma. Diffuse p53 immunostaining and elevated proliferative indices are helpful in targeting the areas of interest and corroborating the histologic diagnosis (Fig. 21.34a–c).
  • Because a diagnosis of early tubal carcinoma in a BRCA(+) patient may provoke prophylactic chemotherapy, this diagnosis should be confirmed by a second pathologist.

2 Laparoscopy and laparotomy are the surgical modalities of choice to allow inspection of the peritoneal surfaces at time of prophylactic oophorectomy and collect fluid for cytologic evaluation.

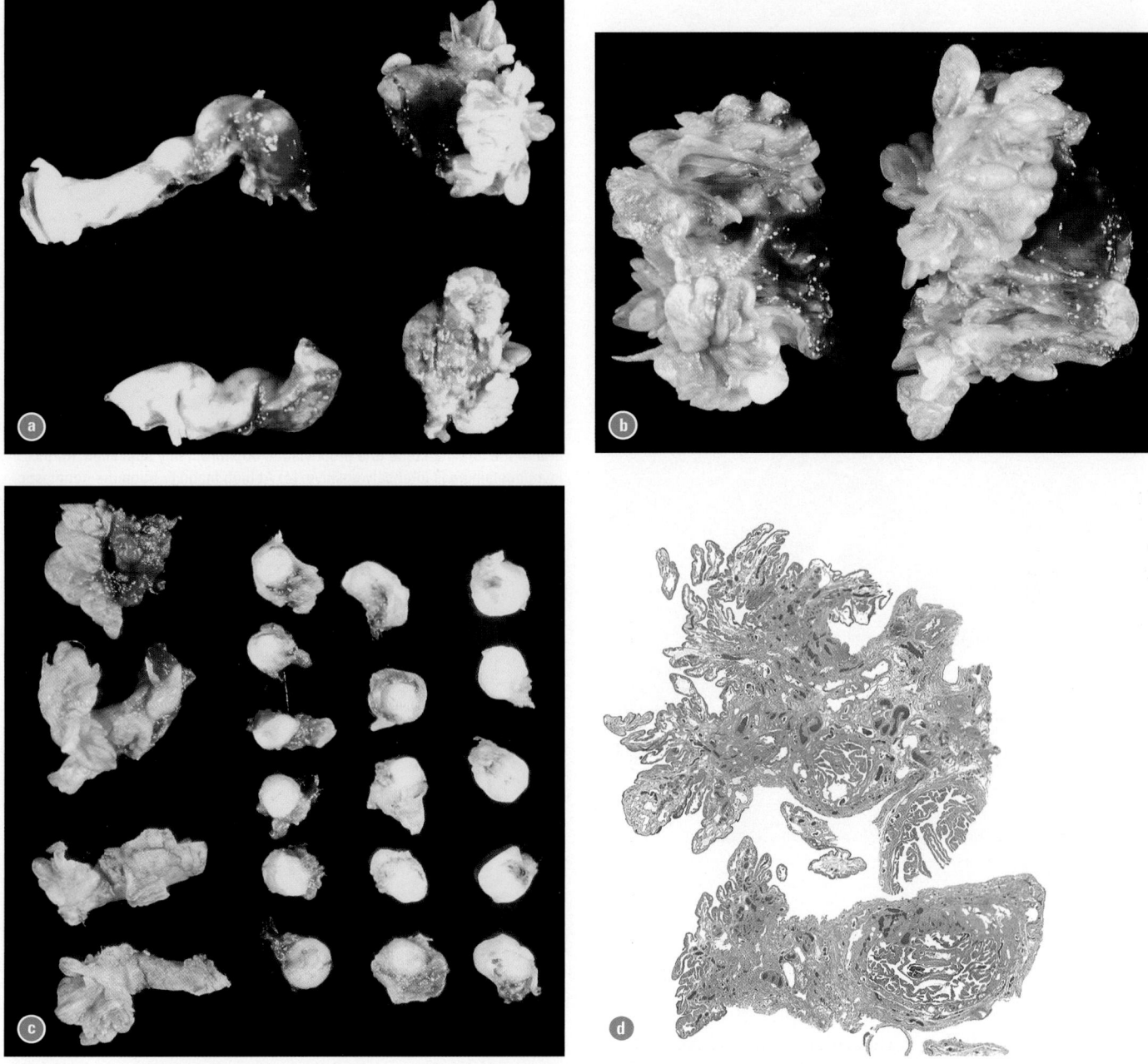

Fig. 21.33 Procedure for sectioning the entire fimbriated end (SEE-FIM protocol) in prophylactic oophorectomy specimens at Brigham and Women's Hospital. Tubes are first fixed for 4 hours, then (a) the fimbriated end is amputated, (b) open-sectioned longitudinally to expose the maximum surface area and (c) submitted in toto with the remainder of the tube sectioned at 2–3 mm intervals. (d) Low-power photomicrograph of tubal segment and fimbria.

The higher frequency of tubal cancers in prophylactic oophorectomy specimens contrasts somewhat with other studies of women with BRCA mutations. In a study of Jewish women, Levine et al. noted that 86% of those with ovarian/peritoneal disease had mutations in BRCA.[92] Conceivably, prophylactic specimens more accurately define the source of the tumor in the setting of minimal disease (favoring tube). Alternatively, the tubal disease that is found is often one of several involved sites. The role of the fallopian tube in the genesis of cancer in genetically susceptible patients will be resolved in part by more lengthy follow-up of these patients to determine if very early tubal cancer behaves as a Stage I or systemic disease.

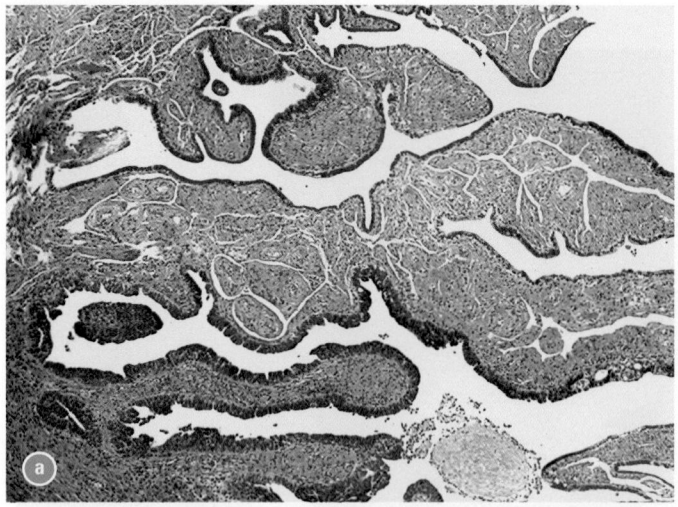

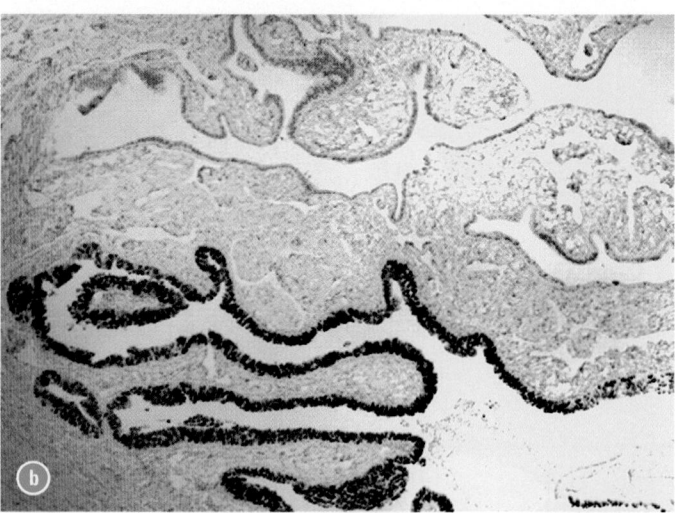

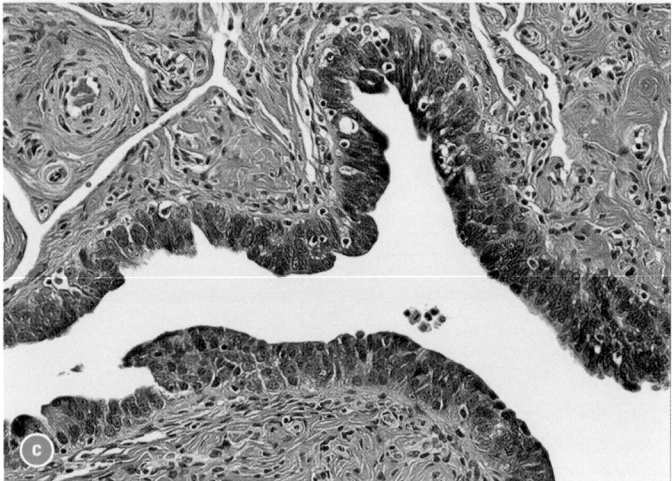

Fig. 21.34 (a) Microscopic focus of intramucosal carcinoma in the fimbriated end of the fallopian tube of a prophylactic oophorectomy specimen. (b) p53 immunostaining is intensely positive. (c) At high magnification the neoplastic epithelium is devoid of cilia and exhibits loss of cell polarity.

PRIMARY CARCINOMA OF THE TUBE

Definition

Primary adenocarcinoma of the fallopian tube is defined as a tumor that fulfills a series of criteria that maximize the odds that the tumor originated in the tube. These include: (1) evidence of origin in the tubal mucosa, ideally in the form of intramucosal carcinoma with or without invasive disease; (2) absence of a coexisting endometrial adenocarcinoma of similar histologic type; and (3) parenchymal involvement of the ovaries is of less magnitude than the tubes and, if present, is largely confined to the surface. These requirements are guidelines and are offered under the assumption that tumors originating in either the ovary or endometrium may implant on the surface of the fallopian tubes. However, the definition presupposes that if a larger tumor is present in the ovary or endometrium, it represents a primary ovarian or endometrial carci-

noma, which is impossible to prove. However, the overall prognosis of any Müllerian primary tumor is similar to others, when staging is taken into account. Thus, the above criteria are followed as much to maintain consistency in the classification and diagnosis of tubal and ovarian carcinomas as to resolve controversies over pathogenesis.

The patient at risk

Primary tubal carcinoma is rare, accounting for less than 1% of female genital tract malignancies. The average patient is postmenopausal, with a mean age of 57 years.[93] In a study of Ashkenazi Jews, BRCA mutations were identified in 5 of 29 patients with fallopian tube carcinoma (17%) and 9 of 22 patients with primary peritoneal carcinoma (41%). Those with mutations presented at a younger mean age than patients without a mutation (60 *vs* 70 years).[93] Meta-analysis revealed a mean age of presentation of 56.7 years, with a nulliparity rate of 27.5% and a mean parity of 1.7.[93] A total of 45% were nulliparous and 22% had evidence of previous pelvic inflammatory disease.[94]

Clinical features

Abnormal vaginal bleeding or discharge (40%), abdominal pain (20–39%) and a palpable mass (24%) are the most common presenting signs and symptoms.[77,93,95] Less than 5% are initially suspected preoperatively.[93] The classically described symptoms attributed to tubal carcinoma – findings of colicky pain and watery discharge followed by relief of the pain (hydrops tubae profluens) – are also uncommon and occur in less than 10%.[93] Cytologic detection is common, but is not specific for the fallopian tube. Depending on the study, the prevalence of a positive vaginal cytology ranges up to 60%.[11,96,97]

Gross examination

The classic appearance of fallopian tube carcinoma is that of a diffusely distended fallopian tube; the fimbriated end is often closed with adhesions (Fig. 21.35a). As stipulated above, the degree of ovarian involvement is low relative to the tube. Cross-sections of the tubal tumor may disclose a friable or fungating luminal mass expanding outward (Fig. 21.35b). Hemorrhage and necrosis are commonly present.

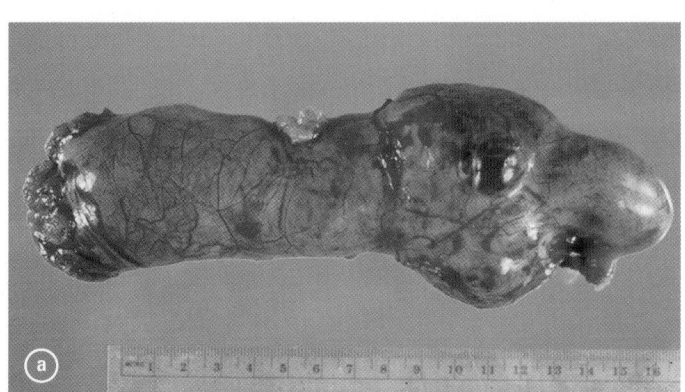

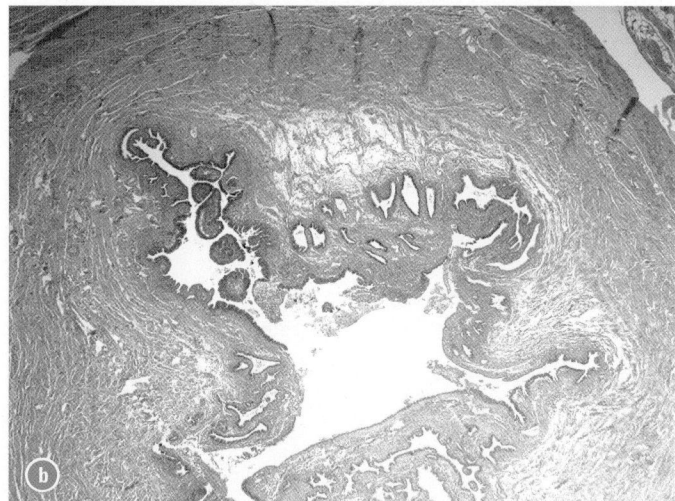

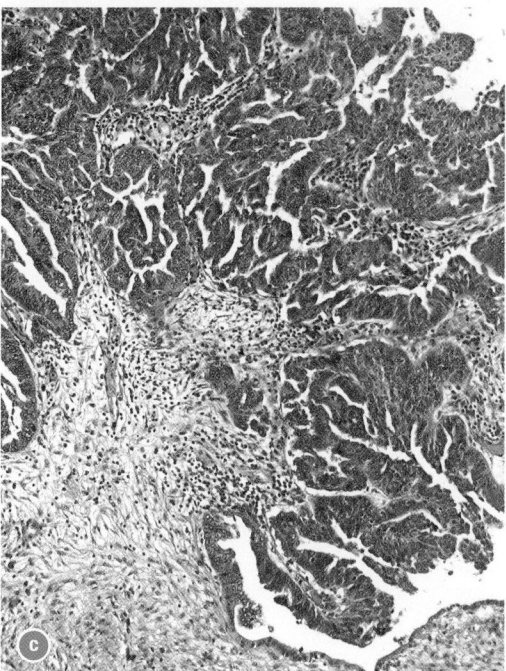

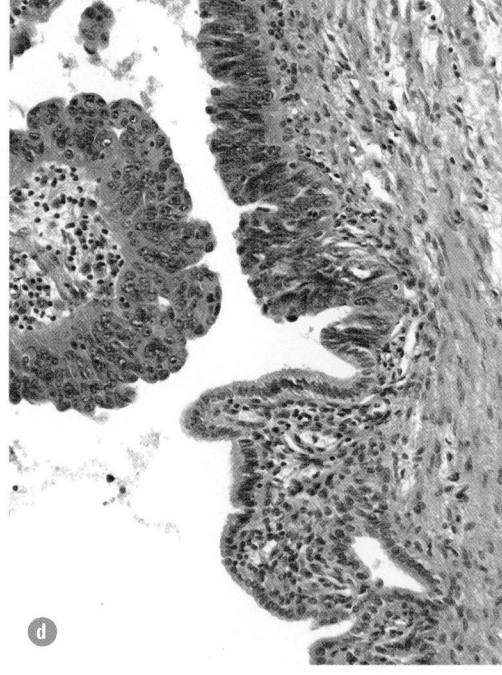

Fig. 21.35 (a) Gross appearance of primary tubal carcinoma. (b) Cross-section of tube involved by carcinoma. Microscopic features of serous tubal cancer. (c) Poorly formed papillae with slit-forming spaces. (d) Early (intraepithelial) carcinoma (upper) adjacent to normal (lower) mucosa.

Histopathology

Approximately two-thirds of primary fallopian tube carcinomas are of the serous type (Fig. 21.35c). The morphology of these tumors is similar to that in other sites, although well-differentiated tumors are underrepresented. Poorly developed papillary architecture with slit-forming lumina and high nuclear grade typify these tumors (Fig. 21.35c). Intramucosal tumor (intra-epithelial carcinoma) is frequently present and may be the only manifestation of tumor in a small number of cases (Fig. 21.35d).[11]

The remainder of tubal carcinomas are divided among endometrioid (Fig. 21.36), transitional (Fig. 21.37), clear cell and other types that are equally uncommon in other sites (Fig. 21.38a,b).[98–100] Some endometrioid tumors have been associated with endometriosis.[11] A proportion of tumors in the endometrioid category have been reported to resemble Wolffian duct tumors, containing small closely arranged uniform glands with dense colloid-like secretions (Fig. 21.38c).[101] Others contain squamous differentiation, including adeno-squamous carcinomas.[102,103]

Staging and management

Overall, a sizable percentage of tubal carcinomas are Stage I when diagnosed. The staging is summarized in Table 21.3. Some 74% were found to be in Stage IA–IIA and 26% in stage III–IV.[94] In a review by Baekelandt et al., one-third were Stage 0 or I.[104] The FIGO (International Federation of Gynecology and Obstetrics) system assigns nearly two-thirds of patients to Stage I or II and is based on surgical staging criteria similar to those for ovarian cancer.[105] However, early spread is the natural course of this disease, with two-thirds of cases with disease present beyond the tube when diagnosed.[104] Survival is summarized in Table

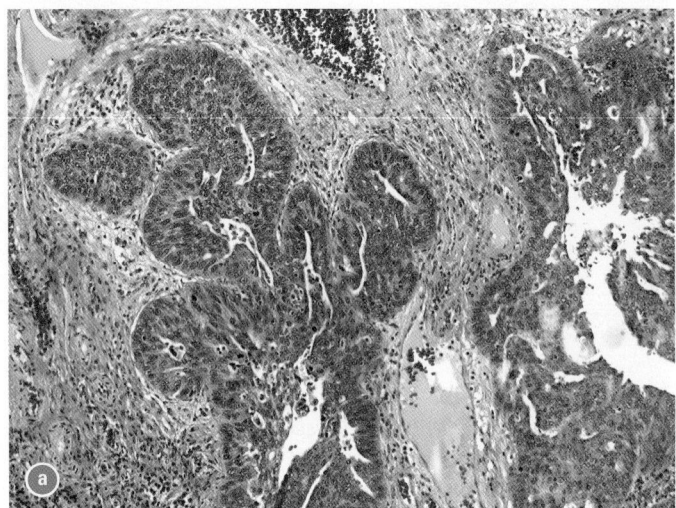

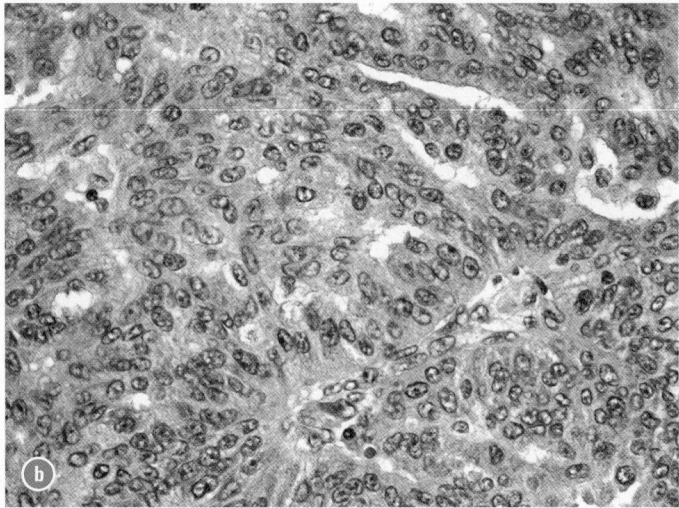

Fig. 21.36 (a) Endometrioid adenocarcinoma of the fallopian tube replacing the tubal plicae. (b) At higher power, exhibiting mild nuclear atypia and mucin droplets. (c) Implant of the tumor on the adjacent ovarian surface.

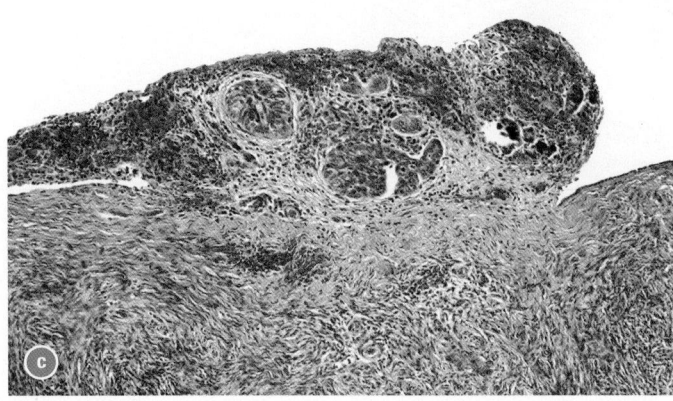

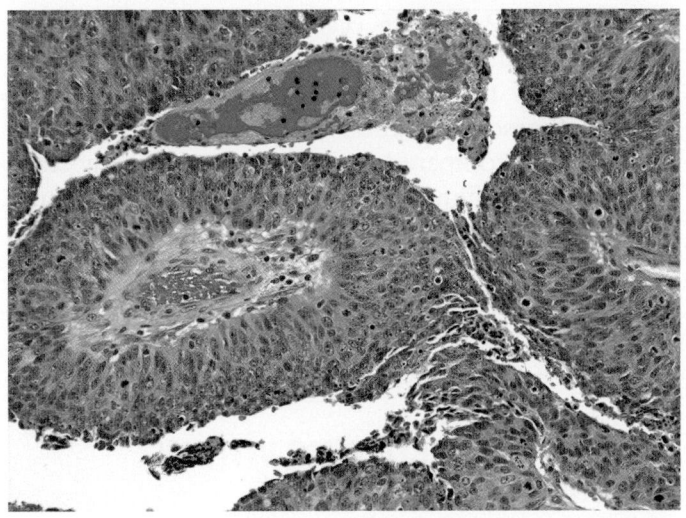

Fig. 21.37 Transitional carcinoma of the tube, with neoplastic papillae lined by stratified neoplastic epithelium. Such neoplasms exhibit a Müllerian (CK7+) rather than transitional immunophenotype and are not considered true transitional carcinomas.

21.4, is consistent across studies and drops precipitously when the tumor involves extratubal structures. Relative to Stage I (73% 5-year survival and a mean survival of 11 years), survival is halved for Stage II and halved again for Stage III/IV. Similar outcomes are seen for all tumors and those with endometrioid histology or other histologic types.[104,106,107] Presence or absence of capillary-lymphatic space invasion and histologic type were not critical variables in one study.[107] At best, tumor grade provides prognostic information of borderline significance.[94,107]

Closure of the fimbriated end has been associated with more favorable outcomes in early-stage tumors and may prevent early spread via direct seeding.[107,108] Depth of invasion and rupture of the tumor at the time of surgery are adverse prognostic indicators.[109] Older age confers an increased mortality, but is of uncertain significance as an independent prognostic indi-

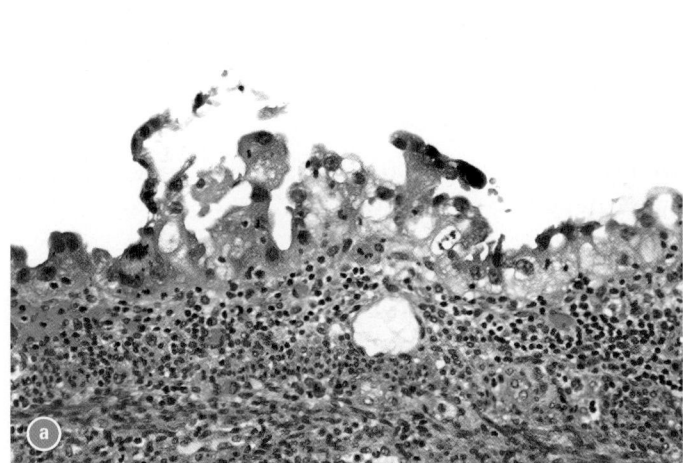

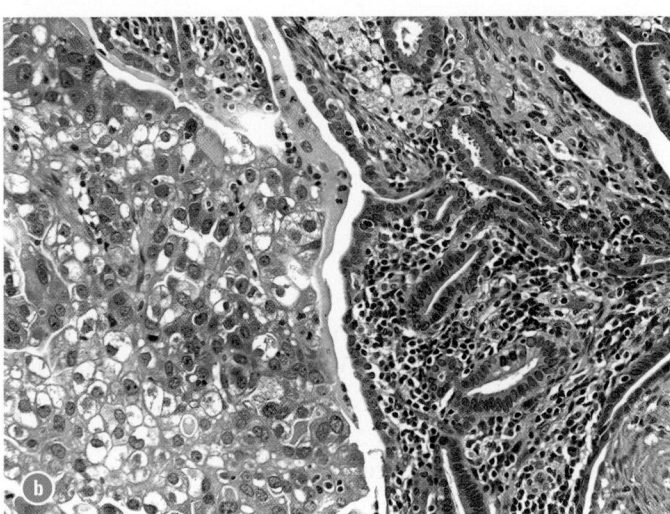

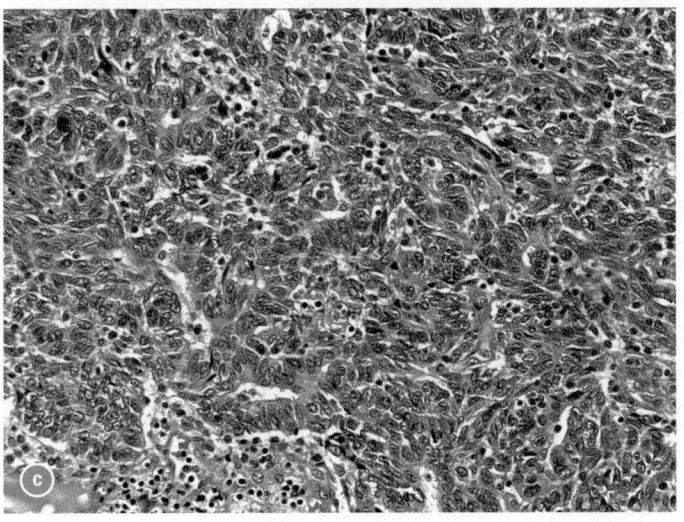

Fig. 21.38 (a) Clear cell carcinoma involving the surface of the endometrium and (b) involving the lumen of the fallopian tube. (c) Endometrioid adenocarcinoma resembling female adnexal tumor of Wolffian origin (FATWO) (photographed from a slide courtesy of Dr Dean Daya) (see Fig. 21.42).

Table 21.3 *Staging of carcinomas of the fallopian tube (FIGO 1994)*[105]

Stage I	Carcinoma confined to fallopian tube(s)
IA	Growth limited to one tube with sparing of the serosal surface, no ascites
IB	Growth limited to both tubes with sparing of the serosa, no ascites
IC	Either IA or IB with serosal involvement or ascites or positive washings
Stage II	Tumor also involves pelvic structures
IIA	Involvement of uterus and/or ovary
IIB	Involvement of other pelvic organs
IIC	Coexisting ascites and/or positive peritoneal washings
Stage III	Carcinoma extends beyond pelvis but remains within the abdominal cavity
IIIA	Histologic confirmation of abdominal involvement only
IIIB	Tumor less than or equal to 2 cm
IIIC	Tumor exceeds 2 cm
Stage IV	Carcinoma extends beyond abdominal cavity, including cytologically positive pleural fluid; parenchymal liver metastases

Table 21.4 *Staging versus survival for fallopian tube carcinoma*[1,104]

Stage	No.	5-year survival (%)
0	8	87.5
1	41	73
2	33	37
3	52	29
4	17	12

cator.[94,107,110] The management of fallopian tube carcinoma is similar to that of ovarian carcinoma, requiring total abdominal hysterectomy, bilateral salpingo-oophorectomy, nodal sampling and aggressive debulking of residual tumor, followed by platinum-based combination chemotherapy. Stage I patients with high-risk disease (poorly-differentiated tumors, capillary-lymphatic space invasion, invasion of the muscularis or subserosa) or unstaged patients may be managed by single-agent chemotherapy. Higher stages require paclitaxel plus carboplatin-based chemotherapy.[111] Patients receiving chemotherapy had superior survival rates compared with those without chemotherapy ($P = 0.0006$) and patients with cisplatin-containing chemotherapy did better than those without cisplatin.[111]

Median follow-up was 70.3 months and the median overall survival was 68.1 months. Surgical Stage I disease ($P = 0.02$) and the absence of residual tumor after operation ($P = 0.03$) were the only factors associated with improved survival. Some 20 of the 36 patients (55%) presented with Stage I disease and

survival was 62.7% at 5 years. No patient with postoperative residual tumor survived. The majority of the patients with fallopian tube carcinoma present with Stage I disease at diagnosis, but their survival probability is low compared with that of other early-stage gynecologic malignancies. If primary surgical debulking cannot achieve macroscopic tumor clearance, the chance of survival is extremely low.[95] Five-year survival for patients with disease confined to the tube at diagnosis (Stage I) is 60–73% and only 10% of patients with advanced disease will be cured.[1,104,105]

CARCINOMA OCCURRING WITHIN ENDOMETRIOSIS

Similar to that seen in other pelvic sites, carcinomas can arise from endometriosis in the fallopian tube (see Chs 23 and 27). Endometrial adenocarcinoma is the most common malignancy arising from endometriosis, but carcinosarcoma, endometrial stromal sarcoma, sex cord tumors and other tumors have been reported (Fig. 21.41a–c).[112–115] Benign and borderline neoplasms arising from endometriosis have also been described.

METASTATIC NEOPLASIA

Metastatic carcinoma to the fallopian tube falls into two categories, as follows:

Müllerian sites

Because of the restrictions imposed on second primaries by classification system and morphologic

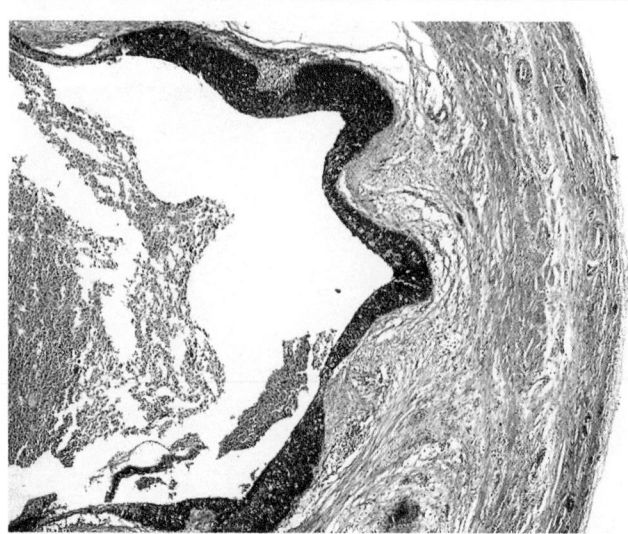

Fig. 21.39 Transgenital tract extension of a cervical intraepithelial neoplasm, including replacement of the tubal lumen.[120]

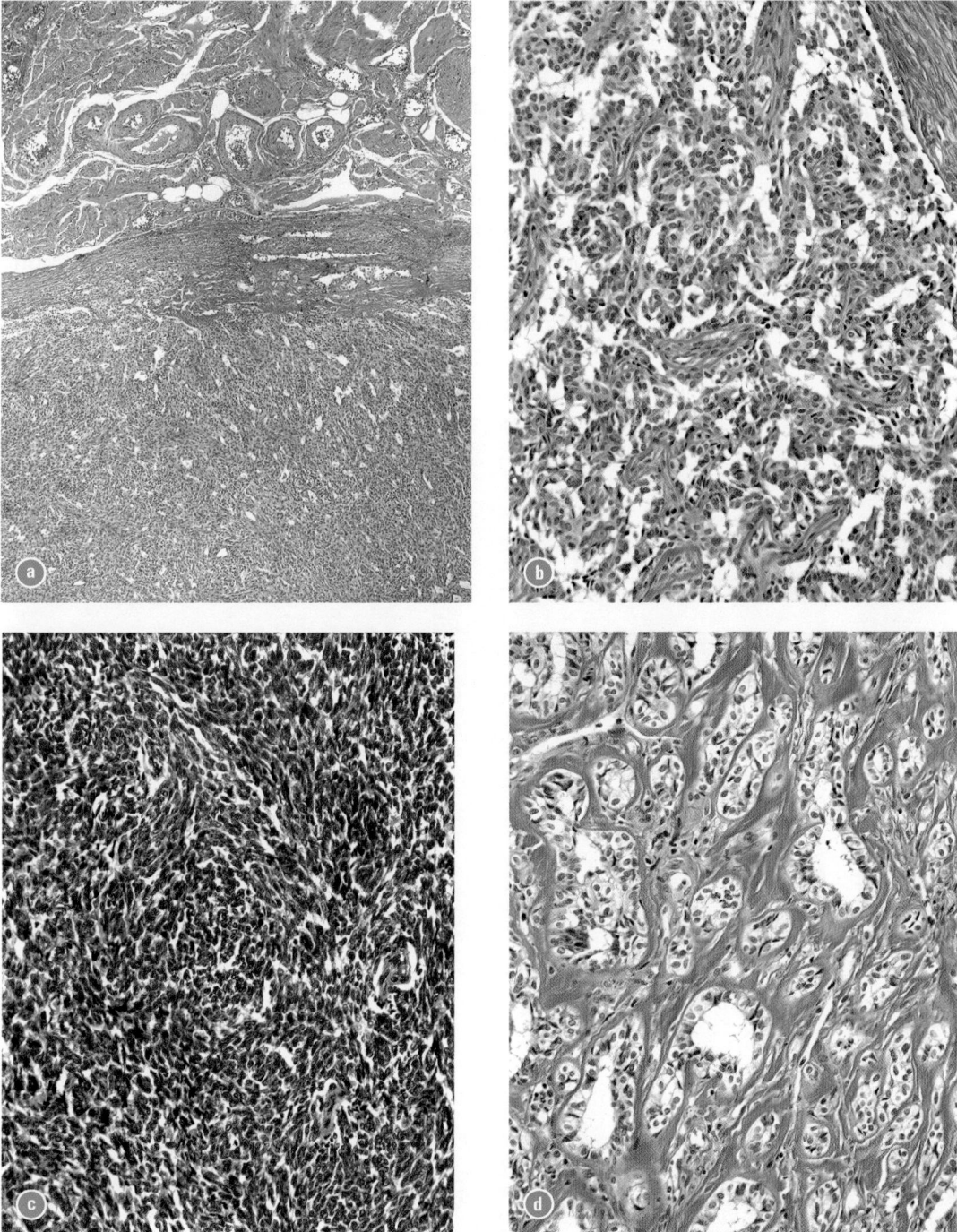

Fig. 21.40 Female adnexal tumor of Wolffian origin (FATWO). (a) The tumor exhibits a uniform interface with the adnexal soft tissue; (b) irregular cleft-like spaces; (c) solid growth with mesenchymal (spindle cell) morphology; and (d) tubules similar to those seen in other mesonephric neoplasms of the genital tract.

similarities between tubal, ovarian and peritoneal cancers, the percentage of fallopian tumors classified as separate primaries is low.[116,117] Tubal washings are not considered prognostically significant.[118] Stage III endometrial carcinomas involving the tube have a better than 80% survival.[119] Rarely, cervical carcinomas can extend into the fallopian tube (Fig. 21.39).[120]

Non-Müllerian sites

Virtually any tumor can metastasize to the fallopian tube, including gastrointestinal tract and breast carcinomas, and rarely, hematopoietic neoplasms and sarcomas (Fig 21.42).[11,121]

TUMORS OF WOLFFIAN ORIGIN (FATWO)

These tumors are rare, and are presumed to originate in the mesonephric remnants in the round ligament. They are characteristically unilateral, variable in size and present as expansile homogeneous tumors suspended in the broad ligament. The cut surface is pale yellow, solid in appearance and rubbery to palpation but may contain small cysts. Microscopically, FATWOs exhibit differentiation analogous to mesonephric tumors of the cervix, which can range from solid with spindled cells to various degrees of tubule formation (Fig. 21.40a–c). Staining for calretinin, cytokeratin and vimentin should be positive, and epithelial membrane antigen and CEA are negative.[11] Glutathione S-transferase mu (GST mu) can distinguish these tumors from Müllerian epithelium.[122–124] Like other mesonephric tumors, FATWOs should be considered low-grade malignancies and monitored closely after removal.[125]

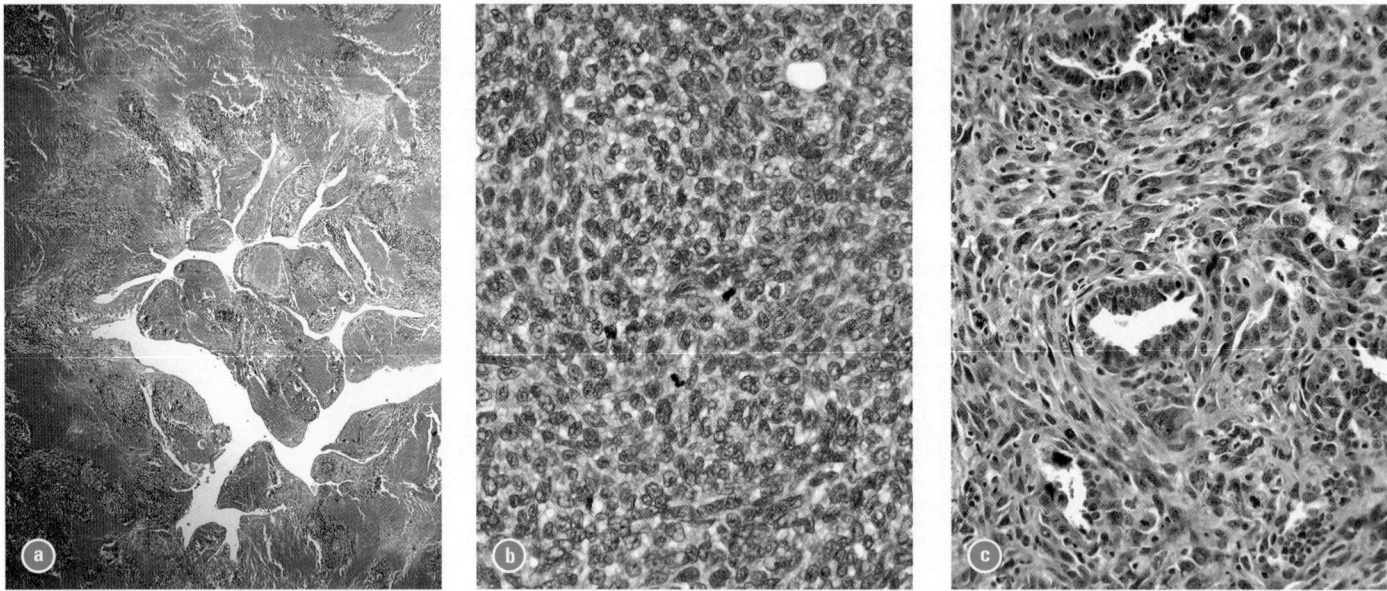

Fig. 21.41 (a) Sarcoma arising in the fallopian tube. The outline of the lumen architecture is partially preserved. (b) At higher power. (c) Carcinosarcoma of the tube.

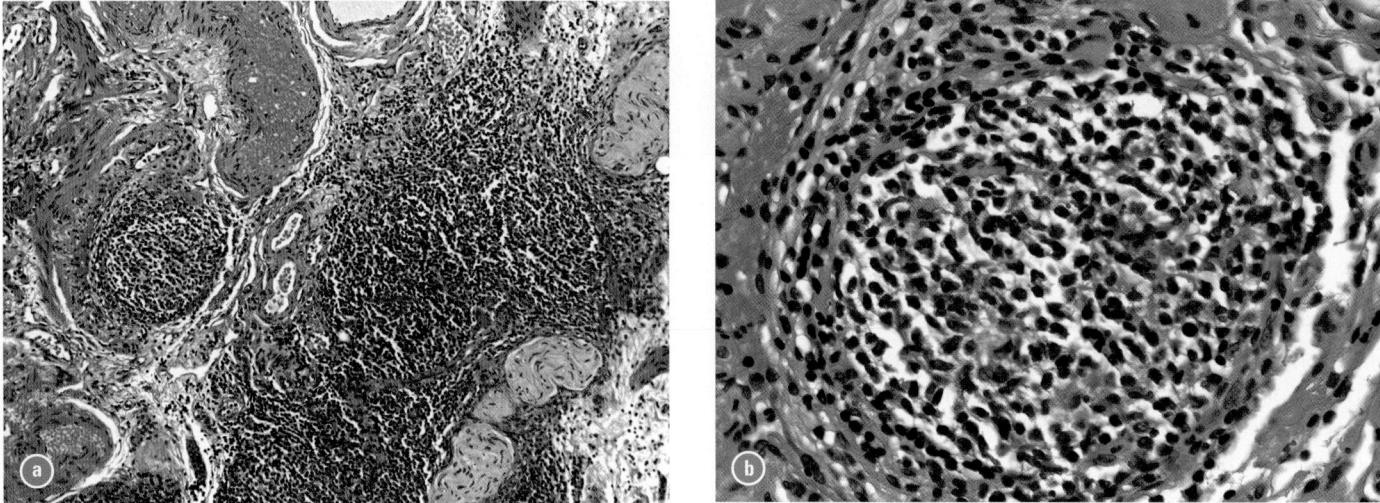

Fig. 21.42 (a) Lymphoma involving the fallopian tube. (b) At higher magnification, germinal centers are not present.

References

1 Wheeler JE. Diseases of the fallopian tube. In: Kurman R, ed. Blaustein's pathology of the female genital tract. New York Springer; 2001.

2 Carcangiu ML, Radice P, Manoukian S, et al. Atypical epithelial proliferation in fallopian tubes in prophylactic salpingo-oophorectomy specimens from BRCA1 and BRCA2 germline mutation carriers. Int J Gynecol Pathol 2004; 23(1):35–40.

3 Piek JM, van Diest PJ, Zweemer RP, et al. Dysplastic changes in prophylactically removed fallopian tubes of women predisposed to developing ovarian cancer. J Pathol 2001; 195(4):451–456.

4 Yanai-Inbar I, Siriaunkgul S, Silverberg SG. Mucosal epithelial proliferation of the fallopian tube: a particular association with ovarian serous tumor of low malignant potential? Int J Gynecol Pathol 1995; 14(2):107–113.

5 Burkman RT. Contraceptive sterilization: trends, options, and surprising new data. Dialogues Contracept 1997; 5(2):5–7.

6 Newton J, McCormack J. Female sterilization: a review of methods, morbidity, failure rates and medicolegal aspects. Contemp Rev Obstet Gynaecol 1990; 2(3):176–182.

7 Mills SE, Fechner RE. Stromal and epithelial changes in the fallopian tube following hormonal therapy. Hum Pathol 1980; 11(5 Suppl):583–585.

8 Cornog JL, Currie JL, Rubin A. Heat artifact simulating adenocarcinoma of fallopian tube. JAMA 1970; 214(6): 1118–1119.

9 Kim SH, Shin CJ, Kim JG, et al. Microsurgical reversal of tubal sterilization: a report on 1,118 cases. Fertil Steril 1997; 68(5):865–870.

10 Samaha M, Woodruff JD. Paratubal cysts: frequency, histogenesis, and associated clinical features. Obstet Gynecol 1985; 65(5):691–694.

11 Scully RE, Young RH, Clement PB. Atlas of tumor pathology, 3rd series, Fascicle 23: tumors of the ovary, maldeveloped gonads, fallopian tube and broad ligament. American Registry of Pathology, Washington DC: AFIP; 1996:169–238.

12 Smith S, Pfeifer SM, Collins JA. Diagnosis and management of female infertility. JAMA 2003; 290(13): 1767–1770.

13 Adamson GD, Baker VL Subfertility: causes, treatment and outcome. Best Pract Res Clin Obstet Gynaecol 2003; 17(2):169–185.

14 Hickman TN. Impact of endometriosis on implantation. Data from the Wilford Hall Medical Center IVF-ET Program. J Reprod Med 2002; 47(10):801–808.

15 Lyons RA, Djahanbakhch O, Saridogan E, et al. Peritoneal fluid, endometriosis, and ciliary beat frequency in the human fallopian tube. Lancet 2002; 360(9341):1221–1222.

16 Fujishita A, Khan KN, Masuzaki H, Ishimaru T. Influence of pelvic endometriosis and ovarian endometrioma on fertility. Gynecol Obstet Invest 2002; 53 (Suppl 1):40–45.

17 Corson SL, Cheng A, Gutmann JN. Laparoscopy in the 'normal' infertile patient: a question revisited. J Am Assoc Gynecol Laparosc 2000; 7(3):317–324.

18 Furuya M, Murakami T, Sato O, et al. Pseudoxanthomatous and xanthogranulomatous salpingitis of the fallopian tube: a report of four cases and a literature review Int J Gynecol Pathol 2002; 21(1):56–59.

19 Gray Y, Libbey NP. Xanthogranulomatous salpingitis and oophoritis: a case report and review of the literature. Arch Pathol Lab Med 2001; 125:260–263.

20 Elliott GB, Brody H, Elliott KA. Implications of 'lipoid salpingitis'. Fertil Steril 1965; 16(4):541–548.

21 Bersi S. Granulomatous salpingitis following hysterosalpingography with 'Lipiodol'. Pathologica 1977; 69(991–992):307–313.

22 Wrork OH Broders AC. Adenomyosis of the fallopian tubes. Am J Obstet Gynecol 1942; 44:412–432.

23 Jenkins CS, Williams SR, Schmidt GE. Salpingitis isthmica nodosa: a review of the literature, discussion of clinical significance, and consideration of patient management. Fertil Steril 1993; 60(4):599–607.

24 Benjamin CL, Beaver DC. Pathogenesis of salpingitis isthmical nodosa. Am J Clin Pathol 1951; 21:212–222.

25 Kutluay L, Vicdan K, Turan C, et al. Tubal histopathology in ectopic pregnancies. Eur J Obstet Gynecol Reprod Biol 1994; 57(2):91–94.

26 Saracoglu FO, Mungan T, Tanzer F. Salpingitis isthmica nodosa in infertility and ectopic pregnancy. Gynecol Obstet Invest 1992; 34(4):202–205.

27 Green LK, Kott ML. Histopathologic findings in ectopic tubal pregnancy. Int J Gynecol Pathol 1989; 8(3):255–262.

28 Punnonen R, Soderstrom KO. Inflammatory etiology of salpingitis isthmica nodosa: a clinical, histological and ultrastructural study. Acta Eur Fertil 1986; 17(3):199–203.

29 Gomel V, Yarali H. Infertility surgery: microsurgery. Curr Opin Obstet Gynecol 1992; 4(3):390–399.

30 Moore SW, Enterline HT. Significance of proliferative epithelial lesions of the uterine tube. Obstet Gynecol 1975; 45:385–390.

31 Saffos RO, Rhatigan RM, Scully RE. Metaplastic papillary tumor of the fallopian tube – a distinctive lesion of pregnancy. Am J Clin Pathol 1980; 74:232–236.

32 Seidman JD. Mucinous lesions of the fallopian tube. A report of seven cases. Am J Surg Pathol 1994; 18:1205–1212.

33 Cheung AN, Young RH, Scully RE. Pseudocarcinomatous hyperplasia of the fallopian tube associated with salpingitis. A report of 14 cases. Am J Surg Pathol 1994; 18(11): 1125–1130.

34 Seidman JD, Sherman ME, Bell KA, et al. Salpingitis, salpingoliths, and serous tumors of the ovaries: is there a connection? Int J Gynecol Pathol 2002; 21:101–107.

35 Sulak PJ. Sexually transmitted diseases. Semin Reprod Med 2003; 21(4):399–413.

36 Westrom L. Incidence, prevalence, and trends of acute pelvic inflammatory disease and its consequences in industrialized countries. Am J Obstet Gynecol 1980; 138:880–892.

37 Quan M. Pelvic inflammatory disease: diagnosis and management. J Am Board Fam Pract 1994; 7(2): 110–123.

38 Curran JW. Economic consequences of pelvic inflammatory disease in the United States. Am J Obstet Gynecol 1980; 138(7 Pt 2):848–851.

39 Shafer MA, Irwin CE, Sweet RL. Acute salpingitis in the adolescent female. J Pediatr 1982; 100:339–350.

40 Chacko MR, Wiemann CM, Smith PB. Chlamydia and gonorrhea screening in asymptomatic young women. J Pediatr Adolesc Gynecol 2004; 17(3):169–178.

41 Eschenbach DA. Acute pelvic inflammatory disease. Urol Clin North Am 1984; 11:65–81.

42 Mishell Dr Jr, Sulak PJ. The IUD: dispelling the myths and assessing the potential. Dialogues Contracept 1997; 5:1–4.

43 Steen R, Shapiro K. Intrauterine contraceptive devices and risk of pelvic inflammatory disease: standard of care in high STI prevalence settings. Reprod Health Matters 2004; 12(23):136–143.

44 Cates W Jr. Contraceptive choice, sexually transmitted diseases, HIV infection, and future fecundity. J Br Fer Soc 1996; 1:18–22.

45 Lee NC. What we've learned about IUDs from the Women's Health Study. Am J Gynecol Health 1989; 3:27–32.

46 Grimes DA. IUDs and pelvic infection. Am J Gynecol Health 1989; 3(3-S):23–26.

47 Rosenberg MJ. Fallout from the STD epidemic: salpingitis, ectopic pregnancy, and infertility. Am J Gynecol Health 1989; 3(3-S):19–22.

48 Henry-Suchet J, Sluzhinska A, Serfaty D. Chlamydia trachomatis screening in family planning centers: a review of cost/benefit evaluations in different countries. Eur J Contracept Reprod Health Care 1996; 1:301–309.

49 Mardh PA. Tubal factor infertility, with special regard to chlamydial salpingitis. Curr Opin Infect Dis 2004; 17:49–52.

50 Zdrodowska-Stefanow B, Ostaszewska-Puchalska I, Pucilo K. The immunology of Chlamydia trachomatis. Arch Immunol Ther Exp (Warsz) 2003; 51(5):289–294.

51 Debattista J, Timms P, Allan J, Allan J. Immunopathogenesis of Chlamydia trachomatis infections in women. Fertil Steril 2003; 79:1273–1287.

52 Taylor-Robinson D. Mycoplasma genitalium – an up-date. Int J STD AIDS 2002; 13:145–151.

53 Sam JW, Jacobs JE, Birnbaum BA. Spectrum of CT findings in acute pyogenic pelvic inflammatory disease. Radiographics 2002; 22:1327–1334.

54 Soper DE. Diagnosis and laparoscopic grading of acute salpingitis. Am J Obstet Gynecol 1991; 164:1370–1376.

55 Guaschino S, De Seta F. Update on Chlamydia trachomatis. Ann N Y Acad Sci 2000; 900:293–300.

56 Westrom LV. Sexually transmitted diseases and infertility. Sex Transm Dis 1994; 21:S32–S37.

57 Peterson HB, Galaid EI, Cates W Jr. Pelvic inflammatory disease. Med Clin North Am 1990; 74:1603–1615.

58 Wiskind AK, Dudley AG, Majmudar B, Masterson KC. Primary fallopian tube carcinoma with coexistent tuberculous salpingitis: a case report. J Med Assoc Ga 1992; 81(2):77–81.

59 Abraham JL, Spore WW, Benirschke K. Cysticercosis of the fallopian tube: histology and microanalysis. Hum Pathol 1982; 13(7):665–670.

60 Brooks JJ, Wheeler JE. Granulomatous salpingitis secondary to Crohn's disease. Obstet Gynecol 1977; 49(1 Suppl):31–33.

61 Wlodarski FM, Trainer TD. Granulomatous oophoritis and salpingitis associated with Crohn's disease of the appendix. Am J Obstet Gynecol 1975; 122:527–528.

62 Antoniou N, Varras M, Akrivis C, et al. Isolated torsion of the fallopian tube: a case report and review of the literature. Clin Exp Obstet Gynecol 2004; 31(3):235–238.

63 Krissi H, Shalev J, Bar-Hava I, et al. Fallopian tube torsion: laparoscopic evaluation and treatment of a rare gynecological entity. J Am Board Fam Pract 2001; 14(4):274–277.

64 Azodi M, Langer A, Jenison EL. Primary fallopian tube carcinoma with isolated torsion of involved tube. Eur J Gynaecol Oncol 2000; 21(4):364–367.

65 Houry D, Abbott JT. Ovarian torsion: a fifteen-year review. Ann Emerg Med 2001; 38(2):156–159.

66 Ganesan R, Ferryman SR, Meier L, Rollason TP. Vasculitis of the female genital tract with clinicopathologic correlation: a study of 46 cases with follow-up. Int J Gynecol Pathol 2000; 19(3):258–265.

67 Pilch H, Schaffer U, Gunzel S, et al. (A)symptomatic necrotizing arteritis of the female genital tract. Eur J Obstet Gynecol Reprod Biol 2000; 91(2):191–196.

68 Meyers KE, Pfieffer S, Lu T, Kaplan BS. Genitourinary complications of systemic lupus erythematosus. Pediatr Nephrol 2000; 14(5):416–421.

69 Azzena A, Altavilla G, Salmaso R, et al. Giant cell arteritis of fallopian tube. Clin Exp Obstet Gynecol 1994; 21(3):184–187.

70 Wilansky R, MacLean JN, Miro R, et al. Necrotizing vasculitis in gynecological surgery. Eur J Obstet Gynecol Reprod Biol 1980; 10(6):401–406.

71 Copeland W Jr, Hawley PC, Teteris NJ. Gynecologic amyloidosis. Am J Obstet Gynecol 1985; 153(5):555–556.

72 Stephenson TJ, Mills PM. Adenomatoid tumours: an immunohistochemical and ultrastructural appraisal of their histogenesis. J Pathol 1986; 148:327–335.

73 Skinnider BF, Young RH. Infarcted adenomatoid tumor: a report of five cases of a facet of a benign neoplasm that may cause diagnostic difficulty. Am J Surg Pathol 2004; 28:77–83.

74 Srigley JR, Colgan TJ. Multifocal and diffuse adenomatoid tumor involving uterus and fallopian tube. Ultrastruct Pathol 1988; 12(3):351–355.

75 Honore LH, Korn GW. Coexistence of tubal ectopic pregnancy and adenomatoid tumor. J Reprod Med 1976; 17(6):342–344.

76 Kayaalp E, Heller DS, Majmudar B. Serous tumor of low malignant potential of the fallopian tube. Int J Gynecol Pathol 2000; 19(4):398–400.

77 Alvarado-Cabrero I, Navani SS, Young RH, Scully RE. Tumors of the fimbriated end of the fallopian tube: a clinicopathologic analysis of 20 cases, including nine carcinomas. Int J Gynecol Pathol 1997; 16:189–196.

78 Sills ES, Kaplan CR, Perloe M, Tucker MJ. Laparoscopic approach to an uncommon adnexal neoplasm associated with infertility: serous cystadenofibroma of the fallopian tube. Am Assoc Gynecol Laparosc 2003; 10:545–547.

79 de la Fuente AA. Benign mixed Mullerian tumour – adenofibroma of the fallopian tube. Histopathology 1982; 6(5):661–666.

80 Quade BJ, McLachlin CM, Soto-Wright V, et al. Disseminated peritoneal leiomyomatosis. Clonality analysis by X chromosome inactivation and cytogenetics of a clinically benign smooth muscle proliferation. Am J Pathol 1997; 150(6):2153–2166.

81 Carinelli I, Senzani F, Bruni M, Cefis F. Lipomatous tumours of uterus fallopian tube and ovary. Clin Exp Obstet Gynecol 1980; 7(4):215–218.

82 Moore JH Jr, Crum CP, Chandler JG, Feldman PS. Benign cystic mesothelioma. Cancer 1980; 45(9):2395–2399.

83 Ross MJ, Welch WR, Scully RE. Multilocular peritoneal inclusion cysts (so-called cystic mesotheliomas). Cancer 1989; 64(6):1336–1346.

84 Piek JM, Kenemans P, Verheijen RH. Intraperitoneal serous adenocarcinoma: a critical appraisal of three hypotheses on its cause. Am J Obstet Gynecol 2004; 191:718–732.

85 Colgan TJ, Murphy J, Cole DE, Narod S, Rosen B. Occult carcinoma in prophylactic oophorectomy specimens: prevalence and association with BRCA germline mutation status. Am J Surg Pathol 2001; 25:1283–1289.

86 Schlosshauer PW, Cohen CJ, Penault-Llorca F, et al. Prophylactic oophorectomy: a morphologic and immunohistochemical study. Cancer 2003; 98(12):2599–2606.

87 Scheuer L, Kauff N, Robson M, et al. Outcome of preventive surgery and screening for breast and ovarian cancer in BRCA mutation carriers. J Clin Oncol 2002; 20:126.

88 Leeper K, Garcia R, Swisher E, et al. Pathologic findings in prophylactic oophorectomy specimens in high-risk women. Gynecol Oncol 2002; 87:52–56.

89 Colgan TJ. Challenges in the early diagnosis and staging of Fallopian-tube carcinomas associated with BRCA mutations. Int J Gynecol Pathol 2003; 22:109–120.

90 Zweemer RP, van Diest PJ, Verheijen RH, et al. Molecular evidence linking primary cancer of the fallopian tube to BRCA1 germline mutations. Gynecol Oncol 2000; 76(1):45–50.

91 Powell CB, Kenley E, Chen LM, et al. Risk-reducing salpingo-oophorectomy in BRCA mutation carriers: role of serial sectioning in the detection of occult malignancy. J Clin Oncol 2005; 23:127–132.

92 Levine DA, Argenta PA, Yee CJ, et al. Fallopian tube and primary peritoneal carcinomas associated with BRCA mutations. J Clin Oncol 2003; 21:4222–4227.

93 Nordin AJ. Primary carcinoma of the fallopian tube: a 20-year literature review. Obstet Gynecol Surv 1994; 49:349–361.

94 Hellstrom AC, Silfversward C, Nilsson B, Pettersson F. Carcinoma of the fallopian tube. A clinical and histopathologic review. The Radiumhemmet series. Int J Gynecol Cancer 1994; 4:395–400.

95 Obermair A, Taylor KH, Janda M, et al. Primary fallopian tube carcinoma: the Queensland experience. Int J Gynecol Cancer 2001; 11:69–72.

96 Takashina T, Ito E, Kudo R. Cytologic diagnosis of primary tubal cancer. Acta Cytol 1985; 29:367–372.

97 Sedlis A. Carcinoma of the fallopian tube. Surg Clin North Am 1978; 58(1):121–129.

98 Chin H, Matsui H, Mitsuhashi A, Nagao K, Sekiya S. Primary transitional cell carcinoma of the fallopian tube: a case report and review of the literature. Gynecol Oncol 1998; 71:469–475.

99 Rabczynski J, Ziolkowski P. Primary endometrioid carcinoma of fallopian tube. Clinicomorphologic study. Pathol Oncol Res 1999; 5:61–66.

100 Herbold DR, Axelrod JH, Bobowski SJ, Freel JH. Glassy cell carcinoma of the fallopian tube. A case report. Int J Gynecol Pathol 1988; 7(4):384–390.

101 Daya D, Young RH, Scully RE. Endometrioid carcinoma of the fallopian tube resembling an adnexal tumor of probable Wolffian origin: a report of six cases. Int J Gynecol Pathol 1992; 11(2):122–130.

102 Moore DH, Woosley JT, Reddick RL, Walton LA, Siegal GP. Adenosquamous carcinoma of the fallopian tube. A clinicopathologic case report with verification of the diagnosis by immunohistochemical and ultrastructural studies. Am J Obstet Gynecol 1987; 157(4 Pt 1):903–905.

103 Imm FC. Primary adenosquamous carcinoma of the fallopian tube. South Med J 1980; 73(5):678–680.

104 Baekelandt M, Kockx M, Wesling F, Gerris J. Primary adenocarcinoma of the fallopian tube. Review of the literature. Int J Gynecol Cancer 1993; 3:65–71.

105 Ng P, Lawton F. Fallopian tube carcinoma – a review. Ann Acad Med Singapore 1998; 27:693–697.

106 Rabczynski J, Ziolkowski P. Primary endometrioid carcinoma of fallopian tube. Clinicomorphologic study. Pathol Oncol Res 1999; 5(1):61–66.

107 Alvarado-Cabrero I, Young RH, Vamvakas EC, Scully RE. Carcinoma of the fallopian tube: a clinicopathological study of 105 cases with observations on staging and prognostic factors. Gynecol Oncol 1999; 72(3):367–379.

108 Green TH, Scully RE. Tumors of the fallopian tube. Clin Obstet Gynecol 1962; 5:886–906.

109 Baekelandt M, Jorunn Nesbakken A, et al. Carcinoma of the fallopian tube. Cancer 2000; 89:2076–2084.

110 Cormio G, Maneo A, Gabriele A, et al. Primary carcinoma of the fallopian tube. A retrospective analysis of 47 patients. Ann Oncol 1996; 7(3):271–275.

111 Gadducci A. Current management of fallopian tube carcinoma. Curr Opin Obstet Gynecol 2002; 14:27–32.

112 Bouraoui S, Goucha A, El Ouertani L, et al. Endometrioid carcinoma of the Fallopian tube arising in tubo-ovarian endometriosis. A case report. Gynecol Obstet Fertil 2003; 31(1):43–45.

113 Lim S, Kim JY, Park K, Kim BR, Ahn G. Mullerianosis of the mesosalpinx: a case report. Int J Gynecol Pathol 2003; 22(2):209–212.

114 Griffith LM, Carcangiu ML. Sex cord tumor with annular tubules associated with endometriosis of the fallopian tube. Am J Clin Pathol 1991; 96(2):259–262.

115 Gaffney EF, Cornog J. Endometrioid carcinoma of the fallopian tube. Obstet Gynecol 1978; 52(1 Suppl):34S–36S.

116 Hovadhanakul P, Nuerenberger SP, Ritter PJ, Taylor HB, Cavanagh D. Primary transitional cell carcinoma of the fallopian tube associated with primary carcinomas of the ovary and endometrium. Gynecol Oncol 1976; 4:138–143.

117   Jordan LB, Abdul-Kader M, Al-Nafussi A. Uterine serous papillary carcinoma: histopathologic changes within the female genital tract. Int J Gynecol Cancer 2001; 11(4):283–289.

118   Mulvany NJ, Arnstein MB, Ryan VA. Prognostic significance of fallopian tube cytology: a study of 99 endometrial malignancies. Pathology 2000; 32:5–9.

119   Mackillop WJ, Pringle JF. Stage III endometrial carcinoma. A review of 90 cases. Cancer 1985; 56:2519–2523.

120   Pins MR, Young RH, Crum CP, Leach IH, Scully RE. Cervical squamous cell carcinoma in situ with intraepithelial extension to the upper genital tract and invasion of tubes and ovaries: report of a case with human papilloma virus analysis. Int J Gynecol Pathol 1997; 16(3):272–278.

121   Mazur MT, Hsueh S, Gersell DJ. Metastases to the female genital tract. Analysis of 325 cases. Cancer 1984; 53(9): 1978–1984.

122   Tiltman AJ, Allard U. Female adnexal tumours of probable Wolffian origin: an immunohistochemical study comparing tumours, mesonephric remnants and paramesonephric derivatives. Histopathology 2001; 38:237–242.

123   Ramirez PT, Wolf JK, Malpica A, et al. Wolffian duct tumors: case reports and review of the literature. Gynecol Oncol 2002; 86(2):225–230.

124   Sheyn I, Mira JL, Bejarano PA, Husseinzadeh N. Metastatic female adnexal tumor of probable Wolffian origin: a case report and review of the literature. Arch Pathol Lab Med 2000; 124:431–434.

125   Atallah D, Rouzier R, Voutsadakis I, et al. Malignant female adnexal tumor of probable wolffian origin relapsing after pregnancy. Gynecol Oncol 2004; 95:402–404.

Benign conditions of the ovary

Alessandra F. Nascimento,

Mark D. Hornstein and

Christopher P. Crum

Introduction

Anatomy of the ovary

Surface, cortex and medulla
Hilus

Common incidental findings seen at hysterectomy

Surface
Ovarian cortex
Hilus

The ovary in pregnancy

Corpus luteum of pregnancy
Theca-lutein hyperplasia
   of pregnancy (including
   so-called pregnancy luteoma)
Hyperreactio luteinalis
Solitary luteinized follicle cyst
Deciduosis (ectopic decidua)

Conditions associated with clinical infertility

Introduction
Premature ovarian failure

Autoimmune disorders and
   autoimmune oophoritis
Polycystic ovarian syndrome
   (PCOS)
Endometriosis

The perimenopausal and postmenopausal ovary

Atrophy
Stromal hyperplasia
Stromal hyperthecosis
Hilus cell hyperplasia
Cortical fibromatosis

Infections of the ovary

Infectious salpingo-oophoritis
Tuberculosis

Benign conditions producing ovarian enlargement

Follicle cyst
Endometriotic cyst
Massive ovarian edema
Ovarian torsion

Ovarian remnant syndrome

Introduction

To the obstetrician-gynecologist, the ovarian examination is a fundamental part of the gynecologic evaluation and, depending on the age of the patient and other risk factors, ovarian enlargement will trigger a series of investigative procedures. The surgical pathologist examines the ovarian specimen for several reasons, including confirming or excluding pathology when the clinical impression is an ovarian abnormality, or examining the ovary for completeness when the uterus and adnexa are removed for other disease. Another possibility is prophylactic oophorectomy in women with a family history of ovarian cancer or documented mutation in a cancer-associated (BRCA) gene (Ch. 27). To perform the examination under any of these circumstances, the pathologist must have a working understanding of the normal ovarian anatomy and the range of findings seen in the age grouping under study.

Anatomy of the ovary

SURFACE, CORTEX AND MEDULLA

The adult ovary has three components, the cortex, subcortical medulla and the hilus. The cortex of the ovary is subdivided into the superficial epithelium and its underlying stroma (Figs 22.1, 22.2). The ovarian surface epithelium (OSE) is composed of a simple

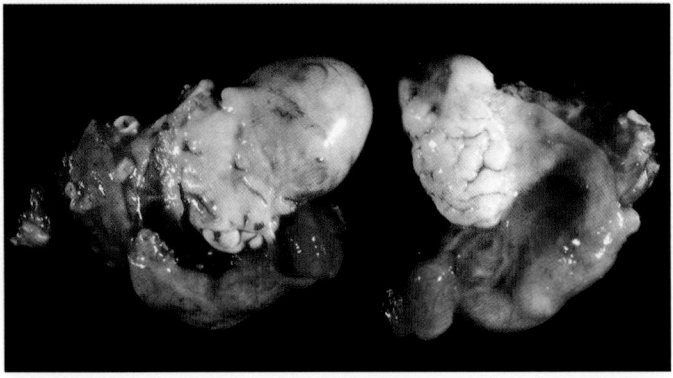

Fig. 22.1 Ovaries from a reproductive-age woman, containing mild surface convolutions. A small fibroma is present on the cortex of the ovary on the left.

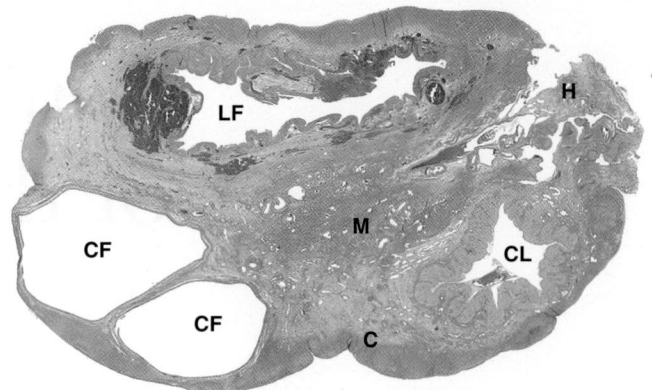

Fig. 22.2 Low-power photomicrograph of the ovarian cortex (C), medulla (M) and hilus (H). CL, corpus luteum; CF, cystic follicle; LF, luteinized follicle.

lining of modified mesothelial cells which are cuboidal to columnar cells with a low nuclear-to-cytoplasmic ratio, inconspicuous nucleoli and a moderate amount of pale cytoplasm (Fig. 22.3). The cells lining the ovarian surface are ultrastructurally related with peritoneal mesothelial cells, including the presence of microvilli, although they tend to be cuboidal when compared with the flattened peritoneal mesothelium.[1] The morphologic and immunophenotypic features of cellular proliferations seen on the ovarian surface are identical to those seen elsewhere (see Ch. 24). In brief, immunohistochemical studies have revealed this epithelium to be positive for cytokeratins, Ber-EP4 and hormone receptors (estrogen and progesterone).[2–5] The OSE lies on a basement membrane and is normally inconspicuous or even absent, particularly if the ovary is handled prior to fixation. Under conditions of stress, such as peritoneal infections or inflammation, the OSE may become prominent and exhibit reactive atypia, with nuclear enlargement, hyperchromasia and prominent nucleoli. The importance of the ovarian surface epithelium lies in its proposed connection to ovarian carcinogenesis, via metaplastic transformation to an epithelial phenotype. This is discussed in greater detail in Chapter 24. Otherwise, it is involved in the formation of adhesions and inclusion cysts.

The underlying stroma is subdivided into cortex and medulla. The cortex is composed of spindled-shaped cells, often arranged in parallel or alternating obliquely arranged bundles in a storiform pattern, with overlapping, tapered nuclei, inconspicuous nucleoli and scant cytoplasm, with a variable amount of stromal

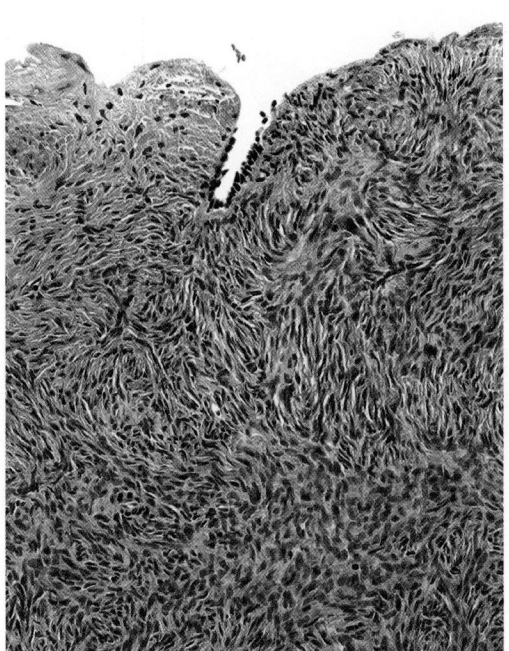

Fig. 22.3 Ovarian cortex with ovarian surface epithelium (center).

Common incidental findings seen at hysterectomy

SURFACE

Adhesions

Periovarian adhesions are fibrous connections that form between the ovary and other organs or peritoneum (Fig. 22.4). These fibrous bands form as a response to intrapelvic injuries, such as bleeding at a site of endometriosis, infection, and abdominal or pelvic surgery. The major consequence of adhesion formation is its association with chronic pelvic pain. The relationship of adhesions to pain is controversial. Although studies have associated various forms of adhesions with different levels of pain, more recent studies have shown no relationship between pelvic pain and adhesions.[7] Histologically, a hypocellular band of fibrous tissue characterizes adhesions with various amount of collagen deposition on the surface of the ovarian cortex.

The differential diagnosis of adhesions includes few entities other than cystic mesothelioma, which conceivably could mimic cystic adhesions. Cystic mesothelioma is a benign recurrent lesion that is characterized by a macroscopic multicystic mass in which the cystic spaces are usually lined by conspicuous mesothelial cells separated by a thick fibrous septae.[8] In contrast, cystic adhesions are small, focal and composed of delicate

collagen. Not surprisingly, these cells are positive for intermediate filament markers such as vimentin and α-smooth muscle actin.[6] The unique attribute of ovarian cortical stroma is the propensity to respond to pituitary or pregnancy hormones, as will be discussed below. Oocytes, Graafian follicles, cystic and atretic follicles, corpora lutea and albicantia are commonly present in various stages of growth and involution in the cortex during reproductive life.

The medulla is composed principally of larger vessels and merges with the hilus. In the reproductive-age ovary, the distinction between cortex and medulla is subtle, due to the abundance of cortical stroma. End-stage corpora lutea (albicantia) are often situated at the interface of the cortex/medulla. After menopause, when the cortex contracts, the medulla will stand out sharply in relief by the presence of corpora albicantia that have not been resorbed.

HILUS

The ovarian hilum is the anatomic site through which blood vessels (ovarian artery and vein) gain access to the ovary and site of attachment of the broad ligament. Embedded within its substance, which is composed of fibroconnective tissue, there are two basic structures: hilar cells and rete ovarii. The latter are mesonephric remnants and are described below.

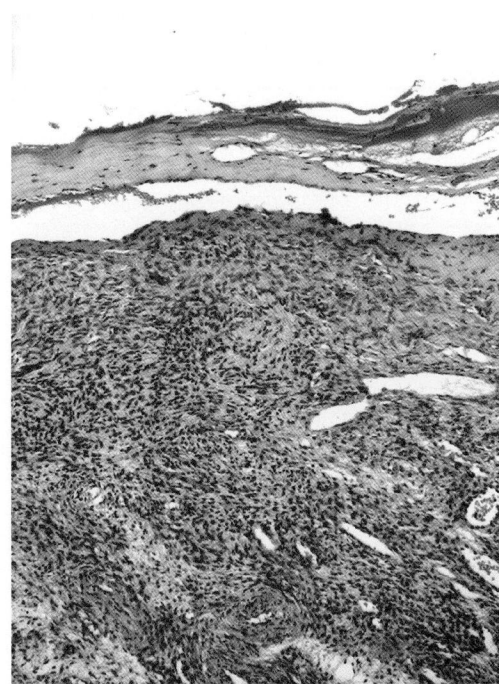

Fig. 22.4 Small fibrovascular adhesions on the ovarian cortex.

715

fibrous strands. Cystic mesothelioma is discussed in greater detail in Chapter 23.

Mesothelial proliferation

Mesothelial proliferations of the ovarian surface include the same spectrum of mesothelial changes seen in other mesothelial-lined surfaces, such as peritoneum, pleura and pericardium, and usually occur in response to pelvic inflammation, local trauma, including torsion or infarction, endometriosis and neoplasia.[9-12] The reactive mesothelial response includes mesothelial hyperplasia, mesothelial-inclusion cysts, and a variable number of macrophages, the latter most conspicuous in endometriosis (Fig. 22.4). Another common, presumably reactive process is micropapillomatosis. Micropapillomatosis is incidental, self-limiting, and consists of small finger-like excrescences composed of a central fibrous core and lined by OSE. Other than the papillary architecture, micropapillomatosis is easily distinguished from surface tumors of serous epithelial origin. The latter are composed of irregular papillae with epithelial differentiation, in contrast to the mesothelial lining of micropapillomatosis (Fig. 22.5).

Much rarer entities are benign papillary mesothelioma and malignant mesothelioma.[9] These are discussed in Chapter 23.

Endosalpingiosis

Endosalpingiosis of the ovary defines epithelial cysts or gland-like structures containing ciliated epithelium. The term endosalpingiosis in this site is best reserved for those epithelial structures that contain not only cilia

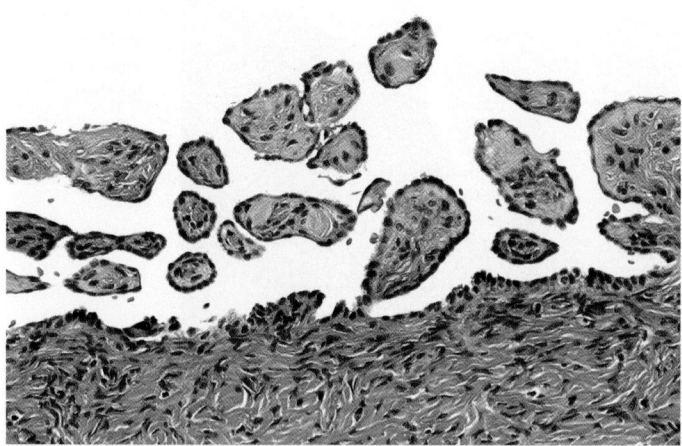

Fig. 22.5 Micropapillomatosis of the ovary, composed of mesothelial-lined fibrous papillae.

but also a pseudostratified epithelium that closely resembles fallopian tube mucosa, with or without supporting stroma typical of that seen in tubal plica (Fig. 22.6). However, if tubal stroma is not present, the term Müllerian (cortical) inclusion cyst is preferred, inasmuch as they conceivably originate from the endometrium, or Müllerian metaplasia of the mesothelium.[11-13]

OVARIAN CORTEX

Cortical inclusion cysts

Cortical inclusion cysts (CICs) originate from the entrapment of epithelium within the cortex of the ovary. This

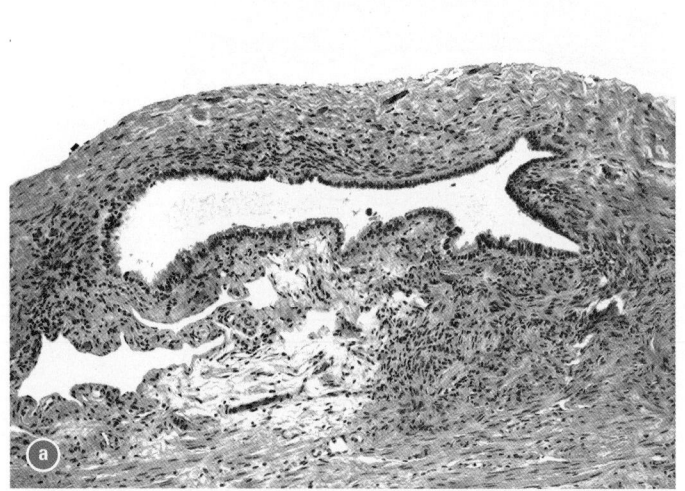

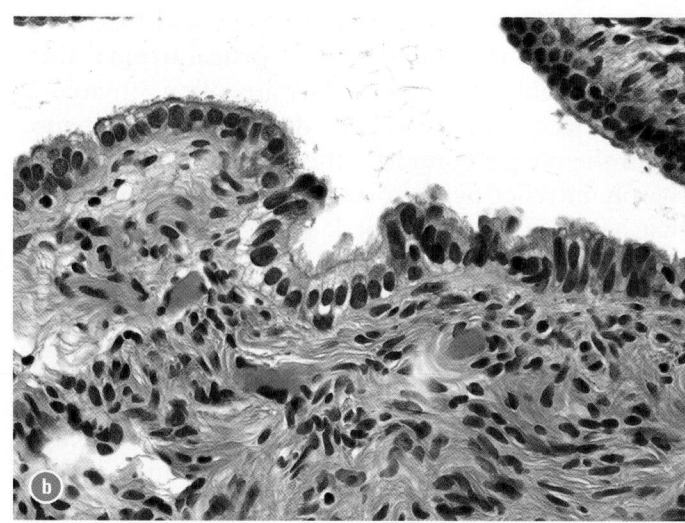

Fig. 22.6 Endosalpingiosis. (a) At low power the impression is that of adhesed tubal epithelium on the ovarian surface. (b) Higher magnification illustrates the prominent cilia.

epithelium may be derived via Müllerian metaplasia of the ovarian surface epithelium, or via transporting of tubal or endometrial epithelium to the ovarian surface. The epithelium lining these CICs may be flat to cuboidal non-ciliated epithelium seen on the surface of the ovary, or exhibit cilia similar to that seen in endosalpingiosis (Fig. 22.7).[14] The mechanisms by which CICs find their way into the ovarian cortex include entrapment within surface adhesions, infolding of surface epithe-lium into the cortex with CICs developing when the folds of the cortex fuse, and repair of ovulation sites, with surface epithelium growing into atretic follicles (see Ch. 24).

Cortical inclusion cysts are considered benign, and are found in the majority of ovaries from postmeno-pausal women. The attention they receive results from their possible role in the pathogenesis of ovarian adeno-carcinomas. This concept continues to evolve as the

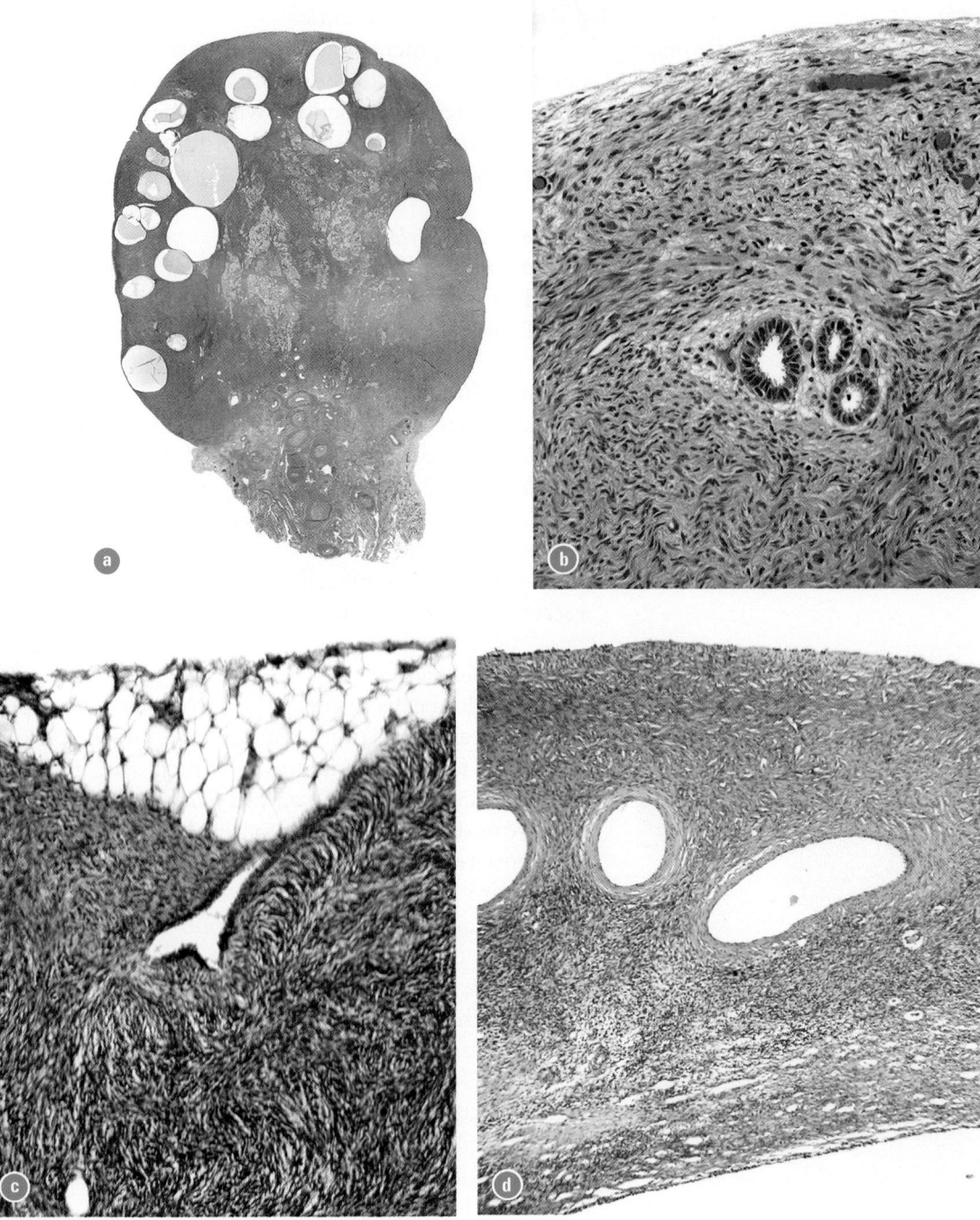

Fig. 22.7 (a) Extensive cortical inclusion cysts (CICs). (b) Higher power of subsurface CICs. (c) CIC forming at interface of peri-ovarian adhesion. (d) Mesothelial-lined atretic follicles are another mechanism for incorporating ovarian surface lining into the ovarian cortex.

relative contributions of the fallopian tube (Ch. 21), endometrium (Ch. 19) and peritoneum (Ch. 23), together with direct transformation of mesothelium to epithelium continue to be resolved.[14] CICs and related Müllerian cysts in the para-ovarian, para-tubal and hilar regions exhibit a wide range of epithelial metaplasias, including mucinous, endometrioid and transitional (Walthard cell rests) type, corresponding to the malignant phenotypes seen in epithelial tumors. The role of CICs in ovarian carcinomas is discussed further in Chapter 24.

Müllerian and simple cysts

Larger cysts of one or more centimeters in diameter may form on the surface of the ovary, within the cortex, or even hilus. The origin of these para-ovarian, intracortical or intra-hilar cysts is presumably similar to that of CICs. The lining of these cysts ranges from flat to cuboidal to pseudostratified columnar. Cysts lined by flat or cuboidal epithelium are termed simple or mesothelial cysts (Fig. 22.8). Those with a distinct epithelial lining are classified as Müllerian cysts or if accompanied by a dense fibrous wall, unilocular serous cystadenomas.

The differential diagnosis of simple cysts includes atretic follicles (residual theca lining cells), senescent endometriosis (hemosiderin and/or rare plasma cells), cystadenomas (dense fibrous capsule and pseudostratified ciliated (serous) epithelium), adhesed hydrosalpinx (smooth muscle wall) and paratubal cyst (continuity with the adnexae).

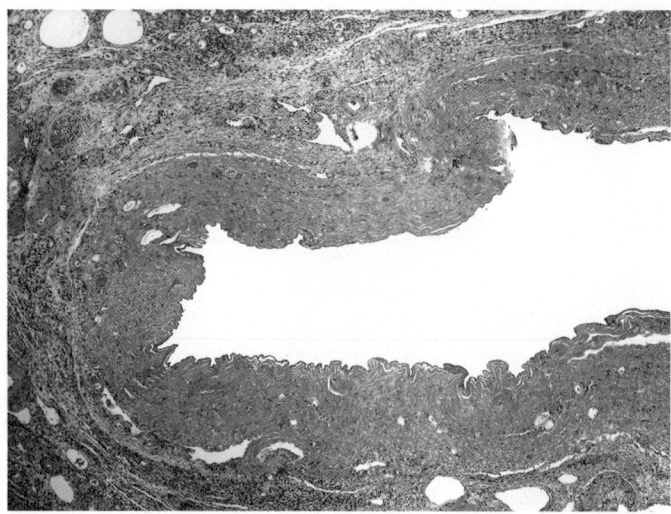

Fig. 22.8 Simple (mesothelial) cyst of the ovary.

Follicles and corpora lutea

Follicle development is a dynamic process that goes on continuously, not only in the reproductive age ovary but also to a lesser degree prior to menarche. Moreover, the preparation of follicles for eventual recruitment and selection and ovulation occurs over an extended period of time and is not confined within the time frame of a single cycle. Accordingly, follicles that are not selected may persist for a period of time prior to atresia. For this reason, the pathologist should expect to see a range of follicle development in otherwise normal ovaries removed incidentally for other reproductive tract abnormalities.

The development of germ cells of the ovary and their embryogenesis are discussed in Chapter 1. In the adult ovary, follicles are embedded within the cortical stroma of the ovary, are classified according to their evolutionary stage and include the following (Fig. 22.9):

Primordial follicles
The *primordial follicles* are present at birth and composed of a primary oocyte and surrounded by a flattened layer of granulosa cells (Fig. 22.9a).

Primary follicles
As the oocyte matures, the granulosa cells increase in size, becoming mitotically active and form the *primary follicle* (Fig. 22.9a).

Secondary follicles
With subsequent stratification of the granulosa cells layer, a *secondary (pre-antral) follicle* is formed (Fig. 22.9b).

Graafian follicles
The granulosa cells forming the secondary follicle produce large amounts of interstitial fluid, which accumulates and form an antrum in which the enlarged, mature oocytes reside (*Graafian follicle*) (Fig. 22.9c).[15]

Surrounding the granulosa cell layer, stromal cells differentiate into an inner and an outer theca layer. This entire process is governed by follicle-stimulating hormone and luteinizing hormone (FSH and LH). Following ovulation, the antrum is filled with fibrin and debris, and starts contracting to form the *corpus luteum*. While a single Graafian follicle (usually) progresses to a corpus luteum, several other follicles may be present throughout the cycle and the pathologist may encounter several follicles in various stages of development and atresia. Some may closely resemble pre-ovulatory follicles, with expanded granulosa and theca cell layers; others will have lost most of their

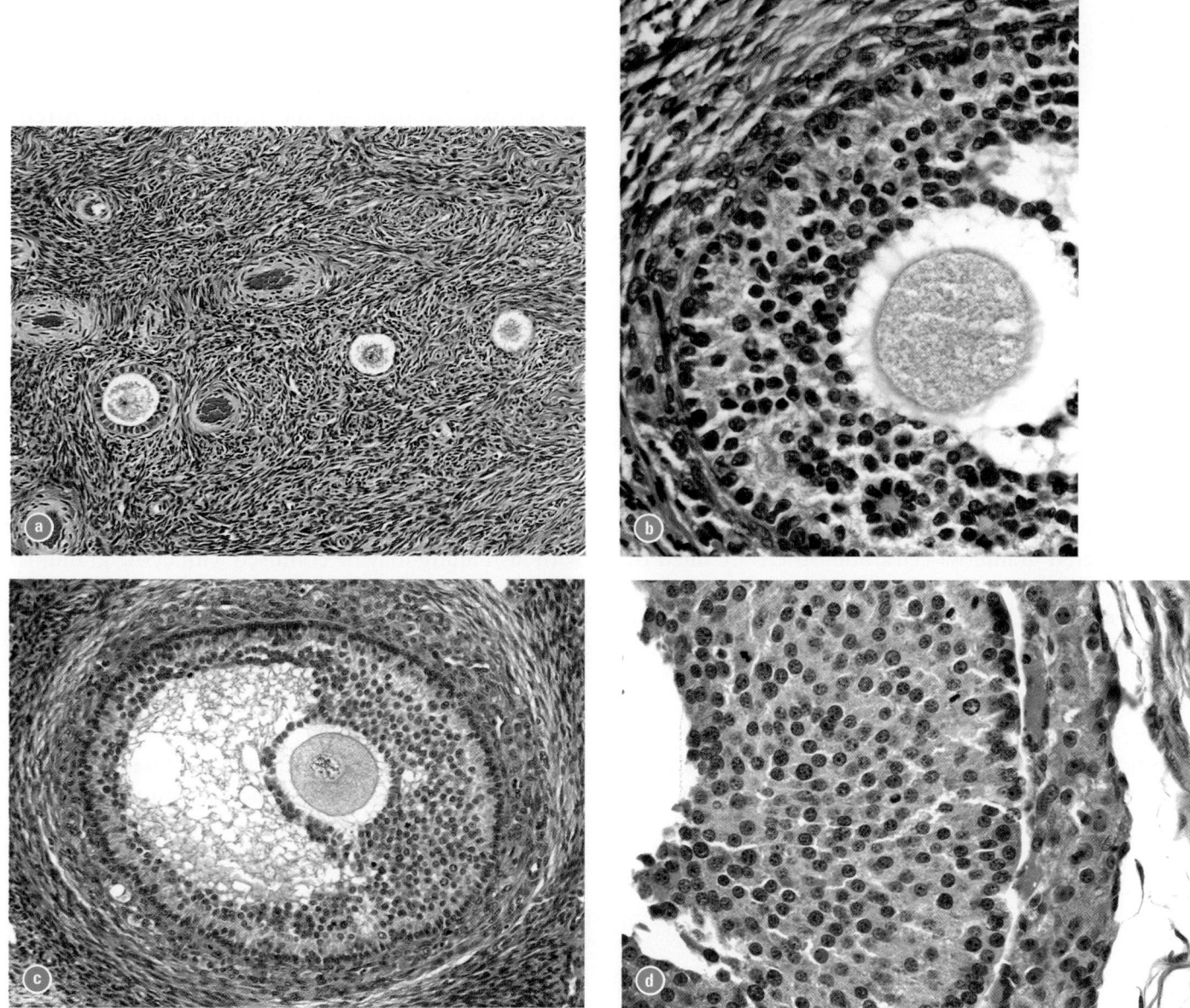

Fig. 22.9 Follicle development. (a) Primordial and primary follicles, the latter exhibiting a single layer of granulosa cells (follicle at left). (b) Secondary follicle demonstrating early peri-oocyte clearing (right) caused by the accumulation of fluid. (c) Early antral (Graafian) follicle, with a distinct zone of fluid accumulation and eccentrically placed oocyte. (d) Luteinized follicle lining cells.

granulosa cells and be in a stage of involution (Fig. 22.9d). If ovulation does not take place, persistent follicle development can lead to an unopposed estrogen effect.

Cystic follicles

Cystic follicles are very commonly encountered in the ovaries of reproductive-age women. They result from Graafian follicles that did not rupture and will eventually undergo reabsorption. Cystic follicles are usually asymptomatic or present with mild, vague pelvic pain. They can be solitary or multiple (Fig. 22.10). Macroscopically, they appear as uniloculated cystic structures on the ovarian surface and cortex, with smooth walls and watery content. They are usually less than 10 mm in diameter.

Cystic follicles vary in their appearance, presumably a function of their age. Some contain a thick layer of partially luteinized granulosa and theca cells and may be mistaken for corpora lutea (Fig. 22.9d). Most are

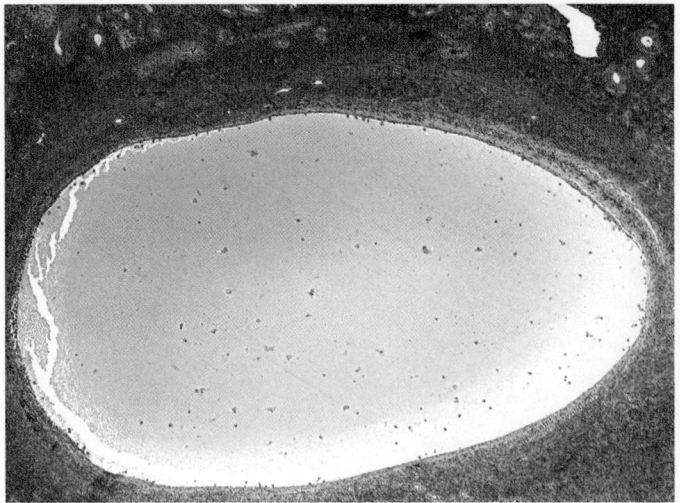

Fig. 22.10 Cystic follicle. Common in reproductive-age women.

composed of a theca layer that is variably luteinized with depleted granulosa cells. Still others are lined by a single layer of luteinized cells, the origin of which are presumably theca. When follicles exceed 3 cm in diameter, they are termed follicle cysts (see below).[15]

Atretic follicles

Atretic follicles are commonly present in the ovary and signify the end stage of follicle involution, cystic or otherwise. Early atretic follicles display a fibrotic rim beneath which the theca cells are slightly dispersed (Fig. 22.11). As atresia progresses, the follicle space disappears, terminating in an indistinct oval to elliptical condensation of stroma with a central crease or slit-like remnant of the original lumen. Atretic follicles are particularly common in polycystic ovarian disease, a sign of increased follicle recruitment (see below).

Differential diagnosis of follicular changes (Fig. 22.12)

The pathologist who routinely examines the ovary is unlikely to confuse follicles with neoplasia, or vice versa, but two pitfalls exist, one common and one rare. (1) Tangentially sectioned theca externa may be misdiagnosed as a stromal neoplasm, particularly because the cells are plump in appearance and mitotically active. This pitfall is avoided by the pathologist familiar with this pattern, coupled with the absence of a discrete cortical mass (Fig. 22.12a,b).[16] (2) Cystic follicles with lush lining may be confused with cystic granulosa cell tumors. The latter are usually multicystic and lined by irregularly arranged neoplastic granulosa cells (Fig. 22.12c).

Recent and degenerating corpora lutea

Gross appearance

Corpora lutea are normal ovarian structures that in the normal cycle are the consequence of ruptured follicles.

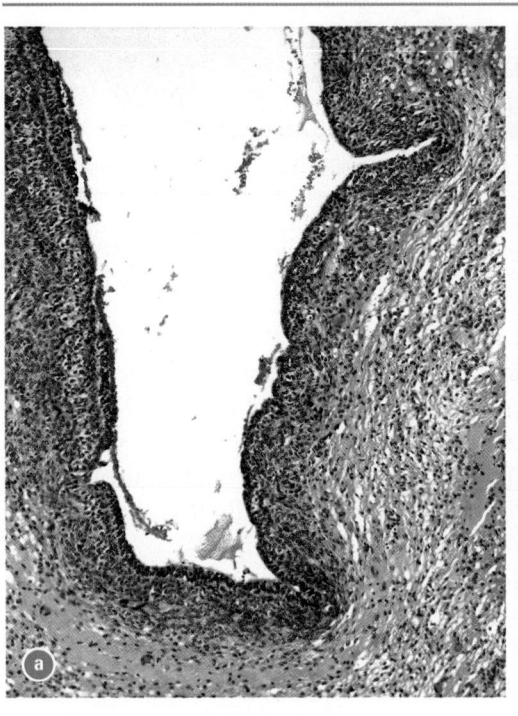

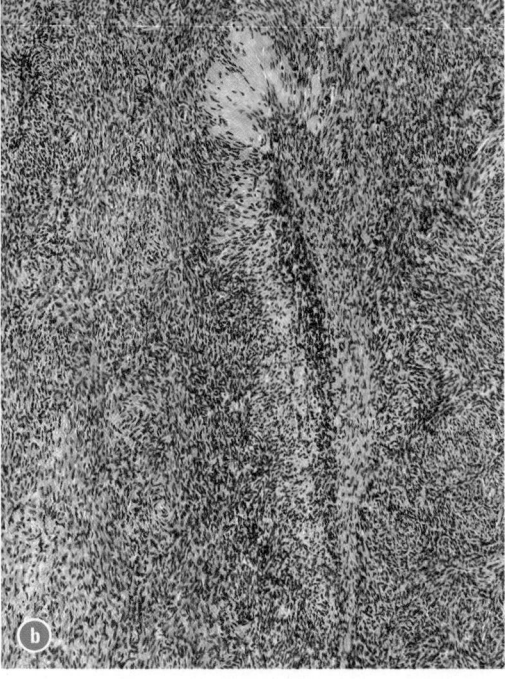

Fig. 22.11 Atretic follicle. (a) Cystic atretic follicle with early sclerosis of the follicle wall and dispersal of the thecal cells. (b) End-stage follicle atresia, with collapse of the follicle space.

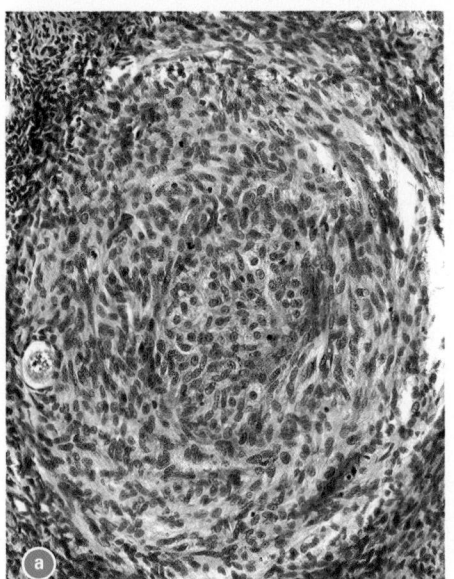
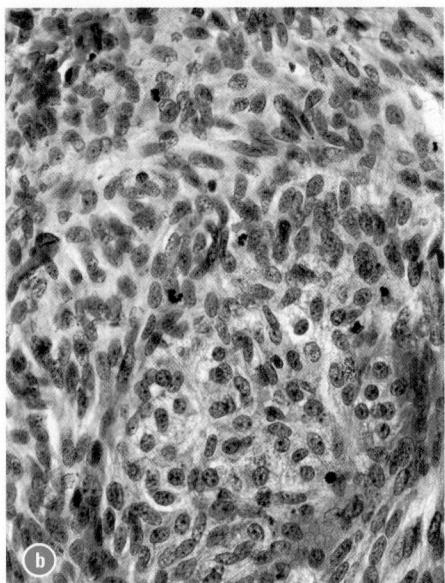
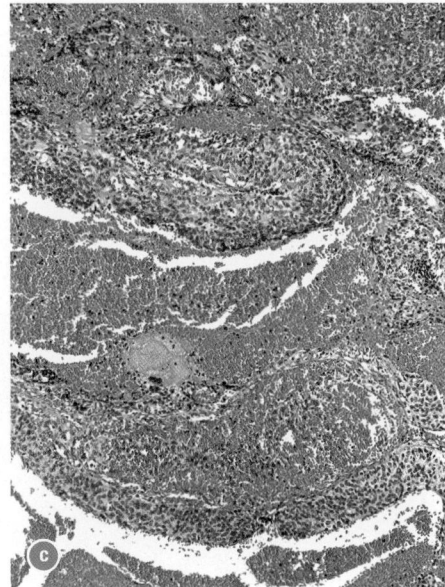

Fig. 22.12 Diagnostic problems in interpreting ovarian follicles. (a) Tangential sectioning of theca mimicking neoplasia. (b) Higher power of mitotic activity. (c) Cystic granulosa cell tumor may mimic follicles.

Macroscopically, these structures are bright yellow masses (recent corpus luteum) or white masses (degenerating corpus luteum) with a small cystic center (Fig. 22.13). A cystic and/or hemorrhagic appearance is common, leading to the common designation of cystic or hemorrhagic corpus luteum. These two characteristics typify most corpora lutea and are not necessary qualifiers; simply qualifying corpora lutea as recent or degenerating will suffice.

Microscopic

The histologic hallmark of a recent corpus luteum is prominent luteinization of the granulosa cell layers, and is synonymous with a 'granulosa-lutein cyst'. The plump granulosa cells are arranged in a cerebriform convoluted mass, with internal folds, the interstices of which contain smaller numbers of smaller luteinized theca cells (Fig. 22.14). Granulosa cells produce progesterone and the theca cells produce the estrogen throughout the cycle. With the onset of menstruation, the granulosa and theca cells undergo apoptosis, with an abrupt drop in progesterone and estrogen production, and by the fifth day of the new cycle (late menstrual phase) have lost their distinct architecture, as the cells become smaller and admixed with mononuclear cells. Within two cycles, the degenerated corpus luteum has contracted to a fraction of its size, the luteal cells are reduced to small rounded nuclei with scant cytoplasm, and the structure is recognized principally by its architectural similarity to the original corpus luteum (Fig. 22.15).[17]

Differential diagnosis

Diagnostic pitfalls associated with corpora lutea include the following: (1) clinical interpretation as an adnexal mass; (2) rarely, misdiagnosis as an ovarian pregnancy during exploratory laparotomy for ectopic pregnancy; and (3) confusion with endometriosis, specifically when the latter consists of a pseudoxanthomatous pseudo-

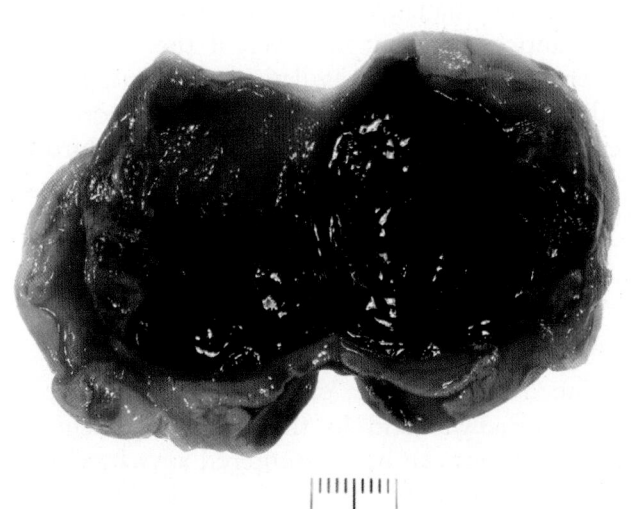

Fig. 22.13 Gross appearance of a recent cystic corpus luteum, with a smooth hemorrhagic lining and yellow rim.

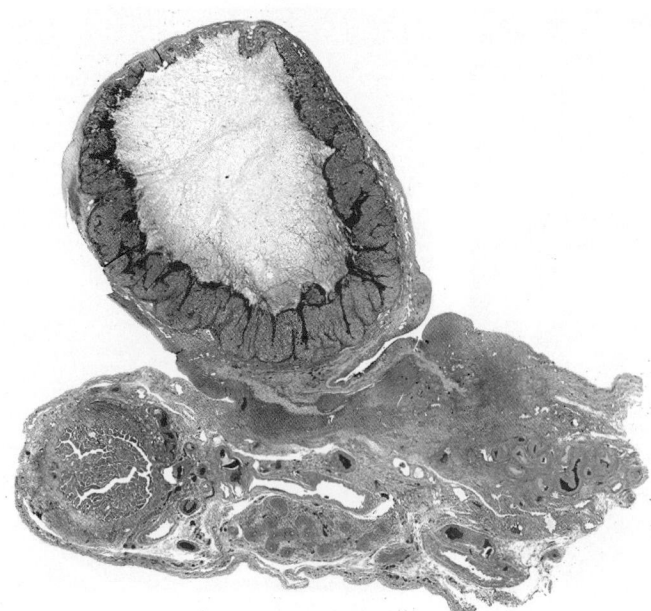

Fig. 22.14 Low power microscopic appearance of a recent corpus luteum accentuates the convoluted appearance.

cyst. The diagnostic confusion stems from interpreting the foamy macrophages lining the pseudocyst as granulosa-lutein cells. The characteristic appearance of foamy histiocytes and the absence of a second theca cell layer characterize the xanthomatous pseudocyst (see below) (Fig. 22.16).

Clinical complications

The most common complication of corpus luteum is massive hemorrhage, the greatest risk factor being anticoagulant therapy or other coagulation disturbance. Some can be managed effectively by rapid reversal of the anticoagulation; however, if the hemorrhage is severe, laparotomy, coagulation or suturing of the bleeding site may be necessary. Rarely, oophorectomy is required. In one study, approximately one-third had recurrent hemorrhage when anticoagulation was resumed.[18]

HILUS

Wolffian remnants

Wolffian remnants are embryologic mesonephric residues usually found in the round ligament and vaginal wall, but can be encountered anywhere in the female genital tract, including the ovaries (see Ch. 1). They are usually incidental microscopic findings. A single layer of cuboidal cells with round nuclei, incon-

spicuous nucleoli and scant cytoplasm lines the glands and ducts of one to several glands. The glands are situated at oblique angles to one another and contain sense eosinophilic intraluminal secretions (Fig. 22.17).

Recognition of Wolffian remnants is important; in certain settings they may be mis-classified as neoplastic. However, the nuclei are generally uniform in appearance and are oriented vertically (see Ch. 30). The major differential diagnosis is with metastatic carcinoma. Nuclear atypia and mitoses are usually absent and aid in the diagnosis.

Hilus cells

Hilus cells are the ovarian counterparts of testicular Leydig cells (Ch. 1). They are found singly or in nests within the hilum of the ovary, present in variable density in the connective tissue spaces between the vessels. In most instances, the cells are present in small groups and require a careful search. However, once found, the cells are distinct, with a moderate amount of cytoplasm, a polygonal shape, round central nuclei, small nucleoli and abundant eosinophilic cytoplasm. Like Leydig cells, hilus cells often contain small round to oval intracytoplasmic droplets. Careful inspection will occasionally disclose crystalloids of Reinke (Fig. 22.18).

Hilus cells are hormone responsive, and become accentuated during pregnancy and at menopause, two conditions associated with increased gonadotropin secretion (see below). Their importance lies in the rare steroid-producing tumors that arise in them, and their close resemblance to and occasional misclassification as lobular carcinoma of the breast.

The ovary in pregnancy

The cells of the ovarian cortex and hilum are uniquely responsive to circulating gonadotropins and steroid hormones, which, apart from the corpus luteum, influence the sub-mesothelial mesenchyme (deciduosis), stromal, follicular and hilus cells. This process is characterized by continued follicle development and regression, upon which a prominent luteinized response in these gonadotropin-sensitive cells is superimposed. The result is general regression of the granulosa cells, expansion and luteinization of the theca interna and interfollicular stromal cells, and coincident hilus cell hyperplasia. The spectrum of pregnancy-related alterations can occasionally cause diagnostic confusion (Table 22.1). The extent of the process varies widely, and gives rise to a continuum of conditions discussed below.

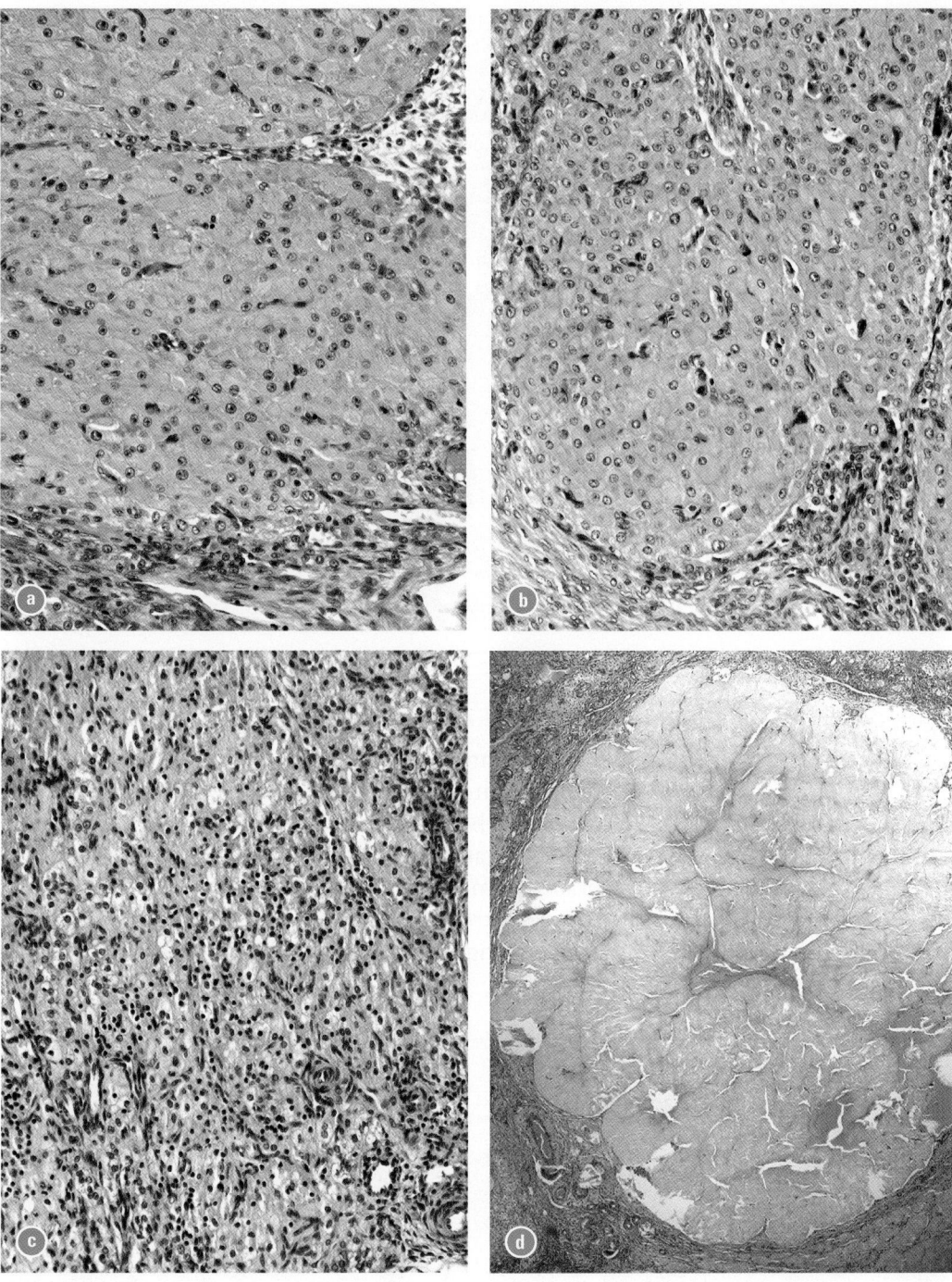

Fig. 22.15 Corpora lutea at different ages: (a) day 24 secretory, (b) day 1 menstrual and (c) late menstrual. (d) Corpus albicans.

CORPUS LUTEUM OF PREGNANCY

The corpus luteum (CL) of pregnancy is simply the persistence of the corpus luteum that accompanied conception. It is most prominent early in pregnancy and is critical to sustaining the gestation in the first 8 weeks, during which the maximum progesterone secretion occurs. As pregnancy evolves, the corpus luteum gradually regresses and plays a negligible role in the final two trimesters. Two histologic features characterize the CL of early pregnancy. The first is enlargement of the granulosa lutein cells. The second is the presence of cytoplasmic vacuoles and droplets of variable size, which persist throughout pregnancy (Fig. 22.19).[19]

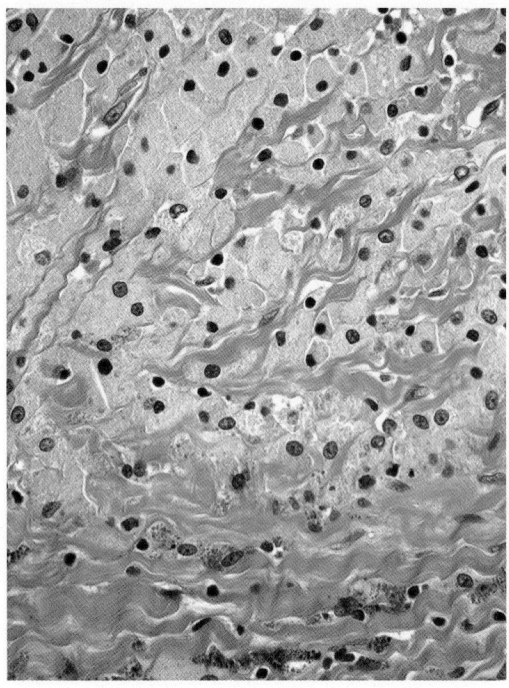

Fig. 22.16
Xanthoma cells lining an endometriotic pseudocyst might mimic luteinized granulosa cells.

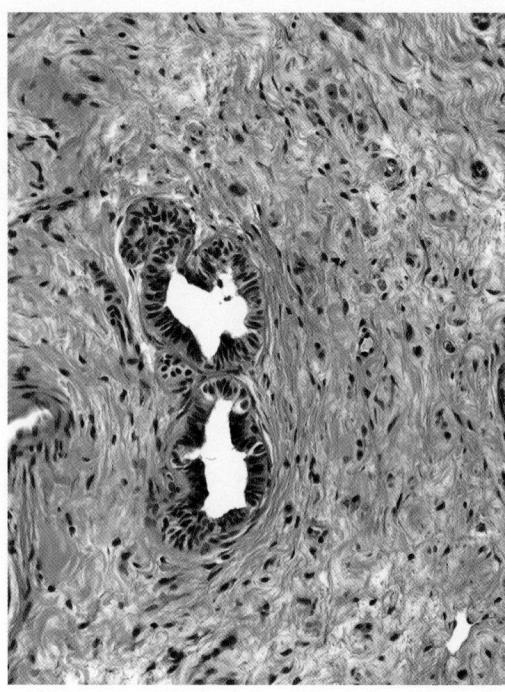

Fig. 22.17
Wolffian remnants in the hilum.

THECA-LUTEIN HYPERPLASIA OF PREGNANCY (INCLUDING SO-CALLED PREGNANCY LUTEOMA)

Ovaries removed incidentally at the time of delivery will display one or more of the following, collectively defined as '*theca-lutein hyperplasia of pregnancy*' (TLHP). This consists of variable numbers of follicles containing an attenuated granulosa cell layer and an expanded luteinized theca (Fig. 22.20). This expansion of the theca is often asymmetric, producing elliptical aggregates of theca cells that merge with the ovarian stroma. The latter frequently contains scattered luteinized stromal cells singly or in clusters, cords or loosely arranged groups. Coincident expansion of the

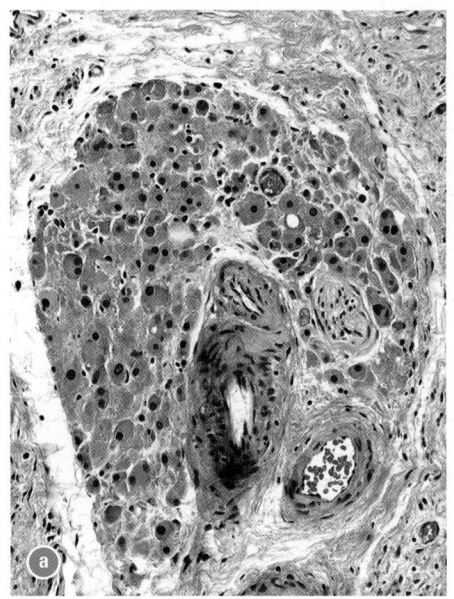
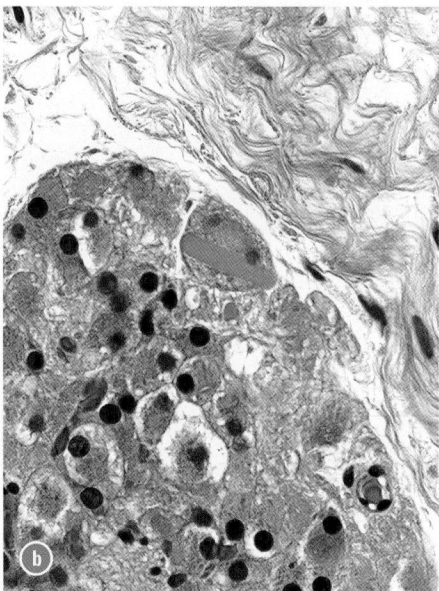
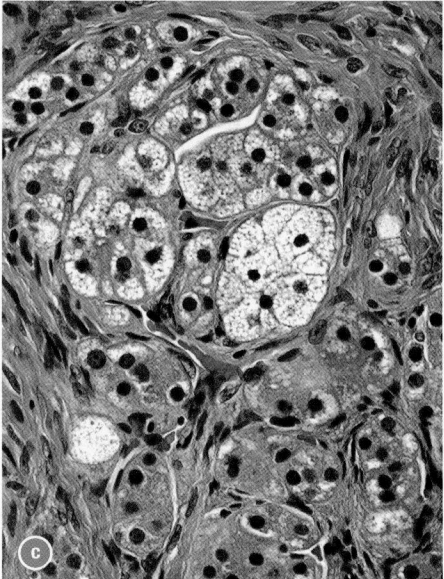

Fig. 22.18 (a) Hilus cells. (b) Reinke crystalloid in a hilus cell (upper center). (c) Lipid-laden hilus cells may mimic an adrenal rest.

Table 22.1 *Pitfalls in the interpretation of the ovary in pregnancy*

Finding	Misclassification as
Luteoma	Metastatic carcinoma
Hyperreactio luteinalis	Cystadenoma
Deciduosis	Mesenchymal tumor
Solitary cyst	Clear cell carcinoma
Decidualized endometrioma	Corpus luteum
	Malignancy (on ultrasound)
	Malignancy (on frozen section)

hilus cells may also be seen. This collective accentuation of luteinized cell growth is not unlike that seen in hyperthecosis (see below), although the pathogenesis is related to the production of chorionic gonadotropins and their effects on the ovary.[20–22]

A more pronounced variation of theca-lutein hyperplasia is *nodular theca-lutein hyperplasia of pregnancy* (NTLHP) (Fig. 22.21).[20–22] NTLHP is characterized by conspicuous expansion of the follicular structures, which coalesce into confluent nodules. These nodules appear to be made up of theca interna, the follicle centers of which are often obliterated by the proliferation of the lining cells. The theca cells are cohesive, but merge peripherally with luteinized cells that stream into the stroma. Whether the latter are derived from theca or stromal cells may be difficult to determine, but their more discohesive appearance and random distribution suggests a stromal origin.

The fate of the granulosa cells in these lesions varies. In most of the follicles undergoing replacement, the granulosa cells are inconspicuous. In others the precise distinction between theca interna and granulosa cells may be difficult to ascertain. The pathologist may initially believe that they are witnessing a granulosa cell proliferation, only to realize that the expanding population of luteinized cells is the only layer present, in which case the logical conclusion is that the granulosa cells have involuted. In others, follicles with preserved, expanded and partially luteinized granulosa cell hyperplasia are occasionally seen (Fig. 22.22).[23] More typically the granulosa cells are attenuated and inconspicuous; in some sites they are incorporated into luminal fibrin. In the latter, the proliferating luteinized theca cells re-populate the follicle surface and residual granulosa cells are present in small linear groups or horizontally arranged tubular structures.

The more extreme form of NTLHP is *pregnancy luteoma*. As strictly defined, pregnancy luteomas are characterized by expansile solitary brown to yellow tumors that displace the ovarian parenchyma (Fig. 22.23). These lesions differ from NTLHP by the greater extent of luteinized cell proliferation and plump, eosinophilic and often vacuolated cells that resemble stromal luteomas or unclassified steroid cell tumors (Fig. 22.24). Experts have traditionally argued that pregnancy luteoma is a more extreme variant of NTLHP and not a neoplasm, due principally to the

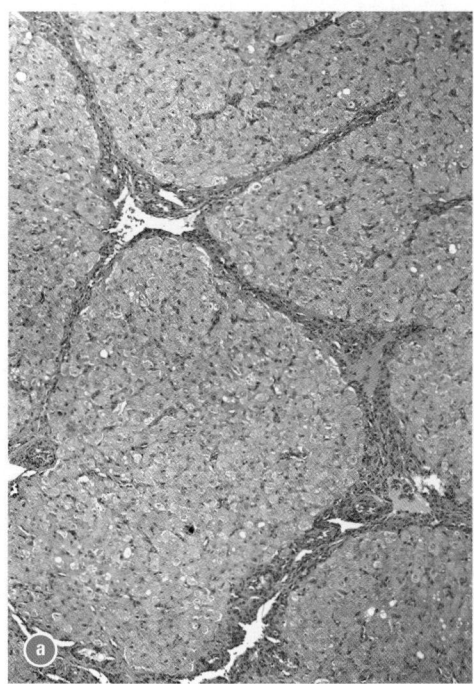
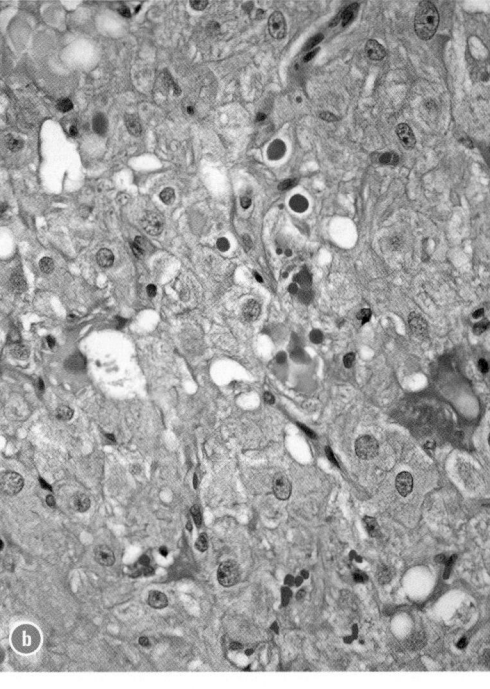

Fig. 22.19 Corpus luteum of pregnancy. (a) Low-power image with cerebriform contour. (b) At higher power the characteristic vacuoles and hyaline droplets are seen.

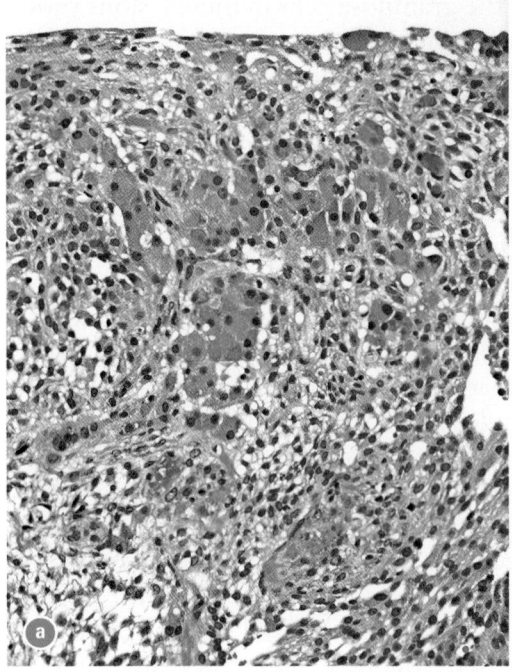

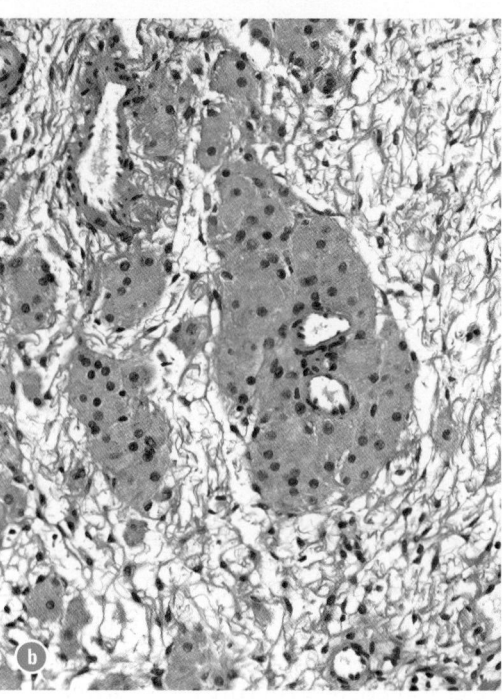

Fig. 22.20 Theca-lutein hyperplasia of pregnancy. (a) Prominent coalescing thecal and stromal luteinized cells. (b) Plump luteinized stromal cells.

tendency for these tumors to spontaneously regress following pregnancy. From a management perspective, this assumption is strongly encouraged, inasmuch as oophorectomy for such tumors should be avoided unless a period of post-partum observation has proven them to be persistent. However, because the hormonal environment that spawns these tumor-like lesions is similar to that seen at menopause (when other steroid-producing tumors develop), it is reasonable to assume that rare solitary luteomas of pregnancy are derived from a clonal population that has a growth advantage realized under the hormonal environment of pregnancy.[21]

Most patients with pregnancy luteoma have a history of multiple pregnancies and up to 80% of cases occur in black women.[21,22] The vast majority of the cases are asymptomatic and the tumor-like mass is incidentally found during prenatal ultrasonographic examination or Cesarean section. However, occasionally the mass may

Fig. 22.1 Nodular theca-lutein hyperplasia of pregnancy, characterized by microscopic nodular aggregates of hyperplastic thecal cells.

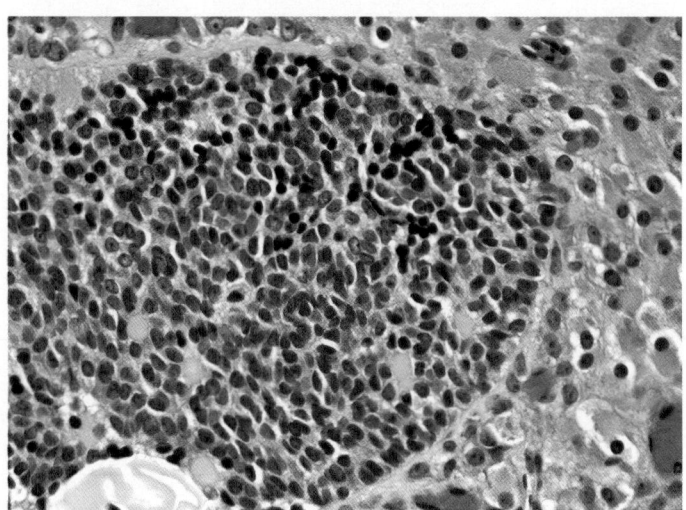

Fig. 22.22 Granulosa cell proliferation in the ovary during pregnancy.

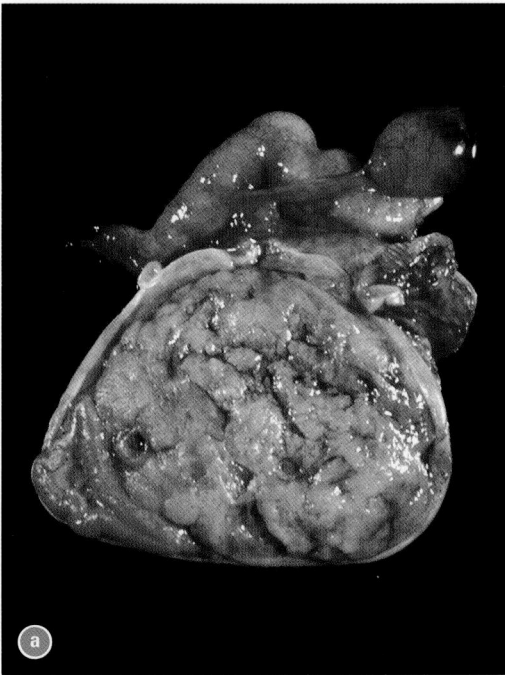

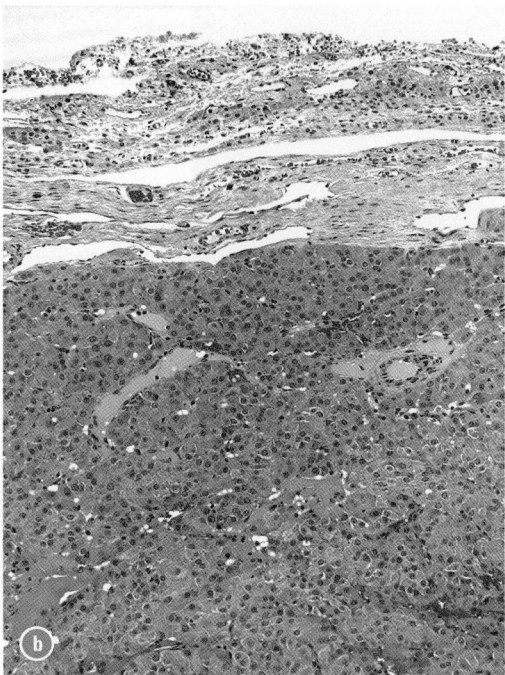

Fig. 22.23 (a) Pregnancy luteoma, manifesting as a dominant ovarian mass in this pregnant patient. (b) Low power of interface between pregnancy luteoma and the ovarian stroma (upper).

grow to a large size and/or is hormonally active leading to virilization of the mother. Rarely, the elevated levels of testosterone may also affect female fetuses, which may also show signs of virilization at birth.[24–29] Hormonal abnormalities in patients with 'pregnancy luteoma' include elevated levels of testosterone, which is seen in most of the patients regardless of the symptomatology.

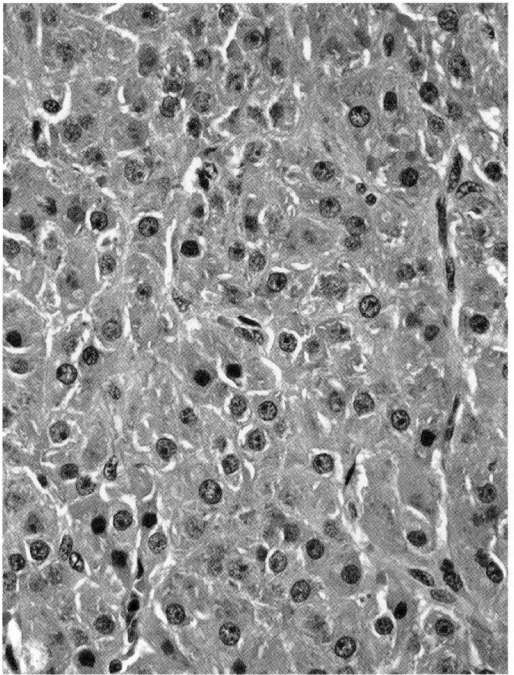

Fig. 22.24 Microscopic view of pregnancy luteoma. The lesion is indistinguishable from a steroid-producing tumor (see Ch. 30).

The differential diagnosis of NTLHP and pregnancy luteoma includes metastatic carcinoma, metastatic melanoma and primary ovarian tumors such as luteinized thecoma, especially on gross examination of the resection specimen. Immunoperoxidase studies in association with a history of pregnancy are the most useful tools in making this differentiation. Carcinomas will be easily differentiated during microscopic examination. In addition, carcinomas will be positive for keratins and the pattern of staining for cytokeratins 7 and 20, in association with other markers (i.e. thyroid transcription factor-1 or CDX-2), can help in the localization of the primary tumor. Amelanotic malignant melanoma can be morphologically very similar to luteoma of pregnancy. It is positive for S-100 protein and other melanocytic markers: such as HMB-45 and Melan-A. Luteoma of pregnancy may be positive for Melan-A and inhibin, but other epithelial and melanocytic markers are negative.[30] As mentioned above, the outcome of pregnancy luteoma is uneventful and the tumor-like mass will typically regress post-partum.[31]

HYPERREACTIO LUTEINALIS

Hyperreactio luteinalis (HRL) is another pregnancy-related ovarian lesion in which numerous follicle cysts are the major manifestation rather than the luteinized thecal-stromal cell expansion of NTLHP (Fig. 22.25). It is associated with physiologic and pathologic states

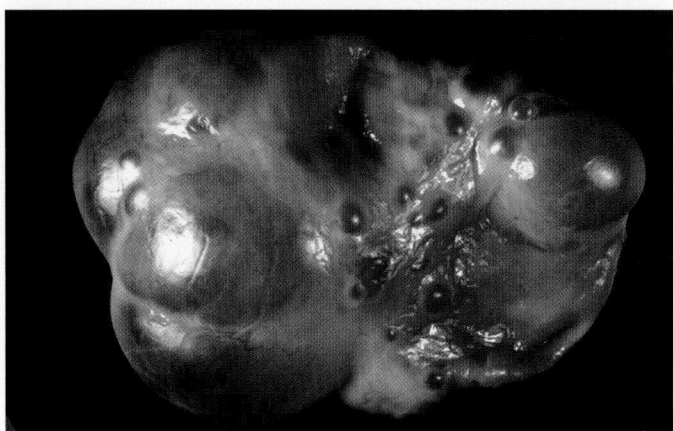

Fig. 22.25 *Hyperreactio luteinalis.* The characteristic features are bilateral expansion of the ovaries by multiple cysts.

of hyperstimulation of the ovaries, such as pregnancies (especially multiple pregnancies), gestational trophoblastic disease and treatment for ovulation induction.[32,33] In all these conditions, ovarian exposure to endogenous or exogenous production of human chorionic gonadotropin (hCG) is present and is believed to be pivotal in the pathogenesis of this condition.

Like other forms of TLHP, HRL may be clinically apparent, may form a palpable mass, may be encountered during a Cesarean section procedure or visualized during ultrasonography examination.[32,34] Pelvic pain, torsion or rupture of cysts with intrapelvic hemor-

rhage can occur but is uncommon.[32] In a smaller percentage of cases, virilization of the mother can be observed.[35]

Grossly, the adnexa are characterized by bilateral cystic expansion of the ovaries by numerous small multiloculated thin-walled cysts (Fig. 22.25). A layer of granulosa cells and a second layer of luteinized theca cells line the cystic cavities (Fig. 22.26). Edema of the ovarian substance can be quite prominent. The principal exclusion is a cystic ovarian neoplasm. Microscopic examination allows immediate discrimination between these two conditions.

The natural history of this condition is post-partum regression of the cysts; however, this process of involution may take up to 6 months.[36] When it is associated with hemorrhage or torsion, surgical removal may be necessary. However, the obstetrician should be aware of this benign condition, particularly in the settings of hydatidiform mole and twin pregnancy, and exercise discretion, particularly when faced with bilateral cystic ovaries.

SOLITARY LUTEINIZED FOLLICLE CYST

Solitary luteinized follicle cyst is a benign condition that affects pregnant females or appears during puerperium. In most cases, the cyst is an incidental finding during Cesarean section or physical or ultrasonographic examination; however, its large dimension may cause

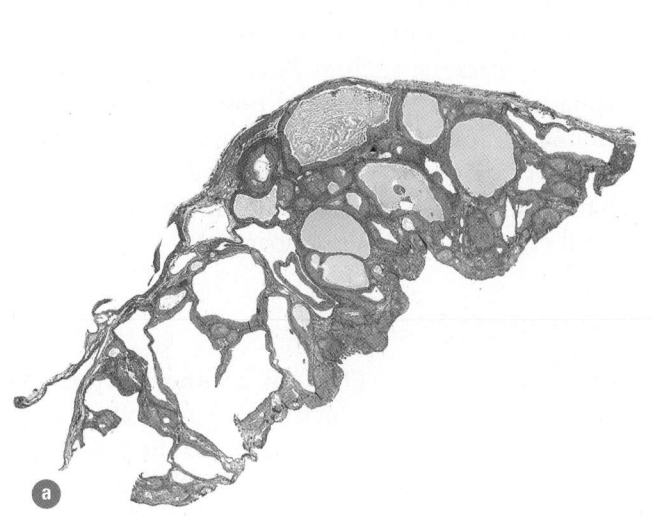

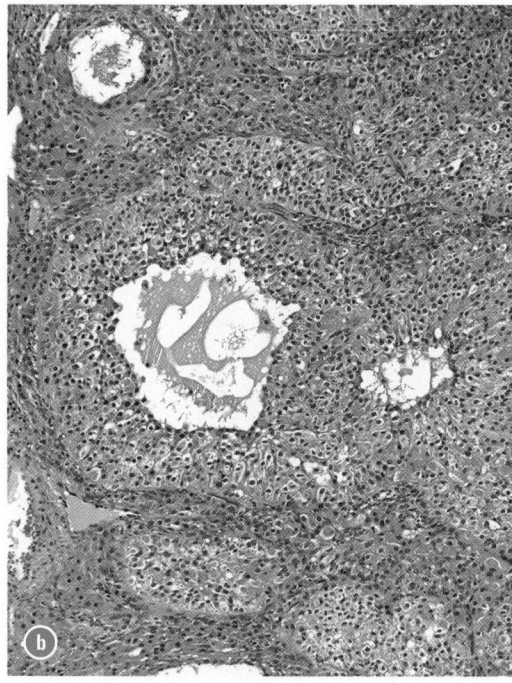

Fig. 22.26 *Hyperreactio luteinalis.* (a) Low-power microphotograph depicts multiple cystic follicles. (b) The follicles are lined by luteinized cells.

an increase in the abdominal size. In the largest series, none of the patients showed hormonal deregulation.[37]

Solitary luteinized follicle cyst is a unilateral, uniloculated cystic mass filled with thin watery fluid. Its median size is of 25 cm in one series.[37] Microscopically, the cyst is lined by luteinized granulosa and theca cells, which show abundant eosinophilic, occasionally vacuolated, cytoplasm and large, hyperchromatic, focally pleomorphic nuclei (Fig. 22.27). Mitoses are absent.

The differentiation between solitary luteinized follicle cyst and a cystic ovarian tumor can be difficult given the amount of nuclear atypia; however, the low nuclear/cytoplasmic ratio, sporadic atypia, absence of mitotic activity, awareness of this entity and clinical setting will minimize the risk of a misdiagnosis.

DECIDUOSIS (ECTOPIC DECIDUA)

Ectopic decidua of the ovary is a common finding during pregnancy and is often present on the ovarian surface and within the ovarian cortex. It is a physiologic response of celomic mesenchyme to increased levels of progesterone during pregnancy or exogenous administration. Ovarian ectopic decidua is an incidental finding in the vast majority of cases.

Macroscopically, ectopic decidua is seen as a tan or red spot on the ovarian surface. At microscopic examination, the cells of ectopic decidua are similar to the cells of decidualized endometrium. The cells form

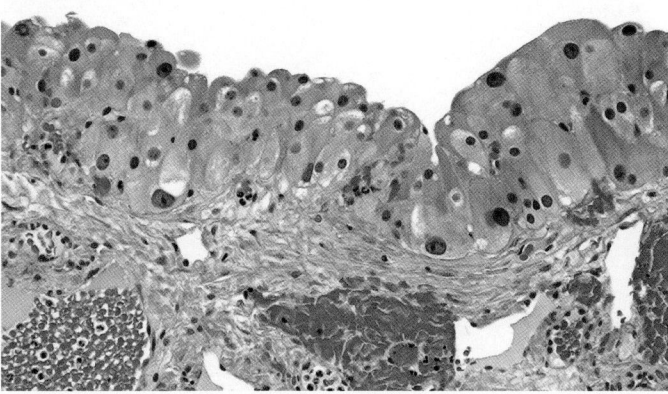

Fig. 22.27 Solitary luteinized follicle cyst of pregnancy. The luteinized lining cells exhibit focal atypia. Similar luteinized cysts may be seen in non-pregnant women.

sheets of large polygonal cells with sharp cell borders, round, centrally placed nuclei, vesicular chromatin, small nucleoli and abundant pale eosinophilic cytoplasm. Occasionally, intercellular edema is conspicuous. Involvement of para-ovarian adhesions and peritoneal surfaces is also common (Fig. 22.28a,b).

In extra-ovarian sites, deciduosis may be mistaken for neoplasms, including mesothelioma (see Ch. 23). This diagnostic error is unlikely in the ovary. Although decidualized endometrium cysts may occasionally be misdiagnosed as neoplasms on ultrasound. The

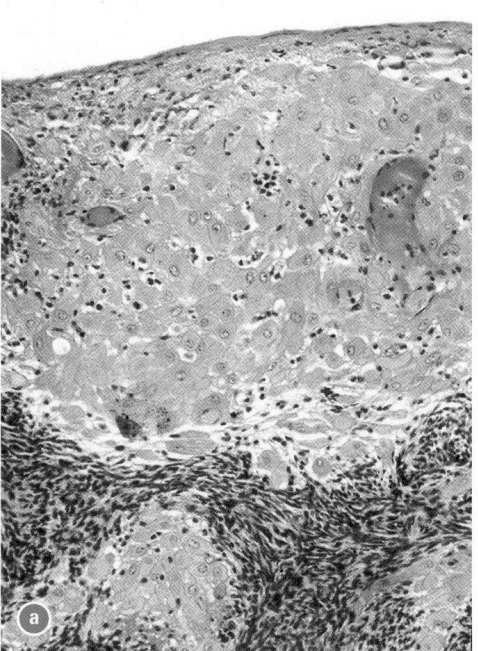
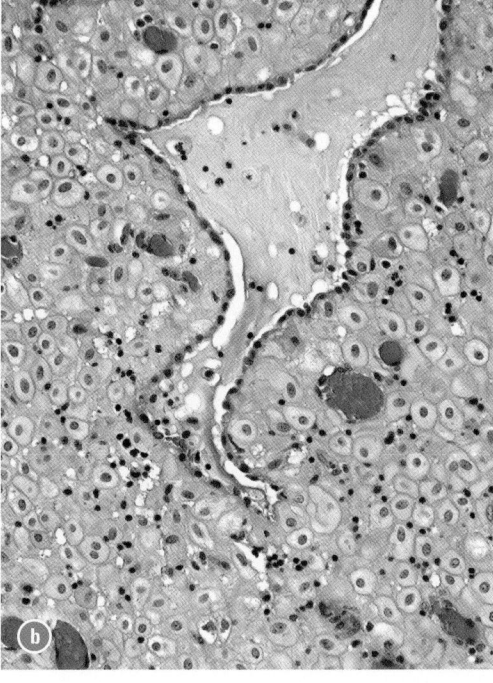

Fig. 22.28 (a) Deciduosis involving the ovarian surface. (b) Involvement of adhesions.

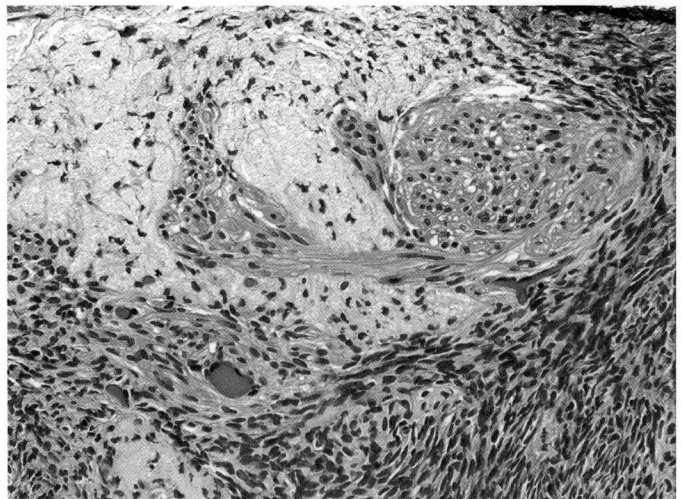

Fig. 22.29 Smooth muscle metaplasia of the ovarian cortex may mimic deciduosis.

principal differential in the ovary is smooth muscle metaplasia (Fig. 22.29).

Conditions associated with clinical infertility

INTRODUCTION

About 12% to 14% of couples are unable to conceive following 1 year of intercourse without contraception. This is attributed to male (30%), female (35%), both (20%) and unknown causes (15%).[38] The most common factors in the woman, in descending order, are ovulatory dysfunction (40%), tubal and pelvic pathology (including endometriosis) (Chs 21 and 23), unexplained (10%) and unusual causes (10%) (Table 22.2). This discussion will address those conditions involving the ovary *per se*. The pathologist is unlikely to receive many ovarian biopsies in the course of an infertility work-up, due largely to the decreasing role of ovarian

Table 22.2 Causes of infertility[38]

Attributed to	(%)	Live births (%)
Ovulation disorders	17.6	41.5
Tubal disease	23.1	21.8
Endometriosis	6.6	6.6
Male factors	16.8	29.8
Unexplained	25.6	32.2
LPD[a], uterine, cervix causes	3.2	41.4

[a]LPD, luteal phase defect.

morphology in the management of this wide array of disorders. Although Stein–Leventhal syndrome (polycystic ovarian syndrome) was previously managed by ovarian wedge biopsy, non-invasive medical treatments are the first line in management. Ovarian biopsy has been proposed in some cases of infertility to ascertain oocyte reserve, but its advantage over biochemical assays is debated.[39,40]

PREMATURE OVARIAN FAILURE

The two major causes of infertility that are attributed to alterations in oocyte development and ovulation are premature ovarian failure (POF) and polycystic ovarian syndrome (PCOS; see below). Menopause typically occurs at a mean age of 51 in Western society, with over 95% occurring between ages 40 and 54. The 5% that fall between age 40 and 45 are termed 'early menopause' and the term 'premature ovarian failure' is reserved for the 1% who enter menopause under age 40 (Table 22.3).[41] Despite the term, POF is not synonymous with permanent sterility, as pregnancies have been documented in a minority of patients.[42] Approximately 5–10% of young women with a diagnosis of POF will eventually become pregnant spontaneously.[43]

POF has been attributed to a variety of causes, including genetic, autoimmune and others, including chemotherapy or radiation therapy and unknown. Premature menopause segregates to some families, supporting a genetic basis for some. Two functioning

Table 22.3 Premature ovarian failure[41]

Genetic
  Familial ovarian failure
  Structural alterations or absence of X chromosome
  Excess of X chromosomes
  Myotonical dystrophica
Enzymatic defects
  17 alpha-hydroxylase deficiency
  Galactosemia
Physical
  Ionizing radiation
  Chemotherapy (alkylating)
  Viral (mumps)
  Cigarette smoking
Immune disturbances
  In association with other autoimmune disorders
  Isolated
  Congenital thymic aplasia
Defects in gonadotropin structure and function
  Abnormal molecular forms of gonadotropin
  Gonadotropin receptor or postreceptor defects
  Circulating FSH-binding inhibitors
Idiopathic

X chromosomes are required to maintain fertility and the most graphic example of genetically programmed ovarian failure is Turner's syndrome, which results in loss of ovarian function prior to menarche. Partial X deletions and fragile X syndrome produce lesser defects. Recently, functional loss of the forkhead transcription factor FOXO3A was shown to precipitate premature ovarian failure in mice, presumably via premature activation and rapid exhaustion of the follicular reserve.[44] Mutation in the FOXL2 gene, another transcription factor, has been implicated in the blepharophimosis-ptosis-epicanthus-inversus syndrome, which is associated with POF. However, neither gene is implicated in cases of POF that are not syndromic.[45] In other studies, women with early menopause are more likely to possess the PVUII polymorphic allele for estrogen receptor alpha. Transgenic murine knockouts of FSH receptor genes, including heterozygous FSH receptor and follistatin knockouts, precipitate ovarian failure.[46]

All of the above avenues of investigation, while providing insights to critical mechanisms involved in ovulation, have not yet divined the pathogenesis of premature menopause in the majority of affected women. Nevertheless, some investigators believe that the genes regulating early (age 40–45) menopause in families are linked to those seen in sporadic cases of POF. If this is the case, studies of kindreds may be useful, either to identify common linkages/polymorphisms or provide common genetic templates to which candidate genes can be referenced.[47]

AUTOIMMUNE DISORDERS AND AUTOIMMUNE OOPHORITIS

The patient at risk and pathogenesis

Approximately 10% of cases of POF are associated with an immune mechanism, which can be appreciated on both a clinical and pathologic level. There is a strong association between ovarian failure and *autoimmune endocrine disease*.[48–50] A wide range of autoimmune disorders, including hypoadrenalism, ITP, hypothyroidism, collagen vascular disease, polyendocrinopathies and others are associated with POF. The relationship between certain autoimmune disorders, such as Addison's disease and POF suggest a causal connection in these patients, including the presence of autoantibodies to steroid-producing cells, shared autoantigens between adrenal and ovarian steroid-producing cells, lymphoplasmacytic infiltrates around ovarian follicles and corpora lutea, and animal models supporting this syndrome (Fig. 22.30). An autoimmune mechanism

for infertility in patients without these other disorders is proposed based on studies of cellular immunity, but less well supported on histologic grounds; less than 3% of the latter have the morphologic correlate of autoimmune ovarian disease – perifollicular lymphoplasmacytic infiltrates – however, it is likely that follicle depletion can occur by immune mechanisms without evidence of conspicuous inflammation.[49]

One presumed mechanism for autoimmune POF is the presence of autoantibodies, which react both against steroid-producing cells (StCA) in adrenal glands and gonad. This has been demonstrated in the polyglandular syndrome, from which antigens have been identified that permit clinicians to predict the development of hypogonadotropic hypogonadism.[50,51] The principal antigens in StCA are P450scc and P450c17. P450c17 is present both in gonads and adrenal glands.[49] Mouse models of the disease permit organ specific autoimmunity following postnatal thymectomy, which is characterized by a reduction in natural killer cell activity and a persistent Th2 response similar to that in the polyglandular type 1 failure in humans.[52] Others have shown no association between MHC genes and autoimmune oophoritis.[53]

Clinical presentation

Autoimmune oophoritis usually presents with symptoms of hypergonadotropic ovarian failure, such as premature menopause, amenorrhea and infertility.[54] Women with autoimmune POF may have had prior successful pregnancies and typically present with secondary infertility or amenorrhea. In other cases, those with polyglandular syndrome, particularly in premenarchal girls, the ovaries cease to function prior to the first menstrual cycle, producing primary amenorrhea. However, in a minority of cases it is an unexpected finding in oophorectomy specimens for other endometrial and/or ovarian pathology.[55] Laboratory studies will often confirm the presence of anti-ovarian autoantibodies. As noted above, some will manifest evidence of other autoimmune diseases, such as Addison's disease or Hashimoto's thyroiditis.

Pathology

Macroscopically, the affected ovaries may be normal is size or enlarged by cystic follicles.[53] On microscopic examination there is a prominent lymphoplasmacytic infiltrate in the ovaries affecting mainly primary and secondary follicle, and corpora lutea (Fig. 22.30). In others eosinophils may be conspicuous; in rare cases a granulomatous infiltrate is present. There is charac-

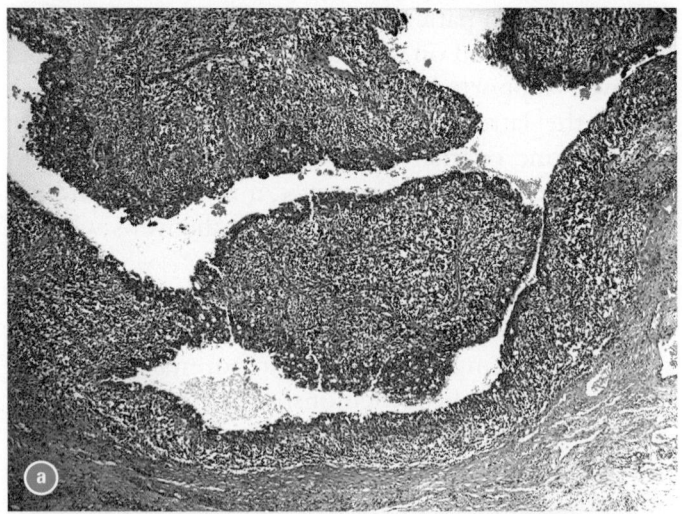

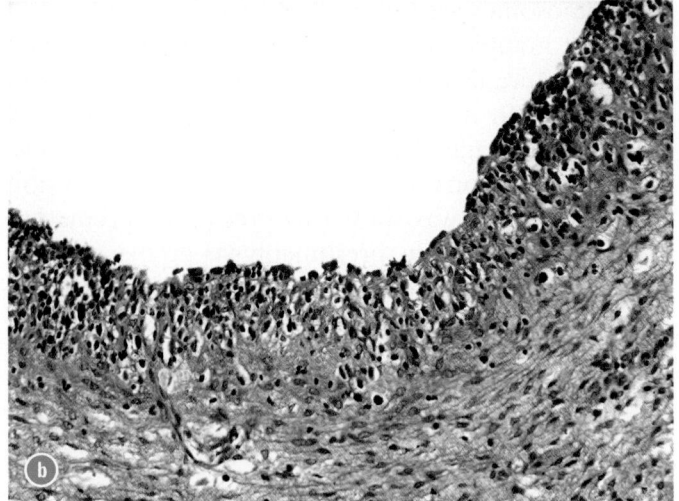

Fig. 22.30 Autoimmune oophoritis. (a) Intense infiltrates in the wall of a cystic follicle. (b) Higher power of follicle lining with lymphocytes. (c) Involvement of both a corpus luteum (left) and follicle (right).

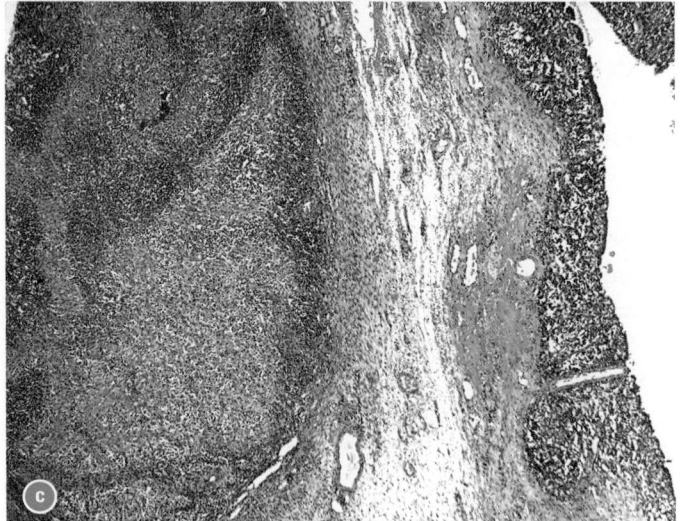

teristic sparing of the primordial follicles with the infiltrates concentrated in mature follicles and in some, corpora lutea.[53] Immunohistochemical studies of the infiltrating lymphocytes have shown a mixture of B and T cells (including CD4+ and CD8+ cells). Perivascular and perineurial chronic inflammatory infiltrates have also been noted.[53]

Differential diagnosis

Other inflammatory conditions, such as acute and chronic salpingo-oophoritis, may produce infiltrates, but the perifollicular distribution is characteristic of autoimmune disease. Similarly, lymphomas of the ovary present with more diffusely distributed infiltrates.

Management

To date, there is no specific therapy for autoimmune oophoritis. Immunosuppression with corticosteroids has been used but not with consistent results and not without complications.[56,57] The prognosis is difficult to evaluate given the rarity of this condition, but some patients may resume normal menses after therapy.[56,57] However, given the fact that some cases spontaneously return to normal menses, cause and effect are difficult to demonstrate.

POLYCYSTIC OVARIAN SYNDROME (PCOS)

Definition and patient at risk

Polycystic ovarian syndrome (also called Stein–Leventhal syndrome) is the most common endocrine disorder of reproductive-age women and one of the most common causes of infertility. PCOS affects between 3–10% of reproductive-age women and possibly more, depending on the population and definitions used.[58,59] PCOS is defined clinically as two of the following three (Table 22.4): oligo- or anovulation; clinical and/or bio-

Table 22.4 *Revised diagnostic criteria of PCOS[59]*

Criteria (both 1 and 2)
1   Chronic anovulation
2   Clinical and/or biochemical signs of hyperandrogenism, and
     exclusion of other etiologies
Revised 2003 criteria (2 out of 3)
1   Oligo- and/or anovulation
2   Clinical and/or biochemical signs of hyperandrogenism
3   Polycystic ovaries and exclusion of other causes (congenital
     adrenal hyperplasias, androgen-secreting tumors, Cushing's
     syndrome)

chemical signs of hyperandrogenism; and polycystic ovaries, exclusion of other entities.[60] Two additional clinical findings that are common if not required are obesity and insulin resistance, with or without clinical diabetes.[59]

Because most patients with the above characteristics have polycystic ovaries, newer definitions permit the diagnosis of PCOS in the presence of polycystic ovaries and either hyperandrogenism or oligo-ovulation. This is a recently approved change in classification and is warranted because while many more women have polycystic ovaries than the syndrome, many of these otherwise normal individuals will display metabolic alterations (albeit less pronounced) similar to those in PCOS. The disorder is classified as a syndrome and not a disease which can be sharply defined to the exclusion of its less severe forms.

Pathogenesis

The pathogenesis of PCOS is not clear and the search for a single initiating factor has parallels to that for toxemia of pregnancy. For example, the key components of PCOS – hyperandrogenism, sustained LH levels and hyperinsulinemia – are interrelated but neither constant nor co-dependent. For example, cultured theca cells from the ovaries of patients with PCOS generate 20-fold higher amounts of androstenedione than normal (Fig. 22.31).[61] This abnormality has not been conclusively identified as the primary cause of PCOS or linked to a specific genetic alteration to which the other components of the syndrome could be anchored. However, the gene encoding p450 (CYP11e) has been implicated by some.[62] The LH pulse amplitude remains high even when ovulation occurs, indicating abnormalities in the feedback mechanism for LH. Some consider hyperinsulinemia a primary causal factor. Others consider insulin resistance a secondary phenomenon associated with body fat distribution, attributing the latter to the abnormal hormonal environment. Analyses of genetic polymorphisms for many of these components have revealed potential targets, but no clear causative path. A recent hypothesis by Abbott et al. proposes that prenatal exposure to androgen excess (via a hyperandrogenic fetal ovary or adrenal) 're-programs' the hypothalamic–pituitary control of LH, permanently altering the ovarian–pituitary axis and explaining the emergence of the syndrome at an early age. Other studies have associated post-term birth or intrauterine growth restriction with PCOS later in life.[63,64]

Another syndrome emphasizing the complexities of insulin resistance, PCOS, and hyperthecosis is the hyperandrogenic-insulin-resistant-acanthosis nigricans

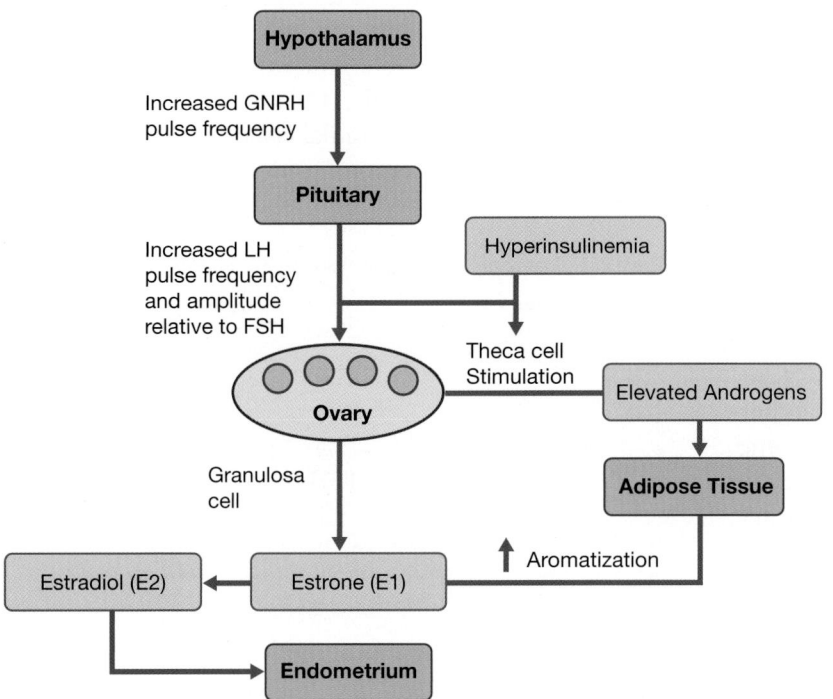

Fig. 22.31 Pathways involved in polycystic ovarian syndrome.

(HAIR-AN) syndrome. In the HAIR-AN syndrome, severe insulin resistance is associated with acanthosis nigricans, and ovarian androgen production is stimulated by hyperinsulinemia. Interestingly, the HAIR-AN syndrome can be subdivided into both insulin-resistant and non-resistant subsets: the former with PCOS and elevated LH, the latter with stromal hyperthecosis and near-normal LH levels.[65]

Familial clustering of cases have been observed, strongly suggesting a genetic basis for this disease; however, the specific mode of inheritance of this condition has not yet been determined.[66,67] No specific genetic abnormality has been shown to be the sole culprit in the development of PCOS, and it appears that this disease is probably a result of a variety of molecular alterations in different genes.[68–70] In addition to infertility, sequelae of this altered hormonal secretion include an increased risk of cardiovascular disease and abnormal lipid profiles.[66–68] A link to other disorders, including epilepsy, has been made in some cases.[71–74]

Clinical presentation and diagnosis

The central disturbance in PCOS is hypersecretion of androgens (hyperandrogenemia) and often, insulin (hyperinsulinemia).[75] The typical patient is in their third or fourth decade with anovulatory bleeding or secondary amenorrhea. Eighty percent present with hyperandrogenism (hirsutism) accompanied by obesity in 50%.[76]

A physical examination and a menstrual history will probably suffice, but the diagnosis is confirmed biochemically by increased serum total testosterone, DHEA sulfate and, in certain ethnic groups, 17-hydroxyprogesterone. Additional assays of fasting glucose, insulin and lipid profiles are often indicated.[77] Ultrasound evaluation of the ovaries is also recommended but not essential, as polycystic ovaries accompany other disorders such as eating disorders, increased output of adrenal androgen and hyperprolactinemia.[78] The ultrasound appearance of the ovary shows peripherally arranged cysts totaling 10 or more and not more than 10 mm in size, coupled with increase in central stroma (Fig. 22.32a).[79] The diagnosis requires that several other disorders be excluded that can cause similar clinical findings, including hyperthecosis (cortical stromal hyperplasia), congenital adrenal hyperplasia, 21-hydroxylase deficiency, Cushing's syndrome, and androgen-producing neoplasms (Sertoli–Leydig cell tumor, steroid-producing tumors of the ovary; Ch. 30).[77]

PCOS overlaps with a disorder termed *the metabolic syndrome*, featuring obesity, insulin resistance and dys-lipidemia, raising concerns about the risk of cardiovascular disease in these patients (Table 22.5).[80,81]

Treatment

PCOS is managed by a variety of means designed to counteract the hyperandrogenism, hyperinsulinemia and infertility. The first is addressed with weight loss and oral contraceptive therapy. Management of hyperinsulinemia is achieved with medications facilitating insulin metabolism, such as metformin. Ovulation induction with clomiphene is the initial therapy for infertile patients.[82] Significant weight loss is estimated to restore menses in nearly 90%, with resulting pregnancy in 30%.[83] Clomiphene is associated with successful ovulation in up to 80%, with pregnancy in up to 50%. In clomiphene-resistant patients, the addition of metformin will produce pregnancy in approximately 25%. Another option for drug-resistant women is ovarian surgery, which has its roots in the early studies of wedge resection for Stein–Leventhal syndrome.[84] With the advent of laparoscopy, more conservative management, including ovarian puncture (drilling), is currently used, with electrocoagulation slightly more effective than laser.[84] From 56 to 94% of patients are clomiphene citrate-resistant ovulate after ovarian puncture (drilling), and at least half of them have become pregnant, particularly those who are younger with a lower body mass index.[85]

Pathology

The pathologist will usually encounter the polycystic ovary in routine hysterectomy specimens or in unusual circumstances when the organ is removed to control the hyperandrogenism. Macroscopically, the ovary of patients is enlarged and smooth, with small bluish-appearing translucences signifying subsurface cortical cystic follicles (Fig. 22.32b). On sectioning, the follicles are typically arranged in a radial fashion along the cortex with 1–2 mm of intervening dense fibrotic stroma

Table 22.5 *Criteria for the metabolic syndrome in women with PCOS[59]*

	Risk factor	Cut-off
1	Abdominal obesity (waist circumference)	>88 cm (>35 in)
2	Triglycerides	150 mg/dl
3	HDL-C	<50 mg/dl
4	Blood pressure	130/85 mmHg
5	Fasting and 2h glucose from OGTT	110–126 mg/dl and/or 2h glucose 140–199 mg/dl

Three out of five qualify for the syndrome.
HDL-C, high-density lipoprotein-cholesterol; OGTT, oral glucose tolerance test.
© European Society of Human Reproduction and Embryology.

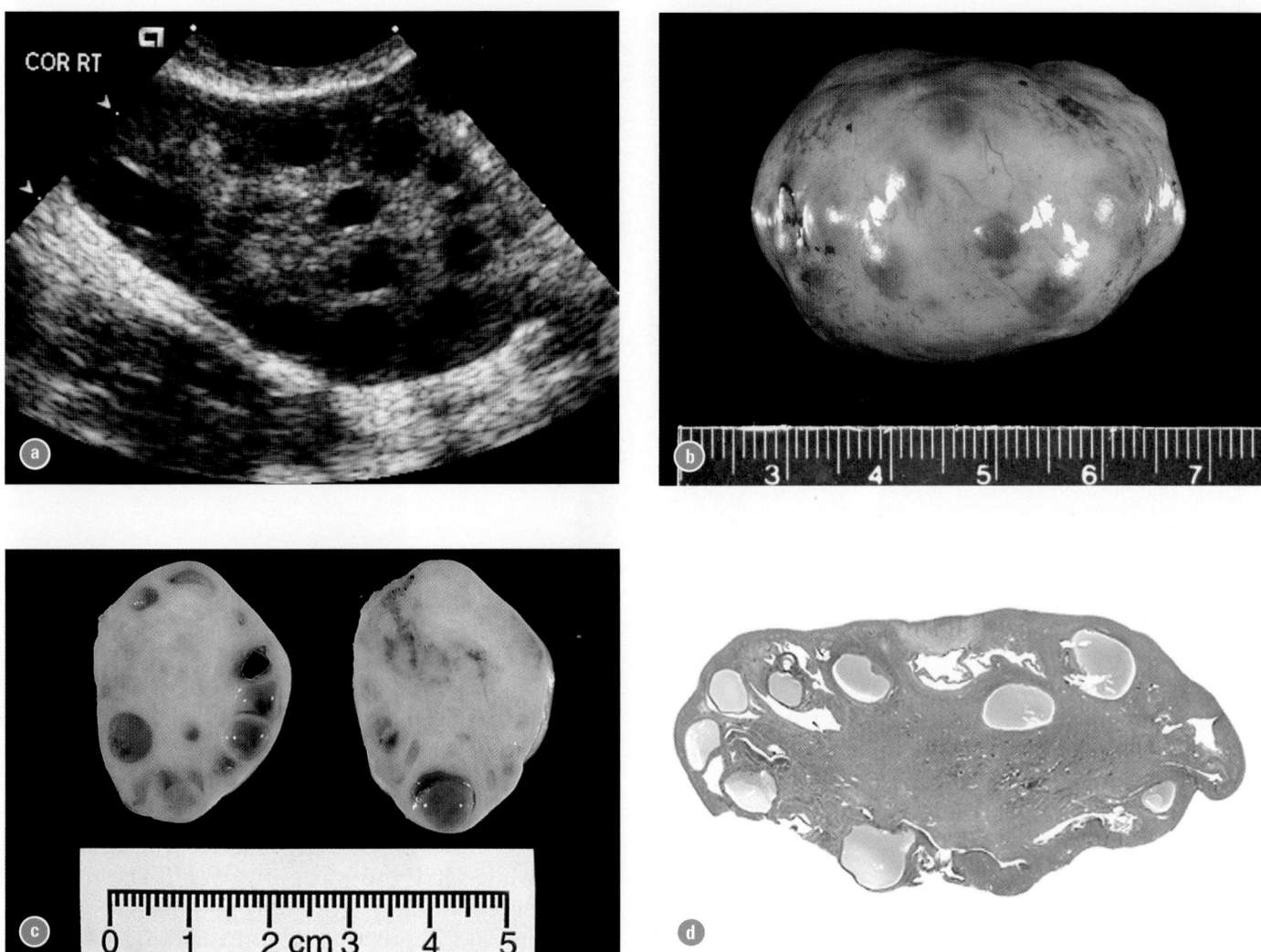

Fig. 22.32 (a) Ultrasound of polycystic ovaries depicting numerous cysts. (b) Gross appearance of polycystic ovaries. (Courtesy of Carol Benson, MD, Brigham and Women's Hospital). Numerous follicles can be appreciated beneath the capsule. (c) Cross-section of (b) illustrates subcortical cystic follicles. (d) Low-power microphotograph exhibits combination of cystic follicles and fibrotic ovarian cortex.

(Fig. 22.32c,d). The classic histologic hallmarks include the following: (1) increased ovarian size (two-fold), including thickness of cortical and subcortical stroma; (2) thickened collagenized tunica (Fig. 22.33a); (3) normal numbers of primordial follicles; (4) twice the expected number of ripening and atretic follicles; and (5) multiple cystic follicles (1–2 mm) with luteinized theca layer (theca-lutein hyperplasia) (Fig. 22.33b). The increased numbers of follicles presumably ensue from biochemical disturbances that promote the excess recruitment of small follicles without emergence of a dominant follicle, coupled with accelerated follicle atresia (Fig. 22.33c).

Additional findings include minimal evidence of ovulation, in the form of recent or degenerating corpora lutea, and increased numbers of hilus cells. However, because it is a disease of variable severity, these findings will vary in their severity and evidence of ovulation does not exclude the diagnosis of PCOS.[86]

In a subset of ovaries from patients with PCOS, stromal hyperplasia with luteinized stromal cells (hyperthecosis) is also present. Luteinized hilus cells may also be present. The coexistence of both follicular and stromal changes warrants a diagnosis of a mixed hyperthecosis.

Other genital tract pathology

Apart from the endocrine and cardiovascular effects of PCOS, these patients have a four-fold increased risk of endometrial neoplasia (see Chs 17 and 19), which

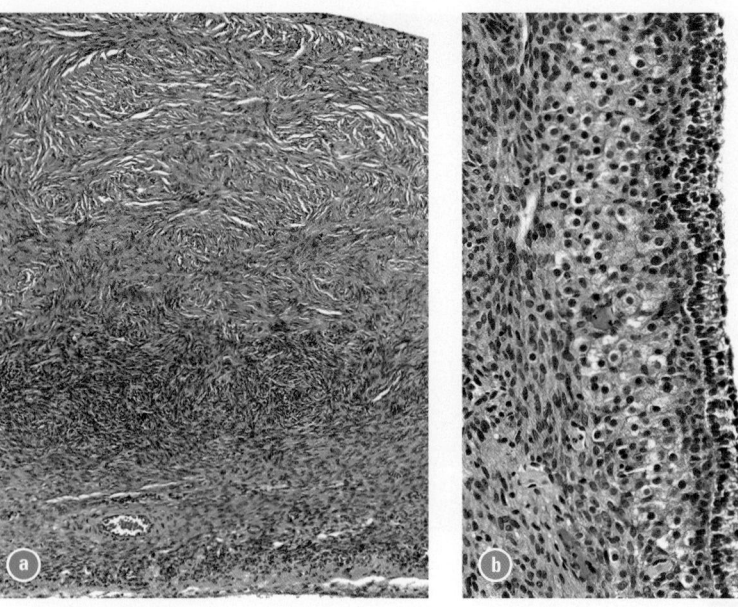
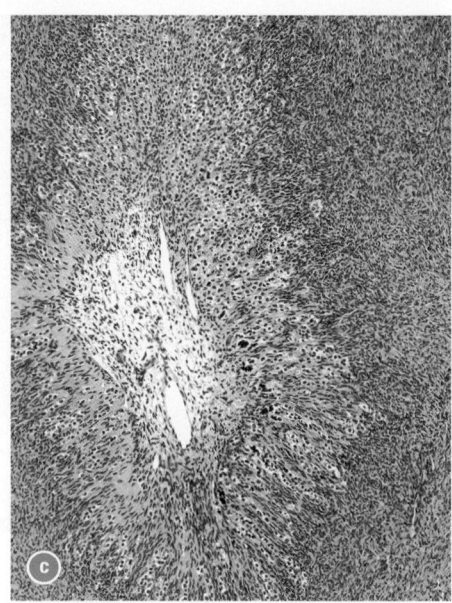

Fig. 22.33 Microscopic features of polycystic ovaries. (a) Collagenized tunica. (b) Theca-lutein hyperplasia in a cystic follicle. (c) Atretic follicle with residual theca-lutein hyperplasia.

occurs in from 5% to 10% of cases. Predictably, the endometrial lesions fall into the more type I (endometrioid) category, including endometrial intraepithelial neoplasia and endometrial adenocarcinoma (Fig. 22.34a,b). The mortality from endometrial cancer for this group is low.

ENDOMETRIOSIS

Risk factors and pathogenesis

Endometriosis is relatively common in the ovary, as is endometriosis of the fallopian tube, peritoneum and cul de sac, and may be asymptomatic. The incidence of endometriosis in asymptomatic women undergoing tubal ligation was 3.7% in one study.[87] Factors associated with an increased risk for endometriosis included advanced age, Asian race, long cycle length, one live birth, use of IUCDs, uninterrupted menstrual cycles, while OCP use was protective.[87] The relationship between various factors and endometriosis appears to be site and depth specific. In one study, ovarian, peritoneal and rectovaginal endometriotic lesions were compared by morphology, morphometry and histochemistry.[88] They found a similarity between eutopic

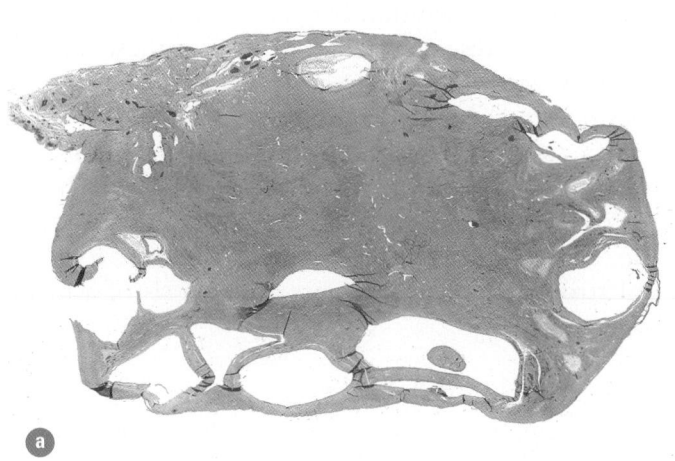
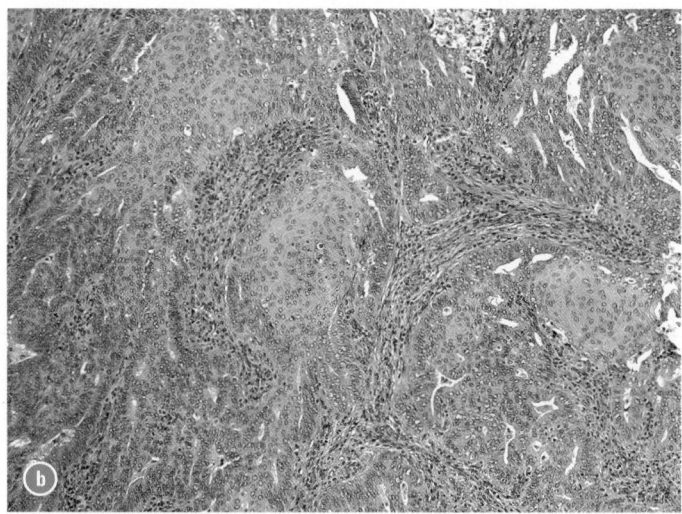

Fig. 22.34 (a) Low-power photomicrograph of polycystic ovary. (b) Coexisting well-differentiated endometrial adenocarcinoma.

endometrium and red peritoneal lesions, suggesting that the latter are the first stage of early implantation of endometrial glands and stroma. In contrast, recto-vaginal endometriotic nodules were classified as adeno-myomas, consisting of smooth muscle with active glandular epithelium and minimal endometrial stroma.[88] The pathogenesis of ovarian endometriomas remains controversial, with a persisting debate over whether these lesions are derived from endometrial tissue or via metaplasia of the ovarian surface epithelium.[89]

Two features distinguish endometriosis from normal endometrium: (1) endometriosis is considered a clonal event and (2) it produces its own estrogen via aromatase activity.[90,91] Aromatase regulates estrogen formation in tissues and is not detected in normal endometrium. In contrast, aromatase is expressed aberrantly in endome-triosis and is stimulated by PGE2. Moreover, not only is the endometriotic stroma a ready source of its own stimulatory hormone, it is deficient in 17beta-hydroxysteroid dehydrogenase (17beta-HSD) type 2 expression required for inactivation of estradiol. This explains both the autonomous behavior of endome-triosis and its response to aromatase inhibitors.

Relationship to infertility

The relationship between even endometriosis and infer-tility is clear in severe cases in which anatomic distortion caused by adhesions and endometriosis leads to infer-tility. In milder cases, the connection between the two is more obscure. Approximately one-quarter of women in their fourth and fifth decades have endometriosis and half of these are infertile.[92] Fertilization rates are reduced by about one-fourth over controls, even following FSH and hCG stimulation. A slight reduction in implantation rate has also been demonstrated. This has been correlated with disturbances in reductions in circulating estradiol concentrations and LH surge, possibly linked to altered follicular function.[93]

Pathology

Endometriosis is manifest in three often coexisting patterns. The most conspicuous is the endometriotic cyst, which is discussed below under benign ovarian masses. The second is surface endometriosis, in which endometrial stroma and /or glands are admixed with adhesions, hemosiderin-laden macrophages and reactive mesothelial cells on the ovarian surface. The amount of stroma varies according to the age of the lesion. Early lesions contain recognizable stroma and glands; older lesions contain minimal stroma or are limited to cuboidal to columnar epithelium with subjacent hemosiderin-

laden macrophages. As in other sites (Chs 21 and 23), the diagnosis of endometriosis requires one of the following combinations: endometrial stroma or Müllerian epithelium and old hemorrhage (hemosiderin). Frequently, the pathologist will encounter hemosiderin-laden macrophages on the ovarian surface, within adhesions. This finding alone is not diagnostic of endometriosis, but should be mentioned in the diagnostic report.

The third form of ovarian endometriosis is cortical endometriosis, arguably the most problematic form of the disease. Cortical endometriosis may be classic, with discrete clusters of small gland and variable stroma and/or hemosiderin (Figs 22.35, 22.36). However, in some cases, the pathologist may not be able to ascertain with certainty whether the glands signify endometriosis or cortical inclusion cysts of generic Müllerian epithelium. This is due in part to the fact that immunostains directed against endometrial stroma (CD10) often reveal a narrow rim of positive stroma around these glands. Whether this CD10-positive stroma signifies induction of endometrial stromal differentiation from the ovarian cortex, or residual endometrial stroma carried with the glands from the uterine lining is not clear. Suffice it to say that the spectrum of epithelial changes containing cortical inclusion cysts, endosalpingiosis and endometriosis includes a subset that cannot be readily assigned to one of these categories (Fig. 22.37).

The perimenopausal and postmenopausal ovary

Physiologic menopause is defined as a period in women's life marked by a natural and permanent cessation of

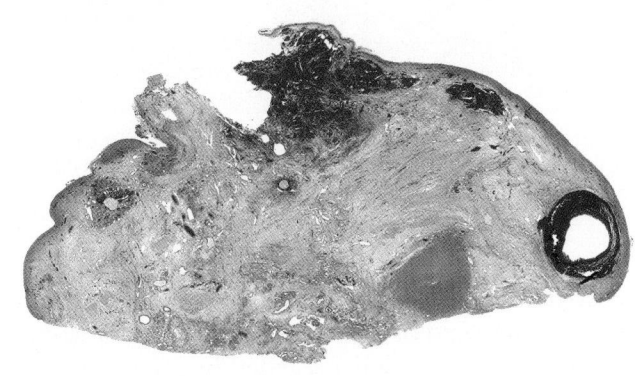

Fig. 22.35 Low-power image of an ovary with surface (center) and intraparenchymal (left) endometriosis.

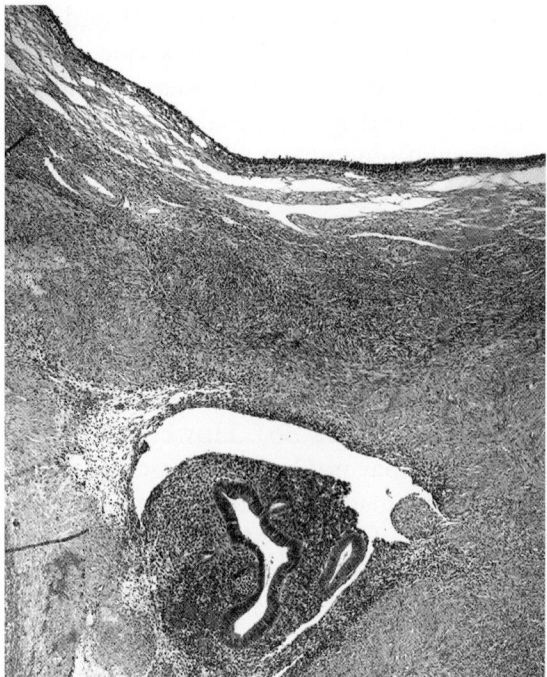

Fig. 22.36 Focus of intraparenchymal endometriosis adjacent to a cystic follicle.

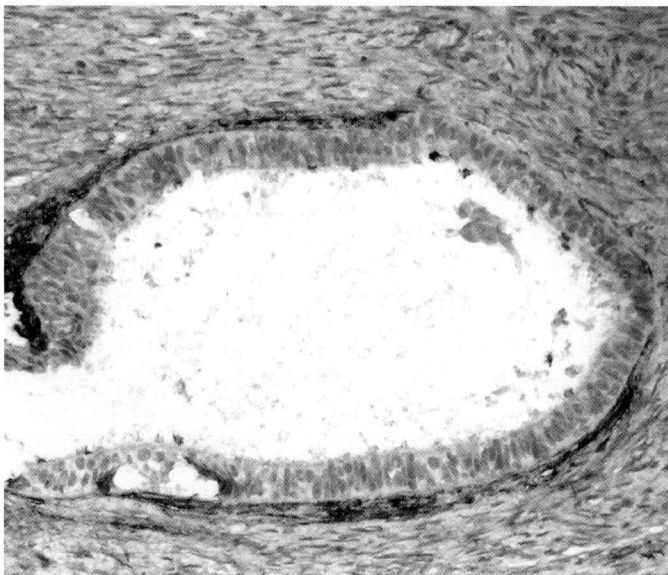

Fig. 22.37 Cortical inclusion cyst with prominent staining for CD10. While not specific for endometriosis, the presence of CD10 staining suggests that CICs and endometriotic glands share morphologic features.

menstruation, absence of ovarian function, and, therefore, marks the end of the reproductive phase of women's life. This event is usually preceded by an interval (premenopause) that is characterized by irregularity of the menstrual cycle and climacteric symptoms, namely, hot flushes, external genitalia dryness and headache.

Menopause can also be artificially or iatrogenically induced, such as consequence of oophorectomy, radiation therapy, oophoritis, etc. In the latter case, climacteric systemic symptoms may also be present, since these are result of the decreased availability of the ovarian hormones. The average age of physiologic menopause in the USA is 51 years of age; however, great individual variability can be appreciated. Apart from benign and malignant neoplasms seen in menopausal women, the most common patterns include the following.

ATROPHY

Atrophy of the ovary is characterized by the contraction of the ovarian cortex, the development of a convoluted cortical surface and progressive reduction in the amount of cortical stroma. This process begins prior to the cessation of ovulation and can be appreciated in ovaries removed during the fifth decade. As the cortex contracts, the vessels in the medulla and hilus become pronounced. Corpora albicantia, which are customarily inconspicuous in the reproductive-age ovary, typically occupy a large percentage of the ovarian volume, lying just beneath the cortex. These structures become less prominent over time and by the seventh decade the ovary is reduced to less than one-third of its premenopausal volume, consisting of a fibrotic cortex with variable amounts of recognizable stroma, overlying the vascular and sclerotic medulla (Fig. 22.38).

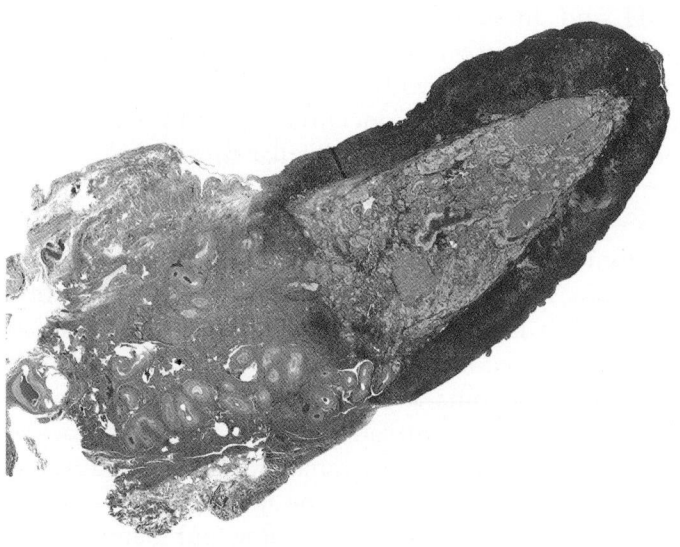

Fig. 22.38 Ovarian atrophy, characterized by marked contraction of the ovarian cortex, accentuating the distinction between cortex and medulla.

Because the cortex is condensed and convoluted, the relative amounts of cortex and medulla are best appreciated in cross section similar to the cuts on a loaf of bread. If the ovary is bivalved longitudinally and the cortex is over-represented in the section, the abundance of stroma may be misinterpreted as cortical stromal hyperplasia.

STROMAL HYPERPLASIA

Definition and patient at risk

Stromal hyperplasia (SH) is defined as an expansion of the cortex and medulla of the ovary by an excess of stromal cells. Stromal hyperthecosis is characterized by the presence of luteinized stromal cells, usually in the presence of a variable degree of stromal hyperplasia. Although the distinction between stromal hyperplasia and hyperthecosis is based on the presence of luteinized stromal cells in the latter, careful inspection of the cortices of ovaries with stromal hyperplasia will often reveal luteinized cells. Thus, the two entities are likely components of a morphologic continuum.

Most patients with these conditions are approaching, in or just beyond menopause. Less commonly are cases of pronounced hyperthecosis that are similar in presentation to, often overlap with, and are considered part of the spectrum of PCOS. Presumably, the ovarian stroma is stimulated by the sustained levels of gonadotropins that characterize menopause. The spectrum of changes that result include stromal hyperplasia and hilus cell hyperplasia. A logical extension of this dynamic is proliferation of fibroblasts, commonly seen in these ovaries, and fibromas.

Clinical features

The majority of patients with cortical stromal hyperplasia are asymptomatic. However, two subsets of patients deserve mention. The first is a small group that present with evidence of androgen excess and virilization. The second and more common group suffers from hyperestrogenic sequelae, specifically abnormal bleeding, endometrial intraepithelial neoplasia and endometrial adenocarcinoma. Predictably, some of these patients display evidence of obesity and adult-onset diabetes mellitus.[94]

Pathology

The hallmark of stromal hyperplasia is uniform expansion of both ovaries. The cortical convolutions that typify atrophy are less conspicuous, the cortical surface is more uniform and smooth in texture, and the ovary varies from the size of a normal reproductive age ovary to

approximately two-fold. To the trained eye, this appearance will immediately distinguish most cases of stromal hyperplasia from atrophy. On sectioning, the surface will vary from a mild increase in representation of the ovarian cortex, with a nodular consistency, to a conspicuous homogeneous tan to a brown surface with a firm to soft texture (Fig. 22.39a).

At low power, the usually condensed cortex of atrophy is not seen, and the medulla and hilus are less conspicuous (Fig. 22.39b). Rather, a variable amount of stroma in a faintly nodular pattern occupies most of the ovary. In extreme examples, the entire ovary is expanded by this cortical proliferation. The color will vary from basophilic when the nuclear density is high and collagen is inconspicuous, to a paler or eosinophilic appearance. At high power, the nodules are characterized by a proliferation of spindle-shaped stromal cells with overlapping, elongated nuclei, inconspicuous nucleoli and scant cytoplasm, identical to the cells that compose the ovarian cortex. Little admixed stromal collagen is present (Fig. 22.39c). Mitoses are not common.

Treatment

Most cases are diagnosed as incidental findings during oophorectomy performed for other reasons. Cases associated with endocrine manifestations require medical and, possibly, surgical intervention; however, given the rarity of this finding, little data exist regarding therapeutic options.

STROMAL HYPERTHECOSIS

Epidemiology

In contrast to cortical stromal hyperplasia, in stromal hyperthecosis the stromal proliferation is accompanied by a proliferation of luteinized cells. Most of the patients diagnosed with stromal hyperthecosis are more likely to be premenopausal. Both hyperthecosis and stromal hyperplasia are less common as a function of increasing number of years postmenopause.[95,96]

Clinical features

Stromal hyperthecosis is among the most common benign causes of virilization. In addition, it is associated with obesity, hypertension, acanthosis nigricans and decreased glucose tolerance.[97,98] Other manifestations such as ascitis and pleural effusions (Meigs' syndrome) have rarely been described in patients with stromal hyperthecosis.[95] The main laboratory finding in patients with stromal hyperthecosis is an increased plasma level of testosterone.[99,100]

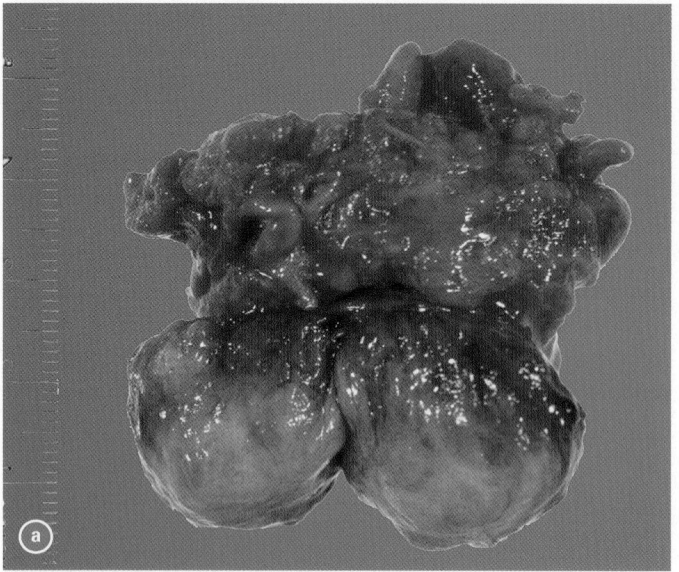

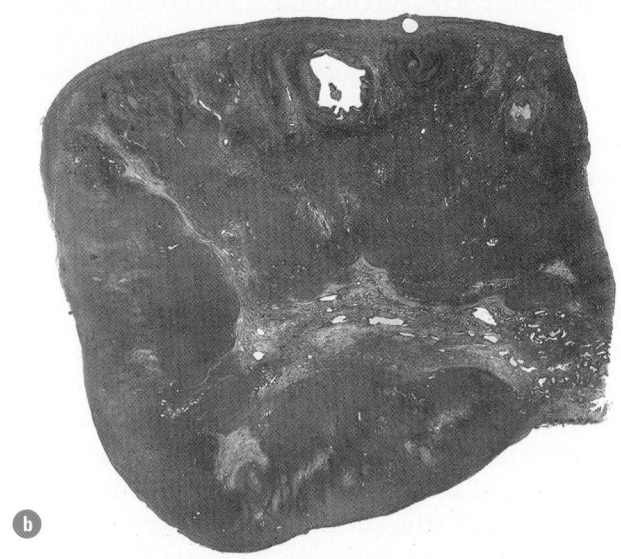

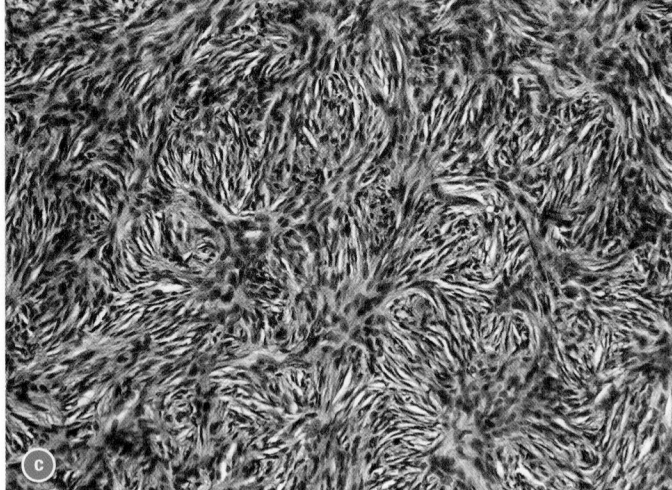

Fig. 22.39 (a) Gross appearance of stromal hyperplasia (SH), seen here as up to 2-fold enlargement of the ovary with a tan to yellow appearance.
(b) Low-power photomicrograph of SH, showing expanded cortical stroma.
(c) The dense stroma in SH is indistinguishable from that seen in the atrophic ovary.

Pathology

Both ovaries are usually affected in stromal hyperthecosis and bilateral enlargement of the ovaries is usually observed. The cut surface of the ovaries shows tan or yellow firm stroma (Fig. 22.40a). Microscopically, ovaries affected by stromal hyperthecosis reveals a hyperplastic stroma with admixed luteinized cells. The hyperplastic stroma is microscopically identical to the stroma seen in cortical stromal hyperplasia. The luteinized cells are usually found singly or arranged in small groups or nests, and are characterized by large cells with vacuolated or clear abundant cytoplasm, central small nuclei and conspicuous nucleoli (Fig. 22.40b,c). Occasionally, residual follicles are noted. Similar to pregnancy, stromal proliferations may distinguish themselves apart, giving rise to luteomas.[101]

In less than 10% of cases, there is a coexisting well-differentiated endometrial adenocarcinoma (Fig. 22.40d).

Treatment

Treatment of hyperthecosis centers on counteracting the androgenic effects of this disorder, including androgen inhibitors, desensitizers, DHT inhibitors, gonadotropin-releasing hormone (GnRH) agonists and oral contraceptives.

HILUS CELL HYPERPLASIA

Hilus cell hyperplasia is common at menopause or during pregnancy and is characterized by an expansion of the hilus cell population. Presumably, this occurs as

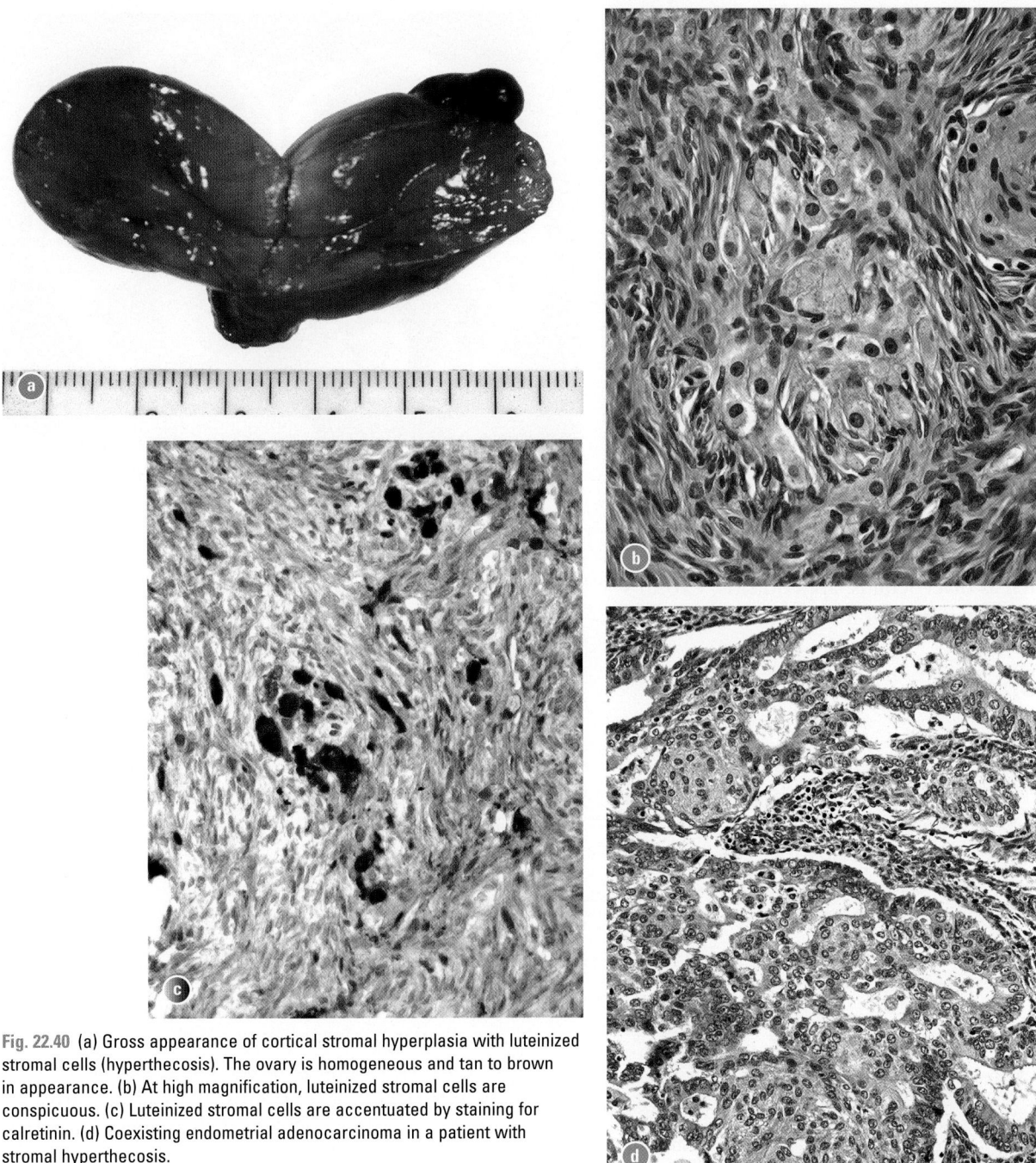

Fig. 22.40 (a) Gross appearance of cortical stromal hyperplasia with luteinized stromal cells (hyperthecosis). The ovary is homogeneous and tan to brown in appearance. (b) At high magnification, luteinized stromal cells are conspicuous. (c) Luteinized stromal cells are accentuated by staining for calretinin. (d) Coexisting endometrial adenocarcinoma in a patient with stromal hyperthecosis.

a generalized stromal response to an altered pituitary–ovary hormonal axis; it often accompanies both cortical stromal hyperplasia, hyperthecosis and cortical fibroma (Fig. 22.41). The differential diagnosis of hilus cell hyperplasia includes hilus cell tumors, which are distinguished by the formation of a mass lesion. Ectopic adrenal may be considered if the cells contain marked vacuoles; however, this entity is never reported in the ovarian hilus (see Ch. 21). Metastatic lobular breast carcinoma is similar in appearance, and might confuse the unwary in the appropriate setting and clinical history.

CORTICAL FIBROMATOSIS

Some degree of cortical stromal proliferation accompanies the entire spectrum of polycystic ovaries, stromal hyperthecosis, stromal hyperplasia and cortical fibromas.

The ovarian cortex is occasionally expanded (but not altered structurally) by a prominent fibrotic process in which the more closely packed stromal cells are replaced by a fibrocyte-like proliferation with abundant collagen. In pure form (as opposed to the fibrotic changes seen in these other entities) it is rare, and seen in the menopausal ovary.

Infections of the ovary

INFECTIOUS SALPINGO-OOPHORITIS

Acute and/or chronic oophoritis is normally seen under two circumstances. The first is a common feature of infectious salpingitis (see Ch. 21), and may manifest as a suppurative inflammation with abscess formation, terminating in extensive tubo-ovarian adhesions (Fig. 22.42). The second is a consequence of infections of a more remote origin such as diverticulitis, appendicitis, Crohn's disease or other intraperitoneal inflammatory process.

TUBERCULOSIS

Epidemiology

Genital involvement by tuberculosis is rare, accounting for approximately 1–2% of all case of tuberculosis.[102] In one series, secondary involvement of genital organs by this infection was seen in up to 60% of patients with pulmonary tuberculosis.[103] Most patients diagnosed with genital tuberculosis are young (mean age 30.4 years).[102]

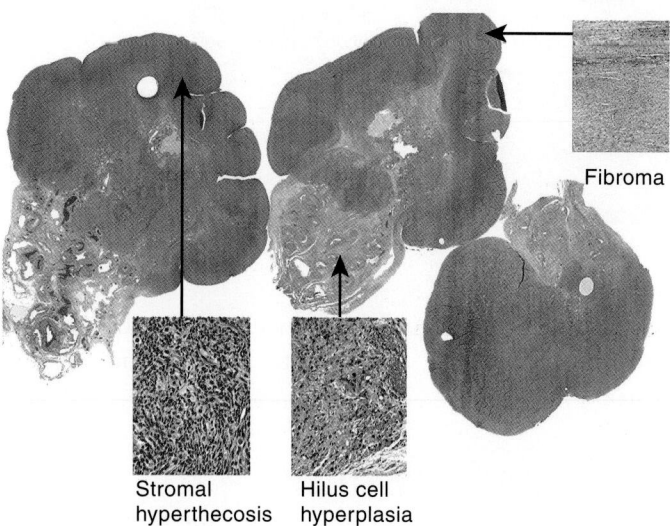

Fig. 22.41 Coordinated hyperplasia of steroid-producing cells is common in the menopausal ovary, often including (a) microscopic cortical fibroma or localized fibromatosis, (b) luteinized stromal cells and (c) hilar cell hyperplasia.

Stromal hyperthecosis

Hilus cell hyperplasia

Fibroma

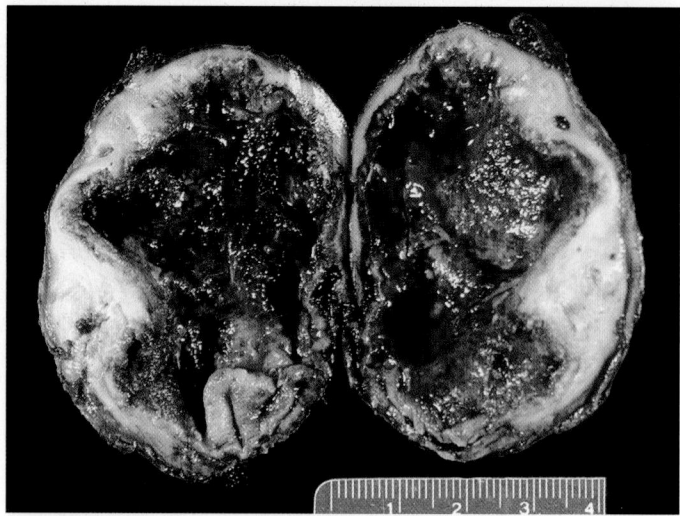

Fig. 22.42 Ovarian abscess, characterized by an irregular fibrous wall with central necrosis and hemorrhage.

In the largest series of genital tuberculosis, the ovaries were involved by the infection in about 13% of the cases, behind endometrial (72%) and fallopian tube (34%) tuberculosis.[103] Cervical tuberculosis was seen in 2.4% of cases.[102]

Clinical features

Most patients (75%) are diagnosed with genital tuberculosis at the time of gynecologic work-up for infertility. Occasionally, these patients will seek medical attention due to abdominal or pelvic pain.[102]

Pathology

Macroscopically, there is often an obliteration of the anatomic relationship between the ovary and fallopian tube fimbria. The histologic findings of genital tuberculosis are similar to those seen elsewhere in the body. Formation of caseating granulomata with a rim of palisading histiocytes should automatically be studied with stains for acid-fast bacilli as well as silver stains for fungal organisms (Fig. 22.43). Granulomata may not be well formed in patients with acquired immunodeficiency syndrome (AIDS). These small organisms may be difficult to visualize and staining of multiple tissue sections may be necessary. In addition, submission of a representative fragment of fresh tissue to microbiologic cultures and/or polymerase chain reaction (PCR) studies may be helpful for the diagnosis and further sub-speciation of the organism.

Treatment

The treatment of genital tuberculosis should follow the guidelines of the World Health Organization (WHO).

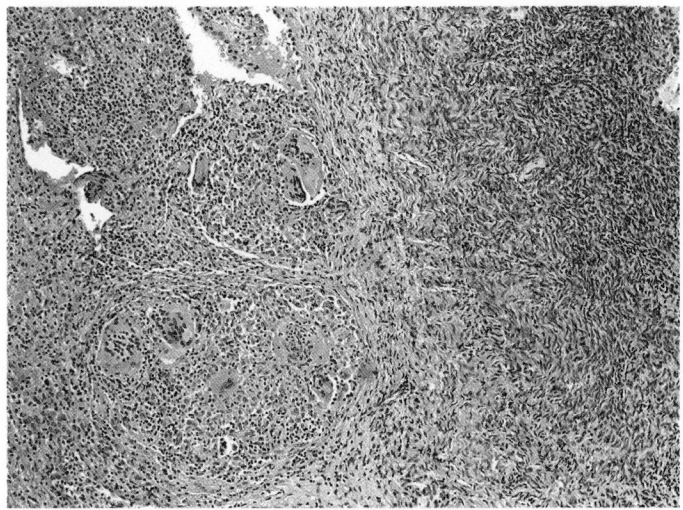
Fig. 22.43 Tuberculosis of the ovary. At the left is a granuloma with giant cells.

There are few data, however, on patients' outcome and future fertility in patients with genital tuberculosis.

Benign conditions producing ovarian enlargement

A variety of benign conditions cause ovarian enlargement and, in some instances, might be confused with neoplasia. These are detailed in Table 22.6 and discussed below.

FOLLICLE CYST

Follicle cysts are defined as functional cysts that exceed 2 cm in diameter. They are most commonly encountered clinically on physical examination in reproductive-

Table 22.6 *Non-neoplastic causes of ovarian enlargement in the non-pregnant patient*

Functional
  Hemorrhagic corpus luteum
  Follicle cyst
  Cortical stromal hyperplasia (hyperthecosis)
  Polycystic ovarian syndrome
Mesothelial/Müllerian
  Endometriotic cyst
  Xanthomatous pseudotumor
  Cystic adhesions/cystic mesothelioma
  Simple cyst
Vascular
  Ovarian torsion/infarction
  Massive ovarian edema

age women and are not usually removed unless persistent. They may develop *de novo*, or as a consequence of gonadotropin administration, and during pregnancy. Because these cysts are typically benign appearing on ultrasound (Fig. 22.44a,b), they are managed with attention to ovarian preservation. The most common approach is aspiration cytology.[104] Mulvany noted that aspiration cytology was highly specific for a diagnosis but had a sensitivity of only 83% for neoplasia (Fig. 22.44c).[105] In an analysis of 151 aspirated cysts analyzed by cytology and histology, the same authors identified follicle cysts in one-third, and 90% had E2 content >20 nmol/l. Some 99% of the non-follicular cystic lesions had E2 levels under 20 nmol/l. Progesterone content did not distinguish the two groups.[106]

The characteristic histologic features of follicle cyst are of a cyst that exceeds 2 cm in diameter, lined by attenuated granulosa cell and a theca layer with variable luteinization (Fig. 22.44d).

ENDOMETRIOTIC CYST

Definition and clinical significance

Endometriotic cysts (endometriomas or 'chocolate cysts') are an extreme form of endometriosis, by which one (usually) or more cysts are formed leading to ovarian enlargement. Endometriotic cysts are among the more common causes of ovarian enlargement in the fourth and fifth decades.[107,108] Excluding their association with endometriosis and infertility, the clinical importance of endometriotic cysts lies in the following, from the most to the least common:

1 Association with chronic hemorrhage, adhesions, tubo-ovarian adhesions and inflammation and pelvic pain. This constellation of features may result in a complex ovarian mass and necessitate surgery to exclude a neoplasm (Figs 22.45, 22.46).
2 Potential misclassification as a malignant tumor on ultrasound. This can rarely occur if the endometrial lining undergoes extensive decidual change, leading to a complex-appearing cyst on ultrasound evaluation (Fig. 22.47).
3 Association with malignancy. The risk of concomitant malignancy in an endometriotic cyst increases with age, and presents a diagnostic challenge during the intraoperative evaluation (see below and Chs 26 and 27).

Intraoperative evaluation

The gross examination of the endometriotic cyst typically takes place during surgery if the latter is performed

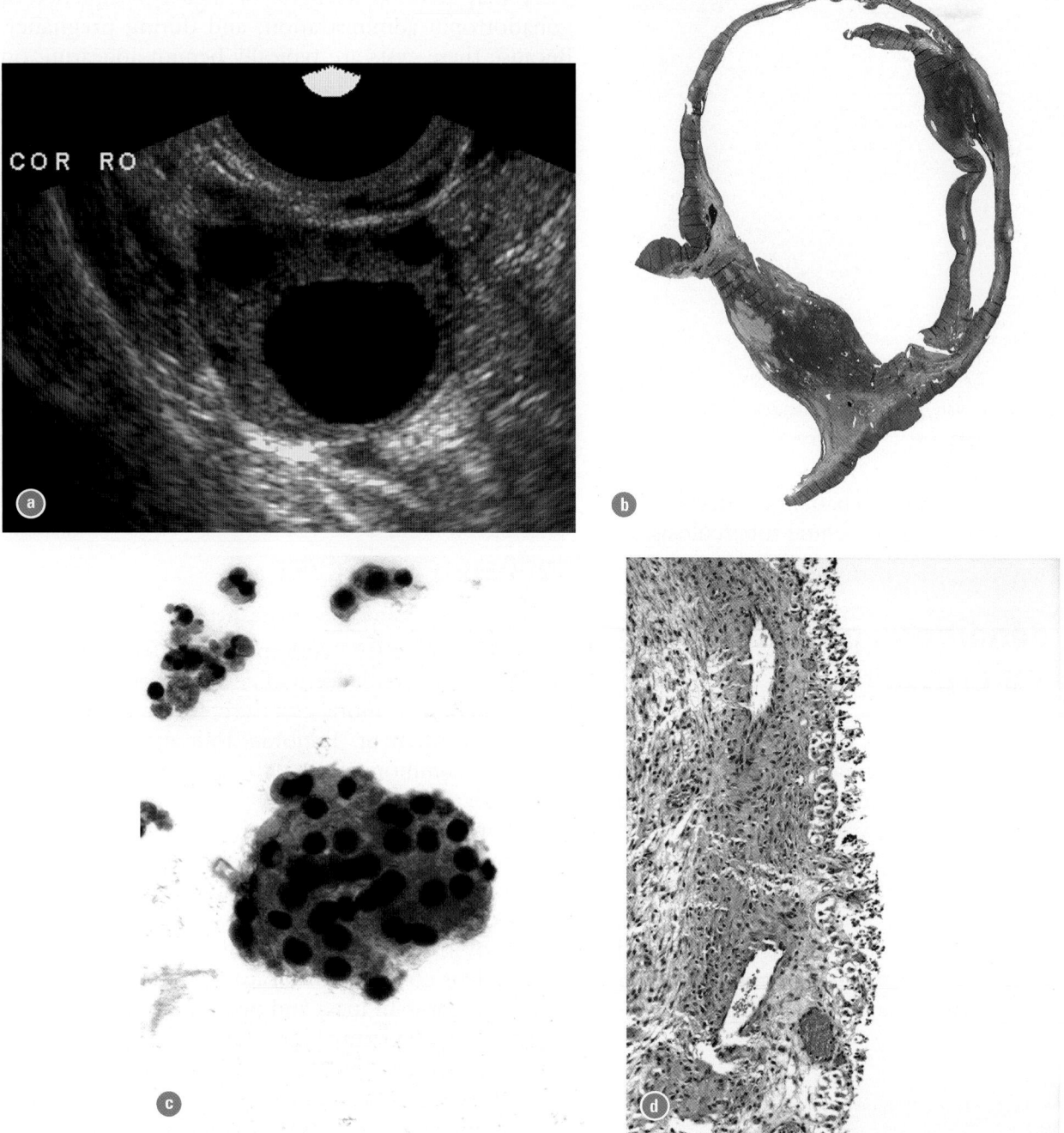

Fig. 22.44 (a) Ultrasound of a follicle cyst. (Courtesy of Carol Benson, MD, Brigham and Women's Hospital.) (b) Low-power image of a follicle cyst of the ovary. (c) Aspirate of cyst showing granulosa cells. (d) Histopathology of follicle cyst, with sparse granulosa cells and partially luteinized theca.

for an ovarian mass. These tumors can present in a variety of gross appearances. Endometriotic cysts range from a few millimeters to over 15 cm in diameter. The typical endometriotic cyst consists of a cyst of variable thickness containing old hemorrhage. The cyst wall may be smooth and glistening or thickened with a rough texture and patches of discoloration. The contents may be viscous and dark brown (chocolate cyst) or only slightly discolored and watery. In rare instances the lining may have a soft, cobblestone appearance if heavily decidualized (Figs 22.46–22.48).

The above descriptions apply to endometriotic cysts that are easily identified on gross examination. An equally common presentation is that of a complex cystic mass

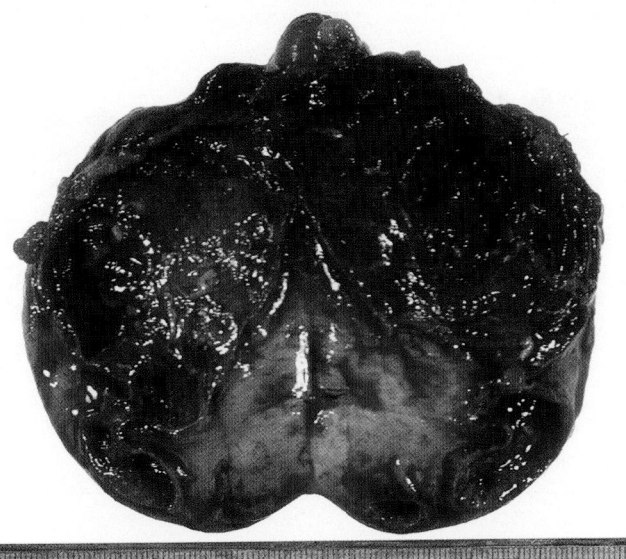

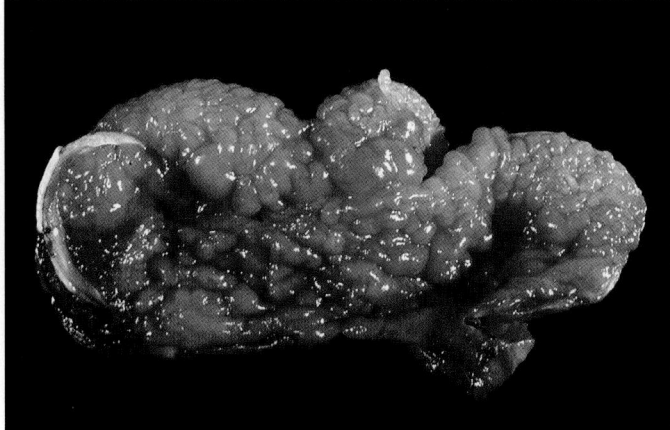

Fig. 22.47 Decidualized endometriotic cysts can be confused with a neoplasm on ultrasound or gross examination.

Fig. 22.45 Endometriotic cyst presents as an irregular cystic mass with dark hemorrhagic material.

composed of extensive adhesions and evidence of recent or old hemorrhage. This may present more of a challenge and requires judicious sampling to identify or exclude masses that might represent neoplasia. The latter may consist of an adenofibroma, Müllerian cystadenoma or, less commonly, carcinoma.

Microscopic evaluation

With the exception of the most thin-walled cysts, the surgeon and pathologist should consider a frozen section to exclude neoplasia. Several sections of the endometriotic cyst should be submitted to ensure representative sampling. The classic hallmarks of endometriotic cysts include endometrial glands, stroma and evidence of prior hemorrhage in stromal macrophages (hemosiderin) (Fig. 22.48). In actuality, the classic textbook presentation occurs in a minority, and the pathologist is faced with a fibrotic cyst wall of variable thickness with an ill-defined lining that is not readily oriented. In this setting the following patterns are common:

1 A nondescript lining with hemosiderin, macrophages and occasional Müllerian lining cells. Confirmation of the endometrioid origin of the cyst often requires a prolonged search for the combination of either Müllerian lining and hemosiderin,

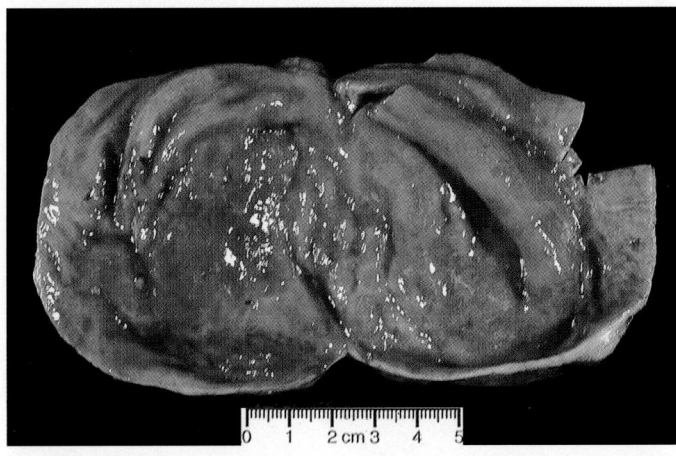

Fig. 22.46 Xanthomatous pseudocyst, consistent with an end-stage endometrioma. The lining is yellow, corresponding to the abundant xanthoma cells in the lining.

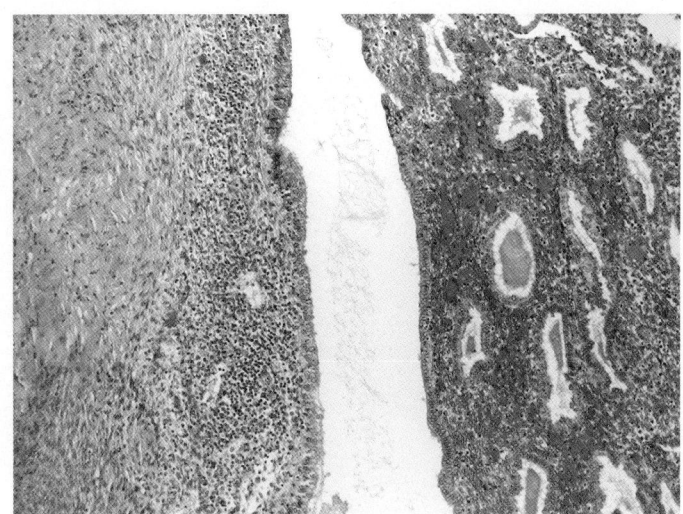

Fig. 22.48 Typical endometriotic cyst lining containing endometrial glands (right) or a more attenuated lining with sparse stroma (left).

or either with stroma. If epithelium and stroma cannot be identified, the term 'hemorrhagic cyst of undetermined origin' is permitted.

2 Prominent xanthoma cells, also referred to as xanthomatous pseudotumor. This process, when present in the ovary, is presumed to be late-stage endometriosis, in which glands and stroma are no longer identifiable and have been replaced by foamy macrophages (Fig. 22.49a).

3 Decidualized changes. These may be confused with either xanthomatous change or a corpus luteum (Fig. 22.49b,c)

4 Epithelial cell atypia, characterized by sporadic nuclear enlargement and hyperchromasia, with preservation of a low nuclear/cytoplasmic ratio. These ostensibly reactive epithelial changes have been discussed repeatedly in the literature and are not associated with risk of subsequent neoplasia. Similar changes may be encountered during pregnancy in the form of Arias-Stella reaction, with hyperchromatic, large nuclei (Fig. 22.50).[109,110] However, if the pathologist identifies atypia, he or she should submit additional tissue.

5 Metaplastic epithelial changes, most typically characterized by mucinous and/or ciliated metaplasia. These epithelial changes typically merge with more classic endometrioid lining epithelium and presumably signify the early stages of metaplastic transformation that characterize Müllerian cystadenomas (see Ch. 27)(Fig. 22.51).[111]

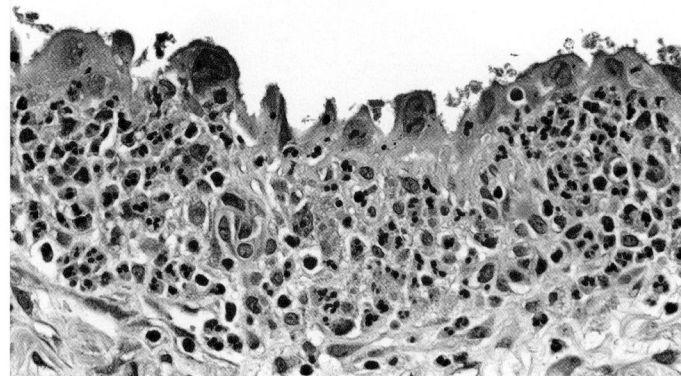

Fig. 22.50 Reactive atypia in an endometrioma.

6 Benign and malignant neoplasms, including adenofibroma and malignancies (Fig. 22.52).[112] (These are discussed further in Ch. 27.)

Management of endometriosis and endometriotic cyst

Endometriosis is usually managed medically with the intent to counteract the estrogenic environment. While oral contraceptives were a traditional mainstay in management, a wide range of drugs with a more narrow range of action are coming into use, including progesterone receptor modulators, GnRH antagonists, aromatase inhibitors and others. Surgery is reserved for severe disease, including ovarian masses (endometriotic cysts) and rectovaginal adenomyotic nodules.[113–116]

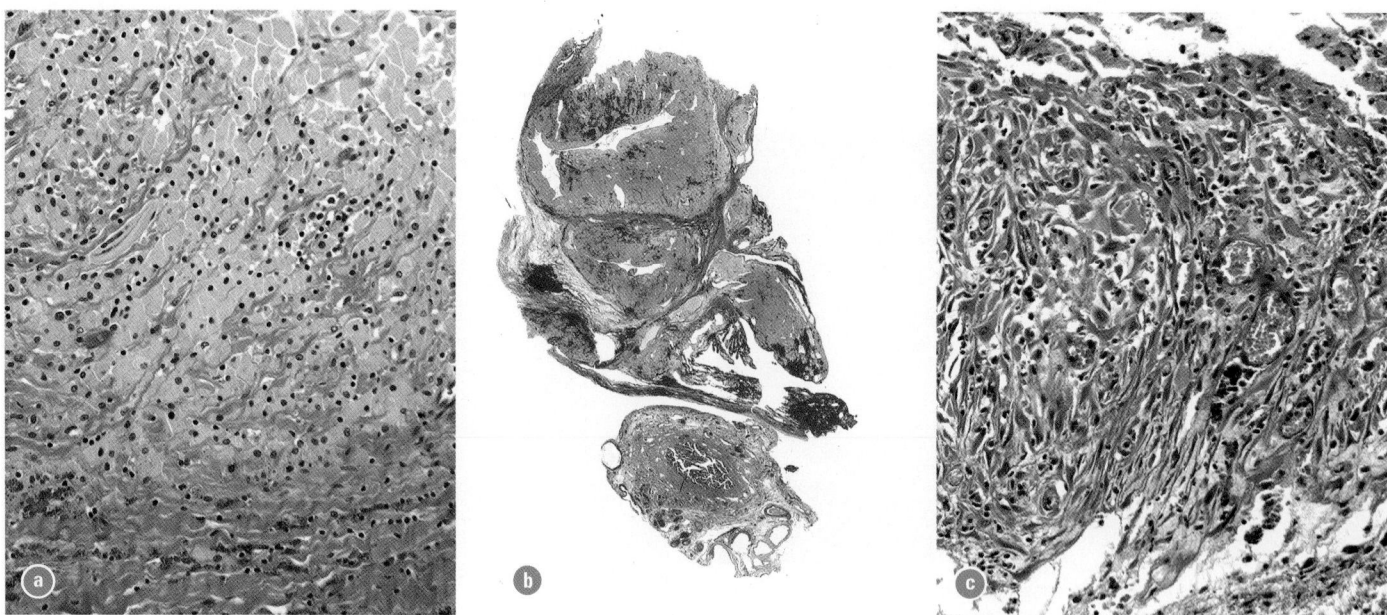

Fig. 22.49 (a) Xanthomatous pseudocyst. (b,c) Lower- and higher-power photomicrographs of decidualized endometrioma.

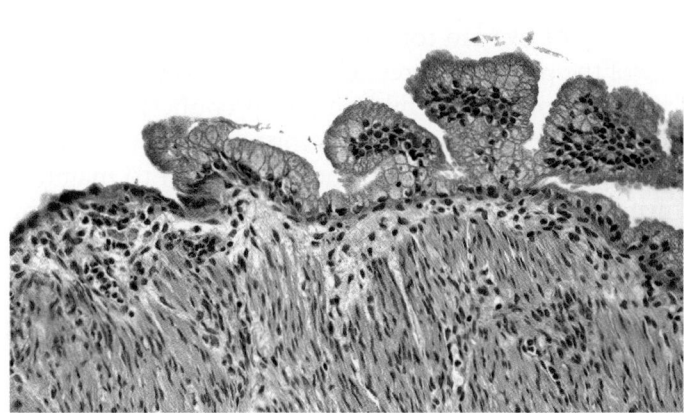

Fig. 22.51 Mucinous metaplasia in an endometriotic cyst. These metaplasias likely represent the earliest neoplastic changes predating the development of Müllerian mucinous cystadenomas.

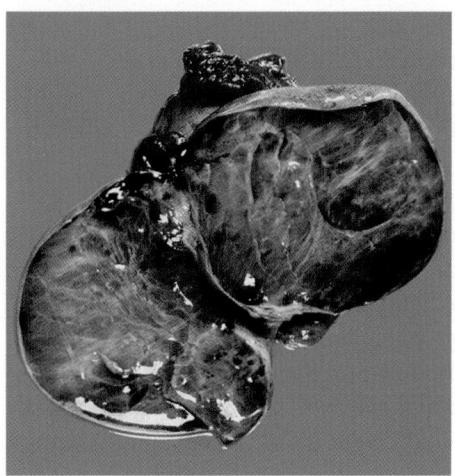

Fig. 22.53 Massive ovarian edema, seen here as homogeneous expansion of the ovary with a glistening appearance on sectioning. An important exclusion is metastatic mucinous carcinomas (Krukenberg's tumor), which can produce a similar appearance.

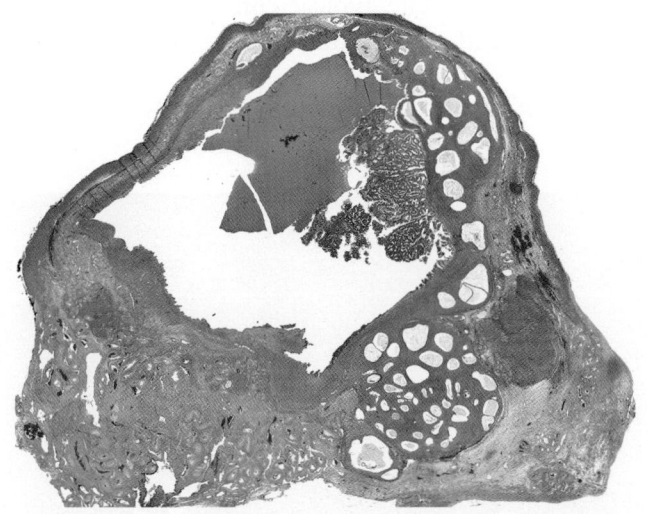

Fig. 22.52 An endometriotic cyst displays a combination of benign endometrial lining (lower left), an endometrioid cystadenofibroma (right) and a well-differentiated endometrioid adenocarcinoma (upper center).

MASSIVE OVARIAN EDEMA

Epidemiology

Massive ovarian edema is a non-neoplastic condition affecting primarily young patients, with a median age of 20 years.[117-119] The majority of the patients seek medical attention due to abdominal and/or pelvic pain, followed by menstrual abnormalities. Occasionally, ovarian torsion and its symptoms may accompany this entity.[117]

The most common scenario is unilateral enlargement of the ovary.[117] Macroscopically, the involved ovary is soft, with a gelatinous or watery cut surface (Fig. 22.53).

Microscopic examination reveals massive edema of the ovarian stroma with pale stroma surrounding native ovarian structures. Luteinized cells may be focally present in clusters. Foci of ovarian fibromatosis are occasionally identified. The pathogenesis is unknown but it is hypothesized that obstruction of the venous and lymphatic drainage underlies the development of massive ovarian edema.[116]

Surgical removal is usually necessary to exclude a neoplasm and to address the possibility of an acute ischemic event (torsion).

OVARIAN TORSION

Epidemiology

Ovarian torsion is defined by rotation of the adnexa on its fibrovascular pedicle, compromising the blood flow to the organ and leading, in some cases, to infarction of the adnexa. It occurs in two distinct clinical settings. In adults, ovaries that undergo torsion usually show evidence of a cyst or a tumor (benign or malignant).[120-122] In infants and children, the twisted ovary is usually normal.[123] The former clinical situation is more frequently encountered. There is also an association with ovarian hyperstimulation, including *hyperreactio luteinalis*.

Clinical features

Most patients present with acute abdominal pain simulating acute appendicitis as well as nausea and vomiting.[124] A mass may be palpable in cases where torsion is associated with an ovarian mass. Intermittent abdominal pain may be present in chronic torsions. The use of imaging techniques such as ultrasonography or magnetic resonance may be helpful in the preoperative diagnosis of these patients.

Pathology

Macroscopically, the ovary is usually enlarged and its surface is usually dark red. The cut surface shows edema and accumulation of blood and fluid (Fig. 22.54a,b). Careful examination is needed to entirely exclude the presence of a neoplasm, which may become masqueraded by the adnexal enlargement. Necrosis may be appreciated in infarcted cases.

The non-neoplastic torsed ovary shows large accumulation of blood and edema in its stroma (Fig. 22.54c). Areas of infarction may be present. In cases where a neoplasm is the inciting event, careful examination of the specimen is needed. Most often, it is a cyst or a benign neoplasm, such as a dermoid tumor.[124] However, malignant tumors are sometimes seen. The pathologist may encounter difficulties in diagnosing the underlying pathologic process due to the obscuring nature of the blood and infarction of the adnexa. Pathologic features of these tumors are described elsewhere in this book.

Treatment

Therapy of ovarian torsion is highly dependent on the age of the patient, degree of adnexal damage and underlying pathology. In children and prepubertal females, laparoscopy with manual detorsion of the ovary is usually attempted, due to the expectation to maintain future fertility. This is particularly important given the possibility of subsequent torsion of the contralateral ovary.[124] In older females, excision of the ovary is most likely necessary to exclude an underlying neoplasm.

Ovarian remnant syndrome

Ovarian remnant syndrome is defined as the presence of symptomatic residual ovarian tissue, usually following a complete hysterectomy and bilateral salpingo-oophorectomy.[125] The typical clinical presentation is pelvic pain and a palpable mass, often following

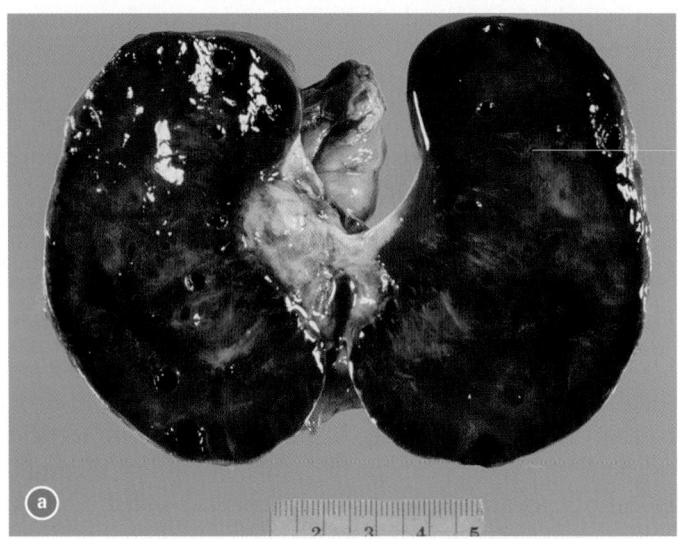

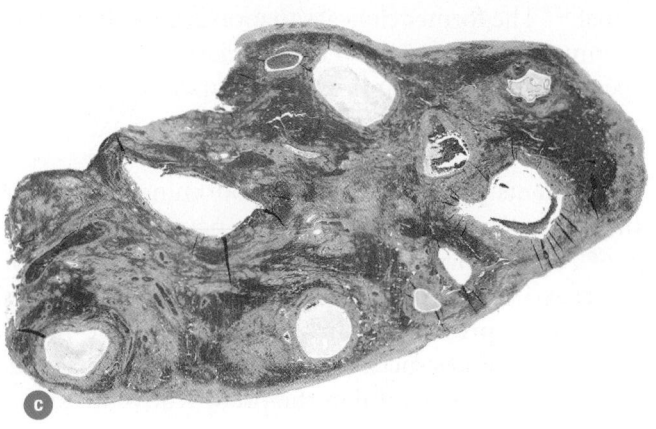

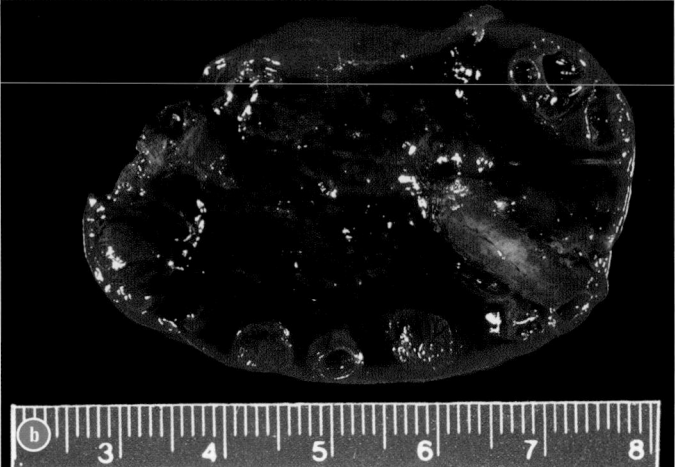

Fig. 22.54 Ovarian torsion. (a) Grossly the ovary is distended and diffusely hemorrhagic. Residual normal structures may be identified. (b) Torsed ovary with theca-lutein hyperplasia of pregnancy, showing diffuse interstitial hemorrhage. (c) Low-power photomicrograph of (b) depicting interstitial congestion and hemorrhage.

multiple prior pelvic surgical procedures. The actual incidence is not known, but in one study, over 20% of patients undergoing post-hysterectomy laparoscopy for persistent pain and a mass were found to have residual ovarian tissue.[126] Residual ovarian tissue is removed by either laparoscopy or laparotomy and may require multiple procedures. Rarely, malignancies have been documented in ovarian remnants.[127]

References

1 Blaustein A. Peritoneal mesothelium and ovarian surface cells – shared characteristics. Int J Gynecol Pathol 1984; 3(4):361–375.

2 Benjamin E, Law S, Bobrow LG. Intermediate filaments cytokeratin and vimentin in ovarian sex cord-stromal tumours with correlative studies in adult and fetal ovaries. J Pathol 1987; 152(4):253–263.

3 Isola J, Kallioniemi OP, Korte JM, et al. Steroid receptors and Ki-67 reactivity in ovarian cancer and in normal ovary: correlation with DNA flow cytometry, biochemical receptor assay, and patient survival. J Pathol 1990; 162(4):295–301.

4 Latza U, Niedobitek G, Schwarting R, Nekarda H, Stein H. Ber-EP4: new monoclonal antibody which distinguishes epithelia from mesothelial. J Clin Pathol 1990; 43(3): 213–219.

5 Rodriguez GC, Berchuck A, Whitaker RS, et al. Epidermal growth factor receptor expression in normal ovarian epithelium and ovarian cancer. II. Relationship between receptor expression and response to epidermal growth factor. Am J Obstet Gynecol 1991; 164(3):745–750.

6 Miettinen M, Lehto VP, Virtanen I. Expression of intermediate filaments in normal ovaries and ovarian epithelial, sex cord-stromal, and germinal tumors. Int J Gynecol Pathol 1983; 2(1):64–71.

7 Swank DJ, Swank-Bordewijk SC, Hop WC, et al. Laparoscopic adhesiolysis in patients with chronic abdominal pain: a blinded randomised controlled multi-centre trial. Lancet 2003; 361:1247–1251. Erratum in: Lancet 2003; 361:2250.

8 Moore JH Jr, Crum CP, Chandler JG, Feldman PS. Benign cystic mesothelioma. Cancer 1980; 45(9):2395–2399

9 Clement PB, Young RH, Scully RE. Malignant mesotheliomas presenting as ovarian masses. A report of nine cases, including two primary ovarian mesotheliomas. Am J Surg Pathol 1996; 20(9):1067–1080.

10 Clement PB, Young RH. Florid mesothelial hyperplasia associated with ovarian tumors: a potential source of error in tumor diagnosis and staging. Int J Gynecol Pathol 1993; 12(1):51–58.

11 Biscotti CV, Hart WR. Peritoneal serous micropapillomatosis of low malignant potential (serous borderline tumors of the peritoneum). A clinicopathologic study of 17 cases. Am J Surg Pathol 1992; 16(5):467–475.

12 Okamura H, Katabuchi H. Detailed morphology of human ovarian surface epithelium focusing on its metaplastic and neoplastic capability. Ital J Anat Embryol 2001; 106(2 Suppl 2):263–276.

13 McCaughey WT, Kirk ME, Lester W, Dardick I. Peritoneal epithelial lesions associated with proliferative serous tumours of ovary. Histopathology 1984; 8(2):195–208.

14 Dubeau L. The cell of origin of ovarian epithelial tumors and the ovarian surface epithelium dogma: does the emperor have no clothes? Gynecol Oncol 1999; 72(3):437–442.

15 Fortune JE. The early stages of follicular development: activation of primordial follicles and growth of preantral follicles. Anim Reprod Sci 2003; 78(3–4):135–163.

16 Scully RE, Young RH, Clement PB. Atlas of tumor pathology. Tumors of the ovary, maldeveloped gonads, fallopian tube and broad ligament. American Registry of Pathology; 1998:409–442.

17 Clement PB. Nonneoplastic lesions of the ovary. In: Kurman RJ, ed. Blaustein's pathology of the female genital tract, 5th edn. New York: Springer; 2002:675–728.

18 Peters WA 3rd, Thiagarajah S, Thornton WN Jr. Ovarian hemorrhage in patients receiving anticoagulant therapy. J Reprod Med 1979; 22:82–86

19 Nelson WW, Green RR. Some observations on the histology of the human ovary during pregnancy. Am J Obstet Gynecol 1958; 76:66–89.

20 Cronje HS. Luteoma of pregnancy. S Afr Med J 1984; 66:59–60.

21 Norris HJ, Taylor HB. Nodular theca-lutein hyperplasia of pregnancy (so-called 'pregnancy luteoma'). A clinical and pathologic study of 15 cases. Am J Clin Pathol 1967; 47:57–66.

22 Garcia-Bunuel R, Berek JS, Woodruff JD. Luteomas of pregnancy. Obstet Gynecol 1975; 45:407–414.

23 Clement PB, Young RH, Scully RE. Ovarian granulosa cell proliferations of pregnancy: a report of nine cases. Hum Pathol 1988; 19:657–662

24 Patterson, R., Hirsutism in pregnancy. Obstet Gynecol 1985; 66:738–740.

25 Wolff E, Glasser M, Gordon GG, Olivo J, Southren AL. Virilizing luteoma of pregnancy. Report of a case with measurements of testosterone and testosterone binding in plasma. Am J Med 1973; 54:229–233.

26 Zander J, Mickan H, Holzmann K, Lohe KJ. Androluteoma syndrome of pregnancy. Am J Obstet Gynecol 1978; 130:170–177.

27 Verkauf BS, Reiter EO, Hernandez L, Burns SA. Virilization of mother and fetus associated with luteoma of pregnancy: a case report with endocrinologic studies. Am J Obstet Gynecol 1977; 129:274–280.

28 Cohen DA, Daughaday WH, Weldon VV. Fetal and maternal virilization associated with pregnancy. A case report and review of the literature. Am J Dis Child 1982; 136:353–356.

29 Hensleigh PA, Woodruff JD. Differential maternal-fetal response to androgenizing luteoma or hyperreactio luteinalis. Obstet Gynecol Surv 1978; 33: 262–271.

30 Yao DX, Soslow RA, Hedvat CV, Leitao M, Baergen RN. Melan-A (A103) and inhibin expression in ovarian neoplasms. Appl Immunohistochem Mol Morphol 2003; 11:244–249.

31 Hatjis CG. Nonimmunologic fetal hydrops associated with hyperreactio luteinalis. Obstet Gynecol 1985; 65(3 Suppl): 11S–13S.

32 Wajda KJ, Lucas JG, Marsh WL Jr. Hyperreactio luteinalis. Benign disorder masquerading as an ovarian neoplasm. Arch Pathol Lab Med 1989; 113:921–925.

33 Curry SL, Hammond CB, Tyrey L, Creasman WT, Parker RT. Hydatidiform mole: diagnosis, management, and long-term follow-up of 347 patients. Obstet Gynecol 1975; 45:1–8.

34 Quereda F, Acien P, Hernandez A. Hyperreactio luteinalis: intraoperative finding during a cesarean section in a twin pregnancy. Eur J Obstet Gynecol Reprod Biol 1996; 66(1):71–73.

35 Berger NG, Repke JT, Woodruff JD. Markedly elevated serum testosterone in pregnancy without fetal virilization. Obstet Gynecol 1984; 63:260–262.

36 Barclay DL, Leverich EB, Kemmerly JR. Hyperreactio luteinalis: postpartum persistence. Am J Obstet Gynecol 1969; 105:642–644.

37 Clement PB, Scully RE. Large solitary luteinized follicle cyst of pregnancy and puerperium: a clinicopathological analysis of eight cases. Am J Surg Pathol 1980; 4(5):431–438.

38 Collins JA, Burrows EA, Wilan AR. The prognosis for live birth among untreated infertile couples. Fertil Steril 1995; 64:22–28.

39 Sharara FI, Scott RT. Assessment of ovarian reserve. Is there still a role for ovarian biopsy? First do no harm! Hum Reprod 2004; 19:470–471.

40 Lass A. Assessment of ovarian reserve: is there still a role for ovarian biopsy in the light of new data? Hum Reprod 2004; 19:467–469.

41 Santoro N. Mechanisms of premature ovarian failure. Ann Endocrinol (Paris) 2003; 64(2):87–92.

42 Rebar RW. Hypergonadotropic amenorrhea and premature ovarian failure: a review. J Reprod Med 1982; 27:179–186.

43 Kalantaridou SN, Davis SR, Nelson LM. Premature ovarian failure. Endocrinol Metab Clin North Am 1998; 27(4): 989–1006.

44 Castrillon DH, Miao L, Kollipara R, Horner JW, DePinho RA. Suppression of ovarian follicle activation in mice by the transcription factor Foxo3a. Science 2003; 301:215–218.

45 Bodega B, Porta C, Crosignani PG, Ginelli E, Marozzi A. Mutations in the coding region of the FOXL2 gene are not a major cause of idiopathic premature ovarian failure. Mol Hum Reprod 2004; 10:555–557.

46 Jorgez CJ, Klysik M, Jamin SP, Behringer RR, Matzuk MM. Granulosa cell-specific inactivation of follistatin causes female fertility defects. Mol Endocrinol 2004; 18(4):953–967.

47 Vegetti W, Marozzi A, Manfredini E, et al. Premature ovarian failure. Mol Cell Endocrinol 2000; 161(1–2): 53–57.

48 Forges T, Monnier-Barbarino P, Faure GC, Bene MC. Autoimmunity and antigenic targets in ovarian pathology. Hum Reprod Update 2004; 10:163–175.

49 Kauffman RP, Castracane VD. Premature ovarian failure associated with autoimmune polyglandular syndrome: pathophysiological mechanisms and future fertility. J Womens Health (Larchmt) 2003; 12(5):513–520.

50 Maclaren N, Chen QY, Kukreja A, et al. Autoimmune hypogonadism as part of an autoimmune polyglandular syndrome. J Soc Gynecol Investig 2001; 8(1 Suppl Proc):S52–S54.

51 Riley WJ. Autoimmune polyglandular syndromes. Horm Res 1992; 38(Suppl 2):9–15.

52 Nelson LM. Autoimmune ovarian failure: comparing the mouse model and the human disease. J Soc Gynecol Investig 2001; 8(1 Suppl Proc):S55–S57.

53 Nair S, Caspi RR, Nelson LM. Susceptibility to murine experimental autoimmune oophoritis is associated with genes outside the major histocompatibility complex (MHC). Am J Reprod Immunol 1996; 36(2):107–110.

54 Sedmak DD, Hart WR, Tubbs RR. Autoimmune oophoritis: a histopathologic study of involved ovaries with immunologic characterization of the mononuclear cell infiltrate. Int J Gynecol Pathol 1987; 6(1):73–81.

55 Biscotti CV, Hart WR, Lucas JG. Cystic ovarian enlargement resulting from autoimmune oophoritis. Obstet Gynecol 1989; 74(3 Pt 2):492–495.

56 Rabinowe SL, Berger MJ, Welch WR, Dluhy RG. Lymphocyte dysfunction in autoimmune oophoritis. Resumption of menses with corticosteroids. Am J Med 1986; 81:347–350.

57 Kalantaridou SN, Braddock DT, Patronas NJ, Nelson LM. Treatment of autoimmune premature ovarian failure. Hum Reprod 1999; 14(7):1777–1782.

58 Hull MG. Epidemiology of infertility and polycystic ovarian disease: endocrinological and demographic studies. Gynecol Endocrinol 1987; 1(3):235–245.

59 The Rotterdam ESHRE/ASRM-Sponsored PCOS Consensus workshop group. Revised 2003 consensus on diagnostic criteria and long term health risks related to polycystic ovary syndrome. Fertil Steril 2004; 81:19–25.

60 Polson DW, Adams J, Wadsworth J, Franks S. Polycystic ovaries – a common finding in normal women. Lancet 1988; 1(8590):870–872.

61 Solomon CG. The epidemiology of polycystic ovary syndrome. Prevalence and associated disease risks. Endocrinol Metab Clin North Am 1999; 28(2):247–263.

62 Wilson EA, Erickson GF, Zarutski P, et al. Endocrine studies of normal and polycystic ovarian tissues in vitro. Am J Obstet Gynecol 1979; 134:56–63

63 Abbott DH, Dumesic DA, Franks S. Developmental origin of polycystic ovary syndrome – a hypothesis. J Endocrinol 2002; 174:1–5

64 Ibanez L, Valls C, Potau N, Marcos MV, de Zegher F. Polycystic ovary syndrome after precocious pubarche: ontogeny of the low-birthweight effect. Clin Endocrinol (Oxf) 2001; 55:667–672.

65 Barbieri RL, Hornstein MD. Hyperinsulinemia and ovarian hyperandrogenism. Cause and effect. Endocrinol Metab Clin North Am 1988; 17(4):685–703.

66 Lunde O, Magnus P, Sandvik L, Hoglo S. Familial clustering in the polycystic ovarian syndrome. Gynecol Obstet Invest 1989; 28(1):23–30.

67 Jahanfar S, Eden JA, Nguyen T, Wang XL, Wilcken DE. A twin study of polycystic ovary syndrome. Fertil Steril 1995; 63(3):478–486.

68 Legro RS, Strauss JF. Molecular progress in infertility: polycystic ovary syndrome. Fertil Steril 2002; 78(3):569–576.

69 Roldan B, San Millan JL, Escobar-Morreale HF. Genetic basis of metabolic abnormalities in polycystic ovary syndrome: implications for therapy. Am J Pharmacogenomics 2004; 4(2):93–107.

70 Escobar-Morreale HF, Luque-Ramirez M, San Millan JL. The molecular-genetic basis of functional hyperandrogenism and the polycystic ovary syndrome. Endocr Rev 2005; 26(2):251–282.

71 Duncan S. Polycystic ovarian syndrome in women with epilepsy: a review. Epilepsia 2001; 42(Suppl 3):60–65.

72 Meo R, Bilo L. Polycystic ovary syndrome and epilepsy: a review of the evidence. Drugs 2003; 63:1185–1227.

73 Rasgon N. The relationship between polycystic ovary syndrome and antiepileptic drugs: a review of the evidence. J Clin Psychopharmacol 2004; 24:322–334.

74 Morrell MJ, Montouris GD. Reproductive disturbances in patients with epilepsy. Cleve Clin J Med 2004; 71(Suppl 2):S19–S24.

75 van der Spuy ZM, Dyer SJ. The pathogenesis of infertility and early pregnancy loss in polycystic ovary syndrome. Best Pract Res Clin Obstet Gynaecol 2004; 18:755–771.

76 Lord J, Wilkin T. Metformin in polycystic ovary syndrome. Curr Opin Obstet Gynecol 2004; 16:481–486.

77 Chang RJ. A practical approach to the diagnosis of polycystic ovary syndrome. Am J Obstet Gynecol 2004; 191:713–717.

78 Buccola JM, Reynolds EE. Polycystic ovary syndrome: a review for primary providers. Prim Care 2003; 30:697–710.

79 Fraser IS, Kovacs G. Current recommendations for the diagnostic evaluation and follow-up of patients presenting with symptomatic polycystic ovary syndrome. Best Pract Res Clin Obstet Gynaecol 2004; 18:813–823.

80 Balen AH, Laven JS, Tan SL, Dewailly D. Ultrasound assessment of the polycystic ovary: international consensus definitions. Hum Reprod Update 2003; 9:505–514.

81 Balen AH, Conway GS, Kaltsas G, et al. Polycystic ovary syndrome: the spectrum of the disorder in 1741 patients. Hum Reprod 1995; 10:2107–2111.

82 Practice Committee of the American Society for Reproductive Medicine. Use of insulin sensitizing agents in the treatment of polycystic ovary syndrome. Fertil Steril 2004; 82(Suppl 1):S181–S183.

83 Saleh AM, Khalil HS. Review of nonsurgical and surgical treatment and the role of insulin-sensitizing agents in the management of infertile women with polycystic ovary syndrome. Acta Obstet Gynecol Scand 2004; 83(7):614–621.

84 Farquhar CM. The role of ovarian surgery in polycystic ovary syndrome. Best Pract Res Clin Obstet Gynaecol 2004; 18(5):789–802.

85 Gomel V, Yarali H. Surgical treatment of polycystic ovary syndrome associated with infertility. Reprod Biomed Online 2004; 9(1):35–42.

86 Hughesdon PE. Morphology and morphogenesis of the Stein–Leventhal ovary and of so-called 'hyperthecosis'. Obstet Gynecol Surv 1982; 37(2):59–77.

87 Sangi-Haghpeykar H, Poindexter AN 3rd. Epidemiology of endometriosis among parous women. Obstet Gynecol 1995; 85(6):983–992.

88 Nisolle M, Donnez J. Peritoneal endometriosis, ovarian endometriosis, and adenomyotic nodules of the rectovaginal septum are three different entities. Fertil Steril 1997; 68:585–596.

89 Zheng W, Li N, Wang J, et al. Initial endometriosis showing direct morphologic evidence of metaplasia in the pathogenesis of ovarian endometriosis. Int J Gynecol Pathol 2005; 24:164–172.

90 Thomas EJ, Campbell IG. Molecular genetic defects in endometriosis. Gynecol Obstet Invest 2000; 50(Suppl 1):44–50.

91 Bulun SE, Gurates B, Fang Z, et al. Mechanisms of excessive estrogen formation in endometriosis. J Reprod Immunol 2002; 55(1–2):21–33.

92 Gianetto-Berrutti A, Feyles V. Endometriosis related to infertility. Minerva Gynecol 2003; 55(5):407–416.

93 Cahill DJ, Hull MG. Pituitary-ovarian dysfunction and endometriosis. Hum Reprod Update 2000; 6(1):56–66.

94 Boss JH, Scully RE, Wegner KH, Cohen RB. Structural variations in the adult ovary. Clinical significance. Obstet Gynecol 1965; 25:747–764.

95 Honore LH, Chari R, Mueller HD, Cumming DC, Scott JZ. Postmenopausal hyperandrogenism of ovarian origin. A clinicopathologic study of four cases. Gynecol Obstet Invest 1992; 34(1):52–56.

96 Krug E, Berga SL. Postmenopausal hyperthecosis: functional dysregulation of androgenesis in climacteric ovary. Obstet Gynecol 2002; 99(5 Pt 2):893–897.

97 Dunaif A, Hoffman AR, Scully RE, et al. Clinical, biochemical, and ovarian morphologic features in women with acanthosis nigricans and masculinization. Obstet Gynecol 1985; 66(4):545–552.

98 Karam K, Hajj S. Hyperthecosis syndrome. Clinical, endocrinologic and histologic findings. Acta Obstet Gynecol Scand 1979; 58(1):73–79.

99 Ramondetta LM, Carlson JA. Jr, Schwarting R. Atypical Meigs' syndrome and bilateral ovarian stromal hyperplasia. A case report. J Reprod Med 1997; 42(9):603–605.

100 Nagamani M, Lingold JC, Gomez LG, Garza JR. Clinical and hormonal studies in hyperthecosis of the ovaries. Fertil Steril 1981; 36(3):326–332.

101 Hayes MC, Scully RE. Stromal luteoma of the ovary: a clinicopathological analysis of 25 cases. Int J Gynecol Pathol 1987; 6(4):313–321.

102 Namavar Jahromi B, Parsanezhad ME, Ghane-Shirazi R. Female genital tuberculosis and infertility. Int J Gynaecol Obstet 2001; 75(3):269–272.

103 Tripathy SN. Laparoscopic observations of pelvic organs in pulmonary tuberculosis. Int J Gynaecol Obstet 1990; 32(2):129–131.

104 Dejmek A. Fine needle aspiration cytology of an ovarian luteinized follicular cyst mimicking a granulosa cell tumor. A case report. Acta Cytol 2003; 47(6):1059–1062.

105 Mulvany NJ. Aspiration cytology of ovarian cysts and cystic neoplasms. A study of 235 aspirates. Acta Cytol 1996; 40(5):911–920.

106 Mulvany N, Ostor A, Teng G. Evaluation of estradiol in aspirated ovarian cystic lesions. Acta Cytol 1995; 39(4):663–668.

107 Egger H, Weigmann P. Clinical and surgical aspects of ovarian endometriotic cysts. Arch Gynecol 1982; 233(1):37–45.

108 Tsukahara Y, Satoh M, Kato J, et al. Clinicopathologic investigation of ovarian endometriosis: a comparative study of cystic and non-cystic types. Nippon Sanka Fujinka Gakkai Zasshi 1985; 37(5):751–757.

109 Moller NE. The Arias-Stella phenomenon in endometriosis. Acta Obstet Gynecol Scand 1959; 38:271–274.

110 Sakaki M, Hirokawa M, Sano T, et al. Ovarian endometriosis showing decidual change and Arias-Stella reaction with biotin-containing intranuclear inclusions. Acta Cytol 2003; 47(2):321–324.

111 Stern RC, Dash R, Bentley RC, et al. Malignancy in endometriosis: frequency and comparison of ovarian and extraovarian types. Int J Gynecol Pathol 2001; 20(2):133–139.

112 Leiserowitz GS, Gumbs JL, Oi R, et al. Endometriosis-related malignancies. Int J Gynecol Cancer 2003; 13(4): 466–471.

113 Olive DL, Pritts EA. The treatment of endometriosis: a review of the evidence. Ann N Y Acad Sci 2002; 955:360–372; discussion 389–393, 396–406.

114 Martin DC, O'Conner DT. Surgical management of endometriosis-associated pain. Obstet Gynecol Clin North Am 2003; 30(1):151–162.

115 Olive DL, Lindheim SR, Pritts EA. New medical treatments for endometriosis. Best Pract Res Clin Obstet Gynaecol 2004; 18(2):319–328.

116 Fedele L, Bianchi S, Zanconato G, Bettoni G, Gotsch F. Long-term follow-up after conservative surgery for rectovaginal endometriosis. Am J Obstet Gynecol 2004; 190(4):1020–1024.

117 Young RH, Scully RE. Fibromatosis and massive edema of the ovary, possibly related entities: a report of 14 cases of fibromatosis and 11 cases of massive edema. Int J Gynecol Pathol 1984; 3(2):153–178.

118 Roth LM, Deaton RL, Sternberg WH. Massive ovarian edema. A clinicopathologic study of five cases including ultrastructural observations and review of the literature. Am J Surg Pathol 1979; 3(1):11–21.

119 Kanbour AI, Salazar H, Tobon H. Massive ovarian edema: a nonneoplastic pelvic mass of young women. Arch Pathol Lab Med 1979; 103(1):42–45.

120 Lee CH, Raman S, Sivanesaratnam V. Torsion of ovarian tumors: a clinicopathological study. Int J Gynaecol Obstet 1989; 28(1):21–25.

121 Houry D, Abbott JT. Ovarian torsion: a fifteen-year review. Ann Emerg Med 2001; 38(2):156–159.

122 Varras M, Tsikini A, Polyzos D, et al. Uterine adnexal torsion: pathologic and gray-scale ultrasonographic findings. Clin Exp Obstet Gynecol 2004; 31(1):34–38.

123 Mordehai J, Mares AJ, Barki Y, Finaly R, Meizner I. Torsion of uterine adnexa in neonates and children: a report of 20 cases. J Pediatr Surg 1991; 26(10):1195–1199.

124 Beaunoyer M, Chapdelaine J, Bouchard S, Ouimet A. Asynchronous bilateral ovarian torsion. J Pediatr Surg 2004; 39(5):746–749.

125 Webb MJ. Ovarian remnant syndrome. Aust N Z J Obstet Gynaecol 1989; 29(4):433–435.

126 Abu-Rafeh B, Vilos GA, Misra M. Frequency and laparoscopic management of ovarian remnant syndrome. J Am Assoc Gynecol Laparosc 2003; 10:33–37.

127 Dereska NH, Cornella J, Hibner M, Magrina JF. Mucinous adenocarcinoma in an ovarian remnant. Int J Gynecol Cancer 2004; 14:683–686.

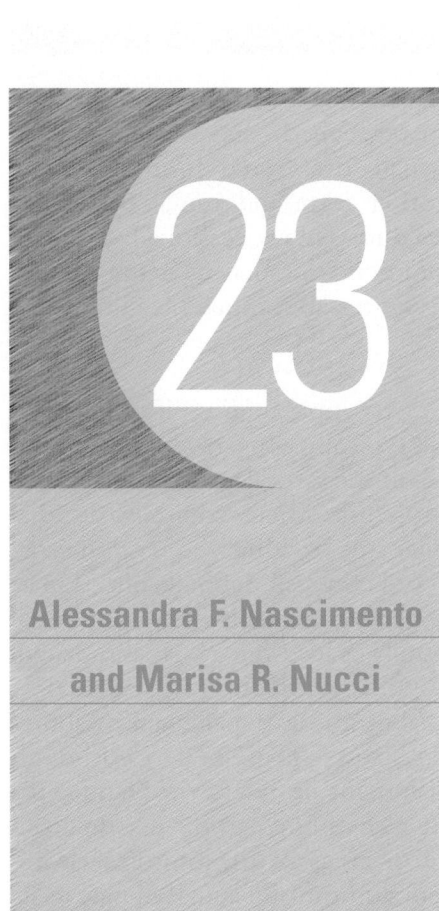

23

Disorders of the peritoneum

Alessandra F. Nascimento
and Marisa R. Nucci

Introduction

**Müllerian-derived lesions
of the peritoneum**

Ectopic decidua (deciduosis)
Endosalpingiosis
Endocervicosis
Endometriosis (conventional
    type)
Polypoid endometriosis
Müllerian neoplasms

**Mesenchymal lesions
of the peritoneum**

Smooth muscle neoplasms
Endometrial stromal sarcoma
Solitary fibrous tumor
Calcifying fibrous tumor
Inflammatory myofibroblastic
    tumor (IMT)
Gastrointestinal stromal tumor
    (GIST)
Peripheral nerve sheath tumors
Desmoid fibromatosis

Liposarcoma
Desmoplastic small round cell
    tumor

**Mesothelial lesions
of the peritoneum**

Mesothelial hyperplasia
Cystic mesothelioma
Well-differentiated papillary
    mesothelioma
Adenomatoid tumor
Malignant mesothelioma

**Miscellaneous lesions
of the peritoneum**

Myxoid hamartoma
Infarcted appendix epiploica
Sclerosing mesenteritis

Implants of the peritoneum

Pseudomyxoma peritonei
Strumosis
Peritoneal gliomatosis

Introduction

The practice of gynecologic pathology often entails the evaluation of abnormalities in the peritoneal cavity and determining their relationship to the reproductive tract. This exercise requires that the pathologist distinguish which peritoneal disorders are Müllerian-derived versus originating from other organs. Diseases affecting the peritoneal cavity and the intra-abdominal organs include entities originating from elements native to the peritoneal cavity (secondary Müllerian system, mesenchymal and mesothelial proliferations), as well as neoplastic and non-neoplastic entities of metastatic nature, or controversial/uncertain origin. Most of these diseases affect males and females; however, for the purpose of this book, emphasis will be given to the disorders occurring mainly in women.

Müllerian-derived lesions of the peritoneum

ECTOPIC DECIDUAS (DECIDUOSIS)

Background

The presence of ectopic decidua in the peritoneal cavity is a relatively common finding in pregnant females, found in up to 97% of pregnant women and focally involving the omentum in one series.[1] It appears to be associated with a physiologic metaplastic response of the subcelomic mesenchymal cells to the elevated levels of circulating progesterone hormone during pregnancy. Another possible explanation is that the systemic hormonal response affects pre-existing foci of endometriosis and that the ectopic endometrial tissue shows an analogous response to that seen in the uterine endometrium. It usually involutes within 4–6 weeks post-partum.[1]

Its occurrence in non-pregnant women is a rare event and this diagnosis should trigger an active search for a source of hormone production, such as exogenous administration of progesterone or a hormone-producing tumor. In this setting, this benign reaction is best regarded as 'pseudodecidualized' tissue.

Clinical features

Ectopic decidual tissue typically occurs on the surface of the pelvic organs, such as the ovarian or tubal serosal surfaces.[2] However, involvement of the peritoneum,[3]

serosa of the gastrointestinal tract,[4,5] omentum[6] and mesentery[1] may also be seen. In most cases, it is an incidental finding, usually discovered during Cesarean section or during other intra-abdominal operation. However, ectopic deciduosis may occasionally simulate acute abdominal emergencies, such as acute appendicitis,[7,8] or may cause intra-abdominal bleeding.[5,9–11]

Pathology

Although usually a microscopic finding, if grossly evident, ectopic decidua typically appears as white or red small nodules located on the serosal surfaces of abdominal organs and peritoneum. Microscopically, decidua shows features similar to decidualized endometrial stroma, being composed of a well-defined collection of bland-appearing large polygonal cells with distinct cell borders, round, centrally placed nuclei, small nucleoli and abundant eosinophilic cytoplasm (Fig. 23.1a).

The main differential diagnosis is malignant mesothelioma with deciduoid features (Fig. 23.1b). Although the latter entity is malignant, it may show bland cytologic features, closely resembling ectopic decidualized tissue. The presence of areas of the tumor showing nuclear pleomorphism and mitotic activity helps in its distinction from ectopic decidua (Fig. 31.1c). The clinical setting of the development of deciduoid mesothelioma is controversial; although the initial descriptions regard this malignant neoplasm as a disease of young women with no history of asbestos exposure,[12] other authors believe that the epidemiology of this tumor follows that of conventional epithelial mesothelioma: namely, it is a disease of older male adults.[13] Immunoperoxidase studies show positivity of neoplastic cells in mesothelioma for keratins, calretinin and WT-1. A more detailed immunoprofile of mesothelial proliferations is discussed below. The immunoperoxidase profile is yet unclear for decidua; however, presumably this process will not be keratin positive.

Treatment and prognosis

The prognosis is excellent for cases of ectopic decidua not complicated by bleeding. Surgical ablation suffices the treatment requirements. The potential for recurrence of this condition is unknown but presumably it may recur during subsequent pregnancies.

ENDOSALPINGIOSIS

Background

Endosalpingiosis is defined by the presence of foci of epithelium resembling fallopian tube lining outside

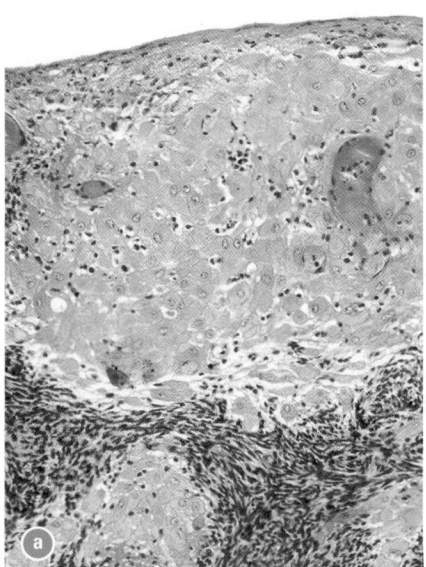
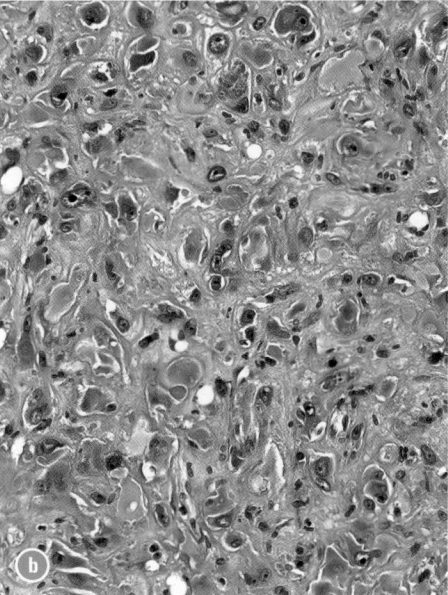
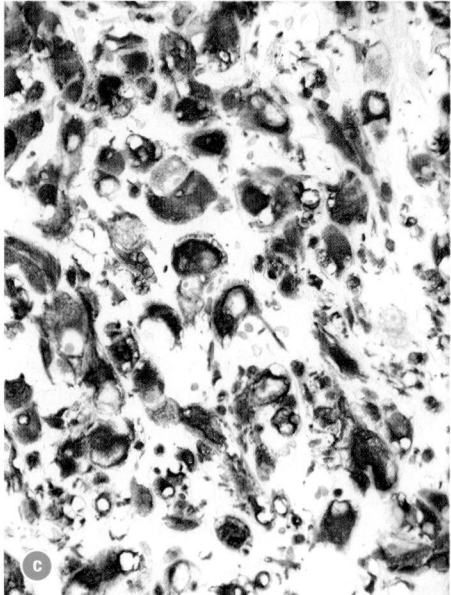

Fig. 23.1 (a) Ectopic decidua (deciduosis) involving the peritoneal surface. (b) Malignant mesothelioma with deciduoid features. (c) A cytokeratin stain distinguishes this process from decidua.

this anatomic location. It affects approximately 7% of the female population in the reproductive age.[14]

Clinical features

Although some authors believe that endosalpingiosis may be a source of abdominal pain, it is more often an incidental finding during abdominal surgery and is frequently seen in association with other pelvic pathologic findings, such as endometriosis, leiomyomata, hydrosalpinx and ovarian neoplasms.[14,15]

Pathology

Macroscopic evidence of endosalpingiosis is rarely seen involving the peritoneum, omentum, retroperitoneal and abdominal lymph nodes, wall of abdominal organs and on the surface of pelvic organs. Most commonly, endosalpingiosis is a microscopic finding, consisting of glandular and tubular structures lined by low cuboidal ciliated epithelium (Fig. 23.2). No endometrial stromal cells, hemosiderin deposition or desmoplastic tissue reaction is present in association with these nests. Although these findings may raise the concern of metastasis, especially when present in a lymph node, the appearances are quite bland, with no mitotic figures or necrosis. Rarely, this ectopic tissue might assume a florid constitution with large cystic spaces that may mimic metastatic carcinoma.[16]

Treatment and prognosis

Due to the benign nature of this finding, surgical biopsy for diagnosis confirmation suffices. The prognosis is excellent.

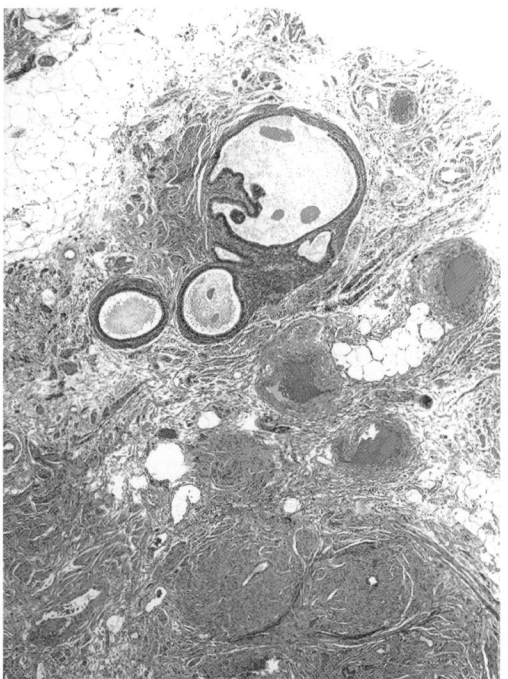

Fig. 23.2 Endosalpingiosis involving the mesosalpinx.

ENDOCERVICOSIS

Background

Endocervicosis is defined by the presence of ectopic endocervical-like glands, i.e. glands lined by columnar cells with mucinous cytoplasm akin to that seen in the endocervix. This condition is encountered in females in the reproductive age.

Clinical features

The vast majority of cases of endocervicosis have been described affecting the wall of the urinary bladder.[17–23] Most patients present with urinary symptoms such as pain, dysuria, frequency and hematuria, clinically mimicking a urinary bladder neoplasm or infection.[17] Rare cases of endocervicosis involving the outer wall of the uterine cervix have been described.[24]

Pathology

Endocervicosis may form large masses, measuring up to 5 cm, and thus may mimic a neoplasm. The tumor-like prominence is usually located in the posterior bladder wall or dome and may project into the bladder cavity.

Microscopically, glands, some of which show cystic dilation, lined by endocervical-like cells, characterize this entity. The cells are columnar in appearance with evidence of mucin production. Mild atypia as well as cilia may be seen. In most cases, ruptured glands with extravasation of mucin into the surrounding stroma, eliciting a stromal reaction, are present. However, mitoses are rare, if present at all.

The major differential diagnosis is with metastatic well-differentiated adenocarcinoma. Neoplasms typically show more pronounced nuclear atypia, stromal desmoplasia and mitotic figures are more easily identified. Careful clinical correlation should be considered.

Treatment and prognosis

The prognosis is excellent and surgical excision should be curative.[17]

ENDOMETRIOSIS (CONVENTIONAL TYPE)

Background

Endometriosis is one of the most common gynecologic diseases. It is defined by occurrence of endometrial-like epithelium and stroma outside the uterine cavity. This condition is seen in reproductive-age females. In asymptomatic women, endometriosis is present in up to 20% of patients.[25,26] In patients being treated for infertility, endometriosis is much more common and can be encountered in up to 60% of the cases.[25] Risk factors for the development of endometriosis appear to be nulliparity and irregular menstrual cycles.[27]

Clinical features

Most cases of endometriosis will involve the pelvic organs and are associated with chronic pelvic pain (not related with the menstrual cycle), dyspareunia, dysmenorrhea and infertility (i.e. ovarian endometriosis). When affecting peritoneal-lined organs, females with endometriosis may be asymptomatic or present with chronic, vague abdominal pain. Diagnosis depends on identification of endometriotic lesions by laparoscopy or laparotomy, with confirmatory biopsy.

Pathology

Macroscopically, endometriosis might present as small dark red, black or bluish cysts or nodules on the surface of peritoneal and pelvic organs (Fig. 23.3a); occasionally, the focus of endometriosis may appear whitish and be associated with adhesions. In cases of extensive involvement of the ovary, bleeding may lead to the formation a cystic mass, or endometrioma.

Histologically, endometriosis is characterized by (1) the ectopic presence of endometrial-like glands (i.e. pseudostratified columnar glandular epithelium), which may show similar alterations when compared with the glands topically located in the uterine cavity; (2) spindled endometrial stroma; and (3) hemosiderin deposition either within the macrophages or in the stroma (Fig. 23.3b–d). In many instances, the classic diagnostic triad of these components is not present or the endometrial glands and stroma may be obscured by hemorrhage, foamy cells and hemosiderin-laden macrophages such that the diagnosis may be suggested but histologic confirmation may not be possible. Endometriosis can be considered superficial if endometriotic foci are located less than 5 mm from the peritoneal surface. However, if the foci extend deeper than 5 mm from the surface, it can be considered deeply infiltrating. Awareness of this distinction is important because deeply infiltrating foci of endometriosis may simulate a neoplasm, may be missed during surgical exploration or may be incompletely excised giving rise to possible recurrent disease.

Atypia, metaplasia, hyperplasia and neoplasia have been reported to occur in the setting of endometriosis.[28,29] The presence of atypia in foci of endometriosis have been associated with aneuploid DNA content and,

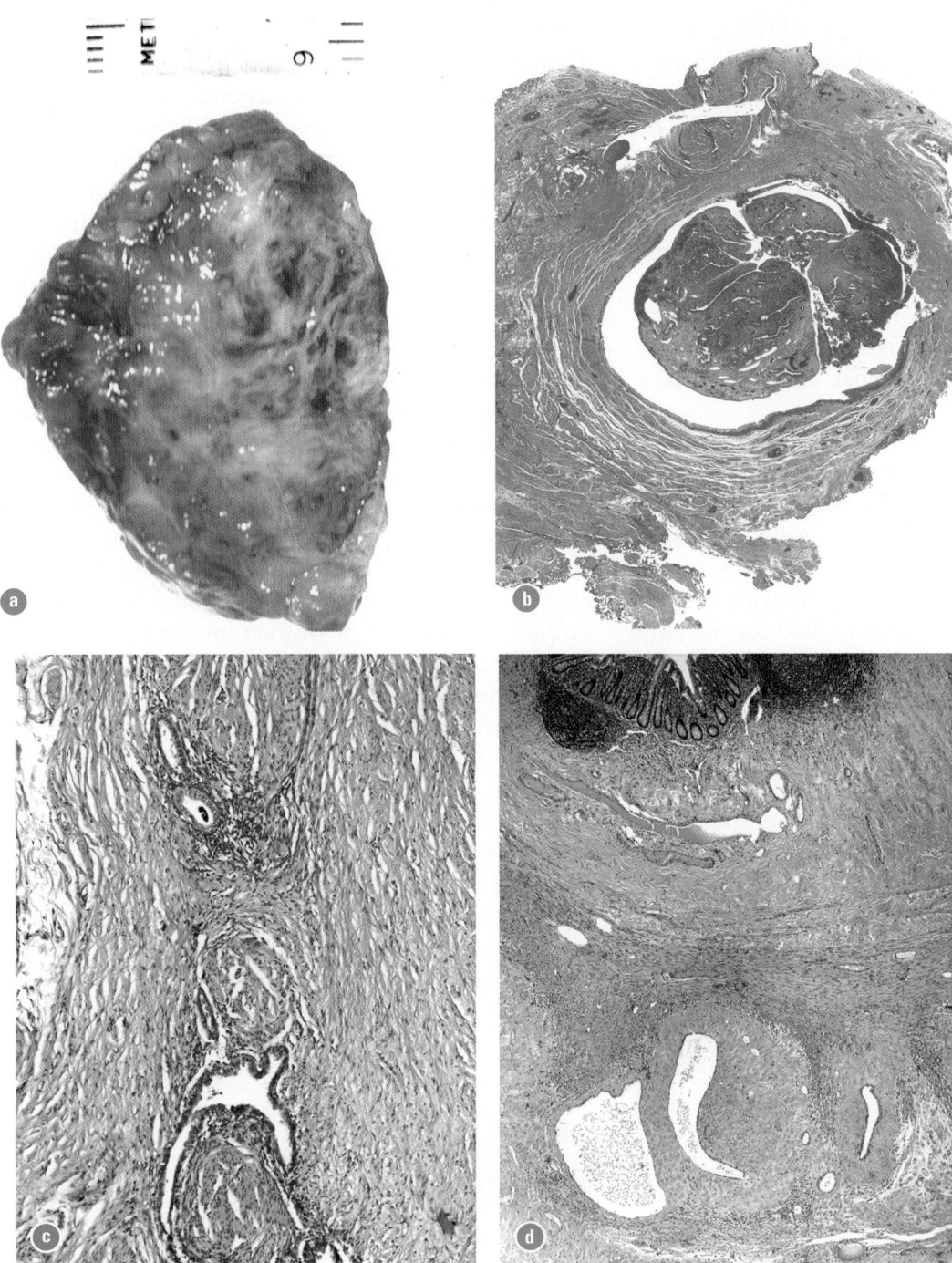

Fig. 23.3 (a) Macroscopic appearance of endometriosis involving the abdominal wall. (b) Low-power image of endometriosis of the ureter. (c) Endometriosis of the mesentery, with reactive fibrosis. (d) Decidualized endometriosis (lower) involving the appendix.

because it has been seen in association with malignancy arising in endometriosis, nuclear atypia is thought by some authors to represent a possible precursor lesion of carcinoma.[30,31] For practical purposes, the presence of nuclear atypia in the absence of architectural complexity (cribriforming, papillary structures) is likely reactive/degenerative in nature; in these cases the atypical cells have enlarged nuclei with smudgy chromatin and abundant vacuolated to eosinophilic cytoplasm. Hobnail cells with enlarged nuclei with prominent nucleoli should raise the possibility of malignancy (clear cell/papillary serous differentiation); in these instances, the presence of diffuse nuclear reactivity for p53 would support a neoplastic process. Adenocarcinoma arising in the setting of ovarian endometriosis is seen in premenopausal women and is not associated with hormone replacement therapy (HRT), while extra-ovarian adenocarcinoma arising in association with endometriosis tends to occur in postmenopausal females and have higher correlation with HRT.[32] The most common histologic subtypes of adenocarcinoma encountered in these patients are endometrioid and clear cell subtypes, which account for 90% of the cancers (Fig. 23.4a,b).[30,32] Similarly, cases of extra-uterine endometrial stromal sarcoma arising from endometriotic foci have been reported and show the typical permeative growth pattern and cytomorphologic features of those tumors that arise within the uterus.[33]

The pathogenesis of endometriosis is unclear and a matter of much debate. The most accepted theory is that viable endometrial cells gain access to the peritoneum via retrograde flow through fallopian tubes during menstruation and attach to the peritoneal surface of pelvic and abdominal organs with the aid of adhesion molecules.[34,35] Other theories include the possibility that endometriosis arises from metaplastic changes of the peritoneum and of the surface epithelial cells of the ovary.[36] In addition, some authors suggest that cells composing superficial and deeply infiltrating endometriosis are distinct and are dependent on different sources of nutrition. It is suggested that superficial endometriosis would be regulated and supported by the microenvironment created by the peritoneal fluid, while deeply infiltrating endometriosis would be more dependent on the blood flow to the involved organ.[37]

Treatment and prognosis

Treatment of endometriosis, including medical and/or surgical therapies, is highly dependent on the presence of symptoms, being reserved mainly for symptomatic patients and those with extensive disease. Surgical options include laser coagulation and resection. Medical interventions include the use of drugs that function as estrogen antagonists, such as oral contraceptives, progesterone, danazol and gonadotropin-releasing hormone (GnRH) agonists.[38] Other newer approaches, such as progesterone receptor modulators, GnRH antagonists, aromatase inhibitors, tumor necrosis factor-alpha inhibitors, angiogenesis inhibitors, matrix metalloproteinase inhibitors and estrogen receptor ß-agonists, are under investigation.[39]

The prognosis is variable and related to the extent of involvement of the ovaries and peritoneal cavity by endometriosis and the depth of infiltration. Recurrence may be seen, especially in cases initially associated with extensive peritoneal or ovarian involvement or deeply infiltrating disease. *In vitro* fertilization may be necessary to overcome infertility associated with extensive endometriosis.[40]

POLYPOID ENDOMETRIOSIS

Background

Polypoid endometriosis is a variant of endometriosis that has a tendency to mimic a neoplasm clinically, surgically and by pathologic examination. The lesions tend to grow as polypoid masses: hence the term

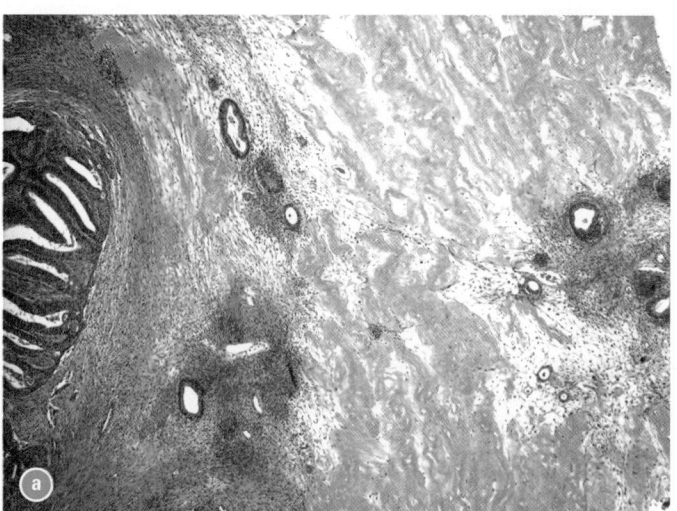
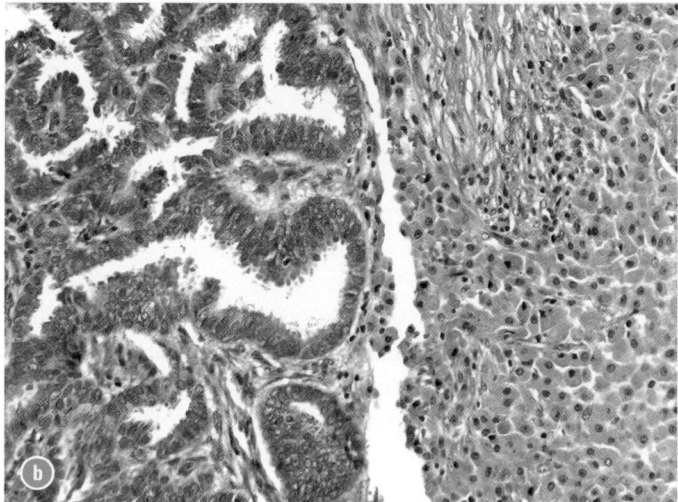

Fig. 23.4 (a) Endometriosis (right) associated with endometrioid adenocarcinoma (left). (b) Focus of early adenocarcinoma (left) adjacent to old hemorrhage (right) in the cul-de-sac.

'polypoid endometriosis', with only a subset of examples showing histologic features of polyps (prominent thick-walled vessels, fibrous stroma, irregularly spaced and cystic glands) (Fig. 23.5a). From a historical perspective, the term 'polypoid endometriosis' was first used by Mostoufizadeh and Scully in their description of a variant of endometriosis that shared histologic features with endometrial polyps.[41] Since their original description, there have been only a handful of case reports, with the largest series on the subject recently reported by Parker et al.[42–51]

Clinical features

In this series of 24 women, patients ages ranged from 23 to 78 years (median 55) with 60% of the patients being older than 50 years. A little less than half of the patients were taking exogenous hormones, possibly a contributing factor to the occurrence of endometriosis in older (peri- and postmenopausal) women. Patients most commonly present with symptoms related either to a pelvic mass, vaginal mass (with associated bleeding) or large bowel obstruction. Practically any site of the abdominal cavity may be affected, with involvement of the colon, pelvic structures, vaginal mucosa, omentum and retroperitoneum having been described in descending order of frequency.

Pathology

On gross examination, lesions may be of varying size, ranging from 0.4 to 14 cm in maximal dimension. They tend to appear as tan/brown, white/grey or pink/red polypoid masses involving mucosal or serosal surfaces or within an endometriotic cyst.

Histologically, the lesions are composed of an admixture of endometriotic glands and stroma, of which the former may show varying degrees of proliferation and metaplastic change (Fig. 23.5b), including tubal, mucinous, squamous and papillary syncytial metaplasia. The stroma typically resembles proliferative phase endometrial stroma without stromal cytologic atypia. In the majority of the cases, stromal fibrosis and numerous thick-walled vessels are present, similar to that seen in endometrial polyps. In some, a discrete endometrial polyp is present (Fig. 23.5c).

Treatment and prognosis

Polypoid endometriosis is benign. In the series by Parker et al., follow-up in 17 (of 24) patients showed that 15 patients were alive without evidence of disease (range of follow-up 1–20 years with mean of 5.9), one patient was alive with endometriosis at 18 months and

one patient died of unrelated causes. Similar to typical endometriosis, malignant transformation may potentially occur, with epithelial, mesenchymal and mixed epithelial-mesenchymal tumors arising out of this lesion.[42]

The principal differential diagnostic consideration is the distinction of polypoid endometriosis from Müllerian adenosarcoma, particularly since the latter can arise from peritoneal endometriosis.[52] Müllerian adenosarcoma can be distinguished from polypoid endometriosis by: (1) the presence of stromal papillae and frond-like proliferations that project into glandular or cystic spaces, (2) mild stromal atypia (at least) and (3) periglandular cellular stromal cuffing. Also within the differential diagnosis is endometrial stromal sarcoma with glandular differentiation,[53] which can be distinguished from polypoid endometriosis by: (1) its characteristic finger-like permeative growth pattern, (2) its propensity for lymphatic/vascular invasion and (3) usually only the focal presence of endometrioid-type glands.

MÜLLERIAN NEOPLASMS

Background

Primary Müllerian neoplasms of the peritoneum include papillary serous tumors, endometrial stromal sarcoma, Müllerian adenosarcoma and malignant mixed Müllerian tumor (MMMT). Extra-uterine endometrial stromal sarcoma is discussed elsewhere in this chapter.

Primary peritoneal papillary serous tumors, the most common of the Müllerian neoplasms of the peritoneum, include borderline or serous tumors of low malignant potential and papillary serous adenocarcinoma. It occurs over a wide age range; however, females with borderline papillary tumors are usually younger, with a median age of 30 years at diagnosis, while most patients diagnosed with papillary serous adenocarcinoma are peri- or postmenopausal.[54–58] These are discussed in greater detail in Chapter 27.

Extra-uterine Müllerian adenosarcomas are rare. Affected females are in the fifth to eighth decades of life and tumors arise in the omentum, ovary and pelvis.[59,60] Occurrence of Müllerian adenosarcoma in a 20-year-old patient has been described.[61] Likewise, MMMT has also been described occurring outside the uterus. In one series, patients with extra-uterine MMMT varied in age from 33 to 67 years.[62]

Clinical features

The clinical presentation of all the primary peritoneal Müllerian neoplasms is quite similar and usually charac-

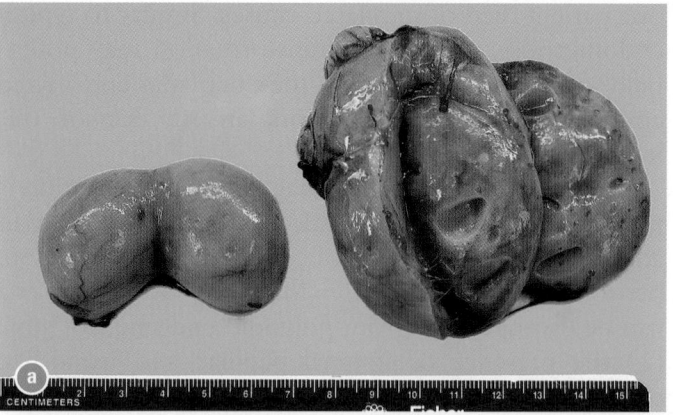

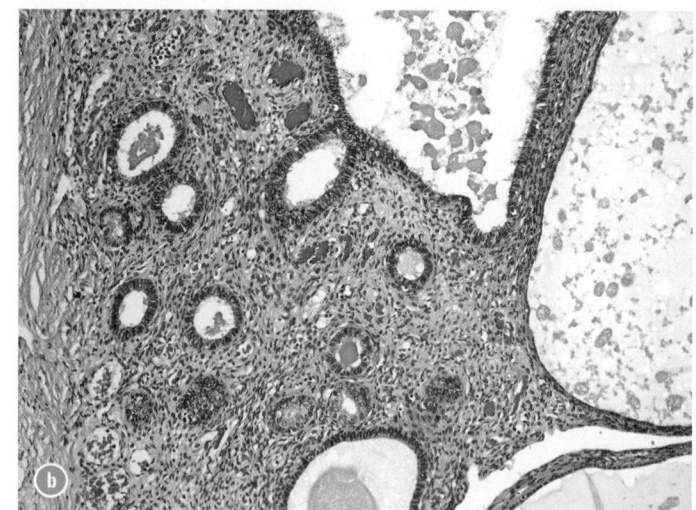

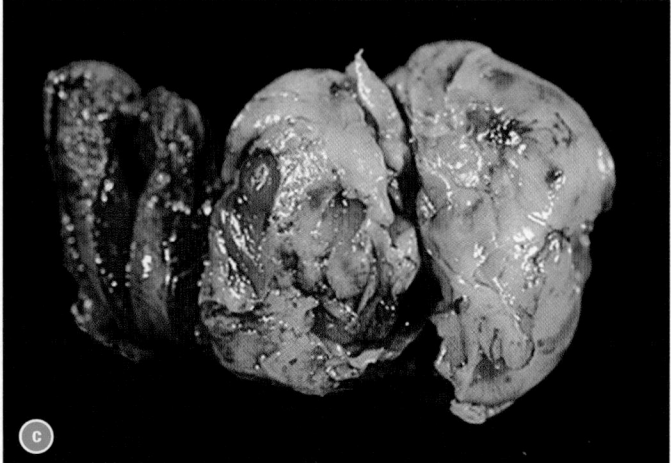

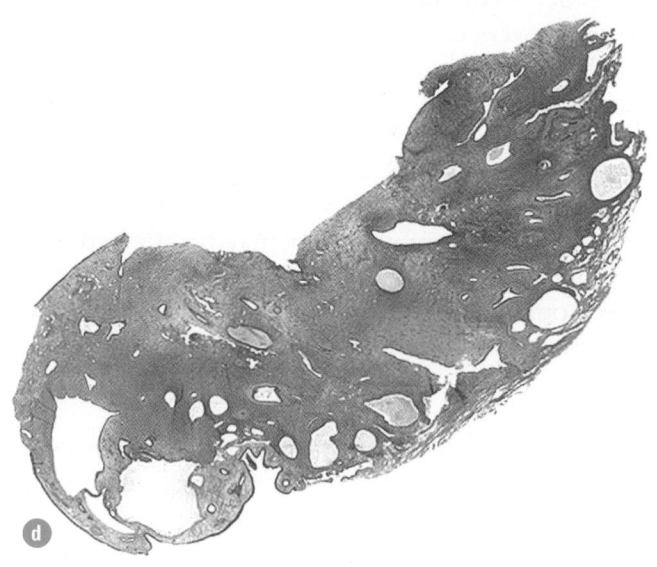

Fig. 23.5 (a) Gross appearance of polypoid endometriosis involving the omentum. (b) Polypoid endometriosis. (c) Endometrial polyp in a focus of pulmonary endometriosis; a small amount of lung tissue is on the left. (d) Microscopically, the lesion is indistinguishable from an endometrial polyp.

terized by symptoms related to large, frequently cystic abdominal and pelvic masses that may show involvement of multiple organs at time of diagnosis. Pain, abdominal distention and intestinal obstruction might develop in the setting of bulky tumors. Malignant peritoneal effusions may be present.

Pathology

Primary papillary serous tumors of the peritoneum resemble their ovarian counterparts. These tumors often form large and multiloculated cystic masses with solid foci and/or papillary excrescences in the wall of the cystic cavities, which are filled with a watery fluid. Seeding and extensive involvement of the peritoneal lining and omentum may be seen at surgery.

Microscopically, papillary serous adenocarcinomas are usually high-grade tumors, characterized by complex and interconnecting papillary formations lined by cuboidal cells showing moderate or marked cytologic atypia, high nuclear-to-cytoplasmic ratio, cellular stratification, increased mitotic activity, including atypical figures, necrosis and invasion of the underlying stroma (Fig. 23.6d). Psammoma bodies are often present and, when predominant, the tumor may be classified as psammocarcinoma (Fig. 23.6c). The latter is a rare variant of papillary serous adenocarcinoma that is characterized by low to moderate nuclear grade, local invasiveness and a somewhat more indolent behavior.[63]

Tumors placed in the borderline or low malignant potential category are distinguished from carcinoma on the basis of blander histologic features and lack of invasive growth (Fig. 23.6c). The diagnosis of a primary peritoneal papillary neoplasm requires careful examination of the ovaries for exclusion of a concur-

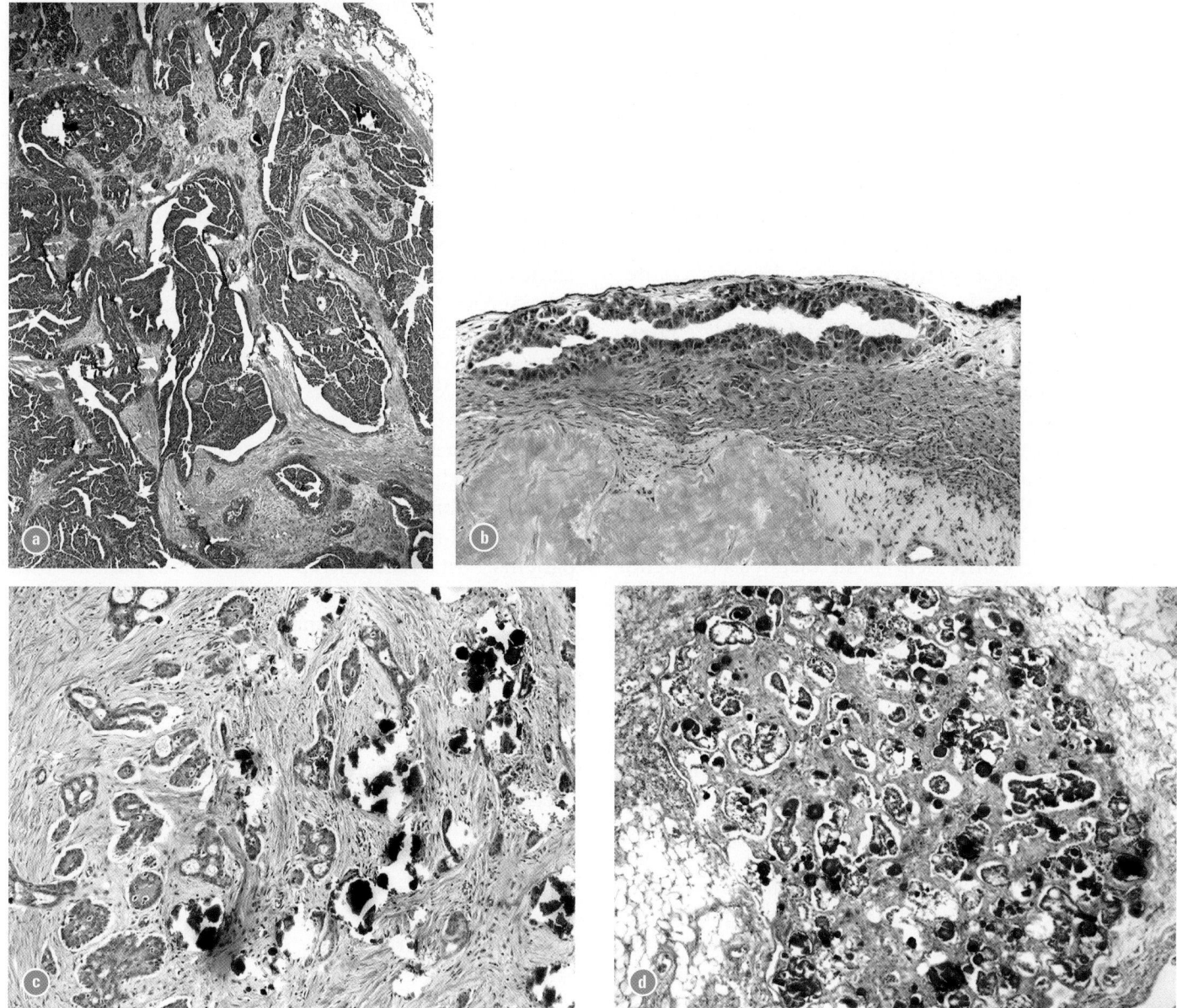

Fig. 23.6 (a) Primary peritoneal serous carcinoma. (b) Focal ovarian surface involvement by the tumor in (a). (c) Borderline tumor of peritoneal origin. (d) Psammocarcinoma.

rent ovarian primary. The presence of an ovarian primary with involvement of the peritoneal surface is regarded as FIGO Stage III.

Müllerian adenosarcoma of the peritoneal cavity also shares morphologic similarities with its uterine counterpart. Morphologically, these tumors are composed of glandular and mesenchymal elements, but only the latter is morphologically malignant. These tumors are composed of benign-appearing neoplastic glands set within a proliferation of the surrounding low-grade sarcomatous stroma, which usually resembles endometrial stromal sarcoma.

MMMT is characterized by proliferation of neoplastic epithelial and mesenchymal elements, both of which are unambiguously malignant. The sarcomatous element often does not show any particular line of differentiation and appears as an unclassified spindle cell sarcoma; however, identifiable foci of heterologous differentiation into rhabdomyosarcomatous, chondrosarcomatous, liposarcomatous or osteosarcomatous elements may be present. Regarding the carcinomatous element, glandular differentiation (adenocarcinoma) is most often seen, such as endometrioid and papillary serous subtypes, but squamous differentiation or undifferentiated carcinoma can also be present. Thorough search for the glandular element is required for the diagnosis in cases where the sarcomatous component is dominant; otherwise, the neoplasm is best classified as a high-grade undifferentiated sarcoma. Mitoses are frequent and necrosis is often present.

Immunoperoxidase studies are ineffective in differentiating between ovarian and primary peritoneal papillary serous adenocarcinomas. In both instances, the neoplastic cells will show reactivity for cytokeratins, epithelial membrane antigen (EMA), B72.3, carcinoembryonic antigen (CEA), WT-1 and Leu-M1.[64] However, immunostains might be extremely useful in the differential diagnosis with malignant mesothelioma. Although both neoplasms are positive for WT-1 (monoclonal antibody) and cytokeratins, calretinin is exclusively expressed in malignant mesothelioma, while Ber-EP4 has 95% sensitivity and 91% specificity for carcinoma.[65] On the other hand, immunoperoxidase stains are of very little help in the diagnosis of adenosarcomas and MMMT. The glandular component will express cytokeratins; however, the sarcomatous component of these lesions may also be positive, with focal positivity for markers such as α-smooth muscle actin (SMA) and vimentin, or express more specific markers when heterologous elements are present (e.g. desmin and myf-4 are positive in rhabdomyosarcomatous elements).

Molecular analysis of papillary serous carcinomas arising from the peritoneal surface has led to the discovery of its association with germline mutations of BRCA1 gene, in rates similar to those noted in ovarian counterparts.[66] Therefore, women with known mutations of this gene should undergo thorough follow-up not only for breast and ovarian carcinomas but also for primary peritoneal papillary serous carcinomas. Also evidenced by molecular studies is the fact that primary peritoneal papillary serous carcinoma has a multifocal origin in some cases, as substantiated by loss of heterozygosity (LOH) at the multiple allelic loci such as androgen receptor (AR) locus, WT-1 gene and of 6q.[67-69] LOH of AR gene is more often seen in patients harboring germline mutations of the BRCA-1 gene.[67] Similarly to papillary serous carcinoma arising in the ovary, serous carcinomas of the peritoneal surface also showed LOH at the p53 loci, located on chromosome 17, in 75–100% of cases.[70]

MMMT are not associated with mutations in BRCA-1 gene.[62] Data regarding cytogenetic or molecular abnormalities in Müllerian adenosarcomas are as yet unclear.

Treatment and prognosis

Primary papillary serous tumors of borderline or low-grade malignant potential have a good prognosis and require conservative therapy. Biscotti and Hart showed that of 14 patients who underwent treatment, which included surgery and adjuvant chemotherapy, only one patient died of complication related to therapy.[56] None of the patients died of disease.[56]

Primary peritoneal papillary serous carcinoma is clinically comparable to advanced-stage ovarian papillary serous carcinomas. Therapy options include cisplatin-based chemotherapy and surgery. Surgical approach encompasses cytoreductive technique and less aggressive, debulking operations. In one series, patients who underwent cytoreductive surgery appeared to have a longer overall survival, suggesting that the amount of residual disease is a prognostic factor.[71] In another series, combination of chemotherapy and cytoreductive surgical technique had a 5-year survival of 27% of patients.[58] In a recently reported series of patients with advanced and recurrent ovarian and peritoneal surface papillary serous carcinomas, the prior surgical score, completeness of cytoreduction and response to chemotherapy prior to surgery were statistically significant prognostic factors.[72]

Extra-uterine Müllerian adenosarcoma has a poor prognosis, with three of five patients developing recurrences and metastasis in one series.[59] MMMT is an extremely aggressive neoplasm with a likewise poor prognosis. To date, there are no large series with long-term follow-up defining therapy guidelines for these two entities; options certainly include chemotherapy, radiation and surgery.

Mesenchymal lesions of the peritoneum

SMOOTH MUSCLE NEOPLASMS

Background

Smooth muscle neoplasms of the peritoneal cavity encompass two main entities: leiomyoma and leiomyosarcoma. Another condition that is included under the designation of smooth muscle neoplasms is leiomyomatosis peritonealis disseminata (LPD); this entity is discussed in Chapter 20. To be considered a primary peritoneal neoplasm, a thorough examination of the uterus has to be performed to exclude 'metastatic' disease. Leiomyomata originating in the retroperitoneum and abdomen are rare, but unquestionably exist and are more often encountered in the female population. Most often they are encountered as a tumor mass arising in the wall of the gastrointestinal tract, mainly colon and rectum. Patients in this latter group are usually within the fifth and sixth decades, and males are more commonly affected than females. Leiomyosarcomas of the abdominal cavity are more often encountered in the retroperitoneum and show female preponderance affecting patients in the sixth and seventh decades of life.[73–75]

Clinical features

Smooth muscle neoplasms of the abdominal cavity and retroperitoneum may be asymptomatic or present as a mass that might impinge an abdominal organs, causing obstruction. In addition, when these tumors arise from the gastrointestinal tract, they may protrude into the bowel, cause obstruction of the lumen, mimic carcinoma and lead to ulceration of the mucosa with gastrointestinal bleeding. Leiomyomata are usually smaller than leiomyosarcomas, which might reach large proportions.

Pathology

Macroscopically, benign smooth muscle neoplasms (leiomyomata) usually have well-defined contours, with a firm, whorled, tan to white cut surface. Foci of hemorrhage may be present as well as focal cystic degeneration. In cases of leiomyosarcoma, malignant features, such as necrosis and invasion of surrounding structures, are often seen. Occasionally, leiomyomata and leiomyosarcomas can be seen in close association with a vascular structure, such as inferior vena cava, and the morphologic features are consistent with origin from the vessel wall.[76–78] When the diagnosis of a leiomyosarcoma is rendered in a retroperitoneal or abdominal mass, origin from a uterine primary should be excluded.

Microscopically, these benign and malignant neoplasms are usually characterized by the typical features associated with smooth muscle neoplasms, being composed of a proliferation of spindle cells arranged in long fascicles with elongated, cigar-shaped nuclei, vesicular chromatin, variably prominent nucleoli and moderate amounts of brightly eosinophilic cytoplasm (Fig. 23.7a,b). Rarely, cells with epithelioid morphology are present and, exceptionally, this morphology may predominate in the neoplasm, imitating an epithelial neoplasm and often making the histologic recognition challenging. Leiomyomata can undergo several degenerative phenomena, including infarction, cystic changes, hydropic or edematous degeneration and stromal hyalinization.

The current accepted criterion for malignancy for smooth muscle neoplasms occurring in the abdominal cavity or retroperitoneum of females is the presence of greater than 10 mitoses per 50 high power fields.[79] Although not indicative of malignancy, hypercellularity is a worrisome feature. The presence of atypical hyperchromatic nuclei should also trigger a more extensive search for diagnostic malignant features (necrosis, mitotic activity).

Although the morphologic features of smooth muscle neoplasms may allow an accurate diagnosis, immunoperoxidase studies are helpful in confirming

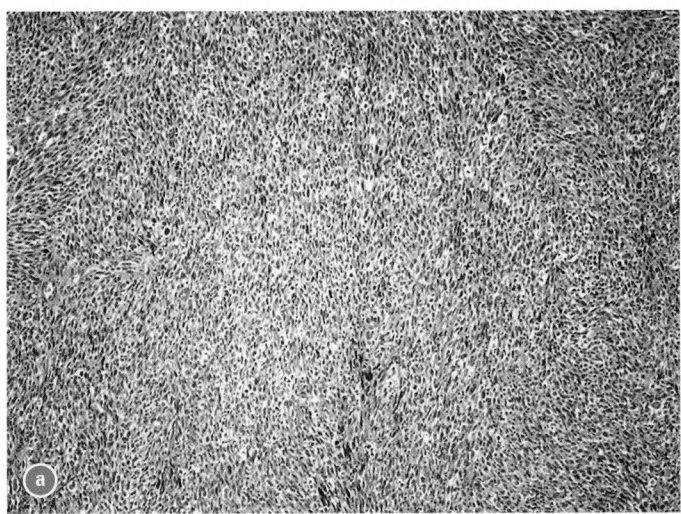 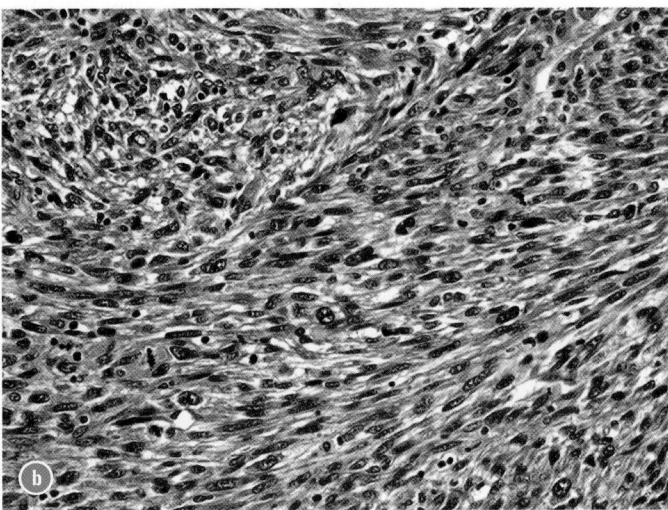

Fig. 23.7 (a) Leiomyosarcoma of the retroperitoneum presenting as a spindle cell neoplasm; (b) with cigar-shaped nuclei and eosinophilic cytoplasm.

the smooth muscle origin in less typical cases or small core needle biopsies. Table 23.1 shows the immuno-phenotypic characteristic of mesenchymal neoplasms of the peritoneum. Smooth muscle tumors are classically positive for SMA, desmin and h-caldesmon. The extent of expression of these markers by tumor cells varies from diffuse to focal, and this variability in expression, not surprisingly, might impact interpretation of small core needle biopsies. One should keep in mind that the morphology, if characteristic, should govern the diagnosis. Malignant tumors, for example, might have decreased expression or even lose expression of these markers. Other markers that can be expressed by smooth muscle tumors include cytokeratins and epithelial membrane antigen, which can be encountered in up to 40% of these tumors. Estrogen and progesterone receptors are often positive in leiomyomata, occurring in reproductive-age females; however, leiomyosarcomas appear to have significantly less expression of ER and PR.[80] S-100 protein, glial fibrillary acidic protein and c-kit are negative.

The differential diagnosis of smooth muscle tumors includes other mesenchymal neoplasms that are often encountered in the abdomen, such as gastrointestinal stromal tumor (GIST), desmoid fibromatosis and nerve sheath tumors, such as schwannomas and malignant peripheral nerve sheath tumor (MPNST). In GISTs, the tumor cells are uniform and show a palely eosinophilic cytoplasm with a syncytial appearance. Immunoperoxidase studies in GIST are somewhat overlapping with smooth muscle neoplasms; however, desmin is only rarely positive in GIST (less than 5% of the cases), whilst c-kit is characteristically positive in the majority of these tumors and negative in smooth muscle neoplasms (Table 23.1). Desmoid fibromatosis shows long hypocellular fascicles composed of cells with tapered ends. Occasionally, this neoplasm may show positivity for SMA and desmin in a very focal pattern, consistent with their myofibroblastic origin; h-caldesmon is negative. Neoplasms of nerve sheath origin (schwannoma and MPNST) usually show fascicles formed by elongated cells with tapered nuclei and display variable positivity for S-100 protein and glial fibrillary acidic protein (GFAP). They are negative for SMA and desmin.

Treatment and prognosis

The treatment of leiomyomata consists of simple excision. There is a very small risk of recurrence.

Leiomyosarcomas carry a poor prognosis with high incidence of recurrence and metastasis. The preferential sites of development of metastatic disease include lungs and liver. Therapy should include surgery with adjuvant chemotherapy and irradiation. The 5-year survival is approximately 30%.[81]

ENDOMETRIAL STROMAL SARCOMA

Epidemiology and clinical features

Endometrial stromal sarcoma (ESS) located in the abdominal cavity may be seen *de novo* or in association with a primary uterine endometrial stromal sarcoma. The former is believed to arise from endometriotic foci,[33,82-85] whereas the latter is due to metastasis or direct extension through the uterine wall. Regardless of the origin, primary peritoneal ESS is a rare phenomenon. The epidemiology of extra-uterine ESS is similar to the primary uterine neoplasm, affecting females in the fourth and fifth decades of life. These tumors may present as a palpable mass or give rise to obstructive symptoms of other intra-abdominal organs.

Table 23.1 Immunohistochemical profile of mesenchymal neoplasms of the peritoneal cavity

	SMA[a]	Desmin	h-Caldesmon	CD10	c-kit	Keratin	WT-1[b]
Smooth muscle neoplasms	+	+	+	±	−	±	
Endometrial stromal sarcoma	+	±	−	+	−	−	
Gastrointestinal stromal tumor	±	±	±		+	−	
Peripheral nerve sheath tumor	−	−	−		−	−	
Desmoplastic round cell tumor	−	+			−	+	+

[a]α-smooth muscle actin; [b]polyclonal antibody.

Pathology

The microscopic appearance of extra-uterine ESS is similar to its uterine counterpart. At low magnification, one can appreciate the characteristic infiltrative growth pattern of these tumors, which invade adjacent tissues with 'finger-like' projections.

Cytologically, they are composed of a uniform cellular proliferation of spindle cells with poorly defined cell borders, short, ovoid nuclei, inconspicuous nucleoli and scant pale cytoplasm, recapitulating non-neoplastic endometrial stroma in the uterus. Admixed within the tumor, foamy histiocytic cells may be present. In the background, frequent small-caliber arteries, reminiscent of spiral arteries of the endometrium, are present. Mitotic figures are rare, often numbering less than 5 mitoses per 10 high-power fields. Necrosis and pleomorphism are not features of these tumors, and neoplasms showing these features are best regarded as high-grade sarcomas, rather than endometrial stromal sarcomas. Glandular[53,83,86] and mesenchymal heterologous differentiation is occasionally seen and includes sex cord stromal elements,[87-90] smooth muscle,[91,92] bone and skeletal muscle.[93-96]

Similar to uterine neoplasms, extrauterine ESS may share morphologic similarities with smooth muscle neoplasms, mainly highly cellular leiomyoma and leiomyosarcoma. ESS are mainly positive for SMA, desmin, CD10 and progesterone receptor.[97,98] In contrast, smooth muscle neoplasms are positive for desmin, SMA and h-caldesmon.[98]

Cytogenetically, most ESS, including metastatic and primary extra-uterine tumors, are characterized by a recurrent chromosomal translocation, the t(7;17).[99] This translocation fuses the 5′ end of *JAZF1* gene on chromosome 7p15 and the 3′ end of *JJAZ1* gene on chromosome 17q21.[100]

Treatment and prognosis

The most common therapeutic modality offered to patients with ESS is cisplatin-based chemotherapy with or without associated radiotherapy. Uterine ESS is low-grade neoplasm that may metastasize many years after the initial diagnosis. The preferential sites of metastatic deposits are pelvis, intra-abdominal organs and lungs. Hence, the presence of a mass of extra-uterine ESS should trigger the search for a concurrent or prior uterine primary. The 5-year survival for uterine ESS is quite variable but approaches 80%. Primary extra-uterine ESS is likewise a low-grade neoplasm, but little data exist regarding the response to treatment and prognostic factors. In one series, extra-uterine ESS showed an intermediate behavior between uterine ESS and high-grade uterine sarcomas, with 8 of 20 patients showing tumor recurrences; five patients died of the disease.[101]

SOLITARY FIBROUS TUMOR

Epidemiology

Solitary fibrous tumor (SFT; *synonym*: hemangiopericytoma, fibrous mesothelioma) occurs over a wide range of ages, but is predominantly seen in adulthood. Males and females are equally affected. Initially SFT was believed to be a pleural-based disease; however, to date, SFT may affect several extra-pleural anatomic locations, including intra-abdominal organs and peritoneum.[102-105]

Clinical features

Frequently SFT will be an incidental finding. When symptomatic, patients will complain of a palpable mass, which is usually slowly growing, and/or sign and symptoms of mass effect on adjacent structures. Rarely, patients will seek medical attention due to symptoms related with hypoglycemia – Doege–Potter syndrome – attributed to elevated levels of insulin-like growth factor II produced by tumor cells.[106] Other systemic symptoms, such as fever and malaise can also be seen.

Pathology

Grossly, SFTs are well-circumscribed tumors with a firm, tan to white, cut surface that may reach considerably large sizes. Histologically, SFT is characterized by a proliferation of spindle cells arranged in a 'patternless' pattern, i.e. with no specific appearance (e.g. fascicular, storiform), with alternating zones of hypocellular myxoid stroma and hypercellular areas of fibrous stroma (Fig. 23.8). The neoplastic cells are small and oval to spindled with limited amount of pale cytoplasm. Scattered thick fibers of collagen and staghorn or 'hemangiopericytoma (HPC)'-like thin-walled branching vessels with hyalinization are frequently present. Most tumors show clear demarcation from the surrounding tissues, with a delicate fibrous capsule. Focal areas of adipocytic differentiation can be present (fat-forming SFT) within the tumor.[107]

Malignant SFT comprises approximately 10% of the cases of SFT.[108] It is characterized by hypercellularity (either diffuse or focal). Necrosis and pleomorphism may be encountered, but the single most widely accepted criterion of malignancy is the presence of more than 4 mitoses per 10 high-power microscopic

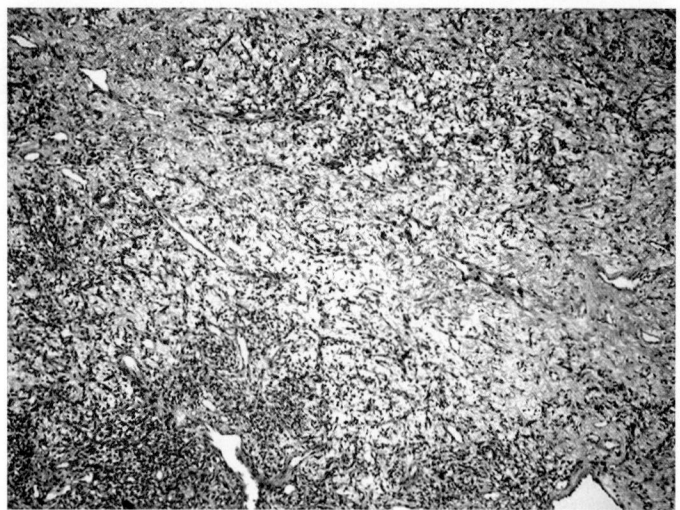
Fig. 23.8 Solitary fibrous tumor with a 'patternless' growth pattern and a combination of hypocellular and hypercellular areas.

fields. Often, areas of 'benign'-appearing SFT are present; however, when no areas of conventional SFT are noted because of predominance of malignant-appearing, unclassified, high-grade sarcoma areas, the diagnosis of SFT is one of exclusion.

SFT is characterized by immunoreactivity for CD34, and variable expression of bcl-2 and cytoplasmic O13 (CD99). Reactivity for CD34 may be partially or entirely lost in malignant SFT. Notably, since none of the above immunoperoxidase stains are specific for this entity, the diagnosis relies mostly on a correct morphologic identification with immunoperoxidase staining as adjunctive support.

The main differential diagnosis is with synovial sarcoma (SS), which carries a worse prognosis. SS differs morphologically from SFT because it is a fascicular cellular spindle cell neoplasm that shows focal immunoreactivity for keratins and EMA. Occasionally, reactivity for O13 and S-100 protein can be observed in SS. SFT should also be differentiated from fibrous mesothelioma. Table 23.2 shows the immunohistochemical profile of malignant mesothelioma and other entities in the differential diagnosis.

The latter is characterized by positivity for calretinin, WT-1 and keratins. Malignant mesothelioma is negative for CD34.[109]

Treatment and prognosis

Benign SFT can be cured by local surgical excision. Occasionally, tumors may recur. Malignant SFT carries a poor prognosis and should be excised with an ample surrounding margin, possibly with consideration of adjuvant chemo- and radiotherapy.

CALCIFYING FIBROUS TUMOR

Epidemiology

Calcifying fibrous tumor (CFT; *synonym*: calcifying fibrous pseudotumor) is a rare neoplasm that was initially described in the pediatric population in 1988 by Rosenthal and Abdul-Karim.[110] In 1993, Fetsch et al. reported the first series of tumors and coined the name of calcifying fibrous pseudotumor.[111] They observed the occurrence of this tumor in children and young adults; however, since the original description, cases affecting older adults have been described. The largest series of CFT included patients with ages ranging from 1 to 65 years.[112]

Clinical features

There appears to be no gender predilection, with a male:female ratio of 1:1.[112] Tumor can present as a subcutaneous mass or be deep in location. The anatomic distribution of this neoplasm is wide and includes head and neck, pleura, mediastinum, inguinal region, axillary area, extremities, and intra-abdominal, including mesentery, omentum, peritoneum and organ walls. Although most tumors are small in size, they can attain sizes up to 25 cm. Most patients present with complaints of a mass and local pain.

Pathology

Macroscopically, these tumors show defined circumscription and may have a thin fibrous capsule. Microscopically, the neoplasm is markedly hypocellular and

Table 23.2 *Immunoprofile of malignant mesothelioma and entities included in the differential diagnosis*

	AE1/AE3	WT-1	Calretinin	TTF-1	CD34
Malignant mesothelioma	+	+	+	–	–
Solitary fibrous tumor	–		–	–	+
Papillary serous carcinoma	+	+	–	–	–

composed of small, inconspicuous spindle cells embedded in a markedly hyalinized stroma (Fig. 23.9). A characteristic finding is the presence of a nodular lymphoplasmacytic infiltrate, sometimes forming germinal centers. Stromal calcifications are present and may be irregular in shape or may be psammomatous, varying from focal to massive. Regardless of the macroscopic appearance, some tumors may microscopically show peripheral entrapment of small vascular elements and small peripheral nerves. Occasionally, foci resembling inflammatory myofibroblastic tumor (IMT) – hypercellularity with prominent lymphoplasmacytic inflammatory infiltrate – are present.[113,114]

Immunoperoxidase studies are of little help in the diagnosis of CFT. The small spindle cells are usually positive for CD34 and may show focal expression of smooth muscle actin and desmin, confirming its myofibroblastic derivation.[112]

Due to the clinical and sometimes morphologic overlap between CFT and IMT, some authors suggest that CFT is in the spectrum of IMT, representing a 'burnt-out' or sclerosing phase.[112,113,115,116] Comparative immunoperoxidase studies have shown that the vast majority of CFT do not express anaplastic lymphoma kinase-1 (ALK-1), which is often expressed in IMTs (see below), suggesting that CFT probably represents a distinct neoplasm.[112,115,116] There are no studies addressing cytogenetic abnormalities in CFT.

Treatment and prognosis

In some cases of CFT, multicentricity has been noted.[112,114,117] In addition, repeated recurrences have been reported in rare cases.[111,112] There are no exam-ples of metastatic disease. The best approach to this neoplasm should be local excision with uninvolved, albeit modest, margins. The prognosis is excellent.

INFLAMMATORY MYOFIBROBLASTIC TUMOR (IMT)

Epidemiology

IMT is a fibroblastic/myofibroblastic neoplasm first recognized to be clonal by Su et al. in 1998, when three tumors were shown to have clonal cytogenetic abnormalities.[118] Before that, the pathogenesis of IMT was controversial and some authors believed it to represent a pseudotumor, rather than a true neoplasm, because of its rich accompanying inflammatory component.

IMT affects mainly children and young adults, although it may demonstrate quite a wide age range. The largest series published shows a median age of 9 years.[119] It has a slight predominance in female patients (F:M=1.3:1) and is most commonly encountered in the abdomen and retroperitoneum, but other sites such as lung, head and neck, trunk and extremities can also be affected.

Clinical features

IMT often presents as an intra-abdominal tumor mass that may be present in a retroperitoneal, mesenteric, omental, or intestinal location. Not uncommonly it will be coupled with systemic symptoms, such as fever, weight loss and pain, and laboratory abnormalities (anemia, thrombocytosis, polyclonal hyperglobulinemia and increased erythrocyte sedimentation rate).[119]

Pathology

Macroscopically, IMT has a tan, fleshy appearance due to the extensive inflammatory infiltrate, similar to the gross appearance of lymphomatous processes. Tumor size is quite variable; however, IMTs tend to be bulky masses when present intra-abdominally. Additionally, this neoplasm may present as multiple tumoral masses.

IMT is characterized by a fascicular proliferation of spindle cells, with indistinct cell borders, elongated nuclei, vesicular chromatin, small nucleoli and scant amounts of pale cytoplasm. Typically, there is an accompanying component of chronic inflammation that is composed mainly of lymphocytes and plasma cells. Often, the inflammatory component may be intense and obscure the neoplastic spindle cells, imparting a pseudotumoral appearance. In addition, the prominent infiltrate of inflammatory cells also may raise the possi-

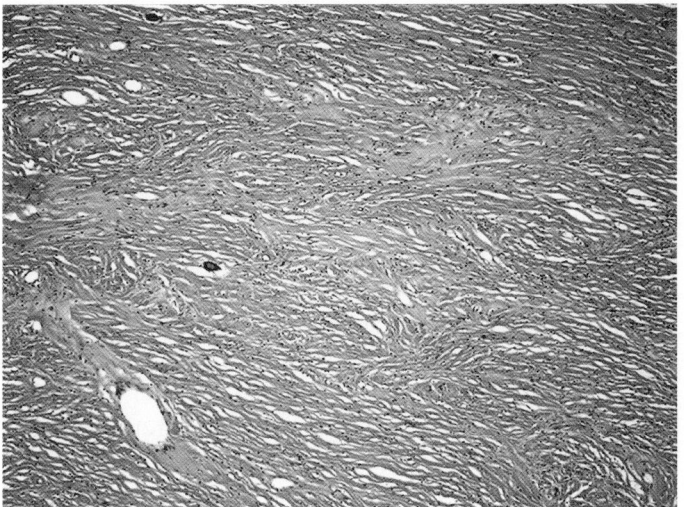

Fig. 23.9 Calcifying fibrous tumor (inflammatory myofibroblastic tumor?).

bility of involvement by a lymphomatous process. Areas of calcification and necrosis may be seen. Rarely, IMT may show intense hyalinization with a minor inflammatory component.

Immunoperoxidase studies will demonstrate the myofibroblastic differentiation of the spindle cells, with focal, non-specific positivity for α-smooth muscle actin and desmin. Occasionally, the tumor cells may be positive for keratins. However, unlike other myofibroblastic proliferations, 40–60% of IMTs are distinguished by positive staining for anaplastic lymphoma kinase-1 (ALK-1) protein that is more commonly seen in pediatric cases.[120-122] Immunoperoxidase studies will also demonstrate a mixed population of T- and B-lymphocytes, and the polyclonal nature of the plasma cells (immunostains for immunoglobulins kappa and lambda light chains).

The expression of the ALK-1 is due to the cytogenetically detectable abnormalities of chromosome 2q23, where the ALK gene is mapped to.[123] Translocation between chromosome 2 and various partners may be seen. The reported partners in this translocation include tropomyosin-3 and 4 (TPM3 and TPM4), clathrin heavy chain (CTLC), cysteinyl-tRNA synthetase (CARS) and Ran-binding protein 2 (RANBP2) genes, all of which have been reported to exchange material with chromosome 2 in IMTs.[124] The presence of the translocation can be suggested in conventional karyotype examination, and confirmed by fluorescence *in situ* hybridization (FISH) utilizing a 'split-apart' probe for chromosome 2.

The differential diagnosis of IMT includes nodular fasciitis (particularly if accompanied by a brisk inflammatory infiltrate), desmoid fibromatosis and CFT. Nodular fasciitis is a benign, self-limited, subcutaneous spindle cell proliferation which, if left untreated, regresses spontaneously. It is characterized by a bland spindle cell proliferation with variable amounts of inflammation and extravasated red blood cells. It is ALK-1 protein negative. Desmoid fibromatosis should be included in the differential of hypocellular, hyalinized IMTs. The cells composing desmoid tumors are usually more elongated. The absence of staining is not contributory; however, ALK-1 protein positivity excludes desmoid tumor. CFT is also in the differential diagnosis of hypocellular IMTs. CFTs are even less cellular and more hyalinized than IMTs. CFTs have also been shown to be negative for ALK-1 protein immunostains.

Treatment and prognosis

The overall prognosis is good. Local recurrence is noted in a small subset of patients (up to 20% of cases), with potential for local aggressive behavior.[125] However, these tumors rarely give rise to metastasis. Morphologically, it is not possible to predict which tumors will have an aggressive clinical course.

Surgery remains the main therapeutic modality for the treatment of IMT.[125] Chemotherapy may be used to manage aggressive and recurrent forms of the disease, decrease tumor burden and facilitate resection. Radiation does not appear to be effective.

GASTROINTESTINAL STROMAL TUMOR (GIST)

Epidemiology

Gastrointestinal stromal tumor (GIST) is an uncommon neoplasm that accounts for only 3% of all gastrointestinal neoplasms; however, these tumors constitute the most common mesenchymal neoplasm of the gastrointestinal tract. They are believed to originate from the interstitial cells of Cajal, the pacemaker cells for the tubular gastrointestinal tract, responsible for its peristalsis.[126] It was not until recently, with the systematic use of immunostains for c-kit, that gastrointestinal mesenchymal tumors that in the past were considered smooth muscle neoplasms (i.e. leiomyosarcoma and leiomyoma) and gastrointestinal autonomic nerve tumors (GANT) were found to in fact represent GISTs.

GIST affects mainly adults with no gender predilection; rarely children may be affected.[127,128] GIST may present as one of the components of Carney's triad, which is additionally composed of (extra-adrenal) paragangliomas and pulmonary chondromas.[129-131] Patients affected by Carney's triad appear to be younger than the usual population of sporadic GISTs.[131]

Clinical features

GIST occurs most often in the stomach (50% of cases), followed by small intestine and, less often, colon and esophagus.[132] When present outside the tubular gastrointestinal tract, such as liver, retroperitoneum and peritoneal or mesenteric surfaces, these tumors are believed to represent metastatic disease. However, it is not infrequent that a primary is never definitively identified, posing the possibility of an extra-gastrointestinal origin.

Pathology

These tumors are often large and well circumscribed. The cut surface is usually lobulated and homogenous, and well demarcated by a thin transparent fibrous capsule. Bulky masses may ulcerate into the tubular gastrointestinal tract, and present with gastrointestinal bleeding. Tumors may show hemorrhage, necrosis or cystic changes, especially after therapy with Gleevec® (see below).

Microscopically, most cases of GIST are distinguished by a monomorphic proliferation of spindled cells arranged in short fascicles (Fig. 23.10a); however, partial or complete epithelioid morphology may be present in a subset of cases (Fig. 23.10b,c). Commonly, a combination of the two cell types is noted, either intermixed or present as distinct areas of the tumor. The vast majority of GISTs have a bland cytomorphologic appearance, with ovoid to spindled nuclei, small to inconspicuous nucleoli and moderate amount of palely eosinophilic cytoplasm. Cell borders are indistinct and the cytoplasm of adjacent cells merges together forming a syncytial appearance. Occasionally,

clear perinuclear punched-out cytoplasmic vacuoles can be appreciated and are a hallmark of GIST. Also skenoid fibers may be present, which are amorphous extracellular eosinophilic deposits of abnormal collagen. Less than 5% of cases of GIST have nuclear pleomorphism.[132]

The vast majority of GISTs are reactive for c-kit, which can be cytoplasmic and/or dot-like positivity adjacent to the cell nucleus (Fig. 23.10d).[132] Furthermore, this positivity can vary from weak to strong and from focal to diffuse. Expression of this marker reflects the different patterns of mutation of Kit tyrosine kinase.[132] Notably, a very small percentage of GISTs are negative for c-kit immunostains.[133] These tumors are more often epithelioid and the diagnosis of GIST relies on exclusion of other neoplasms.[133] Other markers, which are less reliably positive in GISTs, include CD34

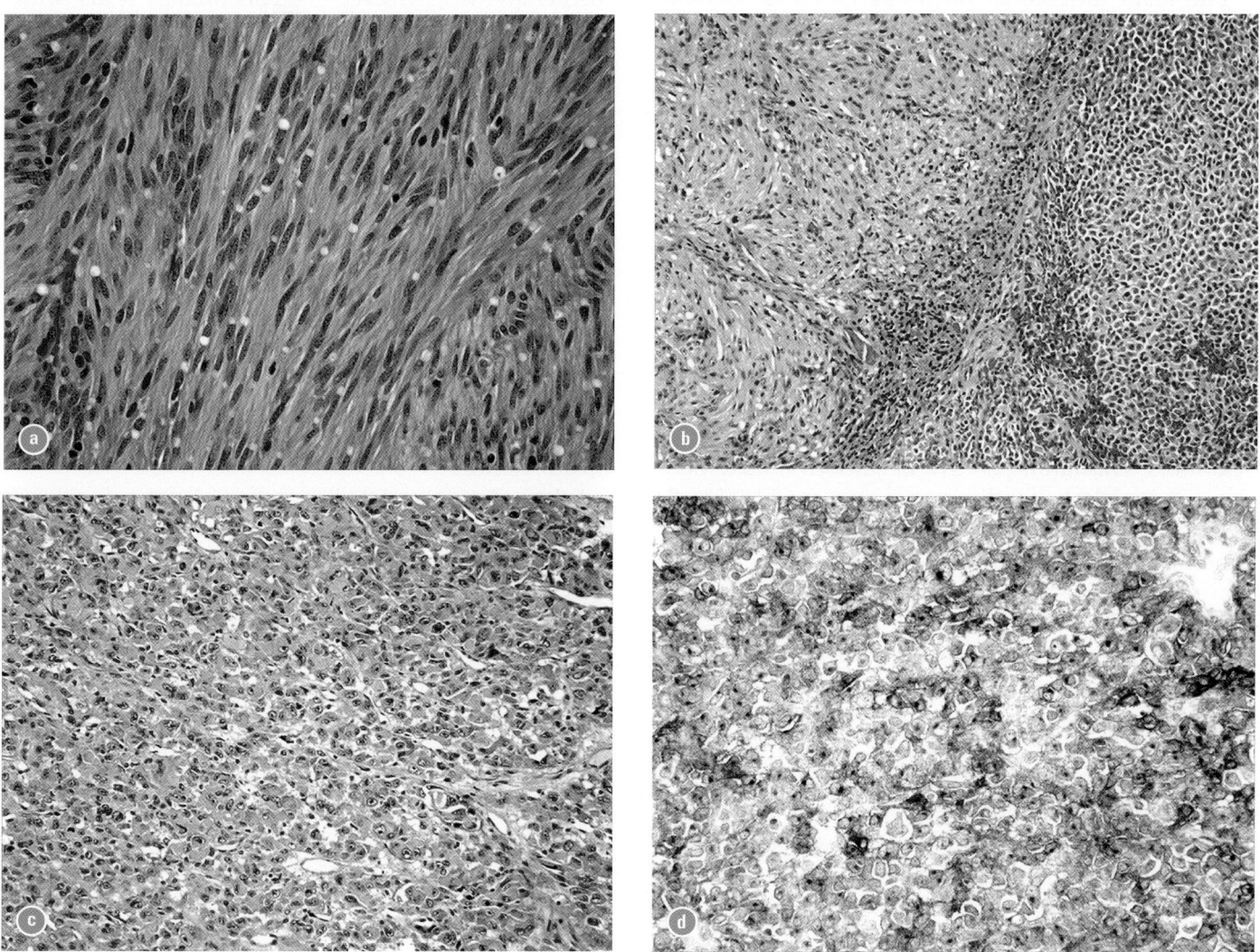

Fig. 23.10 Morphologic variants of gastrointestinal stromal tumor (GIST): (a) Spindle cell GIST, (b) mixed conventional (left) and epithelioid (right) GIST, (c) epithelioid GIST, (d) immunohistochemical study for c-kit showing dot-like positivity.

(60–70% of cases), α-smooth muscle actin and h-caldesmon. None of these are specific of GIST. In less than 5% of the cases, these tumors can express desmin.

The underlying pathogenesis of most cases of GIST is the constitutive activation of c-kit tyrosine kinase, which, independent to its binding to stem cell factor (SCF), will activate cell cycle pathways within the neoplastic cells, favoring proliferation and inhibiting apoptosis. In the majority of the cases (approximately 70%) this phenomenon is due to an in-frame mutation of exon 11 of the c-kit gene (chromosome 4), which encodes the juxtamembrane domain of the c-kit tyrosine kinase.[134] The other possible mutations observed include point mutations in exon 13 and 17, and an in-frame duplication of exon 9.[134] In a subset of cases where mutation in the kit gene cannot be detected, abnormalities in another tyrosine kinase, platelet-derived growth factor receptor alpha (PDGF-α), may be seen.[135]

The main differential diagnosis of GIST includes desmoid fibromatosis, schwannoma and leiomyosarcoma. Although morphologic differences distinguish between these entities, immunoperoxidase stains can easily confirm the diagnosis (see Table 23.2). The spindle cell fascicles forming desmoid tumors are longer that in GIST and the cells are more flattened, whereas the cells composing schwannomas show a more tapered cytomorphology, are usually arranged in Antoni A and Antoni B areas and are accompanied by thick-walled, hyalinized blood vessels. In contrast to GIST, leiomyosarcomas are composed of long fascicles of spindle cells showing plumper cells usually with more cytologic pleomorphism. CD34, once believed to be specific for GIST, can be expressed in a variety of tumors. Desmin is positive in smooth muscle neoplasm and might be focally expressed in myofibroblastic neoplasms, such as desmoid fibromatosis. However, none of these neoplasms will express c-kit.[136]

Treatment and prognosis

In the current accepted consensus, the prognosis of GIST is based on the combination of two pathologic parameters: mass size and number of mitoses (Table 23.3).[132] Based on these parameters, the patient can be grouped into one of four possible clinical outcome categories: very low, low, intermediate and high risk.[132] This system was designed because it was appreciated that tumors that in the past were classified as 'benign' based on macroscopic (i.e. small sizes) and cytomorphologic appearance, were still capable of giving rise to metastatic disease and, eventually, leading to the patient's death.

Table 23.3 Risk assessment of clinical behavior for gastrointestinal stromal tumors[a]

	Tumor size (cm)	Mitotic count (per 50 hpf)
Very low risk	<2	<5
Low risk	2–5	<5
Intermediate risk	<5	6–10
	5–10	<5
High risk	>5	>5
	>10	Any mitotic rate
	Any size	>10

[a]Reproduced from Fletcher et al.[132]

A breakthrough in the treatment of this disease is its response to the small molecule STI-571 (commercially known as Gleevec®). This drug acts by binding to the ATP-binding sites of the tyrosine kinase receptor and inactivating c-kit. Furthermore, some GISTs that have mutations of PDGFRa also appear to be responsive to therapy with Gleevec®.[137] This therapy leads to the often striking shrinkage of the tumor mass with hyalinization and necrosis. However, resistance to this compound has emerged and clinical trials with alternative drugs are in progress.

PERIPHERAL NERVE SHEATH TUMORS

Epidemiology

The list of neoplasms included in the group of peripheral nerve sheath tumors is rather long. However, for the purpose of discussing neoplasms that affect the peritoneal cavity, the focus will be on two distinct entities that occur with increased frequency in this anatomic location: schwannoma and malignant peripheral nerve sheath tumor.

Schwannomas and malignant peripheral nerve sheath tumor (MPNST) are diseases that occur in adults and show no gender predilection. Schwannomas may be seen in association with neurofibromatosis type 2 (NF2); however, in that situation, they usually affect the 8th cranial nerve bilaterally. MPNSTs occur in two distinct settings: sporadic or in association with neurofibromatosis type 1 (NF1). In the latter circumstance the patients are usually younger and there is a distinct male predominance.[138] MPNSTs can rarely be seen arising in patients with history of radiation therapy for other benign or malignant diseases;[139,140] tumors arising in this setting might show a latency period as long as 20 years.

Clinical features

Schwannomas are benign neoplasms that occur in the wall of the tubular gastrointestinal organs, especially the stomach.[141] They may also occur in the retroperitoneum, in association with paraspinal nerves. These tumors are usually incidental findings.

MPNST more frequently presents as a mass affecting an extremity, but it may also present as an intra-abdominal tumor. Very frequently, these tumors are seen in association with, and deforming, a nerve.

Schwannoma

Schwannomas occurring outside the tubular GI tract are characterized by a well-circumscribed tumor mass with a thick fibrous capsule. Within the GI tract these lesions have smooth contours and are well demarcated, but a well-defined capsule is not present. The cut surface is firm, tan to white and whorled, and may show foci of hydropic or edematous changes, cystic degeneration, hemorrhage and infarction.

Histologically, the classic appearance of schwannomas is that of a spindle cell neoplasm composed of short, intersecting fascicles, which have alternating areas of hypercellularity (designated Antoni A areas) and hypocellularity (designated Antoni B areas). The cells show elongated, tapering nuclei, inconspicuous nucleoli, poorly defined cell borders and pale, fibrillary cytoplasm. Frequently, tumor cells form palisading arrangements surrounding a core of fibrillary syncytial cytoplasm (Verocay body). Throughout the tumor there are frequent blood vessels that show hyalinization of their wall, giving them a thick appearance. Usually, in the capsule and within the tumor one can appreciate foci of chronic inflammation composed of plasma cells and small lymphocytes.

Occasionally, schwannomas may be entirely composed of Antoni A type areas, i.e. formed by cellular fascicles of spindle cells with no intervening hypocellular areas, and have no Verocay bodies. These neoplasms are designated cellular schwannomas. This variant is particularly common in the retroperitoneum.[142] Another infrequent variant of schwannoma is melanotic schwannoma, in which tumor cells show deposition of melanin pigment and demonstrate the presence of melanosomes in all stages of differentiation by electron microscopy examination.[143] Not infrequently, focal or diffuse cytologic atypia with large, bizarre nuclei and blotched chromatin are noted. This atypia is characterized by smudged nuclei and is due to degeneration of tumor cells, characterizing an ancient schwannoma, and should not be interpreted as malignant transformation. Malignant transformation of schwannomas is exceedingly rare, and is usually in the form of epithelioid MPNST or angiosarcoma.[144]

MPNST

Grossly, MPNSTs form large masses that show entrapment of adjacent tissues and organs and demonstrate a tan, firm cut surface that often shows evidence of hemorrhage and tumor necrosis. Origin in a large peripheral nerve is quite often easy to determine at macroscopic inspection. In patients with NF1, the entire peripheral nerve appears enlarged and abnormal at macroscopic examination, with areas of more typical neurofibromatous tissue.

At low-power examination, these tumors are characterized by hypercellular long fascicles of spindle cells, which alternate with areas of lower cellular density. Perivascular accentuation, with increased compactness of tumor cells surrounding blood vessels, is a characteristic feature of these tumors (Fig. 23.11a,c). Extensive areas of hemorrhage and necrosis are often present. At higher magnification, the tumor cells show tapered and vesicular nuclei, with small amount of pale cytoplasm (Fig. 23.11b). Mitoses may be quite numerous. Hypercellularity, nuclear atypia and necrosis are criteria for grading these neoplasms in low-, intermediate- and high-grade tumors.

Occasionally, heterologous differentiation, (osteosarcomatous, chondrosarcomatous, angiosarcomatous and rhabdomyosarcomatous, among others) are focally identified and are more frequently seen in tumors arising in the setting of NF-1.[145] Of these, rhabdomyosarcomatous differentiation appears to correlate with a worse prognosis. These tumors are known as 'malignant Triton tumors'. MPNSTs may also show variant morphologies, such as epithelioid and glandular differentiation. However, these variants are quite rare.

Immunoperoxidase studies may be of importance in the diagnosis of schwannomas, especially cellular variants and tumors showing degenerative atypia. These neoplasms are strongly and diffusely positive for S-100 protein and glial fibrillary acidic protein (GFAP).[141] Immunostains for neurofilaments are negative, in accordance with the absence of axons within these neoplasms. In addition, epithelial membrane antigen highlights the tumor capsule. Muscle markers, such as α-smooth muscle actin and desmin, and c-kit are negative.

Immunostains for MPNSTs, however, are not as reliable. These neoplasms are positive for S-100 protein and glial fibrillary acidic protein in approximately 30% of cases (Fig. 23.11d). However, the expression of these markers is usually focal or even absent.[146] In the latter case, the diagnosis relies on morphologic features

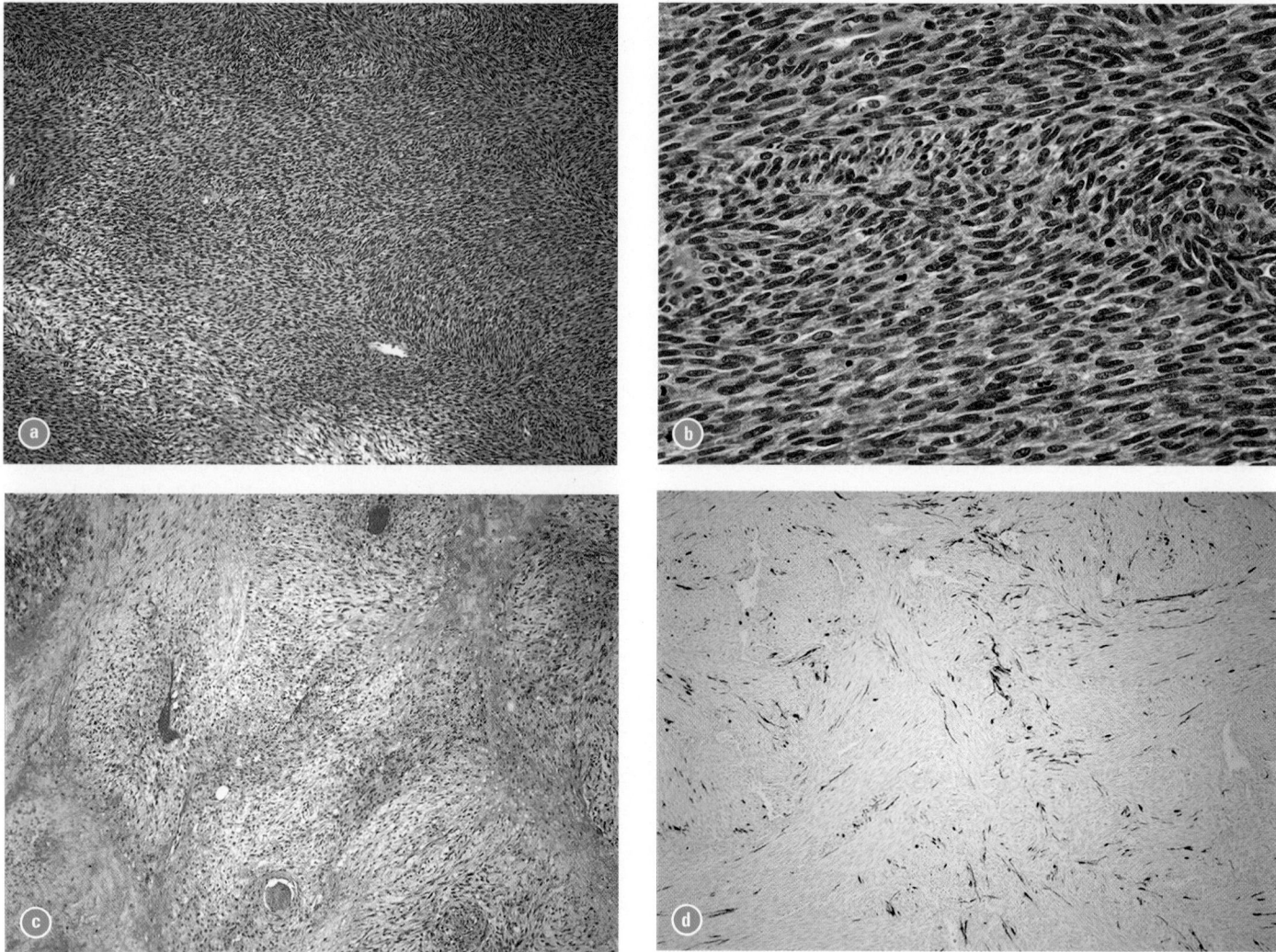

Fig. 23.11 (a) Malignant peripheral nerve sheath tumor at low magnification showing a hypercellular spindle cell neoplasm with intervening areas of hypocellularity; (b) at higher power showing the spindled cell population with tapered nuclear morphology and abundant mitoses. (c) In areas, MPNST may show increased cellularity around blood vessels. (d) S-100 protein stain may display positivity in some tumor cells.

and in excluding other entities, such as smooth muscle tumors. Logically, tumors arising in the setting of NF1 are more likely to be MPNST, even without immunomarkers.

The differential diagnosis of schwannoma and MPNST includes smooth muscle neoplasms and GIST. The immunohistochemical profile of these entities is discussed elsewhere in this chapter. Also important to consider in the differential with MPNST is synovial sarcoma. Synovial sarcomas are positive for keratins and EMA. S-100 protein is positive in a subset of cases; however, GFAP is negative.

Schwannomas are characterized by a few simple chromosomal abnormalities, including loss of material

from the long arm of chromosome 22, loss of a sex chromosome and trisomy of chromosome 7.[147] Most of the MPNSTs analyzed revealed a clonal complex karyotype.[147]

Treatment and prognosis

Schwannomas have an excellent prognosis. A simple surgical excision is curative. They do not recur or metastasize.

MPNSTs carry a poor prognosis, which does not necessarily correlate with tumor grade. The overall 5-year survival is approximately 50%.[148] Surgical excision, preferentially with wide surrounding margins, associated with chemo- and radiotherapy remains the main therapeutic option. Tumors showing rhab-domyosarcomatous differentiation and those occurring in NF1 patients have an even worse clinical outcome, with only 20% of the patients alive at 5 years.[148] MPNSTs show a high recurrence rate and frequently metastasize, particularly to lungs.

DESMOID FIBROMATOSIS

Epidemiology

Desmoid fibromatosis is a bland-appearing, locally aggressive spindle cell proliferation that is commonly encountered in the abdominal wall and in intra-abdominal locations. It commonly affects adults and shows a slight female predilection. Not infrequently, this tumor arises in association with a scar related to a prior abdominal surgery, such as Cesarean section. Extra-abdominal tumors involving head and neck and extremities are also commonly encountered.

Clinical features

The typical clinical presentation is that of an infiltra-tive, painless mass. Tumors arising within the abdomi-nal cavity can potentially cause obstruction of hollow organs. Desmoid tumors can reach proportionally large sizes, particularly when occurring intra-abdominally. Desmoid fibromatosis may occur sporadically, in a familial setting and as an extra-colonic manifestation of familial adenomatous polyposis (FAP). In the latter setting, tumors are frequently located within the abdominal cavity.[149,150]

Pathology

Grossly, desmoid tumors are firm tan, white masses that may show entrapment of normal tissues and structures at the periphery, although a thin fibrous pseudocapsule may be present. The cut surface is firm, shows a whorled aspect and may have small foci of cystic or mucinous change.

Microscopically, these neoplasms are characterized by a relatively hypocellular, fascicular proliferation of bland-appearing spindle cells. In the background a variable amount of collagen fibers, which can amount to keloid-like hyalinization, can be seen (Fig. 23.12). The neoplastic cells show variable cytologic character-istics with elongated tapered or rounder nuclei with small nucleoli and moderate amounts of palely eosinophilic cytoplasm. The cell borders are indistinct. Mitoses may be seen but are usually quite scarce. Necrosis is not a feature of desmoid tumors. Occasion-ally, tumors (particularly those arising in the abdomen),

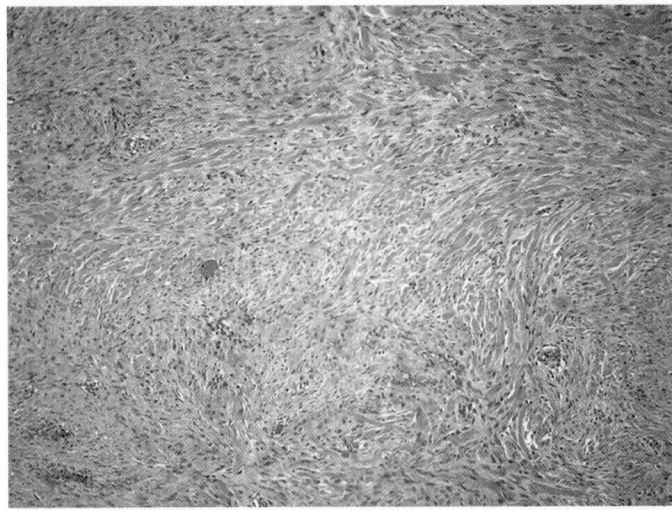

Fig. 23.12 Desmoid fibromatosis is composed of long fascicles of spindle cells. Intra-abdominal examples often show keloidal hyalinization.

may resemble nodular fasciitis, with shorter, inter-secting fascicles associated with extravasated red blood cells.

Immunoperoxidase studies are of very little aid in the diagnosis of desmoid fibromatosis. These tumors may show focal staining with α-smooth muscle actin and desmin, supporting its myofibroblastic derivation. These neoplasms may also be positive for β-catenin (nuclear staining).[151–154] Focal positivity for S-100 protein may be seen in occasional cases. Epithelial markers, such as keratins and epithelial membrane antigen, are negative.

Desmoid tumors are definitively clonal neoplasms, with reported trisomies of chromosomes 8 and 20, and loss of material from 5q.[155–157] Desmoid tumors arising in a familial setting and in patients with FAP show mutations in the adenomatous polyposis coli (APC) gene (5q15-q22).[158–160]

The differential diagnosis includes scar tissue, smooth muscle neoplasms, nodular fasciitis and fibrosarcoma. Hypertrophic scar tissue can simulate a tumor mass; however, usually, there is a clear-cut history of surgery or trauma to the area. Although scars are not encap-sulated or well-circumscribed processes, they will not be as infiltrative when compared with desmoids, with very little or no entrapment of adjacent structures and tissues.

Cells with elongated, oval, cigar-shaped nuclei and brightly eosinophilic cytoplasm characterize leiomyoma and leiomyosarcoma. In addition, immunoperoxidase studies such as SMA, desmin and h-caldesmon can help in the differentiation between desmoid fibromatosis and smooth muscle neoplasms. Nodular fasciitis is a self-limited myofibroblastic lesion encountered in subcutaneous tissue and is distinguished by a cellular proliferation of 'tissue-culture-like' spindle cells with intersecting fascicles interspersed with red blood cells. Keloidal hyalinization is also a feature seen in fasciitis. Mitoses are common. A history of trauma is often present and the lump usually shows a rapid growth over a couple of weeks.

Treatment and prognosis

Desmoid fibromatosis is locally aggressive, with a tendency for local recurrence; however, it does not metastasize. The cornerstone of treatment is surgical resection with a wide margin of uninvolved tissue. The latter may be somewhat difficult to attain because of the locally infiltrative nature of the tumor and, therefore, numerous surgical procedures might be necessary.

Intra-abdominal tumors may represent a therapeutic challenge. Local radiation therapy may be necessary in areas of limited surgical access to decrease the likelihood of local recurrences, whereas chemotherapy may be necessary for local control of lesions that are difficult to remove surgically.

LIPOSARCOMA

Epidemiology

Liposarcoma (LPS) is the most common sarcoma in adults, with no gender predilection. There are three main subgroups: well-differentiated, myxoid and pleomorphic. Myxoid and pleomorphic LPS are more generally encountered involving the limbs, while well-differentiated LPS account for most cases of intra-abdominal liposarcoma. Given the purpose of this chapter, only well-differentiated LPS will be discussed.

Its nomenclature is dependent on the location of the tumor mass. Tumors located in areas amenable to complete surgical excision (i.e. lower extremities) are designated atypical lipomatous tumors (ALT), while those located in areas where surgical access is more difficult (i.e. abdomen and retroperitoneum) are called LPS.

Clinical features

Commonly, LPS presents as a painless mass. It may be discovered incidentally on abdominal scans for unrelated reasons or it may cause symptoms of compression of adjacent organs. It can grow to large proportions to occupy the entire abdominal cavity. Not uncommonly, patients will perceive an enlargement of their abdominal circumference and/or weight gain.

Radiologically, LPS most commonly has signal intensity identical to adipose tissue. When dedifferentiation occurs (see below), a mass with a hyperintense signal will be visualized within the adipocytic tumor.

Pathology

Grossly, well-differentiated LPS is usually a mass or multiple tumor masses composed of yellow adipose tissue, with a thin transparent fibrous capsule that is slightly firmer when compared with non-neoplastic adipose tissue. It usually shows areas with thick fibrous bands transversing the tissue, and may show areas of myxoid degeneration. Occasionally, areas of dedifferentiation are noted and are composed of tan/gray firm areas within the adipocytic tumor, with distinct separation from the adipocytic component.

Microscopically, adipocytic or lipoma-like well-differentiated LPS shows remarkable resemblance to normal adipose tissue. Therefore, identification of variation in adipocyte size and shape is crucial for the diagnosis (Fig. 23.13a,b). In addition, bizarre, hyperchromatic stromal cells should be present. These atypical cells are more frequently noted within the thick fibrous bands that are characteristically present in the tumor, and in vessel walls. Although once a prerequisite for the diagnosis of LPS, lipoblasts may or may not be present and are no longer required for the diagnosis of this entity. Occasionally, sclerosing areas and spindle cell morphology may be noted. The former is characterized by hypocellular fibrous tissue with admixed occasional large, bizarre cells. In the absence of lipoma-like LPS, this variant may be very difficult to recognize. In the inflammatory variant of well-differentiated LPS, the adipocytic nature of the tumor is obscured by the dense chronic inflammatory component and the diagnosis will rely on identification of scattered abnormal stromal tumor cells and occasional lipoblasts.[161] The presence of myxoid changes and heterologous elements such as cartilage or bone may be seen within the tumor.

Dedifferentiation of LPS is a relatively uncommon phenomenon and can occur *de novo* or may be seen in recurrent tumors.[162] Areas showing dedifferentiation are characterized by an abrupt transition from the adipocytic neoplasm into a non-lipogenic spindle cell proliferation that usually shows a 'malignant fibrous histiocytoma'-like appearance, most commonly resembling an unclassified sarcoma. There are no specific morphologic characteristics to dedifferentiated LPS

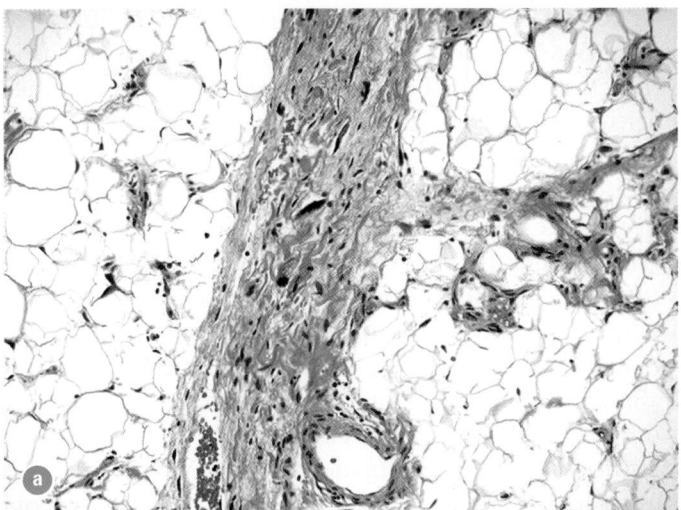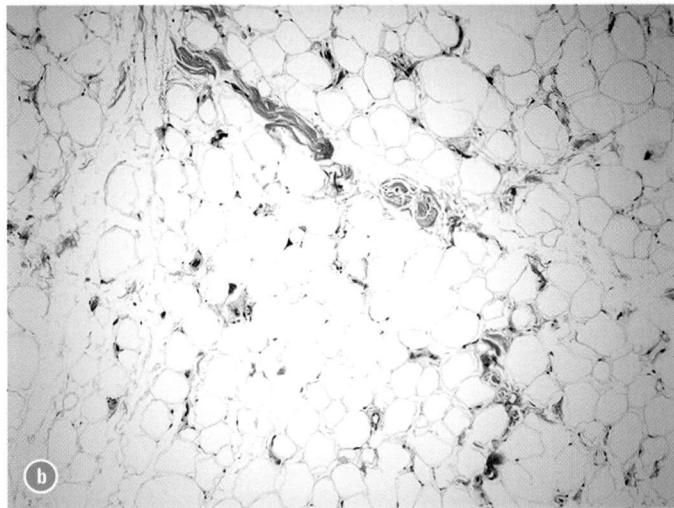

Fig. 23.13 (a) Well-differentiated liposarcomas show thick fibrous septae with conspicuous atypia. (b) Variation of adipocyte size and shape is characteristic.

and, not uncommonly, it may resemble other low- and high-grade sarcomas. However, recognition of certain patterns, such as a peculiar nodular whorling architecture, morphologically resembling perineuriomas, can aid in the diagnosis of dedifferentiated LPS.[163] In cases of recurrent LPS with dedifferentiation, the sharp interface between the well- and dedifferentiated component may be lost and co-mingling of them is usually seen. Immunoperoxidase stains are of no help in the diagnosis of dedifferentiated LPS. Because of its indistinct morphologic appearance, the diagnosis of dedifferentiated LPS requires extensive sampling and recognition of the well-differentiated component.

Cytogenetically, these tumors, both well-differentiated and its variants, and dedifferentiated LPS, are characterized by the presence of a supranumerary ring chromosome or giant marker derived from material from 12q13-15.[164,165]

Treatment and prognosis

The treatment is largely surgical. Although well-differentiated, LPS does not have metastatic potential, its rate of local recurrence is rather high and patients will often succumb to uncontrolled local recurrences.[166]

When a diagnosis of dedifferentiated LPS is made, patients risk of metastasis increases to 20%.[167] The most likely site of metastatic disease is the lung. The metastatic tumor masses may be composed of dedifferentiated LPS or may be identical to the well-differentiated component. Surgery in association with

chemotherapy and radiation are the mainstays of treatment.

DESMOPLASTIC SMALL ROUND CELL TUMOR

Epidemiology

Desmoplastic small round cell tumor (DSRCT) is a highly aggressive small round blue cell tumor of unknown origin, characterized by its marked predilection for adolescents and young adults. Males are by far more frequently affected than females.

Clinical features

Most tumors occur in the abdominal cavity, with rare cases affecting extra-abdominal locations. Pain, weight loss and complaints of a mass are the most common symptoms.[168]

Pathology

Grossly, this tumor is characterized by a firm and lobulated cut surface. Tumor size is variable, but may be as large as 20 cm.

Microscopically, the tumor is composed of a proliferation of small, uniform ovoid cells with indistinct cell borders arranged in sheets, nests and cords, with hyperchromatic nuclei, small nucleoli and small amount of cytoplasm (Fig. 23.14). Characteristically, this tumor is distinguished by a prominent desmoplastic stromal reaction. However, cellular cases showing little desmoplasia are recognized and, in these cases, the diagnosis

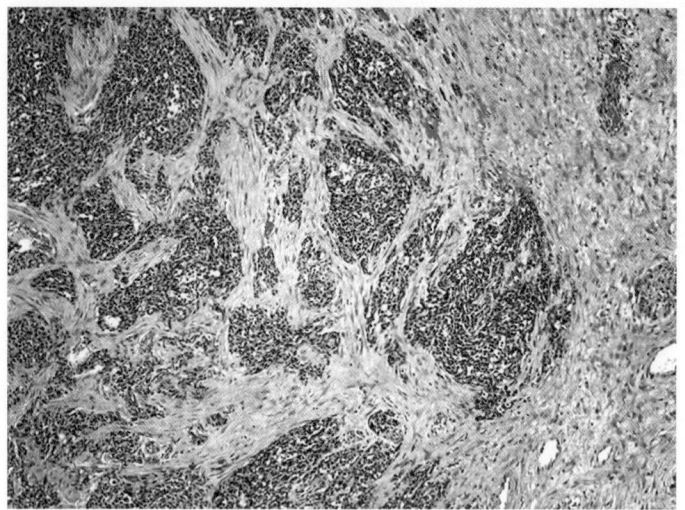

Fig. 23.14 Desmoplastic small round cell tumor is characterized by cohesive nests of small round blue cells within dense desmoplastic stroma.

relies on the typical cytomorphology in combination with immunoperoxidase and cytogenetic findings (see below). Mitotic figures can be numerous and necrosis is usually present. Rarely, glandular and rosette-like structures can be identified.

The characteristic immunoperoxidase profile of DSRCT consists of reactivity for cytokeratins, desmin (in a characteristic perinuclear dot-like pattern) and WT-1 (polyclonal antibody). Other markers such as O13 (also known as CD99 and mic-2) and neuron-specific enolase (NSE) are usually positive, but are neither sensitive nor specific in the absence of reactivity for the former markers.

Cytogenetically, the vast majority of these tumors are characterized by the presence of a reciprocal translocation t(11;22)(p13;q12) that juxtaposes the EWS gene on chromosome 22 and WT-1 gene on chromosome 11.[169] The chimeric EWS-WT-1 protein acts as a transcription factor.

The differential diagnosis of DSRCT includes numerous entities characterized by the neoplastic proliferation of small round blue cells. This list includes entities such as small cell carcinoma, Ewing's sarcoma/PNET, lymphoma, neuroblastoma and rhabdomyosarcoma. Precise diagnosis is of crucial importance because most of these diseases are treated with specific chemotherapeutic regimens. Table 23.4 shows the immunoprofile of the main entities included in the differential diagnosis. Immunoperoxidase and cytogenetics studies help in this differentiation.

Small cell carcinoma may show desmoplasia, frequent mitoses and extensive necrosis. However, small cell carcinoma is negative for desmin and WT-1. Ewing's sarcoma/PNET is another disease of young patients with cells that are round with defined cell borders and its most characteristic finding is a strong, membranous staining pattern for O13. Cytogenetically, it is also characterized by a balanced translocation between chromosomes 11 and 22. However, the gene involved in chromosome 11 is FLI-1 gene, rather than WT-1. Neuroblastoma is mainly a disease of infancy that shows positivity for other neural markers, such as NSE, neurofilament and protein gene product 9.5 (PGP 9.5), and is negative for keratins and desmin. Rhabdomyosarcoma, which include embryonal, alveolar and pleomorphic subtypes, usually has admixed large rhabdomyoblasts that have ample brightly eosinophilic cytoplasm and also shows positivity for desmin and other skeletal muscle markers such as myogenin (Myf-4).

Treatment and prognosis

DSRCT is characterized by a highly aggressive clinical course. Initial response to high-dose chemotherapy can be seen in some patients, but 5-year survival is dismal. In one series, 70% of patients died of uncontrolled disease or widespread metastasis in a mean period of 20 months.[170]

Table 23.4 Immunohistochemical stains for small round blue cell neoplasms

	WT-1[a]	O13 (CD99)	LCA[b]	Desmin	myf-4	NSE[c]
DSRCT[d]	+	+	−	+	−	+
Small cell carcinoma	−	±	−	−	−	+
Ewing's/PNET[e]	−	+ (membranous)	−	−	−	+
Lymphoma	−	−	+	−	−	−
Neuroblastoma	−	−	−	−	−	+
Rhabdomyosarcoma	−	−	−	+	+	−

[a]WT-1, polyclonal antibody; [b]LCA, leukocyte common antigen; [c]NSE, neuron-specific enolase; [d]DSRCT, desmoplastic small round cell tumor, [e]Peripheral neuroectodermal tumor.

Mesothelial lesions of the peritoneum

MESOTHELIAL HYPERPLASIA

Epidemiology

Mesothelial hyperplasia is a benign, reactive condition with no neoplastic potential that is associated with a variety of chronic and acute injuries to the mesothelial surface. The inciting injury can be of inflammatory, infectious or neoplastic nature, with direct or indirect effect on the superficial mesothelial cells. Examples of settings in which mesothelial hyperplasia is often encountered include inflammatory pelvic disease with tubo-ovarian abscess, ovarian neoplasms (malignant or benign) and peritoneal effusion due to cardiac, renal or hepatic insufficiency.

Clinical features

Mesothelial hyperplasia is usually an incidental finding during examination of peritoneal washings or ascites, or in biopsy specimens of the peritoneum at the time of laparotomy/laparoscopy.

Pathology

If grossly evident, mesothelial hyperplasia is characterized by the presence of small white nodules or flat plaques on the surface of the peritoneum. Microscopically, a variety of architectural patterns may be seen, including solid, papillary and tubulo-papillary. The cytologic features of the proliferation of mesothelial cells resemble normal mesothelium with polygonal cells with round nuclei, vesicular chromatin, one to three small nucleoli and ample eosinophilic cytoplasm. The cell borders are usually well defined with spaces or 'windows' between cells that are determined by the ultrastructural presence of microvilli on the cell surface. This feature is more readily appreciated in cytologic preparations. Prominent reactive features, such as nuclear enlargement, increase of nuclear-to-cytoplasm ratio and prominent nucleoli may be seen. Mitoses are a frequent finding. Necrosis is not seen.

The immunoperoxidase pattern of staining of benign mesothelial cells is identical to that seen in malignant mesothelioma (see below).

The main differential diagnosis is with malignant mesothelioma. In florid cases of mesothelial hyperplasia, this differentiation can be difficult; however invasion of underlying adipose tissue is often seen in malignant processes, while absent in mesothelial hyperplasia. In cytologic preparations, malignant mesothelioma is usually characterized by the formation of large, three-dimensional groups, while benign mesothelial cells are usually arranged in flat sheets. The nuclear features are helpful if the mesothelioma is poorly differentiated; however, in well-differentiated cases, malignant mesothelioma may show features identical to benign and reactive mesothelial cells. Psammomatous calcifications can be seen in both conditions. There is a controversial debate regarding the utility of epithelial membrane antigen (EMA) in this important distinction. Although some authors believe that EMA is a useful diagnostic tool, being positive in malignant cases, in our experience, this marker is positive in benign and malignant proliferations, in diverse staining patterns, and does not aid in this dilemma.[171,172] The most reliable tool for the distinction between mesothelial hyperplasia and malignant mesothelioma is the presence of karyotypic abnormalities by conventional cytogenetics, FISH studies or other molecular diagnostic studies. These studies can be carried out on fresh specimens (including peritoneal fluid) or in sections derived from paraffin-embedded, formalin-fixed tissue. Since mesothelial hyperplasia is a reactive condition, it should not have cytogenetic aberrations, while a number of alterations are seen in malignant mesothelioma.

Treatment and prognosis

Mesothelial hyperplasia is a benign, reactive condition. It requires no clinical and/or surgical intervention, and treatment and prognosis are directly related to the underlying condition.

CYSTIC MESOTHELIOMA

Epidemiology

Cystic mesothelioma is a rare disease that involves the peritoneal cavity of females, predominantly in the reproductive-age group.[173–177] Children, males and postmenopausal women are rarely affected. Very often these patients have a history of prior surgery to the abdominal cavity, raising the possibility of a reactive process rather than a true neoplasia.[177,178]

Clinical features

Most patients present with symptoms including abdominal pain with associated clinical and radiologic evidence of a peritoneal mass.

Pathology

At surgery, cystic masses varying in size are noted, and frequently are attached to the peritoneum, and to the surface of abdominal and pelvic organs. The masses may reach quite large dimensions and are composed of thin-walled, multiloculated cystic spaces filled with clear, watery fluid. Careful macroscopic examination searching for the presence of solid areas must be performed.

Microscopically, the cysts are formed by a thin fibrous wall and lined by flattened or cuboidal mesothelial cells (Fig. 23.15a–c). Hobnail appearance of the lining epithelium may be seen. Nuclear atypia is not uncommonly encountered. Rarely, mitotic activity may be seen. Focal squamous metaplasia may be appreciated.

Immunohistochemistry is useful to demonstrate the mesothelial nature of the cells lining the cystic spaces. The cells will have a profile identical to that seen in mesothelial cells in other benign and malignant conditions. Similarly, electron microscopy can show the presence of microvilli and confirm the mesothelial derivation of these cells.

The differential diagnosis includes malignant mesothelioma with cystic degeneration and benign serous cysts of the peritoneal cavity. Although the cytologic features of cystic mesothelioma and malignant mesothelioma might be indistinguishable, the latter will usually be evident by recognition of a solid component with stromal invasion in addition to the cystic components. Benign serous cysts can be morphologically identical to mesothelial-lined cysts. The identification of cilia on the cyst-lining cells favors a diagnosis of serous cyst. In addition, although serous cysts are positive for cytokeratins and WT-1, they are negative for calretinin.

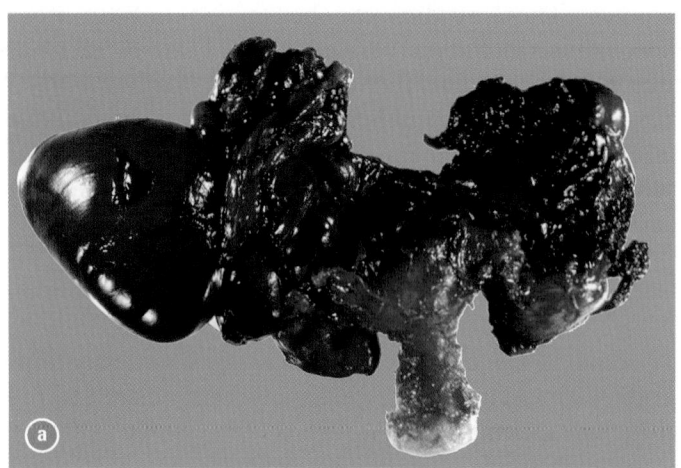

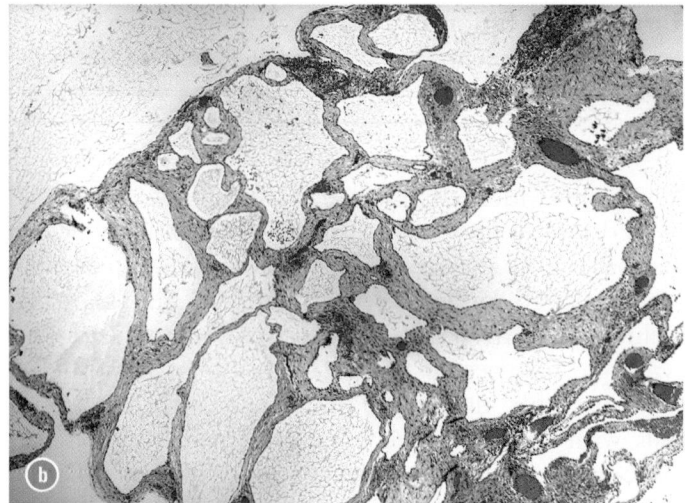

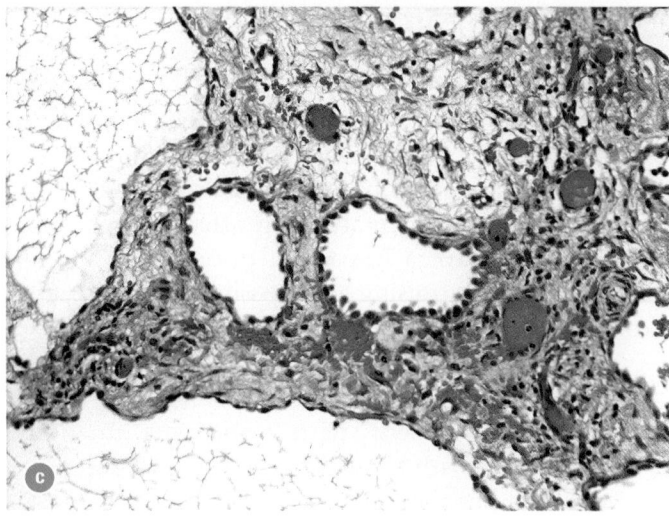

Fig. 23.15 Cystic mesothelioma (formerly benign cystic mesothelioma). (a) This variant extensively involves the uterine serosa, mesosalpinx and meso-ovarium. (b,c) the tumor forms cystic spaces lined by plump mesothelial cells within an organized fibrous stroma.

Treatment and prognosis

Cystic mesothelioma is a benign disease with a tendency to recur, especially if the inciting factor is not removed or discontinued. Of the cases described in the literature, patients showed multiple recurrence of this condition over extended periods of time; however, patients did not die of disease.[176,178] Given this fact, some have suggested that therapy should be somewhat aggressive, with resection of visible peritoneal disease and adjuvant chemotherapy.[176]

WELL-DIFFERENTIATED PAPILLARY MESOTHELIOMA

Epidemiology

This is an uncommon disease that can affect the peritoneal or pleural spaces, and tunica vaginalis in males.[179] In the largest published series of papillary mesothelioma affecting the peritoneal cavity, approximately 82% of the cases occurred in women.[180] The relationship of well-differentiated papillary mesothelioma of the peritoneum with occupational exposure to asbestos is yet unclear. However, recently, Galateau-Salle et al. reported a large series of pleural papillary mesotheliomas where patients in half of the cases had a history of exposure to asbestos fibers.[181]

Clinical features

Well-differentiated papillary mesothelioma is usually an incidental finding at time of surgery; patients may occasionally have symptomatic presentation, with abdominal pain, ascites and an abdominal mass; however, in this instance most pathologists would be compelled to diagnose this entity as malignant mesothelioma. Patients are found to have multifocal nodules involving peritoneal and omental surfaces.

Pathology

Macroscopically, white firm multifocal nodules that are usually smaller than 2 cm characterize this lesion. Upon microscopic examination, papillary formations composed of loose fibrous tissue are noted to be covered by a single layer of benign-appearing mesothelial cells, similar to cells seen in mesothelial hyperplasia (Fig. 23.16a,b). Nuclear atypia and mitoses are not features of well-differentiated papillary mesothelioma. Psammoma bodies may be seen. Additionally, invasion of the underlying tissue is not seen. Immunohistochemical studies show a profile identical to that seen in other mesothelial benign and malignant conditions.

Progression to malignant mesothelioma is not seen. Morphologic distinction of these two entities is of maximal importance since treatment and prognosis differ considerably. No definitive adjunctive tools for this differentiation exist, since both entities are derived from mesothelial cells. Although malignant mesothelioma has well-described cytogenetic abnormalities, there are no data in the literature regarding clonality or cytogenetic alterations in well-differentiated papillary mesothelioma.

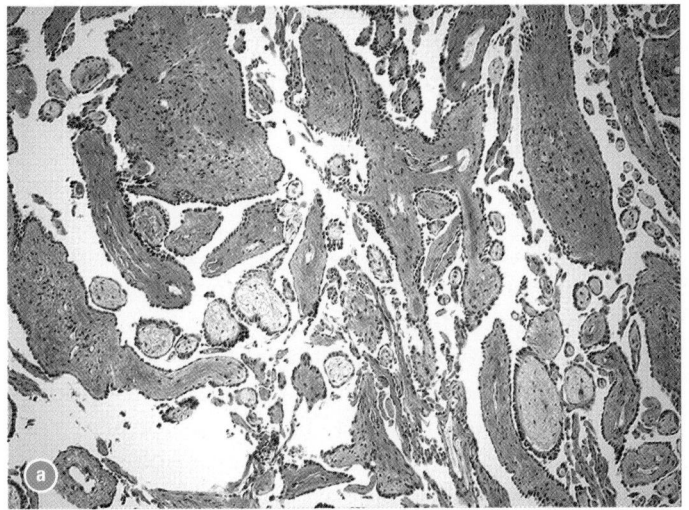
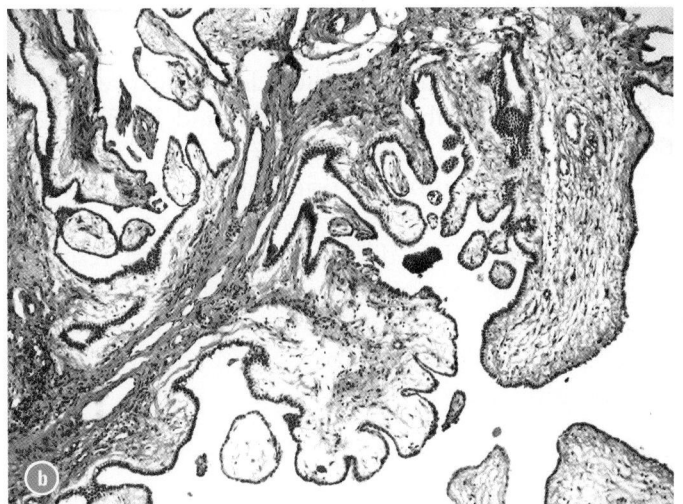

Fig. 23.15 (a,b) Well-differentiated papillary mesothelioma: papillary fronds of mesothelial cells with no invasion of underlying stroma.

Treatment and prognosis

Because papillary mesothelioma appears to have an indolent clinical course, with a much longer overall survival rate when compared with malignant mesothelioma and only rare cases showing aggressive behavior, therapy should include surgical resection of the mass, with close follow-up and possible adjuvant chemotherapy in more aggressive cases.[179]

ADENOMATOID TUMOR

Epidemiology

Adenomatoid tumor is a small lesion mainly found in the uterine wall, but that can also be encountered in the peritoneum, omentum, mesentery, wall of abdominal organs, and male genital tract (epididymis). It can affect males and females in any age range.

Clinical features

In the vast majority of cases, the patients are asymptomatic and the nodules are an incidental finding during surgery for other conditions. However, reported cases of large adenomatoid tumors have been reported in the literature.[182]

Pathology

Grossly, these lesions are small, measuring up to 2.0 cm, and appear to be firm and white at examination. Histologically, adenomatoid tumors are ill-circumscribed and composed of small cystic spaces lined by cuboidal or flat mesothelial cells, with round, regular nuclear contours, fine chromatin, small to inconspicuous nucleoli and a small amount of pale cytoplasm. The stroma between the cysts can vary from a scant myxoid tissue, to fibrous and smooth muscle tissue. Hyperplasia of smooth muscle in the stroma may overgrow the cystic spaces.

Immunohistochemically, these lesions express WT-1 (monoclonal antibody), calretinin and HBME-1.[182] However, EMA is usually negative.[182]

Differential diagnosis is principally with metastatic adenocarcinoma since the cystic spaces can simulate glandular lumina. This dilemma can usually be resolved by the use of immunostains since carcinomas are typically negative for calretinin, while positive for other markers such as Leu-M1 (or CD15) and carcinoembryonic antigen (CEA).

Treatment and prognosis

These lesions carry an excellent prognosis. Excision is curative.

MALIGNANT MESOTHELIOMA

Epidemiology

Malignant mesothelioma is an uncommon entity that most often affects the pleural cavity, but is also well-recognized to occur in the peritoneal cavity. Males appear to be much more often affected, with women accounting for approximately 8% of cases.[183,184] Although exceptionally rare cases of pediatric malignant mesothelioma[185] have been described in the world literature, malignant mesothelioma occurs predominantly in older adults, between the sixth and ninth decades of life. The most important risk factor for the development of malignant mesothelioma appears to be exposure to asbestos, even though the clinical history of contact to this carcinogen is not always known or obvious. In one series analyzing 1517 cases of malignant mesothelioma, Suzuki observed that patients with tumors involving the peritoneal cavity appeared to have a stronger association to exposure to asbestos, in contrast to patients with pleura disease.[183] The time interval between exposure and development of malignant mesothelioma in most cases is longer than 20 years.[183] Infrequently, other cancers, such as carcinomas, can also affect these patients.[183]

Clinical features

Most patients with mesothelioma involving the peritoneal cavity will present with an effusion (ascites) and an abdominal mass. Symptoms related to mass effect on other intra-abdominal organs might be present.

Pathology

Malignant mesothelioma presents as plaques, nodules and/or masses. Often, a combination of presentations is seen in a given patient. Tumor size can vary from microscopic involvement up to coalescing tumor nodules forming large masses. Hemorrhage and necrosis are frequently present. Occasionally, macroscopic invasion of organs can be noted.

Architecturally, malignant mesothelioma can have numerous growth patterns: solid, papillary, tubular and tubulo-papillary (Fig. 23.17a–d). In examination of cytologic preparations, malignant mesothelioma may show large three-dimensional papillary formations or large sheets of atypical mesothelial cells. Tumors may vary from well-differentiated neoplasms to poorly-differentiated mesothelioma. The vast majority of cases of malignant mesothelioma show an epithelial cytology with cells that usually have a round to oval nuclear contour, clumped chromatin, prominent single nucleoli and moderate to small amounts of palely eosinophilic cytoplasm. The nuclear/cytoplasmic ratio can be increased, but the cell borders are well defined with evidence of microvilli ('windows'). Mitoses, including atypical forms, can be numerous. Necrosis may be present. Psammoma bodies can be encountered, including in cytology specimens. One of the most important features of these tumors is the presence of invasion of the underlying tissues. Biphasic tumors, i.e. tumors showing features of epithelial and spindle cell (or sarcomatoid) mesothelioma, have the second most common tumor pattern.[183]

Vacuoles containing hyaluronic acid are frequently seen in neoplastic cells. They have a bluish tinge on hematoxylin-eosin stain and very often mimic mucin. Special stains using Alcian blue histochemistry will highlight this polypeptide. In addition, hyaluronic acid shows absence of reactivity with periodic acid–Schiff (PAS) when pretreated with hyaluronidase, whereas mucin is PAS positive. However, one must be aware of very rare cases of mucin-producing mesothelioma.[186]

Rarer variants of malignant mesothelioma exist and diagnosis will depend on awareness of these variants and supportive immunoperoxidase stains. Pure sarcomatoid or spindle cell malignant mesothelioma is composed of atypical spindle cells and closely resembles a spindle cell sarcoma. Lymphohistiocytic malignant mesothelioma requires identification of malignant cells amidst an intense mixed inflammatory infiltrate, including small lymphocytes, plasma cells and epithelioid histiocytes, giving an appearance of a 'pseudotumor'. The differential diagnosis of this variant should include other tumors with a prominent inflammatory component such as IMT and non-neoplastic

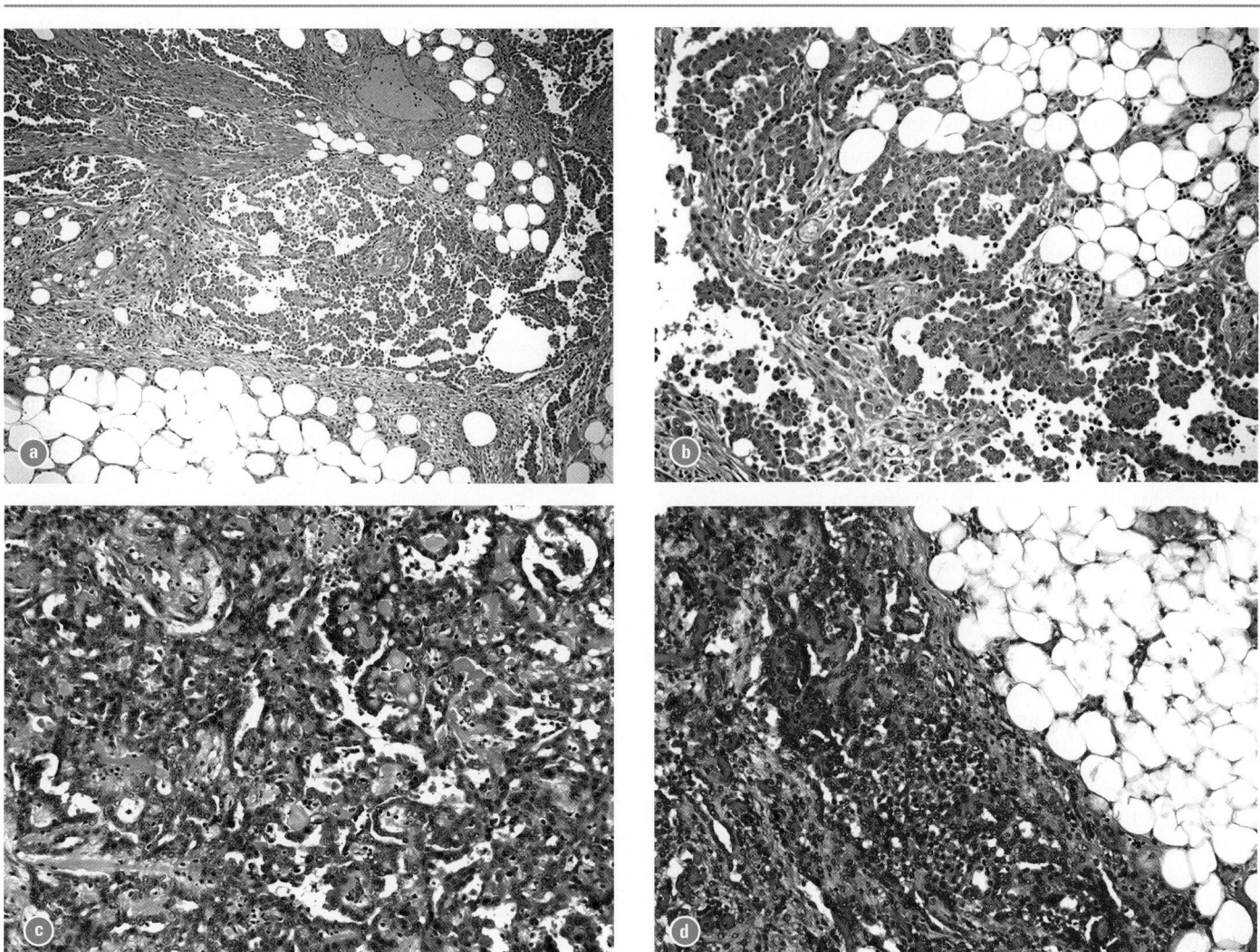

Fig. 23.17 (a–d) Malignant mesothelioma showing papillary structures layered by epithelial cells with inconspicuous nuclear atypia and invasion of underlying adipose tissue.

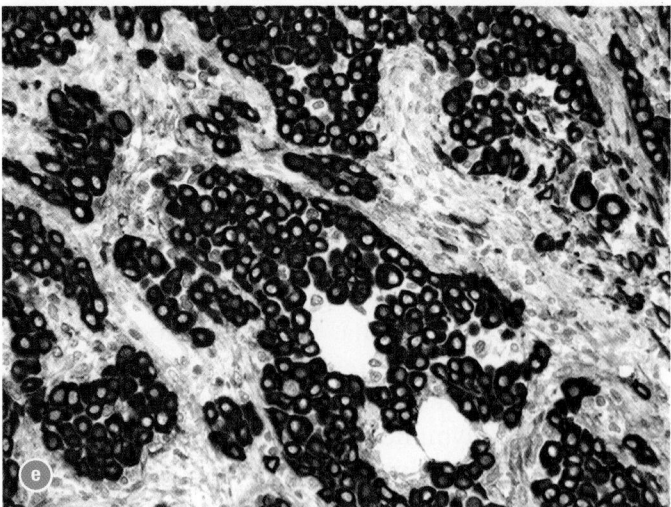

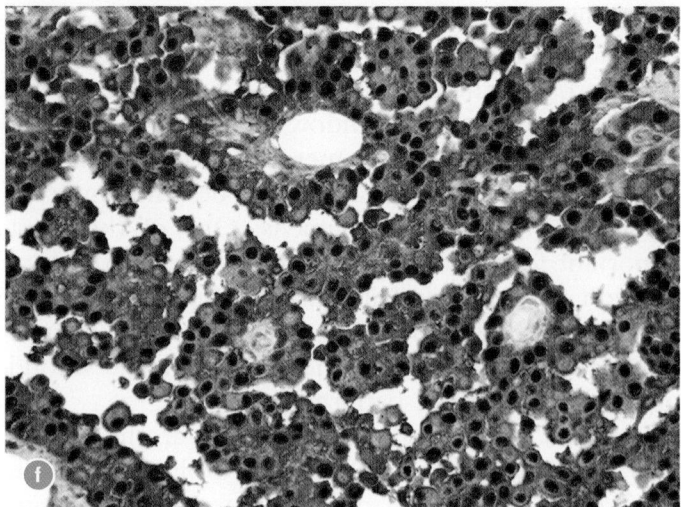

Fig. 23.17 **Cont'd** (e) Immunoperoxidase stain for AE1/AE3 showing strong cytoplasmic reactivity with perinuclear accentuation. (f) Immunoperoxidase stain for calretinin is positive in malignant mesothelioma and is helpful in the differential diagnosis with adenocarcinoma.

inflammatory and infectious conditions. Deciduoid mesothelioma is a rare variant of malignant mesothelioma in which tumor cells have a polygonal shape with abundant eosinophilic cytoplasm that mimics ectopic decidua. This variant was initially reported to affect young females;[12] however, older patients and males have also been seen to develop this variant.[187]

The immunoprofile of malignant cells is identical to that seen in non-neoplastic mesothelial cells and benign mesothelial diseases. The characteristic staining pattern includes expression of cytokeratins (Fig. 23.17e), calretinin (Fig. 23.17f), WT-1 (monoclonal antibody) and variable HBME-1. The positivity for cytokeratins is typically cytoplasmic with a perinuclear enhancement. Staining with calretinin shows a cytoplasmic and nuclear pattern and must be present in the majority of the neoplastic cells to be considered compatible for mesothelioma. WT-1 is a nuclear stain that is helpful in the diagnosis of malignant mesothelioma in conjunction with the other cited markers, since it is also positive in other neoplasms of non-mesothelial origin. Likewise, HBME-1 is also positive in other tumors and expression of this marker is only significant in the presence of the other stains.

A recent development in the diagnosis of malignant mesothelioma is the detection by conventional cytogenetics and/or FISH studies of karyotypic abnormalities. Although there are no constant specific karyotypic aberrations in malignant mesothelioma, a number of alterations are more frequently encountered including loss of chromosomes 4 and 22, polysomy for chromosomes 5, 7 and 20 and loss of material from chromosomes 1p, 3p, 6q, 9p, 13q, 14q and 15q.[188]

Treatment and prognosis

Malignant mesothelioma carries a dismal prognosis. The most important prognostic factors are patient's age, extent of disease, histologic findings and completeness of surgery.[189] Mesotheliomas showing sarcomatoid, lymphohistiocytic or deciduoid features appear to behave poorly. The most common approach to the treatment of this highly aggressive disease is debulking surgery associated with intraoperative and postoperative intraperitoneal chemotherapy.[189] This approach in one institution led to a median survival of 67 months.[189,190]

Miscellaneous lesions of the peritoneum

MYXOID HAMARTOMA

Myxoid hamartoma is a benign condition of infancy first described in 1983 by Gonzalez-Crussi et al.[190] Clinically, it presents as multiple peritoneal nodules arising in the omentum and mesentery. It is composed of a hamartomatous proliferation of spindled mesenchymal cells, probably of fibroblastic origin, amidst a vascularized background. Rare reported cases show evidence of neural-like structures by electron microscopy and immunohistochemical positivity for

S-100 protein.[191] All cases reported in the English literature show a favorable outcome.[190–192]

INFARCTED APPENDIX EPIPLOICA

Although infarction of the appendices epiploicae is not a neoplastic condition, it can imitate a tumor mass by the formation of an abscess[193] or calcification.[194] Torsion with subsequent infarction of the appendices epiploicae due to mechanical limitation of the vascular supply can present itself as a surgical emergency, often mimicking acute appendicitis.[195–198] Histologically, these benign lesions are characterized by fibroadipose tissue with fat necrosis and dystrophic calcification. Surgical excision with drainage of abscesses and appropriate antimicrobial therapy is curative.

SCLEROSING MESENTERITIS

Epidemiology

Sclerosing mesenteritis is a poorly defined benign entity of unknown etiology that has received several different names in the literature over the years, including mesenteric panniculitis, mesenteric lipodystrophy, retractile mesenteritis, xanthogranulomatous mesenteritis, inflammatory pseudotumor, mesenteric lipogranuloma, etc. As its name implies, it is reactive in nature.

Most patients diagnosed with sclerosing mesenteritis are in their seventh decade of life, and there appears to be no gender predilection.[199] Most patients have no prior history of trauma to the abdomen.

Clinical features

Clinically, sclerosing mesenteritis can mimic a malignant process. It may present as a single large mass, multiple masses or diffuse thickening of the mesentery. The most common symptomatology in one large series was abdominal pain, which is seen in association with a mass and/or bowel obstruction.[199] Patients also show evidence of vague systemic symptoms such as weight loss, anorexia and fatigue.

Pathology

The macroscopic presentation is variable; however, most patients will present with one abdominal mass, involving most often the small bowel mesentery and mesocolon.

Likewise, the microscopic appearance is quite variable and probably reflects the different stages of the disease. The morphology includes uneven proportions of fibrous and adipose tissue with fat necrosis, and a mild to marked chronic inflammatory infiltrate composed mainly of small lymphocytes, plasma cells and foamy histiocytes. Calcifications may be present. Immunostains do not help in this diagnosis.

Sclerosing mesenteritis is a diagnosis of exclusion. One should include several entities in the differential diagnosis: desmoid fibromatosis, IMT, lymphoma, reaction to perforation of the intestines (due to benign or malignant causes) and metastatic carcinoma. Immunoperoxidase studies are helpful in this distinction. Fibromatosis will not be accompanied by a prominent inflammatory component. In contrast, IMT is characterized by a marked lymphoplasmacytic infiltrate; however, careful examination of the tumor reveals a population of neoplastic spindle cells in the background. In addition, IMT should not have admixed adipose tissue with fat necrosis and, in a subset of cases, positive immunostains for ALK-1 are noted. Lymphoma can be excluded by demonstrating a mixed lymphoid population, composed of T and B cells, and polyclonal plasma cells in sclerosing mesenteritis. The diagnosis of metastatic carcinoma relies on the demonstration of malignant keratin-positive cells. Close examination of the tubular GI tract for evidence of perforation should be performed. Initially, inflammatory reaction to perforation is limited to the site of tear, in an attempt to contain the extravasation of bowel contents into the peritoneum.

Treatment and prognosis

The treatment of sclerosing mesenteritis is excision of the 'tumor mass'. In symptomatic patients, one study has shown that thalidomide is efficacious.[200] The prognosis is good.

Implants of the peritoneum

PSEUDOMYXOMA PERITONEI

Epidemiology

In the literature, the clinical definition of pseudomyxoma peritonei (PP) is not homogeneously defined. Some authors define PP as the presence of abundant mucin within the peritoneal cavity, with or without the evidence of an associated neoplasm;[201] others believe that the term PP should be used to describe a condition of free mucin within the peritoneal cavity in the presence of a mucinous adenocarcinoma, generally of appendiceal origin.[202,203] In addition, females with PP have to be investigated for the presence of an ovarian tumor (borderline mucinous tumor or mucinous adenocarcinoma).[204] Regardless, the term pseudomyxoma peritonei is a clinical term and should not be used in pathologic reports.

Clinical features

Patients with PP usually present with increased abdominal size due to accumulation of large quantities of mucinous fluid. However, the associated tumor producing the mucin is not always immediately obvious. In fact, it may be quite small, requiring extensive histologic sample of potential sites (appendix, bowel) for the diagnosis.

Pathology

The gastrointestinal tract (appendix, large intestine, pancreas) and ovaries are the most common sites for the presence of a tumoral mass in association with PP.

The appendix is usually, but not always, enlarged and filled with mucin (Fig. 23.18a) and the ovaries may be unilaterally or bilaterally involved by a mucinous tumor, which is usually cystic (uniloculated or multiloculated), filled with mucinous fluid and may have solid projections from the wall of the cysts (Fig. 23.18b).

Microscopically, the presence of neoplastic epithelium free-floating in the mucin arranged singly or in small clusters is characteristic of PP (Fig. 23.18c). Appendiceal and colonic adenocarcinomas are characterized by glands with stratified columnar epithelium composed of hyperchromatic cells showing frequent mitoses. Although infrequent, signet-ring cell phenotype may be present.

The immunohistochemical profile may help in the differentiation between possible sites of origin for the tumor. Cytokeratins (CK) 7 and 20 are the most helpful. Colonic and appendiceal adenocarcinomas are typically positive for CK20 and negative for CK7,

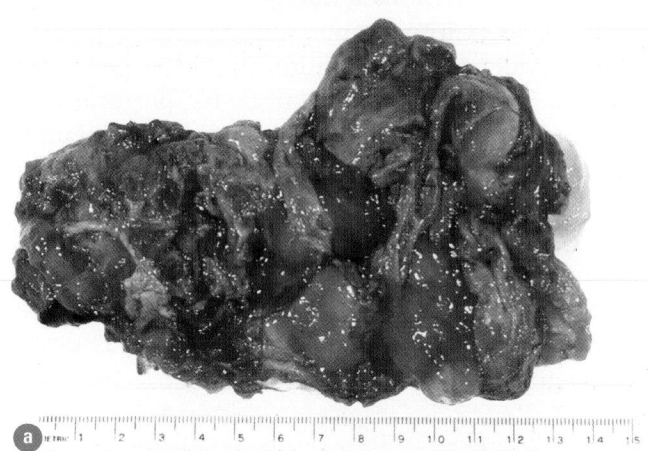

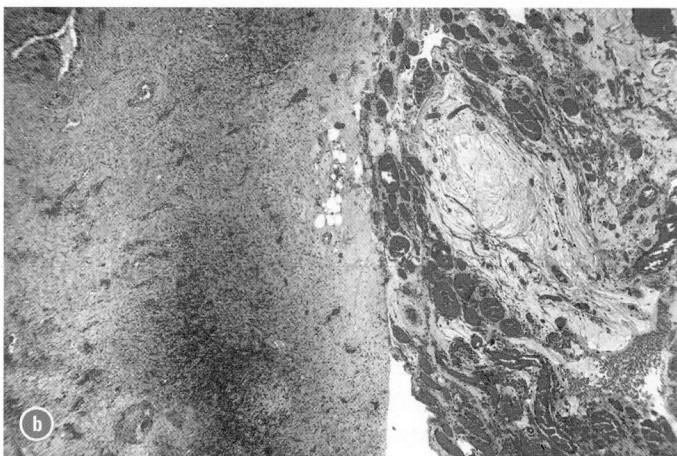

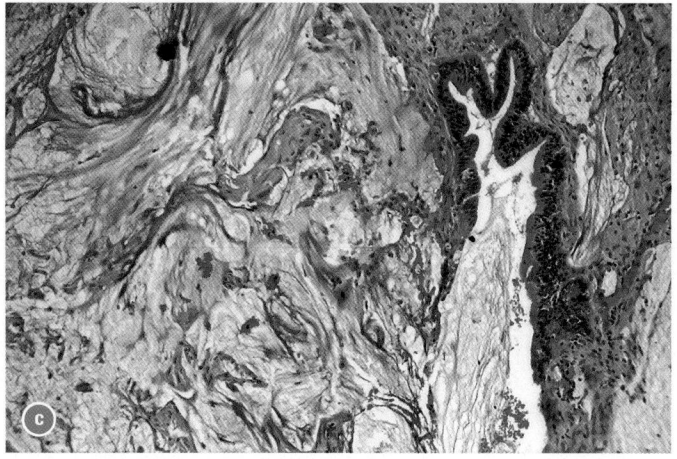

Fig. 23.18 (a) Pseudomyxoma: gross appearance of appendiceal resection specimen with multiple mucin-filled cysts. (b) Pseudomyxoma peritonei (right) on the surface of an ovary (left). (c) Admixture of mucin and neoplastic intestinal epithelium.

while ovarian mucinous adenocarcinomas show the opposite phenotype (CK20 negative and CK7 positive). Additionally, a new marker CDX-2 is positive in gastrointestinal tumors.

Treatment and prognosis

The cornerstone of management of patients with PP is surgical excision of the tumor and drainage of the mucinous ascites associated with intraperitoneal chemotherapy.[205] When considering females with ovarian carcinoma with PP, tumor stages other than Stage I are characterized by recurrence and often pursue a fatal course.[206]

STRUMOSIS

Strumosis is a poorly-defined condition that is associated with struma ovarii, i.e. ovarian teratomas composed entirely of thyroid tissue that presents as peritoneal and omental implants of thyroid tissue (Fig. 23.19). Controversies exist regarding its pathogenesis. While most believe that it is related to rupture of an ovarian teratoma, others report strumosis as a metastatic disease in the setting of a well-differentiated follicular carcinoma arising in teratomas.[207,208]

PERITONEAL GLIOMATOSIS

This is a rare benign condition that is closely related to mature ovarian teratomas. It presents as small nodular lesions on the peritoneal or omental surfaces that vary from a few to numerous. Most authors believe that the ectopic glial tissue is derived from the teratoma,

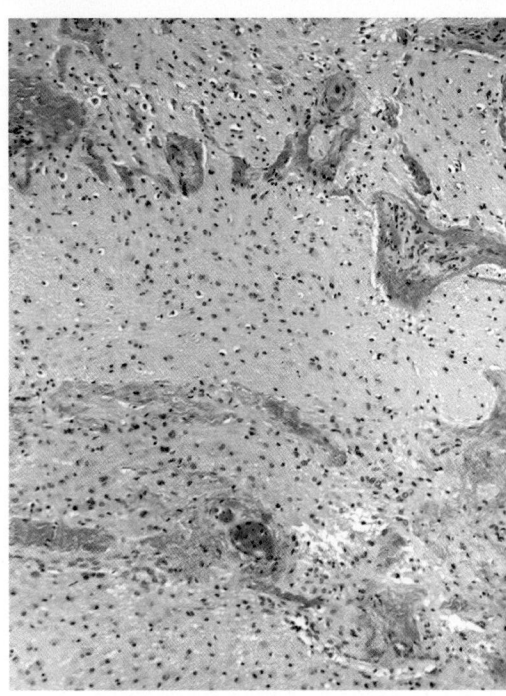

Fig. 23.20 Peritoneal gliomatosis, composed of bland-appearing glial tissue on the peritoneal surface.

while others speculate a possible metaplastic origin in the subcelomic mesenchymal cells.[209] Morphologically, it is composed of mature glial tissue (Fig. 23.20). Although there is no evidence of malignancy, confirmatory biopsy should be performed to exclude implants of malignant elements of teratomas, which will carry a worse prognosis.

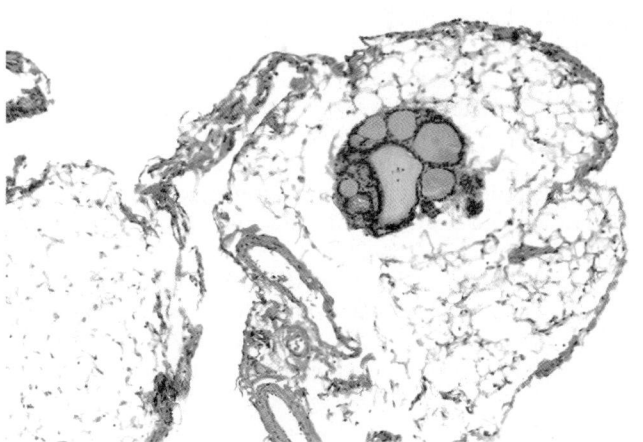

Fig. 23.19 Strumosis of the peritoneum, consisting of small clusters of thyroid follicles. This case persisted over several years with no clinical consequence.

References

1 Buttner A, Bassler R, Theele C. Pregnancy-associated ectopic decidua (deciduosis) of the greater omentum. An analysis of 60 biopsies with cases of fibrosing deciduosis and leiomyomatosis peritonealis disseminata. Pathol Res Pract 1993; 189(3):352–359.

2 Clement PB. Tumor-like lesions of the ovary associated with pregnancy. Int J Gynecol Pathol 1993; 12(2): 108–115.

3 Piccinni DJ, Spitale LS, Cabalier LR, Dionisio de Cabalier ME. Decidua in the peritoneal surface mimicking metastatic nodules. Findings during cesarean section. Rev Fac Cien Med Univ Nac Cordoba 2002; 59(1):113–116.

4 Suster S, Moran CA. Deciduosis of the appendix. Am J Gastroenterol 1990; 85(7):841–845.

5 Bashir RM, Montgomery EA, Gupta PK, et al. Massive gastrointestinal hemorrhage during pregnancy caused by ectopic decidua of the terminal ileum and colon. Am J Gastroenterol 1995; 90(8):1325–1327.

6 Zaytsev P, Taxy JB. Pregnancy-associated ectopic decidua. Am J Surg Pathol 1987; 11(7):526–530.

7 Hauptmann J, Mechtersheimer G, Blaker H, Schaupp W, Otto HF. Deciduosis of the appendix. Differential diagnosis of acute appendicitis. Chirurg 2000; 71(1):89–92.

8 Packeisen J, Knieriem H. Acute appendicitis caused by pregnancy-associated ectopic decidua. Case report and discussion of pathogenesis. Pathologie 1999; 20(6):355–358.

9 Garcia H, Fodor M, Giovannoni A, Gidekel L. Deciduosis of the appendix as cause of acute abdomen in pregnancy. Medicina (B Aires) 2001; 61(2):185–186.

10 Richter MA, Choudhry A, Barton JJ, Merrick RE. Bleeding ectopic decidua as a cause of intraabdominal hemorrhage. A case report. J Reprod Med 1983; 28(6):430–432.

11 Sabatelle R, Winger E. Postpartum intraabdominal hemorrhage caused by ectopic deciduosis. Obstet Gynecol 1973; 41(6):873–875.

12 Nascimento AG, Keeney GL, Fletcher CD. Deciduoid peritoneal mesothelioma. An unusual phenotype affecting young females. Am J Surg Pathol 1994; 18(5):439–445.

13 Ordonez NG. Epithelial mesothelioma with deciduoid features: report of four cases. Am J Surg Pathol 2000; 24(6):816–823.

14 Hesseling MH, Wilde RL De. Endosalpingiosis in laparoscopy. J Am Assoc Gynecol Laparosc 2000; 7(2):215–219.

15 Heinig J, Gottschalk I, Cirkel U, Diallo R. Endosalpingiosis – an underestimated cause of chronic pelvic pain or an accidental finding? A retrospective study of 16 cases. Eur J Obstet Gynecol Reprod Biol 2002; 103(1):75–78.

16 Clement PB, Young RH. Florid cystic endosalpingiosis with tumor-like manifestations: a report of four cases including the first reported cases of transmural endosalpingiosis of the uterus. Am J Surg Pathol 1999; 23(2):166–175.

17 Clement PB, Young RH. Endocervicosis of the urinary bladder. A report of six cases of a benign mullerian lesion that may mimic adenocarcinoma. Am J Surg Pathol 1992; 16(6):533–542.

18 Seman EI, Stewart CJ. Endocervicosis of the urinary bladder. Aust N Z J Obstet Gynaecol 1994; 34(4):496–497.

19 Parivar F, Bolton DM, Stoller ML. Endocervicosis of the bladder. J Urol 1995; 153(4):1218–1219.

20 Young RH, Clement PB. Mullerianosis of the urinary bladder. Mod Pathol 1996; 9(7):731–737.

21 Rodriguez R, Alfert H. Endocervicosis of the bladder: a rare mucinous analogue of endometriosis. J Urol 1997; 157(4):1355.

22 Nada W, Parker J, Wong F, Cooper M, Reid G. Laparoscopic excision of endocervicosis of the urinary bladder. J Am Assoc Gynecol Laparosc 2000; 7(1):135–137.

23 Kim HJ, Lee TJ, Kim MK, et al. Mullerianosis of the urinary bladder, endocervicosis type: a case report. J Korean Med Sci 2001; 16(1):123–126.

24 Young RH, Clement PB. Endocervicosis involving the uterine cervix: a report of four cases of a benign process that may be confused with deeply invasive endocervical adenocarcinoma. Int J Gynecol Pathol 2000; 19(4):322–328.

25 Strathy JH, Molgaard CA, Coulam CB, Melton LJ 3rd. Endometriosis and infertility: a laparoscopic study of endometriosis among fertile and infertile women. Fertil Steril 1982; 38(6):667–672.

26 Noller KL, Melton LJ 3rd, Selwyn BJ, Hardy RJ. Incidence of pelvic endometriosis in Rochester, Minnesota, 1970–1979. Am J Epidemiol 1987; 125(6):959–969.

27 Candiani GB, Danesino V, Gastaldi A, Parazzini F, Ferraroni M. Reproductive and menstrual factors and risk of peritoneal and ovarian endometriosis. Fertil Steril 1991; 56(2):230–234.

28 Czernobilsky B, Morris WJ. A histologic study of ovarian endometriosis with emphasis on hyperplastic and atypical changes. Obstet Gynecol 1979; 53(3):318–323.

29 Fukunaga M, Ushigome S. Epithelial metaplastic changes in ovarian endometriosis. Mod Pathol 1998; 11(8):784–788.

30 Fukunaga M, Nomura K, Ishikawa E, Ushigome S. Ovarian atypical endometriosis: its close association with malignant epithelial tumours. Histopathology 1997; 30(3):249–255.

31 Ballouk F, Ross JS, Wolf BC. Ovarian endometriotic cysts. An analysis of cytologic atypia and DNA ploidy patterns. Am J Clin Pathol 1994; 102(4):415–419.

32 Modesitt SC, Tortolero-Luna G, Robinson JB, Gershenson DM, Wolf JK. Ovarian and extraovarian endometriosis-associated cancer. Obstet Gynecol 2002; 100(4):788–795.

33 Kondi-Paphitis A, Smyrniotis B, Liapis A, Kontoyanni A, Deligeorgi H. Stromal sarcoma arising on endometriosis. A clinicopathological and immunohistochemical study of 4 cases. Eur J Gynaecol Oncol 1998; 19(6):588–590.

34 Linden PJ van der. Theories on the pathogenesis of endometriosis. Hum Reprod 1996; 11(Suppl 3):53–65.

35 Witz CA, Allsup KT, Montoya-Rodriguez IA, et al. Pathogenesis of endometriosis – current research. Hum Fertil (Camb) 2003; 6(1):34–40.

36 Matsuura K, Ohtake H, Katabuchi H, Okamura H. Coelomic metaplasia theory of endometriosis: evidence from in vivo studies and an in vitro experimental model. Gynecol Obstet Invest 1999; 47(Suppl 1):18–22.

37 Koninckx PR, Kennedy SH, Barlow DH. Pathogenesis of endometriosis: the role of peritoneal fluid. Gynecol Obstet Invest 1999; 47(Suppl 1):23–33.

38 Olive DL. Medical therapy of endometriosis. Semin Reprod Med 2003; 21(2):209–222.

39 Olive DL, Lindheim SR, Pritts EA. New medical treatments for endometriosis. Best Pract Res Clin Obstet Gynaecol 2004; 18(2):319–328.

40 Olive DL, Lindheim SR, Pritts EA. Endometriosis and infertility: what do we do for each stage? Curr Womens Health Rep 2003; 3(5):389–394.

41 Mostoufizadeh M, Scully RE. Malignant tumors arising in endometriosis. Clin Obstet Gynecol 1980; 23:951–963.

42 Parker RL, Dadmanesh F, Young RH, Clement PB. Polypoid endometriosis: a clinicopathologic analysis of 24 cases and a review of the literature. Am J Surg Pathol 2004; 28(3):285–297.

43 Benz EJ, Dockerty MB, Dixon CF. Polypoid endometrioma of the colon: report of case in which unusual pathologic features were present. Mayo Clin Proc 1952; 27:201–208.

44 Chang A, Natarajan S. Polypoid endometriosis. Arch Pathol Lab Med 2001; 125:1257.

45 Crum CP, Wible J, Frick HC, et al. A case of extensive pelvic endometriosis terminating in endometrial sarcoma. Am J Obstet Gynecol 1981; 140(6):718–719.

46 Ferraro LR, Hetz H, Carter H. Malignant endometriosis; pelvic endometriosis complicated by polypoid endometrioma of the colon and endometriotic sarcoma; report of a case and review of the literature. Obstet Gynecol 1956; 7:32–39.

47 Grouls V, Berndt R. Endometrioid adenoma (polypoid endometriosis) of the omentum maius. Pathol Res Pract 1995; 191:1049–1052.

48 Jimenez RE, Tiguert R, Hurley P, et al. Unilateral hydronephrosis resulting from intraluminal obstruction of the ureter by adenosquamous endometrioid carcinoma arising from disseminated endometriosis. Urology 2000; 56:331.

49 Kano H, Kanda H. Cervical endometriosis presented as a polypoid mass of portio cervix uteri. J Obstet Gynaecol 2003; 23:84–84.

50 Othman NH, Othman MS, Ismail AN, Mohammad NZ, Ismail Z. Multiple polypoid endometriosis – a rare complication following withdrawal of gonadotrophin releasing hormone (GnRH) agonist for severe endometriosis: a case report. Aust N Z J Obstet Gynaecol 1996; 36(2):216–218.

51 Schlesinger C, Silverberg SG. Tamoxifen-associated polyps (basalomas) arising in multiple endometriotic foci: a case report and review of the literature. Gynecol Oncol 1999; 73(2):305–311.

52 Yantiss RK, Clement PB, Young RH. Neoplastic and pre-neoplastic changes in gastrointestinal endometriosis: a study of 17 cases. Am J Surg Pathol 2000; 24:513–524.

53 Clement PB, Scully RE. Endometrial stromal sarcomas of the uterus with extensive endometrioid glandular differentiation: a report of three cases that caused problems in differential diagnosis. Int J Gynecol Pathol 1992; 11(3):163–173.

54 Raju U, Fine G, Greenawald KA, Ohorodnik JM. Primary papillary serous neoplasia of the peritoneum: a clinicopathologic and ultrastructural study of eight cases. Hum Pathol 1989; 20(5):426–436.

55 Fromm GL, Gershenson DM, Silva EG. Papillary serous carcinoma of the peritoneum. Obstet Gynecol 1990; 75(1):89–95.

56 Biscotti CV, Hart WR. Peritoneal serous micropapillomatosis of low malignant potential (serous borderline tumors of the peritoneum). A clinicopathologic study of 17 cases. Am J Surg Pathol 1992; 16(5):467–475.

57 Rothacker D, Mobius G. Varieties of serous surface papillary carcinoma of the peritoneum in northern Germany: a thirty-year autopsy study. Int J Gynecol Pathol 1995; 14(4):310–318.

58 Zhou J, Ywasa Y, Konishi I, et al. Papillary serous carcinoma of the peritoneum in women. A clinicopathologic and immunohistochemical study. Cancer 1995; 76(3):429–436.

59 Clement PB, Scully RE. Extrauterine mesodermal (mullerian) adenosarcoma: a clinicopathologic analysis of five cases. Am J Clin Pathol 1978; 69(3):276–283.

60 Visvalingam S, Jaworshi R, Blumenthal N, Chan F. Primary peritoneal mesodermal adenosarcoma: report of a case and review of the literature. Gynecol Oncol 2001; 81(3):500–505.

61 Kato N, Zhe J, Endoh Y, Motoyama T. Extrauterine Mullerian adenosarcoma of the peritoneum with an extensive rhabdomyosarcomatous element and a marked myxoid change. Pathol Int 2000; 50(4):347–351.

62 Shen DH, Khoo US, Xue WC, et al. Primary peritoneal malignant mixed Mullerian tumors. A clinicopathologic, immunohistochemical, and genetic study. Cancer 2001; 91(5):1052–1060.

63 Gilks CB, Bell DA, Scully RE. Serous psammocarcinoma of the ovary and peritoneum. Int J Gynecol Pathol 1990; 9(2):110–121.

64 Wick MR, Mills SE, Dehner LP, Bollinger DJ, Fechner RE. Serous papillary carcinomas arising from the peritoneum and ovaries. A clinicopathologic and immunohistochemical comparison. Int J Gynecol Pathol 1989; 8(3):179–188.

65 Attanoos RL, Webb R, Dojcinov SD, Gibbs AR. Value of mesothelial and epithelial antibodies in distinguishing diffuse peritoneal mesothelioma in females from serous papillary carcinoma of the ovary and peritoneum. Histopathology 2002; 40(3):237–244.

66 Bandera CA, Muto MG, Schorge JO, et al. BRCA1 gene mutations in women with papillary serous carcinoma of the peritoneum. Obstet Gynecol 1998; 92(4 Pt 1):596–600.

67 Schorge JO, Miller YB, Qi LJ, et al. Molecular evidence for multifocal papillary serous carcinoma of the peritoneum in patients with germline BRCA1 mutations. J Natl Cancer Inst 1998; 90(11):841–845.

68 Huang LW, Garrett AP, Muto MG, et al. Identification of a novel 9 cM deletion unit on chromosome 6q23-6q24 in papillary serous carcinoma of the peritoneum. Hum Pathol 2000; 31(3):367–373.

69 Schorge JO, Miller YB, Qi LJ, et al. Genetic alterations of the WT1 gene in papillary serous carcinoma of the peritoneum. Gynecol Oncol 2000; 76(3):369–372.

70 Bandera CA, Muto MG, Welch WR, Berkowitz RS, Mok SC. Genetic imbalance on chromosome 17 in papillary serous carcinoma of the peritoneum. Oncogene 1998; 16(26):3455–3459.

71 Taus P, Petru E, Gucer F, Pickel H, Lahousen M. Primary serous papillary carcinoma of the peritoneum: a report of 18 patients. Eur J Gynaecol Oncol 1997; 18(3):171–172.

72 Look M, Chang D, Sugarbaker PH. Long-term results of cytoreductive surgery for advanced and recurrent epithelial ovarian cancers and papillary serous carcinoma of the peritoneum. Int J Gynecol Cancer 2004; 14(1):35–41.

73 Wile AG, Evans HL, Romsdahl MM. Leiomyosarcoma of soft tissue: a clinicopathologic study. Cancer 1981; 48(4):1022–1032.

74 Hashimoto H, Tsuneyoshi M, Enjoji M. Malignant smooth muscle tumors of the retroperitoneum and mesentery: a clinicopathologic analysis of 44 cases. J Surg Oncol 1985; 28(3):177–186.

75 Shmookler BM, Lauer DH. Retroperitoneal leiomyosarcoma. A clinicopathologic analysis of 36 cases. Am J Surg Pathol 1983; 7(3):269–280.

76 Brewster DC, Athanasoulis CA, Darling RC. Leiomyosarcoma of the inferior vena cava. Diagnosis and surgical management. Arch Surg 1976; 111(10):1081–1085.

77 Hines OJ, J, Nelson S, Quinones-Baldrich WJ, Eilber FR. Leiomyosarcoma of the inferior vena cava: prognosis and comparison with leiomyosarcoma of other anatomic sites. Cancer 1999; 85(5):1077–1083.

78 Norris HJ, Parmley T. Mesenchymal tumors of the uterus. V. Intravenous leiomyomatosis. A clinical and pathologic study of 14 cases. Cancer 1975; 36(6):2164–2178.

79 Hornick JL, Fletcher CD. Criteria for malignancy in nonvisceral smooth muscle tumors. Ann Diagn Pathol 2003; 7(1):60–66.

80 Leitao MM, Soslow RA, Nonaka D, et al. Tissue microarray immunohistochemical expression of estrogen, progesterone, and androgen receptors in uterine leiomyomata and leiomyosarcoma. Cancer 2004; 101(6):1455–1462.

81 Massi D, Beltrami G, Mela MM, et al. Prognostic factors in soft tissue leiomyosarcoma of the extremities: a retrospective analysis of 42 cases. Eur J Surg Oncol 2004; 30(5):565–572.

82 Mourra N, Tiret T, Parc Y, et al. Endometrial stromal sarcoma of the rectosigmoid colon arising in extragonadal endometriosis and revealed by portal vein thrombosis. Arch Pathol Lab Med 2001; 125(8):1088–1090.

83 Levine PH, Abou-Nassar S, Mittal K. Extrauterine low-grade endometrial stromal sarcoma with florid endometrioid glandular differentiation. Int J Gynecol Pathol 2001; 20(4):395–398.

84 Bosincu L, Massarelli G, Cossu Rocca P, Issac MA, Nogales FF. Rectal endometrial stromal sarcoma arising in endometriosis: report of a case. Dis Colon Rectum 2001; 44(6):890–892.

85 Fukunaga M, Ishihara A, Ushigome S. Extrauterine low-grade endometrial stromal sarcoma: report of three cases. Pathol Int 1998; 48(4):297–302.

86 Ohta Y, Suzuki T, Kojima M, Shiokawa A, Mitsuya T. Low-grade endometrial stromal sarcoma with an extensive epithelial-like element. Pathol Int 2003; 53(4):246–251.

87 McCluggage WG, Date A, Bharucha H, Toner PG. Endometrial stromal sarcoma with sex cord-like areas and focal rhabdoid differentiation. Histopathology 1996; 29(4):369–374.

88 Fukunaga M, Miyazawa Y, Ushigome S. Endometrial low-grade stromal sarcoma with ovarian sex cord-like differentiation: report of two cases with an immunohistochemical and flow cytometric study. Pathol Int 1997; 47(6):412–415.

89 Pang LC. Endometrial stromal sarcoma with sex cord-like differentiation associated with tamoxifen therapy. South Med J 1998; 91(6):592–594.

90 Vaideeswar P, Madhiwale CV, Sharma JH, Desai AP, Kane S. Endometrial stromal sarcoma with sex-cord like features. Indian J Pathol Microbiol 2001; 44(1):55–56.

91 Khalifa MA, Montgomery EA, Azumi N, et al. Endometrial stromal sarcoma with focal smooth muscle differentiation: recurrence after 17 years: a follow-up report with discussion of the nomenclature. Int J Gynecol Pathol 1996; 15(2):171–176.

92 McCluggage WG, Cromie AJ, Bryson C, Traub AI. Uterine endometrial stromal sarcoma with smooth muscle and glandular differentiation. J Clin Pathol 2001; 54(6):481–483.

93 Fitko R, Brainer J, Schink JC, August CZ. Endometrial stromal sarcoma with rhabdoid differentiation. Int J Gynecol Pathol 1990; 9(4):379–382.

94 Lloreta J, Prat J. Endometrial stromal nodule with smooth and skeletal muscle components simulating stromal sarcoma. Int J Gynecol Pathol 1992; 11(4):293–298.

95 Kim YH, Cho H, Kyeom-Kim H, Kim I. Uterine endometrial stromal sarcoma with rhabdoid and smooth muscle differentiation. J Korean Med Sci 1996; 11(1):88–93.

96 Tanimoto A, Sasaguri T, Arima N, et al. Endometrial stromal sarcoma of the uterus with rhabdoid features. Pathol Int 1996; 46(3):231–237.

97 Zhu XQ, Shi YF, Cheng XD, Zhao CL, Wu YZ. Immunohistochemical markers in differential diagnosis of endometrial stromal sarcoma and cellular leiomyoma. Gynecol Oncol 2004; 92(1):71–79.

98 Oliva E, Young RH, Amin MB, Clement PB. An immunohistochemical analysis of endometrial stromal and smooth muscle tumors of the uterus: a study of 54 cases emphasizing the importance of using a panel because of overlap in immunoreactivity for individual antibodies. Am J Surg Pathol 2002; 26(4):403–412.

99 Dal Cin P, Aly MS, De Wever I, Moerman P, Van Den Berghe H. Endometrial stromal sarcoma t(7;17)(p15-p21;q12-q21) is a nonrandom chromosome change. Cancer Genet Cytogenet 1992; 63(1):43–46.

100 Koontz JI, Soreng AL, Nucci M, et al. Frequent fusion of the JAZF1 and JJAZ1 genes in endometrial stromal tumors. Proc Natl Acad Sci USA 2001; 98(11): 6348–6353.

101 Chang KL, Crabtree GS, Lim-Tan SK, Kempson RL, Hendrickson MR. Primary extrauterine endometrial stromal neoplasms: a clinicopathologic study of 20 cases and a review of the literature. Int J Gynecol Pathol 1993; 12(4):282–296.

102 Young RH, Clement PB, McCaughey WT. Solitary fibrous tumors ('fibrous mesotheliomas') of the peritoneum. A report of three cases and a review of the literature. Arch Pathol Lab Med 1990; 114(5):493–495.

103 Hardisson D, Limeres MA, Jimenez-Heffernan JA, De La Rosa P, Burgos E. Solitary fibrous tumor of the mesentery. Am J Gastroenterol 1996; 91(4):810–811.

104 Adachi T, Sugiyama Y, Saji S. Solitary fibrous benign mesothelioma of the peritoneum: report of a case. Surg Today 1999; 29(9):915–918.

105 Kubota Y, Kawai N, Tozawa K, et al. Solitary fibrous tumor of the peritoneum found in the prevesical space. Urol Int 2000; 65(1):53–56.

106 Lloyd RV, Erickson LA, Nascimento AG, Kloppel G. Neoplasms causing nonhyperinsulinemic hypoglycemia. Endocr Pathol 1999; 10(4):291–297.

107 Folpe AL, Devaney K, Weiss SW. Lipomatous hemangiopericytoma: a rare variant of hemangiopericytoma that may be confused with liposarcoma. Am J Surg Pathol 1999; 23(10):1201–1207.

108 Vallat-Decouvelaere AV, Dry SM, Fletcher CD. Atypical and malignant solitary fibrous tumors in extrathoracic locations: evidence of their comparability to intra-thoracic tumors. Am J Surg Pathol 1998; 22(12):1501–1511.

109 Flint A, Weiss SW. CD-34 and keratin expression distinguishes solitary fibrous tumor (fibrous mesothelioma) of pleura from desmoplastic mesothelioma. Hum Pathol 1995; 26(4):428–431.

110 Rosenthal NS, Abdul-Karim FW. Childhood fibrous tumor with psammoma bodies. Clinicopathologic features in two cases. Arch Pathol Lab Med 1988; 112(8):798–800.

111 Fetsch JF, Montgomery EA, Meis JM. Calcifying fibrous pseudotumor. Am J Surg Pathol 1993; 17(5):502–508.

112 Nascimento AF, Ruiz R, Hornick JL, Fletcher CD. Calcifying fibrous 'pseudotumor': clinicopathologic study of 15 cases and analysis of its relationship to inflammatory myofibroblastic tumor. Int J Surg Pathol 2002; 10(3):189–196.

113 Dorpe J Van, Ectors N, Geboes K, D'Hoore A, Sciot R. Is calcifying fibrous pseudotumor a late sclerosing stage of inflammatory myofibroblastic tumor? Am J Surg Pathol 1999; 23(3):329–335.

114 Chen KT. Familial peritoneal multifocal calcifying fibrous tumor. Am J Clin Pathol 2003; 119(6):811–815.

115 Hill KA, Gonzalez-Crussi F, Chou PM. Calcifying fibrous pseudotumor versus inflammatory myofibroblastic tumor: a histological and immunohistochemical comparison. Mod Pathol 2001; 14(8):784–790.

116 Sigel JE, Smith TA, Reith JB, Goldblum JR. Immunohistochemical analysis of anaplastic lymphoma kinase expression in deep soft tissue calcifying fibrous pseudotumor: evidence of a late sclerosing stage of inflammatory myofibroblastic tumor? Ann Diagn Pathol 2001; 5(1):10–14.

117 Hainaut P, Lesage V, Weynand B, Coche E, Noirhomme P. Calcifying fibrous pseudotumor (CFPT): a patient presenting with multiple pleural lesions. Acta Clin Belg 1999; 54(3): 162–164.

118 Su LD, Atayde-Perez A, Sheldon S, Fletcher JA, Weiss SW. Inflammatory myofibroblastic tumor: cytogenetic evidence supporting clonal origin. Mod Pathol 1998; 11(4):364–368.

119 Coffin CM, Watterson J, Priest JR, Dehner LP. Extrapulmonary inflammatory myofibroblastic tumor (inflammatory pseudotumor). A clinicopathologic and immunohistochemical study of 84 cases. Am J Surg Pathol 1995; 19(8):859–872.

120 Coffin CM, Patel A, Perkins S, et al. ALK1 and p80 expression and chromosomal rearrangements involving 2p23 in inflammatory myofibroblastic tumor. Mod Pathol 2001; 14(6):569–576.

121 Cook JR, Dehner LP, Collins MH, et al. Anaplastic lymphoma kinase (ALK) expression in the inflammatory myofibroblastic tumor: a comparative immunohistochemical study. Am J Surg Pathol 2001; 25(11):1364–1371.

122 Cessna MH, Zhou H, Sanger WG, et al. Expression of ALK1 and p80 in inflammatory myofibroblastic tumor and its mesenchymal mimics: a study of 135 cases. Mod Pathol 2002; 15(9):931–938.

123 Griffin CA, Hawkins AL, Dvorak C, et al. Recurrent involvement of 2p23 in inflammatory myofibroblastic tumors. Cancer Res 1999; 59(12):2776–2780.

124 Ma Z, Hill DA, Collins MH, et al. Fusion of ALK to the Ran-binding protein 2 (RANBP2) gene in inflammatory myofibroblastic tumor. Genes Chromosomes Cancer 2003; 37(1):98–105.

125 Karnak I, Senocak ME, Ciftci AO, et al. Inflammatory myofibroblastic tumor in children: diagnosis and treatment. J Pediatr Surg 2001; 36(6):908–912.

126 Sircar K, Hewlett BR, Huizinga JD, et al. Interstitial cells of Cajal as precursors of gastrointestinal stromal tumors. Am J Surg Pathol 1999; 23(4):377–389.

127 Cypriano MS, Jenkins JJ, Pappo AS, Rao BN, Daw NC. Pediatric gastrointestinal stromal tumors and leiomyosarcoma. Cancer 2004; 101(1):39–50.

128 Haider N, Kader M, McDermott M, et al. Gastric stromal tumors in children. Pediatr Blood Cancer 2004; 42(2):186–189.

129 Carney JA, Stratakis CA. The triad of gastric leiomyosarcoma, functioning extra-adrenal paraganglioma and pulmonary chondroma. N Engl J Med 1977; 296(26):1517–1518.

130 Carney JA. The triad of gastric epithelioid leiomyosarcoma, functioning extra-adrenal paraganglioma, and pulmonary chondroma. Cancer 1979; 43(1):374–382.

131 Carney JA. The triad of gastric epithelioid leiomyosarcoma, pulmonary chondroma, and functioning extra-adrenal paraganglioma: a five-year review. Medicine (Baltimore) 1983; 62(3):159–169.

132 Fletcher CD, Berman JJ, Corless C, et al. Diagnosis of gastrointestinal stromal tumors: a consensus approach. Int J Surg Pathol 2002; 10(2):81–89.

133 Medeiros F, Corless CL, Duensing A, et al. KIT-negative gastrointestinal stromal tumors: proof of concept and therapeutic Implications. Am J Surg Pathol 2004; 28(7):889–894.

134 Rubin BP, Singer S, Tsao C, et al. KIT activation is a ubiquitous feature of gastrointestinal stromal tumors. Cancer Res 2001; 61(22):8118–8121.

135 Heinrich MC, Corless CL, Duensing A, et al. PDGFRA activating mutations in gastrointestinal stromal tumors. Science 2003; 299(5607):708–710.

136 Hornick JL, Fletcher CD. Validating immunohistochemical staining for KIT (CD117). Am J Clin Pathol 2003; 119(3): 325–327.

137 Heinrich MC, Corless CL, Demetri GD, et al. Kinase mutations and imatinib response in patients with metastatic gastrointestinal stromal tumor. J Clin Oncol 2003; 21(23):4342–4349.

138 Chang SM, Ho WL. Malignant peripheral nerve sheath tumor: a study of 21 cases. Zhonghua Yi Xue Zhi (Taipei) 1994; 54(2):122–130.

139 Newbould MJ, Wilkinson N, Mene A. Post-radiation malignant peripheral nerve sheath tumour: a report of two cases. Histopathology 1990; 17(3):263–265.

140 Foley KM, Woodruff JM, Ellis FT, Posner JB. Radiation-induced malignant and atypical peripheral nerve sheath tumors. Ann Neurol 1980; 7(4):311–318.

141 Daimaru Y, Hashimoto H, Enjoji M. Benign schwannoma of the gastrointestinal tract: a clinicopathologic and immunohistochemical study. Hum Pathol 1988; 19(3):257–264.

142 Lodding P, Kindblom LG, Angervall L, Stenman G. Cellular schwannoma. A clinicopathologic study of 29 cases. Virchows Arch A Pathol Anat Histopathol 1990; 416(3):237–248.

143 Mennemeyer RP, Hallman KO, Hammar SP, et al. Melanotic schwannoma. Clinical and ultrastructural studies of three cases with evidence of intracellular melanin synthesis. Am J Surg Pathol 1979; 3(1):3–10.

144 McMenamin ME, Fletcher CD. Expanding the spectrum of malignant change in schwannomas: epithelioid malignant change, epithelioid malignant peripheral nerve sheath tumor, and epithelioid angiosarcoma: a study of 17 cases. Am J Surg Pathol 2001; 25(1):13–25.

145 Ducatman BS, Scheithauer BW. Malignant peripheral nerve sheath tumors with divergent differentiation. Cancer 1984; 54(6):1049–1057.

146 Wick MR, Swanson PE, Scheithauer BW, Manivel JC. Malignant peripheral nerve sheath tumor. An immunohistochemical study of 62 cases. Am J Clin Pathol 1987; 87(4):425–433.

147 Mertens F, Dal Cin P, De Wever I, et al. Cytogenetic characterization of peripheral nerve sheath tumours: a report of the CHAMP study group. J Pathol 2000; 190(1):31–38.

148 Fletcher CD. Peripheral neuroectodermal tumors. In: Fletcher CD, ed. Diagnostic histopathology of tumors. Hong Kong: Churchill Livingstone; 2002:1695–1698.

149 Jones IT, Jagelman DG, Fazio VW, et al. Desmoid tumors in familial polyposis coli. Ann Surg 1986; 204(1):94–97.

150 Clark SK, Neale KF, Landgrebe JC, Phillips RK. Desmoid tumours complicating familial adenomatous polyposis. Br J Surg 1999; 86(9):1185–1189.

151 Li C, Bapat B, Alman BA. Adenomatous polyposis coli gene mutation alters proliferation through its beta-catenin-regulatory function in aggressive fibromatosis (desmoid tumor). Am J Pathol 1998; 153(3):709–714.

152 Tejpar S, Nollet F, Li C, et al. Predominance of beta-catenin mutations and beta-catenin dysregulation in sporadic aggressive fibromatosis (desmoid tumor). Oncogene 1999; 18(47):6615–6620.

153 Saito T, Oda Y, Tanaka K, et al. beta-Catenin nuclear expression correlates with cyclin D1 overexpression in sporadic desmoid tumours. J Pathol 2001; 195(2):222–228.

154 Montgomery E, Tobenson MS, Kaushal M, Fisher C, Abraham SC. Beta-catenin immunohistochemistry separates mesenteric fibromatosis from gastrointestinal stromal tumor and sclerosing mesenteritis. Am J Surg Pathol 2002; 26(10):1296–1301.

155 De Wever I, Dal Cin P, Fletcher CD, et al. Cytogenetic, clinical, and morphologic correlations in 78 cases of fibromatosis: a report from the CHAMP Study Group. CHromosomes And Morphology. Mod Pathol 2000; 13(10): 1080–1085.

156 Qi H, Dal Cin P, Hernandez JM, et al. Trisomies 8 and 20 in desmoid tumors. Cancer Genet Cytogenet 1996; 92(2): 147–149.

157 Fletcher JA, Naeem R, Xiao S, Corson JM. Chromosome aberrations in desmoid tumors. Trisomy 8 may be a predictor of recurrence. Cancer Genet Cytogenet 1995; 79(2):139–143.

158 Miyaki M, Konishi M, Kikuchi-Yanoshita R, et al. Coexistence of somatic and germ-line mutations of APC gene in desmoid tumors from patients with familial adenomatous polyposis. Cancer Res 1993; 53(21): 5079–5082.

159 Nugent KP, Phillips RK, Hodgson SV, et al. Phenotypic expression in familial adenomatous polyposis: partial prediction by mutation analysis. Gut 1994; 35(11): 1622–1623.

160 Eccles DM, van der Luijt R, Breukel C, et al. Hereditary desmoid disease due to a frameshift mutation at codon 1924 of the APC gene. Am J Hum Genet 1996; 59(6):1193–1201.

161 Kraus MD, Guillou L, Fletcher CD. Well-differentiated inflammatory liposarcoma: an uncommon and easily overlooked variant of a common sarcoma. Am J Surg Pathol 1997; 21(5):518–527.

162 McCormick D, Mentzel T, Beham A, Fletcher CD. Dedifferentiated liposarcoma. Clinicopathologic analysis of 32 cases suggesting a better prognostic subgroup among pleomorphic sarcomas. Am J Surg Pathol 1994; 18(12): 1213–1223.

163 Nascimento AG, Kurtin PJ, Guillou L, Fletcher CD. Dedifferentiated liposarcoma: a report of nine cases with a peculiar neurallike whorling pattern associated with metaplastic bone formation. Am J Surg Pathol 1998; 22(8):945–955.

164 Rosai J, Akerman M, Dal Cin P, et al. Combined morphologic and karyotypic study of 59 atypical lipomatous tumors. Evaluation of their relationship and differential diagnosis with other adipose tissue tumors (a report of the CHAMP Study Group). Am J Surg Pathol 1996; 20(10): 1182–1189.

165 Dei Tos AP, Doglioni C, Piccinin S, et al. Coordinated expression and amplification of the MDM2, CDK4, and HMGI-C genes in atypical lipomatous tumours. J Pathol 2000; 190(5):531–536.

166 Lucas DR, Nascimento AG, Sanjay BK, Rock MG. Well-differentiated liposarcoma. The Mayo Clinic experience with 58 cases. Am J Clin Pathol 1994; 102(5):677–683.

167 Henricks WH, Chu YC, Goldblum JR, Weiss SW. Dedifferentiated liposarcoma: a clinicopathological analysis of 155 cases with a proposal for an expanded definition of dedifferentiation. Am J Surg Pathol 1997; 21(3):271–281.

168 Lae ME, Roche PC, Jin L, Lloyd RV, Nascimento AG. Desmoplastic small round cell tumor: a clinicopathologic, immunohistochemical, and molecular study of 32 tumors. Am J Surg Pathol 2002; 26(7):823–835.

169 Sawyer JR, Tryka AF, Lewis JM. A novel reciprocal chromosome translocation t(11;22)(p13;q12) in an intraabdominal desmoplastic small round-cell tumor. Am J Surg Pathol 1992; 16(4):411–416.

170 Quaglia MP, Brennan MF. The clinical approach to desmoplastic small round cell tumor. Surg Oncol 2000; 9(2):77–81.

171 Attanoos RL, Griffin A, Gibbs AR. The use of immunohistochemistry in distinguishing reactive from neoplastic mesothelium. A novel use for desmin and comparative evaluation with epithelial membrane antigen, p53, platelet-derived growth factor-receptor, P-glycoprotein and Bcl-2. Histopathology 2003; 43(3):231–238.

172 Cury PM, Butcher DN, Corrin B, Nicholson AG. The use of histological and immunohistochemical markers to distinguish pleural malignant mesothelioma and in situ mesothelioma from reactive mesothelial hyperplasia and reactive pleural fibrosis. J Pathol 1999; 189(2):251–257.

173 Schneider V, Partridge JR, Gutierrez F, et al. Benign cystic mesothelioma involving the female genital tract: report of four cases. Am J Obstet Gynecol 1983; 145(3): 355–359.

174 Villaschi S, Autelitano F, Santeusanio G, Balistreri P. Cystic mesothelioma of the peritoneum. A report of three cases. Am J Clin Pathol 1990; 94(6):758–761.

175 Sawh RN, Malpica A, Deavers MT, Liu J, Silva EG. Benign cystic mesothelioma of the peritoneum: a clinicopathologic study of 17 cases and immunohistochemical analysis of estrogen and progesterone receptor status. Hum Pathol 2003; 34(4):369–374.

176 Sethna K, Mohamed F, Marchettini P, Elias D, Sugarbaker PH. Peritoneal cystic mesothelioma: a case series. Tumori 2003; 89(1):31–35.

177 McFadden DE, Clement PB. Peritoneal inclusion cysts with mural mesothelial proliferation. A clinicopathological analysis of six cases. Am J Surg Pathol 1986; 10(12): 844–854.

178 Ross MJ, Welch WR, Scully RE. Multilocular peritoneal inclusion cysts (so-called cystic mesotheliomas). Cancer 1989; 64(6):1336–1346.

179 Butnor KJ, Sporn TA, Hammar SP, Roggli VL. Well-differentiated papillary mesothelioma. Am J Surg Pathol 2001; 25(10):1304–1309.

180 Daya D, McCaughey WT. Well-differentiated papillary mesothelioma of the peritoneum. A clinicopathologic study of 22 cases. Cancer 1990; 65(2):292–296.

181 Galateau-Salle F, Vignaud JM, Burke L, et al. Well-differentiated papillary mesothelioma of the pleura: a series of 24 cases. Am J Surg Pathol 2004; 28(4):534–540.

182 Nogales FF, Isaac MA, Hardisson D, et al. Adenomatoid tumors of the uterus: an analysis of 60 cases. Int J Gynecol Pathol 2002; 21(1):34–40.

183 Suzuki Y. Pathology of human malignant mesothelioma – preliminary analysis of 1,517 mesothelioma cases. Ind Health 2001; 39(2):183–185.

184 Roggli VL, Oury TD, Moffatt EJ. Malignant mesothelioma in women. Anat Pathol 1997; 2:147–163.

185 Brenner J, Sordillo PP, Magill GB. Malignant mesothelioma in children: report of seven cases and review of the literature. Med Pediatr Oncol 1981; 9(4):367–373.

186 Cook DS, Attanoos RL, Jalloh SS, Gibbs AR. 'Mucin-positive' epithelial mesothelioma of the peritoneum: an unusual diagnostic pitfall. Histopathology 2000; 37(1):33–36.

187 Shanks JH, Harris M, Banerjee SS, et al. Mesotheliomas with deciduoid morphology: a morphologic spectrum and a variant not confined to young females. Am J Surg Pathol 2000; 24(2):285–294.

188 Sandberg AA, Bridge JA. Updates on the cytogenetics and molecular genetics of bone and soft tissue tumors. Mesothelioma Cancer Genet Cytogenet 2001; 127:93–110.

189 Sugarbaker PH, Welch LS, Mohamed F, Glehen O. A review of peritoneal mesothelioma at the Washington Cancer Institute. Surg Oncol Clin N Am 2003; 12(3):605–621.

190 Gonzalez-Crussi F, deMello DE, Sotelo-Avila C. Omental-mesenteric myxoid hamartomas. Infantile lesions simulating malignant tumors. Am J Surg Pathol 1983; 7(6):567–578.

191 Henriquez A, Latorre JJ, Gonzalez S. Mesocolic myxoid hamartoma showing neural differentiation: an ultrastructural and immunohistochemical study. Pediatr Pathol 1989; 9(5):559–566.

192 Vyas MC, Mathur DR, Ramdeo IN, Rohitasvadana. Omento-mesentral myxoid hamartoma – a case report. Indian J Cancer 1994; 31(3):212–214.

193 Romaniuk CS, Simpkins KC. Case report: pericolic abscess secondary to torsion of an appendix epiploica. Clin Radiol 1993; 47(3):216–217.

194 Borg SA, Whitehouse GH, Griffiths GJ. A mobile calcified amputated appendix epiploica. AJR Am J Roentgenol 1976; 127(2):349–350.

195 Craig RD. Torsion of an appendix epiploica simulating appendicitis. Br J Clin Pract 1962; 16:123–124.

196 Legome EL, Belton AL, Murray RE, Rao PM, Novelline RA. Epiploic appendagitis: the emergency department presentation. J Emerg Med 2002; 22(1):9–13.

197 Manheimer LH. Massive intraperitoneal hemorrhage from appendix epiploica; report of a case. N Engl J Med 1956; 255(12):570–571.

198 Pavone E, Mehta SN, Trudel J, et al. Torsion of an appendix epiploica: a nonsurgical cause of acute abdomen. Dig Dis Sci 1997; 42(4):851–852.

199 Emory TS, Monihan JM, Carr NJ, Sobin LH. Sclerosing mesenteritis, mesenteric panniculitis and mesenteric lipodystrophy: a single entity? Am J Surg Pathol 1997; 21(4):392–398.

200 Ginsburg PM, Ehrenpreis ED. A pilot study of thalidomide for patients with symptomatic mesenteric panniculitis. Aliment Pharm Ther 2002; 16(12):2115–2122.

201 Ronnett BM, Shmookler BM, Sugarbaker PH, Kurman RJ. Pseudomyxoma peritonei: new concepts in diagnosis, origin, nomenclature, and relationship to mucinous borderline (low malignant potential) tumors of the ovary. Anat Pathol 1997; 2:197–226.

202 Sugarbaker PH. Pseudomyxoma peritonei. Cancer Treat Res 1996; 81:105–119.

203 Moran BJ, Cecil TD. The etiology, clinical presentation, and management of pseudomyxoma peritonei. Surg Oncol Clin N Am 2003; 12(3):585–603.

204 Ronnett BM, Kurman RJ, Zahn CM, et al. Pseudomyxoma peritonei in women: a clinicopathologic analysis of 30 cases with emphasis on site of origin, prognosis, and relationship to ovarian mucinous tumors of low malignant potential. Hum Pathol 1995; 26(5):509–524.

205 Glehen O, Mithieux F, Osinsky D, et al. Surgery combined with peritonectomy procedures and intraperitoneal chemohyperthermia in abdominal cancers with peritoneal carcinomatosis: a phase II study. J Clin Oncol 2003; 21(5):799–806.

206 Lee KR, Scully RE. Mucinous tumors of the ovary: a clinicopathologic study of 196 borderline tumors (of intestinal type) and carcinomas, including an evaluation of 11 cases with 'pseudomyxoma peritonei'. Am J Surg Pathol 2000; 24(11):1447–1464.

207 Balasch J, Pahisa J, Marquez M, et al. Metastatic ovarian strumosis in an in-vitro fertilization patient. Hum Reprod 1993; 8(12):2075–2077.

208 Karseladze AI, Kulinitch SI. Peritoneal strumosis. Pathol Res Pract 1994; 190(11):1082–1085.

209 Ferguson AW, Katabuchi H, Ronnett BM, Cho KR. Glial implants in gliomatosis peritonei arise from normal tissue, not from the associated teratoma. Am J Pathol 2001; 159(1):51–55.

24

Pathogenesis of ovarian cancer

Ronny L. Drapkin and

Jonathan L. Hecht

Introduction

Emergence of ovarian surface epithelium and 'transformation' from the mesothelial to epithelial phenotype

The normal to dysplasia to carcinoma pathway

Morphologic evidence
Genetic pathways
Defining precursors in BRCA1, BRCA2 carriers

Differentiation-specific pathways and their precursors

Serous carcinoma
Mucinous carcinomas

Endometrioid carcinomas
Clear cell carcinomas

Integrative models for ovarian cancer

Ovarian cancer divergent pathways
Ovarian cancer as a multiplicity of integrated pathways

Summary

Introduction

The purpose of this chapter is to describe proposed mechanisms by which epithelial cancers arise in the ovary. We will discuss the morphologic and molecular changes associated with the transformation of normal cells of the ovary to precancer lesions and their progression to cancer. We will discuss experimental and animal cancer models with relevance to cancer risk factors and prevention.

Epithelial malignancies are thought to arise through a well-defined progression of genetic and histologic changes leading from normal tissues to a dysplastic or in-situ precursor lesion, to invasive and metastatic cancer. This model is rooted in the study of gastrointestinal cancers where such a progression has been observed at the tissue and molecular levels (Fig. 24.1a).[1,2] Ovarian cancer does not readily fit into this model because it typically presents at an advanced clinical stage and has no consistently defined precursor lesion. In addition, the histologic appearance of ovarian carcinoma is heterogeneous including serous, endometrioid, mucinous and clear cell morphologies and there are no 'normal' mucosal analogues to these histologies in the adult ovary.

Therefore, application of a Vogelstein-type model of ovarian cancer development must:

1 Define a 'transformation zone' on which the neoplastic events are superimposed.

2 Provide a mechanism for and definition of, precursor lesions arising in this zone.

3 Correlate the known genetic changes in ovarian cancer with their histology, clinical presentation and epidemiology.

4 Recognize that the model may fail to be satisfactory for many cancers seen in daily practice that have mixed, divergent differentiation or which are poorly differentiated.

The inevitable failures of such a model reflect a complexity of ovarian tumor biology that is not readily apparent in colon cancers. First, while clinicians tend to group the various histologies (serous, clear cell, endometrioid) together, and treat patients based on grade and stage, these tumors carry distinct molecular defects. Secondly, there is a range of morphologic intermediates that can precede and accompany each histology (Table 24.1). For example, serous cancers can arise from ovarian surface, regions of ciliated epithelium in cortical inclusion cysts (CICs), from implants of the fallopian tube epithelium, from micropapillary serous borderline tumors or even within serous cystadenomas; endometriosis can give rise to or be associated with both clear cell and endometrioid carcinoma, or borderline mucinous tumors (endocervical type). Thirdly, on critical examination, the criteria that are often cited to differentiate serous from endometrioid adenocarcinomas often fail to make this distinction. The degree of overlap in histology and precursor lesions reflects a limited scope in the cell

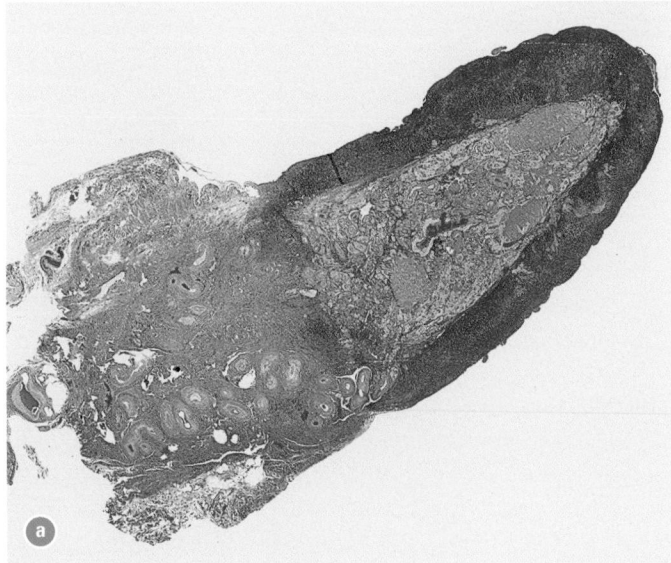

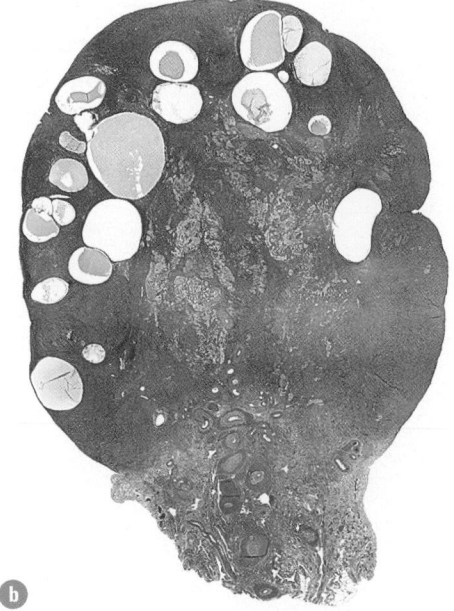

Fig. 24.1 (a) Normal postmenopausal ovary with cortical atrophy. (b) Extensive cortical inclusion cysts in a postmenopausal ovary.

Table 24.1 Pathways to ovarian cancer

Differentiation	Proposed origin (decreasing order of frequency)	Precursor	Molecular alterations	Transit
Serous (poorly differentiated)	OSE CIC Endosalpingiosis Endometriosis	CIC with atypia Cystadenofibroma	p53	Rapid
Serous (well differentiated)	OSE CIC Endosalpingiosis Endometriosis	Borderline serous cystadenoma Cystadenofibroma	K-ras, BRAF	Variable
Endometrioid	Endometriosis CIC OSE	Endometriosis with atypia Endometrioid adenofibroma Endometrioids polyp	PTEN microsatellite instability (MSH2) Beta-catenin	Slow
Clear cell	Endometriosis CIC	None demonstrated	PTEN	Unknown
Carcinosarcoma	Endometriosis CIC	None demonstrated		
Mucinous	CIC	Borderline mucinous (intestinal type) Mucinous cystadenoma	K-ras	Slow
Transitional	OSE Walthard rests Endometriosis	Benign Brenner tumor Borderline Brenner tumor Mucinous cystadenoma Teratoma Endometrioid adenocarcinoma		Unknown
Mixed epithelial	CIC Endometriosis	None demonstrated		

OSE, ovarian surface epithelium; CIC, cortical inclusion cyst.

of origin, not unlike the shared origins of a wide spectrum of endometrial cancers.

Emergence of ovarian surface epithelium and 'transformation' from the mesothelial to epithelial phenotype

Müllerian epithelium is unique to women. The Müllerian duct is formed by an invagination of coelomic epithelium, which eventually forms the fallopian tubes, uterus and endocervix. The development of this system requires that the 'mesothelium' undergo a transformation to the requisite tubal (serous), endometrial (endometrioid) and cervical (mucinous) epithelia. In adult women, the majority of ovarian surface and inclusions in the superficial cortex remain lined by 'mesothelium', but tumors are presumed to derive from regions that have similarly acquired a Müllerian phenotype; a process that appears to be enriched in cortical cysts (Figs. 24.1–24.3).

There are two sources of Müllerian epithelium in the ovary. Either endometrial or tubal epithelium is relocated to the ovarian surface by exfoliation, direct contact or adhesions (the 'transfer model') or the surface cells are induced to transform via metaplasia (the 'metaplasia model') (Fig. 24.2).[3–6]

The metaplasia model has compelling support from both embryogenesis and molecular studies. Although continuous with the mesothelial lining of the peritoneal cavity, ovarian surface epithelium (OSE) shares a common embryologic origin with epithelia of Müllerian duct-derived tissues;[7,8] they both arise from the coelomic epithelium in the area of the gonadal ridge. This common origin is manifest in non-neoplastic adult ovaries as a commonly observed histologic transformation of the OSE to a columnar and ciliated cell type (Fig. 24.3), a process referred to as Müllerian metaplasia. The adult ovarian surface has a phenotypic plasticity that can be demonstrated by its reactivity (immunostaining) with antibodies to both epithelial (cytokeratin, laminin and collagen IV) and mesothelial (vimentin, collagen I and III) antigens. In-vitro (cell culture), OSE cells can be induced to shift between epithelial and mesenchymal morphology,[9,10] The resulting surface epithelia express estrogen, progesterone and androgen receptors.[11] Carcinoma is presumed to arise in metaplastic epithelium

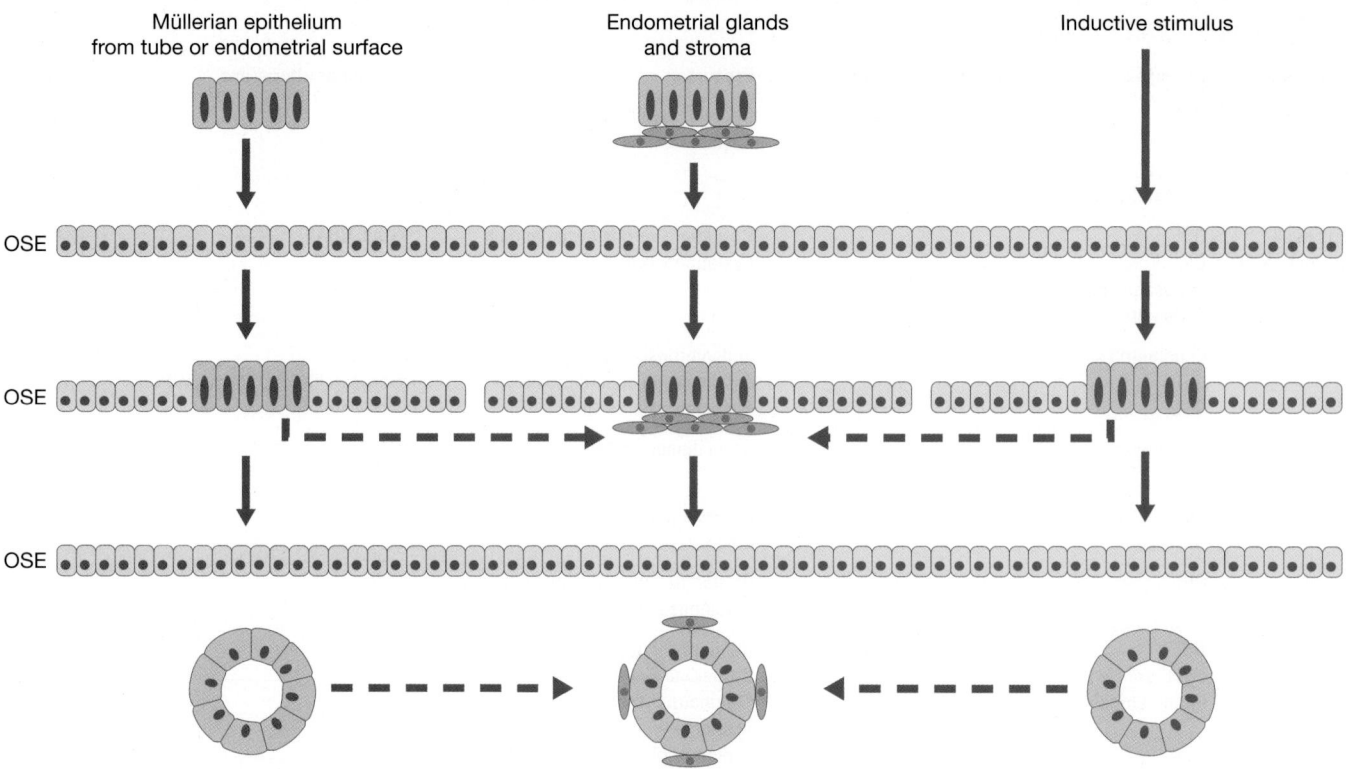

Fig. 24.2 Schematic of the potential origins of ovarian surface Müllerian epithelium and inclusions. These include implantation of salpingeal- or endometrial-lining epithelium on the ovarian surface epithelium (OSE) with subsequent development of cortical inclusion cysts (CICs, left); implantation of both endometrial glands and stroma forming endometriotic cysts (center); and transformation of the OSE to form Müllerian epithelium. In the first and third scenarios, induction of the underlying or adjacent cortical stroma (dotted lines) could lead to the production of endometrial stroma.

through additional, possibly hormonally driven, events (Fig. 24.3).[12–14] Either tubal or endometrial metaplasia or transfer could account for similarities of ovarian carcinoma to other gynecologic cancers, including basal and endometrial.

Animal models of ovarian cancer have focused on the ovarian surface epithelium as the cell of origin of ovarian carcinomas. Murine models of ovarian cancer[15–17] rely on xenografts (reimplanting genetically altered mouse ovarian epithelial cells into the ovarian bursa (site of the ovaries) of adult mice.[17] These models can account for the effects of the local ovarian milieu since they develop within the ovarian bursa. All of these models have been able to generate epithelial tumors with either viral oncoproteins[15] or mutation and/or elimination of human oncogenes and tumor suppressors that arise from the implanted OSE.[16,17]

In humans, the triggers for metaplasia and neoplasia are not known, but CICs commonly harbor metaplastic change and may offer insight into the mechanism. Models of CIC formation include repair of ovulation sites, formation of fibrous or salpingeal adhesions or

cortical invaginations of OSE with aging (Fig. 24.4). In ovulation, the OSE overlying a maturing follicle is subjected to apoptotic signals that ultimately aid in the rupture of the ovum through the ovarian surface. During the repair of the resulting gap in the OSE, some cells become entrapped within the cortex, giving rise to CICs. Adhesions are an obvious mechanism for incorporation of either susceptible OSE or salpingeal epithelium. Aging likely accounts for a third mechanism of CIC generation. As the ovary ages it becomes atrophic and cerebriform on the surface. This process leads to invaginations of the OSE into the ovarian cortex and the formation of CICs. The common element in CIC formation is the entrapment of OSE in a stroma-rich environment, and stroma may be the source of the metaplastic trigger.

CICs may be increased or altered by ovulatory cycles. Epidemiologic studies demonstrate a decreased risk of epithelial ovarian cancer by factors that suppress ovulation, including pregnancy, lactation and oral contraceptives.[18,19] Further support for a causative role of ovulation in cancer comes from the observation that

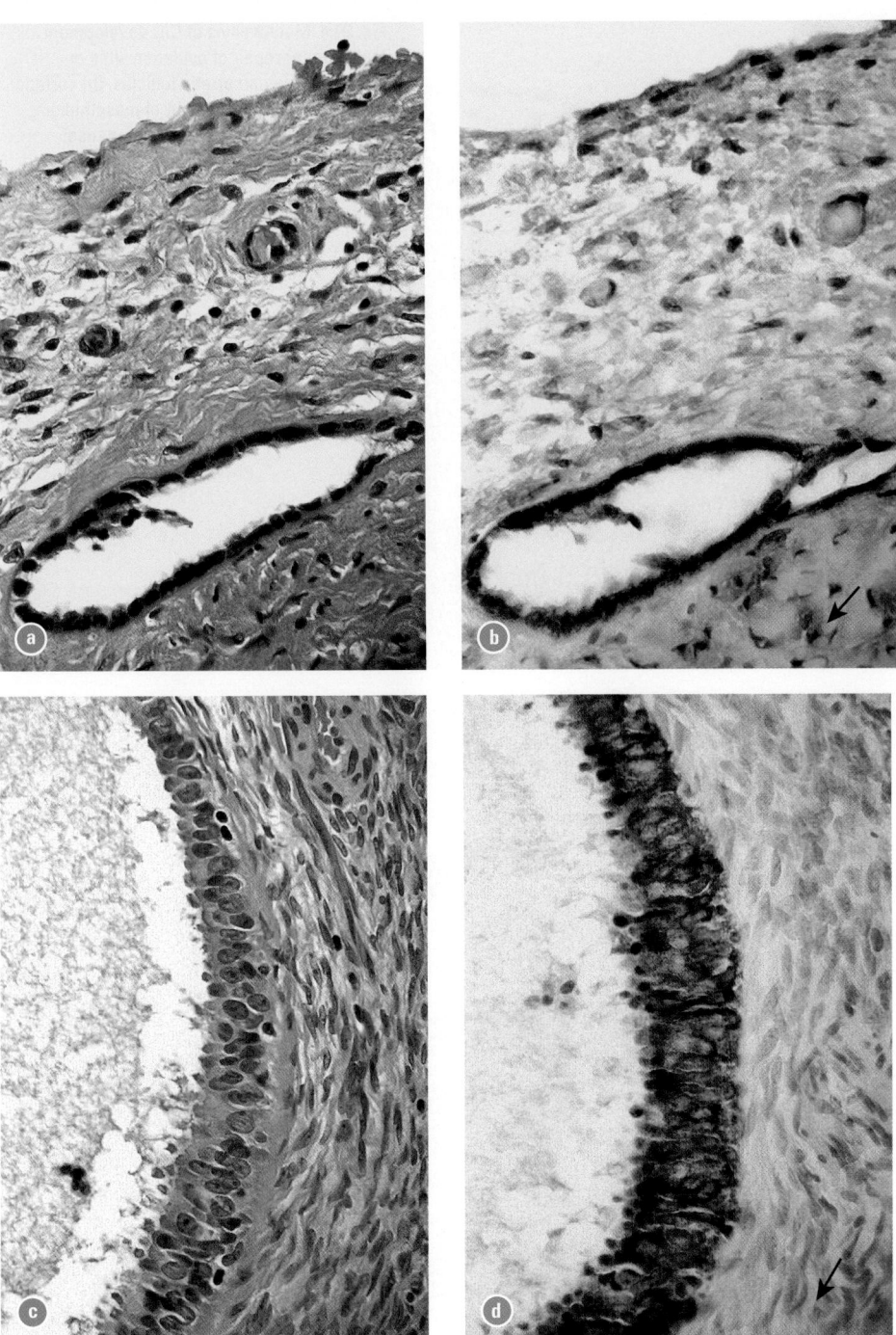

Fig. 24.3 Different ovarian cell phenotypes, including mesothelium (a), expressing calretinin (arrow) (b), and ciliated inclusions (c), expressing epithelial membrane antigen (EMA) (arrow) (d). Presumably the latter are targets for molecular events leading to neoplasia.

cancer of the OSCE is rare in animal species that ovulate infrequently, whereas it is common in hens, which, like humans, are frequent ovulators.[20,21]

Ovulation cannot be the whole explanation and inclusion cysts, while an attractive target for genetic mutations per se, may not be a mandatory precursor. Some serous carcinomas arise directly from the ovarian surface.

Also, intraparenchymal tumors can arise in endometriotic cysts rather than CICs. In addition, some serous and mucinous tumors arise from slow-growing surface neoplasms (adenofibroma or cystic borderline tumor) that not linked to ovulation.

The transfer model is compelling on grounds of tumor morphology. Ovarian tumors are histologically similar

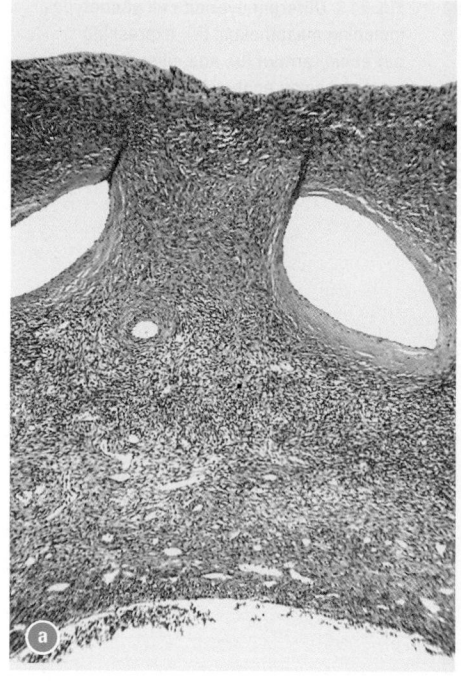
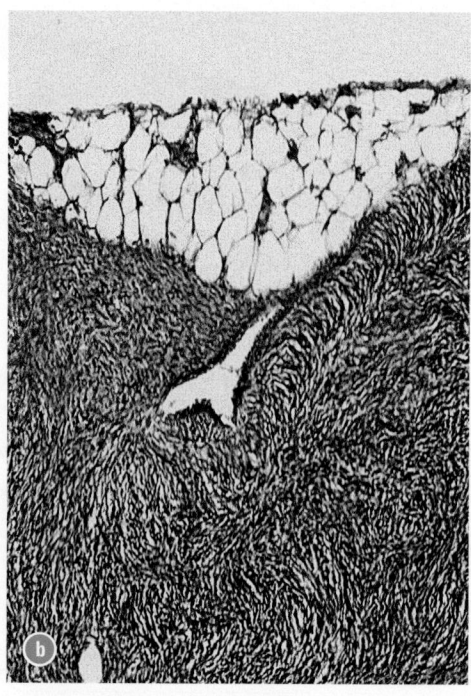

Fig. 24.4 Mechanisms of CIC development, including (a) repair of ovulation sites or entrapment within atretic follicles, (b) surface adhesions with entrapment of mesothelium, (c) invaginations in the postmenopausal atrophic ovary, leading to encysted OSE, and (d) adhesions with entrapment of salpingeal epithelium (endosalpingiosis).

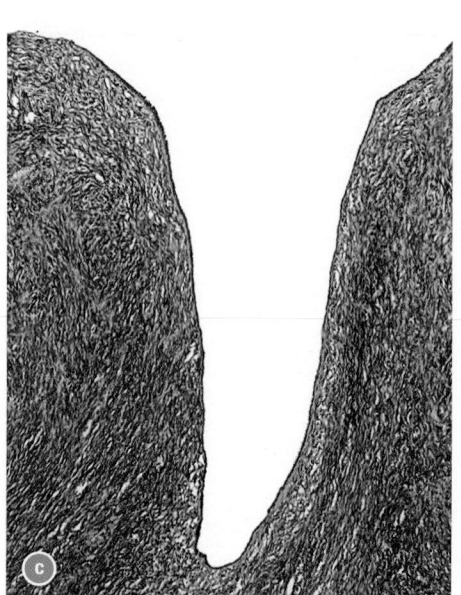
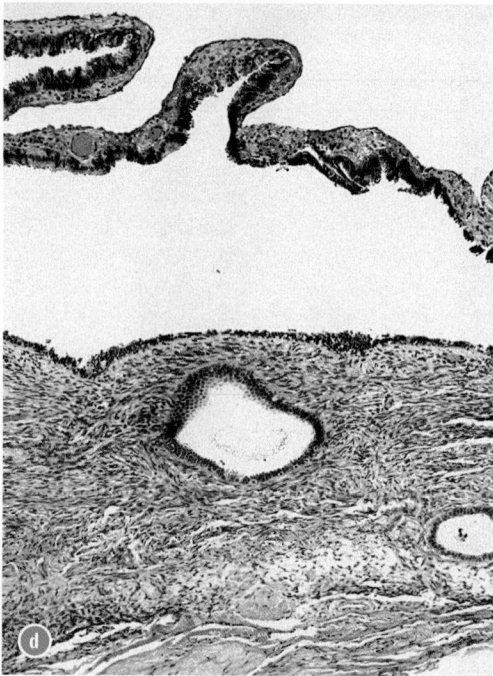

to those arising in the tube and endometrium. Like ovarian cancer, the majority of carcinomas attributed to the ciliated epithelium of the tube, including those associated with BRCA1 mutations, are poorly differentiated carcinomas. Ovarian carcinomas, like those in the endometrium, comprise two major biologic subsets, endometrioid and papillary serous types. The former may be associated with estrogen-responsive pre-existing hyperplasia and the latter appear to arise in the surface endometrial-lining epithelium, often in association with endometrial polyps unrelated to estrogen. Thus, it is not inconceivable that epithelium from these multiple sources could be transported to the ovarian surface, each with its own tumor phenotype. Experimental evidence supports trans-tubal migration of endometrium and concurrent primary tumors are often reported in the ovary and endometrium.[21]

The normal to dysplasia to carcinoma pathway

MORPHOLOGIC EVIDENCE

Several pathways to ovarian cancer are observed in surgical resections.

Direct transformation of OSE or CIC epithelium to high-grade carcinomas (Fig. 24.5)

This is the pathway for the development of the most lethal tumors, papillary serous carcinomas. Notwithstanding occasional juxtaposition of normal and abnormal epithelium in the same histologic field, in this pathway an intermediate lesion is not readily observed. Presumably a series of molecular events mediates a rapid evolution from morphologically benign epithelium to malignancy.

The association between metaplastic/ciliated OSE or CIC and serous carcinoma is largely circumstantial and contradictory. Associations between inclusion cysts and cancer have been based on evaluation of contralateral ovaries of patients with ovarian cancer.[12] Studies have reported increased inclusion cysts, tubal metaplasia and similar alterations in the fallopian tube. Some argue that a subset of serous carcinoma arises from occult tubal primaries (see Chapter 21).[3,66] Westhoff et al. compared the normal contralateral ovaries of 37 ovarian cancer patients with those of 148 non-cancer patients. They reported a similar frequency of inclusions (2.7 and 3.6) per ovary and concluded that increased formation of inclusions was not a risk factor for ovarian cancer.[22] However, Werness et al. reported a comparison of 64 consecutive patients undergoing prophylactic oophorectomy for a strong family history of ovarian cancer, with 30 women with no known family history of ovarian cancer, and found more cortical inclusion cysts in the prophylactically removed than controls' ovaries. Interestingly, although no significant differences were seen at the light microscopic level, the cysts from the cases contained nuclei with greater chromatin heterogeneity.[23] Deligdisch also proposed ovarian dysplasia based on alterations in the chromatin pattern of cortical epithelium detected by image analysis.[24,25] Bell and Scully examined 14 cases of early-stage epithelial ovarian carcinoma; dysplastic change in the adjacent surface epithelium was identified in only three cases and most tumors were

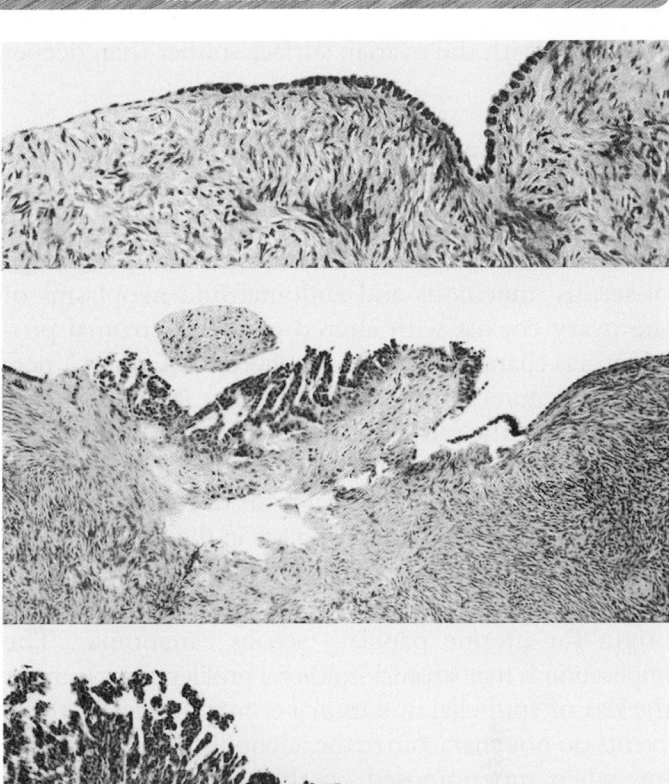
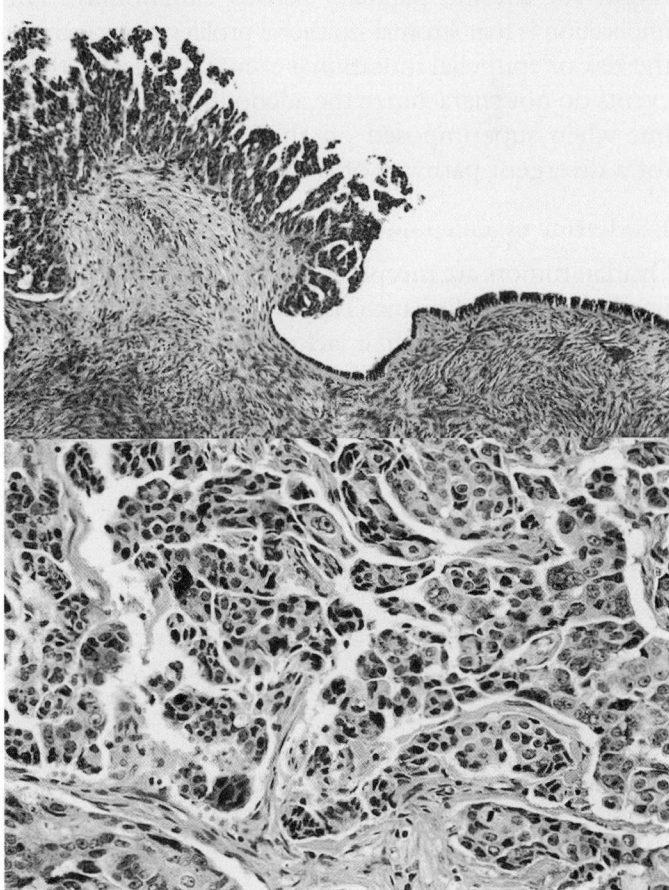

Fig. 24.5 A popular explanation for the development of most serous carcinomas is direct transformation from OSE or CIC epithelia, progressing in order from the top to bottom of the figure. In this model, an intermediate lesion (such as a cystadenoma, adenofibroma or borderline tumor) is uncommon.

associated with the ovarian surface, rather than deeper cortex.[26]

Evolution of cancers in association with pre-existing adenofibromas

Although it is assumed that most ovarian carcinomas do not arise from benign cystadenomas, a small percentage of serous, mucinous and endometrioid neoplasms of the ovary coexist with altered epithelial stromal proliferations characterized as adenofibroma (Crum C, personal communication)(Fig. 24.6). These lesions are often distinct from the carcinomas and do not show cytologic atypia, but indicate that stromal epithelial interactions are at play during the interval prior to cancer development. A similar scenario takes place in the endometrium in the form of endometrial polyps. Polyps are not considered precancers per se, but are frequently the site of origin for uterine papillary serous carcinomas. The implication is that stromal–epithelial proliferations increase the risk of epithelial mutational events. Logically, these events do not characterize the adenofibromas or polyps, but when superimposed on these processes, provide for a divergent pathway of tumor growth.

Borderline cystadenomas as precursors

Ovarian tumors are morphologically classified as benign, borderline or malignant. Tumors of borderline malignancy are defined by their lack of 'obvious invasion' of stroma and are characterized by a better prognosis than invasive carcinoma.[27] Epidemiologically, borderline and invasive serous tumors appear related because there is a 10–15 year time lag between their peak incidences, there are similar epidemiologic risk factors for benign, borderline and invasive lesions and there is an increased incidence of benign and borderline tumors in women at familial/genetic risk for ovarian cancer.[28] However, only a minority of patients with carcinoma will have a preceding borderline lesion,[29] and it is exceedingly rare to find histologic transition from borderline histology to invasive carcinoma in a single tumor (Fig. 24.7).[30,31]

In fact, serous-type borderline lesions have been shown to be genetically distinct from their high-grade invasive counterpart. For example, serous 'borderline' tumors typically contain different genetic changes than carcinomas. Serous borderline tumors show an absence of p53 mutations, loss of heterozygosity (LOH) on the long arm of the inactivated X chromosome and microsatellite instability. In contrast, invasive carcinomas have frequent p53 mutation, LOH on multiple somatic chromosomes (1p, 3p, 5q, 6q, 7p, 8p, 9q, 11p, 13q, 14q, 17q, 18q, 21q, 22q) and lack microsatellite instability.[32–37]

In contrast to high-grade serous tumors, the connection between benign or borderline mucinous tumors and mucinous carcinomas of the ovary is much stronger (Fig. 24.8, see below).

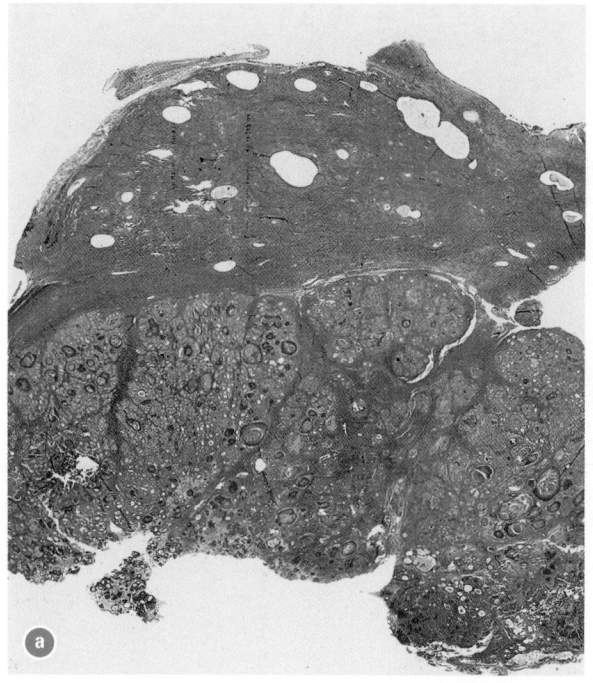
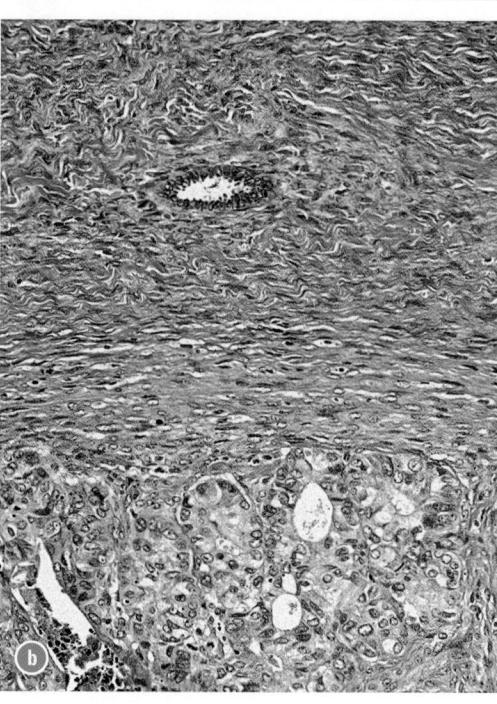

Fig. 24.6 (a) Endometrioid adenofibroma (upper) immediately adjacent to endometrioid adenocarcinoma (lower). (b) Juxtaposed benign epithelium in adenofibroma (upper) and carcinoma (lower).

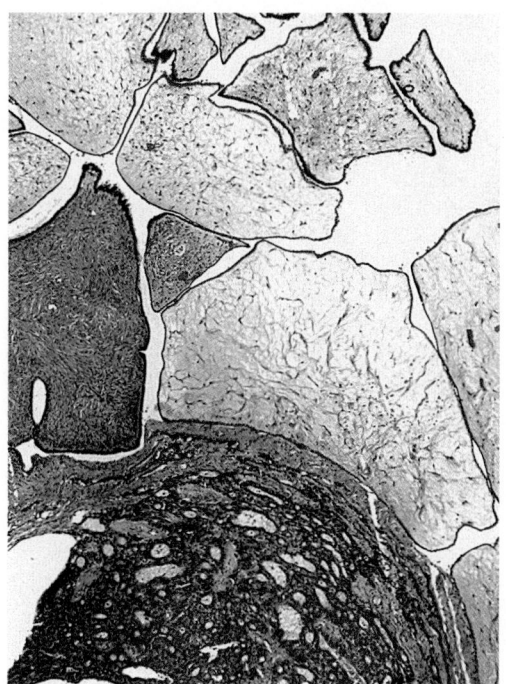

Fig. 24.7 Uncommon scenario where a well-differentiated serous cancer (lower) arises within a borderline tumor (upper).

Low-grade carcinomas (Fig. 24.9)

Serous carcinomas are predominantly high-grade tumors but rarely may be low grade. The low-grade serous carcinomas (and serous borderline tumors) frequently have mutations in BRAF and K-ras, which are rarely encountered in the high-grade carcinoma.[38–40] They also lack p53 mutations, which are very common in high-grade serous carcinoma.[41]

Low-grade serous carcinomas show fewer molecular abnormalities by both cytogenetic[42] and single nucleotide polymorphism analysis in comparison to high-grade serous carcinomas.[43] Gene expression profiling also allows separation of both low-grade serous carcinomas and serous borderline tumors.[43–46] Based on the work of Singer et al., only tumors with grade 1 nuclear atypia, low-grade architecture (typically micropapillary) and low mitotic activity fall into the low-grade group, with respect to their genetic profile.[47]

GENETIC PATHWAYS

Like other solid tumors, ovarian cancer is thought to result from a sequential accumulation of genetic changes in tumor suppressor genes and oncogenes, because consistent abnormalities are present in the mature carcinoma. For example, mutations in p53 and c-Myc are commonly detected in serous carcinomas.[48,49] However, the particular early molecular and genetic events associated with neoplastic transformation of the OSE on the surface or in CICs are still largely unknown. Study of early changes is made difficult by the lack of obvious morphologic precursors.

The problem of oncogenesis has been approached by studying ovarian cancer cell lines and primary tumors using gene-expression profile technologies (differential display, serial analysis of gene expression (SAGE), differential cDNA array, comparative hybridization of cDNA arrays, two-dimensional gel electrophoresis of cellular proteins),[44,50–57] and more recently, proteomic serum patterns.[51,53,57,58] As might be expected, each study has identified a unique set of genes whose expression is altered in the transition from benign OSE to carcinoma. Interestingly, like colonic cancers, the majority of up-regulated genes identified are either surface antigens or secreted protein.[59] Such studies using tissue from carcinoma and related cell lines have not identified at which stage in oncogenesis these genes are involved.

Barkat et al.[60] analyzed groups of high-risk women (BRCA1 heterozygotes) to test the hypothesis that this group would be enriched for premalignant histologic or genetic changes in the ovarian surface epithelium. They assayed a range of epithelial changes, including surface epithelial pseudostratification, inclusion cysts, deep cortical invaginations of surface epithelium, increased stromal cell activity and surface papillomatosis. In addition they immunophenotyped these changes with antibodies to BRCA1, p53 and ERBB-2, quantified proliferative activity with Mib-1 staining (for Ki-67) and assessed the apoptotic index. Like others, they noted some morphologic differences in inclusion cysts; however, there was no molecular difference between the two groups, indicating that if a transition from inclusion cyst to cancer occurs, it is a hidden event.[23–25]

More recently, we have investigated the proteins most commonly reported to be overexpressed in ovarian tumors (HE4, EpCAM, EMA/MUC1, mesothelin and CD9) by immunoperoxidase in normal human ovarian tissues. In non-neoplastic ovary, both surface cells (OSE) and cortical cysts (CICs) ranged from flat to cuboidal to stratified and ciliated in histologic appearance. OSE had a similar staining pattern to omental peritoneum, expressing calretinin and CD9. In contrast, CICs had expression patterns similar to fallopian tube; they frequently expressed HE4, EMA and mesothelin, but lacked CD9. HE4, EMA and mesothelin expression were strongest in stratified and ciliated epithelium. Expression of tumor-associated proteins in metaplastic ovarian surface cells and cysts suggests that either these genes are involved early in the neoplastic process

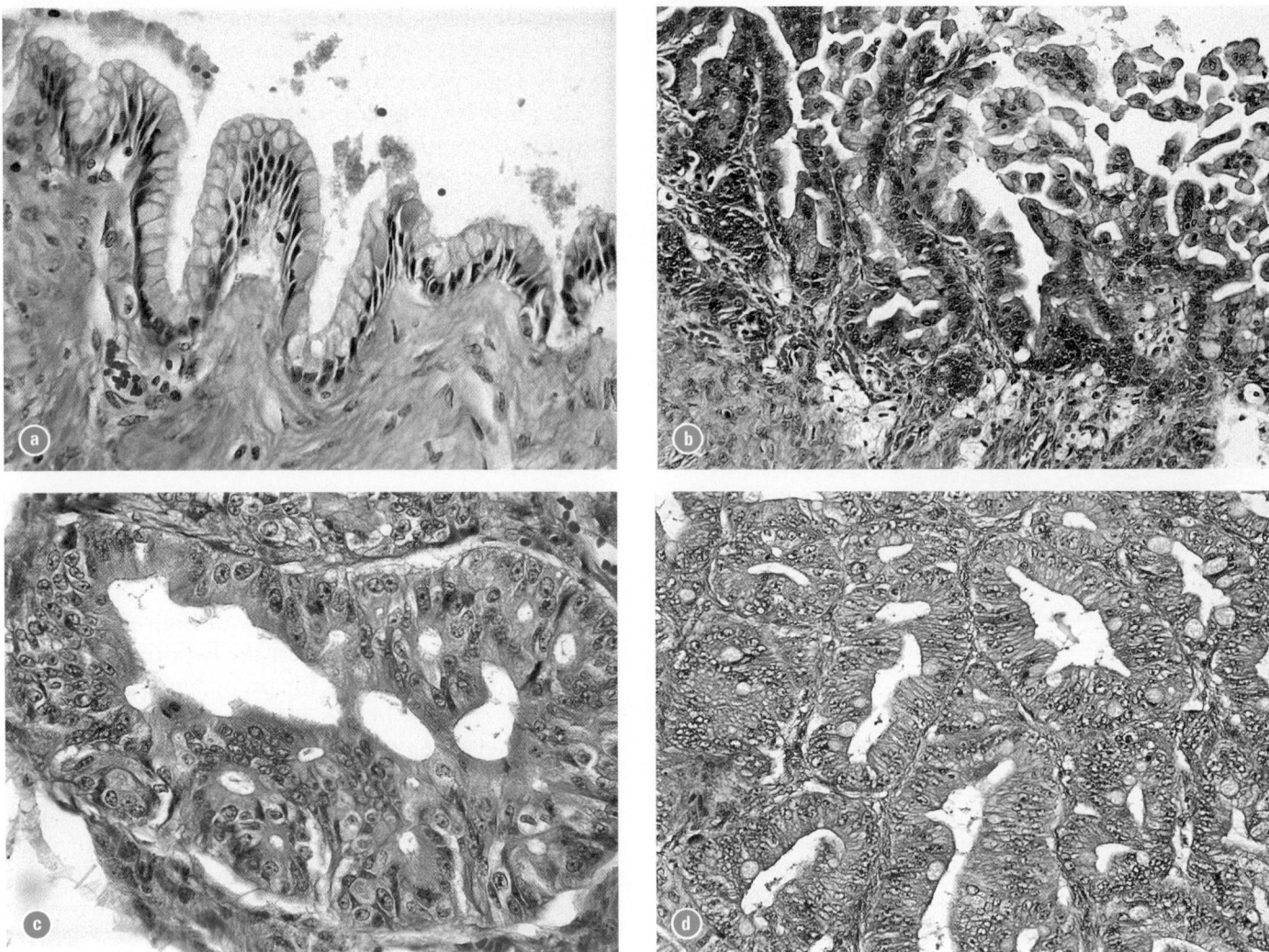

Fig. 24.8 Mucinous tumors are closely related to their benign and borderline counterparts. These come from a case that was diagnosed as a mucinous tumor of borderline malignancy, intestinal type. Much of the tumor (a) had a bland appearance with cuboidal epithelium but several areas (b) contained complex architecture with nuclear stratification. Other areas (c) contained sufficient atypia to warrant a diagnosis of adenocarcinoma, supported by invasion in adjacent foci (d).

or, more likely, that most of the genes consistently overexpressed in carcinoma merely reflect a shift from the mesothelial to epithelial phenotype in the precursor cells of the ovarian surface.[6]

DEFINING PRECURSORS IN BRCA1, BRCA2 CARRIERS

An 'experimental' approach to defining early neoplasia has been to study ovaries from women predisposed to carcinoma. Patients with mutations in the tumor suppressor genes, BRCA1 and BRCA2, have predisposition to breast and ovarian carcinoma. Ovarian carcinomas associated with germline BRCA1 or BRCA2 mutations are indistinguishable from sporadic high-grade, late-stage ovarian carcinomas, based on morphology, gene expression profiling and p53 mutation analysis,[61–66] but prophylactic oophorectomies in high-risk women detect occult early-stage carcinoma in 8–12%.[67,68] As discussed above, the presence of histologic precancer lesions such as epithelial multi-layering or tufting in these patients is controversial.[25,60,69–70] However, molecular abnormalities including LOH for BRCA1 and mutations of p53 gene have been shown to occur prior to detectable cancer (Figs 24.6, 24.10).

The relevance of BRCA1 mutations to sporadic cancers has been questioned since the estimated BRCA1 gene frequency in the general population is 0.15%, accounting for 5.7% of ovarian cancers in women below age 40 and 2.1% in women between 50 and 70.[71] How-

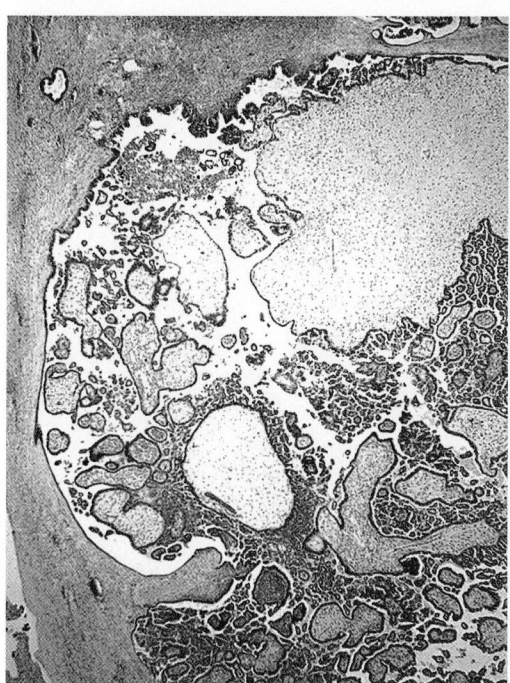

Fig. 24.9 So-called low-grade micropapillary serous carcinoma, another form of low-grade serous carcinoma that is associated with a spectrum of borderline changes.

ever, inactivation of BRCA1 and/or BRCA2 through genetic and epigenetic (promoter hypermethylation) mechanisms can be shown in the majority of sporadic cancers.[72,73] In addition, recent studies have shown that EMSY, a gene encoding a protein that binds and inactivates BRCA2, is amplified in 17% of high-grade ovarian cancers, thus identifying a relatively common genetic mechanism unrelated to the BRCA2 locus that can result in loss of BRCA2 function.[74–76] EMSY amplification was not seen in grade 1 carcinomas, borderline tumors or mucinous carcinomas. Functional loss of BRCA1/BRCA2 with resulting inability to repair double-strand DNA breaks might explain the complex karyotypes typical of high-grade ovarian carcinomas.[42]

Differentiation-specific pathways and their precursors

Surface epithelial carcinomas are typically subclassified based on histologic pattern and grade into serous, endometrioid, mucinous, clear cell, transitional and undifferentiated.[5] Each morphology is associated with specific clinical presentation and genetics.

SEROUS CARCINOMA

Serous carcinoma is, by far, the most common histologic subtype.[77] A prevalent belief is that these tumors arise from the OSE. Studies of patients with BRCA1 mutations have also supported origin in tubal epithelium with subsequent surface ovarian spread.[3,66] However, there is no reason to exclude an origin from CICs or endometriotic foci in some instances. This is supported by the intra-parenchymal confinement of some serous carcinomas.

As discussed previously in this chapter, most high-grade serous carcinomas are not associated with a pre-existing benign or borderline lesion. This lack of defined precursor is sometimes dismissed with the fact that most carcinomas present at high stage when they have presumably overgrown their precursor, but such precursors are only rarely found in the absence of cancer. Screening and prevention of both ovarian and uterine serous carcinomas is a distinctly different challenge relative to other tumors, such as colon cancer, where adenomatous polyps are a detectable risk factor that can guide subsequent triage.[78] Moreover, due to their surface involvement, early detection of surface serous carcinomas may have little impact on their natural history.

Low-grade serous carcinomas (so-called micropapillary carcinomas) may arise in association with borderline tumors. However, these tumors appear genetically distinct from the higher-grade serous tumors.

MUCINOUS CARCINOMAS

Mucinous cystadenocarcinomas differ sharply from serous tumors by the defined relationship between benign, borderline and invasive carcinoma. Mucinous-type tumors comprise less than 15% of ovarian tumors. Approximately 75% are benign and the majority of the remainder are borderline. Primary invasive mucinous carcinoma is exceedingly rare and the large majority are stage I tumors. Such carcinomas more often represent metastases from the appendix and GI tract[79,80] or over-diagnosis of borderline tumors. In borderline mucinous tumors, the epithelium varies from atypical to adenomatous. This has been referred to as 'intraepithelial carcinoma.' Also, true mucinous carcinomas with extensive stromal invasion are often associated with a low-grade component containing areas of intraepithelial carcinoma.[81] Molecular studies have demonstrated a genetic link between benign borderline and invasive mucinous tumors (Fig. 24.8).[82]

Mucinous borderline tumors of intestinal type and mucinous carcinomas show an increasing frequency of K-ras mutations[83] and, unlike the situation for serous tumors, individual tumors frequently show intratumoral heterogeneity with benign, borderline and frankly malignant areas.[84–87]

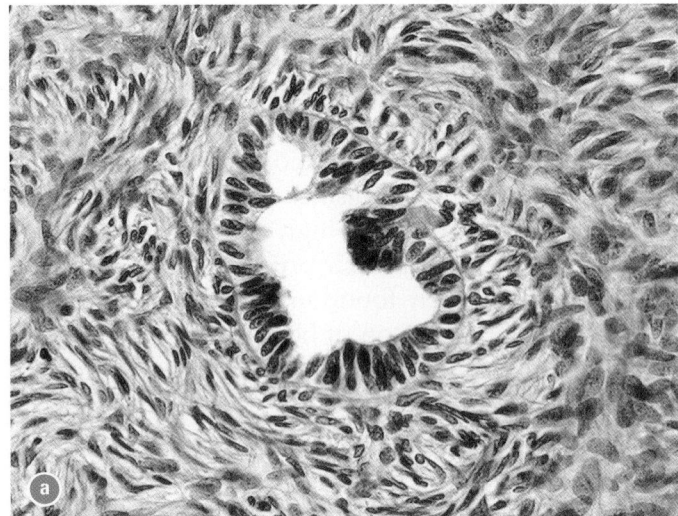

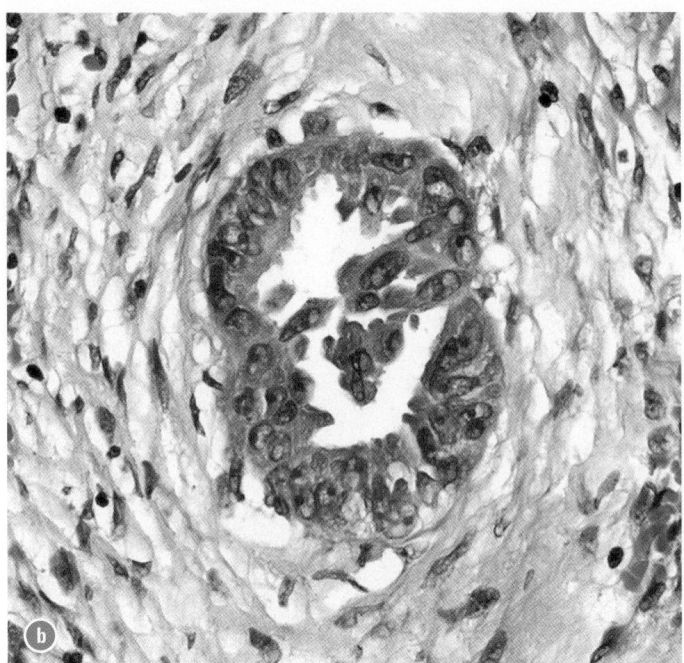

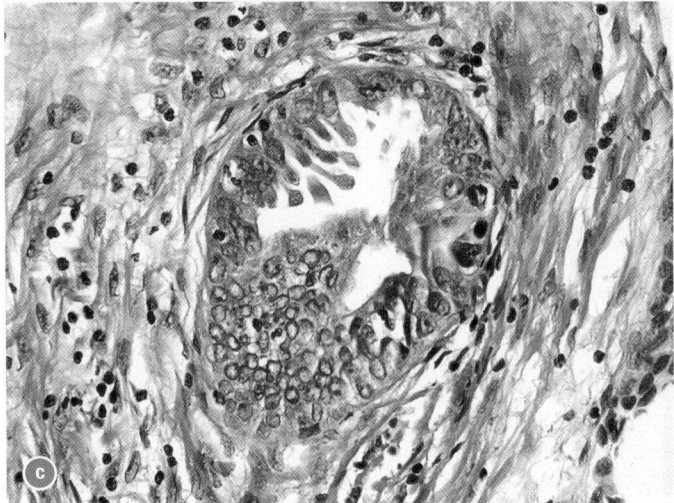

Fig. 24.10 A rarely seen but often speculated pathway to ovarian cancer is the emergence of atypia (dysplasia) within CICs. The cyst in (a) demonstrates ciliated metaplasia typical of CICs. However, the cyst in (b) contains cytologic atypia (nuclear enlargement, vesicular chromatin, enlarged nucleoli) and excessive stratification. These changes are often seen, as in this case, in patients with BRCA mutations and are considered by some to be a progenitor to ovarian cancer. However, a direct relationship of such morphologic changes and cancer has not been established (c).

ENDOMETRIOID CARCINOMAS

Endometrioid carcinomas arise in many instances from extrauterine endometrial tissue (Fig. 24.11). Ovarian cancers with endometrioid and clear cell histologies are associated with endometriosis in 28% and 49% of cases, respectively.[88,89] The risk factors for endometriosis and cancer are similar (early menarche, regular periods, short menstrual cycle and low parity). Moreover, in some studies, tubal ligation is protective for endometrioid and clear cell, but not serous cancers.[90] However, this finding is controversial and there is no evidence that tubal ligation reduces the risk of endometriosis (Mitrovitch and Crum, personal communication).

Adenocarcinomas with endometriosis may develop in association with adenofibromas, proliferative adenofibromas and, in many cases, de-novo malignant transformation of the endometrial-lining epithelium. These tumors and their immediate precursors, like their counterparts in the uterus,[91] carry identical genetic alterations, including PTEN/MMAC genes.[92,93] In cases without carcinoma, endometriosis with cytologic atypia have been shown to be monoclonal, with loss of heterozygosity on chromosomes 9p, 11q and 22q.[92]

The low-grade endometrioid carcinomas of the ovary are characterized by mutations in the beta-catenin gene, an uncommon abnormality in high-grade ovarian

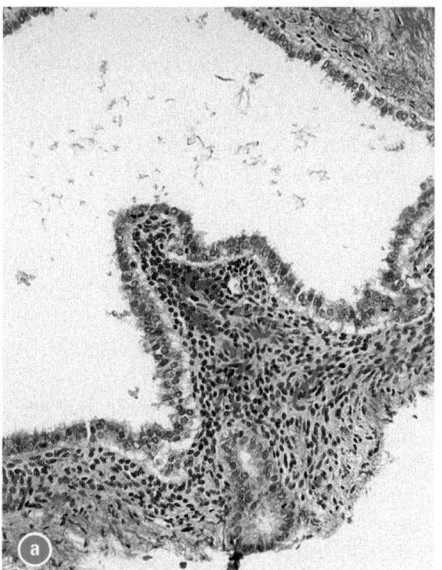 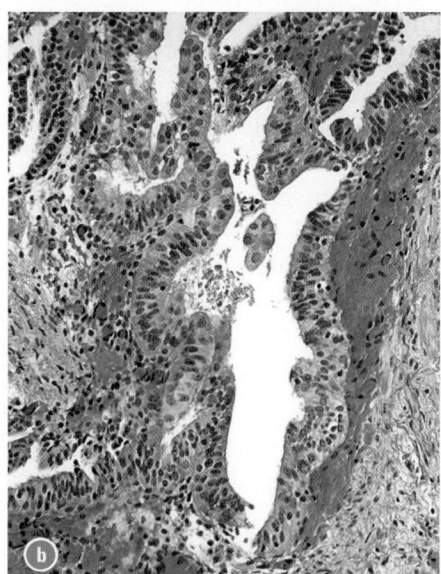 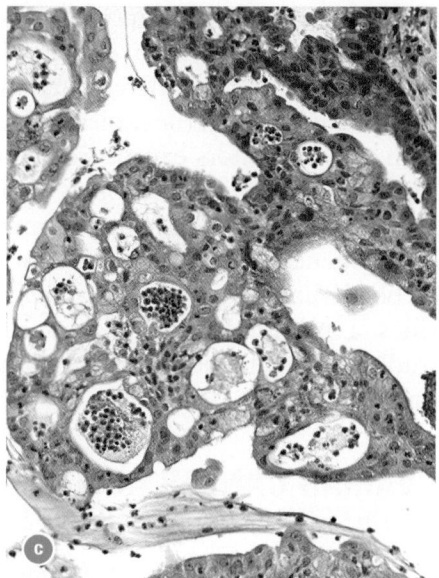

Fig. 24.11 Development of endometrial cancer (b,c) from endometriosis (a). The pathway to neoplasia may conform to the direct transformation model similar to OSE in serous neoplasia.

carcinoma.[94–96] Also, altered beta-catenin expression and microsatellite instability (MSI) are not typically seen together in endometrial carcinoma, suggesting several pathways that generate similar morphology.[94] These low-grade endometrioid tumors typically present with early-stage disease and have a favorable prognosis. The diagnosis of high-grade endometrioid carcinomas is somewhat irreproducible, with considerable morphologic overlap with high-grade serous carcinomas. This may be why high-grade endometrioid carcinomas of the ovary are not separable from high-grade serous carcinomas based on either studies of genetic events or gene expression profiling,[97] and PTEN mutations in endometrioid tumors.[98]

CLEAR CELL CARCINOMAS

Clear cell carcinomas are uncommon, often occur in association with endometriosis and not infrequently are observed to arise in endometriotic cysts. Although included in some all-purpose grading schemes, even the 'borderline' tumors show high-grade cytologic features. These tumors have a relatively low mitotic rate compared with other high-grade ovarian carcinomas and it is doubtful whether grading is relevant to their prognosis. The gene expression profile of clear cell carcinomas is distinct from other types of ovarian carcinomas.[99]

Integrative models for ovarian cancer (Table 24.1)

OVARIAN CANCER DIVERGENT PATHWAYS

As mentioned previously, it is not possible to determine the precise differentiation pathway responsible for all epithelial neoplasms. Efforts to resolve the morphologic spectrum within a molecular definition have centered on dualistic and integrative models of ovarian epithelial neoplasia. The first divides the spectrum of ovarian epithelial neoplasia into two broad categories, designated type I and type II tumors.[100] This approach parallels that in the uterus. Type I tumors tend to be low-grade neoplasms that arise in a stepwise manner from benign or borderline tumors. These include borderline tumors, endometrioid carcinomas, clear cell carcinomas, mucinous carcinomas and low-grade serous carcinomas arising in association with borderline tumors. Type I tumors are associated with distinct molecular changes that are rarely found in type II tumors, such as BRAF and K-ras mutations for serous tumors, K-ras mutations for mucinous tumors and beta-catenin and PTEN mutations and microsatellite instability for endometrioid tumors.

In contrast, type II tumors are high-grade neoplasms for which morphologically recognizable precursor lesions have not been identified, so-called de-novo development. Type II tumors include high-grade serous carcinoma, malignant mixed mesodermal tumors (carcinosarcoma) and undifferentiated carcinoma. There are very limited data on the molecular alterations associated with type II tumors except frequent p53 mutations in high-grade serous carcinomas and malignant mixed Müllerian tumors (carcinosarcomas). This model of carcinogenesis attempts to reconcile the relationship of borderline tumors to invasive carcinoma and provides a morphologic and molecular framework for studies aimed at elucidating the pathogenesis of ovarian cancer.

OVARIAN CANCER AS A MULTIPLICITY OF INTEGRATED PATHWAYS

A second approach does not contradict the first, but adds another layer of complexity, viewing ovarian cancer within a dynamic range of contiguous differentiation pathways. This model holds that the two parameters involved in neoplasia – type of epithelium involved and genetic events in play – are not always aligned. One constant is intestinal-type mucinous tumors, where the genetic changes may be intimately tied to the shift in epithelial differentiation to a mucinous phenotype. Both borderline and malignant epithelial tumors may derive from a range of pre-existing epithelial phenotypes, with classic serous and endometrioid carcinomas occupying the poles of a spectrum, not unlike that seen in the uterus. Undifferentiated carcinomas, 'transitional' carcinomas and carcinosarcomas occupy a place between these poles, arising in association with either serous or endometrioid neoplasia.

Summary

Every practicing pathologist struggles at times in classifying epithelial ovarian cancer. The relevance of pathogenesis lies in both the sub-classification of these neoplasms for prognostic purposes and the recognition of gaps in our understanding. Although pathogenesis has little influence on our ability to treat ovarian cancer, it is critical to understanding the limitations and strengths of screening and constructing a rational approach to ovarian cancer prevention. If therapies are devised that successfully counteract the molecular disturbances that accompany neoplastic transformation and progression, molecular subdivisions will become increasingly germane to ovarian cancer therapy.

References

1 Biankin AV, Kench JG, Dijkman FP, et al. Molecular pathogenesis of precursor lesions of pancreatic ductal adenocarcinoma. Pathology 2003; 35(1):14–24.
2 Vogelstein B, Kinzler KW. The multistep nature of cancer. Trends Genet 1993; 9(4):138–141.
3 Dubeau L. The cell of origin of ovarian epithelial tumors and the ovarian surface epithelium dogma: Does the emperor have no clothes? Gynecol Oncol 1999; 72(3):437–442.
4 Vanderhyden BC, Shaw TJ, Ethier JF. Animal models of ovarian cancer. Reprod Biol Endocrinol 2003; 1(1):67.
5 Drapkin R, Hecht J. The origins of ovarian cancer: hurdles and progress. Women's Oncol Rev 2002; 2:261–268.
6 Drapkin R, Crum C, Hecht J. Expression of candidate tumor markers in ovarian carcinoma and benign ovary: evidence for a link between epithelial phenotype and neoplasia. Hum Pathol 2004; 35(8):1014–1021.
7 Auersperg N, Edelson MI, Mok SC, et al. The biology of ovarian cancer. Semin Oncol 1998; 25(3):281–304.
8 Auersperg N, Wong AS, Choi KC, et al. Ovarian surface epithelium: biology, endocrinology and pathology. Endocr Rev 2001; 22(2):255–288.
9 Papadaki L, Beilby JO. The fine structure of the surface epithelium of the human ovary. J Cell Sci 1971; 8(2):445–465.
10 Blaustein A, Lee H. Surface cells of the ovary and pelvic peritoneum: a histochemical and ultrastructure comparison. Gynecol Oncol 1979; 8(1):34–43.
11 Lau KM, Mok SC, Ho SM. Expression of human estrogen receptor-alpha and -beta, progesterone receptor and androgen receptor MRNA in normal and malignant ovarian epithelial cells. Proc Natl Acad Sci USA 1999; 96(10):5722–5727.
12 Mittal KR, Zeleniuch-Jacquotte A, Cooper JL, Demopoulos RI. Contralateral ovary in unilateral ovarian carcinoma: a search for preneoplastic lesions. Int J Gynecol Pathol 1993; 12(1):59–63.
13 Mittal K. Tumor markers in ovaries at risk of developing carcinoma. Int J Gynecol Pathol 2000; 19(2):191–192.
14 Karlan BY, Jones J, Greenwald M, Lagasse LD. Steroid hormone effects on the proliferation of human ovarian surface epithelium in vitro. Am J Obstet Gynecol 1995; 173(1):97–104.
15 Connolly DC, Bao R, Nikitin AY, et al. Female mice chimeric for expression of the Simian virus 40 tag under control of the MISIIR promoter develop epithelial ovarian cancer. Cancer Res 2003; 63(6):1389–1397.
16 Flesken-Nikitin A, Choi KC, Eng JP, et al. Induction of carcinogenesis by concurrent inactivation of p53 and rb1 in the mouse ovarian surface epithelium. Cancer Res 2003; 63(13):3459–3463.
17 Orsulic S, Soslow R, Vitale-Cross L, et al. Induction of ovarian cancer by defined multiple genetic changes in a mouse model system. Cancer Cell 2002; 1:53–62.
18 Whittemore AS, Harris R, Itnyre J. Characteristics relating to ovarian cancer risk: collaborative analysis of 12 US case-control studies. II. Invasive epithelial ovarian cancers in white women. Collaborative Ovarian Cancer Group. Am J Epidemiol 1992; 136(10):1184–1203.

19 Nieto JJ, Crow J, Sundaresan M, et al. Ovarian epithelial dysplasia in relation to ovulation induction and nulliparity. Gynecol Oncol 2001; 82(2):344–349.

20 Fredrickson TN. Ovarian tumors of the hen. Environ Health Perspect 1987; 73:35–51.

21 Fujii H, Matsumoto T, Yoshida M, et al. Genetics of synchronous uterine and ovarian endometrioid carcinoma: combined analyses of loss of heterozygosity, PTEN mutation, and microsatellite instability. Hum Pathol 2002; 33(4):383–385.

22 Westhoff C, Murphy P, Heller D, Halim A. Is ovarian cancer associated with an increased frequency of germinal inclusion cysts? Am J Epidemiol 1993; 138(2):90–93.

23 Werness BA, Afify AM, Bielat KL, et al. Altered surface and cyst epithelium of ovaries removed prophylactically from women with a family history of ovarian cancer. Hum Pathol 1999; 30(2):151–157.

24 Deligdisch L, Einstein AJ, Guera D, Gil J. Ovarian dysplasia in epithelial inclusion cysts. A morphometric approach using neural networks. Cancer 1995; 76(6):1027–1034.

25 Deligdisch L, Gil J, Kerner H, et al. Ovarian dysplasia in prophylactic oophorectomy specimens: cytogenetic and morphometric correlations. Cancer 1999; 86(8):1544–1550.

26 Bell DA, Scully RE. Early de novo ovarian carcinoma. A study of fourteen cases. Cancer 1994; 73(7): 1859–1864.

27 Silva EG, Kurman RJ, Russell P, Scully RE. Symposium: ovarian tumors of borderline malignancy. Int J Gynecol Pathol 1996; 15(4):281–302.

28 Bourne TH, Whitehead MI, Campbell S, et al. Ultrasound screening for familial ovarian cancer. Gynecol Oncol 1991; 43(2):92–97.

29 Kennedy AW, Hart WR. Ovarian papillary serous tumors of low malignant potential (serous borderline tumors). A long-term follow-up study, including patients with microinvasion, lymph node metastasis and transformation to invasive serous carcinoma. Cancer 1996; 78(2):278–286.

30 Lee KR, Castrillon DH, Nucci MR. Pathologic findings in eight cases of ovarian serous borderline tumors, three with foci of serous carcinoma, that preceded death or morbidity from invasive carcinoma. Int J Gynecol Pathol 2001; 20(4):329–334.

31 Silva EG, Tornos CS, Malpica A, Gershenson DM. Ovarian serous neoplasms of low malignant potential associated with focal areas of serous carcinoma. Mod Pathol 1997; 10(7):663–667.

32 Ortiz BH, Ailawadi M, Colitti C, et al. Second primary or recurrence? Comparative patterns of p53 and K-ras mutations suggest that serous borderline ovarian tumors and subsequent serous carcinomas are unrelated tumors. Cancer Res 2001; 61(19):7264–7267.

33 Kupryjanczyk J, Bell DA, Dimeo D, et al. P53 gene analysis of ovarian borderline tumors and stage I carcinomas. Hum Pathol 1995; 26(4):387–392.

34 Cheng PC, Gosewehr JA, Kim TM, et al. Potential role of the inactivated X chromosome in ovarian epithelial tumor development. J Natl Cancer Inst 1996; 88(8):510–518.

35 Tangir J, Loughridge NS, Berkowitz RS, et al. Frequent microsatellite instability in epithelial borderline ovarian tumors. Cancer Res 1996; 56(11):2501–2505.

36 Halperin R, Zehavi S, Dar P, et al. Clinical and molecular comparison between borderline serous ovarian tumors and advanced serous papillary ovarian carcinomas. Eur J Gynaecol Oncol 2001; 22(4):292–296.

37 Wang VW, Bell DA, Berkowitz RS, Mok SC. Whole genome amplification and high-throughput allelotyping identified five distinct deletion regions on chromosomes 5 and 6 in microdissected early-stage ovarian tumors. Cancer Res 2001; 61(10):4169–4174.

38 Singer G, Oldt R 3rd, Cohen, Y, et al. Mutations in BRAF and KRAS characterize the development of low-grade ovarian serous carcinoma. J Natl Cancer Inst 2003; 95(6):484–486.

39 Singer G, Kurman RJ, Chang HW, et al. Diverse tumorigenic pathways in ovarian serous carcinoma. Am J Pathol 2002; 160(4):1223–1228.

40 Singer G, Shih IeM, Truskinovsky A, et al. Mutational analysis of K-ras segregates ovarian serous carcinomas into two types: invasive MPSC (low-grade tumor) and conventional serous carcinoma (high-grade tumor). Int J Gynecol Pathol 2003; 22(1):37–41.

41 Katabuchi H, Tashiro H, Cho KR, et al. Micropapillary serous carcinoma of the ovary: an immunohistochemical and mutational analysis of p53. Int J Gynecol Pathol 1998; 17(1):54–60.

42 Pejovic T. Genetic changes in ovarian cancer. Ann Med 1995; 27(1):73–78.

43 Jazaeri AA, Lu K, Schmandt R, et al. Molecular determinants of tumor differentiation in papillary serous ovarian carcinoma. Mol Carcinog 2003; 36(2):53–59.

44 Ono K, Tanaka T, Tsunoda T, et al. Identification by cDNA microarray of genes involved in ovarian carcinogenesis. Cancer Res 2000; 60(18):5007–5011.

45 Schwartz DR, Kardia SL, Shedden KA, et al. Gene expression in ovarian cancer reflects both morphology and biological behavior, distinguishing clear cell from other poor-prognosis ovarian carcinomas. Cancer Res 2002; 62(16):4722–4729.

46 Alaiya AA, Franzen B, Hagman A, et al. Molecular classification of borderline ovarian tumors using hierarchical cluster analysis of protein expression profiles. Int J Cancer 2002; 98(6):895–899.

47 Singer G, Shih IeM, Truskinovsky A, et al. Mutational analysis of K-ras segregates ovarian serous carcinomas into two types: invasive MPSC (low-grade tumor) and conventional serous carcinoma (high-grade tumor). Int J Gynecol Pathol 2003; 22(1):37–41.

48 Berchuck A, Kohler MF, Marks JR, et al. The p53 tumor suppressor gene frequently is altered in gynecologic cancers. Am J Obstet Gynecol 1994; 170(1):246–252.

49 Tashiro H, Miyazaki K, Okamura H, et al. C-Myc over-expression in human primary ovarian tumours: its relevance to tumour progression. Int J Cancer 1992; 50(5):828–833.

50 Wang K, Gan L, Jeffery E, et al. Monitoring gene expression profile changes ovarian carcinomas using cDNA microarray. Gene 1999; 229(1/2):101–108.

51 Schummer M, Ng WV, Bumgarner RE, et al. Comparative hybridization of an array of 21,500 ovarian cDNAs for the discovery of genes overexpressed in ovarian carcinomas. Gene 1999; 238(2):375–385.

52 Hough CD, Cho KR, Zonderman AB, et al. Coordinately up-regulated genes in ovarian cancer. Cancer Res 2001; 61(10):3869–3876.

53 Hough CD, Sherman-Baust CA, Pizer ES, et al. Large-scale serial analysis of gene expression reveals genes differentially expressed in ovarian cancer. Cancer Res 2000; 60(22):6281–6287.

54 Welsh JB, Sapinoso LM, Su AI, et al. Analysis of gene expression identifies candidate markers and pharmacological targets in prostate cancer. Cancer Res 2001; 61(16):5974–5978.

55 Wong KK, Cheng RS, Mok SC. Identification of differentially expressed genes from ovarian cancer cells by micromax cDNA microarray system. Biotechniques 2001; 30(3):670–675.

56 Shridhar V, Lee J, Pandita A, et al. Genetic analysis of early-versus late-stage ovarian tumors. Cancer Res 2001; 61(15):5895–5904.

57 Petricoin EF, Ardekani AM, Hitt BA, et al. Use of proteomic patterns in serum to identify ovarian cancer. Lancet 2002; 359(9306):572–577.

58 Jones MB, Krutzsch H, Shu H 3rd, et al. Proteomic analysis and identification of new biomarkers and therapeutic targets for invasive ovarian cancer. Proteomics 2002; 2(1):76–84.

59 Buckhaults P, Rago C, St Croix B, et al. Secreted and cell surface genes expressed in benign and malignant colorectal tumors. Cancer Res 2001; 61(19):6996–7001.

60 Barakat RR, Federici MG, Saigo PE, et al. Absence of premalignant histologic, molecular, or cell biologic alterations in prophylactic oophorectomy specimens from brca1 heterozygotes. Cancer 2000; 89(2):383–390.

61 Zweemer RP, Shaw PA, Verheijen RM, et al. Accumulation of p53 protein is frequent in ovarian cancers associated with brca1 and brca2 germline mutations. J Clin Pathol 1999; 52(5):372–375.

62 Narod SA, Boyd J. Current understanding of the epidemiology and clinical implications of brca1 and brca2 mutations for ovarian cancer. Curr Opin Obstet Gynecol 2002; 14(1):19–26.

63 Boyd J, Sonoda Y, Federici MG, et al. Clinicopathologic features of BRCA-linked and sporadic ovarian cancer. JAMA 2000; 283(17):2260–2265.

64 Shaw PA, McLaughlin JR, Zweemer RP, et al. Histopathologic features of genetically determined ovarian cancer. Int J Gynecol Pathol 2002; 21(4):407–411.

65 Werness BA, Ramus SJ, DiCioccio RA, et al. Histopathology, FIGO stage and BRCA mutation status of ovarian cancers from the Gilda Radner Familial Ovarian Cancer Registry. Int J Gynecol Pathol 2004; 23(1):29–34.

66 Jazaeri AA, Yee CJ, Sotiriou C, et al. Gene expression profiles of BRCA1-linked, BRCA2-linked and sporadic ovarian cancers. J Natl Cancer Inst 2002; 94(13):990–1000.

67 Colgan TJ, Murphy J, Cole DE, et al. Occult carcinoma in prophylactic oophorectomy specimens: prevalence and association with BRCA germline mutation status. Am J Surg Pathol 2001; 25(10):1283–1289.

68 Lu KH, Garber JE, Cramer DW, et al. Occult ovarian tumors in women with brca1 or brca2 mutations undergoing prophylactic oophorectomy. J Clin Oncol 2000; 18(14):2728–2732.

69 Casey MJ, Bewtra C, Hoehne LL, et al. Histology of prophylactically removed ovaries from brca1 and brca2 mutation carriers compared with noncarriers in hereditary breast ovarian cancer syndrome kindreds. Gynecol Oncol 2000; 78(3):278–287.

70 Stratton JF, Buckley CH, Lowe D, Ponder BA. Comparison of prophylactic oophorectomy specimens from carriers and noncarriers of a BRCA1 or BRCA2 gene mutation. United Kingdom Coordinating Committee on Cancer Research (UKCCCR) Familial Ovarian Cancer Study Group. J Natl Cancer Inst 1999; 91(7):626–628.

71 Ford D, Easton DF, Peto J. Estimates of the gene frequency of brca1 and its contribution to breast and ovarian cancer incidence. Am J Hum Genet 1995; 57(6):1457–1462.

72 Hilton JL, Geisler JP, Rathe JA, et al. Inactivation of BRCA1 and BRCA2 in ovarian cancer. J Natl Cancer Inst 2002; 94(18):1396–1406.

73 Geisler JP, Hatterman-Zogg MA, Rathe JA, Buller RE. Frequency of brca1 dysfunction in ovarian cancer. J Natl Cancer Inst 2002; 94(1):61–67.

74 Haber DA. The BRCA2-EMSY connection: implications for breast and ovarian tumorigenesis. Cell 2003; 115(5):507–508.

75 Hughes-Davies L, Huntsman D, Ruas M, et al. EMSY links the BRCA2 pathway to sporadic breast and ovarian cancer. Cell 2003; 115(5):523–535.

76 Livingston DM. EMSY, a Brca-2 partner in crime. Nat Med 2004; 10(2):127–128.

77 Mink PJ, Sherman ME, Devesa SS. Incidence patterns of invasive and borderline ovarian tumors among white women and black women in the United States. Results from the SEER Program, 1978–1998. Cancer 2002; 95(11):2380–2389.

78 Lieberman DA, Weiss DG, Bond JH, et al. Use of colonoscopy to screen asymptomatic adults for colorectal cancer. Veterans Affairs Cooperative Study Group 380. N Engl J Med 2000; 343(3):162–168.

79 Lee KR, Scully RE. Mucinous tumors of the ovary: a clinicopathologic study of 196 borderline tumors (of intestinal type) and carcinomas, including an evaluation of 11 cases with 'pseudomyxoma peritonei'. Am J Surg Pathol 2000; 24(11):1447–1464.

80 Seidman JD, Horkayne-Szakaly I, Haiba M, et al. The histologic type and stage distribution of ovarian carcinomas of surface epithelial origin. Int J Gynecol Pathol 2004; 23(1):41–44.

81 Hoerl HD, Hart WR. Primary ovarian mucinous cystadenocarcinomas: a clinicopathologic study of 49 cases with long-term follow-up. Am J Surg Pathol 1998; 22(12):1449–1462.

82 Garrett AP, Lee KR, Colitti CR, et al. K-ras mutation may be an early event in mucinous ovarian tumorigenesis. Int J Gynecol Pathol 2001; 20(3):244–251.

83 Enomoto T, Weghorst CM, Inoue M, Tanizawa O, Rice JM. K-ras activation occurs frequently in mucinous adenocarcinomas and rarely in other common epithelial tumors of the human ovary. Am J Pathol 1991; 139(4):777–785.

84 Cuatrecasas M, Villanueva A, Matias-Guiu X, Prat J. K-ras mutations in mucinous ovarian tumors: a clinicopathologic and molecular study of 95 cases. Cancer 1997; 79(8):1581–1586.

85 Mok SC, Bell DA, Knapp RC, et al. Mutation of K-ras protooncogene in human ovarian epithelial tumors of borderline malignancy. Cancer Res 1993; 53(7):1489–1492.

86 Mandai M, Konishi I, Kuroda H, et al. Heterogeneous distribution of K-ras-mutated epithelia in mucinous ovarian tumors with special reference to histopathology. Hum Pathol 1998; 29(1):34–40.

87 Garrett AP, Lee KR, Colitti CR, et al. K-ras mutation may be an early event in mucinous ovarian tumorigenesis. Int J Gynecol Pathol 2001; 20(3):244–251.

88 McMeekin DS, Burger RA, Manetta A, et al. Endometrioid adenocarcinoma of the ovary and its relationship to endometriosis. Gynecol Oncol 1995; 59(1):81–86.

89 Sainz Cuesta R de la, Eichhorn JH, Rice LW, et al. Histologic transformation of benign endometriosis to early epithelial ovarian cancer. Gynecol Oncol 1996; 60(2):238–244.

90 Rosenblatt KA, Thomas DB. Reduced risk of ovarian cancer in women with a tubal ligation or hysterectomy. The World Health Organization Collaborative Study of Neoplasia and Steroid Contraceptives. Cancer Epidemiol Biomarkers Prev 1996; 5(11):933–935.

91 Prefumo F, Todeschini F, Fulcheri E, Venturini PL. Epithelial abnormalities in cystic ovarian endometriosis. Gynecol Oncol 2002; 84(2):280–284.

92 Thomas EJ, Campbell IG. Molecular genetic defects in endometriosis. Gynecol Obstet Invest 2000; 50(Suppl)(1):44–50.

93 Obata K, Hoshiai H. Common genetic changes between endometriosis and ovarian cancer. Gynecol Obstet Invest 2000; 50(Suppl)(1):39–43.

94 Gamallo C, Palacios J, Moreno G, et al. Beta-catenin expression pattern in stage I and II ovarian carcinomas: relationship with beta-catenin gene mutations, clinicopathological features and clinical outcome. Am J Pathol 1999; 155(2):527–536.

95 Palacios J, Gamallo C. Mutations in the beta-catenin gene (ctnnb1) in endometrioid ovarian carcinomas. Cancer Res 1998; 58(7):1344–1347.

96 Wu R, Zhai Y, Fearon ER, Cho KR. Diverse mechanisms of beta-catenin deregulation in ovarian endometrioid adenocarcinomas. Cancer Res 2001; 61(22):8247–8255.

97 Schwartz DR, Wu R, Kardia SL, et al. Novel candidate targets of beta-catenin/T-cell factor signaling identified by gene expression profiling of ovarian endometrioid adenocarcinomas. Cancer Res 2003; 63(11):2913–2922.

98 Obata K, Morland SJ, Watson RH, et al. Frequent PTEN/MMAC mutations in endometrioid but not serous or mucinous epithelial ovarian tumors. Cancer Res 1998; 58(10):2095–2097.

99 Schaner ME, Ross DT, Ciaravino G, et al. Gene expression patterns in ovarian carcinomas. Mol Biol Cell 2003; 14(11):4376–4386.

100 Schwartz DR, Kardia SL, Shedden KA, et al. Gene expression in ovarian cancer reflects both morphology and biological behaviour, distinguishing clear cell from other poor-prognosis ovarian carcinomas. Cancer Res 2002; 62(16):47722–4729.

101 Shimizu M, Nikaido T, Toki T, et al. Clear cell carcinoma has an expression pattern of cell cycle regulatory molecules that is unique among ovarian adenocarcinomas. Cancer 1999; 85(3):669–677.

102 Shih IeM, Kurman RJ. Ovarian tumorigenesis: a proposed model based on morphological and molecular genetic analysis. Am J Pathol 2004; 164(5):1511–1518.

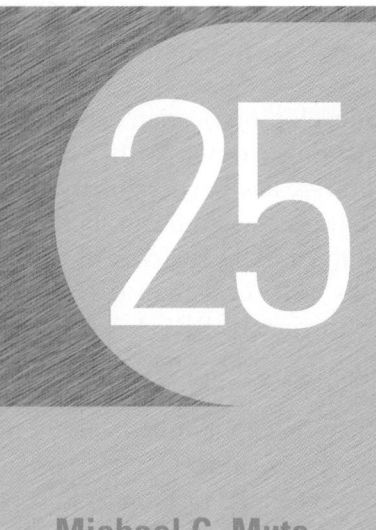

25

The patient at risk of ovarian cancer

Michael G. Muto

Introduction

Predisposing risk factors

Genetic ovarian cancer syndromes
Other risk factors
  for ovarian cancer

Factors reducing risk

Oral contraceptives
Tubal ligation
Prophylactic surgery

Screening for ovarian cancer

Pelvic examination
Biomarkers
Ultrasound and other imaging
  techniques
Ultrasound and biomarkers

Presenting signs and symptoms

**Ultrasound evaluation and risk
(malignancy) assessment**

Introduction

Ovarian cancer is the fourth leading cause of cancer deaths in women. Approximately 70% present at high stage (III or IV). Each year, nearly 25 000 women develop ovarian cancer and over 14 000 die of the disease. Surgery and chemotherapy will produce a complete response in 70%; however, relapse rates are high, often occurring after a relatively brief respite and overall long-term survival rates have not improved appreciably in the past 30 years. The number of cancers and cancer-related deaths in the past decade has increased 30 and 18%, respectively.[1,2]

The 5-year survival for stages I and IV disease are 88 and 18%, indicating that early detection may improve survival.[1] This may be true for those tumors (such as endometrioid, mucinous or serous tumor arising in the ovarian parenchyma) that are stage I at their inception. The impact of early detection on tumors arising on the surface of the ovaries or tube is less certain. Preventing death due to this disease is thus a three-tiered process, including: (1) identifying patients at risk who have not developed cancer and reducing their risk; (2) early detection of patients with cancer at lower and more curable stages; and (3) more effective management schemes. This chapter addresses the first two variables and summarizes the existing knowledge on ovarian cancer prevention and early detection.

Predisposing risk factors

GENETIC OVARIAN CANCER SYNDROMES

There are three well-recognized genetic syndromes that account for the vast majority of familial ovarian cancer and approximately 10% of all ovarian cancers. These are the breast ovarian cancer syndrome (BOCS), the site specific ovarian cancer syndrome (SSOCS) and the hereditary non-polyposis colorectal cancer syndrome (HNPCC) (Lynch II syndrome).[3] Both BOCS and SSOCS are caused by inherited mutations in the BRCA1 and BRCA2 genes. In fact, although often described as separate entities, these two syndromes are most likely phenotypic variants of the same genetic mutations. BRCA1 and BRCA2 function as classic tumor suppressor genes and are inherited in an autosomal dominant fashion. HNPCC is caused by mutations in a series of genes responsible for repairing errors in DNA replication. Inactivation of these so-called mismatch repair genes result in a high incidence of right-sided colon cancer, endometrial cancer and ovarian cancer.[4]

The lifetime risk of developing ovarian cancer in the USA is about 1.8%. Among women with BRCA1 or BRCA2 mutations, the risk has been estimated to be 20–60%.[5] These genes impart a significant lifetime risk of breast cancer in women and, in the case of BRCA2, in male breast cancer as well. Less than 0.15% of the general population are carriers of BRCA 1 or BRCA2 mutations; however, the carrier rate is dependent upon ethnic background.[6]

Founder mutations have been identified among multiple unrelated families in Iceland, The Netherlands, Sweden and among Jews of Central or Eastern European (Ashkenazi) descent. The best-described founder mutations are the 185delAG and 5382insC mutations in BRCA1 and the 6174delT mutation in BRCA2 occurring in Ashkenazi Jews at a carrier rate of 2%.[7] Although no more likely to develop ovarian cancer than a non-carrier, if an Ashkenazi woman develops ovarian cancer, it is far more likely to be genetic, rather than sporadic. Consequently, if a woman of Ashkenazi Jewish descent develops ovarian cancer, there is a 40% chance she carries a mutation in one of these two genes.[8] The implications for her first-degree relatives (mother, sisters, daughters) are that they have a 20% risk for being gene carriers (given autosomal dominant transmission). Therefore, a Jewish woman needs only one first-degree relative with ovarian cancer to be considered for further genetic counseling.[9]

HNPCC is defined by the 3-2-1 rule, the so-called modified Amsterdam criteria: three affected individuals with either colorectal or ovarian cancer in two successive generations with at least one individual who developed cancer under the age of 50 years. Women with documented HNPCC have a 70% lifetime risk of developing endometrial cancer and at least an 11% lifetime risk of ovarian cancer. Testing for mutation in mismatch repair genes can be performed on peripheral leukocytes. Alternatively, the primary tumor from affected individuals can be assessed for the presence of microsatellite instability, a consequence of defective mismatch repair.[10]

From a practical standpoint, identifying women at risk for ovarian cancer can be achieved with attention to four familial risk factors, including age of onset, number of family members affected, ethnicity (Ashkenazi Jewish descent) and breast cancer in males (Table 25.1).[11,12] Additional web-based resources are also available.[12–15]

Table 25.1 *Parameters for assigning an increased risk for ovarian cancer*[11]

1 Personal or family history of breast cancer before age 50 or ovarian cancer at any age
2 Two or more primary diagnoses of breast and/or ovarian cancer
3 Ashkenazi Jewish descent with a personal or family history of breast cancer before age 50 or ovarian cancer at any age
4 Familial history of male breast cancer

OTHER RISK FACTORS FOR OVARIAN CANCER

Dietary factors

Obesity has recently been reported to be associated with an increased risk of ovarian cancer mortality. There may also be an increased risk in women eating a diet high in saturated fat and low in vegetable fiber. In 1989, the observation that Swedes had both a high risk of ovarian cancer and the highest per capita dairy consumption in the world led some investigators to postulate a relationship between lactose consumption and ovarian cancer risk. Specifically, ovarian cancer cases were more likely to have high levels of galactose, a component sugar of the disaccharide lactose and a known oocyte toxin, than matched controls.[16] This observation, however, has been inconsistent. Therefore no specific dietary strategy for ovarian cancer risk reduction can be recommended.

Talc exposure

Talc placed on the perineum may enter the vagina and ascend the upper genital tract. Structurally similar to asbestos, there is theoretical concern that talc may potentially increase ovarian cancer risk. In addition, women who undergo tubal sterilization procedures or hysterectomy have a lower risk of ovarian cancer, supporting the ascending carcinogen hypothesis. Multiple case-control studies have shown a small but consistent increased risk (OR = 1.3, 95% CI 1.1–1.6).[17] The risk appears to be time- and dose-dependent with greater risk associated with more frequent application of perineal talc over a long duration. Given the widespread availability and quality of cornstarch-based dusting powders, the practice of applying genuine talc to the perineum should be discouraged.

Infertility drugs

One of the most difficult issues to study is the association of infertility drugs and the risk of ovarian cancer. It is known, for example, that unexplained infertility is an independent risk factor for the development of ovarian cancer. One retrospective study claimed an association between prolonged clomiphene exposure and an increased risk of ovarian cancer. This study, however, was not restricted to invasive epithelial ovarian cancers but also included granulosa cell tumors.[18] These estrogen-secreting neoplasms of stromal origin may contribute to infertility directly by disrupting normal follicular maturation and the menstrual cycle.

There are, however, a number of studies, including a large collaborative analysis of 12 case-control studies that have reported an association between fertility drugs and invasive epithelial ovarian cancer.[19] In addition, many of the theoretical models of epithelial ovarian cancer pathogenesis implicate both incessant ovulation and high gonadotropin levels as important steps in malignant transformation of ovarian epithelium. Oral contraceptives which reduce ovulatory events and moderate gonadotropin levels are associated with a consistent and significant protective effect. It therefore seems prudent, in the absence of convincing data, to use fertility medication only when absolutely indicated, at the lowest effective dose and for the shortest duration possible without compromising successful fertility treatment. Prior exposure to these agents should not be considered an indication for increased surveillance or prophylactic surgery.

Hormone replacement therapy

There appears to be an increased risk of ovarian cancer among women on estrogen replacement therapy (ERT). When compared with non-users, users of ERT had a relative risk of ovarian cancer of 2.2 (95% CI 1.53–3.17).[20] This risk increased with the duration of use. Long-term users, defined as at least 20 years of ERT use, had a relative risk of 3.2 (95% CI 1.7–5.7).[21] Although some studies suggest a protective effect of combination replacement regimens including both estrogen and progesterone this observation has not been confirmed. Based upon these observations, long-term users of ERT should consider an increased risk of developing ovarian cancer as a factor in whether or not to initiate or continue ERT.

Factors reducing risk (Table 25.2)[22,23]

ORAL CONTRACEPTIVES

Oral contraceptive pills (OCPs) significantly reduce the risk of developing ovarian cancer. A number of studies have demonstrated a 10% per year risk reduction up to

Table 25.2 Preventive strategies for ovarian cancer[22,23]

Preventive method	Odds ratio
Oral contraceptives	0.11–0.80
Tubal ligation	0.33–0.72
Prophylactic oophorectomy[a]	0.15[b]

[a]For high-risk women; [b]expressed as hazard ratio.

5–7 years of use.[24] This effect seems to persist for at least 10 years after OCPs are discontinued. This protective effect has also been observed in patients known to be carriers of the BRCA1 and BRCA2 genes and is the basis for recommending OCPs as a chemoprophylactic agent in known carriers who wish to retain their fertility.[25] There has recently been some controversy about the protective effects of OCPs in BRCA patients. An Israeli population-based study of OCPs and ovarian cancer demonstrated a protective effect of pregnancy but not of OCPs. It is unclear why the Israeli data are inconsistent with prior published reports.[26]

TUBAL LIGATION

Tubal ligation reduces risk by more than half and may be effective in subsets of women with BRCA mutations and family history of ovarian cancer.[27,28] The mechanism by which this procedure reduces risk is unknown, but the popular theory is the transfer of growth factors or carcinogens is interrupted.

PROPHYLACTIC SURGERY

Prophylactic surgery may reduce, but not completely eliminate, the risk of ovarian cancer in high-risk individuals. Bilateral salpingo-oophorectomy (BSO) in BRCA carriers reduces ovarian cancer risk by over 90% and breast cancer risk by more than 50%.[22,29] The operation should be reserved for women with known mutations in BRCA 1 or 2, or who have a family history consistent with one of the genetic syndromes associated with ovarian cancer and should include an evaluation by an genetic counselor.[23] The addition of hysterectomy does not appear to increase the efficacy of the operation and should be performed only for concurrent gynecologic indications or if the patient has HNPCC. Patients should be informed that prophylactic surgery does not protect them against the subsequent development of papillary serous carcinoma of the peritoneum. They should also be warned that about 7% of prophylactic operations detect occult ovarian or tubal carcinoma and that these lesions may not be appreciated until final pathology reports are available.[30] Pathologists should be instructed to submit the entire specimen for sectioning, so as to reduce the risk of missing a microscopic occult malignancy. Finally, the patient should be prepared for the consequences of surgical menopause.

Screening for ovarian cancer

There are two obvious reasons for ovarian cancer screening. The first is that tumors arising in the ovary begin as true stage I (A or B) tumors and early detection will predate de-differentiation or extra-ovarian spread. The second is that (at least theoretically) small neoplasms originating within the tubal mucosa or the ovarian surface epithelium that are detected when the tumor burden is low are more amenable to treatment. Five-year survival rates for stage IA ovarian carcinoma approach 90%.[1] Limited data suggest that some occult neoplasms detected during prophylactic (salpingo)tubo-oophorectomy are curable. Data in support of the latter are from the prophylactic salpingo-oophorectomy studies in which removal of microscopic tumor is associated with prolonged disease-free intervals in some. In one study, 5-year cancer-free rates for BRCA-1 and BRCA-2 mutation carriers were 96% and 69% for those with prophylactic oophorectomy versus intensive surveillance. Three stage I tumors were diagnosed in the former group at the time of surgery.[31] Colgan implied that similar benefits might be obtained in the prevention of carcinomas that might arise from the fallopian tube.[32] Favorable short-term outcomes in small studies raise the prospect that removal of early disease will enhance survival.[33] However, some of these patients have positive peritoneal fluid cytology, indicating early dissemination of malignant cells presumably came from occult tubal or ovarian primary neoplasms.[34,35]

PELVIC EXAMINATION

Pelvic examination is a central component of gynecologic care and permits the evaluation of potential abnormalities throughout the reproductive tract. However, the sensitivity of pelvic exam for a tumor of 6×4 cm is estimated at only 67%. A 15-year study of pelvic exam alone uncovered only one ovarian cancer in over 18 000 exams of 1319 women.[1,36]

BIOMARKERS (Table 25.3)[1,36–40]

CA125 is a high molecular weight glycoprotein that is elevated above 35 IU/ml in 85% of all epithelial carcinomas but in only 50% of women with stage I disease.[1] Moreover, CA125 elevations are associated with a range of other intra-abdominal disorders. By virtue of its relatively lower sensitivity and specificity, CA125 is not by itself a credible marker for population screening.

Zhang et al. evaluated a combination of four markers, including CA125II, CA72-4, CA15-3 and lipid-associated sialic acid and analyzed the data using an artificial neural network (ANN). They first standardized their classifier with an established dataset of benign and malignant tumors, followed by an analysis of a second dataset. Compared with CA125 alone, this approach produced a specificity of 87.5% (*vs* 68.4%) and sensitivity of 79.0% (*vs* 82.4%) in distinguishing ovarian cancer from other disorders. The authors subsequently prospectively screened healthy women, producing a specificity of 100.0% compared with 94.8% CA125II alone.[41] In a recent study evaluating prostasin and CA125, Mok et al. demonstrated a combined sensitivity and specificity of 92 and 94%, respectively.[37] Other markers, such as osteopontin, are currently being evaluated.[42]

Despite the relatively high sensitivity and specificities of some markers under evaluation, it is important to emphasize that a test with a 99% specificity will still necessitate as many as 25 laparotomies to uncover one case of cancer.[1]

A variety of new technologies are emerging in the detection of ovarian cancer markers, including proteomic analysis, protein microarrays and assays targeting unique spectrographic signatures (SELDI-TOF). These are in the process of development and appear promising. However, they must meet the same criteria as the above markers to fulfill expectations for screening. An additional benefit will be the identification of tumor antigens or products that can be used as therapeutic targets.[43,44]

ULTRASOUND AND OTHER IMAGING TECHNIQUES (Table 25.4)[45–47]

There is mounting evidence that transvaginal sonography (TVS) will improve early detection of ovarian cancer and possibly influence mortality. Van Nagell et al. scored ovaries as abnormal if they exceeded 10 and 20 cubic cm from post- and premenopausal women, respectively. In a study of 8500 women who underwent TVS, 121 were abnormal and underwent surgery. A total of 57 had serous cystadenomas and eight had ovarian cancers, six of which were stage IA. Only one each had an enlarged ovary by palpation or an elevated CA125.[47] The implication from studies of this type is that TVS will downstage a proportion of tumors and permit improved survival.[39] Despite the above results, this group found that TVS had a sensitivity of 98.7, but a positive predictive value (PPV) of only 6.8%. Partridge and Barnes recently summarized five studies of 11 283 women, noting a PPV of only 3.1% for ovarian cancer.[1]

In a study of TVS encompassing[42] 113 screening years, van Nagell et al. defined an ovarian volume exceeding 10 cm in postmenopausal women or 20 cm in premenopausal women, or papillary or complex architecture as abnormal. Some 17 of 180 patients with persisting TVS abnormalities who underwent exploratory laparoscopy or laparotomy had cancer, 11 of which were stage I. Eight of the 11 did not have a palpable mass. TVS screening in this setting had a PPV of 9.4% with a negative

---

Table 25.3 Sensitivity and specificity of ovarian cancer screening methods

Method	Sensitivity	Specificity	PPV	Reference
Theoretical ideal	–	99.0%	4.0%	(1)
Pelvic examination	67%	–	–	(36)
CA125	68.4%	82.4%	–	(37)
4 markers	79.5%	87.5%	–	(37)
TVS[a]	81.0	98.5	9.4%	(38)
TVS	98.7	–	6.8	(39)
Ultrasound[b]	–	95.8%	3.1	(40)

[a]Persistently abnormal TVS; [b]summary of five studies.

Table 25.4 Controlled trial of screening for ovarian cancer with CA125 and ultrasound[45]

Group	Control	Screened
Number	10 958	10 977
Screening		TVS + CA125
Referral		CA125 >30 U/ml; ovary vol. >8.8 ml
Raised CA125 (no)		458
Vol. >8.8 ml		29
Negative laparotomy		23
Ovarian cancers		6
Pos. pred. value		20.7
Total cancers (7 years)	20	17
Median survival (months)	41.8	72.9 (*P* <0.01)
Deaths	18	9 (RR = 2.0)

predictive value of 99.97%. When non-epithelial tumors were excluded, the survival of ovarian cancer patients in the annually screened population was 92.9% at 2 years and 83.6% at 5 years. The authors cautioned that while the improved detection and reduced mortality were associated with screening, this benefit did not apply to women whose cancers occurred in the setting of a normal ovarian volume.[47]

ULTRASOUND AND BIOMARKERS

Einhorn et al. reported on a long-term follow-up study of women who underwent screening for ovarian cancer using a combination of CA125 and ultrasound. Based on cancer registry data, 20 ovarian cancer patients were diagnosed subsequent to the screening study and were compared with those that emerged in an unscreened population. Twelve of the 20 died of their disease and six were disease free. Median survivals for screened and unscreened individuals were 100 and 20 months, respectively, which was significant at $P = 0.059$. However, overall survival was not. The authors concluded that larger and longer-term studies were needed to establish the impact of screening on ovarian cancer mortality.[38] Jacobs et al. evaluated over 20 000 cases and controls, combining ultrasound (volume exceeding 8.8 ml) and elevated CA125 levels to guide therapy. This approach yielded a PPV of over 20% for malignancy, improved median survival and a modest reduction in risk of death.[45] However, the large-scale impact of this approach on the overall death rate due to ovarian cancer cannot be ascertained.

Presenting signs and symptoms

Clinical presentations with borderline early and advanced cancer will vary. Webb et al. examined patients in these groups and noted 16, 7 and 4% of patients with borderline disease, early and advanced ovarian cancer were symptom free. Abdominal pain 44% and swelling 39% were the most common symptoms as opposed to abdominal mass and gynecologic symptoms (12% each). Gastrointestinal problems and malaise were more common in advanced disease.[48]

Ultrasound evaluation and risk (malignancy) assessment

In patients with a suspected pelvic mass, TVS, with or without CA125 assessments, is of considerable value in segregating low- versus high-risk patients and can be used as a guide to intervention (Figs 25.1, 25.2).[1,49] The presence of a mass with conspicuous calcium supports the diagnosis of teratoma. In contrast, any solid tumor is of concern. Scoring systems have been proposed by a number investigators, and depend on specific characteristics of tumors that predict risk.

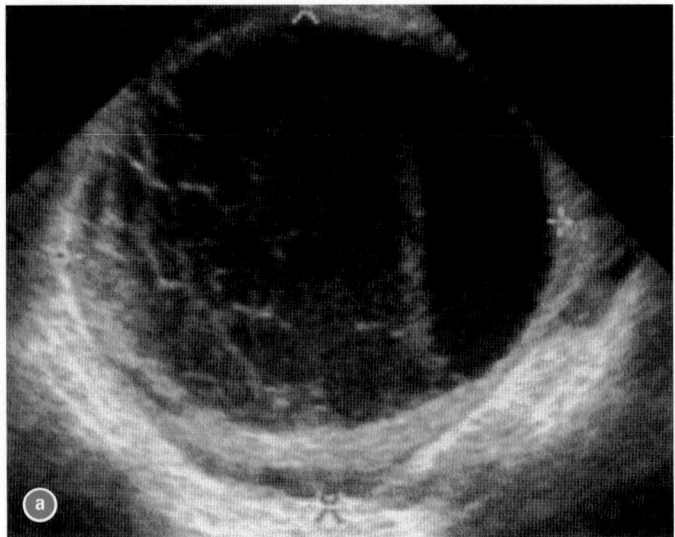
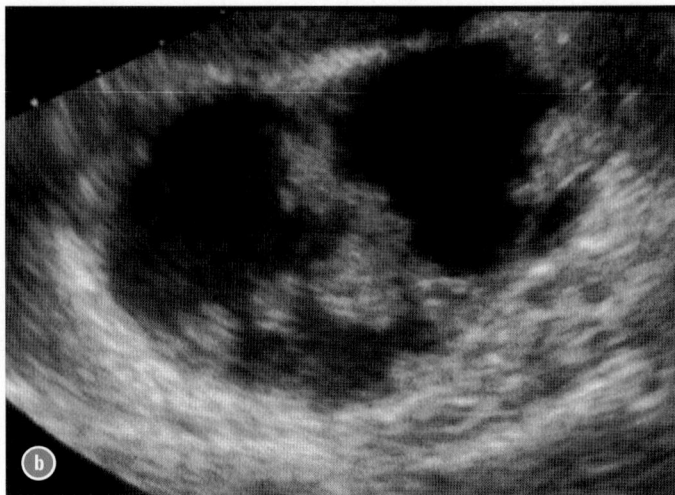

Fig. 25.1 Ultrasound evaluation of benign and malignant ovarian cysts. (a) Hemorrhagic smooth-walled cyst. (b) Ovarian cancer with irregular wall thickness, lining surface and septation. (Courtesy of Beryl Bennaceraf, Boston, Massachusetts.)

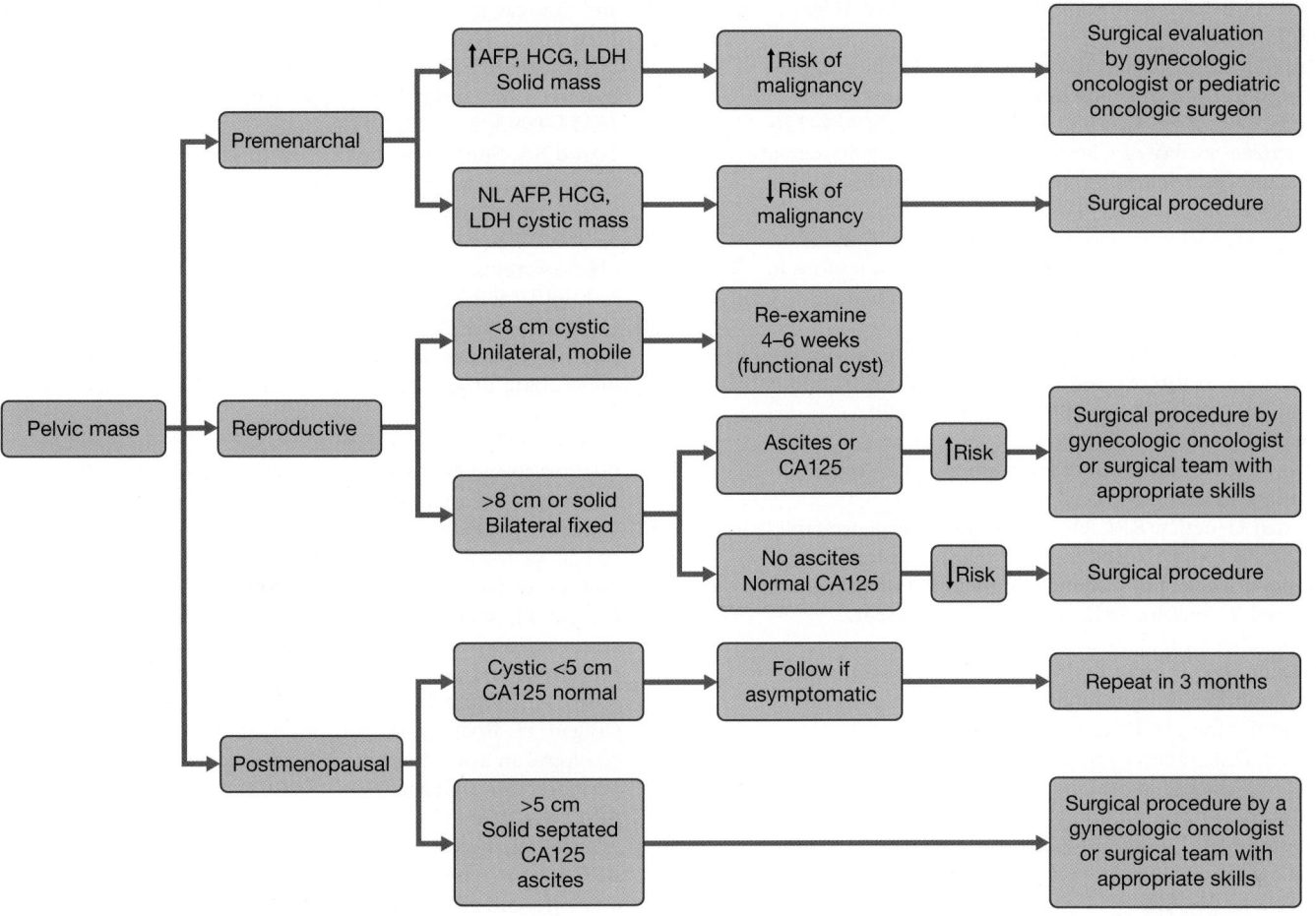

Fig. 25.2 Algorithm for evaluating the patient with a suspected ovarian mass. (From Partridge and Barnes, copyright 1999 Lippincott, Williams and Wilkins, with permission.)[1]

Certain groups can be identified with a strikingly low risk. Bailey et al. showed that none of unilocular cysts under 10 cm in diameter proved to be malignant.[50] Half resolved spontaneously; many of the rest were cystadenomas. In contrast, complex cysts had a similar resolution rate but seven out of 114 proved to be malignant.[50] Overall, ovarian volume is expected to decrease with age.[51] In a study of over 3200 unilocular cysts, nearly 70% resolved spontaneously. Of the remainder, 16.5 (of the total) developed septation, 5.8% a solid area and 6.8% persisted as a unilocular lesion. Of 27 cancers emerging in the persistent group, 10 were associated with the unilocular lesions, underscoring the need to follow all patients with a persistent ovarian lesion.[52]

References

1 Partridge EE, Barnes MN. Epithelial ovarian cancer: prevention, diagnosis, and treatment. CA Cancer J Clin 1999; 49(5):297–320.

2 American Cancer Society. Cancer facts and figures 2003. Atlanta, GA: American Cancer Society; 2003.

3 Trimble EL, Karlan BY, Lagasse LD, et al. Diagnosing the correct ovarian cancer syndrome. Obstet Gynecol 1991; 78(6):1023–1026.

4 Vasen HFA, Watson P, Mecklin J-P. Lynch HT, and the ICG-HNPCC. New clinical criteria for hereditary nonpolyposis colon cancer (HNPCC, Lynch Syndrome): proposed by the International Collaborative Group on HNPCC. Gastroenterology 1999; 116:1453–1456.

5 Easton DF, Ford D, Bishop DT. Breast and ovarian cancer incidence in BRCA1-mutation carriers. Breast Cancer Linkage Consortium. Am J Hum Genet 1995; 56(1):265–271.

6 Antoniou A, Pharoah PD, Narod S, et al. Average risks of breast and ovarian cancer associated with BRCA1 or BRCA2 mutations detected in case series unselected for family history: a combined analysis of 22 studies. Am J Hum Genet 2003; 72(5):1117–1130.

7 Struewing JP, Hartge P, Wacholder S, et al. The risk of cancer associated with specific mutations of BRCA1 and BRCA2 among Ashkenazi Jews. N Engl J Med 1997; 336(20):1401–1408.

8 Lu K, Muto MG, Cramer DW, et al. Prevalence of BRCA mutations among women of Ashkenazi Jewish descent

with epithelial ovarian cancer. Obstet Gynecol 1999; 93(1):34–37.

9 Parent ME, Ghadirian P, Lacroix A, et al. The reliability of recollections of family history: implications for the medical provider. J Cancer Educ 1997; 12(2):114–120.

10 American Society of Clinical Oncology Policy Statement Update. Genetic testing for cancer susceptibility. J Clin Oncol 2003; 21(12):1–10.

11 Frank TS, Deffenbaugh AM, Reid JE, et al. Clinical characteristics of individuals with germline mutations in BRCA1 and BRCA2: analysis of 10,000 individuals. J Clin Oncol 2002; 20(6):1480–1490.

12 Frank TS. Clinical characteristics of individuals with germline mutations in BRCA1 and BRCA2: analysis of 10,000 individuals. Clin Oncol 2002; 20:1480–1490.

13 Ovarian Cancer (PDQ). Prevention of Ovarian Cancer. http://www.cancer.gov/cancerinfo/pdq/prevention/ovarian/healthprofessional

14 Myriad Genetics. BRCA1/2 mutation prevalence tables. http://www.myriadtests.com/provider/mutprevo.htm

15 National Society of Genetic Counselors. Locate a genetic counselor specializing in cancer risk assessment. http://www.nsgc.org/resourcelink.asp

16 Cramer DW, Harlow BL, Willett WC, et al. Galactose consumption and metabolism in relation to the risk of ovarian cancer. Lancet 1989; 2(8654):66–71.

17 Gertig DM, Hunter DJ, Cramer DW, et al. Prospective study of talc use and ovarian cancer. J Natl Cancer Inst 2000; 92(3):249–252.

18 Rossing MA, Daling JR, Weiss NS, et al. Ovarian tumors in a cohort of infertile women. N Engl J Med 1994; 331(12):771–776.

19 Whittemore AS, Harris R, Itnyre J. Characteristics relating to ovarian cancer risk: collaborative analysis of 12 US case studies II. Invasive epithelial cancers in white women. Collaborative Ovarian Cancer Group. Am J Epidemiol 1992; 136(10):1184–1203.

20 Rodriguez C, Patel AV, Calle EE, et al. Estrogen replacement therapy and ovarian cancer mortality in a large prospective study of US women. JAMA 2001; 285(11):1460–1465.

21 Lacey JV Jr, Mink PJ, Jubin JH, et al. Menopausal hormone replacement therapy and risk of ovarian cancer. JAMA 2002; 288(3):334–341.

22 Kauff ND, Satagopan JM, Robson ME, et al. Risk-reducing salpingo-oophorectomy in women with a BRCA1 or BRCA2 mutation. N Engl J Med 2002; 346(1609):1609–1615.

23 Barnes MN, Grizzle WE, Grubbs CJ, Partridge EE. Paradigms for primary prevention of ovarian carcinoma. CA Cancer J Clin 2002;. 52(4):216–225.

24 The Cancer and Steroid Hormone Study of the Centers for Disease Control and the National Institute of Child Health and Human Development. The reduction in risk of ovarian cancer associated with oral contraceptive use. N Engl J Med 1987; 316(11):650–655.

25 Narod SA, Risch H, Moslehi R, et al. Oral contraceptives and the risk of hereditary ovarian cancer. Hered Ovarian Cancer Study Group. N Engl J Med 1998; 339(7):424–428.

26 Modan B, Hartge P, Hirsh-Yechezkel G, et al. Parity, oral contraceptives and the risk of ovarian cancer among carriers and non-carriers of a BRCA1 or BRCA2 mutation. N Engl J Med 2001; 345(4):235–240.

27 Hankinson SE, Hunter DJ, Colditz GA, et al. Tubal ligation, hysterectomy, and risk of ovarian cancer. A prospective study. JAMA 1993; 270(23):2813–2818.

28 Narod SA, Sun P, Ghadirian P, et al. Tubal ligation and risk of ovarian cancer in carriers of BRCA1 or BRCA2 mutations: a case-control study. Lancet 2001; 357(9267):1467–1470.

29 Rebbeck TR, Lynch HT, Neuhausen SL, et al. Prophylactic oophorectomy in carriers of BRCA1 or BRCA2 mutations. N Engl J Med 2002; 346:1616–1622.

30 Lu KH, Garber JE, Cramer DW, et al. Occult ovarian tumors in women with BRCA1 or BRCA2 mutations undergoing prophylactic oophorectomy. J Clin Oncol 2000; 18:2728.

31 Olopade OI, Artioli G. Efficacy of risk-reducing salpingo-oophorectomy in women with BRCA-1 and BRCA-2 mutations. Breast J. 2004; 10(Suppl)(1):S5–S9.

32 Colgan TJ. Challenges in the early diagnosis and staging of Fallopian-tube carcinomas associated with BRCA mutations. Int J Gynecol Pathol 2003; 22(2):109–120.

33 Colgan TJ, Murphy J, Cole DE, Narod S, Rosen B. Occult carcinoma in prophylactic oophorectomy specimens: prevalence and association with BRCA germline mutation status. Am J Surg Pathol 2001; 25(10):1283–1289.

34 Colgan TJ, Boerner SL, Murphy J, et al. Peritoneal lavage cytology: an assessment of its value during prophylactic oophorectomy. Gynecol Oncol 2002; 85(3):397–403.

35 Agoff SN, Mendelin JE, Grieco VS, Garcia RL. Unexpected gynecologic neoplasms in patients with proven or suspected BRCA-1 or -2 mutations: implications for gross examination, cytology, and clinical follow-up. Am J Surg Pathol 2002; 26(2):171–178.

36 McFarlane, D, Sturgis MD, Fetterman FC. Results of an experience in the control of cancer of the female pelvic organs. A report of a 15 year research. Am J Obstet Gynecol 1956; 69:294–301.

37 Mok SC, Chao J, Skates S, et al. Prostasin, a potential serum marker for ovarian cancer: identification through microarray technology. J Natl Cancer Inst 2001; 93(19):1458–1464.

38 Einhorn N, Bast R, Knapp R, et al. Long-term follow-up of the Stockholm screening study on ovarian cancer. Gynecol Oncol 2000; 79(3):466–470.

39 van Nagell JR Jr, Gallion HH, Pavlik EJ, DePriest PD. Ovarian cancer screening. Cancer 1995; 76(10):2086–2091.

40 Grover S, Quinn MA, Weideman P, et al. Screening for ovarian cancer using serum CA125 and vaginal examination: report on 2550 females. Int J Gynecol Cancer 1995; 5(4):291–295.

41 Zhang Z, Barnhill SD, Zhang H, et al. Combination of multiple serum markers using an artificial neural network to improve specificity in discriminating malignant from benign pelvic masses. Gynecol Oncol 1999; 73(1):56–61.

42 Kim JH, Skates SJ, Uede T, et al. Osteopontin as a potential diagnostic biomarker for ovarian cancer. JAMA 2002; 287(13):1671–1679.

43 Alexe G, Alexe S, Liotta LA, et al. Ovarian cancer detection by logical analysis of proteomic data. Proteomics 2004; 4(3):766–783.

44 Wulfkuhle JD, Aquino JA, Calvert VS, et al. Signal pathway profiling of ovarian cancer from human tissue specimens

using reverse-phase protein microarrays. Proteomics 2003; 3(11):2085–2090.

45 Jacobs IJ, Skates SJ, MacDonald N, et al. Screening for ovarian cancer: a pilot randomised controlled trial. Lancet 1999; 353(9160):1207–1210.

46 Karlan BY, Platt LD. Ovarian cancer screening. The role of ultrasound in early detection. Cancer 1995; 76(10):2011–2015.

47 Nagell JR Jr, DePriest PD, Reedy MB, et al. The efficacy of transvaginal sonographic screening in asymptomatic women at risk for ovarian cancer. Gynecol Oncol 2000; 77(3):350–356.

48 Webb PM, Purdie DM, Grover S, et al. Symptoms and diagnosis of borderline, early and advanced epithelial ovarian cancer. Gynecol Oncol 2004; 92(1):232–239.

49 Benjapibal M, Sunsaneevitayakul P, Phatihattakorn C, et al. Sonographic morphological pattern in the pre-operative prediction of ovarian masses. J Med Assoc Thai 2003; 86(4):332–337.

50 Bailey CL, Ueland FR, Land GL, et al. The malignant potential of small cystic ovarian tumors in women over 50 years of age. Gynecol Oncol 1998; 69(1):3–7.

51 Pavlik EJ, DePriest PD, Gallion HH, et al. Ovarian volume related to age. Gynecol Oncol 2000; 77(3):410–412.

52 Modesitt SC, Pavlik EJ, Ueland FR, et al. Risk of malignancy in unilocular ovarian cystic tumors less than 10 centimeters in diameter. Obstet Gynecol 2003; 102(3):594–599.

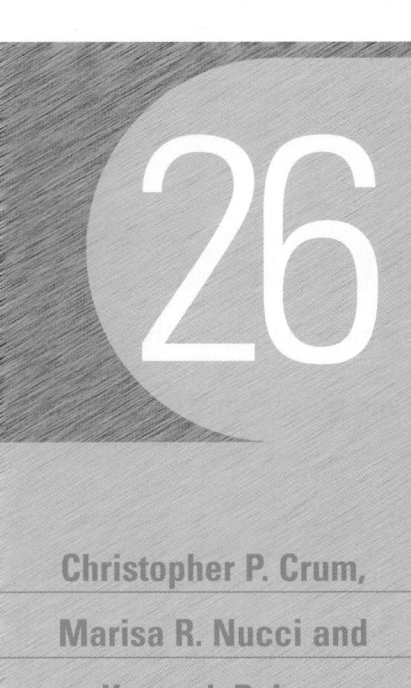

26

Intraoperative evaluation of ovarian tumors

Christopher P. Crum,

Marisa R. Nucci and

Kenneth R. Lee

Introduction

General frequencies of ovarian tumors

Clinical history

The age of the patient
Unilateral versus bilateral
Is there disease elsewhere?

Gross examination

Ovarian tumor weight
Ovarian enlargement with
 preservation of ovarian
 architecture
Cystic ovarian masses
Tumors with a dominant solid
 component
Yellow tumors
Tumors with somatic (hair, etc.)
 elements

Intraoperative frozen section evaluation

Intraoperative gross and microscopic pitfalls

Misclassification based on
 confusing gross appearance
Misclassification due to similarities
 in cell appearance or structure
Pitfalls encountered due to an
 under-appreciation of the
 limitations of intraoperative
 gross evaluation and/or
 limitations in sampling

Summary

Introduction

Once an ovarian mass has been identified and characterized by noninvasive imaging, the next step in management is usually surgery. The critical intermediate between surgery and final diagnosis and one that is particularly germane to the proper clinical management of ovarian masses, is the intraoperative pathology consultation. This process can be subdivided into four components, including: (1) knowledge of the general frequencies of ovarian tumors, (2) relevant clinical history, (3) gross examination and (4) histologic assessment. The reader is forewarned that the gross assessment of a tumor is a guide to sampling, not a diagnostic exercise per se. The conclusion of this chapter will summarize our experience with errors that may occur during both gross and microscopic intraoperative examination of the ovaries.

We emphasize that the figures and percentages discussed below apply to intraoperative evaluation. Estimates of the relative frequency of ovarian pathology depend heavily on whether they are derived from ultrasound, intraoperative and autopsy material.[1] The following addresses the procedures for intraoperative evaluation of ovarian neoplasia stressing in particular the pitfalls that might be encountered. Many of these images have been selected from succeeding chapters.

General frequencies of ovarian tumors

The frequencies with which benign and malignant ovarian tumors are encountered are given in Tables 26.1 and 26.2.[2] Overall, 90% of benign tumors are either benign cystic teratomas, or serous and mucinous cystadenomas (Table 26.1).[2,3] Nearly 85% of malignant tumors are epithelial (Table 26.2).[4]

Clinical history

Three important facts must be known before examining the ovary: the age of the patient; unilateral or bilateral distribution; and the presence (or absence) of disease elsewhere.

THE AGE OF THE PATIENT

Excluding endometriotic and other non-neoplastic cysts, the proportion of ovarian tumors that are malignant is highly age dependent, ranging from a low of 2.1% in the third decade to nearly 50% in the seventh (Table 26.3).[2]

Tumors in women under age 30

The following primary tumors and tumor-like masses of the ovary are found in women under age 30 (Tables 26.4, 26.5):

Table 26.1 Frequency of benign and borderline ovarian tumors (total 681)[2]

Tumor	(%)
Benign cystic teratoma	55.4
Serous cystadenoma	24.0
Mucinous cystadenoma	11.0
Fibroma thecoma	3.7
Borderline serous	2.8
Borderline mucinous	1.6
Brenner tumor	1.0
Struma	0.4
Borderline endometrioid	0.1

Table 26.2 Frequency of malignant ovarian tumors (total 180)[2]

Tumor	(%)
Serous or mixed epithelial carcinomas	47.2
Undifferentiated carcinomas	13.8
Endometrioid	11.0
Mucinous carcinoma	9.4
Sex-cord/stromal	7.2
Clear cell carcinomas	3.8
Germ cell	6.6

Table 26.3 Proportion of ovarian tumors that are malignant as a function of age (excludes endometriotic and benign cysts)[2]

Age range	Malignant (%)
<20	8.1
20–29	2.1
30–39	14.0
40–49	35.1
50–59	46.2
60–69	49.4
70+	29.2

Table 26.4 *Distribution of ovarian neoplasms by age*[2]

Tumor	Percentage of tumor category in each age group						
	<20	20–29	30–39	40–49	50–59	60–69	70+
Benign							
Serous	20	15	17	43	46	59	53
Mucinous	11	11	12	8	14	11	24
Cystic teratoma	70	72	67	43	21	16	0
Fibroma-thecoma	0	1	4	3	17	11	12
Borderline							
Serous	–	86	67	38	50	67	
Mucinous	–	14	33	50	50	33	
Endometrioid	–	0	0	13	0	0	
Malignant							
Serous/mixed/undifferentiated	0	17	58	66	69	64	61
Mucinous	0	8	4	9	6	21	9
Endomat/clear cell	0	8	8	18	19	16	15
Sex-cord/stromal	20	33	21	4	2	0	7
Germ cell	80	33	8	2	2	0	7

Table 26.5 *Histologic type by age, ovarian cancers, 1988 and 1993*[4]

Histologic type	Age at diagnosis (years)		
	Under age 30	Age 30–64	Age 65+
Borderline epith.	28.3	12.3	4.4
Malignant epith.	33.4	83.7	92.2
Sex-cord/stroma	2.3	1.4	0.8
Germ cell	33.6	1.6	0.3
Other soft tissue	0.9	0.3	0.3
Lymphoma	1.1	0.1	0.2
Unclassified	0.4	0.6	1.8

1 More common:
- *Mature cystic teratoma.* This is the most common ovarian tumor, comprising 70% of benign tumors in this age group.[2]
- *Functional cysts.* Functional (follicle) cysts are the most common and do not usually necessitate laparotomy and are less likely to come to frozen section evaluation.[5]
- *Benign or borderline epithelial tumors.* These comprise the other 30% of benign tumors in young women.[2]

2 Less common:
- *Malignant germ cell tumors.* These comprise 80% of malignant tumors in the under 20 age group and one-third in the 20–29 age group.
- *Juvenile granulosa cell and Sertoli–Leydig cell tumors.* This group comprises 20 and 33% of malignancies in the above groups, respectively.
- *Malignant epithelial tumors* comprise the other third of malignancies in this age group.[2]

- *Small cell carcinoma of the hypercalcemic type.* This is a rare tumor, but predominates in women under age 30.[6]

It should be stressed that while uncommon, epithelial, sex-cord stromal and germ cell tumors each comprise a significant minority of the malignancies in women under age 30. In general, ovarian tumors in young women are unilateral and benign. Nowak et al. reviewed 326 patients, defining the 'reproductive age group' as between age 18 and 39. A total of 93% were benign epithelial tumors; 88% were unilateral benign cysts. Only 4.6% were malignant.[7]

Uncommon tumors in women over age 30

The following primary tumors are uncommon in women over age 30:

1 Malignant germ cell tumors, including immature teratoma, dysgerminoma, yolk sac carcinoma and embryonal carcinoma. Malignant germ cell tumors comprise only 8% of malignancies in the 30–39 age group and 2% or less beyond age 40.[2]

Benign tumors in women under age 30

The following benign tumors and tumor-like lesions are uncommon in women under age 30:

1 Brenner tumor
2 Fibroma
3 Endometriotic cyst.

Less than 10% each of Brenner tumors, fibromas and endometriotic cysts occur prior to age 30 (Table 26.6).[2,8–11]

In addition to tumors found in young women, the following tumors/conditions are seen in pregnancy.[12–14]

Table 26.6 *Age range and average age for 1019 benign ovarian lesions*[9]

Tumor type	Average age	Age range
Simple cyst(oma)	38	16–66
Serous cystadenoma	40	15–82
Benign cystic teratoma	43	13–90
Fibroma	45	23–69
Cystadenofibroma/Adenofibroma	42–45	22–75
Brenner tumor	45	29–61
Endometriotic cyst*	42	18–75

*Data on endometriotic cyst are from 73 consecutive cases recorded at Brigham and Women's Hospital (Crum CP, unpublished, 2004).

1 Theca-lutein hyperplasia of pregnancy
2 Giant follicular cyst of pregnancy (similar cysts may be seen in non-pregnant women).
3 Pregnancy luteoma.
It should be emphasized that malignancies of the ovary during pregnancy are most commonly of the epithelial type.[15] However, they are rare. In one study, less than 19/1000 ovaries inspected at Caesarean section were neoplastic and only 5/100 000 were malignant.[16]

UNILATERAL VERSUS BILATERAL (TABLE 26.7)[17]

If the tumor is bilateral it is unlikely to be:
1 Sex cord stromal tumor, excepting fibromas. Some 13% of fibromas are bilateral. Granulosa cell and Sertoli cell tumors are rarely bilateral.

Table 26.7 *Frequency of bilateral ovarian tumors*[17]

Tumor	Bilateral (%)
Mixed epithelial malignancy	41.7
Serous carcinoma	38.5
Serous borderline	33.3
Endometrioid	21.4
Serous cystoma	20.5
Mucinous carcinoma	16.7
Fibroma	12.8
Thecoma	9.1
BCT	8.7
Mucinous cystoma	4.1
Brenner (benign)	0
Clear cell	0
Mucinous borderline	0

2 Primary mucinous tumor, excepting endocervical-like (Müllerian) tumors, which are frequently associated with endometriomas. Less than 5% of intestinal mucinous tumors are bilateral. Older studies recording bilateral primary intestinal mucinous tumors may bear review to exclude metastatic disease.
3 Brenner tumors are rarely bilateral (<1%).
4 Malignant germ cell tumors are virtually always unilateral, excepting dysgerminomas (bilateral in 15%).
5 A primary (teratoma-associated) carcinoid tumor is rarely bilateral, although the opposite ovary may contain a benign cystic teratoma.[17]

Primary tumors that are frequently bilateral include:
1 Most epithelial tumors, including benign and borderline serous and endometrioid lesions; serous and endometrioid carcinomas are bilateral in 20–42% of cases.
2 Endocervical-like (Müllerian – mucinous or seromucinous) mucinous tumors (30–40%)
3 Benign cystic teratomas (15%).

Metastatic tumors are frequently bilateral, including:
1 Gastric
2 Pancreatico-biliary
3 Colonic
4 Small intestine (carcinoid)
5 Appendiceal.
Over 66% of metastatic tumors are bilateral.[18,19]

IS THERE DISEASE ELSEWHERE?

The following must be considered if a neoplasm is identified elsewhere, concurrently or by history:
1 *Uterine carcinoma.* The most common explanation for the ovarian tumor in the presence of a concurrent uterine carcinoma is separate uterine and ovarian primary neoplasms. However, this is highly dependent on histology and other factors.[20]
2 *Extensive omental involvement.* This is almost always a sign of a primary malignant ovarian neoplasm, but rarely may be due to metastases from the colon, appendix or breast.
3 *Colonic mucosal involvement.* This usually indicates a primary colon tumor. However, we have encountered several cases of serous, mucinous and endometrioid tumors with not only external colonic metastases but also extension to the colonic mucosa.

4 *History of breast carcinoma.* In most cases the tumor will be of ovarian origin, especially if large.[21]

5 *History of melanoma, lung carcinoma.* Both can metastasize to the female genital tract.[22,23]

Gross examination

Upon arrival in the frozen section suite the tumor should be measured, weighed, carefully examined externally, photographed if time permits, inked along any sectioning margins (India ink is swabbed on followed by rapid fixing in methanol) and opened. The latter should be done with care. If the tumor contains fluid, it should be described, collected and measured. Once the tumor is opened, various scenarios may be encountered, including the following.

OVARIAN TUMOR WEIGHT

The weight of the ovarian tumor will influence diagnostic outcome, both in terms of risk and sampling. Puls et al. reviewed 294 patients, sub-dividing tumors into less than 450 g, 450–1360 g and over 1360 g. Sensitivity and specificity fell from 96 and 75 to 92 and 67%, respectively, as a function of increasing tumor size. Predictably, borderline epithelial tumors, and mucinous tumors in general, were subject to the greatest disparity from frozen to permanent section interpretation, with 50% of the largest mucinous tumors originally considered benign upgraded following more extensive sampling.[24] This is discussed in greater detail later.

OVARIAN ENLARGEMENT WITH PRESERVATION OF OVARIAN ARCHITECTURE

If the ovary is enlarged but maintains its normal contour without a discrete mass displacing the parenchyma, possibilities include:

1 *Stromal hyperplasia.* This condition produces a uniform expansion of the ovarian medulla and/or cortex with a consistency that ranges from firm and rubbery to brown and soft (Fig. 26.1).

2 *Polycystic ovarian disease.* These 2–4 mm cysts are uniformly arranged in the cortex, in contrast to cortical inclusion cysts, simple cysts or cystadenomas, where the cysts are variably sized and unevenly distributed (Fig. 26.2a).

3 *Theca-lutein hyperplasia* (or its extreme variant, *hyperreactio luteinalis*) of pregnancy. Depending

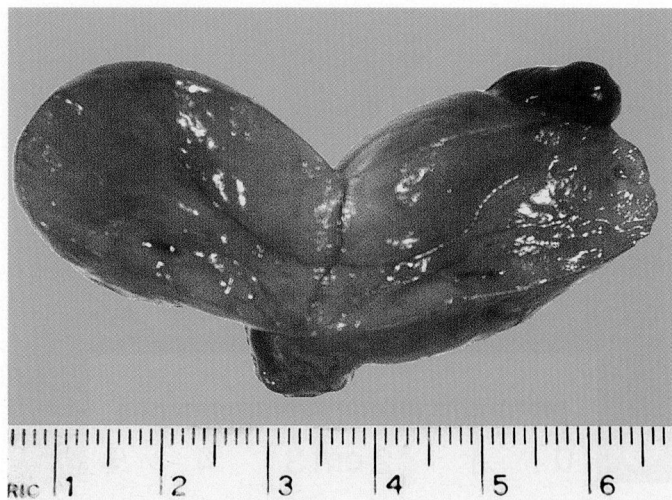

Fig. 26.1 Sectioned ovary with cortical stromal hyperplasia, showing uniform ovarian expansion.

on the size of the cystic changes preservation of ovarian architecture may or may not be conspicuous (Fig. 26.2b,c).

4 *Ovarian edema.* The ovary may be uniformly expanded and edematous (Fig. 26.3).[25]

5 *Ovarian infarction or torsion* (see below). Torsion may cause massive expansion of the ovary and tube and, depending on the degree of parenchymal preservation, the prosector may or may not be able to verify the presence of cortical structures.[26] If preserved, the ovary will contain appropriately distributed follicular and other functional components.

6 *Some infiltrating metastatic tumors,* such as lobular carcinoma of the breast and signet ring carcinomas, may uniformly expand the ovary. The gross distinction from cortical stromal hyperplasia may be difficult (Fig. 26.4a,b).

7 *Primary surface carcinomas with minimal mass.* Early serous surface carcinomas or metastatic tumors to the ovarian cortex might not efface the ovarian architecture and may be confused with adhesions or other benign conditions (Fig. 26.4c) (see Ch. 27).[27]

CYSTIC OVARIAN MASSES

Excluding polycystic ovarian disease, this category pertains to conspicuous ovarian enlargement due to one or more cystic lesions. The index of suspicion generated by an evaluation of the cystic ovarian mass parallels that following ultrasound examination, i.e. the index increases in the progression from a solitary

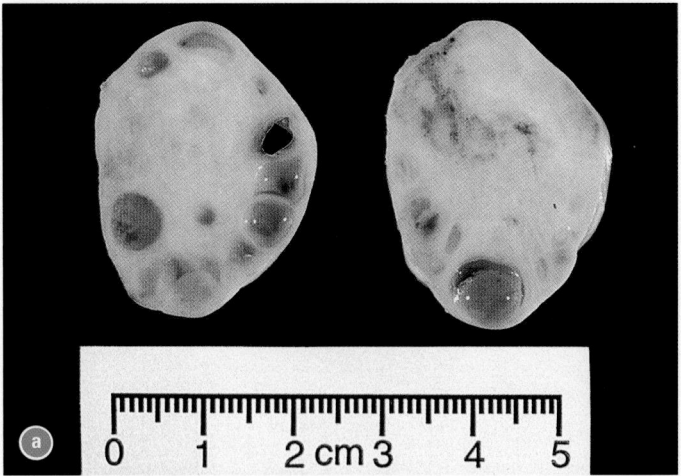

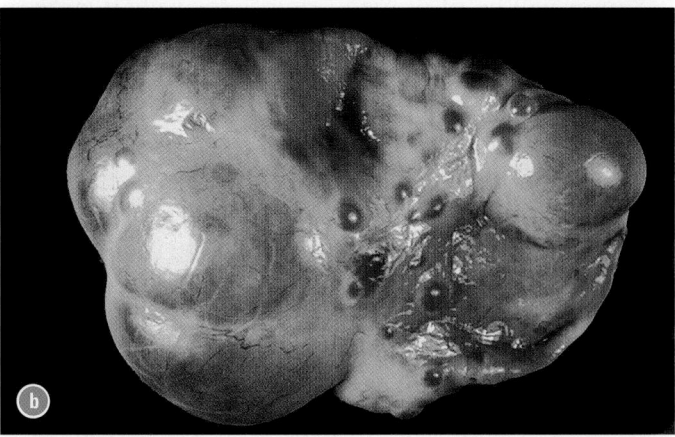

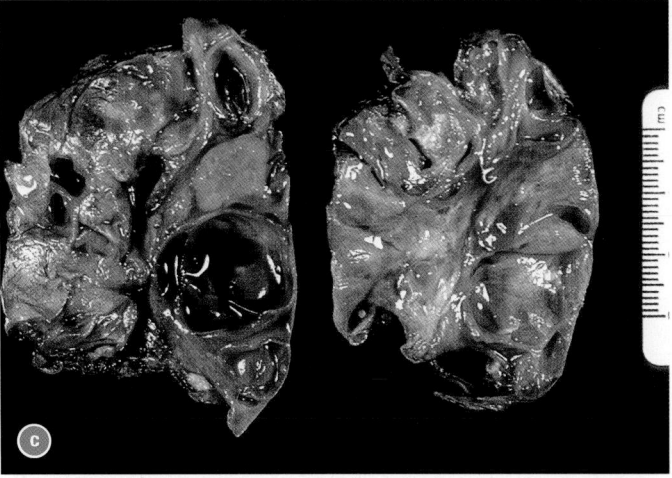

Fig. 26.2 (a) Polycystic ovaries preserve the normal ovarian cortical relationships. (b,c) Symmetrical expansion of the ovaries with multiple theca-lutein cysts associated with pregnancy. These may resemble cystadenomas but should be recognized in the setting of pregnancy.

simple cyst to a multicystic tumor, to the presence of papillary structures to solid components. In one study, completely cystic tumors were benign in over 96% of instances; in contrast, solid and cystic tumors were malignant in 69%.[28] This progression in risk as a function of increasing complexity imposes a responsibility to differentiate simple Müllerian cyst or cystadenoma, borderline tumors and ultimately malignancies.

1 Single smooth-walled, translucent cysts are typically:
- Serous cysts (or unilocular serous cystadenomas)(Fig. 26.5)
- Para-ovarian cysts or paratubal cysts (Fig. 26.6a,b)
- Hydrosalpinx (Fig. 26.6c)
- Others include follicle cysts (exceeding 3 cm). These are encountered uncommonly as a cause for laparotomy and frozen section consultation.

2 Smooth-walled hemorrhagic cysts include:
- Endometriotic cyst (Fig. 26.7a)
- Degenerated corpus luteum (Fig. 26.7b)
- Endocervical-like (sero)mucinous borderline tumor (Fig. 26.8).

Generally, we do not perform a frozen section on thin, unilocular smooth-walled cysts from women of any age. The findings of chocolate material reflecting hemorrhage merits a comment regarding possible endometrioma. Any irregularity or thickening of the cyst wall warrants frozen section.

3 If the tumor consists of a unilocular cyst with an irregular or thickened lining the possibilities include:
- Endometriotic cysts with xanthoma cells and organizing hemorrhage (Fig. 26.9)
- Decidualized endometriotic cysts (Fig. 26.10)
- Mullerian seromucinous tumors arising in endometriosis (Fig. 26.8)
- Rarely, poorly-differentiated carcinomas.

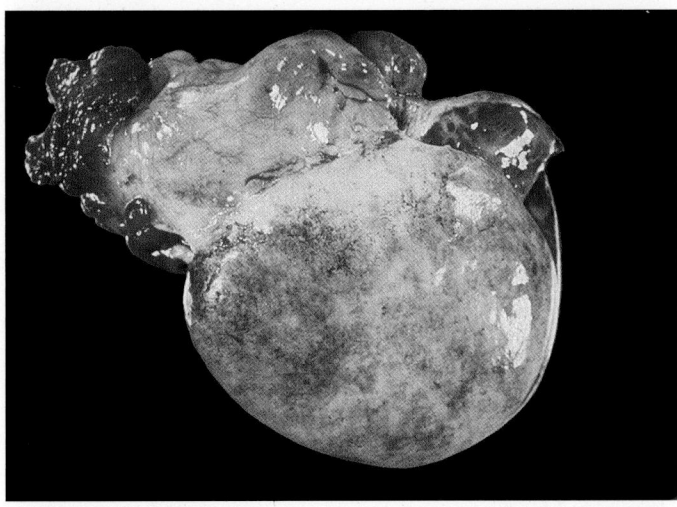

Fig. 26.3 Ovarian edema, with uniform expansion of the ovary.

4 If the cyst lining contains a protrusion or papillary excrescences, consider:
  - Serous or mucinous borderline tumor (Fig. 26.11)
  - Proliferative Brenner tumor (rare, see Ch. 27)
  - Cystic struma ovarii (rare, see Ch. 28).
5 If the cysts are single or multiple and/or combined with a thick mucinous or oily content, consider:
  - Mucinous cystadenoma or borderline tumor (usually unilateral)(Fig. 26.12a)
  - Endocervical-like mucinous cystadenoma (may be bilateral)
  - Metastatic mucinous carcinoma (often bilateral).
6 If the cystic mass is huge and unilateral, a mucinous tumor is most likely (Fig. 26.12b).[29,30]

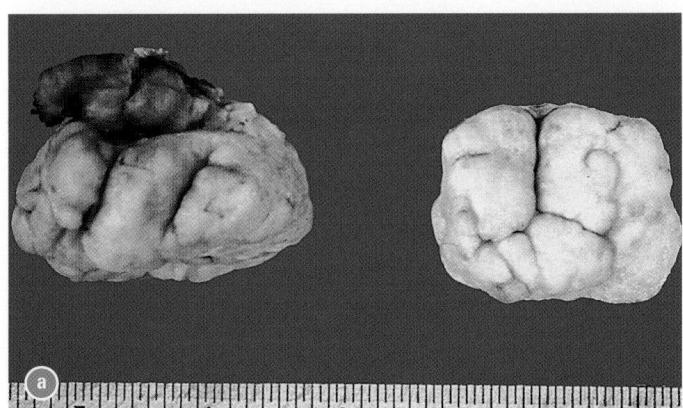

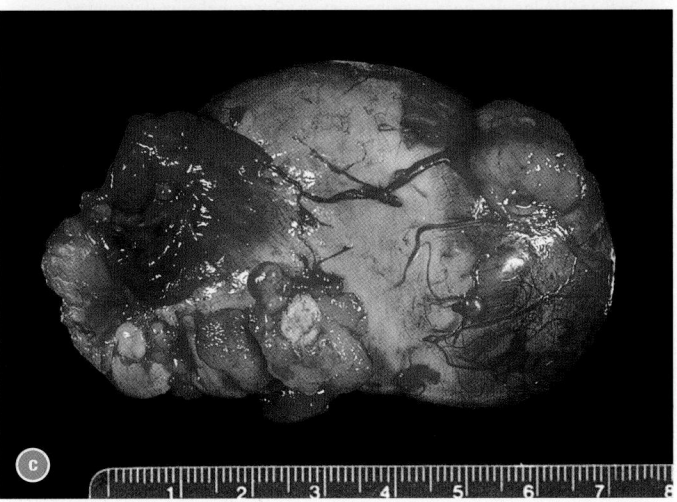

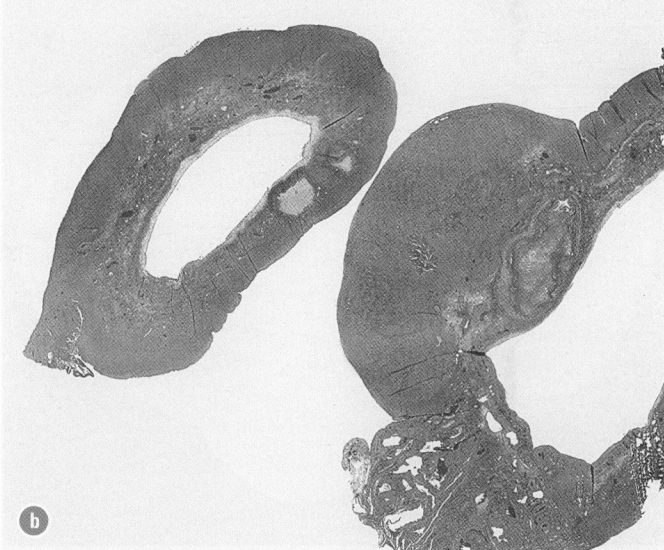

Fig. 26.4 Metastatic breast carcinoma. (a) Bilateral ovarian enlargement with general preservation of the cortical architecture. (b) At low power, mild cortical thickening associated with infiltrating lobular carcinoma (center) overlying a follicle cyst (right). (c) Small deposits of serous carcinoma on the ovarian surface may not be readily appreciated as malignant by gross exam alone.

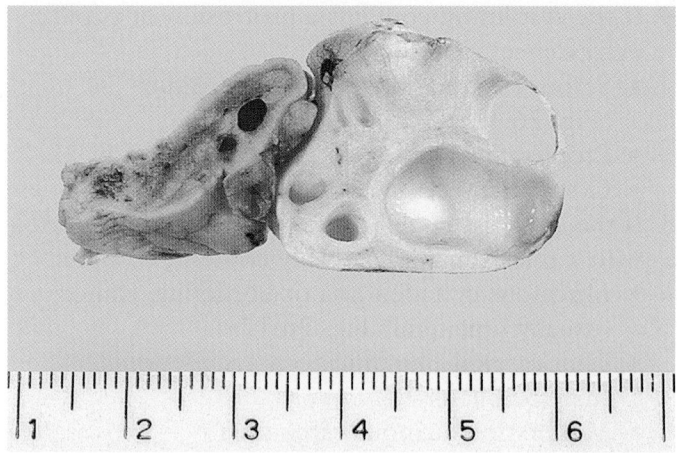

Fig. 26.5 Small parvilocular serous cystadenoma.

TUMORS WITH A DOMINANT SOLID COMPONENT

Friable and necrotic tumors

Tumors combining a cystic architecture with solid, friable and necrotic areas are usually malignant epithelial tumors (Fig. 26.13). Less commonly, malignant germ cell, granulosa and Sertoli–Leydig cell tumors can have this appearance. Epithelial malignancies are not easily distinguished from one another unless they coexist with a benign (e.g. mucinous or serous borderline) component (Figs 26.14, 26.15). Metastatic tumors with this appearance are often from the colon, particularly if they exhibit extensive cystic necrosis (Fig. 26.16).[20]

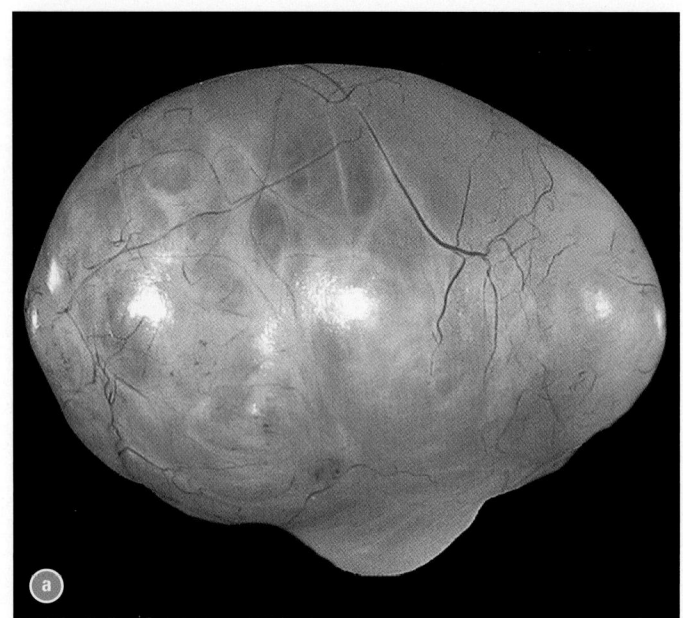

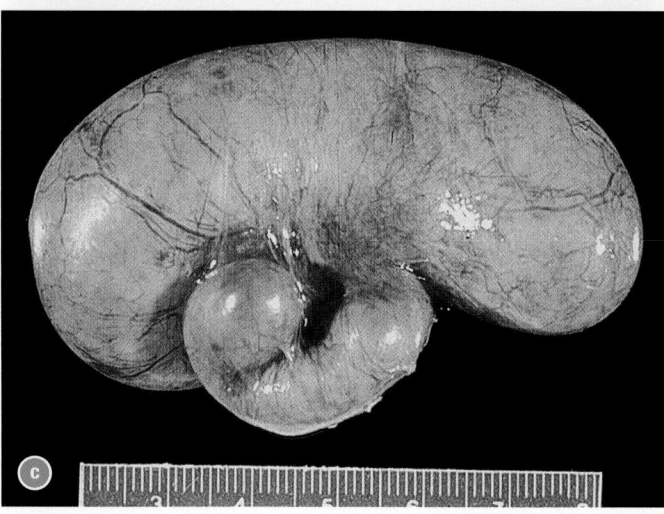

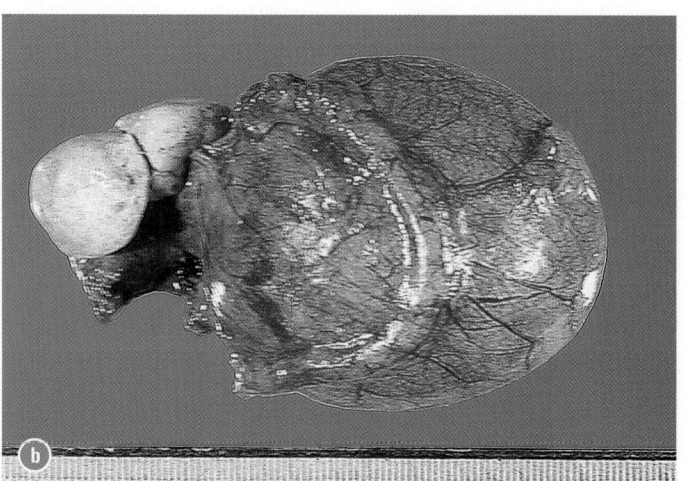

Fig. 26.6 (a) Unilocular para-ovarian cyst. (b) Paratubal cyst (hydatid of Morgagni), presenting as a translucent thin-walled cyst attenuating the overlying fallopian tube. (c) Hydrosalpinx, with uniform expansion of the fallopian tube.

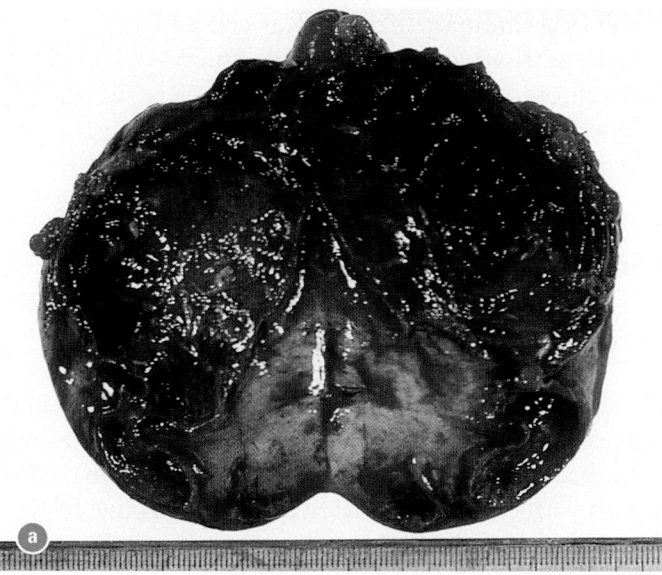

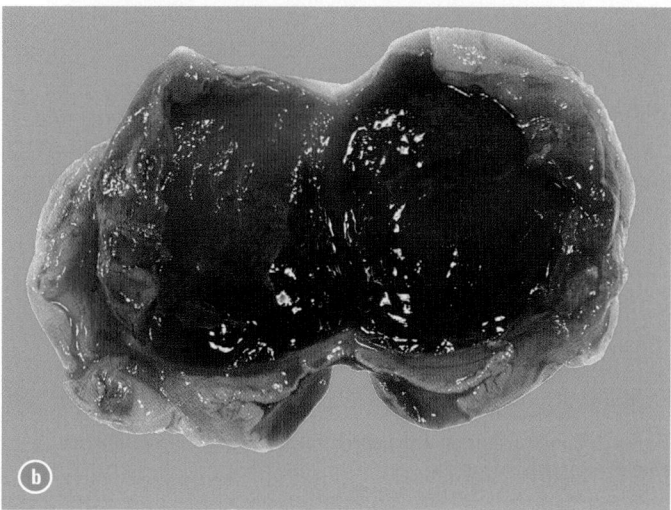

Fig. 26.7 (a) Typical endometriotic cyst presenting as a hemorrhagic cyst. (b) Cystic corpus luteum with hemorrhage. Note the glistening interior and thin orange rim corresponding to residual luteinized cells.

Solid, firm, white to tan tumors

1. Fibroma (Fig. 26.17)
2. Brenner tumor (Fig. 26.18)
3. Leiomyoma (Fig. 26.19)
4. Disseminated peritoneal leiomyomatosis (DPL, rare) (see Ch. 20)
5. Metastatic gastrointestinal stromal tumor (GIST, rare).

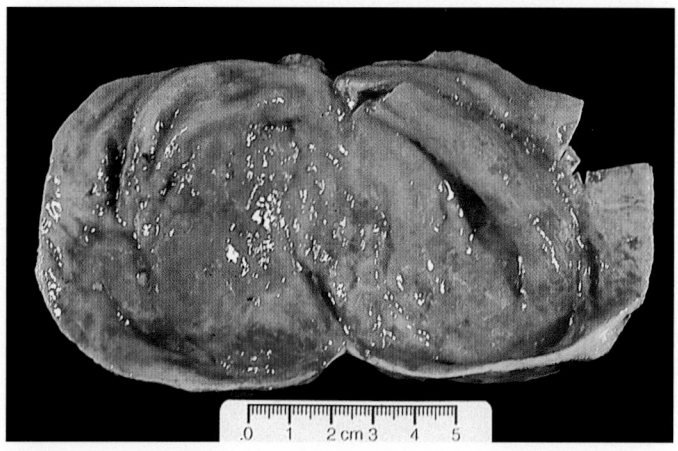

Fig. 26.9 Xanthogranulomatous pseudocyst, arising in association with endometriosis.

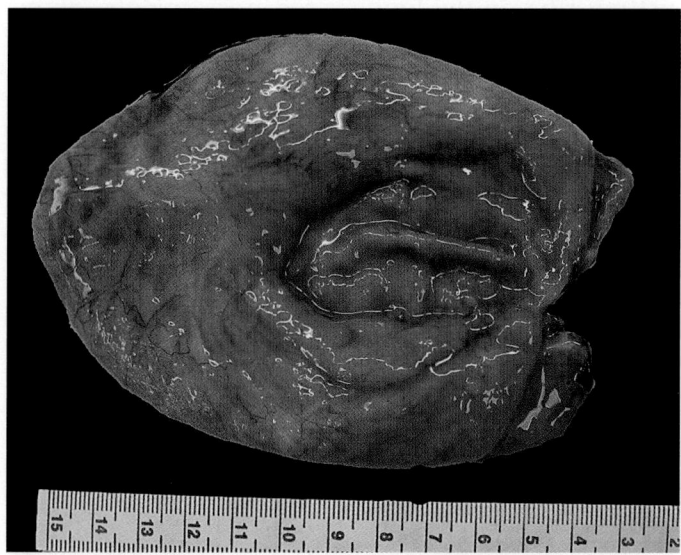

Fig. 26.8 Müllerian mucinous cystadenoma. When lacking epithelial growth and complexity, these tumors are indistinguishable from endometriotic cysts. There is a small amount of mucin present.

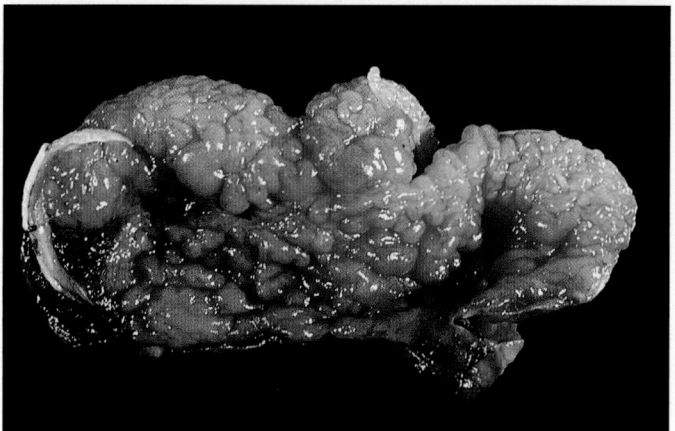

Fig. 26.10 Decidualized endometriotic cyst from a pregnant woman, producing a lush, cobblestone cystic lining.

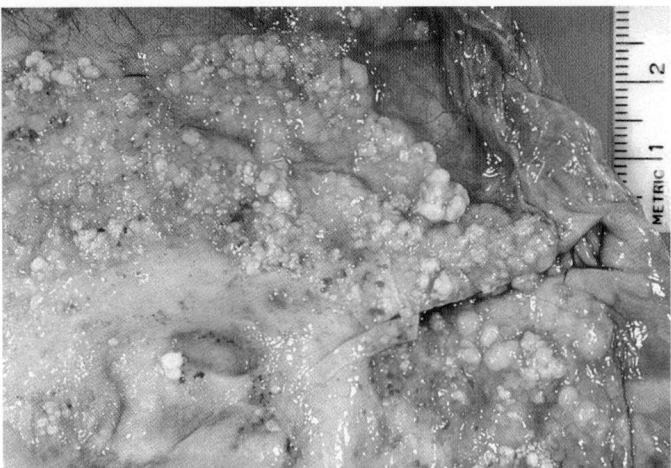

Fig. 26.11 Parvilocular cyst with papillary excrescences characterizes a borderline serous neoplasm.

Solid, soft or fleshy, tan, gray or yellow tumors

1 Primary or metastatic leiomyosarcoma (rare)
2 Endometrial stromal tumors
3 Fibrosarcoma (rare) (Fig. 26.20)
4 Granulosa cell tumor (rare) (Fig. 26.21)
5 Well-differentiated Sertoli cell tumors
6 Small cell carcinomas (hypercalcemic type)
7 Some metastatic carcinomas with minimal supporting stroma (Fig. 26.22)
8 Metastatic carcinoid tumors (usually bilateral).

Solid, soft to necrotic, hemorrhagic tumors

1 Granulosa or poorly differentiated Sertoli–Leydig cell tumors (Fig. 26.23)
2 Small cell carcinomas (Fig. 26.24)

3 Solid carcinomas, such as clear cell and endometrioid carcinomas (Fig. 26.25)
4 Carcinosarcomas
5 Lymphomas (Fig. 26.26)
6 Dysgerminoma (Fig. 26.27).

Dark brown multicystic, cystic or fleshy tumors

1 Struma ovarii (Fig. 26.28).

YELLOW TUMORS

A bright yellow to orange appearance may be attributed to steroid-producing tumors or steroid-producing stromal cells adjacent to tumors. A similar appearance may also be seen with cortical stromal hyperplasia (stromal hyperthecosis) although the latter are typically tan.[20]

1 Luteinized thecoma (Fig. 26.29)
2 Sertoli cell tumor (Fig. 26.30)
3 Brenner tumor (Fig. 26.31).
4 Granulosa-theca cell tumor (Fig. 26.22).
5 Steroid cell tumor (Fig. 26.32).
6 Metastatic carcinoma (Fig. 26.33).

TUMORS WITH SOMATIC (HAIR, ETC.) ELEMENTS

The vast majority of tumors with somatic elements are benign cystic teratomas, which may contain a variety of elements. These are discussed in greater detailed in Chapter 29. Most consist of a parvilocular cyst with hair and/or a necrotic yellow to brown liquid with an oily or waxy consistency (Fig. 26.34a,b). The pathologist must be on the lookout for more complex archi-

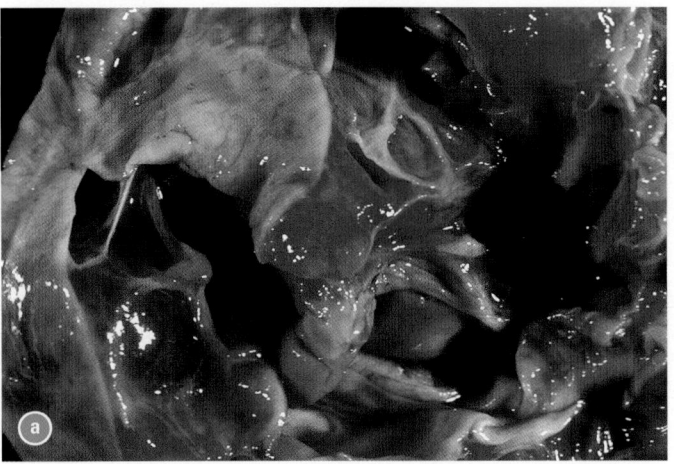

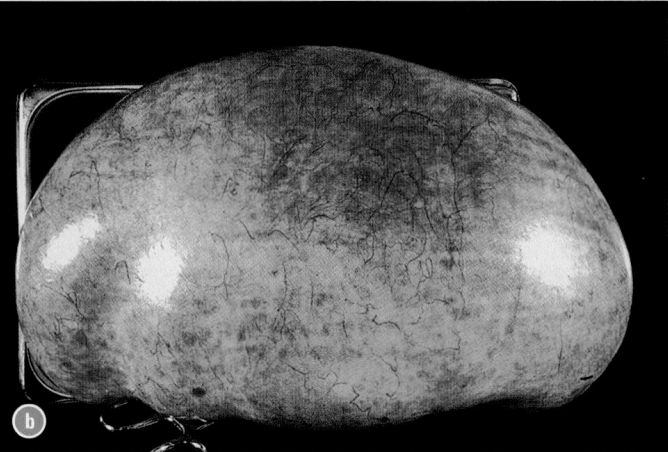

Fig. 26.12 (a) Mucinous cystadenoma with thick mucinous cyst contents. No solid tumor growth is seen. (b) Large cystic mass that proved to be a borderline mucinous cystadenoma.

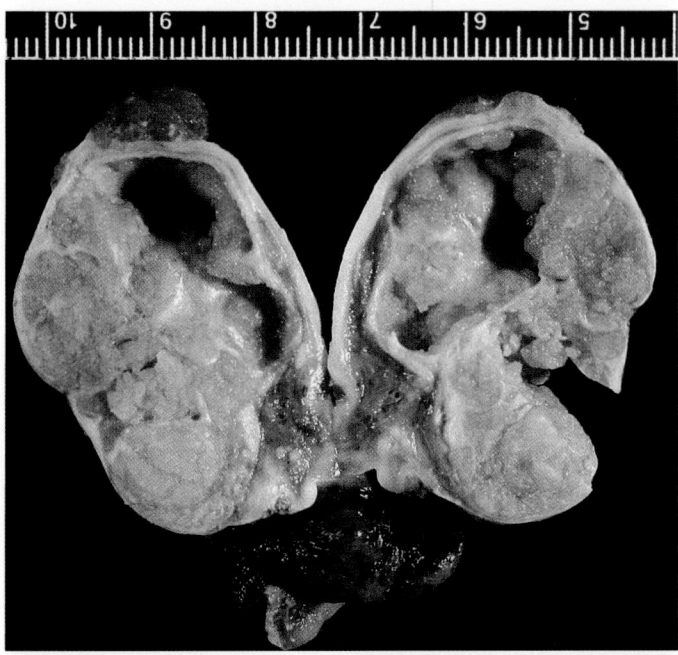

Fig. 26.13 A solid friable ovarian mass characterizes a typical epithelial ovarian malignancy. This is a serous neoplasm.

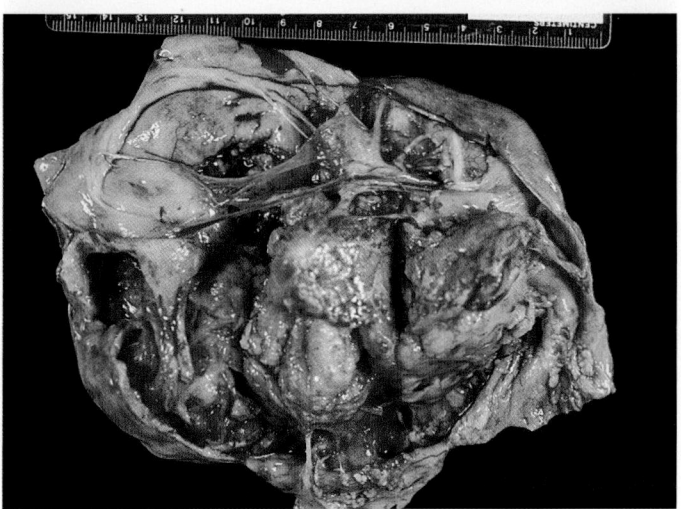

Fig. 26.14 Endometrioid adenocarcinoma presenting as a multicystic and solid tumor mass.

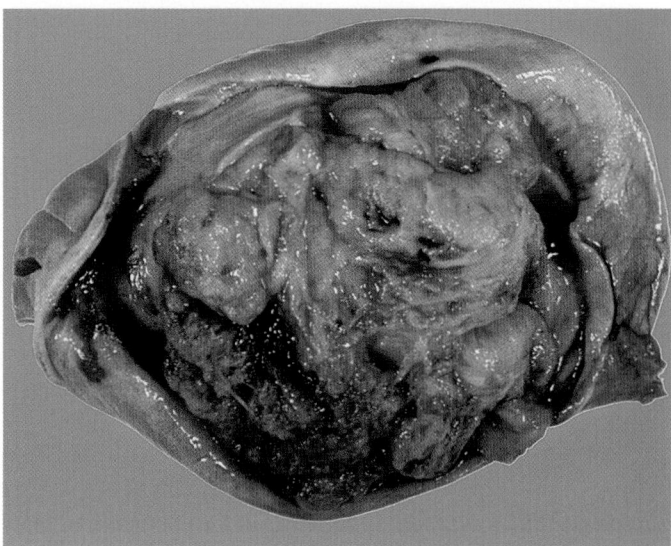

Fig. 26.15 Mucinous cystadenocarcinoma, arising in a unilocular cyst.

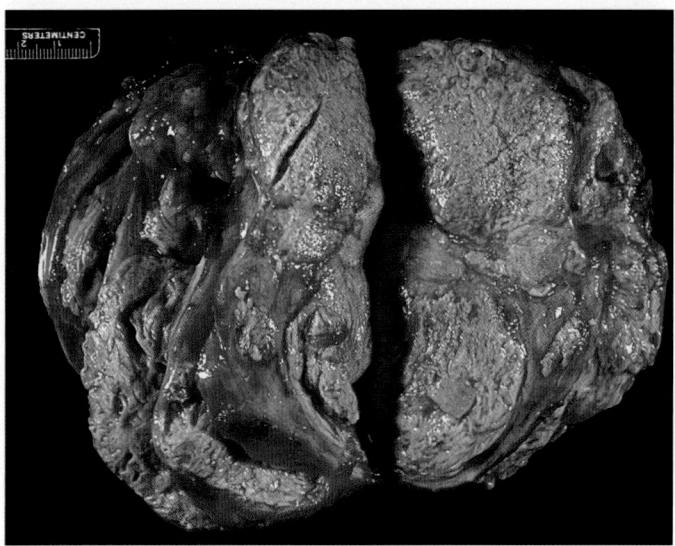

Fig. 26.16 Metastatic colonic carcinoma; this sectioned specimen contains extensive necrosis, in evidence by the friable appearance and yellow discoloration.

tecture that may signal the presence of immature or malignant elements (Fig. 26.35). The latter may prompt a more detailed staging procedure.

Intraoperative frozen section evaluation

By most accounts, the accuracy of the intraoperative frozen section evaluation is high, ranging above 90% in most studies; results are summarized in Table 26.8.[30–39] Positive predictive values (PPVs) for both malignant and benign diagnoses approach 100% with the exception of borderline tumors, including large apparently benign or borderline mucinous cystadenomas. A diagnosis of borderline is unlikely to be downgraded, but an appreciable minority will be upgraded on permanent sections.[30–38]

Errors in frozen section interpretation are typically due to sampling, as were eight of 13 errors in one study.[36]

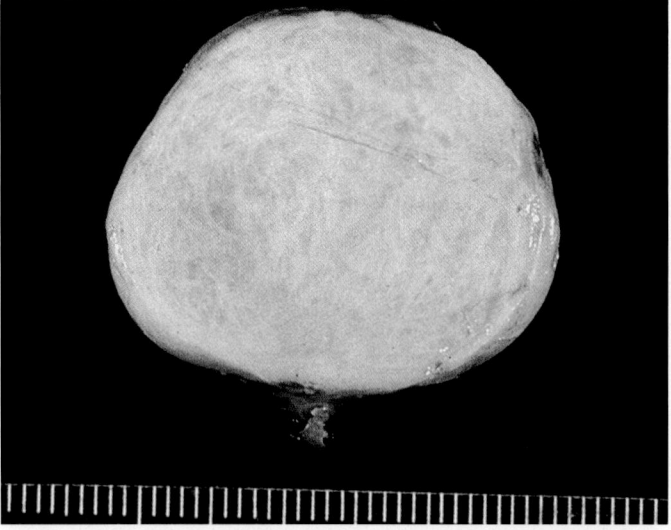

Fig. 26.17 Ovarian fibroma. The white appearance and firm consistency are typical of tumors with a predominant fibrous component.

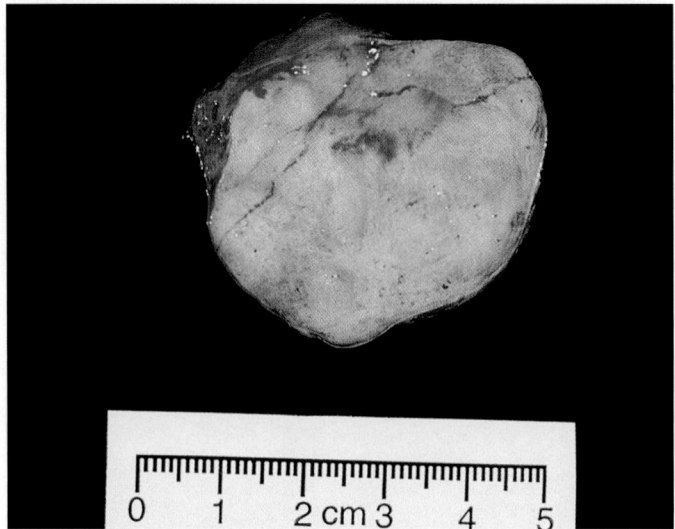

Fig. 26.18 Brenner tumor. These tumors vary in appearance from firm and white to yellow (see Fig. 26.31).

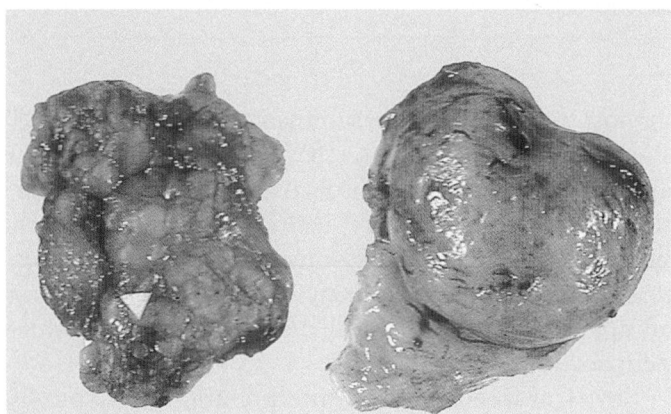

Fig. 26.19 Leiomyoma of the ovary. This tumor is typically tan in appearance and will vary in consistency depending on cellularity.

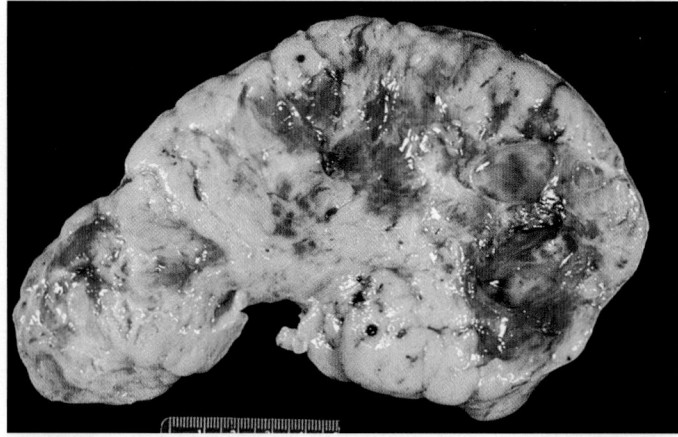

Fig. 26.20 Fibrosarcoma of the ovary. The tumor lacks the uniform firm consistency of the fibroma (Fig. 26.16). It is soft, pale yellow and focally hemorrhagic.

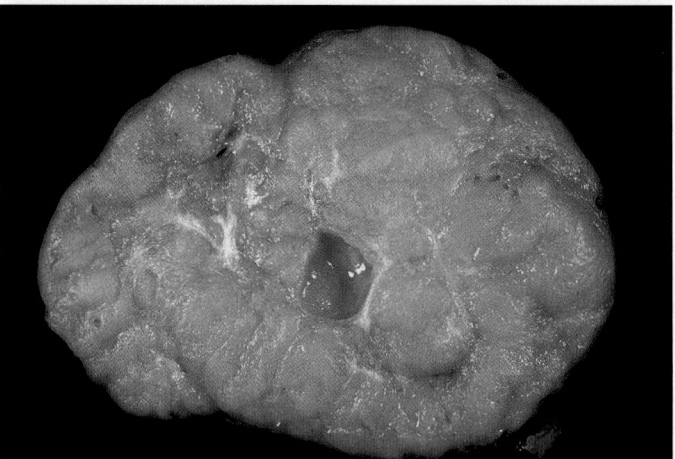

Fig. 26.21 Granulosa cell tumor. This tumor has a uniform appearance and displays broad admixed yellow lobules.

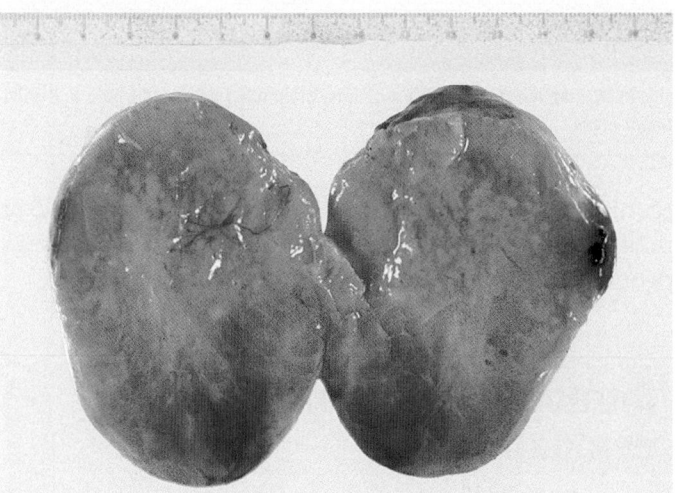

Fig. 26.22 Metastatic gastric carcinoma. The tumor is uniform, glistening (due to mucin content) and soft.

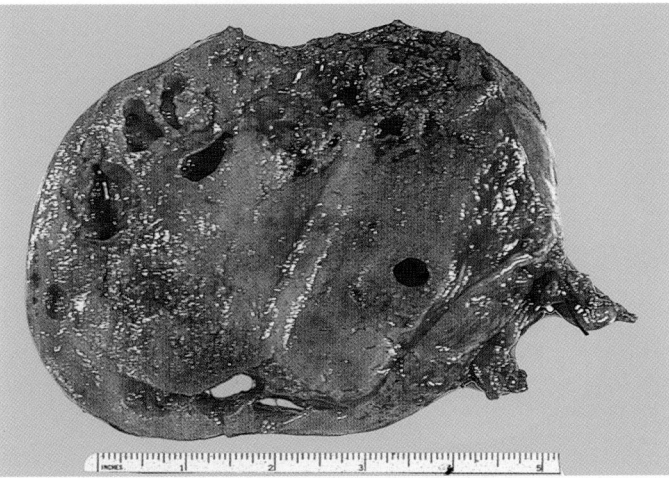

Fig. 26.23 Granulosa cell tumor. These tumors not infrequently combine a golden brown appearance with both hemorrhage and cysts.

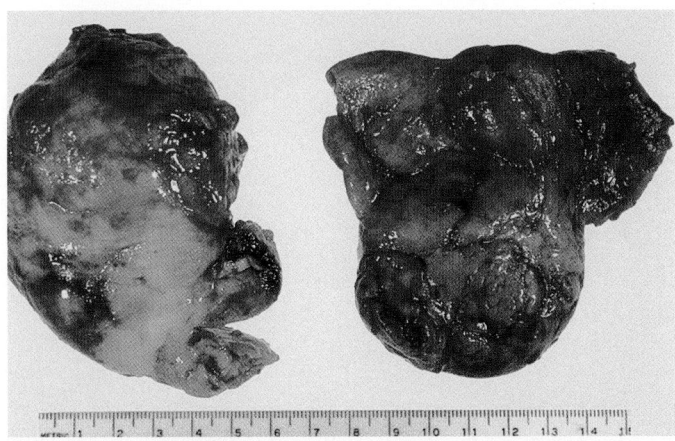

Fig. 26.26 Bilateral lymphomas of the ovary. These tumors cannot be distinguished from other solid ovarian tumors (see Figs 26.20, 26.24, 26.25, 26.27).

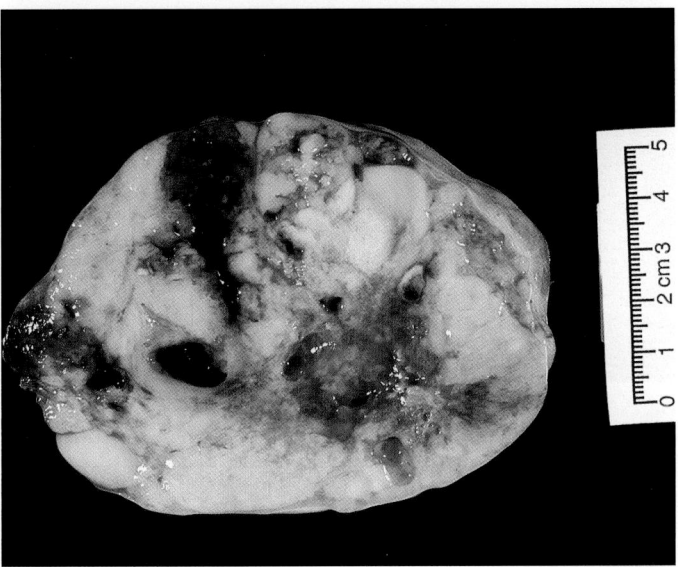

Fig. 26.24 Small cell carcinoma of hypercalcemic type, combining a soft yellow to white appearance with focal hemorrhage.

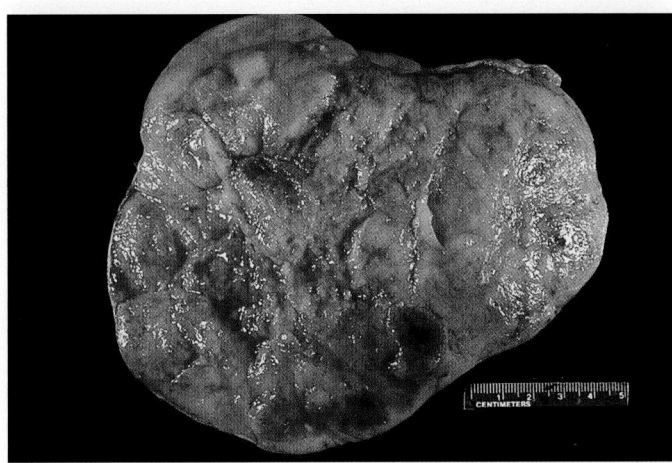

Fig. 26.27 Dysgerminoma of the ovary. These tumors typically are homogeneous, soft and may be confused with lymphomas.

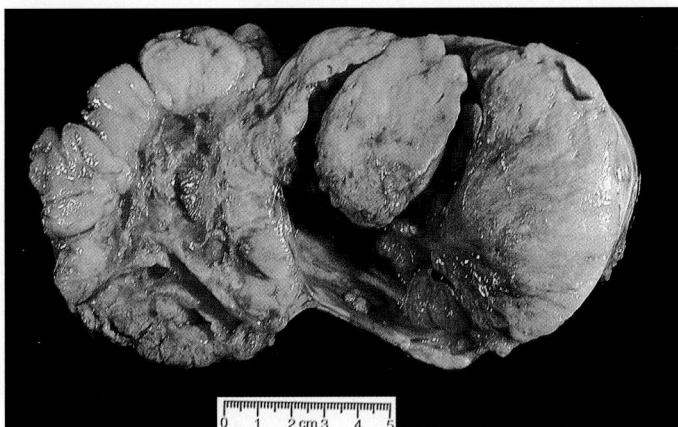

Fig. 26.25 Clear cell carcinoma. The solid components of these tumors are often gray to white with a fleshy consistency.

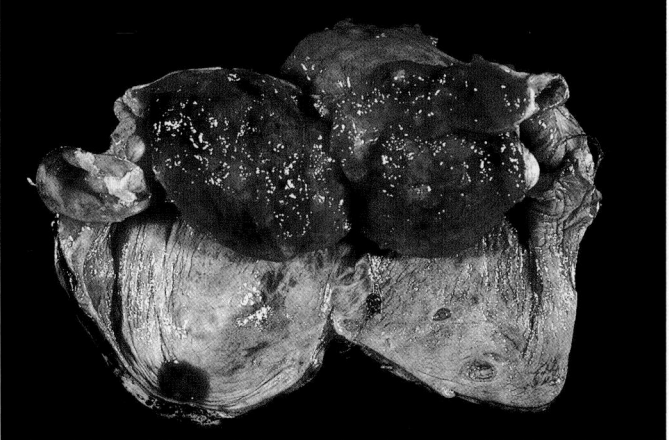

Fig. 26.28 Struma ovarii presenting as a distinct 'cordovan brown' mass within a cystic teratoma.

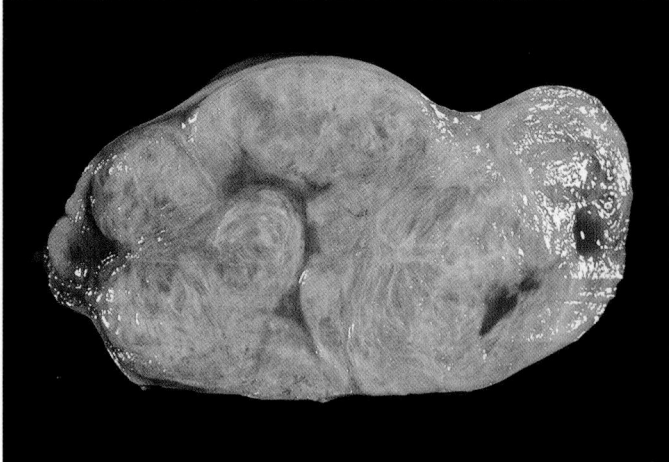

Fig. 26.29 Fibroma-thecoma with partial luteinization imparting a yellow appearance.

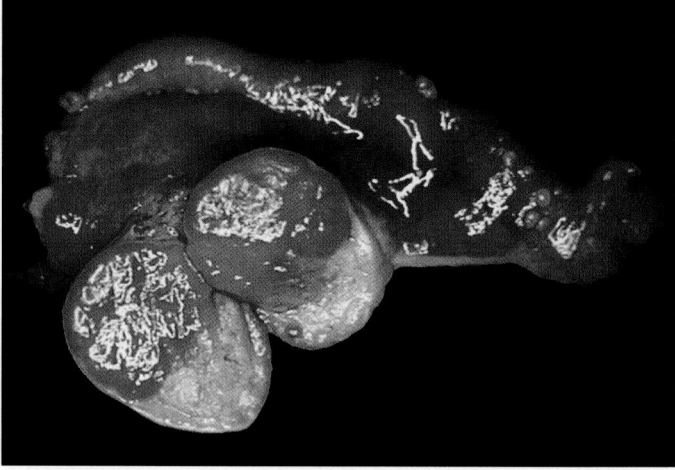

Fig. 26.32 Steroid cell tumors are typically discrete and brown or yellow in color.

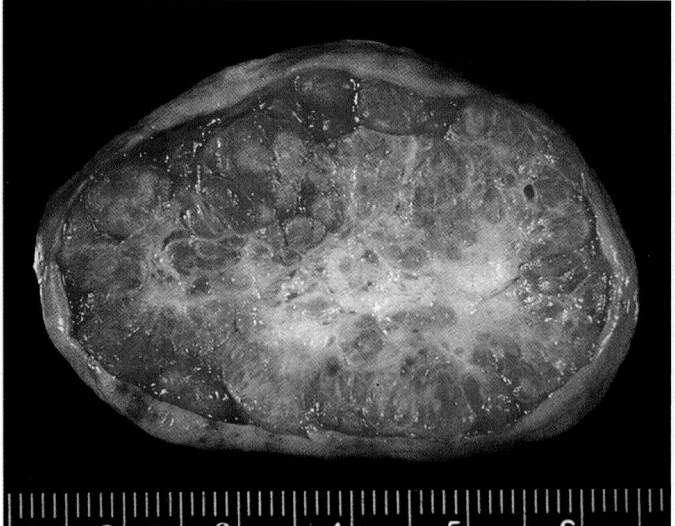

Fig. 26.30 Sertoli–Leydig cell tumors typically present with a golden-brown color.

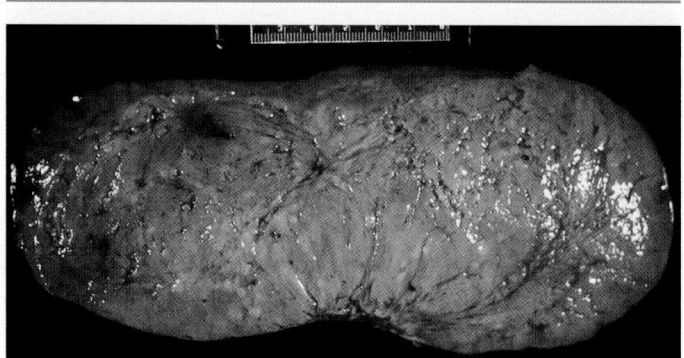

Fig. 26.33 Metastatic gastric carcinoma, with a golden-brown appearance. This may result from luteinized stromal reaction.

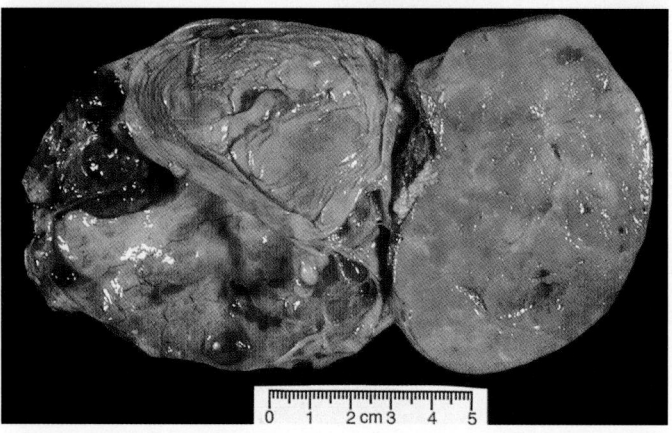

Fig. 26.31 Brenner tumor (right) associated with mucinous cystadenoma (left). This Brenner tumor exhibits prominent yellow to golden brown coloration.

Intraoperative gross and microscopic pitfalls

MISCLASSIFICATION BASED ON CONFUSING GROSS APPEARANCE

1 Papillary adenofibromas have a complex surface architecture, may adhere to pelvic structures and are firm and gritty to feel and on sectioning, suggesting a malignancy (Fig. 26.36a,b).
2 Misinterpretation of an abscess, focal infarct or ischemic (torsed) ovary as tumor (Fig. 26.37).
3 Decidualized endometriotic cyst misinterpreted as neoplasia.
4 Pregnancy-related ovarian changes misclassified as a cystic tumor.
5 Borderline clear cell adenofibroma classified as a fibroma due to inconspicuous cystic architecture.

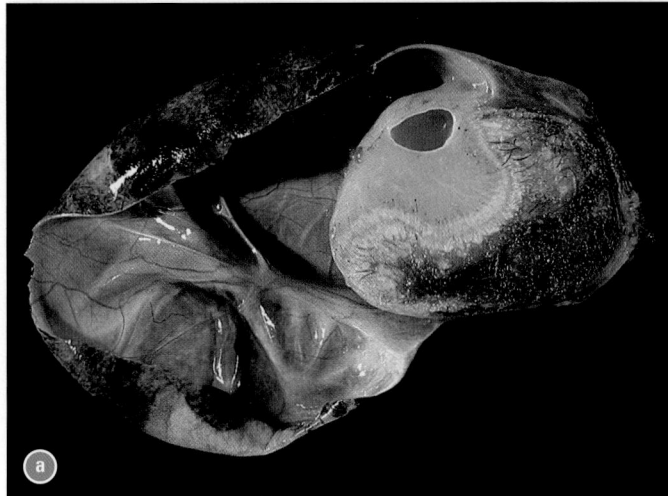
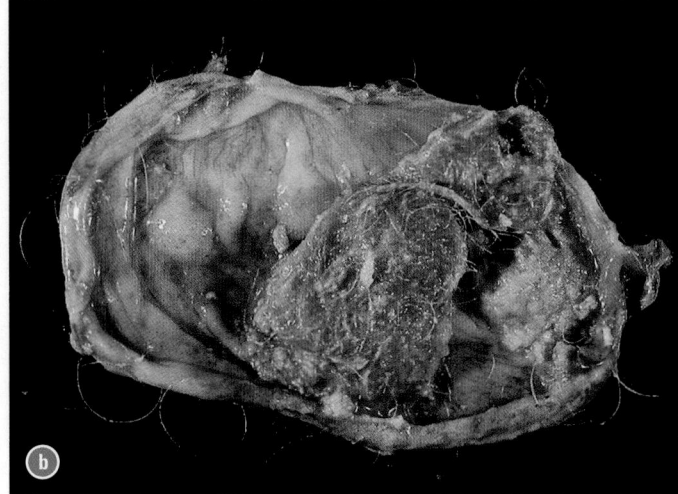

Fig. 26.34 (a) Benign cystic teratoma, containing abundant hair. (b) Benign cystic teratoma, containing matted hair and brown debris.

6 Yellow-appearing endometrioid adenocarcinoma (with sex-cord-like differentiation histologically) misinterpreted as a sex-cord stromal tumor.

7 Primary peritoneal serous carcinoma misclassified on gross exam as chronic salpingitis or tubo-ovarian adhesions.

MISCLASSIFICATION DUE TO SIMILARITIES IN CELL APPEARANCE OR STRUCTURE

1 *Mucinous tumors.* Misclassifying mucinous tumors (as either primary or metastatic) is a pitfall that can not always be avoided but can be minimized if the following are kept in mind: Large, unilateral mucinous tumors without surface involvement are almost always primary ovarian tumors.[29,39] Endocervical-like (Müllerian mucinous) tumors may be bilateral and thus misinterpreted as metastatic.[20] Conversely, mucinous tumors may metastasize to the gastrointestinal tract and histologically resemble a primary colonic carcinoma. In general, ovarian surface involvement signals a metastasis to the ovary with extra-ovarian primary mucinous neoplasia, most commonly from the appendix.

2 Metastatic carcinoid interpreted as a Brenner tumor (metastatic carcinoids are usually bilateral).

3 Mesothelioma classified as serous carcinoma.

4 Poorly-differentiated stromal (or small cell) tumor misclassified as lymphoma.

5 Endometrioid carcinoma misclassified as sex-cord tumor,[40] and rarely, as metastatic colon cancer in patients with prior colonic neoplasia.

6 Follicular salpingitis misclassified as tubal or endometrioid adenocarcinoma.

7 Gastrointestinal stromal tumor (GIST) misclassified as leiomyoma.

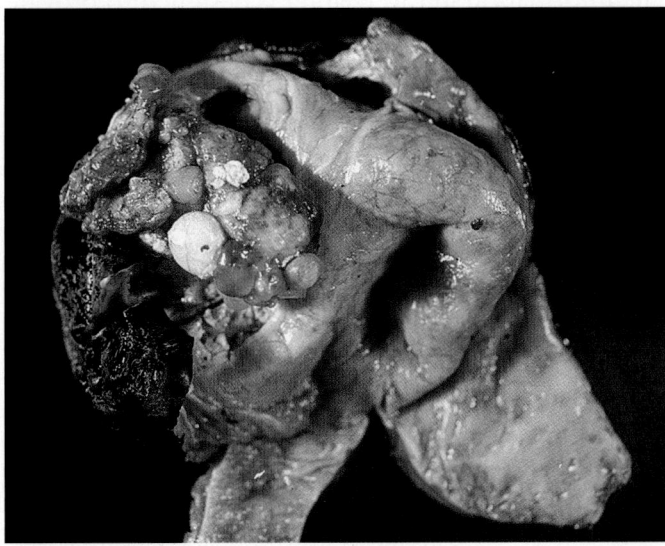

Fig. 26.35 A grade 1 immature teratoma. In addition to hair and one tooth, the cyst wall contains less well-characterized solid growth.

Table 26.8 Accuracy of frozen section diagnosis (%) relative to final[30–38]

	Benign	Borderline	Malignant
Sensitivity	93–98	61–84	84–98
PPV*	92	62–65	98–100

*Positive predictive value

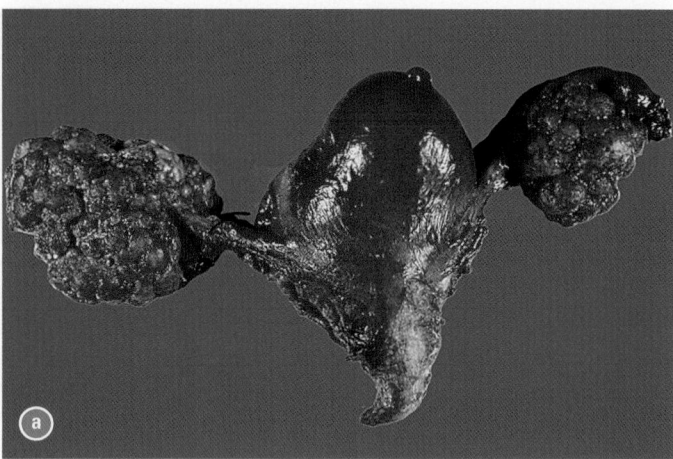
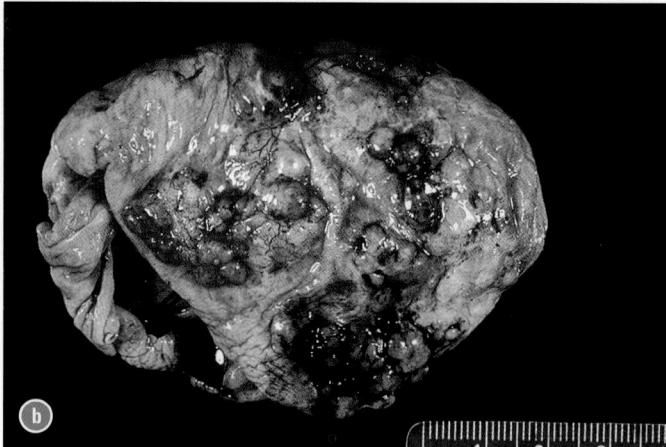

Fig. 26.36 (a) Bilateral adenofibromas of the ovary. (b) Adenofibroma with firm nodular surface may mimic surface serous carcinoma.

8 Desmoplastic noninvasive borderline implants misclassified as malignant.

9 Metastatic gastric carcinoma mimicking massive ovarian edema.[41]

PITFALLS ENCOUNTERED DUE TO AN UNDER-APPRECIATION OF THE LIMITATIONS OF INTRAOPERATIVE GROSS EVALUATION AND/OR LIMITATIONS IN SAMPLING

1 Classifying a complex intestinal (or Müllerian) mucinous carcinoma as borderline. Invasive cancer may be focal and unrecognized until more extensive sampling is performed.[39,42]

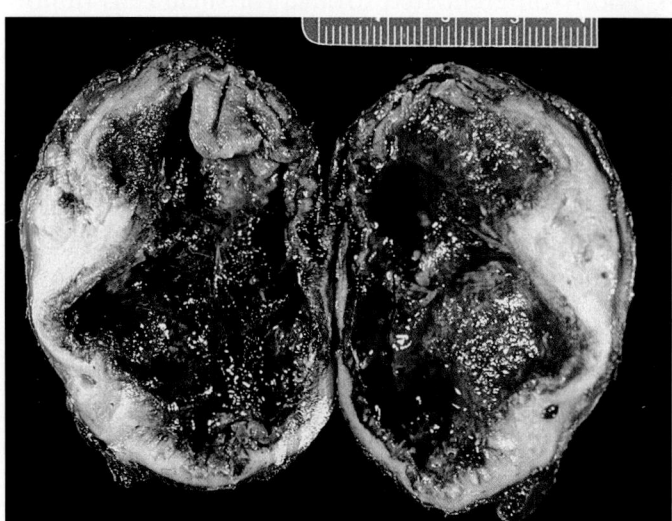

Fig. 26.37 Hemorrhagic infarction of the ovary with a pseudocyst.

2 Classifying a complex cystic and solid teratoma as a mature teratoma. Immature elements, particularly those that are non-neuroepithelial, may be subtle and may require extensive sampling with careful evaluation.[43]

3 Classifying a serous tumor with surface involvement as a benign cystoma. Tumors with surface involvement are typically borderline (occasional stage I cystadenomas on frozen section can become stage III borderline tumors on the final report).[34,35]

4 Undersampling small endometrioid carcinomas or borderline tumors within endometriotic cysts.[44]

Summary

The information in this chapter is designed to provide a template for the intraoperative evaluation of ovarian tumors. However, the reader can appreciate how complex the exercise is and how successful execution is highly dependent on experience. The best approach to this responsibility is to: (1) be cognizant of the tumors or conditions that are most likely to be present based on history, distribution and gross exam; (2) compulsively avoid being unduly biased by the gross exam when reviewing the histopathology; and (3) always be prepared for exceptions to the rule.

References

1 Valentin L, Skoog L, Epstein E. Frequency and type of adnexal lesions in autopsy material from postmenopausal women: ultrasound study with histological correlation. Ultrasound Obstet Gynecol 2003; 22:284–289.

2 Koonings PP, Campbell K, Mishell DR Jr, Grimes DA. Relative frequency of primary ovarian neoplasms: a 10-year review. Obstet Gynecol 1989; 74:921–926.

3 Tuncer ZS, Gunalp S, Aksu T, Ayhan A. Benign epithelial ovarian tumors. Eur J Gynaecol Oncol 1998; 19:391–393.

4 Partridge EE, Phillips JL, Menck HR. The National Cancer Database Report on ovarian cancer treatment in United States hospitals. Cancer 1996; 78:2236–2246.

5 Wilde R De, Bordt J, Hesseling M, Vancaillie T. Ovarian cystostomy. Acta Obstet Gynecol Scand 1989; 68:363–364.

6 Young RH, Oliva E, Scully RE. Small cell carcinoma of the hypercalcemic type in the ovary. Gynecol Oncol 1995; 57:7–8.

7 Nowak M, Szpakowski M, Malinowski A, et al. Ovarian tumors in the reproductive age group. Ginekol Pol 2002; 73:354–358.

8 Westhuizen NG van der, Tiltman AJ. Brenner tumours – a clinicopathological study. S Afr Med J 1988; 73:98–101.

9 Beck RP, Latour JP. Review of 1019 benign ovarian neoplasms. Obstet Gynecol 1960; 16:479–482.

10 Sangi-Haghpeykar H, Poindexter AN 3rd. Epidemiology of endometriosis among parous women. Obstet Gynecol 1995; 85:983–992.

11 Roth MS, Goodner DM. Large endometrioma occurring in an adolescent. Obstet Gynecol 1977; 49:364–366.

12 Joshi R, Dunaif A. Ovarian disorders of pregnancy. Endocrinol Metab Clin North Am 1995; 24:153–169.

13 Clement PB. Tumor-like lesions of the ovary associated with pregnancy. Int J Gynecol Pathol 1993; 12:108–115.

14 Wajda KJ, Lucas JG, Marsh WL Jr. *Hyperreactio luteinalis*. Benign disorder masquerading as an ovarian neoplasm. Arch Pathol Lab Med 1989; 113:921–925.

15 Sayedur Rahman M, Al-Sibai MH, Rahman J, et al. Ovarian carcinoma associated with pregnancy. A review of 9 cases. Acta Obstet Gynecol Scand 2002; 81:260–264.

16 Szpakowski M, Wilczynski JR, Wieczorek A, et al. The number and histopathologic type of ovarian tumors operated during cesarean section at the Polish Mother's Health Institute between 1990-2000. Ginekol Pol 2002; 73:379–385.

17 Katsube Y, Berg JW, Silverberg SG. Epidemiologic pathology of ovarian tumors: a histopathologic review of primary ovarian neoplasms diagnosed in the Denver Standard Metropolitan Statistical Area, 1 July–31 December 1969 and 1 July–31 December 1979. Int J Gynecol Pathol 1982; 1:3–16.

18 Moore RG, Chung M, Granai CO, et al. Incidence of metastasis to the ovaries from nongenital tract primary tumors Gynecol Oncol 2004; 93:87–91.

19 Robboy SJ, Scully RE, Norris HJ. Carcinoid metastatic to the ovary. A clinicopathologic analysis of 35 cases. Cancer 1974; 33:798–811.

20 Scully RE, Young RH, Clement PB. Tumors of the ovary, maldeveloped gonads, fallopian tube and broad ligament. Atlas of tumor pathology. Washington DC: American Registry of Pathology; 1998.

21 Ulbright TM, Roth LM. Stehman FB. Secondary ovarian neoplasia. A clinicopathologic study of 35 cases. Cancer 1984; 53:1164–1174.

22 Remadi S, McGee W, Egger JF, Ismail A. Ovarian metastatic melanoma. A diagnostic pitfall in histopathologic examination. Arch Anat Cytol Pathol 1997; 45:43–46.

23 Householder J, Han A, Edelson MI, et al. Immunohistochemical confirmation of pulmonary papillary adenocarcinoma metastatic to ovaries. Arch Pathol Lab Med 2002; 126:1101–1103.

24 Puls L, Heidtman E, Hunter JE, et al. The accuracy of frozen section by tumor weight for ovarian epithelial neoplasms. Gynecol Oncol 1997; 67:16–19.

25 Friedrich M, Ertan AK, Axt-Fliedner R, et al. Unilateral massive ovarian edema (MOE): a case report. Clin Exp Obstet Gynecol 2002; 29(1):65–66.

26 Varras M, Tsikini A, Polyzos D, et al. Uterine adnexal torsion: pathologic and gray-scale ultrasonographic findings. Clin Exp Obstet Gynecol 2004; 31:34–38.

27 Bell DA, Scully RE. Early de novo ovarian carcinoma. A study of fourteen cases. Cancer 1994; 73:1859–1864.

28 Lim FK, Yeoh CL, Chong SM, Arulkumaran S. Pre and intraoperative diagnosis of ovarian tumours: how accurate are we? Aust N Z J Obstet Gynaecol 1997; 37:223–227.

29 Lee KR, Scully RE. Mucinous tumors of the ovary: a clinicopathologic study of 196 borderline tumors (of intestinal type) and carcinomas, including an evaluation of 11 cases with 'pseudomyxoma peritonei'. Am J Surg Pathol 2000; 24:1447–1464.

30 Gol M, Baloglu A, Yigit S, et al. Accuracy of frozen section diagnosis in ovarian tumors: Is there a change in the course of time? Int J Gynecol Cancer 2003; 13:593–597.

31 Pinto PB, Andrade LA, Derchain SF. Accuracy of intraoperative frozen section diagnosis of ovarian tumors. Gynecol Oncol 2001; 81:230–232.

32 Acs G. Intraoperative consultation in gynecologic pathology. Semin Diagn Pathol 2002; 19:237–254.

33 Robinson WR, Curtin JP, Morrow CP. Operative staging and conservative surgery in the management of low malignant potential ovarian tumors. Int J Gynecol Cancer 1992; 2:113–118.

34 Menzin AW, Rubin SC, Noumoff JS, LiVolsi VA. The accuracy of a frozen section diagnosis of borderline ovarian malignancy. Gynecol Oncol 1995; 59:183–185.

35 Rose PG, Rubin RB, Nelson BE, et al. Accuracy of frozen-section (intraoperative consultation) diagnosis of ovarian tumors. Am J Obstet Gynecol 1994; 171:823–826.

36 Spann CO, Kennedy JE, Musoke E. Intraoperative consultation of ovarian neoplasms. J Natl Med Assoc 1994; 86:141–144.

37 Twaalfhoven FC, Peters AA, Trimbos JB, et al. The accuracy of frozen section diagnosis of ovarian tumors. Gynecol Oncol 1991; 41:189–192.

38 Gramlich T, Austin RM, Lutz M. Histologic sampling requirements in ovarian carcinoma: a review of 51 tumors. Gynecol Oncol 1990; 38:249–256.

39 Seidman JD, Kurman RJ, Ronnett BM. Primary and metastatic mucinous adenocarcinomas in the ovaries: incidence in routine practice with a new approach to improve intraoperative diagnosis. Am J Surg Pathol 2003; 27:985–993.

40 Young RH, Prat J, Scully RE. Ovarian endometrioid carcinomas resembling sex cord-stromal tumors. A clinicopathological analysis of 13 cases. Am J Surg Pathol 1982; 6:513–522.

41 Bazot M, Detchev R, Cortez A, et al. Massive ovarian edema revealing gastric carcinoma: a case report. Gynecol Oncol 2003; 91:648–650.

42 Rodriguez IM, Prat J. Mucinous tumors of the ovary: a clinicopathologic analysis of 75 borderline tumors (of intestinal type) and carcinomas. Am J Surg Pathol 2002; 26:139–152.

43 Steeper TA, Mukai K. Solid ovarian teratomas: an immunocytochemical study of thirteen cases with clinicopathologic correlation. Pathol Annu 1984; 19:81–92.

44 McCluggage WG, Bryson C, Lamki H, Boyle DD. Benign, borderline and malignant endometrioid neoplasia arising in endometriosis in association with tamoxifen therapy. Int J Gynecol Pathol 2000; 19:276–279.

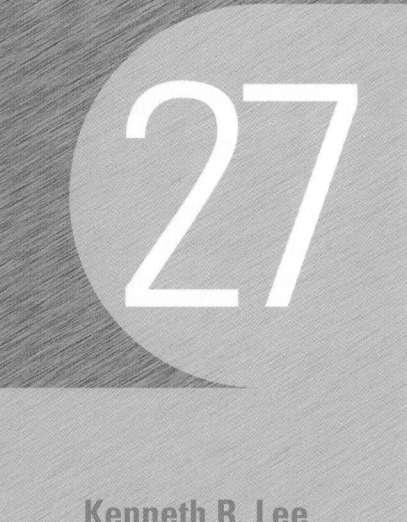

27

The pathology of surface epithelial-stromal tumors of the ovary

Kenneth R. Lee

Epithelial-stromal tumors

Terminology and classification
The concept of ovarian borderline tumors
Histologic grading of epithelial-stromal carcinomas

Serous tumors

General features and clinical aspects
Gross examination
Examination of prophylactic oophorectomy specimens from high-risk patients
Microscopic findings
Differential diagnosis
Etiology, genetics and biomarkers

Mucinous tumors

General features and clinical aspects
Gross examination
Microscopic examination
Mucinous tumors and pseudomyxoma peritonei
Differential diagnosis
Etiology, genetics and biomarkers

Endometrioid tumors

General features and clinical aspects
Gross examination
Microscopic examination
Differential diagnosis
Etiology, genetics and biomarkers

Tumors with a sarcomatous component and endometrioid stromal sarcoma

Clear cell tumors

General features and clinical aspects
Gross examination
Microscopic examination
Differential diagnosis
Etiology, genetics and biomarkers

Transitional cell tumors

General features and clinical aspects
Gross examination
Microscopic examination
Differential diagnosis
Etiology, genetics and biomarkers

Squamous cell tumors

General features and clinical aspects
Gross examination
Microscopic examination
Differential diagnosis
Etiology

Mixed-epithelial tumors and undifferentiated carcinoma

General features and clinical aspects
Gross examination
Microscopic examination
Differential diagnosis

Epithelial-stromal tumors

TERMINOLOGY AND CLASSIFICATION

Tumors in the surface epithelial-stromal category constitute about 50% of all ovarian tumors and, in the USA, 91% of ovarian cancers.[1] The use of the term 'surface epithelial' follows from the theory that tumors in this category originate from the specialized peritoneal cells lining the ovarian surface or their derivatives, the epithelial (cortical) inclusion cysts.[2] The addition of the term 'stromal' reflects the fact that many of them have a conspicuous stromal component that is derived from the specialized stroma of the ovary, which, unlike the nonspecific stroma within most other epithelial tumors, is capable of hormone synthesis, sometimes inducing a paraneoplastic syndrome, usually related to hyperestrogenism.[3,4]

Epithelial-stromal tumors are subdivided into serous, mucinous, endometrioid, clear cell, transitional cell, squamous, mixed epithelial and undifferentiated types. Except for squamous and undifferentiated tumors, there are benign, borderline and malignant subcategories within all of these divisions. The designation 'borderline' is unique in the nosology of human tumors. Use of the term is controversial and merits some introductory remarks.

THE CONCEPT OF OVARIAN BORDERLINE TUMORS

The 'borderline' concept arose from the observations reported by Taylor in 1929 on the experience with ovarian tumors at New York Hospital.[5] He noted that some tumors, primarily in the serous category, had spread beyond the ovaries but their clinical behavior was benign. This was in marked contrast to the behavior of most other serous carcinomas, which were rapidly fatal after peritoneal spread. Taylor noted that the benign-behaving tumors were also less atypical histologically and designated them 'semi malignant'. Subsequently, others confirmed Taylor's observations and noted that tumors with intermediate histologic findings could also be found in other epithelial subtypes. The terms 'borderline', 'of low malignant potential' and 'proliferative', were coined by various authors. The World Health Organization (WHO) selected the designation 'tumors of borderline malignancy' in 1973 and applied it to all epithelial types, defining border-

line tumors as those with epithelial atypicality but without obvious stromal invasion.[6]

However, although they have often been considered as a single entity in clinical follow-up studies, borderline tumors of different epithelial types are not equivalent. In the most frequently encountered borderline tumors, those of the serous type, the intermediate microscopic appearance correlates with a clinical behavior that is also somewhere between benign and malignant. That is, there may be peritoneal implants, but most of the time they do not harm the patient, or do so only after a prolonged period. However, in the second most common, mucinous borderline category, most cases previously thought to have spread to the peritoneum (usually in the form of pseudomyxoma peritonei) are now felt by most pathologists to have been metastases to both the ovaries and the peritoneum from a gastrointestinal (usually appendiceal) primary and are not ovarian tumors at all. The remaining borderline-appearing mucinous tumors that are not associated with a gastrointestinal tumor, and that have implanted outside of the ovary, are thought to actually be carcinomas of which the invasive areas were unsampled. They generally result in high mortality, similar to overt mucinous carcinomas that have also metastasized. Thus, the existence of primary mucinous ovarian tumors that are borderline in both appearance and clinical behavior is uncertain. Finally, the much less common endometrioid, clear cell and transitional cell borderline tumors have only rarely been reported to have metastasized and, even when they have, their clinical behavior has been benign.

On the basis of these observations and to discourage an overly aggressive clinical response to tumors that behave in a benign fashion in the great majority of cases, some authorities recommend that the category of borderline tumors be abandoned.[7,8] They proffer the alternative designation 'atypical proliferative tumors' (and also propose that a small subset in the serous category, the 'micropapillary/cribriform' type, be upgraded to carcinomas). The term 'atypical proliferative', rather than 'borderline', has been adopted in major textbooks of gynecologic pathology.[9,10]

Other experts argue that a change in terminology invites unnecessary confusion.[8,11,12] Since the borderline category has existed for so long, they believe that clinicians understand its implications and are not prone to treat patients unnecessarily. They also argue that borderline tumors do carry a very small risk for recurrence and even death and patients warrant close clinical observation. Further, even borderline tumors that do not cause harm belong to a unique class of neoplasms, many of them premalignant, and further studies to elucidate their nature and risk factors for poor outcomes are needed. Neither of these will be done, they argue, if cases are diagnosed as 'atypical proliferative' tumors and thus considered essentially benign by clinicians and tumor registries.

The most recent (2003) WHO classification designates tumors in this category simply as 'borderline tumors', rather than 'of borderline malignancy'.[13] Thus, they retain a simple and familiar term, yet recognize these tumors as a special subset. This seems to us to be a reasonable compromise and we adhere to the WHO terminology.

Whatever terms one uses in clinical practice, it is very important that pathologists be familiar with the gross and microscopic appearances of borderline tumors so that an erroneous intraoperative diagnosis of carcinoma on a frozen section is avoided. Many borderline tumors can be safely treated with unilateral oophorectomy or cystectomy in young patients who wish to retain their fertility.[14–16] An intraoperative report that a tumor is borderline will then lead to thorough operative staging and generous sampling of the tumor for permanent sections.

HISTOLOGIC GRADING OF EPITHELIAL-STROMAL CARCINOMAS

Although the grade of an ovarian carcinoma is broadly predictive of its behavior, a standard method of grading has not been universally adopted. Thus, the contribution of tumor grade to outcome in an individual patient is imprecise. There are two internationally recognized grading systems: those of the International Federation of Gynecology and Obstetrics (FIGO)[17] and the WHO.[13] In the former, tumor architecture is the sole determinant of grade (<5% solid growth = grade 1, >50% solid growth = grade 3). The WHO system uses both architectural and cytologic features but does not give details, relying on the pathologist's impression to determine grade in a three-tier system. In the USA, the Gynecologic Oncology Group employs a modified FIGO system wherein grade is determined by differing criteria depending on the epithelial subtype.[18] Silverberg and Shimizu have proposed a system of grading for all cell types, modeled on the Nottingham system for grading breast cancer, using architectural features (glandular, papillary, solid), nuclear grade and mitotic count with each scored as 1 to 3 and then the

total score determining the grade.[19] Its predictive value has been validated and proven superior to the FIGO system in at least one study.[20] Recently, Malpica et al.[21] studied serous carcinomas using a simplified two-grade system (high-grade and low-grade) and found grade to be an independent prognostic indicator in a multivariate analysis. In this study, the Silverberg and Shimizu system correlated closely with their two grades (very few Silverberg grade 2 tumors were found). The FIGO system, however, correlated poorly.

Evolving molecular and genetic analyses of ovarian carcinomas support the morphologic system used to separate the various epithelial subtypes. For the most part, these analyses correlate with differences among them at a more fundamental level. Based on this, it seems to us that a grading system ought to take into account the unique histologic features of the individual subtypes, rather than being applied across all subtypes. However, a problem in applying any grading system is that morphologic differences among carcinoma subtypes are most obvious in low-grade tumors; they become less distinct in high-grade tumors with serous, endometrioid, transitional and undifferentiated carcinomas becoming more difficult to reproducibly separate. Thus, it is likely that that a two-tier system, such as that advocated by Malpica and her associates[21] for serous tumors, would be more reproducible and clinically applicable for all epithelial subtypes than the various three-tier systems currently used.

However, until a standard two-tier system is validated and universally adopted, we adhere to the three-tier grading system as recommended by the WHO. We take into account the tumor subtype as follows: (1) We grade serous carcinomas almost entirely on the basis of their nuclear features. Accordingly, most will be grade 3 and the remainder almost all grade 1; often the latter are associated with borderline tumors.[21] (2) We grade endometrioid carcinomas as we do in the uterus, using the FIGO system of architectural grading[17] and upgrading FIGO grade I and grade 2 tumors by one grade on the basis of high nuclear grade.[18] (3) We determine whether mucinous carcinomas have infiltrative or expansile invasion. If the latter, we grade based on cytology. If there is infiltrative invasion, even focally, we grade the entire tumor based on this component using the same system as for endometrioid carcinomas. (4) Clear cell carcinomas are all high grade in theory and we rarely classify them as grade 1; we generally consider those without any solid areas as grade 2, unless the nuclear features are markedly atypical. (5) We grade transitional cell carcinomas on the basis of their nuclear features.

Serous tumors

GENERAL FEATURES AND CLINICAL ASPECTS

Serous tumors are composed of cells and patterns of growth that resemble those of the fallopian tube. They are the most common subtype of epithelial-stromal tumor. In the West, they account for about 30% of all ovarian neoplasms,[22–24] but are relatively less frequent in Asia.[11] Approximately 60% are benign, 10% borderline and 30% malignant. Benign serous tumors occur across the age spectrum but are most common in the fourth to sixth decades. The average age of patients with borderline tumors is approximately 45 years, but these tumors may occur in women in their late teens and early 20s. The average age of patients with serous carcinoma is the mid-to-late 50s;[1,23,25] they are very rare in teenagers and uncommon in patients under 30 years old.

About 70% of patients with serous borderline tumors have no evidence of spread beyond the ovary at the time of initial staging; the disease-free survival in these patients is 98.2%.[26] The remaining 30% of patients have pelvic and/or abdominal peritoneal implants upon initial staging. These account for the great majority that suffer serious morbidity or death. However, in marked contrast to serous carcinomas, only 15–30% of these higher-stage tumors recur and, even when they do, many of them still do not cause harm. Thus, over the past 30 years, the primary focus of research on serous borderline tumors has been to discover predictors of a poor outcome in these higher-stage cases. Studies have examined the prognostic significance of: the histopathologic features of the primary tumor,[27,28] the morphology of the implants,[29–31] lymph node metastases,[32–35] minor foci of invasion in the ovarian tumor,[36–39] flow cytometry,[40,41] and p53 expression in the tumor cells.[42]

By the 1990s it had been generally accepted that the only finding that predicted prognosis in higher-stage serous borderline tumors was the type of extra-ovarian peritoneal implants: whether they were 'invasive' or 'noninvasive'. The 7-year disease-free survival in patients with noninvasive implants is 95.3%; with invasive implants it is 66%.[26]

However, criteria to distinguish the two types of implants were not always the same in the various studies that assessed their predictive value. For this reason and because experience with this distinction by most pathologists is limited, it has been difficult to apply these criteria in clinical cases. In addition, since the mid-1990s, other features, particularly the morphology of the primary tumor, have been revisited and have provoked additional controversies and difficulties, such that the evaluation of serous borderline tumors has become rather complex and is currently in a state of flux. The various issues and current recommendations are addressed below in the microscopic description of borderline tumors.

Serous carcinomas account for 39% to 62% of all epithelial-stromal carcinomas.[22–25,43] Approximately 15% are stage I, 6% stage II, 49 % stage III and 30% stage IV.[44] Five-year disease-free survival in stages I and II combined is in the 80% range, whereas overall survival in stages III and IV is about 20%.[45] These statistics apply primarily to high-grade serous carcinomas, which constitute the great majority of cases. It has been recognized only recently that low-grade serous carcinomas may be fundamentally different in their pathogenesis and natural history. This subject is addressed below in the sections on the microscopic description and etiology of serous carcinomas.

GROSS EXAMINATION

Benign serous tumors are bilateral in 10–20% of cases. Most are either partially or completely cystic. A cystadenoma is arbitrarily distinguished from a cortical inclusion cyst if it exceeds 1 cm in diameter.[11] Entirely cystic tumors may be unilocular or multilocular. Most of them range from 3 to 10 cm and are oval with a smooth, shiny surface. The cyst cavity is usually filled with watery or pale yellow fluid, but it is sometimes viscous and mucoid. The internal cyst lining is smooth. Adenofibromas contain solid areas that range from multiple smooth, knobby papillae lining the surface of a cyst, to confluent firm white to pale yellow areas that may contain smaller cysts (Fig. 27.1), to tumors that are essentially entirely solid-appearing.

Serous borderline tumors are bilateral in about 25% of cases. They are usually partly cystic with watery or mucinous cyst fluid and contain intracystic and/or surface soft white to tan cauliflower-like papillary projections (Fig. 27.2). The papillae are usually more extensive than the firmer, smooth, bosselated papillae of benign tumors. However, one cannot reliably predict the histologic findings on the basis of the gross appearance and frozen section examination of either type of projection is warranted. Sometimes borderline tumors are limited to surface excrescences on an otherwise normal-appearing ovary.

Serous carcinomas are bilateral in approximately 70% of cases. They range from a few cm up to approximately 20 cm. They are much more variable grossly than benign or borderline tumors. Most are both cystic and solid, with a variable predominance of one or the other. The surface may be smooth or contain papillary projections. There may be intracystic or surface papillary areas similar to those of borderline tumors, but often these areas are more lush and extensive. The solid regions are soft and tan and may have areas of hemorrhage and necrosis (Fig. 27.3). Rare carcinomas are almost entirely confined to the surface, sometimes appearing as velvety patches or hard plaques[11] (Fig. 27.4).

EXAMINATION OF PROPHYLACTIC OOPHORECTOMY SPECIMENS FROM HIGH-RISK PATIENTS

Very small serous carcinomas may be present in grossly normal ovaries or fallopian tubes of women with a high risk for ovarian cancer. In 60 grossly normal bilateral

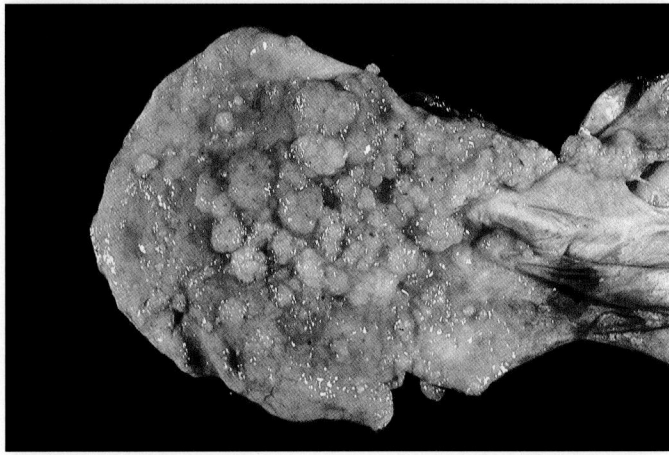

Fig. 27.2 Serous borderline tumor. An opened cyst contains myriad small papillae.

adnexal specimens from high-risk women, five occult carcinomas were found (three ovarian, two tubal) (Fig. 27.5). All five patients had BRCA1 mutations.[46] In another report, seven occult carcinomas, five of which occurred in the fallopian tube, were found in women with suspected or proven BRCA1 or BRCA2 mutations. In two of these cases a positive peritoneal washing, the only initial finding, led to additional fallopian tube tissue being submitted, where the cancers were eventually found.[47] These reports emphasize the importance of obtaining cytologic washings and sectioning the entire ovaries and fallopian tubes from all prophylactic oophorectomy specimens. We breadloaf these specimens at 1–2 mm intervals, and sagittally section the distal fallopian tubes.

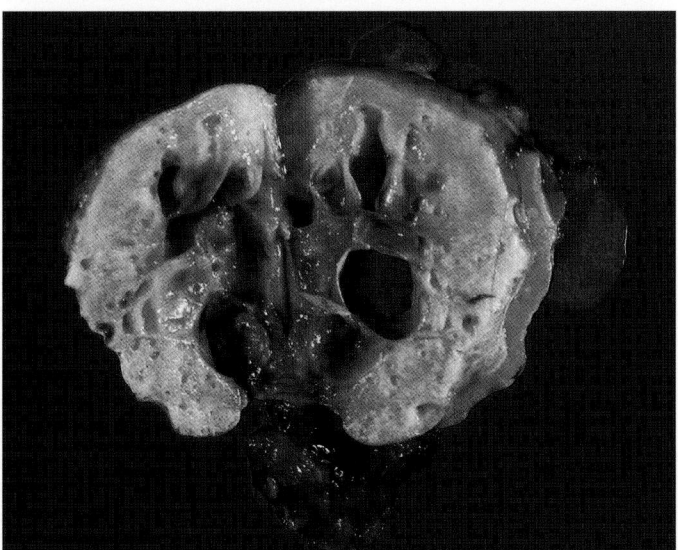

Fig. 27.1 Serous cystadenofibroma. The tumor was egg-shaped. In this bivalved cross-section it is fibrous with small cysts in the interior and on the surface.

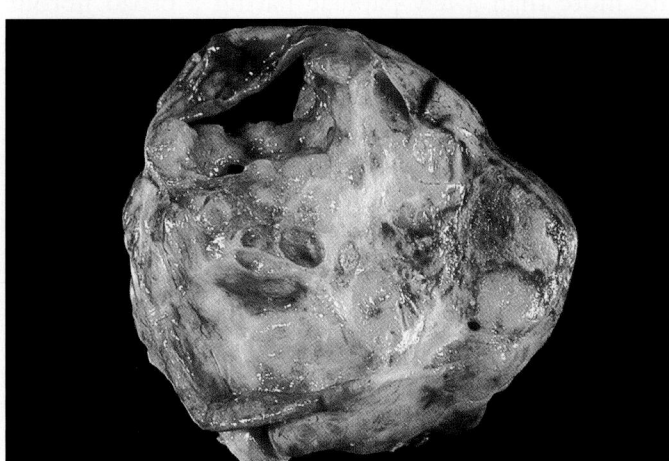

Fig. 27.3 Serous carcinoma. The cut surface is mostly solid, soft and tan.

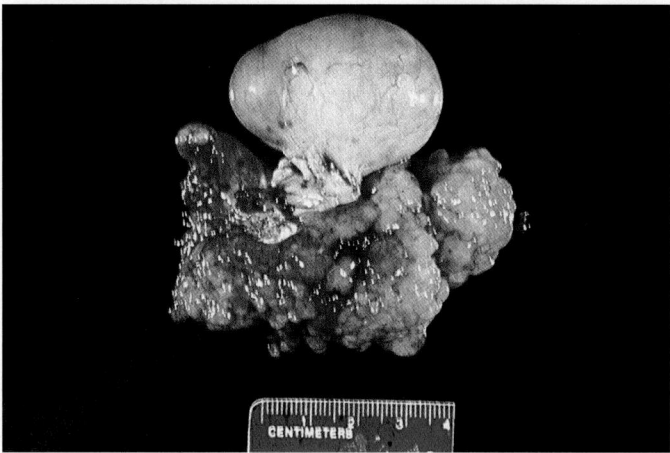

Fig. 27.4 Serous surface carcinoma. The tumor is attached to the ovary (above) only at one pole.

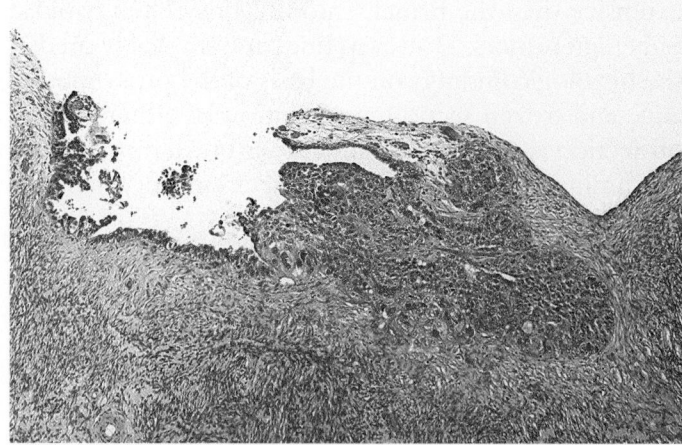

Fig. 27.5 Occult high-grade carcinoma in a prophylactic oophorectomy specimen. The tumor occupies the superficial cortex and extends along the adjacent surface. The entire tumor is present in this field.

MICROSCOPIC FINDINGS

Benign serous tumors – cystadenomas, cystadenofibromas, adenofibromas, papillary adenofibromas, surface papillary adenofibromas

The appropriate term for each of the various benign serous tumors depends on the relative proportion of the cystic and solid components and whether or not the tumor is confined primarily to the surface of the ovary. The 'cyst' prefix is generally used if there are grossly observable cysts. The amount of fibrous stroma required to distinguish a cystadenoma from a cystadenofibroma is arbitrary, since a small amount of stroma surrounds the cyst lining even in tumors that are purely cystic on gross examination. We use the 'fibroma' suffix if there are more than a few papillae having a broad fibrous stromal core (Fig. 27.6). Surface papillary adenofibromas are lesions in which a confluent polypoid growth coats the external surface of the ovary. Small polypoid surface irregularities are commonly present on the ovaries and do not qualify as surface papillary adenofibromas.

The glands, cysts and broad-based papillae of benign serous tumors are lined by focally ciliated columnar epithelium with limited stratification. The epithelial cells have scant eosinophilic or pale cytoplasm and oval to elongated nuclei, some with small nucleoli and with rare or no mitotic figures (Fig. 27.7). The stroma is fibrous-appearing, variably cellular and may be focally calcified. In some adenofibromas the epithelium is cuboidal and without cilia, resembling the ovarian surface epithelium. These cases are customarily included in the serous category.

In some cases the epithelial cells are slightly stratified and one is faced with the distinction between a benign and a borderline tumor. Although there are no strict criteria for this distinction, there should be more than a small focus with hierarchical branching of the papillae, pronounced epithelial cell stratification and budding

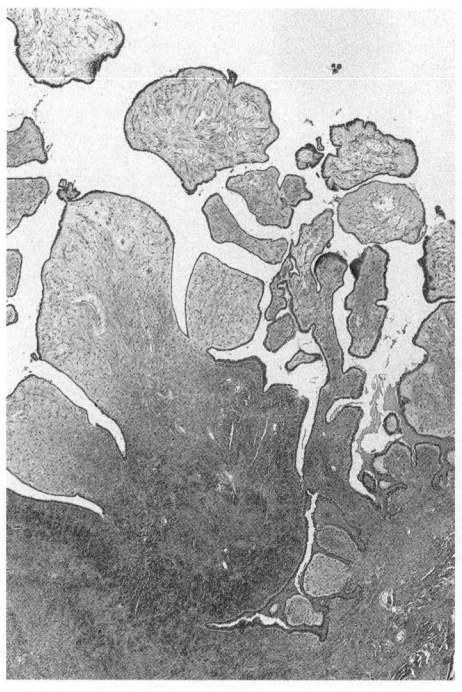

Fig. 27.6 Serous papillary adenofibroma. Broad fibrous papillae project into a cystic space.

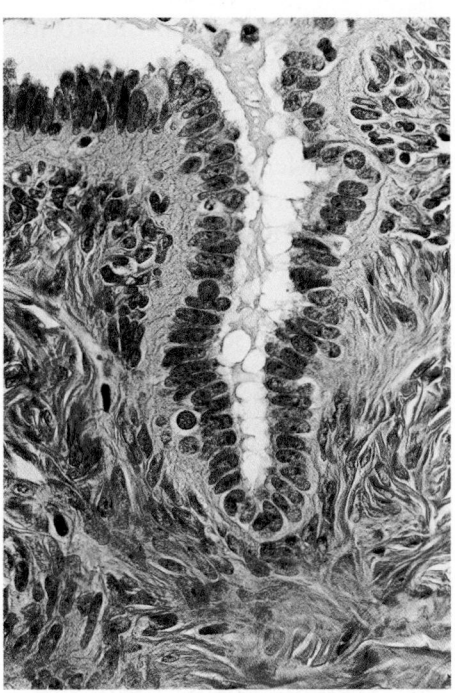

Fig. 27.7 Serous papillary adenofibroma. The epithelial cells are columnar, nonstratified and benign-appearing.

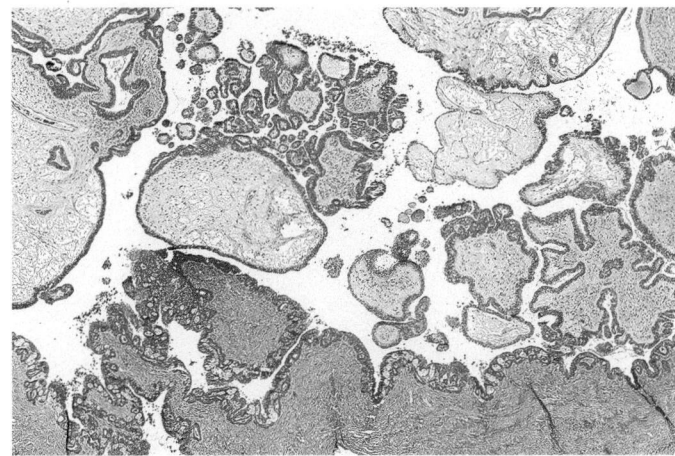

Fig. 27.8 Serous borderline tumor. Broad, edematous papillae with numerous smaller daughter papillae project into a cystic space.

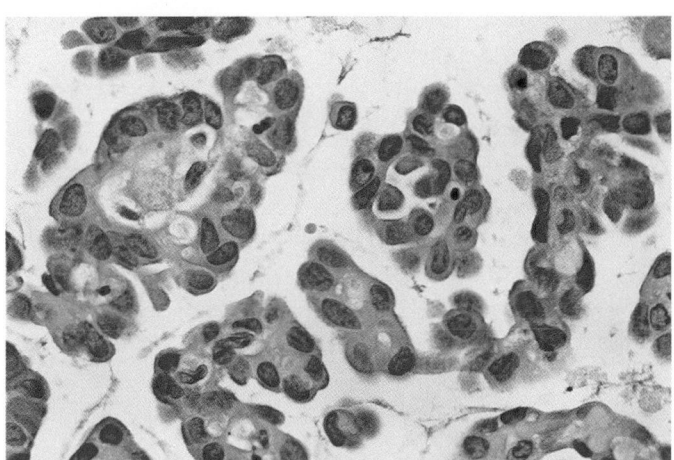

Fig. 27.9 Serous borderline tumor. Bland epithelial cells around the smaller papillae appear to be free-floating in the extracellular space.

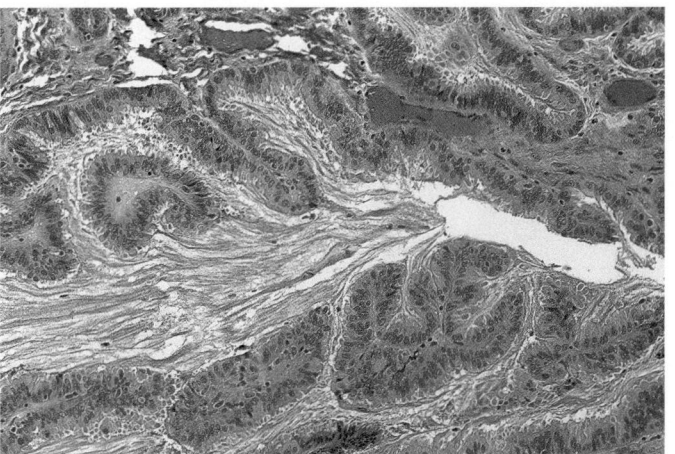

Fig. 27.10 Serous borderline tumor. Stringy mucinous material occupies the extracellular space around the papillae.

of cells into the extrapapillary space before a borderline tumor is considered. We designate tumors with a few foci with minimal stratification and budding as cystadenomas with focal atypia.

Serous borderline tumors

Diagnosis

Serous borderline tumors are characterized by broad, branching papillae focally covered with highly stratified epithelial cells, some of which appear to be free-floating in the extracellular space (Figs 27.8, 27.9). This space is usually clear, but may contain mucin (Fig. 27.10). The epithelial cells are polygonal or columnar, with eosinophilic cytoplasm that is sometimes ciliated or has surface blebs (Figs 27.9, 27.11). In some cases the cytoplasm is abundant, especially in tumors from pregnant women (Figs 27.12, 27.13).[48] Nuclear atypia varies between and within cases from mild to moderate, but it is generally less severe than that of low-grade serous carcinomas (Figs 27.9, 27.11, 27.13). Mitotic figures are infrequent. The stroma is fibrous and variably cellular; it may be edematous, particularly in the papillary cores. There may be few or many psammoma bodies. Benign-appearing areas, either cystadenomatous or adenofibromatous, are often present and may account for the majority of the tumor.

Borderline tumors are distinguished from low-grade carcinomas by the absence of stromal invasion. Due to oblique sectioning of complex papillae, there are areas

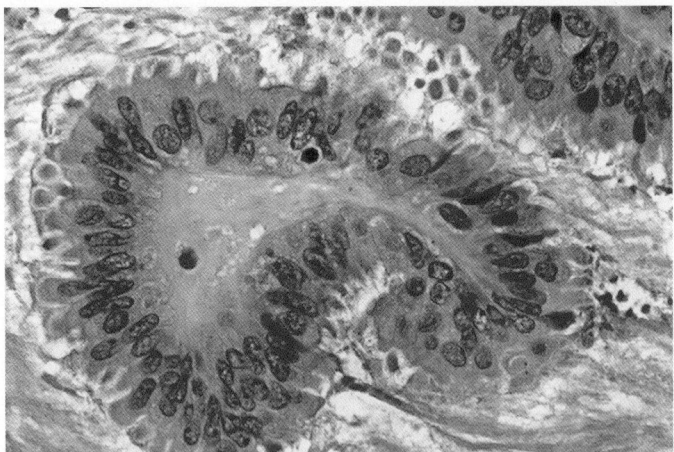

Fig. 27.11 Serous borderline tumor. Bland columnar cells with surface blebs surround the papilla.

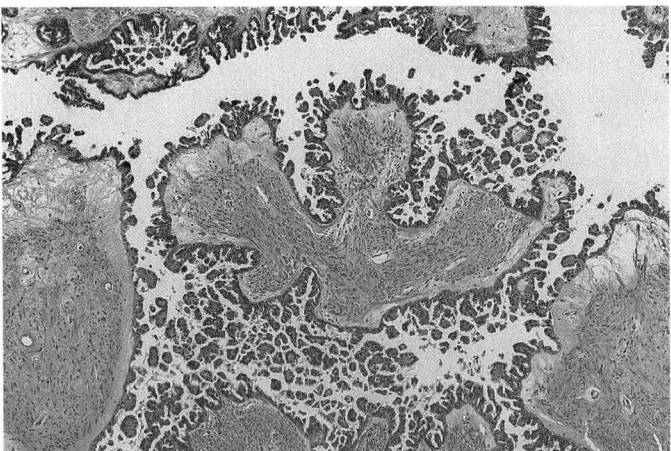

Fig. 27.12 Serous borderline tumor in a pregnant woman. There is exuberant epithelial growth around the papillae.

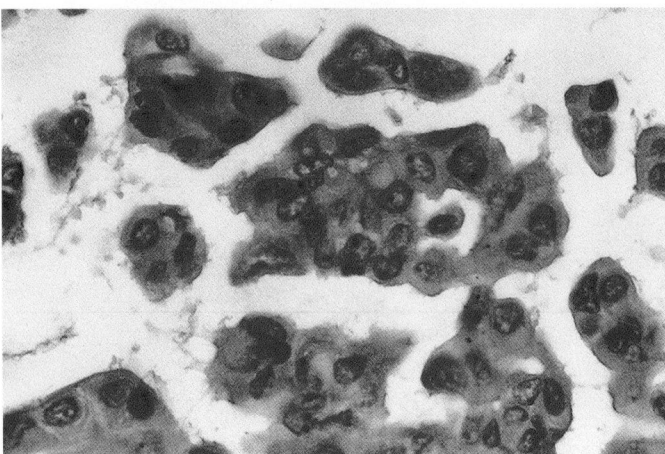

Fig. 27.13 Serous borderline tumor in a pregnant woman. The epithelial cells are large with abundant eosinophilic cytoplasm.

where epithelial cells are included within the stroma. This appearance should not be mistaken for invasion, as there is no stromal reaction and one can easily conceptualize the included areas as secondary to the plane of section. It must be acknowledged that, aside from tumors that have the micropapillary/cribriform patterns described below, there are occasional low-grade serous tumors that lack obvious stromal invasion but have a particularly exuberant epithelial growth pattern.[11] Experienced pathologists may differ on whether to interpret these as borderline tumors or as low-grade serous carcinomas.

Having diagnosed a serous borderline tumor, the pathologist needs to consider five possible additional findings: (1) surface involvement, (2) stromal microinvasion, (3) a micropapillary/cribriform growth pattern, (4) nodal metastases and (5) invasive or noninvasive peritoneal implants. The last of these is the most important, as it will largely determine the prognosis and is a key factor in decisions regarding further treatment.

Surface involvement has been associated with a higher frequency of peritoneal implants.[49] Its exclusion depends on a careful gross examination and orientation such that the surface is evident on the slide, usually by its being inked. The presence or absence of surface involvement should be included in the final report.

Assessing stromal invasion

Most serous borderline tumors are homogeneous. However, generous and judicious sampling is required to exclude focal areas of invasion. In most cases this requires at least one section per cm of tumor diameter. Small areas of invasion consist either of dyshesive eosinophilic cells in the cores of the papillae (Fig. 27.14) or small aggregates of cells with a cribriform or microcystic pattern, usually with a reactive-appearing stroma (Fig. 27.15). Invasive foci measuring less than 10 mm² and less than 3 mm in greatest dimension are present in up to 10% of cases.[36,37] These should be reported as foci of microinvasion. Microinvasion does not alter the overall designation as a borderline tumor, since it has not been shown to alter behavior. Vascular space invasion has also been observed in a few cases with microinvasion, but thus far has not been demonstrated to worsen the prognosis.

Sometimes the surface of the tumor or the lining of a cyst may have plaques of reactive-appearing fibrous stroma containing psammoma bodies and epithelial cells lying singly or in small groups. These have a 'stuck on' appearance and are identical to extraovarian

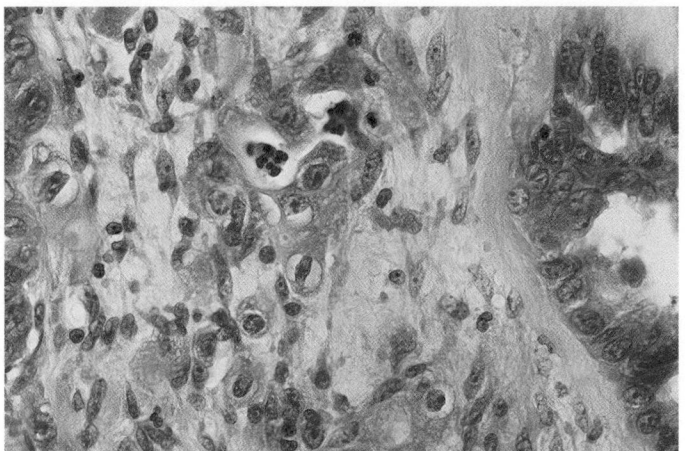

Fig. 27.14 Microinvasion in a serous borderline tumor. Several round cells, some with a peripheral space, percolate through the stroma of a papilla. As in this example, they are often inconspicuous and easily overlooked. They may be highlighted with a keratin stain.

Micropapillary/cribriform architecture

Women with serous borderline tumors that contain extensive areas of micropapillary and/or cribriform epithelial overgrowth have an increased frequency of bilateral tumors and invasive peritoneal implants, with the attendant risk of the latter for subsequent recurrence and death (see below). In the micropapillary pattern, epithelial cells surround a prominent, nonbranching fibrous stalk and protrude radially as long, thin micropapillae without stromal cores so that the low-power appearance resembles a Medusa head (Fig. 27.16). When the micropapillae merge, they take on a ramifying cribriform appearance (Fig. 27.17). The epithelial cells are monomorphous and 'clonal-appearing' with scant cytoplasm. They are mostly cuboidal, but may also have a hobnail, columnar, or flattened appearance.

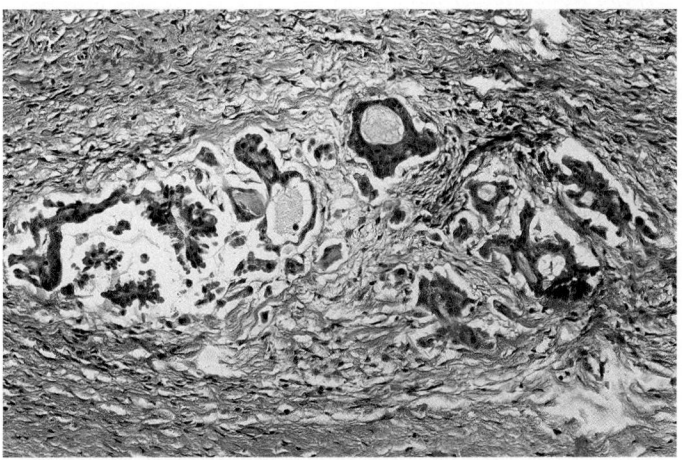

Fig. 27.15 Microinvasion in a serous borderline tumor. Irregular epithelial islands in a reactive-appearing stroma.

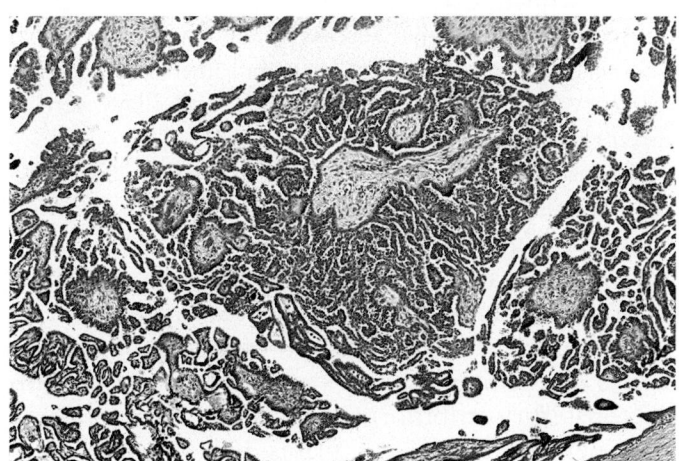

Fig. 27.16 Micropapillary growth pattern in a serous borderline tumor. Long slender papillae radiate from a large central core.

noninvasive desmoplastic implants (see below). These 'auto implants' are associated with an increased frequency of high-stage tumors, but they do not alter the prognosis in stage I and are not currently considered to represent invasion.

A borderline tumor with invasive areas that are larger than microinvasive should be reported as a low-grade serous carcinoma associated with a serous borderline tumor. Patients with these tumors often have invasive extraovarian implants and a high mortality, albeit sometimes only after many years.[21,50–52]

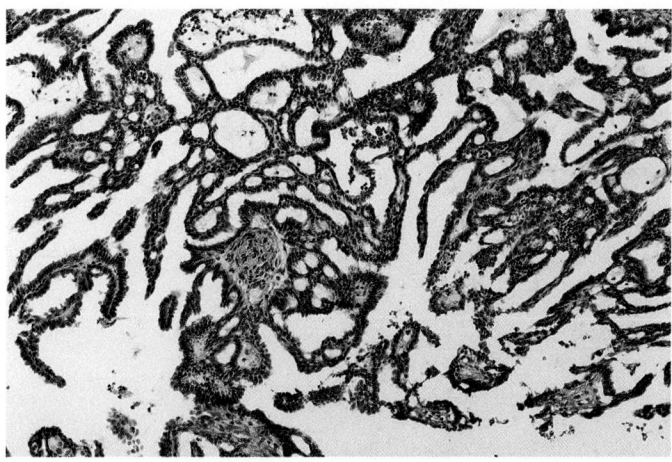

Fig. 27.17 Cribriform growth pattern in a serous borderline tumor. Complex ramifying cords and slim papillae are evident.

Nuclei are round and slightly more hyperchromatic than in the usual borderline tumor (Fig. 27.18).[53]

In a study examining 400 borderline tumors and well-differentiated carcinomas, 17 borderline tumors had micropapillary/cribriform foci at least 5 mm in extent. Of the 13 patients with follow-up data in this group, three had no implants and none recurred; three had noninvasive implants and one had a recurrence; six had invasive implants (defined so as to include micropapillarity in the implant itself as invasive), four of these patients had a recurrence and two died of their tumors.[53]

In a companion study of 65 advanced-stage borderline tumors, 11 ovarian tumors had micropapillary/cribriform areas, in 10 of which there were invasive implants. Seven of the 10 patients had recurrences and four died of their tumors.[54] The frequency of invasive implants and recurrences in this group was much greater than in the remaining cases. Because of these findings and subsequent correlative molecular analyses,[55,56] these authors concluded that serous borderline tumors with micropapillary/cribriform areas belong in a separate category that they designated 'micropapillary serous carcinoma'.

Four subsequent studies of tumors with micropapillary/cribriform areas totaling 59 cases[39,57–59] recorded noninvasive implants in 28 cases, three of which recurred and invasive implants in five cases, all of which recurred. There were no recurrences in the 26 cases without implants. Another study of 99 advanced-stage serous borderline tumors contained 18 cases with micropapillary/cribriform areas. Only three of these 18 patients had invasive implants, but 14 of them had disease progression or recurrence and five of them died. This compared with 25 recurrences and 12 deaths

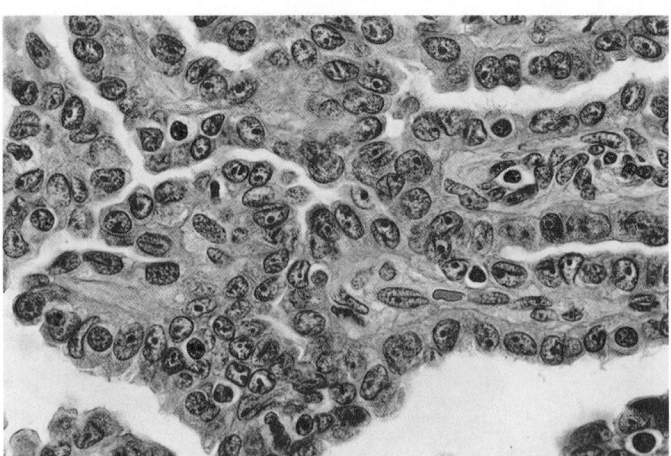

Fig. 27.18 Micropapillary growth pattern in a serous borderline tumor. The nuclei are monomorphous. In this case they are vesicular with small nucleoli.

in 81 patients without micropapillary/cribriform areas in their ovarian tumors.[60]

Taken together, these observations indicate that patients with micropapillary/cribriform foci in a serous borderline tumor have a higher risk than those with ordinary serous borderline tumors for both non-invasive and invasive implants and thus for subsequent recurrence. However, patients with stage I borderline tumors with micropapillary/cribriform foci have the same low risk as those with ordinary borderline tumors. Therefore, until more data are accrued, we adhere to the WHO classification by placing these cases in the borderline category rather than calling them micropapillary serous carcinomas. However, we section cases with micropapillary/cribriform areas thoroughly to exclude invasion within the ovarian tumor and we extensively sample the omentum. Moreover, we append a note to the diagnostic report indicating the presence of micropapillary/cribriform foci.

Lymph node metastases

Pelvic and paraortic lymph node metastases are found in up to 20% of cases in which nodes are examined.[32–35] These metastases are present in sinusoidal spaces, rather than in the substance of the node, distinguishing them from Müllerian rests (endosalpingiosis) that may also be present. The presence of lymph node metastases has not been shown to alter the prognosis of serous borderline tumors.[35] However, lymph nodes are not examined in many cases and the true significance of nodal metastases of serous borderline tumors is not known.

Assessment of peritoneal implants

Introduction Peritoneal deposits are present in approximately 30% of cases of ovarian serous borderline tumors.[26] Tumors with surface involvement are associated with a much higher frequency of these foci than those without surface involvement,[49] which suggests that the extraovarian deposits are derived from the ovarian tumor. Thus, by convention they are designated as 'implants'. However, the following observations indicate that at least some of them are independent *in situ* peritoneal lesions: (1) Borderline tumors can arise in the peritoneum without any ovarian involvement.[61] (2) X chromosome inactivation studies, comparing the implants with the ovarian tumor, have documented clonality differences between them.[62,63] (3) Rarely, low-grade serous carcinomas develop in the abdomen following borderline serous tumors that are confined to the ovaries at initial staging, often after many years.[64] (4) p53 and K-ras mutations in ovarian borderline tumors and subsequent peritoneal serous carcinomas tend to differ, suggesting that the carcinomas and the borderline tumors arise independently.[65] In this sense, one might think of a serous borderline tumor as a marker for a patient at increased risk for the development of peritoneal carcinoma, rather than the cause of it, at least in some cases.

Regardless of their derivation, the presence of peritoneal implants and whether or not they are invasive are the most important indicators of outcome in serous borderline tumors.

Implants *vs* benign mimics Implants must be distinguished from florid mesothelial hyperplastic reactions,[66] which may form gland-like structures, contain psammoma bodies and be associated with a fibrous reaction, similar to true implants. Mesothelial cell nuclei are paler than epithelial cell nuclei and when lining a surface hyperplastic mesothelial cells often have a hobnail arrangement with spaces between them (Fig. 27.19). Although usually not necessary, a positive calretinin stain will confirm their mesothelial nature.

Glandular, cystic, or small papillary inclusions, sometimes with psammoma bodies, are not uncommonly present on peritoneal surfaces, in lymph nodes,[67] and in the omentum[68] (Fig. 27.20) in women with or without borderline tumors. Although some have questioned the benign nature of these foci in lymph nodes,[69] their presence has not been shown to alter the prognosis of a serous borderline tumor and they should not be diagnosed as implants or metastases.[70] True implants have a more exuberant and complex epithelial cell proliferation than do these foci of endosalpingiosis.

Invasive *vs* noninvasive implants Implants may or may not invade pelvic or abdominal structures. On the basis of this distinction, implants are divided into invasive and noninvasive types. These may coexist. Criteria

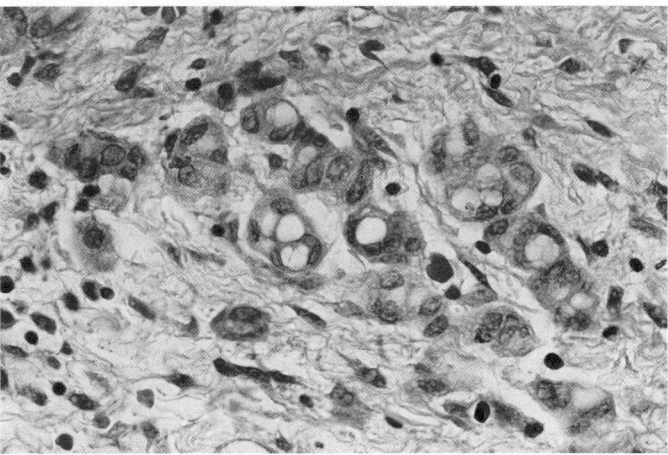

Fig. 27.19 Reactive mesothelial cells in the peritoneum. The formation of small gland-like structures and cytoplasmic vacuoles is distracting, but the nuclei are bland.

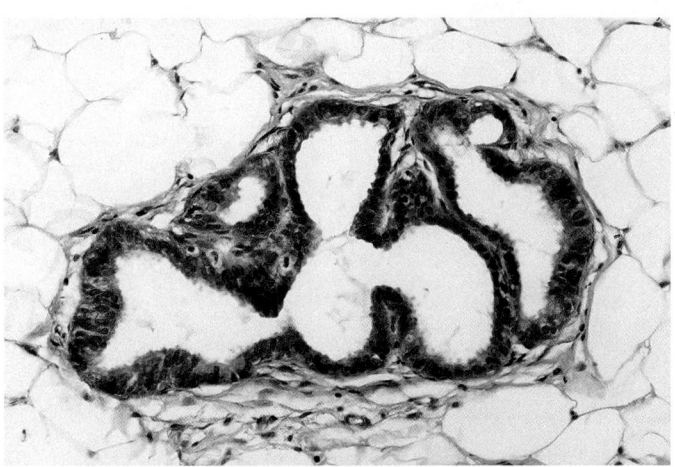

Fig. 27.20 Omentum with endosalpingiosis. There is benign Müllerian inclusion without papillarity or nuclear atypia within the omental fat.

to distinguish the implant types are given below and summarized in Table 27.1.

Noninvasive implants consist of two subtypes, epithelial and desmoplastic. *Epithelial implants* are composed

---

Table 27.1 Invasive versus noninvasive implants of serous borderline tumors

Noninvasive[a]		Invasive	
Epithelial	**Desmoplastic**	**Accepted criteria[13]**	**Proposed additional qualifying criteria[31]**
Papillary epithelium similar to that of the usual borderline tumor in submesothelial invaginations or between lobules of adipose tissue	Papillae, glands, cell clusters, or single cells within inflamed, reactive-appearing fibrous tissue that appears to be 'plastered on' to serosal surfaces or in fibrous septae of adipose tissue	Proliferative epithelium resembling low-grade serous carcinoma invading abdominal/pelvic organs or omental fat, usually with a desmoplastic reaction and an infiltrative margin.	Micropapillary architecture whether or not there is obvious invasion, or solid epithelial nests with surrounding clefts in a fibrous stroma

[a]If underlying tissue is not present in the biopsy, the implant is considered noninvasive.

of papillae resembling those within a borderline tumor. They are found either in mesothelial-lined invaginations of a peritoneal surface or between lobules of fat (Fig. 27.21). *Desmoplastic noninvasive implants* consist of single cells, small epithelial islands, papillae, or cribriform glands encased in stroma, usually with inflammatory cells and psammoma bodies. The entire implant appears well circumscribed and has a 'plastered on', rather than invasive appearance (Fig. 27.22). Early in their evolution desmoplastic noninvasive implants may appear necrotic and inflammatory.[11]

Invasive implants are composed of cells and cell patterns similar to those of well-differentiated serous carcinomas. They are almost always associated with stromal desmoplasia but, in addition, have an irregular, infiltrative-appearing border. They appear to invade underlying structures or replace fatty tissue rather than sitting indolently on the peritoneal surface or between fat lobules (Fig. 27.23).

If underlying tissue is absent in a biopsy, the lesion is classified as noninvasive by default.[11] However, because this is a frequent scenario, one report of implant morphology added the findings of either a micropapillary pattern alone or solid epithelial nests surrounded by clear spaces or clefts in a fibrous stroma (Fig. 27.24) as sufficient to consider an implant invasive in the absence of an obvious infiltrative pattern.[31] Using their expanded criteria, these authors found

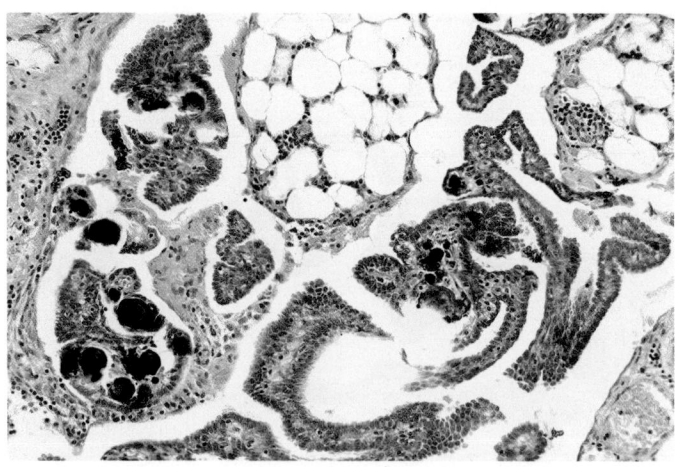

Fig. 27.21 Epithelial, noninvasive implant of a serous borderline tumor. Papillae with psammoma bodies, similar to those of an ovarian borderline tumor, appear to be free-floating in the interstices of the omental fat. There is no stromal reaction.

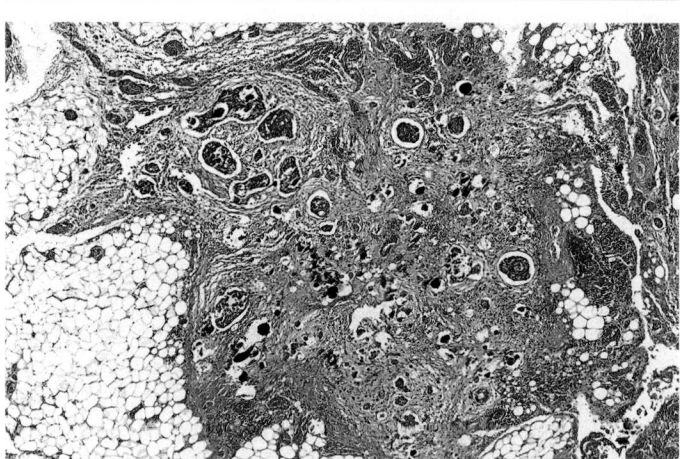

Fig. 27.23 Invasive implant from a serous borderline tumor. Numerous epithelial islands are present in a fibrous and edematous stroma. The lesion appears to be expanding into and replacing the omental fat.

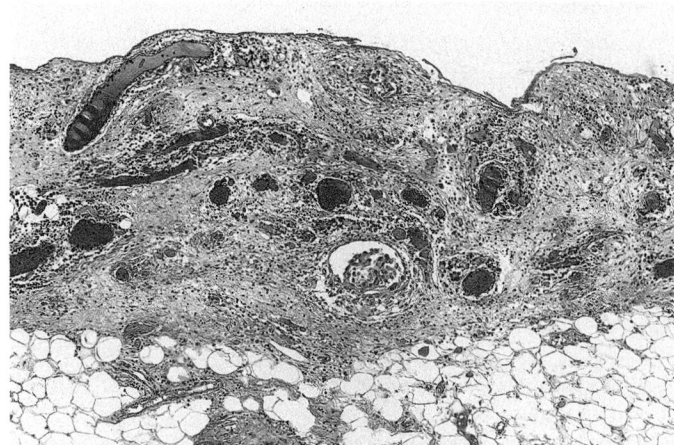

Fig. 27.22 Desmoplastic noninvasive implant from a serous borderline tumor. Two small islands of epithelial cells are present in a fibrovascular stroma that appears 'plastered on' to the surface of the omentum.

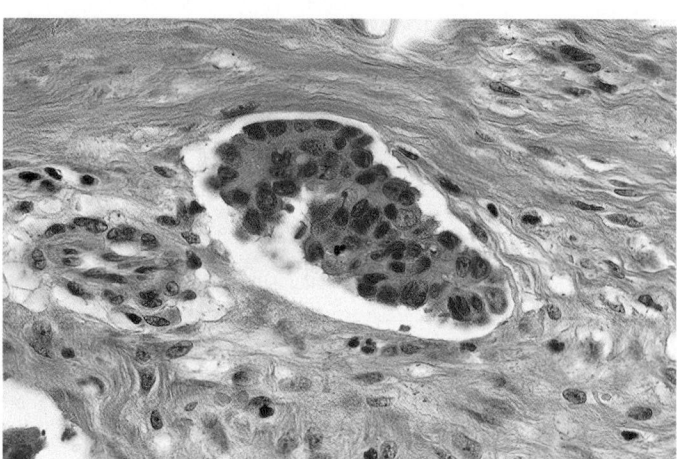

Fig. 27.24 Peritoneal implant with retraction artifact from a serous borderline tumor. This finding, by itself, is considered evidence of invasion by some authors.

that of 60 patients with implants, 31 had the invasive type. Nineteen of these 31 patients had progressive disease and six of them died. Of the 29 remaining patients, three had progression and two died. A caveat is that 27 of the 60 patients (45%) had micropapillary/cribriform areas in their primary tumor. This is a higher frequency than was found in two other studies of high-stage borderline tumors (where micropapillary/cribriform foci were present in only 21% of 146 ovarian tumors),[60,71] indicating that case selection may have skewed the data towards the finding of micropapillary foci in the implants. Nevertheless, these results suggest that an expanded definition of invasive implants, if confirmed in other studies, is warranted.

Serous carcinomas

On the basis of their nuclear features, almost all serous carcinomas can be divided into low-grade and high-grade types (grade 1 or grade 3), with the latter constituting the great majority of cases.

Low-grade serous carcinomas are often associated with serous borderline tumors (Fig. 27.25); they are extensively papillary and often contain many psammoma bodies. The papillae may project into a space (Fig. 27.26) or be embedded in a fibrous stroma that may also contain glands, cysts, irregular islands of tumor cells, or cribriform glands (Fig. 27.27). Often the invasive papillae are surrounded by a clear space, possibly caused by fluid secreted by tumor cells (Fig. 27.24). Nuclei are uniform, round or oval with evenly distributed chromatin, with or without a prominent nucleolus (Fig. 27.28). The mitotic index is usually <10 per 10 high-power fields. A variant of low-grade carcinoma, 'psammocarcinoma', contains a marked preponderance

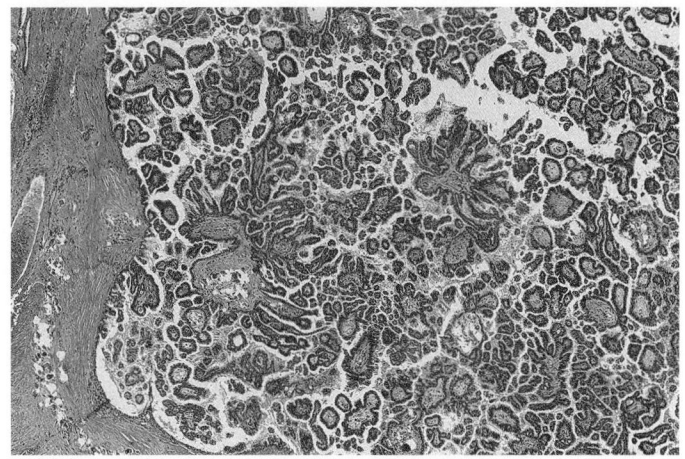

Fig. 27.26 Low-grade papillary serous carcinoma. The extensive proliferation of epithelium and small size of the papillae differ from a borderline tumor.

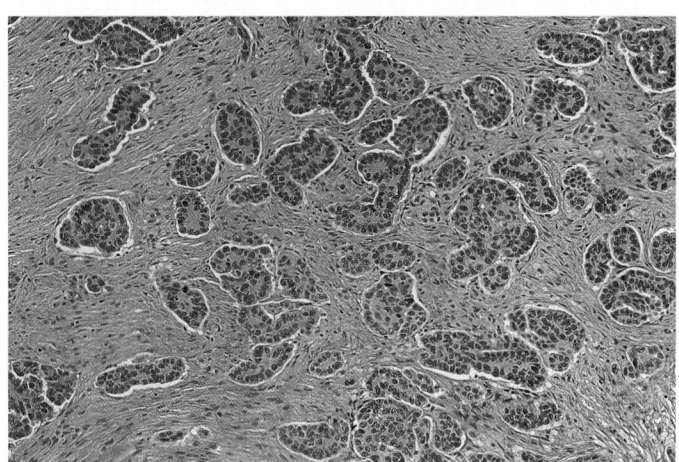

Fig. 27.27 Low-grade serous carcinoma. In this case the tumor is solid with papillae embedded in a desmoplastic stroma.

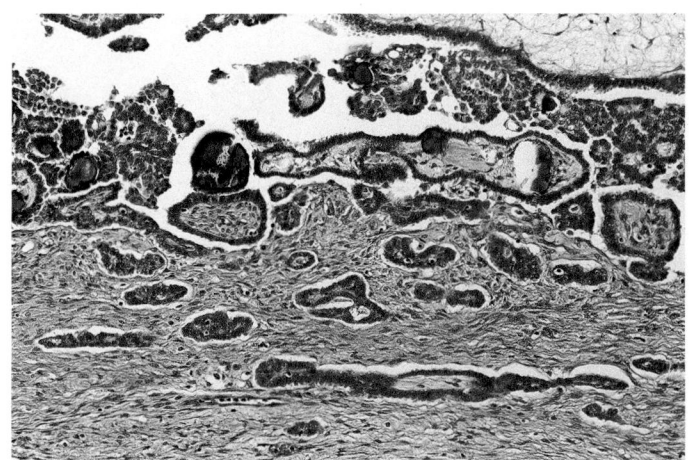

Fig. 27.25 Low-grade serous carcinoma arising in a serous borderline tumor. An invasive focus underlies the borderline tumor above.

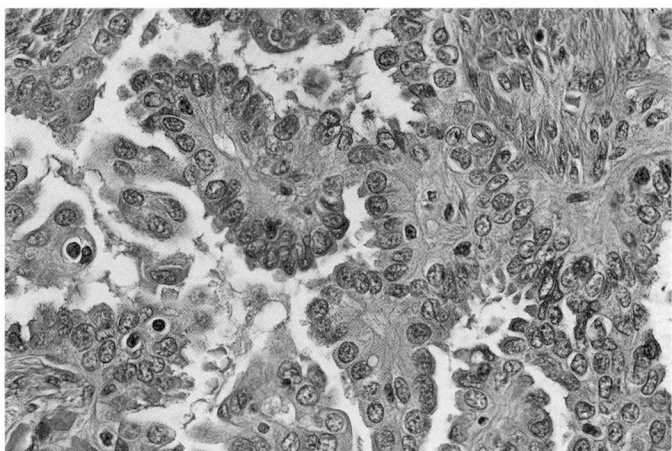

Fig. 27.28 Low-grade papillary serous carcinoma. The papillae are lined by nuclei with only slight atypia. Mitotic figures are absent in this field.

of psammoma bodies to the point where the epithelial cells may be overlooked.[72] Peritoneal metastases from a psammocarcinoma can mimic adhesions or non-invasive implants from a borderline tumor, except for the finding of invasion into underlying tissues.

We very infrequently encounter grade 2 serous carcinomas. They may or may not have an associated borderline component. Nuclei are intermediate between grades 1 and 3 (Fig. 27.29). High-grade serous carcinomas contain enlarged, pleomorphic nuclei, usually with prominent nucleoli and many mitoses. Sometimes bizarre pleomorphic cells and abnormal mitotic figures are present (Figs 27.30–27.32). Papillae may be frequent or sparse, small, or large (Fig. 27.33). Incompletely papillary foci with slit-like fenestrations are common (Fig. 27.34). The stroma is fibrous, desmoplastic, edematous, or myxoid. Psammoma bodies may be plentiful, infrequent, or absent. There may be extensive necrosis. Variations include: foci of squamous differentiation,[73] osseous metaplasia,[74] intracytoplasmic lumina with mucinous inclusions,[75] a microcystic appearance (Fig. 27.35),[76] intracellular or extracellular hyaline globules,[77] multinucleated cells sometimes resembling syncytiotrophoblasts (often B-hCG positive),[11] an adenoid cystic-like pattern,[78] a yolk sac tumor-like reticular pattern[11] and mural nodules of sarcoma or anaplastic carcinoma.[79,80]

In some tumors the serous foci blend with an endometrioid or transitional pattern.[81] We do not designate these as 'mixed epithelial' unless these foci are distinct from the serous component and constitute at least 10% of the tumor area. Similarly, we include solid tumors that have only a minor serous component in the serous rather than the 'undifferentiated' category.

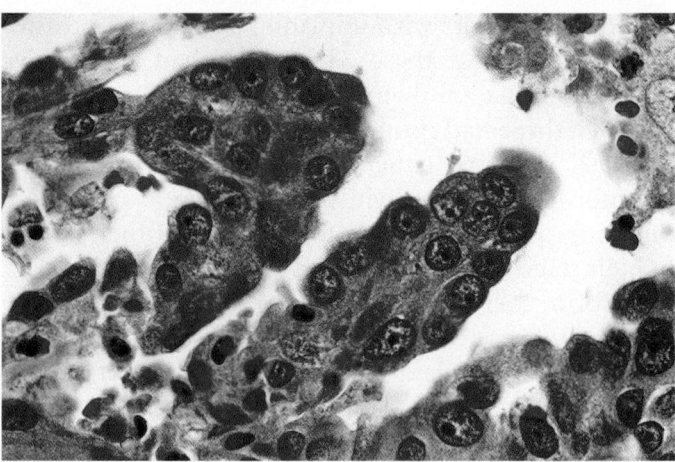

Fig. 27.30 High-grade serous carcinoma. The nuclei are large with prominent nucleoli. Figures 27.30–27.32 illustrate the spectrum of pleomorphism within high-grade serous tumors.

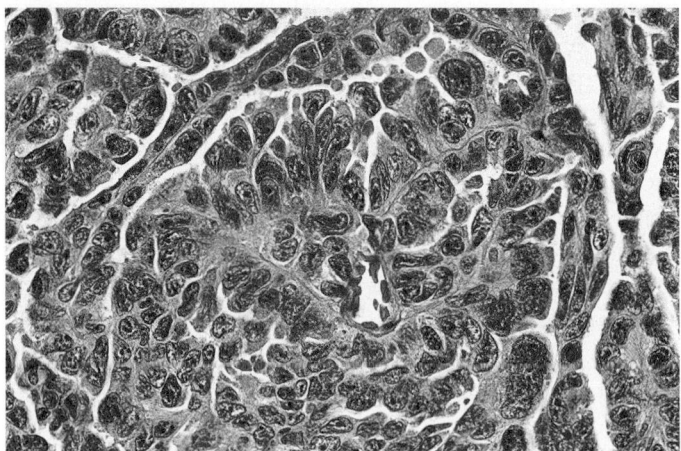

Fig. 27.31 A high-grade serous carcinoma. This figure illustrates a moderate degree of pleomorphism.

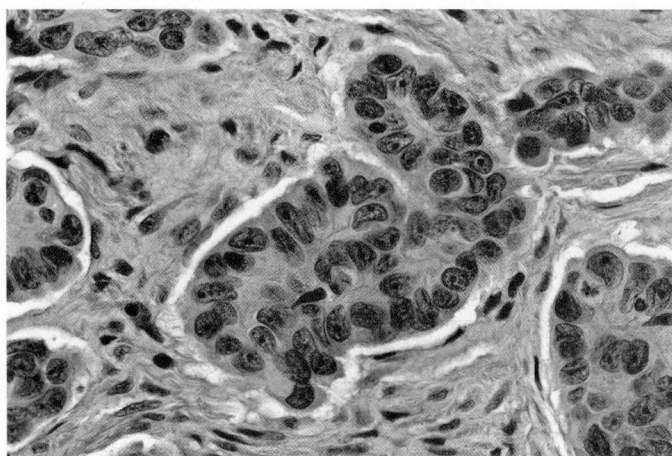

Fig. 27.29 Moderately differentiated (grade 2) serous carcinoma. The nuclei fall on a spectrum between those of Figures 27.28 and 27.30.

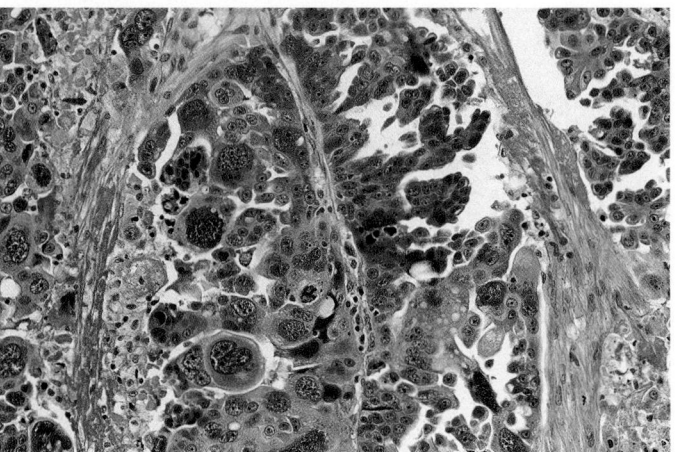

Fig. 27.32 A further example of a high-grade serous carcinoma. In this case there is extreme pleomorphism with bizarre, convoluted nuclear shapes.

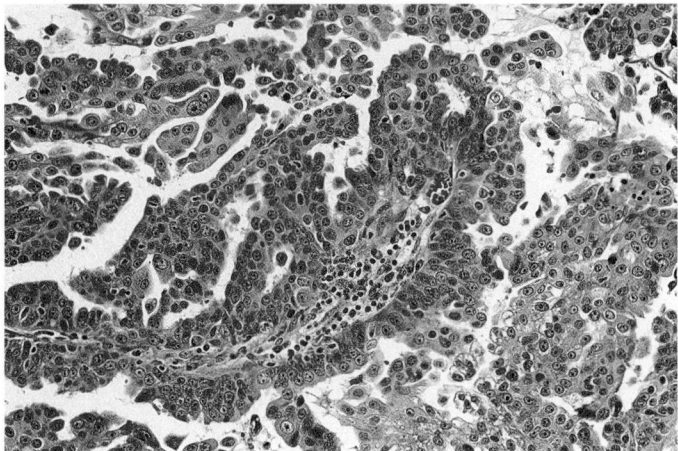

Fig. 27.33 Papillary serous carcinoma. Papillary architecture and high-grade nuclei are evident.

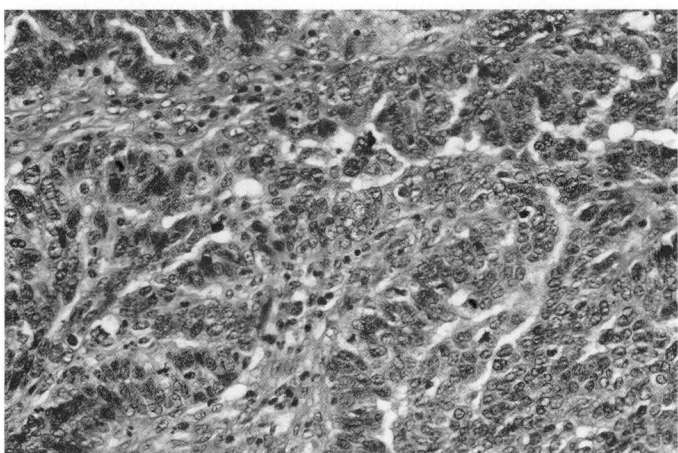

Fig. 27.34 Papillary serous carcinoma. Papillae are less evident and growth is more solid with interspersed ramifying slit-like spaces.

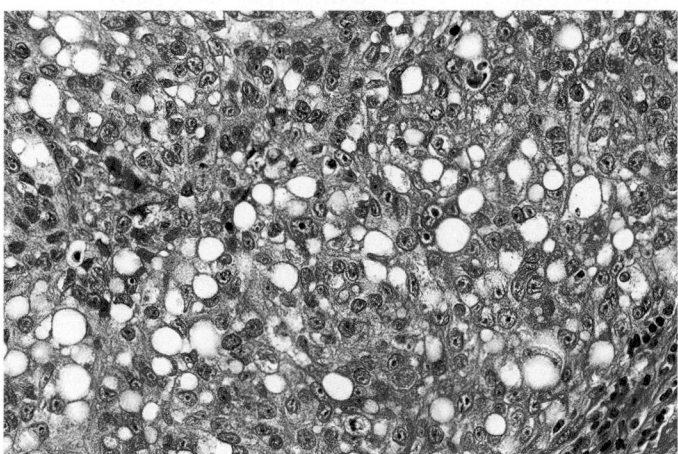

Fig. 27.35 Serous carcinoma. Numerous microcysts are present.

Serous surface carcinomas are usually papillary but may be predominantly solid. There is usually evidence of superficial invasion into the substance of the ovary. In most cases there are also peritoneal implants.[82] Thus, it may be difficult to distinguish between a primary peritoneal serous carcinoma with ovarian implants and a serous surface carcinoma. Arbitrarily, the carcinoma is considered to be of ovarian origin if the bulk of the tumor volume in either ovary is greater than that in the extraovarian sites and if there is at least some ovarian stromal invasion.[83]

DIFFERENTIAL DIAGNOSIS

Benign serous tumors

Serous surface papillary adenofibromas should be at least 1 cm in greatest extent to be considered neoplastic.[11] Small knobby fibrous protrusions on the surface of the ovary are common. Sometimes they are submitted for frozen section with the clinical suspicion of an implant or small carcinoma.

The rare *rete cystadenoma* resembles a serous cystadenoma. However, it is located in the ovarian hilus and lined by nonciliated cuboidal, columnar, or flattened epithelial cells, often forming an undulating or creviced appearance. There is smooth muscle in the wall and hilus cells are often present.[11]

The lining of an *endometrioid adenofibroma* can resemble serous epithelium except for the lack of cilia. The distinction in some cases is arbitrary.

Serous borderline tumors

Endocervical-like (Müllerian) mucinous and mixed epithelial borderline tumors have a papillary architecture that is similar on low-power examination to that of serous borderline tumors. However, their constituent epithelial cells have mucinous, squamous, endometrioid and indifferent differentiation. They are often associated with ovarian endometriosis, contrary to serous tumors.[84,85]

The *retiform variant of Sertoli–Leydig cell tumor* is papillary and may simulate a serous borderline tumor or low-grade serous carcinoma. However, it contains other features of a Sertoli–Leydig cell tumor, is usually found in teenagers and young women and may be androgenic.[86]

Serous carcinomas

Because of overlapping features, serous carcinomas are most commonly confused with other epithelial-stromal tumors, either of the endometrioid, clear cell, or transitional cell types.[87] Less frequently, other papillary neoplasms such as the retiform Sertoli-Leydig cell tumor (see above), mesothelioma,[88] metastatic serous carcinomas from elsewhere in the female genital tract, or papillary carcinomas from distant sites such as the breast[11] can mimic ovarian serous carcinoma.

Unlike serous carcinomas, low-grade endometrioid carcinomas may have squamous foci or aggregates of low-grade spindle cells without obvious keratinization blending with gland-like spaces. Psammoma bodies are rare in endometrioid carcinomas and endometrioid papillary areas are usually villous rather than broad-based and complex as in serous carcinomas. Endometriosis may accompany endometrioid tumors but is only rarely found with serous tumors. In high-grade tumors the distinction may be more difficult. Immunostaining for the Wilms tumor gene, WT1, may be of assistance. There is strong WT1 nuclear staining in most serous carcinomas,[89–93] but endometrioid carcinomas stain only weakly or not at all.[89,91,93] In ambivalent cases we defer to the serous type.

Papillary clear cell carcinomas can resemble serous carcinomas. However, most of the epithelial cells have either clear or oxyphilic cytoplasm and a characteristic nucleus with an angular periphery and a prominent nucleolus. The papillary cores are often hyalinized in clear cell carcinomas and there are almost always other characteristic patterns. As with endometrioid carcinomas, residual endometriosis may be present.

Transitional cell carcinomas have broad papillae lined by highly stratified malignant cells, rather than the branching and budding papillae of serous carcinomas. If minor transitional-like foci are present in a serous carcinoma, we generally consider the entire tumor to be serous, since the two are closely related (see discussion of transitional carcinomas).

Malignant mesotheliomas may sometimes be primarily or exclusively confined to the ovaries.[88] They are often both papillary and solid and may simulate either a serous borderline tumor or a carcinoma. The papillae of mesotheliomas have hyaline cores and are less complex than those of serous tumors. Although there are exceptions, mesothelioma cells are usually less stratified and pleomorphic than those of serous carcinomas. They have a round to oval nucleus with fine chromatin, a small nucleolus and densely eosinophilic cytoplasm. Mesotheliomas mark for calretinin, thrombomodulin and CK 5/6, whereas they are negative for the epithelial markers B72.3, Ber-EP4, CA19-9, Leu-M1 and MOC-31, separating them from Müllerian-derived neoplasms.[94]

Serous carcinomas of the endometrium may metastasize to the ovaries, bringing up the question of origin when both organs are involved. These cases are best evaluated by assessing the volume of tumor, depth of penetration and vascular invasion in the uterus compared with the location and extent of the tumor in the ovaries. WT1 immunostaining may be helpful. It is generally strongly and diffusely positive in primary ovarian serous carcinomas and either negative or only focally positive in uterine serous carcinomas.[90–92]

ETIOLOGY, GENETICS AND BIOMARKERS

The cell of origin and pathway of development of serous carcinomas are still unknown. The ovarian surface epithelial cells or those of their derivatives, the cortical inclusion cysts, are felt most likely to be the progenitor cells.[2,11] However, there is conflicting evidence as to whether serous carcinomas evolve through transformation of benign or borderline tumors or arise de novo as high-grade carcinomas. Support for the former possibility comes from morphologic studies such as those of Puls et al.[95] These investigators found benign-appearing residual areas in 15 of 32 high-grade serous carcinomas and noted direct transformation from these foci to carcinoma in 7 of the 15. Others speculate that the benign-appearing areas represent maturation of malignant cells, rather than being truly benign.[11] Further, although carcinoma *in situ* of the ovary has been difficult to certify,[96,97] support for the *de novo* transformation hypothesis comes from reports of very small high-grade serous cancers occurring in ovaries that appeared grossly normal.[47,98,99]

It may be that both theories are correct. A growing body of evidence supports the idea that low-grade and high-grade serous carcinomas are separate entities, rather than variants of the same process. For example: (1) Low-grade carcinomas often have a borderline component, the latter frequently with a micropapillary pattern.[21,51,52] However, in spite of studies such as those noted above,[95] high-grade carcinomas usually do not have an identifiable noninvasive precursor or a low-grade component.[98] (2) Patients with low-grade carcinomas generally have a more protracted clinical course than those with high-grade carcinomas.[21,50–52] (3) The genetic pathway leading to each appears to be different: low-grade serous carcinomas have a high frequency of K-ras mutations and lack p53 mutations,[100] whereas high-grade serous carcinomas generally exhibit wild type K-ras and commonly have mutant p53.[101,102] Moreover, serous borderline tumors, the presumed precursors to low-grade carcinomas, also differ genetically from high-grade serous carcinomas in that most of them lack p53 mutations, have loss of heterozygosity (LOH) of Xq and exhibit microsatellite instability. High-grade carcinomas, on the other hand, have p53 mutations, have LOH of multiple chromosomes but not of Xq and do not exhibit microsatellite instability.[2]

The majority of serous carcinomas mark positively for a variety of epithelial markers, including epithelial membrane antigen (EMA), CAM5.2, AE1/AE3, CK 7, B72.3, LeuM1, CA125,[13] and the Wilms tumor antigen WT1 (nuclear staining).[89–93] They are negative for CK 20, calretinin and other mesothelial markers.[13]

Mucinous tumors

GENERAL FEATURES AND CLINICAL ASPECTS

Mucinous tumors are those in which most or all of the epithelial cells contain mucin. In well-differentiated tumors the cells may resemble those of the endocervix, gastric pylorus, or intestine. Mucinous tumors are the second most frequent type of epithelial-stromal tumor after the serous type. In the West they account for 12 to 15% of all ovarian tumors.[22,23,25] About 80% are benign, 10% borderline and 10% malignant.[23,103,104] Mucinous carcinomas have been reported to account for from 9 to 13% of epithelial-stromal carcinomas.[22–25] However, the relative and absolute frequencies of both borderline and malignant mucinous tumors are uncertain because of differing criteria that have been used to distinguish them and the likelihood that many mucinous carcinomas that were metastatic to the ovaries were considered to be primary tumors before criteria to separate these two possibilities were better understood.[105] For instance, in a recent report in which the authors took these more recent insights into account, mucinous carcinomas accounted for only 2.4% of 124 ovarian surface epithelial carcinomas in Washington, DC.[106]

The average age of patients with carcinomas and borderline tumors is the early to mid-50s. Those with benign mucinous tumors are somewhat younger. Although still rare, all variants of mucinous tumors are more commonly seen in teenagers and young adults than are other epithelial-stromal tumors.[103]

Mucinous tumors usually cause signs and symptoms that are similar to those of ovarian tumors in general. However, they are the most common of the nonendocrine-cell ovarian tumors to be accompanied by hormonal manifestations, most often estrogenic or androgenic. This is likely to be caused by activation of tumor stromal cells to produce steroids.[103] Rarely, neoplastic neuroendocrine cells from the cyst lining may secrete gastrin or serotonin, causing the Zollinger–Ellison[9,107] or carcinoid syndrome.[103]

About 5% of mucinous tumors have a separate component of dermoid cyst;[24,104,108] less commonly, they are associated with a Brenner tumor.[104] Benign mucinous tumors comprise cystadenomas (by far the most common), adenofibromas and cystadenofibromas. There are two borderline tumor variants: the intestinal type, accounting for about 85% of the total, and the endocervical-like (Müllerian) type.[103] The intestinal-type borderline tumor is further divided into those with mild cytologic atypia only and those with a component of intraepithelial carcinoma.

In stage I cases borderline tumors (with atypia only) are almost all benign, with a recorded recurrence rate of less than 1%.[109] Almost all cases higher than stage I at the time of initial staging have had the clinical appearance of pseudomyxoma peritonei. However, in the large majority of these cases, the ovarian tumor(s) are likely to be metastatic from the appendix or, less commonly, from elsewhere in the gastrointestinal tract (see below under pseudomyxoma peritonei for further discussion).

In stage I cases of borderline tumors with intraepithelial carcinoma, the recurrence rate has been 6.5%.[109] In cases with recurrence, or cases that are higher than stage I, the metastases have been in the form of invasive abdominal implants (rather than pseudomyxoma peritonei) and the prognosis has been poor, similar to that of high-stage invasive mucinous carcinomas.[109,110] In these cases it is likely that areas of invasion in the primary tumor were not sampled.[109,111]

Stage I mucinous carcinomas have recurred in 10.8% of cases, whereas persistence or recurrence and often a fatal outcome have been reported in 92% of higher stage cases.[109]

Serum CA125 levels have not been as sensitive for mucinous carcinomas as for other epithelial malignancies; in one study only 6 of 17 patients with both advanced stage and localized mucinous carcinomas had elevated CA125 levels.[112] Conversely, serum carcinoembryonic antigen (CEA) CA 19-9 and CA 72.4 were more sensitive for mucinous carcinomas than for other types.[112,113]

GROSS EXAMINATION

Mucinous tumors are the largest of all ovarian tumors. One was reported to weigh over 300 pounds.[114] Only about 5% of cystadenomas and intestinal-type borderline tumors are bilateral[115] and stage I mucinous carcinomas are almost always unilateral.[105,109,110,116–122] However, endocervical-like borderline tumors are bilateral in 30–40% of cases. They are smaller than other mucinous tumors and may be adjacent to or within an endometriotic cyst.[84]

Most mucinous tumors are smooth-surfaced, multicystic masses with variable solid areas (Figs 27.36, 27.37). They may also be unilocular cysts, sometimes with a solid nodule in the cyst wall (Fig. 27.38). The cysts are filled with translucent viscous fluid. Since mucinous tumors are often highly variable histologically, with malignant foci sometimes only a small component, it is important to select the areas most likely to be malignant, especially for frozen section. Each cyst must be opened and carefully examined. Malignant foci are

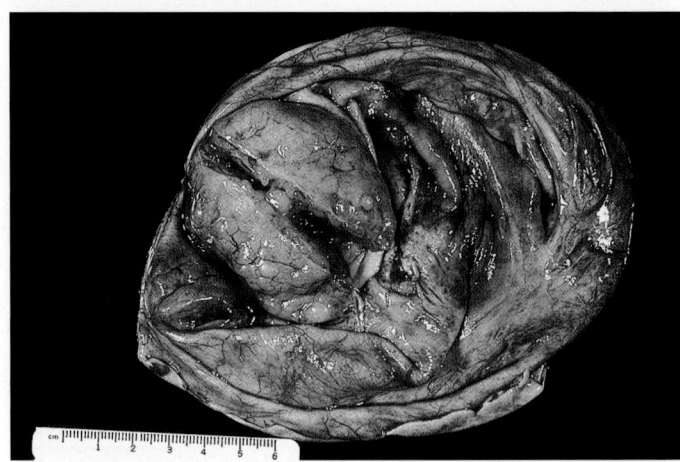

Fig. 27.38 Mucinous cystic tumor with a solid nodule in the wall. In this case the solid area was a borderline tumor. (Courtesy of Dr Robert H. Young, Massachusetts General Hospital.)

usually solid or papillary. Borderline foci may be finely papillary, velvety excrescences on the cyst wall (Fig. 27.39). Entirely malignant tumors may be predominantly solid with only small cysts (Fig. 27.40). If the tumor appears grossly benign and only benign foci are found in one or two frozen sections, we report it as a 'mucinous cystadenoma'. However, if the frozen sections contain borderline areas, it is understood that foci of carcinoma may be discovered on permanent sections and a thorough intraoperative examination of the pelvis and abdomen for potential metastases is initiated. The decision to remove the uterus and opposite ovary depends on the clinical circumstances. At least

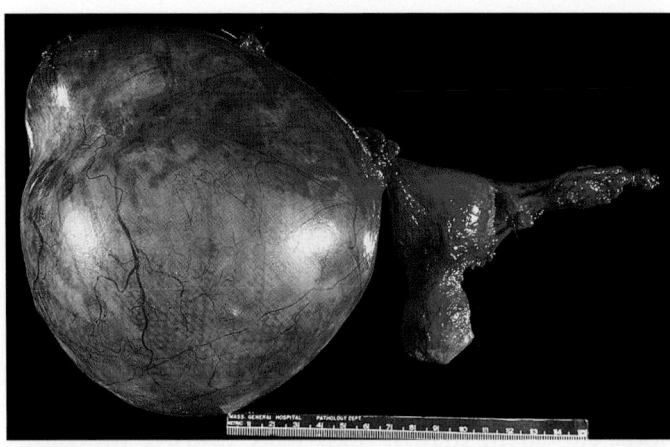

Fig. 27.36 Mucinous cystadenoma. A huge unilateral, smooth-surfaced cystic tumor has replaced the ovary. (Courtesy of Dr Robert H. Young, Massachusetts General Hospital.)

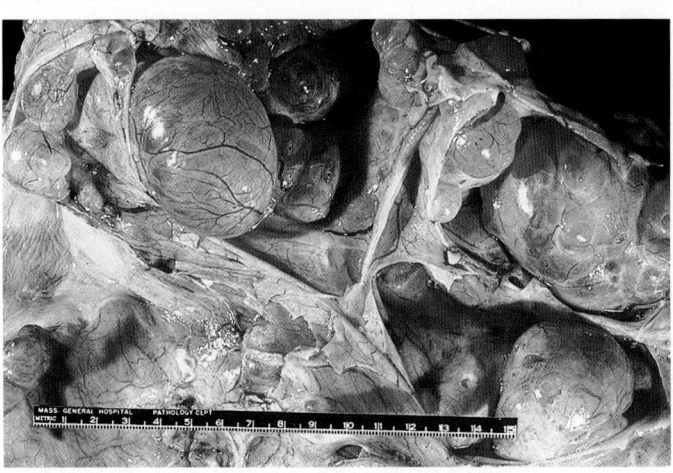

Fig. 27.37 Mucinous cystadenoma. The interior contains numerous smooth cysts of varying sizes. (Courtesy of Dr Robert H. Young, Massachusetts General Hospital.)

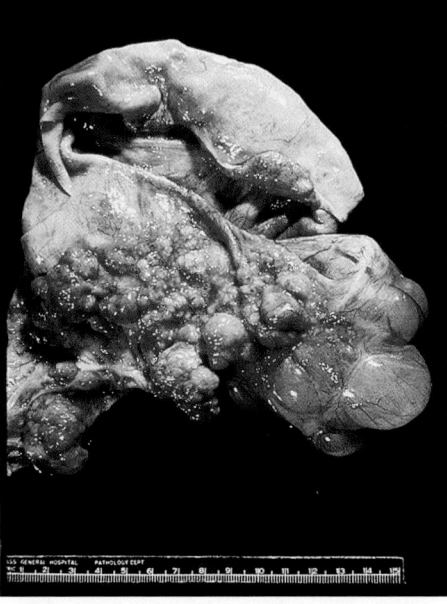

Fig. 27.39 Mucinous borderline tumor, intestinal type. The interior of a cyst is roughened and granular. (Courtesy of Dr Robert H. Young, Massachusetts General Hospital; with permission from AFIP 3rd series, fascicle No. 23.)

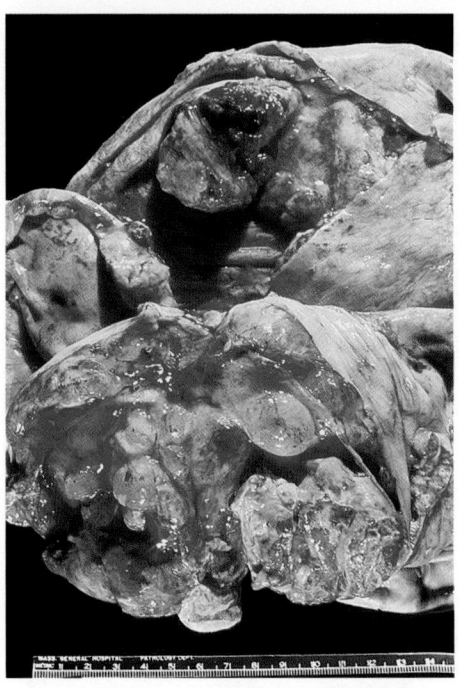

Fig. 27.40 Mucinous carcinoma. The tumor is mostly solid with focal hemorrhage and necrosis. (Courtesy of Dr Robert H. Young, Massachusetts General Hospital.)

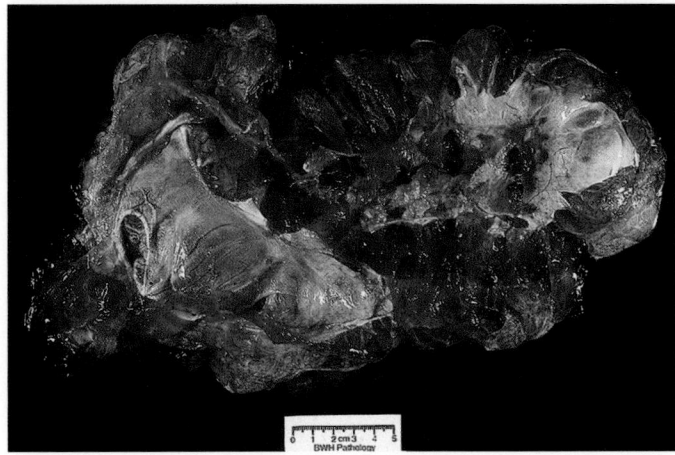

Fig. 27.41 Mucinous cystic tumor in the setting of pseudomyxoma peritonei. The tumor is gelatinous with adherent blobs of mucin on the surface.

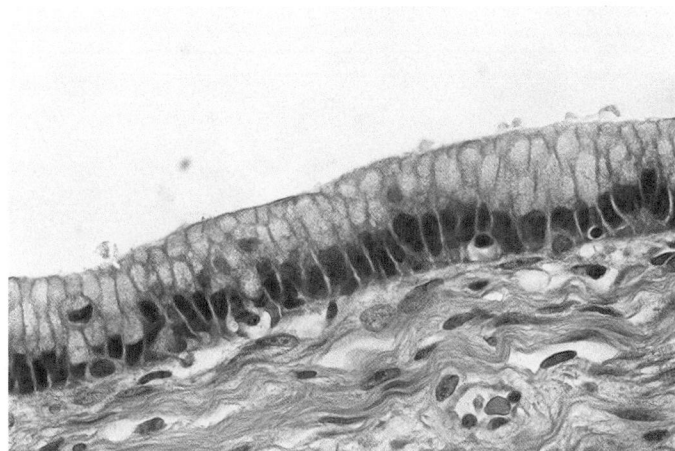

Fig. 27.42 Mucinous cystadenoma. The cyst lining cells are columnar with pale cytoplasm and basal nuclei.

two permanent sections per cm of maximal tumor diameter has been recommended to adequately sample mucinous tumors.[110] This may be excessive, however, if the tumor is entirely cystic with smooth cyst walls throughout.

Cystic ovarian mucinous tumors are sometimes a component of the clinical syndrome of pseudomyxoma peritonei. In this setting, they are more frequently bilateral; they may be grossly similar to the usual mucinous tumor, but are sometimes gelatinous, thin-walled, multicystic masses that differ from the tumors described above (Fig. 27.41). In either case the ovarian tumors are almost always metastatic, the primary most often residing in the appendix, which should be removed and completely examined microscopically in all cases of pseudomyxoma peritonei (see below for further discussion).

MICROSCOPIC EXAMINATION

Benign mucinous tumors – cystadenomas, cystadenofibromas and adenofibromas

These three tumors form a spectrum with varying proportions of epithelial-lined cysts, glands and stroma. The cystadenoma is by far the most common. It is composed of thin-walled cysts that are lined by a single layer of mucinous columnar cells with benign-appearing, basally located nuclei (Fig. 27.42). Mitotic figures may be present. There may also be occasional

goblet cells and neuroendocrine cells, the latter requiring special stains for visualization. Sometimes small papillae with fibrous cores project into the cysts. The stroma may be fibrous or resemble ovarian stroma. It may contain smooth muscle, luteinized cells (Fig. 27.43) and calcifications. Due to cyst rupture and mucin extravasation, large areas of necrosis accompanied by histiocytes and inflammatory cells may be present. Adenofibromas[123] and cystadenofibromas contain a grossly observable solid stromal component. Microscopically, they contain mucinous glands and small cysts uniformly distributed in a fibrous stroma (Fig. 27.44).

Borderline mucinous tumors – intestinal and endocervical-like types

About 85% of mucinous borderline tumors are of the intestinal type.[103] These in turn comprise two subtypes:

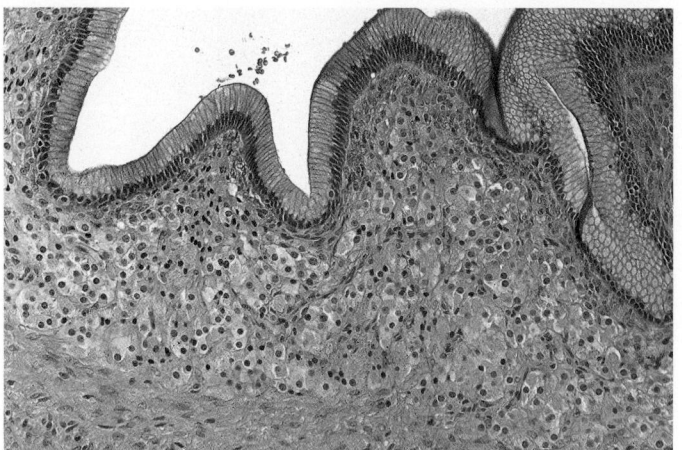

Fig. 27.43 Mucinous cystadenoma with stromal luteinization. The pale luteinized stromal cells cling to the periphery of the epithelial lining cells. These cells may sometimes be the source of hormone production in mucinous tumors.

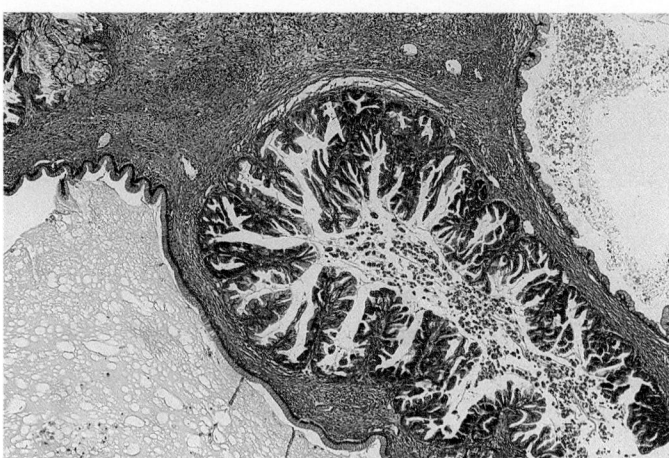

Fig. 27.45 Mucinous borderline tumor, intestinal type. Two benign cysts flank a cyst lined with proliferative epithelium.

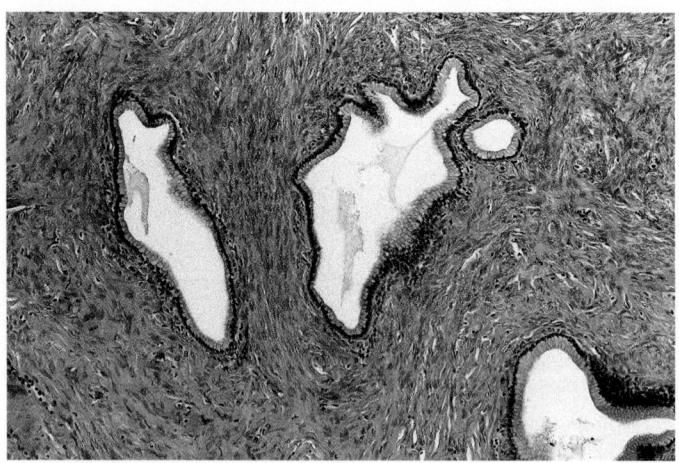

Fig. 27.44 Mucinous adenofibroma. Benign-appearing glands are present in a fibrous stroma.

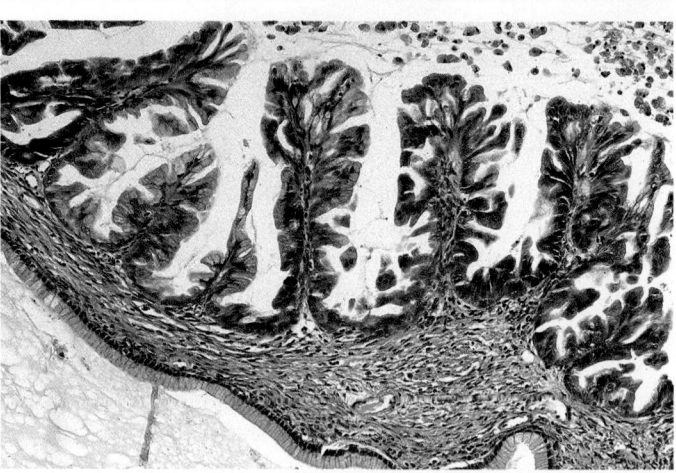

Fig. 27.46 Mucinous borderline tumor, intestinal type. The proliferative cells line papillae with thin fibrous cores.

(1) with atypia only, referred to simply as 'borderline' and (2) with intraepithelial carcinoma.

Intestinal-type mucinous borderline tumors (with atypia only)

Borderline tumors differ from benign tumors in that, in addition to benign-appearing areas, the epithelial cells are focally crowded and stratified and form papillae with thin fibrous cores (Figs 27.45, 27.46). In these foci the nuclei are slightly enlarged and hyperchromatic and have increased mitotic activity, most noticeable at the base of the papillae (Fig. 27.47). The epithelium is intestinal-like with goblet cells (Fig. 27.48) and sometimes Paneth's cells.[111,124,125] Neuroendocrine cells are also present but may require special stains for visuali-

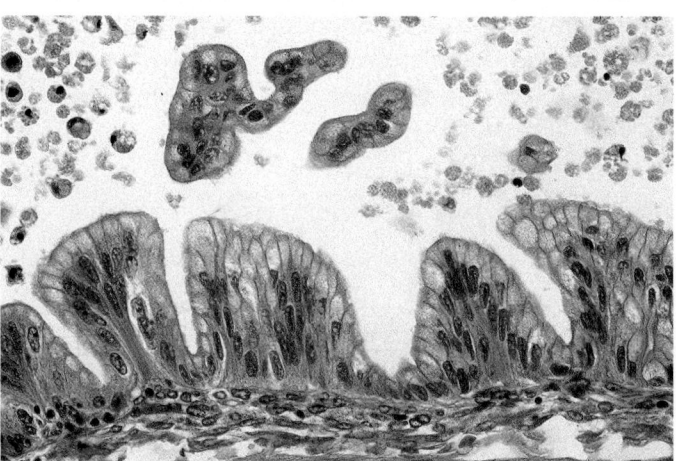

Fig. 27.47 Mucinous borderline tumor, intestinal type. Low-grade mucinous epithelial cells with pseudostratification due to the plane of sectioning of the papillae.

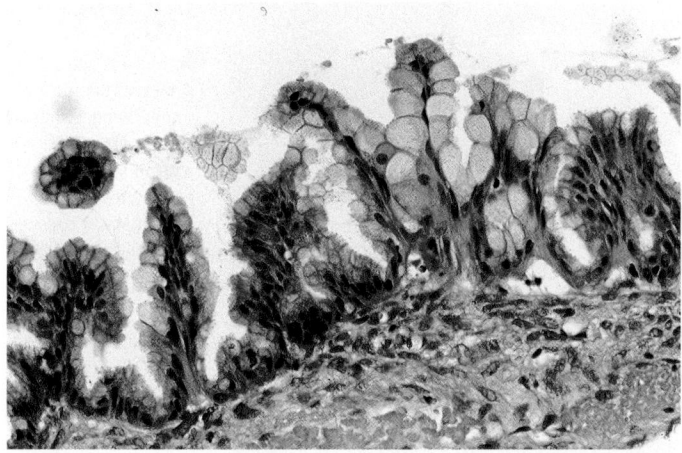

Fig. 27.48 Mucinous borderline tumor, intestinal type. Columnar cells and goblet cells are present.

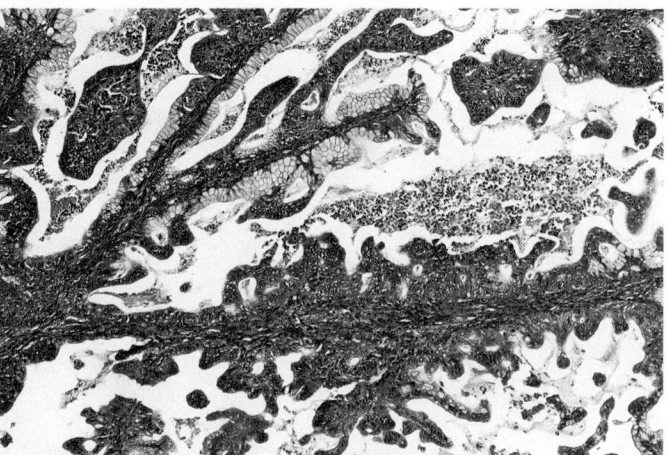

Fig. 27.50 Mucinous borderline tumor with intraepithelial carcinoma. At low power the cysts are lined with mucinous cells and stratified epithelium without mucin.

zation. The gland and cyst lumens contain mucin, sometimes mixed with histiocytes and inflammatory cells. There may be areas of necrosis secondary to mucin extravasation.

Intestinal-type mucinous borderline tumors with intraepithelial carcinoma

If the epithelial cell nuclei appear cytologically malignant (significant enlargement, hyperchromasia and usually with prominent nucleoli) (Fig. 27.49) and there is no obvious stromal invasion, the suffix 'with intraepithelial carcinoma' should be added to the diagnosis of mucinous borderline tumor.[103] In most cases, there is prominent stratification of the malignant-appearing cells.[111] with stroma-free papillae or a cribriform pattern of growth (Figs 27.50–27.52).

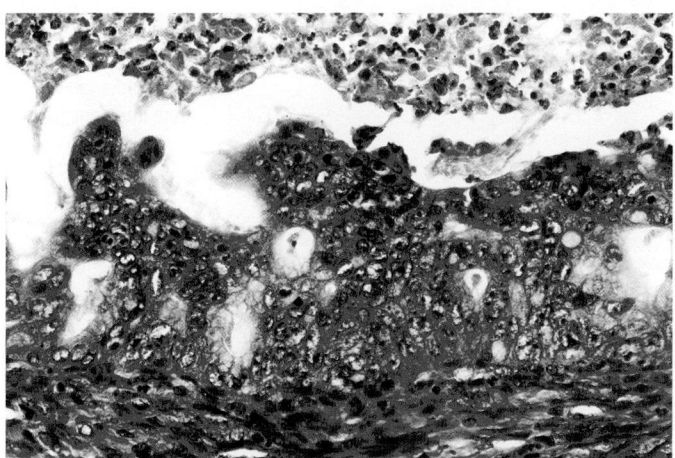

Fig. 27.51 Mucinous borderline tumor with intraepithelial carcinoma. There is marked stratification of crowded, malignant-appearing cells.

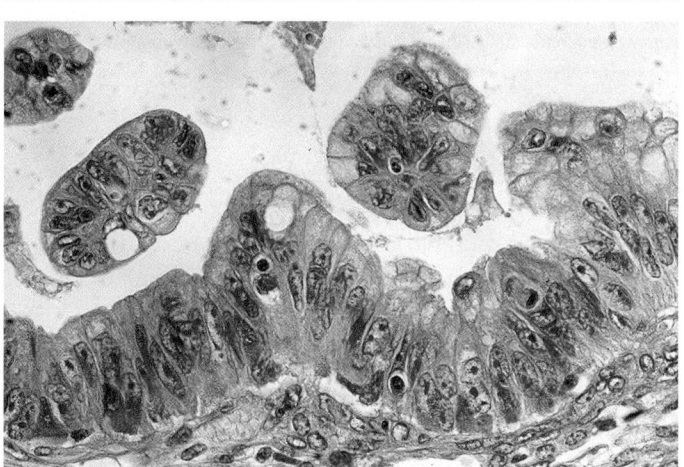

Fig. 27.49 Mucinous borderline tumor with intraepithelial carcinoma. Malignant-appearing epithelial cells with only minimal stratification.

Intestinal-type mucinous borderline tumors with microinvasion

One or several small foci of stromal invasion, often inciting a desmoplastic response, may be present in a borderline tumor (Fig. 27.53). If the invasive areas are all less than 10 mm² and less than 3 mm in any linear dimension, the tumor should be interpreted as 'borderline with focal microinvasion', further specifying the number of invasive foci. Areas of mucin extravasation with a fibrous and histiocytic response containing entrapped benign epithelial cells may be misinterpreted as invasion (Fig. 27.54). Generally, true invasion will have more developed desmoplasia, fewer histiocytes and more obviously malignant epithelial cells arranged in an infiltrative pattern. All reported stage I cases with microinvasion have had a benign clinical behavior.[38,109,120,126]

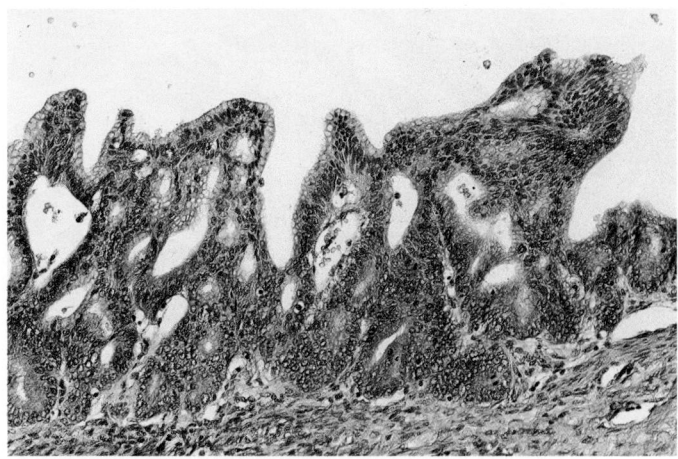

Fig. 27.52 Mucinous borderline tumor with intraepithelial carcinoma. A cribriform intracystic growth pattern is present.

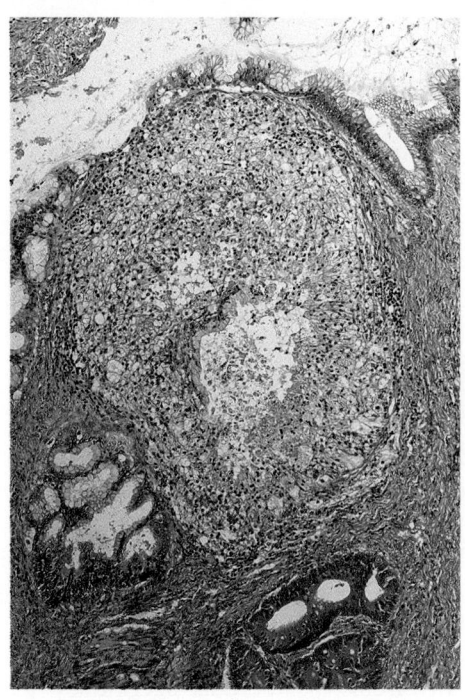

Fig. 27.54 Mucinous borderline tumor with pseudoinvasion. A strip of benign-appearing mucinous cells is present in a large field of histiocytes secondary to cyst rupture and mucin extravasation.

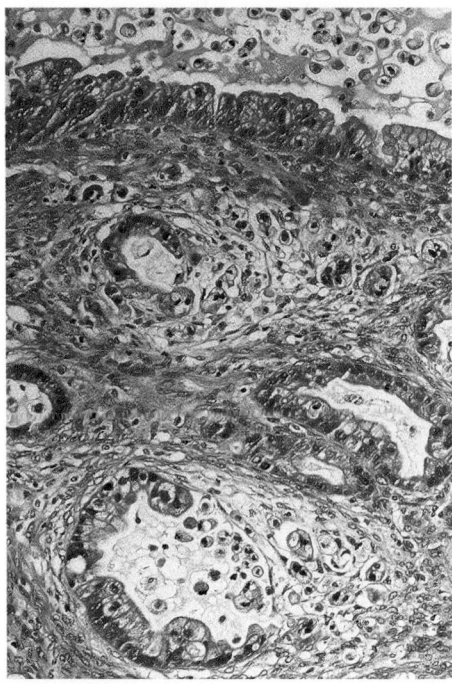

Fig. 27.53 Mucinous borderline tumor with microinvasion. Single cells appear to break off into the stroma from adjacent glands.

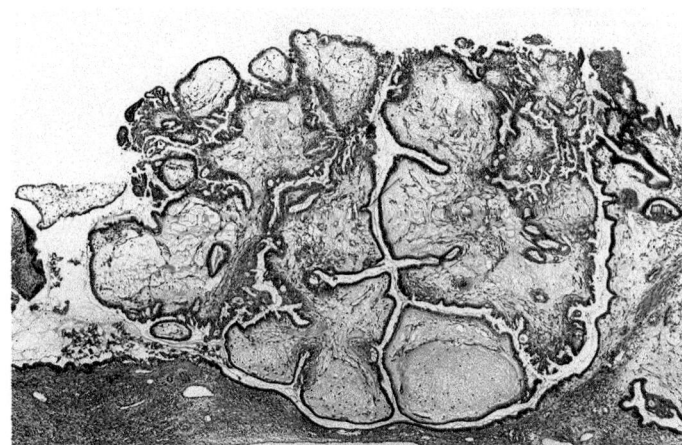

Fig. 27.55 Endocervical-like mucinous borderline tumor. The low-power appearance mimics a serous borderline tumor with bulbous papillae.

Endocervical-like borderline tumors

The low-power microscopic appearance, with broad bulbous papillae and cell stratification, is similar to that of serous rather than intestinal-type mucinous borderline tumors (Fig. 27.55). The papillae, however, are lined by both mucinous columnar cells resembling those of the endocervix and stratified polygonal eosinophilic cells (Figs 27.56, 27.57). Characteristically, many acute inflammatory cells are present in the epithelial cell cytoplasm and in the extracellular mucin (Fig. 27.57). Adjacent endometriosis may be present and sometimes the tumor appears to arise from an endometriotic cyst.[84] Nuclei are usually only slightly atypical, but rare cases with areas of intraepithelial carcinoma or microinvasion have been reported; the behavior of these has been benign.[127] Even in the absence of identifiable stromal invasion, approximately 6% of endocervical-like borderline tumors have had either noninvasive or invasive-appearing abdominal and peritoneal implants (Figs 27.58, 27.59) and rarely lymph node metastases. These have not, however, led to recurrences.[84,128]

The comparative features of the various types of mucinous borderline tumors are given in Table 27.2.

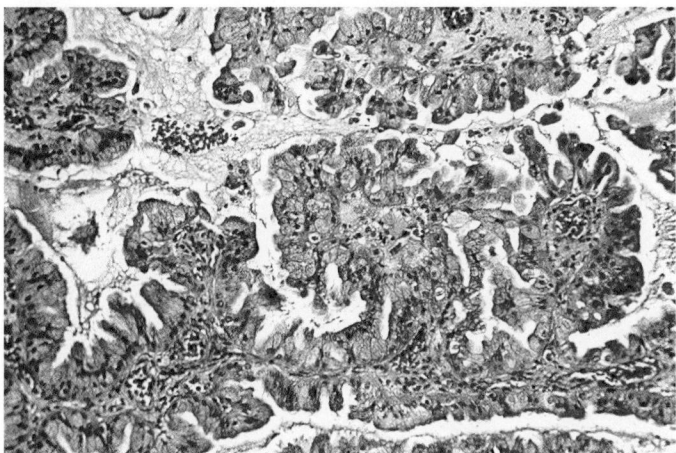

Fig. 27.56 Endocervical-like mucinous borderline tumor. The papillae are lined by benign-appearing mucinous cells that resemble those of the endocervix.

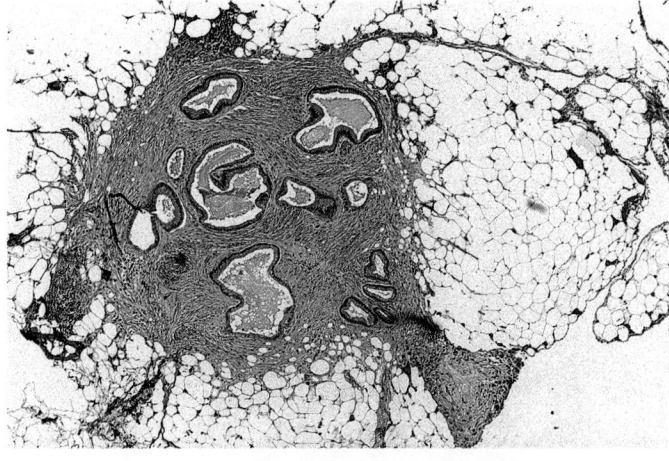

Fig. 27.58 Omental implant from an endocervical-like mucinous borderline tumor. Cysts and glands are set in a desmoplastic stroma. The overall appearance is that of an invasive implant.

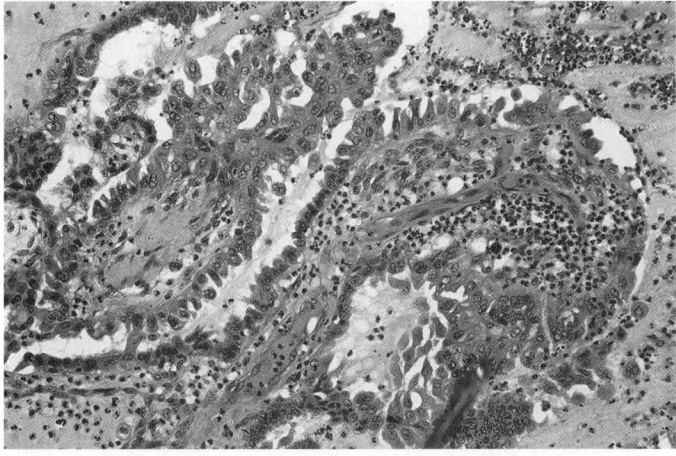

Fig. 27.57 Endocervical-like mucinous borderline tumor. In this focus, the papillae are lined by highly stratified eosinophilic cells. There are numerous leukocytes in the papillae and in the mucin.

Mucinous carcinomas

Only 5–10% of mucinous carcinomas are entirely malignant; the rest have a benign and borderline component. Within this background, there are two forms of invasion: the expansile and the infiltrative types, the former being more common.[109]

In expansile (confluent) invasion, glands and cysts lined by malignant-appearing cells have little or no intervening stroma so that they appear to have invaded by expanding into and replacing the stroma across a broad, sharply demarcated front. The invasive areas may be composed of back-to-back glands, ramifying channels lined by epithelial cells, or cystic spaces lined by complex papillae and containing eosinophilic material and nuclear debris (Figs 27.60, 27.61). The epithe-

Table 27.2 Comparative features of ovarian mucinous borderline tumors

	Intestinal type (with atypia only)	Intestinal type with intraepithelial carcinoma	Endocervical-like
Gross	Large, smooth-surfaced multilocular cyst, cyst linings smooth to rough, bilateral in 5%	Same	Smaller, fewer cysts, may be associated with endometriosis, bilateral in 40%
Microscopic	Cysts or glands lined with slightly stratified mucinous cells and goblet cells, thin papillae with stromal cores, mild nuclear atypia	Same, with foci of malignant-appearing nuclei, often highly stratified, papillary or cribriform	Cysts with broad papillae lined by endocervical-like mucinous cells and stratified eosinophilic cells, numerous neutrophils
Appearance of extraovarian disease	Pseudomyxoma peritonei (PP)[a]	Invasive peritoneal implants without PP[b]	Noninvasive or invasive peritoneal implants, no PP
Usual behavior in cases with extraovarian disease	Variable. Usually persistent or recurrent over many years, eventually fatal in 40–50%	Similar to carcinomas, most are fatal in a few years or less	Benign[c]

[a]Most cases with PP are in fact metastases to the ovaries. See discussion under 'Pseudomyxoma Peritonei'.
[b]Cases with implants likely have invasive areas in the ovarian tumor that are not sampled.
[c]Only a few cases with implants have been reported.

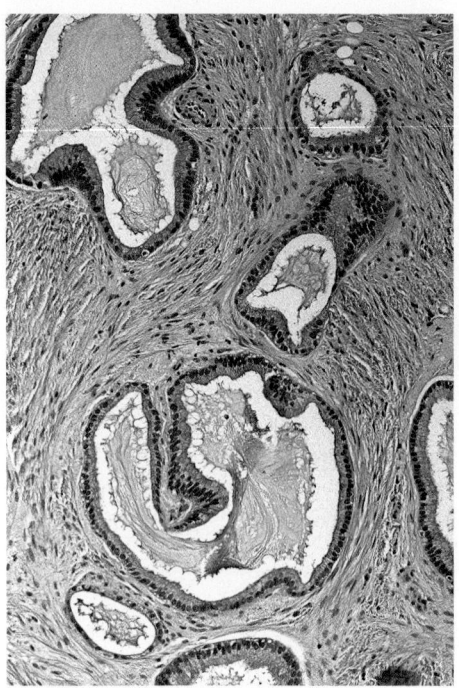

Fig. 27.59 Omental implant from an endocervical-like mucinous borderline tumor. At high magnification the epithelial cells are benign-appearing.

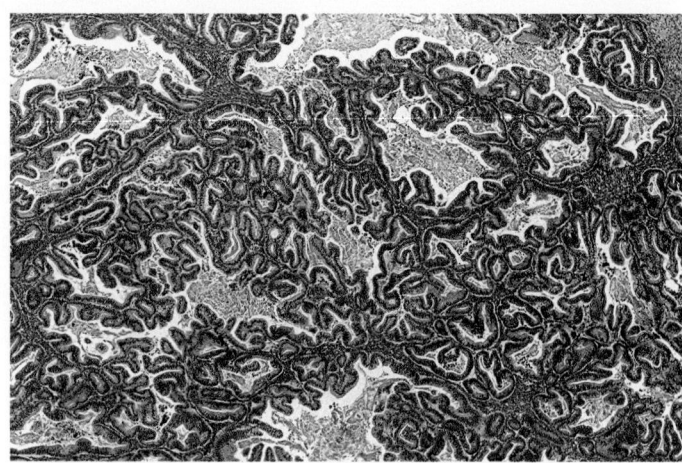

Fig. 27.61 Mucinous carcinoma with expansile invasion. Complex spaces with little intervening stroma occupy the entire field.

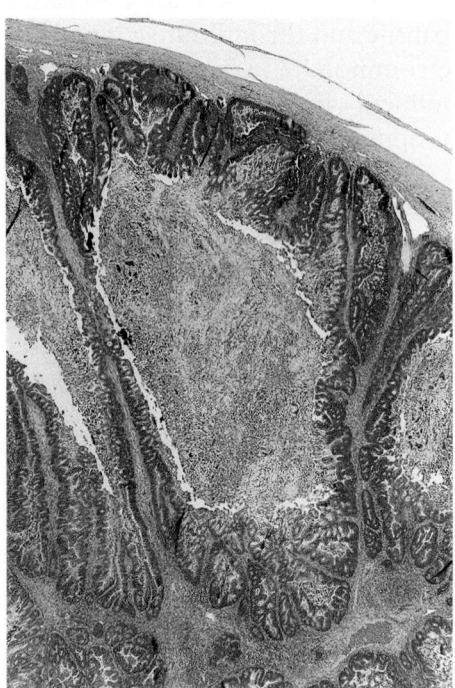

Fig. 27.60 Mucinous carcinoma with expansile invasion. Numerous cysts are lined by papillary epithelium. The cysts are sharply demarcated and do not extend to the overlying ovarian surface.

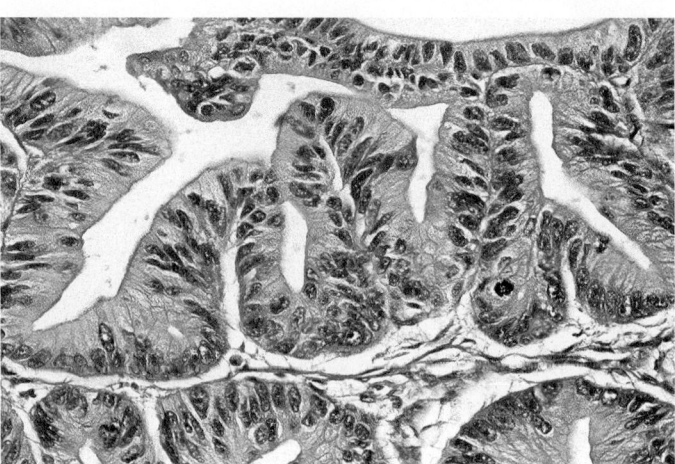

Fig. 27.62 Mucinous carcinoma with expansile invasion. The epithelial cells lining the spaces are mucinous-appearing.

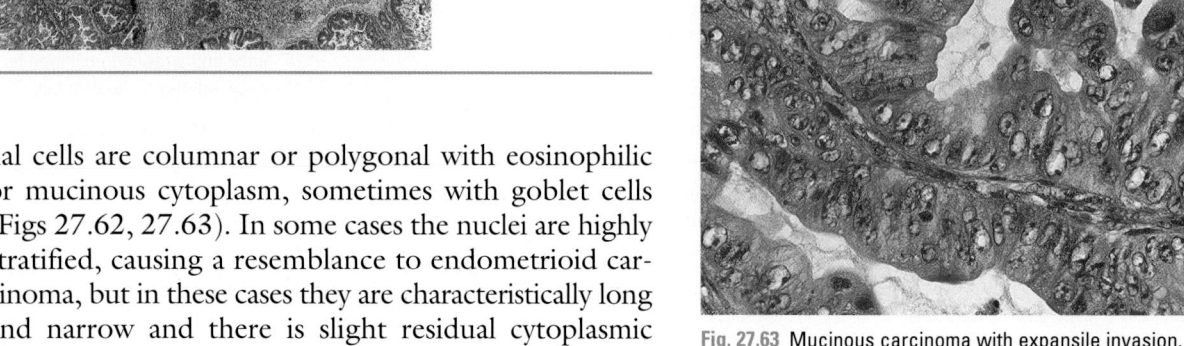

Fig. 27.63 Mucinous carcinoma with expansile invasion. The epithelial cells in this case have a nondescript eosinophilic cytoplasm.

lial cells are columnar or polygonal with eosinophilic or mucinous cytoplasm, sometimes with goblet cells (Figs 27.62, 27.63). In some cases the nuclei are highly stratified, causing a resemblance to endometrioid carcinoma, but in these cases they are characteristically long and narrow and there is slight residual cytoplasmic mucin (Fig. 27.64). Since small confluent areas are

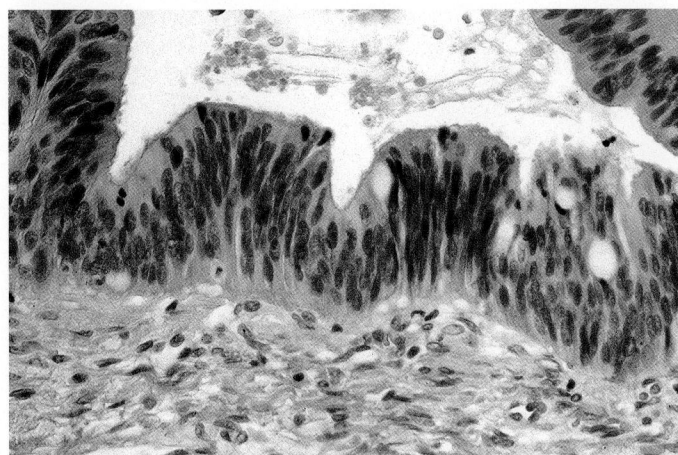

Fig. 27.64 Mucinous carcinoma with expansile invasion. The epithelial cells appear somewhat endometrioid. The slender nuclei and surface cytoplasmic mucin are consistent with a mucinous tumor.

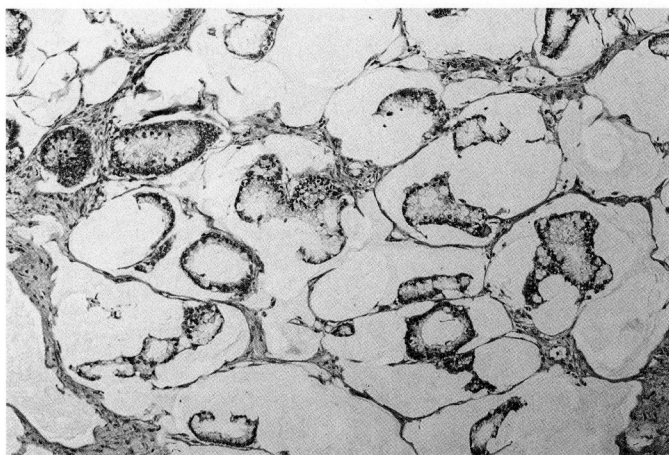

Fig. 27.66 Mucinous carcinoma with infiltrative invasion. Abundant extracellular mucin imparts a colloid carcinoma-like appearance.

difficult to certify as invasive, expansile invasion should not be considered unless the area exceeds 10 mm² and is at least 3 mm in each of two linear dimensions.

In infiltrative invasion, glands sheets, or single epithelial cells haphazardly invade the stroma (Fig. 27.65). The invasive cells may appear endocervical or intestinal, but usually have a nondescript eosinophilic cytoplasm. Occasional mucinous carcinomas have colloid carcinoma-like foci (Fig. 27.66). Signet ring cells may be present, but abundant signet ring cells should raise the question of a metastasis.[105,106] The stroma may be desmoplastic with or without inflammatory cells,[103] or it may be cellular and fibromatous. In the latter instance, an invasive carcinoma may be mistaken for a borderline tumor, especially if the infiltrative glands are large and

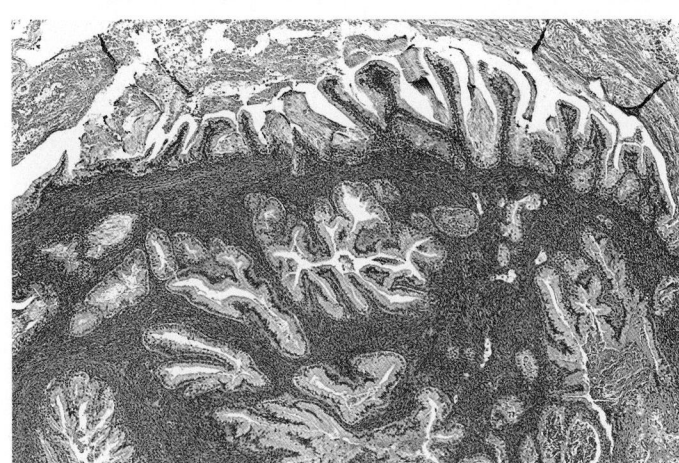

Fig. 27.67 Mucinous carcinoma with infiltrative invasion. The glands are widely spaced and the stroma is cellular and fibromatous, which might cause confusion with a borderline tumor with intraepithelial carcinoma.

evenly distributed (Fig. 27.67). However, in carcinomas the glands are entirely lined by malignant cells, rather than the mixture of benign, atypical and malignant-appearing cells seen in borderline tumors (Fig. 27.68). Tumors with infiltrative invasion are biologically more aggressive and spread beyond the ovary more readily than those with purely expansile invasion.[109,117,119,121]

A rare subtype of mucinous carcinoma, the endocervical-like (Müllerian) type, has recently been described.[129] It has a papillary, cystic and glandular growth pattern with abundant mucin in the extracellular spaces (Fig. 27.69). Most of the epithelial cells are well-differentiated columnar cells, similar to those of the endocervix (Fig. 27.70). There may be minor components of endometrioid (Fig. 27.71), serous, or squamous

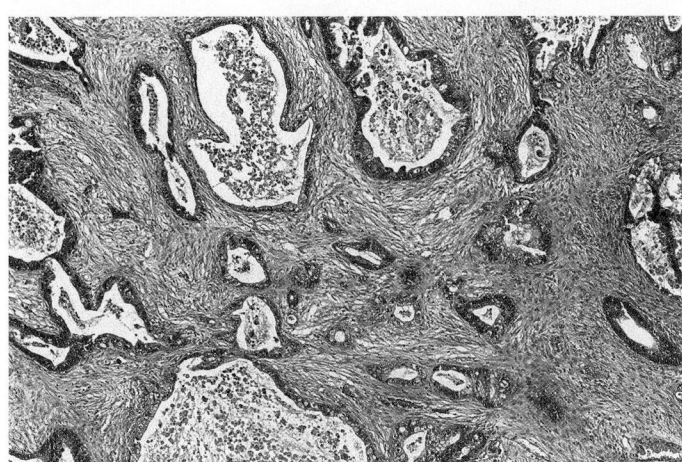

Fig. 27.65 Mucinous carcinoma with infiltrative invasion. Irregularly shaped glands and cysts are set in a desmoplastic stroma.

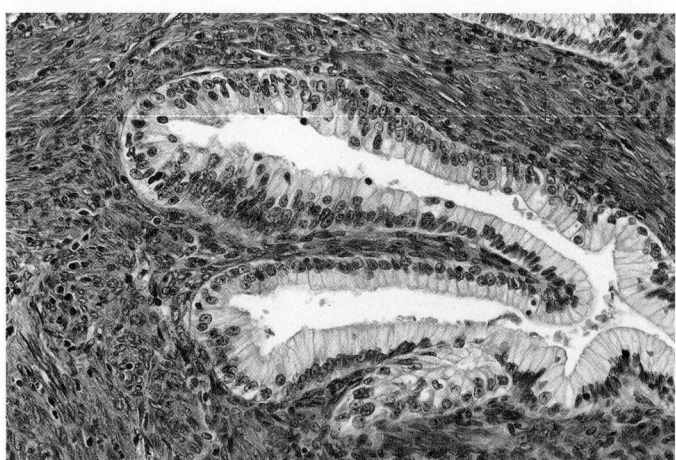

Fig. 27.68 Mucinous carcinoma with infiltrative invasion. A high-magnification view of the tumor in Figure 27.67. This well-differentiated carcinoma with a fibromatous stroma might be confused with a borderline tumor with intraepithelial carcinoma.

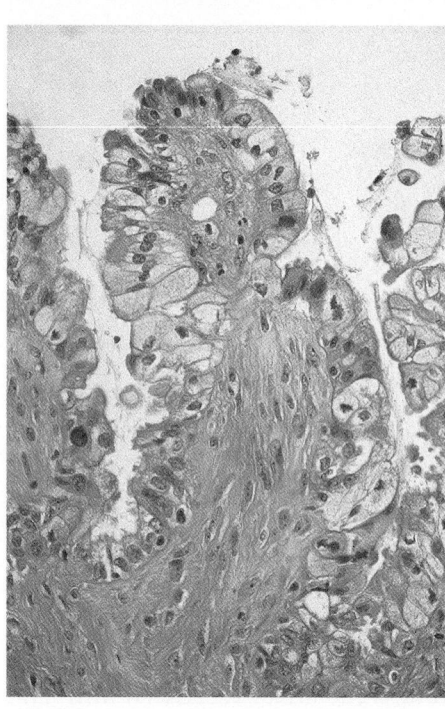

Fig. 27.70 Mucinous carcinoma of the endocervical-like type (seromucinous carcinoma). The epithelial lining cells are well differentiated and resemble those of the endocervix.

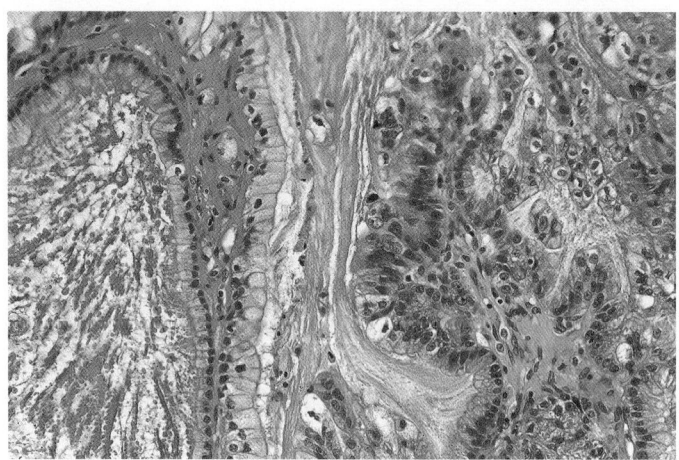

Fig. 27.69 Mucinous carcinoma of the endocervical-like type (seromucinous carcinoma). At low power the spaces are filled with pale mucinous material. The glands and papillae are lined by benign-appearing and only mildly atypical mucinous epithelial cells.

that are widely divergent microscopically from the remainder of the tumor, which is either a borderline tumor or a carcinoma. Grossly, mural nodules may appear uniform, or variegated, yellow, pink, or red; sometimes they have hemorrhage and necrosis; they may be single or multiple and range from <1 cm up to 30 cm.[79,103,130–135] Mural nodules may be benign or malignant; the latter may be an anaplastic carcinoma, a sarcoma, or a carcinosarcoma.[79,131–133]

Three varieties of benign mural nodules have been described.[134,135] In the pleomorphic and epulis-like type,

cell types. When the serous component is prominent, these tumors have been termed 'seromucinous' carcinomas.[127] Endocervical-like mucinous carcinomas may be bilateral and associated with endometriosis. It may be that these and the seromucinous carcinomas are the malignant counterpart of endocervical-like and mixed-epithelial borderline tumors, but this remains to be established.

Mucinous tumors with mural nodules

Ordinary mucinous tumors may have one or more solid areas in the wall of a cyst. The term 'mural nodule', however, is reserved for those very uncommon nodules

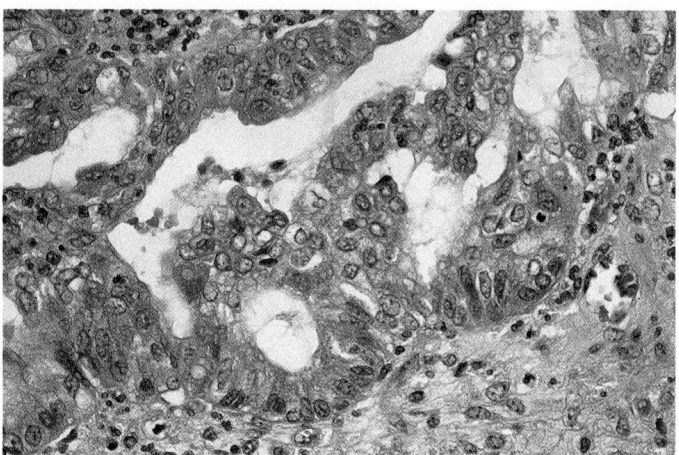

Fig. 27.71 Mucinous carcinoma of the endocervical-like type (seromucinous carcinoma). The cells here have less cytoplasm and are stratified, appearing more endometrioid.

osteoclast-like multinucleated giant cells and extravasated red blood cells are present among pleomorphic spindle cells, similar to an aneurysmal bone cyst or giant cell reparative granuloma of bone (Fig. 27.72). A second variant contains a purely spindle cell population with no or only a few giant cells. The third pattern consists almost entirely of groups of large multinucleated cells with abundant ground-glass cytoplasm separated by thin fibrous bands. Some benign mural nodules have been called 'sarcoma-like' because the cells may be quite pleomorphic and there may be numerous mitotic figures, including atypical forms. However, benign nodules are distinguished from sarcomatous or carcinomatous nodules by their grossly and microscopically sharply circumscribed borders and an absence of vascular invasion. They also tend to be smaller than malignant nodules (1–6 cm) and occur in younger women. There have been no recurrences in any of the 26 cases with follow-up data.[79,134]

Mural nodules with anaplastic carcinoma contain pleomorphic large cells with markedly enlarged nuclei with prominent nucleoli and abundant eosinophilic cytoplasm, the latter sometimes imparting a rhabdoid appearance (Figs 27.73, 27.74). There may be a background of spindle cells or spindle cells may predominate.[79,132,133] Both the epithelioid and spindled malignant cells stain strongly with cytokeratin antibodies, a helpful confirmatory finding. However, focal or weak keratin staining in spindle cells is nonspecific and one must be cautious not to interpret a pseudosarcomatous nodule with focal keratin positivity as an anaplastic carcinoma with spindle cells. Patients with mural nodules composed of anaplastic carcinoma have been reported

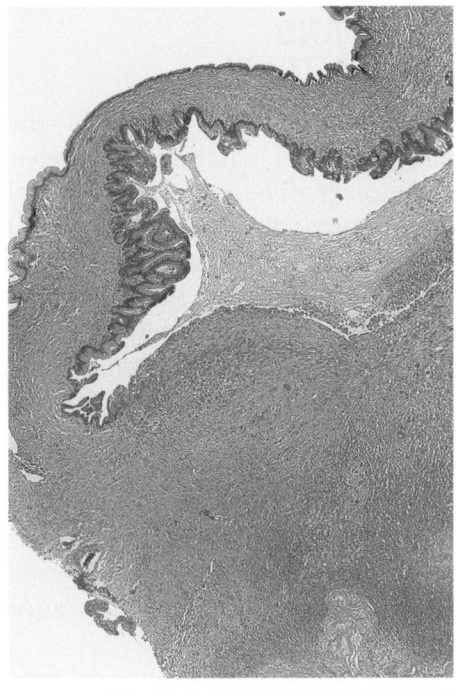

Fig. 27.73 A mural nodule with anaplastic carcinoma in a mucinous tumor. The wall of a cyst is replaced by a solid cellular proliferation.

to have a high risk of metastatic carcinoma and its attendant dire prognosis.[79,132,133] However, in a recent study of 34 patients with mural nodules, all nine stage IA patients with anaplastic carcinoma were alive and clinically free of disease after a median follow-up time of 5 years.[133]

Sarcomatous and carcinosarcomatous mural nodules are rare. Fibrosarcomas, rhabdomyosarcomas and pleomorphic undifferentiated sarcomas have been reported. The prognosis is poor, with six of nine patients dead with metastases.[79,131]

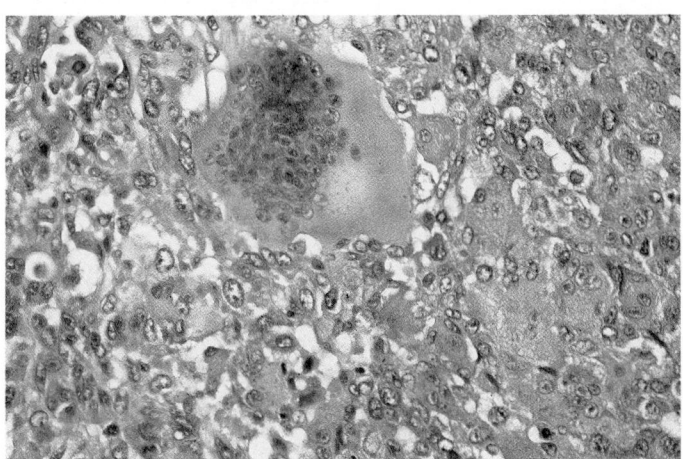

Fig. 27.72 A pseudosarcomatous mural nodule in a mucinous tumor. A large multinucleated cell is a feature of this benign mural nodule.

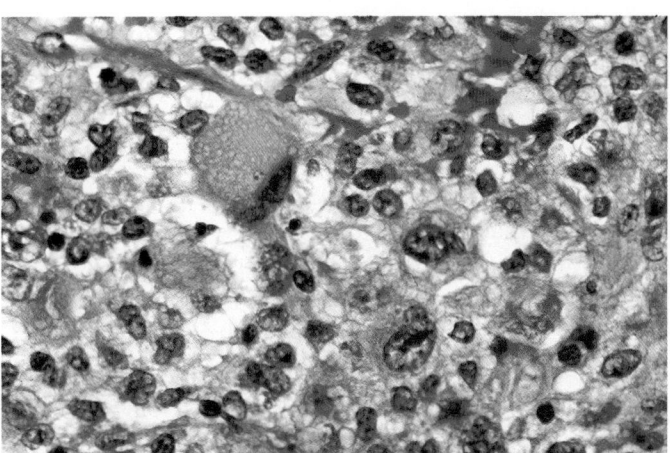

Fig. 27.74 A mural nodule with anaplastic carcinoma in a mucinous tumor. At high power the nodule is composed of anaplastic cells, some with a rhabdoid appearance.

MUCINOUS TUMORS AND PSEUDOMYXOMA PERITONEI

The term pseudomyxoma peritonei refers to the presence of abundant mucinous material in the pelvis or in the pelvis and abdomen. The mucinous material may be relatively liquid (also called mucinous ascites) or gelatinous. The latter may form tumor-like masses that are adherent to visceral organs or the abdominal wall. Pseudomyxoma peritonei is most often the result of spread of a mucin-producing tumor of the appendix and, less commonly, from elsewhere in the gastrointestinal tract. However, when pseudomyxoma is present along with a cystic mucinous ovarian tumor, the pathologist is presented with the dilemma of distinguishing a primary ovarian tumor with peritoneal spread *vs* simultaneous metastatic spread to the ovary(ies) and the peritoneum from an occult tumor of the appendix or elsewhere.

In almost all reported cases of ovarian intestinal-type borderline tumors (without intraepithelial carcinoma) that have peritoneal spread at the time of initial staging, the extraovarian deposits have been in the form of pseudomyxoma peritonei.[109] However, recent studies have presented strong arguments that the great majority of mucinous cystic ovarian tumors associated with pseudomyxoma peritonei are in fact themselves metastases, usually from a histologically similar tumor in the appendix.[136–138] This argument is supported by the fact that an appendiceal neoplasm (often quite small and possibly not obviously invasive) will be found in almost all cases in which the appendix is removed and entirely examined microscopically. Furthermore, the ovarian tumors in such instances differ morphologically and immunohistochemically from borderline ovarian mucinous tumor without associated pseudomyxoma in that they have unusually tall columnar cells, surface implants, extensive mucin extravasation into the ovarian stroma (pseudomyxoma ovarii) and are mostly cytokeratin 7-negative.[139,140] Finally, in all six cases tested, identical c-Ki-ras mutations were found in both the appendiceal and the ovarian tumors.[141]

In spite of the above arguments, it is possible that in some cases the tumors arise synchronously in the appendix and the ovary.[142] This hypothesis is supported by the finding of different loss of heterozygosity patterns in the appendiceal and ovarian tumors in some cases.[143] It is also clear that at least some ovarian tumors with pseudomyxoma peritonei do originate in the ovary. These include those with an ipsilateral dermoid cyst,[109,144] and possibly some of those in which

the appendix did not appear to contain a mucinous tumor (about one-third of reported cases). A caveat is that in some of these cases the appendix was only grossly examined or only partially examined microscopically,[103] potentially allowing a small mucinous tumor to be overlooked.

Given the above uncertainties, it follows that in all cases of cystic mucinous ovarian tumors complicated by pseudomyxoma peritonei, the appendix should be removed and completely examined microscopically. Although still a controversial point,[103] if the appendix contains a mucinous tumor, we feel that it should be considered the primary and the ovarian tumor(s) metastatic (even if the appendiceal wall is not obviously invaded.[109] The peritoneal mucinous material should also be generously sampled. The pathologic diagnosis on this material should not be limited to the term 'pseudomyxoma peritonei', but should state whether or not the mucin contains epithelial cells, whether they appear benign, borderline, or malignant and, if possible, whether the mucin dissects into tissues with a fibrous reaction or is merely adherent to the surface with organizing fibroblasts and endothelial cells.

In cases of pseudomyxoma peritonei in both men and women where the epithelial cells in the mucin appear benign or borderline, the diagnostic term 'disseminated peritoneal adenomucinosis' has been proposed.[145] Follow-up of cases in this category showed 5-year and 10-year survival rates of 75% and 68%, respectively; whereas patients in whom the epithelial cells appeared malignant, designated 'peritoneal mucinous carcinomatosis', have usually had mucinous carcinomas of the intestines and a rapidly fatal course.[145]

Finally, if a low-grade mucinous tumor of the appendix with microscopic features similar to those of the ovarian mucinous tumor(s) is present (the most likely scenario), its pathologic designation is problematic. The current terminology for appendiceal tumors does not include a borderline category and they are diagnosed either as adenomas or carcinomas based strictly on whether or not the wall of the appendix is invaded.[146] Although spread to the ovaries and peritoneum is clearly not benign behavior, neither is it fully malignant in the sense of the usual metastatic gastrointestinal mucinous carcinoma with its dire prognosis. Thus, in this situation, both the adenoma and carcinoma designations are confusing. We agree with others[147] that it is preferable in these cases to use the designation 'low-grade mucinous neoplasm' for the appendiceal tumor and 'metastatic low-grade mucinous neoplasm' for the ovarian tumor(s).

DIFFERENTIAL DIAGNOSIS

Mucinous carcinomas must be distinguished from other primary ovarian carcinomas with epithelial cells that contain mucin. These include endometrioid carcinomas, Sertoli-Leydig cell tumors and mucinous (goblet cell) carcinoid tumors. However, the most common, and often the most difficult differential diagnosis, is that of mucinous carcinoma metastatic to the ovaries.

Metastatic mucinous carcinoma

Metastatic mucinous carcinomas from the cervix, pancreas, gall bladder, appendix, colon, or stomach can form cystic or partially cystic ovarian masses that may be mistaken both clinically and pathologically for primary mucinous tumors.[105,148–155] Table 27.3 summarizes the most useful findings in distinguishing these tumors. Primary mucinous carcinomas are almost always large and unilateral with a smooth external surface. The average maximal dimension of ovarian mucinous carcinomas has been remarkably similar in several reports (around 20 cm), whereas most metastatic mucinous carcinomas measure less than 10 cm.[105,106] Some 34% of colon cancers and 75% of those from a variety of other organs were bilateral.[105,149,150] Therefore, in the frozen section room, receipt of bilateral mucinous carcinomas, mucinous carcinomas less than 10 cm, or those with obvious surface involvement should initiate an inquiry as to whether the patient has a current or previous carcinoma elsewhere.

Microscopic clues favoring metastatic carcinoma, aside from the surface implants previously mentioned, include a nodular growth pattern with intervening areas of residual normal ovarian tissue, a variable pattern of growth from one area to another and vascular space invasion[105] (Table 27.3). Importantly, metastatic mucinous carcinomas may contain deceptively bland epithelial cells that mimic the benign and borderline areas that are commonly present in primary carcinomas.

Immunohistochemistry, primarily using cytokeratins (CK) 7 and 20, may be useful in the distinction from metastatic colon carcinoma: most colon carcinomas are CK 7 negative and CK 20 positive, whereas primary ovarian mucinous tumors are predominately CK 7 positive and are CK 20 variable.[129,156–159] However, occasional primary ovarian mucinous carcinomas are CK 7 negative and CK 20 positive[156,157] and one must be wary of this. Differential cytokeratins are not useful in the distinction from noncolonic mucinous carcinomas.[159,160]

Cdx-2, a homeobox gene transcription factor expressed in almost all colorectal carcinomas, is not expressed in the usual types of ovarian carcinoma. However, Cdx-2 was positive in all 25 mucinous ovarian tumors in two reports,[161,162] negating its value in this distinction when the ovarian tumor is mucinous.

Dpc4, a tumor suppressor gene, is inactivated in ~55% of pancreatic ductal adenocarcinomas, whereas it is expressed in almost all mucinous ovarian carcinomas. Hence, negative staining for this marker in a mucinous ovarian tumor is suggestive of pancreatic origin.[163]

Endometrioid carcinomas with mucinous differentiation

As in primary endometrioid carcinomas of the endometrium, there may be varying degrees of mucinous differentiation in endometrioid ovarian carcinomas. Usually the ovarian carcinomas are well differentiated and the mucinous epithelium appears endocervical. When mucinous epithelium is a minor component, it should be classified as 'endometrioid carcinoma with focal mucinous differentiation', rather than a mixed epithelial carcinoma.

Rare endometrioid ovarian carcinomas have cytoplasmic clearing due to lipid accumulation that may be confused with mucin.[103] The microvesicular or bubbly-appearing cytoplasm is a clue, as is the endometrioid appearance in areas without cytoplasmic lipid.

Sertoli–Leydig cell tumors with heterologous gastrointestinal epithelium

Sertoli–Leydig cell tumors may contain heterologous elements such a cartilage, skeletal muscle and gastrointestinal epithelium.[164] If gastrointestinal epithelium

Table 27.3 Primary versus metastatic mucinous ovarian carcinomas

Findings favoring primary	Findings favoring metastatic	Noncontributory
• Unilateral	• Bilateral	• Benign-appearing or borderline-appearing areas[a]
• Large size, smooth surface	• Known nonovarian primary mucinous carcinoma	
• Expansile (confluent) growth pattern	• Grossly friable and necrotic	
• Complex papillary pattern	• Surface involvement	• Grade
• Luminal necrotic debris[b]	• Variable or nodular growth pattern	
	• Vascular invasion	
	• Cytokeratin 7-negative	

[a]Although most often this feature is seen in primary tumors.
[b]Although seen more often in primary (*vs* metastatic) *mucinous* carcinomas, this feature is often present (along with epithelial cell necrosis) in metastatic colorectal carcinomas. However, the latter more frequently mimic ovarian endometrioid carcinomas rather than mucinous carcinomas.

is a prominent component of a Sertoli–Leydig tumor, it may resemble a mucinous epithelial tumor. The mucinous epithelium lining the glands and cysts of a Sertoli–Leydig tumor is usually benign or borderline-appearing; there may be interspersed goblet cells and neuroendocrine cells as in mucinous tumors. Characteristically, the cytoplasm and the mucin within the gland lumens are densely eosinophilic, differing from the pale or basophilic mucin in mucinous epithelial tumors. Other helpful findings include: (1) solid yellow areas between and apart from the cystic mucinous foci on gross examination, (2) the presence of other, more usual Sertoli–Leydig cell elements and (3) androgenic clinical manifestations (although these may rarely also occur secondary to mucinous epithelial tumors owing to hormonal activity of luteinized stromal cells).

Mucinous (goblet cell) carcinoid tumor

Primary ovarian mucinous carcinoid tumors are rare; in the ovary they are more often metastatic from the appendix. Mucinous carcinoids may be mistaken for a mucinous surface epithelial tumor by those unaware of its characteristic features. They are either pure or associated with a dermoid cyst.[165] Grossly they are solid, soft and tan. Microscopically small glands or nests of epithelial cells permeate a fibrous stroma. Sometimes the cell nests float in pools of mucin. Most of the epithelial cells have either large cytoplasmic mucin vacuoles or granular and eosinophilic cytoplasm, the latter positive for neuroendocrine markers. The nuclei are small and minimally atypical. Ovarian mucinous carcinoids are potentially malignant; 2 of 15 patients with follow-up data died from metastatic spread.[165]

ETIOLOGY, GENETICS AND BIOMARKERS

Although mucinous tumors are classified in the epithelial-stromal category, there is circumstantial evidence that they may be of germ cell origin. The mucinous epithelium often has a gastric, pancreaticobiliary, or intestinal rather than a Müllerian phenotype[166,167] and 3–5% of cases are associated with a dermoid cyst, a tumor of germ cell origin. Furthermore, ovarian cortical inclusion cysts having a mucinous epithelial lining (the hypothetical precursor to an epithelial-derived mucinous tumor) are very uncommon. Against a germ cell derivation is the fact that the large majority of mucinous tumors do not have a component of dermoid cyst (although this does not exclude a mono-dermal teratomatous lineage). Also, a mucinous tumor

might theoretically develop from a nonmucinous precursor cell in a cortical inclusion cyst that undergoes gastrointestinal metaplasia along with neoplastic transformation.[103]

Mucinous carcinomas are genetically distinct from the more common serous carcinomas and, unlike the latter, many of them appear to be to be derived from benign or borderline precursors. K-ras mutations are commonly found in mucinous but not in serous carcinomas. These mutations may be present in benign and borderline foci, indicating that they are an early event in mucinous tumor development.[168–171] Loss of heterozygosity in a variety of chromosome regions also differs between serous and mucinous tumors, yet similar patterns are seen when borderline and malignant mucinous tumors are compared.[171–173] p53 mutations, on the other hand, are rare in mucinous carcinomas, but are common in serous types.[169]

Risk factors for the development of mucinous carcinomas appear to differ from those of serous carcinomas. Studies suggest that increased parity or oral contraceptive use does not reduce the risk for mucinous carcinomas as it does for serous carcinomas,[174] and cancers that develop in women with a family history of ovarian cancer are serous, not mucinous.[99]

Endocervical-like mucinous borderline tumors and carcinomas appear to arise from endometriosis,[84,129] whereas endometriosis is not present in the more common intestinal mucinous borderline tumors or the usual type of mucinous carcinoma.

Approximately 90% of mucinous carcinomas are reactive for cytokeratin (CK) 7, while 50–60% are positive for CK 20.[129,158–160] Endocervical-like mucinous carcinomas are often negative for CK 20 and express vimentin and estrogen and progesterone receptors, findings that distinguish them from the usual type of mucinous carcinoma.[129] Carcinoembryonic antigen positivity is a feature of intestinal-type borderline tumors, but not of endocervical-like borderline tumors.[103,175]

Endometrioid tumors

GENERAL FEATURES AND CLINICAL ASPECTS

Endometrioid epithelial-stromal tumors are composed of epithelial cells and patterns of growth that are similar to common hyperplastic and neoplastic proliferations of the endometrium. Tumors with a sarcomatous component and pure endometrioid stromal sarcomas of the ovary are also included in this category.

Endometrioid ovarian carcinomas are the second most frequent after the serous type. In different series they constitute 8–21% of cases in the epithelial-stromal category.[22,23,25,43,176–180] In contrast, benign endometrioid tumors are rare, accounting for less than 1% of all benign ovarian tumors[22,23,181] and only seven series of endometrioid borderline tumors, totaling 136 cases, have been reported.[181–187] Most patients with endometrioid tumors in all three categories are either postmenopausal or in the late reproductive years, with an average age in the early to mid-50s.

With rare exceptions no reported benign-appearing or borderline endometrioid tumors have recurred after surgical removal. A single endometrioid cystadenofibroma was reported to have recurred in the vagina, possibly due to implantation at the time of initial surgery.[188] The vaginal mass was not removed and it had remained stable at last follow-up 6.4 years later. There have been two borderline endometrioid tumor cases reported with peritoneal 'implants' at the time of diagnosis.[181,185] The authors could not exclude autochthonous foci of endometriosis with atypia, rather than implants in these cases. There were no adverse effects in the single case with follow-up data.[185]

Endometrioid carcinomas are more frequently discovered at an earlier stage than are serous carcinomas, being either stage I or II in 36–67% of cases.[176–178,189] Thus, they have a better overall prognosis. However, when patients are matched for age, stage, grade and level of surgical cytoreduction, those with endometrioid carcinomas and serous carcinomas have similar clinical outcomes.[190] Five-year survival by stage in two relatively recent series of endometrioid carcinomas was: stage I 87 and 89%; stage II 48 and 65%; stage III 41 and 27%; and stage IV, 20 and 7%.[176,178] Among stage I patients, those with grade I tumors appear to have a particularly favorable prognosis. In 31 such patients followed at least 5 years, survival was 97%.[186]

Endometrioid tumors are much more frequently associated with endometriosis than are serous or mucinous tumors. Benign and borderline endometrioid tumors are accompanied by endometriosis, in either the ipsilateral or the contralateral ovary, in approximately 25% and 36% of cases, respectively.[181–188] Residual ipsilateral endometriosis is present in approximately 13% of endometrioid carcinomas.[176–178,189,191]

GROSS EXAMINATION

Benign and borderline endometrioid tumors are grossly similar. They are only occasionally bilateral and vary from a few cm up to 25 cm in greatest dimension. The outer surface is smooth. The cut surface is firm and solid, or variegated with foci of necrosis. Interspersed cysts ranging up to 7 cm may be present. The cyst fluid is clear, mucoid, or hemorrhagic (Fig. 27.75).

Early-stage endometrioid carcinomas are bilateral in 17% of cases.[115] They are variably cystic and solid and not grossly distinct from other carcinomas, except that foci of residual endometriosis are more often present (Fig. 27.76). Uncommonly, the carcinoma is a fleshy mass within an endometrioma (Fig. 27.77).

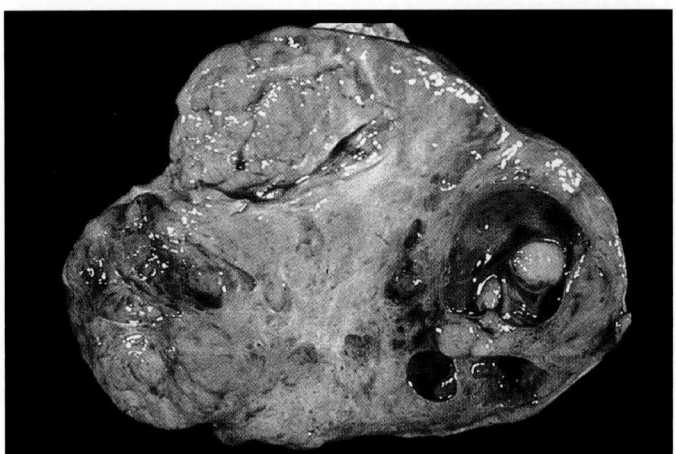

Fig. 27.75 Endometrioid borderline adenofibroma. The tumor is solid and cystic with focal hemorrhage.

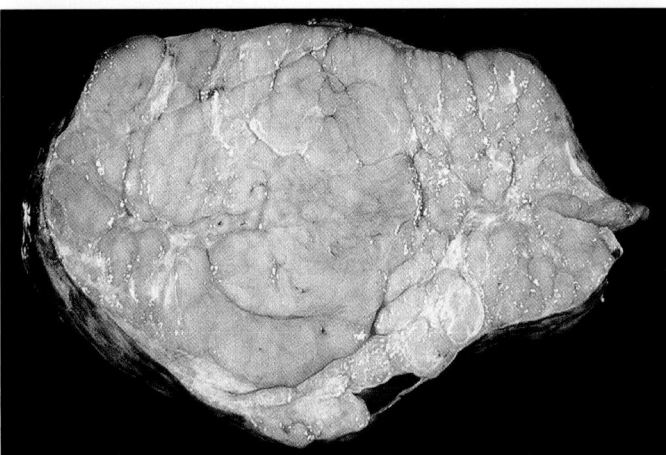

Fig. 27.76 Endometrioid carcinoma. The tumor is lobulated, solid, fleshy and tan, an appearance similar to tumors in the sex cord-stromal category.

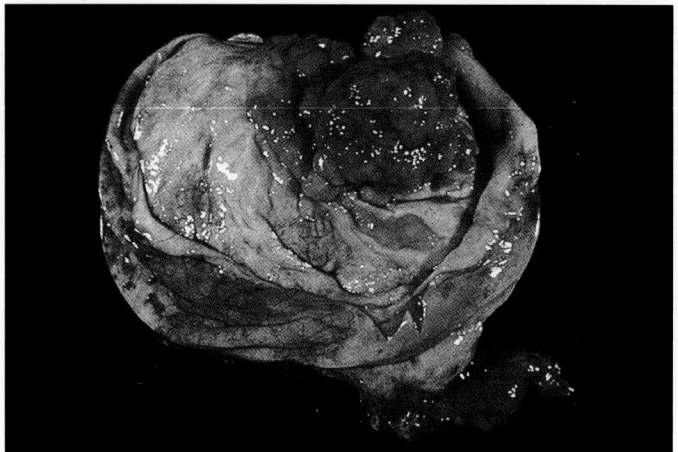

Fig. 27.77 Endometrioid carcinoma. The tumor forms a bulbous mass in the wall of a cyst.

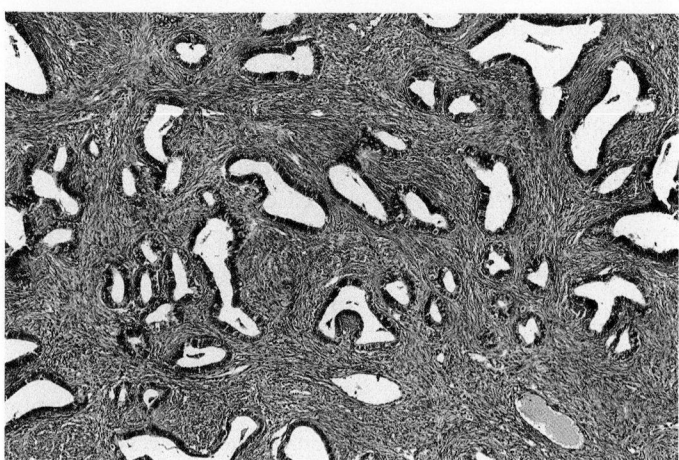

Fig. 27.78 Endometrioid adenofibroma. Irregular spaces uniformly distributed in a fibrous stroma.

MICROSCOPIC EXAMINATION

Benign endometrioid tumors – adenofibroma, cystadenofibroma

Endometrioid (cyst)adenofibromas contain variably shaped glands and cysts lined predominately by stratified columnar or cuboidal epithelial cells resembling endometrial cells. A minority of cells may have ciliated or mucinous cytoplasm. Squamous morules may be present. The glands and cysts may have mucin in the lumen and are uniformly distributed in a fibrous or cellular stroma which may be focally calcified or contain psammoma bodies.[188] There is no nuclear atypia and only occasional mitotic figures (Figs 27.78, 27.79).

'Proliferative', borderline and microinvasive endometrioid tumors

Epithelial proliferations occurring within areas of ovarian endometriosis are distinguished from the tumors discussed in this section by the presence within them of residual endometrial stroma. Rather than forming a mass, they are usually only incidental microscopic findings. They are diagnosed using the same terms that are used for noninvasive endometrial proliferations.[192]

Apart from these nonneoplastic proliferations and distinct from uniformly benign endometrioid neoplasms, there exists a spectrum of architectural and cytologic abnormalities in noninvasive endometrioid neoplasms. Authors have used different terms for the benign end of this spectrum and have differed in defining the threshold for a borderline designation and on whether that term should be used at all.[181–187] We diagnose proliferative tumors with only mild nuclear

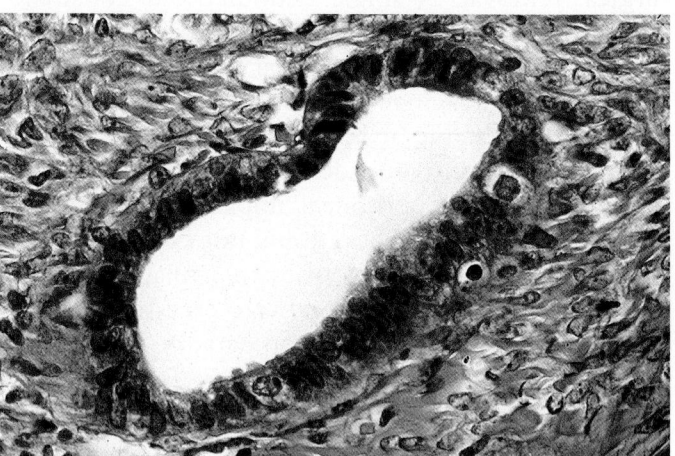

Fig. 27.79 Endometrioid adenofibroma. The space is lined by benign-appearing, crowded, columnar cells.

atypia as 'proliferative endometrioid adenofibromas with atypia'. Proliferative tumors with nuclear atypia that is equivalent to that seen in cases of atypical hyperplasia of the endometrium are considered 'borderline'. Those with more severe nuclear atypia are designated 'borderline with intraepithelial carcinoma'.

The patterns of growth may be glandular (often with squamous differentiation) (Figs 27.80, 27.81), papillary (Fig. 27.82), or a mixture of the two. The glandular areas may be adenofibromatous or consist of closely packed glands in a cribriform arrangement. Papillae project into cystic spaces and are mostly villous without extensive branching. Cellular stratification and nuclear atypia range from mild to severe.

By definition, infiltrative invasion with a stromal response is absent in a borderline tumor. However, it is difficult to exclude invasion in cases in which the

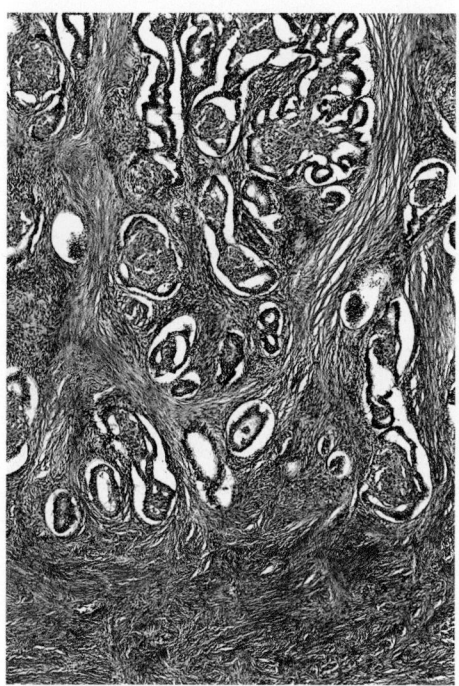

Fig. 27.80
Endometrioid borderline tumor. There is a lobular pattern of glandular and squamous cells that are sharply demarcated at the periphery.

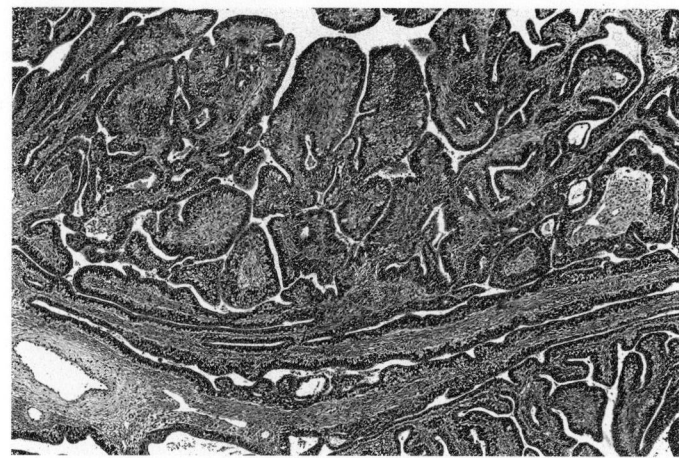

Fig. 27.82 Endometrioid borderline tumor. A complex papillary arrangement is shown. There was no evidence of stromal invasion.

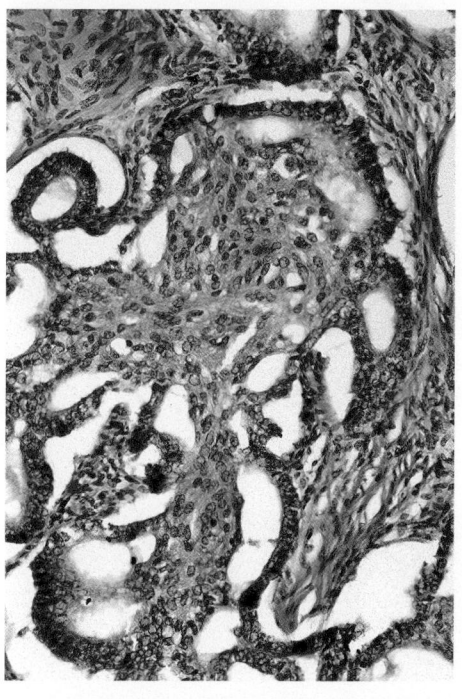

Fig. 27.81
Endometrioid borderline tumor. Bland central squamous cells are surrounded by a garland of low-grade endometrioid glands.

proliferating epithelium occupies a large area without intervening stroma. Some consider cases with confluent growth from 1 to 5 mm in one or more foci to be microinvasive. Using this definition, none of seven cases with microinvasion recurred.[186,187] Others limit microinvasion to cases with small foci (not further specified) of irregular glands inciting a desmoplastic stromal reaction.[184,185] Confluent growth by itself (even in excess of 5 mm) is not considered by them to be evidence of invasion.[185] By this definition there were also no recurrences, in cases with either a confluent growth pattern or infiltrative microinvasion.

On the basis of these results and until more cases are studied, we diagnose invasion if there is either an obviously infiltrative pattern or confluent growth that in the pathologist's judgment is likely to be invasive. Cases with one or more invasive foci <10 mm^2 are reported as 'borderline with microinvasion'.

Endometrioid carcinoma

Well-differentiated endometrioid carcinomas grow in a back-to-back pattern of glands or variably spaced glands in a fibrotic stroma. The glands are lined by stratified epithelial cells with scant eosinophilic cytoplasm resembling those of well-differentiated endometrial carcinomas. Squamous differentiation in the form of morules or larger sheets, sometimes with central necrosis, is common. The cytoplasm may be focally mucinous and there may be mucin or eosinophilic colloid-like material within gland lumens. A villous papillary pattern may be present. In less well-differentiated tumors the glands merge to form solid growth patterns; the cells usually have larger, more pleomorphic nuclei with prominent nucleoli. Central necrosis containing pyknotic nuclear fragments may be present (Figs 27.83–27.89). In some cases the solid pattern contains small rosette-like gland openings, suggesting the Call–Exner bodies of a granulosa cell tumor (Figs 27.90, 27.91). The stroma may be cellular, densely fibrotic, or desmoplastic (Fig. 27.92). Early endometrioid carcinomas may be situated within or adjacent to areas of endometriosis.

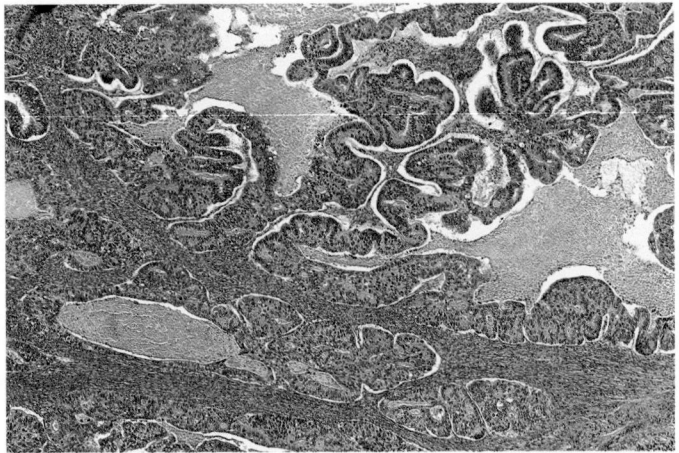

Fig. 27.83 Endometrioid carcinoma. Cystic spaces lined by a cribriform gland arrangement are present.

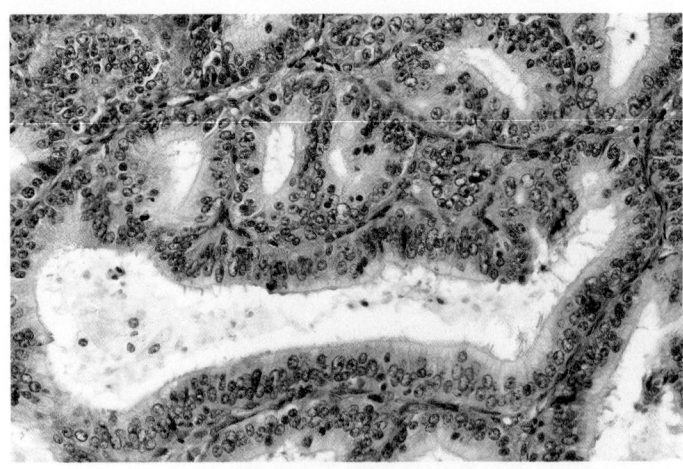

Fig. 27.80 Endometrioid carcinoma. This grade 1 carcinoma is entirely gland forming.

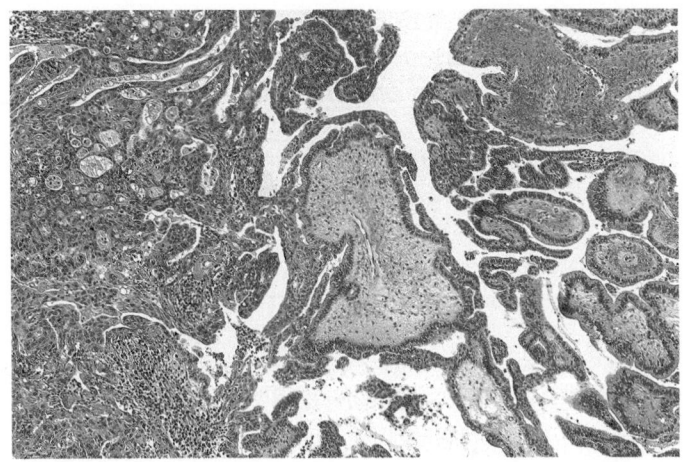

Fig. 27.84 Endometrioid carcinoma. Back-to-back glands on the left merge with a papillary pattern on the right.

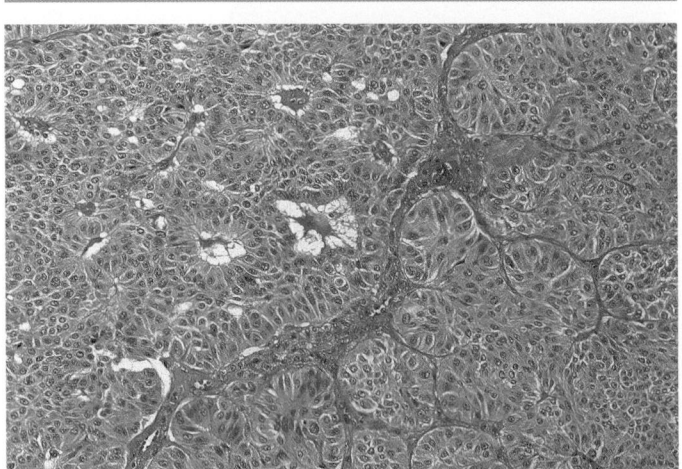

Fig. 27.87 Endometrioid carcinoma. Glands become confluent and partially disappear in this grade 2 carcinoma.

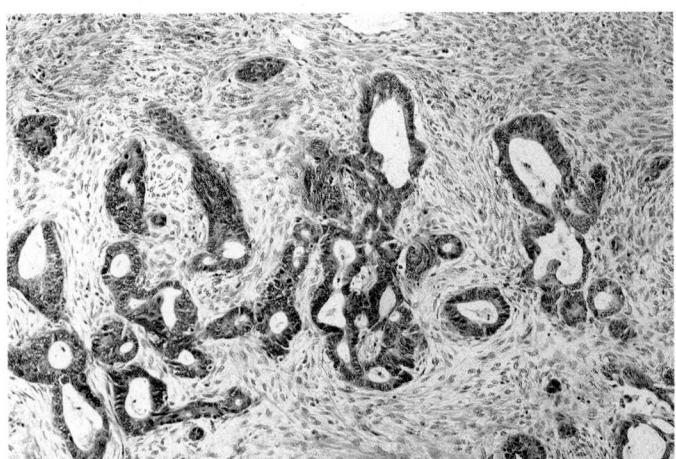

Fig. 27.85 Endometrioid carcinoma. Irregularly spaced glands occupy a desmoplastic stroma.

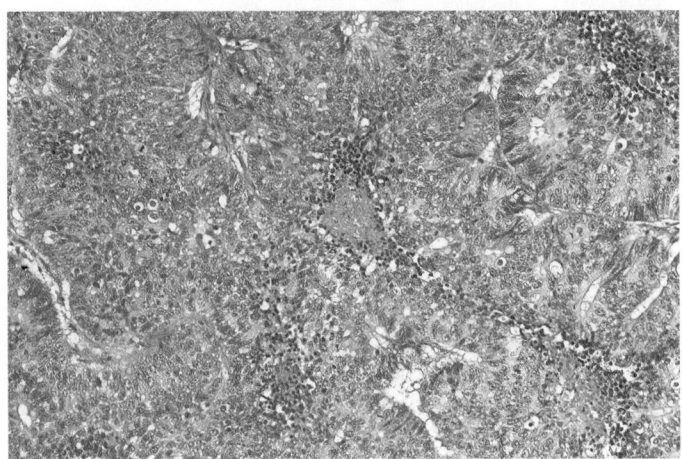

Fig. 27.88 Endometrioid carcinoma. Grade 3 carcinoma with only a few residual glands and extensive necrosis.

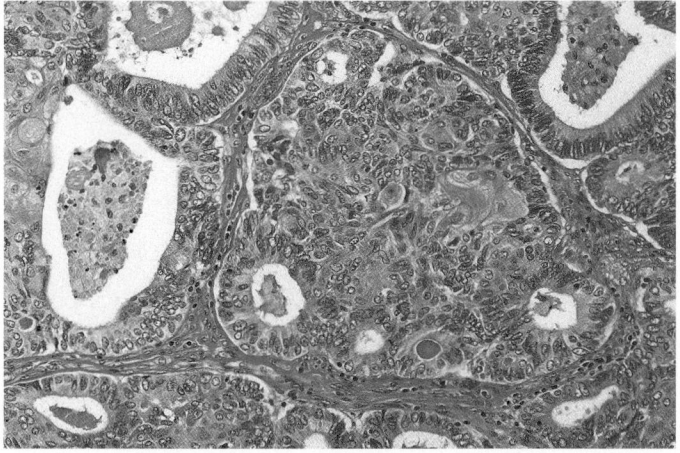

Fig. 27.89 Endometrioid carcinoma. Squamous differentiation is present. The latter is not considered solid in the grading of composite tumors.

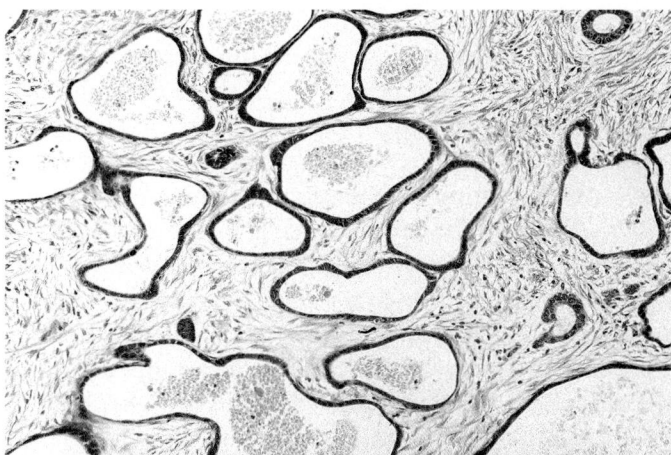

Fig. 27.92 Endometrioid carcinoma. In this case the glands are dilated and the epithelium is attenuated. This tumor might be mistaken for an adenofibroma, except that the stroma appears desmoplastic.

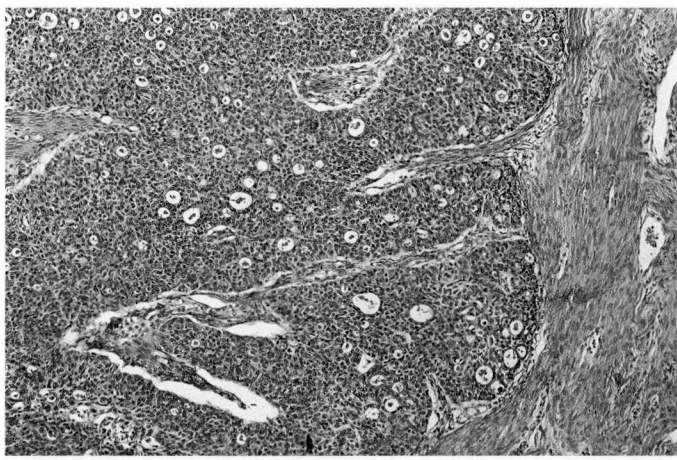

Fig. 27.90 Endometrioid carcinoma. A solid pattern with numerous small spaces. This pattern suggests a granulosa cell tumor with Call-Exner bodies.

We grade endometrioid carcinomas as we do primary carcinomas of the endometrium: excluding squamous areas, grade 1 tumors have <5% solid growth, grade 2 have 5–50% and grade 3 have >50%. Very high nuclear grade elevates a grade 1 or grade 2 tumor by one grade.

Variant cytologic features are: secretory, similar to early secretory endometrial glands,[193] oxyphilic,[194] ciliated,[195] balloon-like[193] and spindle-cell (Fig. 27.93).[196] These variants may mimic a variety of nonendometrioid tumors such as clear cell carcinomas, sex cord tumors, carcinosarcomas, or tumors of probable Wolffian origin (see differential diagnosis below). In all of them, the presence of foci of typical endometrioid carcinoma facilitates a correct interpretation.

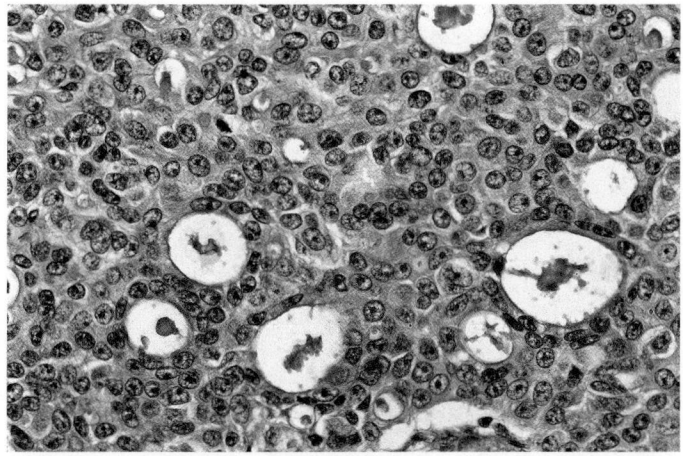

Fig. 27.91 Endometrioid carcinoma. Higher power of the tumor in Figure 27.90. The nuclei are rounder and slightly more atypical than those of the usual granulosa cell tumor. The spaces contain dense eosinophilic material.

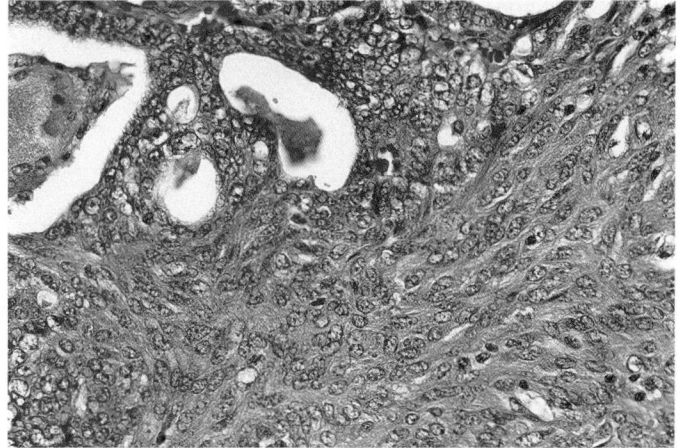

Fig. 27.93 Endometrioid carcinoma. A spindle cell component is present. The spindle cells are bland and should not be considered as solid foci in grading tumors with this appearance.

A variant that has drawn particular attention is the endometrioid carcinoma mimicking Sertoli cell and Sertoli-Leydig cell tumors.[197,198] In these the epithelial cells form small glands, hollow tubules or elongated solid tubular structures in a fibromatous background, the latter sometimes containing luteinized cells (Figs 27.94–27.96). The epithelial cells in the small glands are cuboidal to low columnar with eosinophilic cytoplasm and round/oval nuclei, usually with a single prominent nucleolus.[197] Those in the solid tubules sometimes have polarized basal nuclei arranged around the periphery. In some cases the cells are oxyphilic.[194] In all cases the sex cord-like areas merge with glands that are more typical of well-differentiated endometrioid carcinomas. Further, the epithelial cells are reactive by immunohistochemistry with keratins, including CK 7 and epithelial membrane antigen and are nonreactive with alpha-inhibin, distinguishing them from true sex cord tumors.[199–201]

Rare endometrioid carcinomas with a yolk sac tumor component have been described.[202] These combine typical endometrioid carcinoma with the microcystic and glandular pattern of yolk sac tumor; the latter is positive for alpha-fetoprotein. In six reported cases the average age of the patients was 53 years. Five of the six patients died and one had only a brief follow-up period.

In assessing the peritoneum for extraovarian spread of endometrioid carcinomas, one should be aware of the phenomenon of peritoneal granulomas that may be found in cases of endometrioid ovarian or primary endometrial carcinomas with squamous differentiation.[203] These granulomas are devoid of viable-appearing epithelial cells but have either ghosts of squamous cells or keratin debris surrounded by histiocytes and multinucleated cells. This finding should stimulate a search for viable tumor cell implants but by itself does not change the stage or prognosis.

DIFFERENTIAL DIAGNOSIS

Metastatic endometrial carcinoma

From 15 to 23% of all metastatic carcinomas involving the ovaries originate in the endometrium.[204,205] Further, approximately 12% of patients who present clinically with ovarian endometrioid carcinomas are discovered to also have primary endometrial carcinomas.[176–178,189,191] Hence, the distinction between synchronous endometrial and ovarian endometrioid carcinoma and endometrial carcinoma metastatic to the ovary is a common problem for pathologists.

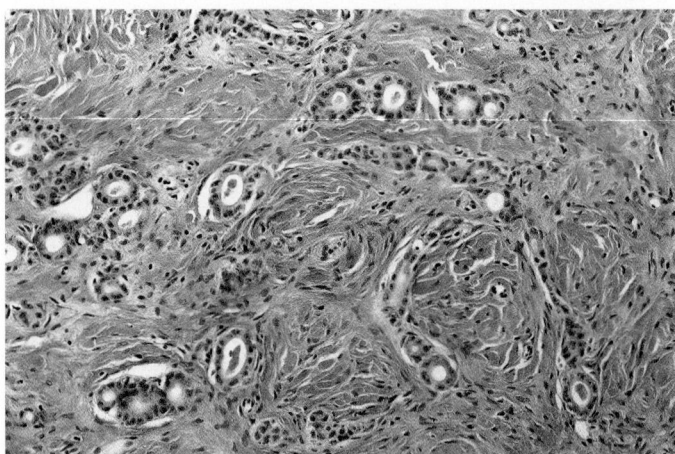

Fig. 27.94 Endometrioid carcinoma mimicking a Sertoli cell tumor. Small, widely spaced well-differentiated glands are seen.

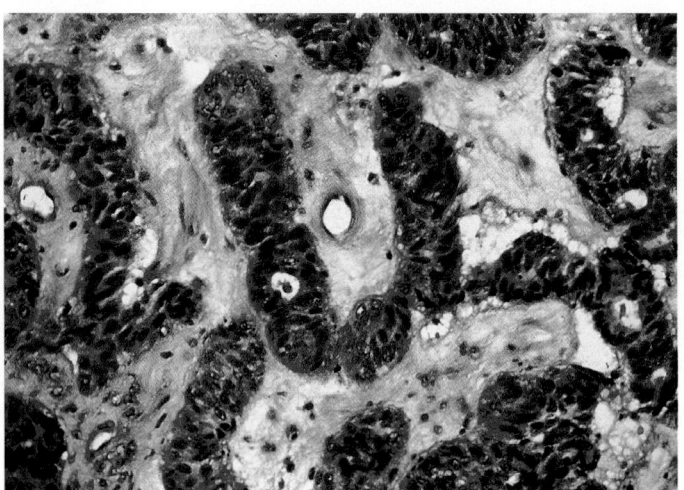

Fig. 27.95 Endometrioid carcinoma mimicking a Sertoli cell tumor. Solid tubules with small openings are seen.

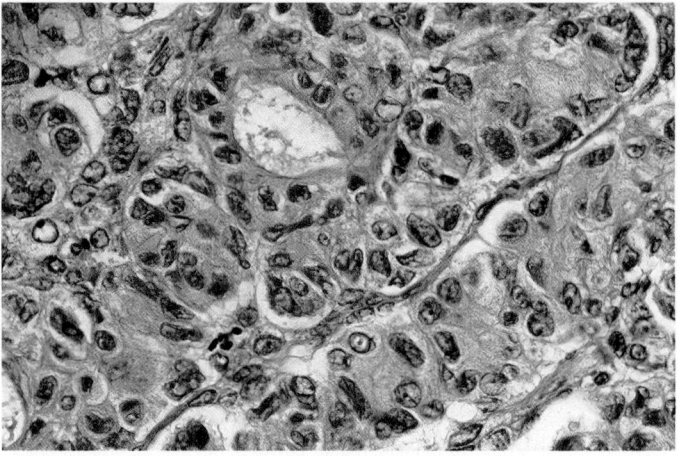

Fig. 27.96 Endometrioid carcinoma mimicking a Sertoli cell tumor. Glands and tubules, the latter with mostly eccentrically placed nuclei, are present.

When the carcinomas are both of the endometrioid type and confined to the uterus and one or both ovaries, the clinical outcome has been the same as if they were separate stage I endometrial and ovarian carcinomas.[206–208] In most of these cases the endometrial carcinomas do not invade deeply into the myometrium. The ovarian carcinomas are often associated with ipsilateral ovarian endometriosis and are bilateral in the same proportion of cases as ovarian endometrioid carcinomas without concomitant endometrial cancers (about 17%). Therefore, it is likely that in most cases the carcinomas have arisen synchronously in both the ovary(ies) and the endometrium. There is further support for this conclusion from molecular and immunohistochemical differences between the ovarian and endometrial tumors in most cases.[209–215] Thus, in this situation, we use diagnostic terminology as though both the ovarian and uterine tumors were primary carcinomas. We often append a note of explanation and cite appropriate references.

When the endometrial carcinoma invades deeply into the myometrium or is present in myometrial vessels, or when metastases are present in lymph nodes or in the pelvis or abdomen, the presumption that the ovarian tumor is a synchronous primary carcinoma is not as obvious. Findings that favor ovarian metastases are: (1) high-grade histologic features in both sites, (2) bilaterality of the ovarian tumors, (3) ovarian surface, vascular, or hilar involvement, (4) a multinodular pattern of ovarian growth and (5) an absence of ovarian endometriosis. Although judgment and common sense are important, the most likely origin of the ovarian tumor may still not be obvious. If available, comparative cytogenetic or molecular analysis of both tumors may be more definitive.[210–215] However, identical genetic profiles can be found in tumors of independent origin and conversely the profiles may differ in tumors of the same origin due to tumor heterogeneity or progression. Thus, clonality analysis is most helpful if it does not rely on a single result and is interpreted in light of the concomitant clinical and pathologic findings.

Metastatic colorectal carcinoma

It has been estimated that up to 7% of all ovarian masses clinically initially considered to be primary tumors are actually metastases, mostly from the gastrointestinal tract.[216] Further, in approximately 3% of all women with colon carcinoma, an ovarian mass is the initial sign.[217] Even after microscopic examination, metastatic colonic carcinomas are often misdiagnosed as primary ovarian cancers, usually of the endometrioid type.[149–151]

Metastatic large-intestinal carcinomas are usually large masses with a smooth external surface and a cystic and soft solid interior that is focally hemorrhagic and necrotic. They are bilateral in about one-third of cases. Microscopically they often contain 'garlands' of glands that encircle large areas of 'dirty necrosis' (granular amorphous material containing abundant nuclear debris). Partially necrotic glands, large areas of confluent epithelial necrosis and a cribriform pattern of back-to-back glands are all commonly present. Usually the nuclei are larger, coarser and more pleomorphic than those of primary endometrioid carcinomas and there is a lack of squamous differentiation, the latter often present in primary tumors.[150,151] However, some endometrioid ovarian carcinomas also grow in a cribriform pattern and contain areas of dirty necrosis.[218] Conversely, occasional large-intestinal metastases do not have the typical garland pattern surrounding areas of dirty necrosis.[151]

Immunohistochemistry can be very useful. Some 80–90% of metastatic colon and rectal carcinomas are negative with CK 7 and approximately 90% are positive with CK 20, whereas endometrioid ovarian carcinomas are CK 7 positive in 95% and CK 20 negative in 80–90%.[157–159,219] In one report, Cdx2 stained all 15 metastatic colon carcinomas and none of 15 primary endometrioid carcinomas.[163] Thus, one can achieve almost 100% certainty in this differential diagnosis by using a panel of these three antibodies along with the clinical and morphologic findings.

Mucinous ovarian carcinoma

Mucin in gland lumens and/or confined to the apical cytoplasm is present in many endometrioid tumors. Also, as in primary endometrial carcinomas, endometrioid ovarian carcinomas may have cells with mucinous cytoplasm resembling endocervical cells. Usually these are minor foci and in these cases we append the phrase 'with mucinous differentiation' to the diagnosis. If the mucinous foci are distinct and comprise more than 10% of the tumor, the tumor is designated 'mixed endometrioid and mucinous carcinoma' and the relative proportion of each component is specified.

Granulosa cell, Sertoli cell and Sertoli–Leydig cell tumor

Endometrioid carcinomas are sometimes yellow with hemorrhagic cystic areas, grossly similar to granulosa cell tumors. Microscopically they can also simulate granulosa cell tumors, forming trabeculae or solid sheets punctuated by small round openings resembling the

Call–Exner bodies of a granulosa cell tumor. Although endometrioid carcinomas may have cells with nuclear grooves, the nuclei are usually rounder and more hyperchromatic than those of a granulosa cell tumor. The Call–Exner-like areas may contain mucin, not a feature of granulosa cell tumors. Inhibin and calretinin are negative in endometrioid carcinomas and epithelial membrane antigen is positive, distinguishing them from granulosa cell tumors.

Ovarian clear cell carcinoma, metastatic intestinal clear cell carcinoma

Mixed-epithelial carcinomas of the ovary often contain the combination of endometrioid and clear cell carcinomas, so that one should not be surprised to find the two together. The epithelial cells of the secretory variant of endometrioid carcinoma have cytoplasmic vacuoles, causing them to resemble a pure clear cell carcinoma. However, the nuclei are less atypical than those of a clear cell carcinoma and the characteristic papillary and tubulocystic growth patterns of clear cell carcinoma are absent.

Areas of squamous differentiation in an endometrioid carcinoma may also have clear cells, but again the overall pattern is that of endometrioid rather than clear cell carcinoma.

The oxyphilic variant of endometrioid carcinoma may be mistaken for an oxyphilic clear cell carcinoma of the ovary.[220] The finding of other foci characteristic of a clear cell carcinoma in the latter tumor is necessary for this distinction.

Rare clear cell variants of large- and small-intestinal carcinomas metastatic to the ovaries may simulate either the secretory variant of endometrioid carcinoma or clear cell carcinoma of the ovary.[221] In some cases, subnuclear and supranuclear vacuoles in the metastatic tumors may produce a striking similarity to secretory endometrial glands. In these cases the finding of dirty necrosis, an unexpected finding in primary secretory ovarian carcinoma, is an important clue. Immunohistochemical findings confirm the correct diagnosis: the metastatic tumors are negative for CK 7 and CA 125 and positive for CK 20 and carcinoembryonic antigen.[221]

Rare primary ovarian tumors: tumor of probable Wolffian origin, yolk sac tumor, ependymoma

Tumors of Wolffian origin are more common in the broad ligament, but may also arise in the ovary.[222] They have a variety of patterns including cystic, sieve-like, tubular and diffuse. The tubular pattern, in particular, may appear endometrioid. However, the presence of the other patterns, a lack of intraluminal mucin and epithelial cells with only mild nuclear atypia, all distinguish the Wolffian tumor from an endometrioid carcinoma. Although not considered to be of sex cord-stromal origin, the Wolffian tumor stains positively with alpha-inhibin in 70–90% of cases and with calretinin in 90%, also distinguishing it from an endometrioid carcinoma.[223,224]

A variant of ovarian yolk sac tumor has been described as 'endometrioid-like', because it contains areas resembling the secretory type of endometrioid carcinoma.[225] The gland-like growth with vacuolated cytoplasm is attributed to endodermal differentiation in these cases. The patients are usually young and other patterns more characteristic of a yolk sac tumor are usually (but not always) present. These tumors stain with alpha-fetoprotein and the serum α-fetoprotein is also elevated. As noted above, rare endometrioid carcinomas have true yolk sac differentiation, usually with a microcystic and glandular pattern.[202]

Neuroectodermal tumors of the ovary are diverse and may mimic a wide variety of other tumors.[226] Those with ependymal differentiation or that are purely ependymal[227] most closely simulate endometrioid carcinomas. Ependymomas contain cells with characteristic elongated tapering, fibrillary processes and perivascular pseudorosettes, not present in carcinomas. They stain with glial fibrillary acidic protein. The patients are younger than most of those with endometrioid carcinomas.

ETIOLOGY, GENETICS AND BIOMARKERS

An unknown percentage of ovarian endometrioid carcinomas arise from endometriosis. Evidence for this includes the following: (1) Women with endometriosis have a higher than average risk for ovarian carcinomas, almost all of which are either of the endometrioid or the clear cell types.[228–232] (2) Although only approximately 13% of all endometrioid carcinomas have adjacent residual identifiable endometriosis,[176–178,18,189,191] in stage I endometrioid carcinomas it has been found in 39% of cases, a much higher frequency than in stage I tumors of the serous or mucinous types.[230] (3) Ovarian endometriosis can harbor a spectrum of architectural and cytologic changes, some of which are similar to atypical hyperplasia of the endometrium;[192,233] these changes are present much more frequently in ovarian endometriosis that is associated with carcinoma than in ovarian endometriosis without carcinoma,[231] and in some cases they are present immediately adjacent to the carcinoma, suggesting a direct transformation.[230] (4) In one study, severely atypical cells in endometriotic cysts were aneuploid, whereas the normal or only slightly atypical cells were diploid.[234] (5) Both ovarian endometriosis and associated ipsilateral endometrioid carcinomas had a loss of heterozygosity on chromosome 12, X chromosome inactivation and p53 mutations in 9 of 11 cases.[235]

All of the above strongly implicates endometriosis in the genesis of some ovarian endometrioid carcinomas. However, women with endometriosis-associated endometrioid carcinomas are younger and have lower-stage tumors than women with tumors in which endometriosis cannot be found.[191,232] In some of the latter, endometriosis may have been present but was overgrown, but it is likely that a subset of endometrioid carcinomas are not derived from endometriosis, perhaps arising from Müllerian inclusions or ovarian surface epithelium, similar to the presumed origin of serous carcinomas.[193]

Molecular analyses of endometrioid carcinomas have found mutations in the PTEN tumor suppressor gene[236] in about 20% of cases and in the beta-catenin gene[215,237] in from 40–50% of cases. Both of these mutations are found more frequently in early-stage tumors, suggesting that they are an early event in tumor development. Microsatellite instability, frequently present in uterine endometrial carcinomas, leads to promoter methylation of hMLH-1 and other mismatch repair genes and the accumulation of mutations in the coding of mononucleotide tracts. While it also may play a role in the pathogenesis of some ovarian endometrioid carcinomas, it has been found in only 12–20% of cases.[213,238,239]

Endometrioid carcinomas have the same immunoprofile as primary carcinomas of the endometrium. That is, they are positive in most cases, with broad-spectrum cytokeratins, CK 7, epithelial membrane antigen, vimentin and estrogen and progesterone receptors. They are generally negative for CK 20,[157–159,219] WT1[89] and inhibin.[199–201]

TUMORS WITH A SARCOMATOUS COMPONENT AND ENDOMETRIOID STROMAL SARCOMA

Definition, clinical aspects

Ovarian malignant Müllerian mixed tumors (carcinosarcomas), adenosarcomas and endometrioid stromal sarcomas are included in the endometrioid stromal-epithelial tumors category by the WHO.[13] The first of these is very uncommon, the others distinctly rare. They are similar microscopically to their much more common counterparts in the uterus and this aspect is described and illustrated more fully in the chapter on uterine sarcomas and carcinosarcomas.

Malignant Müllerian mixed tumor

These are biphasic neoplasms in which both the epithelial and the stromal components are histologically malignant. Almost all patients are older than 50 and have symptoms similar to those with other ovarian cancers.[240–247] Considering all stages, the tumors are bilateral in about one-third of cases. Approximately 80% are stages III or IV at the time of initial staging and essentially all patients with these high-stage tumors die of their cancer. A few stage I patients have survived >5 years.[242,243] There is a weak correlation between stromal cell type and survival: tumors with a homologous sarcomatous component (fibrosarcoma, endometrial stromal sarcoma, myxoid sarcoma) convey a more favorable prognosis by univariate analysis than those with a heterologous stromal component.[242] There is no correlation between survival and the epithelial or stromal cell type in the metastases.[242,243]

Adenosarcoma (Müllerian adenosarcoma, mesodermal adenosarcoma)

These are biphasic neoplasms in which the epithelial component is benign-appearing. In most cases the stromal component is of a lower-grade malignancy than in malignant Müllerian mixed tumors. The largest series describes 40 cases.[248] The authors note that only 20 other cases had been previously reported, the largest prior report containing 10 cases.[249] In this largest series, the patients' ages ranged from 30 to 84 years. In all but one case the tumors were unilateral; 65% were stage I, 28% stage II and 7% stage III. Only 6 of 26 women who were followed for at least 5 years were free of recurrence and the 5-, 10- and 15-year survival rates were 64%, 46% and 30%, respectively. This behavior is not as favorable as that of the more common primary uterine adenosarcomas. A worse prognosis among these cases was related to high tumor grade, high-grade sarcomatous overgrowth, tumor rupture and patient age younger than 53 years.

Endometrioid stromal sarcoma

These are composed primarily of cells that resemble the stromal cells of the proliferative-phase endometrium. Presumably because of their derivation from endometriosis, endometrioid stromal sarcomas can also arise outside of both the uterus and the ovaries, usually in the peritoneal or abdominal cavity.[250] Of those presumed to have originated within one or both ovaries, the largest series describes 23 cases.[251] The patients' ages ranged from 20 to 76 years; 48% were bilateral; and 17% stage I, 39% stage II, 35 % stage III and two cases stage IV because of pulmonary metastases. Notably, in 40% of the cases there was a prior or synchronous endometrial stromal sarcoma of the uterus, raising the possibility that some of the ovarian cases were metastatic. Five of the 23 patients died of their sarcomas, but the follow-up interval was short in some of the survivors. Survival correlated with low-grade tumors, the grade being based on finding fewer than 10 mitotic figures per 10 high power microscopic fields.

Gross examination

Malignant Müllerian mixed tumors are large solid and cystic masses, usually with a soft interior with areas of necrosis and hemorrhage. In rare cases they arise within an endometriotic cyst.[228]

Adenosarcomas range in size from 5 to 50 cm. Some tumors are predominately cystic. However, most are predominately solid, firm to soft, with small cysts. They may contain areas of hemorrhage or necrosis.

Endometrioid stromal sarcomas range from 4 to 23 cm. They are predominately solid and tan or whitish-yellow. Some have variably sized cysts and a few are predominately cystic.

Microscopic examination

The epithelial component of malignant Müllerian mixed tumors is usually serous, endometrioid, or undifferentiated carcinoma; sometimes there is squamous or clear cell and rarely mucinous or neuroectodermal (glial or neuronal) differentiation.[252] The malignant epithelium is usually sharply demarcated from a stromal component. The latter may appear fibrosarcomatous, myxoid, endometrial stromal-like, cartilaginous, or myoid (Fig. 27.97). Periodic acid–Schiff-positive, diastase-resistant, hyaline cytoplasmic bodies are found in ~ 50% of cases.[245]

Müllerian adenosarcomas appear similar to their uterine counterparts, including the presence in some cases of sex cord-like areas and areas of sarcomatous overgrowth (Figs 27.98, 27.99).

Ovarian endometrioid stromal sarcomas are also similar to those in the uterus with the exception that they often merge with areas that are indistinguishable from an ovarian fibroma.[250]

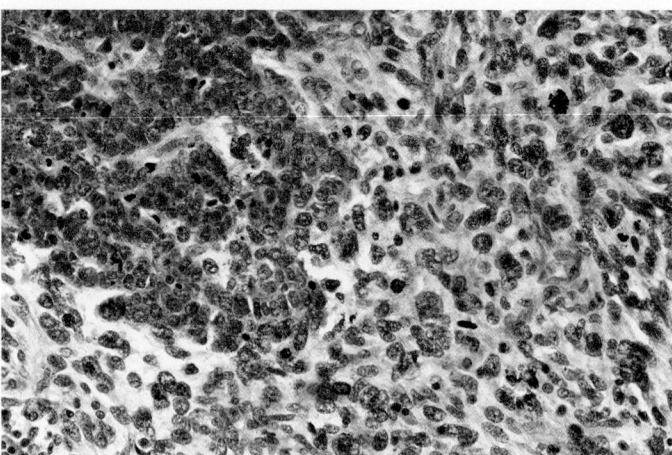

Fig. 27.97 Mixed Müllerian tumor (carcinosarcoma). The epithelial and stromal components are clearly demarcated and both are malignant.

Differential diagnosis

Malignant mixed Müllerian tumors may be mistaken for immature teratoma, poorly differentiated Sertoli–Leydig tumor, endometrioid stromal sarcoma with sex cord-like elements, carcinoma with hypercellular reactive stroma, or spindle cell (sarcomatoid) carcinoma.[193]

Immature teratomas are found in children and young women and contain elements of all three germ layers with a prominent neuroectodermal component. They have an immature, fetal, or embryonal appearance rather

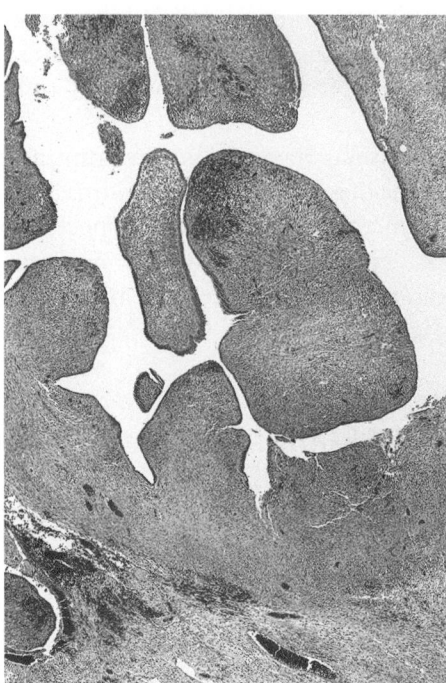

Fig. 27.98 Müllerian adenosarcoma. A broad, polyploid, phyllodes-like growth is seen.

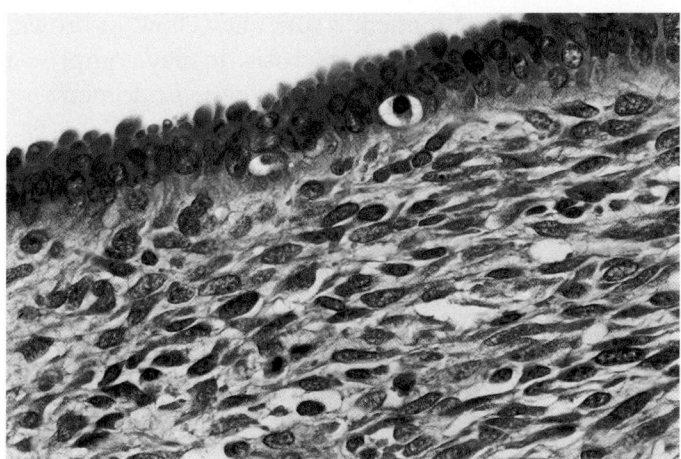

Fig. 27.99 Müllerian adenosarcoma. At high power the epithelium is benign-appearing, whereas the stroma is cellular with mitotic activity, consistent with a low-grade sarcoma.

than the highly malignant epithelial and stromal components of a malignant Müllerian mixed tumor.

Sertoli–Leydig tumors also occur in young women and are often androgenic. Almost all have characteristic Sertoli–Leydig areas and their epithelial-appearing elements usually do not have the high-grade atypia of the epithelial cells of a malignant mixed Müllerian tumor. Sertoli-Leydig tumors are inhibin-positive and EMA-negative, the reverse of malignant Müllerian mixed tumors.

In *endometrioid stromal sarcomas with sex cord-like areas*, both the stromal cells and sex cord-like elements are low grade, unlike the highly malignant appearance of malignant Müllerian mixed tumors.

Some *pure carcinomas* have a spindle cell stroma that is difficult to distinguish from a sarcomatous element. This distinction may be difficult, even arbitrary, in some borderline cases.[193]

Sarcomatoid carcinomas lack the clear-cut boundaries between carcinoma and sarcoma that is present, at least focally, in mixed tumors.

Adenosarcoma can be mistaken for adenofibroma and polypoid endometriosis.

Some *adenofibromas* have a cellular stroma, but pronounced periglandular cuffing, stromal mitotic activity and stromal cell atypia are all absent.

Polypoid endometriosis is an overgrowth of endometrial tissue to form a polypoid mass.[253] It does not possess the broad fronds that project into glandular spaces or from the tumor surface that are characteristic of adenosarcoma. Additionally, nuclear atypia and periglandular cuffing are absent in polypoid endometriosis. However, experience is limited and this distinction is necessarily

arbitrary in some borderline cases. The authors of the *AFIP* fascicle[193] diagnose ovarian adenosarcoma 'if the stroma is unusually cellular, if there is more than minimal stromal nuclear atypia, or if the mitotic count is two or more per ten high power fields'.

Endometrioid stromal sarcoma may be mistaken for granulosa cell tumor of the diffuse type, fibrothecoma, ovarian stromal hyperplasia, or metastatic endometrioid stromal sarcoma of the uterus.[193]

Granulosa cell tumors and fibrothecomas lack the characteristic profusion of spiral arterioles and the tongue-like infiltrative pattern present in endometrioid stromal tumors. The nuclei of granulosa cell tumors are reniform or grooved, unlike the oval or spindled nuclei of stromal sarcomas. Granulosa cell tumors and thecomas are often estrogenic and stain with inhibin, whereas neither are features of stromal sarcoma.

Ovarian stromal hyperplasia does not lead to significant ovarian enlargement and lacks the vascular pattern present in endometrioid stromal sarcoma.

There may be a history of a *uterine stromal sarcoma* in women with an endometrioid stromal sarcoma in the ovary.[251,254] In these cases the ovarian lesion is assumed to be metastatic, unless there is residual endometriosis in continuity with the ovarian tumor. Even without this history, if there has been a prior hysterectomy, it is advisable to review that material before considering a primary ovarian endometrial stromal sarcoma. Uterine endometrial stromal sarcomas can develop ovarian metastases many years after removal and may have been misdiagnosed initially.

Clear cell tumors

GENERAL FEATURES AND CLINICAL ASPECTS

Clear cell tumors are adenocarcinomas in which most or all of the epithelial cells have clear cytoplasm. The cytoplasmic clearing is due to glycogen, although some cells may also contain mucin.[255] In some tumors, the cytoplasm may be focally oxyphilic and in a rare variant it is completely oxyphilic.

Benign and borderline clear cell tumors are rare. The mean age of patients is in the seventh decade.[256,257] Of 14 clear cell borderline tumors, one with microinvasion had a pelvic recurrence and the patient died from her tumor.[257] In an additional case without invasion there was an unconfirmed pulmonary metastasis.[257] In all other cases there have been no recurrences.

Clear cell carcinomas account for 5–12% of carcinomas in the epithelial-stromal category.[22–25,106] The mean patient age is in the sixth decade. The tumors are unilateral in 98% of stage I cases.[115] Clear cell carcinomas have a clinical presentation and pattern of spread similar to other common epithelial tumors. However, similar to endometrioid carcinomas and unlike serous or mucinous carcinomas, clear cell carcinomas are frequently associated with endometriosis.[255,258,259] Rarely, they may give rise to paraneoplastic hypercalcemia.[260]

Approximately 40% of clear cell carcinomas are confined to the ovary at initial staging, a higher frequency than the more common serous carcinomas.[258,259,261–264] Some report a worse prognosis in stage I clear cell carcinomas than in other epithelial tumors, with a 5-year survival of only 50–60%.[258,259,261] Others, however, found outcomes in stage I clear cell carcinomas to be similar to those of other epithelial tumors.[263–265] In some reports high-stage tumors were less responsive to platinum-based chemotherapy than other common epithelial-stromal tumors.[262,264] Others, however, reported 5-year survival in higher-stage cases the same as that associated with other epithelial tumors (~ 20%).[263]

GROSS EXAMINATION

Benign and borderline tumors are solid with variably sized cysts. The solid component is firm; the cysts contain clear fluid. Both are unilateral in over 90% of cases and vary from a few cm up to 20 cm. Some borderline tumors have a unique sponge-like appearance with myriad small, thin-walled cysts throughout (Fig. 27.100).

Carcinomas may be predominantly solid, but are usually partially cystic. The cyst fluid may be serous or mucinous. The solid component is soft, tan, yellow, or brown, often with hemorrhage or necrosis. It may comprise a polypoid mass that projects into a cyst. Endometriosis is often present adjacent to early tumors.

MICROSCOPIC EXAMINATION

Benign and borderline clear cell adenofibromas and cystadenofibromas

The stroma is fibromatous and contains glands and cysts lined by a single layer of cuboidal cells with clear cytoplasm. The tumor is considered borderline if the nuclei of at least some of the epithelial cells appear malignant. The distinction between malignant and merely 'atypical' nuclei in clear cell tumors is somewhat subjective; however, nuclear enlargement, hyperchromasia and a prominent nucleolus are features of malignant clear cells (Figs 27.101, 27.102).

It is important to sample benign and borderline-appearing clear cell tumors generously in order to exclude areas of invasion that are often present if one searches hard enough (Fig. 27.103). Because of their rarity there are no large studies specifying the risk for metastases associated with small areas of invasion in clear cell borderline tumors. As with the more common borderline tumors, we confine the diagnosis of 'borderline with microinvasion' to tumors with less that 10 mm² of invasion in any single focus.

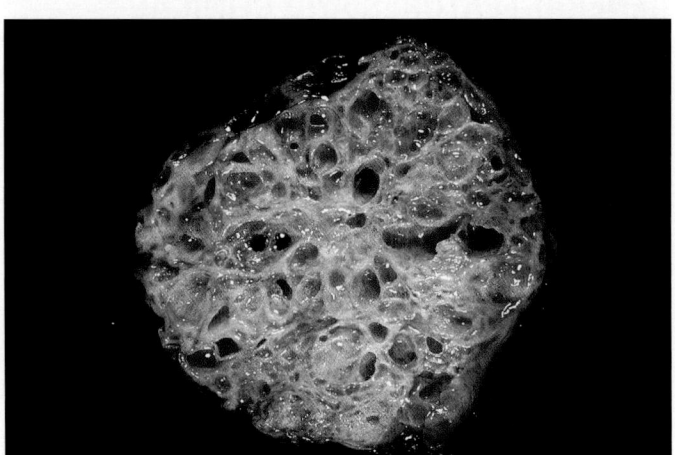

Fig. 27.100 Clear cell borderline tumor. The cut surface has a characteristic spongy appearance.

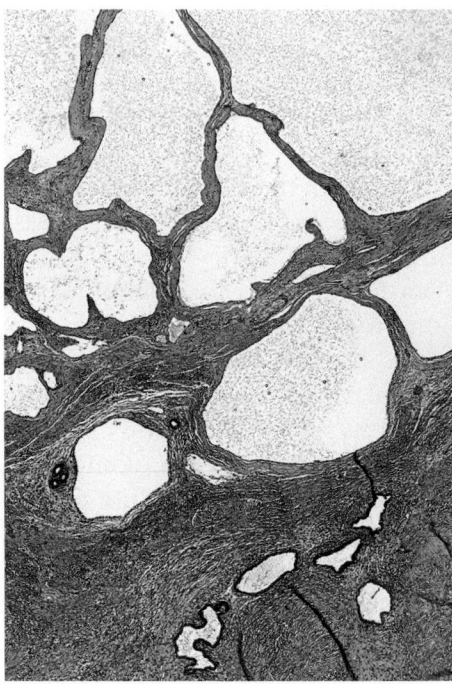

Fig. 27.101 Clear cell borderline tumor. A small focus of endometriosis is present below the cysts of the borderline tumor.

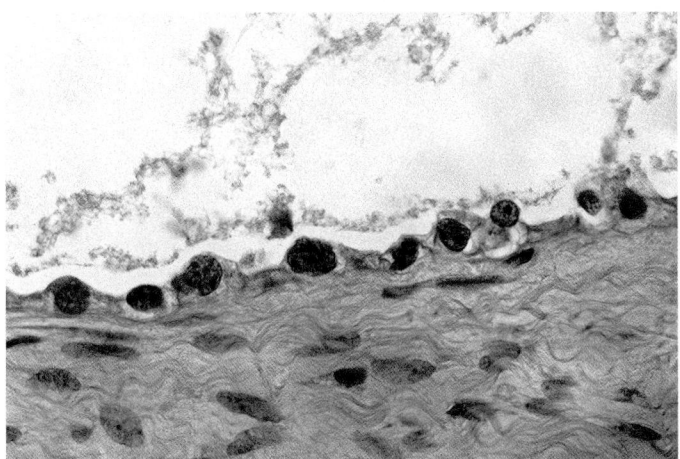

Fig. 27.102 Clear cell borderline tumor. The cyst lining cells are only slightly enlarged. The nuclei are variably shaped with a small nucleolus.

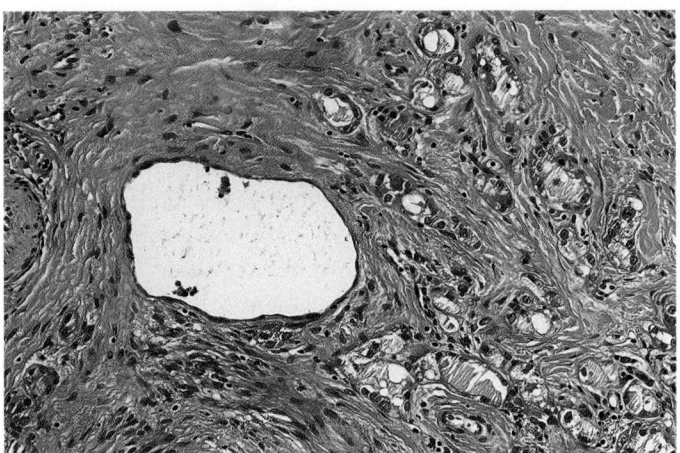

Fig. 27.103 Clear cell borderline tumor with early invasion. Infiltrating tubules of clear cell carcinoma are present adjacent to a residual cyst from a borderline tumor.

Clear cell carcinoma

Most clear cell carcinomas are easily recognizable under low power because of their characteristic architectural patterns. Most apparent is the papillary pattern with its characteristic hyalinized stroma. The papillae have a non-stratified or only minimally stratified epithelial cell lining, as opposed to the marked epithelial cell stratification of papillary serous tumors. Other patterns include cystic, glandular, or solid. These patterns are often mixed and may be accompanied by a fibrous, edematous, or myxoid stroma, sometimes with psammoma bodies. The spaces around the papillae and within the cysts are filled with an eosinophilic or pale blue mucinous fluid. There may be necrosis and hemorrhage. The epithelial cells have abundant cytoplasm that is either clear or bubbly and an enlarged, oval or irregular nucleus with a small to prominent nucleolus. Often the cells lining papillae or cysts have scant cytoplasm and dark nuclei that protrude into the space, causing them to stand out distinctly from one another (hobnail cells). Other cells may be flattened and appear deceptively benign. Foci of endometriosis may be present and in smaller tumors the carcinoma may have arisen within an endometriotic cyst (Figs 27.104–27.109).

Variations include cells with an eosinophilic rather than clear cytoplasm, either as a minor or a major component (oxyphilic variant).[266] There may be foci of mucin-containing signet ring cells that, in rare cases, predominate.[255] Tumors with a reticular pattern resembling a yolk sac tumor,[255] a prominent component of lymphocytes and plasma cells in the stroma,[255] or mixed with rhabdomyosarcoma have been reported.[267]

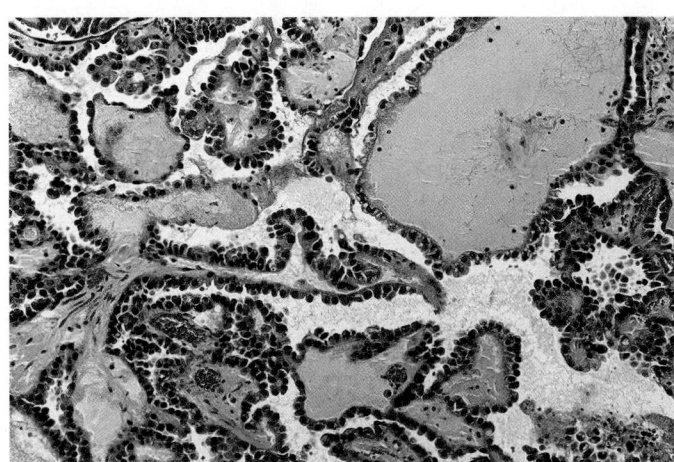

Fig. 27.104 Clear cell carcinoma. A papillary pattern with hyalinized papillary cores is seen. The papillae are lined by nonstratified cells. The hobnail appearance can be appreciated even at low-power magnification.

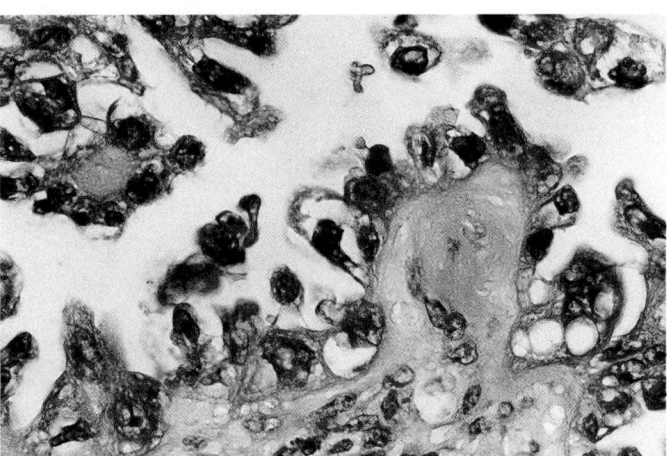

Fig. 27.105 Clear cell carcinoma. Cells with clear or bubbly cytoplasm line papillae with hyaline cores.

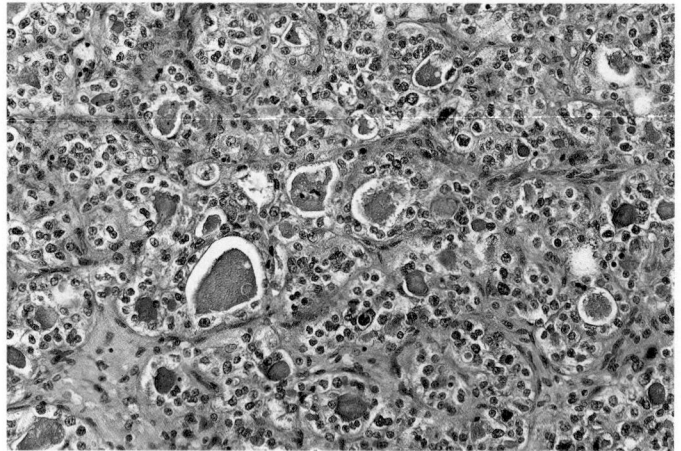

Fig. 27.106 Clear cell carcinoma. A tubulo-glandular appearance is seen.

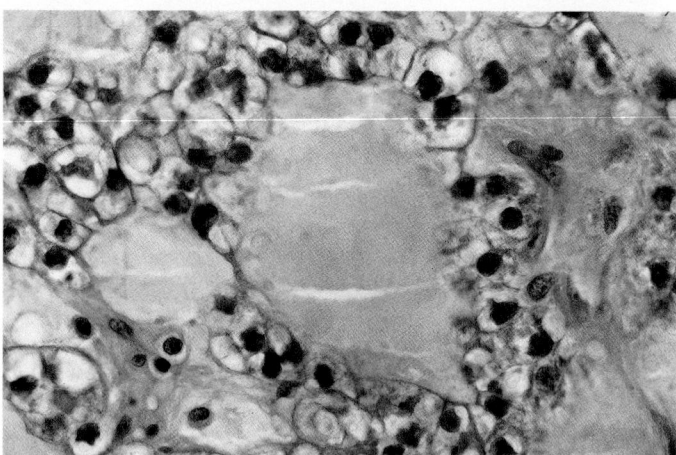

Fig. 27.109 Clear cell carcinoma. The spaces contain a watery, pink fluid. The cytoplasm is clear; the nuclei are only mildly atypical.

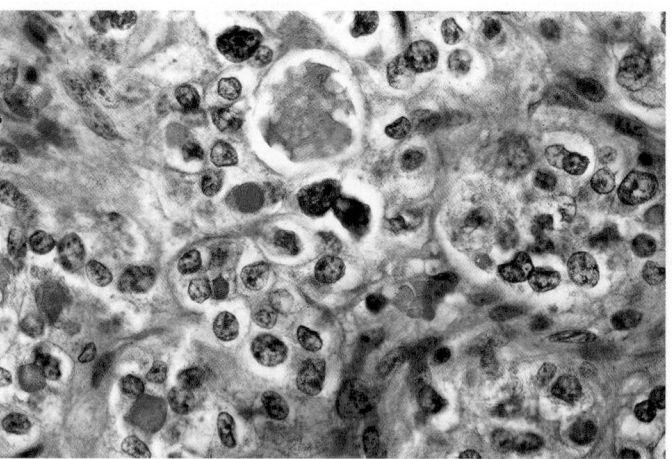

Fig. 27.107 Clear cell carcinoma. The glands are filled with eosinophilic material. The cells have clear cytoplasm and moderately pleomorphic nuclei.

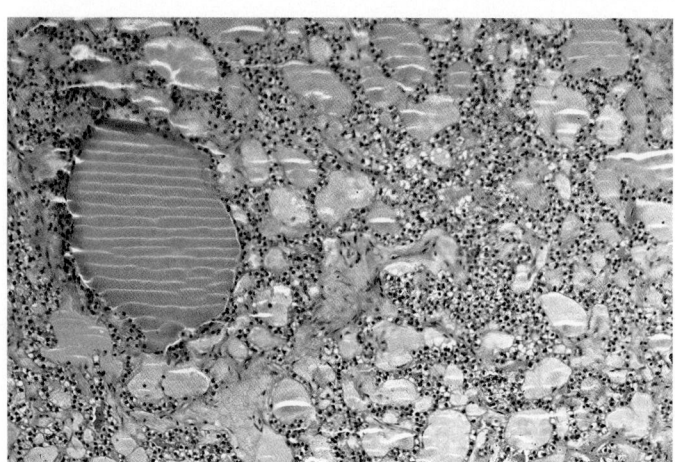

Fig. 27.108 Clear cell carcinoma. A cystic and glandular pattern resembling thyroid follicles is present.

DIFFERENTIAL DIAGNOSIS

Due to the variety of patterns that may be present in clear cell carcinomas, they can be mistaken for serous or endometrioid carcinoma, dysgerminoma, yolk sac tumor, struma ovarii, juvenile granulosa cell tumor, or metastatic clear cell or signet ring cell tumors such as renal carcinoma and Krukenberg tumors.[255]

The rare oxyphilic variant of clear cell carcinoma may mimic a sex-cord-stromal tumor, a hepatoid carcinoma,[268,269] or an endometrioid carcinoma. Since these other entities are more frequently confused with endometrioid carcinomas, they are discussed in the section on endometrioid tumors.

Serous carcinoma

Papillary clear cell carcinomas may have cells with eosinophilic rather than clear cytoplasm, simulating a serous tumor. Usually, however, the cores of the papillae are hyalinized, rather than fibrous or edematous as in a serous carcinoma. Papillary serous carcinomas usually have more stratification and nuclear atypia than clear cell carcinomas. Adjacent endometriosis favors a clear cell carcinoma.

Endometrioid carcinoma

Squamous or secretory areas within an endometrioid carcinoma may have clear cells, potentially mimicking a clear cell carcinoma. Glycogenated squamous cells usually merge with more obvious squamous cells that have dense, eosinophilic cytoplasm. Cytoplasmic vacuoles in secretory endometrioid cells are both sub-nuclear and supranuclear as opposed to the uniformly clear cytoplasm of a clear cell carcinoma. The architectural patterns in both instances are those of an endometrioid rather than a clear cell carcinoma. One should be aware that clear cell and endometrioid carcinomas sometimes coexist and are the most frequent of the mixed-epithelial carcinomas.

Dysgerminoma

Dysgerminoma cells have clear cytoplasm. However, usually the nuclei are central and smooth, rather than eccentric and irregular as in clear cell carcinomas. Dysgerminoma nuclei have a characteristic coarsely granular chromatin and one or several prominent nucleoli. The clear cells of a dysgerminoma are often in groups surrounded by a fibrous stroma containing many lymphocytes. Multinucleated histiocytes, syncytiotrophoblasts and small granulomas can also be present. As opposed to clear cell carcinomas, dysgerminomas do not stain for epithelial membrane antigen,[255] and most are also negative for keratins. They are usually positive for placental alkaline phosphatase, whereas only rare clear cell carcinomas are positive for this antigen.[270] Lastly, dysgerminomas almost always occur in adolescents or women less than 30, younger than almost all patients with clear cell carcinoma.

Yolk sac tumor

Yolk sac tumors almost always occur in children and adolescents. However, they may have clear cytoplasm and suggest a clear cell carcinoma if a reticular and/or solid pattern is dominant, or if papillae with central vessel (Schiller–Duval bodies) are mistaken for the papillae of a clear cell carcinoma. Intracellular and extracellular hyaline globules may be present in both tumors, but are most conspicuous in yolk sac tumors. Alpha-fetoprotein is positive in yolk sac tumors but negative in most clear cell carcinomas. Conversely, Leu-M1 stains most clear cell carcinomas and is negative in yolk sac tumors.[271]

Struma ovarii

The cells of struma ovarii may have clear or oxyphilic cytoplasm and the eosinophilic colloid appears similar to the eosinophilic intraglandular material in a clear cell carcinoma with a tubulocystic pattern. Awareness of this pitfall should lead to a search for other components of a dermoid or a stain for thyroglobulin to document a struma.

Juvenile granulosa cell tumor

The follicle-like spaces of a juvenile granulosa cell tumor can be bounded by hobnail cells or have clear cytoplasm, suggesting a clear cell carcinoma. The background stromal cells, however, are plump and sometimes luteinized and form an integral part of the tumor unlike the fibrous, edematous, or hyalinized stroma that is distinct from the epithelial cells of a clear cell carcinoma. Often there is evidence of hyperestrogenism, a clue to the diagnosis of a juvenile granulosa cell tumor.[272]

Metastatic renal cell carcinoma

Renal cell carcinomas rarely metastasize to the ovaries. However, in a patient with a history of renal carcinoma and a clear cell tumor in the ovary, the distinction from a primary clear cell carcinoma can be very difficult. Findings suggesting a metastasis are a pattern of prominent sinusoidal vessels within the tumor and an absence of hobnail cells, hyaline basement membrane-like material, or the tubulocystic and glandular patterns that are commonly present in primary clear cell carcinomas.[273] Special stains can be very useful. Ovarian clear cell carcinomas are positive for CK 7 and negative for CD 10 and renal cell carcinoma marker,[274] whereas the reverse holds for renal cell carcinoma. 34BE12 and CA 125 are also positive in most ovarian clear cell carcinomas and negative in renal cell carcinomas.[275]

Krukenberg tumor

Clear cell carcinomas can focally contain signet ring cells with intracytoplasmic mucin. If signet ring cells predominate, a Krukenberg tumor is suggested.[255] Krukenberg tumors are usually bilateral, whereas clear cell carcinomas are almost always unilateral. Further, Krukenberg tumors have a characteristic prominent cellular stroma with uniformly distributed signet ring cells.

ETIOLOGY, GENETICS AND BIOMARKERS

Most clear cell carcinomas appear to arise from endometriosis. As discussed in the section on endometrioid carcinomas, there is an increased risk for both endometrioid carcinomas and clear cell carcinomas in women with long-standing ovarian endometriosis.[276] Endometriosis is often present adjacent to these carcinomas in the residual ovarian stroma,[2,277] and there is a suggestion of a direct transformation to malignancy within the endometriosis in up to one-third of such cases.[232,233] Lastly, atypical clear cells can sometimes be found in the lining of an endometrioma in the absence of cancer.

Unlike serous carcinomas, clear cell carcinomas infrequently express p53 by immunohistochemistry.[278,279]

However, p21 and cyclin E expression is enhanced relative to other epithelial tumors, indicative of a different genetic evolution.[278,280] This notion is supported by the detection of loss of heterozygosity on different chromosomes (1p, 19p, 11q)[279] than in other cell types. In addition, unlike serous, mucinous and endometrioid carcinomas, clear cell carcinomas do not express estrogen receptor-alpha, a finding that may be related to their relative chemoresistance.[281]

Clear cell carcinomas stain with common epithelial markers such as keratins AE1/AE3, CAM 5.2 and CK 7, 34BE12, epithelial membrane antigen, Leu M1 and B72.3.[13,174,282] Most cases also mark with CA 125.[275,282] They are negative for CK 20 and CD 10[274,282] and mostly negative for estrogen and progesterone receptors.[282]

Transitional cell tumors

GENERAL FEATURES AND CLINICAL ASPECTS

Tumors in this category have epithelial cells that resemble those of transitional cell neoplasms of the urinary tract. They comprise Brenner tumors (benign, borderline, or malignant) and transitional cell carcinomas.

Brenner tumors, originally described by Fritz Brenner in 1907,[283] account for approximately 5% of benign epithelial ovarian tumors.[22,23] They are often small and only incidentally discovered in an ovary removed for other reasons, but they may be as large as 20 cm. The patients range from 30 to 70 years of age.[284-287] Brenner tumors may be pure or a component of a mixed-epithelial tumor. The other component may be a benign or borderline mucinous tumor, a dermoid cyst, or a serous cystadenoma.

Borderline Brenner tumors are rare. None of the cases reported in five series had recurred or metastasized.[288-292] Malignant Brenner tumors are also rare.[288,290-294] In two reports, 21 of 25 tumors were confined to the ovary at initial staging and 16 of 20 patients with follow-up data were without recurrence.[293,294]

Transitional cell carcinomas account for less than 1% of epithelial-stromal carcinomas.[22,23,25,180,181] A transitional cell appearance is much more frequently encountered as a component of a mixed-epithelial carcinoma that may also have either serous, endometrioid, or undifferentiated elements.[295] In fact, two reviews of high-grade, advanced stage ovarian carcinomas reported a predominant transitional cell component in the ovarian tumors in 34 and 26% of cases.[296,297] Patients with pure transitional cell carcinomas are usually older than 50 years.[294,295] In 60-70% of cases, the tumor has spread beyond the ovary at initial staging. Reports from one center indicate a better response to a variety of chemotherapy regimens[296] and to cisplatin-based regimens[298] for transitional cell-predominant tumors in general and in stage III or IV cases if the metastases were transitional cell carcinomas rather than serous or undifferentiated carcinomas. However, in two other studies outcomes in patients with advanced-stage transitional carcinomas (or mixed carcinomas with either a predominant or focal transitional cell component) treated with either cisplatin-based chemotherapy[297] or a variety of other regimens[81] were poor, similar to those of high-stage serous carcinomas.

GROSS EXAMINATION

Brenner tumors are unilateral in 92% of cases. They are usually well demarcated from residual ovarian tissue and either entirely solid or solid with small or large cysts that contain serous or mucinous fluid. The solid areas are firm and white or tan and often have a gritty consistency due to calcifications (Fig. 27.110). In about one-third of cases there is an adjacent tumor, either a cystic mucinous tumor, a serous tumor, or a dermoid cyst (Fig. 27.111).

Borderline Brenner tumors are almost always unilateral and may be grossly similar to ordinary Brenner tumors, but more often have a cystic component with papillary or polypoid areas in the cyst wall (Fig. 27.112).

Malignant Brenner tumors are unilateral in 88% of cases. They are solid and cystic. The solid areas partially resemble a benign or borderline Brenner tumor and

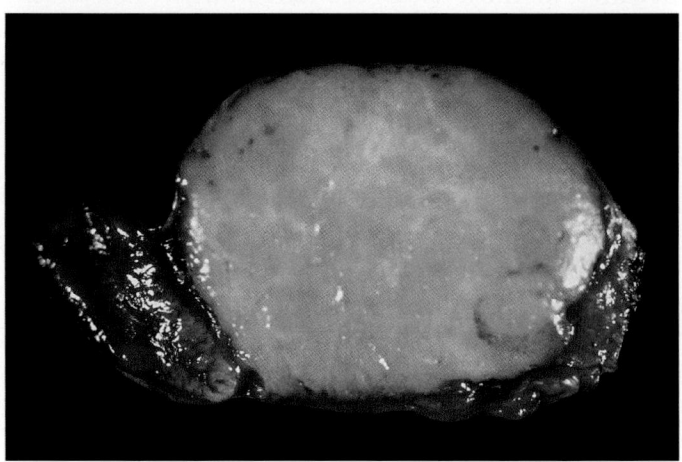

Fig. 27.110 Brenner tumor. The mass displaces most of the ovary. A corpus luteum is present at the lower left.

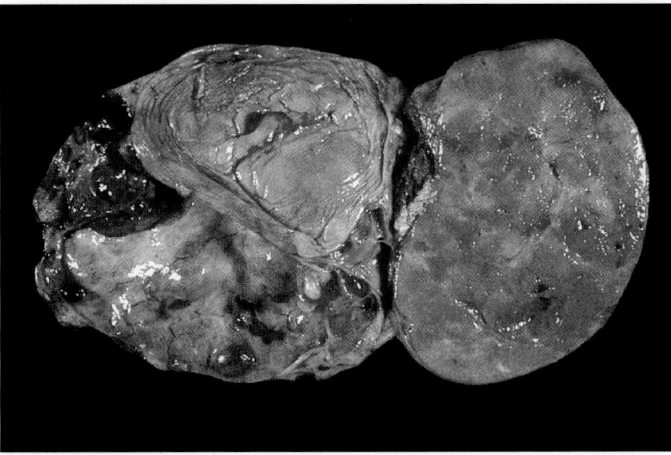

Fig. 27.111 Mixed Brenner tumor and mucinous cystadenoma. The Brenner tumor is at the right. The two components are clearly separate.

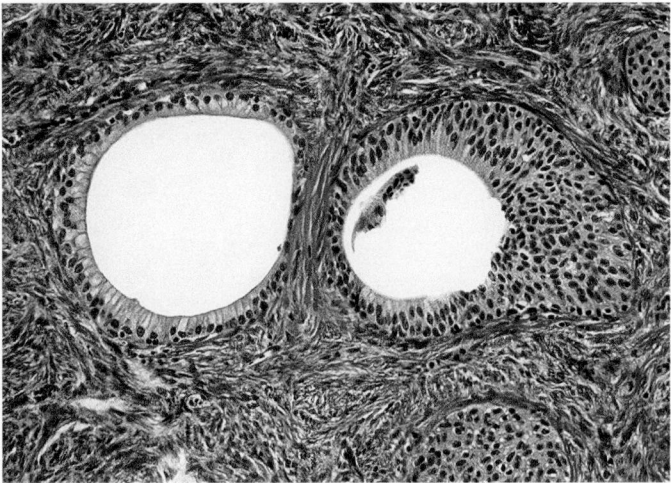

Fig. 27.113 Brenner tumor. A purely mucinous gland on the left is adjacent to an island with mixed transitional and mucinous epithelium.

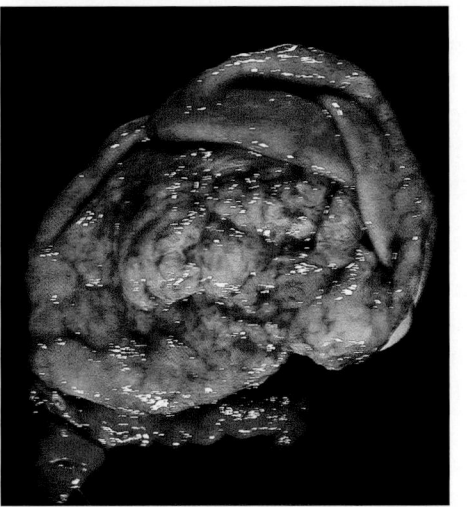

Fig. 27.112 Borderline Brenner tumor. The tumor is cystic. The cyst wall is focally thickened and fleshy with a cobblestone appearance.

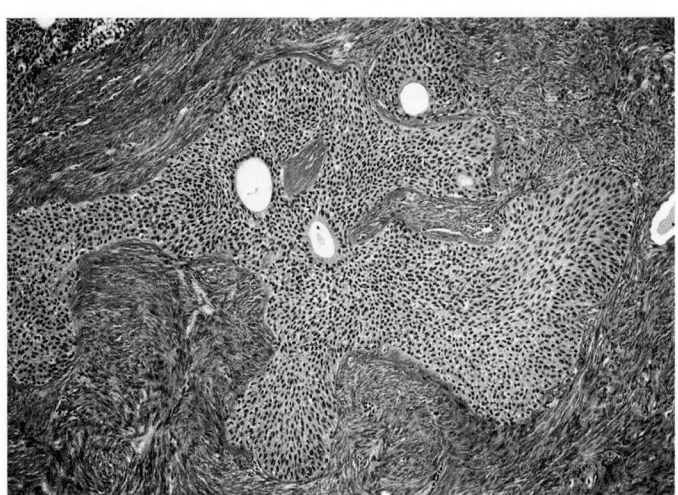

Fig. 27.114 Brenner tumor. Trabeculae of transitional cells with small openings are set in a fibrous stroma.

may have gritty, calcified foci;[294] elsewhere, the solid areas are soft and fleshy or papillary.

Transitional cell carcinomas are bilateral in 15–20% of cases. They resemble other high-grade epithelial-stromal carcinomas, being cystic and solid with soft, fleshy or papillary areas, often with hemorrhage and necrosis.

MICROSCOPIC EXAMINATION

Brenner tumor

Most Brenner tumors have uniformly distributed, small islands of epithelial cells in a fibromatous stroma that often contains spiculated calcium deposits (Fig. 27.113). Sometimes the epithelial cells are arranged in a trabecular pattern (Fig. 27.114) or the stroma has plump, lipid-rich or luteinized cells.[299] The epithelial cells have a characteristic pale, oval or reniform nucleus, often with a longitudinal groove (coffee bean nucleus). The cytoplasm is pale or eosinophilic (Fig. 27.115). Mitoses are rare or absent. Some of the epithelial nests may have a central or eccentric cyst lined by mucinous, ciliated or indifferent glandular cells (Fig. 27.116). Some cysts may be purely glandular and rarely there are large cysts with mixed mucinous and transitional epithelium (meta-plastic Brenner tumor) (Fig. 27.117).[289] Microspaces within the transitional epithelium may be present. A Brenner tumor with an extensive microcystic pattern, almost obscuring the transitional cell nature of the tumor, has been described.[300]

If there is an adjoining mucinous tumor, serous tumor, or dermoid, it usually abuts the Brenner tumor without

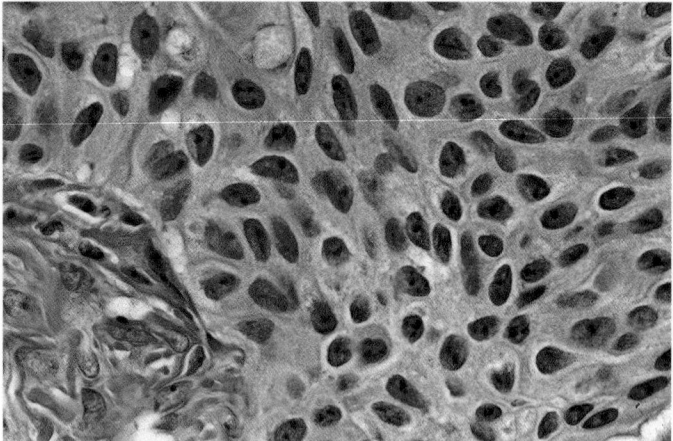

Fig. 27.115 Brenner tumor. The nuclei are pale and oval, sometimes with a longitudinal groove (coffee bean nuclei).

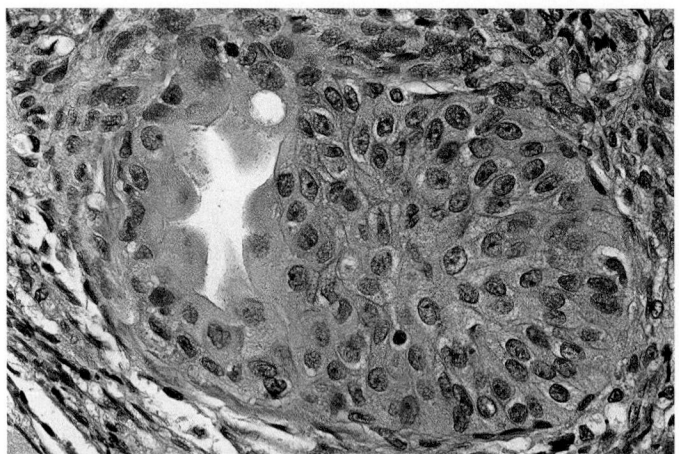

Fig. 27.116 Brenner tumor. Higher power of a mixed-epithelial island.

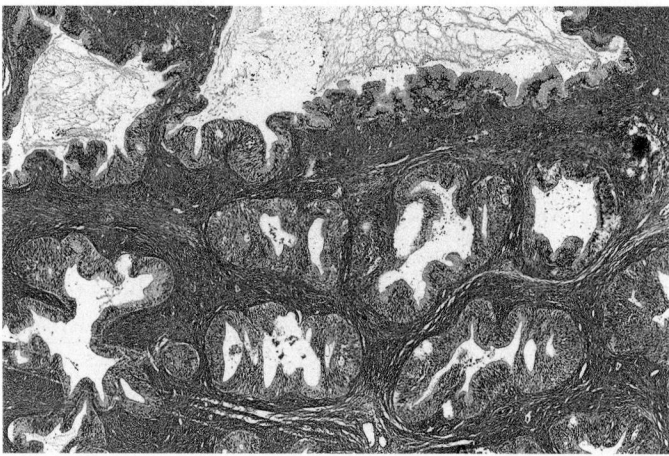

Fig. 27.117 Brenner tumor. This tumor is more cystic than the usual case with a mixture of mucinous and transitional cells within the cysts ('metaplastic' Brenner tumor).

intervening normal ovarian stroma. Because Brenner tumors often have mucinous glands, in order to designate a case as a 'mixed Brenner and mucinous tumor' it should have grossly visible, separate Brenner and mucinous components (Fig. 27.111).[299]

Borderline Brenner tumor

Brenner tumors are considered borderline if there are stratified atypical transitional cells in a papillary arrangement protruding into a cyst (Fig. 27.118) or if a usual-type Brenner tumor has epithelial atypia. In the latter case, the epithelial islands are often larger and more irregular than in benign tumors. In both patterns there is no obvious stromal invasion and usually there is residual ordinary Brenner tumor. The nuclear atypia may range from mild to marked (Fig. 27.119). Some authors refer to those with grades 1 or 2 atypical nuclei as 'proliferative' Brenner tumors, reserving the borderline designation for tumors with grade 3 nuclei.[289,293] Others refer to those with grade 1 atypia as 'borderline' and those with grades 2 or 3 as 'borderline with intraepithelial carcinoma'.[299] We prefer this latter terminology.

Malignant Brenner tumor

This tumor is defined as an invasive carcinoma that contains areas of residual benign or borderline Brenner tumor.[293,294] The invasive areas are either low- or high-grade transitional carcinomas, squamous carcinomas,

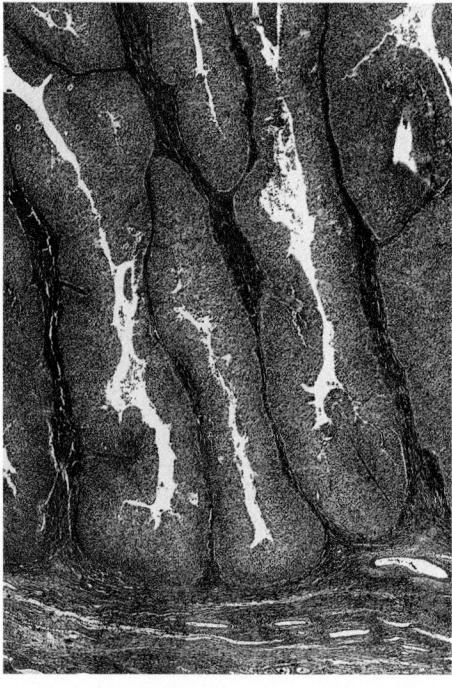

Fig. 27.118 Borderline Brenner tumor. Long slender papillae lined by low-grade transitional cells are present. The growth is sharply demarcated at the base without evidence of invasion.

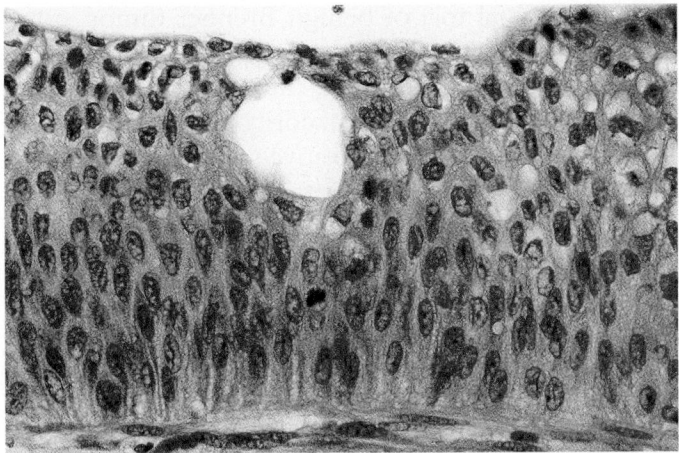

Fig. 27.119 Borderline Brenner tumor. In this case the lining epithelium is similar to that of low-grade papillary transitional cell carcinomas of the bladder.

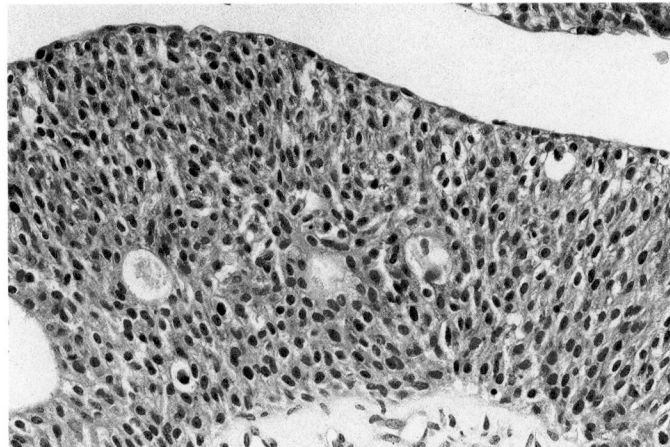

Fig. 27.121 Transitional cell carcinoma. A low-grade tumor. Note the microspaces, a characteristic feature of transitional cell carcinomas.

undifferentiated carcinomas, or a mixture of the three;[293,294,299] commonly the invasive area has focal glandular differentiation and residual calcifications.[294]

Transitional cell carcinoma

By definition transitional carcinomas do not contain any benign or borderline Brenner tumor elements. The low-magnification appearance resembles that of a transitional cell carcinoma of the bladder with broad undulating papillae containing highly stratified epithelial cells (Fig. 27.120). The papillae are usually blunt, but are sometimes slender.[81,294,295–299,301] The lining cells are crowded, highly stratified, polygonal to slightly spindled cells with scant, eosinophilic, or clear cytoplasm; nuclear atypia varies from slight to severe (Figs 27.121, 27.122). The papillae merge with invasive solid islands of malignant

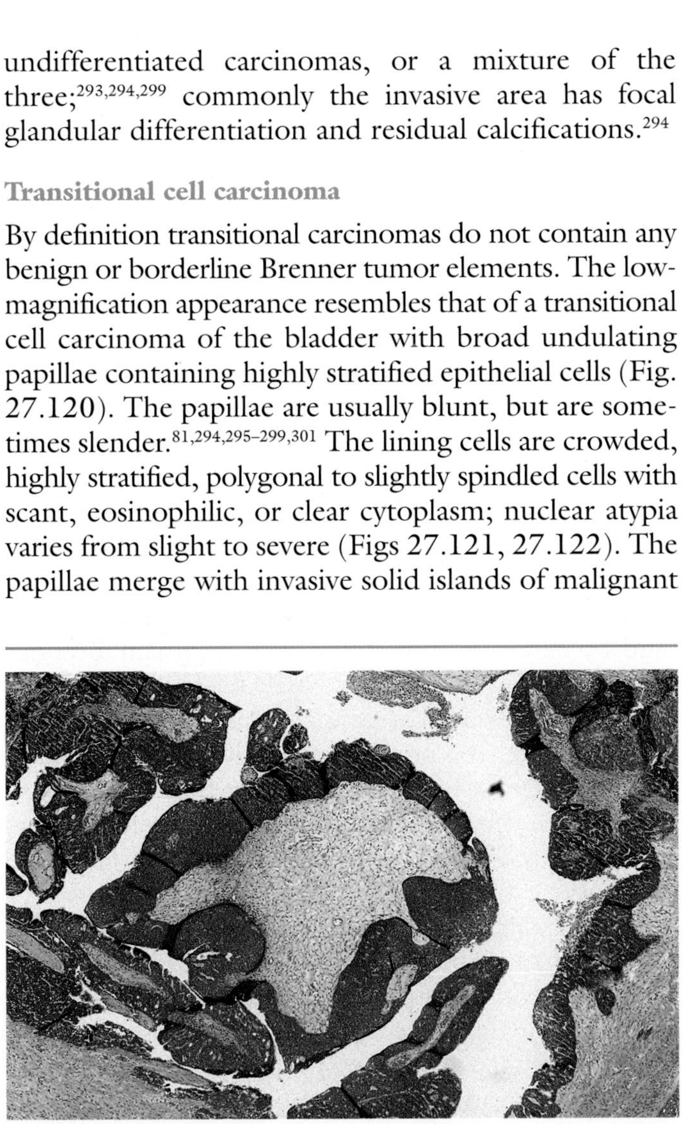

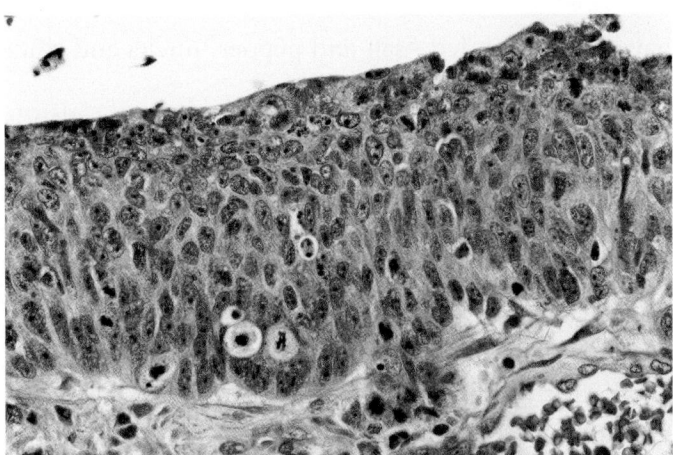

Fig. 27.122 Transitional cell carcinoma. A high-grade tumor.

transitional cells, undifferentiated cells, or squamous cells set in a fibrous stroma. In the majority of cases there are numerous 'microspaces', sometimes containing mucin, uniformly dispersed throughout the epithelium (Fig. 27.123). Occasionally, the spaces are lined by glandular epithelium, or are long and narrow, similar to the slit-like fenestrations seen in serous carcinomas. Psammoma bodies are rarely present. Necrosis is common.[299,301]

DIFFERENTIAL DIAGNOSIS

Brenner tumor

Either granulosa cell tumors or carcinoid tumors with a nested pattern can be confused with a Brenner tumor.[299] Granulosa cell tumors usually have other characteristic patterns, are inhibin positive and may have estrogenic clinical manifestations. Carcinoids

Fig. 27.120 Transitional cell carcinoma. Broad papillae are lined by a uniformly thick band of stratified epithelial cells.

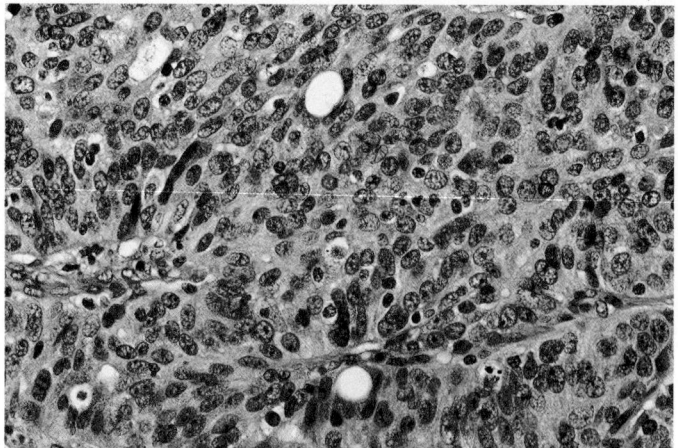

Fig. 27.123 Transitional cell carcinoma. Invasive solid area with high-grade nuclei. Note the microspaces.

have more rounded, 'salt and pepper' nuclei and react with neuroendocrine markers.

A Brenner tumor with extensive mucinous glands might be mistaken for a *mucinous adenofibroma* or even a *mucinous adenocarcinoma*. Awareness of this possibility will initiate a search for the characteristic transitional cells. Stromal calcifications call attention to the possibility of a Brenner tumor.

Mixed-epithelial borderline tumors with a predominance of squamous epithelium might be confused with borderline Brenner tumors. The former are associated with endometriotic cysts and contain a mixture of other types of Müllerian epithelium.[302]

Transitional cell carcinoma, malignant Brenner tumor

Transitional cell carcinoma may be mistaken for either an *endometrioid or a serous carcinoma*.[301] The microspaces commonly present in transitional cell carcinomas confer an endometrioid quality. However, broad undulating papillae are not a feature of endometrioid carcinomas, whereas squamous differentiation and associated endometriosis are much more common in endometrioid than in transitional cell carcinomas. The slit-like fenestrations that may be present in transitional cell carcinoma mimic an appearance often present in serous carcinomas. However, the latter usually have more complex papillae lacking transitional-like cells and often contain psammoma bodies.

Transitional carcinomas of the urinary tract rarely metastasize to the ovaries, but when they do, they can closely mimic both borderline and malignant Brenner tumors and ovarian transitional cell carcinomas.[303] Borderline and malignant Brenner tumors usually contain residual foci of benign Brenner tumor, not a feature of a metastasis. If the ovarian tumor is a pure transitional cell carcinoma, immunohistochemistry can be very useful. The majority of ovarian transitional carcinomas are positive for Wilm's tumor antigen (WT1) and all are negative for CK 20, whereas the reverse is true for urinary transitional cell carcinomas.[304–306]

ETIOLOGY, GENETICS AND BIOMARKERS

Since the embryologic gonadal ridge is close to the mesonephros, part of which eventually forms the bladder, and the two are covered by a continuous mesothelial lining, it is not surprising that the potential for transitional metaplasia exists in gonadal epithelium. On this basis and from their light and electron microscopic features, Brenner tumors are thought to be derived from celomic ovarian surface epithelium or cortical inclusions that have undergone transitional metaplasia and have then progressively grown into the substance of the ovary.[307]

Ordonez and Mackay, however, found only limited ultrastructural similarities between normal urothelium and Brenner tumor epithelium,[308] and Soslow et al.[305] noted that Brenner epithelium and Walthard rests (also presumptively urothelial) are both CK 20 negative, whereas normal bladder epithelium is consistently positive. These observations call into question the derivation of Brenner tumors. However, using the novel urothelial markers thrombomodulin and/or uroplakin[309], three separate groups[304,310,311] reported a high degree of positivity in Brenner tumors, indicative of true urothelial differentiation according to these authors.

While most evidence indicates that Brenner tumors (and by extension borderline and malignant Brenner tumors) are histogenetically closely related to urothelial tumors, it is likely that ovarian transitional cell carcinomas are not. It is also likely that they do not develop from a benign or borderline Brenner tumor precursor. Evidence for this is that most malignant Brenner tumors are discovered at an early stage and have a favorable prognosis, even when the malignant component is of high grade. However, most transitional cell carcinomas in ovarian carcinomas are discovered at an advanced stage and have a poor prognosis. Moreover, transitional-appearing elements are usually only a component of a mixed-epithelial carcinoma that is otherwise of Müllerian derivation. By immunohistochemistry, transitional cell carcinomas (as opposed to Brenner tumors and bladder carcinomas), only infrequently express urothelial-specific markers such as uroplakin and thrombomodulin[304] and are CK 20 negative.[304–306] Furthermore, 82% of 17 transitional cell carcinomas expressed WT1, an antigen frequently also expressed by ovarian serous carcinomas, while none of 15 invasive bladder cancers were positive.[304]

Squamous cell tumors

GENERAL FEATURES AND CLINICAL ASPECTS

Squamous cell tumors of the ovary are rare. In the epithelial-stromal category they include epidermoid cysts and pure squamous cell carcinomas. Patients with epidermoid cysts range from 25 to 57 years of age.[312–314] Epidermoid cysts may be either incidental findings or form an ovarian mass. Their behavior is benign.

Squamous cell carcinoma as the only malignant component of an ovarian carcinoma occurs in various settings: it may be the invasive component of a malignant Brenner tumor or a dermoid cyst; it may be associated with ovarian endometriosis or with squamous carcinoma *in situ* of the cervix; or it may occur without any of the foregoing associations. Squamous cell carcinomas arising in a dermoid cyst are not included in the epithelial-stromal category and are presented in the section on ovarian germ cell tumors.

Patients with ovarian squamous carcinomas were from 29 to 86 years of age (reviewed by Pins et al.).[315] Of 18 cases not associated with a dermoid cyst in the largest series, only two were confined to the ovary at initial presentation; neither patient died of her tumor, although one had a recurrence in the incision. However, of 15 higher-stage cases with follow-up data, 11 patients died from their cancers.[315]

GROSS EXAMINATION

Epidermoid cyst

Epidermoid cysts are unilateral and range from 0.2 to 15 cm. Most are located in the cortex, some in the medulla and one was in the hilus.[314] The cysts are filled with white-gray creamy material. The wall is thin and smooth.

Squamous carcinoma

The gross appearance varies depending on whether or not the tumors arise from a dermoid cyst. If they do, they are usually a mural thickening or polypoid mass in a large cystic cavity. In cases without a dermoid cyst

they are cystic and solid with areas of necrosis. Three of 18 such cases were bilateral.[315]

MICROSCOPIC EXAMINATION

Epidermoid cyst

The cyst is lined by mature squamous epithelium bounded by an outer fibrous wall; sometimes there is a prominent granular layer or basal layer; the latter may have melanin pigment. The interior contains flakes of keratin. By definition there are no adjacent skin appendage structures; however, in some cases small transitional nests are present.[313]

Squamous carcinoma

Various architectural patterns are found, often they coexist: cystic with central necrosis, verrucous (Figs 27.124, 27.125), papillary, insular, diffusely infiltrative, or sarcomatoid.[315] The cytologic features are those of a well to poorly differentiated keratinizing or non-keratinizing squamous carcinoma or a spindle cell carcinoma. Adjacent endometriosis may be present, sometimes with what appears to be a transition from the endometriosis to the carcinoma. Cases of squamous carcinoma *in situ* lining an ovarian cyst have been reported (see discussion below on etiology).[316–319]

DIFFERENTIAL DIAGNOSIS

There may be a component of squamous carcinoma in an endometrioid carcinoma, a transitional carcinoma, or a malignant Brenner tumor. When considering the diagnosis of a pure ovarian squamous carcinoma, a

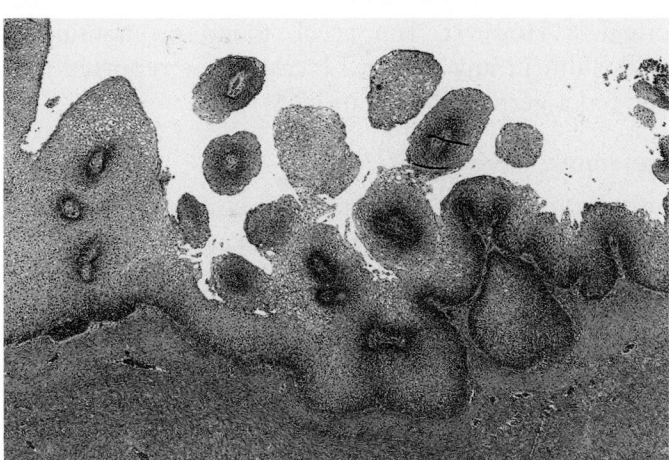

Fig. 27.124 Squamous carcinoma. A condylomatous intracystic growth pattern is present.

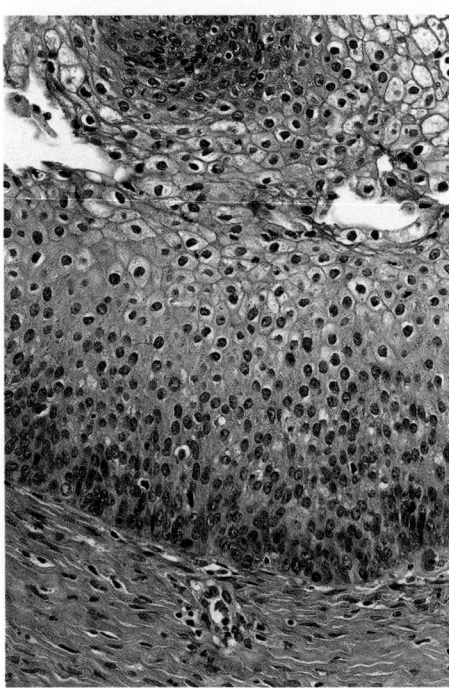

Fig. 27.125
Squamous carcinoma. In this case the tumor is well-differentiated.

very rare tumor, a mixed-epithelial carcinoma should be excluded.

Metastatic squamous carcinoma can usually be excluded on clinical grounds. Residual endometriosis, Brenner tumor, or dermoid cyst strongly favors a primary ovarian origin.

ETIOLOGY

Epidermoid cyst

There are two theories of origin. Young et al. point to the finding of adjacent transitional rests in all three tumors they describe as indicative of ovarian epithelial origin.[313] However, Fan et al. found no transitional epithelium in any of the 11 cases they reported and favored a germ cell derivation.[314]

Squamous carcinoma

Squamous cell carcinomas are associated with endometriosis in about one-third of cases.[315] When one considers that squamous cell carcinoma may be a component of an endometrioid carcinoma and that the latter are often derived from endometriosis, it is probable that some pure squamous carcinomas are also derived from endometriosis.

In cases without endometriosis, transformation from the ovarian surface epithelium or cortical inclusion cyst epithelium or from an epidermoid cyst are all possible etiologies. However, a fascinating finding, present in 10 of 24 cases of ovarian squamous carcinoma without endometriosis, was concomitant squamous carcinoma *in situ* or early invasive squamous carcinoma of the cervix.[315] In some of these cases, the ovarian lesion was also described as *in situ*, as it was confined to the wall of a cyst. Although a single case of contiguous surface spread of squamous carcinoma *in situ* of the cervix to the ovaries via the endometrium and fallopian tubes has been reported,[320] this is unlikely to be the mechanism for the ovarian involvement in most cases. It is also highly unlikely that the ovarian tumors are metastases from the cervix, given the low overall frequency of metastatic squamous carcinoma of the cervix to the ovaries and the fact that no invasion, or only minimal invasion, of the cervix itself was detected in these cases. Thus, this association with cervical carcinoma *in situ* brings up the possibility that the ovarian tumors were induced directly within the ovary by human papillomavirus (HPV). In support of this possibility one case of bilateral ovarian squamous carcinomas with concomitant vulvar and cervical intraepithelial neoplasia in a 40-year-old woman was positive for HPV 16/18 by *in situ* hybridization in the cervix, the vulva and one of the two ovarian tumors.[321] The authors of this report point out that other cases of ovarian squamous carcinoma that had accompanying cervical lesions have occurred in women who were younger than those without cervical lesions and, as in their case, have had an *in situ* component in the ovaries, suggesting that HPV is indeed the etiologic agent in the ovarian tumors, possibly via an ascending infection. The initially infected cell within the ovary remains speculative.

Mixed-epithelial tumors and undifferentiated carcinoma

GENERAL FEATURES AND CLINICAL ASPECTS

Mixed-epithelial tumors

Mixed-epithelial tumors may be benign, borderline, or malignant. Benign mixed epithelial tumors are uncommon. The most frequent combination is the mixed Brenner tumor and mucinous cystadenoma, which is discussed in the section on transitional cell tumors.

Borderline tumors having mixed-epithelial features have been mentioned in several reports of borderline tumors, but have only been separately analyzed in a single study of 36 cases.[85] The average patient age was 35 years. All tumors were stage I; 22% were bilateral and 53% were associated with endometriosis. Three patients developed subsequent pelvic recurrences and one a contralateral ovarian tumor. However, all were successfully treated and none died.

A second study, summarizing 34 patients, combined endocervical-type mucinous borderline tumors (see mucinous tumors section) and mixed-epithelial borderline tumors in the same group, using the designation 'atypical proliferative seromucinous tumors' for all of them.[127] The mean patient age was 38 years: 90% of the tumors were stage I, 3% were stage II and 6% were stage III; 26% were bilateral and 41% were associated with endometriosis. Of 21 stage I and II patients with follow-up data, one had an ovarian recurrence after cystectomy. The two stage III patients had noninvasive peritoneal implants; both were alive without evidence of recurrence after brief follow-up periods.

This report added an additional five cases of mixed-epithelial borderline tumors with intraepithelial carcinoma and eight cases with microinvasion. All eight patients in these two categories combined who had follow-up data were without recurrences, but some follow-up intervals were less than a year.

Mixed-epithelial carcinomas having mixtures of serous, transitional, endometrioid, clear cell, squamous, or undifferentiated elements in various combinations account for up to 5% of carcinomas in the epithelial-stromal category.[23,25,179] However, in our experience mucinous carcinomas other than the uncommon endocervical-like mucinous type are not commonly mixed with other cell types, possibly reflecting a different pathogenesis for mucinous carcinoma than other common epithelial-stromal carcinomas (see discussion under mucinous tumors).

In order to qualify as a mixed-epithelial carcinoma, a second or second and third component must occupy at least 10% of the tumor area.[13] Potential differences in behavior (as opposed to pure carcinomas of the same cell types) has not been extensively studied. The following observations of mixed-epithelial carcinomas have been made:

1 Seven cases of mixed endocervical-type mucinous and serous carcinomas (designated by the authors as seromucinous carcinomas) have been described.[127] The patients' age ranged from 21 to 75 years; in 57% of the cases the tumors were bilateral; four of the seven patients had metastases in the peritoneum upon initial staging and two of them died of their cancers.

2 In one other study of four similar cases, areas of endometrioid and squamous differentiation were also present.[129] The patients' ages ranged from 34–50 years. Three of these four cases were associated with endometriosis; in two cases the tumors were bilateral; in two there were invasive peritoneal metastases. All patients were alive, but follow-up intervals were brief.

3 No difference in behavior or survival was noted in one study based on whether tumors were purely endometrioid, purely clear cell, or a mixture of the two.[322]

4 According to one report,[323] high-stage endometrioid carcinomas that were mixed with even small amounts of serous or undifferentiated elements had a significantly worse prognosis than pure endometrioid carcinomas. The authors recommended extensive sectioning of endometrioid carcinomas to exclude such areas.

5 Silva et al. found that the 5-year survival in patients with tumors containing over 50% undifferentiated carcinoma was worse than that in patients with pure serous or transitional cell carcinomas.[324]

6 Evidence that transitional cell elements may favorably affect the prognosis of high-stage mixed-epithelial carcinomas is conflicting, as discussed in the section on transitional cell tumors.

Undifferentiated carcinomas

Undifferentiated carcinomas have either no differentiating features or only rare minor differentiated areas.[13,325] Probably because the interpretation of what is meant by 'undifferentiated' has varied among observers, undifferentiated carcinomas have been reported to constitute 0.5–16% of epithelial-stromal carcinomas.[23,25,180,181,325] In 35 cases with an undifferentiated component involving more that 50% of the tumor, two were stage I, one was stage II, 26 were stage III and six were stage IV. Thirty-four of the 35 patients died of their cancers in periods from 8 to 108 months (mean, 27 months).[324]

GROSS EXAMINATION

Mixed-epithelial borderline tumors

These tumors are bilateral in about 25% of cases. They range from 2 cm to 25 cm (mean 8 cm). They are predominantly multicystic with occasional solid areas. The cysts contain watery or mucoid yellow, green, or brown fluid. Papillary excrescences on the surface or within the cysts are present in almost all cases.

Mixed-epithelial and undifferentiated carcinoma

The gross features of mixed-epithelial and undifferentiated carcinomas are not different from other high-grade ovarian carcinomas.

MICROSCOPIC EXAMINATION

Mixed-epithelial borderline tumors

The low-power microscopic appearance is similar to that of endocervical-like and serous borderline tumors with a prominent papillary intracystic growth (Fig. 27.55). The papillae are broad with an edematous or fibrous core. There may also be glands and cysts in a fibrous stroma. The papillae, glands and cysts are lined by mucinous columnar cells resembling those of the endocervix (Fig. 27.56), ciliated cells, stratified eosinophilic polygonal cells that are not further differentiated (Fig. 27.57), squamous cells and endometrioid cells in varying proportions. Acute inflammatory cells are often present within the epithelial cells and in the extracellular mucin. Endometriosis, sometimes with atypical epithelial cells, may be present in adjacent areas. Sometimes the tumor appears to arise from endometriosis. Nuclei are usually only slightly atypical, but rare cases have areas that are consistent with intraepithelial carcinoma or have microinvasive foci.

Even in the absence of stromal invasion, rare cases have had extraovarian spread at the time of initial staging or have developed recurrences, usually in the form of noninvasive abdominal and peritoneal implants.

Mixed-epithelial carcinomas

The most frequent combinations are mixed endometrioid and clear cell carcinoma, mixed transitional cell and either serous or endometrioid carcinoma and mixed endometrioid and serous or undifferentiated carcinoma.

Mixed-epithelial carcinomas with endocervical-like mucinous epithelium (also called seromucinous carcinomas) are mostly well-differentiated. They combine papillary, glandular and cystic areas lined mostly by columnar mucinous cells (Figs 27.69–27.71). Ciliated cells, endometrioid and squamous foci are present to a variable degree. There is abundant extracellular pale pink mucinous material.

Undifferentiated carcinoma

Undifferentiated carcinomas grow in solid sheets of moderate to large cells with high-grade nuclei and scant cytoplasm. There is a high mitotic rate and

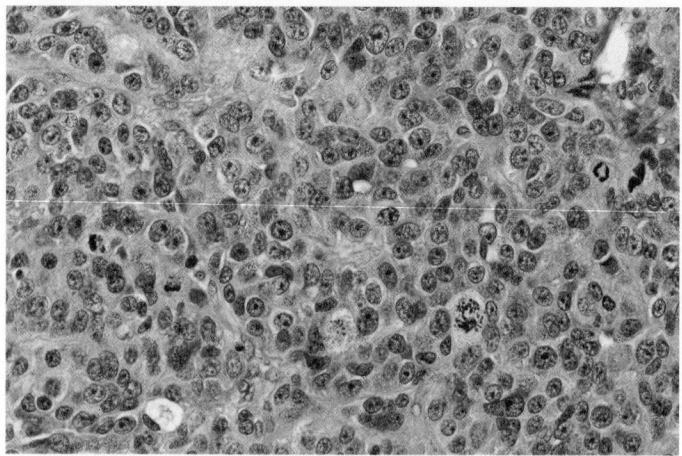

Fig. 27.126 Undifferentiated carcinoma. No differentiating features are present. The cells are large and there are several mitotic figures, including abnormal forms.

necrosis is often present (Fig. 27.126). Occasionally, there is a spindle cell component. Minor foci of gland formation, mucin-filled cells, or psammoma bodies are not specific and do not change the diagnosis.[325] By immunohistochemistry undifferentiated carcinomas stain positively for cytokeratins and epithelial membrane antigen and negatively for vimentin.[326] Undifferentiated carcinomas with areas of choriocarcinoma that produce chorionic gonadotropin have been described.[327]

DIFFERENTIAL DIAGNOSIS

Mixed-epithelial tumors

Mixed-epithelial borderline tumors closely resemble *endocervical-like borderline tumors* and are probably closely related to them. The distinction is in the greater percentage of serous, endometrioid and squamous elements in the mixed-epithelial type.

The minor component of a mixed epithelial carcinoma should be distinct in order for it to qualify. For instance, small gland-like openings within solid areas of a *serous, transitional cell, or undifferentiated carcinoma* do not necessarily signify endometrioid differentiation. Likewise, the presence of a small number of cells with cytoplasmic mucin does not infer a mucinous component.

Squamous differentiation may be a component of an *endometrioid carcinoma, a transitional carcinoma, or a malignant Brenner tumor*. These are not designated as mixed-epithelial carcinomas, but rather as having focal squamous differentiation.

Undifferentiated carcinoma

The diffuse type of *granulosa cell tumor* can mimic an undifferentiated carcinoma. The nuclei in most granulosa cell tumors have fine chromatin and characteristic nuclear folding and grooves. However, rare granulosa cell tumors have foci with bizarre nuclei, causing a closer resemblance to an undifferentiated carcinoma.[328] A positive inhibin and negative epithelial membrane antigen stain are useful in confirming a granulosa cell tumor.

Undifferentiated tumors composed of small cells, or a mixture of small and large cells, evoke the possibility of *ovarian small cell carcinoma*, of either the hypercalcemic or the pulmonary type.[260,329] In the hypercalcemic type, patients are often teenagers and young adults and this diagnosis must be considered when one encounters an undifferentiated-appearing carcinoma in this age group. In the pulmonary type the microscopic appearance is similar to that of pulmonary small cell carcinomas, sometimes with small areas of glandular or squamous differentiation.

Ovarian neuroendocrine carcinomas of non-small cell type have sheets, islands, cords and trabeculae of large malignant cells and might be considered undifferentiated carcinomas. The nuclei are either coarsely granular or vesicular with a prominent nucleolus. The cytoplasm may be scant or abundant and stains positively with neuroendocrine markers. Usually there is an additional component of surface epithelial carcinoma, either endometrioid or mucinous.[330]

An undifferentiated carcinoma with a prominent spindle cell component can be mistaken for a *mixed Müllerian tumor*. In the latter, the epithelial and stromal phenotypes are usually distinct and sharply demarcated, whereas they blend with one another in an undifferentiated carcinoma.

References

1 Goodman MT, Howe HL. Descriptive epidemiology of ovarian cancer in the United States, 1992–1997. Cancer 2003; 97(Suppl):2615–2630.

2 Feeley KM, Wells M. Precursor lesions of ovarian epithelial malignancy. Histopathology 2001; 38:87–95.

3 Wren BG, Frampton J. Oestrogenic activity associated with nonfeminizing ovarian tumors after the menopause. Br Med J 1963; 2:842–844.

4 Rome RM, Fortune DW, Quinn MA, Brown JB. Functioning ovarian tumors in postmenopausal women. Obstet Gynecol 1981; 57:705–710.

5 Taylor HC Jr. Malignant and semimalignant tumors of the ovary. Surg Gynecol Obstet 1929; 48:204–230.

6 Serov SF, Scully RE, Sobin LH. International histology of tumors (no. 9). Histological typing of ovarian tumours. Geneva, Switzerland: World Health Organization; 1973:9.

7 Seidman JD, Ronnett BM, Kurman RJ. Why abandoning the borderline category of ovarian tumors is beneficial. Contemp Ob/Gyn 1997; 66–81.

8 Silva EG, Kurman RJ, Russell P. Scully RE. Symposium: ovarian tumors of borderline malignancy. Int J Gynecol Pathol 1996; 15:281–302.

9 Seidman JD, Russell P, Kurman R. Surface epithelial tumors of the ovary. In: Kurman RJ, ed. Blaustein's pathology of the female genital tract, 5th edn. New York: Springer-Verlag; 2001:791–904.

10 Russell P, Robboy SJ, Anderson MC, eds. Epithelial/stromal ovarian tumors. Serous tumors. In: Pathology of the female reproductive tract. London: Churchill Livingstone; 2002:539–605.

11 Scully RE, Young RH, Clement PB, eds. Surface epithelial-stromal tumors. Serous tumors. Tumors of the ovary, maldeveloped gonads, fallopian tube and broad ligament. In: Atlas of tumor pathology, 3rd series, fascicle 23. Washington, DC: Armed Forces Institute of Pathology; 1998:51–79.

12 Kempson RL, Hendrickson MR. Ovarian serous borderline tumors: the Citadel defended. Hum Pathol 2000; 5(31):525–526.

13 Lee KR, Tavassoli FA, Prat J, et al. Surface epithelial-stromal tumors. In: Tavassoli FA, Devilee P, eds. World Health Organization classification of pathology and genetics of tumours of the breast and female genital Organs. Lyon: IARC Press; 2003:117–145.

14 Lim-Tan SK, Cajigas HE, Scully RE. Ovarian cystectomy for serous borderline tumors: a follow-up study of 35 cases. Obstet Gynecol 1988; 72:775–781.

15 Tazelaar HD, Bostwick DG, Ballon SC, et al. Conservative treatment of borderline ovarian tumors. Obstet Gynecol 1985; 66:417–422.

16 Morris RT, Gershenson DM, Silva EG, et al. Outcome and reproductive function after conservative surgery for borderline ovarian tumors. Obstet Gynecol 2000; 95:541–547.

17 International Federation of Gynecology and Obstetrics. Classification and staging of malignant tumours in the female pelvis. Acta Obstet Gynecol Scand 1971; 50:1–7.

18 Benda JA, Zaino R. GOG pathology manual. Buffalo, NY: Gynecologic Oncology Group; 1994.

19 Silverberg SG. Histopathologic grading of ovarian carcinoma: a review and proposal. Int J Gynecol Pathol 2000; 19:7–15.

20 Shimizu Y, Kamoi S, Amada S, et al. Toward the development of a universal grading system for ovarian epithelial carcinoma: testing of a proposed system in a series of 461 patients with uniform treatment and follow-up. Cancer 1998; 82:893–901.

21 Malpica A, Deavers MT, Lu K. Grading ovarian serous carcinoma using a two-tier system. Am J Surg Pathol 2004; 28:496–504.

22 Katsube Y, Berg JW, Silverberg SG. Epidemiologic pathology of ovarian tumors: a histopathologic review of primary ovarian neoplasms diagnosed in the Denver

Standard Metropolitan Statistical Area, 1 July–31 December 1969 and 1 July–31 December 1979. Int J Gynecol Pathol 1982;1(1):3–16.

23 Koonings PP, Campbell K, Mishell DR, et al. Relative frequency of primary ovarian neoplasms: a 10-year review. Obstet Gynecol 1989; 74:921–926.

24 Russell P. The pathological assessment of ovarian neoplasms: I: introduction to the common epithelial tumours and analysis of benign epithelial tumours. Pathology 1979; 11:5–26.

25 Pecorelli S, Odicino F, Maisonneuve P, et al. Carcinoma of the ovary. J Epidem Biostat 1998; 3:75–102.

26 Seidman JD, Kurman RJ. Ovarian serous borderline tumors: a critical review of the literature with emphasis on prognostic indicators. Hum Pathol 2000; 31(5):539–557.

27 Katzenstein AL, Mazur MT, Morgan TE, Kao MS. Proliferative serous tumors of the ovary. Histologic features and prognosis. Am J Surg Pathol 1978; 2:339–355.

28 Bostwick DG, Tazelaar HD, Ballon SC, et al. Ovarian epithelial tumors of borderline malignancy. A clinical and pathologic study of 109 cases. Cancer 1986; 58:2052–2056.

29 Bell DA, Weinstock MA, Scully RE. Peritoneal implants of ovarian serous borderline tumors: histologic features and prognosis. Cancer 1998; 62:2212–2222.

30 Gershenson DM, Silva EG. Serous ovarian tumors of low malignant potential with peritoneal implants. Cancer 1990; 65:578–585.

31 Bell KA, Smith Sehdev AE, Kurman RJ. Refined diagnostic criteria for implants associated with ovarian atypical proliferative serous tumors (borderline) and micropapillary serous carcinomas. Am J Surg Pathol 2001; 25(4):419–432.

32 Tan LK, Flynn SD, Carcangiu ML. Ovarian serous borderline tumors with lymph node involvement. Am J Surg Pathol 1994; 18:904–912.

33 Kadar N, Krumerman M. Possible metaplastic origin of lymph node 'metastases' in serous ovarian tumor of low malignant potential (borderline serous tumor). Gynecol Oncol 1995; 59(3):394–397.

34 Prade M, Spatz A, Bentley R, et al. Borderline and malignant serous tumor arising in pelvic lymph nodes: evidence of origin in benign glandular inclusions. Int J Gynecol Pathol 1995; 14:87–91.

35 Camatte S, Morice P, Atallah D, et al. Lymph node disorders and prognostic value of nodal involvement in patients treated for a borderline ovarian tumor: an analysis of a series of 42 lymphadenectomies. J Am Coll Surg 2002; 198(3):332–338.

36 Tavassoli FA. Serous tumors of low malignant potential with early stromal invasion. Mod Pathol 1998; 1:407–414.

37 Bell DA, Scully RE. Ovarian serous borderline tumors with stromal microinvasion: a report of 21 cases. Hum Pathol 1990; 21:397–403.

38 Nayar R, Siriaunkgul S, Robbins KM, et al. Microinvasion in low malignant potential tumors of the ovary. Hum Pathol 1996; 27(6):521–527.

39 Prat J, Nictolis M de. Serous borderline tumors of the ovary. A long-term follow-up study of 137 cases, including 18 with a micropapillary pattern and 20 with microinvasion. Am J Surg Pathol 2002; 26:1111–1128.

40 DeNictolis M, Montironi R, Tommasoni S, et al. Serous borderline tumors of the ovary: a clinicopathologic, immunohistochemical and quantitative study of 44 cases. Cancer 1992; 70:152–160.

41 Seidman JD, Norris HJ, Griffin J, Hitchcock CL. DNA flow cytometric analysis of serous ovarian tumors of low malignant potential. Cancer 1993; 71:3947–3951.

42 Gershenson DM, Deavers M, Diaz S, et al. Prognostic significance of P53 expression in advanced-stage ovarian serous borderline tumors. Clin Cancer Res 1999; 5:4053–4058.

43 Seidman JD, Horkayne-Szakaly I, Haiba M, et al. The histologic type and stage distribution of ovarian carcinomas of surface epithelial origin. Int J Gynecol Pathol 2003; 23:41–44.

44 Partridge EE, Phillips JL, Menck HR. The National Cancer Database Report on ovarian cancer treatment in United States hospitals. Cancer 1996; 78:2236–2246.

45 Cannistra SA. Cancer of the ovary. N Engl J Med 1993; 329:1550–1539.

46 Colgan TJ, Murphy J, Cole DEC, et al. Occult carcinoma in prophylactic oophorectomy specimens: prevalence and association with BRCA germline mutation status. Am J Surg Pathol 2001; 25(10):1283–1289.

47 Agoff SN, Menedelin JE, Grieco VS, et al. Unexpected gynecologic neoplasms in patients with proven or suspected BRCA-1 or -2 mutations: implications for gross examination, cytology and clinical follow-up. Am J Surg Pathol 2002; 26(2):171–178.

48 Mooney J, Silva E, Tornos C, et al. Unusual features of serous neoplasms of low malignant potential during pregnancy. Gynecol Oncol 1997; 65:30–35.

49 Segal GH, Hart GH. Ovarian serous tumors of low malignant potential (serous borderline tumors); the relationship of exophytic surface tumor to peritoneal implants. Am J Surg Pathol 1992; 16(8):577–583.

50 Lee KR, Castrillon DH, Nucci MR. Pathologic findings in eight cases of ovarian serous borderline tumors, three with foci of serous carcinoma, that preceded death or morbidity from invasive carcinoma. Int J Gynecol Pathol 2001; 20:329–334.

51 Smith Sehdev AE, Sehdev PS, Kurman RJ. Noninvasive and invasive micropapillary (low-grade) serous carcinoma of the ovary: a clinicopathologic analysis of 135 cases. Am J Surg Pathol 2003; 27(6):725–736.

52 Silva EG, Tornos CS, Malpica A, et al. Ovarian serous neoplasms of low malignant potential associated with focal areas of serous carcinoma. Mod Pathol 1997; 10(7):663–667.

53 Burks RT, Sherman ME, Kurman RJ. Micropapillary serous carcinoma of the ovary: a distinctive low-grade carcinoma related to serous borderline tumors. Am J Surg Pathol 1996; 20(11):1331–1345.

54 Seidman JD, Kurman RJ. Subclassification of serous borderline tumors of the ovary into benign and malignant types: a clinicopathologic study of 65 advanced stage cases. Am J Surg Pathol 1996; 20(11):1331–1345.

55 Katabuchi H, Tashiro H, Cho KR, et al. Micropapillary serous carcinoma of the ovary: an immunohistochemical and mutational analysis of p53. Int J Gynecol Pathol 1998; 17:54–60.

56 Staebler A, Heselmeyer-Haddad K, Bell K, et al. Micropapillary serous carcinoma of the ovary has distinct patterns of chromosomal imbalances by comparative genomic hybridization compared with atypical proliferative serous tumors and serous carcinomas. Hum Pathol 2002; 33(1):47–59.

57 Eichorn JH, Bell DA, Young RH, et al. Ovarian serous borderline tumors with micropapillary and cribriform patterns. Am J Surg Pathol 1999; 23(4):397–409.

58 Goldstein NS, Ceniza N. Ovarian micropapillary serous borderline tumors. Am J Clin Pathol 2000; 114:380–386.

59 Slomovitz BM, Caputo TA, Gretz HF, et al. A comparative analysis of 57 serous borderline tumors with and without noninvasive micropapillary component. Am J Surg Pathol 2002; 26(5):592–600.

60 Deavers MT, Gershenson DM, Tortelero-Luna G, et al. Micropapillary and cribriform patterns in ovarian serous tumors of low malignant potential. A study of 99 advanced stage cases. Am J Surg Pathol 2002; 26:1129–1141.

61 Bell DA, Scully RE. Serous borderline tumors of the peritoneum. Am J Surg Pathol 1996; 14(3):230–239.

62 Lu KH, Bell DA, Welch WR, et al. Evidence for the multifocal origin of bilateral and advanced human serous borderline ovarian tumors. Cancer Res 1998; 58:2328–2330.

63 Gu J, Roth LM, Younger C, et al. Molecular evidence for the independent origin of extra-ovarian papillary serous tumors of low malignant potential. J Natl Cancer Inst 2001; 93(15):1147–1152.

64 Silva E, Tornos C, Zhuang Z, et al. Tumor recurrence in stage I ovarian serous neoplasms of low malignant potential. Int J Gynecol Pathol 1998; 17:1–6.

65 Ortiz BH, Ailawadi M, Colitti C, et al. Secondary primary or recurrence? Comparative patterns of p53 and K-ras mutations suggest that serous borderline ovarian tumors and subsequent serous carcinomas are unrelated tumors. Cancer Res 2001; 61:7264–7264.

66 Clement PB, Young RH. Florid mesothelial hyperplasia associated with ovarian tumors: a potential source of error in tumor diagnosis and staging. Int J Gynecol Pathol 1993; 12:51–58.

67 Kheir SM, Mann WJ, Wilkerson JA. Glandular inclusions in lymph nodes. The problem of extensive involvement and relationship to salpingitis. Am J Surg Pathol 1981; 5:353–359.

68 Zinsser KR, Wheeler JE. Endosalpingiosis in the omentum. A study of autopsy and surgical material. Am J Surg Pathol 1982; 6:109–117.

69 Moore WF, Bentley RC, Berchuck A, et al. Some mullerian inclusion cysts in lymph nodes may sometimes be metastases from serous borderline tumors of the ovary. Am J Surg Pathol 2000; 24:710–718.

70 Copeland LJ, Silva EG, Gershenson DM, et al. The significance of mullerian inclusions found at second-look laparotomy in patients with epithelial ovarian neoplasm. Obstet Gynecol 1988; 71:763–770.

71 Gilks CB, Abdulmohsen A, Yue JW. Advanced-stage serous borderline tumors of the ovary: a clinicopathological study of 49 cases. Int J Gynecol Pathol 2002; 22:29–36.

72 Gilks CB, Bell DA, Scully RE. Serous psammocarcinoma of the ovary and peritoneum. Int J Gynecol Pathol 1990; 9:110–121.

73 Ulbright TM, Roth LM, Sutton GP. Papillary serous carcinoma of the ovary with squamous differentiation. Int J Gynecol Pathol 1990; 9:86–94.

74 Bosscher J, Barnhill D, O'Connor D. Osseous metaplasia in ovarian papillary serous cystadenocarcinoma. Gynecol Oncol 1990; 39:228–231.

75 O'Donnell M, Al-Nafussi AI. Intracytoplasmic lumina and mucinous inclusions in ovarian carcinomas. Histopathology 1995; 26:181–184.

76 Che M, Tornos C, Deavers MT, et al. Ovarian mixed-epithelial carcinomas with a microcystic pattern and signet-ring cells. Int J Gynecol Pathol 2001; 20:232–328.

77 Al-Nafussi AI, Hughes DE, Williams ARW. Hyaline globules in ovarian tumours. Histopathology 1993; 23:563–566.

78 Eichorn JH, Scully RE. 'Adenoid cystic' and basaloid carcinomas of the ovary: evidence for a surface epithelial lineage; a report of 12 cases. Mod Pathol 1995; 8(7):731–740.

79 Baergen RN, Rutgers JL. Mural nodules in common epithelial tumors of the ovary. Int J Gynecol Pathol 1994; 13:62–72.

80 Rosa G De, Donofrio V, Rosa N De, et al. Ovarian serous tumor with mural nodules of carcinomatous derivation (sarcomatoid carcinoma): report of a case. Int J Gynecol Pathol 1991; 10:311–318.

81 Costa MJ, Hansen C, Dickerman A, et al. Clinicopathologic significance of transitional cell carcinoma pattern in nonlocalized ovarian epithelial tumors (stages 2–4). Am J Clin Pathol 1998; 109:173–180.

82 Gooneratne S, Sassone M, Blaustein A, et al. Serous surface papillary carcinoma of the ovary: a clinicopathologic study of 16 cases. Int J Gynecol Pathol 1982; 1:258–269.

83 Bloss JD, Liao S, Buller RE, et al. Extraovarian peritoneal papillary serous carcinoma: a case-control retrospective comparison to papillary adenocarcinoma of the ovary. Gynecol Oncol 1993; 50:347–351.

84 Rutgers JL, Scully RE. Ovarian mullerian mucinous papillary cystadenomas of borderline malignancy: a clinicopathologic analysis. Cancer 1988; 61:340–348.

85 Rutgers JL, Scully RE. Ovarian mixed-epithelial papillary cystadenomas of borderline malignancy of the mullerian type: a clinico-pathologic analysis. Cancer 1998; 61:546–554.

86 Young RH, Scully RE. Ovarian Sertoli-Leydig cell tumors with a retiform pattern: a problem in histopathologic diagnosis. A report of 25 cases. Am J Surg Pathol 1983; 7:755–771.

87 Cramer SF, Roth LM, Ulbright TM, et al. Evaluation of reproducibility of the World Health Organization classification of common ovarian cancers; with emphasis on methodology. Arch Pathol Lab Med 1987; 111:819–829.

88 Clement PB, Young RH, Scully RE. Malignant mesotheliomas presenting as ovarian masses; a report of nine cases, including two primary ovarian mesotheliomas. Am J Surg Pathol 1996; 20(9):1067–1080.

89 Shimizu M, Toki T, Takagi Y, et al. Immunohistochemical detection of Wilms' tumor gene (WT1) in epithelial ovarian tumors. Int J Gynecol Pathol 2000; 19:158–163.

90 Goldstein NS, Uziebo A. WT-1 immunoreactivity in uterine papillary serous carcinomas is different from ovarian serous carcinomas. Am J Clin Pathol 2002; 117:541–545.

91 Al-Hussaini M, Stockman A, Foster H, et al. WT-1 assists in distinguishing ovarian from uterine serous carcinomas and in distinguishing between ovarian and endometrioid ovarian carcinoma. Histopathology 2004; 44:109–115.

92 Hashi A, Yuminamochi T, Murata S-I, et al. Wilms tumor gene immunoreactivity in primary serous carcinomas of the fallopian tube, ovary, endometrium and peritoneum. Int J Gynecol Pathol 2003; 22:374–377.

93 Acs G, Pasha T, Zhang PJ. WT1 is differentially expressed in serous, endometrioid, clear cell and mucinous carcinomas of the peritoneum, fallopian tube, ovary and endometrium. Int J Gynecol Pathol 2004; 23:110–118.

94 Ordonez NG. Role of immunohistochemistry in distinguishing epithelial peritoneal mesotheliomas from peritoneal and ovarian serous carcinomas. Am J Surg Pathol 1998; 22(10):1203–1214.

95 Puls LE, Powell DE, DePreist PD, et al. Transition from benign to malignant epithelium in mucinous and serous ovarian cystadenocarcinoma. Gynecol Oncol 1992; 47:53–57.

96 Deligdisch L. Ovarian dysplasia: a review. Int J Gynecol Cancer 1997; 7:89–94.

97 Brewer MA, Johnson K, Follen M, et al. Prevention of ovarian cancer: intraepithelial neoplasia. Clin Cancer Res 2003; 9:20–30.

98 Bell DA, Scully RE. Early de novo ovarian carcinoma: a study of fourteen cases. Cancer 1994; 73:1859–1864.

99 Shaw PA, McLaughlin JR, Zweener RP, et al. Histopathologic features of genetically determined ovarian cancer. Int J Gynecol Pathol 2002; 21(4):407–411.

100 Singer G, Shih I, Truskinovsky A, et al. Mutational analysis of K-ras segregates ovarian serous carcinomas into two types: invasive MPSC (low-grade tumor) and conventional serous carcinoma (high-grade tumor). Int J Gynecol Pathol 2002; 22:37–41.

101 Berchuck A, Kohler MF, Marks JR, et al. The p53 tumor suppressor gene frequently is altered in gynecologic cancers. Am J Obstet Gynecol 1994; 170:246–252.

102 Wen WH, Reles A, Runnebaum IB, et al. p53 mutation and expression in ovarian cancers: correlation with overall survival. Int J Gynecol Pathol 1999; 18:29–41.

103 Scully RE, Young RH, Clement PB, eds. Mucinous tumors and pseudomyxoma peritonei: tumors of the ovary, maldeveloped gonads, fallopian tube and broad ligament. In: Atlas of tumor pathology, 3rd series, fascicle 23. Washington, DC: Armed Forces Institute of Pathology; 1998:81–105.

104 Cariker M, Dockerty M. Mucinous cystadenomas and mucinous cystadenocarcinomas of the ovary: a clinical and pathological study of 355 cases. Cancer 1954; 7:302–310.

105 Lee KR, Young RH. The distinction between primary and metastatic mucinous carcinomas of the ovary: gross and histologic findings in 50 cases. Am J Surg Pathol 2003; 27:281–292.

106 Seidman JD, Kurman RJ, Ronnett BM. Primary and metastatic mucinous adenocarcinomas in the ovaries. Incidence in routine practice with a new approach to improve intraoperative diagnosis. Am J Surg Pathol 2003; 27:985–993.

107 Hirasawa K, Yamada M, Kitagawa M, et al. Ovarian mucinous cystadenocarcinoma as a cause of Zollinger- Ellison syndrome: report of a case and review of the literature. Am J Gastroenterol 2000; 95:1348–1351.

108 Beck RP, Latour JP. A review of 1019 benign ovarian neoplasms. Obstet Gynecol 1960; 16:479–482.

109 Lee KR, Scully RE. Mucinous tumors of the ovary: a clinicopathologic study of 196 borderline tumors (of intestinal type) and carcinomas, including an evaluation of 11 cases with 'pseudomyxoma peritonei'. Am J Surg Pathol 2000; 24:1147–1464.

110 Guerrieri C, Högberg T, Wingren S, et al. Mucinous borderline and malignant tumors of the ovary. A clinicopathologic and DNA ploidy study of 92 cases. Cancer 1994; 74:2329–1040.

111 Hart WR, Norris HJ. Borderline and malignant mucinous tumors of the ovary: histologic criteria and clinical behavior. Cancer 1973; 31:1031–1045.

112 Tholander B, Taube A, Lindgren A, et al. Pretreatment serum levels of CA-125, carcinoembryonic antigen, tissue polypeptide antigen and placental alkaline phosphatase, in patients with ovarian carcinoma, borderline tumors, or benign adnexal masses: relevance for differential diagnosis. Gynecol Oncol 1990; 39:16–25.

113 Gadducci A, Ferdeghini M, Prontera C, et al. The concomitant determination of different tumor markers in patients with epithelial ovarian cancer and benign ovarian masses: relevance for differential diagnosis. Gynecol Oncol 1992; 44:147–154.

114 O'Hanalan KA. Resection of a 303.2 pound ovarian tumor. Gynecol Oncol 1994; 54:365–371.

115 Pettersson F. Annual report of the results of treatment in gynecological cancer. Stockholm: International Federation of Gynecology and Obstetrics; 1991.

116 Chaitin BA, Gershenson DM, Evans HL. Mucinous tumors of the ovary: a clinicopathologic study of 70 cases. Cancer 1985; 55:1958–62.

117 Hoerl HD, Hart WR. Primary ovarian mucinous cystadenocarcinomas. A clinicopathologic study of 49 cases with long-term follow-up. Am J Surg Pathol 1998; 22:1449–62.

118 Kikkawa F, Kawai M, Tamakoshi K, et al. Mucinous carcinoma of the ovary. Clin Anal Oncol 1996; 53:303–307.

119 Nomura K, Aizawa S. Noninvasive, microinvasive and invasive mucinous carcinomas of the ovary: a clinicopathologic analysis of 40 cases. Cancer 2000; 89:1541–1546.

120 Riopel MA, Ronnett BM, Kurman RJ. Evaluation of diagnostic criteria and behavior of ovarian intestinal-type mucinous tumors. Atypical proliferative (borderline) tumors and intraepithelial, microinvasive, invasive and metastatic carcinomas. Am J Surg Pathol 1999; 23:617–635.

121 Watkin W, Silva EG, Gershenson DM. Mucinous carcinoma of the ovary: pathologic prognostic factors. Cancer 1992; 69:208–12.

122 Rodriguez IM, Prat J. Mucinous tumors of the ovary: a clinicopathologic analysis of 75 borderline tumors (of intestinal type) and carcinomas. Am J Surg Pathol 2002; 26:139–152.

123 Bell DA. Mucinous adenofibromas of the ovary: a report of 10 cases. Am J Surg Pathol 1991; 15:227–232.

124 Hart WR. Ovarian epithelial tumors of borderline malignancy (carcinomas of low malignant potential). Hum Pathol 1977; 8:541–49.

125 Russell P, Merkur H. Proliferative ovarian 'epithelial' tumors: a clinicopathological analysis of 144 cases. Aust NZ J Obstet Gynec 1979; 19:45–51.

126 Khunamornpong S, Russell P. Dalrymple JC. Proliferating (LMP) mucinous tumors of the ovaries with microinvasion: morphologic assessment of 13 cases. Int J Gynecol Pathol 1999; 18:238–246.

127 Shappell HW, Riopel MA, Sehdev AES, et al. Diagnostic criteria and behavior of ovarian seromucinous (endocervical-type mucinous and mixed cell-type) tumors: atypical proliferative (borderline) tumors, intraepithelial, microinvasive and invasive carcinomas. Am J Surg Pathol 2002; 26:1529–1541.

128 Siriaunkgul S, Robbins KM, McGowan L, et al. Ovarian mucinous tumors of low malignant potential: a clinicopathologic study of 54 tumors of intestinal and mullerian type. Int J Gynecol Pathol 1995; 14:198–208.

129 Lee KR, Nucci MR. Ovarian mucinous and mixed epithelial carcinomas of the mullerian (endocervical-like) type: a clinicopathologic analysis of four cases of an uncommon variant associated with endometriosis. Int J Gynecol Pathol 2002; 22:42–51.

130 Nichols GE, Mills SE, Ulbright TM, et al. Spindle cell mural nodules in cystic ovarian mucinous tumors: a clinicopathologic and immunohistochemical study of five cases. Am J Surg Pathol 1991; 15:1055–1062.

131 Prat J, Scully RE. Sarcomas in ovarian mucinous tumors: a report of two cases. Cancer 1979; 44:1327–31.

132 Prat J, Young RH, Scully RE. Ovarian mucinous tumors with foci of anaplastic carcinoma. Cancer 1982; 50:300–304.

133 Provenza C, Prat J, Young RH. Foci/nodules of anaplastic carcinoma in mucinous cystic ovarian tumors: a clinicopathologic study of 34 cases. Mod Pathol 2004; 17:211A.

134 Bague S, Rodriguez IM, Prat J. Sarcoma-like mural nodules in mucinous cystic tumors of the ovary revisited: a clinicopathologic analysis of 10 additional cases. Am J Surg Pathol 2002; 26:1467–1476.

135 Prat J, Scully RE. Ovarian mucinous tumors with sarcoma-like mural nodules: a report of seven cases. Cancer 1979; 44:1332–1344.

136 Prayson RA, Hart WR, Petras RE. Pseudomyxoma peritonei: a clinicopathologic study of 19 cases with emphasis on site of origin and nature of associated ovarian tumors. Am J Surg Pathol 1994; 18:591–603.

137 Young RH, Gilks CB, Scully RE. Mucinous tumors of the appendix associated with mucinous tumors of the ovary and pseudomyxoma peritonei: a clinicopathological analysis of 22 cases supporting an origin in the appendix. Am J Surg Pathol 1991; 15:415–429.

138 Ronnett BM, Kurman RJ, Zahn CM, et al. Pseudomyxoma peritonei in women: a clinicopathologic analysis of 30 cases with emphasis on site of origin, prognosis and relationship to ovarian mucinous tumors of low malignant potential. Hum Pathol 1995; 26:509–524.

139 Guerrieri C, Frånlund B, Boeryd B. Methods in pathology: expression of cytokeratin 7 in simultaneous mucinous tumors of the ovary and appendix. Mod Pathol 1995; 8:573–576.

140 Ronnett BM, Shmookler BM, Diener-West M, et al. Immunohistochemical evidence supporting the appendiceal origin of pseudomyxoma peritonei in women. Int J Gynecol Pathol 1997; 16:1–9.

141 Cuatrecasas M, Matias-Guiu X, Prat J. Synchronous mucinous tumors of the appendix and the ovary associated with pseudomyxoma peritonei. A clinicopathologic study of six cases with comparative analysis of c-Ki-ras mutations. Am J Surg Pathol 1996; 20:739–746.

142 Seidman JD, Elsayed AM, Sobin LH, et al. Association of mucinous tumors of the ovary and appendix: a clinicopathologic study of 25 cases. Am J Surg Pathol 1993; 17:22–34.

143 Chuaqui RF, Zhuang Z, Emmert-Buck MR, et al. Genetic analysis of synchronous mucinous tumors of the ovary and appendix. Hum Pathol 1996; 27:165–171.

144 Ronnett BM, Seidman JD. Mucinous tumors arising in mature cystic teratomas. Relationship to the clinical syndrome of pseudomyxoma peritonei. Am J Surg Pathol 2003; 27:650–657.

145 Ronnett BM, Zahn CM, Kurman RJ, et al. Disseminated peritoneal adenomucinosis and peritoneal mucinous carcinomatosis: a clinicopathologic analysis of 109 cases with emphasis on distinguishing pathologic features, site of origin, prognosis and relationship to pseudomyxoma peritonei. Am J Surg Pathol 1995; 19:1390–1408.

146 Hamilton SR, Aaltonen LA. Pathology and genetics of tumors of the digestive system. World Health Organization classification of tumors. Lyon: IARC Press; 2002.

147 Misraji J, Yantiss RK, Graeme-Cook FM, et al. Appendiceal mucinous neoplasms: a clinicopathologic analysis of 107 cases. Am J Surg Pathol 2003; 27:1089–1103.

148 Young RH, Scully RE. Differential diagnosis of ovarian tumors based primarily on their patterns and cell types. Semin Diagn Pathol 2001; 18:161–235.

149 Lash RH, Hart WR. Intestinal adenocarcinomas metastatic to the ovaries; a clinicopathologic evaluation of 22 cases. Am J Surg Pathol 1987; 11(2):114–121.

150 Daya D, Nazerali L, Frank GL. Metastatic ovarian carcinoma of large intestinal origin simulating primary ovarian carcinoma: a clinicopathologic study of 25 cases. Am J Clin Pathol 1992; 97:751–758.

151 Dionigi A, Facco C, Tibiletti MG, et al. Ovarian metastases from colorectal carcinoma. Clinicopathologic profile, immunophenotype and karyotype analysis. Am J Clin Pathol 2000; 114:111–122.

152 Young RH, Hart WR. Metastases from carcinomas of the pancreas simulating primary mucinous tumors of the ovary: a report of seven cases. Am J Surg Pathol 1989; 13(9):748–756.

153 Young RH, Scully RE. Ovarian metastases from carcinoma of the gallbladder and extrahepatic bile ducts simulating primary tumors of the ovary: a report of six cases. Int J Gynecol Pathol 1990; 9:60–72.

154 Ronnett BM, Kurman RJ, Shmookler BM, et al. The morphologic spectrum of ovarian metastases of appendiceal adenocarcinomas: a clinicopathologic and

immunohistochemical analysis of tumors often misinterpreted as primary ovarian tumors or metastatic tumors from other gastrointestinal sites. Am J Surg Pathol 1997; 21:1144–1155.

155 Young RH, Scully RE. Mucinous ovarian tumors associated with mucinous adenocarcinomas of the cervix: a clinicopathological analysis of 16 cases. Int J Gynecol Pathol 1988; 7:99–111.

156 Wauters CCAP, Smedts F, Gerrits LGM, et al. Keratins 7 and 20 as diagnostic markers of carcinomas metastatic to the ovary. Hum Pathol 1995; 26:852–855.

157 Loy TS, Calaluce RD, Keeney GL. Cytokeratin immunostaining in differentiating primary ovarian carcinoma from metastatic colonic adenocarcinoma. Mod Pathol 1996; 9(11):1040–1044.

158 Lagendijk JH, Mullink H, Diest PJ Van, et al. Tracing the origin of adenocarcinomas with unknown primary using immunohistochemistry: differential diagnosis between colonic and ovarian carcinomas as primary sites. Hum Pathol 1998; 29:491–497.

159 Cathro HP, Stoler MH. Expression of cytokeratins 7 and 20 in ovarian neoplasia. Am J Clin Pathol 2002; 117:944–951.

160 Chu P, Wu E, Weiss LM. Cytokeratin 7 and cytokeratin 20 expression in epithelial neoplasms: a survey of 435 cases. Mod Pathol 2000; 13:962–972.

161 Barbareschi M, Murer B, Colby TV, et al. CDX-2 homeobox gene expression is a reliable marker of colorectal adenocarcinoma metastases to the lungs. Am J Surg Pathol 2003; 27:141–149.

162 Groisman GM, Meir A, Sabo E. The value of Cdx2 immunostaining in differentiating primary ovarian carcinomas from colonic carcinomas metastatic to the ovaries. Int J Gynecol Pathol 2003; 23:52–57.

163 Ji H, Isacson C, Seidman JD, et al. Cytokeratins 7 and 20, Dpc4 and MUC5AC in the distinction of metastatic mucinous carcinomas in the ovary from primary ovarian mucinous tumors: Dpc4 assists in identifying metastatic pancreatic carcinomas. Int J Gynecol Pathol 2002; 21:391–400.

164 Young RH, Prat J, Scully RE. Ovarian Sertoli-Leydig cell tumors with heterologous elements. 1. Gastrointestinal epithelium and carcinoid: a clinicopathologic analysis of thirty-six cases. Cancer 1982; 50:2448–2456.

165 Baker PM, Oliva E, Young RH, et al. Ovarian mucinous carcinoids including some with a carcinomatous component. Am J Surg Pathol 2001; 25:557–568.

166 Tenti P, Aguzzi A, Riva C, et al. Ovarian mucinous tumors frequently express markers of gastric, intestinal and pancreaticobiliary epithelial cells. Cancer 1992; 69:2131–2142.

167 Shiohara S, Shiozawa Y, Shimizu M, et al. Histochemical analysis of estrogen and progesterone receptors and gastric-type mucin in mucinous ovarian tumors with reference to their pathogenesis. Cancer 1997; 80:908–916.

168 Mandai M, Konishi I, Kuroda H, et al. Heterogenous distribution K-ras-mutated epithelia in mucinous ovarian tumors with special reference to histopathology. Hum Pathol 1998; 28:34–40.

169 Caduff RF, Svoboda-Newman SM, Ferguson AW, et al. Comparison of mutations of Ki-ras and p53

170 Garrett AP, Lee KR, Colitti CR, et al. K-ras mutation may be an early event in mucinous ovarian tumorigenesis. Int J Gynecol Pathol 2001; 20:244–251.

171 Pieretti M, Hopenhayn-Rich C, Khattar NH, et al. Heterogeneity of ovarian cancer: relationships among histologic groups, stage of disease, tumor markers, patient characteristics and survival. Cancer Invest 2002; 20:11–23.

172 Lassus H, Laitinen MPE, Anttonen M, et al. Comparison of serous and mucinous ovarian carcinomas: distinct pattern of allelic loss at distal 8p and expression of transcription factor GATA-4. Lab Invest 2001; 81:517–526.

173 Pieretti M, Powell DE, Gallion HH, et al. Genetic alterations on chromosome 17 distinguish different types of epithelial ovarian tumors. Hum Pathol 1995; 26:393–397.

174 Purdie DM, Webb PM, Siskind V, et al. The different etiologies of mucinous and nonmucinous epithelial cancers. Gynecol Oncol 2003; 88:S145–S148.

175 Rutgers JL, Bell DA. Immunohistochemical characterization of ovarian borderline tumors of intestinal and mullerian types. Mod Pathol 1992; 5:367–371.

176 Grosso G, Raspagliesi F, Balocchi G, et al. Endometrioid carcinoma of the ovary: a retrospective analysis of 106 cases. Tumori 1998; 84:552–557.

177 Czernobilsky B, Silverman BB, Mikuta JJ. Endometrioid carcinoma of the ovary: a clinicopathologic study of 75 cases. Cancer 1970; 26:1141–1152.

178 Kline RC, Wharton JT, Atkinson EN, et al. Endometrioid carcinoma of the ovary: retrospective review of 145 cases. Gynecol Oncol 1990; 39(3):337–346.

179 Russell P. The pathological assessment of ovarian neoplasms III: The malignant 'epithelial' tumors. Pathology 1979; 11:493–532.

180 Yoshikawa H, Jimbo H, Okada S, et al. Prevalence of endometriosis in ovarian cancer. Gynecol Obstet Invest 2000; 50(Suppl 1):11–17.

181 Russell P. The pathological assessment of ovarian neoplasms. II: The proliferating 'epithelial tumors'. Pathology 1979; 11:251–282.

182 Kao GF, Norris HJ. Cystadenofibromas of the ovary with epithelial atypia. Am J Surg Pathol 1978; 2(4):357–363.

183 Roth LM, Czernobilsky B, Langley FA. Ovarian endometrioid adenofibromatous and cystadenofibromatous tumors: benign, proliferating and malignant. Cancer 1981; 48:1838–1845.

184 Bell DA, Scully RE. Atypical and borderline endometrioid adenofibromas of the ovary: a report of 27 cases. Am J Surg Pathol 1985; 9(3):205–214.

185 Snyder RR, Norris HJ, Tavassoli F. Endometrioid proliferative and low malignant potential tumors of the ovary: a clinicopathologic study of 46 cases. Am J Surg Pathol 1998; 12(9):661–671.

186 Bell KA, Kurman RJ. A clinicopathologic analysis of atypical proliferative (borderline) tumors and well-differentiated endometrioid adenocarcinomas of the ovary. Am J Surg Pathol 2000; 24(11):1465–1479.

187 Roth LM, Emerson RE, Ulbright TM. Ovarian endometrioid tumors of low malignant potential: a clinicopathologic study of 30 cases with comparison to

well-differentiated endometrioid adenocarcinoma. Am J Surg Pathol 2003; 27:1253–1259.

188 Kao GF, Norris HJ. Unusual cystadenofibromas: endometrioid, mucinous and clear cell types. Obstet Gyn 1979; 54(6):729–736.

189 DePriest PD, Banks ER, Powell DE, et al. Endometrioid carcinoma of the ovary and endometriosis: the association in postmenopausal women. Gynecol Oncol 1992; 47:71–75.

190 Zwart J, Geisler ZJ, Geisler HE. Five-year survival in patients with endometrioid carcinoma of the ovary versus those with serous carcinoma. Eur J Gynecol Oncol 1988; 19(3):225–228.

191 McMeekin DS, Burger RA, Manetta A, et al. Endometrioid adenocarcinoma of the ovary and its relationship to endometriosis. Gynecol Oncol 1995; 59:81–86.

192 Seidman JD. Prognostic importance of hyperplasia and atypia in endometriosis. Int J Gynecol Pathol 1996; 15:1–9.

193 Scully RE, Young RH, Clement PB, eds. Endometrioid tumors: tumors of the ovary, maldeveloped gonads, fallopian tube and broad ligament. In: Atlas of tumor pathology, 3rd series, fascicle 23. Washington, DC: Armed Forces Institute of Pathology; 1998:107–140.

194 Pitman MB, Young RH, Clement PB, et al. Endometrioid carcinoma of the ovary and endometrium, oxyphilic cell type: a report of nine cases. Int J Gynecol Pathol 1994; 13:290–301.

195 Eichhorn JH, Scully RE. Endometrioid ciliated-cell tumors of the ovary: a report of five cases. Int J Gynecol Pathol 1996; 15:248–256.

196 Tornos C, Silva EG, Ordonez NG, et al. Endometrioid carcinoma of the ovary with a prominent spindle-cell component, a source of diagnostic confusion: a report of 14 cases. Am J Surg Pathol 1995; 18(12):1343–1353.

197 Young RH, Prat J, Scully RE. Ovarian endometrioid carcinomas resembling sex cord-stromal tumors: a clinicopathological analysis of 13 cases. Am J Surg Pathol 1982; 6:513–522.

198 Roth LM, Liban E, Czernobilsky B. Ovarian endometrioid tumors mimicking Sertoli and Sertoli-Leydig cell tumors: sertoliform variant of endometrioid carcinoma Cancer 1982; 50:1322–1331.

199 Matias-Guiu X, Pons C, Prat J. Mullerian inhibiting substance, alpha-inhibin and CD99 expression in sex cord-stromal tumors and endometrioid ovarian carcinomas resembling sex cord-stromal tumors. Hum Pathol 1998; 29(8):840–845.

200 Guerriere C, Frånlund B, Malmstrom H, et al. Ovarian endometrioid carcinomas simulating sex cord-stromal tumors: a study using inhibin and cytokeratin 7. Int J Gynecol Pathol 1998; 17:266–271.

201 Ordi J, Schammel DP, Rasekh L, et al. Sertoliform endometrioid carcinomas of the ovary: a clinicopathologic and immunohistochemical study of 13 cases. Mod Pathol 1999; 12(10):933–940.

202 Nogales F, Bergeron C, Carvia RE, Alvaro T, Fulwood HR. Ovarian endometrioid tumors with yolk sac tumor component, an unusual form of ovarian neoplasm. Analysis of six cases. Am J Surg Pathol 1996; 20(9):1056–1066.

203 Kim KR, Scully RE. Peritoneal keratin granulomas with carcinomas of endometrium and ovary and atypical polypoid adenomyoma of endometrium: a clinicopathological analysis of 22 cases. Am J Surg Pathol 1990; 14:925–932.

204 Demopoulos RI, Touger L, Dubin N. Secondary ovarian carcinoma: a clinical and pathological evaluation. Int J Gynecol Pathol 1987; 6:166–175.

205 Yada-Hashimoto N, Yamamoto T, Kamiura S, et al. Metastatic ovarian tumors: a review of 64 cases. Gynecol Oncol 2003; 89:314–317.

206 Eifel P, Hendrickson M, Ross J, et al. Simultaneous presentation of carcinoma involving the ovary and the uterine corpus. Cancer 1982; 50:163–170.

207 Montaya F, Martin M, Schneider J, et al. Simultaneous appearance of ovarian and endometrial carcinoma: a therapeutic challenge. Eur J Gynaecol Oncol 1989; 10(2):135–139.

208 Zaino R, Whitney C, Brady MF, et al. Simultaneously detected endometrial and ovarian carcinomas – a prospective clinicopathologic study of 74 cases: a gynecologic oncology group study. Gynecol Oncol 2001; 83:355–362.

209 Prat J, Matias-Guiu X, Baretto J. Simultaneous carcinoma involving the endometrium and the ovary: a clinicopathologic, immunohistochemical and DNA flow cytometric study of 18 cases. Cancer 1991; 68:2455–2459.

210 Fujita M, Enomoto T, Wada H, et al. Application of clonal analysis. Differential diagnosis for synchronous primary ovarian and endometrial cancers and metastatic cancer. Am J Clin Pathol 1996; 105:350–359.

211 Emmert-Buck MR, Chuaqui R, Zhuang Z, et al. Molecular analysis of synchronous uterine and ovarian endometrioid tumors. Int J Gynecol Pathol 1997; 16:143–148.

212 Caduff RF, Svoboda-Newman SM, Bartos RE, et al. Comparative analysis of histologic homologues of endometrial and ovarian carcinoma. Am J Surg Pathol 1998; 22(3):319–326.

213 Shenson DL, Gallion HH, Powell DE, et al. Loss of heterozygosity and genomic instability in synchronous endometrioid tumors of the ovary and endometrium. Cancer 1995; 76:650–657.

214 Matias-Guiu X, Lagarda H, Catasus L, et al. Clonality analysis in synchronous or metachronous tumors of the female genital tract. Int J Gynecol Pathol 2002; 21(3):205–211.

215 Moreno-Bueno G, Gamallo C, Perez-Gallego L, et al. Beta-catenin expression pattern, beta-catenin gene mutations and microsatellite instability in endometrioid ovarian carcinomas and synchronous endometrial carcinomas. Diagn Mol Pathol 2001; 10(2):116–122.

216 Ulbright TM, Roth LM, Stehman FB. Secondary ovarian neoplasia: a clinicopathologic study of 35 cases. Cancer 1984; 53:1164–1174.

217 Harcourt KF, Dennis DL. Laparotomy for 'ovarian tumors' in unsuspected carcinoma of the colon. Cancer 1968; 21:1244–1246.

218 DeCostanzo DC, Elias JM, Chumas JC. Necrosis in 84 ovarian carcinomas: a morphologic study of primary versus metastatic colonic carcinoma with a selective immunohistochemical analysis of cytokeratin subtypes and carcinoembryonic antigen. Int J Gynecol Pathol 1997; 16:245–249.

219 Berezowski K, Stastny JF, Kornstein MJ. Cytokeratins 7 and 20 and carcinoembryonic antigen in ovarian and colonic carcinoma. Mod Pathol 1996; 9(4):426–429.

220 Young RH, Scully RE. Oxyphilic clear cell carcinoma of the ovary. Am J Surg Pathol 1987; 11(9):661–667.

221 Young RH, Hart WR. Metastatic intestinal carcinomas simulating primary ovarian clear cell carcinoma and secretory endometrioid carcinoma: a clinicopathologic and immunohistochemical study of five cases. Am J Surg Pathol 1998; 22(7):805–815.

222 Young RH, Scully RE. Ovarian tumors of probable wolffian origin: a report of 11 cases. Am J Surg Pathol 1983; 7:125–135.

223 Kommoss F, Olivia E, Bhan AK, et al. Inhibin expression in ovarian tumors and tumor-like lesions: an immunohistochemical study. Mod Pathol 1998; 11(7):656–664.

224 Devouassoux-Shisheboran M, Silver SA, Tavassoli FA. Wolffian adnexal tumor, so-called female adnexal tumor of probable wolffian origin (FATWO): immunohistochemical evidence in support of a wolffian origin. Hum Pathol 1999; 30(7):856–863.

225 Clement PB, Young RH, Scully RE. Endometrioid-like variant of ovarian yolk sac tumor: a clinicopathological analysis of eight cases. Am J Surg Pathol 1987; 11(10):767–778.

226 Kleinman GM, Young RH, Scully RE. Primary neuroectodermal tumors of the ovary: a report of 25 cases. Am J Surg Pathol 1993; 17(8):764–768.

227 Kleinman GM, Young RH, Scully RE. Ependymoma of the ovary: report of three cases. Hum Pathol 1984; 15:632–638.

228 Mostoufizadeh M, Scully RE. Malignant tumors arising in endometriosis. Clin Obstet Gynecol 1980; 23:951–963.

229 Stern RC, Dash R, Bentley RC, et al. Malignancy in endometriosis: frequency and comparison of ovarian and extraovarian types. Int J Gynecol Pathol 2001; 20:133–139.

230 Cuesta RS De La, Eichorn JH, Rice LW, et al. Histologic transformation of benign endometriosis to early epithelial ovarian cancer. Gynecol Oncol 1996; 60:238–244.

231 Fukunaga M, Nomura K, Ishikawa E, et al. Ovarian atypical endometriosis: its close association with malignant epithelial tumours. Histopathology 1997; 30(3):249–255.

232 Modesitt SC, Tortolero-Luna G, Robinson JB, et al. Ovarian and extraovarian endometriosis-related cancer. Obstet Gynecol 2002; 100(4):788–795.

233 Czernobilsky B, Morris WJ. A histologic study of ovarian endometriosis with emphasis on hyperplastic and atypical changes. Obstet Gynecol 1979; 53:318–323.

234 Ballouk F, Ross JS, Wolf BC. Ovarian endometriotic cysts: an analysis of cytologic atypia and DNA ploidy patterns. Am J Clin Pathol 1994; 102:415–419.

235 Jiang X, Morland SJ, Hitchcock A, et al. Allelotyping of endometriosis with adjacent ovarian carcinoma reveals evidence of a common lineage. Cancer Res 1995; 58(8):1707–1712.

236 Obata K, Morland SJ, Watson RH, et al. Frequent PTEN/MMAC mutations in endometrioid but not serous or mucinous epithelial ovarian tumors. Cancer Res 1998; 58(10):2095–2097.

237 Placios J, Gamallo C. Mutations in the beta-catenin gene (CTNNB1) in endometrioid ovarian carcinomas. Cancer Res 1998; 58(7):1344–1347.

238 Gras E, Catasus L, Arguelles R, et al. Microsatellite instability, MLH-1 promoter hypermethylation and frameshift mutations at coding mononucleotide repeat microsatellites in ovarian tumors. Cancer 2001; 92(11):2829–2836.

239 Liu J, Albarracin CT, Chang KH, et al. Microsatellite instability and expression of hMLH1 and hMSH2 proteins in ovarian endometrioid cancer. Mod Pathol 2004; 17:75–80.

240 Shakfeh SM, Woodruff JD. Primary ovarian sarcomas: report of 46 cases and review of the literature. Obstet Gynecol Surv 1987; 42:331–349.

241 Deligdisch L, Plaxe S, Cohen CJ. Extrauterine pelvic malignant mixed mesodermal tumors: a study of 10 cases with immunohistochemistry. Int J Gynecol Pathol 1998; 7:361–372.

242 Barakat RR, Rubin SC, Wong G, et al. Mixed mesodermal tumor of the ovary: analysis of prognostic factors in 31 cases. Obstet Gynecol 1992; 80:660–664.

243 Sood AK, Sorosky JI, Gelder MS, et al. Primary ovarian sarcoma: analysis of prognostic variables and the role of surgical cytoreduction. Cancer 1998; 82(9):1731–1737.

244 Dellers EA, Valente PT, Edmonds PR, et al. Extrauterine mixed mesodermal tumors: an immunohistochemical study. Arch Pathol Lab Med 1991; 115:918–920.

245 Dictor M. Ovarian malignant mixed mesodermal tumor: the occurrence of hyaline droplets containing α-1-antitrypsin. Hum Pathol 1982; 13:930–933.

246 Dinh TV, Slavin RE, Bhagavan BS, et al. Mixed mesodermal tumors of the ovary: a clinicopathologic study of 14 cascs. Obstet Gynecol 1988; 72:409–412.

247 Terada KY, Johnson TL, Hopkins M, et al. Clinicopathologic features of ovarian mixed mesodermal tumors and carcinosarcomas. Gynecol Oncol 1989; 32:228–232.

248 Eichorn JH, Young RH, Clement PB, et al. Mesodermal (Müllerian) adenosarcoma of the ovary: a clinicopathological analysis of 40 cases and a review of the literature. Am J Surg Pathol 2002; 26(10):1243–1258.

249 Kao GF, Norris HJ. Benign and low-grade variants of mixed mesodermal tumor (adenosarcoma) of the ovary and the adnexal area. Cancer 1978; 42(3):1314–1324.

250 Chang KL, Crabtree GS, Lim-Tan SK, et al. Primary extrauterine endometrial stromal neoplasms; a clinicopathologic study of 20 cases and a review of the literature. Int J Gynecol Pathol 1993; 12:282–296.

251 Young RH, Prat J, Scully RE. Endometrioid stromal sarcomas of the ovary: a clinicopathologic analysis of 23 cases. Cancer 1984; 53:1143–1155.

252 Ehrmann RL, Weidner N, Welch WR, et al. Malignant mixed mullerian tumor of the ovary with prominent neuroectodermal differentiation (teratoid carcinosarcoma). Int J Gynecol Pathol 1990; 9:272–282.

253 Parker RL, Dadmanesh F, Young RH, Clement PB. Polypoid endometriosis: a clinicopathologic analysis of 24 cases and a review of the literature. Am J Surg Pathol 2004; 28:285–297.

254 Young RH, Scully RE. Sarcomas metastatic to the ovary: a report of 21 cases. Int J Gynecol Pathol 1990; 9:231–252.

255 Scully RE, Young RH, Clement PB, eds. Clear cell tumors: tumors of the ovary, maldeveloped gonads, fallopian tube and broad ligament. In: Atlas of tumor pathology, 3rd series, fascicle 23. Washington, DC: Armed Forces Institute of Pathology; 1998:141–151.

256 Roth LM, Langley FA, Fox H, et al. Ovarian clear cell adenofibromatous tumors: benign, of low malignant potential and associated with invasive clear cell carcinoma. Cancer 1984; 53:1156–1163.

257 Bell DA, Scully RE. Benign and borderline clear cell adenofibromas of the ovary. Cancer 1985; 56:2922–2931.

258 Montag AG, Jenison EL, Griffiths CT, et al. Ovarian clear cell carcinoma. A clinicopathologic analysis of 44 cases. Int J Gynecol Pathol 1989; 8:85–96.

259 Crozier MA, Copeland LJ, Silve EG, et al. Clear cell carcinoma of the ovary: a study of 59 cases. Gynecol Oncol 1989; 35:199–203.

260 Young RH, Oliva E, Scully RE. Small cell carcinoma of the ovary, hypercalcemic type: a clinicopathological analysis of 150 cases. Am J Surg Pathol 1994; 18:1102–1116.

261 O'Brien MER, Schofiels JB, Tan S, et al. Clear cell epithelial cancer (mesonephroid): bad prognosis only in early stages. Gynecol Oncol 1993; 49:250–254.

262 Goff BA. Sainz de la Cuesta, Muntz HG, et al. Clear cell carcinoma of the ovary: a distinct histologic type with poor prognosis and resistance to platinum-based chemotherapy in stage III disease. Gynecol Oncol 1996; 60:412–417.

263 Kennedy AW, Markman M, Biscotti CV, et al. Survival probability in ovarian clear cell adenocarcinoma. Gynecol Oncol 1999; 74:108–114.

264 Sugiyama T, Kamura T, Kigawa J, et al. Clinical characteristics of clear cell carcinoma of the ovary. Cancer 2000; 88:2584–2589.

265 Leitao MM, Boyd J, Hummer A, et al. Clinicopathologic analysis of early-stage sporadic ovarian carcinoma. Am J Surg Pathol 2004; 28:147–159.

266 Young RH, Scully RE. Oxyphilic clear cell carcinoma of the ovary. A report of nine cases. Am J Surg Pathol 1987; 11(9):661–667.

267 Sant'Ambrogio S, Malpica A, Schroeder B, et al. Primary ovarian rhabdomyosarcoma associates with clear cell carcinoma of the ovary: a case report and review of the literature. Int J Gynecol Pathol 2000; 19:169–173.

268 Ishikura H, Scully RE. Hepatoid carcinoma of the ovary. A newly described tumor. Cancer 1987; 60:2775–2784.

269 Tochigi N, Kishimoto T, Supriatna, et al. Hepatoid carcinoma of the ovary: a report of three cases admixed with a common surface epithelial carcinoma. Int J Gynecol Pathol 2003; 22:266–271.

270 Wick MR, Swanson PE, Manivel JC. Placental-like alkaline phosphatase reactivity in human tumors: an immunohistochemical study of 520 cases. Hum Pathol 1987; 18:946–954.

271 Zirker TA, Silva EG, Morris M, et al. Immunohistochemical differentiation of clear cell carcinoma of the female genital tract and endodermal sinus tumor with the use of alpha-fetoprotein and Leu-M1. Am J Clin Pathol 1989; 91:511–514.

272 Young RH, Dickerson GR, Scully RE. Juvenile granulosa cell tumor of the ovary: a clinicopathological analysis of 125 cases. Am J Surg Pathol 1984; 8:575–596.

273 Young RH, Hart WR. Renal cell carcinoma metastatic to the ovary: a report of three cases emphasizing possible confusion with ovarian clear cell adenocarcinoma. Int J Gynecol Pathol 1992; 11:96–104.

274 Cameron RI, Ashe P, O'Rouke DM, et al. A panel of immunohistochemical stains assists in the distinction between ovarian and renal clear cell carcinoma. Int J Gynecol Pathol 2003; 22:272–276.

275 Nolan LP, Heatley MK. The value of immunohistochemistry in distinguishing between clear cell carcinoma of the kidney and ovary. Int J Gynecol Pathol 2001; 20:155–159.

276 Brinton LA, Gridley G, Persson I, et al. Cancer risk after a hospital discharge diagnosis of endometriosis. Am J Obstet Gynecol 1997; 176:572–579.

277 Vercellini P, Parazzini F, Bolis G, et al. Endometriosis and ovarian cancer. Am J Obstet Gynecol 1993; 169:181–182.

278 Shimizu M, Nikaido T, Toki T, et al. Clear cell carcinoma has an expression pattern of cell cycle regulatory molecules that is unique among ovarian adenocarcinomas. Cancer 1999; 85(3):669–677.

279 Okada S, Tsuda H, Takarabe T, et al. Allelotype analysis of common epithelial ovarian cancers with special reference to comparison between clear cell adenocarcinoma with other histological types. Jpn J Cancer Res 2002; 93:798–806.

280 Werness BA, Jobe JS, DiCioccio RA, et al. Expression of p53 induced tumor suppressor p21wafl/cip1 in ovarian carcinomas: correlation with p53 and Ki-67 immunohistochemistry. Int J Gynecol Pathol 1997; 16:149–155.

281 Fujimura M, Hidaka T, Kataoka K, et al. Absence of estrogen receptor-a expression on human ovarian clear cell adenocarcinoma compared with ovarian serous, endometrioid and mucinous adenocarcinoma. Am J Surg Pathol 2001; 25(5):667–672.

282 Vang R, Whitaker BP, Farhood AI, et al. Immunohistochemical analysis of clear cell carcinoma of the gynecologic tract. Int J Gynecol Pathol 2001; 20:252–259.

283 Brenner F. Das oophorma folliculare. Frankfurt Z Pathol 1907; 1:150–171.

284 Fox H, Agrawal K, Langley FA. The Brenner tumour of the ovary. A clinicopathological study of 54 cases. J Obstet Gynaecol Br Commonw 1972; 79:661–665.

285 Ehrlich CE, Roth LM. The Brenner tumor: a clinicopathologic study of 57 cases. Cancer 1971; 27:332–342.

286 Silverberg SG. Brenner tumor of the ovary: a clinicopathologic study of 60 tumors in 54 women. Cancer 1971; 28:588–596.

287 Waxman M. Pure and mixed Brenner tumors of the ovary: clinicopathologic and histogenetic observations. Cancer 1979; 43:1830–1839.

288 Hallgrimsson J, Scully RE. Borderline and malignant Brenner tumours of the ovary: a report of 15 cases. Acta Path Microbiol Scand [A] 1972; 80(233):56–66.

289 Roth LM, Dallenbach-Hellweg G, Czernobilsky B. Ovarian Brenner tumors. I. Metaplastic, proliferating and of low malignant potential. Cancer 1985; 56:582–591.

290 Miles PA, Norris HJ. Proliferative and malignant Brenner tumors of the ovary. Cancer 1972; 30:174–186.

291 Woodruff JD, Dietrich D, Genadry R, et al. Proliferative and malignant Brenner tumors: review of 47 cases. Am J Obstet Gynecol 1981; 141:118–125.

292 Trebeck CE, Friedlander ML, Russell P, et al. Brenner tumors of the ovary: a study of histology, immunochemistry and cellular DNA content in benign, borderline and malignant ovarian tumors. Pathology 1987; 19:241–246.

293 Roth LM, Czernobilsky B. Ovarian Brenner tumors: II. Malignant. Cancer 1985; 56:592–601.

294 Austin RM, Norris HJ. Malignant Brenner tumor and transitional cell carcinoma of the ovary: a comparison. Int J Gynecol Pathol 1987; 6:29–39.

295 Silva EG, Robey-Cafferty SS, Smoth TL, et al. Ovarian carcinomas with transitional cell carcinoma pattern. Am J Clin Pathol 1990; 93(4):458–465.

296 Robey SS, Silva EG, Gershenson DM, et al. Transitional cell carcinoma in high-grade high-stage ovarian carcinoma: an indicator of favorable response to chemotherapy. Cancer 1989; 63:839–847.

297 Hollingsworth HC, Steinberg SM, Silverberg SG, et al. Advanced stage transitional cell carcinoma of the ovary. Hum Pathol 1996; 27(12):1267–1272.

298 Gershenson DM, Silva EG, Mitchell MF, et al. Transitional cell carcinoma of the ovary: a matched control study of advanced-stage patients treated with cisplatin-based chemotherapy. Am J Obstet Gynecol 1993; 168:1178–1187.

299 Scully RE, Young RH, Clement PB, eds. Transitional and squamous cell tumors: tumors of the ovary, maldeveloped gonads, fallopian tube and broad ligament. In: Atlas of tumor Pathology, 3rd series, fascicle 23. Washington, DC: Armed Forces Institute of Pathology; 1998:153–164.

300 Baker PM, Young RH. Brenner tumor of the ovary with striking microcystic change. Int J Gynecol Pathol 2003; 22:185–188.

301 Eichhorn J, Young RH. Transitional cell carcinoma of the ovary. A morphologic study of 100 cases with emphasis on differential diagnosis. Am J Surg Pathol 2004; 28:453–463.

302 Nagai Y, Kishimoto T, Nikaido T, et al. Squamous predominance in mixed-epithelial papillary cystadenomas of borderline malignancy of mullerian type arising in endometriotic cysts: a study of four cases. Am J Surg Pathol 2003; 27(2):242–247.

303 Young RH, Scully RE. Urothelial and ovarian carcinomas of identical cell types: problems in interpretation. Int J Gynecol Pathol 1988; 7:197–211.

304 Logani S, Olivia E, Amin MB, et al. Immunoprofile of ovarian tumors with putative transitional cell (urothelial) differentiation using novel urothelial markers: histogenetic and diagnostic implications. Am J Surg Pathol 2003; 27(11):1434–1441.

305 Soslow RA, Rouse RV, Hendrickson MR, et al. Transitional cell neoplasms of the ovary and bladder: a comparative immunohistochemical analysis. Int J Gynecol Pathol 1996; 15:257–265.

306 Ordonez NG. Transitional cell carcinomas of the ovary and bladder are immunophenotypically different. Histopathology 2000; 36:433–438.

307 Shevchuk MM, Fenoglio CM, Richart RM. Histogenesis of Brenner tumors, I: histology and ultrastructure. Cancer 1980; 46:2607–2616.

308 Ordonez NG, Mackay B. Brenner tumor of the ovary: a comparative immunohistochemical and ultrastructural study with transitional cell carcinoma of the bladder. Ultrastruct Pathol 2000; 24:157–167.

309 Kaufmann O, Volmerig J, Dietel M. Uroplakin III is a highly specific and moderately sensitive immunohistochemical marker for primary and metastatic urothelial carcinomas. Am J Clin Pathol 2000; 113:683–687.

310 Ogawa K, Johansson SL, Cohen SM. Immunohistochemical analysis of uroplakins, urothelial specific proteins in ovarian Brenner tumors, normal tissues and benign and neoplastic lesions of the female genital tract. Am J Pathol 1999; 155:1047–1050.

311 Riedel I, Czernobilsky B, Lifschitz-Mercer B, et al. Brenner tumors but not transitional cell carcinomas of the ovary show urothelial differentiation: immunohistochemical staining of the urothelial markers, including cytokeratins and uroplakins. Virchows Arch 2001; 438:181–191.

312 Nogales FF, Silverberg SG. Epidermoid cysts of the ovary: a report of five cases with histogenetic considerations and ultrastructural findings. Am J Obstet Gynecol 1976; 124:523–528.

313 Young RH, Prat J, Scully RE. Epidermoid cyst of the ovary: a report of three cases with comments on histogenesis. Am J Clin Pathol 1980; 73:272–276.

314 Fan LD, Zang HY, Zhang XS. Ovarian epidermoid cyst: report of eight cases. Int J Gynecol Pathol 1996; 15:69–71.

315 Pins MR, Young RH, Daly WJ, et al. Primary squamous cell carcinoma of the ovary: a report of 37 cases. Am J Surg Pathol 1996; 20(7):823–833.

316 Black WC, Benitez RE. Non-teratomatous squamous cell carcinoma in situ of the ovary. Obstet Gynecol 1974; 120:556–520.

317 Genadry R, Parmley T, Woodruff JD. Simultaneous malignant squamous metaplasia of the cervix and ovary. Gynecol Oncol 1979; 8:87–91.

318 McGrady BJ, Sloan JM, Lamki H, et al. Bilateral ovarian cysts with squamous intraepithelial neoplasia. Int J Gynecol Pathol 1993; 12:350–354.

319 Sworn MJ, Jones H, Letchworth AT, et al. Squamous intraepithelial neoplasia in an ovarian cyst, cervical intraepithelial neoplasia and human papillomavirus. Hum Pathol 1995; 26:344–347.

320 Young RH, Gersell DJ, Roth LM, et al. Ovarian metastases from cervical carcinomas other than pure adenocarcinomas: a report of 12 cases. Cancer 1993; 71:407–418.

321 Mia KT, Yazdi HM, Bertrand MA, et al. Bilateral primary ovarian squamous cell carcinoma associated with human papilloma virus infection and vulvar and cervical intraepithelial neoplasia: a case report with review of the literature. Am J Surg Pathol 1996; 20(6):767–772.

322 Brescia RJ, Dubin N, Demopoulos RI. Endometrioid and clear cell carcinoma of the ovary. Int J Gynecol Pathol 1989; 8:132–138.

323 Tornos C, Silva EG, Khorana SM, Burke TW. High-stage endometrioid carcinoma of the ovary. Prognostic

significance of pure versus mixed histologic types. Am J Surg Pathol 1994; 18:687–693.

324 Silva EG, Tornos C, Bailey MA, et al. Undifferentiated carcinoma of the ovary. Arch Pathol Lab Med 1991; 115:377–381.

325 Scully RE, Young RH, Clement PB, eds. Mixed epithelial tumors and undifferentiated carcinomas: tumors of the ovary, maldeveloped gonads, fallopian tube and broad ligament. In: Atlas of tumor pathology, 3rd series, fascicle 23. Washington, DC: Armed Forces Institute of Pathology; 1998:165–168.

326 Kuwashima Y, Uehara T, Kishi K, et al. Immunohistochemical characterization of undifferentiated carcinomas of the ovary. J Cancer Res Clin Oncol 1994; 120:672–677.

327 Oliva E, Andrada E, Pezzica E, et al. Ovarian carcinomas with choriocarcinomatous differentiation. Cancer 1993; 72:2442–2446.

328 Young RH, Scully RE. Ovarian sex cord-stromal tumors with bizarre nuclei: a clinicopathologic study of 34 cases. Int J Gynecol Pathol 1983; 1:325–330.

329 Eichhorn JH, Young RH, Scully RE. Primary ovarian small cell carcinoma of pulmonary type: a clinicopathologic, immunohistologic and flow cytometric analysis of 11 cases. Am J Surg Pathol 1992; 16:926–938.

330 Eichhorn JH, Lawrence WD, Young RH, et al. Ovarian neuroendocrine carcinomas of non-small cell carcinoma cell type associated with surface epithelial adenocarcinomas: a study of five cases and review of the literature. Int J Gynecol Pathol 1996; 15:303–314.

28

Pathology-based management and outcome of epithelial tumors of the ovary

Michael G. Muto

Introduction

Staging of ovarian epithelial neoplasia

The staging procedure
FIGO staging classification

Serous neoplasia

Borderline serous neoplasia
Serous tumors with complex (micropapillary) architecture and/or microinvasion
Serous carcinoma

Endometrioid neoplasia

Borderline endometrioid and clear cell tumors

Early carcinomas arising in endometriotic cysts

Mucinous neoplasia

Borderline tumors
Mucinous carcinomas

Primary peritoneal carcinomas

Extraovarian endometrioid carcinoma

Postsurgical management

Lingering controversies

Introduction

The classification of ovarian epithelial neoplasia, with its nuances of origin, cell type, gradations of malignant potential, propensity for extra-ovarian disease (concurrent or metastatic) and variations in type of peritoneal spread renders this disease one of the most complex in the female genital tract. Accordingly, the task of properly managing these patients imposes a significant responsibility on the clinician and pathologist to precisely record the findings in the context of their impact on prognosis and therapy. Although the pathologist should know the pathologic variables critical to the management of every tumor, the shifting trends of ovarian tumor classification and therapy deserve special attention and have been allotted this brief chapter. The important pathologic parameters will be discussed and their impact on therapy detailed.

Staging of ovarian epithelial neoplasia

THE STAGING PROCEDURE

The first step in the management of presumed ovarian cancer is usually exploratory surgery. The goals of primary surgery are to establish a diagnosis, establish a stage and to reduce (de-bulk) the tumor to the lowest possible residual (optimal less than 1 cm largest tumor nodule) disease. Depending on the diagnosis, patient's age and options for preserving fertility, the uterus and contralateral ovary may or may not be spared.[1]

Intermediate-risk and low-risk pelvic masses are now often approached initially by laparoscopic salpingo-oophorectomy, with open surgical staging if the frozen section is positive.[2,3] This approach is recommended for masses 5 cm and smaller. For high-risk or larger ovarian masses, laparotomy is required. High-risk masses are those with solid components, bilateral, with free fluid, elevated tumor markers, high Doppler blood flow or patients with high-risk history. Steps in management include: (1) vertical laparotomy; (2) pelvic-abdominal washings and smear diaphragm; (3) exploration; (4) resection of pelvic mass for frozen section; (5) surgical staging with omentum, and lymph node dissection (6) total abdominal hysterectomy and bilateral salpingo-oophorectomy depending on future fertility, histology and stage.

FIGO STAGING CLASSIFICATION

Tables 28.1–28.4 summarize the International Federation of Gynecology and Obstetrics (FIGO) staging classification for ovarian cancer and morphology-specific outcomes.[4-7] The prognosis for each stage is highly

Table 28.1 The FIGO[4] staging for primary carcinoma of the ovary (1985)

Stage	Description	5-year survival (%)
I	Growth limited to the ovaries	78
IA	Growth limited to one ovary; no ascites. No tumor on the external surface; capsule intact	84
IB	Growth limited to both ovaries: no ascites. No tumor on the external surfaces; capsules intact	79
IC	Tumor either Stage IA or IB but with tumor on surface of one or both ovaries, or with capsule ruptured; or with ascites present containing malignant cells or with positive peritoneal washings	73
II	Growth involving one or both ovaries with pelvic extension	59
IIA	Extension and/or metastases to the uterus and/or tubes	65
IIB	Extension to other pelvic tissues	54
IIC	Tumor either Stage IIA or IIB but with tumor on surface of one or both ovaries: or with capsule(s) ruptured; or with ascites present containing malignant cells or with positive peritoneal washings	61
III	Tumor involving one or both ovaries with peritoneal implants outside the pelvis and/or positive retroperitoneal or inguinale nodes. Superficial liver metastasis equals Stage III. Tumor is limited to the true pelvis but with histologically proven malignant extension to small bowel or omentum	22
IIIA	Tumor grossly limited to true pelvis with negative nodes but with histologically confirmed microscopic seeding of abdominal peritoneal surfaces	52
IIIB	Tumor of one or both ovaries with histologically confirmed implants of abdominal peritoneal surfaces none exceeding 2 cm in diameter. Nodes are negative	29
IIIC	Abdominal implants greater than 2 cm in diameter and/or positive retroperitoneal or inguinale nodes	18
IV	Growth involving one or both ovaries, with distant metastases. If pleural effusion is present, there must be positive cytology. Parenchymal liver metastases equal Stage IV	14

Table 28.2 *Distribution of ovarian carcinomas by stage*[6]

Tumor type	No	Stage (%)			
		I	II	III	IV
Mucinous	123	19.1	23.0	43.1	14.8
Endometrioid	205	50.8	28.7	13.9	6.5
Clear cell	63	47.6	24.5	21.2	6.7
Serous	283	35.2	25.5	27.6	11.7
Undifferentiated	155	57.1	25.4	7.9	9.5

tumor type and grade dependent. Stage I and II tumors that are well-differentiated carry a 91–98% 5-year survival and include those tumors that are amenable to conservative management. Those that are endometrioid or mucinous in differentiation are typically localized to the ovary and do not involve the ovarian surface. Higher-grade tumors with serous morphology, ovarian surface involvement and/or positive washings have a higher risk of extra-ovarian relapse. The 5-year survival with Stage III and IV tumors drops to 20% and the short- to intermediate-term outcome is influenced by degree to which the tumor can be de-bulked and the response to chemotherapy. If optimal de-bulking is not accomplished, long-term survival falls to under 10%.[1,8]

Most of the following discussion will address the management of specific pathologic categories, particularly borderline and low-grade carcinomas. The management of this group is most controversial and is highly dependent on nuances of pathologic interpretation.

Serous neoplasia

The diagnosis of borderline serous cystadenoma is usually not a difficult task for the pathologist. There is some risk that an unusual variant (such as lesions containing micropapillary features or microinvasion) may be overlooked or that a very well-differentiated serous carcinoma will be misclassified. However, the management of these patients hinges almost entirely on whether there is spread beyond the ovary and, if so, the nature of the implants.[9–13] The following are scenarios in management and their rationale.

BORDERLINE SEROUS NEOPLASIA

Stage I borderline serous neoplasms

Stage I borderline serous tumors are treated by removal of the adnexal structures alone. There is no need for chemotherapy and, if fertility is desired, the opposite

ovary may be left *in situ*. If only one ovary is present, cystectomy is adequate therapy in most cases and further surgery to remove the remainder of the reproductive organs is not mandatory after childbearing.[9,11,12,18]

The above approach is rooted in one principle, which is that borderline serous tumors are biologically 'stable' and will not dedifferentiate over time. An outcome of carcinoma occurs in less than 1% of Stage I serous borderline tumors.[14,16,18,27] This is true with some caveats. The first is that the opposite ovary is at risk for either a new primary serous tumor or spread from the first.[14,16,18,27] In addition, if cystectomy is performed, up to one-third may recur in the treated ovary.[2,12] However, the risk of malignancy in the contralateral ovary is remote. The second is that a very small proportion of borderline tumors will be followed by a *bona-fide* carcinoma in an extra-ovarian pelvic site.[16] This can take the form of extra-ovarian invasive implants or (less commonly) frank carcinoma concurrent with or subsequent to a diagnosis of ovarian borderline tumor. However, there is no evidence that the latter scenario can be prevented by removal of all the reproductive organs.[9,18]

Stage II borderline

The management of Stage II borderline is in keeping with the potential for ovarian preservation, which is less feasible than when a small tumor involves a single ovary. While bilateral cystectomies are an option, the patient must be counseled regarding the high rate of expected recurrence. In one study employing conservative surgery, pregnancy was achieved in 14 of 44 patients.[12]

Stage III borderline

Stage III is defined as involvement of not only the ovaries but also the peritoneal, cul-de-sac or omental surfaces. It is this group of borderline tumors that are at the highest risk for persistence, progression, and in some instances, death. In contrast to a greater than 99% 5-year survival for Stage I borderline tumors, the recurrence rates for Stages II–IV are 20–30% and mortality for Stage III or greater is 15–20% (Table 28.4).[17,26,27] Overall, disease-free survival for Stage I, II and III is 99.6, 95.8 and 89%, respectively (Table 28.3).

Several variables influence risk of recurrence and death in serous borderline tumors. As discussed in Chapter 27, the pathologist must make the distinction between conventional non-invasive implants, desmo-

Table 28.3 Pathology-based outcome of borderline tumors

Diagnosis	Stage	No.	Deaths	References
SBT	I/II or not specified	330	0	13–15,18
SBT	I/II microinvasion	39	1	19,20
SBT	I micropapillary/cribriform	56	0	21–24
SBT	II/III non-invasive implants	203	11	26–28
SBT	II/III invasive implants	79	28	26–31
MBT	I	134	2	32,33
MIEC	I	86	3	32,33

SBT, serous borderline tumor; MBT, mucinous borderline tumor; MIEC, mucinous intraepithelial carcinoma.

plastic non-invasive implants and invasive implants. If the disease involves only one ovary and invasive implants are not identified, the uninvolved adnexae and uterus can be saved to preserve fertility. However, current management guidelines mandate that all visible disease be removed. The value of adjunctive chemotherapy is doubtful.

Stage III borderline serous tumors with invasive implants

The management of a Stage III borderline with invasive implants is governed by the fact that most studies link them with adverse outcome relative to non-invasive implants. In contrast to a greater than 80% disease-free survival and 2% risk of progressive disease for non-invasive implants at 5 years, invasive implants confer a more dismal outcome, with over 30% progressing.[17,26–28] Because high-stage tumors with invasive implants carry an approximately 20–50% mortality, the oncologist will consider adjuvant chemotherapy. However, the degree to which this will influence outcome is not known. An important consideration in these instances is *whether all visible disease can be removed.*

The oncologist may do the following: (1) treat all patients, irrespective of respectability; (2) consider chemotherapy if the implants cannot be completely removed and observe the patient if no residual disease is present; and (3) observe all patients. Suffice it to say that any of these choices may invite controversy among oncologists and that treatment must be individualized. However, in general, unless invasive implants are extensive, complete surgical removal is considered adequate therapy.

SEROUS TUMORS WITH COMPLEX (MICROPAPILLARY) ARCHITECTURE AND/OR MICROINVASION

The management of borderline serous tumors with micropapillary architecture (variously termed micropapillary borderline tumors or well-differentiated micropapillary carcinomas) or with microinvasion of the ovarian stroma will depend almost entirely on the stage and whether invasive implants or worse are present on the peritoneum. The risk of death associated with microinvasion is minimal.[19,20] Similarly, the mortality associated with micropapillary or complex architecture is stage dependent. These features are more likely to be associated with a higher stage (II or greater) borderline neoplasm, but do not confer a significant mortality risk in Stage I borderline serous tumors (Table 28.3). In contrast, approximately 50% of micropapillary serous tumors (carcinomas) with stromal invasion and invasive implants are dead within 5 years.[23] The presence of invasive implants in such settings will frequently lead the clinician to consider chemotherapy despite the questionable benefit.

SEROUS CARCINOMA

Stage I

The management of Stage I papillary serous carcinomas is based on grade and substage. Stage I grade 1 tumors can be conservatively managed with unilateral salpingo-oophorectomy and no chemotherapy with preserva-

Table 28.4 Pathology and stage-dependent outcome (5-year survival) of ovarian cancer[47]

Type	Stage			
	I	II	III	IV
Mucinous	83	55	21	9
Endometrioid	78	63	24	6
Clear cell	69	55	14	4
Serous	76	56	25	9
All	78	59	22	14

tion of fertility.[12] However, higher grade (2 or 3) tumors will increase pressure on the surgeon to remove the reproductive organs. The management of Stage IC disease is less clear. If the positive cytology is attributed to intraoperative rupture alone, it may be considered a unique low-risk situation. However, if the rupture is considered the consequence of capsular invasion rather than surgical technique, chemotherapy must be strongly considered.

Stage II

It is often said that there are very few surgical Stage II serous carcinomas, in that they have invariably spread beyond the ovaries and will recur. This is the case for both borderline and malignant serous tumors. The standard management of serous carcinomas will include adjunctive chemotherapy.

Stage III

Management is similar to that outlined at the beginning of the chapter, including staging, removal of visible disease and adjunctive chemotherapy.[1]

Endometrioid neoplasia

The management of endometrioid adenocarcinomas of the ovary is influenced by the fact that these tumors can arise in other Müllerian sites, including endometrial cavity and peritoneal endometriotic foci. For this reason, conservative management must always take into account these additional risks, particularly when conserving the contralateral ovary or uterus.

BORDERLINE ENDOMETRIOID AND CLEAR CELL TUMORS

Stage I or II proliferative endometrioid cystadenomas and cystadenofibromas and borderline clear cell adenofibromas are managed by total abdominal hysterectomy (TAH), bilateral salpingo-oophorectomy (BSO) in postmenopausal patients and by unilateral salpingo-oophorectomy (SO) in premenopausal women who desire to retain their fertility. The risk of spread beyond the ovary is low.[34]

EARLY CARCINOMAS ARISING IN ENDOMETRIOTIC CYSTS

Endometriosis is a common site for ovarian and extra-ovarian endometrial carcinoma.[35–37] Although early

serous carcinomas arising in ovarian cortical inclusion cyst are extremely rare, such transitions are common in endometriosis.[38] Early tumors arising in endometriotic cysts that are non-invasive carry no appreciable risk of metastasizing beyond the ovary and are treated by removal and observation.[39]

The most compelling issue when considering conservative management of endometrioid tumors of the ovary is the risk of multifocal disease, including the endometrium, contralateral ovary and peritoneal surfaces.[36,40]

Stage IA, grade 1–2 endometrioid adenocarcinomas

Postmenopausal patients are typically managed by total hysterectomy and bilateral salpingo-oophorectomy. Women of reproductive age can be treated by unilateral oophorectomy and peritoneal sampling; however, special attention to the endometrial cavity and to any other endometriotic implants in the pelvis is critical. Stage IA grade 3 cancers require chemotherapy. There is no consensus on the management of intermediate-grade lesions. The higher the grade, the less likely the surgeon will adopt a conservative approach to the contralateral ovary.

Stage IA clear cell or grade 3 endometrioid tumors

These tumors are all managed as high-grade ovarian carcinomas. Contralateral ovarian preservation can be considered but chemotherapy is always recommended due to high risk of recurrent disease.

Stage II or greater

In general, Stage II endometrioid carcinoma, regardless of grade, should be managed with surgery and chemotherapy with some exceptions. Once again, concern that concurrent or subsequent neoplasia might develop in previously benign endometriotic implants might prompt the clinician to avoid postoperative hormone replacement therapy or to make certain that replacement therapy includes a progestin.

Stage IA endometrioid adenocarcinoma with coexisting concurrent endometrial cancer can be managed without regard to the endometrial cancer in view of the excellent prognosis reported in the literature. Thus, most can avoid chemotherapy. Conceivably, women with Stage II grade 1 endometrioid ovarian carcinomas – with or without a coexisting endometrial tumor – could avoid chemotherapy, providing there was convincing evidence of two discrete ovarian primary tumors. In such instances, the size and extent of the ovarian tumors would influence the decision.[40]

Mucinous neoplasia

BORDERLINE TUMORS

The most common borderline mucinous tumors are of the intestinal type, of which over 90% are unilateral. Bilateral tumors of intestinal type must be carefully studied with attention to excluding metastatic disease. The Müllerian mucinous tumors are bilateral in approximately 40% of cases (owing to their frequent origins in endometriosis). These tumors are managed by either total abdominal hysterectomy and bilateral salpingo-oophorectomy or, in younger women, unilateral salpingo-oophorectomy, and from 10 to 20% recur on the opposite ovary.[41]

MUCINOUS CARCINOMAS

Stage I grade 1 non-invasive carcinomas (intraepithelial carcinomas)

These tumors are routinely managed by total abdominal hysterectomy and bilateral salpingo-cophorectomy or unilateral oophorectomy. The recurrence rates are less than 5%.[32,33]

Stage I grade 1 invasive tumors

These are managed similar to endometrioid adenocarcinomas. However, in contrast to the latter, mucinous carcinomas of the intestinal type are bilateral in less than 5%. When faced with a mucinous carcinoma, the surgeon should pay close attention to grade when considering conservative management.

Stage I grade 2 invasive tumors

The management of these tumors, like endometrioid adenocarcinomas of similar grade, is problematic and will be determined by the patient's age and desire to preserve fertility.

Stage I grade 3 and Stage II tumors

Stage I grade 3 and Stage II tumors are managed in the same fashion as other epithelial tumors.

Primary peritoneal carcinomas

Primary peritoneal cancer is managed as any advanced ovarian cancer with surgical exploration, cytoreductive surgery and cytotoxic chemotherapy. From the perspective of therapy, we know of no specific features that distinguish these tumors from advanced-stage ovarian serous tumors.

Extraovarian endometrioid carcinoma

Extraovarian endometrioid carcinoma arising in implants of endometriosis is managed like any advanced ovarian cancer medically and surgically. Special attention to resection of other implants and avoidance of estrogen postoperatively are reasonable, but are based on little data. In one study, median survival was 35 months and was dependent on stage and gravidity.[36]

Postsurgical management

Following surgery, CIS-platinum and taxane combination therapy for six cycles is required followed by tumor markers, physical and radiographic follow up every 3 months for 5 years. For patients who are a poor surgical risk, three cycles of chemotherapy precede surgery.

Second-look surgery at completion of primary therapy is not the standard approach unless the patient is enrolled in a research trial. There is no difference in overall survival in women managed with or without second look.[42]

Second-line therapy for recurrent ovarian cancer depends on the disease-free interval (DFI). If the patient is less than 1 year out of primary therapy, the reintroduction of platinum often fails. There is also no good surgical option with a short DFI. Second-line therapy should be conducted with Doxil, Gemzar, etc, or an experimental protocol. If the DFI is greater than 1 year, the reintroduction of platinum-based chemotherapy may re-induce short-term remission, but not cure. Surgery for secondary cytoreduction is best used in selected cases: long DFI or isolated recurrences amenable to surgical extirpation. Overall impact on survival is minimal, but has some impact on the DFI. Investigational protocols are suggested.

Lingering controversies

As discussed above, the more common dilemmas involve whether to spare the uterus and contralateral ovary for fertility purposes and whether or not to institute adjunctive chemotherapy. Additional controversies include the following:

1 In an asymptomatic patient with a rising CA 125, when does the oncologist begin second-line therapy? Many will treat a rising CA 125; others will wait until the patient is symptomatic and treat at that time.

2 Who should be treated with neoadjuvant chemotherapy? What criteria should we use to select patients who should get chemotherapy before attempted cytoreduction?

3 Just how aggressive should one be in attempting to reduce a patient to minimal residual disease? Does removing bowel, ureter, spleen and diaphragm help?

These questions relate to a fundamental issue in the management of ovarian cancer, which is the impact of chemotherapy on outcome. Survival is highly dependent upon stage, grade and the degree to which the tumor can be cytoreduced. The latter property is likely an index of tumor aggressiveness, degree of advancement, or both. For a woman diagnosed today with a poorly differentiated Stage IIIC ovarian cancer, median survival is 30 months, with 5-year survival around 20%. These numbers improve for the subset of women with adequate (<1 cm) residual tumor but are lower with clear cell carcinomas. The addition of Taxol to a platinum-containing regimen has added meaningfully to the DFI and perhaps to overall survival, but comes at the cost of increased toxicity, specifically neurotoxicity. For Stage II cancers, there is marked improvement, with 5-year survivals around 60–74%. Stage IV disease survival is only around 10%. Stage I patients, depending upon histology and grade, can experience a 75–90% 5-year survival. It is important to note that with the increasing use of long-term low-dose chemotherapy, 5-year survival numbers may improve because patients are alive with the disease under treatment. Traditionally, if the patient was alive at 5 years, she was more likely to be disease free. Now, with the current paradigm of managing cancer as a chronic disease state, many patients alive at 5 years are not cured, but continue to live with smoldering disease.

References

1 Cannistra SA. Cancer of the ovary. N Engl J Med 1993; 329:1550–1559.
2 Camatte S, Morice P, Atallah D, et al. Clinical outcome after laparoscopic pure management of borderline ovarian tumors: results of a series of 34 patients. Ann Oncol 2004; 15:605–609.
3 Maneo A, Vignali M, Chiari S, et al. Are borderline tumors of the ovary safely treated by laparoscopy? Gynecol Oncol 2004; 94:387–392.
4 Pettersson F (ed.) Annual report on the results of treatment in gynecologic cancer, Vol. 22. Stockholm: International Federation of Gynecology and Obstetrics; 1991.
5 Seidman JD, Russell P, Kurman RJ. Surface epithelial tumors of the ovary. In: Kurman RJ, ed. Blaustein's pathology of the female genital tract. New York: Springer; 2001:810–863.
6 Aure JC, Hoeg K, Kolstad P. Clinical and histologic studies of ovarian carcinoma. Long-term follow-up of 990 cases. Obstet Gynecol 1971; 37:1–9.
7 Scully RE, Young RH, Clement PB. Atlas of tumor pathology, 3rd series: Tumors of the ovary, maldeveloped gonads, fallopian tube and broad ligament. Washington, DC: AFIP; 1998.
8 Griffiths CT, Parker LM, Lee S, Finkler NJ. The effect of residual mass size on response to chemotherapy after surgical cytoreduction for advanced ovarian cancer: long-term results. Int J Gynecol Cancer 2002; 12:323–331.
9 Gershenson DM. Clinical management potential tumors of low malignancy. Best Pract Res Clin Obstet Gynecol 2002; 16:513–527.
10 Sutton GP, Bundy BN, Omura GA, et al. Stage III ovarian tumors of low malignant potential treated with cisplatin combination therapy: a Gynecologic Oncology Group study. Gynecol Oncol 1991; 41:230–233.
11 Lackman F, Carey MS, Kirk ME, McLachlin CM, Elit L. Surgery as sole treatment for serous borderline tumours of the ovary with noninvasive implants. Gynecol Oncol 2003; 90:407–412.
12 Morice P, Cammatte S, Wicart-Poque F, et al. Results of conservative management of epithelial malignant and borderline ovarian tumours. Hum Reprod Update 2003; 9:185–192.
13 Creasman WT, Park R, Norris H, et al. Stage I borderline ovarian tumors. Obstet Gynecol 1982; 59:93–96.
14 Barnhill DR, Kurman RJ, Brady MF et al. Preliminary analysis of the behavior of stage I ovarian serous tumors of low malignant potential: a Gynecologic Oncology Group study. J Clin Oncol 1995; 13:2752–2756.
15 Young RC, Walton LA, Ellenberg SS, et al. Adjuvant therapy in stage I and stage II epithelial ovarian cancer: results of two prospective randomized trials. N Engl J Med 1990; 322:1021–1027.
16 Zanetta G, Rota S, Chiari S, et al. Behavior of borderline tumors with particular interest to persistence, recurrence, and progression to invasive carcinoma: a prospective study. J Clin Oncol 2001; 19:2658–2664.
17 Gilks CB, Alkushi A, Yue JJ, et al. Advanced-stage serous borderline tumors of the ovary: a clinicopathological study of 49 cases. Int J Gynecol Pathol 2003; 22:29–36.
18 Trope C, Kaern J, Vergote IB, Kristensen G, Abeler V. Are borderline tumors of the ovary over-treated both surgically and systemically? A review of four prospective randomized trials including 253 patients with borderline tumors. Gynecol Oncol 1993; 51:236–243.

19 Tavassoli FA. Serous tumors of low malignant potential with early stromal invasion (serous LMP with microinvasion). Mod Pathol 1988; 1:407–414.

20 Bell DA, Scully RE. Ovarian serous tumors with stromal microinvasion: a report of 21 cases. Hum Pathol 1990; 21:397–403.

21 Eichorn JH, Bell DA, Young RH, et al. Ovarian serous borderline tumors with micropapillary and cribriform patterns: a study of 40 cases and comparison with 44 cases without these patterns. Am J Surg Pathol 1999; 23:397–409.

22 Prat J, De Nictolis M. Serous borderline tumors of the ovary: a long-term follow-up study of 137 cases, including 18 with a micropapillary pattern and 20 with microinvasion. Am J Surg Pathol 2002; 26:1111–1128.

23 Smith Sehdev AE, Sehdev PS, Kurman RJ. Noninvasive and invasive micropapillary (low grade) serous carcinomas of the ovary: a clinicopathologic analysis of 135 cases. Am J Surg Pathol 2003; 27:725–736.

24 Slomovitz BM, Caputo TA, Gretz HF 3rd, et al. A comparative analysis of 57 serous borderline tumors with and without a noninvasive micropapillary component. Am J Surg Pathol 2002; 26:592–600.

25 Deavers MT, Gershenson DM, Tortolero-Luna G, et al. Micropapillary and cribriform patterns in ovarian serous tumors of low malignant potential: a study of 99 advanced stage cases. Am J Surg Pathol 2002; 26:1129–1141.

26 Bell DA, Weinstock MA, Scully RE. Peritoneal implants of ovarian serous borderline tumors: histologic features and prognosis. Cancer 1988; 62; 2212–2222.

27 Seidman JD, Kurman RJ. Ovarian serous borderline tumors: a critical review of the literature and emphasis on prognostic indicators. Hum Pathol 2000; 31:539–557.

28 Gershenson DM, Silva EG, Levy L, et al. Serous borderline tumors with invasive implants. Cancer 1988; 82:1096–1103.

29 De Nictolis M, Montironi R, Tommasoni S, et al. Serous borderline tumors of the ovary: a clinicopathologic, immunohistochemical and quantitative study of 44 cases. Cancer 1994; 70:152–160.

30 McCaughey WTE, Kirk ME, Lester W, et al. Peritoneal epithelial lesions associated with proliferative serous tumors of the ovary. Histopathology 1984; 8:195–208.

31 Russell P, Merkur H. Proliferating ovarian 'epithelial' tumors: a clinico-pathologic analysis of 144 cases. Aust N Z J Obstet Gynecol 1979; 19:45–51.

32 Hart WR, Norris HJ. Borderline and malignant mucinous tumors of the ovary: histologic criteria and clinical behavior. Cancer 1973; 31:1031–1045.

33 Lee KR, Scully RE. Mucinous tumors of the ovary: a clinicopathologic study of 196 borderline tumors (of intestinal type) and carcinomas, including an evaluation of 11 cases of 'pseudomyxoma peritonei'. Am J Surg Pathol 2000; 24:1447–1464.

34 Bell KA, Kurman RJ. A clinicopathologic analysis of atypical proliferative (borderline) tumors and well-differentiated endometrioid adenocarcinomas of the ovary. Am J Surg Pathol 2000; 24:1465–1479.

35 Sainz de la Cuesta R, Eichhorn JH, Rice LW, et al. Histologic transformation of benign endometriosis to early epithelial ovarian cancer. Gynecol Oncol 1996; 60:238–244.

36 Modesitt SC, Tortolero-Luna G, Robinson JB, Gershenson DM, Wolf JK. Ovarian and extraovarian endometriosis-associated cancer. Obstet Gynecol 2002; 100:788–795.

37 Steed H, Chapman W, Laframboise S. Endometriosis-associated ovarian cancer: a clinicopathologic review. J Obstet Gynaecol Can 2004; 26:709–715.

38 Bell DA, Scully RE. Early de novo ovarian carcinoma. A study of fourteen cases. Cancer 1994; 73:1859–1864.

39 Guthrie D, Davy ML, Philips PR. A study of 656 patients with 'early' ovarian cancer. Gynecol Oncol 1984; 17:363–369.

40 Soliman PT, Slomovitz BM, Broaddus RR, et al. Synchronous primary cancers of the endometrium and ovary: a single institution review of 84 cases. Gynecol Oncol 2004; 94:456–462.

41 Rutgers JL, Scully RE. Ovarian Müllerian mucinous papillary cystadenomas of borderline malignancy. A clinicopathologic analysis. Cancer 1988; 61(2):340–348.

42 Friedman JB, Weiss NS. Second thoughts about second-look laparotomy in advanced ovarian cancer. N Engl J Med 1990; 322(15):1079–1082.

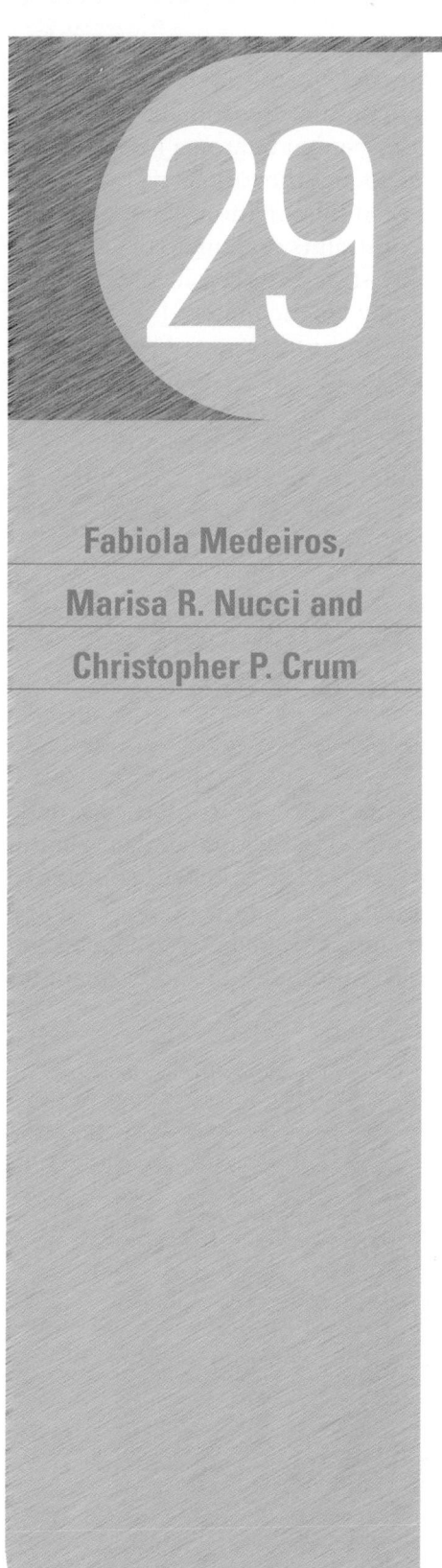

29

Germ cell tumors of the ovary

Fabiola Medeiros,

Marisa R. Nucci and

Christopher P. Crum

Introduction and pathogenesis

Common germ cell tumors encountered in practice

Epidermoid cyst
Benign (mature) cystic teratoma

Monodermal and malignant variants of (mature) cystic teratoma

The patient at risk
Variants
Tumors containing thyroid tissue

Carcinoid tumors
Other malignancies arising
   in teratomas

Rare germ cell tumors with embryonal, extra-embryonal and fetal differentiation

Pathogenesis, classification and
   the patient at risk
Tumor types

Introduction and pathogenesis

Germ cell tumors of the ovary are presumed to derive from the pathogenetic transformation of ovarian germ cells. The tumors that develop from these transformed germ cells are among the most unique in the human body, for the simple reason that they recreate, however imperfectly, aspects of human development. Germ cell neoplasms can be subdivided into three general categories. The first is immature germ cell tumors, which depict a range of differentiation, including immature germ cells (dysgerminoma), early embryonic development (embryonal carcinoma, polyembryoma), extra-embryonic differentiation (choriocarcinoma, yolk sac tumor) and immature somatic tissues (immature teratoma). The second and by far the most common is the mature germ cell tumor, typically a benign cystic teratoma, composed of a wide range of somatic tissues, from simple dermoid cysts to tumors with human form (homunculus). The third is benign cystic teratoma giving rise to a malignant neoplasm, such as squamous carcinoma, carcinoid, malignant struma ovarii (thyroid carcinoma) and other rare neoplasms. The first group predominates in young women under age 20, the second is the most common ovarian tumor in reproductive-age women and the last group is more common in postmenopausal women.

The first group – immature germ cell tumors – is exceedingly rare; the third group – malignancies arising in benign cystic teratomas – is likewise uncommon, occurring in approximately 1% of these tumors.

In the most common practice scenario, the pathologist identifies and samples a benign teratoma for histologic examination, then catalogues the various types of tissue present. The range of differentiation encountered is limited only by the constraints on human tissue differentiation; virtually any structure seen in the developing or adult human may be encountered. While navigating this potentially confusing array of patterns, the pathologist has three tasks. The first is to develop a familiarity with these patterns. The second is to recognize immature (fetal or embryonal) differentiation. The third is to identify malignancies arising in adult tissues. The following discussion will address these tasks in the diagnosis of germ cell neoplasia.

Common germ cell tumors encountered in practice

EPIDERMOID CYST

Epidermoid cysts of the ovary are composed strictly of squamous epithelium, often with abundant keratin debris with variable giant cell reaction. In contrast to benign cystic teratomas, these tumors do not exhibit a Rokitansky's tubercle and are devoid of skin appendages (Fig. 29.1). Theories of origins include squamous

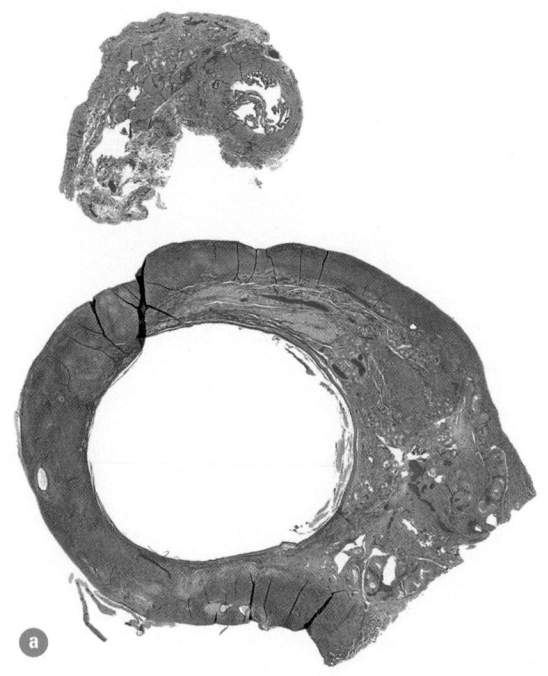

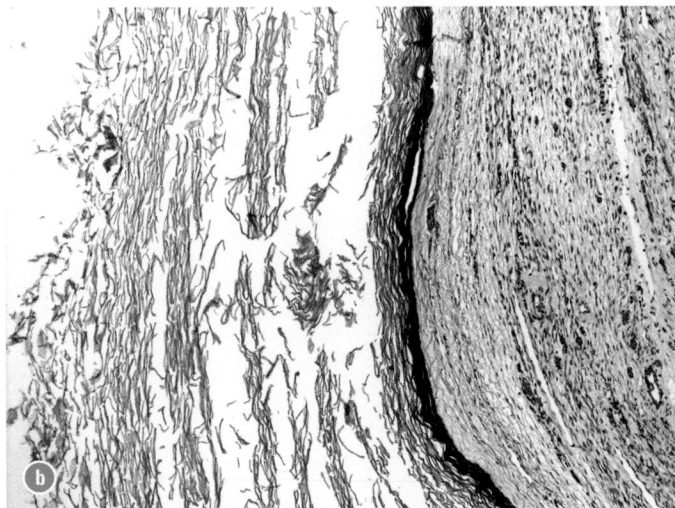

Fig. 29.1 Epidermoid cyst of the ovary. (a) Scanning photomicrograph shows a single unilocular cyst. (b) The squamous epithelium lining the cyst is devoid of skin appendages or other elements.

metaplasia within a mesothelial or Müllerian cyst, and a monodermal teratoma. Similar lesions have been reported in the testis of presumed teratomatous origin.[1–3] We have encountered one case of epidermoid cyst with a contralateral cystic teratoma, supporting a teratomatous origin. However, the capacity of the Müllerian or mesothelium tissue for squamous differentiation is well established and may account for others.

BENIGN (MATURE) CYSTIC TERATOMA

The patient at risk

Benign cystic teratoma is the most common benign tumor in reproductive-age women and the most commonly encountered during pregnancy.[4] Despite the fact that malignant germ cell tumors are most commonly encountered before age 20, benign cystic teratoma is still the more common of the two diagnosed in this age group. De Silva et al. found that in children with ovarian masses, benign cystic teratoma was still five times more likely to be diagnosed than a germ cell malignancy.[5]

Presenting signs and symptoms

Benign cystic teratomas predominate in the reproductive years, with the majority presenting under age 40 and a mean age in the mid-30s. Approximately two-thirds are asymptomatic at the time of discovery and 13% presented with an acute abdomen in one study.[6] The precise proportion with symptoms may be difficult to assess inasmuch as many may be discovered at the time of Cesarean section. Nearly two-thirds contain calcium on X-ray.[7]

Intraoperative evaluation and gross pathology

Approximately 15% of benign cystic teratomas are bilateral. Moreover, the contralateral ovary in cases of other germ cell tumors will contain a benign cystic teratoma at a similar frequency. The gross picture can be classic or extremely variable. The most common (classic) appearance of a cystic teratoma is that of a smooth cyst containing a mixture of hair and oily brown to tan sebaceous material (Fig. 29.2). A raised protuberance (Rokitansky's tubercle) containing adipose tissue and overlying skin is often present (Fig. 29.3). However, the cyst contents may appear hemorrhagic, similar to an endometriotic cyst; alternatively, the tumor may be multicystic. As a rule, the more complex the lesion, the more likely other elements will be detected. For example, thyroid tissue will appear characteristically solid and brown (Fig. 29.4). Teeth

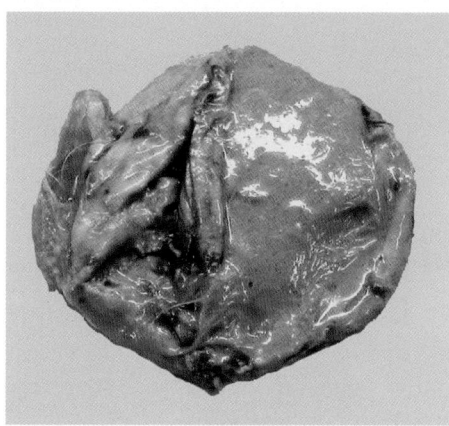

Fig. 29.2 Benign cystic teratoma with scant hair and a viscid oily material content.

are present in a minority but are dramatic (Fig. 29.5). A rare variant of teratoma of which fewer than 200 have been reported in the world literature exhibits a human-like appearance on gross examination, with a rudimentary head, hair and appendages (Fig. 29.6). These tumors may initially be mistaken for ovarian pregnancies, but are recognized by the absence of umbilical cord and normal extremities. Another extremely rare entity that may be confused with fetiform teratoma is *fetus in fetu*, wherein a left-over twin of the patient has been ensconced in the pelvic cavity for years.[8] Because these are not typically in the ovary, they should be easily distinguished, particularly with the presence of a normal human form.

The principal tasks for the pathologist in the frozen section or gross room are as follows:

1 Exclude immature teratoma. If the patient is over 30, the risk of immature teratoma is low.

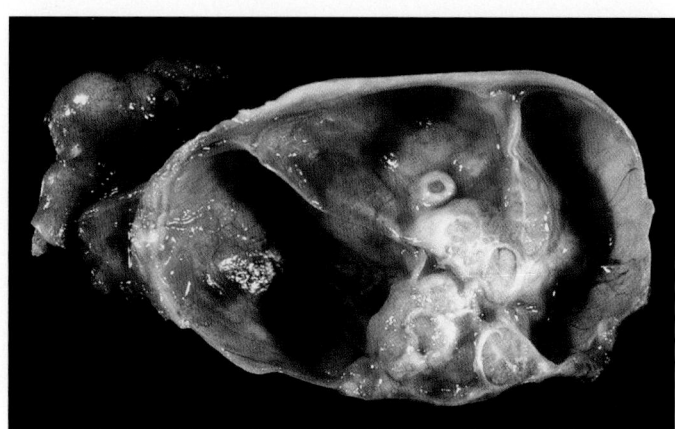

Fig. 29.3 Benign cystic teratoma. The cyst contains a condensed mass from which the skin and appendages arise (Rokitansky's tubercle).

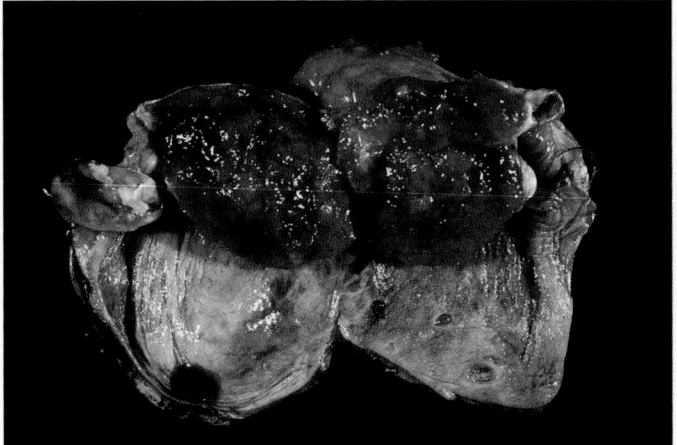

Fig. 29.4 Benign cystic teratoma containing thyroid tissue, seen here as a red-brown gelatinous mass.

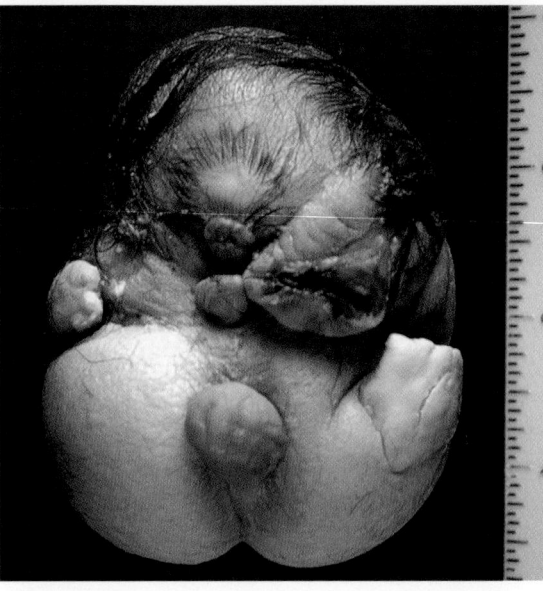

Fig. 29.6 Fetiform teratoma (homunculus). Note the tumor is more differentiated in its caudal aspects.

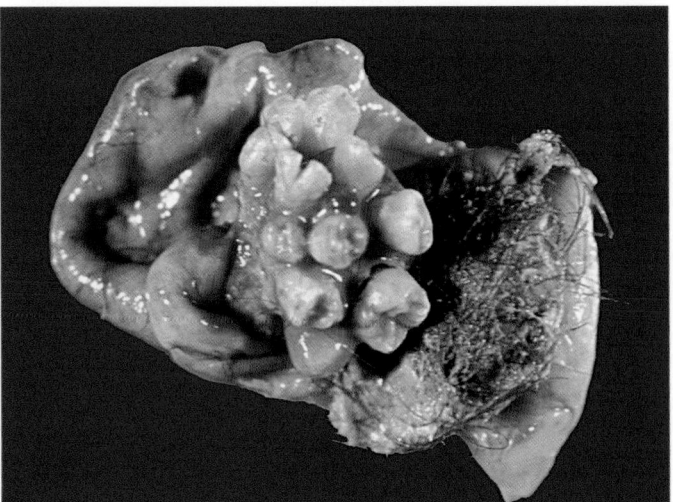

Fig. 29.5 Teeth and a portion of jaw in a benign cystic teratoma.

Less than 10% of immature teratomas occur above this age. Findings that support immature teratoma are greater percentage of solid tumor, particularly if it is not readily identified as skin, thyroid, or another mature element. The pathologist should exercise care in interpreting immature elements on frozen section. If an immature germ cell tumor is suspected, the surgeon should be advised to carefully stage the tumor. The risk of contralateral ovarian involvement is negligible, although a contralateral benign teratoma is present in up to 15% of cases.

2 Exclude a carcinoma arising in a mature cystic teratoma. A coexisting epithelial malignancy is more commonly encountered in postmenopausal women. The most common carcinomas arising in cystic teratomas are squamous carcinomas, carcinoids and thyroid carcinomas. These tumors will usually manifest as cystic masses with a fungating tumor or a solid nodule. Although frozen section is not required to verify a hair-filled cyst with a Rokitansky tubercle, suspicious masses or lesions should be evaluated by frozen section to ensure that further staging is not necessary.

Histopathology

In keeping with the wide variety of tissues that may be seen grossly, an even wider range of differentiation can be appreciated on histologic examination of cystic teratomas. Figures 29.7 and 29.8 depict these; the most common include skin, skin appendages, adipose tissue, respiratory epithelium, cerebral cortex (including ventricles and chorioid plexus), cerebellum, peripheral nerve, bone and cartilage. The principal task of the pathologist is to catalogue these patterns of differentiation, learn to recognize the diverse appearances and exclude both malignancy and immaturity, either of which can place the patient at risk for recurrence.

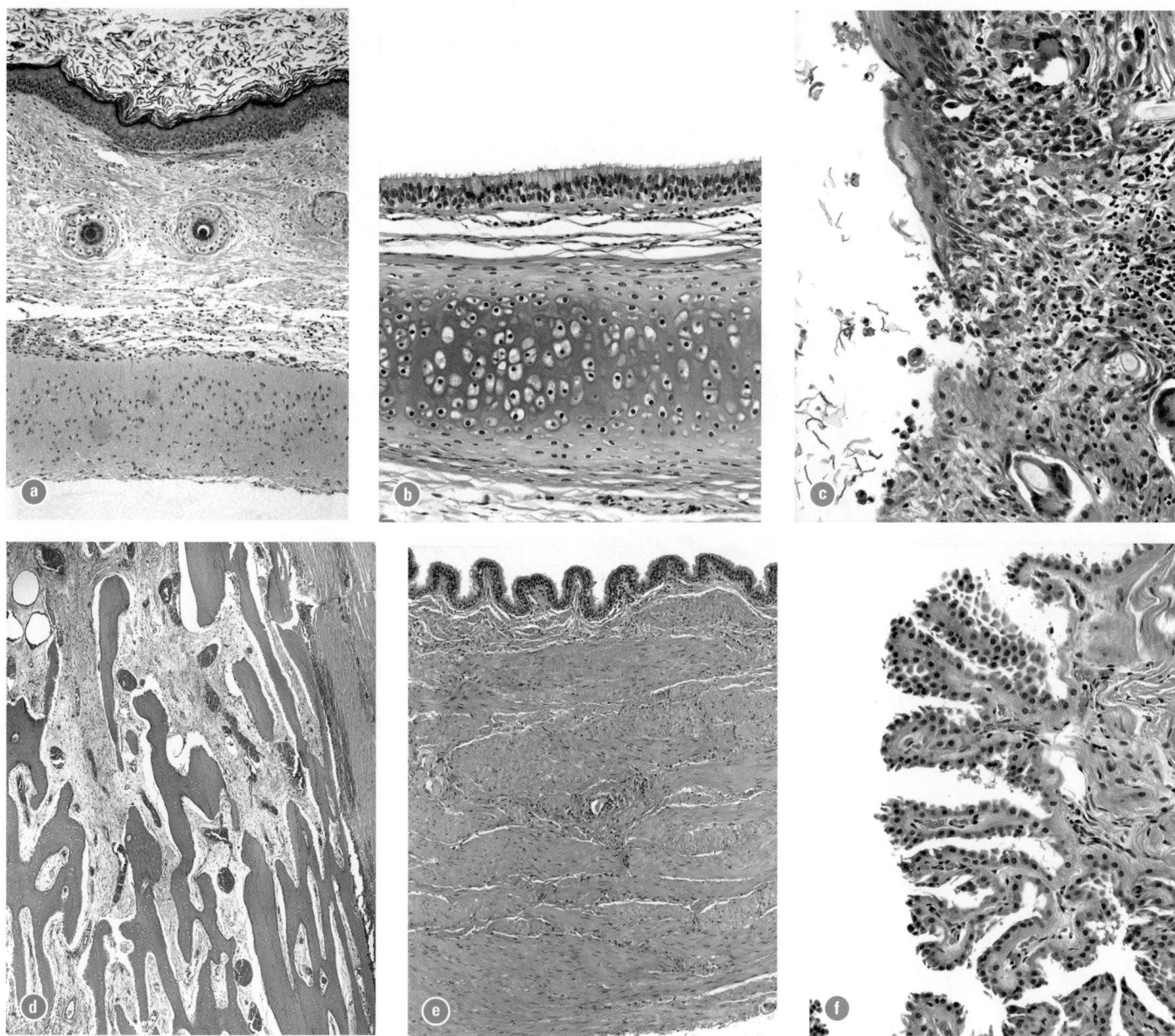

Fig. 29.7 Components of benign cystic teratoma: (a) skin (above) and cerebral cortex (below), (b) respiratory epithelium and underlying cartilage, (c) giant cell reaction to keratin, (d) bone, (e) columnar epithelium over smooth muscle (viscus) and (f) choroid plexus.

Management and outcome

Management of benign cystic teratoma is influenced by the risk of malignancy – a function of the age of the patient – and the desire to minimize surgical trauma. Typically, cystectomy is performed to preserve ovarian function; however, follow-up is necessary to exclude recurrence. Because the latter is typically asymptomatic, a periodic ultrasound examination is recommended. Laparoscopy is acceptable provided strict guidelines are followed that pertain to any ovarian mass. For younger patients, preoperative serologic studies to exclude a malignant germ cell tumor are indicated and every patient must be aware of the small risk of malignancy, which would necessitate a second surgical procedure.[7]

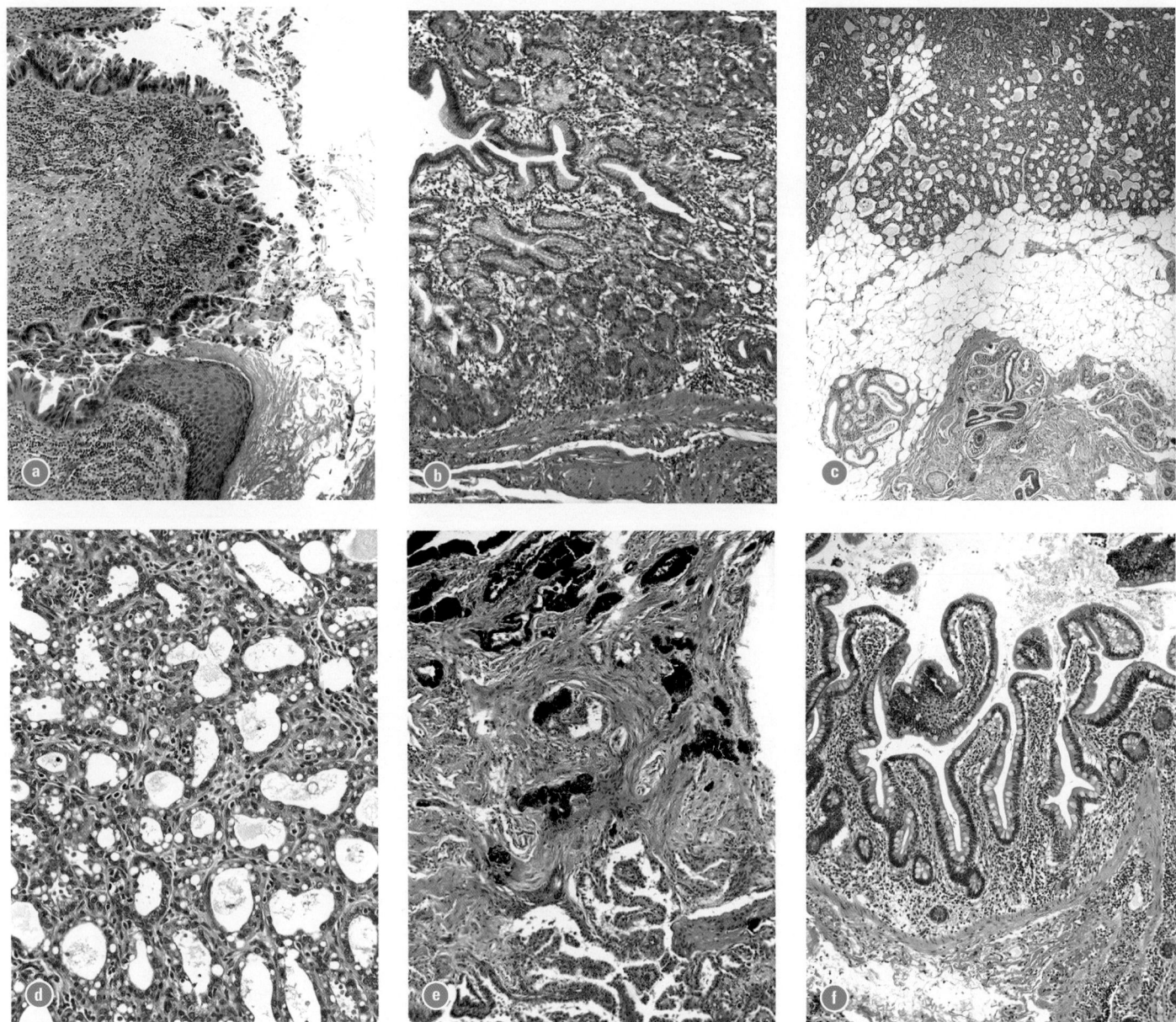

Fig. 29.8 Components of benign cystic teratoma. (a) Gastroesophageal junction (Barrett's-like). (b) Gastric mucosa. (c) Salivary gland. (d) Higher power of (c). (e) Choroid plexus (lower) with pigmented choroids (upper). (f) Small intestine.

Monodermal and malignant variants of (mature) cystic teratoma

THE PATIENT AT RISK

Malignancy is rare in a cystic teratoma and occurs in approximately 1% of tumors. Over 90% are epithelial and of these 80–90% are squamous carcinomas.[9]

VARIANTS

Squamous carcinoma

Squamous carcinoma is the most common form of malignant transformation in cystic teratomas, comprising approximately 80% of cases with an epithelial malignancy (Fig. 29.9). They can occur at any age but the mean age is approximately 20 years older than benign cystic teratoma, with most cases occurring in the sixth decade.[10–13]

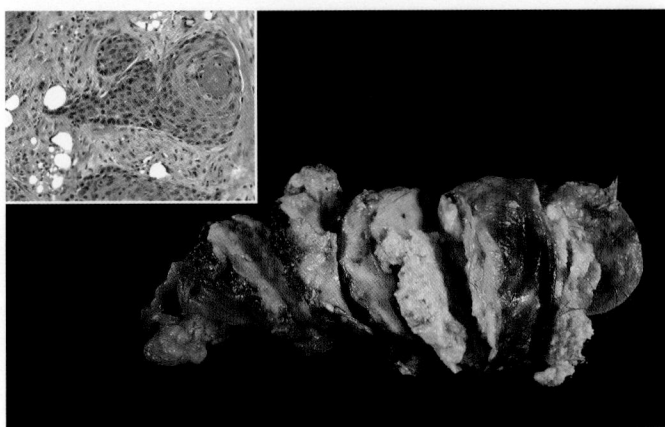

Fig. 29.9 Squamous carcinoma in a teratoma. Hair is present on the left. The remainder of the mass is composed of keratin debris and fibrosis, with focal squamous carcinoma (inset).

TUMORS CONTAINING THYROID TISSUE

Excluding those with focal thyroid differentiation, tumors of the ovary containing thyroid tissue fall into three categories.

Struma ovarii

Struma ovarii are monodermal ovarian teratomas predominately composed of thyroid tissue that occur most frequently in the fifth decade. Approximately one-fifth of cystic teratomas contain microscopic thyroid tissue; about 5% are composed primarily or entirely of thyroid. Like all specialized patterns of differentiation, these tumors are unilateral; however, like all teratomas, the frequency of a contralateral cystic teratoma is approximately 10–15%.

Unlike classic cystic teratoma, struma ovarii may not be diagnosed preoperatively, inasmuch as the ultrasound appearance is not as specific, appearing as a hetero-geneous solid mass.[14] Clinicians are advised to proceed cautiously if a suspected teratoma contains a complex ultrasonographic picture, as a benign struma may be the cause.[15] Clinical evidence of hyperthyroidism occurs in less than 5% of cases;[16] rarely pseudo-Meigs' syndrome,[17] and hyperemesis gravidarum (in pregnancy).[18]

On gross examination, the thyroid component has the characteristic appearance of normal thyroid, present-ing as a greenish-brown, firm to slightly gelatinous tissue, either solid or mixed with cystic and fibrous areas; it may be subtle if focal but classic if comprising the bulk of the tumor. The histologic appearance varies from a classic arrangement of prominent macro- and microfollicles with abundant colloid to a fibrotic cyst with inconspicuous small tubules (Figs 29.10, 29.11).

Solid patterns lacking colloid with oxyphilic or clear cells also may be present.[19] The solid patterns include trabeculae that may be confused with (or merge with) carcinoid (see below). Struma may also coexist with both benign and malignant tumors, including Brenner tumor and mucinous cystadenomas.[20,21]

The differential diagnosis of struma ovarii includes sex cord-stromal neoplasms, carcinoid and epithelial tumors, particularly if the follicles are inconspicuous and the epithelial cells are arranged in tubules or cell cords. The key to diagnosis is an index of suspicion, particularly if other components of teratoma are present. Immunostaining for thyroglobulin is diagnostic.[22]

Removal of the tumor is followed by cure, with the exception of rare instances when small foci of struma persist on the peritoneal surface in the form of *strumosis*. Strumosis presumably develops when the thyroid tissue gains access to the peritoneal surface via rupture (Fig. 29.12). The process can persist for years but is self-limited and considered benign.[23]

Strumal carcinoid

Strumal carcinoid is defined simply as the coexistence of struma ovarii and a carcinoid tumor. The latter is always a trabecular carcinoid and, in 60% of cases, there is a coexisting benign cystic teratoma and, like other teratomas, a contralateral cystic teratoma is present in about 10%. A small percentage (less than 10%) display evidence of increased thyroid hormone production; none were associated with the carcinoid syndrome in one study.[24]

Grossly, strumal carcinoids usually associate with a mature teratoma and may exhibit both the solid white-to-yellow appearance of carcinoid and brown areas signifying thyroid differentiation. Histologically, the trabeculae of the carcinoid often merge abruptly with the thyroid follicles, but in many cases, the two elements are not readily distinguished by hematoxylin and eosin staining. More subtle transitions, in which small colloid-producing lumina emerge within the trabeculae are common (Figs 29.13, 29.14). Ultrastructural studies and immunostaining for thyroid transcription factor-1 (TTF-1) have sharply distinguished the thyroid from carcinoid components.[25,26] Other studies have identified cells with both thyroid and neuroendocrine charac-teristics considered to be cells with capacity for bidirec-tional differentiation.[27,28] Immunohistochemical stains will identify thyroglobulin and chromogranin within the same foci if not the same cells. Areas of trabecular morphology that are devoid of either also raise questions about differentiation patterns that exclude both thyroid and neuroendocrine differentiation.

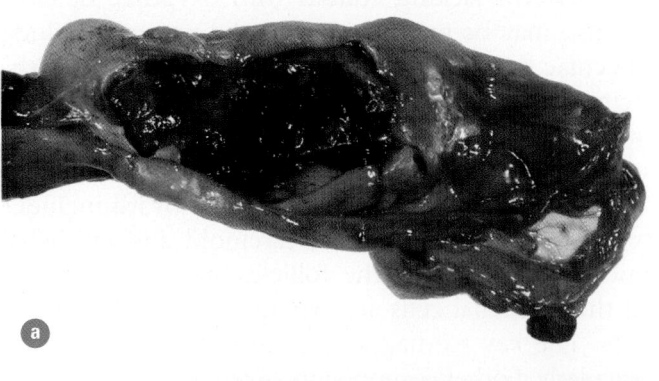

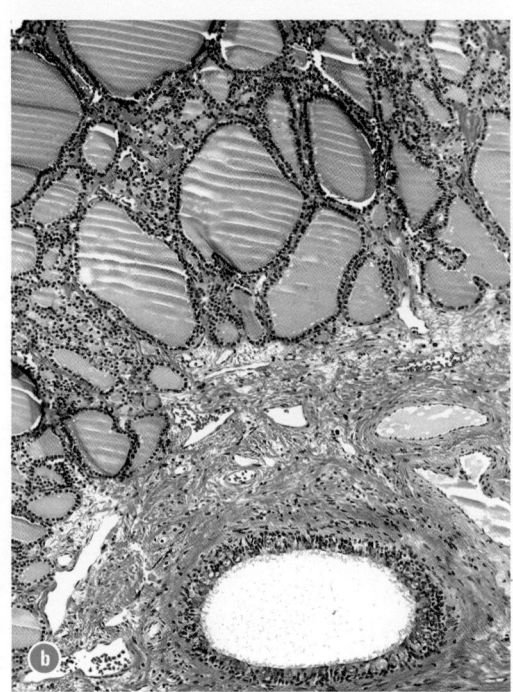

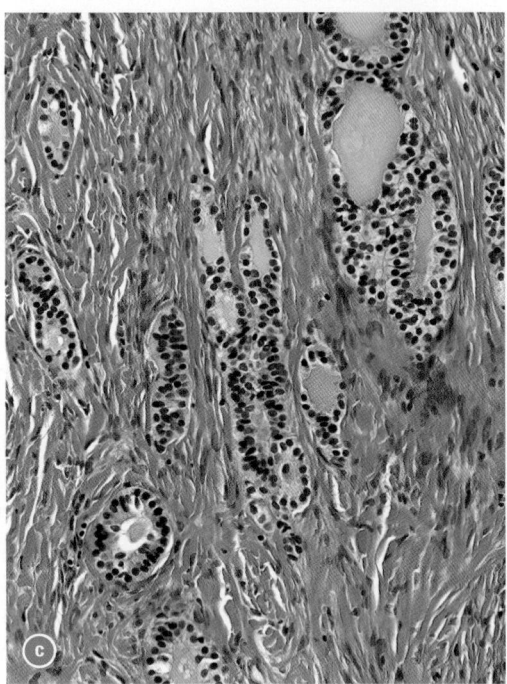

Fig. 29.10 Struma ovarii. (a) Classic appearance of thyroid tissue in a cyst. (b) Struma, with variably sized follicles and cords. (c) Immunostaining for thyroglobulin.

Strumal carcinoids are universally benign, with rare exceptions, and a minority are associated with increased thyroid production.[28,29]

Malignant struma (thyroid carcinoma)

Malignant struma (thyroid carcinoma) in the ovary is rare and can be seen in struma ovarii or in strumal carcinoid tumors, where thyroid tissue is usually present. In strumal carcinoid tumors there is thyroid tissue and carcinoid intimately admixed, and other teratomatous elements may be present.

Less than 10% of strumas have been considered malignant; however, a small number of these tumors have spread beyond the ovary. Most malignant struma ovarii have the histopathologic features of papillary thyroid carcinoma (PTC). The nuclear features of PTC are the only criteria to establish the diagnosis of malignancy in struma ovarii: nuclear crowding, nuclear clearing ('Orphan Annie eyes'), nuclear grooves, nuclear membrane irregularities and nuclear pseudo inclusions. The subtypes of thyroid carcinoma usually identified are classical variant with prominent papillae, and follicular variant of PTC. The diagnosis of follicular carcinoma in struma ovarii cannot be established, since struma ovarii generally lacks a capsule and no other criteria for malignancy is determined. Some recurrent tumors can be a poorly-differentiated thyroid carcinoma, and immunostains may be necessary to confirm the diagnosis (Figs 29.15–29.17).

The presence of thyroglobulin and TTF-1 within less-differentiated tumors establishes the diagnosis of

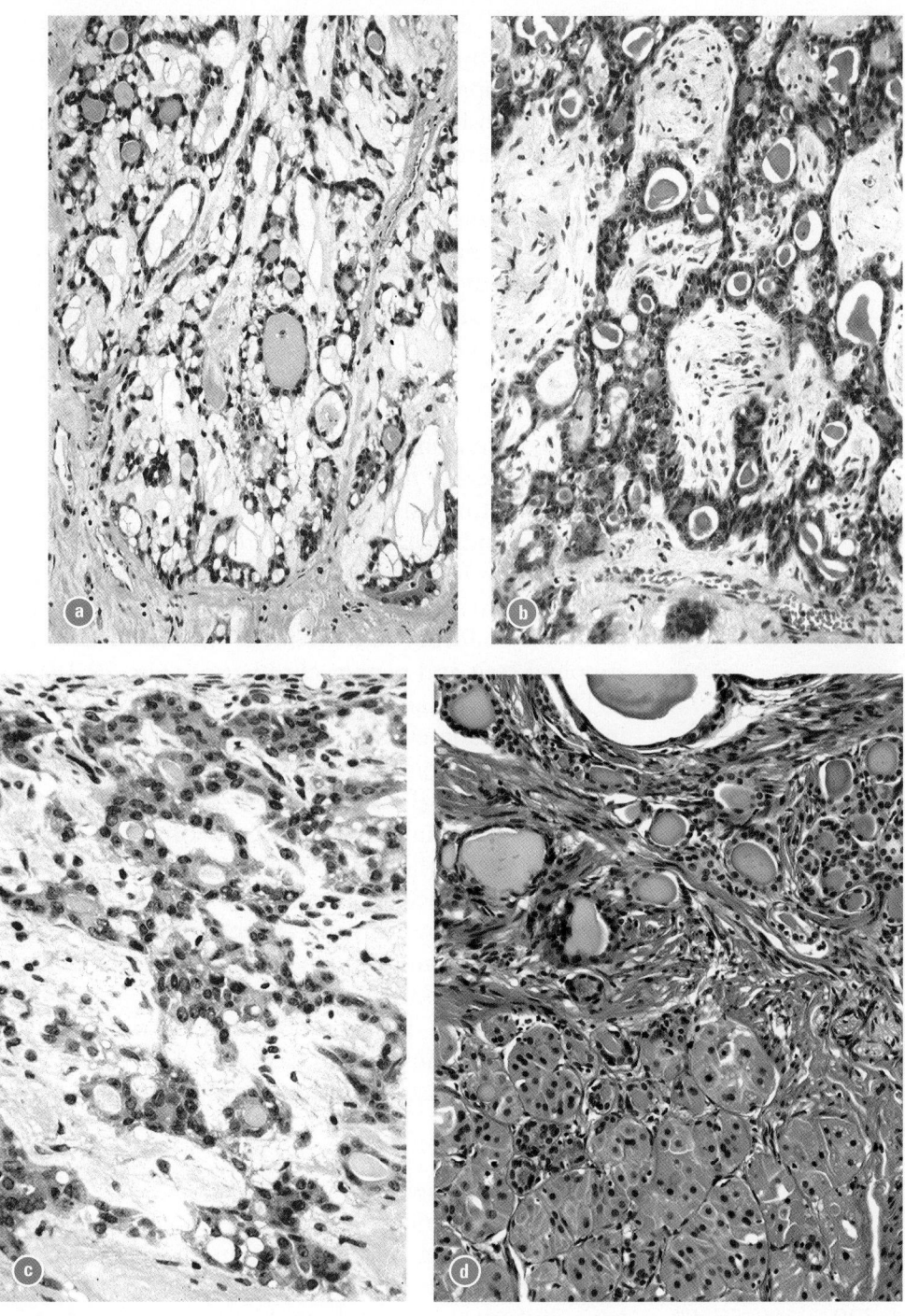

Fig. 29.11 Variants of struma. (a–c) Variable lumen formation, including interconnecting cords of epithelium. (d) Hürthle cells in struma.

a thyroid follicular origin. HBME1 and Galectin-3 immunostains may be useful in differentiating benign thyroid proliferations from papillary thyroid carcinoma within a struma ovarii or strumal carcinoid. Papillary thyroid carcinomas in struma ovarii can be associated with RET, RAS and BRAF mutations, similar to those observed in papillary thyroid carcinoma. Mutations in the RET/RAS/BRAF pathway are not found in benign struma ovarii.[30–35]

CARCINOID TUMORS

Carcinoid tumors are neuroendocrine neoplasms that arise in a minority of cystic teratomas. In approximately 80%, a concurrent teratoma can be identified. These tumors can be divided into five categories, four primary and one metastatic. The latter will be discussed briefly, and is also addressed in Chapter 31. Primary carcinoids fall into four categories, comprising insular, trabecular, strumal (see above) and goblet cell.

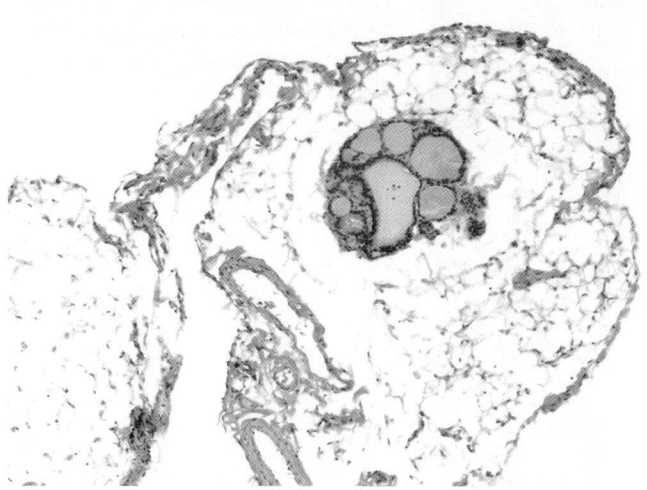

Fig. 29.12 Strumosis of the peritoneum years after removal of a struma ovarii.

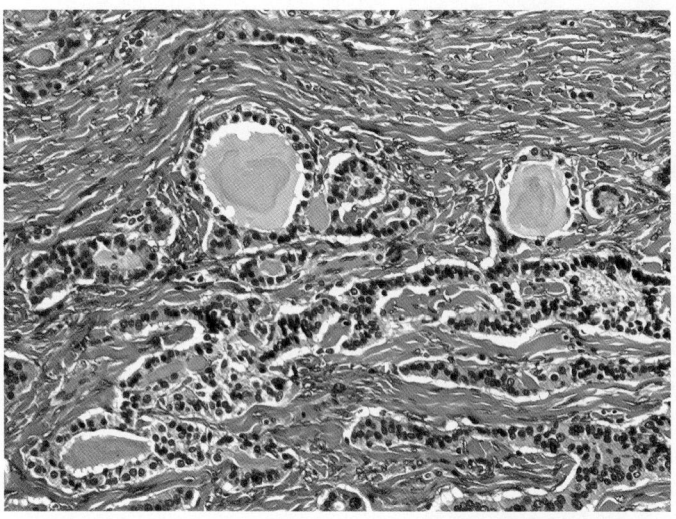

Fig. 29.13 Strumal carcinoid, seen here as a mixture of colloid-filled spaces and cords.

In a large study from Japan of 329 cases, 57.4% were associated with a cystic teratoma. Tumors unassociated with a teratoma were twice as large (9.0 cm) and were more likely to be associated with metastases (22.1 *vs* 5.8), hepatic involvement (15.0% *vs* 2.1%) and higher incidence of carcinoid syndrome (22.9 *vs* 13.8%). The 5-year survival rate for those unassociated and associated with a teratoma was 93.7% and 84.0%, respectively. Insular and trabecular carcinoids comprised 22% and 26% of tumors recorded; carcinoid syndrome occurred in 39% and 8% of these two types, respec-

tively.[36] Not all studies specify whether the tumors are primary or not. Those confined to the ovary have a survival approaching 100%. Those bilateral are presumed to be metastatic and studies with advanced (>Stage I) disease report a poor outcome.[37,38]

Insular carcinoids

Insular carcinoids are the most common pattern.[39,40] In one study of 48 tumors, one-third were associated with carcinoid syndrome, which was linked to tumor size. One-third was associated with a contralateral cystic teratoma or mucinous ovarian tumor. Two-thirds of tumors over 7 cm were associated with carcinoid syndrome.[39]

Histologically, insular carcinoids are characterized by two distinguishing features. The first is simple tubular glands arranged in garland-like patterns or small groups in a fibrous stroma, with sharply defined central lumina and, frequently, retraction artifact. The second is uniform rounded nuclei with fine chromatin stippling (salt and pepper chromatin) (Fig. 29.18).

The differential diagnosis of insular carcinoid includes endometrioid adenocarcinoma (Ch. 27), metastatic gastrointestinal carcinoma (Ch. 31) and sex-cord stromal tumor, either Sertoli cell or granulosa cell tumors (Ch. 30). Because of fixation artifacts, the pathologist may not always appreciate the stippled nuclear features of insular carcinoid (Fig. 29.19). However, the above can be excluded by appropriate immunohistochemical stains that confirm carcinoid (chromogranin) or sex cord-stromal tumors (inhibin). If the tumor is bilateral, associated with carcinoid syndrome, or unaccompanied by a cystic teratoma, a metastatic mid-gut carcinoid must always be considered.

Trabecular carcinoids

Trabecular carcinoids are similar in appearance to fore- and hind-gut carcinoids and display discrete linear cords and trabeculae (Fig. 29.20). Some reports have linked them to bronchial tissue in adjacent teratomas. None had carcinoid syndrome and only one died of the disease.[41-44]

The differential diagnosis of trabecular carcinoid includes strumal carcinoid (see above), struma ovarii, Sertoli cell tumor (Ch. 30) and epithelial or stromal tumors with prominent sex cord-like differentiation (Chs 19 and 27). A combination of chromogranin and thyroid staining will distinguish these patterns. The outcome of trabecular carcinoids is favorable, with no deaths reported in the larger studies.

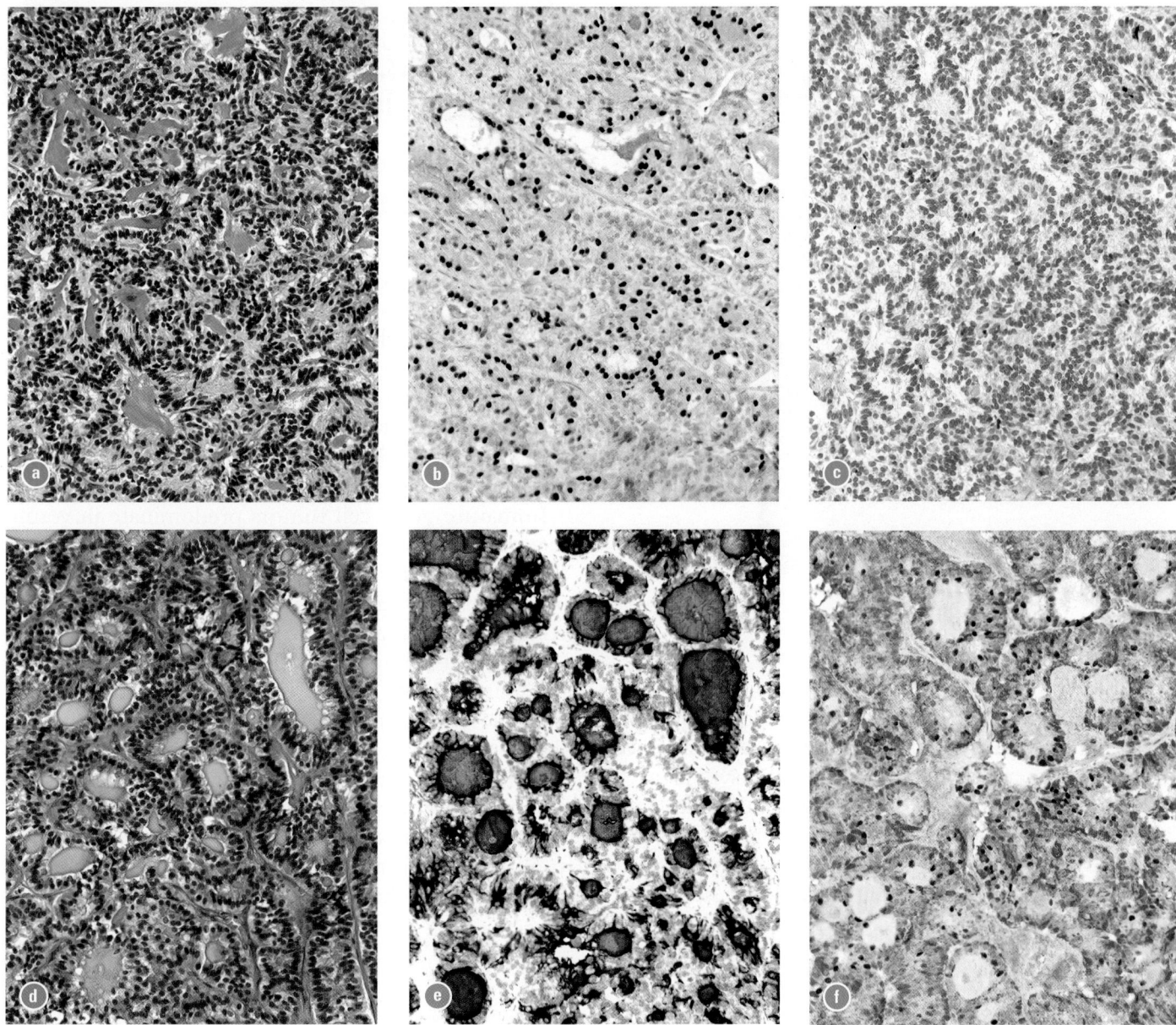

Fig. 29.14 Strumal carcinoid. Thyroid differentiation (a) following immunostaining for TTF-1 (b) and chromogranin (c). Mixed differentiation (d) following staining for thyroglobulin (e) and double staining for TTF-1 (nuclear) and chromogranin (cytoplasm) (f). This illustrates the immunophenotypic overlap in these tumors.

Goblet cell carcinoids

Goblet cell carcinoids are rare, with the largest study consisting of 17 cases.[45] These tumors coexist with a recognizable teratoma in less than one-third of cases and exhibit a range of differentiation, including relatively well-differentiated tumors with small glands lined by goblet or columnar cells in a mucinous background, atypical with crowded or confluent glands, including cribriform or microcystic patterns and frank carcinomas associated with the carcinoid. The diagnosis is based on the coexistence of both neuroendocrine and mucinous differentiation. Approximately 85% were Stage I in the largest study, all were unilateral and 80% were alive and free of tumor a mean of 4.7 years later. Poor outcome correlated with the presence of frank carcinoma. Features supporting a primary ovarian origin included coexisting teratoma, absence of capillary-lymphatic space invasion and confinement to a single ovary. Similar features help to distinguish mucinous carcinoids from Krukenberg tumors.

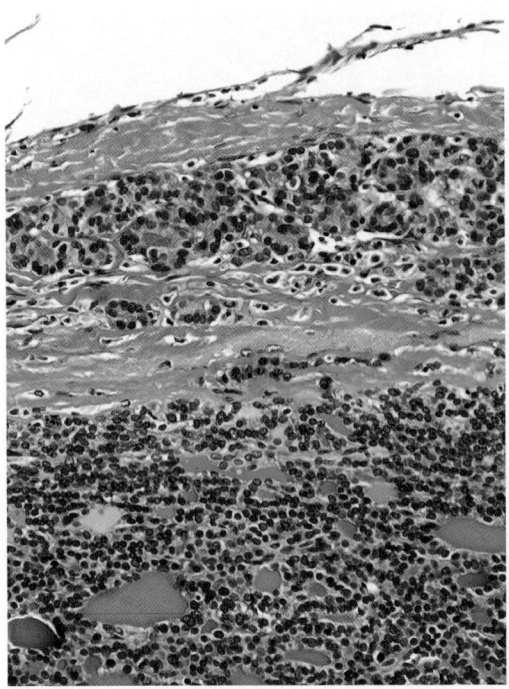

Fig. 29.15 Low power of malignant struma, seen here as a follicular variant of papillary carcinoma.

Rare germ cell tumors with embryonal, extra-embryonic and fetal differentiation

PATHOGENESIS, CLASSIFICATION AND THE PATIENT AT RISK

Immature germ cell tumors are an extremely rare group of neoplasms that recapitulate stages of early development. With rare exceptions, they arise via neoplastic transformation of germ cells. One theory poses that benign cystic teratomas arise from benign germ cells via parthenogenesis, whereas immature germ cell tumors arise from malignant germ cells that subsequently undergo a spectrum of differentiation (Fig. 29.22). The pathway and degree of differentiation governs the ultimate phenotype(s).[60]

Immature germ cell tumors predominate in young persons, with 80% occurring prior to the age of 30. The mean age for all of these tumors is between 15 and 20 years of age. Despite the early age and origin from germ cells, familial syndromes are uncommon.[61]

Germ cells recapitulate differentiation as described in Figure 29.22. The most primitive is the dysgerminoma, which shares an appearance and immunophenotype with germ cells. Choriocarcinoma and yolk sac carcinomas signify extra-embryonic differentiation, whereas the embryonic pathway progresses through embryonal carcinoma to immature teratoma. Common to all of these tumors is a pattern of differentiation that is similar to that seen in early human development.

TUMOR TYPES

The clinical presentation of germ cell tumors varies somewhat according to the tumor. The following is a summary of the individual tumors and their unique characteristics.

Dysgerminoma

The patient at risk

Dysgerminoma is a malignant germ cell neoplasia of the ovary, believed to arise from primordial germ cells similar to the testicular seminoma counterpart. These are uncommon neoplasms that correspond to about 1% of all ovarian germ cell tumors. Dysgerminoma is considered the most common malignant ovarian germ cell neoplasm to occur in pure form.[62] Most cases occur in the second and third decades of life. The tumor may arise before puberty but is very rare after menopause.

Metastatic carcinoids

Metastatic carcinoids are typically insular and are distinguished from primary carcinoids by the following: (1) bilateral ovarian involvement, (b) larger size, (c) absence of coexisting teratoma and (d) carcinoid syndrome.[46] The typical pattern is that of an insular carcinoid (Fig. 29.21). The outcome is poor and a primary mid-gut carcinoid is most likely. Tumors with a prominent signet-ring cell component may signify metastatic mucinous carcinoids from the appendix.[47,48]

Carcinoids arising in association with mucinous neoplasms

A small percentage of carcinoids in the ovary coexist with other tumors, specifically mucinous neoplasms.[49,50]

OTHER MALIGNANCIES ARISING IN TERATOMAS

A variety of other tumors have been reported to arise within teratomas, including sebaceous carcinomas, adenocarcinomas of respiratory epithelium, small cell carcinomas, primitive neuroectodermal tumors, other neural tumors, including glioblastoma, paragangliomas, melanomas, and even osteosarcomas.[51–59] The pathologist should maintain an index of suspicion for a teratomatous origin when faced with any unusual ovarian tumors in a reproductive-age or postmenopausal patient, particularly if associated with a contralateral teratoma.

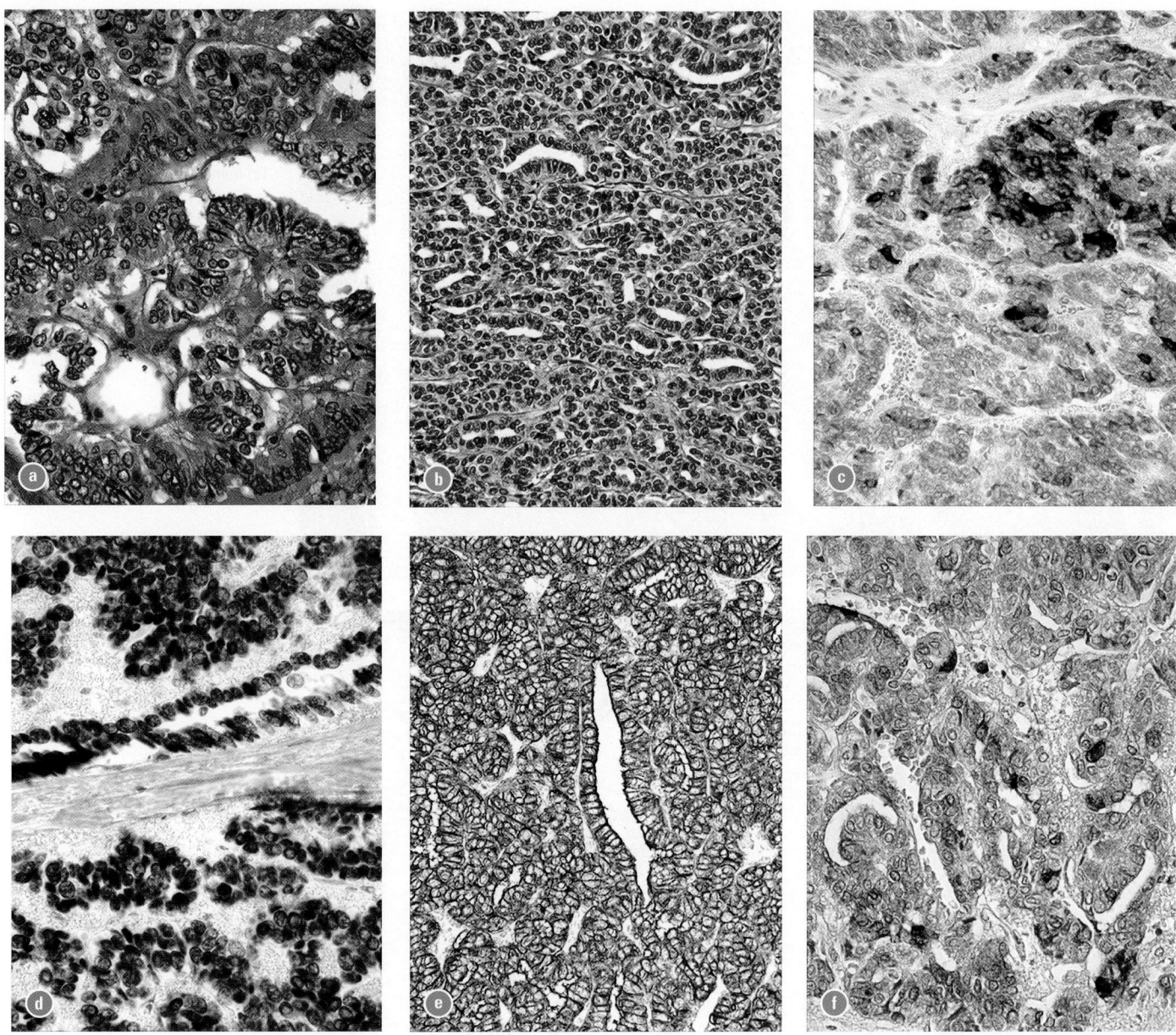

Fig. 29.16 Recurrent/metastatic malignant struma ovarii. (a) Classical variant features: papillary projections, marked nuclear crowding, nuclear grooves and nuclear clearing. (b) Areas of poorly-differentiated thyroid carcinoma, with poorly-formed follicles, prominent nuclear grooves and nuclear crowding. (c) Areas of poorly-differentiated thyroid carcinoma, with focal immunoreactivity for thyroglobulin. (d) Diffuse nuclear staining for TTF-1 in the poorly-differentiated areas, indication thyroid origin. (e) Diffuse membranous staining for HBME1 in the poorly-differentiated areas. (f) Immunoreactivity for Galectining 3 in the poorly-differentiated areas of the papillary thyroid carcinoma. (Courtesy of Dr Vânia Nosé, Brigham and Women's Hospital.)

Dysgerminoma is one of the most common neoplasms observed during pregnancy.[63]

Presenting signs and symptoms

Dysgerminomas are rapidly growing tumors, which are bilateral in 15% of the cases. Unilateral tumors have a slight tendency to be right sided.[64] Infrequently, dysgerminoma is found incidentally as a small tumor in patients with gonadal dysgenesis that almost invariably arises from a gonadoblastoma. Most often, however, dysgerminomas occur in normal females with a non-distinct symptomatology related to an enlarging mass. In the great majority of cases, dysgerminoma is not associated with endocrine manifestations. Up to 95% of patients with dysgerminoma have an elevated serum level of lactic dehydrogenase at presentation. Serum levels of alkaline phosphatase, neuron-specific enolase (NSE) and CA 125 can also be increased in some patients.[65]

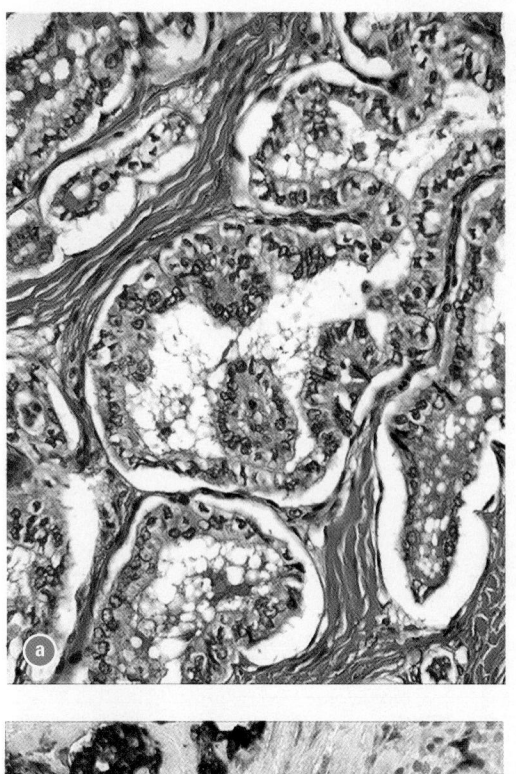

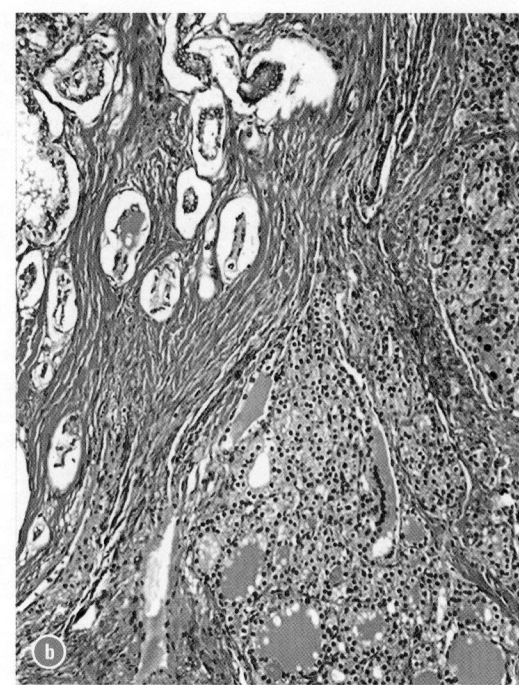

Fig. 29.17 Papillary thyroid carcinoma in struma ovarii. (a) Follicular variant with fibrosis, with prominent nuclear clearing and nuclear grooves. (b) Papillary thyroid carcinoma (left) with adjacent thyroid tissue (right upper). (c) Immunoreactivity for Galectin-3 in papillary thyroid carcinoma areas (upper), and not in the normal thyroid tissue (lower). (d) Immunoreactivity for HBME1 in papillary thyroid carcinoma areas, with sparing of normal thyroid tissue. (Courtesy of Dr Vânia Nosé, Brigham and Women's Hospital.)

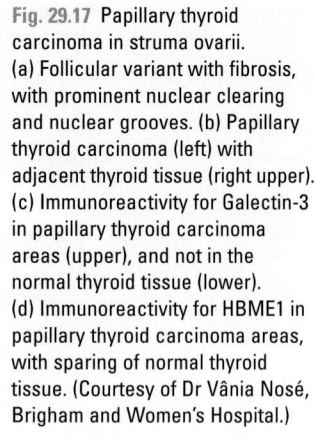

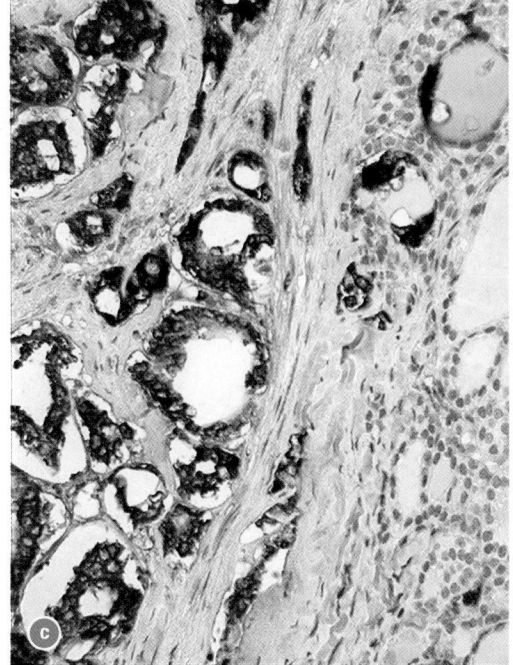

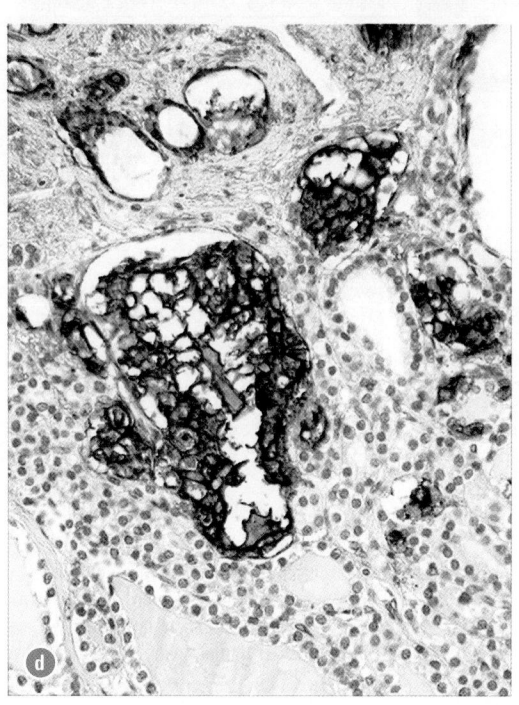

Gross pathology

Dysgerminomas are usually solid and firm with a uniform pale tan to grey-pink cut surface (Figs 29.23, 29.24). The size is highly variable with a median diameter of 15 cm. Hemorrhage and necrosis can be present, forming areas of cystic degeneration. However, distinct cystic structures within the tumor warrant the search for other neoplastic elements as teratoma. Large areas of calcification are seen in dysgerminomas arising from gonadoblastomas.

Histopathology

The tumor is composed of nests or cords of large, uniform, polyhedral cells separated by fibrous tissue septa with lymphocytes (Fig. 29.25). Rarely, the tumor cells line irregular or rounded gland-like spaces or

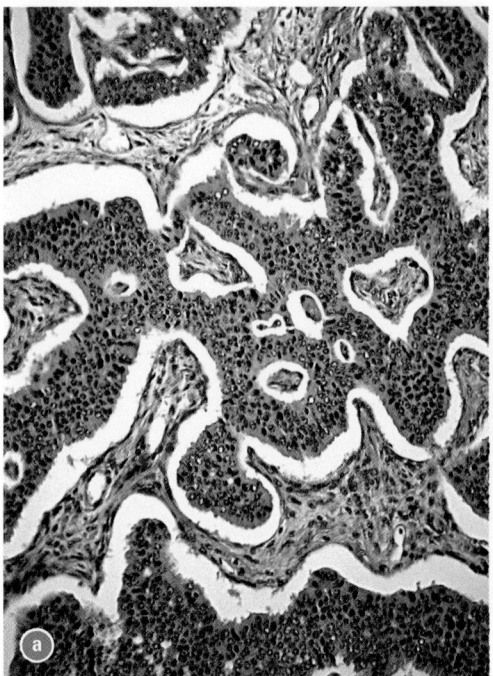

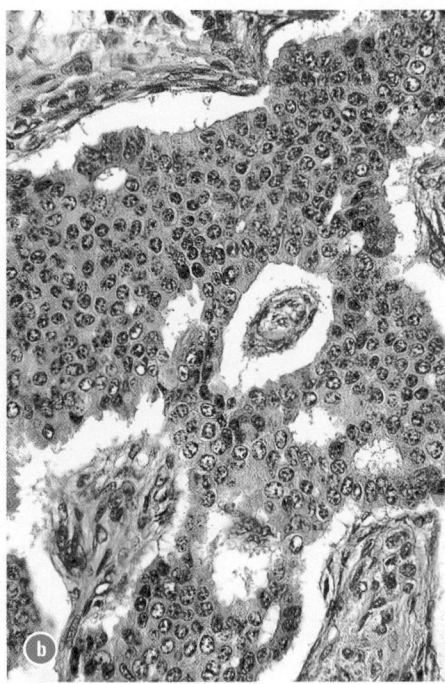

Fig. 29.18 Insular carcinoid. (a) The tumor forms broad interconnected sheets at low power. (b) At higher power the tumor cells display the characteristic granular (salt and pepper) chromatin.

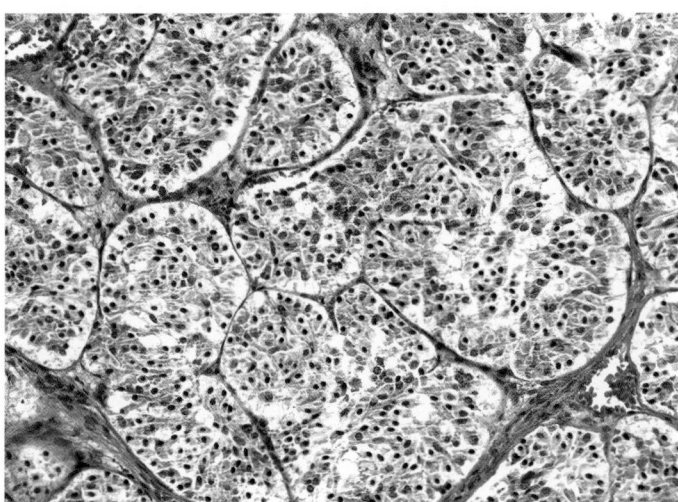

Fig. 29.19 Metastatic insular carcinoid with fixation artifact. The nuclei are small and dense-appearing.

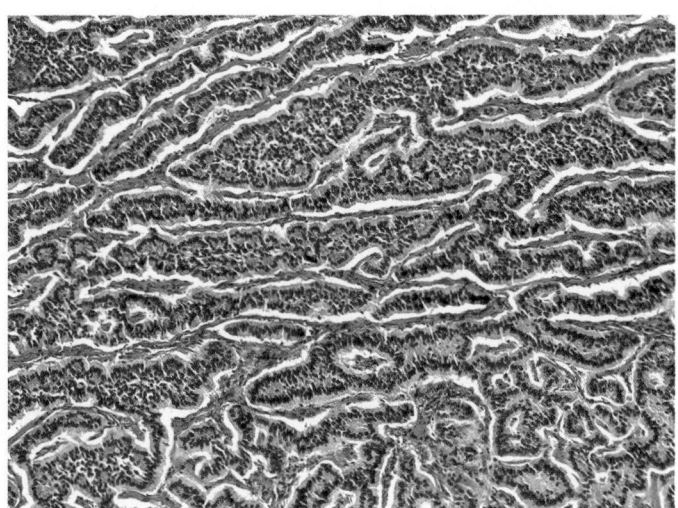

Fig. 29.20 Trabecular carcinoid.

form solid tubular structures (Fig. 29.26). Tumor cells have abundant pale or eosinophilic cytoplasm. Nuclei are large, vesicular round to oval, and centrally located with finely granular chromatin and sharp nuclear membrane (Fig. 29.27). Nucleoli are typically prominent and eosinophilic (Fig. 29.28). Some variation in nuclear size is usually present and giant mononucleate tumor cells, resembling typical dysgerminoma

cells, may be seen. Mitotic activity is variable, even within different areas of the same tumor. Giant cells, histiocytic or syncytiotrophoblastic, can be seen in some cases. The latter may be present in groups or in isolation and are found in about 3% of cases and should not be considered to be evidence of concomitant choriocarcinoma if not accompanied by cytotrophoblast.[64] The syncytiotrophoblastic compo-

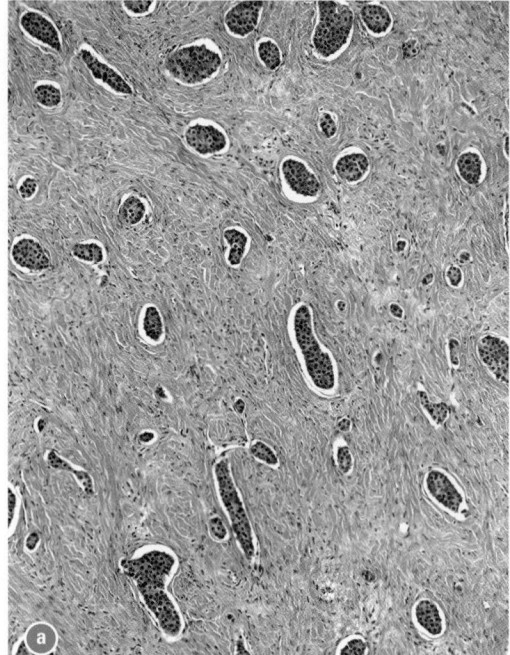
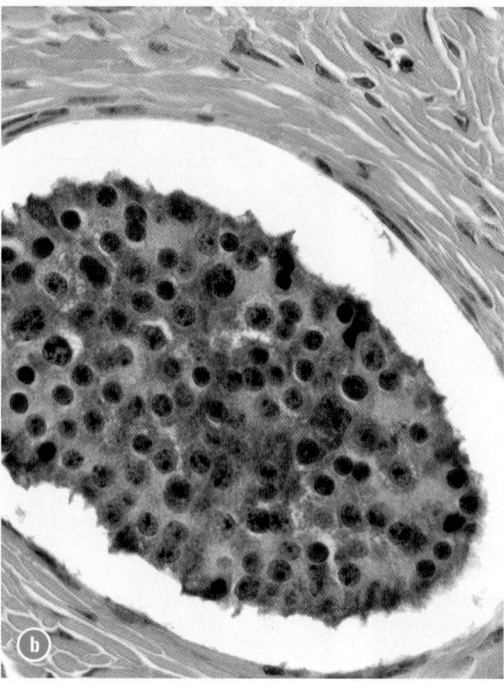

Fig. 29.21 (a) Metastatic carcinoid infiltrating a fibrotic stroma; (b) at higher magnification.

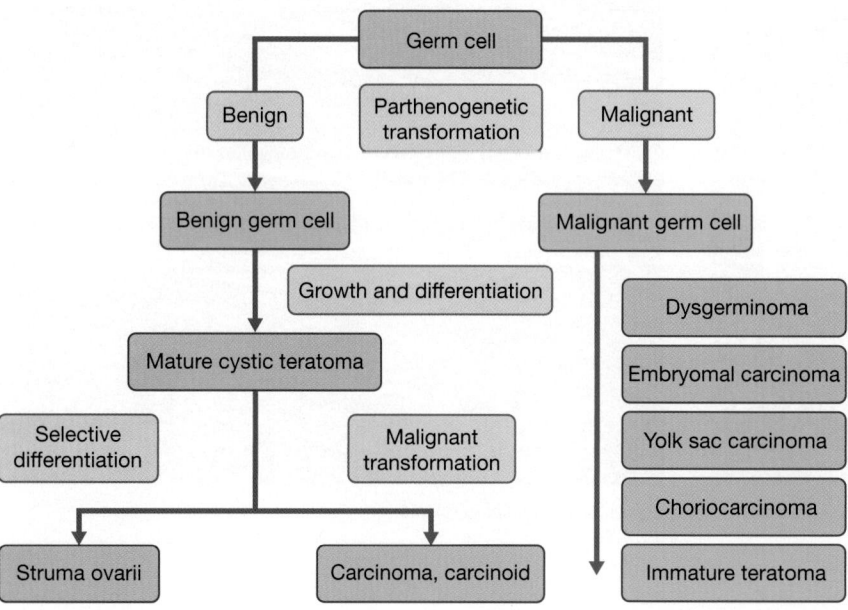

Fig. 29.22 Diagram of differentiation patterns in benign and malignant germ cell tumors.

nent may produce gonadotropin and these patients may have elevated levels of human chorionic gonadotropin (hCG).[66] Extensive sampling of tumors associated with hCG production is important to exclude foci of choriocarcinoma and embryonal carcinoma.

The stromal network is usually delicate and loose but may be dense and hyalinized and represent the predominant component in some cases. Areas of myxoid and luteinized stroma can be present, including occasional Leydig-like cells. Infiltrating lymphocytes are

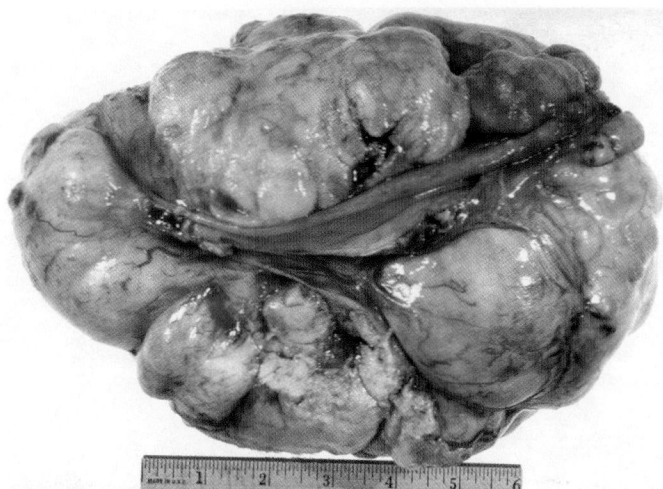

Fig. 29.23 Dysgerminoma. The tumor has a cerebriform architecture. The fallopian tube is attenuated along the surface.

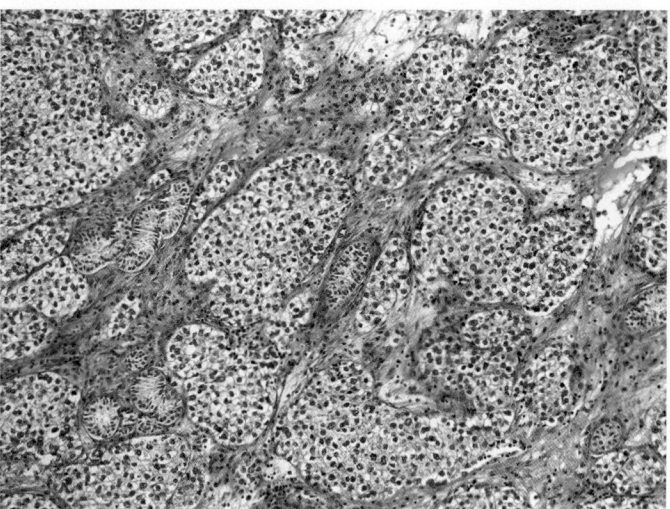

Fig. 29.25 Dysgerminoma. At low power this tumor contains lobular units of uniform tumor cells separated by a delicate stroma.

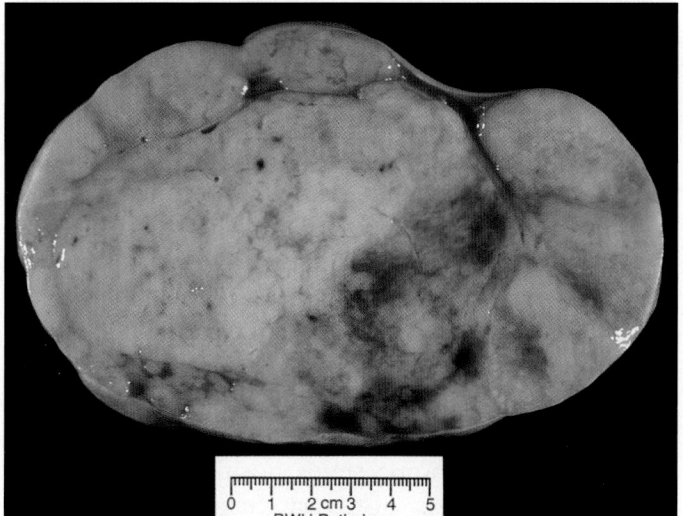

Fig. 29.24 Dysgerminoma. On sectioning, the surface is tan-yellow with focal hemorrhage.

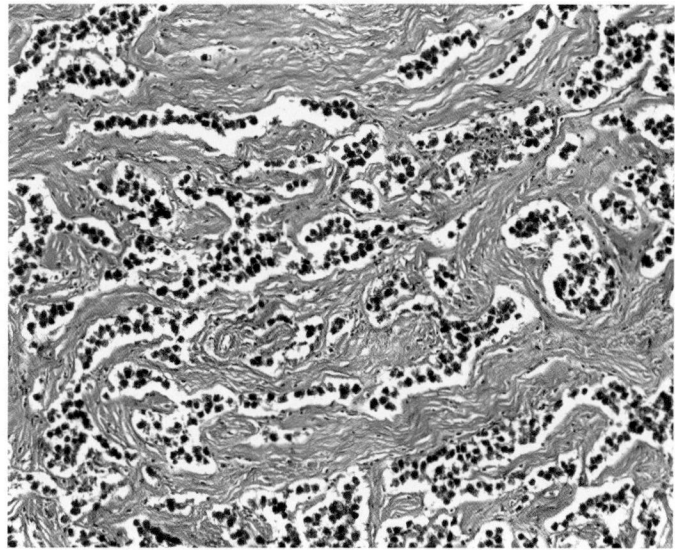

Fig. 29.26 Dysgerminoma. This tumor has linear arrays of neoplastic cells in a fibrous stroma.

predominantly of T-cell lineage (Fig. 29.29). The amount of lymphocytes is variable and may include lymphoid follicles with germinal centers. Less commonly, histiocytes, eosinophils and plasma cells are identified. When prominent, the histiocytic component may form granulomas. Necrosis and hemorrhage can be marked in large tumors. Microscopic foci of calcification can be seen in the absence of gonadoblastoma as a precursor lesion. These are usually dystrophic and associated with areas of tumor degeneration, in contrast to the more rounded and obvious foci seen in

gonadoblastoma. Aberrant follicles may be eventually found at the periphery of dysgerminomas in karyotypically normal females and should not be mistaken for gonadoblastoma nests.

Dysgerminomas are typically immunoreactive for placental alkaline phosphatase (PLAP) and vimentin. Other markers frequently positive are lactic dehydrogenase, neuron-specific enolase, Leu-7, cytokeratins, desmin and GFAP.[67–69] The tumor cells are reportedly negative for EMA and CEA. Syncytiotrophoblastic cells are positive for hCG and keratins, but, in rare cases of

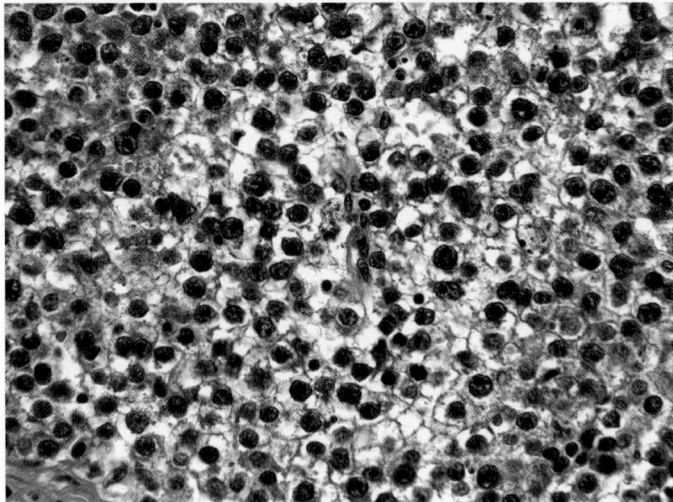

Fig. 29.27 Dysgerminoma. At higher power the tumor cells display centrally placed nuclei with delicate cytoplasmic membranes.

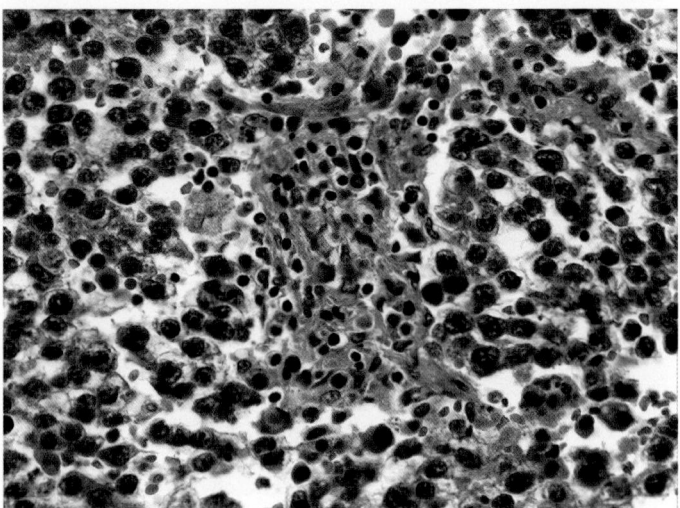

Fig. 29.29 Dysgerminoma with inflammatory (mononuclear) cells.

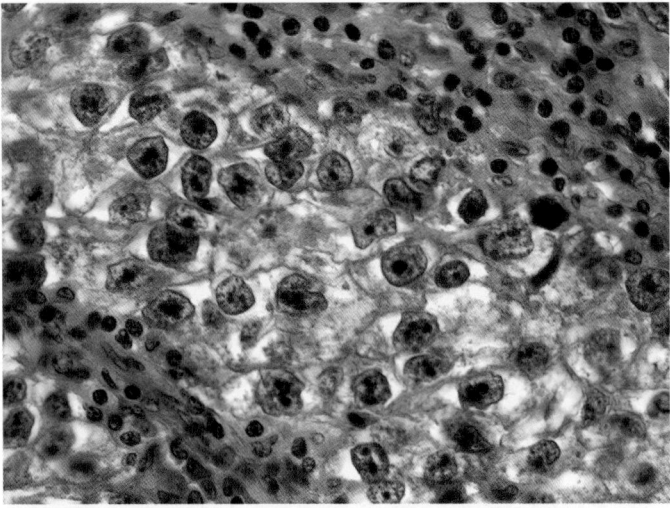

Fig. 29.28 Dysgerminoma. High magnification illustrates the prominent violaceous nucleoli.

hCG-secreting dysgerminomas in which these cells are not identified, the cytoplasm of dysgerminoma cells may be hCG positive.[66]

Differential diagnosis

The principal diagnostic challenge in classifying germ cell tumors in general, and particularly dysgerminoma, is assuring that the tumor is present in its pure form. Dysgerminoma may be associated with teratoma, yolk sac tumor, embryonal carcinoma and choriocarcinoma. Yolk sac tumor is distinguished by more marked nuclear size variation and fewer or absent lymphocytes, presence of hyaline bodies and AFP immunoreactivity. Embryonal

carcinomas have larger cells with hyperchromatic nuclei. Most dysgerminomas do not stain with cytokeratins, a feature helpful in their distinction from embryonal carcinoma and yolk sac tumor.[68]

The cytoplasm of the tumor cells contains glycogen, which is removed by diastase reaction. PAS staining will vary from weak to strong. Immunohistochemical staining for placenta-specific alkaline phosphatase (PLAP) usually shows a membranous pattern.[67,69] It may be useful in the differential diagnosis with clear cell carcinoma, lymphoma and granulosa cell tumor. However, as PLAP also positively stains other malignant germ cell tumors, it cannot be used to differentiate dysgerminoma from other malignant germ cell tumors. Dysgerminoma stains positively with c-KIT, but this reaction is not very helpful in diagnosis because a variety of tumors are c-KIT positive.

Management and outcome

Dysgerminoma is a malignant neoplasm capable of metastatic and local spread. However, it is generally less aggressive than other malignant germ cell tumors. About two-thirds are confined to the ovary at the time of diagnosis. Lymphatic spread affects first the common iliac nodes and then the mediastinal and supraclavicular nodes. Distant metastases occur later and affect liver, lungs, bone and kidneys. Metastasis to the contralateral ovary are typically microscopic in the form of small cords or individual neoplastic cells infiltrating the ovarian stroma, emphasizing the importance of biopsy examination of both ovaries in patients for whom conservative surgery is planned.

It has been suggested that cellular tumors with minimal stromal and lymphocytic component, marked nuclear pleomorphism and high mitotic rate will behave more aggressively.[62,63] Vascular invasion and capsular involvement may also adversely alter the prognosis. However, none of these variables have proved to be independent of tumor stage. The presence of other neoplastic germ cell tumor elements has an adverse effect on prognosis.

A conservative approach involving unilateral oophorectomy is currently advocated for tumors confined to the ovary. The neoplasm is highly radiosensitive and it also responds well to combination chemotherapy.[70] These later two options are usually reserved for patients with more advanced disease. Hysterectomy and bilateral salpingo-oophorectomy is performed in patients with dysgenic gonads in view of the high risk for the development of bilateral neoplasms in these patients. Therefore, karyotypic evaluation of patients with dysgerminoma is recommended. The prognosis of patients with pure dysgerminoma is favorable, with a 5-year survival of 75–90%. Most recurrences occur in the first 2 years after diagnosis.

Yolk sac tumor

The pataient at risk

Yolk sac tumors, also termed endodermal sinus tumors, are believed to develop as a result of differentiation of primitive malignant germ cell elements in the direction of yolk sac or vitelline structures. It is the second most common malignant ovarian germ cell neoplasm after dysgerminoma. Yolk sac tumor is encountered most frequently in the second and third decades and followed by the first and fourth.[71,72]

Presenting signs and symptoms

Most patients have symptoms of abdominal enlargement and pain and present with a pelvic mass. Alpha-fetoprotein (AFP) is a constituent of the normal human fetal serum and is produced by the yolk sac, liver and upper gastrointestinal tract. Germ cell tumors in patients with elevated serum AFP will usually contain yolk sac tumor elements. Yolk sac tumor is usually not associated with endocrine-related symptoms.

Gross pathology

Yolk sac tumor is almost always unilateral and involvement of both ovaries is typically a manifestation of metastatic disease. The tumor is usually large, most measuring more than 10 cm (Fig. 29.30).[73] The tumor

is usually oval shaped, encapsulated, firm and gray-yellow. It is frequently solid and cystic with necrosis and hemorrhage.

Histopathology

Yolk sac tumors exhibit a wide range of histologic patterns:

1 *Microcystic*: composed of a loose network of small cystic spaces forming a honeycomb pattern. The microcysts are lined by flat cells with pleomorphic, hyperchromatic nuclei (Fig. 29.31).
2 *Macrocystic*: the tumor exhibits larger cyst in contrast to microcysts (Fig. 29.32).

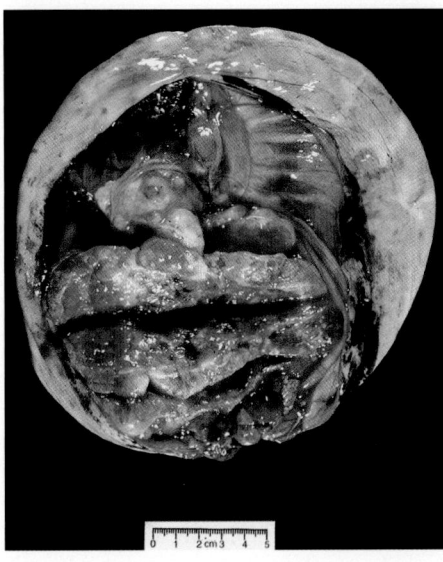

Fig. 29.30 Gross appearance of yolk sac tumor.

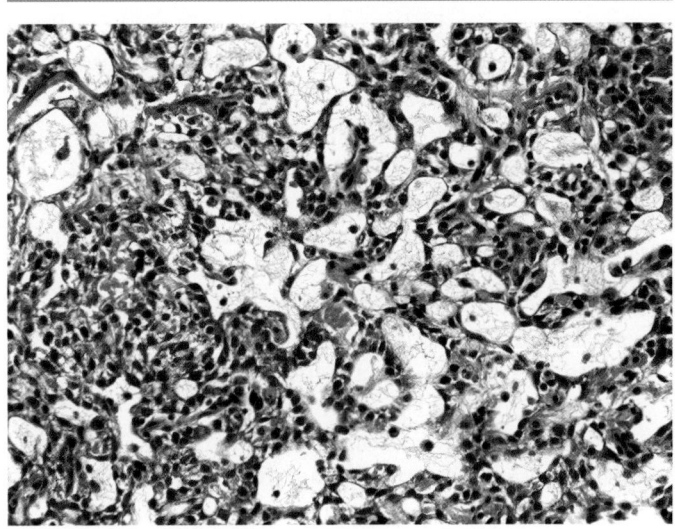

Fig. 29.31 Yolk sac tumor. Microcystic pattern.

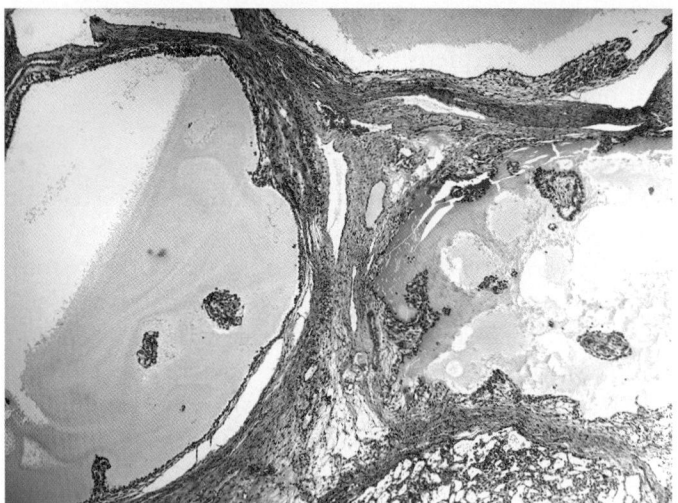

Fig. 29.32 Yolk sac tumor. Macrocystic pattern.

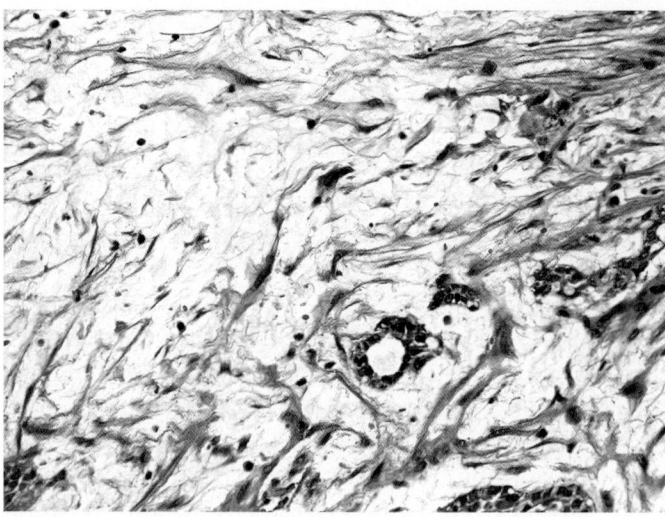

Fig. 29.33 Yolk sac tumor. Scant tumor cells in a myxoid background.

3 *Myxomatous*: small collections of epithelial-like cells forming strands or gland-like structures are seen within abundant myxomatous tissue (Fig. 29.33).

4 *Solid*: aggregates of small epithelial-like polygonal cells with clear cytoplasm and large vesicular or pyknotic nuclei. Occasional microcysts are usually present.

5 *Endodermal sinus*: composed of perivascular formations, consisting of a narrow band of connective tissue with a capillary in the center and lined by a layer of cuboidal or low columnar epithelial-like cells (Fig. 29.34). The cells have large, vesicular nuclei and prominent nucleoli. These structures are known as sinuses of Duval or Schiller–Duval bodies. The presence of these structures can be considered diagnostic of yolk sac tumor but their absence does not exclude the diagnosis.

6 *Alveolar-glandular*: composed of alveolar, gland-like spaces lined by one or more layers of flat, cuboidal or columnar cells with large nuclei, surrounded by myxomatous stroma or cellular aggregates.

7 *Polyvesicular*: numerous cysts and vesicles surrounded by compact connective tissue stroma. The vesicles are lined partially by columnar and partially by flat cells, the transition occasionally marked by a constriction, recapitulating the embryologic conversion of the primary into the secondary yolk sac (Fig. 29.35).

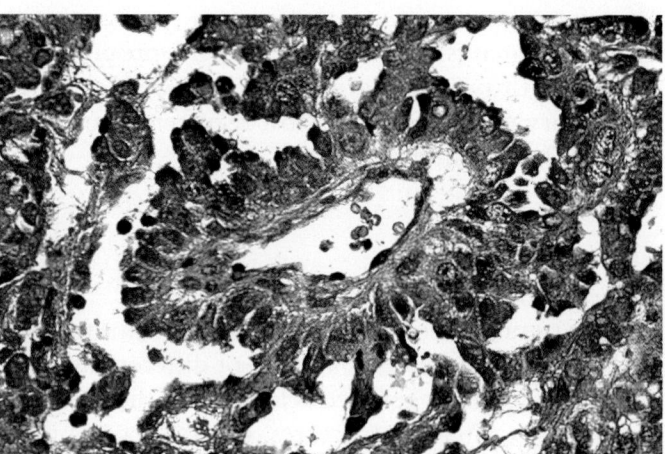

Fig. 29.34 Yolk sac tumor. Schiller–Duval body, consisting of a central vessel surrounded by primitive cells within a second ill-defined space.

8 *Papillary*: papillary structures consisting of connective tissue cores lined by epithelial-like cells with marked pleomorphism.

9 *Hepatoid*: solid aggregates or cords of polygonal cells with eosinophilic, granular cytoplasm, and well-defined cells borders, resembling hepatocytes. Small areas of hepatoid differentiation are seen in one-third to one-half of yolk sac tumors, but this pattern is rarely the predominant one.[74]

10 *Glandular or primitive endodermal (intestinal)*: the tumor is composed of nests of primitive endodermal cells forming glands or solid aggregates and surrounded by connective tissue. The glands are usually sparsely distributed within the tumor, only rarely being the predominant

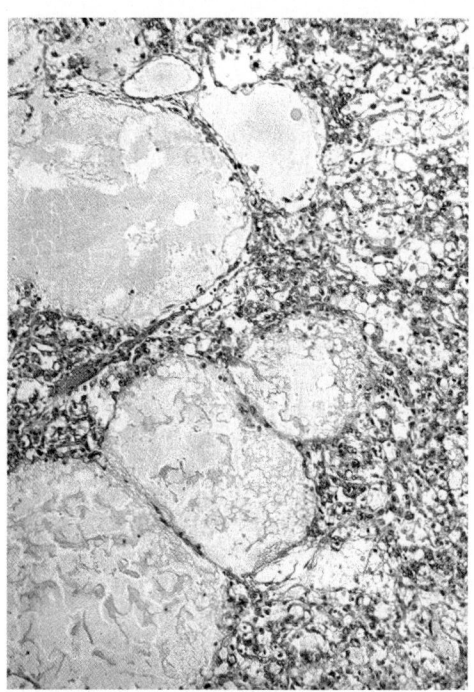

Fig. 29.35 Yolk sac tumor. Attenuated cystic spaces characterize the polyvesicular-vitelline pattern.

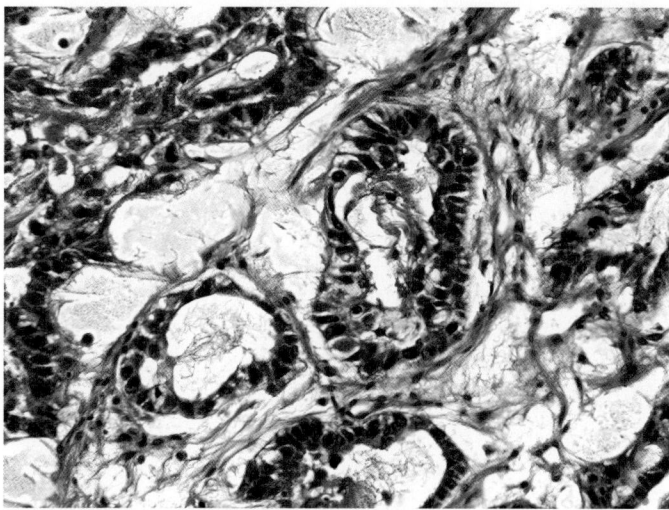

Fig. 29.36 Yolk sac tumor. Glandular differentiation.

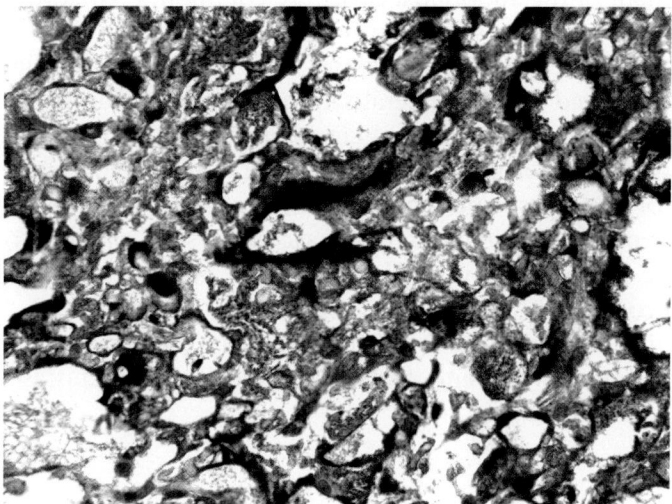

Fig. 29.37 Yolk sac tumor, immunopositive for alpha-fetoprotein.

pattern (Fig. 29.36). The degree of differentiation varies from primitive to well-differentiated with cytoplasmic vacuoles, which may resemble mature enteric epithelium.[75] When the appearance is similar to secretory endometrium, the designation 'endometrioid' variant has been described.[76] Eosinophilic hyaline droplets that are PAS-positive and diastase-resistant may be present either within the tumor cells or outside of them. The droplets may be observed in all the histologic patterns and their identification is a helpful diagnostic feature. However, their presence is not diagnostic of yolk sac tumor because they are observed in other malignant neoplasms. Some tumors have accumulation of basement membrane material in the form of extracellular deep eosinophilic linear structures. These have been designated parietal differentiation.[74]

Yolk sac tumor is usually positive for AFP, keratin and alpha-1-antitrypsin.[77] The tumor is negative for EMA (Fig. 29.37). CEA is usually positive in areas of enteric differentiation.

Differential diagnosis

The differential diagnosis includes clear cell carcinoma, embryonal carcinoma and dysgerminoma.

Clear cell carcinomas occur in older patients (Ch. 27). They show a more regular tubular pattern, lacking the honeycomb network of yolk sac tumors. The tubular spaces are usually lined by hobnail cells. Also, most clear cell carcinomas will have solid areas composed of large cells with clear cytoplasm, and small hyperchromatic nuclei.

Embryonal carcinomas lack the characteristic patterns observed in yolk sac tumors. The tumor cells are larger with a more granular cytoplasm and the nuclei are more pleomorphic with prominent nucleoli. In contrast to dysgerminomas, yolk sac tumors are keratin and AFP positive.[68]

Yolk sac tumors can also be confused with vascular tumors but careful examination reveals cystic spaces rather than vessels. Immunostains for vascular markers such as CD31 and CD34 may be used to make this distinction.

Retiform Sertoli–Leydig cell tumors and juvenile granulosa cell tumors should also be considered in the differential diagnosis. The absence of the various patterns of yolk sac tumor, presence of inhibin, the absence of immunostaining for AFP and the lack of elevated levels of serum AFP are useful features in this differential.

Hepatoid yolk sac tumors must be differentiated from both primary and metastatic lesions that have large cells with eosinophilic cytoplasm, including steroid cell tumor, clear cell carcinoma, melanoma and hepatocellular carcinoma.

Management and outcome

Yolk sac tumor is a highly malignant neoplasm, with early metastasis and invasion of surrounding structures. Lymphatic spread affects first the para-aortic and common iliac lymph nodes. Recurrences in the pelvis and involvement of the abdominal cavity are common. Hematogenous metastases frequently occur to lungs and liver.

In recent years, outcomes have been substantially improved with unilateral salpingo-oophorectomy and adjuvant combination chemotherapy that includes cisplatinum, etoposide and bleomycin. Complete cure for all stages is now possible in more than 80%.[70] Pure hepatoid and glandular yolk sac tumors are claimed to be more resistant to chemotherapy and have a worse prognosis.

Serial serum AFP measurements are used for monitoring therapy and for early detection of metastasis and recurrences.

Embryonal carcinoma

The patient at risk

Embryonal carcinomas are rare tumors in the ovary. They occur from the first to third decades of life. Mean age of the patients at presentation is 12 years.[78]

Presenting signs and symptoms

Patients usually present with a pelvic mass. Endocrine symptoms are present in about half of the time and include isosexual pseudoprecocity and irregular bleeding. Serum levels of hCG and AFP are usually elevated.[79]

Gross pathology

The tumor is large and unilateral. It has a variegated appearance with alternating gray, tan and yellow colors and cysts with mucous material. Hemorrhage and necrosis are frequent.

Histopathology

Embryonal carcinomas are composed of solid sheets of large primitive cells with amphophilic to clear cytoplasm and delineated cell boarders. The nuclei are round with coarse chromatin and prominent nucleoli (Fig. 29.38). The tumor usually shows admixed papillary areas and focal slit-like spaces. Mitosis and necrosis are marked. Eosinophilic droplets, as seen in yolk sac tumors, can be seen. Syncytiotrophoblastic giant cells are typically numerous and stain for hCG (Fig. 29.39).

Embryonal carcinomas are positive for cytokeratins, PLAP and NSE. EMA is almost always negative. One-third of tumors are AFP positive.[69]

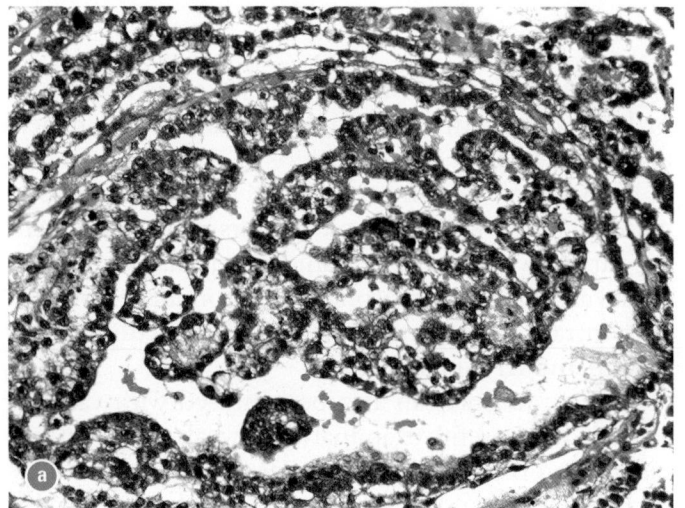 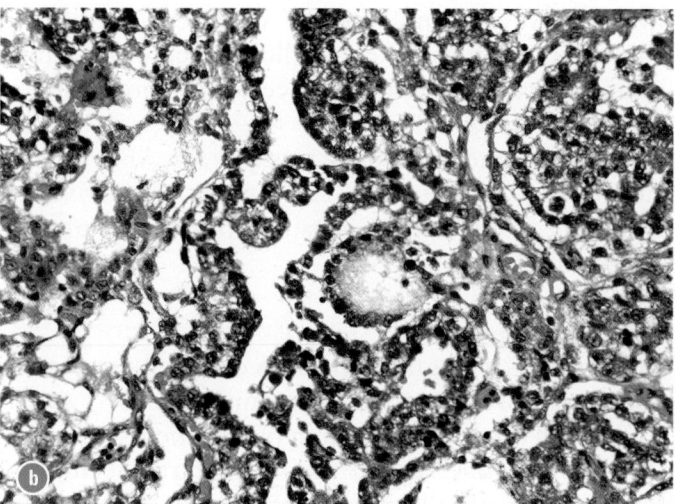

Fig. 29.38 Embryonal carcinoma. (a,b) Primitive germ cells forming epithelial-lined structures.

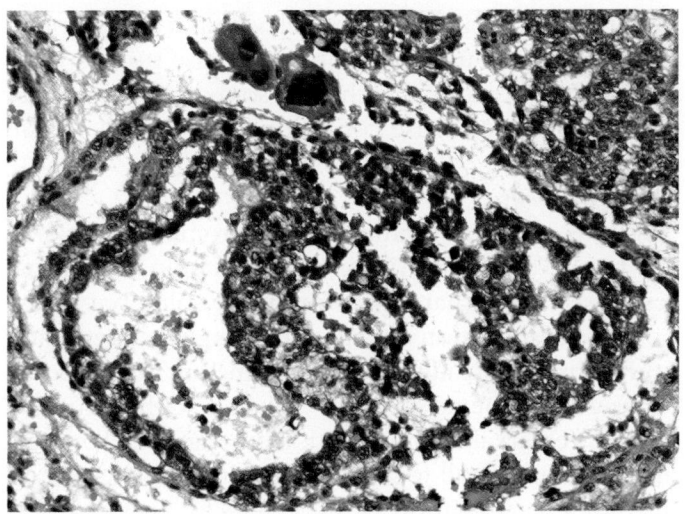

Fig. 29.39 Syncytial cells in embryonal carcinoma (top).

Differential diagnosis

The differential diagnosis includes dysgerminoma and yolk sac tumor, as discussed above. Rarely, it may be confused with ovarian adenocarcinomas. These tumors, however, occur in older patients, do not show trophoblastic giant cells or AFP expression and are frequently positive for EMA.

Management and outcome

Patients undergo unilateral salpingo-oophorectomy, debulking of extra-ovarian disease and combination chemotherapy. Almost half of the patients have extra-ovarian disease at the time of diagnosis. Serum levels of AFP and hCG are useful in determining the response to treatment.

Polyembryoma

The patient at risk

Polyembryomas are very rare ovarian germ cell tumors characterized by the presence of embryoid bodies, which resemble early embryos in various stages of development. Less than 20 cases have been reported in the literature, most being the predominant component of mixed malignant germ cell tumors such as immature teratoma and embryonal carcinoma.[80,81]

Presenting signs and symptoms

The patients are typically children or young adults and present with symptoms related to a pelvic mass.

Gross pathology

Polyembryomas form large unilateral solid masses. The cut surface is usually soft and red to brown with microcystic and hemorrhagic areas.

Histopathology

The tumor is composed of myriads of small struc-tures resembling normal or abnormal early embryos ranging from 15 to 18 days of development. The embryoid bodies include an embryonic disc, amniotic cavity and yolk sac with surrounding trophoblastic elements and extra-embryonic mesenchyme.[82] The embryoid bodies are embedded in a fibrous or edematous stroma. Mature and immature teratomatous elements are usually present. The yolk sac component of the embryoid body and the teratomatous hepatic tissue stain for AFP. The syncytiotrophoblastic elements are reactive to hCG.[83]

Management and outcome

Polyembryomas tend to behave aggressively. In most patients the tumor invades adjacent structures and produces intraperitoneal metastases at the time of diagnosis. The main therapeutic measure consists of surgical removal of the tumor. Most cases with disseminated disease have responded to chemotherapy.[84]

Choriocarcinoma

The patient at risk

Choriocarcinomas are composed of an admixture of cytotrophoblast and syncytiotrophoblast. Pure primary ovarian choriocarcinomas account for less than 1% of malignant ovarian germ cell tumors.[85,86] However, choriocarcinomatous elements are encountered in up to 20% of mixed germ cell tumors. Gestational ovarian choriocarcinomas are almost always metastatic from the uterus.

Presenting signs and symptoms

The tumor affects children and young adults who present with a pelvic mass. Elevated hCG causes various manifestations as isosexual pseudoprecocity and menstrual abnormalities.[87–89]

Gross pathology

The tumor is usually large, solid and unilateral. The cut surface is friable and hemorrhagic.

Histopathology

The presence of both the cytotrophoblastic and syncytiotrophoblastic cells is required for the diagnosis, although the proportion of each of these elements varies within the same tumor. Cytotrophoblastic cells have a polygonal, amphophilic cytoplasm with a single nucleus. Syncytiotrophoblastic cells are multinucleated with frequent cytoplasmic vacuolation. Multiple dilated sinusoids are usually present and vascular invasion can be prominent.[90]

Cytotrophoblastic cells stain for keratins. Syncytiotrophoblastic cells are positive for hCG, keratin and hPL.

Differential diagnosis

Syncytiotrophoblastic giant cells can be encountered in various germ cell tumors as dysgerminomas, embryonal carcinomas and yolk sac tumors and also in undifferentiated carcinomas that occur in older women. For the diagnosis of choriocarcinoma or mixed germ cell tumor with choriocarcinomatous component to be made, an intimate admixture of both the cytotrophoblast and syncytiotrophoblast must be identified.[91]

Management and outcome

Choriocarcinomas frequently invade surrounding structures and produce early lymphatic or hematogenous metastases. Currently, the treatment consists of cytoreductive surgery and combination chemotherapy.[70] Non-gestational choriocarcinomas are believed to be less responsive to chemotherapy than the gestational counterpart.[89,92]

Immature teratoma

Introduction and the patient at risk

Immature teratoma is defined as a malignant germ cell neoplasm containing patterns of differentiation that recapitulate that seen in embryonic and fetal tissues. Together with dysgerminoma, yolk sac carcinoma and mixed germ cell tumors, immature teratomas account for over 80% of all malignant germ cells tumors. The ranking of each tumor varies, depending on the study, but immature teratomas are always among the three most common, accounting for from 20% to 50%. Immature teratomas are less than 3% of teratomas in general and less than 1% of all ovarian malignancies. Like the other germ cell tumors, they may coexist with a concurrent or prior contralateral cystic teratoma in approximately 10% of cases.

Like other malignant germ cell tumors, immature teratomas predominate in the second and third decades and less than 10% are seen above age 30. The mean age of approximately 19 years is identical to other malignant germ cell tumors.

Presenting signs and symptoms

Immature teratomas typically present as a pelvic mass, increased abdominal girth and vaginal bleeding. Isosexual precocity is uncommon, but serum markers, specifically AFP and hCG, are elevated in the majority. Ultrasound will usually distinguish these tumors from benign cystic teratoma, although some solid derivatives such struma may cause confusion.[14]

Gross pathology

The gross findings in immature teratoma vary according to the degree of tissue differentiation. The usual result is a tumor that is predominately solid, but which on gross examination contains areas vaguely resembling normal tissue, including neural and mesenchymal (bone, cartilage) elements (Figure 29.40). Other tumors exhibit remarkable preservation of mature elements, in which only small foci of immaturity are detected on histologic examination (Figure 29.41). In the latter, thorough sampling is indicated, particularly tumors from younger patients.

Histopathology

The pathologic and clinical management of immature teratoma involves the following tasks:

1. Exclusion of benign solid teratomas and tumors with minor foci of immaturity. This is achieved by confirming the presence of immature tissues (Fig. 29.42).
2. Determining the grade of the tumor. Tumor grading systems used in the past have been tailored to estimate the amount of immature tissue in the teratoma. Assessments of grade were based on

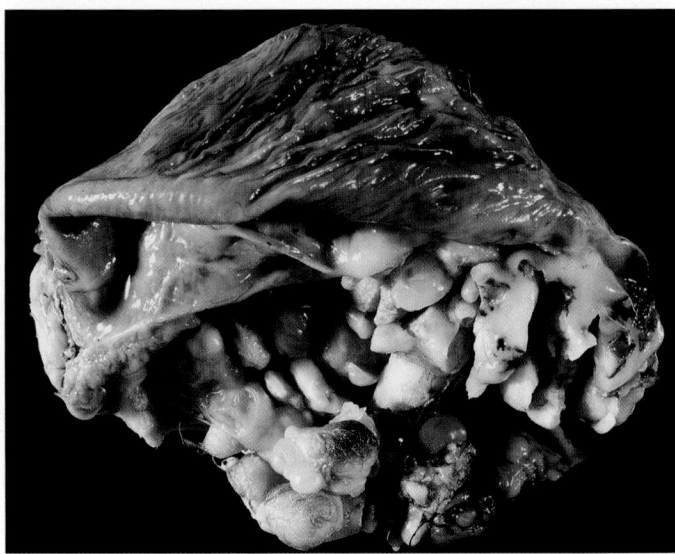

Fig. 29.40 Immature teratoma. The tumor is a large encapsulated mass containing tissues of different consistency, some of which resemble cartilage. A small amount of hair is seen (bottom center).

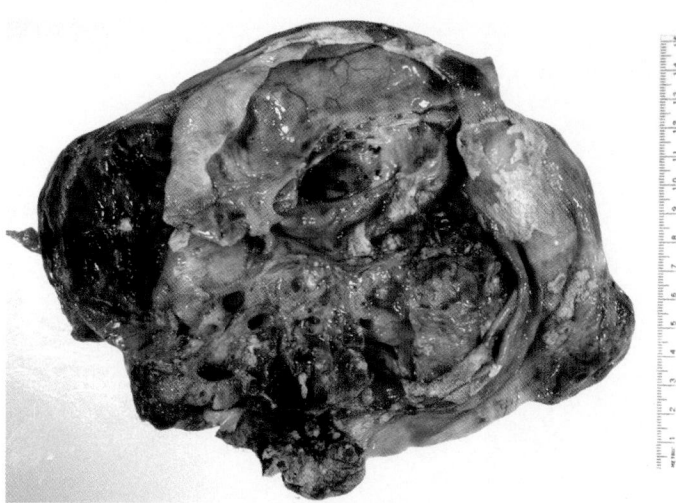

Fig. 29.41 Sectioned immature teratoma reveals a variety of solid and cystic components. This tumor displayed mostly mature elements on histologic examination.

the overall extent of immature neuroepithelium. In retrospect, the selection of neuroepithelium as the barometer of malignancy was due to the fact that this tissue was the most recognizable and increased reproducibly in the grading system. The grading was as follows: grade 1 tumors had occasional foci of immature neuroepithelium such that they did not occupy more than one low power (×40) field in a given slide; grade 2 tumors occupied from 1–4 low power fields per slide; and grade 3 tumors exceeded this limit.[92] In a follow-up report, O'Connor and Norris proposed a two-grade system, in which any tumor with immature elements exceeding one low power field per slide was classified as a high-grade tumor, without separating grades 2 and 3.[93] This approach is supported by both the cut-point for aggressive behavior (grade 2) and the traditional clinical management guidelines for Stage I immature teratomas, which recommended chemotherapy for both grades 2 and 3.[94–96] Thus, the critical decision is determining the extent of immature teratomatous elements in the tumor in question (Fig. 29.43a–c).

Differential diagnosis

The following must be excluded when considering the diagnosis of immature teratoma: (1) Mature solid teratomas with minimal immaturity. Such tumors are not classified as immature teratomas.[97] (2) Thurlbeck

and Scully showed that immature cartilage and developing cortex were not sufficient, because these elements were present after fetal life.[98] (3) Carcinosarcomas contain a mixture of primitive-appearing tissues but these do not organize into coordinated tissue units with recognizable embryonal or fetal structures. (4) In mixed germ cell tumors, exclusion of other elements is important, as they may contribute to recurrences, particularly in the pediatric age group. Heifetz et al. observed that central pathology review of immature pediatric teratomas uncovered subtle patterns such as hepatoid and lung or intestine-like glandular differentiation in yolk sac tumors. Exclusion of these subtle components of mixed germ cell tumor was important from a prognostic perspective.[99,100]

Tumor spread, peritoneal implants and gliomatosis peritoneii

Approximately one-third of immature teratomas have spread beyond the ovary at the time of diagnosis.[9] Overall, higher stage is associated with an unfavorable outcome, with the following caveats:

1 Extra-ovarian immature tumor, including lymph node metastases and peritoneal implants, are associated with poorer survival.

2 Peritoneal implants may convert from immature to mature tissues. Numerous studies have reported the finding of mature glial implants on the peritoneum following chemotherapy. The mechanism for this phenomenon is controversial. The traditional theory held that this phenomenon was due to the effects of chemotherapy on the tumor, favoring the retention of mature elements. In fact, 'retroversion' of immature to mature implants has been documented in one study using CT scan. In their study, Moskovic et al. noted a reduction in mass size following chemotherapy, with mature tissue only found on histologic examination.[101] However, even these elements did not adversely affect prognosis.

Despite the above observations, gliomatosis peritonei has been shown by molecular studies to be an independent phenomenon that accompanies immature teratomas but is not genetically related. First shown by Ferguson et al. and later confirmed by others, gliomatosis peritonei appears to represent the emergence of gliomatous differentiation from the surface of the peritoneum.[102–104] The precise mechanism by which this occurs remains obscure, but may be related to growth factors liberated by the teratoma.

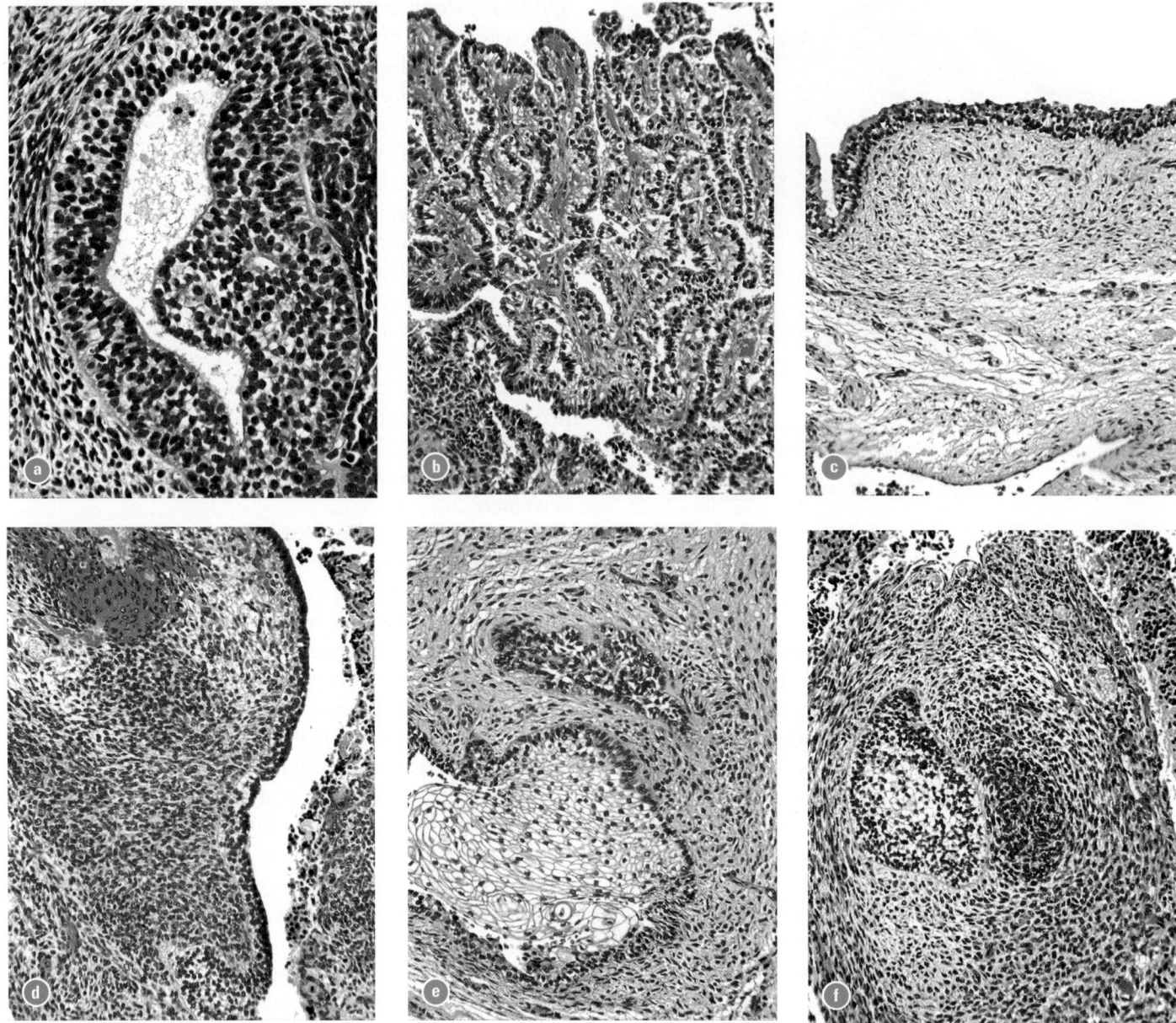

Fig. 29.42 Immature teratoma. (a) Primitive epithelium. (b) Immature choroids plexus. (c) Immature surface epithelium and stroma. (d) Immature mesenchyme. (e) Immature squamous epithelium. (f) Immature cartilage.

Management and outcome

The management of grade 1, Stage I tumors is unilateral oophorectomy. Chemotherapy, including bleomycin, etoposide and platinum, is recommended for Stage I tumors exceeding grade 1. This has achieved a near 95% cure rate for Stage I and 75% cure rate for higher-stage disease.[96] There is no evidence that contralateral oophorectomy, hysterectomy or radiation therapy will improve survival.[105,106]

In addition to the finding of gliomatosis peritonei, another post-therapy complication that has been reported is the 'growing teratoma syndrome'. This is characterized by the persistence and continued growth of mature teratomatous tissue despite chemotherapy.[107]

Mixed germ cell tumors

Mixed germ cell tumors are responsible for from 10 to 20% of immature germ cell tumors of the ovary and are the fourth most common after dysgerminomas, yolk sac carcinoma and immature teratoma. The computed frequency of these tumors is dependent on sampling and observer skill in identifying subtle forms

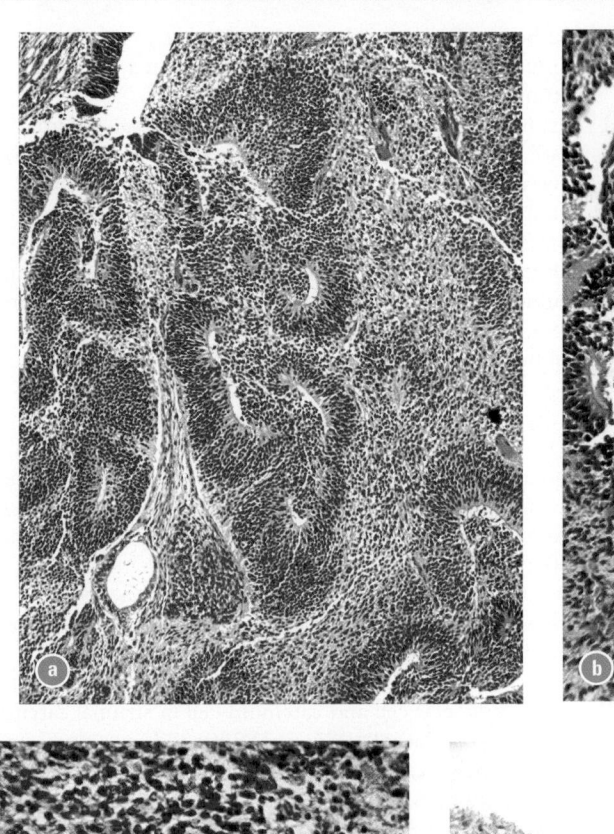
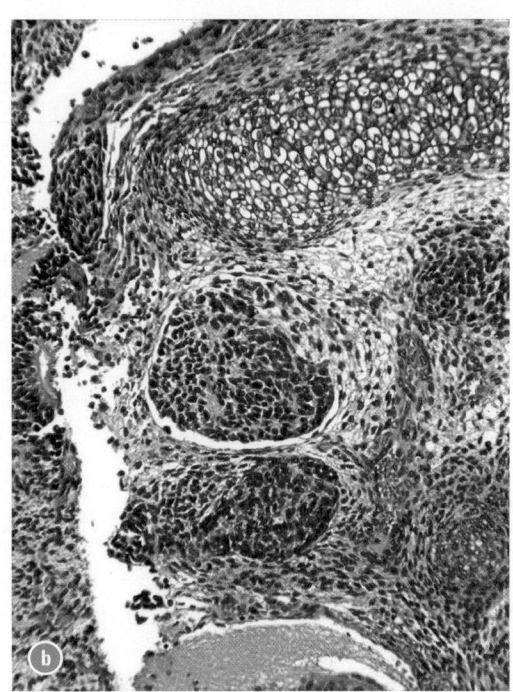
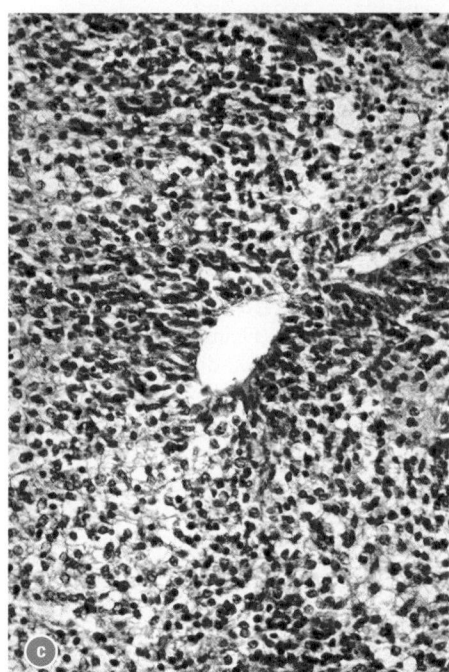
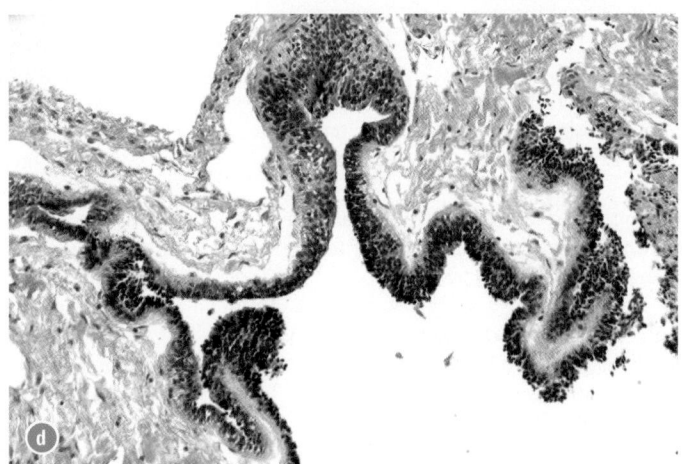

Fig. 29.43 Immature neuroepithelium in an immature teratoma. (a) Typical immature neuroepithelium, seen here as gland-like structures with palisaded nuclei. (b) Fetal ganglia. (c) Immature neuroepithelium resembling neuroblasts. (d) Normal neuroepithelium, sometimes found in mature cystic teratomas, must be excluded.

of non-teratomatous components, such as hepatoid yolk sac carcinomas and others. Previously, mixed germ cell tumors were assigned a more guarded prognosis because of these more aggressive components. Currently, in view of the success of combination chemotherapy, the outlook is excellent for these tumors, particularly those of low stage.[108–113]

References

1 Shah KH, Maxted WC, Chun B. Epidermoid cysts of the testis: a report of three cases and an analysis of 141 cases from the world literature. Cancer 1981; 47(3):577–582.
2 Young RH, Prat J, Scully RE. Epidermoid cyst of the ovary. A report of three cases with comments on histogenesis. Am J Clin Pathol 1980; 73(2):272–276.

3 Nogales FF Jr, Silverberg SG. Epidermoid cysts of the ovary: a report of five cases with histogenetic considerations and ultrastructural findings. Am J Obstet Gynecol 1976; 124(5):523–528.

4 Khong KG. Peripartum ovarian masses. J Obstet Gynaecol 1997; 17(6):531–534.

5 de Silva KS, Kanumakala S, Grover SR, Chow CW, Warne GL. Ovarian lesions in children and adolescents – an 11-year review. J Pediatr Endocrinol Metab 2004; 17(7):951–957.

6 Bloomfield TH. Benign cystic teratomas of the ovary: a review of seventy-two cases. Eur J Obstet Gynecol Reprod Biol 1987; 25(3):231–237.

7 Templeman CL, Fallat ME, Lam AM, et al. Managing mature cystic teratomas of the ovary. Obstet Gynecol Surv 2000; 55:738–745.

8 Kuno N, Kadomatsu K, Nakamura M, et al. Mature ovarian cystic teratoma with a highly differentiated homunculus: a case report. Birth Defects Res A Clin Mol Teratol 2004; 70(1):40–46.

9 Scully RE, Clement P, Young R. Atlas of tumor pathology. tumors of the ovary. Washington DC: AFIP; 1993.

10 As K, Webb JB, Wijesinghe D. Advanced squamous cell carcinoma developing in a mature cystic teratoma (dermoid) of the ovary in a young woman: a diagnostic and therapeutic challenge. J Obstet Gynaecol 1997; 17(6):598–599.

11 Bontis J, Vakiani M, Vavilis D, Agorastos T, Dragoumis K. Squamous cell carcinoma arising from mature cystic teratoma: a report of three cases. Eur J Gynaecol Oncol 1996; 17(1):49–52.

12 Krumerman MS, Chung A. Squamous carcinoma arising in benign cystic teratoma of the ovary: a report of four cases and review of the literature. Cancer 1977; 39(3):1237–1242.

13 Ulbright TM. Germ cell tumors of the gonads: a selective review emphasizing problems in differential diagnosis, newly appreciated, and controversial issues. Mod Pathol 2005; 18(Suppl 2):S61–S79.

14 Outwater EK, Siegelman ES, Hunt JL. Ovarian teratomas: tumor types and imaging characteristics. Radiographics 2001; 21:475–490.

15 Van de Moortele K, Vanbeckevoort D, Hendrickx S. Struma ovarii: US and CT findings. JBR-BTR 2003; 86:209–210.

16 Ciccarelli A, Valdes-Socin H, Parma J, et al. Thyrotoxic adenoma followed by atypical hyperthyroidism due to struma ovarii: clinical and genetic studies. Eur J Endocrinol 2004; 150(4):431–437.

17 Zannoni GF, Gallotta V, Legge F, et al. Pseudo-Meigs' syndrome associated with malignant struma ovarii: a case report. Gynecol Oncol 2004; 94(1):226–228.

18 Haddad LC. Struma ovarii presenting as hyperemesis gravidarum in pregnancy. J Obstet Gynaecol 2000; 20(3):310.

19 Loughrey MB, McCusker G, Heasley RN, Alkalbani M, McCluggage WG. Clear cell struma ovarii. Histopathology 2003; 43(5):495–497.

20 Burg J, Kommoss F, Bittinger F, Moll R, Kirkpatrick CJ. Mature cystic teratoma of the ovary with struma and benign Brenner tumor: a case report with immunohistochemical characterization. Int J Gynecol Pathol 2002; 21(1):74–77.

21 Utsunomiya D, Shiraishi S, Kawanaka K, et al. Struma ovarii coexisting with mucinous cystadenoma detected by radioactive iodine. Clin Nucl Med 2003; 28(9):725–727.

22 Young RH. New and unusual aspects of ovarian germ cell tumors. Am J Surg Pathol 1993; 17(12):1210–1224.

23 Balasch J, Pahisa J, Marquez M, et al. Metastatic ovarian strumosis in an in-vitro fertilization patient. Hum Reprod 1993; 8(12): 2075–2077.

24 Robboy SJ, Scully RE. Strumal carcinoid of the ovary: an analysis of 50 cases of a distinctive tumor composed of thyroid tissue and carcinoid. Cancer 1980; 46(9): 2019–2034.

25 Hamazaki S, Okino T, Tsukayama C, Okada S. Expression of thyroid transcription factor-1 in strumal carcinoid and struma ovarii: an immunohistochemical study. Pathol Int 2002; 52(7):458–462.

26 Tsubura A, Sasaki M. Strumal carcinoid of the ovary. Ultrastructural and immunohistochemical study. Acta Pathol Jpn 1986; 36(9):1383–1390.

27 Kimura N, Sasano N, Namiki T. Evidence of hybrid cell of thyroid follicular cell and carcinoid cell in strumal carcinoid. Int J Gynecol Pathol 1986; 5(3):269–277.

28 Braunschweig R, Hurlimann J, Gloor E, et al. Ovarian carcinoid tumors: immunohistochemical and ultrastructural study of 8 cases Ann Pathol 1994; 14:155–162.

29 Armes JE, Ostor AG. A case of malignant strumal carcinoid. Gynecol Oncol 1993; 51(3):419–423.

30 Young RH. New and unusual aspects of ovarian germ cell tumors. Am J Surg Pathol 1993; 17(12):1210–1224.

31 Makani S, Kim W, Gaba AR. Struma ovarii with a focus of papillary thyroid cancer: a case report and review of the literature. Gynecol Oncol 2004; 94(3):835–839.

32 Sussman SK, Kho SA, Cersosimo E, Heimann A. Coexistence of malignant struma ovarii and Graves' disease. Endocr Pract 2002; 8(5):378–380.

33 DeSimone CP, Lele SM, Modesitt SC. Malignant struma ovarii: a case report and analysis of cases reported in the literature with focus on survival and I131 therapy. Gynecol Oncol 2003; 89(3):543–548.

34 Oestreicher-Kedem Y, Halpern M, Roizman P, et al. Diagnostic value of galectin-3 as a marker for malignancy in follicular patterned thyroid lesions. Head Neck 2004; 26(11):960–966.

35 Kimura ET, Nikiforova MN, Zhu Z, Knauf JA, et al. High prevalence of BRAF mutations in thyroid cancer: genetic evidence for constitutive activation of the RET/PTC-RAS-BRAF signaling pathway in papillary thyroid carcinoma. Cancer Res 2003; 63(7):1454–1457.

36 Soga J, Osaka M, Yakuwa Y. Carcinoids of the ovary: an analysis of 329 reported cases. J Exp Clin Cancer Res 2000; 19(3):271–280.

37 Davis KP, Hartmann LK, Keeney GL, Shapiro H. Primary ovarian carcinoid tumors. Gynecol Oncol 1996; 61(2):259–265.

38 Robboy SJ, Scully RE, Norris HJ. Carcinoid metastatic to the ovary. A clinicopathologic analysis of 35 cases. Cancer 1974; 33(3):798–811.

39 Robboy SJ, Norris HJ, Scully RE. Insular carcinoid primary in the ovary. A clinicopathologic analysis of 48 cases. Cancer 1975; 36(2):404–418.

40 Talerman A. Carcinoid tumors of the ovary. J Cancer Res Clin Oncol 1984; 107(2):125–135.

41 Robboy SJ, Scully RE, Norris HJ. Primary trabecular carcinoid of the ovary. Obstet Gynecol 1977; 49(2):202–207.

42 Ren JH, Chang DY, Huang SC. Primary trabecular carcinoid tumor of the ovary. Int J Gynaecol Obstet 1996; 52(2):195–196.

43 Tsubura A, Sasaki M. Strumal carcinoid of the ovary. Ultrastructural and immunohistochemical study. Acta Pathol Jpn 1986; 36(9):1383–1390.

44 Talerman A, Evans MI. Primary trabecular carcinoid tumor of the ovary. Cancer 1982; 50(7):1403–1407.

45 Baker PM, Oliva E, Young RH, Talerman A, Scully RE. Ovarian mucinous carcinoids including some with a carcinomatous component: a report of 17 cases. Am J Surg Pathol 2001; 25(5):557–568.

46 Robboy SJ, Scully RE, Norris HJ. Carcinoid metastatic to the ovary. A clinicopathologic analysis of 35 cases. Cancer 1974; 33(3):798–811.

47 Ikeda E, Tsutsumi Y, Yoshida H, Yanagi K. Goblet cell carcinoid of the vermiform appendix with ovarian metastasis mimicking mucinous cystadenocarcinoma. Acta Pathol Jpn 1991; 41(6):455–460.

48 Mandai M, Konishi I, Tsuruta Y, et al. Krukenberg tumor from an occult appendiceal adenocarcinoid: a case report and review of the literature. Eur J Obstet Gynecol Reprod Biol 2001; 97(1):90–95.

49 Kim SM, Choi HS, Byun JS, et al. Mucinous adenocarcinoma and strumal carcinoid tumor arising in one mature cystic teratoma of the ovary with synchronous cervical cancer. J Obstet Gynaecol Res 2003; 29(1):28–32.

50 Robboy SJ. Insular carcinoid of ovary associated with malignant mucinous tumors. Cancer 1984; 54(10): 2273–2276.

51 Ribeiro-Silva A, Chang D, Bisson FW, Re LO. Clinicopathological and immunohistochemical features of a sebaceous carcinoma arising within a benign dermoid cyst of the ovary. Virchows Arch 2003; 443(4):574–578.

52 Sumi T, Ishiko O, Maeda K, et al. Adenocarcinoma arising from respiratory ciliated epithelium in mature ovarian cystic teratoma. Arch Gynecol Obstet 2002; 267(2):107–109.

53 Lim SC, Choi SJ, Suh CH. A case of small cell carcinoma arising in a mature cystic teratoma of the ovary. Pathol Int 1998; 48(10):834–839.

54 Ueda G, Fujita M, Ogawa H, et al. Adenocarcinoma in a benign cystic teratoma of the ovary: report of a case with a long survival period. Gynecol Oncol 1993; 48(2):259–263.

55 Olah KS, Needham PG, Jones B. Multiple neuroectodermal tumors arising in a mature cystic teratoma of the ovary. Gynecol Oncol 1989; 34(2):222–225.

56 Bjersing L, Cajander S, Rogo K, Ottosson UB, Stendahl U. Glioblastoma multiform in a dermoid cyst of the ovary. Eur J Gynaecol Oncol 1989; 10(6):389–392.

57 Mahdavi A, Silberberg B, Malviya VK, Braunstein AH, Shapiro J. Gangliocytic paraganglioma arising from mature cystic teratoma of the ovary. Gynecol Oncol 2003; 90(2):482–485.

58 Vimla N, Kumar L, Thulkar S, Bal S, Dawar R. Primary malignant melanoma in ovarian cystic teratoma. Gynecol Oncol 2001; 82(2):380–383.

59 Aygun B, Kimpo M, Lee T, et al. An adolescent with ovarian osteosarcoma arising in a cystic teratoma. J Pediatr Hematol Oncol 2003; 25(5):410–413.

60 Ulbright TM. Gonadal teratomas: a review and speculation. Adv Anat Pathol 2004; 11(1):10–23.

61 Stettner AR, Hartenbach EM, Schink JC, et al. Familial ovarian germ cell cancer: report and review. Am J Med Genet 1999; 84(1):43–46.

62 Bjorkholm E, Lundell M, Gyftodimos A, Silfversward C. Dysgerminoma. The Radiumhemmet series 1927–1984. Cancer 1990; 65:38–44.

63 De Palo G, Lattuada A, Kenda R, et al. Germ cell tumors of the ovary: the experience of the National Cancer Institute of Milan. I. Dysgerminoma. Int J Radiat Oncol Biol Phys 1987; 13:853–860.

64 Gordon A, Lipton D, Woodruff JD. Dysgerminoma: a review of 158 cases from the Emil Novak Ovarian Tumor Registry. Obstet Gynecol 1981; 58:497–504.

65 Kawai M, Kano T, Kikkawa F, et al. Seven tumor markers in benign and malignant germ cell tumors of the ovary. Gynecol Oncol 1992; 45:248–253.

66 Mullin TJ, Lankerani MR. Ovarian dysgerminoma: immunocytochemical localization of human chorionic gonadotropin in the germinoma cell cytoplasm. Obstet Gynecol 1986; 68:80S–83S.

67 Lifschitz-Mercer B, Walt H, Kushnir I, et al. Differentiation potential of ovarian dysgerminoma: an immunohistochemical study of 15 cases. Hum Pathol 1995; 26:62–66.

68 Eglen DE, Ulbright TM. The differential diagnosis of yolk sac tumor and seminoma. Usefulness of cytokeratin, alpha-fetoprotein, and alpha-1-antitrypsin immunoperoxidase reactions. Am J Clin Pathol 1987; 88:328–332.

69 Niehans GA, Manivel JC, Copland GT, Scheithauer BW, Wick MR. Immunohistochemistry of germ cell and trophoblastic neoplasms. Cancer 1988; 62:1113–1123.

70 Segelov E, Campbell J, Ng M, et al. Cisplatin-based chemotherapy for ovarian germ cell malignancies: the Australian experience. J Clin Oncol 1994; 12:378–384.

71 Fujita M, Inoue M, Tanizawa O, et al. Retrospective review of 41 patients with endodermal sinus tumor of the ovary. Int J Gynecol Cancer 1993; 3:329–335.

72 Gershenson DM, Del Junco G, Herson J, Rutledge FN. Endodermal sinus tumor of the ovary: the M. D. Anderson experience. Obstet Gynecol 1983; 61:194–202.

73 Kurman RJ, Norris HJ. Endodermal sinus tumor of the ovary: a clinical and pathologic analysis of 71 cases. Cancer 1976; 38:2404–2419.

74 Ulbright TM, Roth LM, Brodhecker CA. Yolk sac differentiation in germ cell tumors. A morphologic study of 50 cases with emphasis on hepatic, enteric, and parietal yolk sac features. Am J Surg Pathol 1986; 10:151–164.

75 Cohen MB, Friend DS, Molnar JJ, Talerman A. Gonadal endodermal sinus (yolk sac) tumor with pure intestinal differentiation: a new histologic type. Pathol Res Pract 1987; 182:609–616.

76 Clement PB, Young RH, Scully RE. Endometrioid-like variant of ovarian yolk sac tumor. A clinicopathological analysis of eight cases. Am J Surg Pathol 1987; 11:767–778.

77 Kawai M, Furuhashi Y, Kano T, et al. Alpha-fetoprotein in malignant germ cell tumors of the ovary. Gynecol Oncol 1990; 39:160–166.

78 Kurman RJ, Norris HJ. Embryonal carcinoma of the ovary: a clinicopathologic entity distinct from endodermal sinus tumor resembling embryonal carcinoma of the adult testis. Cancer 1976; 38:2420–2433.

79 Morris HH, La Vecchia C, Draper GJ. Endodermal sinus tumor and embryonal carcinoma of the ovary in children. Gynecol Oncol 1985; 21:7–17.

80 King ME, Hubbell MJ, Talerman A. Mixed germ cell tumor of the ovary with a prominent polyembryoma component. Int J Gynecol Pathol 1991; 10:88–95.

81 Tsukahara Y, Fukuta T, Yamada T, Nakai I. Retroperitoneal giant tumor formed by migrating polyembryoma with numerous embryoid bodies from an ovarian mixed germ cell tumor. Gynecol Obstet Invest 1991; 31:58–60.

82 Nakashima N, Murakami S, Fukatsu T, et al. Characteristics of 'embryoid body' in human gonadal germ cell tumors. Hum Pathol 1988; 19:1144–1154.

83 Takeda A, Ishizuka T, Goto T, et al. Polyembryoma of ovary producing alpha-fetoprotein and HCG: immunoperoxidase and electron microscopic study. Cancer 1982; 49:1878–1889.

84 Chapman DC, Grover R, Schwartz PE. Conservative management of an ovarian polyembryoma. Obstet Gynecol 1994; 83:879–882.

85 Axe SR, Klein VR, Woodruff JD. Choriocarcinoma of the ovary. Obstet Gynecol 1985; 66:111–114.

86 Gerbie MV, Brewer JI, Tamimi H. Primary choriocarcinoma of the ovary. Obstet Gynecol 1975; 46:720–723.

87 Jacobs AJ, Newland JR, Green RK. Pure choriocarcinoma of the ovary. Obstet Gynecol Surv 1982; 37:603–609.

88 Vance RP, Geisinger KR. Pure nongestational choriocarcinoma of the ovary. Report of a case. Cancer 1985; 56:2321–2325.

89 Vogler C, Schmidt WA, Edwards CL. Primary ovarian nongestational choriocarcinoma. Report of a case in a young woman of childbearing age. Diagn Gynecol Obstet 1981; 3:331–336.

90 Wheeler CA, Davis S, Degefu S, Thorneycroft IH, O'Quinn AG. Ovarian choriocarcinoma: a difficult diagnosis of an unusual tumor and a review of the hook effect. Obstet Gynecol 1990; 75:547–549.

91 Axe SR, Klein VR, Woodruff JD. Choriocarcinoma of the ovary. Obstet Gynecol 1985; 66:111–114.

92 Norris HJ, Zirkin HJ, Benson WL. Immature (malignant) teratoma of the ovary: a clinical and pathologic study of 58 cases. Cancer 1976; 37(5):2359–2372.

93 O'Connor DM, Norris HJ. The influence of grade on the outcome of stage I ovarian immature (malignant) teratomas and the reproducibility of grading. Int J Gynecol Pathol 1994; 13(4):283–289.

94 Gershenson DM. Management of early ovarian cancer: germ cell and sex cord-stromal tumors. Gynecol Oncol 1994; 55(3 Pt 2):S62–S72.

95 Aziz MF. Current management of malignant germ cell tumor of the ovary. Gan To Kagaku Ryoho 1995; 22(Suppl 3):262–276.

96 Carinelli SG, Senzani F, Luzzani S, Carinelli I, Cefis F. Immature teratoma of the ovary stage IA(i) treated with conservative surgery alone. Tumori 1981; 67:575–580.

97 Yanai-Inbar I, Scully RE. Relation of ovarian dermoid cysts and immature teratomas: an analysis of 350 cases of immature teratoma and 10 cases of dermoid cyst with microscopic foci of immature tissue. Int J Gynecol Pathol 1987; 6:203–212.

98 Thurlbeck WM, Scully RE. Solid teratoma of the ovary. A clinicopathological analysis of 9 cases. Cancer 1960; 13:804–811.

99 Heifetz SA, Cushing B, Giller R, et al. Immature teratomas in children: pathologic considerations: a report from the combined Pediatric Oncology Group/Children's Cancer Group. Am J Surg Pathol 1998; 22:1115–1124.

100 Cushing B, Giller R, Ablin A, et al. Surgical resection alone is effective treatment for ovarian immature teratoma in children and adolescents: a report of the pediatric oncology group and the children's cancer group. Am J Obstet Gynecol 1999; 181:353–358. .

101 Moskovic E, Jobling T, Fisher C, Wiltshaw E, Parsons C. Retroconversion of immature teratoma of the ovary: CT appearances. Clin Radiol 1991; 43:402–408.

102 Ferguson AW, Katabuchi H, Ronnett BM, Cho KR. Glial implants in gliomatosis peritonei arise from normal tissue, not from the associated teratoma. Am J Pathol 2001; 159(1):51–55.

103 Best DH, Butz GM, Moller K, Coleman WB, Thomas DB. Molecular analysis of an immature ovarian teratoma with gliomatosis peritonei and recurrence suggests genetic independence of multiple tumors. Int J Oncol 2004; 25(1):17–25.

104 Kwan MY, Kalle W, Lau GT, Chan JK. Is gliomatosis peritonei derived from the associated ovarian teratoma? Hum Pathol 2004; 35(6):685–688.

105 Gallion H, van Nagell JR Jr, Donaldson ES, Hanson MB, Powell DF. Immature teratoma of the ovary. Am J Obstet Gynecol 1983; 146(4):361–365.

106 Koulos JP, Hoffman JS, Steinhoff MM. Immature teratoma of the ovary. Gynecol Oncol 1989; 34(1):46-49.

107 Itani Y, Kawa M, Toyoda S, Yamagami K, Hiraoka K. Growing teratoma syndrome after chemotherapy for a mixed germ cell tumor of the ovary. J Obstet Gynaecol Res 2002; 28(3):166–171.

108 Skof E, Grasic Kuhar C, Cerar O, Zakotnik B. Survival and fertility of patients with malignant ovarian germ cell tumours. Eur J Gynaecol Oncol 2004; 25(6):702–706.

109 Schultz KA, Sencer SF, Messinger Y, Neglia JP, Steiner ME. Pediatric ovarian tumors: a review of 67 cases. Pediatr Blood Cancer 2005; 44(2):167–173.

110 Zuntova A, Sumerauer D, Teslik L, Kabickova E, Koutecky J. Mixed germ cell tumours of the ovary in childhood and adolescence. Cesk Patol 2004; 40(3):92–101.

111 Curtin JP, Morrow CP, D'Ablaing G, Schlaerth JB. Malignant germ cell tumors of the ovary: 20-year report of LAC-USC Women's Hospital. Int J Gynecol Cancer 1994; 4(1):29–35.

112 Low JJ, Perrin LC, Crandon AJ, Hacker NF. Conservative surgery to preserve ovarian function in patients with malignant ovarian germ cell tumors. A review of 74 cases. Cancer 2000; 89(2):391–398.

113 Tewari K, Cappuccini F, Disaia PJ, et al. Malignant germ cell tumors of the ovary. Obstet Gynecol 2000; 95(1):128–133.

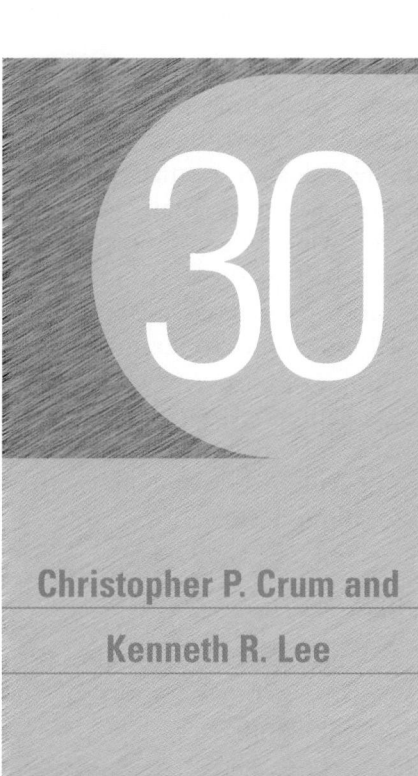

30

Sex cord-stromal and miscellaneous tumors of the ovary

Christopher P. Crum and

Kenneth R. Lee

Introduction

Histogenesis
Frequency and clinical
significance
The patient at risk

A histopathologic algorithm of sex cord-stromal tumors

Classification of sex cord-stromal tumors

Fibroma
Cellular fibroma and fibrosarcoma
Thecomas
Granulosa and granulosa-theca
cell tumors

Sertoli and Sertoli–Leydig cell
tumors
Gynandroblastoma
Sex cord tumor with annular
tubules (SCTAT)
Sex cord-stromal tumor
unclassified
Steroid cell tumors
Other stromal tumors

Other ovarian tumors

Poorly-differentiated (small round
cell) tumors of the ovary
Other rare ovarian neoplasms
of uncertain classification

Introduction

HISTOGENESIS

Sex cord-stromal tumors of the ovary comprise a diverse collection of tumors that are derived from the ovarian cortical and hilar cells (Fig. 30.1). These cells form during embryogenesis as condensations of sub-coelomic mesenchyme, in the form of the 'sex cords', which ultimately differentiate into the supporting stroma of the cortex and the granulosa-theca cells of the developing follicle in the adult ovary. The same pro-genitor cells diverge to form the Sertoli and Leydig cells of the testis and a subset closely resembling Leydig cells form the hilar cells of the ovary. The range of embryonic and adult differentiation seen in these stromal and supporting cells explains the complexity of tumor phenotypes attributed to them (Fig. 30.2).[1,2]

FREQUENCY AND CLINICAL SIGNIFICANCE

As a group, with the exception of highly malignant small cell carcinomas of the ovary which are of uncertain histogenesis, sex cord-stromal tumors behave as benign tumors (fibromas, thecomas) or low-grade malignancies (granulosa, Sertoli–Leydig cell tumors, steroid cell tumors). The principal diagnostic problems attributed to sex cord-stromal tumors are due to their rarity. Sex cord-stromal tumors constitute less than 10% of all ovarian tumors.[2] Moreover, of these, nearly 90% are common fibromas (or fibrothecomas) which are easily recognized. This leaves a small group of tumors that account for no more than 1% of all ovarian tumors that have a wide range of morphologic presentations. More than half of these are granulosa cell tumors. Hence, most patients dying of a sex cord-stromal tumor will succumb to granulosa cell tumor.

The purpose of this chapter is to organize these tumors into groups that can be readily recognized by the pathologist and to provide diagnostic alternatives to minimize the chance of misclassification.

THE PATIENT AT RISK

Table 30.1 outlines the clinical features associated with the more common sex cord-stromal tumors of the ovary.[3] They include the following:

Frequency

Fibromas, thecomas and fibroma-thecomas account for approximately 87% of all tumors in the sex cord-stromal group. These, along with adult granulosa cell tumors, Sertoli–Leydig cell tumors and sclerosing stromal tumors, account for approximately 99% of sex cord-stromal tumors. The remaining are exceedingly rare and, with the exception of those encountered by

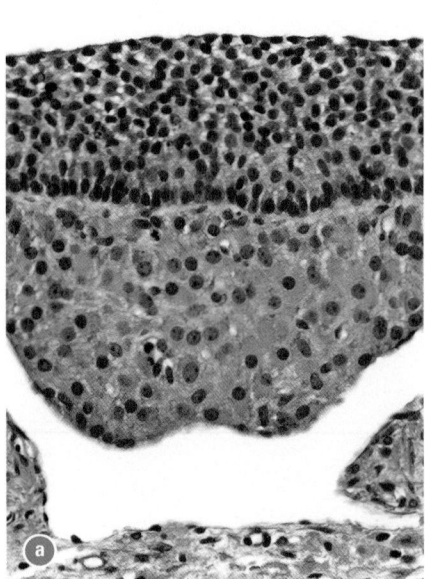 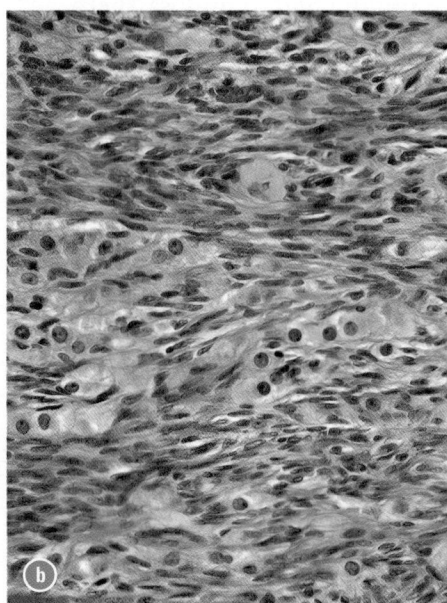 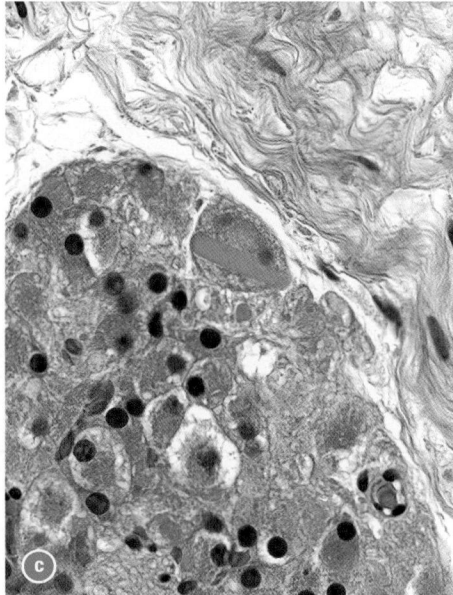

Fig. 30.1 Normal ovarian counterparts of sex cord-stromal tumors. (a) Granulosa (upper) and theca cells (lower) of the normal ovarian follicle. (b) Ovarian stroma containing luteinized stromal cells. (c) Hilar cells. A Reinke crystalloid is present (center).

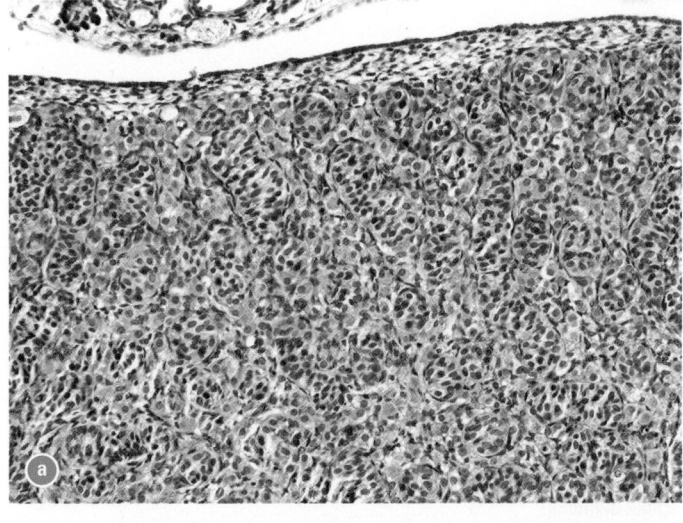

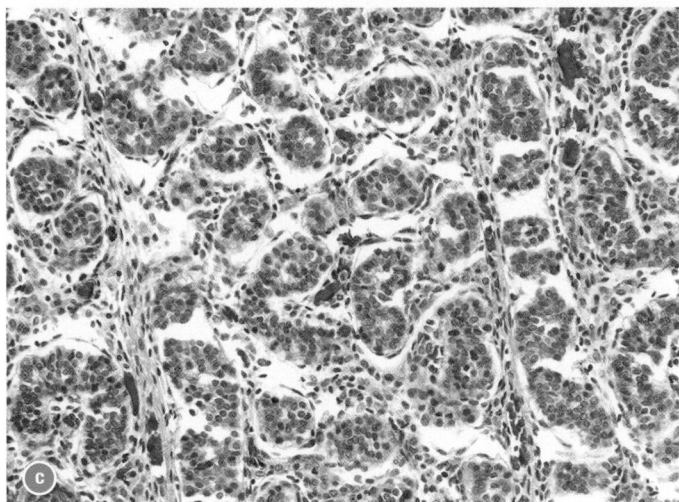

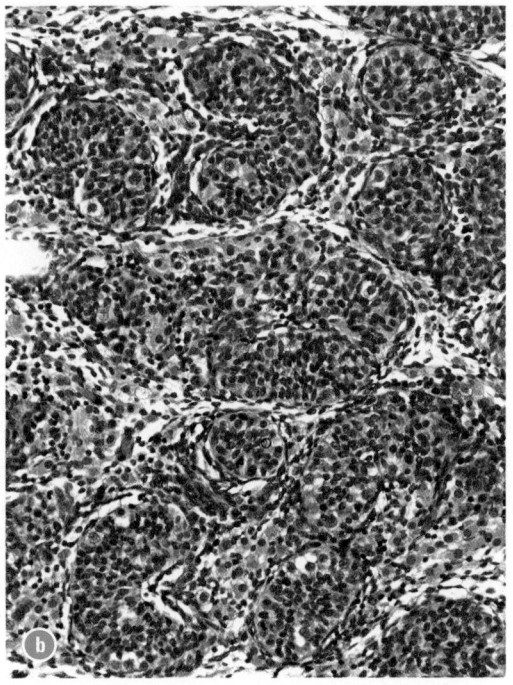

Fig. 30.2 Normal testicular counterparts to sex cord-stromal tumors. Normal Sertoli (tubules or cords) and Leydig (pink cells) cells at (a) 15, (b) 22 and (c) 36 weeks' gestation.

authors with a larger referral base, are the subject of case reports and small series.[2]

Age

Different subsets of sex cord-stromal tumors predominate in women of four age ranges. These include: premenarchal, under 25 years, 25–50 years and postmenopausal. Those most likely to occur in premenarchal girls are the juvenile granulosa cell tumors (JGCTs). Between menarche and 25 years, JGCT and Sertoli–Leydig cell tumors predominate. In the 25–50 year age group fibroma-thecomas and granulosa cell tumors are found. Beyond menopause, in addition to fibromas and steroid cell tumors, rare malignancies such as fibrosarcomas emerge. Age incidence is a useful guideline to the pathologist who is faced with a stromal tumor on frozen section. However, all of these tumors can be seen over a wide age range.[2]

Presenting signs and symptoms

The most common tumors (fibromas) present simply as a mass. Granulosa-theca and Sertoli–Leydig cell tumors may, in addition, cause symptoms referable to hyperestrinism and hyperandrogenism (virilization), respectively, or to either of these (steroid cell tumors). Some are associated with specific syndromes or other tumors, such as Meigs' or Gorlin's syndrome (fibroma), Ollier's disease or Maffucci's syndrome (granulosa-theca cell tumor) and either Peutz–Jeghers syndrome or minimal deviation carcinoma of the cervix (sex cord-stromal tumor with annular tubules).[2]

Outcome

Table 30.2 summarizes the outcomes associated with sex cord-stromal tumors. These tumors are generally benign or behave as lower-risk malignancies with long natural histories relative to epithelial tumors. The low-

Table 30.1 *Frequency and presentation of sex cord-stromal tumors[3]*

Type	Frequency[a]	Mean age (range)	Presenting symptoms	Bilateral (%)	Other
Fibroma	70	48 (17–79)	Mass	8	Meigs', Gorlin's syndromes
Thecoma-fibrothecoma	17	59(19–80)	PMB, mass	3	EM Hyper EMCA (20%)
GTCT (A)	7	57(40–83)	PMB, mass	9	EM Hyper EMCA (7%)
GTCT (J)	<1	12(0–67)	Isosexual precocity, abnormal bleeding	1–2	Ollier's disease Maffucci's syndrome
SLCT	3	25(2–75)	Virilizing (38%) amenorrhea, abnormal bleeding	1–2	
Sex cord tumor unclassified	<1	49(12–83)	Mass, PMB	1–2	
Sclerosing stromal tumor	2	27(14–51)	Mass, vaginal bleeding	0	
Stromal luteoma	<1	47(3–80)	Virilizing, hyperestrinism	0	
Hilar, stromal Leydig CT	<1	58(32–82)	Virilizing	Rare	
Steroid CT NOS	<1	43(3–80)	Virilizing Estrogen Cushing's syndrome	6%	
SCTAT (+)PJS	<1	27(4–57)	Asymptomatic	50	Adenoma malignum
SCTAT (–)PJS	<1	34(6–76)	Mass, abnormal bleeding	0	

[a]As percentage of sex cord-stromal tumors. PMB, postmenopausal bleeding; GTCT, granulosa-theca cell tumor – (A) adult, (J) juvenile; SLCT, Sertoli–Leydig cell tumor; CT, cell tumor; NOS, not otherwise specified; SCTAT, sex cord tumor with annular tubules; PJS, Peutz–Jeghers syndrome; EM, endometrium(al); EM Hyper, endometrial hyperplasia; EMCA, endometrial carcinoma.

Table 30.2 *Initial stage and outcome of sex cord-stromal tumors*

Type	Stage I (%)	Recurrence (%)	Comments	Ref.
Fibroma	100	<1	Rare recurring cellular fibroma	4, 6
Thecoma-fibroma	100	<1	Rare reports of metastasizing thecoma	8
Fibrosarcoma	100	100	Few reported cases	6
GTCT (A)	93	20–30	Late metastases	20, 21, 23
GTCT (J)	96	7		15, 16
SLCT (WD)	100	0		25, 26
SLCT (MD)	91	10		24, 25
SLCT (PD)	93	50		24, 25
SLCT (retiform)	100	22		33, 34
SLCT (heterologous elements)	85	21		35, 36
SCT NOS	100	11		40
Sclerosing ST	100	0	Few reported cases	53
Stromal luteoma	100	0		44
Leydig CT	100	0		45
Steroid CT NOS	82	36		44
SCTAT PJ (+)	100	0		37
SCTAT PJ (–)	85	15		37

GTCT, granulosa-theca cell tumor – (A) adult, (J) juvenile; SLCT, Sertoli–Leydig cell tumor; CT, cell tumor; NOS, not otherwise specified; PJ, Peutz–Jeghers syndrome; SCTAT, sex cord tumor with annular tubules.

risk group includes granulosa-theca cell tumors, the more poorly-differentiated Sertoli–Leydig tumors, unclassified sex cord-stromal tumors, steroid cell tumors, and sex cord tumors with annular tubules that are not associated with Peutz–Jeghers syndrome (Table 30.2).

A histopathologic algorithm of sex cord-stromal tumors

Although the classification of sex cord-stromal tumors includes a defined set of entities, these generally may be included within larger morphologic categories allowing a rational approach to diagnosis:

1 Tumor types fall into four general categories: well-differentiated epithelioid or stromal lesions, moderately differentiated mixed epithelioid-stromal lesions, predominately mesenchymal-appearing tumors and tumors with prominent Leydig, lutein or steroid cells.

2 Many tumor types with a defined histogenesis (such as granulosa cell tumor) may fall into more than one of these categories. Thus, recognition of a given tumor depends on not only identifying its cell type but also on distinguishing it from other tumors that may share similar cellular features (such as luteinized fibrothecoma and luteinized granulosa cell tumor).

3 Many primary ovarian and metastatic malignant tumors of epithelial or mesenchymal origin may be confused with sex cord-stromal tumors. This is of particular importance, inasmuch as the natural history of and therapy for these will differ from those of sex cord tumors.

Figures 30.3–30.6 outline the range of diagnostic choices encountered with these tumors and serve as a reference point when considering the differential diagnosis of a given morphologic pattern.

Classification of sex cord-stromal tumors

FIBROMA

Definition

Fibromas are defined as tumors composed of fibrocytes with variable collagen deposition and minimal theca cell-like or luteal differentiation. Fibromas, along with tumors showing partial thecomatous differentiation (fibrothecomas), comprise the largest group of sex

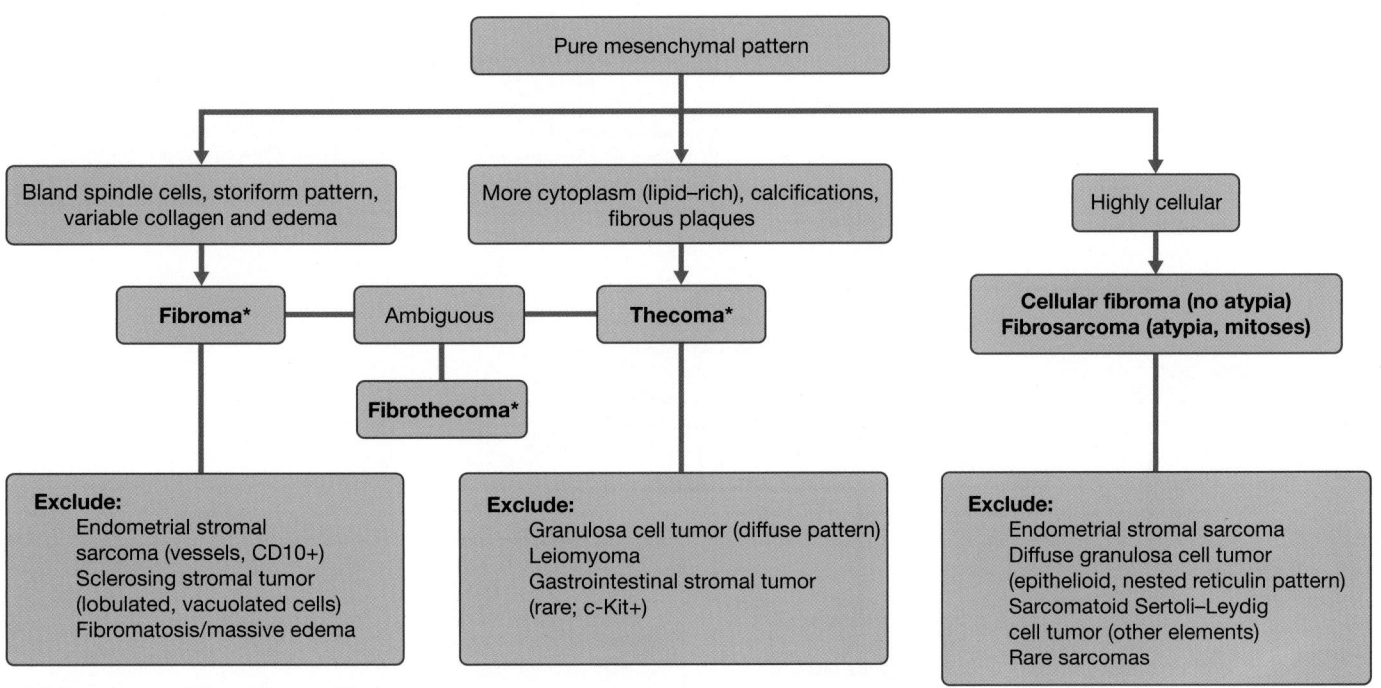

*Minor sex cord elements permitted

Fig. 30.3 Differential diagnosis of pure mesenchymal sex cord-stromal tumors.

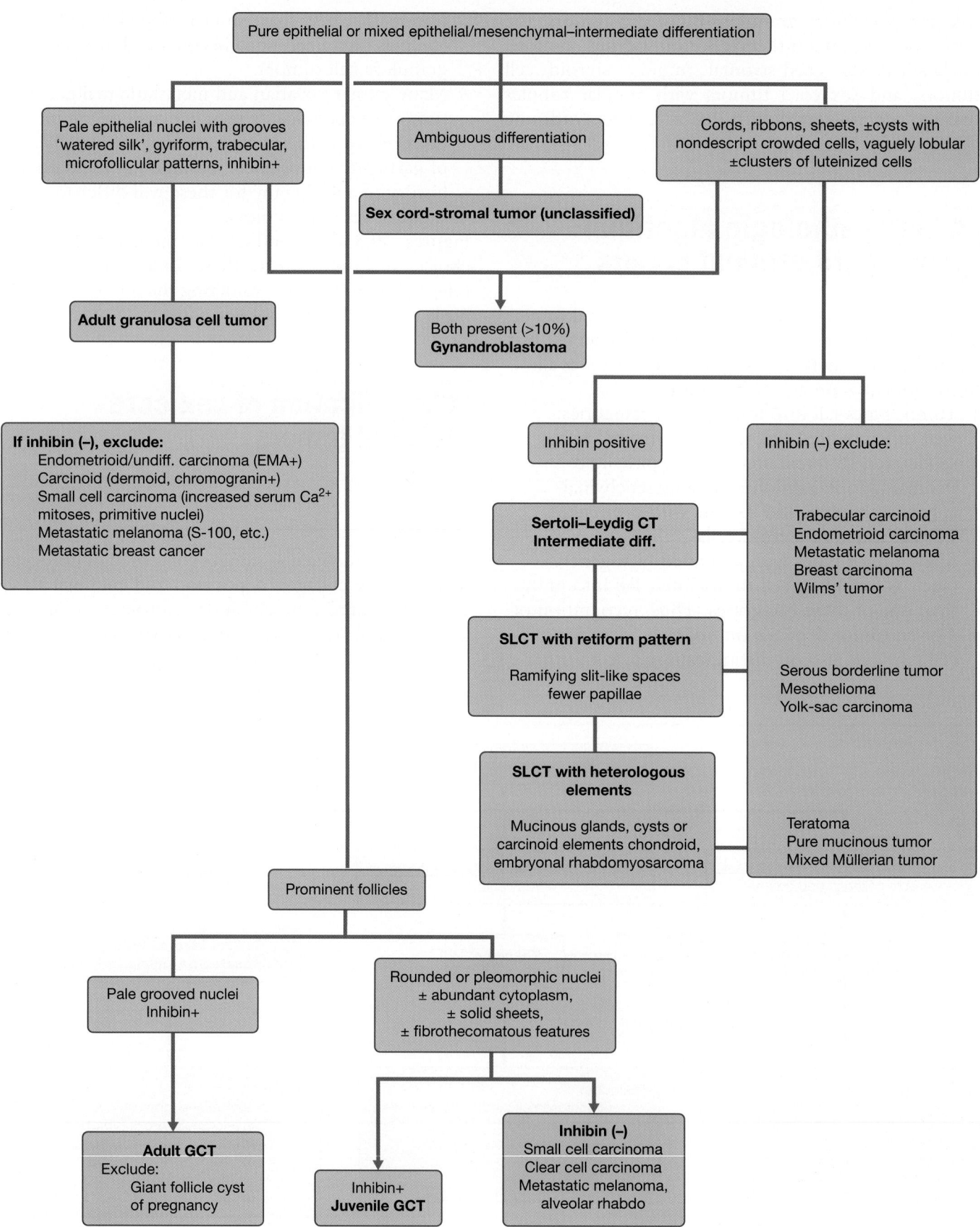

Fig. 30.4 Differential diagnosis of intermediately differentiated sex cord-stromal tumors

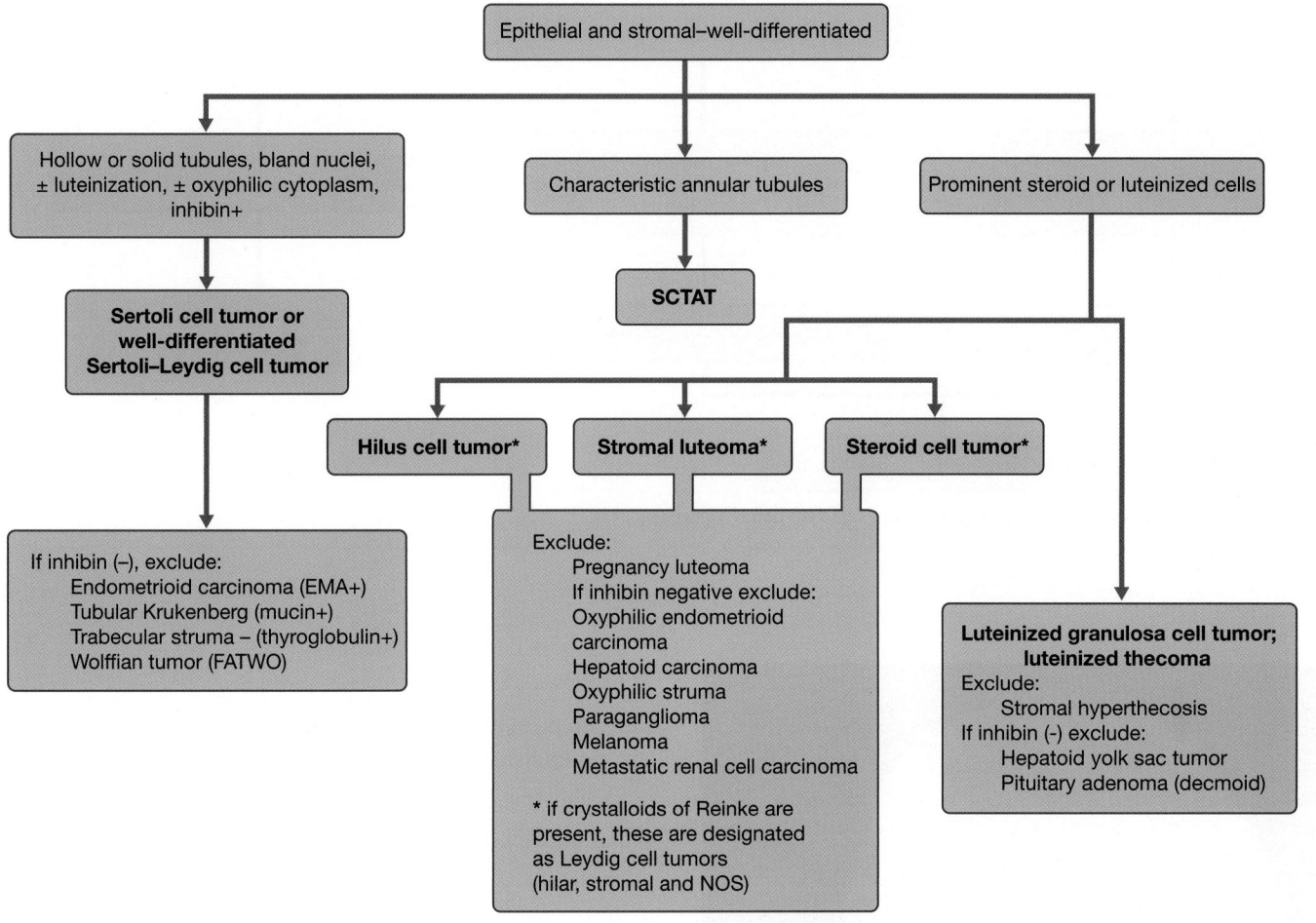

Fig. 30.5 Differential diagnosis of well-differentiated sex cord-stromal tumors

cord-stromal tumors, accounting for approximately 80% of this group.

The patient at risk

Fibromas are uncommon in women under age 30, predominating in the fifth decade, with a mean age of 48 years. Fibromas may be associated with Meigs' syndrome (ascites and pleural effusion) and nevoid basal cell syndrome, but are not linked to appreciable hormonal activity.

Gross features

Fibromas are the most common sex cord-stromal tumor to involve both ovaries (8%). The tumors are predominately smooth-surfaced, solid, firm to rubbery, white to tan, and in some instances, edematous. Infarction and hemorrhage may be present, but is discrete (Fig. 30.7).

Histopathology

The spindled tumor cells of some fibromas are uniformly distributed with moderate cellularity; others may be interrupted by zones of cell-poor collagen.[2] The cells are often arranged in a swirling (storiform) pattern. Nuclei are elongated, small and with inconspicuous nucleoli. Mitotic figures are infrequent in most cases. (Fig. 30.8).

A rare finding of fibroma-thecomas is the presence of minor sex cord elements, presenting as discrete tubules or epithelioid cords that appear abruptly within the spindled stroma (Fig. 30.9a,b). Although a potential cause of confusion in diagnosis, these features do not alter the outcome of these benign tumors.[4]

Differential diagnosis

Typical fibromas are easily recognized, although small ones may be confused with the hypercellularity of

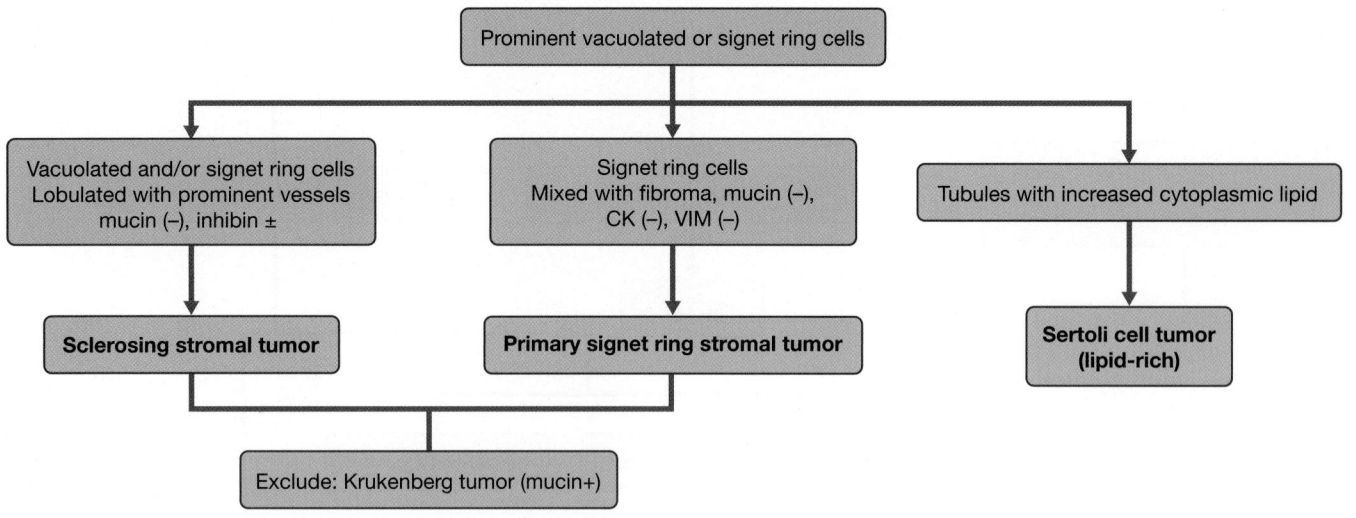

Fig. 30.6 Differential diagnosis of sex cord-stromal tumors with lipid-rich or signet-ring cells.

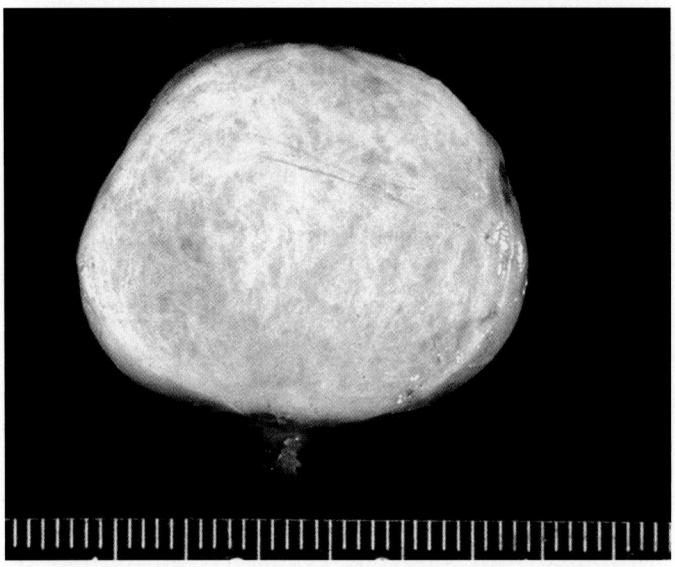

Fig. 30.7 Gross appearance of ovarian fibroma, typically a smooth well-circumscribed mass with a firm consistency and white to tan appearance on sectioning.

the ovarian cortex (fibromatosis) seen in polycystic ovarian disease or stromal hyperthecosis. In some instances it may be impossible to distinguish these from early microscopic fibromas (Fig. 30.10). The preservation of ovarian architecture and atretic follicles in stroma of the latter entities will distinguish them. However, the pathologist may occasionally render a diagnosis of 'microscopic cortical fibroma' if the changes are discrete.

Management and outcome

Fibromas typically do not recur and are cured by simple excision.

CELLULAR FIBROMA AND FIBROSARCOMA

Definition and background

Cellular fibromas and fibrosarcomas will be discussed together, inasmuch as the pathologist must distinguish the two whenever he or she encounters a 'fibroma' with increased cellularity and mitotic activity. Like fibromas,

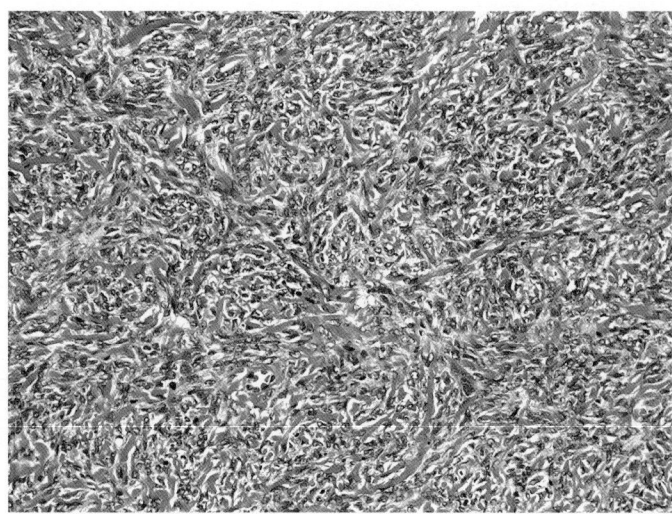

Fig. 30.8 Fibroma with characteristic spindled stromal cells, fibroblasts and abundant collagen matrix.

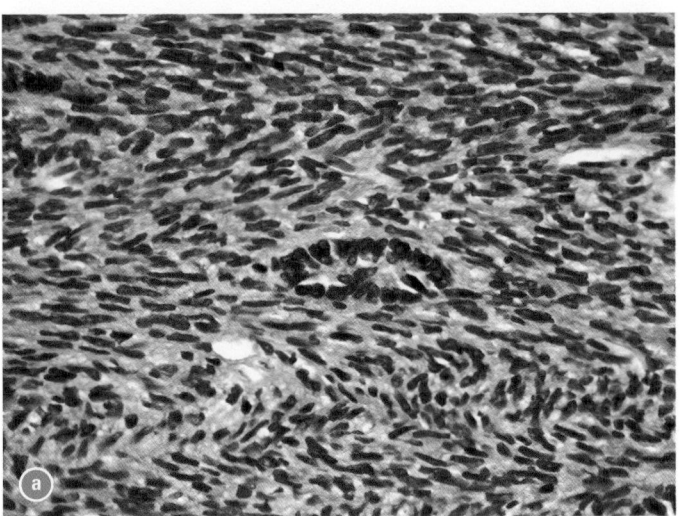 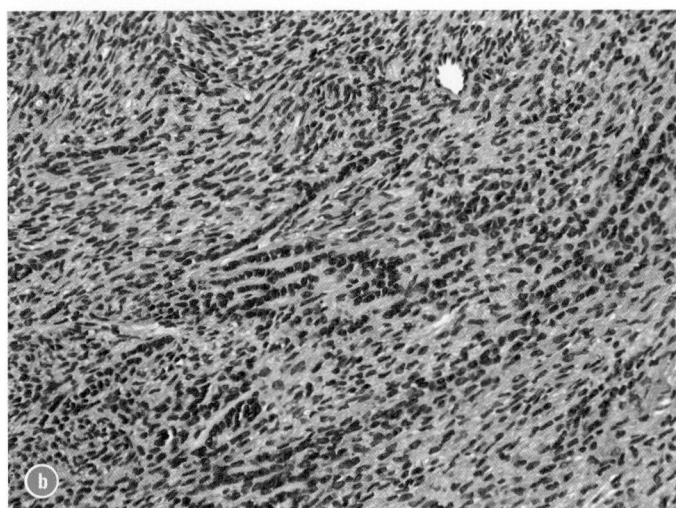

Fig. 30.9 Fibroma with minor sex cord elements. The latter appear as (a) scattered small tubules or (b) cords, in an otherwise conventional-appearing fibromatous stroma.

cellular fibromas and fibrosarcomas predominate in the fifth decade, although sarcomas tend to occur in older women; one fibrosarcoma in a child has been linked to the basal cell nevus syndrome.[5] Both tumors are typically unilateral, and are not readily distinguished on gross examination, although the diameter of cellular fibroma tends to be larger than ordinary fibromas (mean 12 cm in one series, 8 cm in another) and fibrosarcomas even larger (mean 17 cm).[6] Tumors can be solid or partially cystic, soft or rubbery and may contain hemorrhage or necrosis (Fig. 30.11).

Histology

Cellular fibromas and fibrosarcomas are composed of spindle cells arranged in bundles or fascicles, often in a herringbone or storiform pattern (Fig. 30.12a,b). The histologic diagnosis of either requires attention to the following.

Distinguishing between cellular fibroma and fibrosarcoma

Relative to cellular fibromas, fibrosarcomas are very uncommon. In the initial study by Prat and Scully these were distinguished from cellular fibromas based

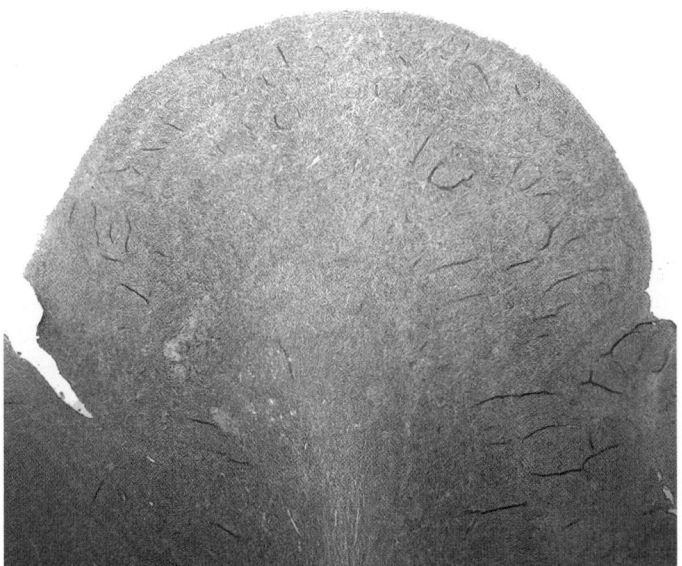

Fig. 30.10 The differential diagnosis of fibroma includes condensations of fibrotic cortical stroma associated with hyperthecosis. In fact, these may be early fibromas.

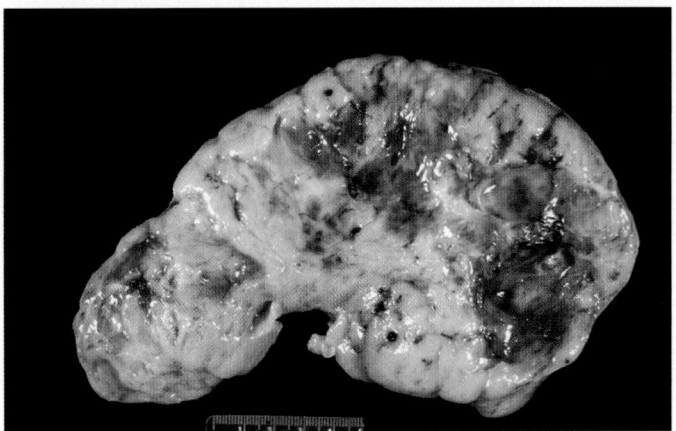

Fig. 30.11 Gross appearance of fibrosarcoma. The consistency is typically softer than fibroma and foci of hemorrhage or necrosis are common.

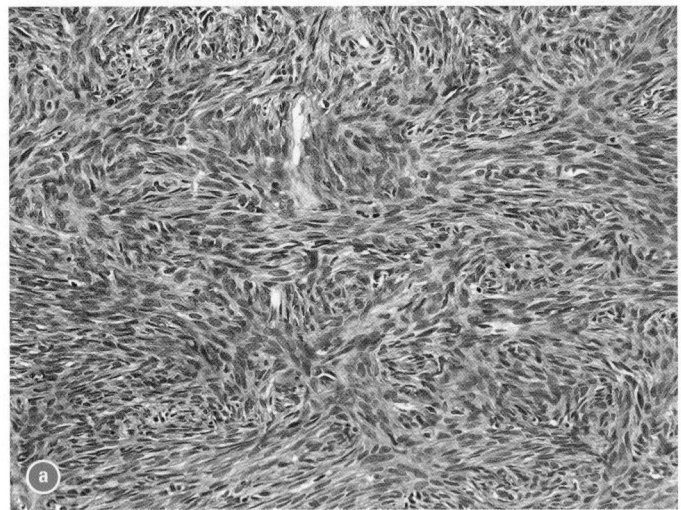

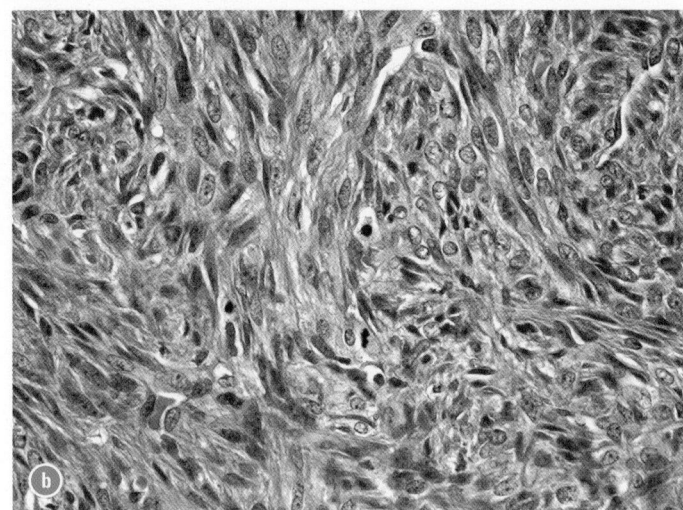

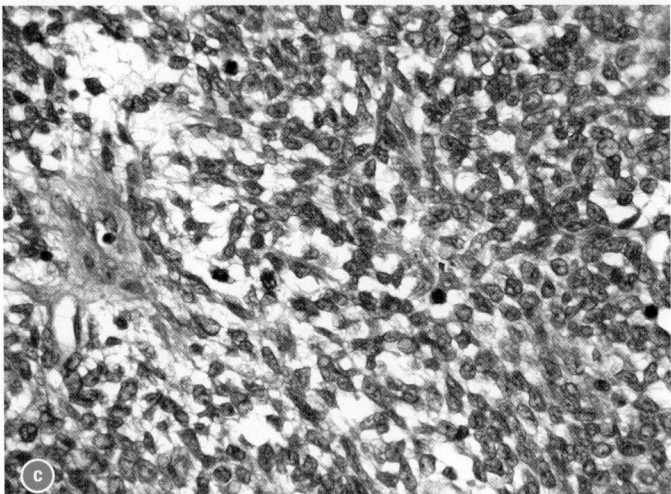

Fig. 30.12 (a) Cellular fibroma. (b) At higher power increased mitotic activity is present (lower middle). (c) Fibrosarcoma, with increased nuclear atypia and mitoses.

on mitotic index (those with >3/10 HPFs (high-power fields) considered sarcomas). The outcome for patients with sarcomas was dismal, all six of them dying from their tumors. However, all cases in this series with recurrences or metastases (including cases classified as cellular fibromas) had either moderate or severe cytologic atypia (Fig. 30.12c).[6] A more recent report of 62 cellular fibromas with bland nuclei disclosed a benign behavior in all 16 of these cases that had a mitotic index >3/10 HPFs (several with >10/10 HPFs).[7] Thus, it appears that mitotically active cellular fibromas without nuclear atypia are essentially benign, although more cases with long-term follow-up are needed.

Exclusion of other mimics

These include diffuse granulosa cell tumor, sarcoma-toid (poorly-differentiated) Sertoli–Leydig cell tumor, endometrial stromal sarcoma leiomyosarcoma (Fig. 30.13a,b) and metastatic gastrointestinal stromal tumor (Fig. 30.13c,d).

Outcome

As above, based on the limited number of reports, fibrosarcoma, defined as a cellular tumor with moderate or severe nuclear atypia and a mitotic index >3/10 HPFs, has a poor prognosis. All of the six cases in the study by Prat and Scully either died or recurred with distant metastases.[6] However, two of 11 patients with cellular fibroma also succumbed, both displaying moderate atypia, but fewer than four mitoses/10 HPFs. However, these cases were also complicated by higher stage and management by limited (oophorectomy) or incomplete removal.[6] Based on this experience, both pathologists and clinicians should carefully review the histologic diagnosis and management options when

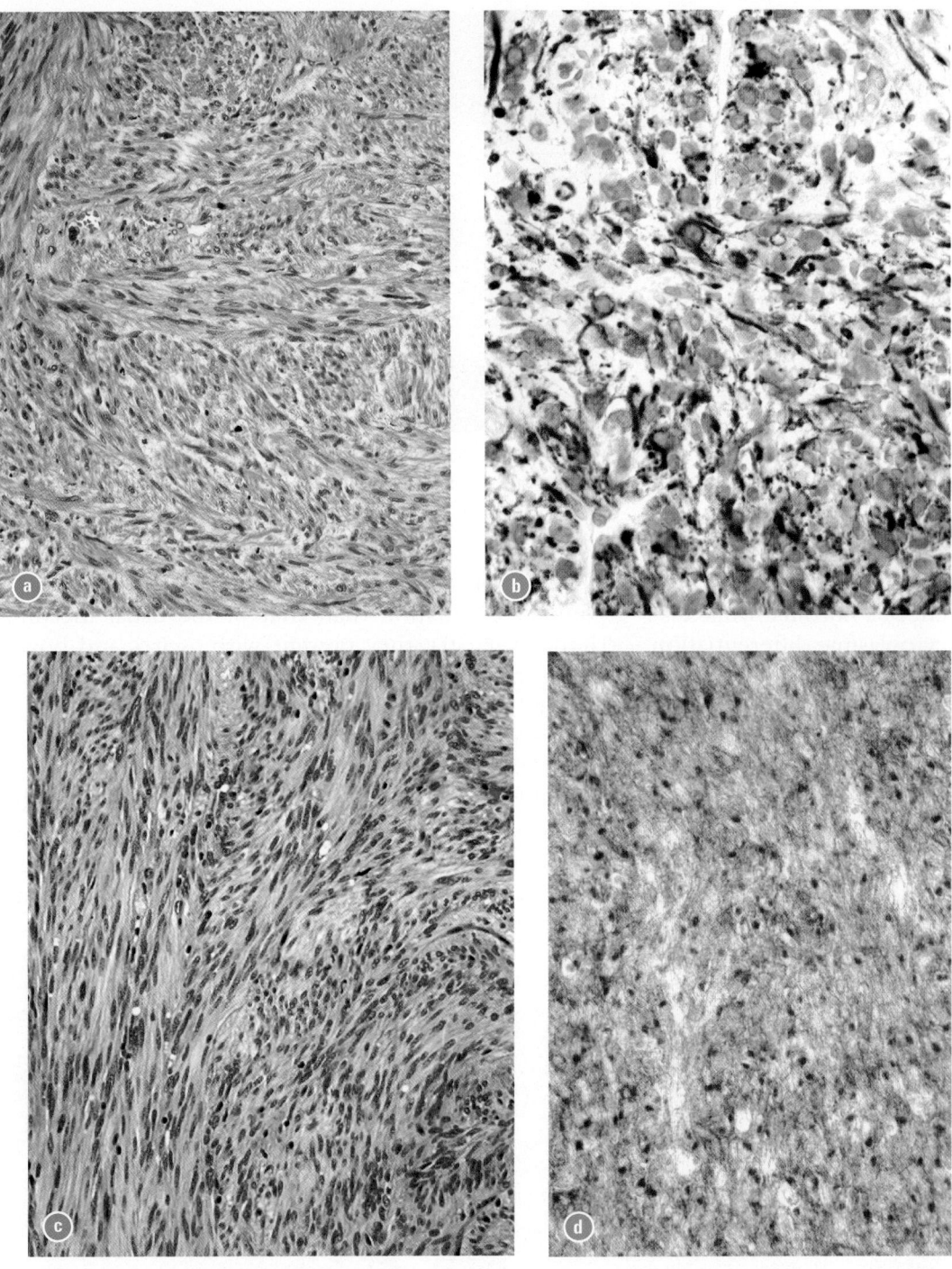

Fig. 30.13 Mimics of cellular fibroma/ fibrosarcoma include (a) leiomyosarcoma. (b) Following staining for desmin. (c) Gastrointestinal stromal tumor. (d) Following staining for c-Kit.

faced with any fibromatous tumor that appears aggressive despite a low mitotic index.

THECOMAS

Definition

Thecomas are defined as tumors that recapitulate the thecal cells of the follicle and are composed of a minimum (less than 10%) of cells with granulosa cell differentiation. Pure thecomas, lacking either a significant fibromatous or granulosa cell component (classified as fibrothecomas or granulosa-theca cell tumors, respectively), are rare. They are only one-third as common as granulosa cell tumors, and account for less than 1% of all ovarian tumors. Much more common are so-called fibrothecomas, made up of mixtures of the two tumor patterns.

The patient at risk

The typical patient with a thecoma is approximately 10 years older than that those with fibromas, with a mean age of 59. At least one-half of cases are associated with hyperestrinism, usually in the form of abnormal uterine bleeding; one-fifth are associated with endometrial adenocarcinoma.[8]

Gross features

Thecomas, as is the case with all of the sex cord-stromal tumors (excepting fibroma), are rarely bilateral (less than 5%).[8] They present as firm, smooth-surfaced, homogeneous tan to yellow tumors (Fig. 30.14).

Histopathology

Thecomas form an intermediate in a morphologic spectrum, bridging fibromas and the diffuse variant of granulosa cell tumor. The tumor cells are fusiform, forming parallel arrangements in dense collagen, often with calcifications, reminiscent of a fibroma, while displaying a higher degree of cytoplasmic differentiation and vesicular nuclei with delicate nuclear membranes akin to those of granulosa cell tumors (Fig. 30.15).

A proportion of thecomas are luteinized. In this variant, a variable proportion of the cells exhibit a lower nuclear/cytoplasmic ratio (Fig. 30.16). These tumors are associated with hyperestrinism in 50% of cases and in a small percentage, hyperandrogenism.[9,10] A rare condition coexisting with luteinized thecomas

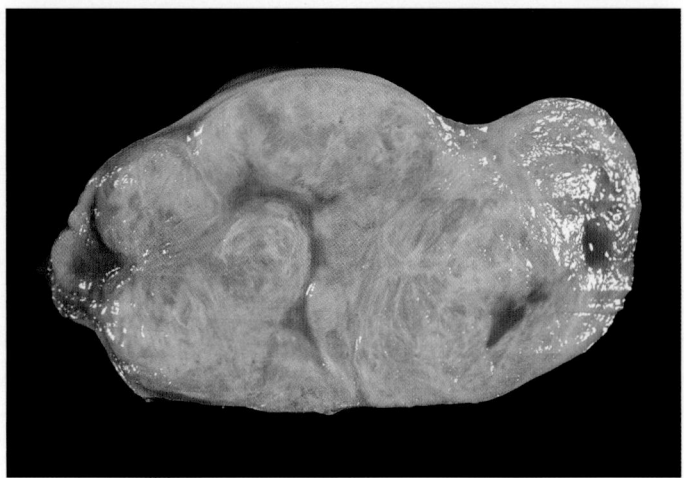

Fig. 30.14 Gross appearance of fibrothecoma. These tumors typically are firm and have a tan to yellow appearance.

is *sclerosing peritonitis*.[11] This process is found in a younger population than that of the usual thecoma (under age 30); they present with ascites and bowel symptoms. The peritoneal surfaces exhibit fibrosis and a mixed inflammatory cell infiltrate (Fig. 30.17).

Differential diagnosis

The differential diagnosis of thecoma includes the following (summarized in Fig. 30.3): (1) Granulosa cell tumors with a diffuse pattern of growth. Although there is some overlap, reticulin stains will delineate

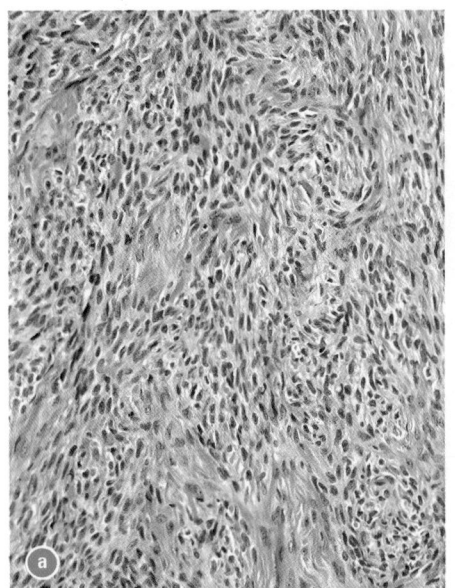
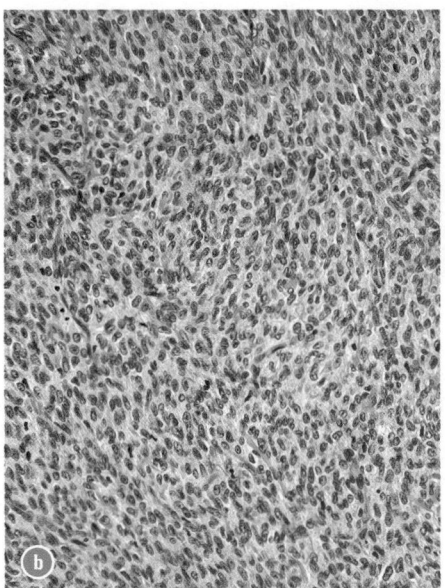
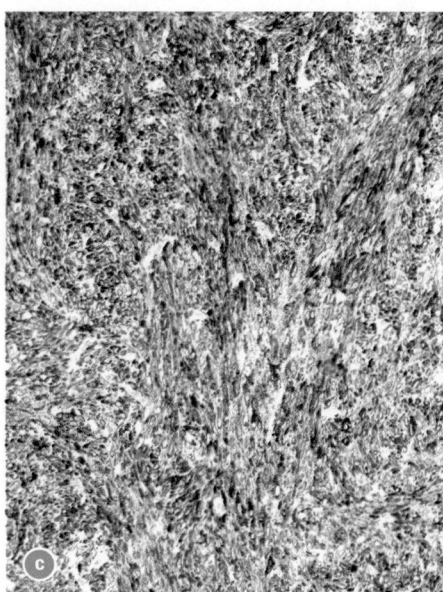

Fig. 30.15 Microscopic views of thecoma. (a) Dense arrangements of plump fusiform stromal cells alternating with fibroblasts characterize fibrothecoma. (b) Homogeneous populations of thecal cells in a thecoma. (c) The cells are strongly inhibin positive.

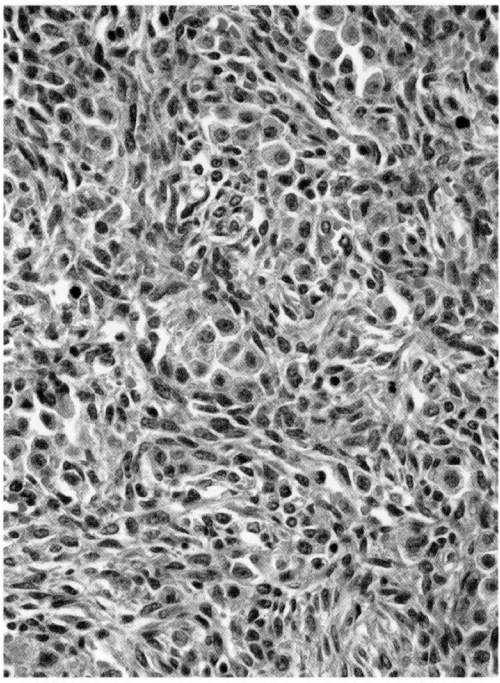

Fig. 30.16 Luteinized thecoma. The tumor contains spindled theca cells with prominent clusters of luteinized cells that are ovoid and contain more abundant cytoplasm.

individual cells in thecomas and cell clusters in granulosa cell tumors. However, luteinized granulosa cell tumors lacking characteristic granulosa cell tumor architectural definition and are extremely difficult to distinguish on histologic grounds alone from a thecoma. (2) Smooth muscle neoplasia. The distinction between thecoma and leiomyoma can usually be made by the classic fascicle formation of leiomyomas.[12]

Outcome

Thecomas are benign tumors.[13] Rare malignant thecomas have been described; however, these may have actually been fibrosarcomas or variants of granulosa cell tumor.[14] The latter may occur when the primary tumor is heterogeneous in appearance and the granulosa cell component is inconspicuous. We have seen one tumor that was initially classified as a thecoma based on histologic examination and reticulin staining and that recurred in the lung as a classic granulosa cell tumor several years later.

GRANULOSA AND GRANULOSA-THECA CELL TUMORS

Definition

Granulosa cell tumors are defined as those in which at least 10% of the cells fall within a defined morphologic range that closely resembles the granulosa cells of the developing follicle. These tumors are uncommon, comprising 1–2% of all ovarian tumors; however, they are the most common sex cord-stromal tumor after fibromas and fibrothecomas. In the Women's and Perinatal Division at Brigham and Women's Hospital, approximately one granulosa cell tumor is encoun-

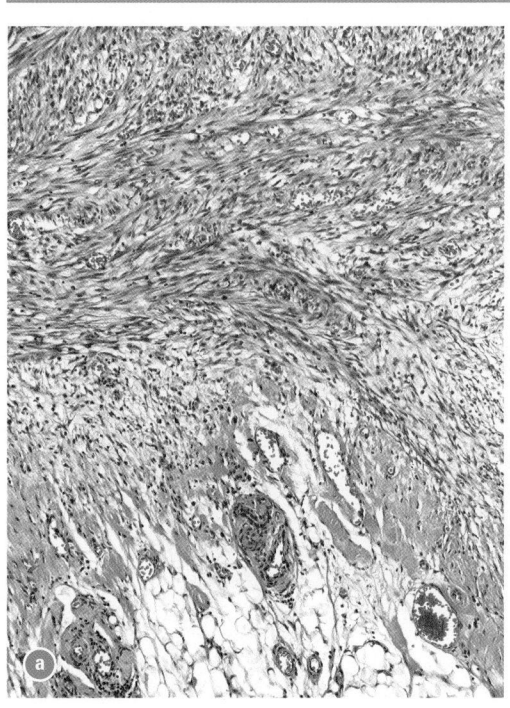

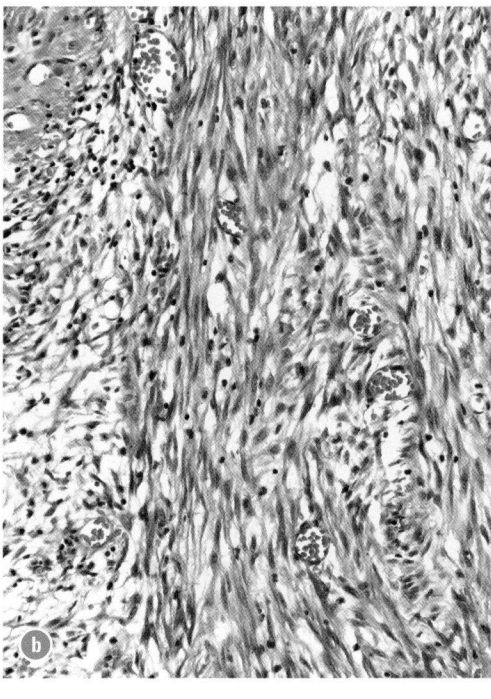

Fig. 30.17 Sclerosing peritonitis associated with luteinized thecoma. (a) Dense fibrosis replaces the peritoneal adipose tissue (below). (b) Immature fibroblasts are admixed with mononuclear cells.

tered for every 50 epithelial tumors; the vast majority are received in consultation.

Clinical features

Granulosa cell tumors can be divided into adult and juvenile types.[15-23] The adult type predominates in menopausal or postmenopausal women, with a mean age in the mid-50s. Because the cells are steroidogenic, they can elicit either estrogenic or androgenic effects, including uterine bleeding. The classically described endometrial lesion is an anovulatory pattern (cystic hyperplasia), although atypical hyperplasia or cancer have also been reported; endometrial carcinomas have been associated with approximately 5% of tumors.[2]

Gross findings

Granulosa cell tumors are almost always unilateral; approximately 9% occur in both ovaries. Approximately 93% present as Stage I. The gross appearance varies widely, often depending on the percentage of theca cells or luteinized cells, and the presence or absence of necrosis. Tumors are typically solid, variably cystic and not uncommonly hemorrhagic (Figs 30.18–30.20). Tumors with a prominent theca cell component or a luteinized quality are often yellow and firm. Some 10–15% are found to have ruptured at the time of surgery.

Histology

The histopathologic appearance of granulosa cell tumors varies from a conspicuous epithelioid or organoid pattern to solid and mesenchymal-appearing. The epithelioid

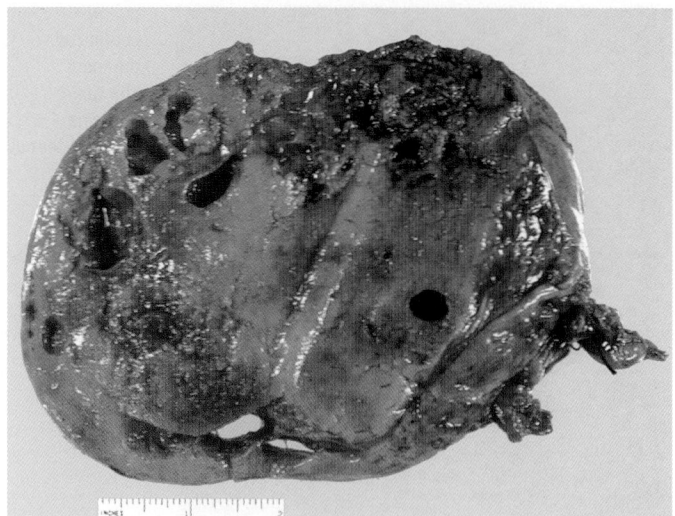

Fig. 30.19 Granulosa cell tumor. This tumor is a solid yellow-brown mass with small cysts and focal necrosis.

patterns include trabecular (Fig. 30.21a), insular (Fig. 30.21b), gland-like (Fig. 30.21c), microfollicular (Fig. 30.22a), macrofollicular, disaggregated (Fig. 30.22b) and 'watered silk' arrangements (Fig. 30.22c). Some are diffusely cellular, in which case the diagnosis and distinction from other tumors is more difficult. Less than 5% are luteinized; these may mimic luteinized thecomas.

The nuclei of granulosa cell tumors are typically uniform, with minimal chromatin complexity and delicate nuclear membranes. Folds or grooves in the nuclei are touted as an important feature, albeit vari-

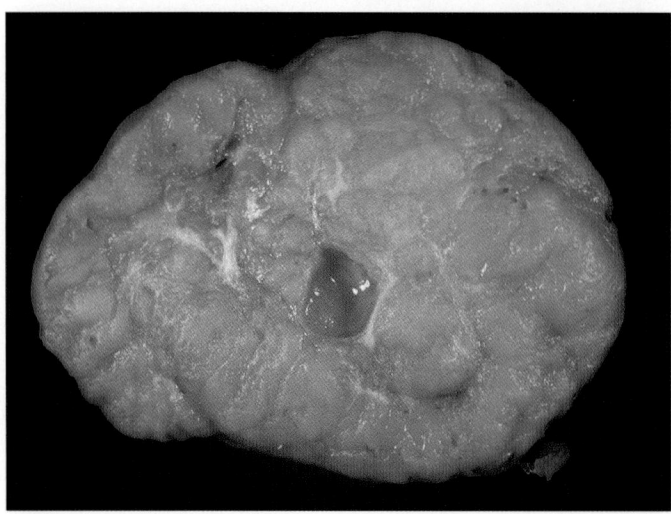

Fig. 30.18 Granulosa cell tumor. This tumor presents as a homogeneous yellow, circumscribed mass.

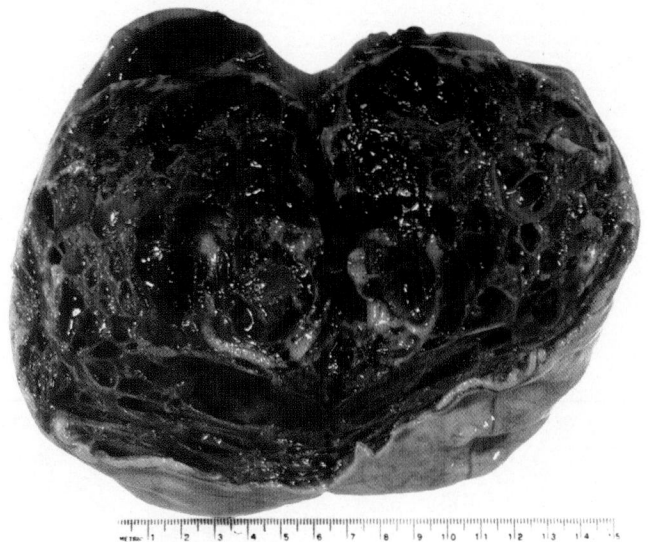

Fig. 30.20 Granulosa cell tumor. This tumor exhibits two common features, cystic necrosis and hemorrhage.

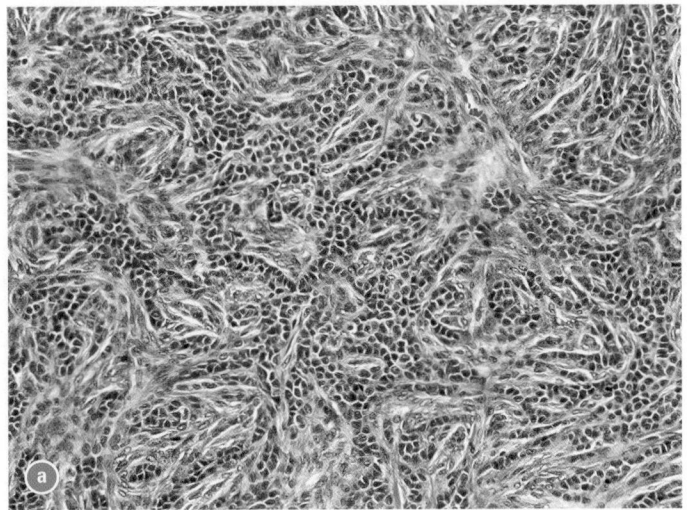

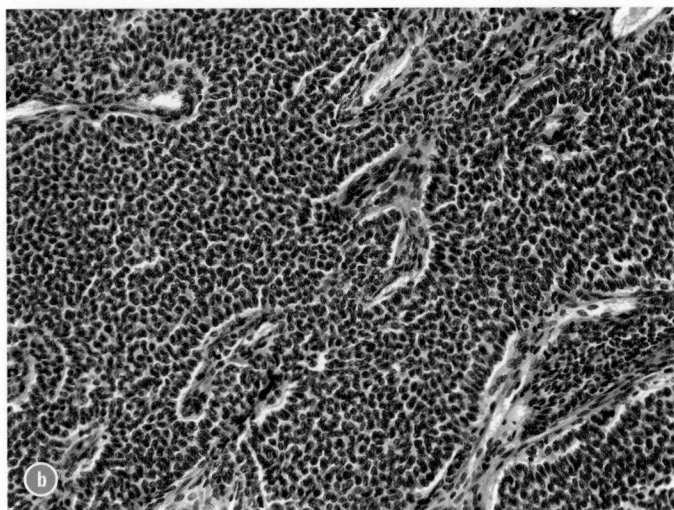

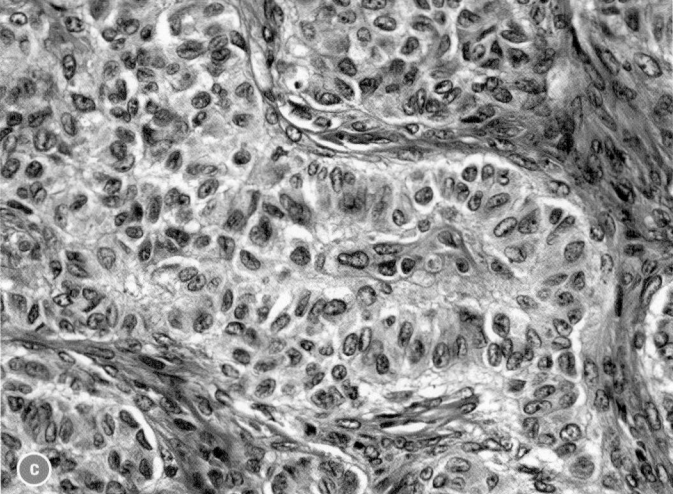

Fig. 30.21 Histologic patterns of granulosa cell tumor. (a) Trabecular or cord-like pattern. (b) Insular or nesting pattern. (c) Gland-like pattern.

able in frequency (Fig. 30.23a) and not specific for granulosa cell tumors. In the diffuse variant the cells are actually arranged in a nested pattern that may be highlighted by reticulin staining, whereas reticulin invests single cells in a thecoma. Granulosa and thecal cell elements may coexist in the same tumor; if either occupies at least 10% of the tumor the term granulosa-theca cell tumor is used. Some tumors contain focal marked atypia (Fig. 30.23b,c), although this is more common in juvenile granulosa cell tumors (see below); others are partially or almost completely luteinized, displaying cells with a decreased nuclear/cytoplasmic ratio and pale cytoplasm (Fig. 30.23d).[22]

Juvenile granulosa cell tumor is a rare variant (less than 5% of all granulosa cell tumors) that predominates in a younger age group; 97% of patients are less than 30 years of age (Fig. 30.24).[15,16] The histology departs from that seen in adult granulosa cell tumors

as follows: (1) nuclei are larger, slightly more hyperchromatic, and usually lacking in conspicuous grooves, and cytoplasm is more eosinophilic or sometimes vacuolated; (2) architecturally, there are nodules of cells and variably-sized follicles containing proteinaceous material within solid sheets of tumor cells with variable cellularity (Fig. 30.25a); (3) cytologic atypia may be striking, with bizarre nuclei (Fig. 30.25b).

Differential diagnosis

The differential diagnosis of granulosa cell tumors includes the following:

1 *Adenocarcinoma*: tumors exhibiting an organoid arrangement may be confused with poorly-differentiated endometrioid carcinoma of the ovary. However, the latter contains cells with a higher nuclear grade that are positive for epithelial membrane antigen. Breast carcinomas, particularly

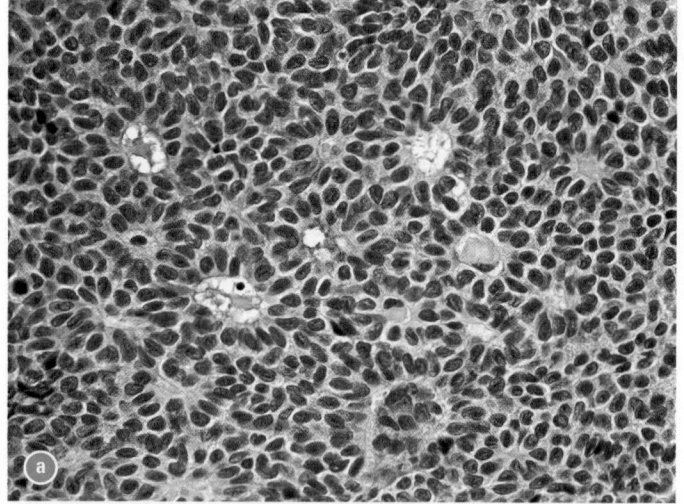

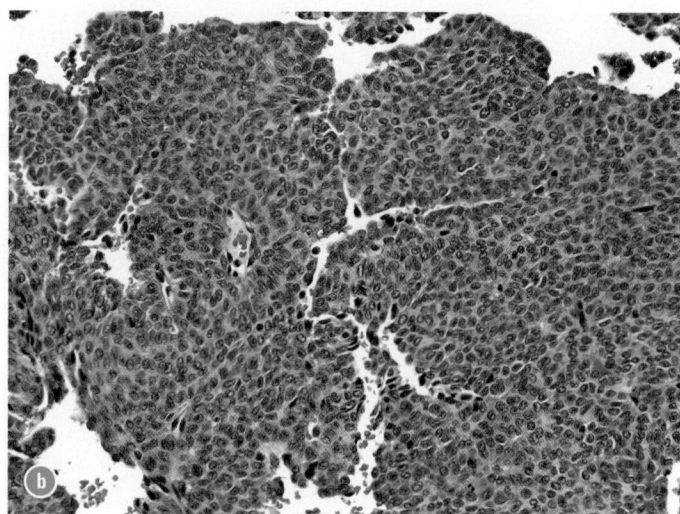

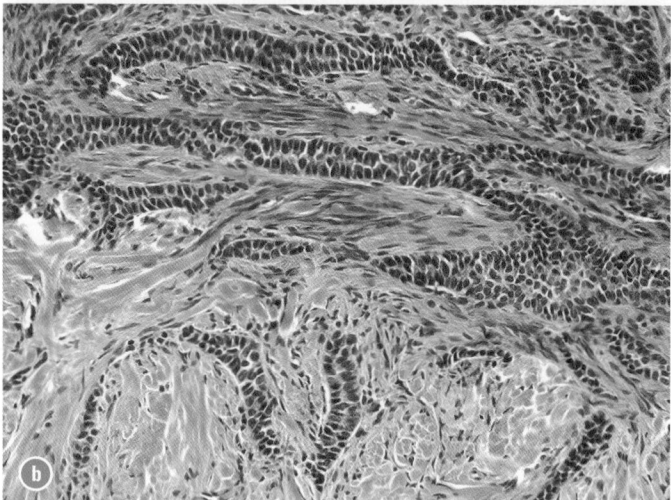

Fig. 30.22 (a) GCT with microfollicular pattern and Call–Exner bodies. (b) Disaggregated clusters of cohesive tumors cells. (c) 'Watered silk pattern', characterized by branching 'rivulets' of tumor.

lobular carcinoma, will produce cord-like arrangements reminiscent of GCT. However, they are typically bilateral and inhibin negative.

2 *Carcinoid tumor*: an insular carcinoid is typically unilateral and may exhibit a low-power appearance that is strikingly similar to a GCT. However, a coexisting teratoma is often present and the nuclear chromatin is typically granular. Inhibin and chromogranin stains will exclude or confirm carcinoid.

3 *Small cell carcinomas*: these are among the more problematic because they are typically unilateral and composed of a homogeneous population of epithelioid cells with a high nuclear/cytoplasmic ratio. However, the cells are typically more primitive without the characteristic pale nuclei of GCTs. They can be further distinguished by lack of inhibin staining and the finding of hypercalcemia in about half of the patients (see below).

4 *Luteinized granulosa cell tumors* must be distinguished from luteinized thecomas (reticulin stain) and rarely hepatoid yolk-sac carcinomas (younger patients, alpha-fetoprotein (AFP) positive) and rare pituitary tumors arising in teratomas.

Juvenile granulosa cell tumors evoke a different set of diagnostic possibilities; in addition to small cell carcinoma, these include clear cell carcinoma, dysgerminoma and metastatic tumors, such as melanoma. When any of these tumors is considered in a woman under age 30, the possibility of juvenile granulosa cell tumor must be excluded due to the radically different prognostic implications (see Fig. 30.2).

Management and outcome

Over 90% of granulosa cell tumors are Stage I when diagnosed and the 10-year survival is 85–90%.[17–21]

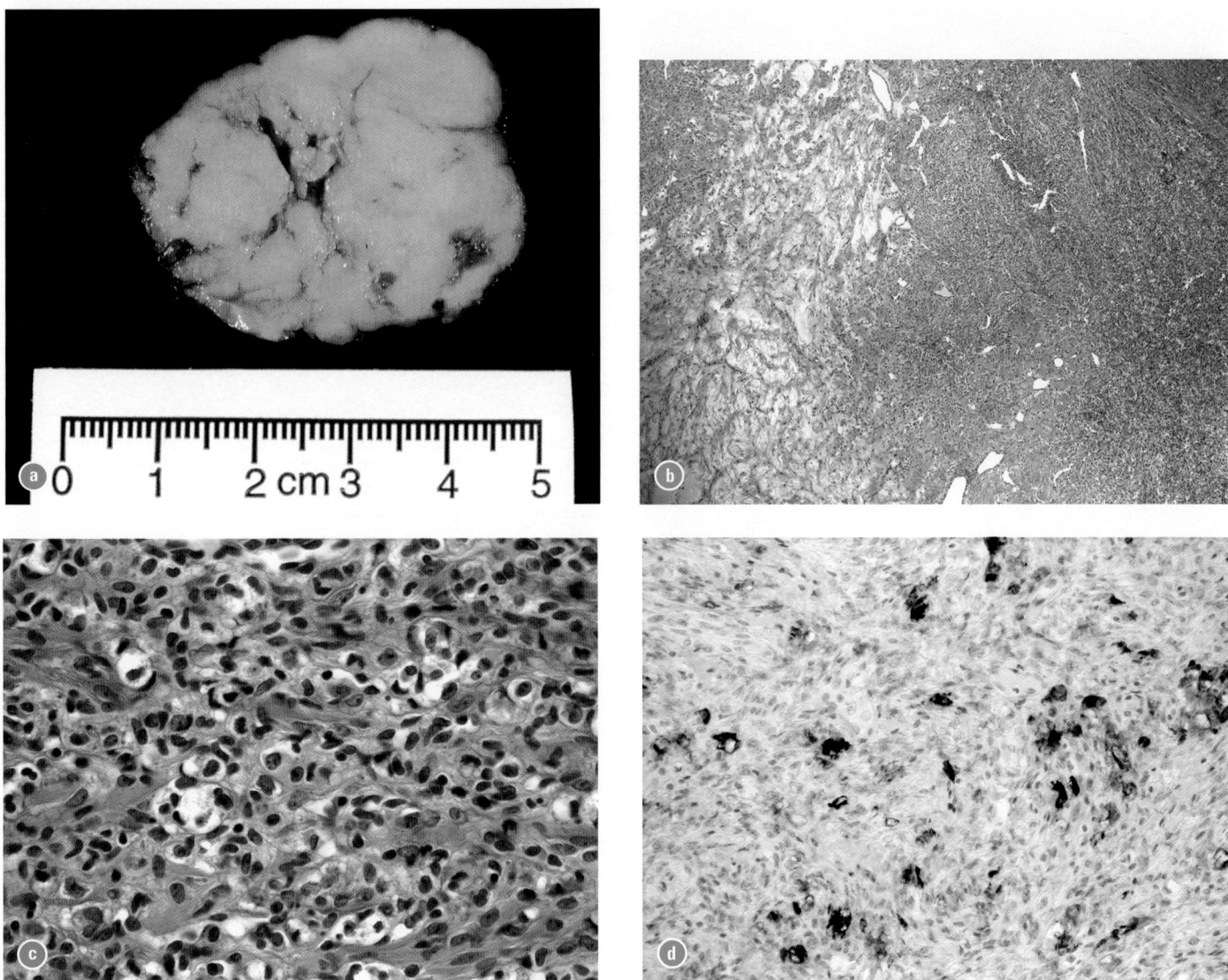

Fig. 30.41 (a) Gross appearance of a sclerosing stromal cell tumor (SSCT). (b) Histology of an SSCT, with ill-defined nodular groups of cells showing a range of stromal cell differentiation within a collagenized background. (c) Higher magnification of luteinized stromal cells. (d) Following immunostaining for inhibin.

tumors are rarely familial and have the following characteristics: (1) unilateral ovarian involvement; (2) elevated calcium level (62%); and (3) extra-ovarian involvement in one-half.[54]

The gross features are typically a solid, lobulated cream-colored tumor with necrosis and hemorrhage (Fig. 30.42a). Histologically, the tumor is composed of diffusely distributed, closely packed round tumor cells with a high nuclear/cytoplasmic ratio and a high mitotic rate. The diffuse pattern may be punctuated by follicle-like architecture, islets of cells and cords or trabeculae (Fig. 30.42b,c). Cytoplasmic differentiation

also varies, including cells with prominent eosinophilic cytoplasm. One report described a large cell variant.[55] Other elements including mucinous glands and mucin deposition may be present. The differential diagnosis includes lymphoma (which will not display the epithelioid features, see below), metastatic small cell carcinoma to the ovary (see Ch. 31) and the entities discussed below.[56]

The mortality for small cell tumor of hypercalcemic type is high, with the majority dying of their disease. Occasional cases in each series have an extended survival with combination radiotherapy and chemotherapy.

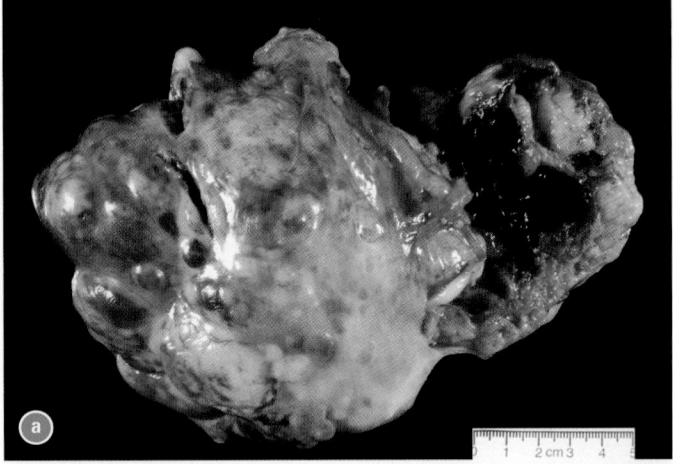

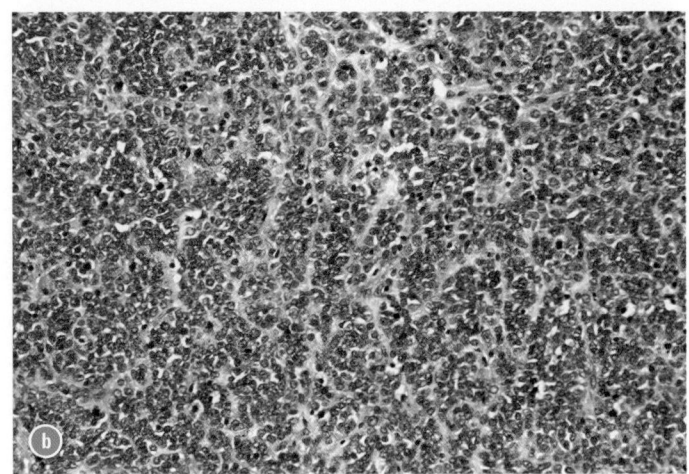

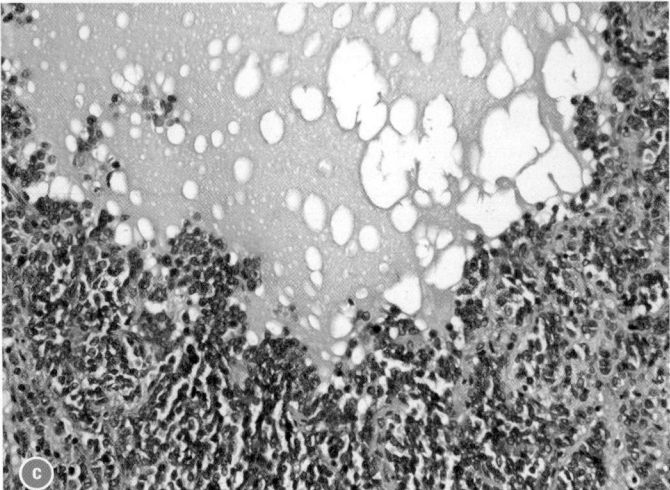

Fig. 30.42 (a) Gross appearance of small cell hypercalcemic tumor of the ovary. (b) Histopathology of small cell hypercalcemic tumor with small closely packed tumor cells and focal epithelioid arrangements. (c) An ill-defined space with eosinophilic contents.

Small cell carcinoma of pulmonary (neuroendocrine) type

This tumor is the subject of few reports and is distinguished from the small cell carcinoma of hypercalcemic type by the following: (1) a mean age of 59 years and (2) bilateral ovarian involvement in one-half. The microscopic appearance is similar to other small cell carcinomas of the lung and includes a large cell variant (Fig. 30.43). Like the tumor of hypercalcemic type, the pulmonary type may be associated with other elements. In the study by Eichhorn et al., additional elements included endometrioid carcinoma, squamous and mucinous differentiation and Brenner tumor. These would suggest an origin in a more conventional tumor, with neuroendocrine differentiation and overgrowth.[57,58]

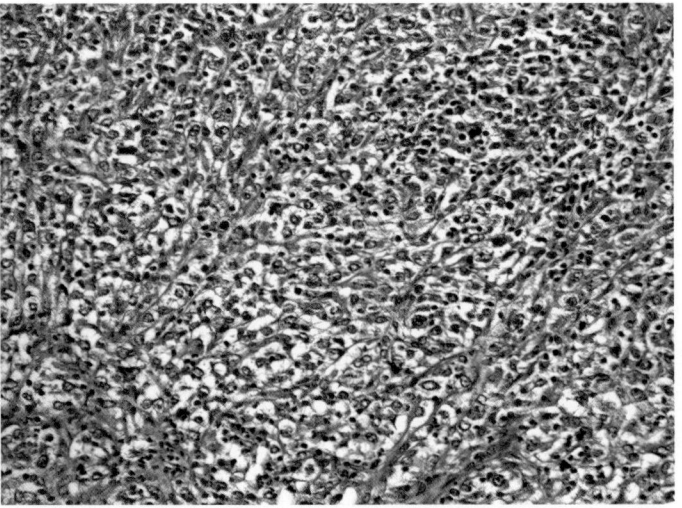

Fig. 30.43 Large cell variant of small cell hypercalcemic carcinoma.

Like the hypercalcemic type, the neuroendocrine variant has a poor prognosis, with a high mortality. This has led some to recommend chemotherapeutic protocols targeting pulmonary carcinomas.[59]

Intra-abdominal desmoplastic small round cell tumor

This tumor is discussed in Chapters 23 and 31 and is assumed to arise in the peritoneum with secondary ovarian involvement.[59,60] The tumors present histologically as solid nests of tumor in a desmoplastic stroma. The differential diagnosis is in the Table 30.3.

Primitive neuroectodermal tumor (PNET)

PNETs are discussed in Chapters 9, 15 and 31. They are poorly-differentiated neuroectodermal tumors that either metastasize to or sometimes arise in benign cystic teratomas (see Ch 29).[61-63] Histologically, they consist of a monomorphic tumor cell population of sheets and nests of cells with variable rosette-like structures. These tumors contain a unique t(111:22)(q24:q12) translocation that is specific for the PNET/Ewing sarcoma family. Consequently, they can be identified by the presence of either the EWS?FLI-I chimeric mRNA (by RTPCR) or expression of the LFI-1 protein.[64]

Prognosis of ovarian PNETs cannot be determined with certainty due to the small number of reports. However, long-term survivals have been reported with chemotherapy. Studies of similar tumors occurring in either children or adults at other sites report an approximately 60% 5-year survival for tumors presenting as a localized mass *vs* 33% if the tumor had spread. The relative values of surgery, radiation therapy and chemotherapy have been debated.[65]

Endometrial stromal cell sarcoma (ESS)

These tumors are also discussed in Chapters 20 and 23 and are included for completion. The distinguishing features of ESS of the ovary include a uniform population of fusiform nuclei with a prominent network of arterioles. Endometriosis is the likely origin and, if evident, facilitates the diagnosis. CD10 staining is particularly helpful in distinguishing ESS from the other small round cell tumors.[59,66]

Lymphoma and leukemia

Primary lymphomas of the ovary are rare and encompass a wide range of phenotypes, including Burkitt's lymphoma, T- and B-cell types. The tumors occur over a wide age range, are typically unilateral, present with a pelvic mass or are discovered incidentally. Grossly, uniform expansion of the ovary is seen in smaller tumors (Fig. 30.44). The histologic picture is of a diffuse lymphoid infiltrate replacing the parenchyma of the ovary while sparing the structures (Fig. 30.45a,b). The outcome is favorable in primary tumors.[67]

Granulocytic sarcomas typically occur in the ovary as a manifestation of relapsing myeloid leukemia. These tumors diffusely replace the ovarian parenchyma and can be distinguished by immunostaining for CD68, CD44 and myeloperoxidase. These markers may be helpful in excluding mimics such as granulosa cell tumor

Table 30.3 Clinically significant pitfalls associated with sex cord-stromal tumors

Tumor	Pitfall (misclassified as)
GTCT (spindled)	Benign thecoma
GTCT (other)	Endometrioid CA, carcinoid, small cell CA
GTCT (juvenile)	Germ cell tumor, epithelial malignancy, small cell carcinoma
Retiform SLCT	Serous carcinoma
Oxyphilic SLCT	Clear cell carcinoma
Well-diff. SLCT	Endometrioid carcinoma
SLCT (heterologous)	Carcinosarcoma or immature teratoma
Steroid cell tumor	Metastatic renal cell carcinoma
SLCT (intermediate)	Metastatic carcinoma, melanoma
SSCT; SRCT	Metastatic gastrointestinal carcinoma (Krukenberg), adenomatoid tumor
Cellular fibroma	Fibrosarcoma, other sarcoma

CA, carcinoma; GTCT, granulosa-theca cell tumor; SLCT, Sertoli–Leydig cell tumor; SRCT, signet-ring cell stromal tumor; SSCT, sclerosing stromal cell tumor.

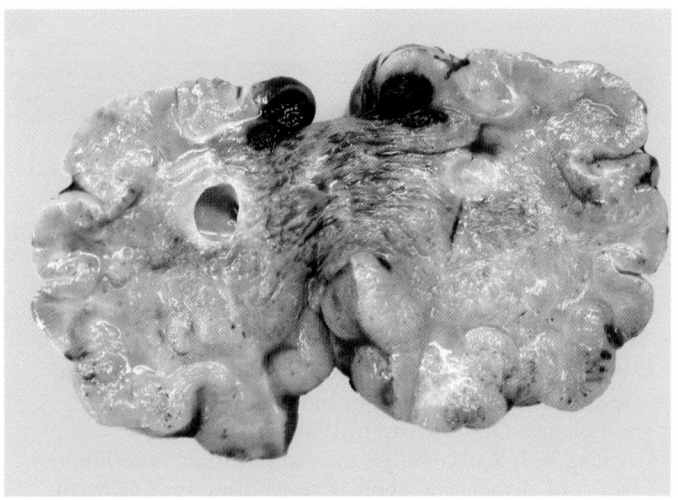

Fig. 30.44 Gross appearance of ovarian lymphoma.

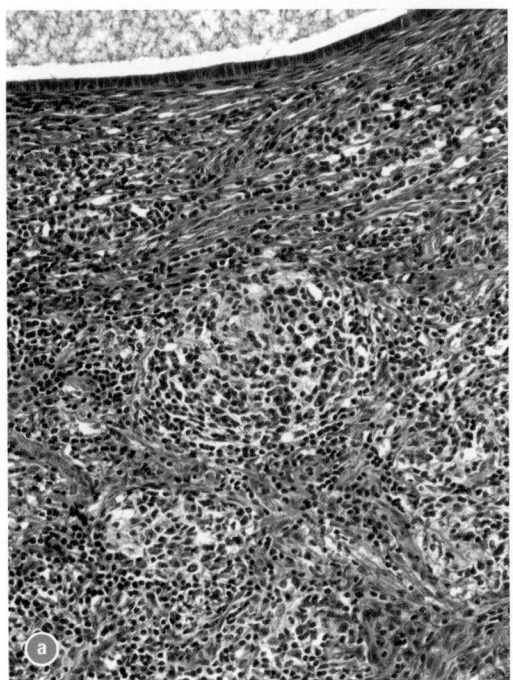
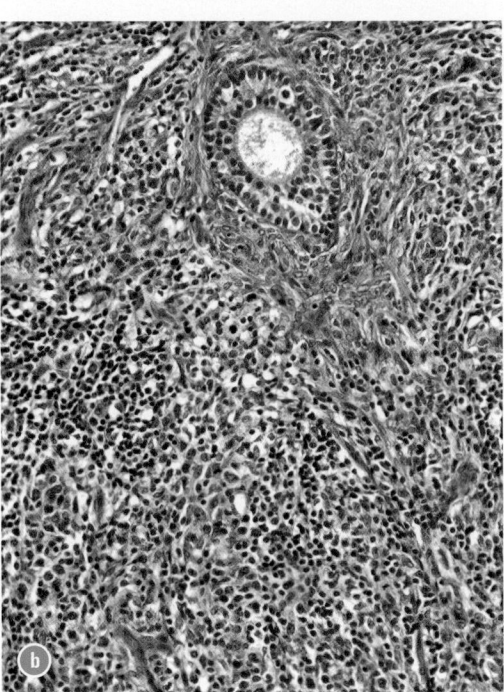

Fig. 30.45 Ovarian lymphoma. (a) Diffuse and (b) nodular arrangements of neoplastic lymphoid cells are distributed in the ovarian stroma. Note the preservation of other ovarian architecture.

and other poorly-differentiated neoplasms of the ovary. Overall, prognosis is poor, but prolonged remissions have been achieved.[68]

OTHER RARE OVARIAN NEOPLASMS OF UNCERTAIN CLASSIFICATION

Additional tumors reviewed in greater detail in other publications include hepatoid carcinomas, basaloid carcinomas with adenoid cystic features,[69] adenomatoid tumors (see Ch. 21), tumors of probably Wolffian origin (Ch. 21), oncocytomas,[70] paragangliomas[71] and Wilms' tumors (Ch. 19).

References

1 Langman J. Medical embryology. Philadelphia, PA: Lippincott, Williams and Wilkins; 1970.

2 Scully RE, Young RH, Clement PB. Atlas of tumor pathology, 3rd series, Fascicle 23: Tumors of the ovary, maldeveloped gonads, fallopian tube and broad ligament. American Registry of Pathology, Washington DC: AFIP; 1996:169–238.

3 Bennington JL, Ferguson BR, Haber SL. Incidence and relative frequency of benign and malignant ovarian neoplasms. Obstet Gynecol 1968; 32:627–632.

4 Young RH, Scully RE. Ovarian stromal tumors with minor sex cord elements: a report of seven cases. Int J Gynecol Pathol 1983; 2(3):227–234.

5 Kraemer BB, Silva EG, Sneige N. Fibrosarcoma of ovary. A new component in the nevoid basal-cell carcinoma syndrome. Am J Surg Pathol 1984; 8(3):231–236.

6 Prat J, Scully RE. Cellular fibromas and fibrosarcomas of the ovary: a comparative clinicopathologic analysis of seventeen cases. Cancer 1981; 47(11):2663–2670.

7 Alkushi A, Young RH, Clement PB. Cellular fibromas of the ovary: a study of 62 cases including 24 with ≥4 MFs/10 HFPFs. Mod Pathol 2004; 17:189A.

8 Bjorkholm E, Silfversward C. Theca-cell tumors. Clinical features and prognosis. Acta Radiol Oncol 1980; 19(4): 241–244.

9 Roth LM, Sternberg WH. Partly luteinized theca cell tumor of the ovary. Cancer 1983; 51(9): 1697–1704.

10 Zhang J, Young RH, Arseneau J, Scully RE. Ovarian stromal tumors containing lutein or Leydig cells (luteinized thecomas and stromal Leydig cell tumors) – a clinicopathological analysis of fifty cases. Int J Gynecol Pathol 1982; 1(3):270–285.

11 Clement PB, Young RH, Hanna W, Scully RE. Sclerosing peritonitis associated with luteinized thecomas of the ovary. A clinicopathological analysis of six cases. Am J Surg Pathol 1994; 18(1):1–13.

12 Lerwill MF, Sung R, Oliva E, Prat J, Young RH. Smooth muscle tumors of the ovary: a clinicopathologic study of 54 cases emphasizing prognostic criteria, histologic variants, and differential diagnosis. Am J Surg Pathol 2004; 28(11):1436–1451.

13 Bjorkholm E, Pettersson F. Granulosa-cell and theca-cell tumors. The clinical picture and long-term outcome for the Radiumhemmet series. Acta Obstet Gynecol Scand 1980; 59(4):361–365.

14 McCluggage WG, Sloan JM, Boyle DD, Toner PG. Malignant fibrothecomatous tumour of the ovary: diagnostic value of anti-inhibin immunostaining. J Clin Pathol 1998; 51(11):868–871.

15 Zaloudek C, Norris HJ. Granulosa tumors of the ovary in children: a clinical and pathologic study of 32 cases. Am J Surg Pathol 1982; 6(6):503–512.

16 Young RH, Dickersin GR, Scully RE. Juvenile granulosa cell tumor of the ovary. A clinicopathological analysis of 125 cases. Am J Surg Pathol 1984; 8(8):575–596.

17 Schumer ST, Cannistra SA. Granulosa cell tumor of the ovary. J Clin Oncol 2003; 21(6):1180–1189.

18 Chua IS, Tan KT, Lim-Tan SK, Ho TH. A clinical review of granulosa cell tumours of the ovary cases in KKH. Singapore Med J 2001; 42(5):203–207.

19 Cronje HS, Niemand I, Bam RH, Woodruff JD. Review of the granulosa-theca cell tumors from the emil Novak ovarian tumor registry. Am J Obstet Gynecol 1999; 180(2 Pt 1):323–327.

20 Fontanelli R, Stefanon B, Raspagliesi F, et al. Adult granulosa cell tumor of the ovary: a clinico pathologic study of 35 cases. Tumori 1998; 84(1):60–64.

21 Pankratz E, Boyes DA, White GW, et al. Granulosa cell tumors. A clinical review of 61 cases. Obstet Gynecol 1978; 52(6):718–723.

22 Young RH, Oliva E, Scully RE. Luteinized adult granulosa cell tumors of the ovary: a report of four cases. Int J Gynecol Pathol 1994; 13(4):302–310.

23 Norris HJ, Taylor HB. Prognosis of granulosa-theca tumors of the ovary. Cancer 1968; 21(2):255–263.

24 Zaloudek C, Norris HJ. Sertoli–Leydig tumors of the ovary. A clinicopathologic study of 64 intermediate and poorly differentiated neoplasms. Am J Surg Pathol 1984; 8(6):405–418.

25 Young RH, Scully RE. Ovarian Sertoli–Leydig cell tumors. A clinicopathological analysis of 207 cases. Am J Surg Pathol 1985; 9(8):543–569.

26 Young RH, Scully RE. Well-differentiated ovarian Sertoli–Leydig cell tumors: a clinicopathological analysis of 23 cases. Int J Gynecol Pathol 1984; 3(3):277–290.

27 Ferry JA, Young RH, Engel G, Scully RE. Oxyphilic Sertoli cell tumor of the ovary: a report of three cases, two in patients with the Peutz–Jeghers syndrome. Int J Gynecol Pathol 1994; 13(3):259–266.

28 Bullon A Jr, Arseneau J, Prat J, Young RH, Scully RE. Tubular Krukenberg tumor. A problem in histopathologic diagnosis. Am J Surg Pathol 1981; 5(3):225–232.

29 Roth LM, Anderson MC, Govan AD, et al. Sertoli–Leydig cell tumors: a clinicopathologic study of 34 cases. Cancer 1981; 48(1):187–197.

30 Mooney EE, Nogales FF, Bergeron C, Tavassoli FA. Retiform Sertoli–Leydig cell tumours: clinical, morphological and immunohistochemical findings. Histopathology 2002; 41(2):110–117.

31 Moyles K, Chan YF, Hamill J, Massey R. Ovarian Sertoli–Leydig cell tumor with retiform pattern. Pathology 1995; 27(4):371–373.

32 Talerman A. Ovarian Sertoli–Leydig cell tumor (androblastoma) with retiform pattern. A clinicopathologic study. Cancer 1987; 60(12):3056–3064.

33 Young RH, Scully RE. Ovarian Sertoli–Leydig cell tumors with a retiform pattern: a problem in histopathologic diagnosis. A report of 25 cases. Am J Surg Pathol 1983; 7(8):755–771.

34 Roth LM, Slayton RE, Brady LW, Blessing JA, Johnson G. Retiform differentiation in ovarian Sertoli–Leydig cell tumors. A clinicopathologic study of six cases from a Gynecologic Oncology Group study. Cancer 1985; 55(5):1093–1098.

35 Young RH, Prat J, Scully RE. Ovarian Sertoli–Leydig cell tumors with heterologous elements. I. Gastrointestinal epithelium and carcinoid: a clinicopathologic analysis of thirty-six cases. Cancer 1982; 50(11):2448–2456.

36 Prat J, Young RH, Scully RE. Ovarian Sertoli–Leydig cell tumors with heterologous elements. II. Cartilage and skeletal muscle: a clinicopathologic analysis of twelve cases. Cancer 1982; 50(11):2465–2475.

37 Young RH, Welch WR, Dickersin GR, Scully RE. Ovarian sex cord tumor with annular tubules: review of 74 cases including 27 with Peutz–Jeghers syndrome and four with adenoma malignum of the cervix. Cancer 1982; 50(7): 1384–1402.

38 Young RH, Dickersin GR, Scully RE. A distinctive ovarian sex cord-stromal tumor causing sexual precocity in the Peutz–Jeghers syndrome. Am J Surg Pathol 1983; 7(3):233–243.

39 Young RH, Dudley AG, Scully RE. Granulosa cell, Sertoli–Leydig cell, and unclassified sex cord-stromal tumors associated with pregnancy: a clinicopathological analysis of thirty-six cases. Gynecol Oncol 1984; 18(2):181–205.

40 Seidman JD. Unclassified ovarian gonadal stromal tumors. A clinicopathologic study of 32 cases. Am J Surg Pathol 1996; 20(6):699–706.

41 Seidman JD, Abbondanzo SL, Bratthauer GL. Lipid cell (steroid cell) tumor of the ovary: immunophenotype with analysis of potential pitfall due to endogenous biotin-like activity. Int J Gynecol Pathol 1995; 14(4):331–338.

42 Taylor HB, Norris HJ. Lipid cell tumors of the ovary. Cancer 1967; 20(11):1953–1962.

43 Norris HJ, Taylor HB. Nodular theca-lutein hyperplasia of pregnancy (so-called 'pregnancy luteoma'). A clinical and pathologic study of 15 cases. Am J Clin Pathol 1967; 47(5):557–566.

44 Hayes MC, Scully RE. Stromal luteoma of the ovary: a clinicopathological analysis of 25 cases. Int J Gynecol Pathol 1987; 6(4):313–321.

45 Zhang J, Young RH, Arseneau J, Scully RE. Ovarian stromal tumors containing lutein or Leydig cells (luteinized thecomas and stromal Leydig cell tumors) – a clinicopathological analysis of fifty cases. Int J Gynecol Pathol 1982; 1(3):270–285.

46 Roth LM, Sternberg WH. Ovarian stromal tumors containing Leydig cells. II. Pure Leydig cell tumor, non-hilar type. Cancer 1973; 32(4):952–960.

47 Sternberg WH, Roth LM. Ovarian stromal tumors containing Leydig cells. I. Stromal–Leydig cell tumor and non-neoplastic transformation of ovarian stroma to Leydig cells. Cancer 1973; 32(4):940–951.

48 Hayes MC, Scully RE. Ovarian steroid cell tumors (not otherwise specified). A clinicopathological analysis of 63 cases. Am J Surg Pathol 1987; 11(11):835–845.

49 Chetkowski RJ, Judd HL, Jagger PI, Nieberg RK, Chang RJ. Autonomous cortisol secretion by a lipoid cell tumor of the ovary. JAMA 1985; 254(18):2628–2631.

50 Young RH, Scully RE. Ovarian steroid cell tumors associated with Cushing's syndrome: a report of three cases. Int J Gynecol Pathol 1987; 6(1):40–48.

51 Vang R, Bague S, Tavassoli FA, Prat J. Signet-ring stromal tumor of the ovary: clinicopathologic analysis and comparison with Krukenberg tumor. Int J Gynecol Pathol 2004; 23(1): 45–51.

52 Kawauchi S, Tsuji T, Kaku T, et al. Sclerosing stromal tumor of the ovary: a clinicopathologic, immunohistochemical, ultrastructural, and cytogenetic analysis with special reference to its vasculature. Am J Surg Pathol 1998; 22(1):83–92.

53 Chalvardjian A, Scully RE. Sclerosing stromal tumors of the ovary. Cancer 1973; 31(3):664–670.

54 Young RH, Oliva E, Scully RE. Small cell carcinoma of the ovary, hypercalcemic type. A clinicopathological analysis of 150 cases. Am J Surg Pathol 1994; 18(11):1102–1116.

55 Di Vagno G, Melilli GA, Cormio G, et al. Large-cell variant of small cell carcinoma of the ovary with hypercalcaemia. Arch Gynecol Obstet 2000; 264(3):157–158.

56 Eichhorn JH, Young RH, Scully RE. Nonpulmonary small cell carcinomas of extragenital origin metastatic to the ovary. Cancer 1993; 71(1):177–186.

57 Eichhorn JH, Lawrence WD, Young RH, Scully RE. Ovarian neuroendocrine carcinomas of non-small-cell type associated with surface epithelial adenocarcinomas. A study of five cases and review of the literature. Int J Gynecol Pathol 1996; 15(4):303–314.

58 Eichhorn JH, Young RH, Scully RE. Primary ovarian small cell carcinoma of pulmonary type. A clinicopathologic, immunohistologic, and flow cytometric analysis of 11 cases. Am J Surg Pathol 1992; 16(10):926–938.

59 McCluggage WG. Ovarian neoplasms composed of small round cells: a review. Adv Anat Pathol 2004; 11(6):288–296.

60 Parker LP, Duong JL, Wharton JT et al. Desmoplastic small round cell tumor: report of a case presenting as a primary ovarian neoplasm. Eur J Gynaecol Oncol 2002; 23(3):199–202.

61 Young RH, Kozakewich HP, Scully RE. Metastatic ovarian tumors in children: a report of 14 cases and review of the literature. Int J Gynecol Pathol 1993; 12(1):8–19.

62 Block M, Gilbert E, Davis C. Metastatic neuroblastoma arising in an ovarian teratoma with long-term survival. Case report and review of the literature. Cancer 1984; 54(3):590–595.

63 Reid HA, van der Walt JD, Fox H. Neuroblastoma arising in a mature cystic teratoma of the ovary. J Clin Pathol 1983; 36(1):68–73.

64 Martin RC 2nd, Brennan MF. Adult soft tissue Ewing sarcoma or primitive neuroectodermal tumors: predictors of survival? Arch Surg 2003; 138(3):281–285.

65 Shamberger RC, LaQuaglia MP, Gebhardt MC, et al. Ewing sarcoma/primitive neuroectodermal tumor of the chest wall: impact of initial versus delayed resection on tumor margins, survival, and use of radiation therapy. Ann Surg 2003; 238(4):563–567; discussion 567–568.

66 Young RH, Prat J, Scully RE. Endometrioid stromal sarcomas of the ovary. A clinicopathologic analysis of 23 cases. Cancer 1984; 53(5):1143–1155.

67 Vang R, Medeiros LJ, Warnke RA, Higgins JP, Deavers MT. Ovarian non-Hodgkin's lymphoma: a clinicopathologic study of eight primary cases. Mod Pathol 2001; 14(11):1093–1099.

68 Oliva E, Ferry JA, Young RH, et al. Granulocytic sarcoma of the female genital tract: a clinicopathologic study of 11 cases. Am J Surg Pathol 1997; 21(10):1156–1165.

69 Eichhorn JH, Scully RE. "Adenoid cystic" and basaloid carcinomas of the ovary: evidence for a surface epithelial lineage. A report of 12 cases. Mod Pathol 1995; 8(7): 731–740.

70 Yoshida Y, Tenzaki T, Ishiguro T, Kawanami D, Ohshima M. Oncocytoma of the ovary: light and electron microscopic study. Gynecol Oncol 1984; 18(1):109–114.

71 Fawcett FJ, Kimbell NK. Phaeochromocytoma of the ovary. J Obstet Gynaecol Br Commonw 1971; 78(5):458–459.

31

Metastatic tumors to the ovary

Michelle S. Hirsch and

Kenneth R. Lee

Introduction

Gross evaluation of ovarian masses

Metastatic tumors from the gynecologic tract

Metastatic endometrial carcinoma
Metastatic uterine sarcomas
Metastatic fallopian tube
  carcinomas
Metastatic cervical carcinomas

Metastatic tumors from the gastrointestinal and pancreaticobiliary tracts

Gastric carcinomas
Colorectal carcinomas
Tumors of the small bowel

Appendiceal carcinomas
Pancreatic and biliary tract
  carcinomas

Other secondary tumors of the ovary

Metastatic breast carcinoma
Metastatic lung carcinoma
Metastatic renal cell carcinoma
Metastatic urothelial carcinoma
Malignant melanoma
Metastatic sarcoma
Metastatic small round blue cell
  tumors
Metastatic malignant
  mesothelioma
Lymphoma and leukemia
  involving the ovaries

Introduction

The distinction between primary and secondary tumors of the ovary is one of the more difficult determinations in gynecologic pathology, as there are similarities in both clinical and morphologic features in many cases. The reported frequency of metastatic tumors in the ovary varies with the study design (e.g. autopsy *vs* surgical material) and the country of origin (Table 31.1); however, it ranges between 15% and 25% of all malignancies involving the ovary.[1–3] Among cases that clinically or pathologically mimic a primary ovarian tumor, most originate from the endometrium, the colon, the appendix, the upper gastrointestinal tract, the pancreas and the breast.[4] Metastases to the ovary connote a poor prognosis, with overall 5-year survival of approximately 20%.[1,3]

Gross evaluation of ovarian masses

The gross findings are often helpful in distinguishing a primary from a metastatic tumor. This subject is discussed more fully in Chapter 23. Briefly:

1 Primary mucinous tumors of the ovary are often larger (20–30 cm) than metastatic mucinous tumors, which are often 10 cm or less in greatest dimension.[5,6]

2 Metastatic neoplasms often affect both ovaries. Most primary ovarian neoplasms are unilateral, except for serous carcinomas, which are often bilateral and unlikely to be confused with metastases.

3 A multinodular appearance and surface implants are clues to a metastasis.[4,5]

4 Homogeneous expansion of the ovarian parenchyma without cyst formation occurs with metastatic breast cancer, signet ring cell tumors and lymphomas and is unusual in primary epithelial ovarian carcinomas.

5 Large tumors with conspicuous necrosis and hemorrhage are common in metastatic colonic carcinomas (which are not infrequently unilateral).

Metastatic tumors from the gynecologic tract

METASTATIC ENDOMETRIAL CARCINOMA

Endometrial adenocarcinomas account for 15–20% of all ovarian metastases.[1,3] Difficulty often arises in distinguishing a metastasis from the endometrium from a primary endometrioid tumor of the ovary, since up to 12% of patients who present with an endometrioid-appearing ovarian adenocarcinoma also have a synchronous endometrial carcinoma.[7–11] This subject is reviewed in detail in Chapter 27 in the differential diagnosis of endometrioid carcinomas of the ovary. Briefly, ovarian metastases should be suspected if the endometrial tumor is deeply invasive in the myometrium or invades myometrial vessels. Also, a metastasis is likely if the ovarian tumor involves the ovarian surface or has a multinodular growth pattern and there is no evidence of ovarian endometriosis.

METASTATIC UTERINE SARCOMAS

The frequency of a uterine leiomyosarcoma metastasizing to the ovary is only 3.9%.[12] Further, in a series of 10 metastatic endometrial stromal sarcomas, only one involved the ovary (Fig. 31.1).[13] Nevertheless, if one encounters either a leiomyosarcoma or an endometrial stromal sarcoma in the ovary, a metastasis from the uterus (possibly remote or unrecognized) should always be excluded.[14,15]

Table 31.1 *Frequency of primary sites in metastatic tumors to the ovary in Japan and the USA*

	From Yada-Hashimoto et al.[1]	From Demopoulos et al.[3]
Total cases	64	76
Müllerian	26 (41%)	16 (21%)
Endometrium	15	14
Myometrium		
Fallopian tube	2	
Cervix	9	2
Non-Müllerian	38 (59%)	60 (79%)
Stomach	14	6
Breast	9	32
Colon	7	12
Ileum	2	
Appendix	1	
Biliary duct	1	
Lung	1	
Ureter	2	
Lymphoma	1	
Unspecified	1	8

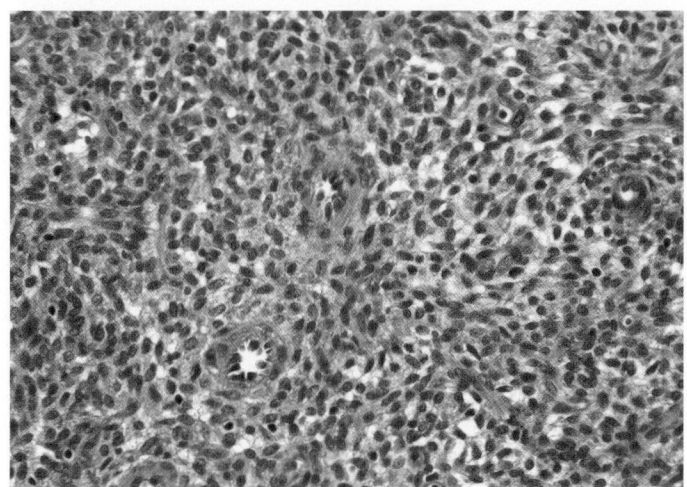

Fig. 31.1 Metastatic low-grade endometrial stromal sarcoma with bland nuclei and prominent spiral arterioles.

METASTATIC FALLOPIAN TUBE CARCINOMAS

The conundrum of distinguishing a primary tubal carcinoma from a metastasis to the tube is discussed in Chapter 21. Based on current classification systems, if the ovary and tube are both involved, the ovary is classified as a metastasis only if the tubal neoplasm is the dominant mass. Whether this classification reflects reality remains unclear.

METASTATIC CERVICAL CARCINOMAS

Cervical carcinomas metastasize to the ovary in less than 5% of cases, the majority of these being adenocarcinomas. However, the possibility of a cervical metastasis should be seriously considered in any ovarian adenocarcinoma following a diagnosis of cervical adenocarcinoma,[16] especially since metastatic cervical adenocarcinomas often resemble endometrioid ovarian carcinomas. Features suggesting a cervical primary include high nuclear grade, luminal cytoplasmic eosinophilia with apically situated mitoses, and minimal stratification (Fig. 31.2a). Patterns resembling mucinous and intestinal carcinomas may also be seen (Fig. 31.2b,c). HPV analysis of the ovarian tumor is a valuable adjunct in difficult cases, as metastatic cervical adenocarcinomas are positive for high-risk HPV, and primary ovarian carcinomas are not.

Additional metastatic tumors reported from the cervix include papillary transitional and undifferentiated carcinomas.

Metastatic tumors from the gastrointestinal and pancreaticobiliary tracts

Gastrointestinal carcinomas and carcinoids commonly metastasize to the ovaries and may be difficult to distinguish from primary tumors, both histologically and immunohistochemically.

GASTRIC CARCINOMAS

The most common pattern of metastatic gastric carcinoma is the signet ring carcinoma (Krukenberg tumor). Krukenberg tumors may also originate in the intestine (including the appendix), breast, pancreas, or biliary tract.[17,18] The majority of cases present with symptoms related to a pelvic mass as the primary lesion may be occult. Tumors are usually bilateral solid masses that grossly may demonstrate a mucoid, glistening cut surface (Fig. 31.3). The signet ring cells are filled with cytoplasmic mucin (Fig. 31.4a) and may be present as scattered single cells, or in tubular or glandular patterns (tubular Krukenberg tumor) (Fig. 31.4b).[19] There may or may not be a prominent spindled cellular stroma. The differential diagnosis for signet ring cell carcinomas in the ovary includes a primary mucinous ovarian carcinoma, which may have focal Krukenberg-like areas, but usually has other more characteristic patterns, and, in cases with a prominent stroma, primary stromal tumors such as a luteinized thecoma or a sclerosing stromal tumor. In difficult cases, a mucin stain is useful to accentuate the malignant cells.

COLORECTAL CARCINOMAS

Colorectal carcinomas are the most common gastrointestinal site of origin for metastatic ovarian carcinomas. They characteristically mimic primary endometrioid carcinomas, and awareness that the colonic tumor may be undiagnosed can help avoid a serious diagnostic error. This topic is reviewed fully in Chapter 27 in the sections on the differential diagnosis of endometrioid and mucinous ovarian carcinomas. Briefly, metastatic colonic tumors are usually large and necrotic (Fig. 31.5); about 50% of cases are bilateral. The characteristic

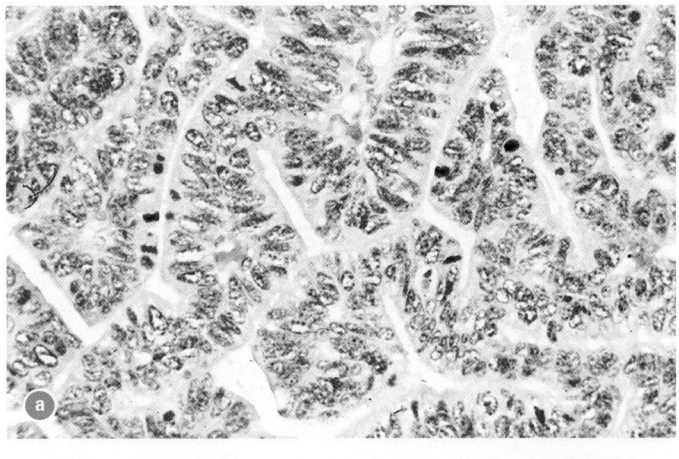

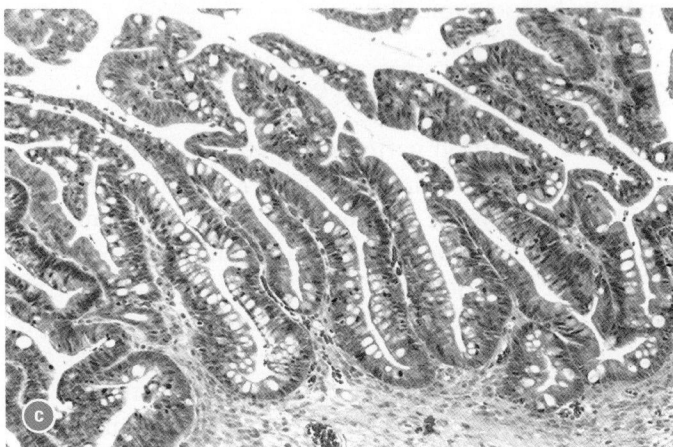

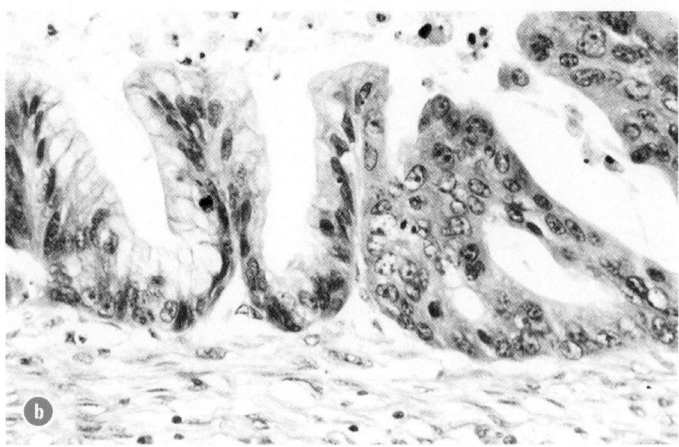

Fig. 31.2 (a) Metastatic cervical carcinoma. Note 'endometrioid' appearance, but with prominent apical mitoses. (b) Metastatic cervical carcinoma. In this case the cells are more endocervical (mucinous) in appearance. (c) Metastatic cervical carcinoma. Here the pattern is of the intestinal type.

histologic findings are garland and cribriform arrangements of pseudostratified epithelial cells with high nuclear grade and segmental epithelial necrosis with nuclear debris in cystic spaces ('dirty necrosis') (Fig. 31.6a).[20] As opposed to primary endometrioid ovarian carcinomas, most colorectal carcinomas are character-

Fig. 31.3 Gross photograph of metastatic gastric carcinoma (Krukenberg tumor).

istically CK7 negative, CK20 positive and cdx2 positive (see Ch. 27). Nuclear staining with beta-catenin is another, more recently introduced marker for colorectal adenocarcinoma (Fig. 31.6b).

TUMORS OF THE SMALL BOWEL

Metastases from the small intestine are most often carcinoid tumors. In the largest series of cases,[21] 40% of the patients had carcinoid syndrome, and most also had extra-ovarian metastases. The tumors are usually bilateral solid masses with a smooth surface and a white or yellow nodular cut surface. Microscopically, metastatic carcinoids are typically of the insular type (Fig. 31.7), but they may also demonstrate other patterns. Acinar-like spaces typically form at the periphery of the islands and in some cases there are rounded nests of cells with many goblet cells accompanying the carcinoid cells (goblet cell carcinoid).[22] A prominent fibromatous stroma is often present. The differential diagnosis includes primary carcinoid tumors, Sertoli cell tumors, granulosa cell tumors, and benign or malignant primary

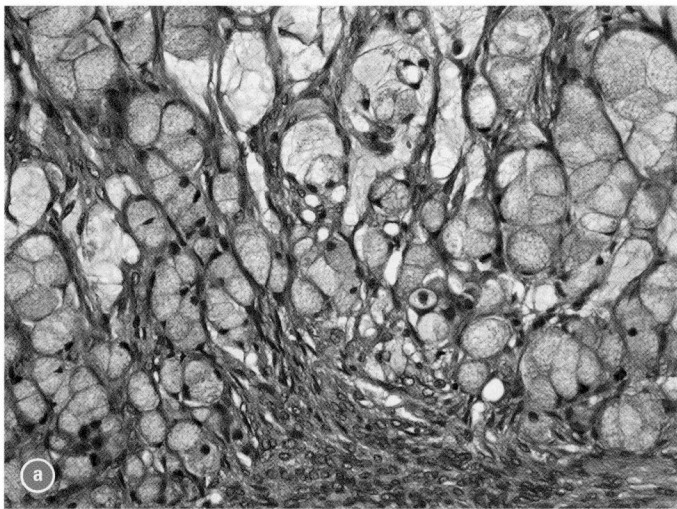

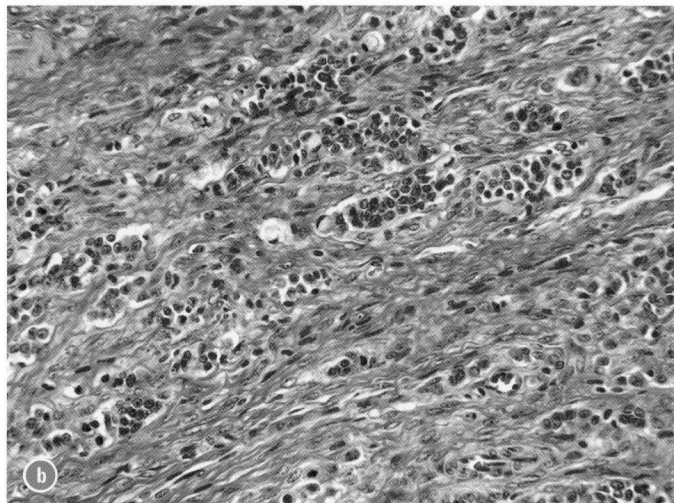

Fig. 31.4 (a) Metastatic gastric carcinoma (Krukenberg tumor) with numerous signet ring cells. (b) Metastatic gastric carcinoma (Krukenberg tumor) with signet ring cells in cords and trabeculae.

ovarian adenofibromas. Special stains for neuroendocrine markers confirm the diagnosis of carcinoid. An absence of other germ cell tumor elements and bilateral tumors strongly indicates a metastatic lesion.

Metastatic small bowel tumors with a prominent clear cell component are a rare source of confusion with a primary clear cell carcinoma or a secretory endometrioid carcinoma of the ovary (Fig. 31.8).[23]

APPENDICEAL CARCINOMAS

The subject of metastatic low-grade appendiceal mucinous tumors to the ovary in the setting of pseudomyxoma peritonei is extensively reviewed in Chapter 27 in the section on mucinous ovarian tumors. In the absence of pseudomyxoma peritonei,

appendiceal tumors that spread to the ovaries range from the goblet cell carcinoid,[22] to intestinal, colloid, or signet ring cell patterns (Fig. 31.9a–c). This diverse array of patterns often leads to confusion with primary ovarian mucinous carcinomas or with metastatic mucinous carcinomas from other sites. This is especially true as appendiceal lesions may be small and occult, even in the presence of large ovarian masses.[24,25] Immunohistochemistry may aid in differentiating secondary appendiceal carcinomas from primary ovarian carcinomas as most ovarian mucinous carcinomas are CK7 positive and CK20 negative, whereas most appendiceal carcinomas are CK20 positive and demonstrate variable (often focal or negative) staining for CK7. In addition, MUC2 and cdx2 are positive in mucinous appendiceal carcinomas and negative or only focally positive in mucinous ovarian carcinomas (Hirsch and Hornick, unpublished data) (Fig. 31.10a,b).

PANCREATIC AND BILIARY TRACT CARCINOMAS

Pancreatic carcinomas that metastasize to the ovary account for about 10% of metastatic tumors that present clinically as ovarian masses. This topic is reviewed more thoroughly in Chapter 27 in the differential diagnosis of primary mucinous ovarian tumors. In brief, they are usually bilateral large cystic masses that can grossly and microscopically closely simulate primary ovarian mucinous carcinomas or even mucinous borderline tumors[26] because the epithelial cells are often low grade and even benign-appearing in focal areas (Fig.

Fig. 31.5 Gross photograph of metastatic colon carcinoma. Note hemorrhagic and focally necrotic cystic and solid mass.

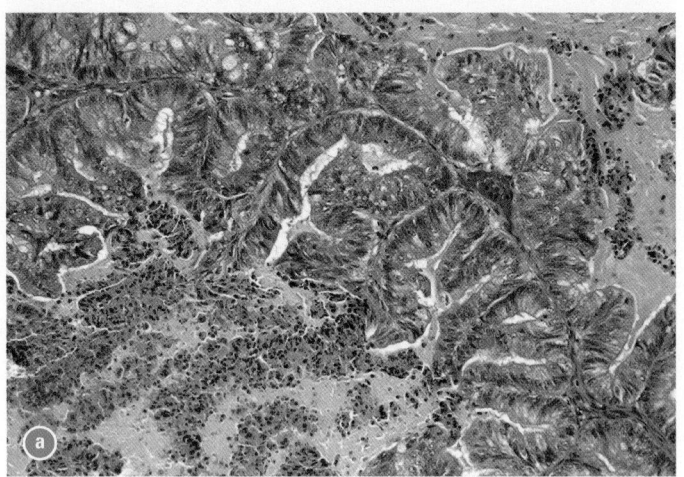
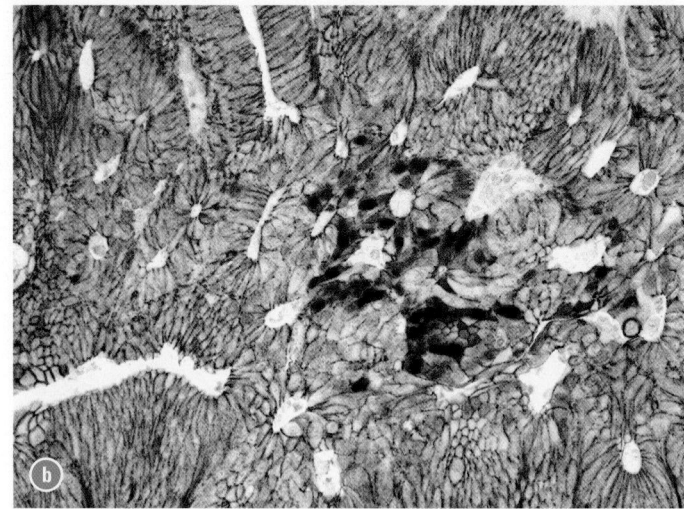

Fig. 31.6 (a) Metastatic colon carcinoma with 'dirty necrosis'. (b) Beta-catenin stain showing focal nuclear positivity in metastatic colon carcinoma (primary ovary carcinoma would have only cell membrane staining).

31.11a). Bilateral ovarian tumors, as well as a variable histologic pattern and surface implants, are clues to the correct diagnosis. Negative staining with dpc4 (smad4) is seen in approximately 50% of pancreatic carcinomas, whereas it is positive in ovarian mucinous carcinomas. Therefore, a negative stain is helpful in confirming a metastasis (Fig. 31.11b).

Metastatic gallbladder or bile duct carcinomas are rare. They are usually solid masses that contain infiltrative small glands (Fig. 31.12) or, sometimes, larger glands or cysts simulating an endometrioid or mucinous ovarian carcinoma.[27]

Other secondary tumors of the ovary

METASTATIC BREAST CARCINOMA

Historically, breast carcinomas have been among the most common primary sites metastasizing to the ovary. Ovarian metastases were estimated to occur in up to one-third of patients with breast carcinoma as determined by autopsy studies.[28] However, symptomatic ovarian metastases or obvious mass-forming lesions in the ovaries that originate from a primary breast carci-

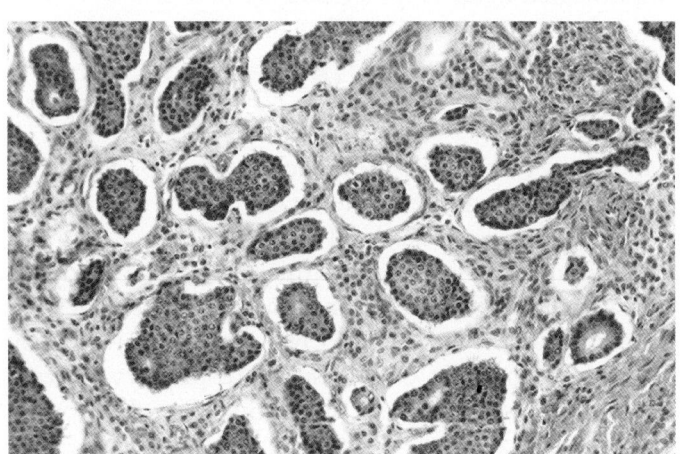

Fig. 31.7 Metastatic insular carcinoid tumor from the small bowel.

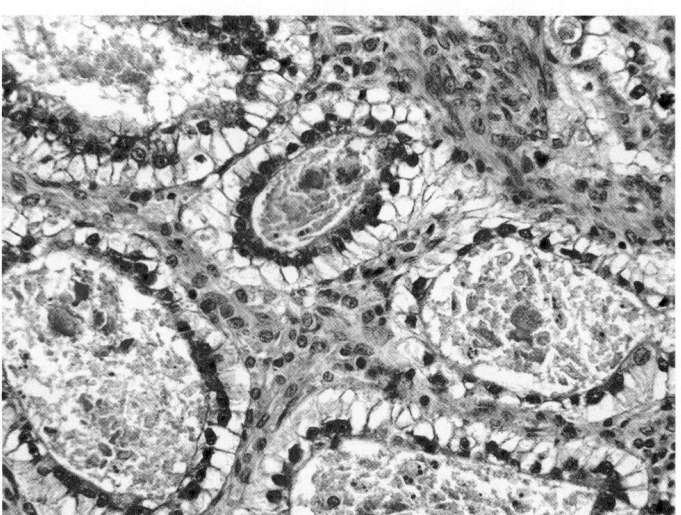

Fig. 31.8 Metastatic clear cell carcinoma from the small bowel. The morphology is similar to early secretory endometrium.

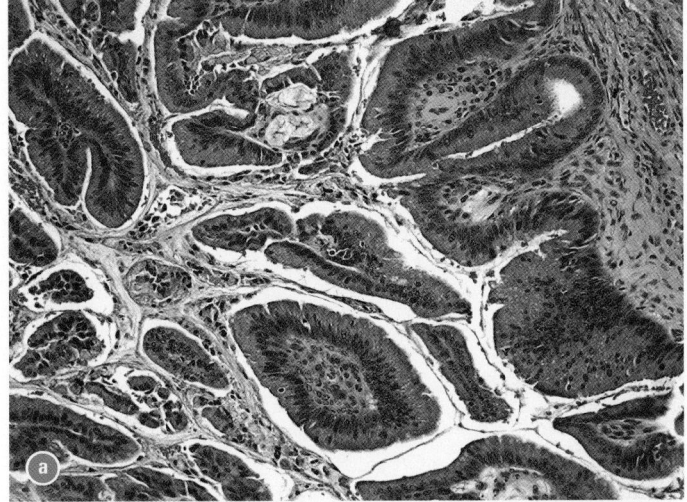

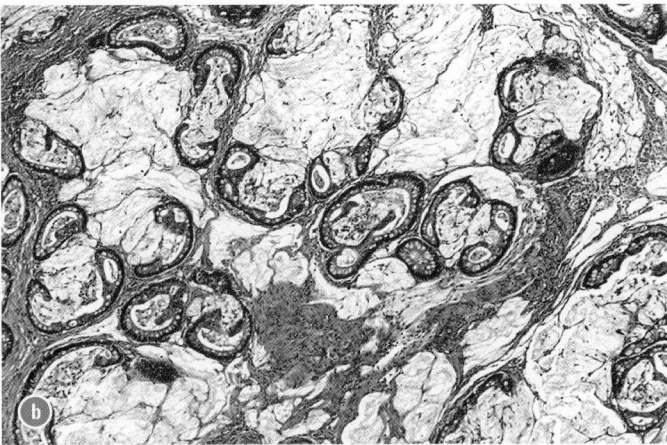

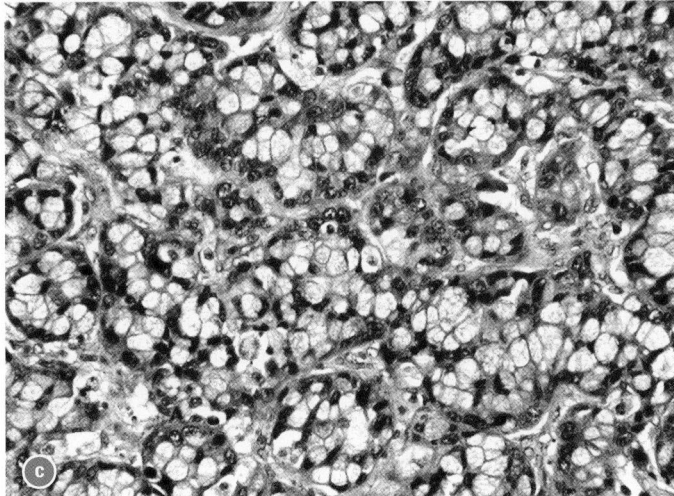

Fig. 31.9 (a) Metastatic appendiceal carcinoma with a villous papillary pattern. (b) Metastatic mucinous (colloid) appendiceal carcinoma. (c) Metastatic appendiceal carcinoma with numerous signet ring cells.

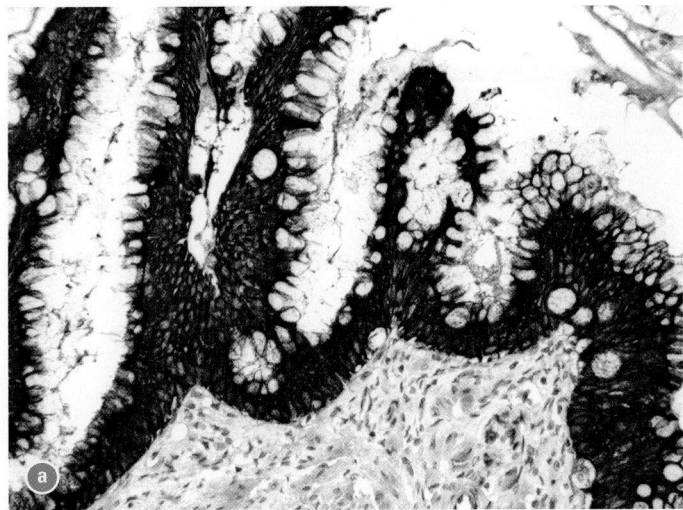

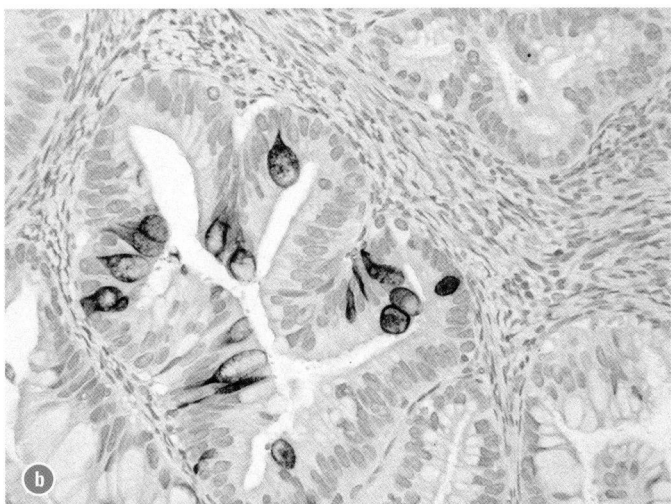

Fig. 31.10 (a) MUC2 is diffusely positive in a metastatic mucinous appendiceal carcinoma. (b) MUC2 in primary ovarian mucinous carcinoma. There is only focal positivity.

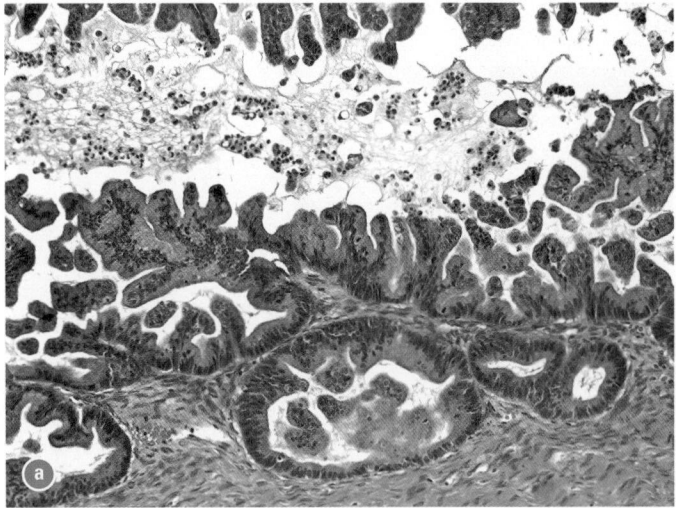

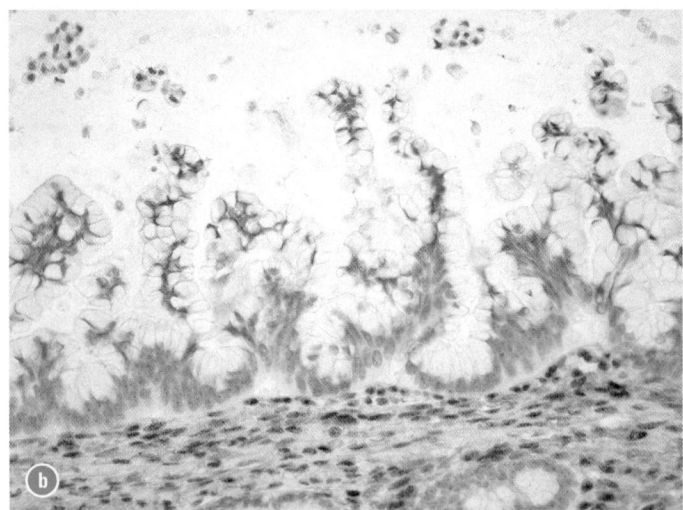

Fig. 31.11 (a) Metastatic pancreatic carcinoma resembling a primary mucinous borderline tumor. (b) dpc4 (smad4) is negative in this metastatic pancreatic carcinoma. Note that the stromal cells are positive in the nuclei; primary ovarian tumors should also be positive in nuclei.

noma are much less common, especially now that breast cancer is detected and treated earlier than when the above data were collected.[29,30] Metastatic breast carcinomas are usually bilateral solid masses that efface the ovarian parenchyma (Fig. 31.13). The diagnostic options that arise in the patient with a history of breast cancer and an ovarian mass include the following:

Metastatic lobular carcinoma

These are easily recognized if history is available. Both ovaries (and other adnexal structures) are commonly involved and the tumor will vary from microscopic to a grossly apparent mass. Occasionally, large omental masses will accompany the ovarian involvement. However, non-lobular-appearing ovarian carcinomas accom-

panied by extensive omental involvement are usually primary ovarian in origin.

Metastatic ductal carcinoma

These tumors are rarely associated with omental involvement. The tumor may, however, simulate an endometrioid carcinoma, carcinoid tumor, or granulosa cell tumor of the ovary (Fig. 31.14a,b).[31] Immunostains for GCDFP may be helpful, although one should keep in mind that this marker is specific but not very sensitive for breast carcinomas.[32]

Primary ovarian carcinoma

Women can present with independent breast and ovarian carcinomas. One study claims that women with an

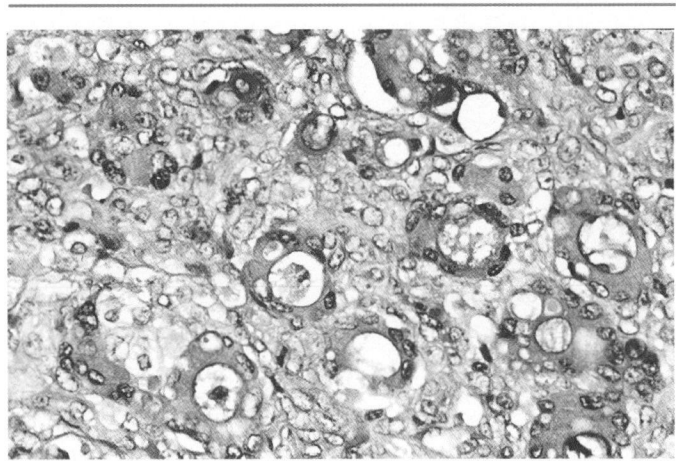

Fig. 31.12 Metastatic tubular adenocarcinoma from the gall bladder.

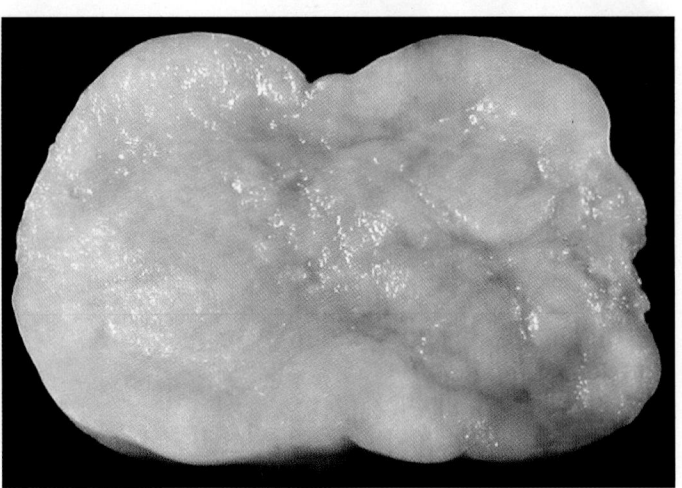

Fig. 31.13 Gross photograph of metastatic breast carcinoma.

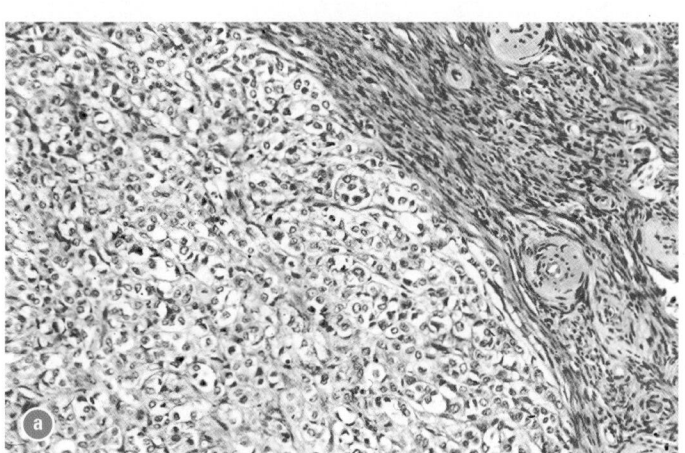
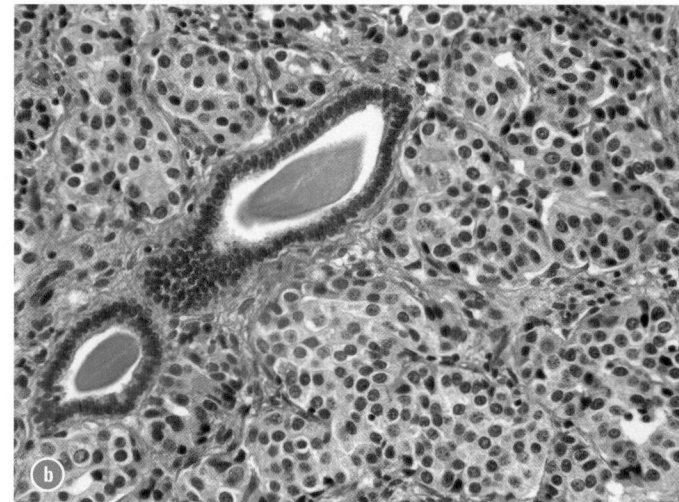

Fig. 31.14 (a) Metastatic breast carcinoma in a solid pattern. (b) Metastatic breast carcinoma involving an ovarian endometrioid adenofibroma. Note the sparing of the ovarian tumor epithelium.

ovarian mass and a history of breast cancer were three times more likely to have a primary ovarian tumor than a metastasis.[33]

METASTATIC LUNG CARCINOMA

Approximately 5% of women with lung carcinoma will have ovarian metastases at autopsy. Lung carcinomas rarely clinically mimic a primary ovarian neoplasm. Nevertheless, cases have been documented in which the initial presentation was a pelvic mass, with the pulmonary neoplasm only appreciated during the subsequent follow-up.[34,35] In a patient with a history of lung cancer, bilateral ovarian tumors, a nodular growth pattern (Fig. 31.15) and lymphovascular invasion strongly suggest metastatic carcinoma. A panel of immunohistochemical markers, including CK7, CK20 and TTF-1, is often useful; TTF-1 is both sensitive and specific for lung adenocarcinomas and small cell carcinomas (Fig. 31.16a,b).[36–38] One should, however, be aware that TTF-1 is also immunoreactive in benign and malignant struma ovarii, metastatic thyroid carcinomas and non-pulmonary neuroendocrine tumors.

METASTATIC RENAL CELL CARCINOMA

Although renal cell carcinoma is known to metastasize to unusual sites throughout the body, fewer than 15 case reports of ovarian metastases have been documented.[39–41] Overlapping morphologic features of primary clear cell carcinomas and metastatic clear cell renal carcinomas include cells with clear cytoplasm

and distinct cell borders, tubulocystic, papillary and solid patterns. Findings in primary ovarian clear cell carcinomas, but not in clear cell renal cell carcinomas, include hobnail cells, PAS-positive luminal mucin and the presence of hyaline basement membrane-like material. Ovarian clear cell carcinomas are also often associated with endometriosis or an endometrioma. Further, many clear cell renal cell carcinomas have low-grade nuclei (Fig. 31.17a). Ovarian clear cell carcinomas nearly always demonstrate significant cytologic atypia (Fig. 31.17b). A panel of immunohistochemical markers can be useful: although not entirely specific, CK7 is highly sensitive for ovarian clear cell

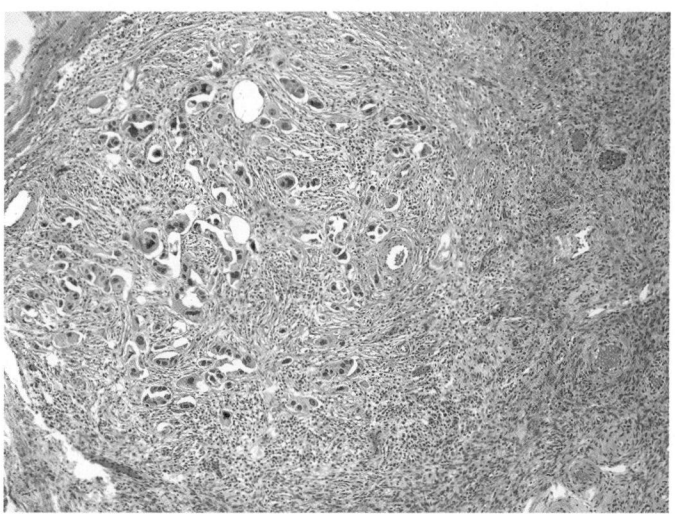

Fig. 31.15 Metastatic lung carcinoma in a well-defined nodule in the ovarian stroma. The cells were TTF-1 positive.

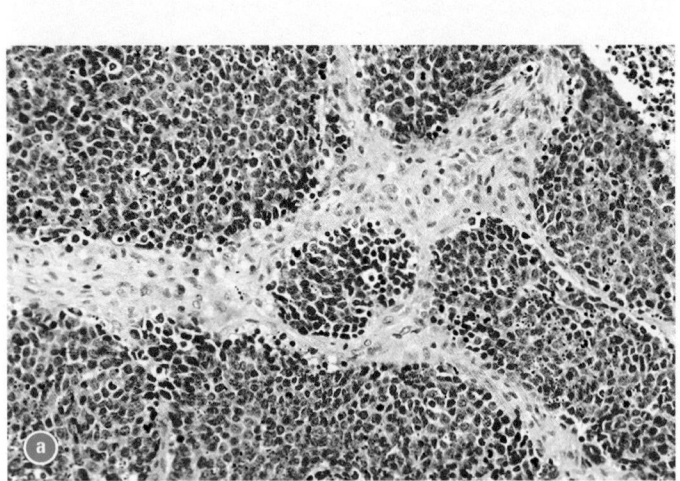

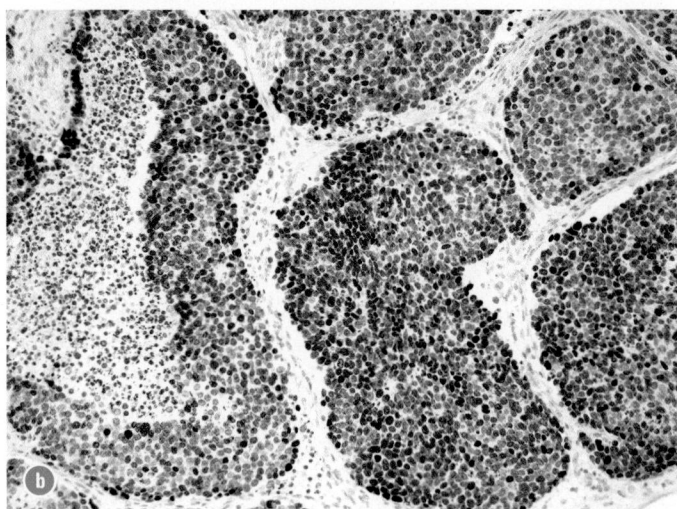

Fig. 31.16 (a) Metastatic small cell carcinoma from the lung. (b) TTF-1-positive metastatic small cell carcinoma of the lung. Primary ovarian small cell carcinomas, both of the pulmonary and hypercalcemic types are negative for TTF-1.

carcinomas, whereas CD10 marks most clear cell renal cell carcinomas.[42–44] Additionally, the monoclonal antibody 'renal cell carcinoma marker' is both specific and sensitive for renal cell carcinomas; however, the sensitivity of this marker can be decreased in metastatic lesions.[45]

METASTATIC UROTHELIAL CARCINOMA

The distinction between a primary transitional cell carcinoma of the ovary and a metastasis from an urothelial carcinoma can be very difficult based solely on histologic findings.[46] Broad undulating papillae with a stratified epithelium and varying degrees of

cytologic atypia are present in primary ovarian transitional cell carcinomas and malignant Brenner tumors, as well as in metastatic urothelial carcinomas. The presence of a benign or borderline Brenner tumor signifies an ovarian primary, whereas bilateral ovarian involvement and a history of invasive urothelial carcinoma would favor a metastasis.

As detailed in Chapter 27, primary transitional cell carcinomas of the ovary have an immunoprofile similar to other ovarian epithelial malignancies, and different from the immunoprofile of urothelial carcinomas. Primary ovarian transitional cell carcinomas are usually CK7 and WT-1 positive, and CK20 and thrombomodulin negative. In contrast, metastatic urothelial

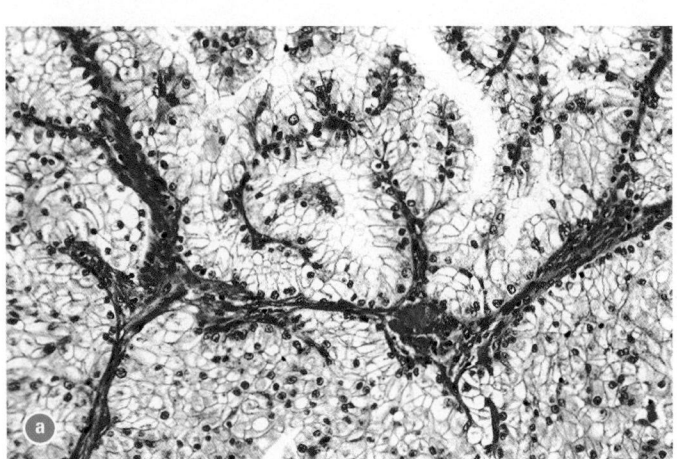

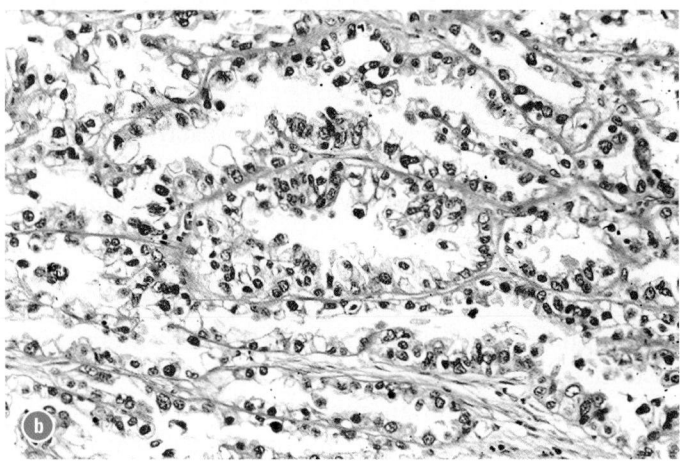

Fig. 31.17 (a) Clear cell renal carcinoma with papillary features. Compare with (b). Notice the bland nuclei without hobnail protrusions. (b) Clear cell carcinoma of the ovary with papillary features. Note atypical nuclei and hobnailing.

carcinomas more commonly demonstrate the presence of CK20 and thrombomodulin, and an absence of WT-1. CK7 can, however, be positive in a minority of urothelial carcinomas.[47–50]

MALIGNANT MELANOMA

Metastatic melanoma to the ovary is rare and carries a high mortality rate. Although usually involvement of the ovary is associated with widely metastatic disease, metastatic melanoma can sometimes mimic a primary ovarian neoplasm. Commonly, the relevant history is lacking, as melanoma metastases may not be clinically evident for many years following diagnosis. In a series of 23 cases, the average lag time until a metastasis was discovered in the ovary was 77 months (range 15–228 months).[51] Further, the majority of cases of metastatic melanoma involve only one ovary[51–53] and the gross findings may include either a cystic or solid mass that may not be pigmented (Fig. 31.18).[52,53] Histologically metastatic melanoma looks similar to primary melanoma, including its well-known heterogeneity. Metastatic melanoma grows in sheets or nests of cells, and follicle-like spaces containing eosinophilic material may also be present.[51–53] Most cases are composed of epithelioid cells with moderate to large amounts of eosinophilic cytoplasm and nuclei with prominent nucleoli (Fig. 31.19a). Occasionally, however, the cells are smaller, with round to oval nuclei, or have a predominant spindle cell appearance. Multinucleated cells, numerous mitoses and necrosis may be present. Nuclear pseudoinclusions may be present and nuclear grooves are infrequent. The presence of melanin pigment is important, but other types of pigment (such as hemosiderin) should not be misinterpreted as melanin.

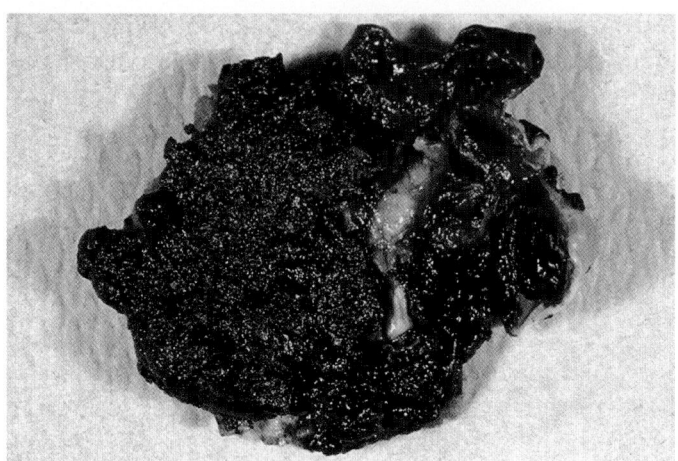

Fig. 31.18 Gross photo of metastatic melanoma.

Because of its multiple guises, the differential diagnosis of metastatic ovarian melanoma is wide and includes primary or metastatic carcinoma, sarcoma, lymphoma, sex cord-stromal tumors, steroid cell tumors (which can show pigmentation), pregnancy luteoma, germ cell tumors (especially a yolk sac tumor) and a primary melanoma arising in association with a teratoma. Suspicion for a metastatic melanoma and the use of immunohistochemistry are pivotal in confirming the diagnosis. Positive immunostaining for S-100, HMB-45 and/or MART-1 is highly sensitive and specific for metastatic melanoma (Fig. 31.19b).[51,53,54] Focal inhibin and calretinin positivity has been shown is a small subset of metastatic melanomas,[51] potentially causing confusion with a sex cord-stromal tumor; however, the latter are characteristically negative for HMB-45 and MART-1 (although they can be immunoreactive for S-100). Negative staining for keratins, leukocyte

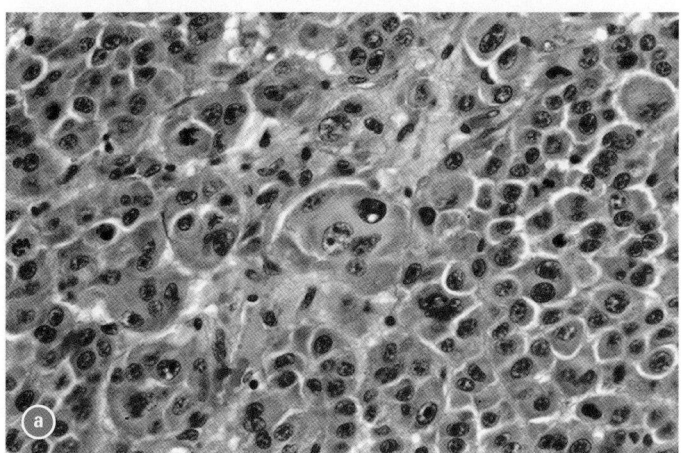

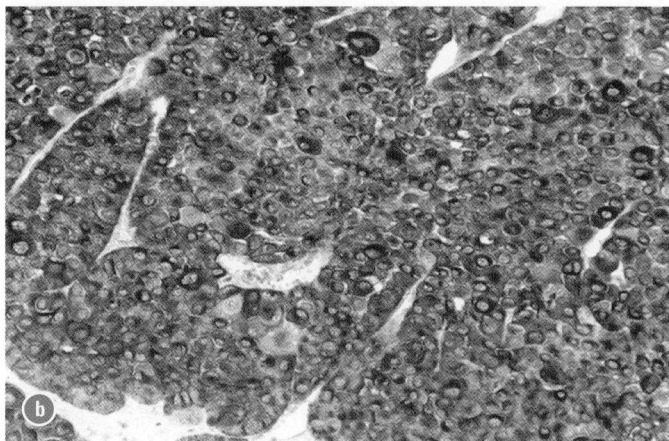

Fig. 31.19 (a) Metastatic melanoma with epithelioid cells; some are multinucleated. (b) Metastatic melanoma positive for HMB-45.

common antigen, placental alkaline phosphatase and alpha-fetoprotein rules out carcinoma, lymphoma and germ cell tumors. A diagnosis of primary melanoma of the ovary in the absence of other teratomatous elements should be made with extreme caution, and only after a metastasis from a recent, remote, or regressed primary melanoma has been excluded.[55]

METASTATIC SARCOMA

Sarcomas metastatic to the ovary are very rare. In the largest series of secondary ovarian sarcomas, three cases presented in the ovary prior to identifying the primary tumour, 11 cases presented at the same time the ovarian metastasis was identified, and in seven cases, the metastasis appeared 7 months to 9 years following the original primary diagnosis.[56] Of these 21 cases, 10 were from extragenital sites, four of which were originally diagnosed as metastatic gastrointestinal leiomyosarcomas,[56] but were likely metastatic gastrointestinal stromal sarcomas (GISTs) (Fig. 31.20a,b).[57–60] The remaining 11 cases metastasized from the uterus and included three leiomyosarcomas and eight endometrial stromal sarcomas.[56] Additional cases of metastatic sarcomas to the ovary include osteosarcoma, chondrosarcoma and angiosarcoma.[61–64]

In addition to the clinical presentation and morphologic findings, immunohistochemistry and cytogenetics are often required to accurately classify and distinguish metastatic sarcomas from other malignancies such as carcinoma, melanoma and lymphoma.[54,65–68] When associated with a teratoma, any sarcoma is more likely a primary malignancy of the ovary.

METASTATIC SMALL ROUND BLUE CELL TUMORS

Metastatic small round blue cell tumors in children and young women have been the subject of multiple case reports and small studies.[56,64,69,70] The differential diagnosis includes rhabdomyosarcoma, intra-abdominal desmoplastic small round cell tumor, Ewing sarcoma/primitive neuroectodermal tumor (PNET) and neuroblastoma. Embryonal rhabdomyosarcoma is the more common of the two subtypes of childhood rhabdomyosarcoma to occur as a primary ovarian tumor.[71] In contrast, of 11 cases of rhabdomyosarcoma metastatic to the ovary over half were of the alveolar subtype.[64,71] Embryonal rhabdomyosarcoma is composed of small round to spindle-shaped cells associated with discernible rhabdomyoblasts, set in a myxoid matrix. Alveolar rhabdomyosarcoma consists of undifferentiated cells with larger nuclei, rhabdomyoblasts, and wreath-like multinucleated giant cells, associated with fibrous septae. Both subtypes of rhabdomyosarcoma are immunoreactive with desmin and the specific skeletal muscle markers myogenin (myf4) and MyoD1.[72,73] Additionally, a translocation between chromosomes 2 (or 1 less frequently) and 13 is found in most alveolar rhabdomyosarcomas, whereas deletions in chromosome 11 are more characteristic of embryonal rhabdomyosarcomas.[68,74]

Metastatic ovarian desmoplastic small round cell tumor and Ewing sarcoma/PNET have been documented in four cases and three cases, respectively.[69,75] Metastases to the ovary in both tumor types appear similar to their primary counterpart. Desmoplastic small round cell tumors are characterized by nests of

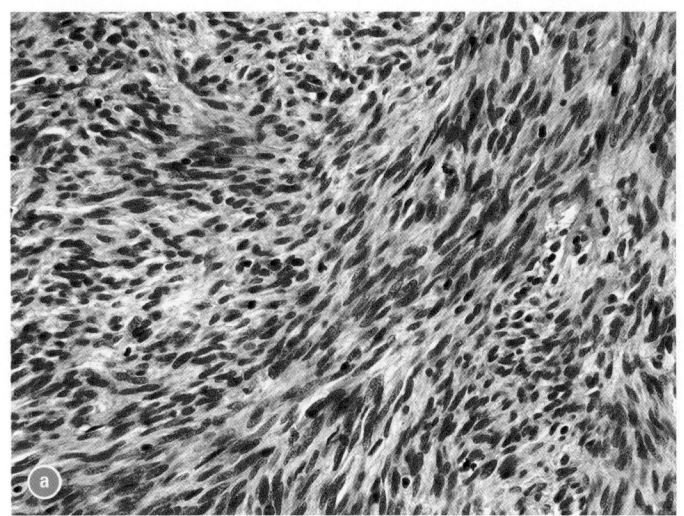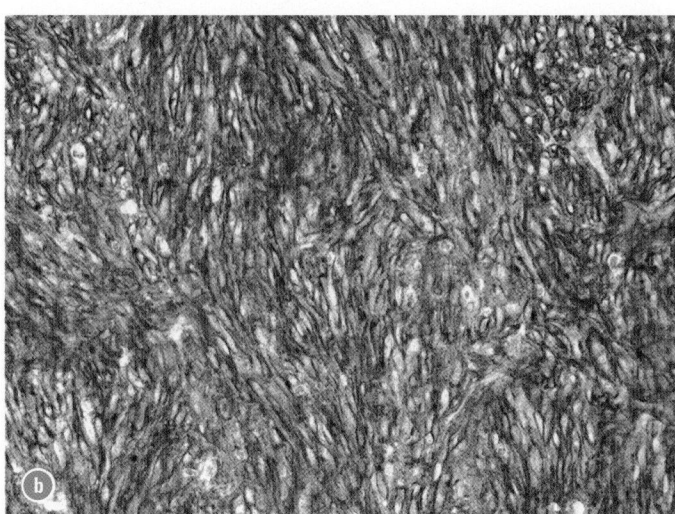

Fig. 31.20 (a) Metastatic gastrointestinal stroma sarcoma (GIST) with fascicles simulating a smooth muscle neoplasm. (b) GIST is positive for c-kit.

small cells with scanty cytoplasm and hyperchromatic nuclei, separated by a prominent desmoplastic stroma. Mitotic figures and necrosis are common. The immunophenotype includes desmin (often with a dot-like staining pattern), keratin, EMA and WT-1 positivity; specific skeletal muscle markers are negative.[54,69] The presence of the chromosomal translocation t(11;22) (p13:q12) (between the EWS and WT1 genes) is diagnostic of intra-abdominal desmoplastic small round cell tumor.[76]

Ewing sarcoma/PNET is also composed of small cells with round to ovoid hyperchromatic nuclei. Rosette-like structures are frequently present, as are mitoses and necrosis. The unique chromosomal translocation for Ewing sarcoma/PNET, t(11;22) (q24;q12), is diagnostic. Although it may exclude other malignancies, immunohistochemical staining is not very useful for confirming Ewing sarcoma/PNET. However, CD99 (MIC2) can be helpful if it is diffusely positive (i.e. in all tumor cells) in a membranous pattern.

Up to 25% of patients with adrenal neuroblastoma have ovarian involvement at autopsy.[77] Rarely an ovarian metastases is discovered along with the primary tumor.[64,78,79] Neuroblastomas are composed of small round cells with hyperchromatic nuclei, arranged in an ill-defined lobular or nested pattern with thin fibrovascular septae and variable amounts of pale fibrillary material between the tumor cells. Rosettes with fibrillary material in their center are sometimes present. These findings, along with immunostaining (i.e. NSE positive, desmin negative), help to distinguish neuroblastomas from other metastatic small round blue cell tumors.

METASTATIC MALIGNANT MESOTHELIOMA

Peritoneal malignant mesothelioma is a rare disease that occurs in men more frequently than women. The distinction between primary ovarian mesothelioma and secondary malignant mesothelioma that also involves the ovary can be very difficult; however, in the latter, the tumor will more often occur as a part of bulky peritoneal disease and involve both ovaries.[80,81] Morphologically and immunophenotypically metastatic malignant mesothelioma resembles the primary lesion, and includes a papillary, tubulocystic or diffuse pattern with bland-appearing epithelioid cells that resemble mesothelial cells. Occasionally malignant mesotheliomas are composed of spindle cells ('sarcomatoid' variant) or a combination of epithelioid and spindle cells (biphasic 'mixed epithelial and spindle cell' variant). Mitoses are often inconspicuous.

The primary differential diagnosis for metastatic mesothelioma to the ovary is the much more common papillary serous carcinoma. However, papillary serous carcinomas have greater cytologic atypia, more necrosis and increased numbers of mitoses as compared with malignant mesothelioma. Clear cell carcinomas, which may be papillary, might also be considered. The greater degree of cytologic atypia, increased number of clear cells and the presence of endometriosis in some cases are keys to the diagnosis.

As outlined in Chapter 27 (the differential diagnosis of serous carcinomas), immunohistochemistry is not very useful in distinguishing metastatic malignant mesothelioma from primary ovarian carcinomas. Mesotheliomas are classically immunoreactive for calretinin, AE1/AE3 (peri-nuclear pattern), EMA (membranous pattern) and WT-1 (nuclear); however, each of these markers can also be positive in primary ovarian serous and clear cell carcinomas. The presence of CEA and Leu-M1 may help distinguish primary tumors of the ovary from mesothelioma, as CEA may be present in a subset of ovarian endometrioid carcinomas, and CEA and/or Leu-M1 may be present in a subset of serous carcinomas, both of which should be negative in malignant mesothelioma. If a sarcomatoid variant of mesothelioma is suspected, sarcoma immunomarkers (such as desmin and ckit) should be used to exclude a metastatic sarcoma.

LYMPHOMA AND LEUKEMIA INVOLVING THE OVARIES

Malignant lymphomas

Up to 25% of disseminated malignant lymphomas are found to involve one or both ovaries at autopsy.[82] However, cases that present with symptoms due to ovarian enlargement are rare. Patients range widely in age from children, to adults in their mid-70s, with most in their third to fifth decades. In countries where Burkitt's lymphoma is endemic the ovary is frequently involved, and the patients are mostly children.[83] Most patients in Western countries with Burkitt-type or undifferentiated lymphomas are also either children or less than 30 years old.[84–87]

Symptoms are non-specific, usually related to the mass effect of the tumor, but sometimes there is acute abdominal pain or ascites.[86] In only a minority of cases has a peripheral nodal lymphoma been diagnosed before exploration, but in most other cases, there is concomitant abdominal, pelvic and internal lymph node involvement so that it is not possible to determine the site of origin.[84–87] In four series totaling 133 cases, 25 cases (19%) were confined to a single ovary without extra-ovarian spread and thus could be considered as having originated in the ovary.[84–87] Some of these were small and asymptomatic incidental findings upon surgical exploration for other gynecologic conditions, but others were large masses.

Lymphomas range in size from small nodules that only partially involve the ovary to 25 cm masses that completely obliterate the ovarian parenchyma;[84,85] about 60% are bilateral.[84,85,87] The surface of the involved ovary is usually smooth or bosselated. The cut surface is white, tan or variegated, sometimes with areas of cystic degeneration, hemorrhage or necrosis, although larger tumors tend to be solid.

In a series of 80 cases that used current terminology, 40% were of the undifferentiated type (either Burkitt or non-Burkitt), 31% were diffuse large cell lymphomas, 15% were immunoblastic, 11% were follicular lymphomas (Fig. 31.21) and 3% were various rare types.[84,85,88] Thirty of 33 cases were of B-cell phenotype and the remaining three were T-cell type.[85] Hodgkin's disease is extremely rare in the ovaries, with only one case reported in the 133 summarized above.[86] Also rarely, plasmacytomas of the ovary have been reported.[89]

Cytologically, lymphomas in the ovary are identical to those in lymph nodes (Fig. 31.21), including a 'starry sky' appearance in the Burkitt and undifferentiated non-Burkitt types. However, an 'indian file' or trabecular pattern may often be present as well as prominent sclerosis, especially in diffuse large cell lymphomas

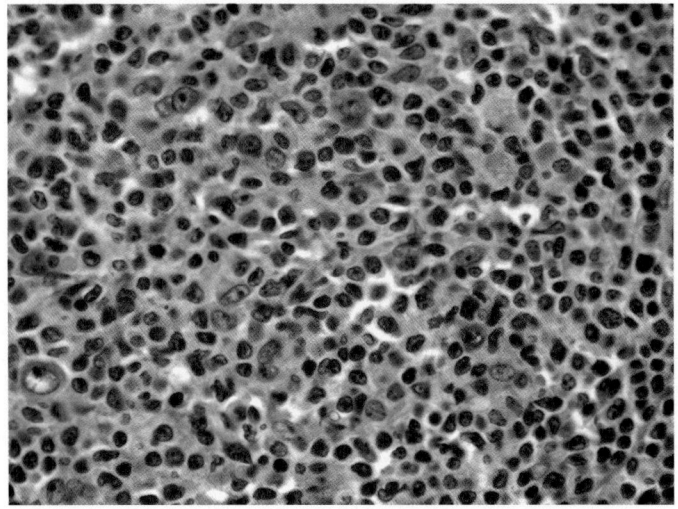

Fig. 31.21 B-cell lymphoma involving the ovary. This case was unusual in that the lymphoma was nodular with both small cleaved and large cells.

separating groups of cells into islands or loose alveolar arrangements.[85] Lymphomas may also diffusely infiltrate while sparing residual ovarian follicles. Vascular space involvement is common along with infiltration of vessel walls.

Although ovarian lymphomas are cytologically similar to their nodal counterparts, the architectural features of ovarian involvement noted above may cause them to appear more epithelioid. Along with their rarity, this may lead to misdiagnosis. Differential considerations include granulosa cell tumor, dysgerminoma, small cell carcinoma of the hypercalcemic type, granulocytic sarcoma, undifferentiated carcinoma and metastatic tumors, including breast carcinoma, melanoma or Krukenberg tumors. All of these are easily excluded using immunohistochemistry if a malignant lymphoma is at least considered.

Since most ovarian lymphomas are a component of disseminated malignant lymphomas, the prognosis is variable and related to the cell type and individual response to radiation and various chemotherapeutic agents. Overall, the outlook is poor, but long-term survival without evidence of recurrence is possible.[84–87] In cases that are confined to a single ovary (Ann Arbor Stage IE), however, the prognosis is favorable. In one study of 10 such cases, all patients were alive and well at intervals from 1.3 to 10 years after receiving various forms of chemotherapy and/or radiation.[88]

Leukemia

In studies that have included both leukemias and lymphomas, there were only three cases of ovarian leukemia within a total of 61 cases (5%).[84,86] However, in an autopsy study of 1206 children and adults with acute and chronic leukemias, the ovary was involved by the leukemic cells in 11% of cases of acute myelogenous leukemia, 9% of cases of chronic myelogenous leukemia, 21% of cases of acute lymphocytic leukemia and 22% of cases of chronic lymphocytic leukemia.[90] In all of these categories the percentage of ovarian involvement decreased over the time period of the study, which ended in 1982, which is indicative of the increasing efficacy of treatment.

In practically all autopsy cases, the ovaries were not enlarged or the cause of clinical symptoms. Rarely however, cases of acute myelogenous leukemia can present with an ovarian mass (i.e. granulocytic sarcoma, see below). In a report containing seven such cases, the patients ranged from 13 to 43 years old, two were bilateral; the tumors ranged from 5 to 14 cm.[91] Six of the seven patients had bone marrow involvement and other evidence of leukemia. However, one patient had a normal bone marrow and peripheral blood count; she was treated with chemotherapy and oophorectomy and was free of disease after 18 months of follow-up.

The gross and microscopic features of granulocytic sarcomas are similar to those of lymphomas of the ovary. In fact, a lymphoma would likely be the initial diagnostic consideration. However, the cells of a granulocytic sarcoma have paler, more finely granular nuclei than do most lymphomas, and either inconspicuous or eosinophilic cytoplasm. Eosinophilic myelocytes are an important clue to the diagnosis. Confirmation, once leukemia is suspected, can be made with a positive chloroacetate esterase, myeloperoxidase, or lysozyme stain. Cells will also be immunoreactive for CD43 and CD68.

Other types of leukemia have not been reported to be the cause of symptomatic ovarian enlargement. However, several cases of acute lymphoblastic leukemia have persisted in the ovaries while in remission at all other sites.

References

1 Yada-Hashimoto N, Yamamoto T, Kamiura S, et al. Metastatic ovarian tumors: a review of 64 cases. Gynecol Oncol 2003; 89:314–317.

2 Fujiwara K, Ohishi Y, Koike H, et al. Clinical implications of metastases to the ovary. Gynecol Oncol 1995; 59:124–128.

3 Demopoulos RI, Touger L, Dubin N. Secondary ovarian carcinoma: a clinical and pathological evaluation. Int J Gynecol Pathol 1987; 6:166–175.

4 Ulbright TM, Roth LM, Stehman FB. Secondary ovarian neoplasia. A clinicopathologic study of 35 cases. Cancer 1984; 53:1164–1174.

5 Lee KR, Young RH. The distinction between primary and metastatic mucinous carcinomas of the ovary: gross and histologic findings in 50 cases. Am J Surg Pathol 2003; 27:281–292.

6 Riolpel MA, Ronnett BM, Kurman RJ. Evaluation of diagnostic criteria and behavior of ovarian intestinal-type mucinous tumors: atypical proliferative (borderline) tumors and intraepithelial, microinvasive, invasive, and metastatic carcinomas. Am J Surg Pathol 1999; 23:617–635.

7 McMeekin DS, Burger RA, Manetta A, et al. Endometrioid adenocarcinoma of the ovary and its relationship to endometriosis. Gynecol Oncol 1995; 59:81–86.

8 Grosso G, Raspagliesi F, Baiocchi G, et al. Endometrioid carcinoma of the ovary: a retrospective analysis of 106 cases. Tumori 1998; 84:552–557.

9 Czernobilsky B, Silverman BB, Mikuta JJ. Endometrioid carcinoma of the ovary. A clinicopathologic study of 75 cases. Cancer 1970; 26:1141–1152.

10 Kline RC, Wharton JT, Atkinson EN, et al. Endometrioid carcinoma of the ovary: retrospective review of 145 cases. Gynecol Oncol 1990; 39:337–346.

11 DePriest PD, Banks ER, Powell DE, et al. Endometrioid carcinoma of the ovary and endometriosis: the association in postmenopausal women. Gynecol Oncol 1992; 47:71–75.

12 Leitao MM, Sonoda Y, Brennan MF, et al. Incidence of lymph node and ovarian metastases in leiomyosarcoma of the uterus. Gynecol Oncol 2003; 91:209–212.

13 Yilmaz A, Rush DS, Soslow RA. Endometrial stromal sarcomas with unusual histologic features: a report of 24 primary and metastatic tumors emphasizing fibroblastic and smooth muscle differentiation. Am J Surg Pathol 2002; 26:1142–1150.

14 Lerwill MF, Sung R, Oliva E, et al. Smooth muscle tumors of the ovary: a clinicopathologic study of 54 cases emphasizing prognostic criteria, histologic variants, and differential diagnosis. Am J Surg Pathol 2004; 28: 1436–1451.

15 Young RH, Prat J, Scully RE. Endometrioid stromal sarcomas of the ovary. A clinicopathologic analysis of 23 cases. Cancer 1984; 53:1143–1155.

16 Young RH, Scully RE. Mucinous tumors of the ovary associated with mucinous adenocarcinomas of the cervix. A clinicopathologic analysis of 16 cases. Int J Gynecol Pathol 1988; 7:99–111.

17 Holtz F, Hart WR. Krukenberg tumors of the ovary. A clinicopathologic analysis of 27 cases. Cancer 1982; 50:2438–2447.

18 Yakushiji M, Tazaki T, Nishimura H, Kato T. Krukenberg tumors of the ovary: a clinicopathologic analysis of 112 cases. Acta Obstet Gynaecol Jpn 1987; 39:479–485.

19 Bullon A, Arseneau J, Prat J, Young RH, Scully RE. Tubular Krukenberg tumor. A problem in histopathologic diagnosis. Am J Surg Pathol 1981; 5:225–232.

20 Lash RH, Hart WR. Intestinal adenocarcinomas metastatic to the ovaries. A clinicopathological evaluation of 22 cases. Am J Surg Pathol 1987; 11:114–121.

21 Robboy SJ, Scully RE, Noroos HJ. Carcinoid metastatic to the ovary. A clinicopathologic analysis of 35 cases. Cancer 1974; 33:798–811.

22 Ikeda E, Tsutsumi Y, Yoshida H, Yanagi K. Goblet cell carcinoid of the vermiform appendix with ovarian metastasis mimicking mucinous cystadenocarcinoma. Acta Pathol Jpn 1991; 41:445–460.

23 Young RH, Hart WR. Metastatic intestinal carcinomas simulating primary ovarian clear cell carcinoma and secretory endometrioid carcinoma. A clinicopathologic and immunohistochemical study of five cases. Am J Surg Pathol 1998; 22:805–815.

24 Merino MJ, Edmonds P, LiVolsi V. Appendiceal carcinoma metastatic to the ovaries and mimicking primary ovarian tumors. Int J Gynecol Pathol 1985; 4:110–120.

25 Ronnett BM, Kurman RJ, Shmookler BM, et al. The morphologic spectrum of ovarian metastases of appendiceal adenocarcinomas: a clinicopathologic and immunohistochemical analysis of tumors often misinterpreted as primary ovarian tumors or metastatic tumors from other gastrointestinal sites. Am J Surg Pathol 1997; 21:1144–1155.

26 Young RH, Hart WR. Metastases from carcinomas of the pancreas simulating primary mucinous tumors of the ovary. A report of seven cases. Am J Surg Pathol 1989; 13:748–756.

27 Young RH, Scully RE. Ovarian metastases from carcinoma of the gallbladder and extrahepatic bile ducts simulating primary tumors of the ovary: a report of six cases. Int J Gynecol Pathol 1990; 9:60–72.

28 Viadana E, Bross ID, Pickren JW. An autopsy study of some routes of dissemination of cancer of the breast. Br J Cancer 1973; 27:336–340.

29 Lumb G, Mackenzie DH. The incidence of metastases in adrenal gland and ovaries removed for carcinoma of the breast. Cancer 1971; 27:1374–1378.

30 Gagnon Y, Tetu B. Ovarian metastases of breast carcinoma. A clinicopathologic study of 59 cases. Cancer 1984; 50:23–30.

31 Young RH, Carey RW, Robboy SJ. Breast carcinoma masquerading as a primary ovarian neoplasm. Cancer 1981; 48:210–212.

32 Monteagudo C, Merino J, Laporte N, Neumann RD. Value of gross cystic disease protein-15 in distinguishing metastatic breast carcinomas among poorly differentiated neoplasms involving the ovary. Hum Pathol 1991; 22:368–372.

33 Curtin JP, Barakat RR, Hoskins WJ. Ovarian disease in women with breast cancer. Obstet Gynecol 1994; 84:449–452.

34 Yeh KY, Chang JW, Hsueh S, et al. Ovarian metastasis originating from bronchioloalveolar carcinoma: a rare presentation of lung cancer. Jpn J Clin Oncol 2003; 33:404–407.

35 Young RH, Scully RE. Ovarian metastases from cancer of the lung: problems in interpretation – a report of seven cases. Gynecol Oncol 1985; 21:337–350.

36 Reis-Filho JS, Carrilho C, Valenti C, et al. Is TTF1 a good immunohistochemical marker to distinguish primary from metastatic lung adenocarcinomas? Pathol Res Pract 2000; 196:835–840.

37 Chang YL, Lee YC, Liao WY, et al. The utility and limitation of thyroid transcription factor-1 protein in primary and metastatic pulmonary neoplasms. Lung Cancer 2004; 44:149–157.

38 Ordonez NG. Value of thyroid transcription factor-1 immunostaining in distinguishing small cell lung carcinomas from other small cell carcinomas. Am J Surg Pathol 2000; 24:1217–1223.

39 Valappil SV, Toon PG, Anandaram PS. Ovarian metastasis from primary renal cell carcinoma: report of a case and review of literature. Gynecol Oncol 2004; 94:846–849.

40 Young RH, Hart WR. Renal cell carcinoma metastatic to the ovary: a report of three cases emphasizing possible confusion with ovarian clear cell adenocarcinoma. Int J Gynecol Pathol 1992; 11:96–104.

41 Insabato L, De Rosa G, Franco R, et al. Ovarian metastasis from renal cell carcinoma: a report of three cases. Int J Surg Pathol 2003; 11:309–312.

42 Cameron RI, Ashe P, O'Rourke DM, et al. A panel of immunohistochemical stains assists in the distinction between ovarian and renal clear cell carcinoma. Int J Gynecol Pathol 2003; 22:272–276.

43 Vang R, Whitaker BP, Farhood AI, et al. Immunohistochemical analysis of clear cell carcinoma of the gynecologic tract. Int J Gynecol Pathol 2001; 20:252–259.

44 Chu P, Arber DA. Paraffin-section detection of CD10 in 505 nonhematopoietic neoplasms. Frequent expression in renal cell carcinoma and endometrial stromal sarcoma. Am J Clin Pathol 2000; 113:374–382.

45 McGregor DK, Khurana KK, Cao C, et al. Diagnosing primary and metastatic renal cell carcinoma: the use of the monoclonal antibody 'Renal Cell Carcinoma Marker'. Am J Surg Pathol 2001; 25:1485–1492.

46 Young RH, Scully RE. Urothelial and ovarian carcinomas of identical cell types: problems in interpretation. A report of three cases and review of the literature. Int J Gynecol Pathol 1988; 7:197–211.

47 Soslow RA, Rouse RV, Hendrickson MR, et al. Transitional cell neoplasms of the ovary and urinary bladder: a comparative immunohistochemical analysis. Int J Gynecol Pathol 1996; 15:257–265.

48 Ordonez NG. Transitional cell carcinomas of the ovary and bladder are immunophenotypically different. Histopathology 2000; 36:433–438.

49 Logani S, Oliva E, Amin MB, et al. Immunoprofile of ovarian tumors with putative transitional cell (urothelial) differentiation using novel urothelial markers: histogenetic and diagnostic implications. Am J Surg Pathol 2003; 27:1434–1441.

50 Riedel I, Czernobilsky B, Lifschitz-Mercer B, et al. Brenner tumors but not transitional cell carcinomas of the ovary show urothelial differentiation: immunohistochemical staining of urothelial markers, including cytokeratins and uroplakins. Virchows Arch 2001; 438:181–191.

51 Gupta D, Deavers MT, Silva EG, et al. Malignant melanoma involving the ovary: a clinicopathologic and immunohistochemical study of 23 cases. Am J Surg Pathol 2004; 28:771–780.

52 Fitzgibbons PL, Martin SE, Simmons TJ. Malignant melanoma metastatic to the ovary. Am J Surg Pathol 1987; 11:959–964.

53 Young RH, Scully RE. Malignant melanoma metastatic to the ovary. A clinicopathologic analysis of 20 cases. Am J Surg Pathol 1991; 15:849–860.

54 McCluggage WG. Ovarian neoplasms composed of small round cells: a review. Adv Anat Pathol 2004; 11:288–296.

55 Vimla N, Kumar L, Thulkar S, et al. Primary malignant melanoma in ovarian cystic teratoma. Gynecol Oncol 2001; 82:380–383.

56 Young RH, Scully RE. Sarcomas metastatic to the ovary: a report of 21 cases. Int J Gynecol Pathol 1990; 9:231–252.

57 Miettinen M, Sarlomo-Rikala M, Lasota J. Gastrointestinal stromal tumours. Ann Chir Gynaecol 1998; 87:278–281.

58 Miettinen M, Sobin LH, Sarlomo-Rikala M. Immunohistochemical spectrum of GISTs at different sites and their differential diagnosis with a reference to CD117 (KIT). Mod Pathol 2000; 13:1134–1142.

59 Miettinen M, Sarlomo-Rikala M, Lasota J. Gastrointestinal stromal tumors: recent advances in understanding of their biology. Hum Pathol 1999; 30:1213–1220.

60 Miettinen M, Monihan JM, Sarlomo-Rikala M, et al. Gastrointestinal stromal tumors/smooth muscle tumors

(GISTs) primary in the omentum and mesentery: clinicopathologic and immunohistochemical study of 26 cases. Am J Surg Pathol 1999; 23:1109–1118.

61 Swift R, Jalleh R, Patel A, et al. Chondrosarcoma from a rib metastasizing to the ovary. Acta Orthop Scand 1991; 62:76.

62 Sedgely MG, Ostor AG, Fortune DW. Angiosarcoma of breast metastatic to the ovary and placenta. Aust N Z J Obstet Gynaecol 1985; 25:299–302.

63 Eltabbakh GH, Belinson JL, Biscotti CV. Osteosarcoma metastatic to the ovary: a case report and review of the literature. Int J Gynecol Pathol 1997; 16:76–78.

64 Young RH, Kozakewich HP, Scully RE. Metastatic ovarian tumors in children: a report of 14 cases and review of the literature. Int J Gynecol Pathol 1993; 12:8–19.

65 Coindre JM. Immunohistochemistry in the diagnosis of soft tissue tumours. Histopathology 2003; 43:1–16.

66 Fletcher CD. Soft tissue tumours: the impact of cytogenetics and molecular genetics. Verh Dtsch Ges Pathol 1997; 81:318–326.

67 Sandberg AA. Cytogenetics and molecular genetics of bone and soft-tissue tumors. Am J Med Genet 2002; 115:189–193.

68 Fletcher JA. Cytogenetics of soft tissue tumors. Cancer Treat Res 1997; 91:9–29.

69 Young RH, Eichhorn JH, Dickersin GR, et al. Ovarian involvement by the intra-abdominal desmoplastic small round cell tumor with divergent differentiation: a report of three cases. Hum Pathol 1992; 23:454–464.

70 McCarville MB, Hill DA, Miller BE, et al. Secondary ovarian neoplasms in children: imaging features with histopathologic correlation. Pediatr Radiol 2001; 31:358–364.

71 Young RH, Scully RE. Alveolar rhabdomyosarcoma metastatic to the ovary. A report of two cases and a discussion of the differential diagnosis of small cell malignant tumors of the ovary. Cancer 1989; 64:899–904.

72 Cessna MH, Zhou H, Perkins SL, et al. Are myogenin and myoD1 expression specific for rhabdomyosarcoma? A study of 150 cases, with emphasis on spindle cell mimics. Am J Surg Pathol 2001; 25:1150–1157.

73 Wang NP, Marx J, McNutt MA, et al. Expression of myogenic regulatory proteins (myogenin and MyoD1) in small blue round cell tumors of childhood. Am J Pathol 1995; 147:1799–1810.

74 Kushner BH, LaQuaglia MP, Cheung NK, et al. Clinically critical impact of molecular genetic studies in pediatric solid tumors. Med Pediatr Oncol 1999; 33:530–535.

75 Parker LP, Duong JL, Wharton JT, et al. Desmoplastic small round cell tumor: report of a case presenting as a primary ovarian neoplasm. Eur J Gynaecol Oncol 2002; 23:199–202.

76 Gerald WL, Rosai J, Ladanyi M. Characterization of the genomic breakpoint and chimeric transcripts in the EWS-WT1 gene fusion of desmoplastic small round cell tumor. Proc Natl Acad Sci USA 1995; 92:1028–1032.

77 Himelstein-Braw R, Peters H, Faber M. Influence of irradiation and chemotherapy on the ovaries of children with abdominal tumours. Br J Cancer 1977; 36:269–275.

78 Somjee S, Kurkure PA, Chinoy RF, et al. Metastatic ovarian neuroblastoma: a case report. Pediatr Hematol Oncol 1999; 16:459–462.

79 Meyer WH, Yu GW, Milvenan ES, et al. Ovarian involvement in neuroblastoma. Med Pediatr Oncol 1979; 7:49–54.

80 Goldblum J, Hart WR. Localized and diffuse mesotheliomas of the genital tract and peritoneum in women. A clinicopathologic study of nineteen true mesothelial neoplasms, other than adenomatoid tumors, multicystic mesotheliomas, and localized fibrous tumors. Am J Surg Pathol 1995; 19:1124–1137.

81 Clement PB, Young RH, Scully RE. Malignant mesotheliomas presenting as ovarian masses. A report of nine cases, including two primary ovarian mesotheliomas. Am J Surg Pathol 1996; 20:1067–1080.

82 Freeman C, Berg JW, Cutler SJ. Occurrence and prognosis of extranodal lymphomas. Cancer 1972; 29:252–260.

83 Halpin TF. Gynecologic implications of Burkitt's tumor. Obstet Gynecol Surv 1975; 30:351–358.

84 Osborne BM, Robboy SJ. Lymphomas or leukemia presenting as ovarian tumors. An analysis of 42 cases. Cancer 1983; 52:1933–1943.

85 Monterroso V, Jaffe ES, Merino MJ, et al. Malignant lymphomas involving the ovary. A clinicopathologic analysis of 39 cases. Am J Surg Pathol 1993; 17:154–170.

86 Chorlton I, Norris HJ, King FM. Malignant reticuloendothelial disease involving the ovary as a primary manifestation: a series of 19 lymphomas and 1 granulocytic sarcoma. Cancer 1974; 34:397–407.

87 Fox H, Langley FA, Govan AD, et al. Malignant lymphoma presenting as an ovarian tumour: a clinicopathological analysis of 34 cases. Br J Obstet Gynaecol 1988; 95:386–390.

88 Vang R, Medeiros LJ, Warnke RA, et al. Ovarian non-Hodgkin's lymphoma: a clinicopathologic study of eight primary cases. Mod Pathol 2001; 14:1093–1099.

89 Cook HT, Boylston AW. Plasmacytoma of the ovary. Gynecol Oncol 1988; 29:378–381.

90 Barcos M, Lane W, Gomez GA, et al. An autopsy study of 1206 acute and chronic leukemias (1958 to 1982). Cancer 1987; 60:827–837.

91 Oliva E, Ferry JA, Young RH, et al. Granulocytic sarcoma of the female genital tract: a clinicopathologic study of 11 cases. Am J Surg Pathol 1997; 21:1156–1165.

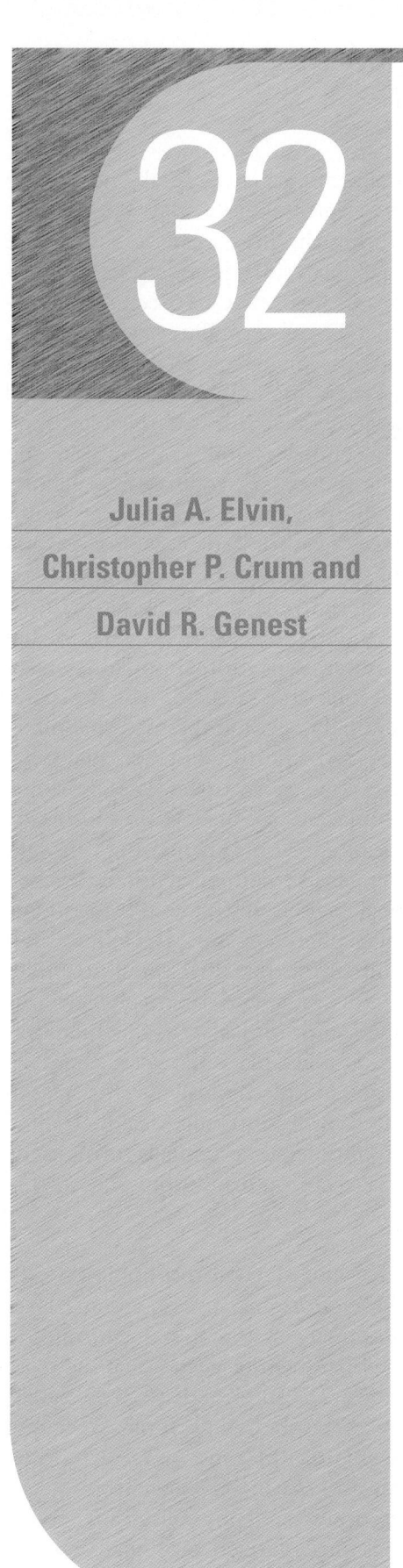

32

Complications of early pregnancy, including trophoblastic neoplasia

Julia A. Elvin,

Christopher P. Crum and

David R. Genest

Introduction

Clinical and pathologic scenarios
The morphology of early
 placental development
Sonographic correlates of early
 gestation
Gross examination of the early
 gestation

Spontaneous abortion

The patient at risk
Early (sporadic) spontaneous
 abortion
Recurrent (habitual) abortion

Ectopic pregnancy

The patient at risk
Clinical presentation
Clinical diagnostic algorithm
 and management

Examination of the curettings
Pitfalls in histologic examination
 of endometrial curettings
Examination of the fallopian tube
Other sites of ectopic gestation

Post-abortal complications

The patient at risk
Clinical presentation
Pathologic findings
Management and outcome

Trophoblastic neoplasia

General
The patient at risk
Molecular pathogenesis
Target tissues
Complete hydatidiform mole
Partial hydatidiform mole
Choriocarcinoma
Placental site trophoblastic tumor

Introduction

CLINICAL AND PATHOLOGIC SCENARIOS

Clinical practitioners and surgical pathologists frequently work together to resolve patient-related questions concerning disorders in early pregnancy. These disorders fall into several categories:

1 *The first is the patient with a spontaneous abortion or habitual abortion.* In most cases, the clinician is eager to identify the causes that would impact on future pregnancies. A pathologic examination may be helpful, but the role of the pathologist is usually to confirm intrauterine pregnancy and secure cytogenetic information.
   In uncommon cases, a pathologic clue may be identified.

2 *The second is the patient with suspected ectopic pregnancy.* In practice, every pathologic examination of a supposed product of conception entails excluding ectopic pregnancy. If this is suspected, the clinician and pathologist are drawn concurrently into a decision-making exercise that requires precise evaluation and an appropriate clinical response.

3 *The third is the exclusion of molar pregnancy or other trophoblastic neoplasm.* Like the other exclusions detailed above, this one must be performed on every specimen from a first trimester fetal loss. In essence, the pathologist examines the specimen, excludes hydatidiform mole and confirms or excludes *current* (not remote) intrauterine pregnancy.

4 *A fourth is the proper disposition of these tissues to comply with the wishes of the families.* In many states, this entails obtaining the necessary permissions to perform examinations and preserving tissues for burial or cremation. This is a complex issue, inasmuch as some persons may wish access to tissues containing minimal or no evidence of fetal parts. Moreover, uterine evacuations for incomplete abortions may take place under circumstances (such as in the emergency room) in which family wishes are not immediately made clear. The pathologist should be mindful of such scenarios, realizing that, in unusual circumstances, families may wish access to embedded tissue from early pregnancy losses for burial. Release of such tissues must be made with care, in accordance with state regulations and with the interests and desires of the family in mind.

THE MORPHOLOGY OF EARLY PLACENTAL DEVELOPMENT

Early development

The oocyte is fertilized near the distal end of the fallopian tube, at approximately day 15 of the menstrual cycle. During the next week, as the zygote travels through the fallopian tube, it undergoes progressive cellular divisions to form first a 16-cell raspberry-like morula and then a 32-cell centrally cystic blastocyst. On days 23 to 26 of the menstrual cycle, the blastocyst attaches to and then implants into the superficial endometrium. The inner cell mass of the blastocyst eventually forms the embryo, yolk sac, amnion and umbilical cord, while the outer, trophoblastic cellular layers will become the placenta and chorionic membrane. The blastocyst's trophoblastic covering consists of the outer mitotically inactive syncytiotrophoblastic layer, and the inner actively proliferating cytotrophoblastic layer, which functions as primordial trophoblast. The outer syncytiotrophoblastic layer develops multiple cytoplasmic lacunae, which expand and coalesce to eventually become the maternal intervillous vascular space (to be perfused by decidual spiral arterioles). Primitive connective tissue, the chorionic stroma, develops subjacent to the cytotrophoblastic layer. As this sphere of chorionic stroma thickens and expands, peripheral finger-like villous extensions develop. Initially the gestational sac is evenly covered by chorionic villi. As the chorionic sphere expands, the villi located furthest from the nurturing decidual spiral arterioles gradually regress, forming the relatively avillous chorionic membrane ('chorion laevae'); this membranous villous regression takes place between 7 and 15 weeks menstrual age. Simultaneously, well-perfused chorionic villi located near nuturing decidual spiral arterioles continue to proliferate, eventually forming the placental parenchyma ('chorion frondosum' Fig. 32.1).[1]

Implantation site

Adjacent to the cyto- and syncytiotrophoblastic cells at the periphery of the chorionic sphere, a dense layer of eosinophilic, proteinaceous, material ('fibrinoid', 'Nitabuch's fibrin') separates the gestational sac from the deciduas (Fig. 32.2). Intermediate trophoblast cells migrate singly through the fibrinoid layer and permeate the adjacent decidua and spiral arterioles. Following vascular invasion by intermediate trophoblast, decidual spiral arterioles are physiologically transformed from normal muscularized resistance arteries, into dilated eosinophilic fibrinous vessels which

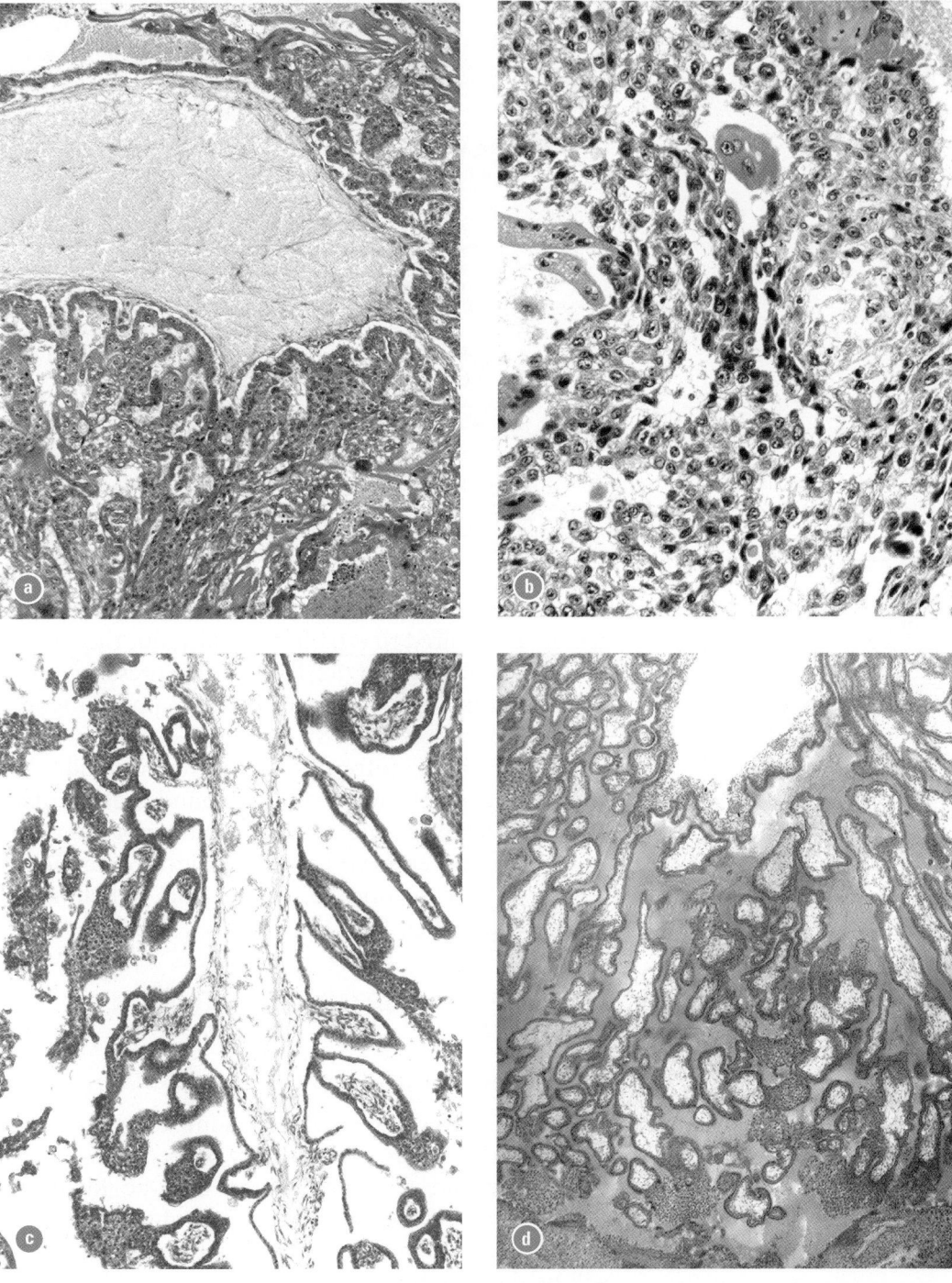

Fig. 32.1 Early placental disc development. The early non-villous chorionic sac (spherical gestational sac) is surrounded by pre-villous trophoblast (a) seen at higher power (b). Villous mesenchyme emanates from the disc and is enveloped by the peripheral trophoblast (c). Subsequent gestational sac (above) with well-developed chorionic villi (d).

passively divert increasingly larger percentages of the maternal cardiac output (up to 25% at term) to the intervillous vascular space.[1]

In the center of the chorionic sphere, the developing inner cell mass forms first a bilayered and then a trilayered embryonic disc

The embryonic disc is laterally contiguous with two cystic structures, the dorsal amniotic sac and the ventral yolk sac. Hematopoiesis begins in the wall of the yolk sac. Eventually, part of the yolk sac is incorporated into the embryonic body (as the gut), while the remainder is exteriorized to form part of the body stalk (the future umbilical cord) or the secondary yolk sac (a vestigial collapsed cyst in the placental chorionic surface). As the amniotic sac expands, its epithelium will cover the ventral body stalk (umbilical cord) and the inner surface of the chorionic sphere (Fig. 32.3).[1]

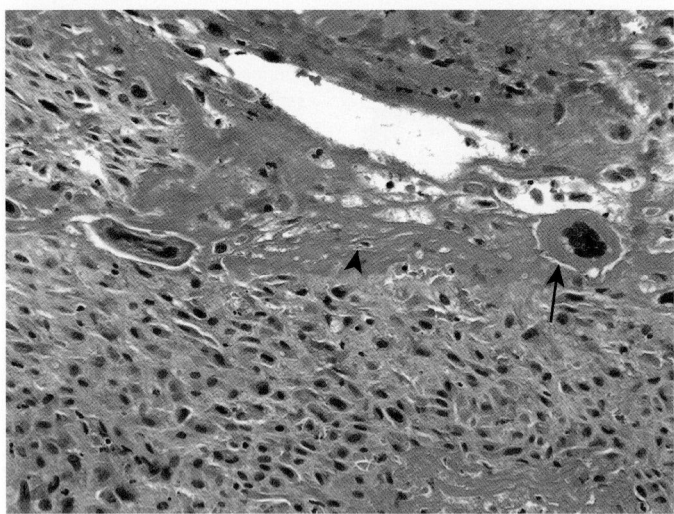

Fig. 32.2 Implantation site and Nitabuch's fibrin, note the mononuclear intermediate trophoblasts (arrowhead), multinucleated syncitiotrophoblasts (arrow).

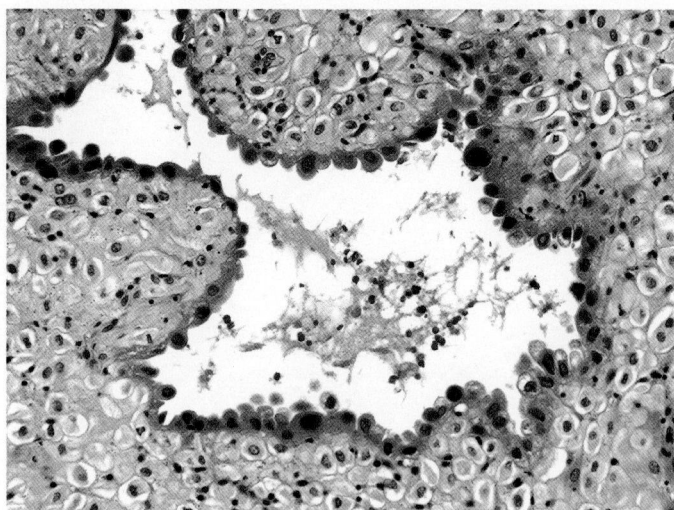

Fig. 32.4 Arias-Stella reaction in a gestational endometrial gland, characterized by hyperchromatic polyploid nuclei.

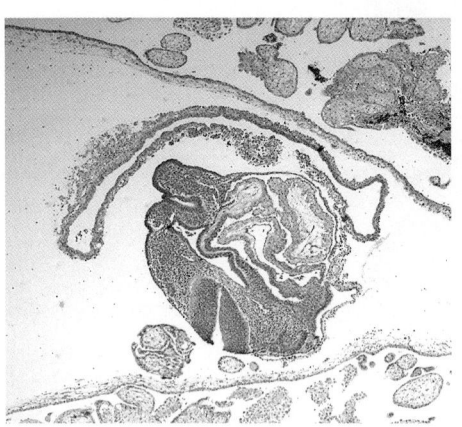

Fig. 32.3 Early embryo (center) and secondary yolk sac within a villous chorionic (gestational) sac (as seen sonographically in Fig. 32.5).

Arias-Stella reaction

Arias-Stella reaction is defined as nuclear enlargement and hyperchromasia of the secretory endometrial lining cells. It is presumably the consequences of hormonal effect and stems from polyploidy in the lining cells. Its presence signifies pregnancy (or high level progestin exposure), but will not establish the site of origin (Fig. 32.4).[1]

SONOGRAPHIC CORRELATES OF EARLY GESTATION

Sonographic evaluations of the conceptus play a dual role of pregnancy confirmation and outcome prediction. Currently, transvaginal ultrasound permits detection of a 2–3 mm gestational sac corresponding to 4.5 weeks. Sac diameter increases at a rate of approximately 1 mm/day from this point in normally progressing pregnancies. The yolk sac is visible at 6 weeks, after

which time cardiac activity should be detected. Cardiac activity is required to establish viability, but the absence of a yolk sac beyond 32 days or the presence of an abnormal (enlarged) yolk sac portend a poor outcome. Heart rates of less than 85 bpm at 6–8 weeks are also associated with a uniformly poor outcome. Additional abnormalities detectable on ultrasound that predict a poor outcome are: the absence of an embryonic pole at 16–18 mm (embryonic size), oligohydramnios in the first and second trimester and subchorionic hemorrhages (Fig. 32.5).[2]

GROSS EXAMINATION OF THE EARLY GESTATION

Identification of placental tissue

Most early abortion specimens are admixtures of decidual and placental tissues; in a minority of specimens (~25%) embryonic and fetal tissues can also be identified. Examination of the early placenta is discussed in the following paragraph, while examination of the embryo will be discussed below.

Placental tissues are grossly identified in abortion specimens as pale pink to tan-white, delicate, velvety fragments with a sponge-like consistency. Vessels are not identified in the chorionic villi, either with the naked eye or with the dissecting microscope; this property distinguishes villi from linear fragments of deciduas or endometrium. Decidual tissue possesses a more uniform consistency to touch. Fragments of implantation site cannot normally be distinguished from deciduas but may have a slightly more rubbery consistency due to

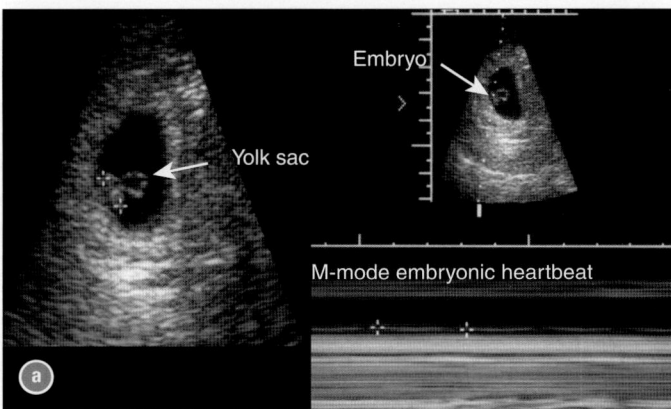

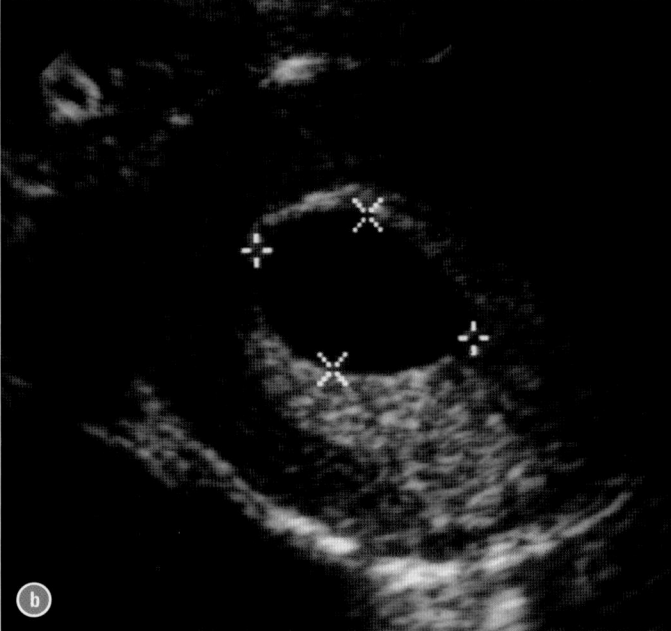

Fig. 32.5 Sonographic findings in early gestation. (a) A 6–7 week live intrauterine pregnancy: the embryo is marked by calipers in the image on the right and with an arrow on the left. The normal yolk sac (arrow, yolk sac) is seen adjacent to the embryo. The M-mode beneath the left image demonstrates embryonic cardiac activity. (b) Empty gestational sac: image of failed intrauterine gestation at approximately 8 weeks' gestation demonstrating a large gestational sac (calipers) within the uterus with no embryo present.

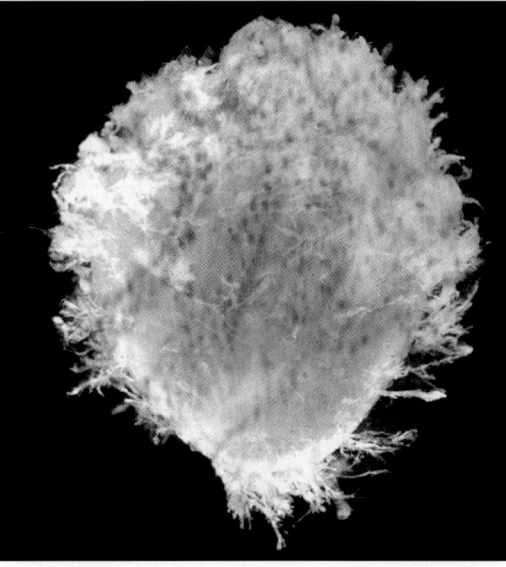

Fig. 32.6 Dissecting microscopic image of an early sac. The chorionic villi emanate as filamentous projections corresponding to histologic images in Figures 32.1(c) and (d).

the presence of abundant Nitabuch's fibrin. Examining the passed or curetted specimen in a petri dish of sterile saline may help identify potential chorionic villi, which expand and float, compared with the more dense deciduas, which settle to the bottom. A cyst-like, intact, collapsed chorionic sac is sometimes found; it will have a roughened, velvety exterior surface and a smooth, shiny interior lining; intact sacs are most commonly seen in spontaneously-passed specimens as opposed to curettings (Fig. 32.6).

For all early abortion specimens, at least 1–2 blocks of villous (and decidual) tissues should be submitted

for histologic assessment. In many specimens, particularly early spontaneous abortions, no grossly identifiable gestational tissue is present and sampling should take this uncertainty into account. When villous and embryonic tissues are not grossly evident, when the specimen is small, or when the clinician raises the suspicion of an ectopic gestation, the entire specimen should be histologically examined. Examination of the tissue through the dissecting microscope may be helpful in selecting the most likely villous tissue, but should be done with care (Fig. 32.7). For larger specimens, particularly if ectopic gestation is not suspected clinically, several blocks of tissue can be submitted initially, to be followed by additional sampling as necessary.

Many specimens submitted to confirm intrauterine pregnancy consist principally of blood clot and, on gross examination, may not appear promising. However, small amounts of gestational tissue can often be found in the center of the blood clot. The pathologist should carefully section these clots and submit sections that contain small cystic or lucent central foci. Microscopic examination may disclose villous tissue in these sites (Fig. 32.8).

Villous hydrops

Gross villous hydrops is characterized by tiny intraplacental cystic structures that resemble clear spheres in

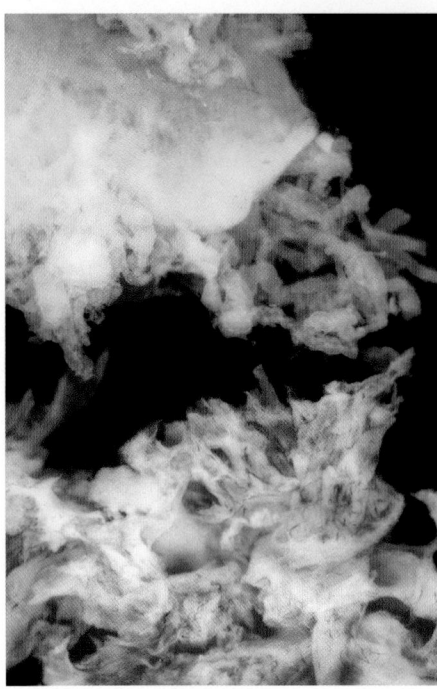

Fig. 32.7 Dissecting microscopic image of early chorionic villi (upper). Note the absence of vessels in contrast to the endometrial tissue (lower).

tissue to distinguish between hydropic abortus, partial and complete mole.

Karyotypic analysis

Karyotypic analysis will be considered in the event of repeated spontaneous abortion (see below). If a karyotype is requested, the unfixed specimen should be dissected sterilely to grossly identify villous tissue samples; disposable suture removal sets work well for this purpose. The sample is subsequently placed into Hanks' balanced salt solution and can be refrigerated for up to 72 h, but never frozen, to maintain optimal viability for culture and preparation of chromosomes. In the cytogenetics laboratory, the submitted specimen is disaggregated and cultured for several days until a sufficient fraction of cells are undergoing mitosis. Mitotic spindle formation is then blocked by adding colcemide to the culture, arresting cells in metaphase. The metaphase chromosomes are spread, stained, counted and analyzed by their characteristic banding patterns. The pathologist's selection of appropriate material for karyotypic analysis is critical to ensure that the results reflect the chromosomal composition of the gestation and not the mother (i.e. from endometrial or decidual tissue). If villous tissue is not apparent to the unaided eye, a dissecting microscope is useful for grossly identifying small fragments of embryonic or placental villous tissues (see Fig. 32.7); ideally, samples of uncertain origin should be divided to allow histologic confirmation of the tissue source.[3]

tapioca, and when present, requires further examination to exclude hydatidiform mole (see below). When gross villous hydrops is present, or if a hydatidiform mole is clinically or sonographically suspected, flow cytometric or cytogenetic studies of villous tissues should be considered if available. In addition, more extensive histologic sampling of 5–10 blocks of villous and decidual tissues is warranted to ensure sufficient villous

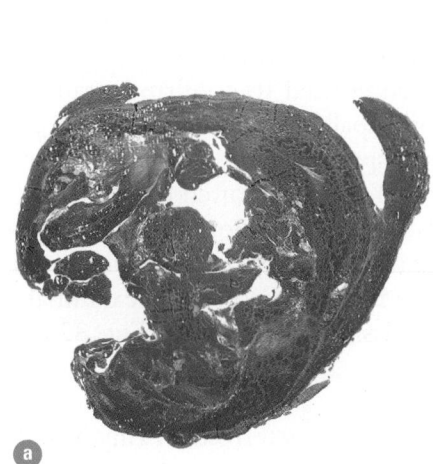

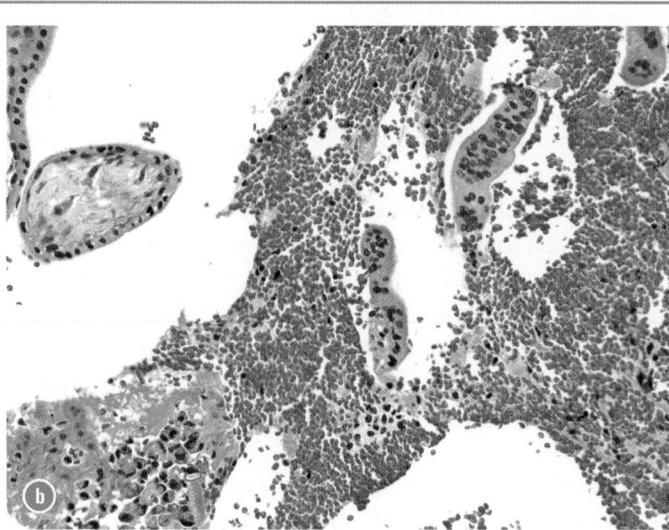

Fig. 32.8 Early pregnancy within a blood clot (a). Attention to the center of the clot will often disclose a few villi and trophoblasts (b).

Spontaneous abortion

THE PATIENT AT RISK

Early spontaneous abortion can be clinically divided into sporadic abortion (97%) and recurrent/habitual abortion (3%). Because early pregnancy loss is relatively common, and subsequent pregnancies are usually normal, most patients are not further assessed following one or two sporadic abortions. However, the odds of having three spontaneous abortions by chance has been calculated as 0.3%.[4] Thus in the 3% of abortions clinically categorized as recurrent, the patient and her pathologic specimens are typically evaluated for cytogenetic, anatomic, hormonal, and/or immunologic abnormalities, which may offer potential treatment options for subsequent gestations.

EARLY (SPORADIC) SPONTANEOUS ABORTION

Clinical

By convention, early spontaneous abortion is defined by pregnancy loss before 13 weeks gestation. Early spontaneous abortion is a common event, complicating 12% to 14% of all recognized pregnancies.[5-7] Using a high-sensitivity serum beta human chorionic gonadotropin (β-hCG) assay to detect very early pregnancy, one group found that approximately two-thirds of all detectable early pregnancies terminate spontaneously.[6] Because of this high frequency of early pregnancy loss, many pathologists regularly encounter early abortion specimens. Karyotypic disorders constitute the major known mechanism of early spontaneous abortion, being responsible for approximately 50–60% of all early abortions. Of karyotypic abnormalities identified, the most common are various trisomies (identified in approximately 30% of early abortions), monosomy X (in 10%) and triploidy (in 2%)(Table 32.1).[8-10] Some authors hypothesize that many of the remaining cases of sporadic spontaneous abortion are also due to chromosomal abnormalities, which include small deletions or rearrangements that cannot be identified by standard karyotyping. Trisomies of every autosome except chromosome 1 have been reported in early spontaneous abortions. Trisomy 16 is most commonly encountered (accounting for 30–50% of all trisomies), and virtually all gestations with this abnormality miscarry. Trisomies of 2, 7, 13, 14, 15, 21 and 22 each account for approximately 5–10% of trisomies. Although chromosomal disorders are the presumptive cause of many (if not most) early abortions, most first-

Table 32.1 Chromosomal abnormalities in spontaneous abortion[10]

Abnormality	(%)
None	56.1
45,X	9.8
Autosomal trisomy	30.9
16	8.6
22	4.3
21	4.9
Others	13.4
Double/triple trisomy	2.0
Triploidy	6.5
Tetraploidy	1.8
Structural rearrangement	2.5
Mosaicisms, XXY, monosomy	<0.2

time abortion specimens in routine practice are not submitted for cytogenetic evaluation (see below).[8-10] In fact, only 4–6% of karyotypically abnormal abortions are due to a parental germline abnormality (such as a balanced reciprocal translocation or Robertsonian translocation). Thus, even when an abnormal karyotype is obtained for an abortion specimen, it is far more likely to represent a sporadic event resulting in a non-viable conceptus, rather than a phenomenon with a high recurrence risk and/or implications for outcomes of future pregnancies.

Pathology

The pathologist should be aware of the following features of spontaneous abortion when examining the curetting:

Changes associated with embryonic death

Spontaneous abortions typically follow death of the embryo. The earliest change is cellular debris within fetal vessels, developing several hours after the fetal death.[11] Several days after fetal death, the chorionic villi will vary from appearing normal, with nucleated red blood cells (Fig. 32.9a), to edematous, with myxoid villous degeneration and villous hydrops (Fig. 32.9b), to eosinophilic, collagenized and avascular, termed villous fibrosis, villous sclerosis and villous avascularity (Fig. 32.9c). In specimens retained for several days to weeks after fetal death, a combination of the two patterns often coexists. These histologic findings are related only to placental retention after the cessation of embryonic development and will not pinpoint the cause of the spontaneous abortion.

Changes that appear abnormal but typify early gestation

A common pattern seen in early gestational tissue is discrete clusters of immature villi with villous degenera-

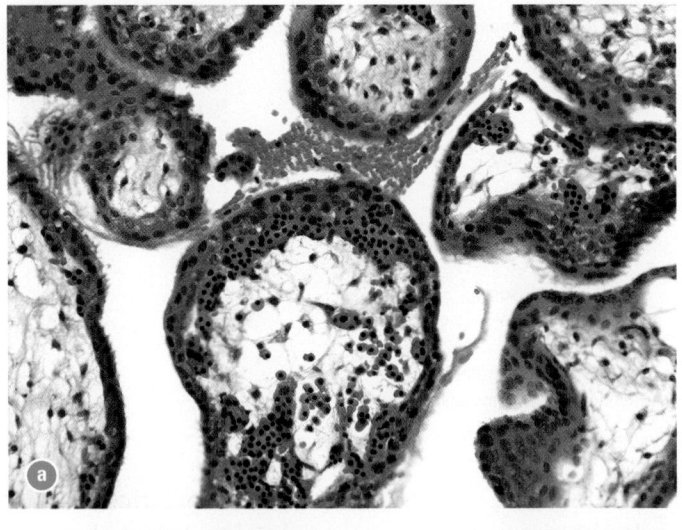

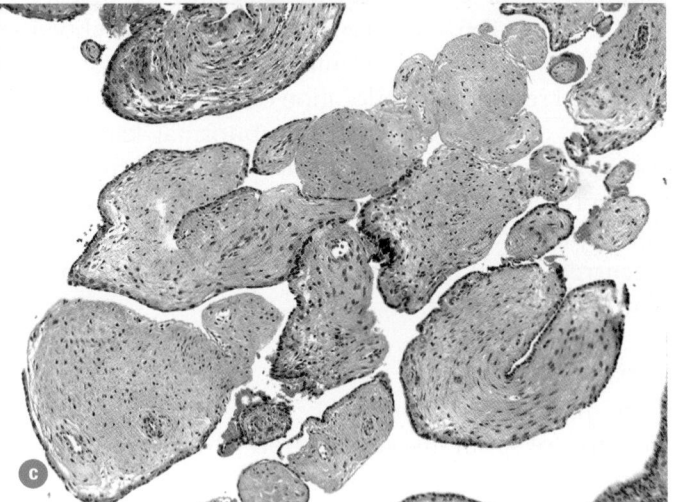

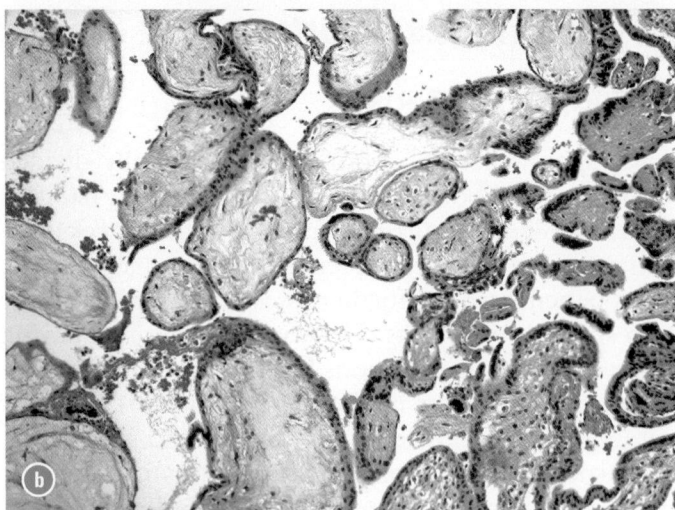

Fig. 32.9 (a) Normal immature chorionic villi at approximately 8 weeks, with nucleated red blood cells; (b,c) Villous changes in early spontaneous abortion, including villous edema (b) and villous sclerosis (c) associated with embryonic death.

tion and prominent perivillous fibrin, suggesting infarct. The pathologist may be tempted to postulate this as a mechanism of early loss; however, such changes are also seen in therapeutic abortions and probably do not contribute to early gestational loss (Fig. 32.10).

Villous edema

Another common pattern seen in early spontaneous abortion is pronounced villous edema (hydropic abortus), which must be distinguished from a molar gestation. The latter will be discussed in detail later. The features characterizing a hydropic abortus include a villous population that is relatively uniform in size, predominately round or oval with gradual differences in diameter and without trophoblastic hyperplasia or cisterns (Fig. 32.11).

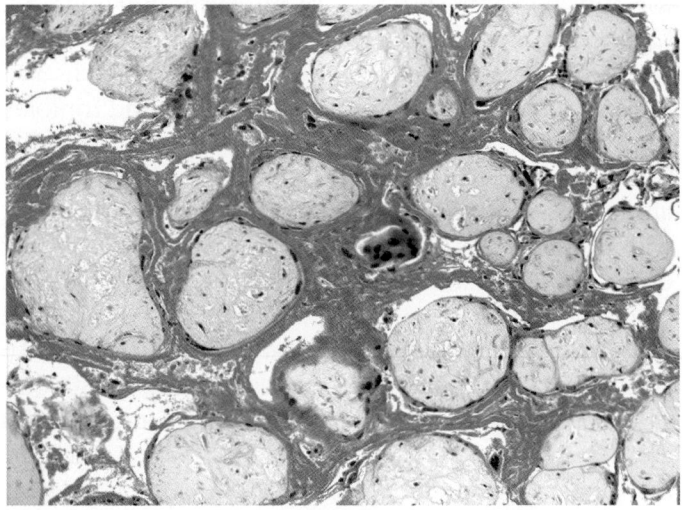

Fig. 32.10 Villous degeneration and perivillous fibrin. A common finding in early gestations.

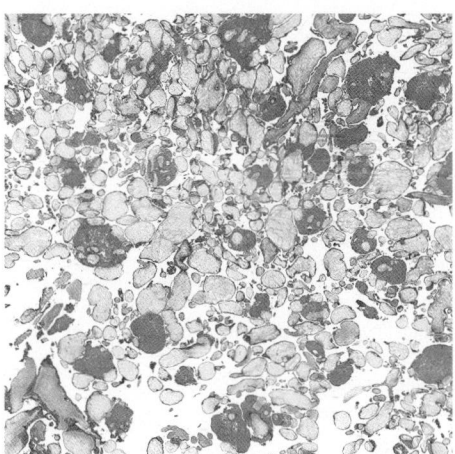

Fig. 32.11 Hydropic abortus, containing diffuse villous edema.

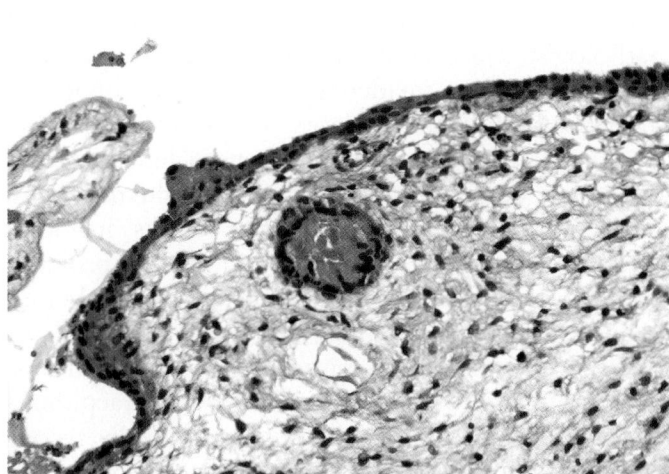

Fig. 32.12 Trophoblastic inclusion. These are commonly seen in partial moles but may be present in other types of gestations.

Histopathologic findings indicative of a specific mechanism of abortion or fetal death

Such findings are very uncommon in early abortion specimens. The only relatively common, well-established histologic and reproducible finding that identifies a specific mechanism is partial or compete hydatidiform mole (discussed below). Rarely, the pathologist will encounter chronic villitis or evidence of viral changes (such as cytomegalovirus or parvovirus).

Mildly dysmorphic villi with trophoblastic hyperplasia may be seen in the case of trisomic gestations, but are not sufficient to warrant a diagnosis without cytogenetic analysis.[12] Another histopathologic finding that has been reported in association with genetic anomalies is intravillous inclusions.[13] Dysmorphic villi and inclusions are commonly seen in partial hydatidiform moles, but may also be seen in other types of non-viable gestations. Thus, although these features may accompany a genetically abnormal conceptus, they have no value in terms of genetic counseling (Fig. 32.12).[14]

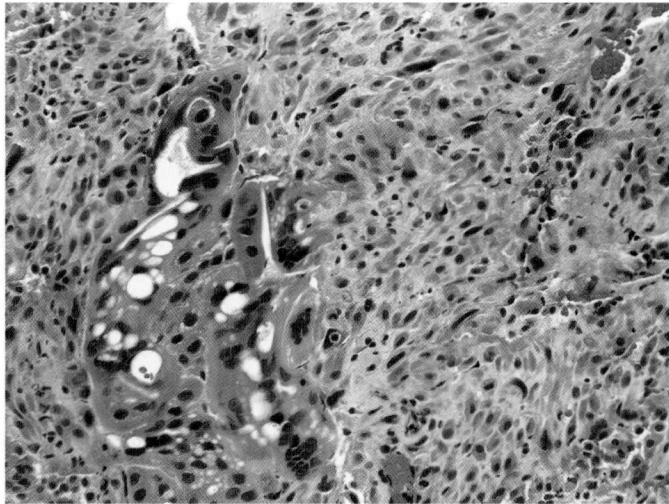

Fig. 32.13 Exaggerated implantation site in moderate intermediate trophoblast hyperplasia and atypia, a normal variant commonly seen in early gestation.

The implantation site

Most abortion specimens contain placental bed tissues (fresh endomyometrial implantation site, discussed above). In some abortion specimens, an exaggerated implantation site reaction is seen, which represents exuberant, non-neoplastic, physiologic, trophoblastic invasion of decidua and myometrium. Histologically, there is moderate hyperplasia or atypia of intermediate trophoblast cells (Fig. 32.13). Most exaggerated implantation site reactions occur concurrently with an early gestation (immature villi are usually present in the specimen), or with a hydatidiform mole (diagnostic villi are usually present in the specimen).

Maternal tissues

The maternal tissues are usually not central to the diagnosis of early spontaneous abortion. Endometrial inflammation and necrosis are common secondary changes; they are usually not causally related to abortion and do not in themselves indicate a septic gestation. Rarely, severe decidual acute inflammation accompanied by chorionic tissue with acute villitis could accompany a 'septic abortion', a post-abortal complication (infected retained tissue), or a primary infectious cause of the abortion (such as group B streptococcal or listerial infection).

Although the maternal components may not be relevant to the etiology of gestational loss, the thorough pathologist will examine the curetting carefully with the possibility of incidental but clinically-important findings. Lesions and tumors which are occasionally encountered in gestational specimens include: (a) endocervical or endometrial polyps; (b) submucus leiomyomas; (c) endometrial proliferative lesions, including localized hyperplasia ('localized endometrial proliferation associated with pregnancy', LEPP) (Fig. 32.14) and endometrial adenocarcinoma; and (d) cervical neoplasms (usually squamous intraepithelial lesions). LEPP may be confused with either endometrial intraepithelial neoplasia or carcinoma; the authors typically recommend a follow-up endometrial sample in 6 months, but follow-up is usually benign.[15]

RECURRENT (HABITUAL) ABORTION

The patient at risk

Recurrent abortion is defined as a history of three spontaneous abortions. Possible etiologies for recurrent abortion are summarized in Table 32.2 and include the following: luteal phase/ovulatory defects (20–40%); uterine anomalies, such as septae, leiomyomas and polyps (10–18%); incompetent cervix (2%); maternal thrombotic or immunologic factors (4–20%); and fetal unbalanced chromosomal translocation, due to a balanced chromosomal translocation in one parent (5%).[16–18]

Table 32.2 List of reported factors associated with recurrent (habitual) abortions

Genetic	Structural chromosomal abnormalities (parental or *de novo* during gametogenesis) Balanced translocations Robertsonian translocation Inversions Single gene mutations (Mendelian disorders) Multifactorial genetic disorders
Endocrine	Luteal phase defect Diabetes mellitus w/ uncontrolled blood glucose or high hemoglobin A1C Hyperprolactinemia Polycystic ovary syndrome
Anatomic	Septate uterus Bicornuate uterus Didelphic uterus Unicornuate uterus Leiomyomas Incompetent cervix Acquired/iatrogenic defects (Asherman's syndrome)
Immunologic	Systemic lupus erythematosus w/ antiphospholipid antibodies (lupus anticoagulant) Antiphospholipid syndrome Autoantibodies: thyroid, anti-SSA, anti-nuclear antibodies
Environmental	Cigarette smoking Alcohol Chemical (arsenic, benzene, aniline, ethylene oxide, formaldehyde, lead)
Not implicated in recurrent abortions (although reported in association with sporadic abortion):	
Infectious	Severe maternal infection (ex. pneumonia) *Toxoplasma gondii* Rubella virus Herpes simplex virus Cytomegalovirus Measles virus Coxsackievirus *Listeria monocytogenes* *Treponema pallidum* *Ureaplasma urealyticum*

Adapted from Roberts and Murphy.[16] A causative relationship between these factors and recurrent abortion has not been unequivocally established for many of the entities listed.

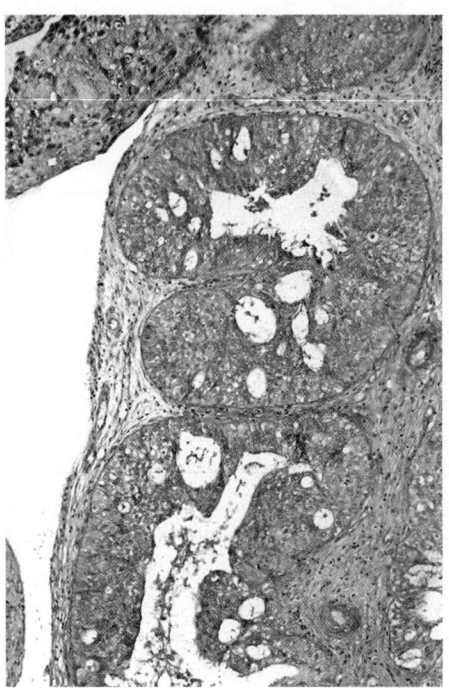

Fig. 32.14 Localized endometrial proliferation of pregnancy (LEPP), consisting of complex glands with stratified lining and cribriform architecture. These changes are characteristically followed by normal curettings postpartum.

Karyotypic analysis

In the case of habitual abortion, a placental or fetal karyotype is usually indicated to identify a possible recurrent abnormality due to germline mutation in one parent (recurrent translocation, Robertsonian translocation). Unfixed villous and fetal tissue fragments to be submitted for cytogenetics should be separated from maternally derived deciduas with the aid of a dissecting microscope under sterile condition, as sample viability and sterility is critical for successful karyotyping (see above). Samples from uncertain tissues should be histologically identified and correlated with cytogenetic findings (i.e. normal karyotype results due to diploid fetus *vs* maternal somatic tissue).[3]

Histologic findings

Uterine and cervical anatomic defects, endometrial luteal phase defect and immunologic/thrombotic factors are usually clinically and pathologically evaluated following the pregnancy, and prior to the next conception. Histologic examination of the products of conception will rarely identify a cause of recurrent abortion in most specimens, but in some instances a cause can be found with examination of the placenta or embryonic tissue.

Chronic intervillositis

This rare placental disorder has recently been associated with first and second trimester recurrent abortion.[19–21] In the third trimester, chronic intervillositis is associated with poor fetal growth (intrauterine growth restriction, IUGR) and stillbirth. An immunologic origin (maternal rejection of the placental allograft) has been postulated for most cases of chronic intervillositis. In rare instances, an infectious origin has been documented, including maternal malaria and recurrent sepsis. Histologically, chronic intervillositis is characterized by numerous maternal mononuclear cells (predominantly histiocytes and scattered lymphocytes) and deposits of fibrin located within the maternal intervillous space (see Ch. 33; Fig. 33.67 and Ch. 34; Fig. 34.12).

Embryonic and fetal tissues

In every early spontaneous abortion specimen, the pathologist should carefully search for embryonic or fetal tissues. In the majority of such specimens, no recognizable embryonic or fetal tissues can be grossly identified. This results either from specimen fragmentation, precluding gross recognition of fetal parts, or from genetically abnormal gestations which cannot form an embryo ('empty sac', 'blighted ovum') (Figs 32.5b, 32.15a,b).[9] When an intact gestational sac is identified, a small, deformed embryo may be found in approximately 25% of specimens (this is variously referred to as a 'nodular', 'amorphous', 'cylindrical', or 'growth disorganized' embryo); in another 25% of intact sacs, a well-formed embryo or fetus may be found (Fig. 32.15c,d). When evaluating relatively normally formed embryos and fetuses, pathologists should determine the gestational age and assess whether landmarks of normal development and growth have been reached (Tables 32.3, 32.4).[22,23] Ten weeks of gestational age divides the embryonic period of organogenesis from the fetal period of growth and differentiation; a crown rump length of 3 cm separates the embryo (<3 cm) from the fetus (>3 cm). In fragmented specimens, foot length is the standard gross pathologic measurement used for estimating gestational age; a foot length of 5 mm distinguishes an embryo (<5 mm) from a fetus (>5 mm) (additional foot length measurements are summarized in Table 32.4). Careful examination, complemented by low-power magnification with a dissecting microscope, will identify congenital malformations in approximately 10% of fetuses in early abortion specimens. The most commonly recognized anomalies include neural tube defects, cyclopia, facial clefts and polydactyly. Because some of these malformations have a risk of recurrence, genetic counseling is warranted when malformations are identified.

Ectopic pregnancy

THE PATIENT AT RISK

Ectopic pregnancies, defined as any implantation of a conceptus outside of the uterus or in an abnormal position within the uterus, have dramatically increased in incidence. Ectopic pregnancies, which two decades ago occurred once in every 250 pregnancies, have increased in frequency six-fold and now account for approximately 2% of all documented pregnancies in the USA.[24,25]

Epidemiologic studies have shown that ectopic pregnancy more commonly occurs in women who are older, urban dwellers, of black race, lower socioeconomic status and of increasing parity. Specifically, ectopic pregnancy is the leading cause of maternal death in the first trimester and accounts for 9–13% of pregnancy-related deaths.[24,26] The mortality in recent years has been low, estimated at 30–40 women in the USA (MMWR).

In a study of 126 consecutive ectopic pregnancies, 35% had a history of infertility; 38% a prior fallopian tube operation; 17% a history of prior pelvic inflammatory disease; 16% prior ectopic pregnancy; and 13% a prior pelvic operation. Importantly, no risk factor was identified in 47% of patients.[27] Table 32.5 summarizes relative risk estimates from a large study. The fallopian tube is the most common site of ectopic implantation, accounting for 97% of all ectopic pregnancies.

Fallopian tube factors, which have been associated with ectopic pregnancy, include congenital abnormalities (diverticula, hypoplasia, accessory ostia, etc.), prenatal DES exposure (causing structural abnormalities),

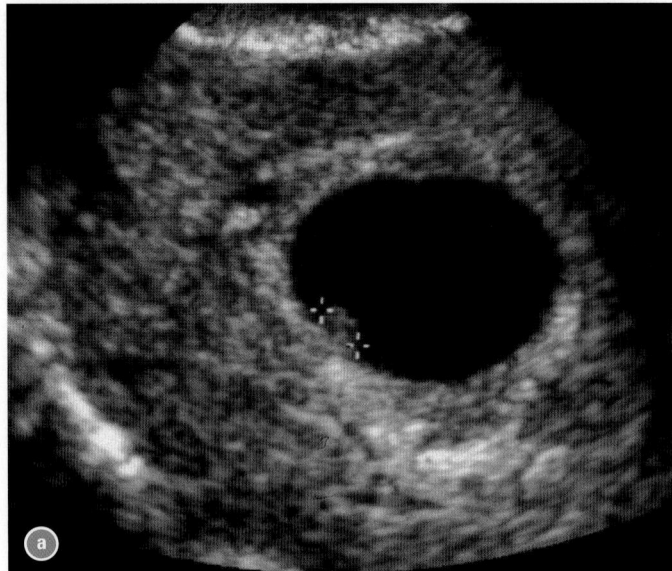

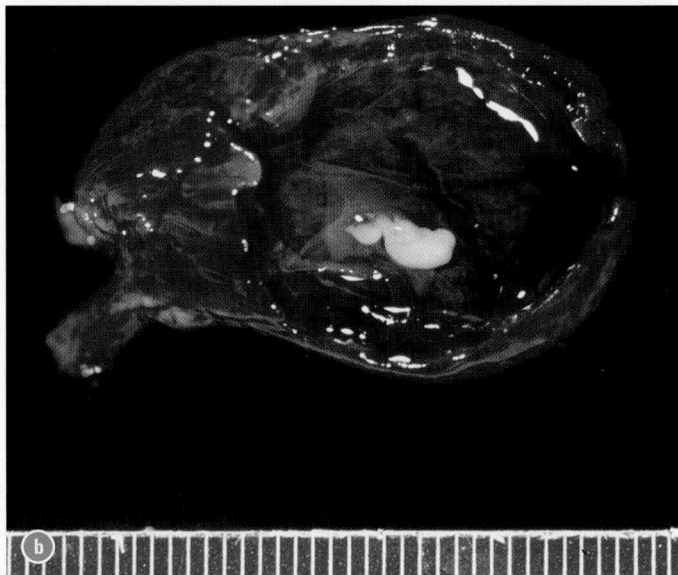

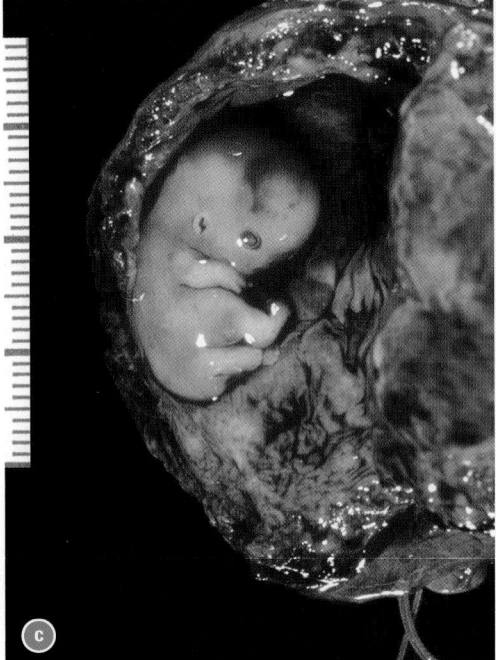

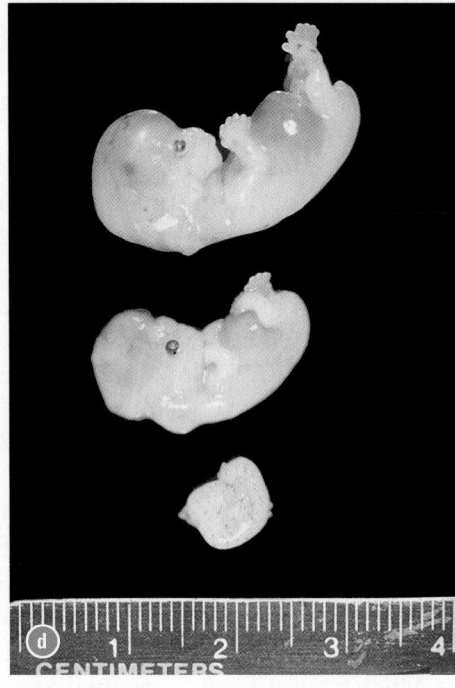

Fig. 32.15 (a) Sonogram of abnormal intrauterine gestation containing a very small embryonic pole (calipers) that had no heartbeat, representing a failed pregnancy. (b) Blighted ovum at 8 weeks gestational age. (c) Normal fetus at approximately 10 weeks gestational age. (d) Embryos at approximately 5, 7 and 8 weeks (bottom to top).

salpingitis isthmica nodosa and tubal neoplasms (very rare). Non-granulomatous (especially *chlamydia trachomatis* and possibly *Mycoplasma hominis*) and granulomatous salpingitis (especially treated *Mycobacterium tuberculosis*) increase the risk of ectopic pregnancy presumably through post-inflammatory scarring and lining epithelial cell cilia dysfunction. In contrast, condom use is associated with a lower incidence of tubal pregnancy. Women who have undergone prior tubal sterilization have an overall lower risk of ectopic pregnancy than the general population. However, post-ligation pregnancies, when they do occur, are much more likely to be ectopic (10–15%). Similarly, following tuboplasty to reverse a tubal ligation, 5–10% of resulting pregnancies implant in the fallopian tube.[27]

Extratubal factors that have been reported to increase ectopic pregnancy rates include smoking and hormonal alterations, such as ovulatory dysfunction and

Table 32.3 *Criteria for estimating developmental stages in human embryos*

Developmental age (days)*	Gestational age (weeks)	No. of somites	Greatest length (mm)	Main characteristics
Embryonic stage				
20–21	5	1–3	1.5–3.0	*Deep neural groove and first somites present.* Head fold evident.
22–23		4–12	2.0–3.5	*Embryo straight or slightly curved.* Neural tube forming or formed opposite somites, but widely open at rostral and caudal neuropores. First and second pairs of branchial arches visible.
24–25		13–20	2.5–4.5	*Embryo curved owing to head and tail folds.* Rostral neuropore closing. Otic placodes present. Optic vesicles formed.
26–27		21–29	3.0–5.0	*Upper limb buds appear.* Caudal neuropore closing or closed. Three pairs of branchial arches visible. Heart prominence distinct. Otic pits present.
28–30	6	30–35	4.0–6.0	*Embryo has C-shaped curve. Upper limb buds are flipper-like.* Four pairs of branchial arches visible. Lower limb buds appear. *Otic vesicles* present. Lens placodes distinct. Attenuated *tail* present.
31–32		33–36	5.0–7.0	*Upper limbs are paddle-shaped.* Lens pits and nasal pits visible. Optic cups present.
33–36	7		7.0–9.0	*Hand plates formed.* Lens vesicles present. Nasal pits prominent. *Lower limbs are paddle-shaped.* Cervical sinus visible.
37–40			8.0–11.0	*Foot plates formed.* Pigment visible in retina. Auricular hillocks developing.
41–43	8		11.0–14.0	*Digital, or finger, rays appear.* Auricular hillocks outline future auricle of external ear. Trunk beginning to straighten. Cerebral vesicles prominent.
44–46			13.0–17.0	*Digital, or toe, rays appearing.* Elbow region visible. Eyelids forming. Notches between finger rays. Nipples visible.
47–48	9		16.0–18.0	*Limbs extend ventrally.* Trunk elongating and straightening. Midgut herniation prominent.
49–51			18.0–22.0	*Upper limbs longer and bent at elbows. Fingers distinct but webbed.* Notches between toe rays. Scalp vascular plexus appears.
52–53			22.0–24.0	*Hands and feet approach each other. Fingers are free and longer. Toes distinct but webbed.* Stubby tail present.
54–55			23.0–28.0	*Toes free and longer.* Eyelids and auricles of external ears are more developed.
Fetal stage begins				
56	10		27.0–31.0	*Head more rounded and shows human characteristics.* External genitalia still have sexless appearance. Distinct bulge still present in umbilical cord; caused by herniation of intestines. *Tail has disappeared.*

From Table 5.1, Moore.[22]

*Age from fertilization (gestational age – 2 weeks).

low-dose progestin only oral contraception, presumably by altering epithelial cilia function.[28] Some 2–10% of assisted reproductive technology (ART)-derived pregnancies implant in the tube, but it is not clear whether this is secondary to exogenous gonadotropin exposure and subsequent hormonal alterations or a manifestation of the underlying process causing infertility.[29–31] In contrast, the overall incidence of ectopic pregnancy is *not* increased in patients using IUDs compared with the non-user population. However, 4–8% of pregnancies which occur when an IUD is in place are ectopic, and 10% of these implant in the ovary, likely reflecting the efficacy of the IUD in preventing intrauterine implantation relative to extrauterine sites.[32,33]

In light of these risk factors, the increased rate of ectopic pregnancy observed in Europe and North America, has been ascribed to the early treatment of salpingitis (preserving fertility but leading to tubal scarring rather than complete occlusion), increased utilization of ART, and wider use of sensitive imaging and laboratory techniques to diagnose early, potentially previously unrecognized ectopic gestations.

CLINICAL PRESENTATION

The initial history and physical examination of a patient later found to have an ectopic pregnancy can be misleading and cause clinical misdiagnosis.[24] The classic presenting symptoms of pelvic or abdominal pain and vaginal bleeding are not consistently present, especially if the ectopic pregnancy has not yet ruptured. Further obscuring the clinical presentation, less than 50% of patients give a history that includes any of the aforementioned ectopic pregnancy risk factors. Additionally, pelvic examination is often not reliable. Furthermore,

Table 32.4 Foot length (FL) at different gestational ages

Gestational age (weeks)	Mean (mm)	Min. FL (mm)	Max. FL (mm)
Embryonic stage			
8.5	4.2	3.8	4.6
9	4.6	4.2	5.0
Fetal stage[a]			
10	5.5	5.0	6.0
11	6.9	6.0	7.8
12	9.1	7.5	10.8
13	11.4	9.8	13.0
14	14.0	12.5	15.5
15	16.8	15.2	18.5
16	19.9	18.2	21.6
17	23.0	21.0	25.0
18	26.8	24.8	28.8
19	30.7	28.5	33.0
20	33.3	31.0	35.7
21	35.2	32.5	38.0
22	39.5	36.0	43.0
23	42.2	39.0	45.5
24	45.2	42.0	48.5

[a]For practical purposes, a foot length of ≥5mm distinguishes a fetus (≥10 weeks) gestational age) from an embryo (<10 weeks). From Streeter.[23]

Table 32.5 Risk factors for ectopic pregnancy[26]

Risk factor	Specific	Relative risk
Prior tubal surgery	Yes	4.0
Smoking	>20 cigarettes/day	3.9
H/O STD	with PID	3.4
Prior SAB	>3	3.0
Age	>40	2.9
Prior TAB	Medical or Surgical	2.8
H/O infertility	>2 years	2.7
Appendectomy	Yes or ruptured	1.4
Prior IUD	Yes	1.3

H/O, history of; STD, sexually transmitted disease; SAB, spontaneous abortion; TAB, therapeutic abortion; IUD, intra-uterine device; PID, pelvic inflammatory disease.

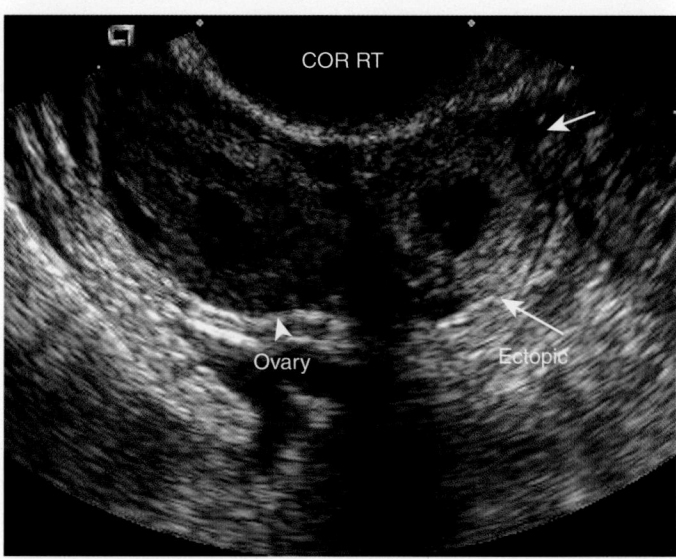

Fig. 32.16 Tubal ectopic pregnancy. Coronal sonographic image of right adnexa demonstrating a well-defined mass (arrows) adjacent to but separate from the ovary (arrowhead). Within the mass was an embryo with a visible heartbeat, confirming the diagnosis of an ectopic pregnancy.

CLINICAL DIAGNOSTIC ALGORITHM AND MANAGEMENT

When there is a high index of suspicion for an ectopic pregnancy and a positive serum β-hCG, the diagnostic algorithm entails a transvaginal ultrasonogram (Fig. 32.16), followed by sampling of the endometrium if no intrauterine gestational sac is seen. With the rare exception of heterotopic gestations (coexisting ectopic and intrauterine pregnancy, incidence estimated at approximately 1 in 4000 pregnancies), the presence of products of conception in the uterine cavity confirms a failed intrauterine pregnancy and effectively excludes an ectopic. When an ectopic pregnancy is confirmed (either clinically or histologically) or an intrauterine pregnancy cannot be confirmed, treatment options include expectant management or methotrexate administration if the patient is stable, and/or surgery.

EXAMINATION OF THE CURETTINGS

General

When the pathologist receives the uterine curettings from the clinical service the first task is to determine if there is a clinical suspicion of ectopic pregnancy. If there is a low index of suspicion, the patient is clinically stable and there are no plans to intervene surgically, the curettings should be grossly examined, the most promising areas culled into a single cassette and the entire specimen

a history of vaginally passed tissue does not distinguish a missed intrauterine abortion from a sloughed decidual cast in a patient with an ectopic pregnancy. A low or slowly increasing serum β-hCG level cannot reliably distinguish an abnormal intrauterine from extrauterine pregnancy. Finally, while transvaginal ultrasound can be very helpful, the results are often indeterminate (Fig. 32.16).

processed for a rush reading the following day. However, if there is a high index of clinical suspicion of ectopic pregnancy, concerns about the stability of the patient's medical condition and/or the specimen cannot be routinely processed and evaluated within 18 h, the specimen should be evaluated thoroughly by frozen section.

Examination of the tissues

As discussed above, careful examination for presence of immature villi, embryonic tissue or fresh implantation site should be made histologically. The tissue should first be examined with the naked eye, preferably while floating in a Petri dish of sterile saline, with attention to the fine spongy features of immature villi. If a dissecting microscope is available, it can be used to identify tissues that may have the highest yield. However, at this point in the examination, the pathologist must be aware of the risk of confusing vascular or glandular epithelial structures emanating from fragments of deciduas with chorionic villi. Evaluation of the former is particularly treacherous for the novice. For this reason, it is prudent to never declare the presence of chorionic villi without histologic verification. One or more of the following features must be identified histologically in the curettings: fetal parts, chorionic villi or implantation site. It should be emphasized that the presence of ectopic gestation does not exclude any form of endometrial histology, which may range from normal cyclic endometrium to gestational endometrium, depending on the timing of the ectopic. In fact, in >60% of cases the endometrium responds to hormones generated by the ectopic gestation, developing hypersecretory glands, deciduas and/or focal Arias-Stella reaction.[34] Thus, observation of Arias-Stella reaction and/or decidualized endometrium alone in the curettage specimen is not sufficient to indicate an intrauterine pregnancy. Moreover, as mentioned above, the absence of any evidence of pregnancy also does not exclude ectopic pregnancy.

PITFALLS IN HISTOLOGIC EXAMINATION OF ENDOMETRIAL CURETTINGS (TABLE 32.6 AND FIGS 32.17, 32.18)

Contaminating tissues or trophoblast that are not diagnostic of current intrauterine pregnancy

Mature villi

When only rare chorionic villi are microscopically found, it is important to confirm that villous morphology is compatible with immature first trimester chorionic villi, rather than contaminating mature villi (from a term

Table 32.6 Pitfalls in the laboratory management of suspected ectopic pregnancy

Floaters or contaminants
  Mature villi
  Implantation site
  Degenerate villi shed from ectopic into endometrial cavity
Misclassification
  Interpreting implantation site nodule as current intrauterine pregnancy
  Interpreting inflamed or degenerating decidual cells as intermediate trophoblast
  Interpreting tangential sectioned Arias-Stella effect as implantation site
Under-appreciating gestational trophoblastic disease
  Very early complete mole
  Placental site trophoblastic tumor
Extraordinary events
  Concurrent tubal and intrauterine pregnancy
False assumptions/caveats
  Excluding or confirming ectopic based on gross examination alone (not recommended)
  Not performing frozen section
  Misclassification of decidual vessels as villous structures
  Instead (recommended):
    If patient is stable and clinician is patient – 'rush' permanent sections for reading within 18–24 h
    If immediate answer needed – gross examination of curettings and frozen section of suspected villous structures. *Caution:* bloody, degenerated specimens are particularly treacherous to freeze and interpret due to the delicate nature of the chorionic villi

placenta of another patient processed at the same bench). Third trimester placental 'floats' are scattered, small villi with syncytial knots and no nucleated fetal red blood cells (Fig. 32.17a). When immature chorionic villi cannot be identified, a current or very recent intrauterine pregnancy can still be confirmed if fresh implantation site tissue is present in the endometrial curettings

Shed immature villi

It should always be remembered that shedding of villi from a degenerating tubal pregnancy could result in a few degenerating immature villi in an endometrial curetting. Thus, it is important for the pathologist and treating physician to always integrate the pathologic and clinical information available to direct management. Only the finding of a fresh implantation site absolutely confirms the presence of an intrauterine gestation (and essentially excludes an ectopic gestation except in the very rare scenario of heterotopic twin gestations).

Implantation site

The authors have seen one example in which fragments of contaminating implantation site were transported to a sample from an ectopic pregnancy. In this case, a single fragment of implantation site was present on the periphery of the specimen. A high degree of skepticism

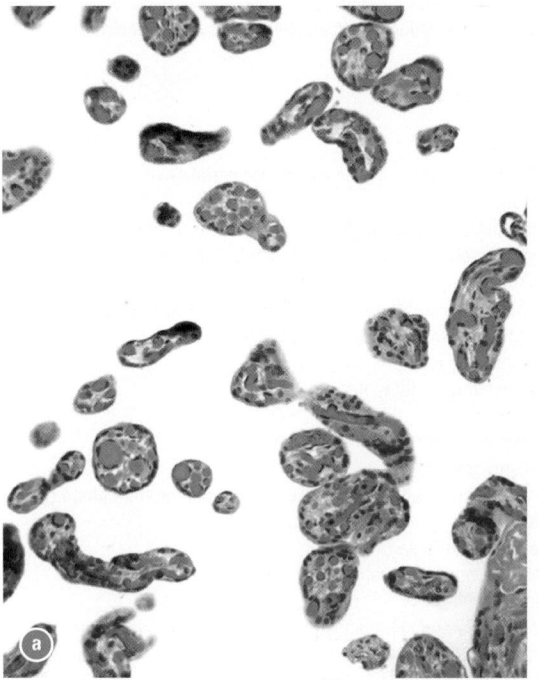
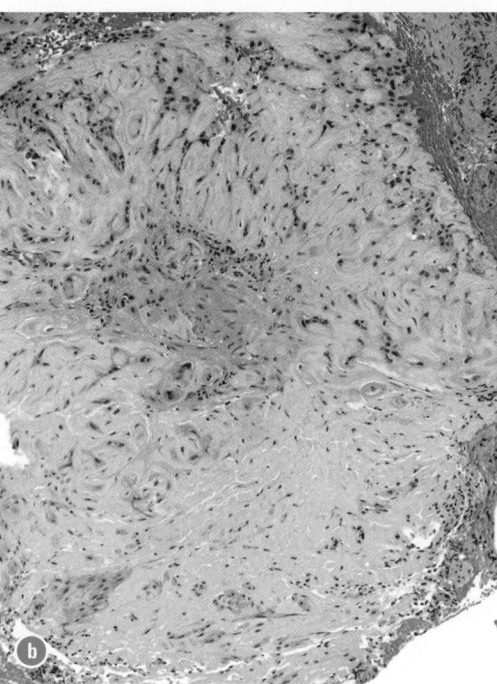

Fig. 32.17 Pitfalls in excluding ectopic pregnancy: (a) mature chorionic villi from term pregnancy may contaminate the specimen and must be distinguished from early pregnancy; (b) implantation site nodule from prior intrauterine pregnancy may occasionally be present in the curettings from a current ectopic pregnancy.

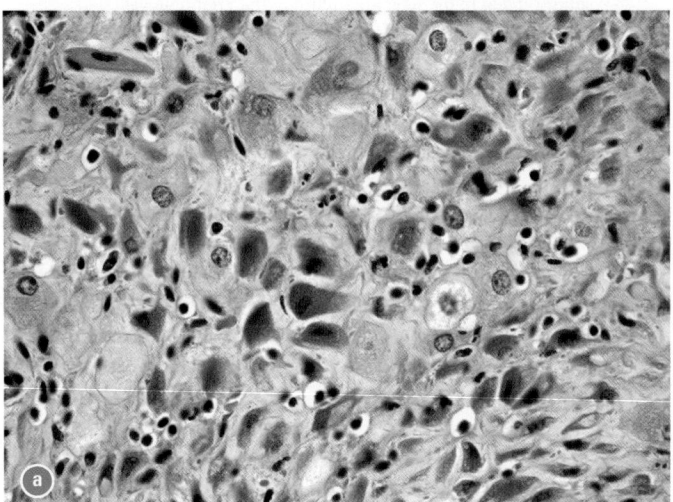
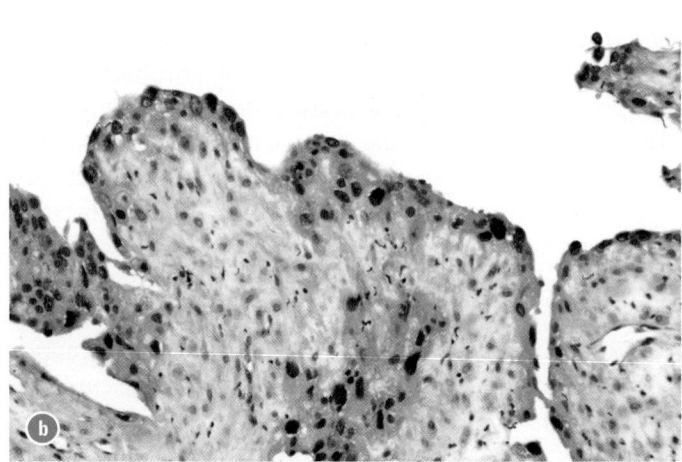

Fig. 32.18 Mimics of implantation site include: (a) inflamed or degenerating decidua with pyknotic nuclei; (b) Arias-Stella change near the endometrial surface may resemble intermediate trophoblasts and be confused with implantation site.

about isolated villi or fragments of implantation site should be maintained.

Implantation site nodule from prior pregnancy (Fig. 32.17b)

Placental implantation site nodules (ISN) or plaques are small, intra-endometrial, well-circumscribed hyalinized eosinophilic nodules, with scattered degenerated-appearing intermediate trophoblastic cells, without cytologic atypia or mitoses. Fibrin is not localized on the decidual surface, as in fresh implantation site. Placental site nodules occur several months to many years after the antecedent pregnancy. This lesion can be identified in both endometrial and endocervical curettings.

Placental site trophoblastic tumors (PSTTs)

These are very rare tumors composed of a monophasic proliferation of intermediate trophoblastic cells (see below) and are highly unlikely to be identified in a specimen taken to exclude ectopic pregnancy. However, we have experienced a single instance when a patient with a history of a prior term delivery several months earlier presented with a persistent low β-hCG level. She underwent dilatation and curettage to exclude an ectopic gestation and was discovered to have a PSTT. In contrast to an early implantation site, there is no histologic evidence of a recent pregnancy in the form of superficial placental bed fibrin or chorionic villi, and the cytologically-atypical, mitotically-active, neoplastic trophoblasts infiltrate myometrium as small groups or single cells.

Molar pregnancy

We include molar pregnancy to emphasize that this entity must always be excluded. In particular, a small amount of molar trophoblast can produce HCG levels in the range of an ectopic pregnancy and yet not be visualized in the uterine cavity by ultrasound. The reader is cautioned to scrutinize carefully even scant villous tissue to ensure that an early complete mole is not overlooked.

Mimics of implantation site

These include: (a) Reactive or inflammatory change in decidua (Fig. 32.18a). Inflammatory or degenerative changes in decidual tissue may produce minor alterations in nuclear morphology, including hyperchromasia. However, the nuclei are typically uniform in contour. (b) Arias-Stella effect. This change is usually easily identified within secretory glands, and consists of polyploid hyperchromatic and enlarged nuclei. Much less commonly, Arias-Stella effect will either involve the surface epithelium, mimicking implantation site, or be sectioned obliquely, giving the impression of implantation site (Fig. 32.18b). The practitioner should be aware of these pitfalls to avoid misclassifying such cases as intra-uterine pregnancies.

Combined intrauterine and ectopic pregnancies

The incidence of coexisting pregnancies of both the tube and ovary is now reported to be approximately 1 in every 4000 pregnancies.[35] The risk of this event is expected to be increased with the use of ART causing multiple ovulations or when multiple embryos are transferred. However, we have diagnosed only one case of this type in the past 14 years at Brigham and Women's Hospital (BWH delivery rate ~10 000/year), suggesting that the incidence is much lower.

Pitfalls to be avoided by both clinician and pathologist

1 *Assuming that the pregnancy is an ectopic one based on gross or dissecting microscopic examination only.*

This is to be avoided. If the surgeon is prepared to perform a laparotomy based on the outcome of the examination, frozen section is mandatory.

2 *Assuming a pregnancy is not an ectopic one based on gross or dissecting microscopic examination.*
As above, if the pathologic examination is required to dictate immediate therapeutic decisions, frozen section is required.

3 *Making an unequivocal diagnosis of intrauterine pregnancy based on a small number of villi or a single fragment of implantation site situated at the periphery of the specimen.* Further tissue should be submitted for examination. Ideally, both implantation site and villi are present.

4 *Making a diagnosis of intrauterine pregnancy based on the identification of placental implantation site nodule (ISN).* ISN is characteristic of prior (not current) pregnancy. We have seen examples of ISN in the curettings of patients with current ectopic pregnancy.

5 *Making a diagnosis of ectopic pregnancy exclusively from the lack of villi in the endometrial curetting.* Instead, this may be due to an inadequately sampled or previously expelled intrauterine pregnancy. In these circumstances, a diagnostic comment stating that an ectopic pregnancy cannot be excluded on the basis of the tissue examined is clear and appropriate.

EXAMINATION OF THE FALLOPIAN TUBE

Confirmation of ectopic pregnancy

In salpingectomy specimens, the fallopian tube should be examined in its entirety, with notation of intact versus ruptured status (Fig. 32.19). Typically, focal to general tubal distention, serosal congestion and possible fimbrial ostia occlusion by blood clot is seen. Around 60% of tubal pregnancies rupture before evacuation. If the tube is ruptured, blood clot or placental tissue protrudes from the site of rupture. This blood clot, when present, should be thinly sectioned and examined carefully with attention to the presence of any sac-like or fetal structures. Implantation can occur anywhere along the length of the tube at varying frequency: involving the ampulla, isthmus, fimbria (often difficult to differentiate from ovarian implantation) in decreasing order of frequency. It is important to remember that the site of rupture does not necessarily correspond to the implantation site.[34]

If enough space is available within the tube lumen, quasi-normal implantation occurs; anchoring villi and cytotrophoblast columns are present (Fig. 32.20).

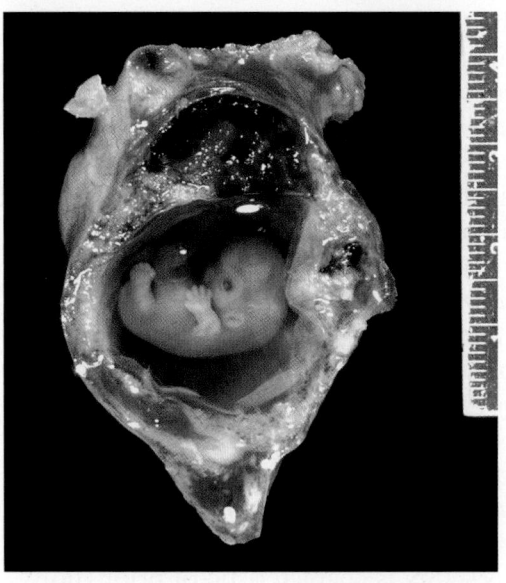

Fig. 32.19 Gross examination of tubal ectopic pregnancy distending the tube. An intact embryo, gestational sac and placental tissues are present within the lumen.

Frequently, trophoblasts infiltrate between smooth muscle fascicles of the tube wall to subserosa and may invade and replace salpingeal vessel walls with fibrinoid (as seen in endometrial spiral arterioles). Ectopic chorionic villi in approximately one-third of tubal pregnancies have normal morphology, particularly if detected and evacuated early while still viable. In the remaining cases the villi show changes consistent with fetal death (stromal fibrosis, villous vessel sclerosis, hydropic changes).

Establishing possible causes

Attention should be paid to the presence or absence of structural abnormalities of the tube, acute or chronic salpingitis, salpingitis isthmic nodosum, endometriosis, hydrosalpinx, neoplasia and other tubal abnormalities (Fig. 32.20; see also Ch. 21). With regard to evaluating acute or chronic salpingitis, it is important to remember that a mixed inflammatory infiltrate in the tubal wall similar to that seen in normal deciduas is very common and should not be overinterpreted as evidence of previous tubal infection.

Differential diagnosis

Retained trophoblastic material from a prior unsuspected and undiagnosed ectopic pregnancy can form a nodular mass, consisting of intermediate trophoblasts, hyalinized villi and other hyalinized material, or form a placental site nodule, which can persist for an extended period of time. Other entities that may distend the tube and/or clinically mimic ectopic pregnancy include hematosalpinx, hematometra, acute or chronic salpingitis, hydrosalpinx, ectopic molar pregnancy (Figs 32.21, 32.22), torsion and benign or malignant neoplasms of the fallopian tube (see Ch. 21).

OTHER SITES OF ECTOPIC GESTATION

Approximately 97% of ectopic gestations occur in the fallopian tube. Other sites, which have been reported include the ovary, cervix, abdominal cavity and, very rarely, vagina, liver and spleen. Most of these sites are not as sensitive to conceptus size as the fallopian tube, and the duration of gestation survival depends instead on the adequacy of the blood supply established.

Ovary

Ovarian implantation of an ectopic pregnancy accounts for approximately 1% of all ectopics in non-IUD users (Fig. 32.23). In IUD users, 10–30% of ectopic pregnancies are reported to occur in the ovary.[36] The conceptus may result from fertilization of the ovum within the ovarian follicle or the conceptus may implant on the ovarian surface primarily or secondarily after fallopian tube rupture. In order to diagnose a primary ovarian ectopic pregnancy, the ipsilateral fallopian tube must be normal and separate from the ovary, the gestational sac must occupy the normal position of the ovary, and be connected to the uterus by ovarian ligaments, and ovarian tissue must be present in the wall of the gestational sac.

Cervix

Cervical pregnancy accounts for ~1% of all ectopic gestations and is reportedly more common in patients with Asherman's syndrome.[37] Hypotheses regarding the mechanism of cervical implantation include increased speed of conceptus transport, delayed maturation of conceptus, endometrial cavity hostility and low placement of embryos after IVF procedures. An enlarged cervix with a normal uterine size and spontaneous abortion is the most commonly reported clinical scenario.

Abdomen

The estimated frequency of an abdominal ectopic pregnancy is 1 in 10 000 pregnancies and can be either primary or secondary following fallopian tube rupture or tubalectomy.[38]

Post-hysterectomy pregnancy

This is a very uncommon occurrence, with less than 50 reported in the world literature. Most have occurred due to conception immediately prior to hysterectomy, when the fertilized ovum becomes trapped in the

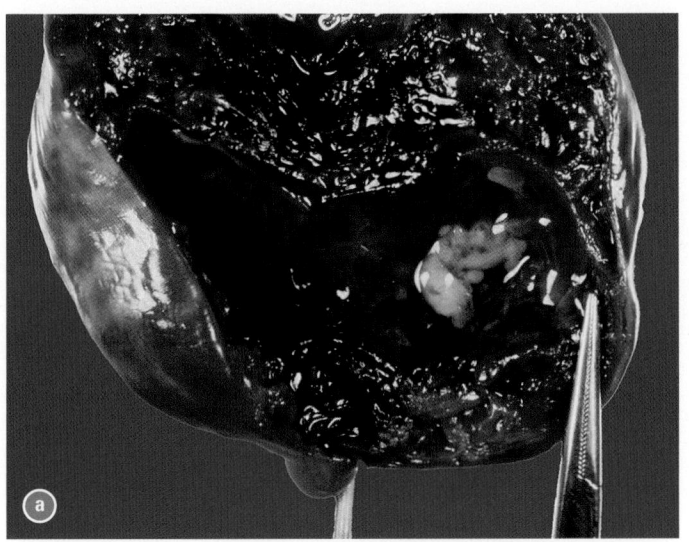

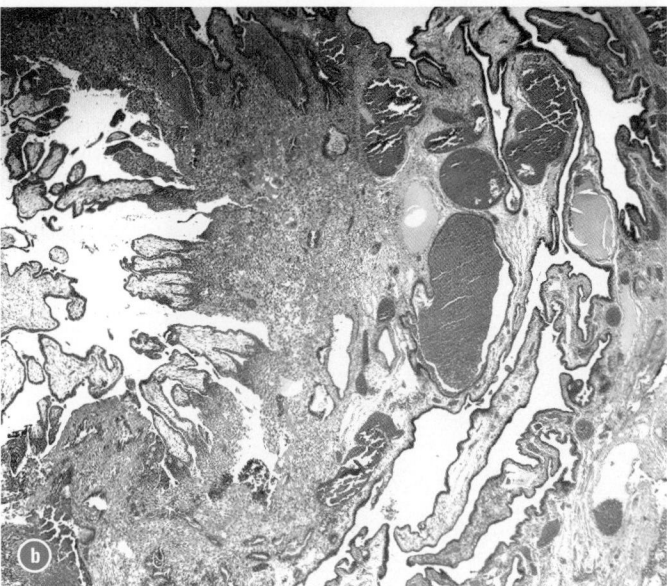

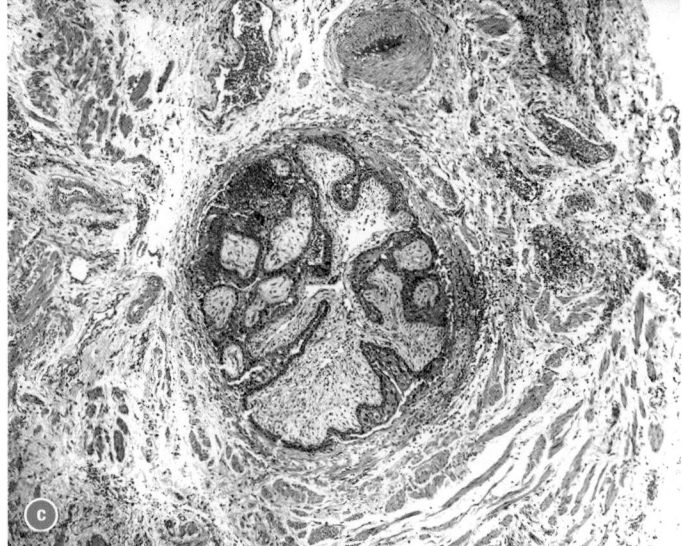

Fig. 32.20 Histologic findings in ectopic pregnancy. (a) At low power the tube is distended with blood clot. (b) An ectopic pregnancy has implanted on the tubal plicae. Note the presence of fused plicae characteristic of prior follicular salpingitis (right). (c) Villi within the tubal wall.

fallopian tube.[35,38] Alternatively, case reports of ectopic pregnancy occurring in patients with a remote history of hysterectomy are attributed to sperm passage through a vaginal-peritoneal fistula.

Post-abortal complications

THE PATIENT AT RISK

Although uncommon in the USA, abortion-related deaths account for nearly 50% of maternal morbidity worldwide.[39] Post-abortal complications may arise from both spontaneous and induced abortions, and include retained products of conception, infection, sepsis, hemorrhage, uterine perforation, intra-abdominal injury and cervical or bowel damage. In the USA, a rapid decline in deaths due to post-abortal complications coincides with the antibiotic era, legalization of therapeutic abortion, and the more effective use of contraception to prevent unplanned pregnancies. In 1987 the total number of deaths following over 1.3 million legal abortions was six, in contrast to over 1000 deaths (following presumably a much smaller number of illegal pregnancy terminations) in the 1940s.[40] In contrast, in underserved countries, as many as one-quarter of a million women die each year following illegal abortion.[41] In Romania, a 10-fold increase in maternal mortality

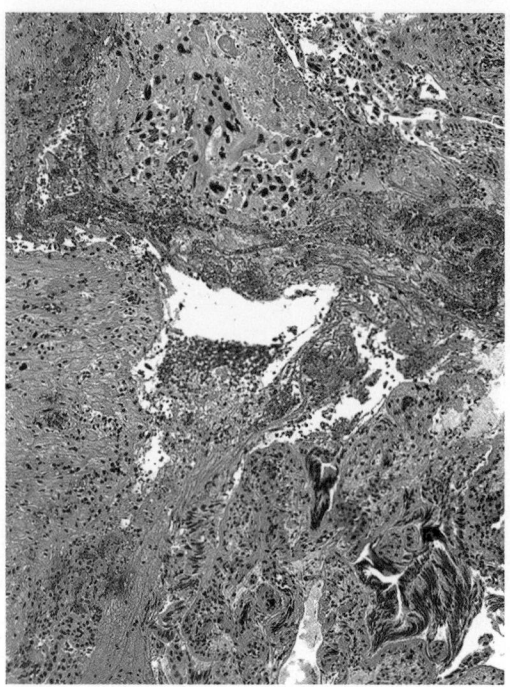

Fig. 32.21 Ectopic molar pregnancy with juxtaposition of normal tubal mucosa (lower) with molar implantation site (upper).

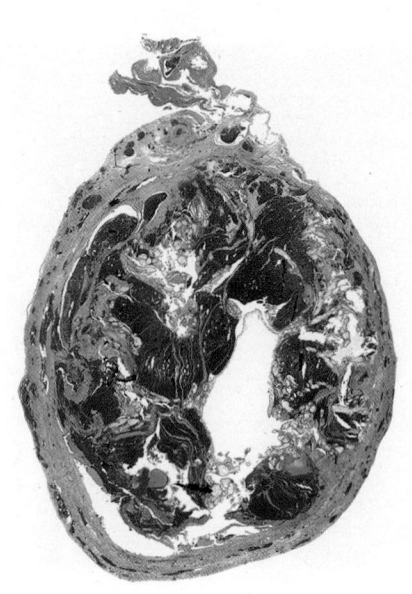

Fig. 32.23 Ectopic ovarian pregnancy. Note the presence of ovarian stroma in the wall.

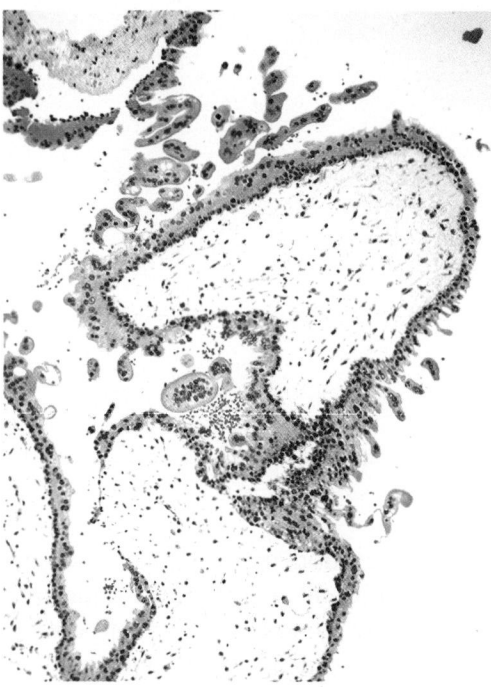

Fig. 32.22 Molar villi characteristic of early complete mole, with moderate villous enlargement, stromal hypercellularity and concentric trophoblastic hyperplasia, are seen in this ectopic molar pregnancy.

Table 32.7 Post-abortal complications

Risk factors
  Non-hygienic technique
  Long interval between initiation of abortion and care
  Limited provider skill
  Inadequate examination of extracted tissue
  Coexisting gonorrhea or pelvic infection

Complications
  Retained products of conception
  Infection/sepsis
  Bleeding/hemorrhage/anemia
  Cervical trauma/tear
  Uterine perforation
  Intra-abdominal injury/bowel perforation

Critical early symptoms
  Heavy or persistent vaginal bleeding
  Lower abdominal pain with enlarged/tender uterus on pelvic examination
  Foul-smelling vaginal discharge
  Fever/chills

followed the outlawing of abortion, which reversed when abortion was legalized.[42] Factors which increase the likelihood of complications from abortion include unhygienic techniques to initiate abortion, a long interval between initiation of abortion and post-abortal care, limited provider skill, inadequate examination of removed uterine contents and the presence of gonorrhea or other pelvic infections prior to the procedure (Table 32.7).

CLINICAL PRESENTATION

The most important presenting symptoms for retained products of conception are heavy or persistent vaginal bleeding, lower abdominal pain and, possibly, an enlarged or tender uterus on pelvic examination. Infection can develop in this setting ('septic abortion'), particularly when instrumentation of the uterus was utilized to induce abortion, and is heralded by the additional symptoms of fever, chills, foul-smelling vaginal discharge and uterine and/or adnexal tenderness. Cultures obtained from septic abortions are usually polymicrobial, and may include Gram-positive (including group B streptococcus, enterococci and *Staphylococcus epidermidis*) and Gram-negative aerobes (especially *Gardnerella vaginalis* and *Escherichia coli*), mycoplasma (especially *Ureaplasma urealyticum*), anaerobes, *Neisseria gonorrheaoeae* and *Chlamydia*.[43] Thus, culture of uterine contents is not generally useful to direct subsequent therapy.

The range of symptoms and severity of illness will vary as will the speed and appropriateness of the clinical response. Ultimately, the outcome can be resolution of symptoms with early antibiotic therapy and uterine evacuation, hysterectomy if the progression of the disease process cannot be controlled, and death if the delay from infection to medical attention results in irreversible septic shock. It is also important to recognize that many of the symptoms of a septic abortion are identical to those of an ectopic pregnancy and thus should be considered in the clinical and pathologic differential diagnosis

PATHOLOGIC FINDINGS

The pathology of septic abortion is of relatively little consequence, as management is based almost entirely on clinical presentation. The uterus, when removed, may appear relatively normal or, in extreme cases of sepsis, may be discolored. Retained products of conception with abundant bacterial growth are commonly seen. A hysterectomy which follows instrumentation should also be evaluated for procedure-related damage to the uterus and cervix; the identification of a uterine perforation may signal other potentially catastrophic intra-abdominal injuries such as bowel perforation.

MANAGEMENT AND OUTCOME

The key to managing septic abortion lies in its prevention, in terms of proper patient education, post-abortal care and aggressive management of post-partum or post-abortal patients who are suspected of having retained products of conception or intrauterine infection.

Trophoblastic neoplasia

GENERAL

Gestational trophoblastic disease (GTD) is defined as a spectrum of abnormal gestations and neoplasms arising from villous or extra-villous trophoblast that are associated with pregnancy. As discussed below, GTD may take several forms, each with its own risk of mortality and responsiveness to chemotherapy. The gestational nature of these disorders justifies their discussion in the context of pregnancy evaluation as (a) most cases are directly related to a pregnancy, (b) the evaluation of each pregnancy requires the exclusion of trophoblastic neoplasia and (c) a high percentage of hydatidiform moles are discovered in the first trimester. The most common types of trophoblastic lesions occur primarily in the first trimester of pregnancy and consist (in descending order of frequency) of partial hydatidiform mole, complete hydatidiform mole, placental site trophoblastic tumor and choriocarcinoma.[44-47] The best studied are the complete hydatidiform moles, which are genetically abnormal gestations carrying a significant risk of subsequently developing gestational trophoblastic neoplasia, including choriocarcinoma. A pathologic diagnosis of hydatidiform mole should prompt the clinician to serially monitor the patient's serum β-hCG for regression. The clinical features of these tumors, histopathology and management are detailed in Tables 32.8–32.10.

THE PATIENT AT RISK

Risk factors for gestational trophoblastic disease include a range of epidemiologic and genetic parameters (Table 32.11)[48] and are most strongly associated with subtypes of GTD at greatest risk for either persisting or evolving into malignancy. The principal risk factors are advanced maternal age, Asian ethnicity, lower socioeconomic status (in selected populations) and one or more prior molar pregnancy. Two types of molar gestations have been recognized and their incidence varies widely worldwide: complete hydatidiform mole (CHM–prevalence approximately 1 per 1000 pregnancies) and partial hydatidiform mole (PHM–prevalence approximately 1 per 100 pregnancies).

Age

Molar gestations occur in women of all reproductive ages, but the highest incidence (per pregnancy) occurs in women over 40 years of age, where the relative risk increases to over five. Women less than 20 years of age have a slightly increased risk as well (relative risk = 1.5).

Ethnicity

Another major risk factor for molar pregnancy is maternal Asian race. In Indonesia, the rate is more than 1 molar

Table 32.8 Clinico-radiologic and gross pathologic presentation of trophoblastic neoplasia

Disorder	Clinico-radiologic features	β-hCG	Endometrial curettings/hysterectomy (gross)	Exclude
Partial mole (PHM)	• 11–25 weeks gestation • ± fetal cardiac activity • Vaginal bleeding • Missed/incomplete Ab.	Variable	• Moderate amount of tissue • Hydropic and normal villi • Sac/membranes • ± Fetal parts (esp. syndactyly)	• SAB • CHM
Complete mole (CHM)	• 'Snowstorm' U/S. • Vaginal bleeding • Toxemia • Hyperemesis • Thyrotoxicosis[a]	High (>100K mIU/ml)	• Voluminous grape-like, transparent vesicles • Mild diffuse swelling under dissecting microscope (early CHM)	• SAB • Ectopic pregnancy • PHM
Persistent GTD/invasive mole	• Vaginal bleeding • Prior CHM or PHM	Plateau (<10% drop in 14 days) or rising (>10% increase ×3 weeks)	• Minimal residual villous tissue • Subtle, sometimes hemorrhagic myometrial nodule	• Choriocarcinoma • Unsuspected degenerating intra-uterine pregnancy (IUP)
ChorioCa Choriocarcinoma	• Irregular/severe bleeding • Recent CHM or normal pregnancy • Pulmonary, neurologic or gastrointestinal symptoms	• Rising, 2 weeks after delivery • After CHM: plateau (<10% drop in 14 days) or rising (>10% incr. ×3 weeks)	Hemorrhagic tumor nodules in endomyometrium	• Persistent mole • PSTT • Unsuspected degenerating IUP
PSTT	• Irregular vaginal bleeding • Pregnancy months to years earlier	Persistent, low <50	Discrete polypoid or endophytic, tan, fleshy mass in endomyometrium	• Placental site nodule • Ectopic pregnancy • Unsuspected IUP
Spontaneous abortion	Vaginal bleeding, 1st–2nd trimester	Declining	Minimal villous edema (not typically grossly evident; by dissecting microscope or histology usually)	• CHM • PHM • Ectopic pregnancy

[a]With 1st trimester ultrasound screening and quantitative β-hCG, complete hydatidiform moles are most often diagnosed before clinical manifestations are evident.

PHM, partial hydatidiform mole; CHM, complete hydatidiform mole; GTD, gestational trophoblastic disease; ChorioCa, choriocarcinoma PSTT, placental site trophoblastic tumor; U/S, ultrasound; SAB, spontaneous abortion; β-hCG, human chorionic gonadotropin.

gestation in 100 non-molar pregnancies. The socioeconomic status of women within this population is also an important factor in some studies; poor individuals show a 10-fold greater risk of GTD than wealthy individuals from the same Asian population.

Nulliparity and prior spontaneous abortion

Nulliparity is associated with a slightly less than two-fold increased risk of GTD. In one study, two or more spontaneous abortions conferred a 32-fold increase in risk of GTD.

Prior hydatidiform mole

Approximately 1% of pregnancies following a single hydatidiform mole will be a recurrent hydatidiform mole. If the patient has had two prior molar pregnancies, the risk is increased to 16–28%.[48]

MOLECULAR PATHOGENESIS

Complete and partial moles have different genetic, clinical and pathologic features (Fig. 32.24). Complete hydatidiform mole develops when an empty (i.e. no female pronucleus) egg is fertilized by one or two spermatozoa, resulting in two complete male-derived haploid chromosomal sets (diandry). In 90% of complete moles a single 23,X spermatozoa duplicates its chromosomes, resulting in a 46,XX complete mole; in the remaining 10% of complete moles, two spermatozoa fertilize an empty egg, resulting in 46,XX or 46,XY molar karyotypes. Partial hydatidiform moles result from two potential scenarios. In approximately three-quarters of the partial mole cases, a normal egg is fertilized by two spermatozoa, resulting in diandric, monogynic triploidy (70% 69,XXY; 27% 69,XXX; 3% 69,XYY).[49] In the second scenario, non-disjunction in meiosis I or meiosis II of spermatogenesis results in an extra set of paternal chromosomes in one sperm (diandric), which fertilizes a haploid (monogynic) egg. It is important to realize that not all triploid gestations are partial moles; cases which have two haploid sets of maternal chromosomes resulting from non-disjunction in meiosis I or meiosis II of oogenesis and one haploid set of paternal chromosomes (monoandric and dygynic)

Table 32.9 Trophoblastic neoplasia, histologic classification, diagnosis and exclusions

Disorder	Villi	Trophoblast	Exclusions	Ancillary studies
Partial mole (PHM)	• Both large and normal • Scalloped contours • Cisterns (variable) • Nucleated RBCs	• Focal mild syncytial T'blast hyperplasia • T'blast inclusions	• Hydropic abortus • Beckwith–Wiedemann syndrome • Trisomic gestations with mild villous irregularity	• Flow: triploid. • Karyotype: 70% 69 XXY; 27% 69 XXX; 3% 69 XYY • Immunostain: p57^{KIP2} (present)
Complete mole (CHM)	• Diffusely and variably enlarged • Focal prominent cisterns	• Diffuse triphasic T'blast hyperplasia and atypia • Atypical implantation site	• Hydropic abortus • ChorioCa • Collapsed gestational sac	• Flow: diploid • Immunostain: p57^{KIP2} (absent)
Early CHM	• Scattered, slightly enlarged • Subtle cavitation • Hypercellular stroma in blue myxoid matrix • Stromal karyorrhexis	• Focal to diffuse T'blast hyperplasia and atypia • Atypical implantation site	• Hydropic abortus • PHM	• Flow: diploid • Immunostain: p57^{KIP2} (absent)
ChorioCa	None present	• Dimorphic/biphasic T'blast atypia • Hemorrhage and necrosis	• Persistent CHM • PSTT • Extra-villous T'blast	• Immunostain: strongly β-hCG positive
PSTT	None present	• Sheets of mononuclear atypical intermediate T'blast • Dissection between muscle fibers • Mitoses	• Extravillous T'blast • Exaggerated implantation site • ChorioCa • Persistent CHM	• Immunostain: hPL +; β-hCG +/– • Keratin +; ≥15% MIB-1 fraction • Tap63+ (epithelioid PSTT)
Hydropic abortus	Gradual differences in villous size with edema	• Minimal or polar T'blast proliferation only • No T'blast atypia	• Early CHM • PHM • Twin (CHM and normal)	• Flow: diploid • Immunostain: p57^{KIP2} (present)

PHM, partial hydatidiform mole; CHM, complete hydatidiform mole; hPL, human placental lactogen; β-hCG, beta human chorionic gonadotropin; PSTT, placental site trophoblastic tumor; T'blast, trophoblast; RBCs, red blood cells; ChorioCa, choriocarcinoma; Flow, flow cytometry.

are abnormal but non-molar (accounting for ~10% of all triploid gestations); see below.

As will be discussed further below and is detailed in Table 32.12, the diagnosis, classification and differential diagnosis of gestational trophoblastic disease has undergone a major renaissance in the past 25 years, due to the genetic information obtained from these abnormal conceptuses combined with new biomarkers used for their diagnosis.

TARGET TISSUES

Three distinct types of trophoblast are found in the human placenta. Associated with chorionic villi are cytotrophoblasts and syncytiotrophoblasts, while intermediate trophoblasts are found in the endomyometrial implantation site and in placental membranes (Fig. 32.25).

Cytotrophoblast

The precursor of intermediate and syncytiotrophoblast, cytotrophoblast consists of small, polyhedral cells with clear cytoplasm, distinct cell borders and single, central vesicular nuclei; mitoses are occasionally seen. This cell type is found at the periphery of villi, beneath the syncytiotrophoblast. Cytotrophoblast is also present in 'cell columns', eccentric clumps of trophoblastic cells adherent to villi, which are prominent in early gestations. Because such eccentric trophoblast proliferations tend to occur at one 'pole' of a villus, this growth pattern is termed 'polar' trophoblast proliferation. The cytotrophoblast is strongly immunoreactive for cytokeratins, but essentially non-reactive for human chorionic gonadotropin (hCG) and human placental lactogen (hPL).

The cytotrophoblast plays a major role in both complete hydatidiform mole and choriocarcinoma. The diagnosis of both is predicated on the identification of both cytotrophoblastic proliferation and atypia. This is in contrast to partial hydatidiform mole and tumors of placental site trophoblast.

Syncytiotrophoblast

This terminally-differentiated, mitotically inactive, functional trophoblast is a syncytium with amphophilic to

Table 32.10 Management and outcome of trophoblastic neoplasia

Disorder	Therapy	Risk of progression	Comments/caveats
Partial mole (PHM)	1. Suction curettage 2. Follow β-hCG q. week until <5 mIU/ml × 3 weeks, then q. month × 6 months, then q. year × 1–3 years 3. Contraception × 1 year	Persistent GTD = 4–15% ChorioCa = essentially 0%	Confusion with a twin complete and normal gestation (rare)
Complete mole (CHM)	Low-risk; same as PHM High-risk; chemoprophylaxis (see Tables 32.13 and 32.14)	Persistent GTD = 10–30% Invasive mole = 15% ChorioCa: 2–3%	If persistently elevated β-hCG: 75% have persistent GTD; 25% risk of chorioCa
Persistent invasive mole	1. Evaluate for metastatic disease 2. Single-agent chemo until β-hCG <5 mIU/ml 3. Contraception for 1 year 4. Hysterectomy for local control (optional) or bleeding complications		'Persistent GTD' is a clinical diagnosis applied to persistently elevated serum β-hCG following molar pregnancy and often treated empirically w/o pathologic sampling to distinguish persistent/invasive mole *vs* chorioCa
Choriocarcinoma	1. Evaluate for metastatic disease 2. Single-agent chemo if low risk 3. Multiagent chemo if high risk 4. Hysterectomy for local control (optional) (see Tables 32.13 and 32.14)	Based on FIGO staging and WHO score. Remission: No metastases = 80% Metastases = 67% Overall disease-free survival w/single agent chemo = 87%	
PSTT	1. Hysterectomy (therapy of choice) 2. Evaluate for metastatic disease 3. Multiagent chemo	Non-metastatic disease: cured by surgery Metastases = >30% at diagnosis Recurrence = 30% Mortality: 21–36%	Poor prognosis: >5 mitoses/10 hpf (recurrence), pulmonary metastases, antecedent pregnancy >4 years prior

PHM, partial hydatidiform mole; CHM, complete hydatidiform mole; GTD, gestational trophoblast disease; β-hCG; beta human chorionic gonadotropin; ChorioCa, choriocarcinoma; PSTT, placental site trophoblastic tumor; FIGO; International Federation of Gynecology and Obstetrics; WHO, World Health Organization; chemo, chemottherapy.

Table 32.11 Risk factors for trophoblastic neoplasia

Factor	Qualifier	Relative risk
Maternal age	<20 years	1.5
	>40	5.2
Prior SAB	1.9–3.3	
Parity	>1	0.4
Vitamin A	Consumption > median	0.6
		Incidence
Race	Indonesia	1:85
	Japan	1:522
	Sweden	1:1560
	USA	1:1724
Socioeconomic status	Philippines (wealthy)	1:2000
	Philippines (poor)	1:200
Prior molar pregnancy	1	1:100
	>1	1:6 to 1:4
		Trend
Smoking	>15 cigarettes/day	Increasing
Infertility		Increasing
Theca-lutein cyst	> 6 cm by ultrasound	Increasing (GTD subsequently develops in up to 50%)

SAB, spontaneous abortion; GTD, gestational trophoblastic disease.

eosinophilic cytoplasm and multiple, small, hyperchromatic nuclei. The syncytiotrophoblast cytoplasm may be finely to coarsely vacuolated; when multiple large vacuoles ('lacunae') are present, the cytoplasm has an irregular, lacy appearance. Syncytiotrophoblast covers all chorionic structures (i.e. chorionic plate and villi), where it is located peripheral to the cytotrophoblast layer. In this location, syncytiotrophoblast interfaces with the maternal blood, lining the entire maternal intervillous (vascular) space much like an endothelial layer. In the first trimester, syncytiotrophoblast is strongly immunoreactive for hCG and weakly immunoreactive for hPL; in later pregnancy, this staining pattern reverses (i.e. hCG weakens, hPL strengthens). Syncytiotrophoblast is also strongly reactive for cytokeratins.

Syncytial trophoblasts are involved in both complete and partial moles. In the complete mole, this component is distinctly immature, producing a lushly festooned arrangement of concentric syncytiotrophoblast that appears to cascade from the involved villi. In contrast, in the partial mole, the syncytiotrophoblastic proliferation

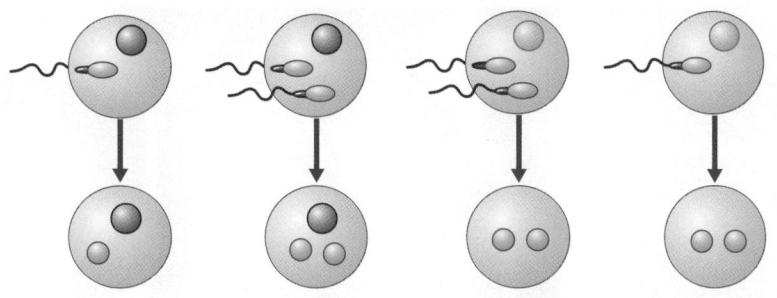

	Normal	Partial mole	Complete hydatidiform mole	
Ploidy	2n	3n	2n	1n>2n (duplication)
Parents	Biparental	Biparental	Paternal	Paternal
Chorio Ca risk	Low	Low	Elevated	Elevated

Table 32.12 *Schematic of changes in classification of trophoblastic neoplasia, including the use of biomarkers*

Decade	Molar categories	Parameters	Differential diagnosis
1970s	Hydatidiform mole grade 1–6	Morphology	Hydropic abortus
1980s	Partial and complete mole	Genetics	Hydropic abortus
1990s	Partial and complete mole	Genetics Morphology	Hydropic abortus Trisomy 18 Beckwith–Wiedemann syndrome Angiomatous malformation Early complete mole Diandric partial mole Digynic triploidy Twin mole–normal gestation
2000s	Partial and complete mole	p57 expression Genetics	Complete mole *vs* other biology

is more subdued, composed of smaller aggregates but still concentrically arranged in some villi.

Intermediate (extra-villous) trophoblast

The intermediate trophoblast is a polyhedral to spindle shaped cell, larger than the cytotrophoblast, with eosinophilic cytoplasm. Most intermediate trophoblasts have a single, central nucleus, but binucleate and multi-nucleated forms ('implantation site giant cells') can be prominent and occasional mitoses are seen. In comparison with syncytiotrophoblast, the nucleus of intermediate trophoblast is larger and more reactive-appearing, with prominent chromatin and nucleolus. Smudging of chromatin and sharp angulations of nuclear shape are common; also characteristic of intermediate trophoblast are intranuclear cytoplasmic 'inclusions'. The most

characteristic feature of intermediate trophoblast is its location: this cell type is usually found within fibrin or within the endomyometrium, particularly in the walls and lumens of spiral arterioles. Intermediate trophoblast is strongly immunoreactive for cytokeratins and hPL, and weakly reactive for hCG.[50]

Intermediate trophoblast can be subdivided into villous intermediate, implantation site and chorionic type. The implantation site trophoblast is distinctly atypical in both complete hydatidiform moles and tumors arising from the placental bed (placental site trophoblastic tumors, PSTTs). In CHM, the intermediate trophoblasts are markedly enlarged and atypical. In PSTTs, the intermediate trophoblasts comprise the tumors. Villous intermediate trophoblast is commonly seen in the mature placenta (see Chs 33 and 34) and is not associated with

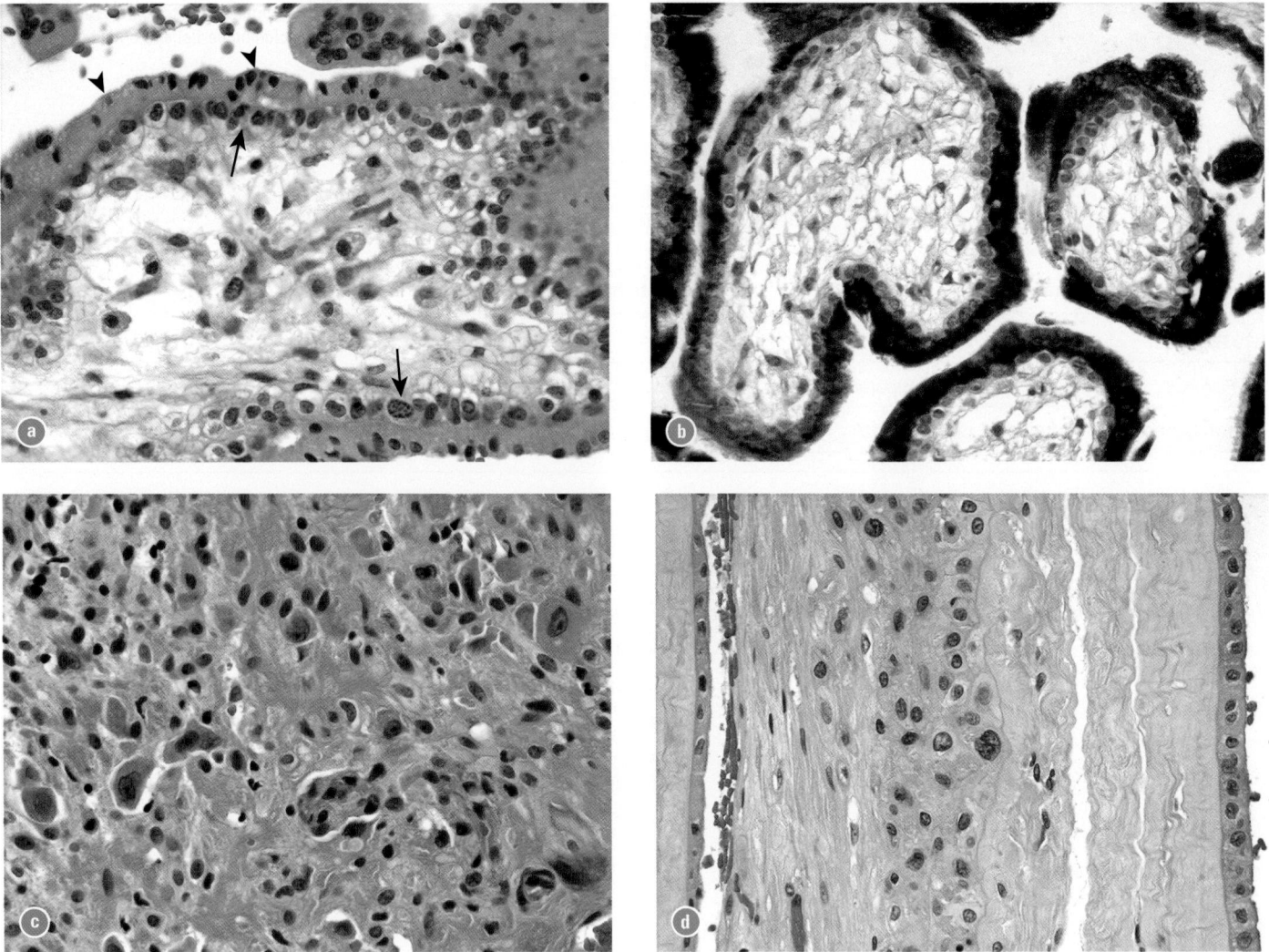

Fig. 32.25 Potential target tissues for trophoblastic neoplasia include (a) cytotrophoblast (arrows) and syncytiotrophoblast (upper layer, arrowheads). (b) The syncytiotrophoblast is highlighted by antibody to human chorionic gonadotropin. (c) Implantation site trophoblast is the origin of placental site trophoblastic tumor. (d) Epithelioid trophoblast from the chorionic membrane is the possible origin of epithelioid trophoblastic tumors.

neoplasia. Chorionic (membranous) trophoblasts are rarely associated with so-called epithelioid trophoblastic tumors (see below).

Recent studies imply that the three types of trophoblast can be distinguished in part by their expression of certain proteins, one of which is p63. p63 is related to both p53 and p73 and encodes two different isoforms, a full-length form resembling p53 (TAp63) and a truncated isoform (ΔNp63) that is commonly expressed in squamous epithelium.[51] Trophoblastic columns adjacent to villous structures in the early placenta, and villous cytotrophoblast strongly express p63. Cells in transition from the cytotrophoblast to mature intervillous trophoblast, and to a lesser extent, cells in similar transition near the maternal surface of the placenta,

express p63, but syncytiotrophoblast and the more mature intervillous and implantation site trophoblast are p63-negative. Interestingly, membranous (chorionic) trophoblast also express p63.[50] The expression patterns of this protein suggest that, like other epithelia, trophoblast expression is a function of both maturation and proximity of the trophoblast to supporting mesenchyme (villi and membranes) (Lee and Crum, unpublished data). Recently, one study reported that differential expression of the two isoforms will distinguish cytotrophoblast (ΔNp63) from membranous trophoblast (TAp63).[50] Other studies using TAp63-specific antibody have shown that the dominant p63 protein in membranous trophoblast is most likely ΔNp63 (Lee, McKeon and Crum, unpublished data).

COMPLETE HYDATIDIFORM MOLE

Classic (late) complete mole

In the past, most complete hydatidiform moles were clinically recognized in the early second trimester because of heavy vaginal bleeding, anemia, marked uterine enlargement, highly elevated β-hCG level and a characteristic ultrasound appearance in which the swollen villi give the appearance of Swiss cheese (Fig. 32.26). Such 'late' complete moles were evacuated at a mean gestational age of 14 weeks. Most complete moles are currently evacuated between 8 and 12 weeks of gestational age ('early' complete moles), because widespread use of ultrasonography now permits early recognition and evacuation of most abnormal gestations. However, early complete moles may not be clinically suspected, because frequently there has been minimal bleeding, uterine enlargement and β-hCG elevation, and because the ultrasonographic features may be subtle. Because of this, the pathologist is often the first to suspect the diagnosis in many current 'early' complete hydatidiform moles.[52,53]

Macroscopically, the complete mole is distinguished by diffuse villous swelling, produced by the influx of fluid into the villi and the absence of any villous vasculature. The fluid distends the villi, producing the appearance of grapes (hence the term hydatidiform). These transparent, swollen chorionic villi (vesicles) measure up to 2 cm in diameter and are distinguished from those in partial moles by their uniformity throughout the specimen (Fig. 32.27). As will be discussed below, the size of these villi and the ease with which the pathologist recognizes a complete mole is determined by the gestational age, with older moles being most conspicuous.

The pathologist can immediately appreciate a well-evolved complete mole on histologic examination.

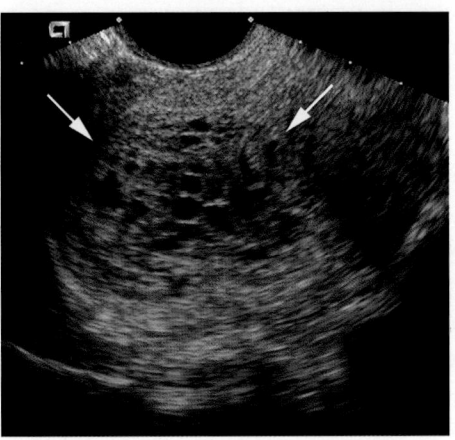

Fig. 32.26 Sonographic findings in complete mole. Transverse image of the uterus demonstrating a complex mass (arrows) filling the uterine cavity. The mass has solid components and small cystic areas, characteristic of a complete hydatidiform mole.

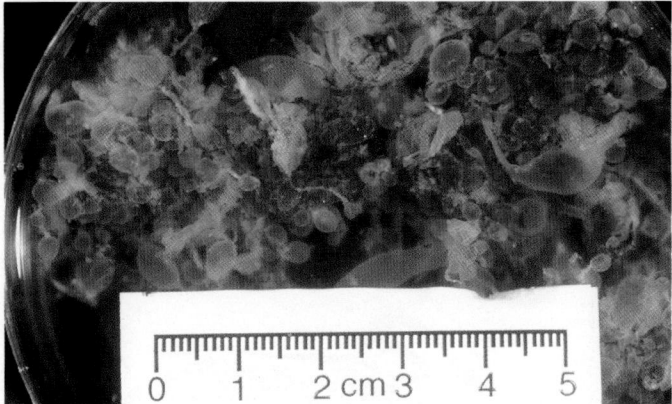

Fig. 32.27 Complete mole as seen through the dissecting microscope. Note the diffuse grape-like villous swelling.

At low power, enlarged hydropic, frequently cavitated villi occupy a large geographic area. The conspicuous cavitations within villi are due to necrosis, forming spaces or cisterns. The other conspicuous finding is the presence of sheets of trophoblast both encircling the villi and bridging one or more villous structures. This villous trophoblastic proliferation is most notable for its concentric distribution on some villi and the participation of both cyto- and syncytiotrophoblast. Often, the syncytiotrophoblast may appear immature and form Medusa-like festoons emanating from the molar villi. The degree of cytologic atypia of the cytotrophoblast and syncytiotrophoblast exceeds that of non-molar pregnancy but is not always conspicuous (Fig. 32.28a–c). Non-villous gestational tissues, including chorionic membrane, amnion, yolk sac and nucleated fetal red blood cells, are typically if not invariably absent. All complete moles (early and late) typically show significant atypia of intermediate trophoblastic cells within the decidual implantation site (Fig. 32.28d).[54] This latter feature is useful in confirming the diagnosis histologically, particularly in small samples or when the differential diagnosis includes partial mole or hydropic abortus.

Early complete mole

The higher surveillance of early gestations has permitted clinicians and pathologists to recognize complete moles earlier in their natural history. These abnormal gestations can be appreciated on ultrasound, by careful gross inspection of the placental villi and attention to subtle but defined histologic parameters that herald the presence of early complete mole. Most early complete moles grossly resemble spontaneous abortion specimens; macroscopic villous edema is usually minimal but may

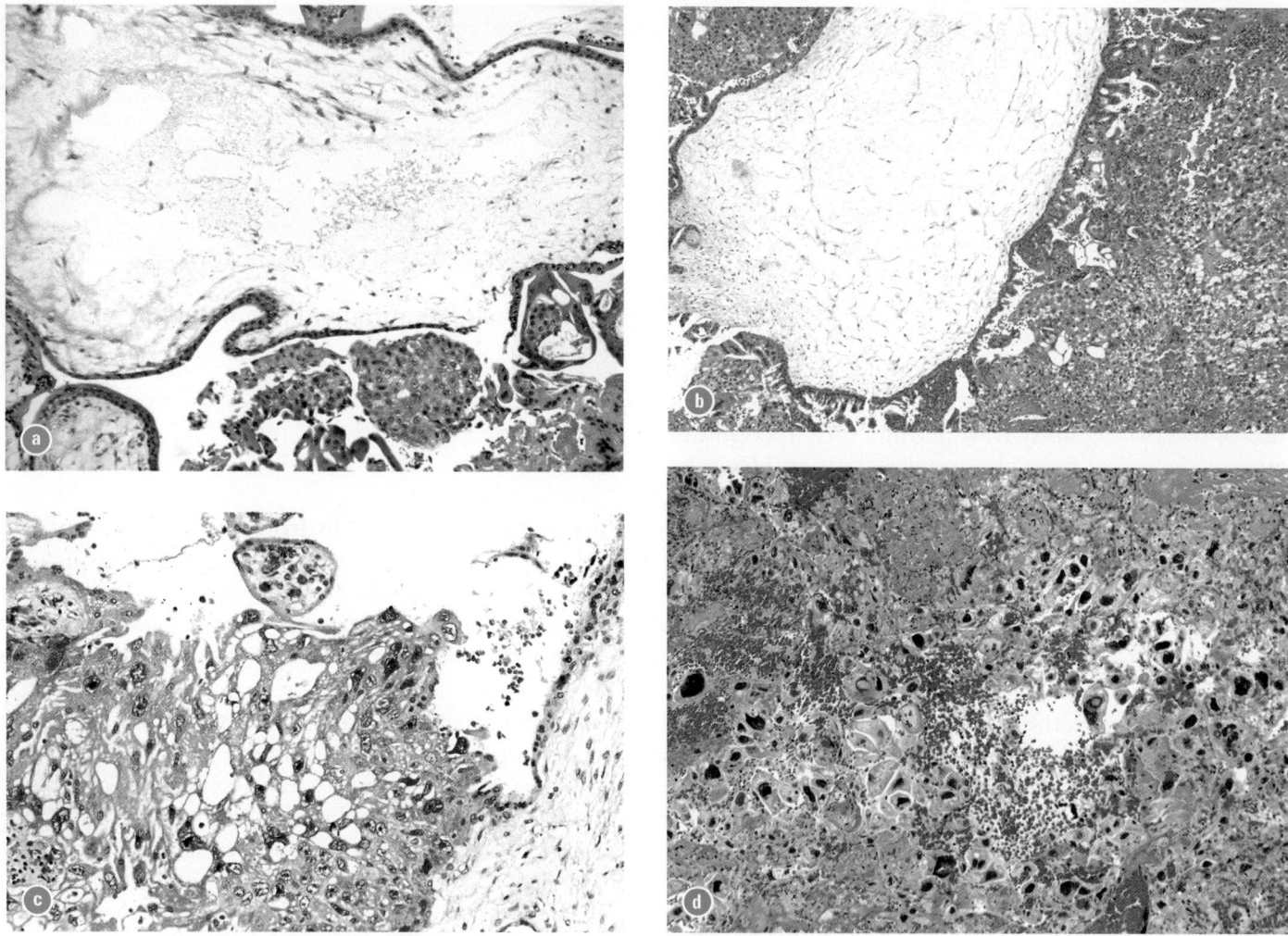

Fig. 32.28 Histologic features of complete mole include: (a) large swollen villi with necrosis of the mesenchyme producing central cavitations (cisterns); (b,c) conspicuous, concentric cyto- and syncytiotrophoblastic hyperplasia; and (d) atypical implantation site.

be appreciated by the trained eye, particularly under the dissecting microscope. However, because many practices do not perform an exhaustive pre-histologic examination of products of conception, most early complete moles are discovered by careful attention to several parameters. (1) Histologically, these specimens typically display scattered cavitated villi (with slight enlargement), and focal to diffuse hyperplasia and atypia of trophoblast. (2) Villous stromal features are highly characteristic, including a hypercellular population of tiny stellate mesenchymal cells in a blue myxoid matrix (resembling a fibroadenoma). (3) Prominent karyor-rhexis is seen in the villous mesenchymal cells. (4) Typical villous morphology includes many 'cauliflower-like' villi, with toe or knuckle-like bulbous protrusions separated by linear slits (Fig. 32.29a–c). (5) An important features confirming the disease is the marked implantation site

atypia (Fig. 32.29d). Because the pathologic features of early complete mole may be subtle, pathologic recognition can be challenging, particularly with limited sampling. Adequate tissue sampling (a minimum of 4–5 paraffin blocks) is warranted whenever a molar gestation is clinically suspected, or when the initial histologic evaluation raises the suspicion of hydatidiform mole.[52,53]

Differential diagnosis and the use of biomarkers

The differential diagnosis of complete mole is similar to partial mole (see below), and includes hydropic abortus, partial mole, villous changes seen with Beckwith–Wiedemann syndrome, an intact gestational sac mimicking a single cavitated villus and others. Most of these entities can be excluded by attention to the histologic criteria, specifically the diffuse enlargement and triphasic

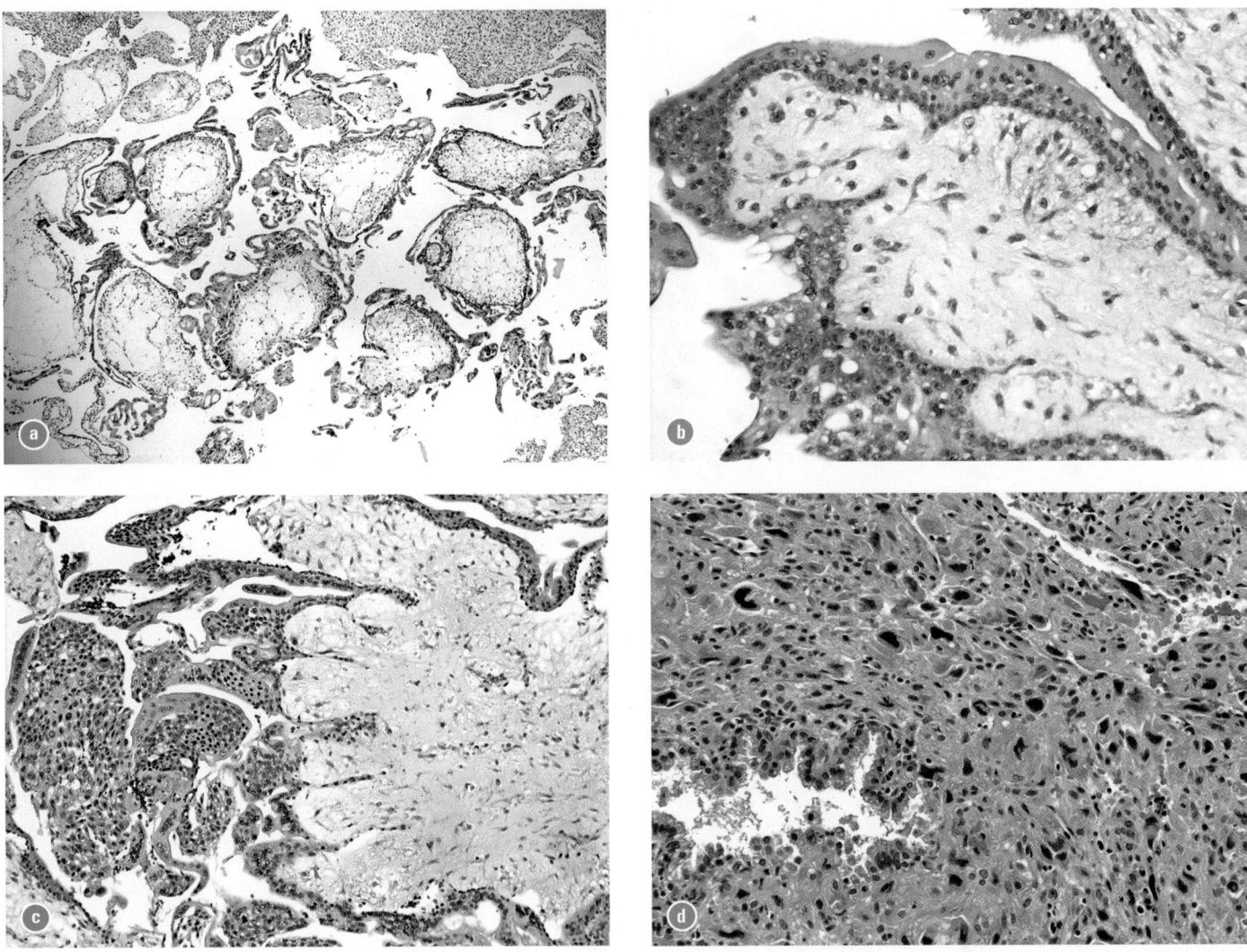

Fig. 32.29 Features of early complete hydatidiform mole include: (a) moderately enlarged villi; cisterns are not prominent, but the concentrically arranged trophoblast is conspicuous; (b) hypercellular, 'fibroadenoma-like' villous stroma with a bluish appearance due to immature fibroblasts, accompanied by modest but often circumferential trophoblastic proliferation; (c) characteristic irregular villous contours resembling knuckles or toes; (d) implantation site trophoblast is often the most conspicuous trophoblastic atypia in early complete mole.

trophoblastic atypia seen in CHM. Recently, biomarkers have emerged that take advantage of imprinted genes to distinguish CHM from other entities. Because complete moles result from diandry (paternal fertilization of an empty egg, which lacks maternal chromosomes), paternally imprinted gene products (i.e. protein) which are normally expressed only from maternally derived chromosomes) should be absent. Studies have recently shown that immunohistochemistry for p57[KIP2] or IPL/PHLDA2 (paternally imprinted, maternally expressed gene products) is useful for confirming the diagnosis of complete moles (both early and late).[55,56] Nuclei of decidua (maternally derived tissue) and extra-villous trophoblast of all types of gestations stain positively for p57[KIP2], serving as an internal control for immuno-reactivity of the specimen (Fig. 32.30a). Almost all complete moles have absent (or near absent) villous stromal and cytotrophoblastic nuclear reactivity for p57[KIP2], while all other types of gestations (including partial moles) show nuclear reactivity in more than 25% of villous stromal and cytotrophoblastic nuclei (Fig. 32.30b–d).[56] Interestingly, very rare exceptions to this rule (complete moles with p57[KIP2] staining) invariably have been shown to carry a retained maternal chromosome 11.[57]

Invasive mole

This is defined as a hydatidiform mole (partial or complete) whose villi are present within the myometrium or its vascular spaces (Figs 32.31, 32.32). Once vascular

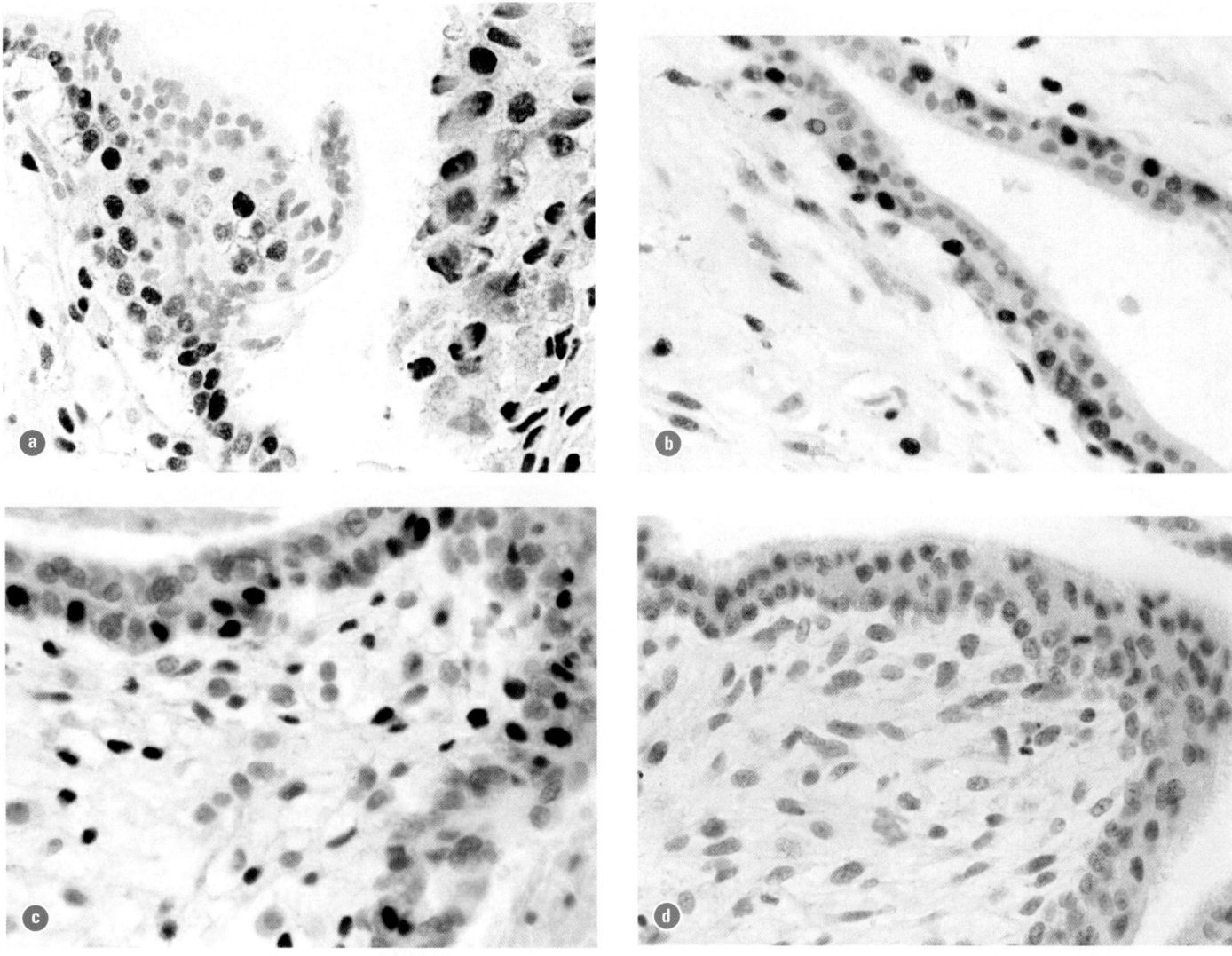

Fig. 32.30 (a) Normal villous (left) and extra-villous (right) trophoblast stained for p57^KIP2. The latter stains in normal and abnormal gestations and serves as a positive control. (b,c) Hydropic gestation and partial mole exhibit staining in both villous mesenchyme and cytotrophoblast. (d) In contrast, complete mole is negative.

invasion has developed, villi may embolize to distant sites, including the vagina, the lung and the brain ('metastatic' invasive mole). Historically, invasive mole was called 'chorioadenoma destruens'.[58] Invasive mole may be clinically suspected when persistent gestational trophoblastic disease develops and the endometrial cavity contains scant tissue (determined by curettage or ultrasound examination). However, in this setting, invasive mole usually cannot be pathologically confirmed from the curettage specimen, even when abundant myometrium is obtained. In general, pathologic documentation of invasive mole (or metastatic invasive mole) necessitates surgical resection (i.e. hysterectomy, lung biopsy). Because such surgical procedures are currently uncommon for treatment of gestational

trophoblastic disease, the pathologic diagnosis of invasive/metastatic mole is currently infrequently made.

When invasive/metastatic molar tissue is available for pathologic assessment, the gross appearance of invasive mole is a hemorrhagic nodule(s), often without easily identifiable villi. The histologic appearance of invasive mole consists of hydropic villi with associated atypical, hyperplastic and degenerating trophoblast, located within myometrium, blood vessels or other site. If the trophoblast is relatively exuberant and the villi relatively scarce, invasive/metastatic mole may be incorrectly diagnosed as choriocarcinoma. Although invasive/ metastatic mole usually responds to chemotherapy, morbidity or mortality can result, generally related to localized hemorrhage (intraperitoneal bleeding with

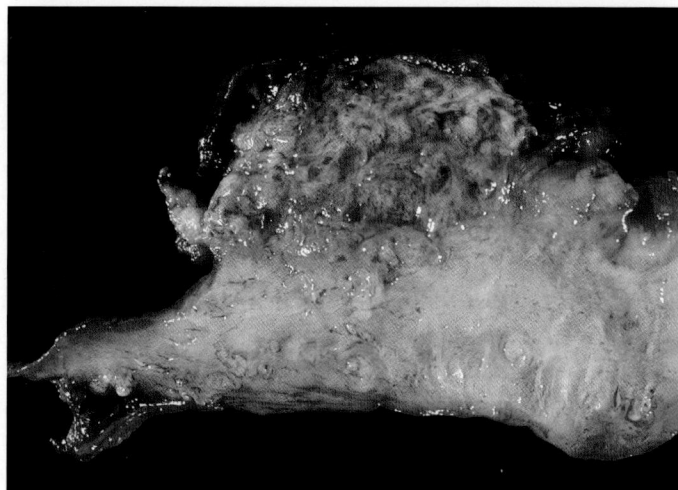

Fig. 32.31 Gross appearance of invasive complete mole extending into the superficial myometrium.

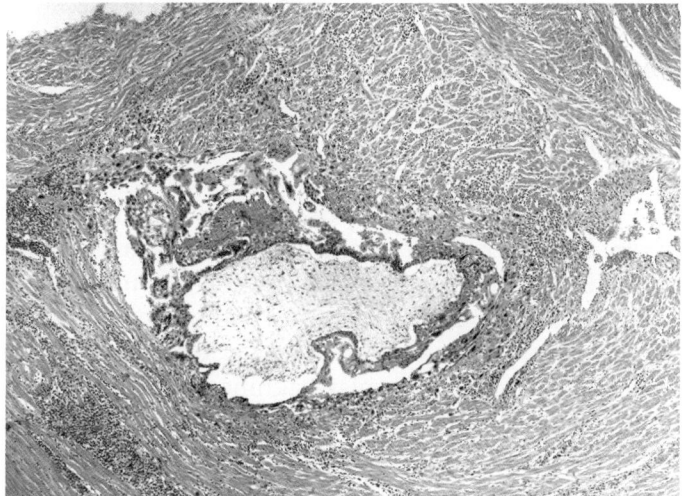

Fig. 32.32 Molar tissue is identified in the myometrium on histologic examination of the invasive complete mole pictures above.

transmural invasive mole; pulmonary hemorrhage); these complications are currently very unusual in the USA, but more common in underdeveloped countries.[59]

Management and outcome

The outcome of a complete mole cannot be predicted in advance by histopathology alone.[60] Interestingly, although complete hydatidiform moles are typically diagnosed earlier due to closer radiologic and hormonal monitoring, there appears to be no reduction in the rate of post-molar tumors.[47] Management and outcome are influenced by two systems of risk assessment. The first system stratifies Stage 1 GTD (confined to the uterus clinically) according to defined risk factors; the presence of any factor significantly increases the risk of recurrence (Tables 32.13, 32.14). The most important variables include the duration from the antecedent pregnancy to the diagnosis of the mole, the size of the uterus and the β-hCG level. Based on these parameters, the patient will either be triaged to follow-up β-hCG measurements or immediate chemotherapy (chemoprophylaxis). Persistent elevations in β-hCG levels and/or clinical, radiologic, or pathologic evidence of persistence or spread of the disease significantly increases the risk of a malignancy (choriocarcinoma)(Table 32.10).[45–47]

Early complete moles with no risk factors may be treated similarly to partial moles, with weekly follow-up β-hCG determinations until three consecutive normal levels are obtained. Higher-risk lesions receive single-agent chemoprophylaxis and, if resistant, are managed by combination chemotherapy and/or hysterectomy. Overall, approximately 92% of Stage 1 complete moles enter remission following chemotherapy, and a majority

Table 32.13 Staging of gestational trophoblastic disease

Stage 1	Persistent elevations of β-hCG levels and tumor confined to uterus
Stage 2	Disease beyond the uterus but localized to vagina or pelvis
Stage 3	Pulmonary metastases by clinical assessment
Stage 4	Brain, liver, kidney, spleen or gastrointestinal involvement

Table 32.14 Risk factors for poor outcome in gestational trophoblastic disease (GTD)[45]

Stage 1 disease[a] Risk factor	Parameter
Interval between antecedent pregnancy and evacuation	≥4 months
Theca-lutein cysts	≥6 cm
Uterine size	Significantly increased
Serum β-hCG	>100K mIU/ml
Maternal age	>40
History of prior GTD	Yes

Stage 2–4 disease Good prognosis	Poor prognosis
<4 months duration	>4 months duration
Serum hCG <40K	Serum hCG >40K
No prior chemotherapy	Prior chemotherapeutic failure
No brain/liver involvement	Brain/liver involvement
Prior spontaneous abortion	Prior term pregnancy

[a]Recurrence with 0 risk factors = 6–9%, 1 risk factor = 31%, >1 risk factor = 45%.
K = thousand

of the remainder can be salvaged by additional rounds of chemotherapy.[45–47,59]

The second classification of GTD subdivides metastatic GTD (Stages 2–4) into good and poor prognostic categories (Tables 32.13, 32.14). Poor outcome is associated with longer (>4 months) duration, higher pre-treatment β-hCG levels, a prior term pregnancy, evidence of brain or liver metastases and a history of failure to chemotherapy. Overall, control of recurrent GTD is successful in over 80% of cases with multi-agent chemotherapy.[45–47,59]

PARTIAL HYDATIDIFORM MOLE

Clinical and histologic features

Clinically, most partial moles present as missed abortions, with late first trimester bleeding and a small uterus. Partial mole specimens grossly mimic spontaneous abortions; however, on careful inspection the placental villous tissue has scattered tiny cysts (1–3 mm diameter tapioca-like spheres, best seen in fresh floated specimens) which correspond to the sonographic findings (Fig. 32.33a–c). Histologically, partial moles are an admixture of two populations of villi: (1) smaller, fibrotic, normal-appearing villi; and, (2) larger, irregularly shaped, hydropic villi with mild degrees of syncytiotrophoblastic hyperplasia. Some enlarged villi have central cisterns (often measuring 2–3 mm in diameter), while other enlarged villi appear dysmorphic, with an irregular, scalloped border, and trophoblastic-lined invaginations and inclusions. Hyperplasia of villous and chorionic plate syncytiotrophoblast is usually mild, primarily consisting of foci of cytoplasmic expansion with prominent lacunae. Significant cytologic atypia is usually absent in syncytiotrophoblast, cytotrophoblast and implantation site intermediate trophoblast (Fig. 32.34a–c). Villous blood vessels often contain nucleated fetal red blood cells; other evidence of fetal development is common, including embryonic/fetal tissue, chorionic membrane, amnion and umbilical cord. When a fetus is available for evaluation, multiple malformations are usually present, especially syndactyly involving the third and fourth finger, (Fig. 32.34d). Additional findings in the fetus may include marked growth retardation, prominent forehead, micrognathia, microphthalmia, hypertelorism, hypogonadism and ambiguous genitalia, and toe syndactyly. However, the absence of fetal tissue does not exclude the diagnosis of a partial mole, as it is not uncommon for villous vessels to collapse and fetal red blood cells (RBCs) to degenerate with a retained partial mole.[61]

Molecular studies

Many studies have demonstrated that ploidy analysis (determined by flow cytometry or image analysis) is complementary to histopathology for properly classifying molar gestations (Fig. 32.35). The vast majority of partial moles (90% to 100%) have a triploid or near-triploid DNA content, while most complete moles (95%) show either a diploid or tetraploid result. Ploidy studies are most valuable when histologic assessment is suggestive of partial mole but not conclusive; in this setting, confirmation of triploidy strongly suggests the diagnosis of partial mole.[62]

In a recent paper, Redline et al. resolved the 20-year question of why only a portion of triploid gestation demonstrates a molar phenotype.[63] They found that when two of the three chromosomal complements were derived from the mother (digynic), partial mole was never diagnosed histologically. This contrasts with triploid gestations in which two of the three were male derived (diandric). Most of these will present as partial moles (Fig. 32.36).[63]

Differential diagnosis

Hydropic abortus and complete mole

Hydropic abortus and complete mole are the major differential diagnostic entities to be considered when the pathologist assesses a possible partial hydatidiform mole. The histopathology of a hydropic abortus is characterized by degenerated-appearing, edematous villi with balloon-like, rounded contours and an attenuated trophoblastic lining (Fig. 32.11). Complete molar specimens typically display significant trophoblastic hyperplasia and atypia (involving cyto-, syncytio- and intermediate trophoblast), and characteristic villous morphology (either diffuse hydrops in late complete moles, or primitive stromal features in early complete mole). In specimens that are difficult to pathologically classify, adequate sampling (at least five blocks of tissue), supplemented by ploidy analysis and/or p57 immunohistochemistry (as discussed above), will disclose the correct diagnosis in most cases.[56]

Beckwith–Wiedemann syndrome

A rare mimic of partial hydatidiform mole is the placenta in Beckwith–Wiedemann syndrome (BWS), a congenital overgrowth syndrome caused by mutation in the chromosome 11p15.5 region (Fig. 32.37a,b). The affected fetus is characterized by omphalocele, macrosomia, macroglossia, visceromegaly, dysplasia of the renal medulla and cytomegaly of the fetal adrenal gland. Adrenal carcinoma, nephroblastoma, hepatoblastoma and rhabdomyosarcoma occur with increased frequency

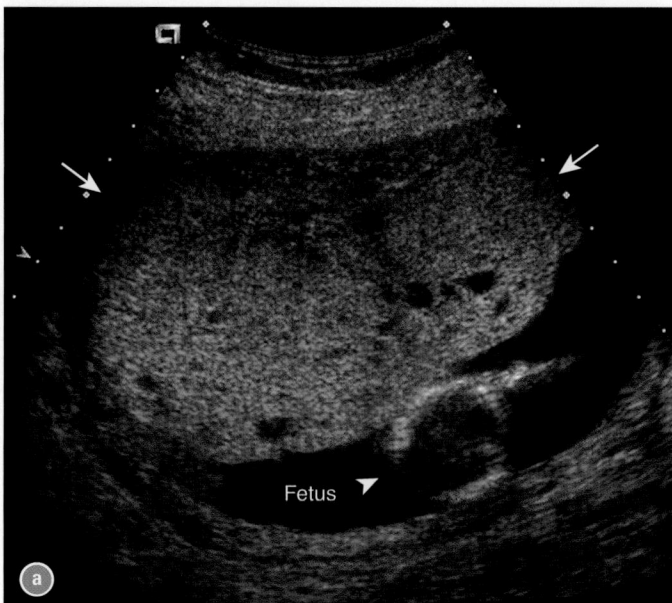

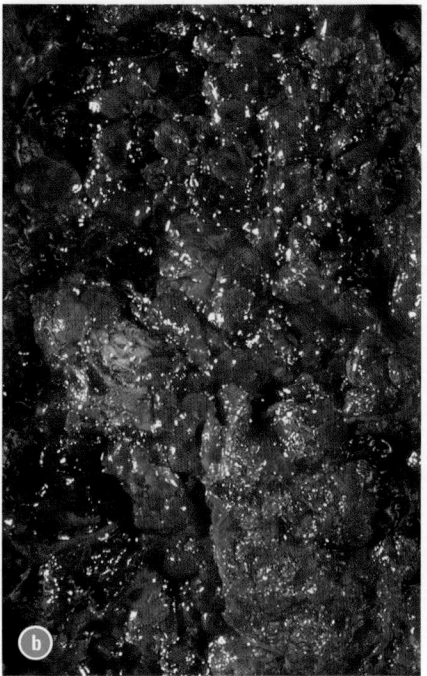

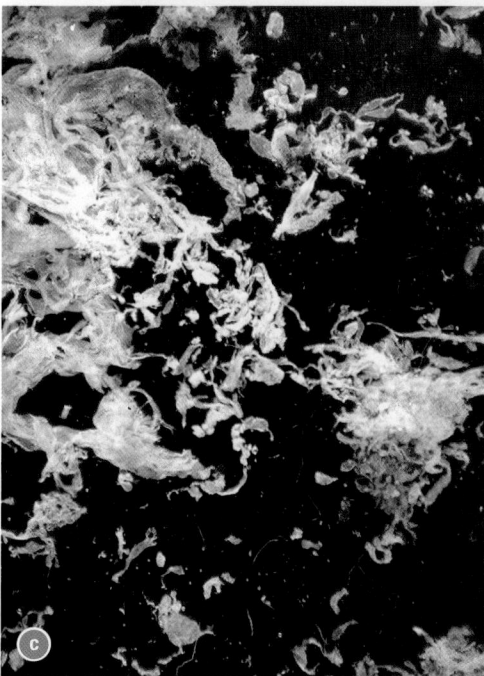

Fig. 32.33 Partial mole. (a) Sonographic image of a 13-week gestation with triploidy demonstrating the placenta (arrows) to be markedly thickened, containing scattered small cystic areas consistent with villous swelling. The fetus (fetus, arrowhead) is seen within the amniotic cavity. (b) Immature placenta with focal villous enlargement. (c) Early partial mole with scattered swollen villi (upper center) seen in the dissecting microscope.

in BWS patients. The placenta displays marked umbilical edema and scattered, enlarged, cavitated stem villi. Histologically, the enlarged stem villi display central cavitation, with prominent muscularized vessels, and a smooth villous contour; no trophoblastic hyperplasia is present.[44] Notably, in contrast to partial hydatidiform mole, syndactyly and triploidy are absent in BWS.

Twin pregnancy with complete mole and normal gestation

Rarely, both a complete mole and normal gestation will coexist (Fig. 32.37c). The differential diagnosis is partial mole and hydropic abortus. A partial mole is excluded by the presence of trophoblastic hyperplasia and homogeneous villous enlargement and cavitation localized to one region of the specimen. Likewise, the

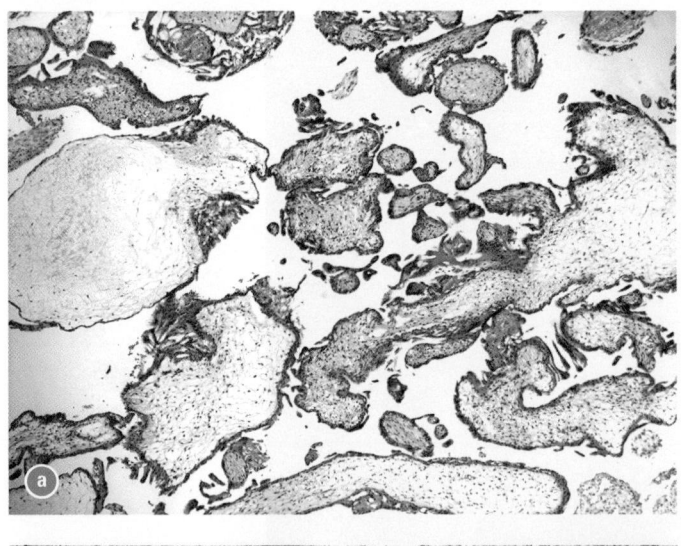
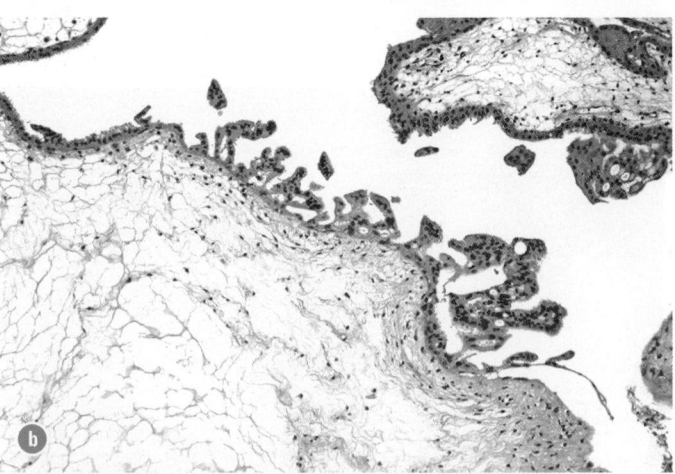
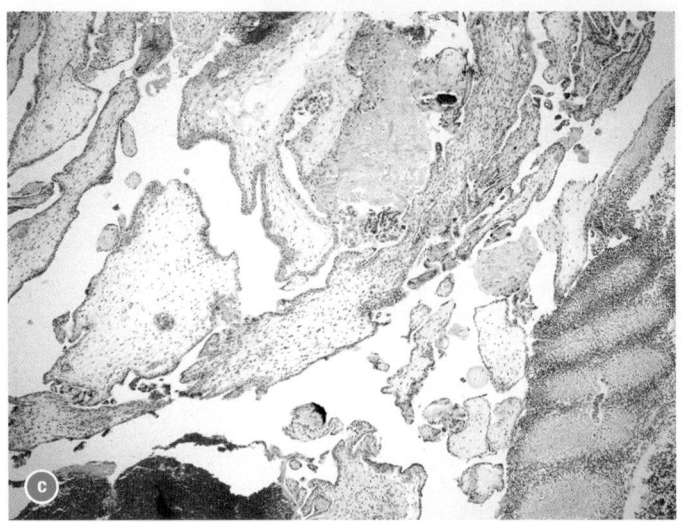
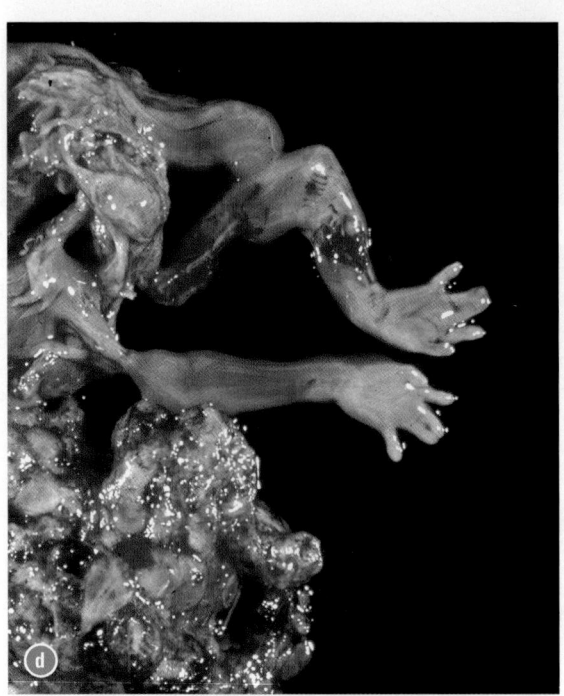

Fig. 32.34 Histologic appearance of partial mole includes: (a) a mixed population of villi with relatively sharp differences in villous size, (b) predominately mild syncytiotrophoblastic proliferation, (c) coexisting fetal tissue (lower right). (d) Characteristic phenotype of 3-4 syndactyly in the triploid fetus.

discrete separation of two components is unusual for a hydropic abortus.[64] Immunostaining with p57 will easily distinguish the two components.

Gestational sac masquerading as a cavitated villous

This should always be suspected in the presence of a single large villous-like structure (Fig. 32.37d).

Management

Partial moles are managed as low-risk disease (Table 32.10), with follow-up to exclude persistent moles. Rare cases of progression to choriocarcinoma have been documented in the literature and remain a source of controversy.

CHORIOCARCINOMA

Clinical features

Gestational choriocarcinoma may occur subsequent to molar pregnancy (50% of instances), abortion (25% of cases), ectopic pregnancy (2.5% of cases) or normal pregnancy (22.5% of cases).[45–47,65] Choriocarcinoma may also be diagnosed *concurrently* with pregnancy, although this is very rare.[66,67] Metastasis of choriocarcinoma to the fetus has infrequently been reported.[68,69] Choriocarcinoma usually follows a recognized pregnancy (molar or other) by an interval of several months; however, prolonged intervals following gestation (up to 14 years) have been reported.[70]

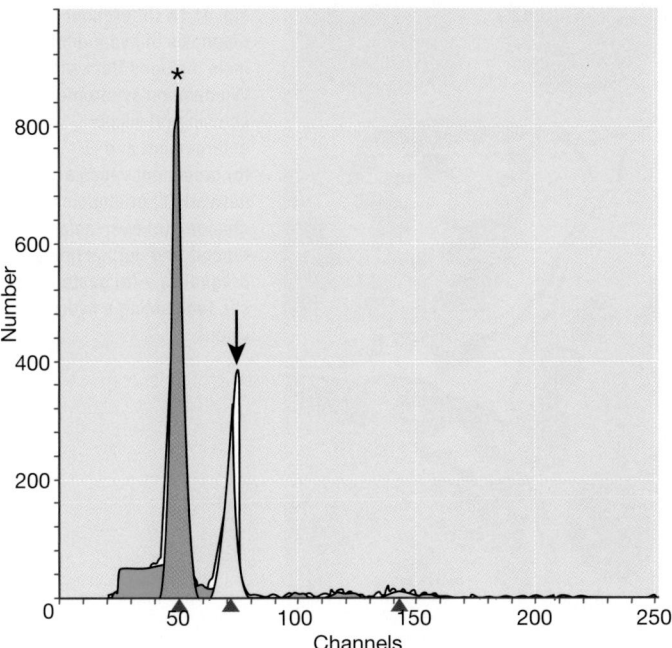

Fig. 32.35 Flow cytometric profile of partial mole with prominent peak at 1.5N (arrow) with background peak of diploid maternal cells (asterisk).

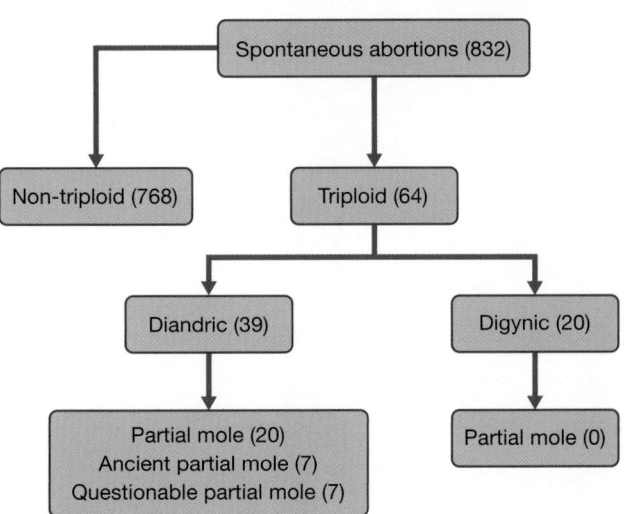

Fig. 32.36 Outcome of a series of 832 spontaneous abortions. Note that digynic triploid gestations do not eventuate in partial moles in contrast to diandric triploid pregnancies.[57]

Choriocarcinoma often presents with abnormal uterine bleeding due to involvement of the endometrium by tumor. Presenting signs of choriocarcinoma may also reflect metastatic disease, such as hemoptysis due to pulmonary involvement, or neurologic abnormalities due to bleeding from a cerebral metastasis. In patients with metastatic disease, the lungs are involved in 90% of cases and the brain and liver are involved in 20–60% of patients. Brain and/or liver metastases in the absence of pulmonary involvement is extremely rare.[71] Choriocarcinoma is usually diagnosed earlier following a molar gestation than a non-molar pregnancy; this is probably due to closer patient surveillance (with gonadotropin screening) following a mole. Possibly for this reason, post-molar choriocarcinomas have a better prognosis than those with non-molar precursors.[72]

Gross and histologic features

Choriocarcinoma in any site (endometrium, myometrium, lung) has a similar gross appearance: one or several well-circumscribed very hemorrhagic nodules (Fig. 32.38). Because of extensive bleeding, such tissues may require extensive sampling to demonstrate the biphasic histology characteristic of these neoplasms. Often, viable tumor is found only at the periphery of a hemorrhagic nodule (at the tumor–host interface), while the center of the nodule is entirely composed of blood clot. Histologically, choriocarcinoma consists of an admixture of syncytiotrophoblast, and either cytotrophoblast, intermediate trophoblast, or both. Hemorrhage and necrosis may predominate and vascular invasion may be prominent (Fig. 32.39a,b). By definition, villi should not be present in choriocarcinoma; however, in rare cases of 'early' choriocarcinoma, which are diagnosed concurrently with an advanced normal pregnancy, villi are seen (discussed below). The trophoblast of choriocarcinoma shows marked cytologic atypia (syncytiotrophoblast – somewhat less than other types of trophoblast); although mitoses are common in cyto- and intermediate trophoblast, they are not seen in syncytiotrophoblast. Although syncytiotrophoblast may be encountered only focally, its identification is necessary for the diagnosis of choriocarcinoma. Syncytiotrophoblast is strongly hCG immunoreactive, and weakly immunoreactive for hPL; intermediate trophoblast stains somewhat weaker for hCG and hPL. All types of trophoblast are strongly immunoreactive for cytokeratins. Choriocarcinoma is usually not given a histologic grade; however, some studies have suggested that tumors with abundant syncytiotrophoblastic differentiation may have a better prognosis than other tumors.[73] A small number of choriocarcinomas, including some fatal cases, have been studied by flow cytometry and all have been reported to be diploid.[74]

Differential diagnosis

The major differential diagnoses for choriocarcinoma include: (1) previllous trophoblast in early gestations; (2) persistent molar tissue following hydatidiform mole; (3) placental site trophoblastic tumor; and (4) undifferentiated carcinoma.

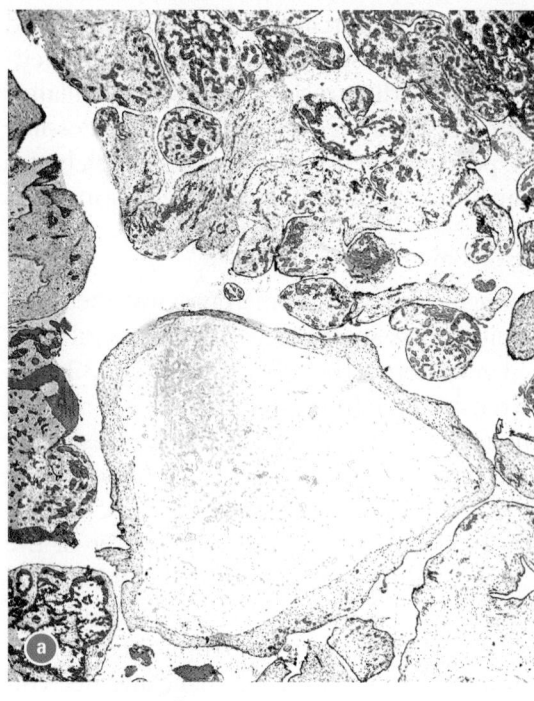

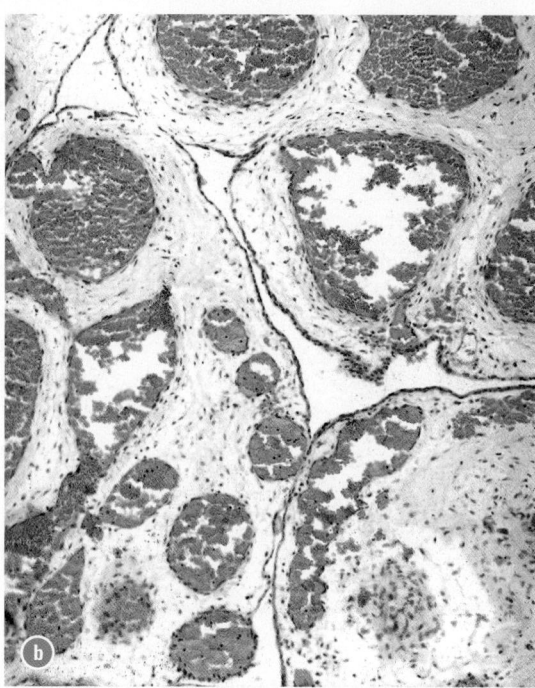

Fig. 32.37 Differential diagnosis of hydatidiform mole includes Beckwith–Wiedemann syndrome, showing (a) villous enlargement and (b) prominent vascular network (choriangiomatoid change), (c) twin molar (upper) and normal (lower) pregnancy – (d) gestational sac resembling a hydropic villous.

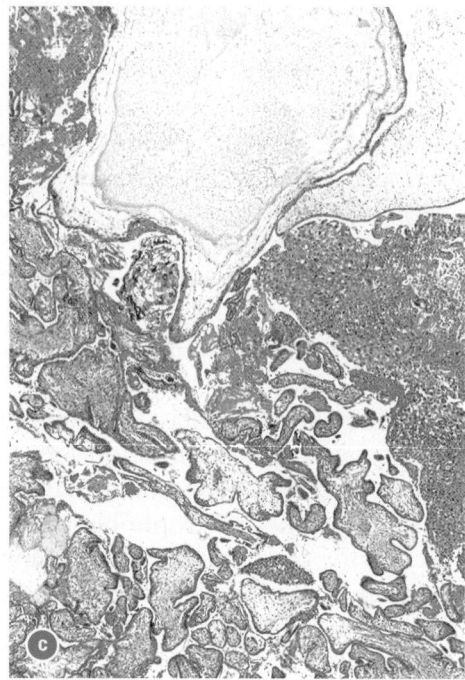

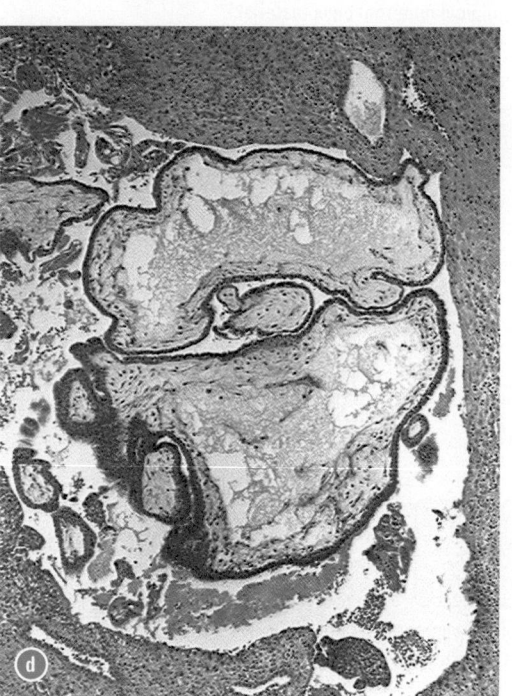

Previllous trophoblast

In very early gestation, prior to the formation of villi, trophoblastic tissue is relatively scant, although striking cytologic atypia may be seen (Fig. 32.40a). In contrast to choriocarcinoma, the β-hCG level of an early gestation is low. If villi are demonstrated, this confirms an early pregnancy and rules out choriocarcinoma.

Post-molar curettings

When 'persistence' develops following hydatidiform mole, a second endometrial curettage is sometimes performed. Often the curettage specimen will have no villi, but may have scattered *microscopic* foci of very atypical, avillous trophoblast. Although this picture after a non-molar pregnancy might strongly suggest choriocarcinoma, following a mole it is possible that this tissue represents

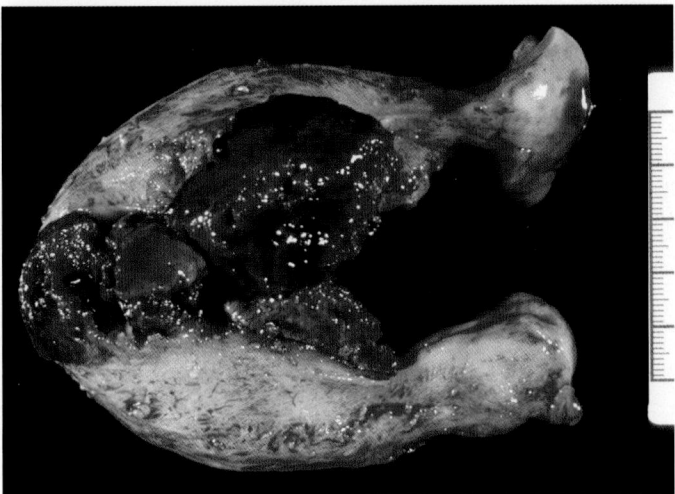

Fig. 32.38 Gross appearance of choriocarcinoma, consisting of a hemorrhagic mass involving the endomyometrium.

residual implantation site or the trophoblastic component of an invasive mole (Fig. 32.40b,c). The presence of any villi will exclude choriocarcinoma (Fig. 32.40d). In the absence of villi, small, scattered clusters of atypical trophoblast may be designated 'Atypical avillous trophoblast, scattered foci; although choriocarcinoma must be excluded, this diagnosis is not confirmed'. In contrast, abundant large *sheets* of markedly atypical, biphasic, mitotically active trophoblast should be diagnosed as choriocarcinoma, particularly when there is evidence of endomyometrial invasion by tumor.[75]

Placental site trophoblastic tumor (PSTT)

Because the PSTT is monophasic (i.e. does not contain syncytiotrophoblast), wide sampling and careful evaluation will discriminate these tumors. In scant curettage specimens, such a distinction is not always possible; under these circumstances, immunohistochemical staining may be helpful. hLAG positivity may confirm the presence of intermediate trophoblast and distinguish from the cyto- and syncytiotrophoblast of choriocarcinoma, but cannot distinguish intermediate trophoblasts of PSTT from those of choriocarcinoma (see below).[76] The intermediate trophoblasts of PSTTs are typically placental lactogen (HPL) positive while chorionic gonadotropin (HCG) is only focal.

Undifferentiated carcinoma

Immunohistochemical staining, wide sampling and clinical context are the best methods to exclude this possibility.

Intraplacental choriocarcinoma

Clinical and histologic features

Usually non-molar gestational choriocarcinoma presents post-partum, after an interval of weeks to months – less commonly after several years. Rarely, choriocarcinoma coexistent with a normal pregnancy is documented; most descriptions are single case reports.[77–79] Such intraplacental choriocarcinomas may be diagnosed antenatally (in cases with symptomatic metastatic disease), or at the time of delivery ('incidental' placental discovery). 'Incidental' choriocarcinoma in a term placenta is usually

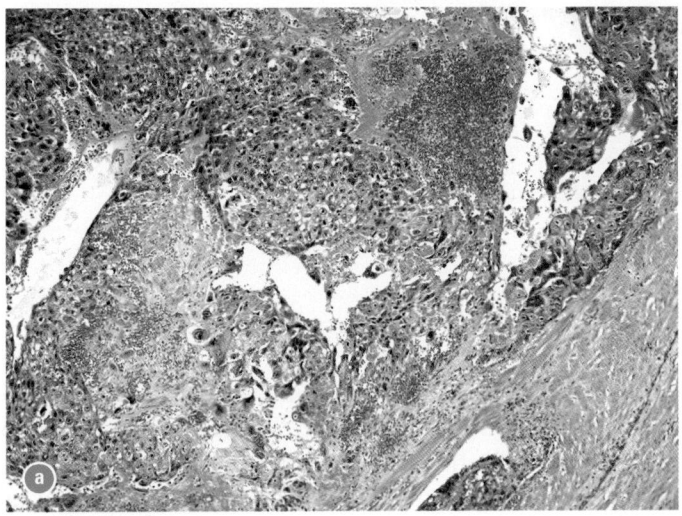
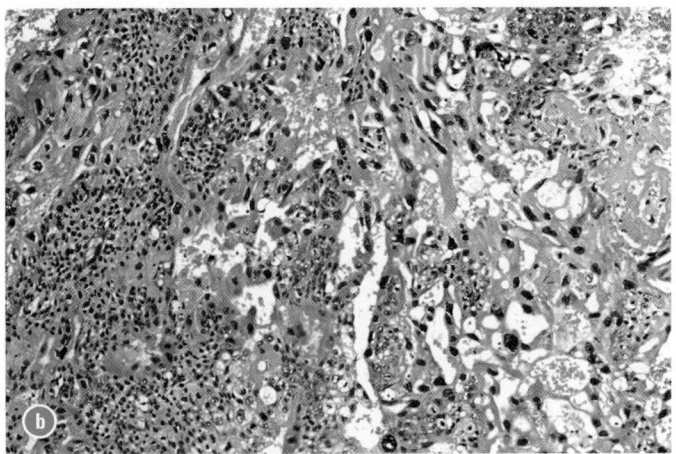

Fig. 32.39 Histologic appearance of choriocarcinoma, with (a) biphasic trophoblastic atypia, hemorrhage and necrosis. (b) Higher-power view depicts marked trophoblastic atypia.

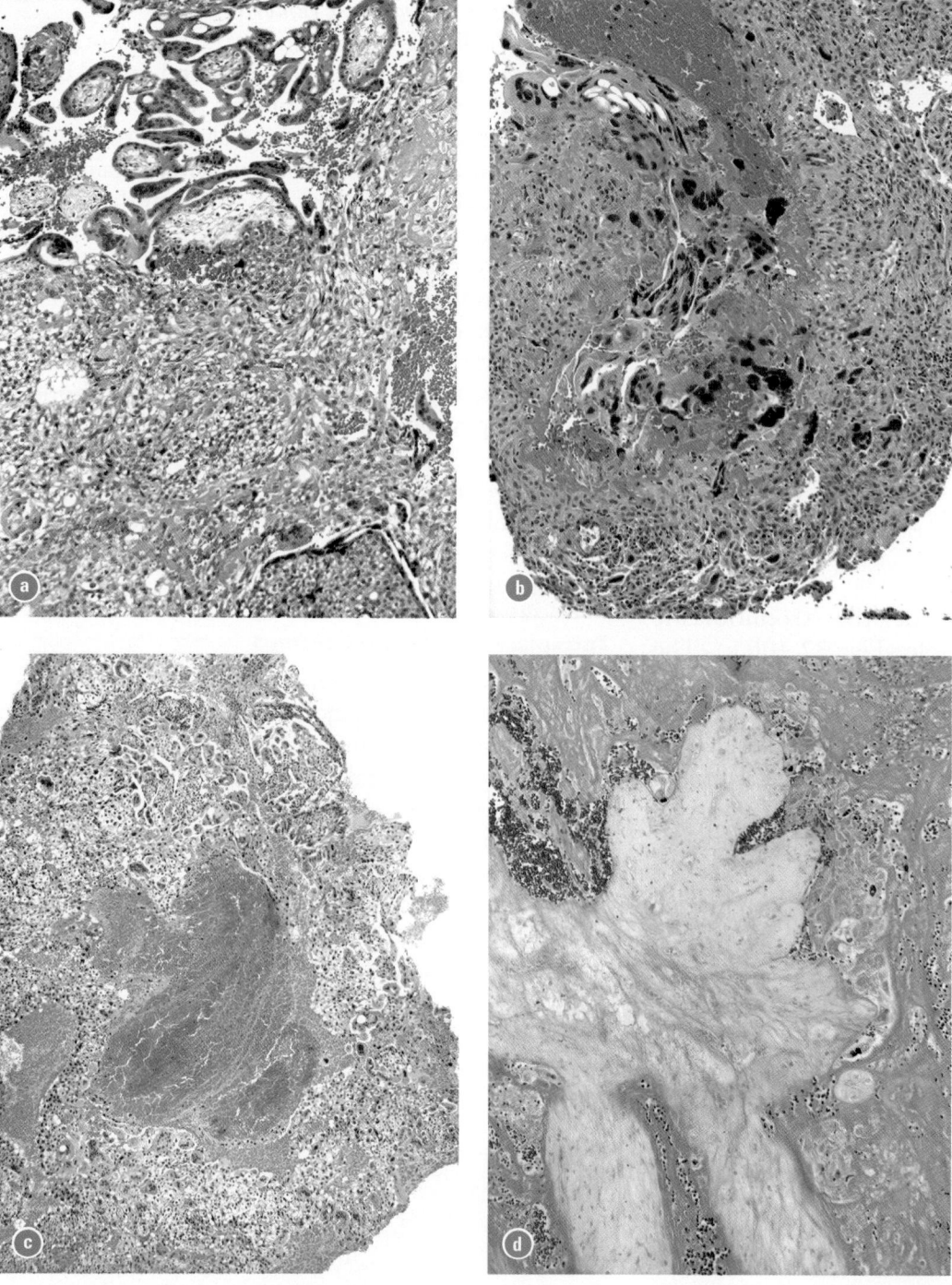

Fig. 32.40 Differential diagnosis of choriocarcinoma includes (a) immature extra-villous trophoblast, (b) molar implantation site and (c and d) end retained complete molar tissue. The presence of residual molar villi (d) excludes choriocarcinoma in this setting.

grossly described as a solitary 'infarct' (less than 1 cm up to several centimeters), or less commonly as multiple, widely dispersed, small white nodules (up to 5 mm in diameter) (see Chs 33 and 34). Histologically, a highly atypical, biphasic, solid trophoblastic proliferation is located in the (maternal) intervillous space, appearing to originate from stem villi. Sheets of hyperchromatic, mitotically active, primitive-appearing cytotrophoblast are admixed with syncytiotrophoblast, the latter having numerous cytoplasmic lacunae (Fig. 32.41). When choriocarcinoma is discovered in a term placenta, β-hCG levels should be measured in mother and infant, to determine whether further metastatic evaluation is indicated. Commonly, maternal metastatic tumor is discovered; rarely, metastases in the infant (some of which have proved fatal) have been seen.

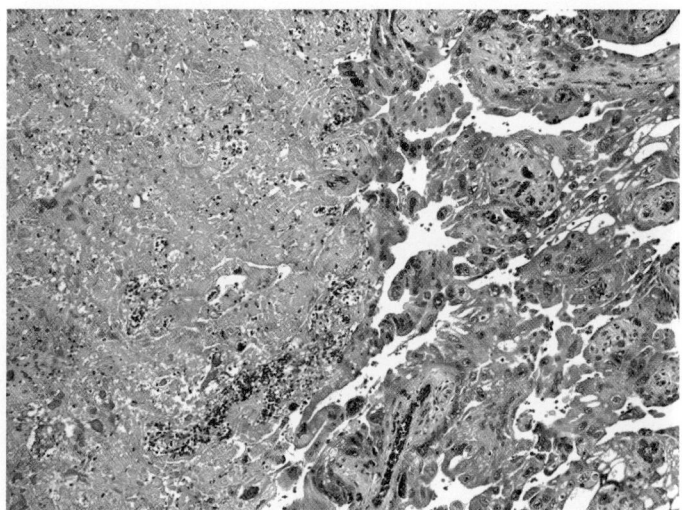

Fig. 32.41 Intraplacental choriocarcinoma (right) associated with infarct (left) in a term pregnancy.

Differential diagnosis

The differential diagnosis of intraplacental chorio-carcinoma includes the following:

1 *Hydatidiform mole.* If extensive villous hydrops or cavitation are found, a biphasic trophoblastic proliferation is likely to represent a hydatidiform mole.

2 *Intraplacental trophoblast proliferation in fibrin.* Extensive perivillous fibrin deposition in a term placenta is often accompanied by a proliferation of mononuclear intermediate trophoblast cells, characterized by eosinophilic cytoplasm, hyperchromatic irregular nuclei and occasional intranuclear cytoplasmic 'inclusions'; rarely, pronounced degrees of degenerative atypia may be seen; despite striking atypia, this phenomenon appears to be degenerative rather than neoplastic.

3 *Trophoblastic hyperplasia accompany in other benign conditions*, including chorangioma (see Ch. 33).

Treatment and follow-up

Choriocarcinoma is managed by chemotherapy with an overall disease-free survival approaching 90% (Table 32.10).

PLACENTAL SITE TROPHOBLASTIC TUMOR

Our understanding of placental site trophoblastic tumor has slowly evolved since its initial description as 'trophoblastic pseudotumor'. Its malignant nature was first reported in 1981 and the tumor was renamed placental site trophoblastic tumor (PSTT).[80]

Risk factors and clinical features

The epidemiology and risk factors of PSTT are not well understood. The disease is seen mostly in reproductive-age women, although cases have been reported in postmenopausal women. The antecedent pregnancy in most cases is a term delivery; however, PSTT may follow SAB, TAB or molar pregnancy. The majority of women present with irregular bleeding months to years following an antecedent pregnancy. Rarely, PSTT presents with nephrotic syndrome; a glomerular lesion has been described and may be secondary to the deposition of immune complexes stimulated by the tumor (PSTT nephrotic syndrome).[81] Classically, CG is only marginally elevated and does not reflect tumor burden. Uterine enlargement may initially suggest pregnancy; however, uterine growth is inappropriate and ultimately work-up for missed abortion leads to diagnosis of PSTT. Ultrasound may disclose an intrauterine mass.

Metastases at presentation were originally believed to occur in 10–15% of patients and recurrences developed in 10%.[80] However, more recent literature suggests that metastases at presentation occur in 30–53% or greater[80,82,83] and recurrences develop in greater than 30% of cases (Table 32.8). The common sites of metastases are the lungs, pelvis and lymph nodes. Less commonly, metastatic sites include the central nervous system, kidney and liver

Gross and histologic features

PSTTs present as discrete masses in the endomyometrium that will produce a sonographic appearance of a complex mass (Fig. 32.42a). The primary tumor is usually confined to the uterus and may be a polypoid mass within the endometrial cavity or an endophytic lesion invading the myometrium. Necrosis is common, but hemorrhage is much less common than in choriocarcinoma (Fig. 32.42b).

Histologically, PSTTs are predominantly composed of intermediate cytotrophoblast cells resembling those arising from the placental implantation site. The pattern of invasion simulates that of physiologic infiltration occurring during normal placentation. The tumor cells are arranged in aggregates of polyhedral, rounded, or occasionally spindle-shaped intermediate trophoblastic cells that dissect between individual and bundles of myometrial fibers. Most of the cells are mononuclear with occasional multinucleated giant cells present. The size and shape of the nuclei vary considerably and nucleoli are prominent (Fig. 32.43a,b). Mitotic count ranges from 1–2 mitotic figures per 10 high-power fields (HPFs) to occasionally 50 mitoses per 10 HPFs.

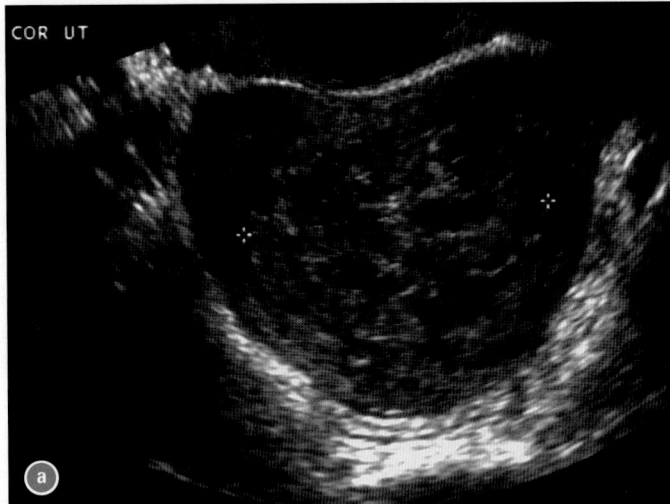

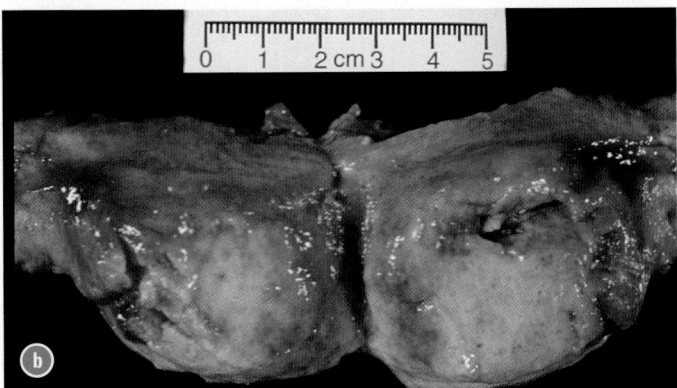

Fig. 32.42 Placental site trophoblastic tumor. (a) Sonographic appearance of PSTT. Coronal image of the uterus demonstrates a complex solid and cystic mass (calipers) in the uterine cavity of a patient who had had a miscarriage several months before. (b) Gross appearance of the tumor discovered in (a), seen here as a discrete non-hemorrhagic mass in the myometrium.

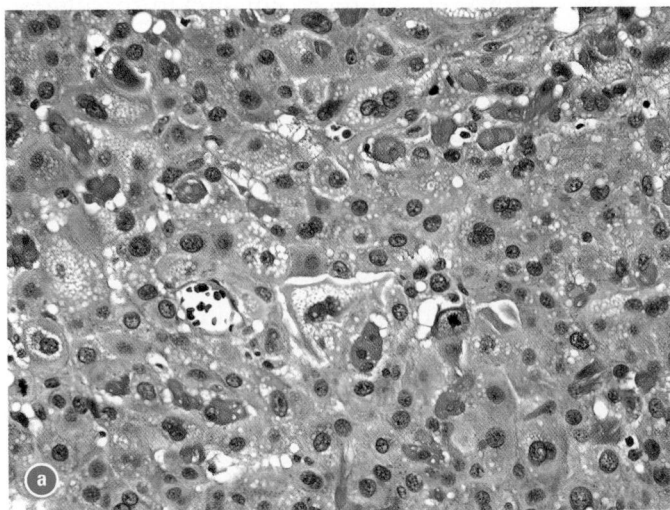

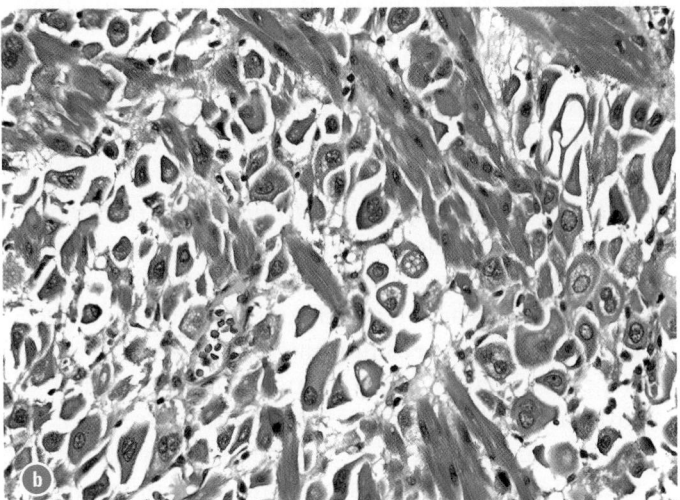

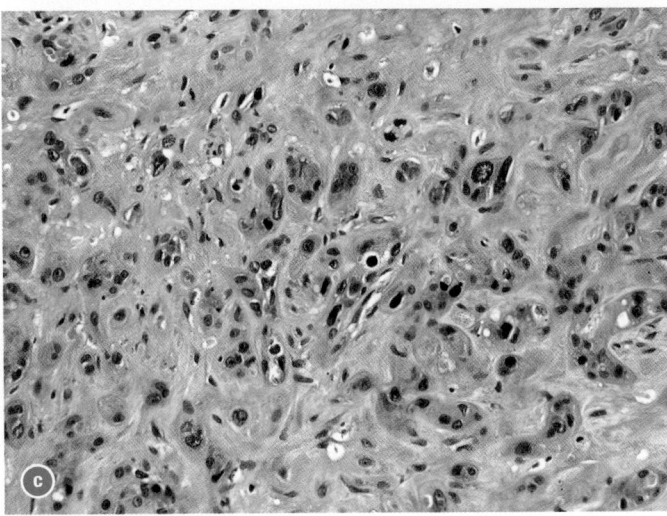

Fig. 32.43 Histologic features of placental site trophoblastic tumor. (a) Sheets of atypical intermediate trophoblast with minimal intervening matrix, (b) Pleomorphic intermediate trophoblastic cells dissecting through muscle fibers. (c) Epithelioid trophoblastic tumor, a subtype of PSTT arising from chorionic type intermediate trophoblast.

Most tumors have less than five mitoses per 10 HPFs. The MIB-1 index of <10% differentiates a benign epithelioid placental site nodule from an ETT (Fig. 32.44).[51] In advanced disease, there can be extensive invasion of blood vessel walls, although the wall integrity itself is maintained. The proportion of syncytiotrophoblastic cells is small; thus, β-hCG production is low and is not a reliable marker for tumor volume.

A subset of PSTTs has been termed epithelioid trophoblastic tumor (ETT). These tumors appear to arise from chorionic-type intermediate trophoblasts, which can be differentiated from implantation site-derived intermediate trophoblasts by their expression of p63 and lack of expression of HPL (Fig. 32.43c). The MIB-1 index of <10% differentiates a benign epithelioid placental site nodule from an ETT (Fig. 32.43c).[51] p63 expression is useful in the distinction of ETTs and PSTTs by profiling trophoblastic subpopulations (Fig. 32.45a–c).[51]

Biomarkers for diagnosis

Immunohistochemistry may be helpful in distinguishing PSTT from benign conditions such as exaggerated placental site and placental site nodule, malignant conditions such as choriocarcinoma and the recently described ETT, as well as other non-trophoblastic tumors such as leiomyosarcoma.[84] In PSTT, cytokeratin and HPL are diffusely present while HCG is only focal. A recent study by Shih et al. utilized immunoperoxi-

dase staining with HPL, Mel-CAM, oncofetal fibronectin, placental alkaline phosphatase, inhibin-alpha and Ki-67 to better characterize the types of intermediate trophoblast (Fig. 32.44a,b).[50]

Antibodies to ΔNp63 (which identify all protein products of p63) reportedly will discriminate between an epithelioid trophoblastic tumor and either choriocarcinoma or conventional PSTT (Fig. 32.45a–c). However, they will not distinguish it from squamous cell carcinoma. This distinction is achieved using antibodies to hLA-G.[50,76]

Molecular studies

There is little information on the cytogenetics of PSTT. Most are diploid.[85] Comparative genomic hybridization profiles of four cases revealed two with a balanced profile, and two with chromosomal gains in the regions of chromosomes 19, 21 and 22.[86] Newlands et al. used polymerase chain reaction allelotyping, which showed that PSTT resulted from biparental pregnancy in four of seven cases and androgenetic monospermic hydatidiform mole in three of seven cases.[87] None of these studies has shown any prognostic value of cytogenetic origin in predicting clinical course or outcome.

Treatment and follow-up

Predicting aggressive tumor behavior at presentation remains problematic but important. Mitotic count has

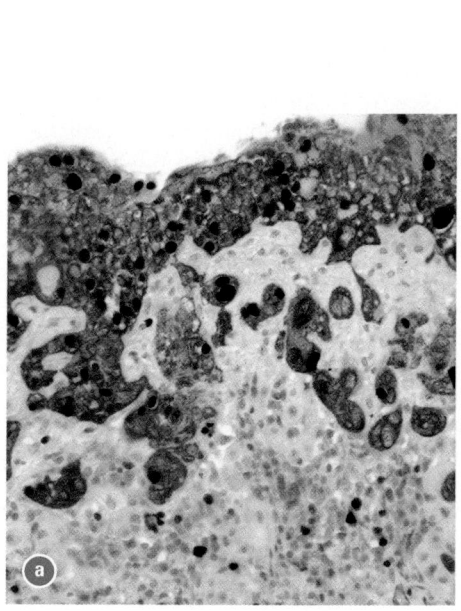

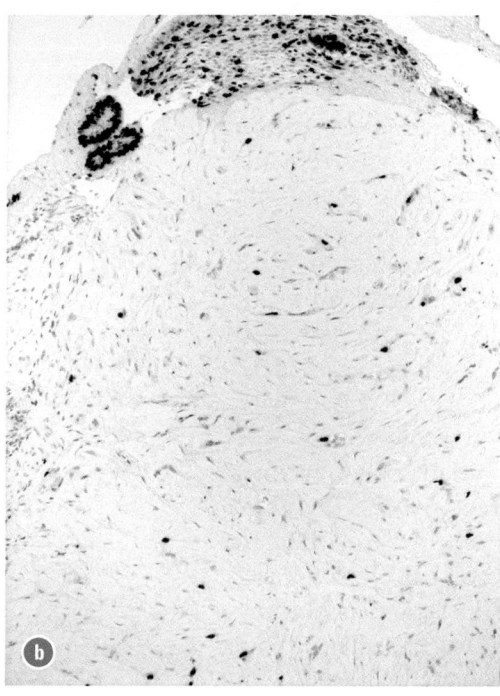

Fig. 32.44 PSTT following combined staining for Ki-67 (nuclear, brown) and Mel-CAM (cytoplasmic, red) (a) which highlights numerous proliferating epithelial (trophoblastic) cells. (b) By comparison, Ki-67 staining of implantation site nodule (bottom) depicts minimal proliferative activity (top – layer of proliferative endometrium).

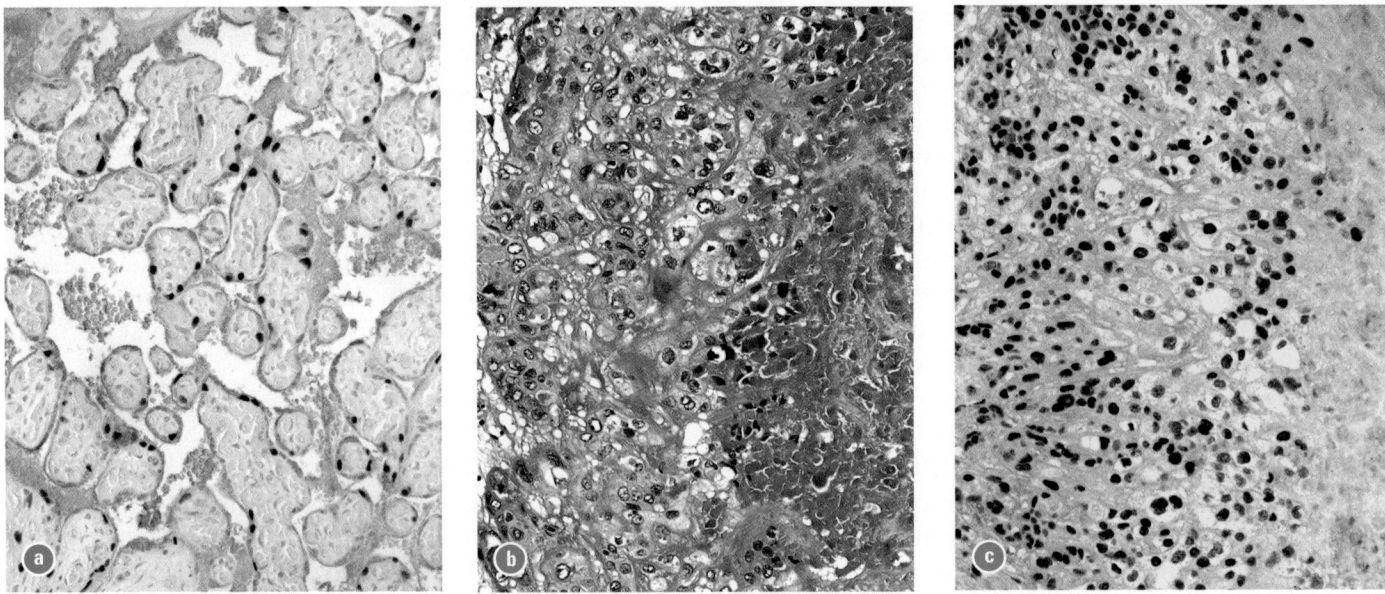

Fig. 32.45 Expression of p63 in trophoblast. (a) Immunostaining for a generic p63 antibody (which detects both TAp63 and ΔNp63) highlights villous cytotrophoblast. (b) Epithelioid trophoblastic tumor (ETT) and (c) following staining for an antibody targeting p63 (Lee and Crum, unpublished data). (Case provided by Dr Yonghee Lee.)

been determined to be a prognostic indicator by several authors. In the most recent study by Feltmate et al. mitotic index >5 mitoses/10 HPFs significantly increased the risk for recurrent disease.[88] Length of time from antecedent pregnancy greater than 2–4 years has also been reported as a negative prognostic indicator. One study reported that when the antecedent pregnancy was less than 2 years all 12 patients with PSTT survived.[89,90] In contrast, when the antecedent pregnancy was greater than 2 years, four of five patients died of their disease. Although there has been a reported case of surgical resection and conservation of the uterus, the mainstay of treatment remains hysterectomy.[90] The most recent data from the Charing Cross Hospital suggests EMA-EP (etoposide, methotrexate and actinomycin D alternating with etoposide and cisplatin) as the preferred adjuvant chemotherapeutic regimen.[91] Three patients with metastatic PSTT, where the interval from the antecedent pregnancy was less than 2 years, were treated with EMA-EP and all achieved complete remission.

In conclusion, PSTT is a rare variant of gestational trophoblastic tumor, and hysterectomy remains the treatment of choice for non-metastatic disease. Adjuvant chemotherapy should be considered in selected cases where poor prognostic indicators exist, including mitotic index >5 mitoses/10 HPFs, time from antecedent pregnancy >2 years and metastases at presentation. EMA-EP is the recommended adjuvant chemotherapy at this time. Serum β-hCG levels should be used in following treatment response and magnetic resonance imaging (MRI) may also be helpful in monitoring disease status. Although radiotherapy has been used with some success in controlling local recurrences, the role of radiation therapy has not been clearly defined.

References

1 Benirschke K, Kaufmann P. Pathology of the human placenta, 4th edn. New York: Springer-Verlag; 2000.

2 Moor KL, Persaud TVN. The developing human: clinically oriented embryology, 5th edn. Philadelphia: WB Saunders; 2004.

3 Winter RM, Knowles SAS, Bieber FR, Baraitser M. The malformed fetus and stillbirth – a diagnostic approach, 1st edn. New York: John Wiley & Sons; 1988.

4 Hataska HH. Recurrent miscarriage: epidemiologic factors, definitions, and incidence. Clin Obstet Gynecol 1994; 37(3):625–634.

5 Miller JF, Williamson E, Glue J, et al. Fetal loss after implantation. A prospective study. Lancet 1980; 2(8194):554–556.

6 Edmonds DK, Lindsay KS, Miller JF, Williamson E, Wood PJ. Early embryonic mortality in women. Fertil Steril 1982; 38(4):447–453.

7 Wilcox AJ, Weinberg CR, Baird DD. Risk factors for early pregnancy loss. Epidemiology 1990; 1(5):382–385.

8 Hassold T, Chen N, Funkhouser J, et al. A cytogenetic study of 1000 spontaneous abortions. Ann Hum Genet 1980; 44(Pt 2):151–178.

9 Kalousek DK. Anatomic and chromosome anomalies in specimens of early spontaneous abortion: seven-year experience. Birth Defects Orig Artic Ser 1987; 23(1):153–168.

10 Kajii T, Ferrier A, Niikawa N, et al. Anatomic and chromosomal anomalies in 639 spontaneous abortuses. Hum Genet 1980; 55(1):87–98.

11 Genest DR. Estimating the time of death in stillborn fetuses: II. Histologic evaluation of the placenta; a study of 71 stillborns. Obstet Gynecol 1992; 80(4):585–592.

12 Redline RW, Hassold T, Zaragoza M. Determinants of villous trophoblastic hyperplasia in spontaneous abortions. Mod Pathol 1998; 11(8):762–768.

13 Kliman HJ, Segel L. The placenta may predict the baby. J Theor Biol 2003; 225(1):143–145.

14 Genest DR, Roberts D, Boyd T, Bieber FR. Fetoplacental histology as a predictor of karyotype: a controlled study of spontaneous first trimester abortions. Hum Pathol 1995; 26(2):201–209.

15 Genest DR, Brodsky G, Lage JA. Localized endometrial proliferations associated with pregnancy: clinical and histopathologic features of 11 cases. Hum Pathol 1995; 26(11):1233–1240.

16 Roberts CP, Murphy AA. Endocrinopathies associated with recurrent pregnancy loss. Semin Reprod Med 2000; 18(4):357–362.

17 Hill JA. Immunological contributions to recurrent pregnancy loss. Baillières Clin Obstet Gynaecol 1992; 6(3):489–505.

18 Plouffe L Jr, White EW, Tho SP, et al. Etiologic factors of recurrent abortion and subsequent reproductive performance of couples: have we made any progress in the past 10 years? Am J Obstet Gynecol 1992; 167(2):313–320; discussion 320-321.

19 Doss BJ, Greene MF, Hill J, et al. Massive chronic intervillositis associated with recurrent abortions. Hum Pathol 1995; 26(11):1245–1251.

20 Jacques SM, Qureshi F. Chronic intervillositis of the placenta. Arch Pathol Lab Med 1993; 117(10):1032–1035.

21 Boyd TK, Redline RW. Chronic histiocytic intervillositis: a placental lesion associated with recurrent reproductive loss. Hum Pathol 2000; 31(11):1389–1396.

22 Moore KL. The developing human. Philadelphia: WB Saunders; 1982.

23 Streeter GL. Weight, sitting height, head size, foot length and menstrual age of the human embryo. Contributions to Embryology. Carnegie Institute of Washington; 1920: XI: Contribution 55.

24 Fylstra DL. Tubal pregnancy: a review of current diagnosis and treatment. Obstet Gynecol Surv 1998; 53(5):320–328.

25 Rajkhowa M, Glass MR, Rutherford AJ, et al. Trends in the incidence of ectopic pregnancy in England and Wales from 1966 to 1996. Br J Obstet Gynaecol 2000; 107(3):369–374.

26 Bouyer J, Coste J, Shojaei T, et al. Risk factors for ectopic pregnancy: a comprehensive analysis based on a large case-control, population-based study in France. Am J Epidemiol 2003; 157(3):185–194.

27 Garrett AM, Vukov LF. Risk factors for ectopic pregnancy in a rural population. Fam Med 1996; 28(2):111–113.

28 Castles A, Adams EK, Melvin CL, Kelsch C, Boulton ML. Effects of smoking during pregnancy. Five meta-analyses. Am J Prev Med 1999; 16(3):208–215.

29 Yang MH, Ng SC, Ratnam SS, et al. Outcome of 143 pregnancies conceived by assisted reproductive techniques. Asia Oceania J Obstet Gynaecol 1992; 18(4):299–307.

30 Lesny P, Killick SR, Robinson J, Maguiness SD. Transcervical embryo transfer as a risk factor for ectopic pregnancy. Fertil Steril 1999; 72(2):305–309.

31 Fernandez H, Gervaise A. Ectopic pregnancies after infertility treatment: modern diagnosis and therapeutic strategy. Hum Reprod Update 2004; 10(6):503–513.

32 Xiong X, Buekens P, Wollast E. IUD use and the risk of ectopic pregnancy: a meta-analysis of case-control studies. Contraception 1995; 52(1):23–34.

33 Ganacharya S, Bhattoa HP, Batar I. Ectopic pregnancy among non-medicated and copper-containing intrauterine device users: a 10-year follow-up. Eur J Obstet Gynecol Reprod Biol 2003; 111(1):78–82.

34 Randall S, Buckley CH, Fox H. Placentation in the fallopian tube. Int J Gynecol Pathol 1987; 6(2):132–139.

35 Bouyer J, Coste J, Fernandez H, Pouly JL, Job-Spira N. Sites of ectopic pregnancy: a 10 year population-based study of 1800 cases. Hum Reprod 2002; 17(12):3224–3230.

36 World Health Organization. WHO Task Force on Intrauterine Devices for Fertility Regulation: a multinational case control study of ectopic pregnancy. Clin Reprod Fertil 1985; 3:131–143.

37 Gun M, Mavrogiorgis M. Cervical ectopic pregnancy: a case report and literature review. Ultrasound Obstet Gynecol 2002; 19(3):297–301.

38 Atrash HK, Friede A, Hogue CJ. Abdominal pregnancy in the United States: frequency and maternal mortality. Obstet Gynecol 1987; 69(3 Pt 1):333–337.

39 Stubblefield PG, Grimes DA. Septic abortion. N Engl J Med 1994; 331(5):310–314.

40 Cates W Jr, Grimes DA, Ory HW, Tyler CW Jr. Publicity and the public health: the elimination of IUD-related abortion deaths. Fam Plann Perspect 1977; 9(3):138–140.

41 Mahler H. On safe motherhood. Nurs J India 1988; 79(5):119–120, 128.

42 Stephenson P, Wagner M, Badea M, Serbanescu F. Commentary: the public health consequences of restricted induced abortion – lessons from Romania. Am J Public Health 1992; 82(10):1328–1331.

43 Gall SA. Infections in the female genital tract. Compr Ther 1983; 9(8):34–47.

44 Genest DR, Berkowitz RS, Fisher RA, Newlands ES, Fehr M. Gestational trophoblastic disease. In: Tavassoli F, Devilee P, eds. Pathology and genetics of tumours of the breast and female genital organs. World Health Organization Classification of Tumours Series. Cambridge, UK: International Agency for Research on Cancer (IARC); 2003:250–254.

45 Goldstein DP, Berkowitz RS. Gestational trophoblastic disease. In: Abeloff MD et al., eds. Clinical oncology. London: Elsevier; 2004.

46 Wang J, Berek JS. Epidemiology and pathology of gestational trophoblastic disease. 2005. Available from Up To Date http://www.utdol.com/application/topic.asp?file=gyne_onc/7618&type=A&selectedTitle=1~15 (Accessed 29 March 2005).

47 Berkowitz RS, Goldstein DP. Gestational trophoblastic disease. In: Hoskins WJ et al., eds. Principles and practice of gynecologic oncology, 4th edn. Philadelphia: Lippincott, Williams & Wilkins; 2005:1055–1076.

48 Buckley JD. The epidemiology of molar pregnancy and choriocarcinoma. Clin Obstet Gynecol 1984; 27(1):153–159.

49 Hemming JD, Quirke P, Womack C, et al. Diagnosis of molar pregnancy and persistent trophoblastic disease by flow cytometry. J Clin Pathol 1987; 40(6):615–620.

50 Shih I-M, Kurman RJ. P63 is useful in the distinction of epithelioid trophoblastic and placental site trophoblastic tumors by profiling trophoblastic subpopulations. Am J Surg Pathol 2004; 28:1177–1183.

51. Yang A, Schweitzer R, Sun D, et al. p63 is essential for regenerative proliferation in limb, craniofacial and epithelial development. Nature 1999; 398:714–718.

52 Mosher R, Goldstein DP, Berkowitz R, Bernstein M, Genest DR. Complete hydatidiform mole. Comparison of clinicopathologic features, current and past. J Reprod Med 1998; 43(1):21–27.

53 Keep D, Zaragoza MV, Hassold T, Redline RW. Very early complete hydatidiform mole. Hum Pathol 1996; 27(7):708–713.

54 Montes M, Roberts D, Berkowitz RS, Genest DR. Prevalence and significance of implantation site trophoblastic atypia in hydatidiform moles and spontaneous abortions. Am J Clin Pathol 1996; 105(4):411–416.

55 Thaker HM, Berlin A, Tycko B, et al. Immunohistochemistry for the imprinted gene product IPL/PHLDA2 for facilitating the differential diagnosis of complete hydatidiform mole. J Reprod Med 2004; 49(8):630–636.

56 Castrillon DH, Sun D, Weremowicz S, et al. Discrimination of complete hydatidiform mole from its mimics by immunohistochemistry of the paternally imprinted gene product p57^{KIP2}. Am J Surg Pathol 2001; 25(10):1225–1230.

57 Fisher RA, Nucci MR, Thaker HM, et al. Complete hydatidiform mole retaining a chromosome 11 of maternal origin: molecular genetic analysis of a case. Mod Pathol 2004; 17(9):1155–1160.

58 Hertig AT, Mansell H. Tumors of the female sex organs part 1: hydatidiform mole and choriocarcinoma. Washington, DC: Armed Forces Institute of Pathology; 1956:13, 18.

59 Schorge JO, Goldstein DP, Bernstein MR, Berkowitz RS. Gestational trophoblastic disease. Curr Treat Options Oncol 2000; 1(2):169–175.

60 Genest DR, Laborde O, Berkowitz RS, et al. A clinicopathologic study of 153 cases of complete hydatidiform mole (1980–1990): histologic grade lacks prognostic significance. Obstet Gynecol 1991; 78(3 Pt 1):402–409.

61 Sebire NJ, Makrydimas G, Agnantis NJ, et al. Updated diagnostic criteria for partial and complete hydatidiform moles in early pregnancy. Anticancer Res 2003; 23:1723–1728.

62 Lage JM, Sheikh SS. Genetic aspects of gestational trophoblastic diseases: a general overview with emphasis on new approaches in determining genetic composition. Gen Diagn Pathol 1997; 143:109–115.

63 Redline RW, Hassold T, Zaragoza MV. Prevalence of the partial molar phenotype in triploidy of maternal and paternal origin. Hum Pathol 1998; 29:505–511.

64 Choi-Hong SR, Genest DR, Crum CP, et al. Twin pregnancies with complete hydatidiform mole and coexisting fetus: use of fluorescent in situ hybridization to evaluate placental X- and Y-chromosomal content. Hum Pathol 1995; 26(11):1175–1180.

65 Berkowitz RS, Goldstein DP. Pathogenesis of gestational trophoblastic neoplasms. Pathobiol Annu 1981; 11:391–411.

66 Brewer JI, Mazur MT. Gestational choriocarcinoma. Its origin in the placenta during seemingly normal pregnancy. Am J Surg Pathol 1981; 5(3):267–277.

67 Driscoll SG. Gestational trophoblastic neoplasms: morphologic considerations. Hum Pathol 1977; 8(5):529–539.

68 Aozasa K, Ito H, Kohro T, et al. Choriocarcinoma in infant and mother. Acta Pathol Jpn 1981; 31(2):317–322.

69 Daamen CB, Bloem GW, Westerbeek AJ. Chorionepithelioma in mother and child. J Obstet Gynaecol Br Emp 1961; 68:144–149.

70 Lathrop JC, Wachtel TJ, Meissner GF. Uterine choriocarcinoma fourteen years following bilateral tubal ligation. Obstet Gynecol 1978; 51(4):477–488.

71 Goldstein DP. Gestational trophoblastic neoplasia in the 1990s. Yale J Biol Med 1991; 64(6):639–651.

72 Soper JT. Gestational trophoblastic neoplasia. Curr Opin Obstet Gynecol 1990; 2(1):92–97.

73 Deligdisch L, Driscoll SG, Goldstein DP. Gestational trophoblastic neoplasms: morphologic correlates of therapeutic response. Am J Obstet Gynecol 1978; 130(7):801–806.

74 Fukunaga M, Ushigome S. Malignant trophoblastic tumors: immunohistochemical and flow cytometric comparison of choriocarcinoma and placental site trophoblastic tumors. Hum Pathol 1993; 24(10):1098–1106.

75 Elston CW, Bagshawe KD. The diagnosis of trophoblastic tumours from uterine curettings. J Clin Pathol 1972; 25(2):111–118.

76 Singer G, Kurman RJ, McMaster MT, Shih IeM. HLA-G immunoreactivity is specific for intermediate trophoblast in gestational trophoblastic disease and can serve as a useful marker in differential diagnosis. Am J Surg Pathol 2002; 26:914–920.

77 Lage JM, Roberts DJ. Choriocarcinoma in a term placenta: pathologic diagnosis of tumor in an asymptomatic patient with metastatic disease. Int J Gynecol Pathol 1993; 12:80–85.

78 Fox H, Laurini RN. Intraplacental choriocarcinoma: a report of two cases. J Clin Pathol 1988; 41:1085–1088.

79 Hustin J, Jauniaux E. Markedly elevated maternal serum alpha-fetoprotein associated with a normal fetus and choriocarcinoma of the placenta. Obstet Gynecol 1991; 77:329–330.

80 Young RH, Scully RE. Placental-site trophoblastic tumor: current status. Clin Obstet Gynecol 1984; 27:248–258.

81 Young RH, Scully RE, McCluskey RT. A distinctive glomerular lesion complicating placental site trophoblastic tumor: report of two cases. Hum Pathol 1985; 16:35–42.

82 Feltmate CM, Genest DR, Wise L, et al. Placental site trophoblastic tumor: a 17-year experience at the New England Trophoblastic Disease Center. Gynecol Oncol 2001; 82(3):415–419.

83 Newlands ES, Bower M, Fisher RA, Paradinas FJ. Management of placental site trophoblastic tumors. J Reprod Med 1998; 43:53–59.

84 Chang YL, Chang TC, Hsueh S, et al. Prognostic factors and treatment for placental site trophoblastic tumor – report of 3 cases and analysis of 88 cases. Gynecol Oncol 1999; 73(2):216–222.

85 Fukunaga M, Ushigome S. Malignant trophoblastic tumors: immunohistochemical and flow cytometric comparison of choriocarcinoma and placental site trophoblastic tumors. Hum Patho 1993; 24:1098–1106.

86 Hui P, Riba A, Pejovic T, et al. Comparative genomic hybridization study of placental site trophoblastic tumour: a report of four cases. Mod Pathol 2004; 17(2):248–251.

87 Newlands ES, Bower M, Fisher RA, Paradinas FJ. Management of placental site trophoblastic tumors. J Reprod Med 1998; 43(1):53–59.

88 Feltmate CM, Genest DR, Goldstein DP, Berkowitz RS. Advances in the understanding of placental site trophoblastic tumor. J Reprod Med 2002; 47:337–341.

89 Bower M, Paradinas FJ, Fisher RA, et al. Placental site trophoblastic tumor: molecular analysis and clinical experience. Clin Cancer Res 1996; 2(5):897–902.

90 Papadopoulos AJ, Foskett M, Seckl MJ, et al. Twenty-five years' clinical experience with placental site trophoblastic tumors. J Reprod Med 2002; 47(6):460–464.

91 Khoo SK. Clinical aspects of gestational trophoblastic disease: a review based partly on 25-year experience of a statewide registry. Aust N Z J Obstet Gynaecol 2003; 43:280–289.

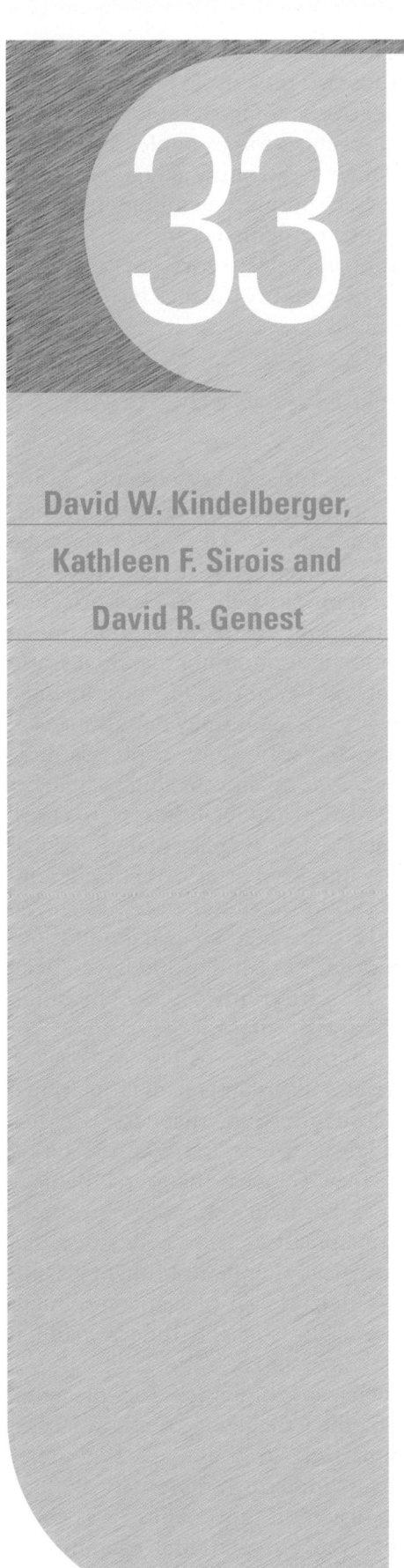

33

Evaluation of the placenta

David W. Kindelberger,

Kathleen F. Sirois and

David R. Genest

General principles

Rationale for placental
   examination
Selection of placentas for tissue
   examination
Fixation and sampling
Special procedures (cultures,
   karyotype, photography)

**Gross examination of the
placenta**

General appearance
Umbilical cord and membranes

Fetal surface
Maternal surface
Sectioned surfaces of the placenta
The placenta from multiple
   gestations

**Microscopic examination
of the placenta**

Umbilical cord and membranes
Chorionic plate
Stem villi
Terminal villi
Intervillous space
Basal plate (maternal surface)

General principles

RATIONALE FOR PLACENTAL EXAMINATION

Gross placental examination is important, (a) as a means of documenting structural abnormalities of the placenta and (b) as a guide for tissue selection for histology. Regarding the former, many structural abnormalities were classified as significant placental disorders by the 1959–1966 Collaborative Perinatal Study, a large prospective study which evaluated relationships between placental pathology and mental, neurologic, or psychological disturbances in childhood (Table 33.1).[1]

Regarding these findings, plausible pathogenetic mechanisms may be proposed for some placental structural abnormalities and their related outcomes. For example, prolonged fetal inactivity (predictive of subsequent neurologic disease or mental retardation) may be associated with a short umbilical cord and absent subchorionic fibrin;[2,3] conversely, excessive fetal movement (predictive of subsequent childhood hyperactivity) may be associated with an abnormally long umbilical cord and increased subchorionic fibrin. For many gross placental lesions listed in Table 33.1, however, the relationship between a placental structural abnormality and an adverse outcome is obscure; for example, why should a bipartite placenta be associated with a subsequent psychological disturbance (more specifically 'fearful', 'apprehensive', 'inflexible' or 'hostile' behavior).[1]

From a practical viewpoint, gross placental examination is important for two reasons: (1) placental gross abnormalities may provide clinicopathologic correlations with obstetric events (for example, very small placental size and infarcts strongly suggest chronic placental ischemia, while ruptured membranous vessels may explain fetal death or neonatal anemia) and (2) gross placental abnormalities represent placental regions which should be studied further histologically (i.e. infarcts, depressions).

SELECTION OF PLACENTAS FOR TISSUE EXAMINATION

Some authors have stated that every placenta should be pathologically examined, at least grossly;[4,5] others have written that a minimum of 10–15% of placentas should be examined.[6] Currently, at the Brigham and Women's Hospital, approximately 20% of placentas are selected by obstetricians for pathologic examination. The most common indications for placental examination at the Brigham and Women's Hospital include: (1) premature delivery, (2) multiple gestations, (3) fetal death, (4) maternal diseases such as preeclampsia and diabetes, (5) fetal abnormalities including malformations, growth retardation and fetal distress, (6) third trimester bleeding and (7) gross placental abnormalities, including single umbilical artery, abnormal cord insertion, cord knots and placental masses.

Over the past 10–15 years, medicolegal implications of placental pathologic examination have been emphasized.[7–11] In obstetrical malpractice litigation involving perinatal death, neurologic damage or mental impairment, the presence of chronic placental abnormalities (such as infarcts, small placental size, membranous cord insertion, maternal decidual vasculopathy, chorangiosis, nucleated fetal red blood cells (RBCs), etc.) may suggest that fetal damage occurred antenatally rather than perinatally.[12] A recent analysis of obstetric malpractice claims concluded that 'many more neurologically impaired infant claims could be successfully defended if placenta specimens were available for evaluation at the time a claim is made'.[13]

Recent comprehensive guidelines for placental selection published by the College of American Pathologists are as summarized in Table 33.2.[4,14] They include circumstances indicting maternal or fetal pathology, visible placental anomalies, or other historical events that warrant placental examination (Table 33.1).

Table 33.1 Gross placental abnormalities associated with abnormal childhood mental, neurologic or psychological outcome

Placental abnormality	Abnormal outcome
Short umbilical cord	MR, neuro, CP
Single umbilical artery	MR, neuro
Velamentous cord insertion	Psych
Green-colored umbilical cord (sugg. of meconium)	Psych
Long umbilical cord	Psych
Opaque fetal surface (sugg. of chorioamnionitis)	MR, neuro, Sz
Circumvallate membrane insertion	Neuro
Meconium-stained amniotic fluid	CP, MR, Sz
Absent subchorionic fibrin	MR, neuro, CP
Succenturiate lobe	MR, Sz
Maternal floor infarct	MR, neuro
Bipartite/tripartite shape	MR, neuro, psych
Diffuse chorionic fibrin	Psych, neuro

MR, mental retardation; neuro, various neurologic disorders – abnormal speech, poor motor coordination; CP, quadriplegic, hemiplegic or paraplegic cerebral palsy; Sz, seizures; Psych, behavior disturbances, attention deficit disorders. Adapted from Naeye.[1]

FIXATION AND SAMPLING

The placenta is optimally examined in the fresh state (with prompt refrigeration, for up to 1 week or more); however, some institutions use formalin fixation before pathologic examination. Figure 33.1 summarizes the steps in a routine singleton placental examination. After gross inspection, a short segment of umbilical cord (including any abnormal regions) and a 'jelly roll' of the membranes (wrapped around a portion of the marginal placenta) are fixed in 10% formalin; in cases of suspected maternal vascular disease (i.e. hypertension, diabetes, systemic lupus, fetal growth retardation, etc.), two membrane rolls are prepared. The remaining membranes and cord are then trimmed from the placental disc and the disc is weighed. Next, with the maternal surface of the placenta facing up, the parenchyma is 'bread-loafed' at 1 cm intervals; two full-thickness cubes of normal parenchyma (2–3 cm²) and representative blocks of lesions (infarcts, intervillous thrombi, chorangiomas, etc.) are fixed in

formalin overnight, before processing and H&E staining. One or two slides of normal parenchyma and of the adnexa (two cord sections and one or two membrane rolls) and additional samples of grossly abnormal areas are assessed histologically (Fig. 33.2). Separated twin placentas are handled exactly like singleton placentas. Additional details concerning fused twin placentas are discussed below.

SPECIAL PROCEDURES (CULTURES, KARYOTYPE, PHOTOGRAPHY)

Bacteriologic cultures need not be performed routinely, even when chorioamnionitis is suspected. However, if a particular pathogen (such as group B streptococcus or *Listeria*) is of special clinical interest, a culture may be taken from the (sterile) chorionic surface, after carefully peeling away the (contaminated) amnion. Viral cultures from sterile villous tissue occasionally yield important information when fetal viral infection is strongly suspected from the history or neonatal exam-

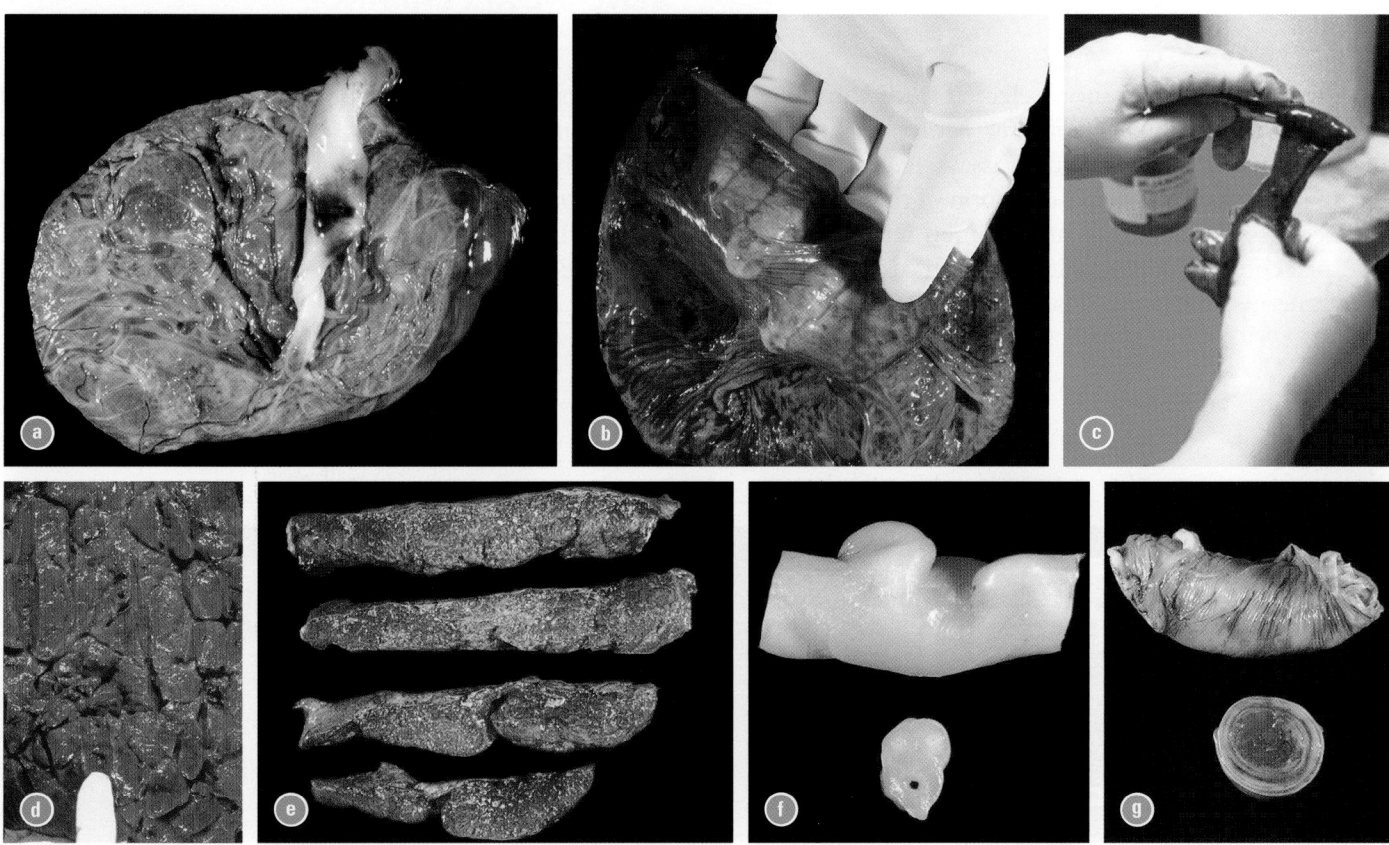

Fig. 33.1 Illustrated outline of placental gross examination (composite), including (a) examination of the surface, (b) membranes, (c) membrane roll, (d) ventral surface, (e) cross-sections, (f) cord and (g) membrane roll.

Table 33.2 Conditions warranting placental examination

Maternal conditions
  Diabetes
  Hypertension

Prior reproductive failure (one or more spontaneous abortions, stillbirths, neonatal deaths, premature births)
  Maternal substance abuse

Prematurity or postmaturity

Peripartum conditions
  Fever
  Suspected or proven infection
  Bleeding
  Suspected abruptio placentae

Fetal/neonatal conditions
  Stillbirth or perinatal death
  Multiple births
  Congenital anomalies
  Fetal growth retardation
  Hydrops
  Meconium
  Neonatal ICU admission
  Apgar scores of <3 at 5 min
  Neurologic problems including seizures
  Suspected infection
  Oligohydramnios

Gross placental anomalies

Other (abnormal delivery, infant, medicolegal concerns)

ination. However, if not selected judiciously, viral cultures will usually be unfruitful. Moreover, immuno-histochemistry and molecular assays have been sufficiently developed to permit detection of these pathogens in fixed tissues including unexplained fetal death.[15]

A placental karyotype is indicated in cases of habitual spontaneous abortion. Placental karyotypes are also useful when chromosomal abnormalities are suspected in macerated stillborn fetuses – in these circumstances, although autolyzed fetal tissues will not grow in tissue culture, villous tissues can often be readily cultured and karyotyped because the placental villi are nourished by maternal blood after fetal death. Karyotypes are performed on sterile dissected villous tissue (disposable suture removal sets work well), placed into Hanks' balanced salt solution (which can be refrigerated for storage, but never should be frozen). Two caveats regarding placental karyotypes should be noted: (1) a karyotype revealing a 46,XX genotype may reflect contamination by maternal tissues; and (2) rarely, the placental karyotype may differ from that of the fetus (confined placental mosaicism).

Photography of any gross placental abnormality is always recommended for both documentation and correlation with the histopathology.

Gross examination of the placenta

GENERAL APPEARANCE

Shape

Variations in placental shape can occur, possibly related to an unusual uterine shape or to incomplete regression of membranous villi. These shape variations include: bilobation (two roughly equal placental masses; Fig. 33.3, either marginally fused or entirely separated, but connected by membranous fetal vessels; trilobation;

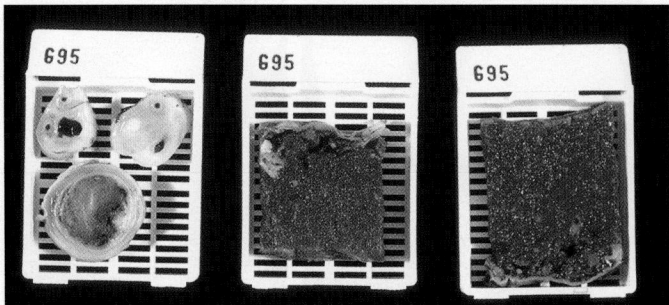

Fig. 33.2 Membrane roll, cord and two full-thickness placenta sections are sent for processing.

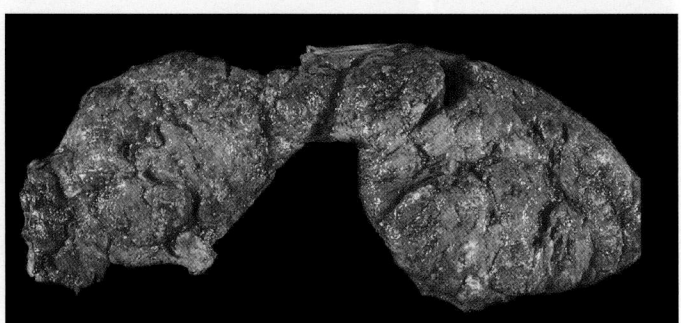

Fig. 33.3 Cross-section of a bilobed placenta.

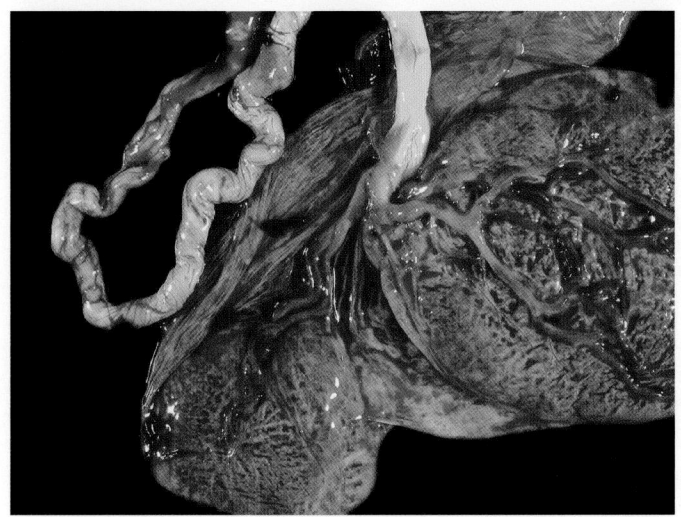

Fig. 33.4 Succenturiate lobe (lower left).

Table 33.3 *Significance of placental weight*

Conditions associated with small placentas (<10th percentile)	Conditions associated with large placentas (>90th percentile)
Chronic placental underperfusion (preeclampsia, etc.)	Maternal diabetes
Fetal growth retardation	Fetal hydrops
Chromosomal disorders (particularly trisomy 18)	Congenital syphilis
Congenital malformations	Villous edema
Poss. abnormal neurologic outcome such as cerebral palsy[56]	Chorangiosis Beckwith–Wiedemann syndrome

accessory or succenturiate lobation (smaller 'islands' of placental tissue connected by membranous vessels; Fig. 33.4) and, very rarely, placenta membranacea (a spherical placenta, due to near total persistence of membranous villi). Although the Collaborative Perinatal Study suggested that some of these abnormal placental shapes may be associated with adverse outcomes (Table 33.1), little literature exists in this area and most general placental texts have minimized the significance of these aberrant placental shapes.[1] Of note however, oddly shaped placentas are often associated with unprotected membranous fetal vessels and these vessels should be carefully examined for thromboses or evidence of rupture. When membranous vessels are identified adjacent to the site of membrane rupture in a placental specimen, this finding suggests vasa praevia (defined as membranous fetal vessels traversing the internal cervical os).

Weight

Placentas should be weighed after removal of the cord, membranes and any attached maternal blood clots. Abnormally small placentas are most commonly associated with chronic uteroplacental hypoperfusion (preeclampsia, etc.) and fetal growth retardation. Other conditions that may be associated with small-for-gestational-age placentas are listed in Table 33.3.[16] Excessively heavy placentas may signify maternal diabetes, severe villous edema, fetal hydrops, or congenital syphilis, among other conditions. Placental weights above the 90th or below the 10th percentile for gestational age should be noted in the pathology report.[17,18]

Color

The membranes and the fetal surface of the placenta are normally clean, shiny and transparent; in a normal placenta, fine ramifications of chorionic plate vessels can be readily visualized through these transparent superficial tissues (Fig. 33.5). A dull, white, opaque appearance develops with acute chorioamnionitis, due to tissue infiltration by acute inflammatory cells; the underlying chorionic vasculature is obscured by the opacity (Fig. 33.6). This appearance is most common in premature placentas, particularly with prolonged rupture of the membranes. In addition to the dull/opaque appearance, the placenta in chorioamnionitis often has a foul odor. Benirschke and Kaufmann describe a characteristic 'fetid' smell with *E. coli* infections and a 'sweet' smell with listerial infections.[18] Brown discoloration of the membranes and chorionic plate suggests hemosiderin deposition, which may be secondary to chronic abruptio placentae. This brown discoloration develops because retroplacental or retromembranous blood seeps through the membranes, discolors the amniotic fluid ('port wine amniotic fluid') and is picked up by chorionic macrophages (see below). A slimy, green appearance suggests meconium staining, a finding most common in term or post-term placentas; gross meconium staining begins at 1–2 hours and is maximal by 3–6 hours after meconium exposure (Fig. 33.7).[19] Prolonged meconium exposure of many hours duration can cause tissue necrosis, with linear fissures and ulcerations of the umbilical cord and microscopic myonecrosis of large fetal vessels of the cord and chorionic plate; it has been estimated to take a minimum of 16 hours for such necrosis to develop.[20] When very prolonged/severe meconium exposure is suspected, extra sampling of the umbilical cord and the chorionic plate is indicated to look for such meconium-induced fetal vascular necrosis (see below).

Fig. 33.5 Outline for inspecting the placental surface.

Cord — Twist / Vessels / Knots / Thrombi

Disc — Weight / Integrity / Lobes

Insertion — Location (Marginal or membranous) / Velamentous

Membranes — Distribution / Opacity / Color / Hemorrhage

UMBILICAL CORD AND MEMBRANES (Fig. 33.5)

Umbilical cord

Cord

The cord should be severed at the insertion to the placental disc and the following should be recorded:

1 *Insertion*: marginal (Fig. 33.8a), in which the cord is inserted at the edge of the placental disc and is seen in approximately 5% of placentas, *vs* central.

2 *Distribution of vessels*: membranous (or velamentous) (Fig. 33.8b), which are encountered in 1% of placentas. Rarely, these vessels rupture causing fetal exsanguinations, especially when located within the membranes near the birth canal ('vasa praevia'). All membranous vessels should be described as 'intact' or 'disrupted'.

3 *Twist* (Fig. 33.9): non-coiled cord (untwisted vessels) *vs* normally coiled (right or left twisted cord); non-coiled suggests prolonged fetal inactivity (muscular disorder, fetal entrapment, etc).

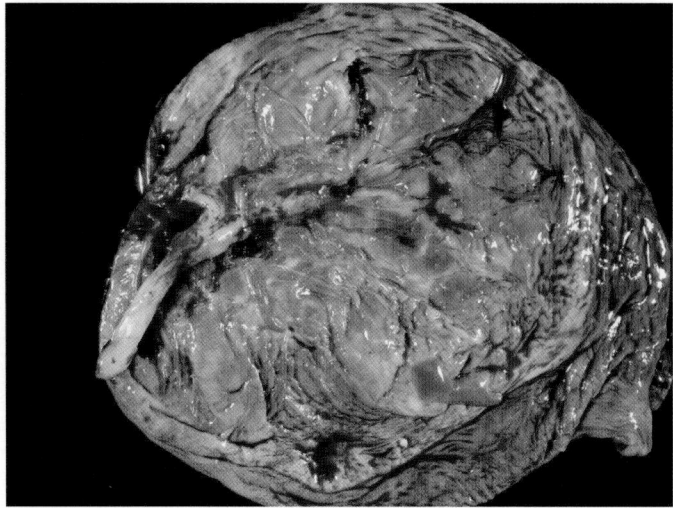

Fig. 33.6 White, semi-opaque membranes in acute chorioamnionitis.

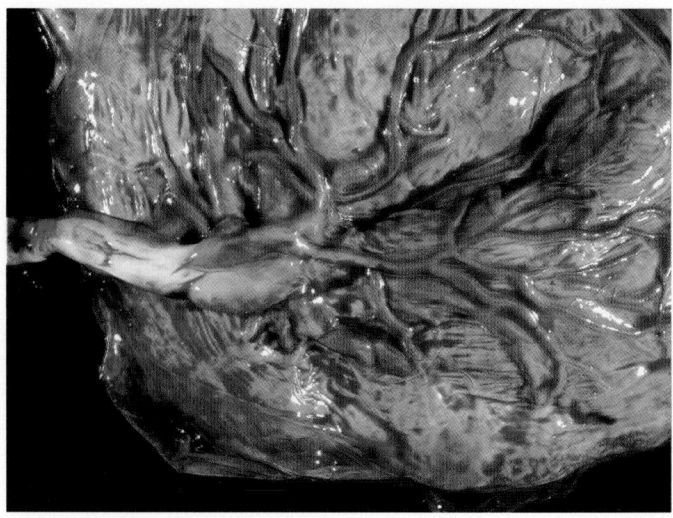

Fig. 33.7 Meconium-stained membranes.

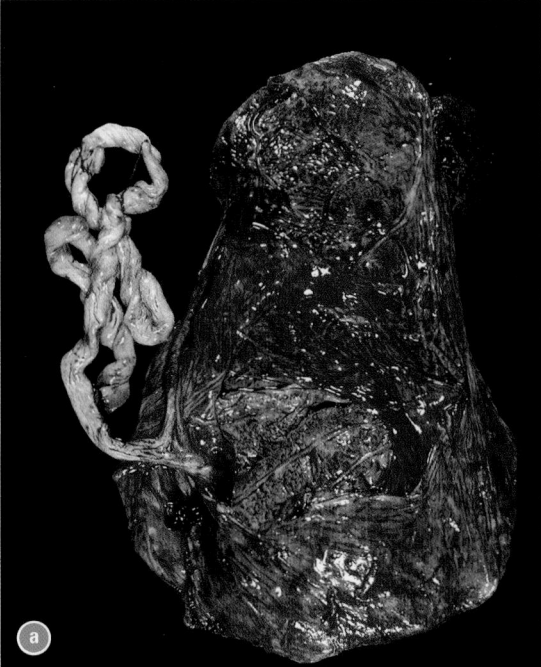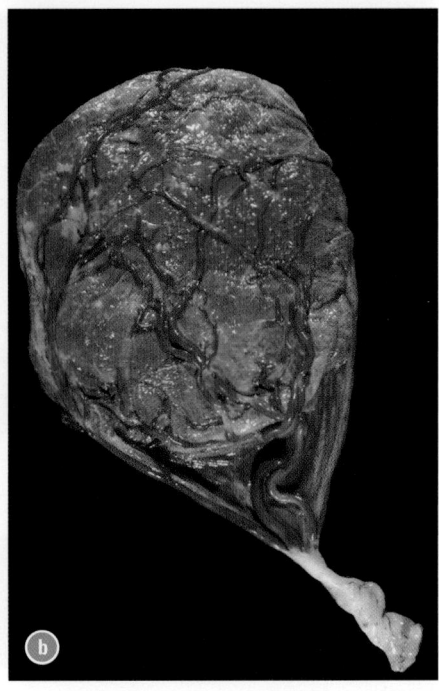

Fig. 33.8 (a) Marginal cord insertion. (b) Membranous cord insertion.

4 *Length*: it is important to remember that the pathologist's measurement is incomplete unless the portion of the cord attached to the fetus is also measured (as at autopsy). If the entire length is assessed and correlated with gestational age, a short cord (<40 cm at term) is associated with prolonged fetal inactivity and an excessively long cord (>90 cm at term) may be a risk factor for fetal death.

5 *Color*: shiny white or tan-white is normal; numerous, tiny white spots (less than 1 mm diameter) suggest fungal (candidal) amniotic fluid infection; yellow-green color suggests meconium exposure (for hours or more before birth); diffuse brown-red discoloration (Fig. 33.10a) suggests fetal retention after death (hemolysis), at least several hours after fetal death (this red-brown discoloration is may incorrectly be designated 'thrombosed' by obstetricians who deliver stillborn fetuses; however, this finding is likely secondary to fetal death, not the cause of fetal death).

6 *Knots*: so-called 'false knots' (Fig. 33.10a) are commonly seen and reflect vascular ectasia within the cord, probably of no clinical significance. True knots (Fig. 33.10b) are much less common and may be incidental, insignificant findings ('loose knot'), or may be significant as a cause of fetal death if they are tight and appear constrictive. Even when tight and lethal, they usually do not demonstrate confirmatory histologic findings (i.e. thrombosis, interstitial hemorrhage and inflammation are not usually demonstrated).

7 *Vessel number* (Fig. 33.10c): single umbilical artery is present in about 1% of placentas and is associated with slightly increased risk of numerous adverse sequelae, including fetal malformations,

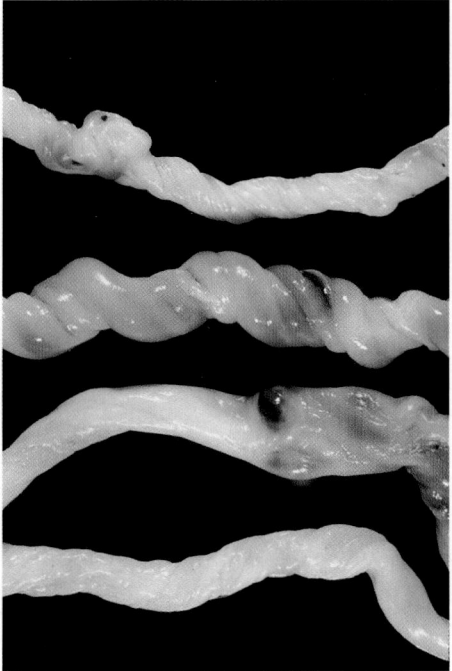

Fig. 33.9 Examples of cord twist.

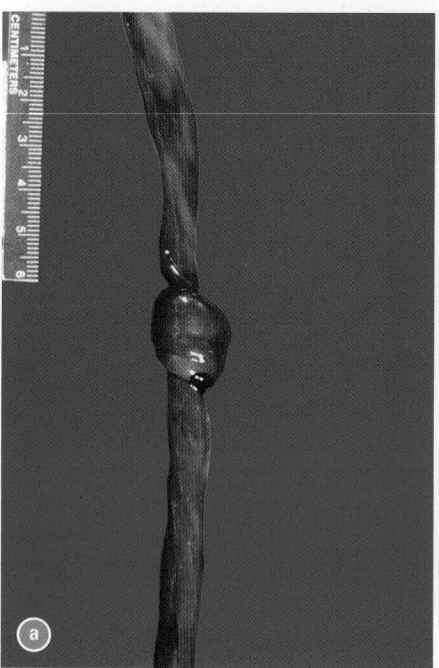
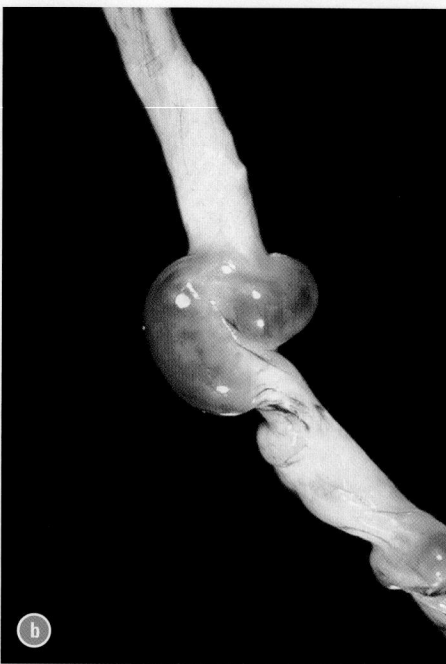
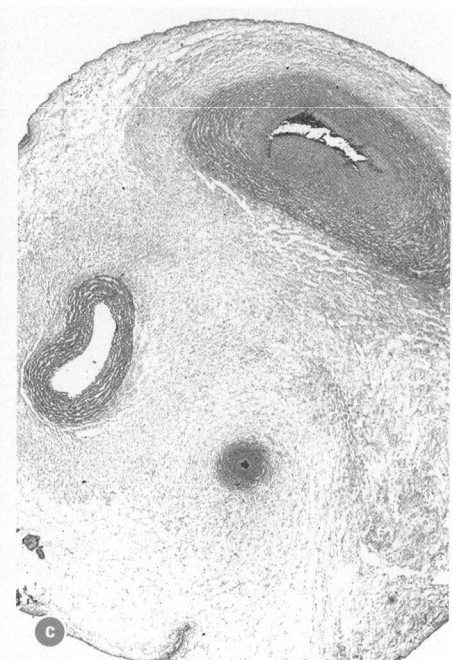

Fig. 33.10 (a) True knot, (b) false knot, (c) single umbilical artery.

fetal aneuploidy and fetal or neonatal death; however, very commonly, there is a healthy outcome.

8 *Vessel patency*: including the exclusion of thrombi (Fig. 33.11a).[18]

9 *Vessel trauma with vessel rupture*: cord trauma is common during delivery and removal of the placenta, often with blood concentrically arranged around the cord vessels in the perivascular space. In live-born infants such changes should be viewed as an incidental finding unless there is a clear history of a cord lesion prior to manipulation. In stillbirths or in circumstances in which *in utero* cord compression or trauma is considered, a diagnosis of prior vascular rupture is supported by evidence of dissecting hemorrhage with collapse of the vein and splitting of the venous wall (Figs 33.11b–d). This may or may not be the cause of death, but may indicate that the cord was compressed *in utero*.

Placental membranes

The membranes should be examined with the following in mind:

1 *Distribution*: including circummarginate (Fig. 33.12a) and circumvallate.

2 *Integrity*: if the amnion is absent, tethered around the cord or present as conspicuous webs (Fig. 33.12b), this may reflect early amnion rupture (amniotic band syndrome), often with destructive, asymmetric fetal abnormalities (extremity and other deformations, Fig. 33.12c); the chorionic surface should be sampled to look for amniotic absence, vernix granulomas and a reactive, chorionic surface. The presence of webs should be excluded.

3 *Opacity and color*: usually parallel that seen on the surface of the disc. Opacity, indicated by inability to delineate fetal vessel branching, is suggestive of acute chorioamnionitis. A greenish color is suggestive of meconium staining and a red-brown color may indicate the presence of hemosiderin, but may also be seen in some cases of acute chorioamnionitis.

4 *Odor*: a foul odor may reflect infection.[18]

FETAL SURFACE

General

The shiny, transparent amnion is normally loosely adherent to the chorion of the placental disc. Branching out from the umbilical cord insertion site, the fetal surface chorionic vessels are arranged such that arteries are the most superficial vessels (i.e. arteries cross over veins). Beneath the chorionic plate, patches of sub-chorionic fibrin are visualized as tan-white regions (Fig. 33.5).

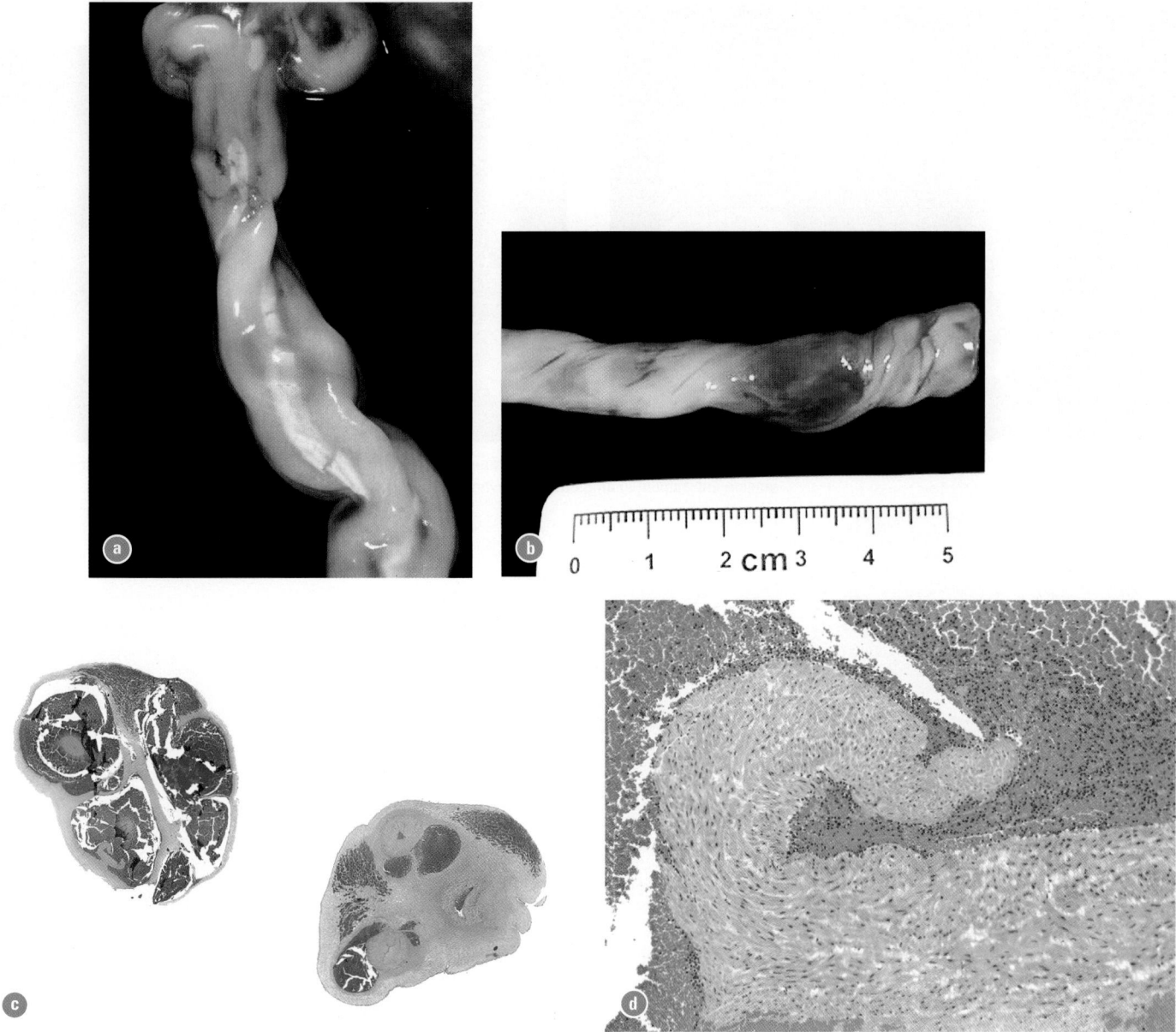

Fig. 33.11 (a) Cord vessel thrombosis, seen as a linear white streak. (b) Focal nodal swelling signifying recent rupture of the umbilical cord vein predating death by minutes. (c) Cross-section of (b) showing extensive dissecting hemorrhage around vessels (upper left) and into Wharton's jelly (lower right). (d) At high power, the umbilical vein has collapsed following segmental rupture.

Thrombi

Thrombosis of chorionic vessels can affect arteries or veins; a dilated, discolored vessel suggests fresh thrombosis; a shrunken, tan-white or yellow fibrosed vessel suggests an older thrombus. Fetal thrombosis is highly associated with fetal growth retardation and occasionally is seen with maternal diabetes or other disorders including fetal chromosomal disorders; fetal death; abnormal cord insertion; viral infection; chorangioma; and fetal hypercoagulation, i.e. protein S or C deficiency.

Cysts

Cysts of the placental surface include thin-walled amniotic cysts and thicker-walled chorionic cysts, both incidental findings (Fig. 33.13); however, the presence of numerous chorionic cysts may be associated with maternal floor infarction.

Small nodules

Tiny nodular lesions on the chorionic surface may represent: (a) amnion nodosum (nodules of fetal vernix adherent to the amniotic surface – this is due to severe

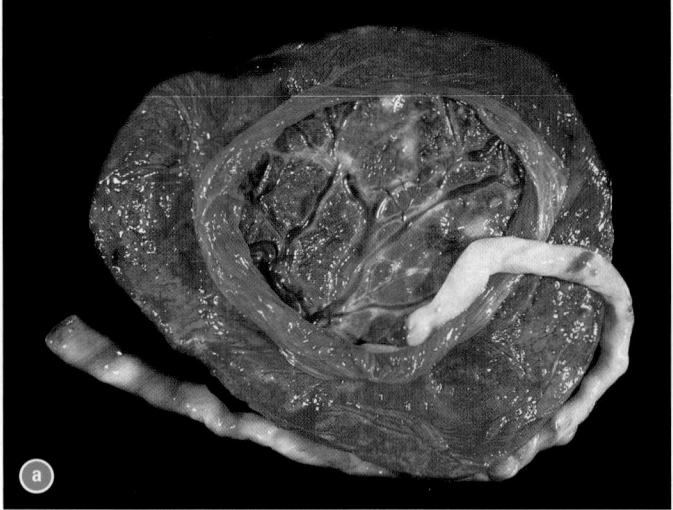

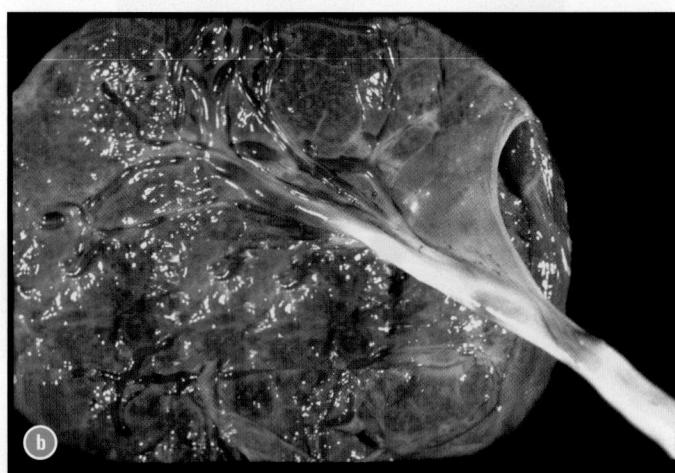

Fig. 33.12 (a) Circummarginate membranes. (b) Amnion web. (c) Constricted terminal digits following amnion entrapment in amniotic band syndrome.

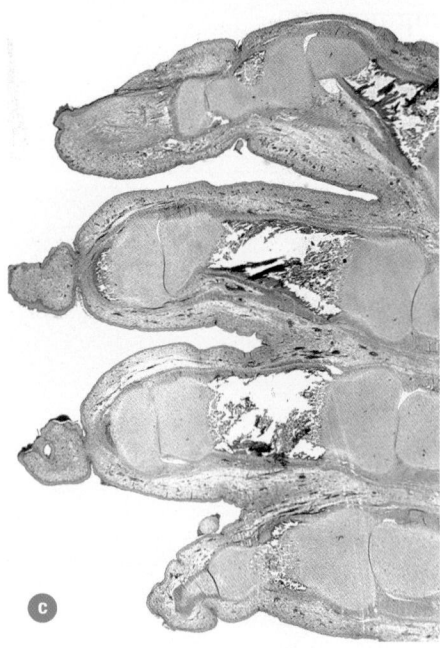

oligohydramnios, classically caused by fetal renal agenesis or renal dysplasia) (Fig. 33.14); or, (b) incidental squamous metaplasia (small plaques, usually localized to the region of cord insertion). Amnion nodosum can be grossly differentiated from squamous metaplasia in that nodules of amnion nodosum can be peeled off the placental surface, while squamous metaplasia cannot.

Large nodules

These include: (a) Chorangiomas or placental capillary hemangiomas (Fig. 33.15a). On cross-section, chorangiomas have a smooth, glistening, tan/red, myxoid consistency (Fig. 33.15b); sometimes, however, they have a uniformly dark red appearance, grossly resembling an old blood clot. Because chorangiomas originate from the chorionic plate or stem villi, they are usually located adjacent to the chorionic surface; in contrast, infarcts are usually basally oriented. (b) Fetus papyraceous (Fig. 33.15c). When present, one or more of these structures are usually located within the membranes, just adjacent to the placental margin and consist of flattened, pale amorphous ellipses with identifiable dots of retinal pigment. (c) Subchorionic hematoma. A nodular mass of subchorionic fibrin, often with a

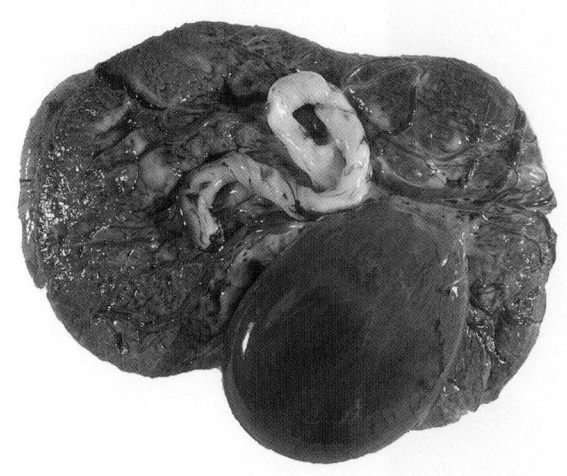

Fig. 33.13 Subchorionic cyst.

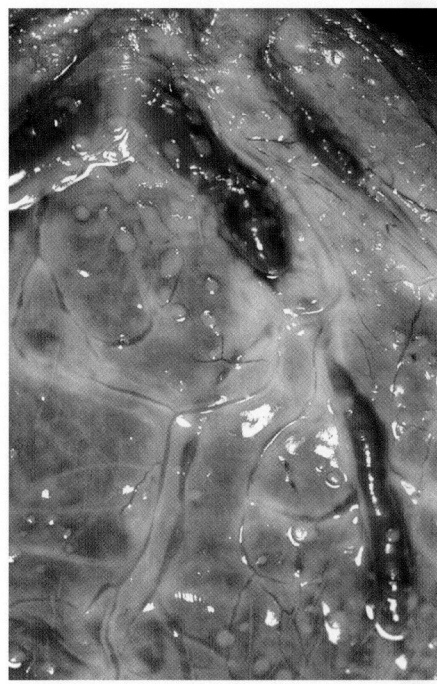

Fig. 33.14 Amnion nodosum.

laminated appearance on cross-section; a large sub-chorionic hematoma (so-called 'Brues' mole') (Fig. 33.15d) may result from rupture of a fetal stem villous vessel and result in stillbirth.[21]

Amniotic absence

Amnion may be totally absent from the placental surface following early rupture of the amniotic sac (so-called 'amniotic band syndrome'). Gross examination may show a sleeve of tissue wrapped around the proximal umbilical cord (formed by the collapsed amniotic sac, see Ch. 34). Alternatively, strands or webs of disrupted amnion may entangle the cord base (Fig. 33.12b). Amniotic band syndrome is clinically suspected when destructive fetal deformities are present (amputations, constriction rings) (Fig. 33.12c). Often gross placental abnormalities are not found; in this circumstance, the placental pathologist's most important task is to adequately sample the chorionic surface, to histologically document changes of the chorionic surface which have resulted from prolonged exposure to amniotic fluid.[18]

Absent subchorionic fibrin

Although very premature placentas have little subchorionic fibrin, it accumulates as gestational age increases. Naeye hypothesized that subchorionic fibrin accumulates from placental trauma due to normal fetal movement and further suggested that the absence of subchorionic fibrin at term may indicate a longstanding decrease in fetal mobility, possibly reflecting a longstanding fetal neurologic impairment.[3]

MATERNAL SURFACE

General

The maternal placental surface has a mosaic pattern composed of 10 to 40 'cotyledons'; each cotyledon has a slightly convex surface and is supported by one or more fetal stem villi (Fig. 33.16). This mosaic pattern is focally or diffusely absent when there is a maternal floor infarct, which obliterates the separation between cotyledons, due to decidual thickening with extensive fibrin deposition within the decidua and basal placenta.

Fragmentation

When the placenta separates from the decidua after birth, 'lacerations' of the maternal surface may develop, usually located between cotyledons (Fig. 33.17). Such localized fragmentation may suggest that the placenta is incomplete (i.e. retained). This issue can usually be resolved by gently molding the placenta back into its original shape; if placental tissue is truly missing, obvious gaps in the maternal surface will appear.

True fragmentation of the placenta is often evident following manual removal of the placenta. This raises the possibility that additional placental tissue may be retained, either due to incomplete placental removal, or due to a placenta creta. Placenta creta usually cannot be confirmed by the pathologist from placental assessment alone, unless histologic assessment of the basal

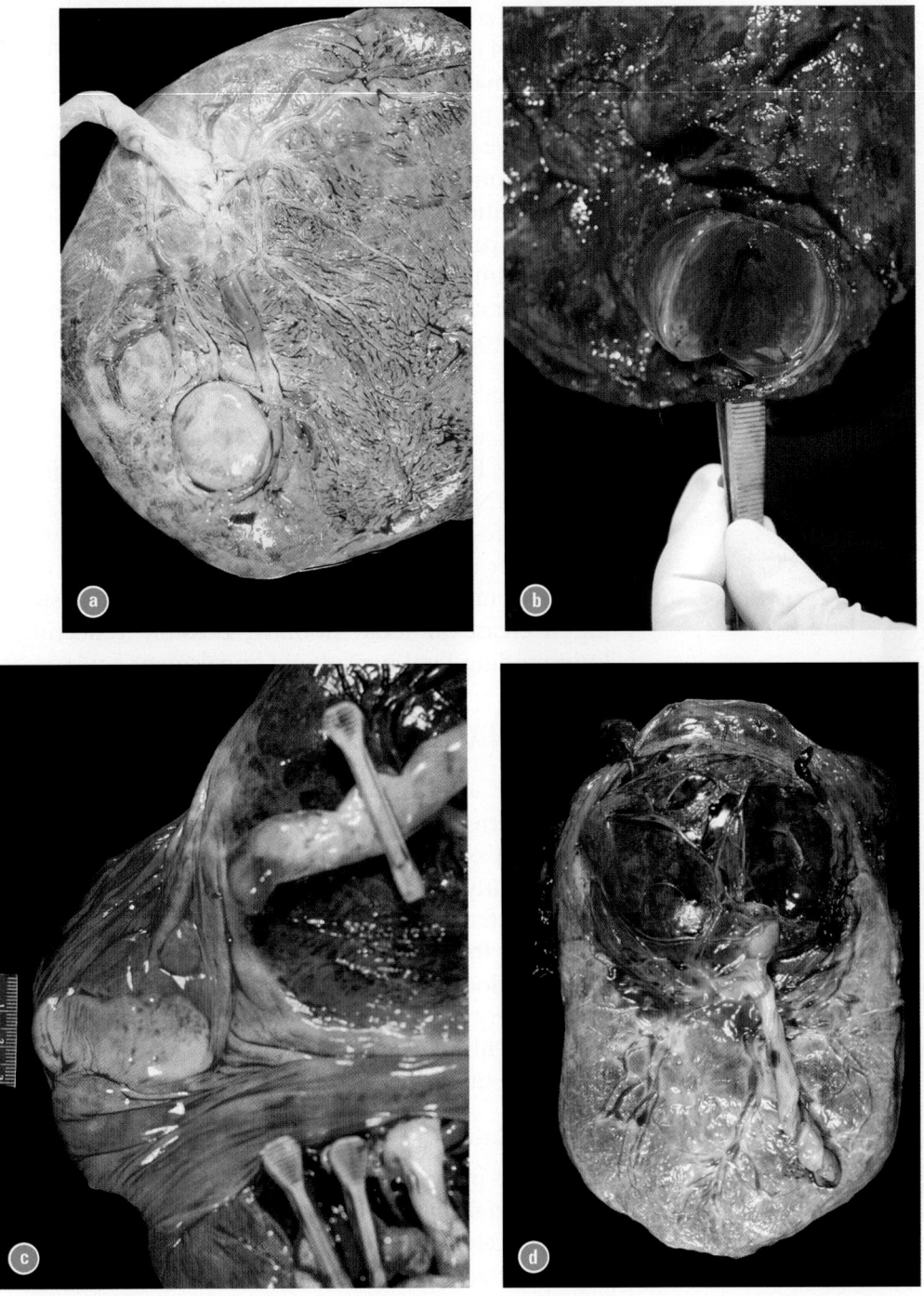

Fig. 33.15 Larger nodules, including (a) chorangioma, (b) sectioned chorangioma, (c) fetus papyraceous and (d) subchorionic hematoma (Breus' mole).

placental villi demonstrates adherence of basal villi to myometrium (without an intervening decidual layer, see Ch. 34).

Retroplacental blood clot

In many placentas, adherent fresh blood clot is attached to the maternal surface; when this fresh clot is removed (easily done), the adjacent maternal surface is unremarkable (Fig. 33.18). With abruptio placentae, an adherent, sometimes grossly laminated, blood clot is found (Fig. 33.19a). Sometimes the clot destructively dissects into the adjacent placental parenchyma (Fig. 33.19b). The blood clots of a remote abruptio placentae become firm, dry and stringy and eventually brown in color. The placenta adjacent to the adherent blood clot may be: (a) dark red (due to villous hemorrhage,

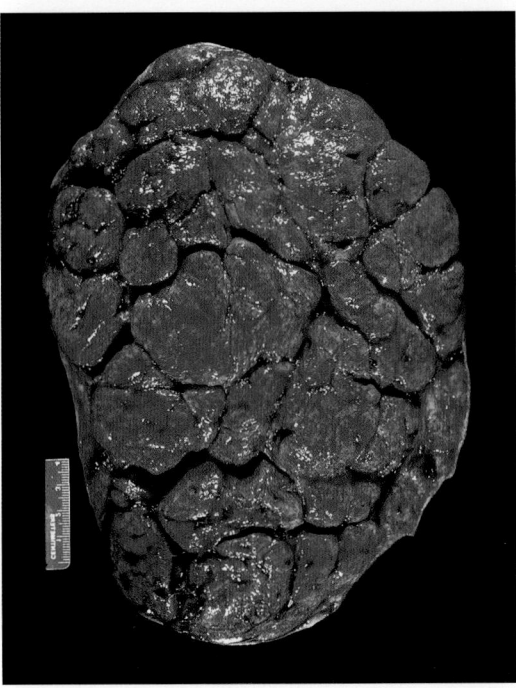

Fig. 33.16 A normal maternal surface.

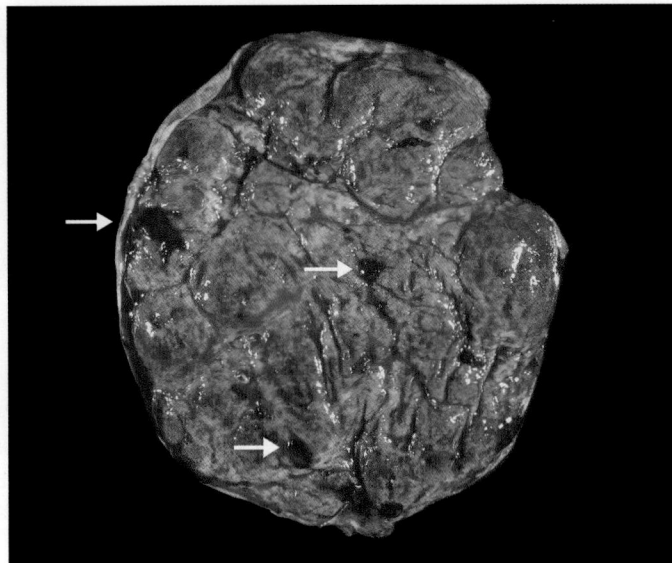

Fig. 33.18 Incidental retroplacental hemorrhage, present as small clots (arrows) on the maternal surface.

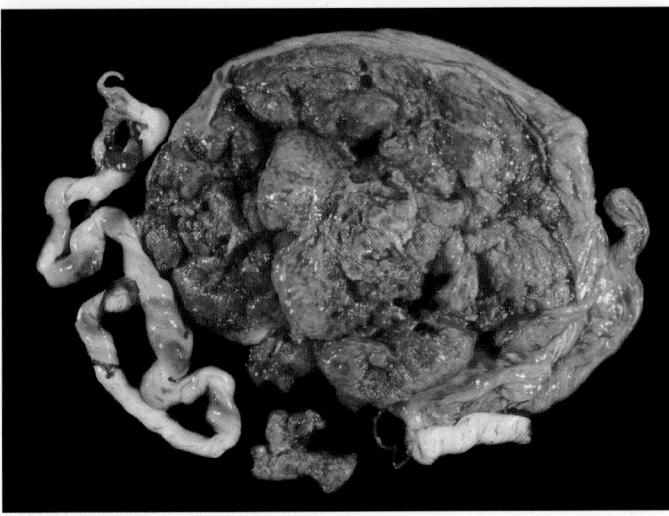

Fig. 33.17 A fragmented maternal surface.

an early hemorrhagic infarction); (b) thinned out (a 'saucer-like' depression is characteristic); or (c) firm and pale (indicating an infarct of several days' duration) (Fig. 33.20). Although in many instances abruptio placentae is clinically silent, the history may be helpful (i.e. second/third trimester bleeding; premature labor; 'port wine' amniotic fluid; passage of a large clot with the placenta; hypertonic contractions; maternal hypertension; fetal death/distress; or, rarely, maternal trauma, such as a fall or a motor vehicle accident).

SECTIONED SURFACES OF THE PLACENTA

General

At term, the typical cut surface of the placenta has a red color, a spongy consistency and a thickness of 1.5 to 3 cm. On cross-section, the following gross findings are evident: stem villi; small areas of tan/shiny fibrin (perivillous fibrin or septae) and laminated, subchorionic fibrin (rare in premature placentas, very common at term) (Fig. 33.21).

Thickness

A diffusely very thin placenta suggests marked prematurity, or poor placental growth due to ischemia (for instance in fetal growth retardation). Localized placental thinning may result from a remote infarct, a retroplacental leiomyoma, retroplacental hematoma (with an attached clot), or from incomplete removal of the placenta (possibly due to placenta creta). Excessive thickness is associated with placentomegaly from hydrops fetalis (most commonly), or from maternal diabetes or congenital syphilis, among other conditions.

Color

A diffuse, dark red color usually indicates congestion of fetal capillaries, a non-specific finding. Less commonly, it may indicate diffuse fetal capillary proliferation (chorangiosis), an abnormality associated with maternal diabetes. A localized dark red area usually indicates an early infarct or a region of villous hemorrhage (the

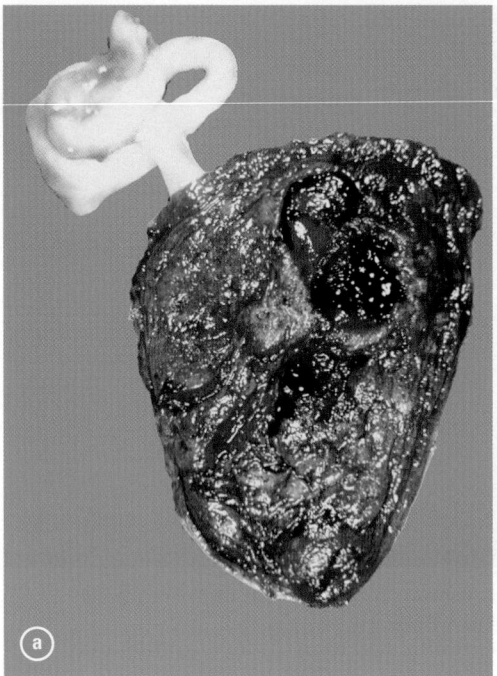
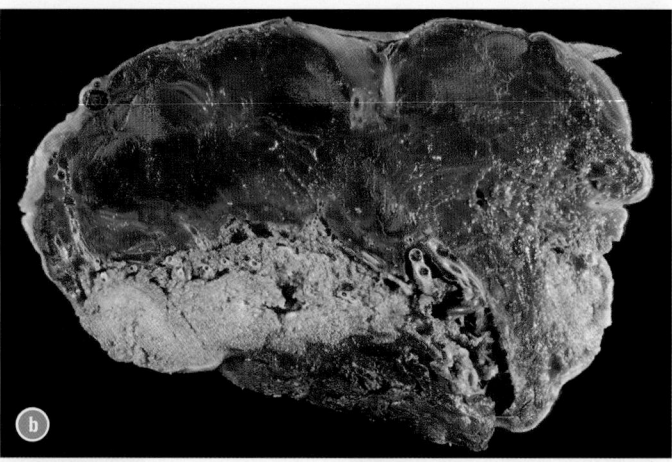

Fig. 33.19 (a) Abruptio placentae, with a retroplacental thrombus and associated depression (upper right). (b) Retroplacental hemorrhage dissecting into parenchyma.

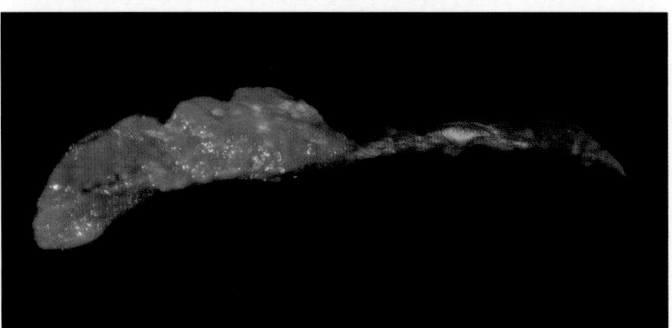

Fig. 33.20 Old abruption with marked thinning of the placental disc (right).

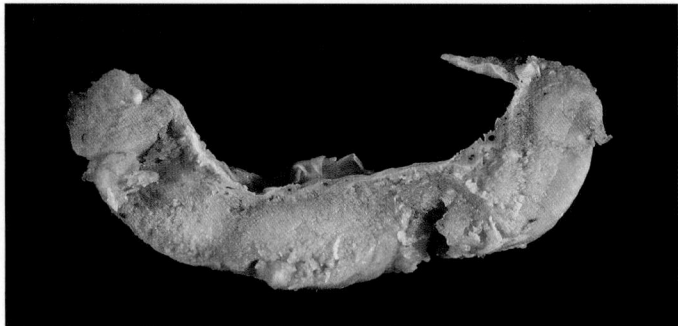

Fig. 33.22 Marked surface pallor associated with fetal death and absence of perfusion.

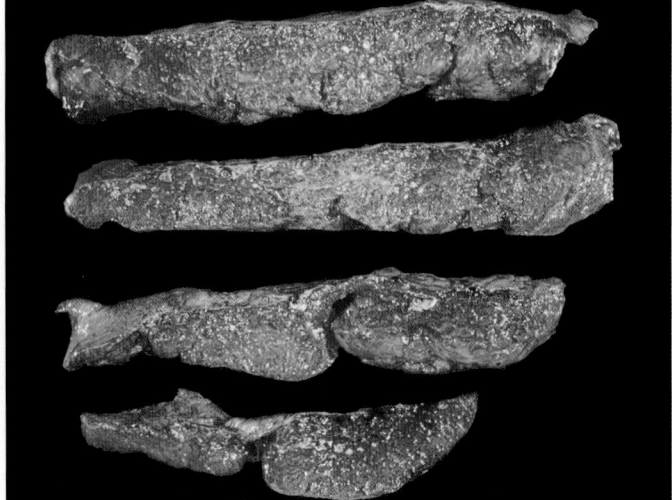

Fig. 33.21 Sectioned surface of term placenta showing homogeneous consistency.

latter is commonly due to abruptio placentae or placental trauma following manual extraction). Diffuse pallor may indicate: (1) remote fetal death (>1–2 weeks before birth) with diffuse villous fibrosis (Fig. 33.22); (2) edema from hydrops fetalis; or (3) marked fetal anemia from any cause; of note, stillbirth from fetal exsanguination related to massive fetal–maternal hemorrhage may be suggested by placental and fetal pallor and can be documented and quantified from a maternal Kleihauer–Betke test. Localized pallor usually indicates intravillous fibrin, infarction, or regional villous fibrosis resulting from a fetal thrombosis ('white infarct').

Masses

Infarcts are best recognized by their gritty, granular consistency, which is related to their villous composition. Infarcts are commonly located close to the maternal–placental surface, reflecting their pathogenesis in diseased maternal spiral arterioles. Recent infarcts are dark red; older infarcts gradually change from brown-red, to tan and finally to a yellow-white color. The entire sequence may take several days to weeks (Fig. 33.23). It is important to record the size of infarcts, as well as the approximate total percentage of placental parenchyma which is involved by infarction. Representative infarcts should always be histologically sampled to document and confirm gross impressions (i.e. primary placental choriocarcinomas have often been described as grossly resembling placental infarcts).

Intervillous thrombi (IVT) are dark red masses, sometimes with white laminations, which have a smooth, glassy consistency. They consist of clotted blood, which displaces the villi peripherally (Fig. 33.24). IVTs are usually at least 1 cm in diameter.

Chorangiomas (placental hemangiomas), as mentioned above, are often located adjacent to the fetal surface of the placenta, usually contiguous with the chorionic plate or large stem villi (Fig. 33.15a,b). Giant chorangiomas (>5 cm) can result in fetal hydrops, congestive heart failure and thrombocytopenia.

Septal cysts are small, smooth-lined structures, usually less than 1 cm in diameter, which are filled with a clear, mucinous fluid. Such structures are formed by cystic degeneration of the fibrinous placental septae. Isolated, small septal cysts are usually insignificant findings; multiple, large septal cysts may be associated with maternal floor infarct or extensive perivillous fibrin deposition.

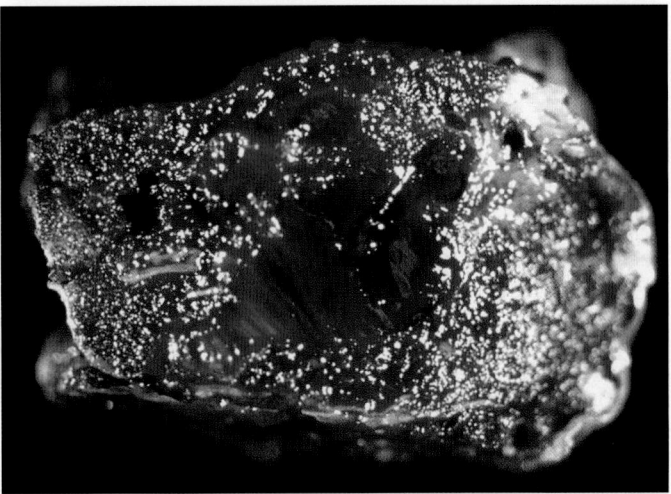

Fig. 33.24 Cross-section of placental disc with fresh intervillous thrombus (center).

Localized fibrin deposition

Small, tan-white, smooth nodules of fibrin (up to 1–2 cm in size) are relatively common findings in several regions: beneath the chorionic plate (except in premature placentas) (Fig. 33.25), at the placental margin and scattered throughout the placental parenchyma. Although most represent incidental, insignificant findings, some may be the sequelae of remote intervillous thrombi or regional retroplacental hematomas.

Extensive fibrin deposition

Although excessive fibrin deposition can represent a truly pathologic process (associated with fetal growth retardation, stillbirth and recurrent poor obstetric outcome), the categorization of placental fibrin as

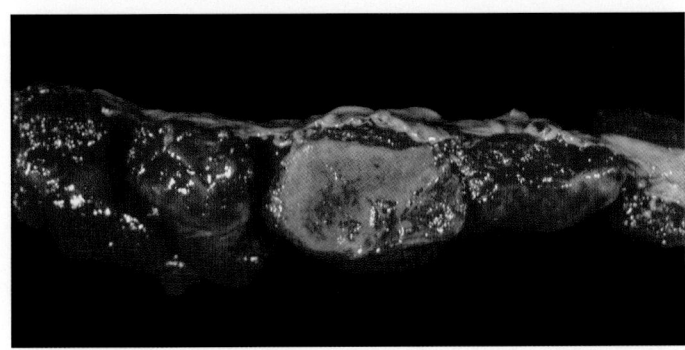

Fig. 33.23 Recent placental infarct (center).

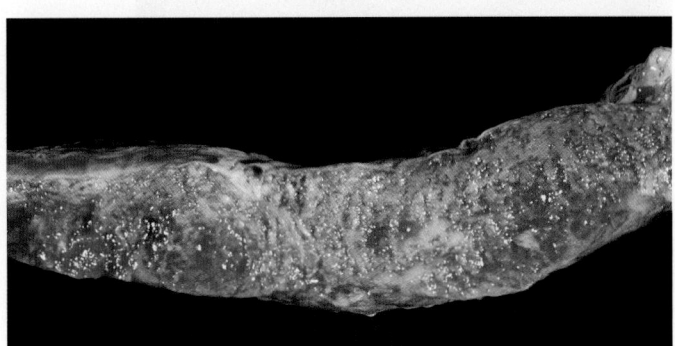

Fig. 33.25 Localized fibrin.

excessive, extensive, or pathologic is subjective. Two general patterns of extensive fibrin deposition have been described: (1) Maternal floor infarction is usually defined as a grossly visible fibrinous plaque occupying much of the maternal surface, which appears as a leathery, basal thickening; histologically, it consists of extensive fibrin deposits within the decidua and the adjacent basal intervillous space (Fig. 33.26).[22] (2) Gitterinfarct ('network of fibrin') consists of diffuse placental parenchymal infiltration by fibrin, forming a dense, netlike patchwork of intervillous/perivillous fibrin occupying a significant percentage of the intervillous space. Both of these conditions are classically described as not involving ischemic necrosis of villi.

In our experience, these two diagnoses are very subjective and they frequently overlap. In addition, contrary to published reports, we have found that these lesions are often histologically composed of an admixture of patterns, including perivillous fibrin deposition, ischemic infarction, chronic villitis, villous fibrosis, hemorrhagic endovasculitis and fetal vascular thrombosis. Although it is usually quite evident that significant placental pathology exists, often there is no single, satisfactory diagnostic term that fits the picture and usually no single pathogenetic processes (ischemic, immunologic, thrombotic) can be invoked.

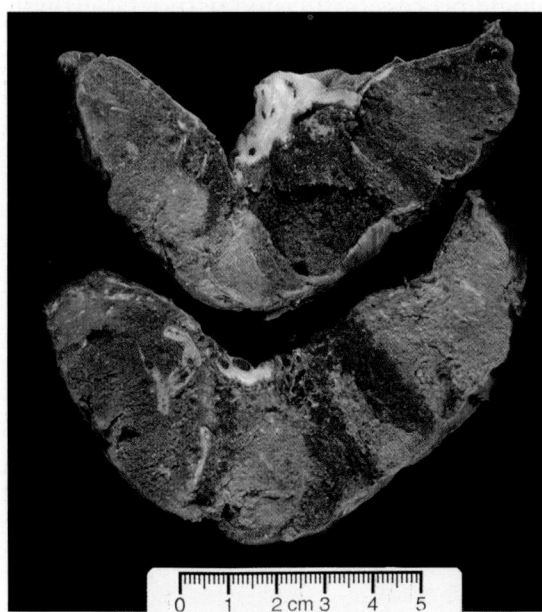

Fig. 33.26 Maternal floor infarct, present as extensive fibrin in the maternal surface and parenchyma.

THE PLACENTA FROM MULTIPLE GESTATIONS

General

One of the goals in examining the twin placenta is establishing zygosity. About 40% of twins are monozygous (identical) and 60% are dizygous (fraternal). A monochorionic placenta is diagnostic of monozygosity; about 30% of twin placentas are monochorionic (2% monoamniotic-monochorionic and 28% diamniotic-monochorionic).[23] Dichorionic twin placentas (70% of twins) can be from either a monozygous or dizygous pregnancy, i.e. zygosity cannot be determined from placental examination. Additional genetic studies of dichorionic gestations will reveal that about 85% are dizygous and 15% are monozygous. Other issues include exclusion of twin-twin transfusion syndrome and other complications of twin pregnancy (see Ch. 34).

Careful gross inspection of the twin placenta is the most important task for the pathologist. A general approach to this is outlined below:

Inspect the cords
1 Hopefully the obstetrician has clearly marked the cords regarding the twins' birth order. Parenthetically, when chorioamnionitis is found, it usually affects placenta No.1 exclusively or most severely; this reflects the fact that chorioamnionitis is caused by an ascending bacterial infection which reaches the presenting sac before the non-presenting sac.
2 Cord anomalies are very common in twins, much more common than in singletons (see later). Their approximate prevalence is shown in Table 33.4.

Are the discs separate or fused?
1 Separate discs indicate dichorionic placentas; such placentas can be pathologically assessed like two singleton placentas (i.e. there is no need to worry about twin transfusion syndrome or intertwin anastomoses, etc.).
2 Fused discs can be either monochorionic or dichorionic (Fig. 33.27). This issue can be resolved by carefully examining the dividing membranes, which are transparent, like cellophane, in monochorionic placentas (Fig. 33.27) and are thicker and translucent in dichorionic placentas (Fig. 33.28). Several cautions apply regarding dividing membrane transparency: (1) in very premature placentas, dichorionic dividing membranes may be nearly transparent, mimicking

Table 33.4 *Approximate prevalence of cord anomalies in single and twin placentas*

	Marginal insertion	Membranous insertion	Single umbilical artery
Twin placenta	10–20%	5–10%	2–3%
Single placenta	5%	1%	1%

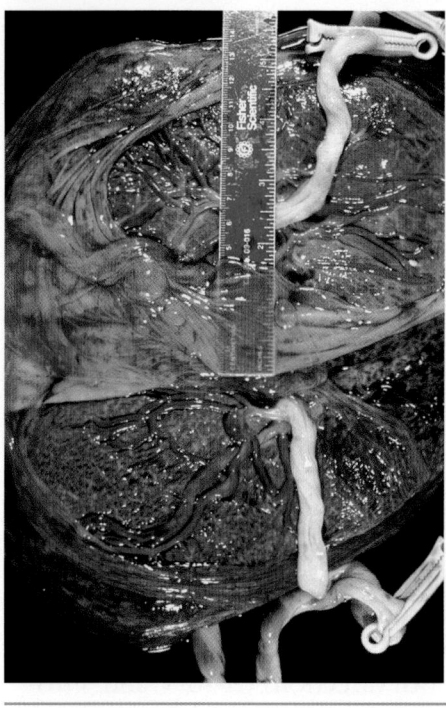

Fig. 33.28 Dividing membrane composed of amnion and chorion (dichorionic diamnionic) is thicker and translucent.

monochorionic dividing membranes and (2) with meconium staining or with acute chorioamnionitis, monochorionic dividing membranes may become opaque. Therefore, a dividing membrane 'jelly roll' should always be histologically assessed, to confirm the gross impression regarding the dividing membrane.

If it is a dichorionic twin placenta...

1 For all practical purposes, there is no need to worry about anastomoses (only very rare anastomoses between dichorionic placentas have been reported).

2 For convenience, once the 'jelly roll' has been made from the dividing membrane, the placental discs can be divided and the placentas can be processed individually, as for singleton placentas. The dividing cut should be made after noting the branching patterns of the two umbilical cords; these demarcate the placental parenchyma supplied by each cord.

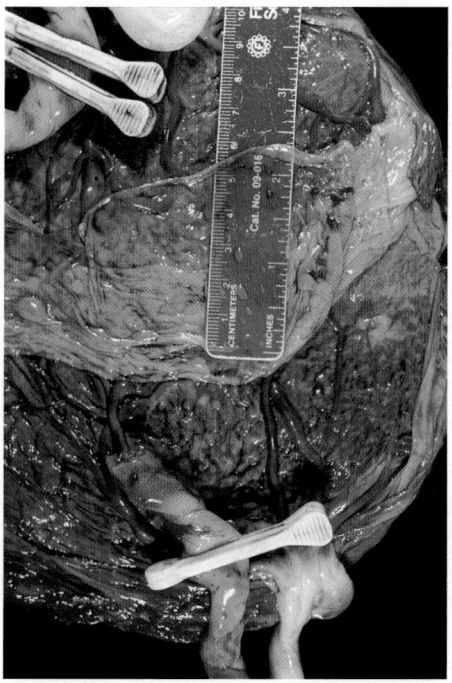

Fig. 33.27 (a) Dividing membrane composed of amnion (monochorionic diamnionic placenta) is transparent.

3 Look for one or more fetus papyracea (Fig. 33.15c). A fetus papyraceous is a common finding in multichorionic gestations resulting from infertility treatment (i.e. pergonal or *in vitro* fertilization, IVF). Such multichorionic gestations may be 'selectively reduced' at approximately 9 to 11 weeks of gestational age. The resulting 'iatrogenic' fetus papyraceous is a small, flat disc measuring approximately 3 × 1 cm (crown–rump length at 10 weeks gestation is 3 cm).

Less commonly, a larger 'iatrogenic' fetus papyraceous is seen following later selective reduction of one twin (usually for a chromosomal or structural anomaly). Because the diagnosis of a fetal anomaly is not made before the second trimester, the resulting fetus papyraceous is large, approximately 8 to 12 cm in length (crown–rump length at 17 weeks is 10 cm). Even though the large fetus papyraceous is markedly flattened and distorted due to prolonged retention, fetal anomalies can occasionally be recognized.

If it is a monochorionic twin placenta...

After the dividing membrane 'jelly roll' has been made, both amniotic membranes are carefully removed from the placental discs to allow optimal visualization of the chorionic vasculature and inspection for anastomoses. The 'vascular equator' between the two fetal circulations should then be carefully scrutinized for the following:

- *Surface vascular anastomoses.* These are either artery-to-artery (AA) or vein-to-vein (VV) anastomoses. The type of anastomosis can be identified, recalling that chorionic arteries cross over veins (Fig. 33.29).[24,25]
- *Deep vascular anastomoses.* These are artery-to-vein (A-V) anastomoses that pass through a capillary bed. Their presence can be inferred when an isolated artery from one twin terminates adjacent to an isolated vein from the co-twin. (Normally, on the fetal surface of the placenta, each superficial terminal artery is paired with a single terminal vein.)

What is the significance of intertwin anastomoses? Superficial anastomoses typically connect vessels with similar pressures (A-A or V-V); equal pressure minimizes shunting. In contrast, 'deep' anastomoses connect vessels of unequal pressure (A-V), allowing shunting to occur. If multiple deep shunts exist in both directions (A-to-V and V-to-A), the shunts tend to balance and blood volume shift may be minimal. However, when deep shunts are unbalanced (particularly when only one deep shunt is present), blood volume will gradually shift from one twin to the other: the chronic twin-to-twin transfusion syndrome (TTTS) (see Ch. 34). This leads to a pale, growth-retarded 'donor' twin (with oligohydramnios due to volume contraction and oliguria) and a larger, plethoric, hydropic 'recipient' twin (with polyhydramnios due to polyuria). The consequences are discussed in Chapter 34.[26-28]

- *Injection studies:* Benirschke and Kaufmann write that 'Once learned, injection studies are rarely necessary. However, they aid in delineating the pattern for the novice and should be performed routinely'.[18] (Although this advice is somewhat confusing, it appears Benirschke and Kaufmann mean that if one strips the amnion from the fetal surface and carefully scrutinizes the inter-twin vascular equator, most twin-twin vascular anastomoses will be obvious.) Because we agree with this reasoning, we do not routinely inject all monochorionic twin placentas at the Brigham and Women's Hospital; instead we follow the procedure outlined above (remove both amnions, then carefully scrutinize the placental vascular equator). However, if one wishes, anastomoses can often be demonstrated by injection (of air, water, dye, milk) if the underlying placental parenchyma and vasculature is intact. The first steps are the same as above (strip the amnion and identify the likely sites of anastomosis). Before injections are attempted, both cords should then be amputated near their placental insertions (to reduce vascular resistance to injection). The vessel(s) in question can then be gently cannulated (fairly near to the suspected anastomosis site) and air or liquid can be gently, slowly infused. Backflow is prevented by compressing the proximal vessel with one's finger, an instrument, or a tie. For such injection studies, Benirschke and Kaufmann recommend using a blunt, large needle (15 gauge) with a small syringe (20 ml). Baldwin prefers using a smaller needle (21–25 gauge) and a larger syringe (50 ml). Such injection procedures often allow confirmation of one's gross impression.[23]

Even more complex injection strategies have been utilized by some investigators to study the entire placental vascular tree in monochorionic twins more thoroughly: (1) the placenta is studied fresh, within minutes of delivery; (2) the cord vessels are cannulated and flushed with a heated, heparinized saline solution, at physiologic pressures; (3) the entire vascular tree is then infused with variously colored dyes (four colors were utilized by one group); and (4) in some cases, the cut parenchyma is then examined to confirm the expected admixtures of dye colors in regions of possible A-V anastomoses. Such elaborate procedures require practice, patience, technical skill, significant time and painstaking effort.

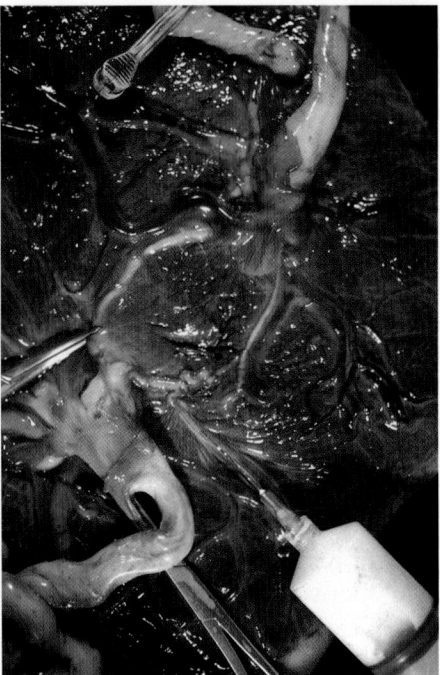

Fig. 33.29 Vascular anastomoses in a twin placenta are highlighted by injection.

Regardless of the specific approach used, the findings should be documented in detail. For example, 'Four inter-twin placental vascular anastomoses were identified, including one superficial A-A anastomosis, two superficial V-V anastomoses and one deep A-V anastomosis (from twin 2 to twin 1)'.

Microscopic examination of the placenta

This discussion will focus on the major histologic features of the placental disc, beginning with the fetal surface and moving to the maternal surface. Each layer will initially be briefly described histologically and major pathologic findings of the various components of each layer will be briefly summarized. As a quick reference, composites summarizing the examination and poten-

tial abnormalities are provided in Figure 33.30 and again later in Figure 33.38.

UMBILICAL CORD AND MEMBRANES (Fig. 33.30)

Cord

The umbilical cord should be examined to confirm or exclude: (1) single umbilical artery, (2) umbilical cord vascular inflammation and its mimics (Fig. 33.31a–c), (3) parenchymal inflammation (funisitis) (Fig. 33.32a), (4) inflammatory exudate on the surface that may signify *Candida* infection (Fig. 33.32b) and, rarely, (5) vascular thrombosis or anomalies. (6) Wharton's jelly may harbor other organisms, including *Toxoplasma* (Fig. 33.33).

Membrane roll

The membrane role should be examined for three pathologic changes. (1) Infections, in the form of

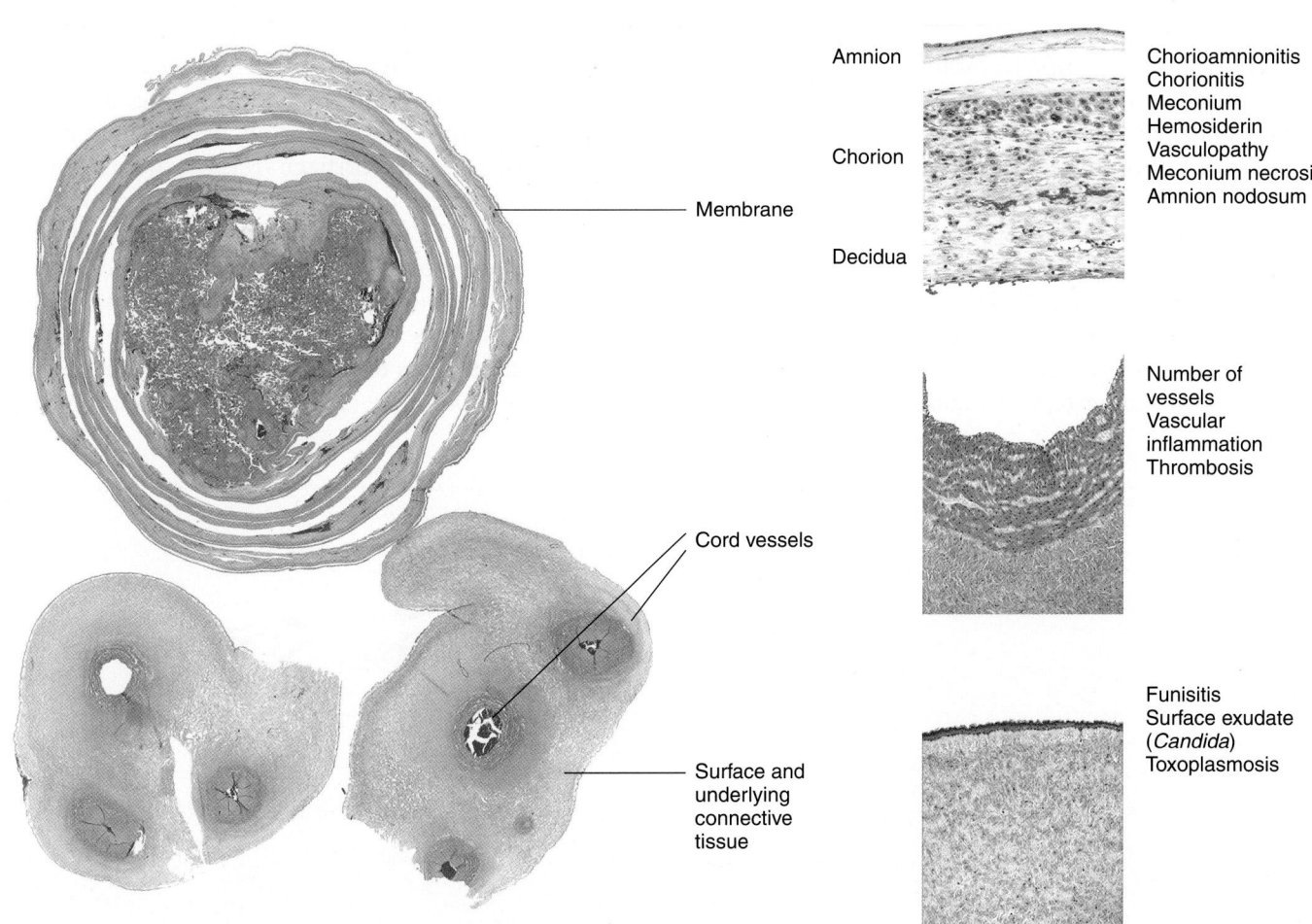

Fig. 33.30 A summary composite of cord and membranes with associated disorders.

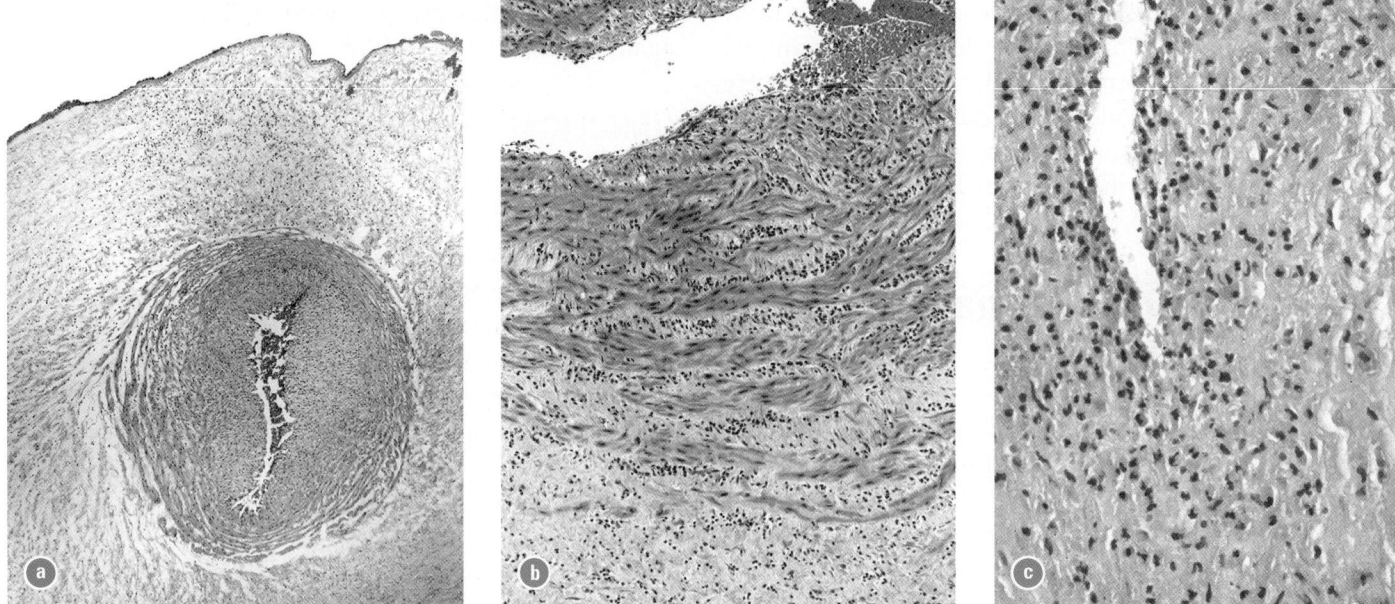

Fig. 33.31 (a) Umbilical cord vascular inflammation with funisitis. (b) At higher power neutrophils can be seen in the spaces between the myofibers in the vessel wall. (c) 'Pseudovasculitis' (due to autolysis of vascular wall and nuclear pyknosis) following fetal death may mimic infection.

acute chorionitis or chorioamnionitis, are characterized by the presence of neutrophils within the chorion or amnion (Fig. 33.34a–d). Neutrophils in the decidua are not specific and may occur in the absence of inflammation. (2) Vascular changes, specifically fibrinoid changes in the small arterioles, may signify either toxemia of pregnancy or be associated with intrauterine growth restriction. The characteristic features are, at the minimum, thickening of the arterioles with homogenous eosinophilic appearance to the media and, in severe cases, these features combined with vascular dilatation, foamy macrophages in the vessel wall and a surrounding infiltrate of lymphocytes (Fig. 33.35a–d). (3) Recent or remote abruption may be detected by retromembranous hemorrhage (recent) or hemosiderin-laden macrophages in any layer of the amnion (hours to days) (Fig. 33.36a). (4) More commonly, pigment in the membranes is associated with meconium. In contrast to the hemosiderin, meconium has a finer texture and ranges from barely imperceptible brown-tinged macrophages to more conspicuous finely distributed brown pigment (Fig. 33.36b). It may be asso-

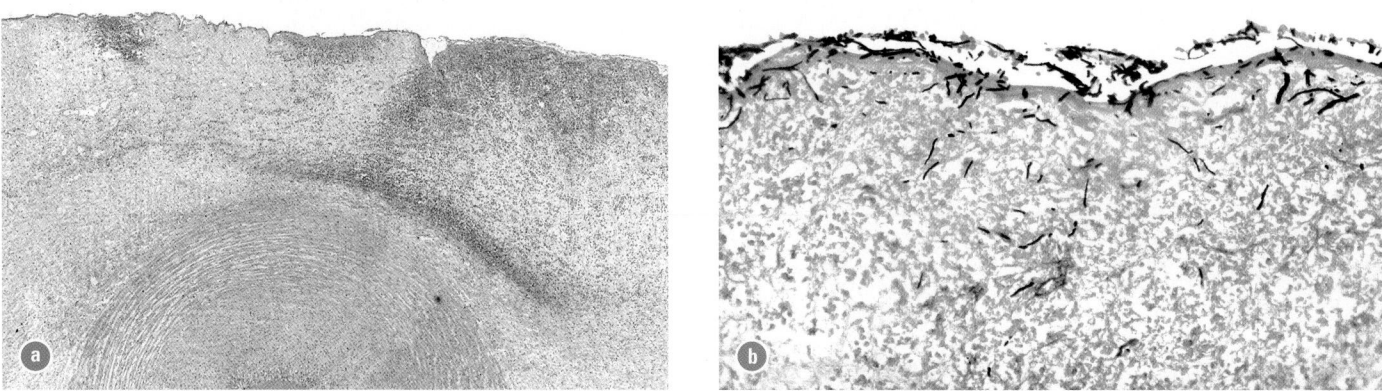

Fig. 33.32 (a) Funisitis with surface exudates, covering the surface of the cord. (b) Yeast forms are associated with surface exudates.

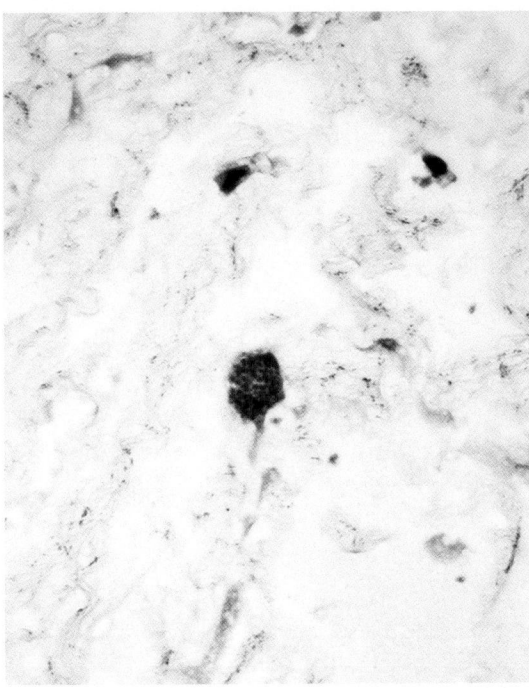

Fig. 33.33 Toxoplasmosis, seen as a single organism in Wharton's jelly (center).

ciated with alterations in the surface amnion character-ized by stratification (dysplastic amnion; Fig. 33.37).

CHORIONIC PLATE (Fig. 33.38)

On the placental disc, there are four layers in the chorionic plate:

Amnion

Definition

The amnion is composed of a cuboidal-to-columnar epithelium, basement membrane and a thin supporting layer of collagenous connective tissue) (Fig. 33.38).

Conditions

1 Amniotic epithelial disorganization (dysplasia, pseudostratification). This usually results from meconium exposure. Amniotic disorganization begins within 1 hour of exposure to meconium.[29] A bizarre amniotic epithelial dysplastic appearance has been associated with fetal gastroschisis (Fig. 33.37).[30]
2 Amniotic epithelial erosion:
   • Acute erosion develops with severe acute chorioamnionitis ('severe necrotizing chorioamnionitis') (Fig. 33.40a,b).
   • Chronic, multifocal erosion develops due to amniotic epithelial debridement by fetal movement in the setting of longstanding, severe oligohydramnios. The amniotic ulcerations are covered over by patches of vernix caseosa (proteinaceous eosinophilic nodules with embedded fetal squamous cells and hairs) (Fig. 33.39).
3 Amniotic stromal pigment deposition (in amniotic macrophages):
   • Pale gold meconium staining is most common; it develops approximately 1 hour after meconium exposure begins (Fig. 33.36b).[29]
   • Refractile, dark, iron-positive hemosiderin staining is less commonly observed; this indicates the presence of intra-amniotic blood, usually due to a previous abruptio placentae ('chronic abruptio placentae') (Fig. 33.36a).
4 Microorganisms. Occasionally bacterial cocci or rods are seen on the surface of the amniotic epithelium or within the amniotic stroma on H&E stain. When surface 'microabscesses' are present, candidal hyphae should be sought in the stroma (special stains are useful) (Fig. 33.32b). The amnion is an excellent place to find toxoplasmosis cysts (within amniotic epithelial cells or in the stroma) (Fig. 33.33).
5 Acute inflammatory cells. Neutrophils may be derived either from the mother (Stage 3 chorioamnionitis) or from the fetus (chorionic vasculitis). Of interest, the fetal inflammatory response often includes numerous eosinophils.

Amniotic-chorionic cleft (potential space between amnion and chorion)

Definition

This cleft is usually apparent histologically, often filled with pockets of amniotic fluid, which may contain:
1 Fetal squames and hairs. These are of no clinical significance (normal amniotic fluid components).
2 Neutrophils. These may be of either maternal or fetal origin. Neutrophils indicate that bacteria are present within the amniotic fluid (i.e. acute chorioamnionitis).
3 Meconium. Pigmented macrophages containing meconium indicate that meconium has been passed by the fetus. If meconium passage occurred many hours before delivery, the amniotic-chorionic cleft will often develop a characteristic bluish, myxoid appearance; this is an excellent low-power 'clue' that meconium-containing macrophages will be

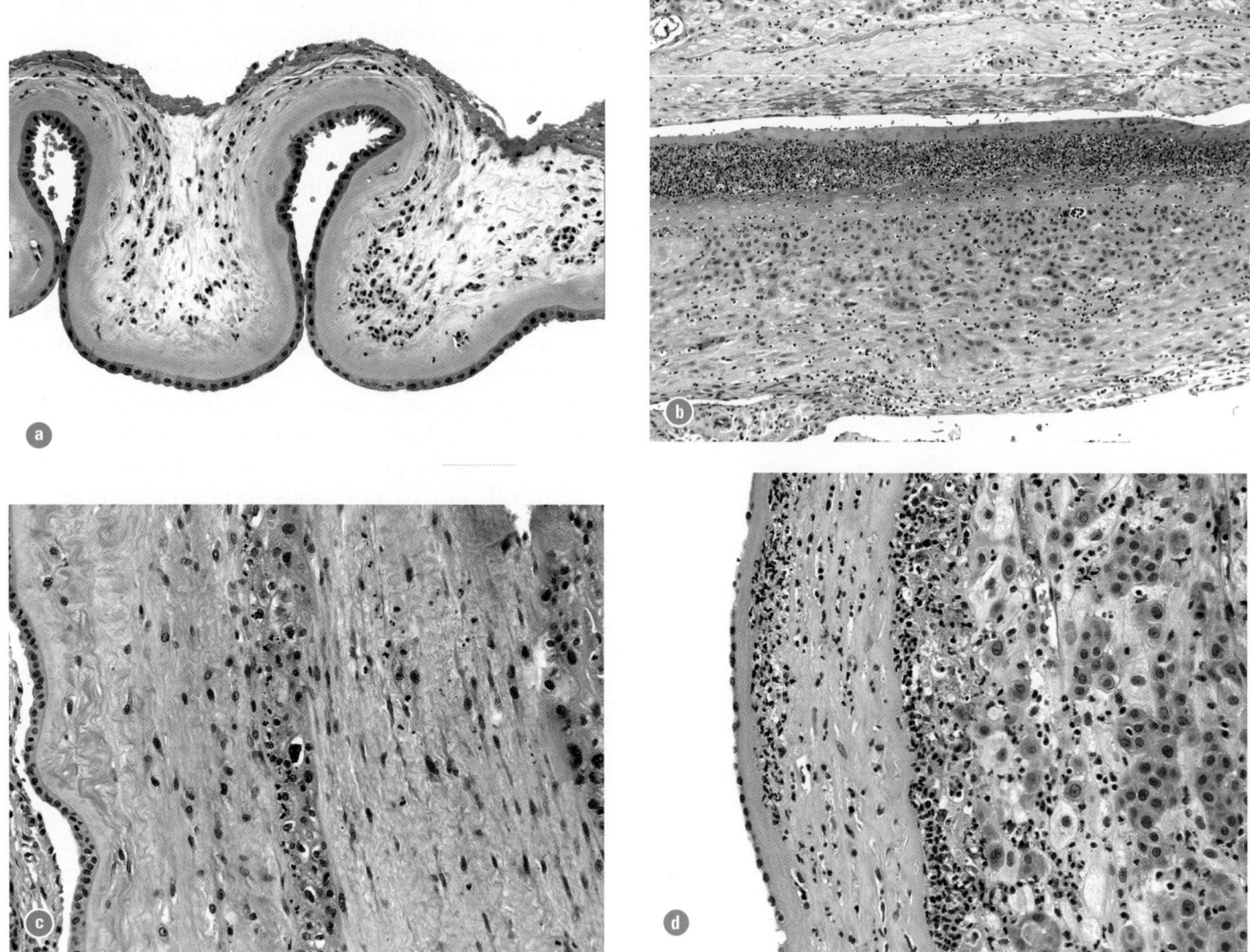

Fig. 33.34 Features and stages of chorioamnionitis include (a) detached amnion with neutrophils, (b) amnion necrosis associated with acute chorioamnionitis (Stage 3), (c) early acute chorionitis (Stage 1) and (d) moderate infection of both amnion and chorion (Stage 2).

found in the tissues and that meconium-induced vascular necrosis may be present.

Chorion

Definition
The chorion consists of a mildly cellular collagenous stroma containing numerous large muscularized fetal vessels.

Conditions
1 Fetal vessels. Although arteries and veins can be histologically differentiated in the umbilical cord, this is not possible in the chorionic plate and the stem villi. Because of this, it is usually not possible to determine whether fetal thrombi are arterial or venous from microscopic sections. Chorionic vessels are frequently dilated; often the superficial half of the vessel wall is eccentrically, markedly attenuated.

2 Pigmented macrophages. Macrophages may contain meconium (after >3 hours of exposure) or hemosiderin (after many hours of exposure, suggesting a chronic abruptio placentae) (Fig. 33.36a,b).[29]

3 Neutrophils. Acute inflammatory cells may be derived from the mother (i.e. Stage 2–3 chorioamnionitis) or from the fetus (i.e. chorionic vasculitis). Chorionic vasculitis is usually not seen in the absence of chorioamnionitis; isolated chorionic vasculitis may signify something other

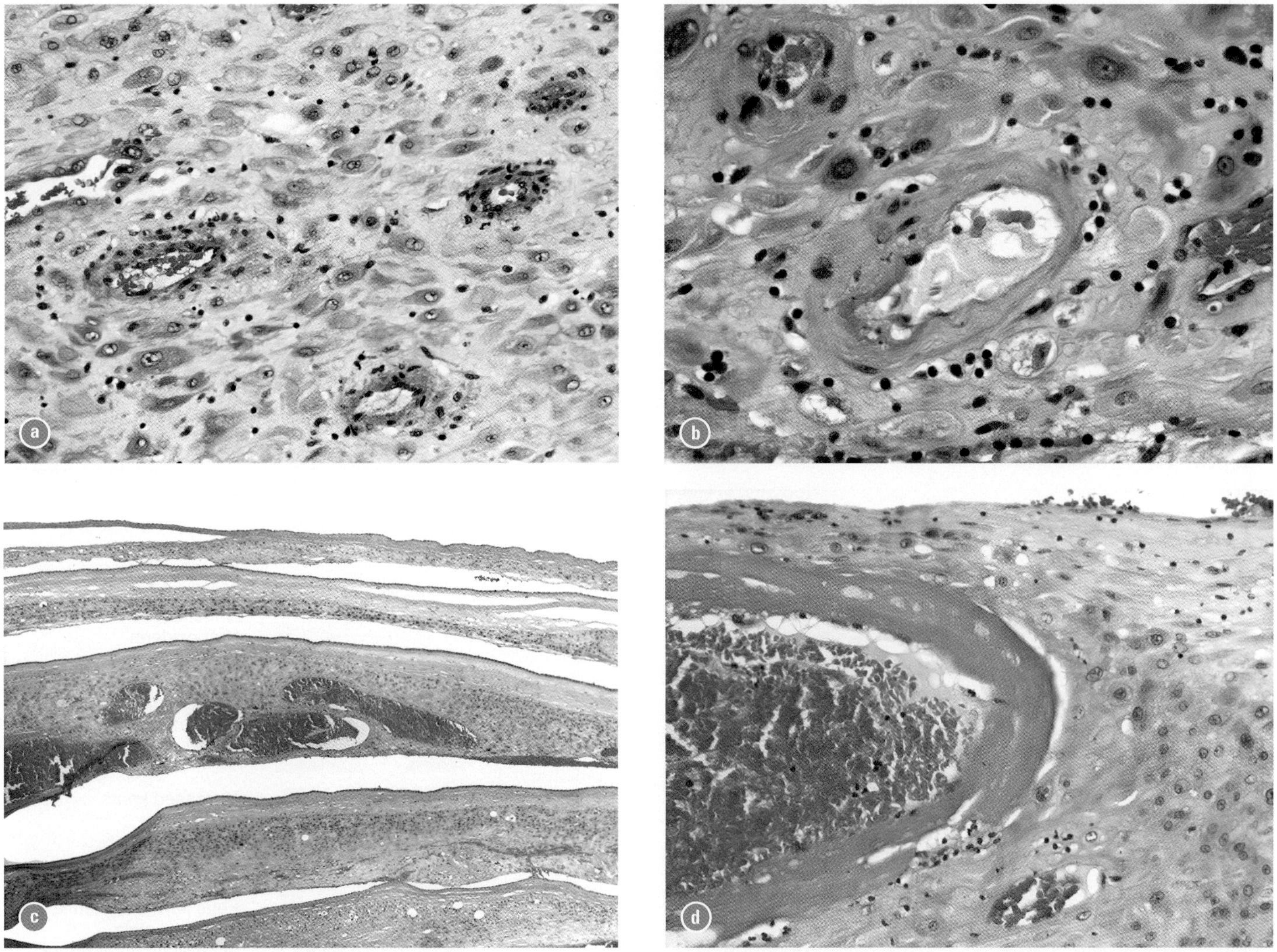

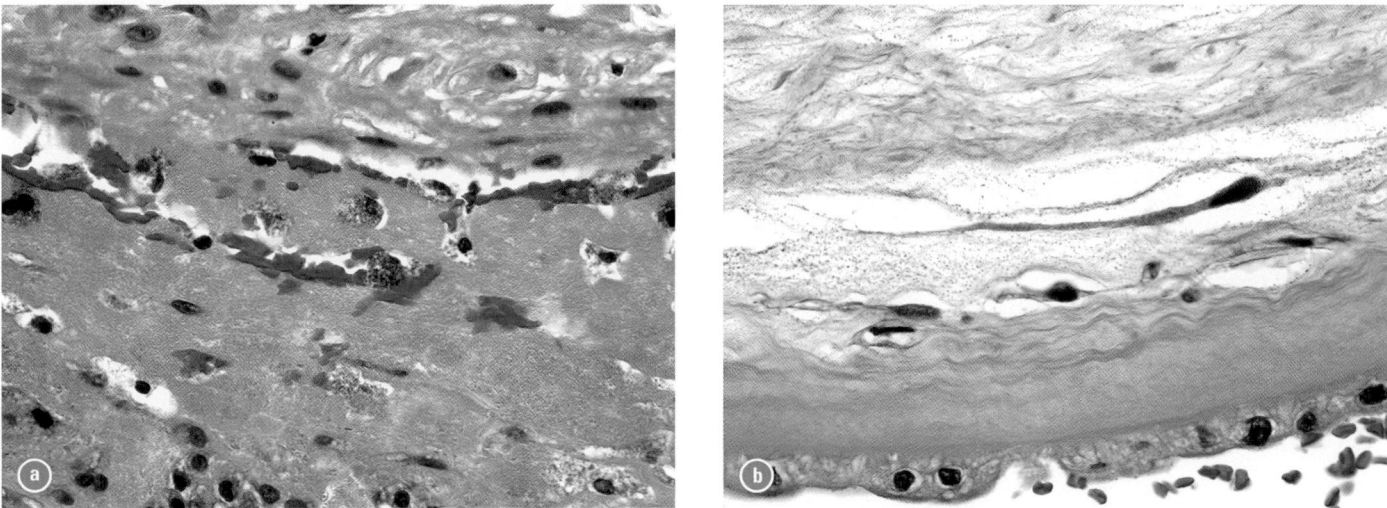

Fig. 33.35 (a) Normal arterioles are frequently present in the decidua vera. (b) Mild decidual vasculopathy displays fibrinoid change in the arterial wall. (c) Severe vasculopathy often displays conspicuous vascular dilatation at low-power magnification. (d) Acute atherosis exhibits marked fibrinoid change and macrophages in the vessel wall (see also Fig. 33.68a).

Fig. 33.36 Pigment in the membranes includes (a) hemosiderin, seen as more coarsely granular, green-brown deposits in macrophages and (b) meconium, seen as a uniformly distributed brown pigment in macrophages.

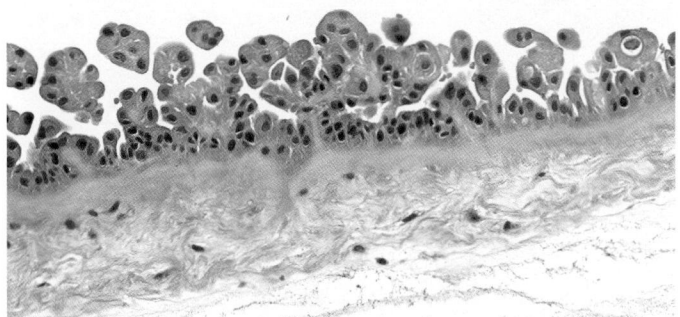

Fig. 33.36 Stratified 'dysplastic' amnion follows exposure to meconium.

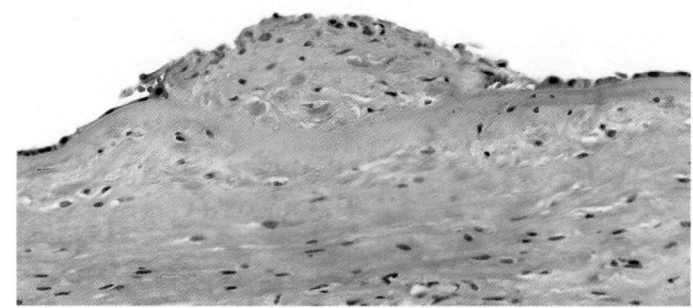

Fig. 33.39 Embedded squames (amnion nodosum) associated with Potter's syndrome.

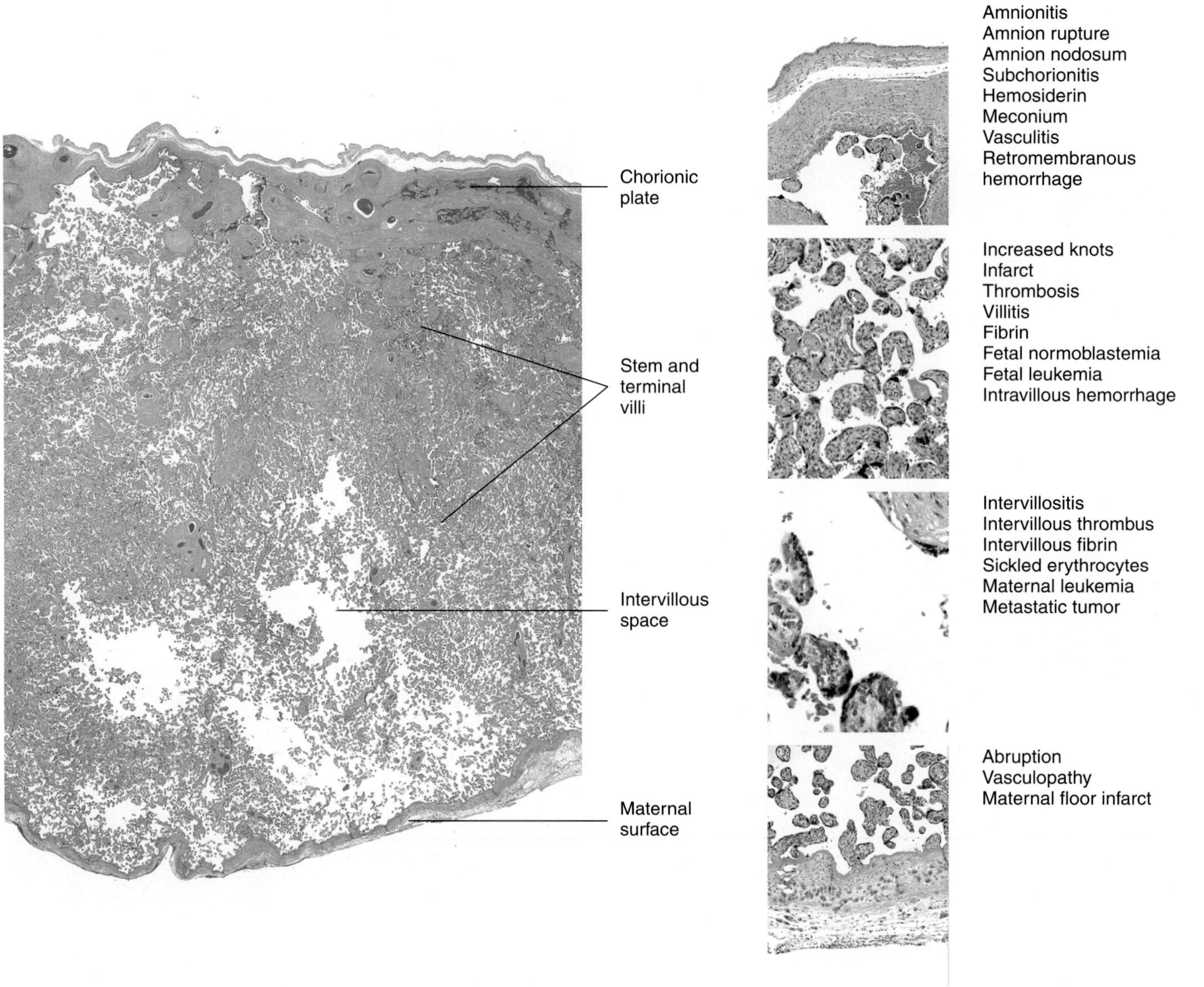

Chorionic plate

Stem and terminal villi

Intervillous space

Maternal surface

Amnionitis
Amnion rupture
Amnion nodosum
Subchorionitis
Hemosiderin
Meconium
Vasculitis
Retromembranous hemorrhage

Increased knots
Infarct
Thrombosis
Villitis
Fibrin
Fetal normoblastemia
Fetal leukemia
Intravillous hemorrhage

Intervillositis
Intervillous thrombus
Intervillous fibrin
Sickled erythrocytes
Maternal leukemia
Metastatic tumor

Abruption
Vasculopathy
Maternal floor infarct

Fig. 33.38 Composite of placental disc, its components and associated conditions.

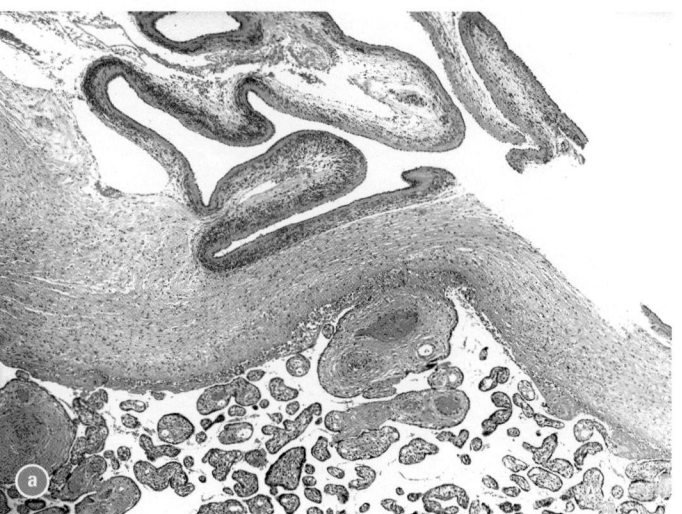 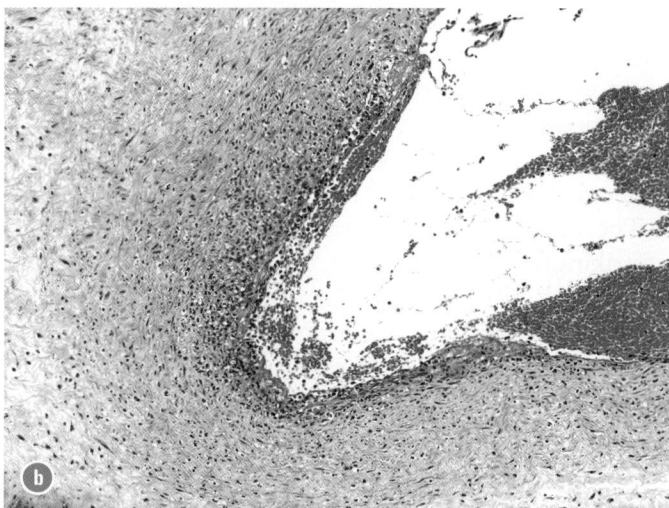

Fig. 33.40 (a) Low-power view of chorionic plate shows acute subchorionitis and amnion necrosis. (b) At high magnification there is inflammation of the chorionic plate with vasculitis (center).

than bacteria in the amniotic fluid (i.e. look carefully for fetal thrombosis or meconium-induced vascular necrosis) (Fig. 33.40b).

4 Chorionic thrombosis. Most fetal chorionic thrombi are non-occlusive (Fig. 33.41a). Non-occlusive fetal thrombi are characterized by a bright eosinophilic intimal plaque; often, mild acute inflammation, karyorrhexis, dystrophic calcification and fibroblast proliferation are also found. Old thrombi may have extensive dystrophic calcification. Occlusive fetal thrombi are characterized by either complete lumenal obliteration, or extensive lumenal septation

(i.e. fibroblast bridges, multiple tiny blood pools, hemosiderin deposition and interstitial hemorrhage with RBC cytoplasmic fragmentation). The latter picture is identical to 'hemorrhagic endovasculitis' as described by Sander (Fig. 33.41b).[31,32] When fetal thrombosis is present, other regions of the placenta should be screened for regional villous fibrosis (eosinophilic, fibrotic, avascular stem villi and terminal villi (see below)).

5 Chorionic meconium-induced vascular necrosis. The portion of the chorionic vessel wall closest to the amniotic surface may show striking single cell

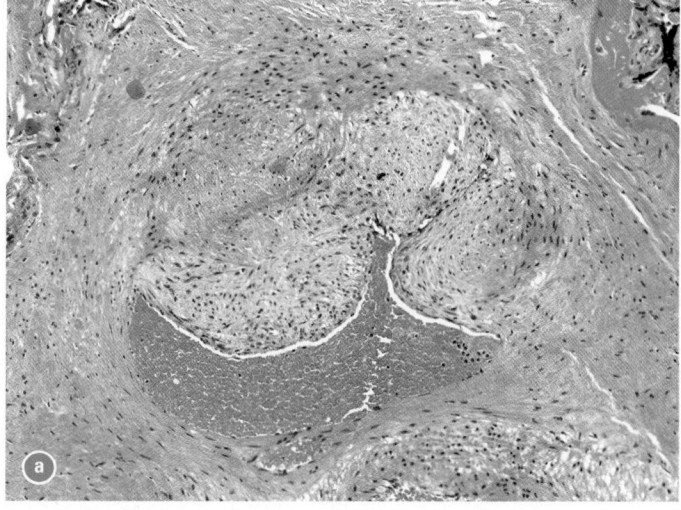 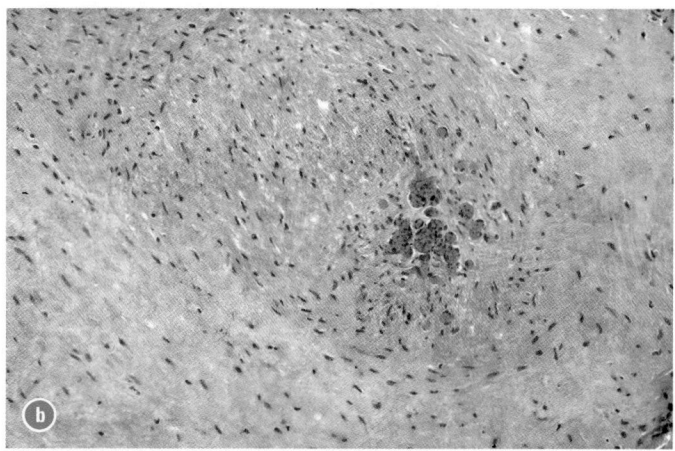

Fig. 33.41 (a) Thrombosis involves a chorionic plate vessel with partial occlusion. (b) Hemorrhagic endovasculitis is characterized by a fine mesh-like network of fibrin in the lumen. This change is not specific but may follow fetal death or fetal thrombosis.

myocyte necrosis (shrunken smooth muscle cells with characteristic cytoplasmic rounding, cytoplasmic hypereosinophilia and nuclear pyknosis).[20] Locally, meconium-pigmented macrophages are prominent, sometimes located deeply within the wall of the necrotic vessel. The vessel undergoing vasonecrosis is often strikingly dilated (a good 'low-power' microscopic clue); in addition, vascular acute inflammation may be prominent. An identical picture can be seen in umbilical cord vessels (Fig. 33.42).

6 Increased neutrophils in fetal vessels. Not infrequently, impressive numbers of fetal neutrophils and band forms are seen intravascularly; because acute chorioamnionitis is usually present, this finding probably reflects a fetal neutrophilic left shift (due to amniotic fluid bacterial infection).

7 Microorganisms. *Toxoplasma* cysts can be found in the chorionic stroma (also look in Wharton's jelly).

Subchorionic trophoblastic/fibrinous layer

Definition

Initially, a complete trophoblastic lining is present (cyto- and syncytiotrophoblast), which is gradually eroded and replaced by subchorionic fibrin. Before 24 weeks the chorionic plate is entirely lined with trophoblast. After 35 weeks most of the trophoblastic lining has been replaced by subchorionic fibrin (up to several mm thick) (Fig. 33.43).

Conditions

1 Massive subchorionic hematoma. Defined as a large plaque of subchorionic fibrin (>1 cm in thickness);[33] this may result from rupture of a chorionic plate

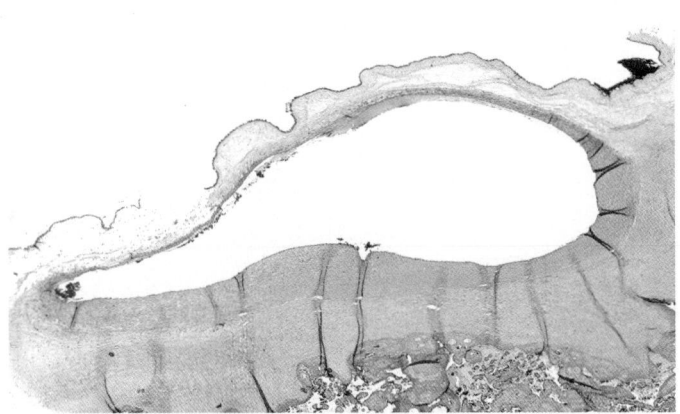

Fig. 33.42 Meconium vasonecrosis involves a chorionic plate vessel.

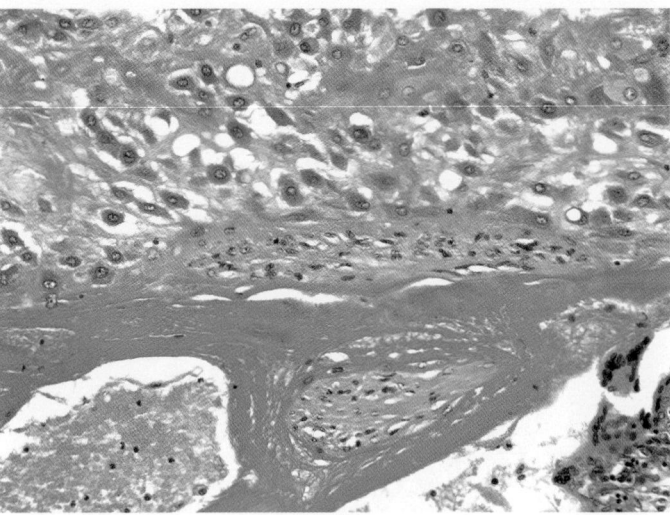

Fig. 33.43 Subchorionic fibrin commonly replaces trophoblast in subchorion.

or stem villous vessel, with subsequent fetal death from exsanguination (Breus' mole) (Fig. 33.15d).

2 Other subchorionic masses with fibrin. The differential diagnosis of these masses includes (1) intervillous thrombus, (2) evolving infarct and (3) intervillous fibrin. Infarcts are typically excluded by their more frequent basal location. Thrombi are typically more discrete, composed of lamellar fibrin and often associated with infarct or ischemic (dusky or hazy) syncytial trophoblast. In contrast, fibrin preserves (encases) the villous structures (the syncytial trophoblast are often inconspicuous or absent) and contains patches or nodules of intermediate trophoblast (Fig. 33.44).

Subchorionic maternal blood (in the intervillous space)

The source of most neutrophils which comprise acute chorioamnionitis (Fig. 33.40b). Other pathologic findings in the maternal blood are discussed below in the 'Intervillous Space' section.

STEM VILLI

Definition

All stem villi have a similar basic anatomy: (1) a trophoblastic covering; (2) a cellular stroma composed of fibroblasts, stromal cells and macrophages; and (3) muscularized fetal vessels (Fig. 33.45). Stem villi are categorized into three groups, based on their size and location: primary stem villi, the largest stem villi, which branch from the chorionic plate at right angles;

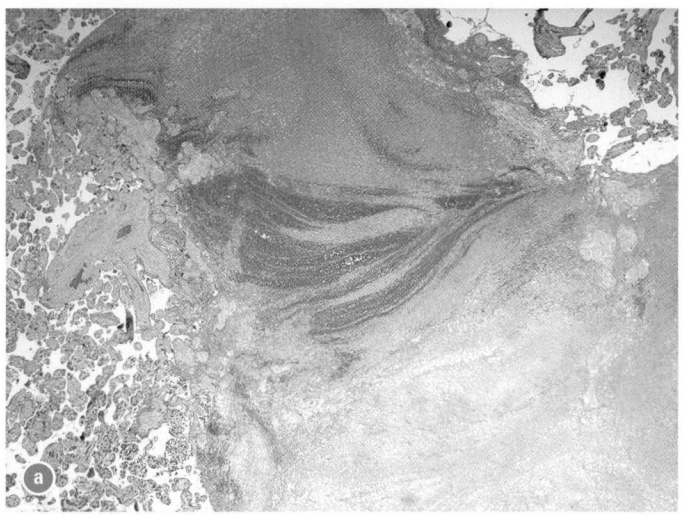

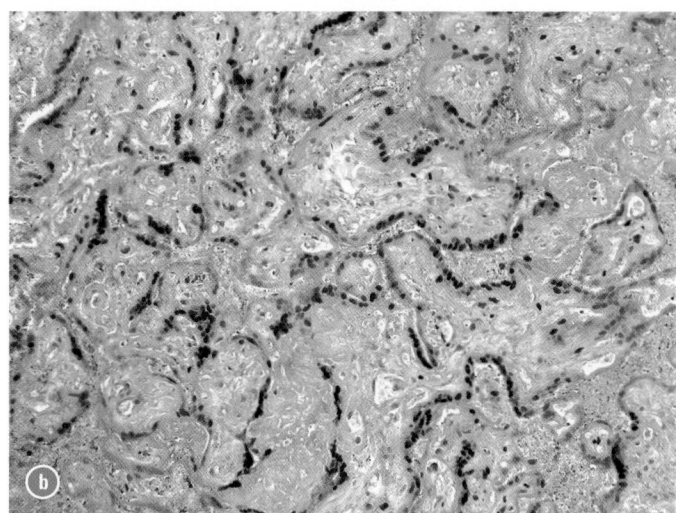

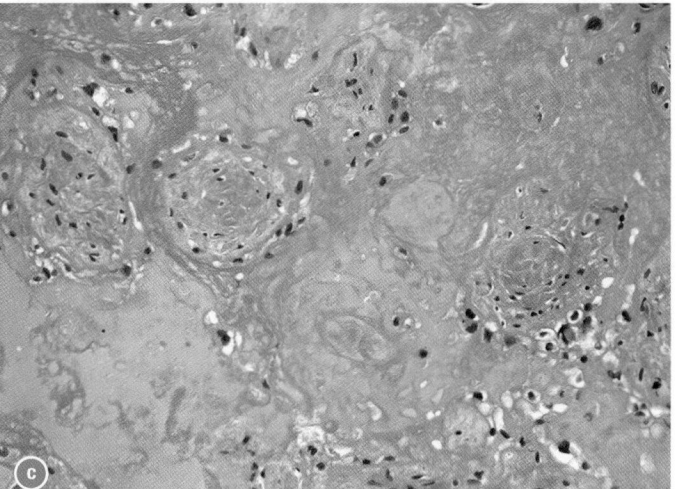

Fig. 33.44 Histologic correlates of intraparenchymal densities include (a) intravillous thrombus with laminated fibrin, (b) recent infarct with early villous necrosis and coalescence of villi and (c) intervillous fibrin encasing villi.

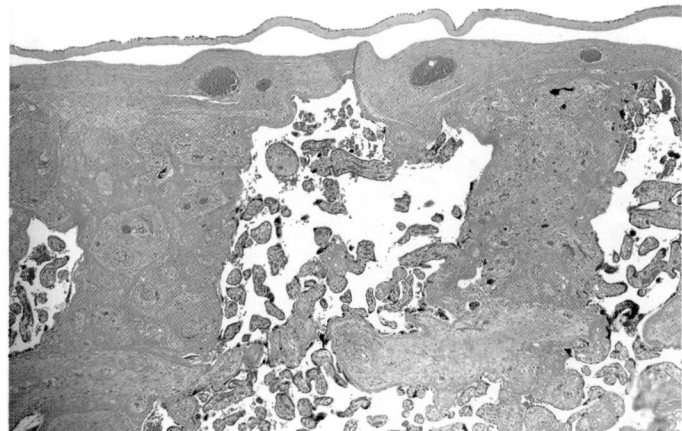

Fig. 33.45 The villous tree emerges from the chorionic plate (upper), beginning with the stem villi.

secondary stem villi, the intermediate generation of stem villi. Tertiary stem villi, the smallest stem villi, which distally connect with the terminal villi; and tertiary stem villi are the smallest villous structures and possess fibrotic stroma and muscularized fetal vessels; in contrast, terminal villi have a looser stroma and contain only capillaries.

Conditions

1 Fetal vascular thrombosis. As described above, thrombi may be non-occlusive or occlusive; occlusive thrombi and 'hemorrhagic endovasculitis' represent closely related (if not identical) processes (Fig. 33.41a,b). Fetal thrombosis is usually a localized process (focal or multifocal). When diffuse thrombosis is found, it suggests prior fetal death

(following fetal asystole, absent placental perfusion results in diffuse placental 'thrombosis'). Under these circumstances, the process should be more properly diagnosed as 'vascular changes consistent with (recent, remote) fetal death' or 'fibromuscular sclerosis, consistent with (recent, remote) fetal death' rather than 'diffuse thrombosis' (which incorrectly implies that the process preceded the fetal death).

2 Microorganisms. Stromal cells may contain cytomegalovirus (CMV) inclusions (see below). Rarely, stromal toxoplasmosis cysts are found. In cases of fetal bacterial sepsis, large numbers of intravascular bacteria may occasionally be visualized; group B streptococcus is the most common organism to cause this finding.

Fetal blood

Increased nucleated RBCs (>5 nucleated RBCs/100 WBCs) indicates either subacute/chronic fetal anemia or subacute/chronic fetal hypoxia. This finding may be seen with Rh erythroblastosis fetalis, massive fetal-to-maternal hemorrhage, fetal thalassemia, chronic fetal hypoxia, maternal diabetes or fetal parvoviral infection (Fig. 33.46a). Violet, glassy intranuclear inclusions in erythroblasts are characteristic of parvoviral infection. The fetal nRBC:WBC ratio is best assessed by examining fetal blood in large vessels (cord and chorionic plate) in areas where the blood is thin and non-clumped to allow clear visualization of individual nuclei (Fig. 33.46a).

Metastatic fetal tumor and fetal leukemia

Rare cases of disseminated fetal neuroblastoma have been reported; neuroblasts (single cells or rosettes) may be seen intravascularly or in the villous stroma. Fetal leukemias are diagnosed in this region by the presence of blasts and immature forms in the larger vessels (Fig. 33.46b).

Capillary proliferation

Chorangiomas are benign vascular tumors of the chorionic stroma; most chorangiomas originate in large stem villi or the chorionic plate. Chorangiomas may be: (1) circumscribed and solitary, (2) locally expansive, involving the contiguous stem villi, or (3) multifocal (very rarely). Chorangiomas are associated with fetal hemangiomas and with twin gestations (Fig. 33.47).

Storage disorders

Trophoblastic and stromal cells of stem and terminal villi may display marked cytoplasmic swelling and fine vacuolization, due to the deposition of storage disease metabolites (Fig. 33.48).[34]

TERMINAL VILLI

Definition

Immature terminal villi are larger, more cellular and more edematous than mature terminal villi (Fig. 33.49a). Fetal capillaries are centrally located, with relatively

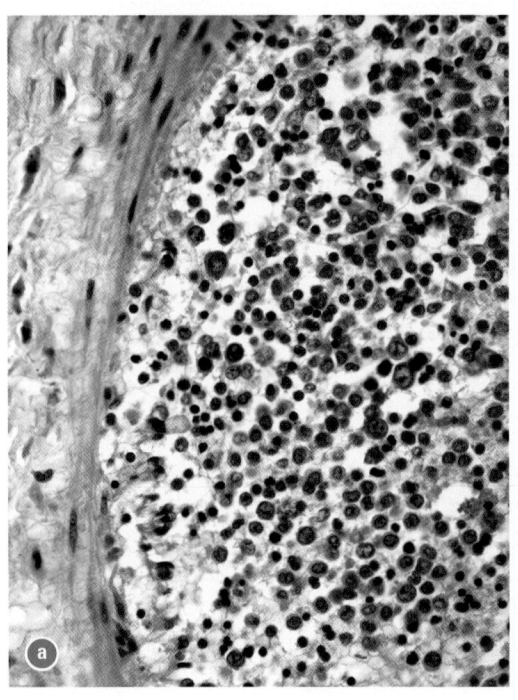
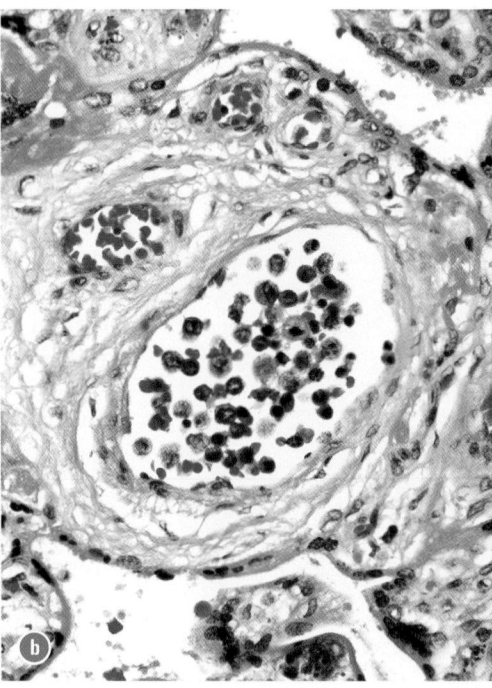

Fig. 33.46 Stem vessels contain (a) marked normoblastemia associated with hydrops fetalis and (b) Blast forms within a stem vessel in fetal leukemia.

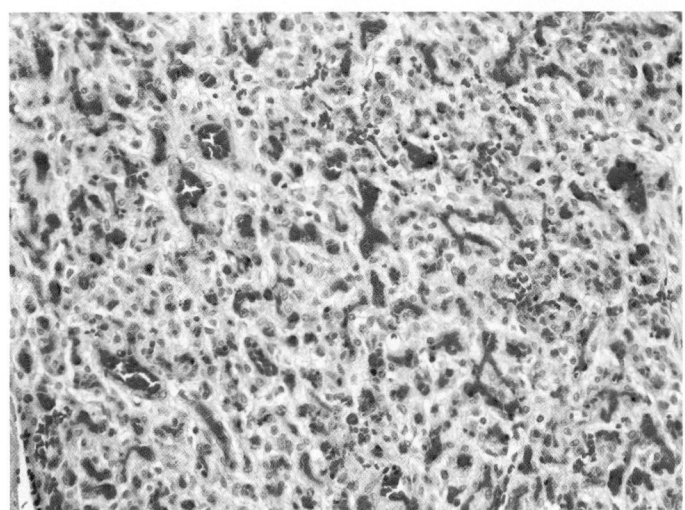

Fig. 33.47 Microscopic view of chorangioma exhibits an angiomatous proliferation similar to hemangiomas.

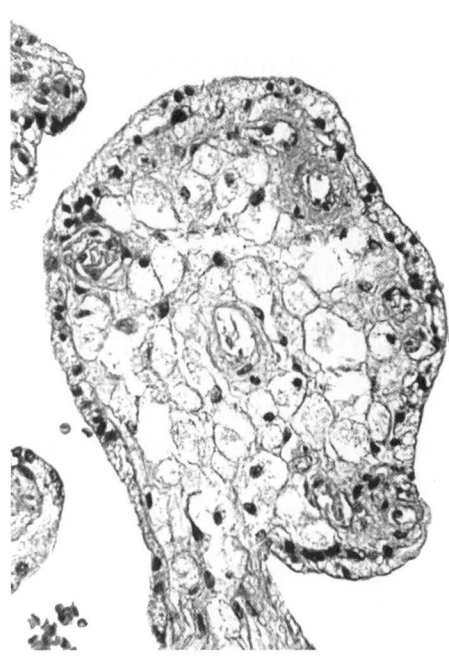

Fig. 33.48 Storage disorders typically are characterized by foamy villous stromal cells and cytotrophoblast.

few 'vasculosyncytial membranes'. The trophoblastic covering is relatively evenly distributed, with a continuous layer of syncytiotrophoblastic nuclei and numerous cytotrophoblastic cells. Immature terminal villi are prevalent in premature placentas (about 25% of villi at 20–25 weeks; about 10% of villi at 26–32 weeks; about 5% of villi at 33–36 weeks; about 1–2% of villi thereafter). Immature terminal villi are increased in hydrops fetalis, maternal diabetes and congenital syphilis, among others.

Mature terminal villi are smaller, less cellular villi; fetal capillaries are located peripherally, with marked attenuation of the adjacent trophoblastic cytoplasm ('vasculosyncytial membrane') (Fig. 33.49b). Cytotrophoblastic cells are very inconspicuous; syncytiotrophoblastic nuclei are found in large aggregates, 'syncytial knots'. Mature terminal villi predominate after

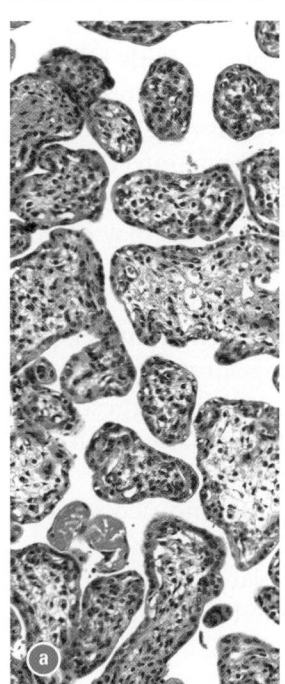

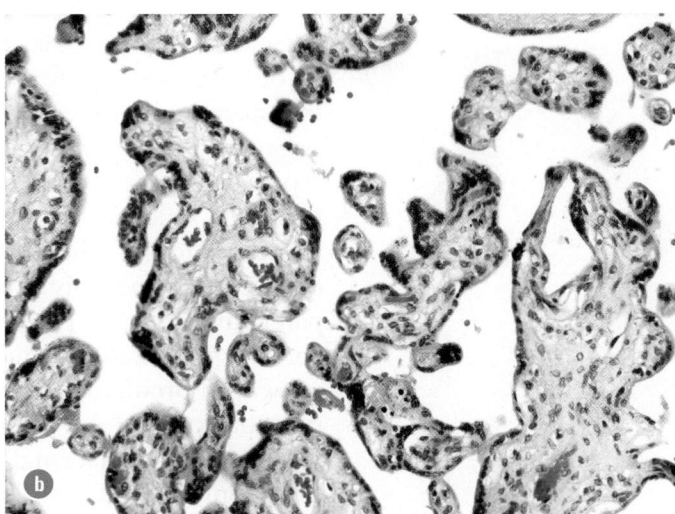

Fig. 33.49 (a) Terminal villi of first trimester pregnancy are slightly enlarged relative to later pregnancy and exhibit few syncytial knots. (b) Third trimester placentas contain smaller villi and prominent knots.

37 weeks, comprising 98–99% of all terminal villi. An increased percentage of mature terminal villi is also seen at younger gestational ages with chronic placental ischemia (i.e. preeclampsia, hypertension, lupus anticoagulant, fetal growth retardation, collagen vascular diseases, etc.).

Conditions

1 Acute villitis is characterized by neutrophils within villi and surrounding villi. This finding strongly suggests maternal or fetal bacteremia. Common pathogens which cause acute villitis include *Listeria monocytogenes*, group B streptococcus, various pathogenic enteric bacteria and *Treponema pallidum*.[35-37] *Listeria*, a small Gram-positive rod, characteristically causes multiple villous microabscesses and severe acute chorioamnionitis (Fig. 33.50); bacteria can be identified in microabscesses and within the chorioamnion. A Gram stain is indicated in all cases of acute villitis; silver stains (Steiner, Dieterle) are also indicated if the mother is VDRL positive or congenital syphilis is suspected.

2 Chronic villitis exhibits perivillous or intravillous chronic inflammation (Fig. 33.51a). Most often, mononuclear histiocytes predominate and there are scattered lymphocytes and rare plasma cells; if histiocytic multinucleated giant cells are prominent, the condition is designated 'granulomatous villitis' (discussed below). In contrast to acute villitis (which suggests fetal and/or maternal bacteremia), chronic villitis suggests either: (1) viral infections such as those in the TORCH (toxoplasmosis, other, rubella, CMV and herpes) group, also designated as 'specific' chronic villitis; or (2) a possible immunologic disorder, also termed 'non-specific' chronic villitis, or 'villitis of unknown etiology' (VUE). Many cases of infectious chronic villitis result from CMV. CMV villitis is variable in histologic appearance, ranging from minimal villous inflammation to an intense histio-lymphoplasmacytic destructive villitis, associated with villous stromal necrosis, fibrosis, calcification and hemosiderin deposition. Characteristic CMV nuclear and cytoplasmic inclusions range from widespread to focal; in some cases, inclusions are identified only after examining numerous blocks of placental parenchyma. Other viral etiologies for chronic villitis usually do not have specific features; however, villitis from HSV may show ground-glass intranuclear inclusions and villitis from varicella may show histiocytic giant cells (Fig. 33.51b, see also Ch. 34).[38] Non-infectious villitis may have an immunologic etiology, maternal–placental graft rejection.[39,40] Recently, Redline and Patterson used *in situ* hybridization to demonstrate that the villous chronic inflammatory cells of VUE are maternal histiocytes and T-lymphocytes.[41]

3 Granulomatous villitis is defined as a severe chronic villitis with numerous multinucleated histiocytic giant cells; well-formed granulomas are not usually present. Granulomatous villitis is non-specific, but has been reported with HSV, varicella, toxoplasmosis, tuberculosis, leprosy, Chagas' disease and blastomycosis (Fig. 33.51c).[42] In our experience, often no specific infectious organism is clinically or pathologically identified, suggesting that granulomatous villitis may often represent severe VUE.

4 Increased syncytial knots containing dozens of nuclei are found adjacent to placental infarcts, or dispersed unevenly throughout the placental parenchyma; either pattern strongly suggests chronic placental ischemia, particularly when present in premature placentas. 'Increased syncytial knots' (also called 'unevenly accelerated maturation' or 'placental hypermaturity') commonly coexist with low placental weight, decidual vasculopathy, placental infarction and maternal preeclampsia (Fig. 33.52).[5] Some authors have noted that increased numbers of

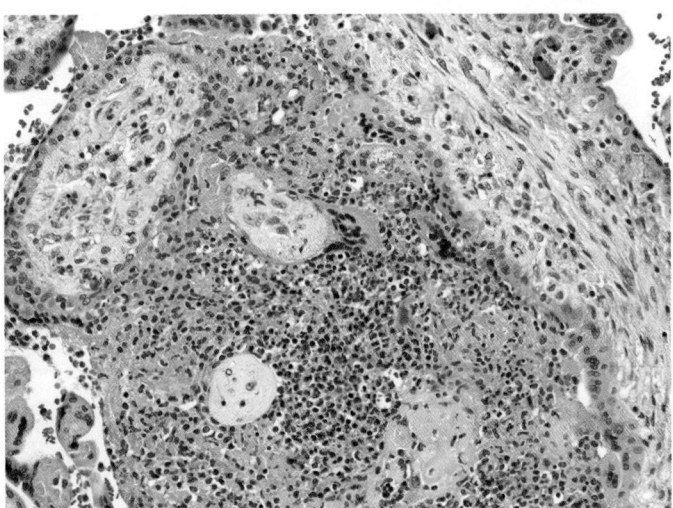

Fig. 33.50 Acute villitis and intervillositis associated with *Listeria*. Note the exudate between villi.

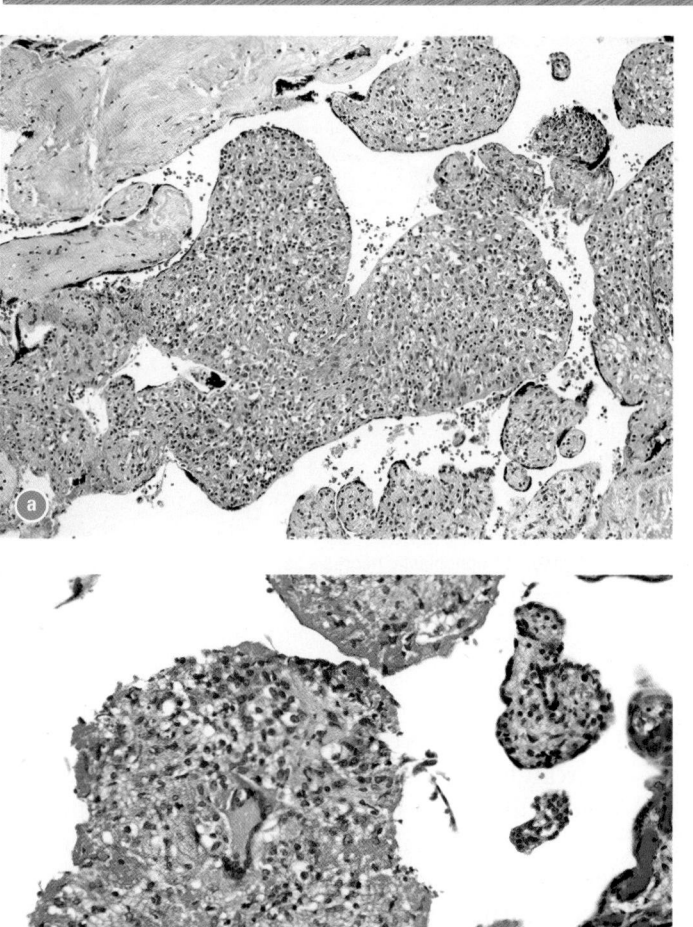

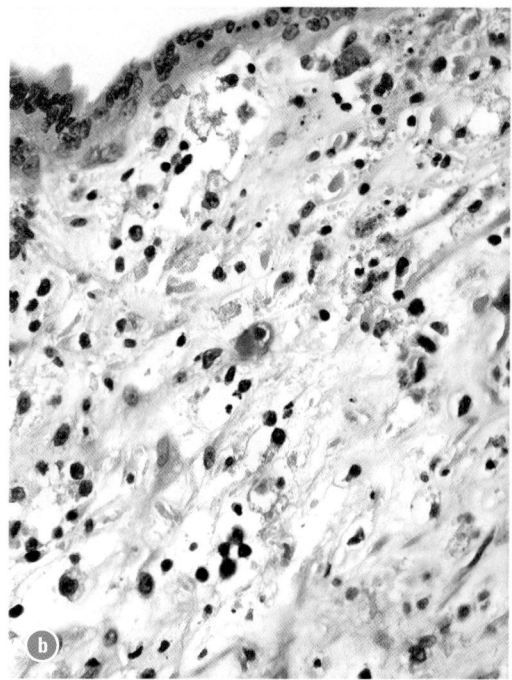

Fig. 33.51 (a) Chronic villitis is characterized by variable increases in mononuclear cells within terminal villi. (b) Cytomegalovirus infection may be subtle. In this case there is a single inclusion (center). (c) Like chronic villitis, granulomatous villitis is often non-specific. A giant cell is seen in the center.

cytotrophoblastic cells are found in terminal villi with chronic placental ischemia.

Trophoblastic necrosis is seen in areas of placental infarction. The earliest finding is syncytiotrophoblastic cytoplasmic eosinophilia; later, nuclear basophilia disappears, resulting in pink 'ghost' nuclei. When the intervillous space is locally collapsed, the presence of trophoblastic necrosis confirms an early infarct, rather than an artifact (Fig. 33.53).

5 Stromal edema in villi has two general appearances: (1) diffuse villous edema (villi are enlarged and edematous, with a clear, watery, relatively hypocellular stroma); and (2) multifocal, 'Swiss cheese' villous edema (scattered villi have multiple, small, round loculations of edema fluid, often containing a central Hofbauer cell in each loculation) (Fig. 33.54a,b). Diffuse villous edema is associated with fetal hydrops. Although the incidence of immune fetal hydrops (erythroblastosis fetalis) has recently sharply declined, occasional cases of immune erythroblastosis (Rh, Kell, Duffy, etc.) are seen. However, most current cases of diffuse placental edema and fetal hydrops are now of the 'non-immune' variety. Many such cases can be classified into one of the following 'top five' etiologies: (1) fetal cardiovascular disease (including arrhythmias); (2) fetal chromosome anomaly (most often trisomy 21 or 45,X); (3) fetal thoracic anomaly (including diaphragmatic hernia and congenital cystic adenomatoid malformation); (4) complications of twinning; and (5) severe fetal anemia (especially thalassemia).[43] Multifocal, 'Swiss cheese' villous edema is more poorly understood; Naeye et al. have proposed that such edema accumulates

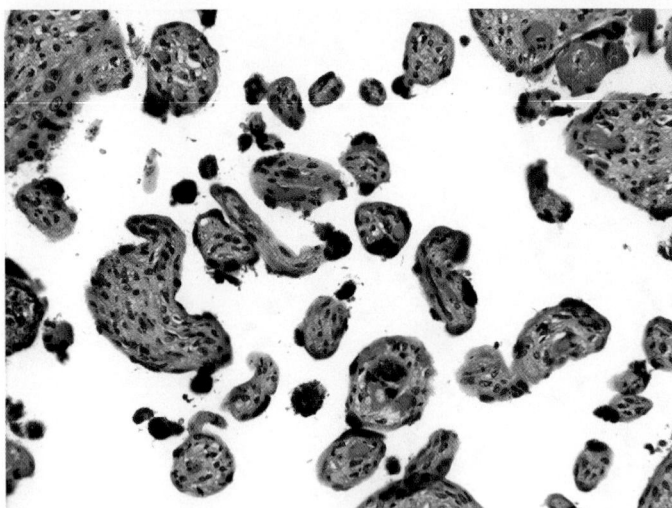

Fig. 33.52 Increased syncytial knots are associated with villous ischemia, including intrauterine growth restriction and toxemia.

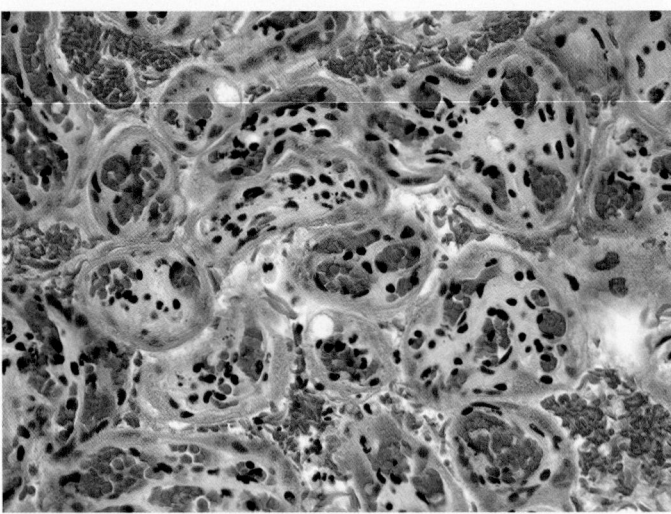

Fig. 33.53 Syncytial trophoblastic necrosis associated with a recent infarct.

rapidly, interferes with fetal oxygenation and may be a placental etiology of subacute or chronic fetal anoxia (Fig. 33.54b).[44]

6 Stromal fibrosis, in the form of increased stromal collagenization and fibroblast proliferation, is associated with interruption of the fetal circulation; the fetal capillaries of fibrotic villi are often collapsed or totally absent. Following vascular injury (thrombosis), villous fibrosis begins to develop after several days and becomes prominent after several weeks (Fig. 33.55). Regional villous fibrosis, suggestive of an upstream fetal thrombus, may be associated with significant fetal morbidity, including neurologic damage.[45] Diffuse villous fibrosis, involving all of the placenta, is strongly associated with remote fetal death.[46] Villous fibrosis is often accompanied by a fine, 'dusty' stromal calcification; although this calcific debris may closely mimic the appearance of bacteria, the absence of neutrophils should suggest that this is an artifact.

7 Stromal calcification can be coarse or fine. Course calcification may be present within villi or adjacent to villi; it has no clinical significance. As previously mentioned, fine calcification is often associated with villous fibrosis, fetal

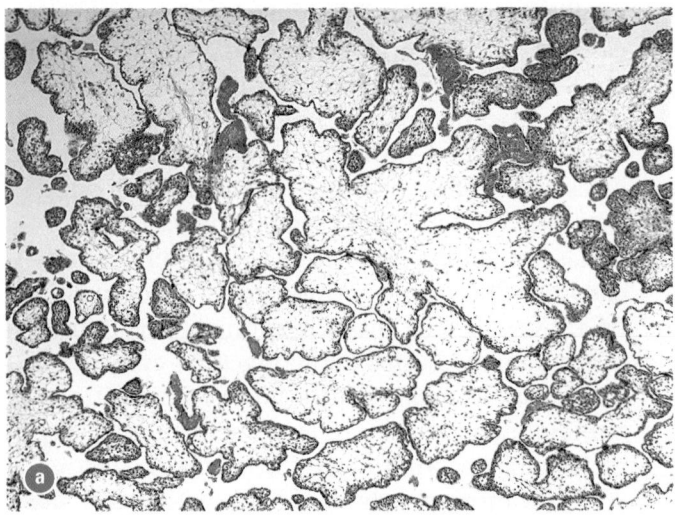

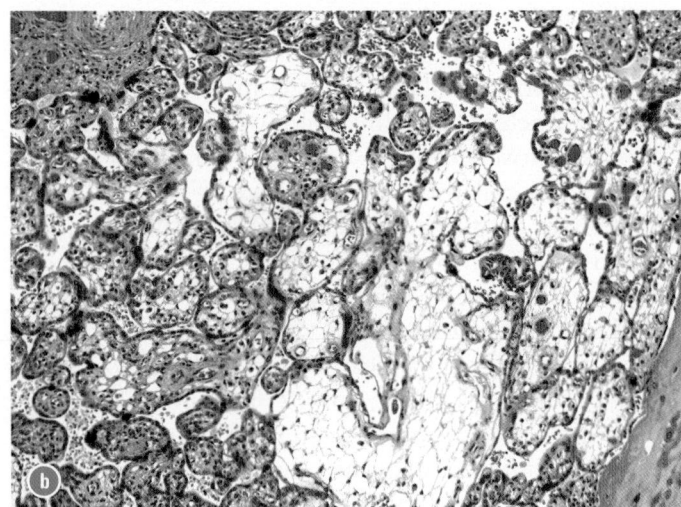

Fig. 33.54 Villous edema. (a) Diffuse edema associated with immune hydrops. (b) Focal edema associated with fetal hypoxia.

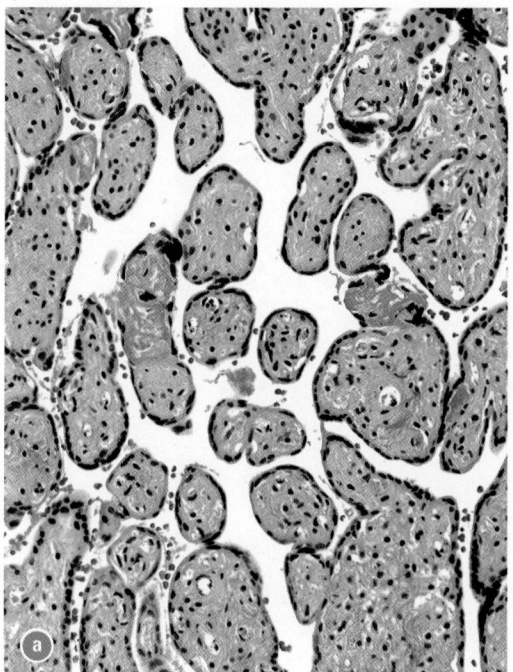
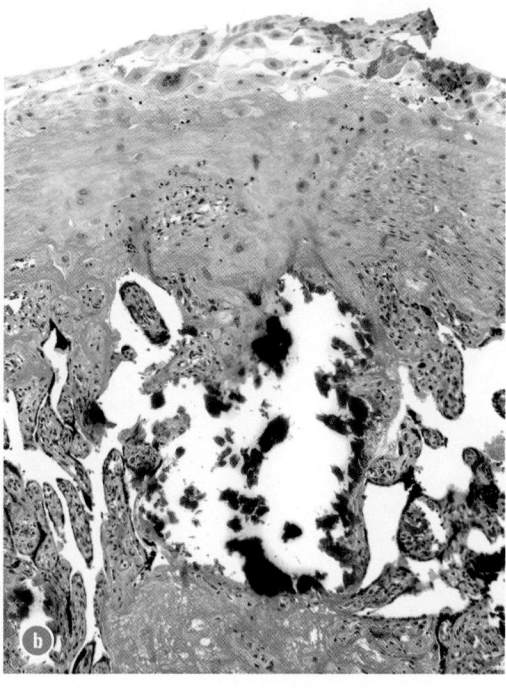

Fig. 33.55 Villous stromal fibrosis associated with fetal death or thrombosis (a) Calcifications are common late in pregnancy (b).

thrombosis, or fetal death. Fine calcification is characteristically distributed either in a linear fashion (along the trophoblastic basement membrane) or in a finely dispersed distribution throughout the villous stroma; its small, regular size can readily mimic bacteria.

8 Fetal capillary contents should always be inspected. As discussed above, fetal blood may contain increased nRBCs, erythroblasts, metastatic neuroblasts, fetal leukemic cells, parvovirally infected erythroblasts, or bacteria (Fig. 33.56).

9 Fetal capillary proliferation (chorangiosis). Chorangiosis is defined by Altshuler and Hyde as more than 10 capillary cross-sections present in more than 10 villi, at 10× magnification, in at least four placental regions. Chorangiosis has been related to maternal diabetes, toxemia, neonatal death, chronic anoxia and congenital anomalies, among other conditions (Fig. 33.57).[47]

10 Fetal capillary rupture (intravillous hemorrhage). With villous interstitial hemorrhage, the terminal villi resemble dilated 'bags of blood'. Villous hemorrhage follows placental trauma (i.e. manual placental extraction). Villous hemorrhage is also highly associated with acute abruptio placentae (Fig. 33.58).[48]

11 Selective fetal capillary obliteration with concentric fibrosis or onion skinning may be seen in association with syphilis (Fig. 33.59).

Additional features, such as enlarged villi with chronic villitis, should also be present.

12 Malignancy (including intraplacental choriocarcinoma) may displace villi or be seen in the intravillous space (see below and Chs 32 and 34) (Fig. 33.60).

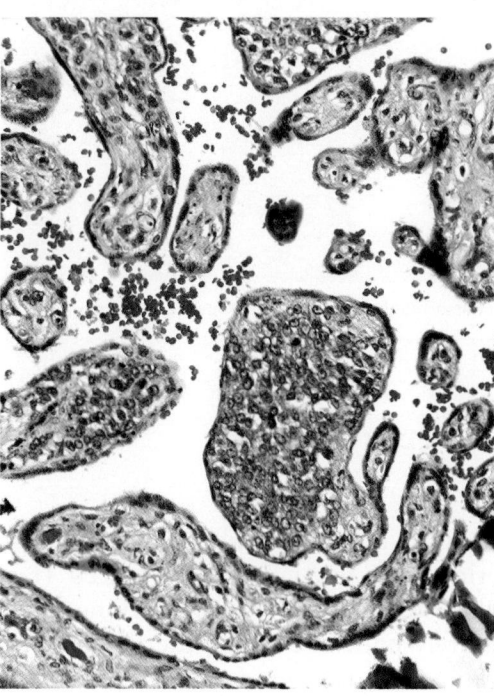

Fig. 33.56 Fetal leukemia present as clusters of blasts infiltrating villous parenchyma.

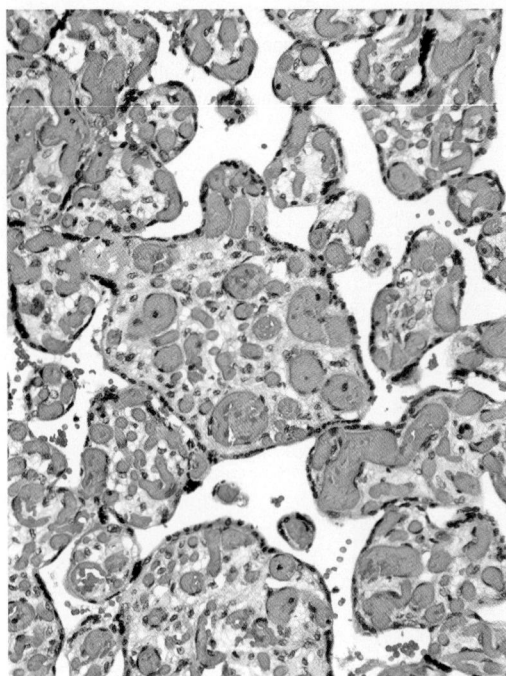

Fig. 33.57 Chorangiosis, seen with a high density of villous vessels.

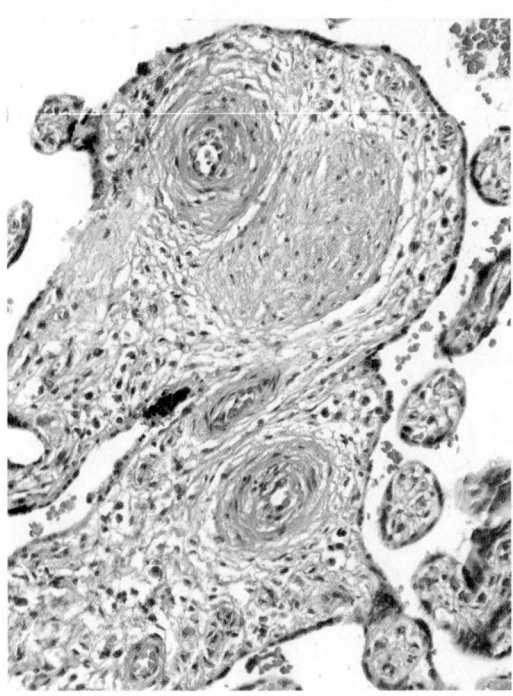

Fig. 33.59 Concentric fibrosis of villous vessels associated with syphilis.

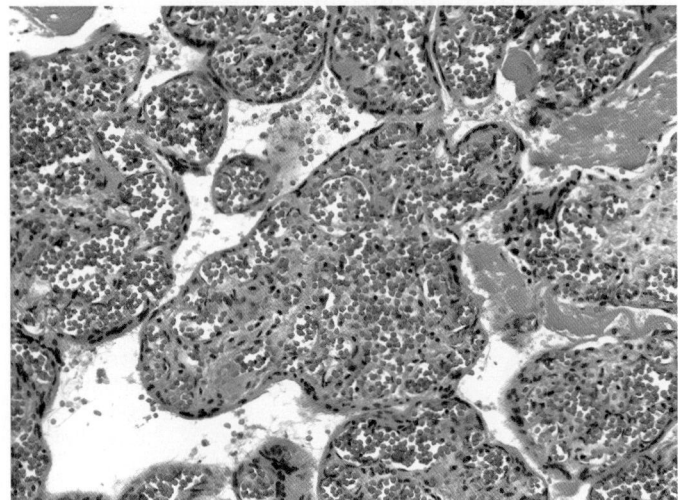

Fig. 33.58 Intravillous hemorrhage associated with recent abruption.

next, the cytotrophoblastic cells differentiate into intermediate trophoblastic cells, which move out into the fibrin layer (much like the intermediate trophoblastic cells of the implantation site permeate through Nitabuch's fibrin) (see below and Fig. 33.43). This is a normal (physiologic) response.

Conditions

1 Collapse of the intervillous space occurs in the setting of infarction, when the neighboring villi become crowded or touch one another.

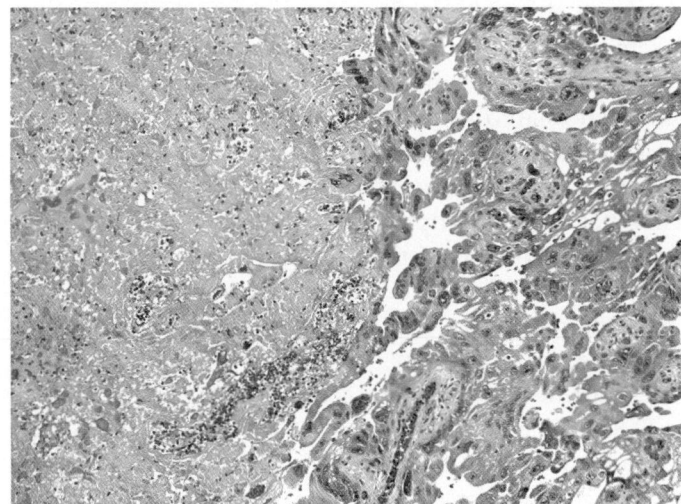

Fig. 33.60 Intraplacental choriocarcinoma (right) adjacent to infarct (left).

INTERVILLOUS SPACE

Definition

The intervillous space is normally filled with maternal blood and fibrin, with the villi evenly spaced (i.e. neighboring villi usually do not touch one another). When fibrin entirely encases a villus, the villous syncytiotrophoblastic covering gradually degenerates;

Eventually, an area of infarction develops. Placental infarcts result from localized interruption of the maternal blood supply, which causes a regional collapse of the intervillous space (Fig. 33.61a–c). The underlying cause may be maternal vascular disease (thrombus in an underlying decidual vessel; vasculopathy) or abruptio placentae. The latter may produce classic 'ball in socket' infarcts composed of a concentric rim of infracteded placenta encasing fibrinous material (Fig. 33.62). Although small infarcts in term placentas are common and possibly 'normal', any infarct in a premature placenta is distinctly abnormal. Large infarcts at term (>3 cm in diameter) are also definitely abnormal and are associated with serious perinatal morbidity and mortality. Extensive placental infarction (10–50% of the parenchyma) may be responsible for fetal death.

2 Fibrin can be seen in the intervillous space in four forms, comprising fresh intervillous thrombi (laminated blood clots which push villi to the periphery); nodular perivillous fibrin deposits; 'extensive' perivillous fibrin deposits (occupying approximately 25–50% of the intervillous space); and placental fibrinous septae (structures contiguous with the basal fibrinous layer) (Fig. 33.63a,b).

- Intervillous thrombi (IVTs) are seen in about one-third of uncomplicated pregnancies (Fig. 33.44a).[49] They apparently result from small, localized fetal-to-maternal hemorrhages (FMHs); admixtures of fetal and maternal blood cells have been documented in IVTs by immunohistochemistry.[50]
- Nodular perivillous fibrin begins as an intravillous, subtrophoblastic fibrinous zone,

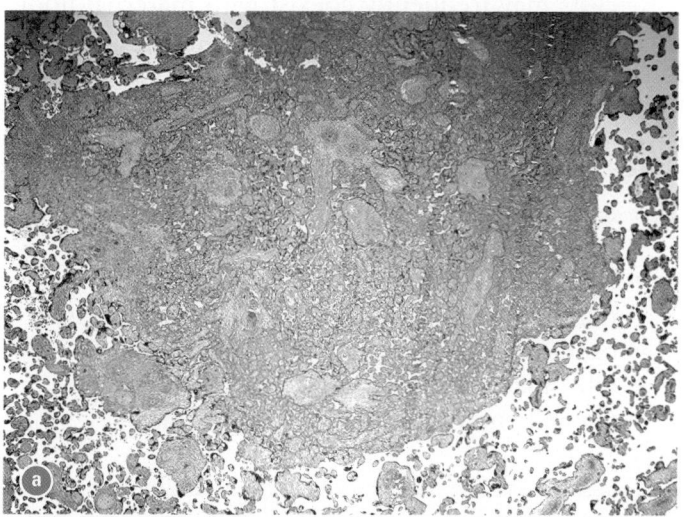
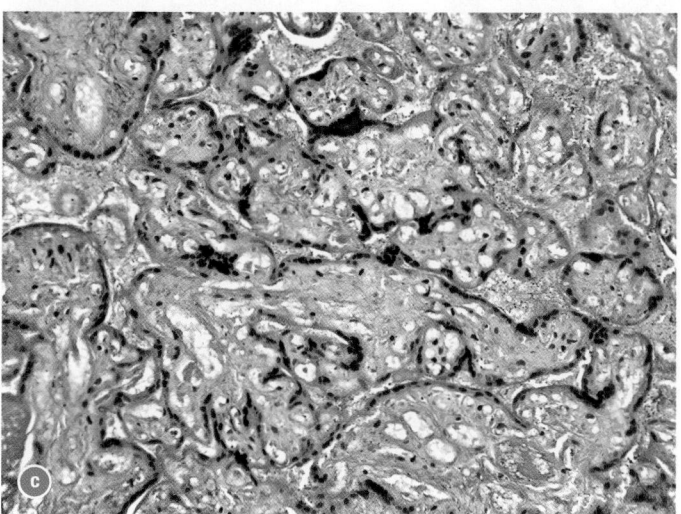
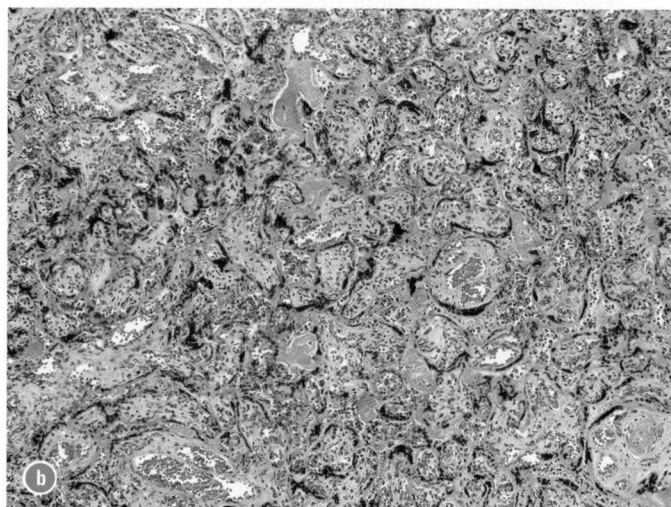

Fig. 33.61 Placental infarcts. (a) Low-power view of discrete infarct. (b,c) Higher-power images illustrate trophoblastic necrosis and collapse of the villi.

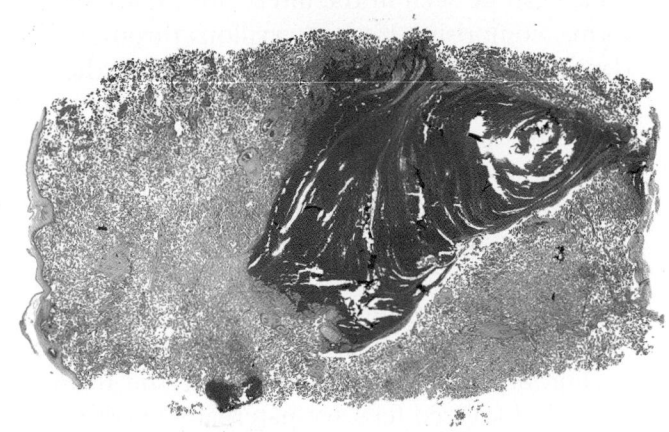

Fig. 33.62 'Ball in socket' infarct associated with abruption and subjacent intervillous thrombus.

which gradually extends to the intervillous space. The syncytiotrophoblastic covering of the adjacent villi degenerates. The intervillous fibrin is eventually invaded by intermediate trophoblastic cells (Fig. 33.63a,b). A small number of such nodular fibrinous regions is normally seen in most placentas. The functional significance (if any) of these areas is unknown. On occasion, very bizarre degenerative atypia is found in the intermediate trophoblastic nuclei; this striking focal finding has not been associated with adverse sequelae.

- Extensive perivillous fibrin is defined as a very significant percentage of the intervillous space (>25–50%) involved by dense perivillous fibrin deposition; maternal placental oxygenation may be compromised (Fig. 33.64a,b). Such extensive perivillous fibrin deposition appears to be related to fetal growth retardation, fetal death and possibly recurrent poor pregnancy outcome. The precise definition of this condition is elusive; however, and its pathogenesis is also uncertain. This is referred to as 'gitterinfarct' by Benirschke and Kaufmann, who regard this condition as closely related to (if not identical to) maternal floor infarction (Fig. 33.64c).

- Placental fibrinous septae. Ribbons of eosinophilic fibrin which are contiguous with Nitabuch's fibrin. Placental septae are diffusely infiltrated by numerous intermediate trophoblastic cells, with clear to eosinophilic cytoplasm (Fig. 33.65). Focal central cystic degeneration of placental septae is common. Placental septae are normal placental structures with no pathologic significance; however, large numbers of septal cysts may frequently coexist with maternal floor infarction.

3 Maternal blood occasionally will yield a specific pathologic diagnosis.

- Sickled maternal RBCs are easily identified with sickle cell trait/disease; malarial parasites can be easily visualized on conventional H&E staining (Fig. 33.66).

- Metastatic tumor rarely may be present in the maternal intervillous space (metastatic breast cancer is most common).

- Chronic intervillositis, also called 'massive chronic intervillositis' (MCI), is a rare

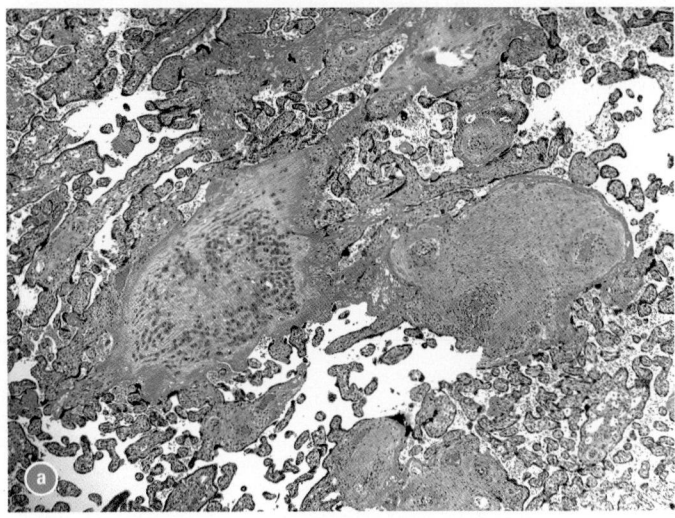
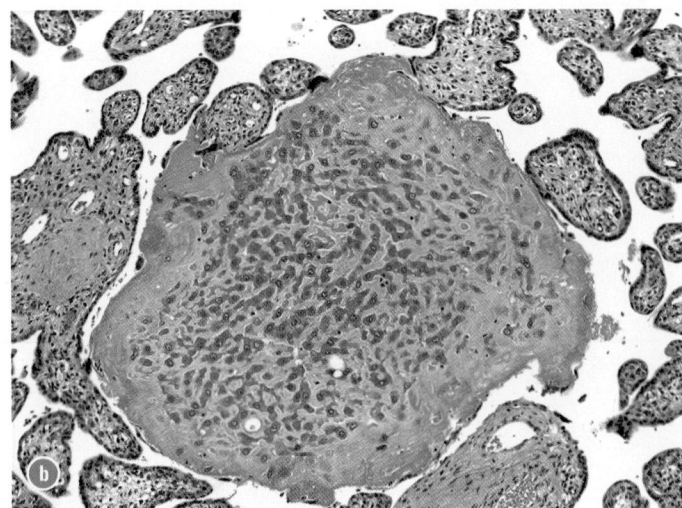

Fig. 33.63 (a) Low- and (b) high-power views of intervillous fibrin with associated intermediate trophoblast, frequently encountered in the normal placental disc.

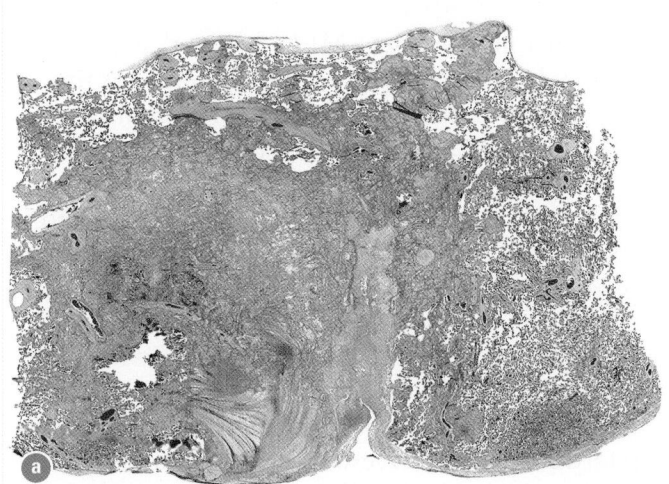

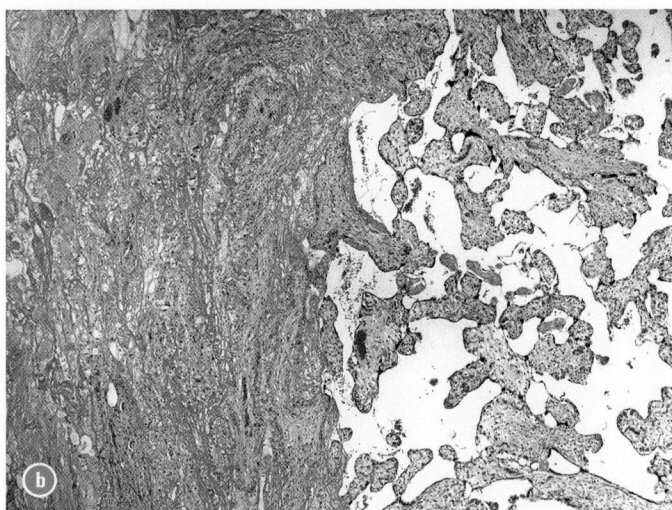

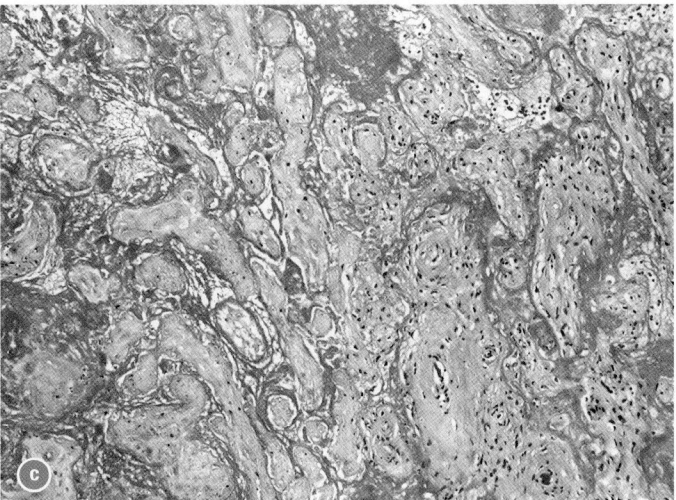

Fig. 33.64 (a) Maternal floor infarct, with extensive intervillous fibrin extending upward from the maternal floor. (b) Interface of normal villi and extensive fibrin, characterizing either maternal floor infarct or massive intervillous fibrin. (c) High power; both are characterized by extensive fibrin deposition with preservation of the villous architecture (compare with Figs 33.61 and 33.62).

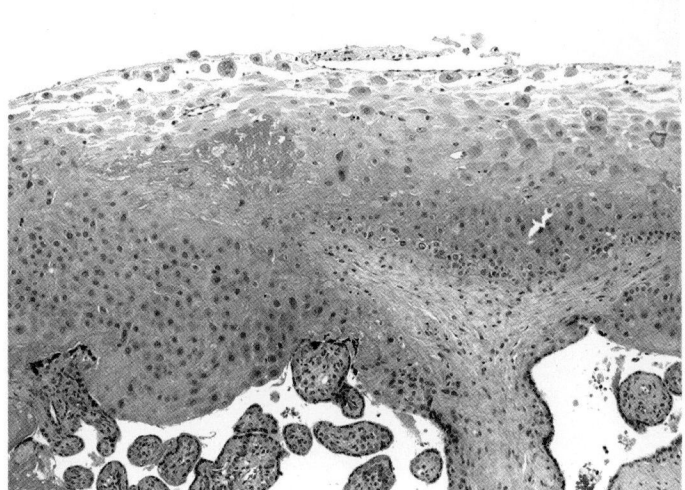

Fig. 33.65 Basal plate (upper) and placental septae.

abnormality characterized by large numbers of mononuclear cells within the maternal intervillous space, often accompanied by abundant fibrin (Fig. 33.67a,b).[51] Mononuclear cells are predominantly monocytes/macrophages with scattered lymphocytes (predominantly T-cells). MCI is highly associated with fetal growth retardation and fetal death; it may also be a cause of recurrent abortion.[52]

BASAL PLATE (MATERNAL SURFACE)

Definition

The layers of the basal plate include: (1) basal 'anchoring' villi, (2) Nitabuch's fibrin (eosinophilic layer between placenta and deciduas) and (3) the deciduas,

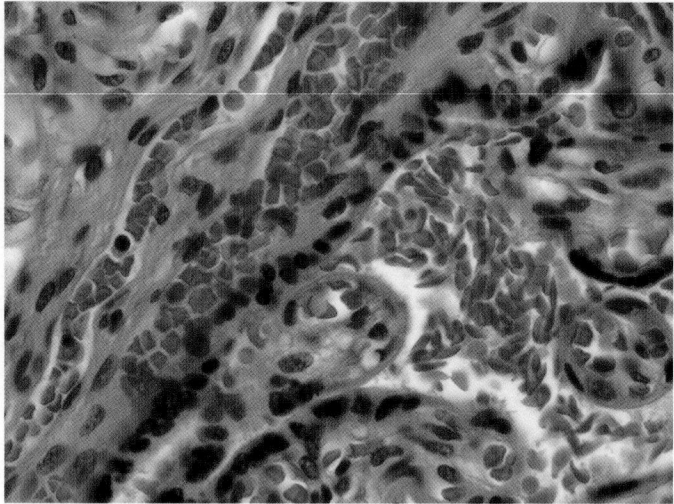

Fig. 33.66 Sickled erythrocytes in the maternal space (center). Compare with erythrocytes in the fetal circulation (left).

ranging from scant to full thickness (with abundant maternal vessels, decidualized stroma, endometrial glands and superficial myometrium). Both Nitabuch's fibrin and the deciduas are diffusely infiltrated by intermediate trophoblastic cells, which are motile, spindle-shaped, predominantly mononuclear cells, with a clear to eosinophilic cytoplasm (mimicking decidual stromal cells); the nuclei are variable, ranging from oval and vesicular to angulated and hyperchromatic. Some trophoblastic cells have multiple nuclei (implantation site giant cells).

Conditions

1 Maternal floor infarct (MFI). Defined as a grossly visible, leathery plaque occupying much of the maternal surface; histologically, MFIs consist of extensive fibrin deposition in the deciduas and the adjacent intervillous space (Figs 33.26, 33.64c). MFI is idiopathic, but has been strongly related to stillbirth, fetal growth retardation and possible recurrence.[22]

2 Maternal vasculopathy. Abnormalities of basal decidual spiral arterioles are associated with preeclampsia, diabetes, collagen vascular diseases, lupus anticoagulant and 'idiopathic' fetal growth retardation. Only severe lesions can be easily recognized in the basal plate (acute atherosis), characterized by marked vascular dilatation, fibrinoid necrosis of the intima and media, numerous lipid-laden macrophages within the vessel wall and perivascular chronic inflammation (Fig. 33.68a).

3 Decidual inflammation is common, variable and usually non-specific. However, severe plasma cell deciduitis may be associated with congenital syphilis (Fig. 33.68b).

4 Decidual hemorrhage. Fresh retroplacental blood clot is common; it is easily detached and is not associated with adjacent placental compression, villous hemorrhage or infarction. Large, firm, adherent blood clots suggest abruptio placentae; often there is a localized placental depression and histologic evidence of ischemia (either acute villous

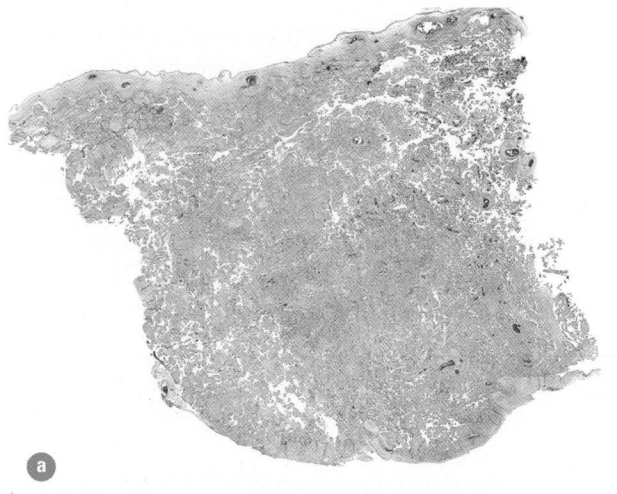

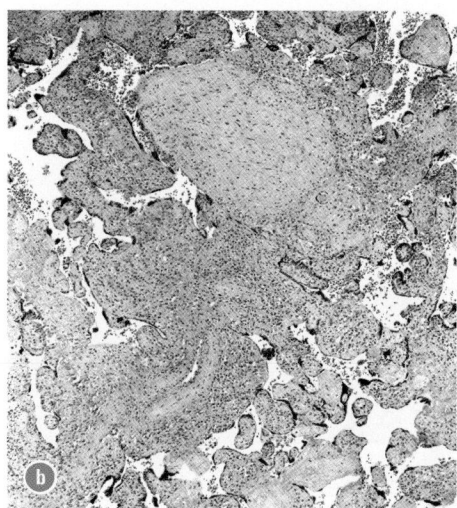

Fig. 33.67 (a) Massive chronic intervillositis. (b) Higher power showing extensive infiltrates of mononuclear cells in the maternal space coalescing with villi.

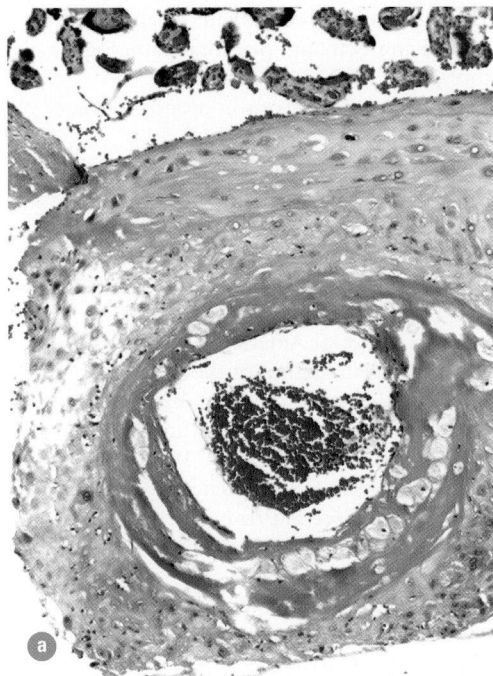

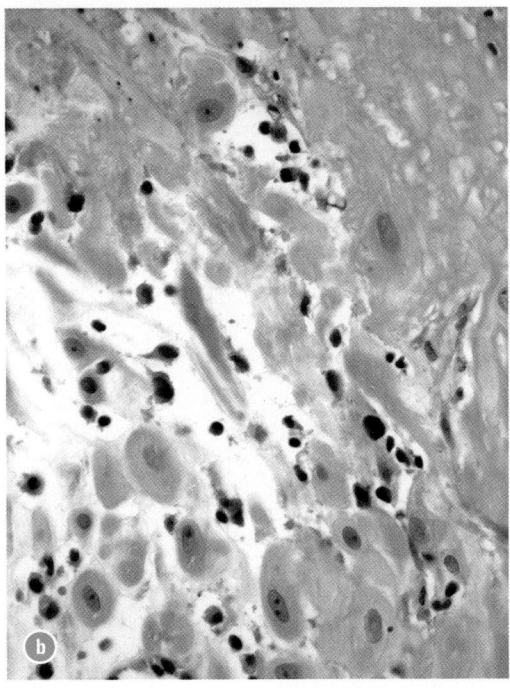

Fig. 33.68 (a) Decidual vasculopathy in the decidua on the maternal surface of the placenta. (b) Like chronic villitis, chronic inflammation with plasma cells (chronic deciduitis) may be associated with infection, but is considered non–specific.

interstitial hemorrhage or placental infarction). With very acute abruptio placenta, there may be no findings in the adjacent placenta (approximately 25–50% of cases). With more remote abruptio placentae, blood enters the amniotic fluid ('port wine' amniotic fluid); eventually, hemosiderin-laden macrophages are present within the amnion and chorion. Abruptio placentae is highly associated with maternal hypertension due to decidual vascular rupture; less commonly, abruptio placentae may follow maternal trauma (particularly automobile accidents) (Fig. 33.69a–c).

5 Decidual absence (placenta creta). With placenta creta, the deciduas is absent (at least focally);

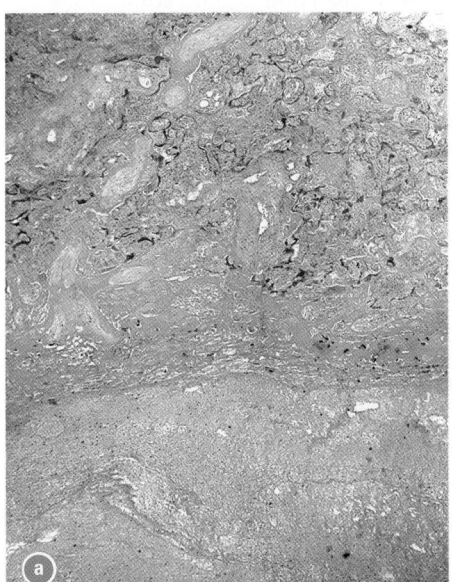

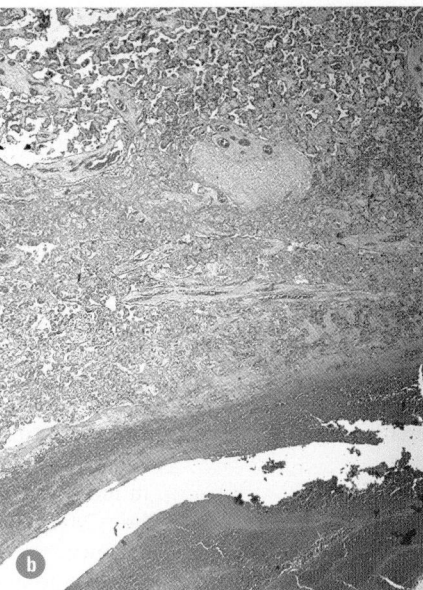

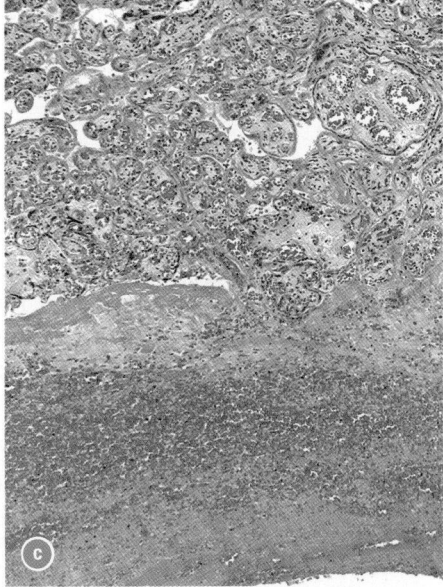

Fig. 33.69 Retroplacental hemorrhage. (a) Recent abruption with hemorrhage (lower) and ischemic adjacent placental parenchyma (upper). (b) Abruption (lower) with subjacent infarct (center) and healthy placental parenchyma (upper). (c) Higher power of the transition between retroplacental thrombus (lower) and recently infarcted placental tissue (upper).

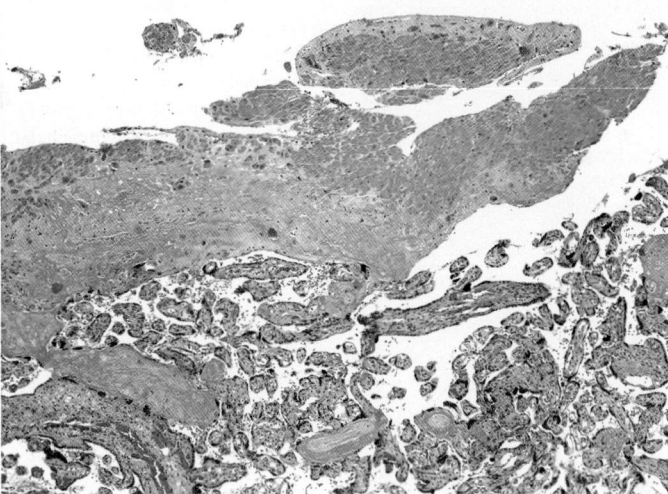

Fig. 33.70 Muscle fibers in basal plate above the maternal surface suggest creta.

histologically, Nitabuch's fibrin and basal villi come into direct contact with the underlying myometrium (Fig. 33.70). Because intermediate trophoblastic cells may closely resemble the appearance of decidualized stromal cells, this diagnosis can be difficult; keratin immunoperoxidase stains can be helpful (all trophoblastic cells are strongly cytokeratin immunoreactive, but decidual stromal cells are negative for cytokeratins).

References

1 Naeye RL. Disorders of the placenta, fetus and neonate: Diagnosis and clinical significance. St Louis: Mosby; 1992.

2 Naeye RL. Umbilical cord length: clinical significance. J Pediatr 1985; 107(2):278–281.

3 Naeye RL. The clinical significance of absent subchorionic fibrin in the placenta. Am J Clin Pathol 1990; 94:196–198.

4 Altshuler G, Deppisch LM. College of American Pathologists Conference XIX on the Examination of the Placenta: Report of the Working Group on Indications for Placental Examination. Arch Pathol Lab Med 1991; 115:701–703.

5 Naeye RL. Functionally important disorders of the placenta, umbilical cord and fetal membranes. Hum Pathol 1987; 18:680–691.

6 Driscoll SG. Placental examination in a clinical setting. Arch Pathol Lab Med 1991; 115:668–671.

7 Cordry RD. Placental evidence in malpractice litigation Plaintiff's case. Arch Pathol Lab Med 1991; 115:682–684.

8 Altshuler G. Placenta within the medicolegal imperative. Arch Pathol Lab Med 1991; 115:688–695.

9 Bejar R, Wozniak P, Allard M, et al. Antenatal origin of neurologic damage in newborn infants. I. Preterm infants. Am J Obstet Gynecol 1988; 159:357–363.

10 Benirschke K. Intrauterine death of a twin: mechanisms, implications for surviving twin and placental pathology. Sem Diagn Pathol 1993; 10:222–231.

11 Grafe MR. Antenatal cerebral necrosis in monochorionic twins. Pediatr Pathol 1993; 13:15–19.

12 Grafe MR. The correlation of prenatal brain damage with placental pathology. J Neuropathol Exp Neurol 1994; 53:407–415.

13 Schindler NR. Importance of the placenta and cord in the defense of neurologically impaired infant claims. Arch Pathol Lab Med 1991; 115(7):685–687.

14 Naeye R, Travers H. College of American Pathologists Conference XIX on the Examination of the Placenta: Report of the Working Group on the Role of the Pathologist in Malpractice Litigation Involving the Placenta. Arch Pathol Lab Med 1991; 115(7):717–719.

15 Genest DR, Granter S, Pinkus GS. Umbilical cord 'pseudo-vasculitis' following second trimester fetal death: a clinicopathological and immunohistochemical study of 13 cases. Histopathology 1997; 30(6):563–569.

16 Torfs CP, van den Berg B, Oechsli FW, Cummins S. Prenatal and perinatal factors in the etiology of cerebral palsy. J Pediatr 1990; 116(4):615–619.

17 Naeye RL. Do placental weights have clinical significance? Hum Pathol 1987; 18:387–391.

18 Benirschke K, Kaufmann P. Pathology of the human placenta, 4th edn. New York: Springer-Verlag; 2000.

19 Miller PW, Coen RW, Benirschke K. Dating the time interval from meconium passage to birth. Obstet Gynecol 1985; 66:459–62.

20 Altshuler G, Arizawa M, Molnar-Nadasdy G. Meconium-induced umbilical cord vascular necrosis and ulceration: a potential link between the placenta and poor pregnancy outcome. Obstet Gynecol 1992; 79:760–766.

21 Shanklin DR, Scott JS. Massive subchorial thrombohaematoma (Breus' mole). Br J Obstet Gynaecol 1975; 82:476–487.

22 Naeye RL. Maternal floor infarction. Hum Pathol 1985; 16:823–828.

23 Baldwin VJ. Pathology of multiple pregnancy. New York: Springer-Verlag; 1993.

24 Bajoria R, Wigglesworth J, Fisk NM. Angioarchitecture of monochorionic placentas in relation to the twin-twin transfusion syndrome. Am J Obstet Gynecol 1995; 172:856–863.

25 Bendon RW. Twin transfusion: pathological studies of the monochorionic placenta in liveborn twins and of the perinatal autopsy in monochorionic twin pairs. Pediatr Pathol Lab Med 1995; 15:363–376.

26 Benson CB, Bieber FR, Genest DR, Doubilet PM. Doppler demonstration of reversed umbilical blood flow in an acardiac twin. J Clin Ultrasound 1989; 1989; 17:291–295.

27 Boyd T, Blatman R, Greene M, Genest DR. Twin-twin transfusion is related to velamentous umbilical cord insertion in monochorionic twins. Mod Pathol 1994; 7:270.

28 Fries MH, Goldstein RB, Kilpatrick SJ, et al. The role of velamentous cord insertion in the etiology of twin-twin transfusion syndrome. Obstet Gynecol 1993; 81:569–574.

29 Miller PW, Coen RW, Benirschke K. Dating the time interval from meconium passage to birth. Obstet Gynecol 1985; 66:459–462.

30 Ariel IB, Landing BH. A possibly distinctive vacuolar change of the amniotic epithelium associated with gastroschisis. Pediatr Pathol 1985; 3(2–4):283–289.

31 Sander CH. Hemorrhagic endovasculitis and hemorrhagic villitis of the placenta. Arch Pathol Lab Med 1980; 104(7): 371–373.

32 Novak PM, Sander CM, Yang SS, von Oeyen PT. Report of fourteen cases of nonimmune hydrops fetalis in association with hemorrhagic endovasculitis of the placenta. Am J Obstet Gynecol 1991; 165:945–950.

33 Shanklin DR, Scott JS. Massive subchorial thrombohaematoma (Breus' mole). Br J Obstet Gynaecol 1975; 82:476–487.

34 Roberts DJ, Ampola MG, Lage JM. Diagnosis of unsuspected fetal metabolic storage disease by routine placental examination. Pediatr Pathol 1991; 11(4):647–656.

35 Singer DB, Campognone P. Perinatal group B streptococcal infection in midgestation. Pediatr Pathol 1986; 5:271–276.

36 Genest DR, Choi-Hong SR, Tate JE, et al. Diagnosis of congenital syphilis from placental examination: comparison of histopathology, Steiner stain, and polymerase chain reaction for *Treponema pallidum* DNA. Hum Pathol 1996; 27(4):366–372.

37 Qureshi F, Jacques SM, Reyes MP. Placental histopathology in syphilis. Hum Pathol 1993; 24:779–784.

38 Kaplan C, Lowell DM, Salafia C. College of American Pathologists Conference XIX on the Examination of the Placenta: Report of the Working Group on the Definition of Structural Changes Associated with Abnormal Function in the Maternal/Fetal/Placental Unit in the Second and Third Trimesters. Arch Pathol Lab Med 1991; 115:709–715.

39 Redline RW, Abramowsky CR. Clinical and pathologic aspects of recurrent placental villitis. Hum Pathol 1985; 16(7):727–731.

40 Labarre C, Sebastiani M, Siminovich M, et al. Absence of Wharton's jelly around the umbilical cord; an unusual cause of perinatal mortality. Placenta 1985; 6:555–559.

41 Redline RW, Patterson P. Villitis of unknown etiology is associated with major infiltration of fetal tissue by maternal inflammatory cells. Am J Pathol 1993; 143:473–479.

42 Popek EJ. Granulomatous villitis due to *Toxoplasma gondii*. Pediatr Pathol 1992; 12:281–288.

43 Machin GA. Hydrops revisited: literature review of 1,414 cases published in the 1980s. Am J Med Genet 1989; 34:366–390.

44 Naeye RL, Maisels J, Lorenz RP, Botti JJ. The clinical significance of placental villous edema. Pediatrics 1983; 71:588–594.

45 Redline RW, Pappin A. Fetal thrombotic vasculopathy: the clinical significance of extensive avascular villi. Hum Pathol 1995; 26:80–85.

46 Genest DR. Estimating the time of death in stillborn fetuses: II. Histologic evaluation of the placenta; a study of 71 newborns. Obstet Gynecol 1992; 80(4):585–592.

47 Altshuler G, Hyde SR. Clinicopathologic implications of placental pathology. Clin Obstet Gynecol 1996; 39(3):549–570.

48 Mooney EE, al Shunnar A, O'Regan M, Gillan JE. Chorionic villous haemorrhage is associated with retroplacental haemorrhage. Br J Obstet Gynaecol 1994; 101(11):965–969.

49 Fox H, Elston CW. Pathology of the placenta. Major Probl Pathol 1978; 7:1–491.

50 Kaplan C, Blanc WA, Elias J. Identification of erythrocytes in intervillous thrombi: a study using immunoperoxidase identification of hemoglobins. Hum Pathol 1982; 13:554–557.

51 Jacques SM, Qureshi F. Chronic intervillositis of the placenta. Arch Pathol Lab Med 1993; 117(10):1032–1035.

52 Genest DR. Massive chronic intervillositis associated with recurrent abortions. Hum Pathol 1995; 26(11):1245–1251.

34

Gestational diseases and the placenta

Mana M. Parast and

David R. Genest

Introduction

Late abortion (13–19 weeks gestation)

Late spontaneous abortion
Second trimester fetal death
Late elective abortion for fetal
  anomalies

Premature birth or accelerated delivery

Acute chorioamnionitis
Abruptio placentae
Cervical incompetence

Operative or induced delivery for maternal or fetal disorders

Toxemia of pregnancy
Intrauterine growth restriction
Maternal diabetes
Immune and non-immune hydrops
Fetal distress

The placenta in the setting of the malformed fetus

Background
Single umbilical artery
Amnion nodosum

The placenta in fetal death

Primary placental disorders
Placental pathology secondary
  to fetal death

The placenta in multiple gestations

Establishing chorionicity
Twin-twin transfusion syndrome
Other complications of twinning

Tumors in the placenta seen at term

Chorangioma
Choriocarcinoma
Placental site trophoblastic tumor
Metastatic carcinoma
Congenital leukemia

Peri- or post-partum hemorrhage (including gravid hysterectomy)

Background and clinical
  presentation
Placenta previa
Creta

Introduction

The purpose of this chapter is to integrate the most common clinical scenarios faced in obstetrical practice with the pathologic examination of the placenta. Because much of this has been covered descriptively in Chapter 33, this chapter will to a limited degree illustrate additional examples of pathologic entities, grouping them together under their respective disorders. In addition, the chapter will outline the expected findings for each disease or constellation of clinical findings.

Late abortion (13–19 weeks gestation)

Semantically, late abortion, which occurs in the first half of the second trimester, appears to be closely related to early, or first trimester, abortion. However, from etiologic and clinicopathologic perspectives, late abortion bears little resemblance to first trimester abortion and more closely resembles premature birth.

First, a chromosomal disorder is the etiology of a large percentage (50–60%) of early abortions, but an infrequent pathogenesis of late abortion, found in less than 5% of cases studied. Secondly, first trimester abortion specimens rarely have histopathologic findings causally related to the abortion and infrequently have evaluable fetuses; in contrast, late abortion specimens always have fetal remains and commonly show placental or fetal abnormalities etiologically related to the pregnancy loss. Clinicopathologic similarities in placentas from late abortions and premature births include high prevalences of acute chorioamnionitis and placental abruption.

Late abortion specimens can be divided into three major groups, based on their clinical presentations (Table 34.1):

1 *Late spontaneous (inevitable) abortions*, which follow unplanned deliveries and frequently contain normally developed, well-preserved (possibly fragmented) fetal tissues.
2 *Intrauterine fetal deaths* (IUFD), usually following induced or instrumented deliveries and typically containing macerated, or autolyzed, fetal remains and
3 *Elective abortions for fetal structural or chromosomal anomalies*, usually following induced or instrumented deliveries and characteristically

containing fetal tissues which are well preserved (possibly fragmented) with identifiable congenital anomalies.

LATE SPONTANEOUS ABORTION

Late spontaneous abortion clinically resembles premature labor, in that patients with both conditions frequently present with symptoms suggestive of chorioamnionitis or abruption, including vaginal bleeding, premature rupture of the membranes, cervical incompetence and maternal sepsis.

Gross fragmentation is characteristic of placentas from late abortions, because of the marked fragility of very immature placentas. Despite fragmentation, it is important to grossly identify and histologically sample the chorionic plate of the placenta, umbilical cord, normal placental parenchyma and any placental regions involved by hematomas or other gross lesions. The most commonly encountered placental pathologic disorders in late spontaneous abortions include acute chorioamnionitis and acute abruptio placentae. The former may be related to a third disorder, cervical incompetence. The pathologic features of these placental disorders are identical to those described in the next section ('Premature Birth'), with some minor but important exceptions.

Second trimester abruption

In instances where placental abruption is suspected clinically (because of vaginal bleeding, or a sonographic finding of retroplacental or subchorionic hematoma), fragmentation of the placenta may preclude gross confirmation. Characteristic features of acute abruption in very early gestations include the following: (a) Dissecting intervillous hematoma distorts the placental villous architecture, as it expands into the placental parenchyma

Table 34.1 Second trimester abortion

Clinical presentation	Condition
Inevitable abortion	Acute chorioamnionitis Abruption
IUFD	Remote abruption Viral infection (TORCH, parvovirus)
Fetal anomalies	Malformations Deformities (amnion rupture)

IUFD, intrauterine fetal deaths; TORCH (*t*oxoplasmosis, *o*ther, *r*ubella, *c*ytomegalovirus and *h*erpes simplex) stands for a series of bacterial, viral and parasitic pathogens that can produce a congenital or perinatally acquired infection.

to sometimes reach and lift the chorionic plate (massive subchorionic hematoma, 'Breus' mole') (Fig. 34.1a). This contrasts with the characteristic depression seen in a late abruption, largely because the immature placenta lacks an established villous support network to discourage upward dissection. (b) Intravillous hemorrhage is another common feature of acute abruption and may aid in distinguishing this condition from incidental hemorrhage (Fig. 34.1b). The reader is reminded that intravillous hemorrhage may be the only finding if the specimen is fragmented or the blood clot is not provided with the specimen. Other histologic features of abruption may also be present, including hemosiderin within the membranes and early infarction. However, these are usually associated with subacute or older retroplacental hemorrhage.[1]

A typical final pathologic diagnosis might read as follows: 'Well-developed, well-preserved female fetus (130 g, 14 cm crown rump length, 1.8 cm foot length), consistent with 18 weeks gestational age; no congenital malformations are identified; fragmented, immature placenta with intraplacental hematoma with adjacent villous infarction, consistent with acute placental abruption'.

Acute chorioamnionitis

The findings in acute chorioamnionitis in the second trimester are similar to those seen later in pregnancy, with the exception that the placenta may be fragmented and less amenable to examination. If membranes and cord are not readily available, examination of the chorionic plate for subchorionitis will confirm amniotic fluid infection. However, a well-preserved stillborn fetus consistent with intra-partum death will provide important clues to the pathogenesis. The pathologist should grossly check the fetus' gender, evaluate the extent of development and look for malformations. Congenital anomalies, extensive maceration and evidence of growth restriction are uncommonly seen in late spontaneous abortion specimens. A variety of fetal tissues should be routinely histologically assessed, including lung, gastrointestinal tract, gonad, liver and kidney. When acute chorioamnionitis is seen in the placenta, histologic assessment of the fetal gut and lungs will usually demonstrate intraluminal/intra-alveolar neutrophils and may occasionally show bacteria. Less commonly, evidence of fetal sepsis, including intravascular bacteria, fetal pneumonia and cutaneous and parenchymal micro abscesses should prompt a search for infections that accompany acute villitis, including listeria, beta strep and others (Fig. 34.2). The surgical pathologic report of a late spontaneous abortion specimen should incorporate information about the fetus (including gender, estimated gestational age (EGA) and malformations) as well as the placenta.

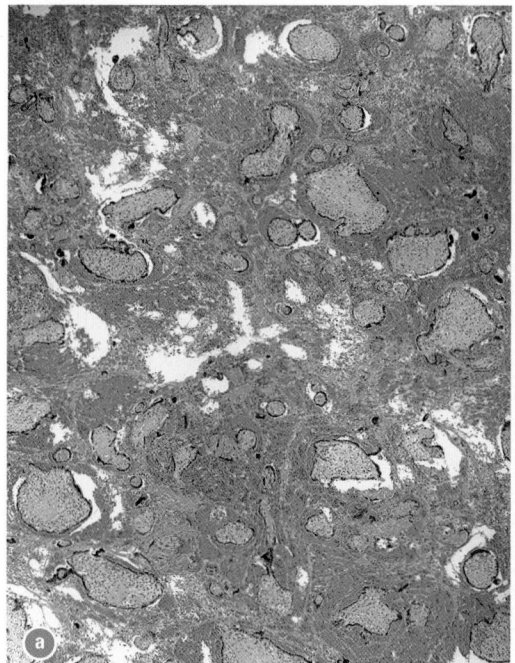 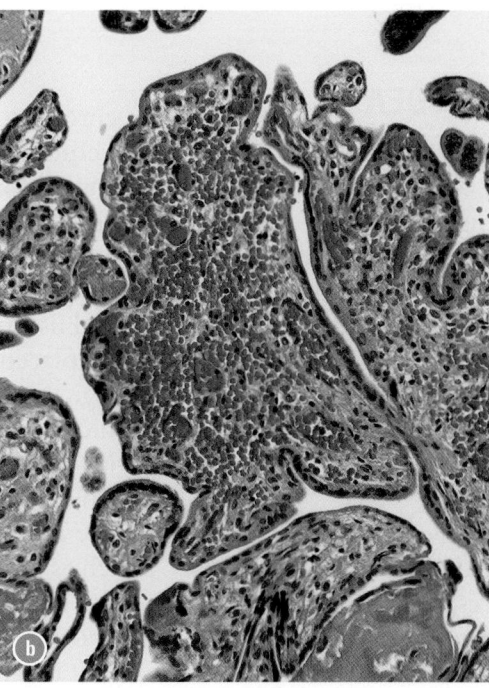

Fig. 34.1 (a) Dissecting intervillous hematoma in a second trimester abruption. (b) Focal intravillous hemorrhage associated with (a).

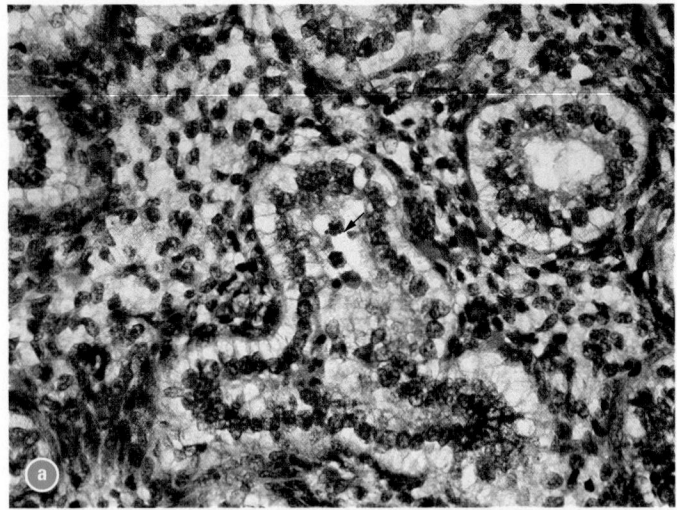

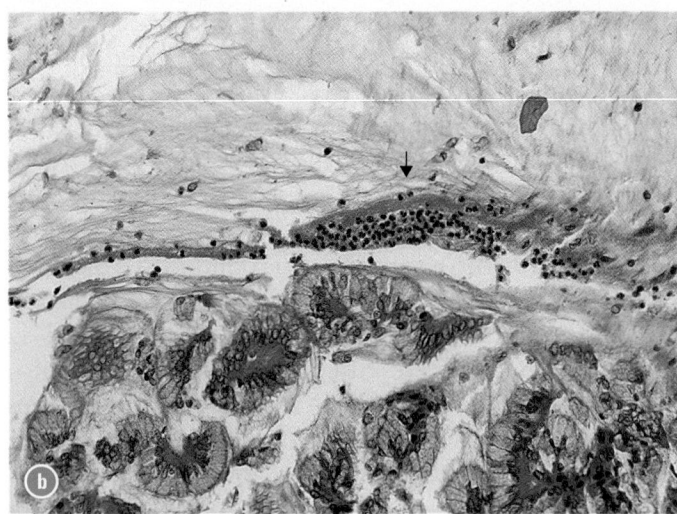

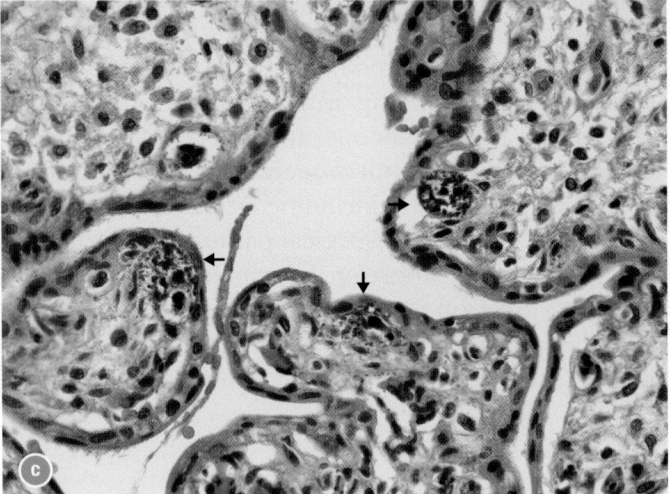

Fig. 34.2 Evidence of fetal exposure to infection includes neutrophils in (a) pulmonary and (b) intestinal lumina spaces (arrow). Intravascular bacteria (c, arrows) indicate fetal sepsis.

SECOND TRIMESTER FETAL DEATH

Clinically, most intrauterine fetal deaths (IUFD) discovered between 14 and 19 weeks of gestation are identified unexpectedly during a routine, monthly, prenatal check. Although a reason for fetal death is not usually clinically suspected, in some instances sonographic findings may suggest a possible cause, such as fetal hydrops, malformations or viral infection. In rare instances, a history such as abdominal trauma (from a fall or motor vehicle accident) or prior amniocentesis may suggest fetal death from direct placental or fetal injury.

The pathologic specimen usually consists of irregular portions of the placenta mixed with macerated fetal tissue fragments. Despite autolysis, the pathologist should pay attention to the following: (a) Gross anomalies prompting exclusion of a chromosomal anomaly. When

a chromosomal abnormality is suspected or a karyotype is requested, placental and fetal tissues should both be sampled for cytogenetics; placental samples will usually yield a karyotype (because chorionic villi continue to be nourished by maternal blood after fetal death), while autolyzed fetal tissues often will not grow in culture. (b) Histopathologic evaluation will be a challenge. The placenta will contain villous sclerosis and hemorrhagic endovasculitis of stem villous vessels, neither of which will be contributory. Evaluation of fetal tissues will usually disclose only advanced autolysis, consistent with remote fetal death; very rarely, a specific histologic finding related to fetal death may be identified, such as (1) parvoviral inclusions in the liver (Fig. 34.3), or (2) CMV inclusions in lung and kidney. However, important placental histopathologic findings are seen, albeit in a minority of instances, including (3) evidence

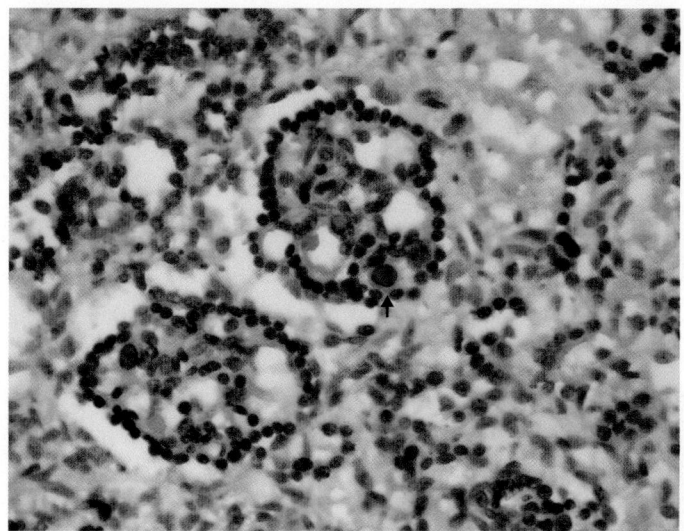

Fig. 34.3 Parvovirus infection, seen as characteristic inclusions (arrow) within normoblasts within fetal glomeruli.

of remote abruption, (4) infarction, (5) chronic villitis, or (6) amnion rupture. Evidence of acute chorioamnionitis is usually not present. However, autolysis will frequently result in (7) 'umbilical pseudovasculitis', in which degenerating umbilical vascular smooth muscle cells mimic the appearance of neutrophils (see Ch. 32).[1,2]

LATE ELECTIVE ABORTION FOR FETAL ANOMALIES

Late elective abortions are frequently performed for abnormal fetal karyotypes, previously diagnosed by chorionic villus sampling or genetic amniocentesis, or for suspected fetal anomalies detected by sonography. Less often, late pregnancy terminations follow possible teratogen exposure, or nonreassuring clinical or sonographic findings, such as fetal growth restriction, oligohydramnios, or abnormal maternal serum alpha-fetoprotein (AFP).

It is beyond the scope of this chapter to discuss in detail the pathologic assessment of fetal chromosomal disorders and congenital anomalies. A general approach to such late elective abortion specimens will be briefly summarized. For intact fetuses, the pathologic assessment closely resembles the autopsy: it includes careful external and internal inspections, routine measurements and weights, precise description of malformations (or documentation of their absence), histologic sampling of multiple organs, evaluation of the number of umbili-

cal vessels and gross and microscopic assessment of the placenta. Possible additional procedures include photographic documentation of gross findings and whole body postero–anterior (P-A) and lateral X-rays when bone defects or dwarfism is suspected. For fragmented fetuses, the foregoing protocol should be followed as far as possible; each fetal fragment should be carefully assessed to determine its anatomic origin and to identify malformations (or normal development) for that region; when an X-ray is warranted, all fetal parts containing bone should be anatomically assembled on X-ray film, oriented with respect to both cranial–caudal and left–right axes.

Many placental disorders are associated with fetal malformations or chromosome anomalies. These include partial hydatidiform mole (see Ch. 32), single umbilical artery and several additional placental disorders (see below). The placental disorder most commonly encountered in late abortion specimens for fetal anomalies is amniotic band syndrome. Amniotic band syndrome, also known as 'early amniotic rupture sequence' and 'extra-amniotic pregnancy', should be suspected when grossly asymmetric fetal deformities are identified, such as amputations, constriction rings, tethering of fingers and toes, irregular defects of the calvarium, unusual facial clefts and large body wall defects. In some cases, thin strands of tissue (so called amniotic bands) may be attached to amputated or disrupted fetal structures (Fig. 34.4a). Although the thin fibrous bands may represent amniotic stroma, residual amniotic epithelium is usually not identified. Therefore, the foregoing findings are usually suggestive of, but not diagnostic for, early amniotic rupture sequence.[1,3,4]

Confirmation of amniotic band syndrome most often relies upon placental pathologic assessment.[4] Characteristic gross placental features include total absence of the amnion, a sleeve of collapsed amniotic membranes wrapped around the proximal umbilical cord (Fig. 34.4b) and a disrupted ring of residual amnion encircling the umbilical cord base. It is important to evaluate the chorionic surface histologically, to look for chorionic features indicative of prolonged exposure to amniotic fluid. Characteristic histologic alterations of the chorionic surface include absence of amnion accompanied by reactive changes of the superficial chorionic stroma (Fig. 34.4c) and 'vernix granulomas' (eosinophilic, proteinaceous debris and fetal squames, adherent to, or embedded in, the superficial chorion) (Fig. 34.4d). Although these placental histopathologic changes are subtle and easily overlooked, they are diagnostic of amnion band syndrome.

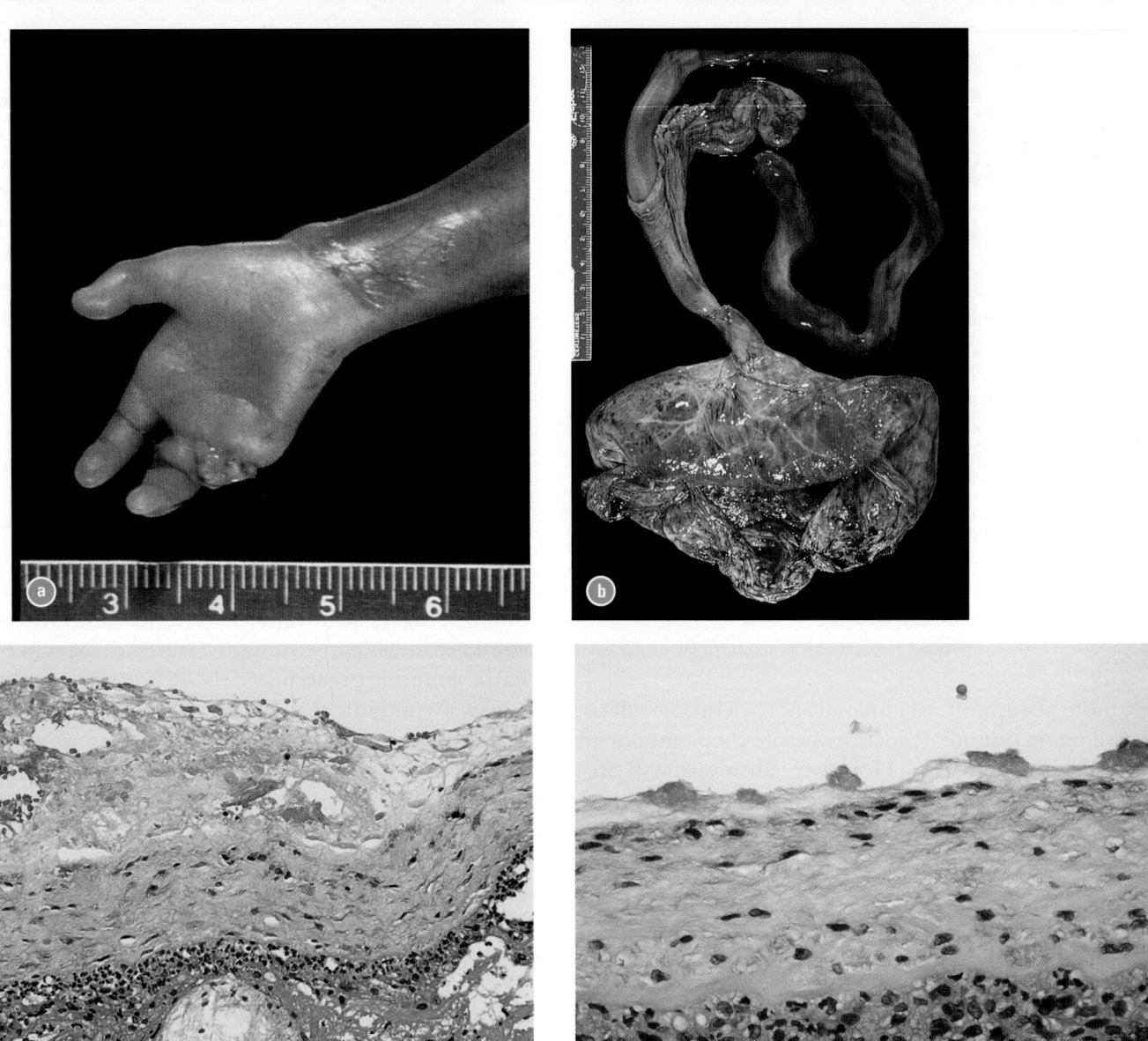

Fig. 34.4 Amniotic band syndrome includes (a) fetal hand deformities, (b) collapse of the amnion around the cord base and (c) absence of amnion accompanied by reactive changes in the chorion. (d) A more subtle example with individual squamous atop denuded chorion with reactive stromal changes.

Premature birth or accelerated delivery

Premature delivery (defined here as in the third trimester) occurs in 10% of pregnancies but is responsible for 80–90% of all perinatal morbidity and mortality. Premature births can be separated into induced premature deliveries (initiated by the obstetrician for significant fetal or maternal disorders) and spontaneous premature births (due to premature labor). Pathologists should examine all preterm placentas, because diagnostic findings that clarify the clinical course are usually present.

Premature delivery can be subdivided into several categories, the distinctions of which have important implications for fetal outcome. The pathologist's major goal following such induced premature births is to document placental findings that contributed to or resulted from the underlying clinical disorder (see below).

Among the most common predisposing factors is maternal hypertension, such as preeclampsia or HELLP syndrome (hypertension, elevated liver enzymes, low platelets), fetal intrauterine growth restriction (IUGR) and non-reassuring fetal testing (Benirschke and Kaufman). These disorders may necessitate terminating the pregnancy. Abruptio placentae is another common factor, occurring in 10% of cases with premature delivery. Both of these conditions may put the fetus at considerable risk due to utero-placental ischemia. In contrast, preterm labor and delivery attributed to acute bacterial chorioamnionitis (sometimes associated with premature rupture of the membranes) is seen in 50% of preterm delivery. The likelihood of chorioamnionitis is further influenced by the clinical setting; the risk is approximately 25% following idiopathic premature delivery, roughly 60% following premature rupture of the membranes and around 80% in premature delivery related to cervical incompetence.[5]

ACUTE CHORIOAMNIONITIS

Cause and clinical presentation

Acute chorioamnionitis is a common placental disorder, found in up to 5% of term placentas and 25–50% of premature placentas. Many studies have established that acute chorioamnionitis is strongly linked to amniotic fluid bacterial infection, typically via an ascending trans-cervical route ('amniotic fluid infection syndrome').[6] Although amniotic fluid infection has several potential clinical consequences, including maternal or fetal sepsis and injury to fetal organs such as lung and brain, premature birth is by far the most significant disorder from an epidemiologic perspective. Chorioamnionitis has been linked to premature labor through uterine contractions caused by leukocytic prostaglandins and cervical dilation caused by bacterial collagenases.[7,8] Recent bacteriologic studies using subamniotic placental and amniotic fluid cultures have isolated one or more infectious organisms in the vast majority of cases of acute chorioamnionitis.[9–11] Among the numerous bacterial species which have been isolated, the most prevalent include *Ureaplasma urealyticum* (11–39%), anaerobic cocci such as peptostreptococci (16–60%), *Staphylococcus epidermidis* (18–24%), *Fusobacterium* sp. (20%) and Group B streptococci (8–25%). The bacterial species most frequently associated with neonatal death from sepsis in premature infants include Group B strep-tococci and *E. coli*. *Candida albicans* and other fungi also may rarely cause acute chorioamnionitis.

Pathology

Very early chorioamnionitis may be grossly unapparent. Nonetheless, macroscopic examination usually suggests the presence of acute chorioamnionitis by the presence of a dull, opaque appearance of the membranes and fetal surface of the placenta, with obscurity of the fetal vessels on the placental surface (Fig. 34.5a). In addition, there may be a foul odor: a characteristic 'fetid' smell with *E. coli* infections and a 'sweet' smell with *Listeria* infections have been described.[1] Microscopically, amniotic fluid infection is characterized by the presence of maternal or fetal neutrophils in various tissues. Maternal acute inflammation is found in the chorioam-niotic membranes or in the superficial chorioamniotic tissues of the placenta. Fetal acute inflammation is seen in the walls or adjacent tissues of umbilical and chorionic vessels (Fig. 34.5b). Maternal acute inflammation may be subdivided into one of three stages, which likely relate to the duration and virulence of infection (Tables 34.2, 34.3): Stage 1, acute subchorionitis (neutrophils in fibrin beneath the chorionic plate); Stage 2, acute chori-onitis (neutrophils in the chorionic stroma of the pla-cental surface or membranes); and Stage 3, acute chorioamnionitis (neutrophils in the chorion and amnion of the chorionic plate or membranes) (Fig. 34.5c–e). Fetal inflammation can display several patterns, including umbilical 'vasculitis' (neutrophils in the umbilical arterial or venous walls); umbilical perivasculitis, extending into Wharton's jelly (funisitis); and chorionic plate 'vasculitis' (neutrophils in fetal chorionic vessel walls).

Any combination of the foregoing patterns of inflam-mation provides strong presumptive evidence for the presence of bacteria or *Candida* within the amniotic fluid. Additional features suggesting *Candida* include acute exudates on the surface of the cord, which should always prompt a PAS stain (Fig. 34.5f). Because maternal acute inflammation may be found without fetal inflam-mation (but usually not the converse), an entirely maternal inflammatory response is thought to suggest the earliest infection. Conversely, a combined maternal and fetal acute inflammatory response suggests a more long-standing infectious process. In addition, in cases

Table 34.2 Histopathology of amniotic fluid bacterial infection

Earliest stage	Mild acute subchorionitis (involving chorionic plate fibrin)
Middle stage	Acute chorioamnionitis Patchy or mild to moderate fetal vascular inflammation (umbilicus, chorion) Umbilical venous inflammation precedes arterial
Advanced stage	Severe necrotizing acute chorioamnionitis with severe fetal vasculitis Necrotizing funisitis (concentric perivascular necrosis and inflammation)

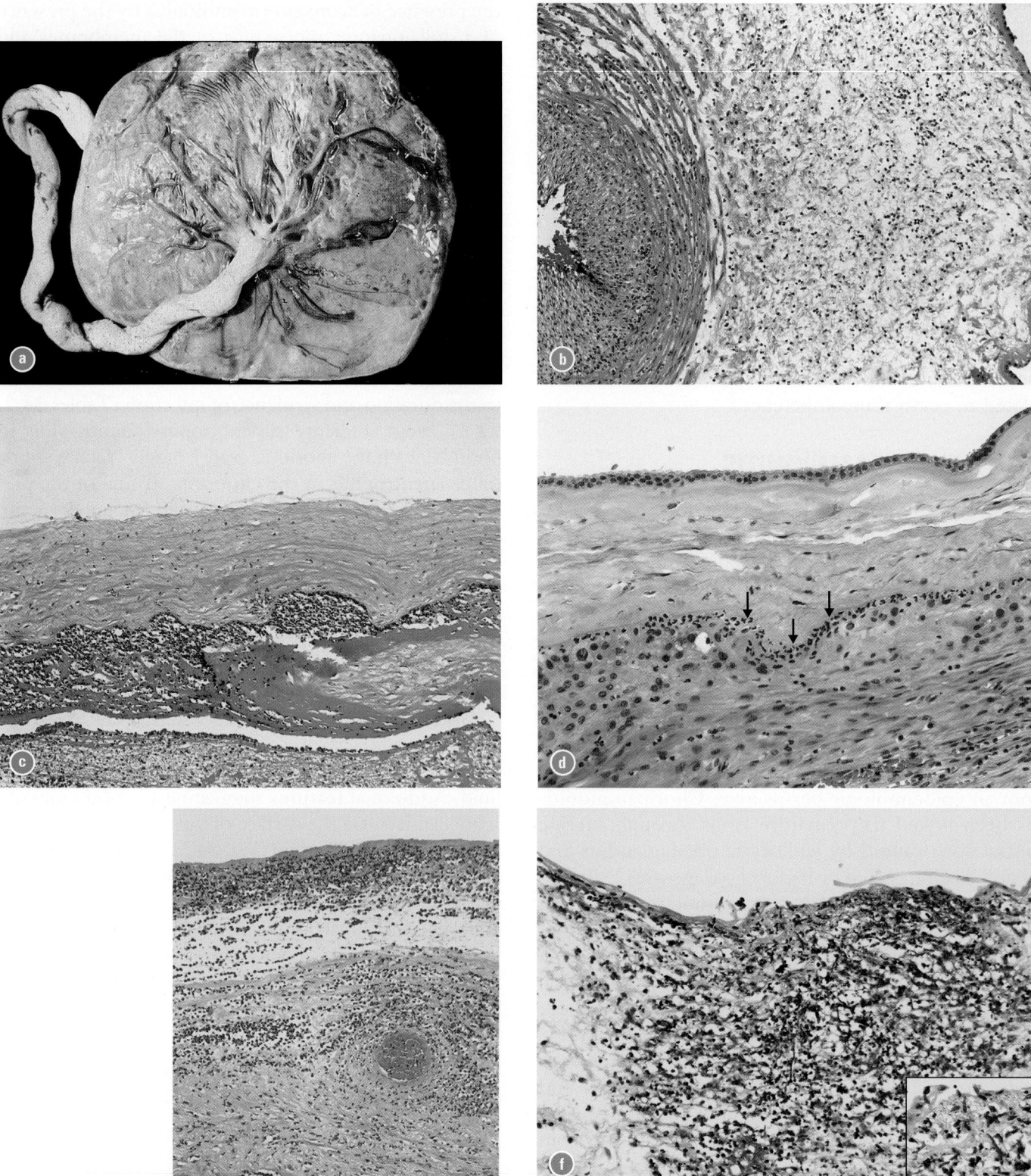

Fig. 34.5 (a) Opaque membranes in acute chorioamnionitis. (b) Umbilical cord vascular inflammation extending into Wharton's jelly (funisitis). (c) Acute subchorionitis. (d) Earliest acute chorionitis (arrows). (e) Advanced necrotizing chorioamnionitis with fetal chorionic vasculitis. (f) Abscess on surface of cord associated with *Candida* (see inset).

Table 34.3 *Clinical and pathologic features of fetal bacterial infection*

Major mechanisms
  Maternal bacteremia seeds placental intervillous space; bacteria invade villous tissue and fetal blood stream producing fetal sepsis
  Intra-amniotic bacteria invade fetal tissue (particularly the lung and bowel), producing localized infection with possible sepsis
Placental findings highly correlated with fetal sepsis:
  Acute villitis (microabscesses involving chorionic villi)
  Bacterial 'overgrowth' within fetal vessels (in placental or autopsy specimens)

of stillbirth, the presence of fetal acute inflammation indicates that intra-amniotic infection developed prior to fetal death; similar inferences can be drawn when aspirated and swallowed amniotic neutrophils are identified within the fetal airways or gastrointestinal lumen at autopsy (Tables 34.2, 34.3).

Whenever acute chorioamnionitis is pathologically identified, the placental villous parenchyma should be carefully assessed for acute inflammation and bacteria, two histologic findings that strongly suggest fetal sepsis (Table 34.2). Acute villitis is characterized by inter- and intravillous acute inflammation. Typically, there are multiple villous micro abscesses, which consist of small aggregates of terminal villi surrounded by fibrin and neutrophils, with intravillous acute inflammation; sometimes, large regions resembling 'septic' infarcts with marked acute inflammation are present. Acute villitis usually indicates either fetal or maternal bacteremia; frequently, positive maternal blood cultures are documented even before the placental pathologic assessment has been completed. Bacterial species most highly associated with acute villitis include *Listeria monocytogenes*, Group B streptococci, *E. coli* and *Treponema pallidum*. In acute villitis associated with *Listeria*, microscopic examination demonstrates small Gram-positive bacilli in tiny clusters resembling 'Chinese writing' within villous microabscess and on the amniotic surface (Fig. 34.6). In addition to Gram stains, a stain for spirochetes is warranted when congenital syphilis is suspected (as discussed below).

In rare cases, severe, diffuse acute villitis may be accompanied by numerous clusters of bacteria present within the fetal vessels of the placenta; although this could be related to placental retention and bacterial overgrowth following fetal death, the intravascular location of bacteria indicates antenatal fetal bacteremia. Intravascular bacterial 'overgrowth' can also be seen within fetal vessels in autopsy tissues. Group B streptococci are the most frequently identified organisms in placental and fetal vessels.

ABRUPTIO PLACENTAE

Cause and clinical presentation

The causes of accelerated delivery will naturally overlap with those of antepartum hemorrhage. The differential diagnosis of antepartum hemorrhage includes: (1) abruptio placentae, (2) placenta accreta, or (3) placenta previa. The latter two entities will be discussed later in this chapter. Abruptio placentae, or premature placental separation, is manifested by significant vaginal bleeding in late second-to-third trimester (Table 34.4). However, abruptions can also be clinically silent, presenting without vaginal bleeding, in up to 20% of cases; this is so called 'concealed abruption'. Bleeding due to placental abruption is not typically life threatening to the mother but may threaten the fetus, causing fetal death in about 35% of such cases. Fetal demise is due to hypoxia secondary to maternal hemorrhage and occurs more frequently with the clinically silent concealed abruptions. Other clinical manifestations of abruption include premature labor, labor with hypertonic uterine contractions, 'port wine' amniotic fluid noted at Caesarean section, fetal death or distress and large clots passed with the placenta following vaginal delivery. While the primary cause is unknown, there are multiple predisposing factors associated with placental abruption, including maternal hypertension, preeclampsia, uterine overdistention (multiple pregnancy or hydramnios), cocaine abuse and maternal trauma (such as a fall or motor vehicle accident).

Pathology

Gross and microscopic features of placental abruption are summarized in Table 34.4. Even when clinical features strongly suggest abruption, characteristic patho-

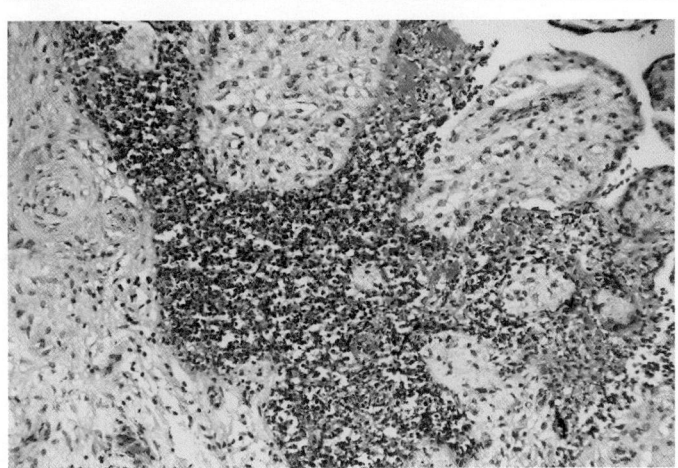

Fig. 34.6 Acute necrotizing intervillositis associated with *Listeria*.

logic findings may be absent; this suggests that abruptions which occur very shortly before delivery may be pathologically unapparent. Typical pathologic findings of abruption include: (1) a detached blood clot submitted with the placenta (solid documentation for abruption, if sent from a Caesarean delivery; a retroplacental hematoma; infarction or 'saucer-like' depression of placental parenchyma adjacent to retroplacental clot (Fig. 34.7a); extensive retromembranous hemorrhage

(Fig. 34.7b) obvious in the membrane role, basal thrombus and intraparenchymal hemorrhagic infarction (Fig. 34.7c) and in some cases, intraplacental dissection by a retroplacental hematoma (ball in socket infarct), sometimes extending to the chorionic surface (see Ch. 33). The villous parenchyma adjacent to retroplacental hematomas may be dark red (from intravillous hemorrhage and congestion) or firm, pale and gritty (indicating infarction). Histologically, intravillous

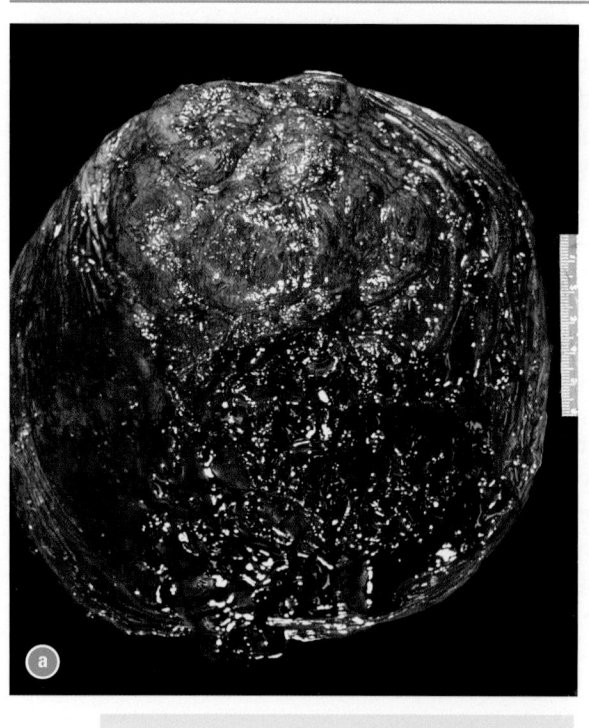

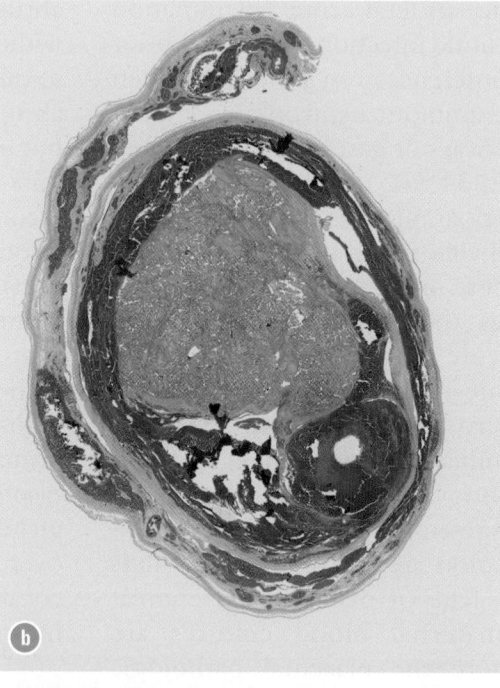

Fig. 34.7 Excluding abruption requires attention to (a) gross evidence of adherent blood clot with depression, (b) extensive retromembranous hemorrhage seen in this membrane role, (c) retroplacental thrombus (lower) associated with hemorrhagic infarct, (d) hemosiderin in placental membranes (arrow) suggesting remote abruption. The latter may have resolved weeks or months prior and not be grossly apparent (see also Fig. 34.1 and Ch. 33).

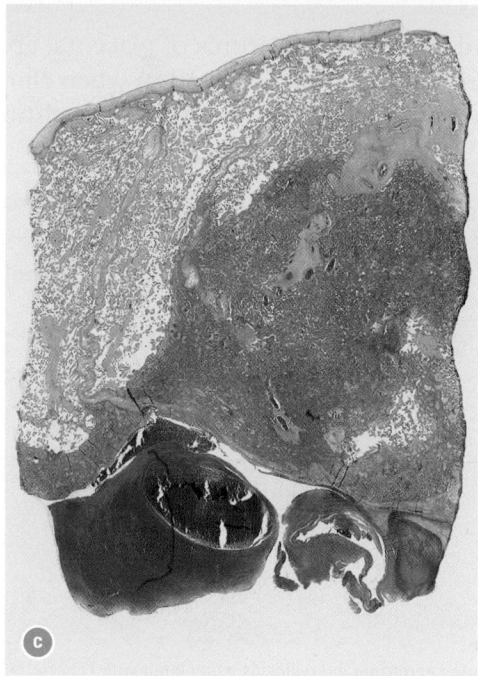

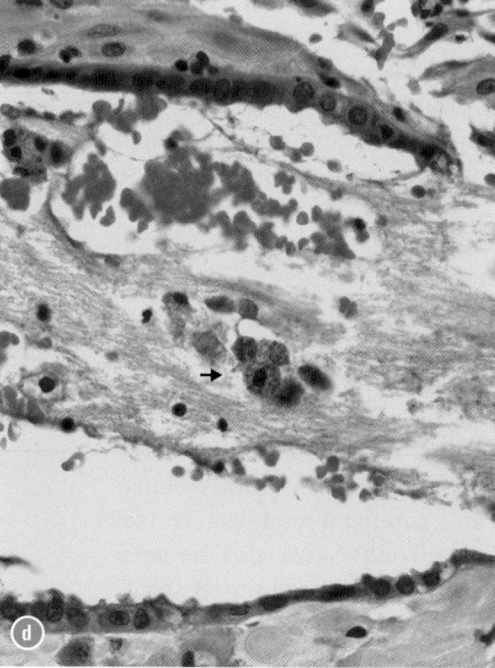

Table 34.4 *Placental pathology in abruptio placentae*

Very recent abruptio placentae (minutes duration):
   Possibly no pathologic findings
   Intravillous hemorrhage
   Adherent blood clot, may dissect into adjacent placenta; no depression
Abruptio placentae of intermediate age (hours duration):
   Adherent blood clot with depressed (compressed) placenta
   Adjacent compression of maternal surface ('saucer-like depression')
Chronic/oldest abruptio placentae (days–weeks duration):
   Lysed clot, placental depression and placental infarction
   Hemosiderin deposition (deep within chorionic plate)

hemorrhage (an early change, which likely develops within minutes) or villous infarction (a later change, which usually takes hours or days to develop) may be found adjacent to a retroplacental hemorrhage (Fig. 34.1a,b). When bloodstained ('port wine') amniotic fluid is present, hemosiderin-laden macrophages may be present in the superficial amnion and chorion; this suggests that retroplacental bleeding began several days, or in some cases weeks, before birth (Fig. 34.7d). In addition to the foregoing findings that are indicative of abruption, abnormalities associated with maternal hypertension and preeclampsia are commonly seen (see below section on 'Toxemia of Pregnancy').

CERVICAL INCOMPETENCE

Cervical incompetence is defined as recurrent second trimester pregnancy loss attributed to the inability of the cervix to retain the pregnancy.[12] It is related to prior traumatic injury to the cervix associated with prior delivery or cone biopsy and with congenital anomalies such as diethylstilbestrol exposure. In general, cervical incompetence is classified as a continuous variable, in that gradations of cervical length may influence risk and risk may vary in a given pregnancy. Sonographic studies have shown a progressive increase in risk as a function of shorter cervix length, with a cut-off point assigned at 3.0–3.5 cm.[13] The typical scenario in preterm delivery associated with cervical incompetence is painless cervical dilatation with protruding membranes and abrupt delivery of a live fetus. Efforts at prevention have focused on the McDonald cerclage, which was initially popular when introduced in the 1950s. However, only a proportion of women with prior early gestational losses have a repeat miscarriage irrespective of management and the value of placing cerclage in a given case has been controversial.[14–16] Currently transvaginal cerclage and bed rest are recommended if the cervical length is less than 25 mm prior to 27 weeks gestation.

Operative or induced delivery for maternal or fetal disorders

TOXEMIA OF PREGNANCY

Physiology and clinical presentation

Toxemia of pregnancy refers to a symptom complex characterized by hypertension, proteinuria and edema (preeclampsia) known as preeclamptic toxemia (PET). It occurs in about 6% of pregnant women, usually in the last trimester and more commonly in primiparous than multiparous women. Certain of these patients become more seriously ill, developing convulsions; this more severe form is termed eclampsia. Patients with eclampsia can develop disseminated intravascular coagulation (DIC) with lesions in the liver, kidneys, heart, placenta and sometimes the brain, although there is no absolute correlation between the severity of eclampsia and the magnitude of the anatomic changes.[17]

The causes of the initial events of toxemia are unknown, but evidence points to an abnormality of placentation, leading to placental ischemia (Table 34.5). This may involve an abnormality in both trophoblast invasion and the development of the physiologic alterations in the placental vessels required to perfuse the placental bed adequately. Immunologic, genetic and other factors have been postulated as causes of these abnormalities. One particular abnormality is in endovascular invasion, the process in which cytotrophoblasts invade and remodel the uterine spiral arterioles.[18,19] This abnormality is manifested by the inability of the invading cytotrophoblast to assume the phenotype of vascular endothelial cells, which normally includes changes in the expression of surface adhesion recep-

Table 34.5 *Potential causes/mechanisms of toxemia of pregnancy*

Abnormal implantation, with defects in:
   cytotrophoblastic differentiation
   endovascular invasion
   spiral arteriole remodeling
Reduced placental blood flow/placental ischemia
Increased maternal vascular resistance (hypertension):
   increased circulating vasoconstrictor substances
   altered renin–angiotensin mechanism
   altered endothelial function
Altered coagulation/platelet function (increased thrombosis/DIC)
Imbalance of angiogenic molecules (increased sVEGFR-1 and decreased P1GF and VEGF)

DIC, disseminated intravascular coagulation; P1GF, placental growth factors; sVEGFR-1, soluble vascular endothelial growth factor receptor-1; VEGF, vascular endothelial growth factors.

tors.[19,20] These defects in cytotrophoblastic differentiation result in shallow implantation, with incomplete conversion of low-capacitance, high-resistance uterine vessels to high-capacitance, low-resistance vessels needed for the pregnancy state.[21,22] The net effect is reduced blood flow and placental ischemia, the basis for the toxemic placenta.[23,24] It is further thought that this decreased uteroplacental perfusion induces stimulation of vasoconstrictor substances (thromboxane, angiotensin, endothelin) and the inhibition of vasodilator influences (prostaglandin I2, prostaglandin E2, nitric oxide) from the ischemic placenta. The end result is DIC, hypertension and organ damage.

As to the pathogenesis of DIC in toxemia, endothelial damage, abnormalities in the level and activities of coagulation factors and primary platelet alteration may play a role.[25] For example, during toxemia, the placental ischemia leads to a higher output of thromboplastic substances and antithrombin III levels are reduced. The characteristic lesions in eclampsia are in large part due to thrombosis of arterioles and capillaries throughout the body, particularly in the liver, kidneys, brain, pituitary and placenta.

The mechanism of toxemic hypertension appears to also involve the renin–angiotensin mechanism and prostaglandins.[25] Normal pregnant women develop a resistance to the vasoconstrictive and hypertensive effects of angiotensin, but women with toxemia lose such resistance, developing a tendency to hypertension. Prostaglandins of the E series, produced in the uteroplacental vascular bed during pregnancy, are thought to mediate the normal resistance of pregnant women to angiotensin and prostaglandin production is indeed decreased in the placenta of toxemic women. Thus, the increase in angiotensin hypersensitivity, characteristic of toxemia, may be due to decreased synthesis of prostaglandin by the toxemic placenta. There is also evidence that renin production by the toxemic placenta is increased, another potentially vasoconstrictive event.

An additional mechanism recently proposed involves circulating soluble vascular endothelial growth factor receptor-1 (sVEGFR-1), which binds both placental growth factors (PlGF) and vascular endothelial growth factors (VEGF).[26] Normally, near term, serum levels of sVEGFR-1 increase and PIGF and VEGF decrease, reflecting a reduction in angiogenic activity. In preeclampsia, this process is initiated much earlier than normal.[26,27] It has been shown that preeclamptic placentas overproduce sVEGFR-1, which, when administered to pregnant rats, produces the characteristic systemic and renal abnormalities seen in humans with this disorder.[26] While the inciting culprit in the development of preeclampsia still remains unknown, it is clear that the premature application of antiangiogenic 'brakes', including sVEGFR-1, is a significant part of this pregnancy-related disorder.[28]

Other disorders which share clinical and pathologic features with preeclampsia include lupus erythematosus; lupus-anticoagulant disorder/antiphospholipid syndrome; hemolysis, elevated liver enzymes and low platelet (HELLP) syndrome and some cases of 'idiopathic' fetal growth restriction.

A high percentage of placentas from pregnancies complicated by preeclampsia show characteristic findings indicative of either chronic placental ischemia or placental abruption. These major gross and histologic findings are summarized in Table 34.4 (abruption) and Table 34.5 (preeclampsia). Because several changes will frequently be identified in each specimen, a pathologic summary stating that 'multiple abnormalities identified in this specimen are consistent with maternal preeclampsia' may be useful.

Pathology

Maternal pathology

Maternal pathology is linked to the vascular injury that ensues and involves the liver, kidney and brain. The liver lesions, when present, take the form of irregular, focal, subcapsular and intraparenchymal hemorrhages (Fig. 34.8a). On histologic examination, there are fibrin thrombi in the portal capillaries with foci of characteristic peripheral hemorrhagic necrosis (Fig. 34.8b). The kidney lesions are variable. Glomerular lesions are diffuse, at least when they are assessed by electron microscopy. They consist of striking swelling of endothelial cells, the deposition of fibrinogen-derived amorphous dense deposits on the endothelial side of the basement membrane and mesangial cell hyperplasia. Immunofluorescent studies confirm the abundance of fibrin in glomeruli. In the more well-defined cases, fibrin thrombi are present in the glomeruli and capillaries of the cortex. When the lesion is far advanced, it may produce complete destruction of the cortex in the pattern referred to as bilateral renal cortical necrosis. The brain may have gross or microscopic foci of hemorrhage along with small vessel thromboses. Similar changes are often found in the heart and the anterior pituitary.

Placental pathology

The placenta is the site of variable changes, most of which reflect ischemia and vessel injury (Table 34.6). A wide range of changes have been described. These

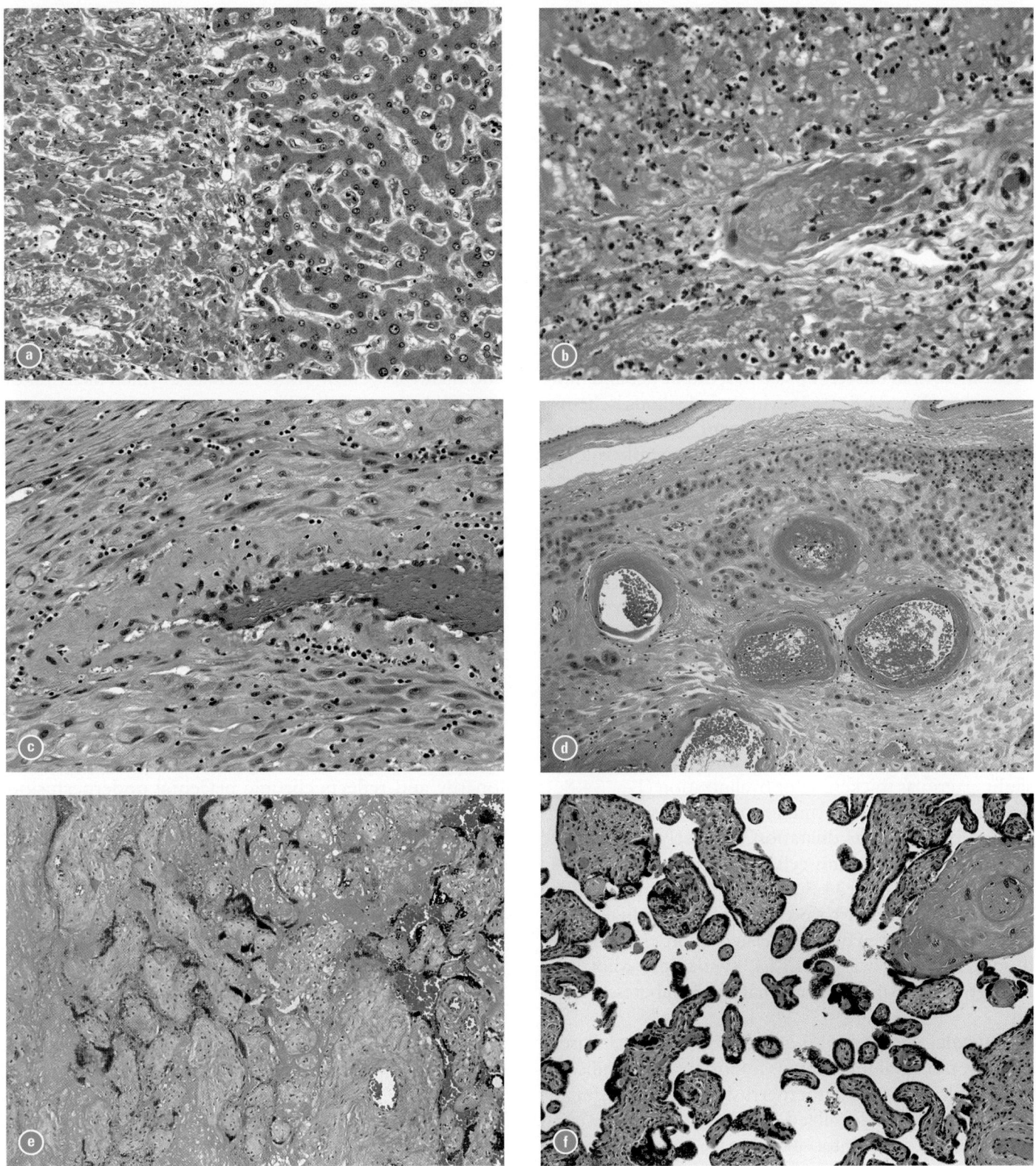

Fig. 34.8 Changes associated with placental ischemia in toxemia. (a) Hepatic necrosis (left) and (b) thrombi in hepatic veins, (c) mild decidual vasculopathy with arteriole thickening, (d) acute atherosis with vascular dilatation and prominent fibrinoid necrosis, (e) multiple infarcts and (f) hypermature villous changes. These findings are not restricted to toxemia and may also be associated with intrauterine growth restriction.

Table 34.6 *Placental pathology in preeclampsia*

Small placenta (<10th percentile by weight)
Increased syncytial knots (unevenly accelerated maturation)
Infarction
Abruptio placentae
Maternal decidual vasculopathy
  Mild: vascular thickening (no vascular dilation)
  Severe: acute atherosis (fibrinoid necrosis with prominent dilation)

changes include: (1) a characteristic finding in the walls of uterine vessels of striking fibrinoid necrosis and intramural lipid deposition (decidual vasculopathy and acute atherosis)(Fig. 34.8c,d), (2) placental infarcts, which occur in normal full term placentas, but larger and more numerous (Fig. 34.8e), (3) evidence of villous ischemia, including formation of prominent syncytial knots, thickening of trophoblastic basement membrane and villous hypovascularity (Fig. 34.8f) and (4) increased frequency of retroplacental hematomas. The former three pathologic changes are discussed in more detail herein.

Decidual vasculopathy Characteristic pathologic changes are seen in maternal decidual spiral arteries in preeclampsia. Because the decidua attached to fetal membranes is the optimal site to identify such changes, it is useful to histologically assess tissue from two membrane rolls. Vasculopathy may have a patchy distribution and maternal decidual vessels are unevenly distributed in the membranes. Mild vasculopathy is characterized by slight arteriolar thickening or hyalinization (Fig. 34.8c). Severe vasculopathy, termed acute atherosis, is characterized by arteriolar dilatation, intensely eosinophilic fibrinoid necrosis, foam cells and perivascular chronic inflammation (Fig. 34.8d); thrombosis may also be present. In addition to preeclampsia, decidual vasculopathy may be seen in other related disorders, including lupus erythematosus, HELLP syndrome, idiopathic fetal growth restriction and maternal diabetes.[29]

Placental infarction Like maternal decidual vasculopathy, placental infarction is important as an indicator of chronic placental underperfusion. Placental infarctions result from localized interruptions of maternal blood flow to the intervillous space due to maternal vascular disease (see also Ch. 33). Infarcts usually result from thrombi in decidual spiral arteries; less commonly, they originate from spiral arteriolar rupture and placental abruption. In premature placentas, infarcts of any size are abnormal. In term placentas, small infarcts are relatively common, particularly at the margin. More centrally located infarcts may indicating maternal vascular disease; however, it has been suggested that only large infarcts (>3 cm in diameter) in term placentas are likely to be associated with serious morbidity and mortality. At any gestational age, extensive placental infarction (25 to 50% of the parenchyma) is significant and may result in fetal death.

Macroscopically, placental infarcts are discrete firm masses with a gritty, granular consistency (related to villous composition) (see Ch. 33). Infarcts are often located near the maternal surface of the placenta, reflecting their pathogenesis in diseased maternal spiral arterioles. Recent infarcts are dark red, while older infarcts progressively change from brown-red, to tan and finally to yellow-white, a change which likely takes several days to weeks. The size and number of infarcts and approximate percentage of involved parenchyma should be recorded.

All placental infarcts should be histologically assessed. The earliest infarct that can be histologically recognized is characterized by collapse of the intervillous space, with villous congestion, trophoblastic nuclear eosinophilia and intravillous debris and scattered neutrophils (Fig. 34.8c). Older infarcts show progressive necrosis, which eventually results in total eosinophilia (see Ch. 33).

Villous ischemia The finding of large numbers of syncytiotrophoblastic knots in a placenta ('increased syncytial knots'; 'accelerated maturation') has the same significance as placental infarction and decidual vasculopathy and reflects chronic placental underperfusion by the mother.[30] Typical histologic findings include tiny terminal villi, with increases in both the number and the size of perivillous syncytial knots (Fig. 34.8d).

Clinical course

Preeclampsia usually starts after the 32nd week of pregnancy but begins earlier in patients with hydatidiform mole or preexisting kidney disease or hypertension. The onset is usually insidious, characterized by hypertension and edema, with proteinuria following within several days. Headaches and visual disturbances are common. Eclampsia is heralded by central nervous system involvement, including convulsions and eventual coma. Mild and moderate forms of toxemia can be controlled by bed rest, a balanced diet and antihypertensive agents, but induction of delivery is the only definitive treatment of established preeclampsia and eclampsia. Proteinuria and hypertension usually disappear within 1 or 2 weeks after delivery except in patients in whom these findings predated the pregnancy.

INTRAUTERINE GROWTH RESTRICTION

Intrauterine growth restriction (IUGR) is an important cause of infant mortality and morbidity. Major causes include obvious fetal disorders such as chromosomal abnormalities and malformations (20%) and maternal vascular disease, including toxemia (30%), chronic hypertension and diabetic vasculopathy. Other causes include maternal and fetal infections, chronic villitis, fetal thrombosis, chronic abruptio placentae and metabolic disorders (Table 34.7).[31–34] In over one-third of IUGR cases, the placenta is small for dates, implying poor perfusion; however, IUGR can also occur in the setting of a clinically unremarkable pregnancy and placenta. Management of these disorders, particularly when the fetus is otherwise normal, requires careful monitoring of fetal and placental development and rapid delivery if placental blood flow appears compromised.

Fetal IUGR is antenatally suspected when sonographically estimated fetal weight is below the 10th percentile. Because IUGR is associated with stillbirth, increased pregnancy surveillance is customary after the diagnosis is sonographically confirmed. Fetuses with progressive IUGR or non-reassuring fetal testing are frequently delivered prematurely (often by Caesarean section).

In cases of IUGR, the pathologist's primary goal is to identify placental disorders that may have contributed to poor fetal growth (Table 34.8). In approximately 50% of instances, placental pathologic findings are present to suggest that the placenta played a significant role in the pathogenesis of IUGR. The most common of placental disorders associated with IUGR include fetal vascular thrombosis (about 40%), chronic ischemic changes (about 30%) and non-infectious chronic villitis (about 10%); less common disorders include maternal floor infarction, chronic intervillositis and infectious chronic villitis (TORCH) (Table 34.8).[33,34]

Fetal thrombosis

Fetal thrombosis is found in approximately 40% of placentas from fetuses with IUGR, as compared with 5% of 'routine' placentas. In addition to its strong association with IUGR, fetal thrombosis is commonly seen with maternal diabetes and less frequently seen with fetal chromosomal disorders, fetal death, abnormal umbilical cord insertion, viral infection or chorangiomas. Fetal thrombosis may also occasionally result from fetal hypercoagulation (secondary to, for example, protein S or protein C deficiency). Several distinctive patterns of placental disease indicative of fetal thrombosis can be seen, including: (1) thrombi in large fetal vessels, (2) clusters of avascular terminal villi and (3) hemorrhagic endovasculitis (Fig. 34.9a–c). Several of these patterns will frequently coexist in one placenta.

Thrombi in umbilical or chorionic surface vessels can occasionally be grossly visualized as dilated dark red vessels (due to recent thrombosis), or as shrunken, tan-white, sometimes calcified vessels (due to remote thrombosis). Histologically, non-occlusive to totally occlusive thrombi may be seen in umbilical vessels, chorionic surface vessels, or muscularized stem villous vessels.

Table 34.7 Causes of intrauterine growth restriction

Maternal
  Maternal vascular disease
    Toxemia (preeclampsia)
    Chronic hypertension
    Collagen vascular diseases
  Coagulopathy
  Infections – viral (TORCH)
  Severe lung disease/hypoxia
  Sickle cell disease
  Renal transplantation
  Nutrition
  Smoking (slight effect, small for gestational age)
Fetal
  Congenital malformations/chromosomal abnormalities
  Fetal thrombosis
  Multiple gestation
Placental
  Chronic villitis (vast majority idiopathic)
  Placental infarction
  Maternal floor infarct
  Fetal placental thrombosis

TORCH, toxoplasmosis, other, rubella, cytomegalovirus and herpes simplex. Adapted from Salafia et al.,[31] Redline and Peppin[32] and Lin.[33]

Table 34.8 Placental pathology in fetal growth restriction

Chronic placental ischemia
Chronic villitis
  Infectious villitis (TORCH)
    Toxoplasmosis
    Rubella
    Cytomegalovirus
    Herpes simplex
    Herpes zoster
    Enteroviruses
  Non-specific villitis (may recur)
  Massive chronic intervillositis
Fetal vasculopathy (including fetal thrombosis, hemorrhagic endovasculitis and diffuse villous fibrosis)
Increased perivillous fibrin/maternal floor infarct
Vascular malformations ('mesenchymal dysplasia' aka 'pseudo-partial mole')

Adapted from Salafia et al.[31] and Redline and Peppin.[32]

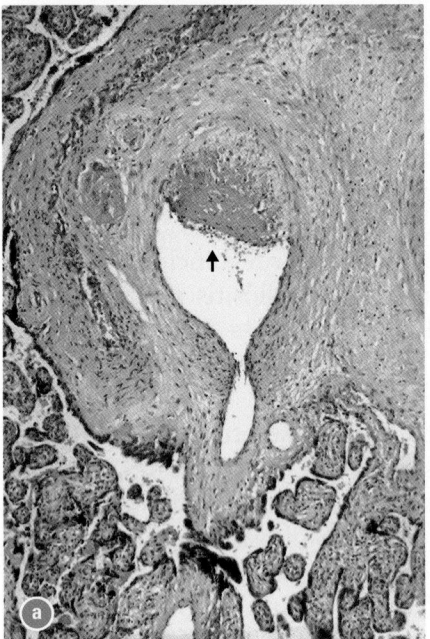 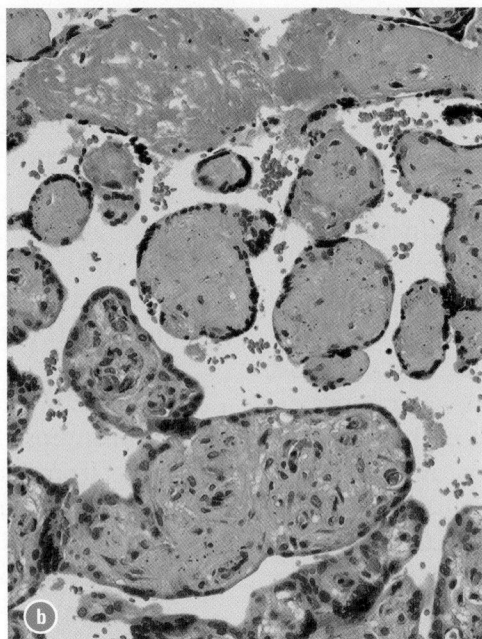 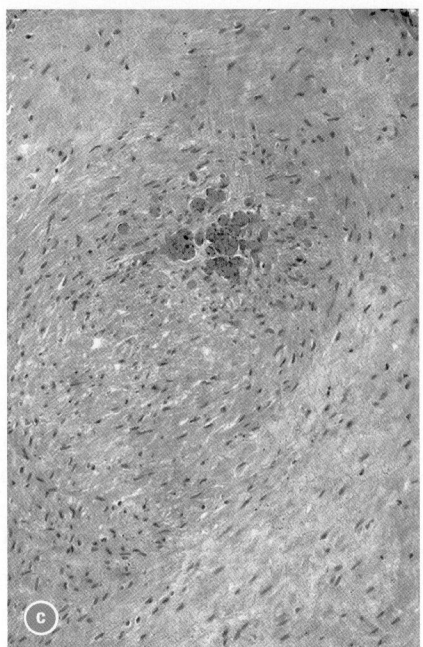

Fig. 34.9 Fetal thrombosis, commonly associated with intrauterine growth restriction (see also Figs 34.8 and 34.10). (a) Thrombus in large vessel (arrow). (b) Avascular villi reflecting loss of circulation. (c) Hemorrhagic endovasculitis (center).

Thrombi in umbilical vessels can be identified as involving arteries or vein; however, in more distal fetal vessels, this is usually not certain from histologic assessment. The earliest lesions are eosinophilic fibrin cushions attached to or embedded within the superficial vascular intima. The oldest lesions are organized thrombi with dystrophic calcification. Hemorrhagic endovasculitis (HEV) is characterized by thrombosis and endothelial degeneration. This lesion can often be confused with post-mortem fetal vascular occlusions due to autolysis of vessel walls. Although controversial, HEV is not representative of a specific disease entity; rather, it has been associated with preeclampsia, post-term pregnancy, meconium staining, as well as IUGR.[1]

Occlusive thrombi are often seen upstream of a cluster of avascular terminal villi ('fetal thrombotic vasculopathy'). When large regions of avascular villi are present, placental cross-sections may show macroscopic pallor (so-called 'white infarct'); this change is poorly appreciated in unfixed specimens, but readily evident in formalin-fixed specimens. It is important to note that such avascular, fibrotic villi represent atrophy and not true infarction, since the latter occurs only when maternal blood supply is interrupted.[1] When fetal thrombotic vasculopathy is extensive, the fetus is likely to have suffered adverse sequelae, including antenatal neurologic injury.[32,35]

Extensive fibrin deposition/maternal floor infarction

Extensive perivillous fibrin deposition (PVF) and maternal floor infarction (MFI) are rare, related, idiopathic pathologic processes associated with fetal growth restriction and other significant adverse outcomes including stillbirth (Fig. 34.10a,b). These placental disorders can recur in subsequent gestations.[36,37] Grossly, MFIs are characterized by a fibrinous plaque partially or completely covering the maternal surface of the placenta, resembling a leathery, 'orange rind'. On cross-section, a band of tan fibrous material is present adjacent to the maternal surface. In extensive fibrin deposition, the placental cut surface shows 'marbling' of the placental parenchyma by tan-white fibrinous material, in a nodular to diffuse pattern. Histologically, MFI shows a band of eosinophilic fibrinoid material occupying the maternal intervillous space near the maternal floor, adjacent to Nitabuch's fibrin (resembling an expansion of the basal fibrin into the basal intervillous space) (Fig. 34.10a). The basal villi are evenly spaced in the fibrinoid; although the perivillous trophoblast disappears, the villous stromal cells appear viable. Features of ischemic infarction are not present (i.e. collapse of the intervillous space, close apposition of terminal villi, with ischemic necrosis). In extensive perivillous fibrin deposition (also termed Gitterinfarct ('network of fibrin'), placental intervillous space is diffusely infiltrated by a dense network of fibrin, occupying a significant percentage of the intervillous space (Fig. 34.10b).

Because some intraplacental fibrin is present in all placentas, the categorization of some cases as excessive, extensive, or pathologic can be subjective and difficult to reproduce.[38] Semiquantitative histologic definitions of MFI and PVF have recently been suggested, with MFI defined as basal intervillous fibrin greater than 3 mm in thickness on one histologic slide and PVF defined as greater than 50% of the intervillous space of one histologic slide occupied by fibrin.[38] Of note, these two lesions are often histologically admixed with one another or with other patterns of disease, including ischemic infarction, chronic villitis, villous fibrosis, hemorrhagic endovasculitis and fetal vascular thrombosis. When this happens, although it may be evident that significant placental pathology exists, often there is no single, satisfactory diagnostic term that fits the picture and often no single pathogenetic processes (ischemic, immunologic, thrombotic) can be invoked with certainty.

Chronic villitis

Chronic villitis is defined as chronic inflammatory cells (usually macrophages and lymphocytes) in terminal villi; most commonly, the villous stroma is abnormally fibrotic and may be totally avascular. Frequently, clusters of involved villi will clump together, with the surrounding maternal vascular space showing monocytosis. In contrast to acute villitis (which as covered above, suggests fetal and/or maternal bacteremia), chronic villitis signifies either viral infection ('specific' or infectious chronic villitis)

or an idiopathic, non-infectious condition ('non-specific' chronic villitis, or 'villitis of unknown etiology', VUE).

Infectious chronic villitis (TORCH)

The acronym 'TORCH' (*t*oxoplasmosis, *o*ther, *r*ubella, *c*ytomegalovirus and *h*erpes simplex) stands for a series of bacterial, viral and parasitic pathogens that can produce a congenital or perinatally acquired infection. The category 'other' includes a growing number of fetal pathogens such as HIV, *Mycobacterium tuberculosis*, hepatitis B and C, varicella zoster, syphilis, parvovirus and enterovirus infections.[1] As will be discussed below, it is important to emphasize that placental infections by these pathogens produce variable morphologic and cellular responses that may not be diagnostic of their presence and will not always produce a conspicuous villitis. Thus, adjunctive special stains may be required for their confirmation. Moreover, placental infections may contribute to not only intrauterine growth restriction but also to intrauterine fetal death (IUFD), spontaneous abortion and neonatal morbidity and should be considered in the differential diagnosis of these conditions.[1]

Toxoplasmosis Most cases of congenital infection by *Toxoplasma gondii* occur when a woman has her primary infection during pregnancy. The rate of infection increases with each trimester, but fetal morbidity is greatest when infection occurs in the first trimester.[39] Fetal infection may cause chorioretinitis, hydrocephalus, central nervous system calcification and hydrops. The organisms in the placenta may be difficult to identify

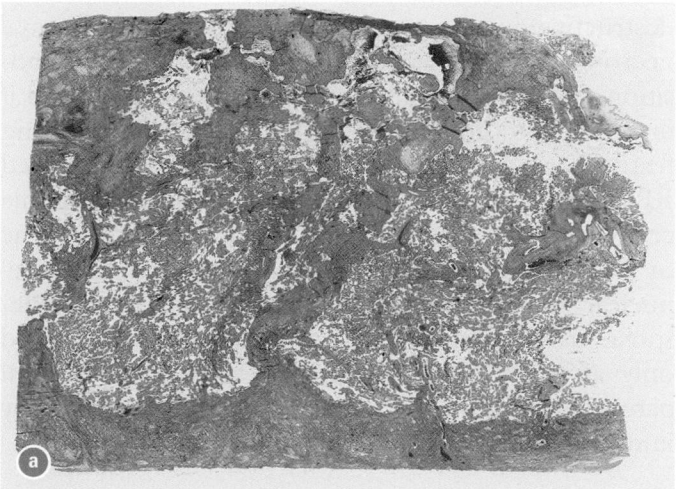 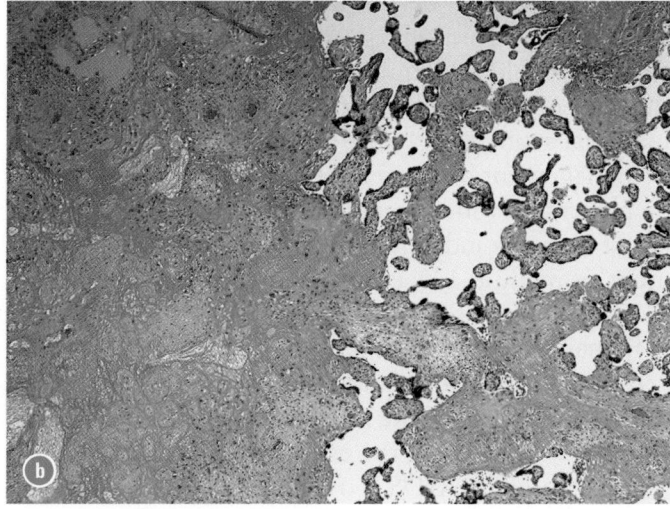

Fig. 34.10 Extensive fibrin deposition in IUGR. (a) Classic maternal floor infarct with linear basal distribution. (b) Focal extensive perivillous fibrin. These two entities are distinguished principally by extent and location (or distribution) of fibrin deposition.

because there is sometimes no associated inflammation; however, chronic villitis, sometimes granulomatous, can be found.[40] Wharton's jelly of the umbilical cord is a good place to search for the 200 μm-diameter encysted organisms; the cysts contain numerous 4 μm-diameter, PAS-positive organisms (Fig. 34.11a). Cysts are also characteristically found in the membranes, but only rarely in villi. A fluorescent antibody test is available for equivocal cases, although polymerase chain reaction (PCR) provides much more specific results.[41,42]

Syphilis Congenital syphilis is uncommon in developed countries but has carried an incidence as high as 10% in sub-Saharan Africa in the mid-1980s with some declines in incidence in the 1990s.[43,44] The disease has increased in frequency with rising drug use and exchange of drugs for sex.[45] It is estimated that approximately 50% of infants born to infected mothers will be premature, stillborn, or die in the neonatal period. Moreover, recent reports suggest an increase in antibiotic resistance.[46]

The histologic features commonly seen in syphilis include the triad of enlarged hypercellular villi, proliferative fetal vascular changes with vascular obliteration and onion-skinning and acute or chronic villitis (Fig. 34.11b,c).[47] Sheffield et al. specified necrotizing funisitis as a common feature and noted that *normoblastemia* was frequent in cases of stillbirth. They also reported an increase in sensitivity for detecting syphilis (from 67–89% in live-born infants) with attention to the above placental findings.[48] Genest et al. noted a strong association between the presence of treponemal DNA by PCR analysis and the above triad, and in a few cases, detected treponemal DNA in the absence of the classic triad.[47] It should be emphasized that enlarged villi and, mild chronic villitis are not specific and vascular changes would be required to suspect this diagnosis in the absence of clinical findings supporting fetal or maternal syphilis.

Management of congenital syphilis hinges principally on prevention with screening in the first trimester, retesting of high-risk individuals and treatment. Despite treatment, as many as 14% of infants may be born infected.[45]

Human immunodeficiency virus (HIV) HIV-induced acquired immunodeficiency syndrome (AIDS) is undoubtedly one of the most alarming health crises of our time. Worldwide, the estimated number of people living with HIV/AIDS is over 36 million, of which 16 million are women of childbearing age, 70% of which live in sub-Saharan Africa.[49] Mother-to-child trans-

mission is generally thought to occur *in utero*, during delivery, or post-partum as a result of breastfeeding.[50] Transmission rate is thought to be at least partially dependent on maternal viremia, since current antiretroviral therapies significantly reduce viral transmission.[50] The presence of the virus has been demonstrated in syncytiotrophoblasts as well as Hofbauer cells of the placenta, although the exact mechanism of infection, particularly the role of various cell surface receptors, remains controversial.[1] Other than CD4 receptor, other cell surface molecules involved in HIV infection have been identified in the placenta. These include the chemokine receptor CCR5, β_2 integrins and the HIV-binding lectins DC-SIGN and DC-SIGNR.[51–53] The latter are expressed by dendritic cells and capillary endothelial cells in the placenta, where they are thought to increase attachment efficiency of the virus and hence its presentation and transmission to receptor-positive cells.[54]

Morphologically, HIV infection does not cause any specific histopathologic abnormalities in the placenta; however, maternal HIV infection is associated with endometritis and fetal prematurity.[1] Furthermore, infants infected with HIV have a greater chance of congenital cytomegalovirus (CMV) co-infection.[55] HIV-infected pregnant women also have increased susceptibility to placental malaria, which is associated with IUGR and prematurity.[56]

Cytomegalovirus CMV infection is a major cause of chronic villitis. Perinatal infection can have devastating effects ranging from hydrops and macerated stillbirth to late-onset manifestations of hearing loss, blindness and cerebral palsy.[1] CMV villitis is variable, ranging from minimal inflammation to an intense lymphoplasmacytic destructive process, associated with villous stromal necrosis, fibrosis, calcification and hemosiderin deposition. CMV inclusions are more likely to be found if in addition to chronic villitis, several of the following features are also present (Fig. 34.11d): fetal nucleated RBCs, villous necrosis and acute inflammation, plasma cells (in villi or decidua), fetal death, IUGR, petechiae or hepatosplenomegaly. The characteristic 'owl-eye' nuclear and cytoplasmic inclusions range from widespread to focal; in some cases, inclusions are identified only after examining numerous blocks of placental parenchyma. The virus can also be identified by immunofluorescence or PCR.[57,58]

Herpes simplex The major route of fetal infection by HSV is through natal transmission in women with active genital herpes lesions, although transplacental and ascending infection can also occur.[1,59] Prenatally-acquired HSV can result in necrotizing deciduitis, amnionitis, chorionic vasculitis and funisitis, as well as severe chronic villitis. None of these features are specific, however, and only rarely are characteristic 'ground-glass' nuclear inclusions identified. Furthermore, the finding of multinucleated giant cells in association with villitis are non-specific; giant cells can be seen in chronic villitis due to HSV, varicella, or toxoplasmosis, but are actually most commonly found in severe, non-infectious villitis (see below).[60] Recent reports have emphasized the fact that HSV may be detected in the absence of morphologic abnormalities, including cases in which poor outcome ensued.[61-63]

Other virus infections Other viral infections of the placenta, including enterovirus, coxsackie, adenoviruses and echoviruses, have been receiving increasing attention in the pathogenesis of stillbirth and poor fetal outcome. The magnitude of the role of these viruses is unclear because the viruses are detected by molecular means and their link to the preceding events is not always possible. However, these viruses are commonly associated with spontaneous abortion and poor fetal outcomes.[64-67] Genen et al. examined 33 infants with evidence of systemic illness and identified coxsackie virus in 46% by *in situ* hybridization.[66] Similarly, Basso et al. isolated enterovirus from cases of spontaneous abortion; both studies linked these infections to these disorders relative to controls.[64-66] The portal of entry has been postulated to be syncytial trophoblast and staining for viral proteins is often identified in the trophoblast or Hofbauer cells (Fig. 34.11e,f).[68] Other infections include varicella-zoster and parvovirus.[69-71]

Clearly, placental examination will aid in the identification of common bacterial infections including undiagnosed acute chorioamnionitis.[72] Precisely how much the diagnostic yield will be increased with viral assays in the setting of IUGR or stillbirth is unclear.[73] This is due in part to the facts that morphologic abnormalities may not be present and the connection between the pathogen detected and the outcome may be uncertain with sensitive assays.[65] Nevertheless, the significant association between the detection of these pathogens and these outcomes warrants their use, particularly when a viral infection is suspected clinically and the histologic findings are unrewarding. The authors of these studies recommend not only Gram stain, but immunohistochemistry for enterovirus, parvovirus and cytomegalovirus for placentas from infants who are stillborn or born with neurologic abnormalities.[65]

Non-infectious chronic villitis (villitis of unknown etiology, VUE)
For the vast majority of chronic villitis, no infectious agent can be identified, even in cases of severe clinical

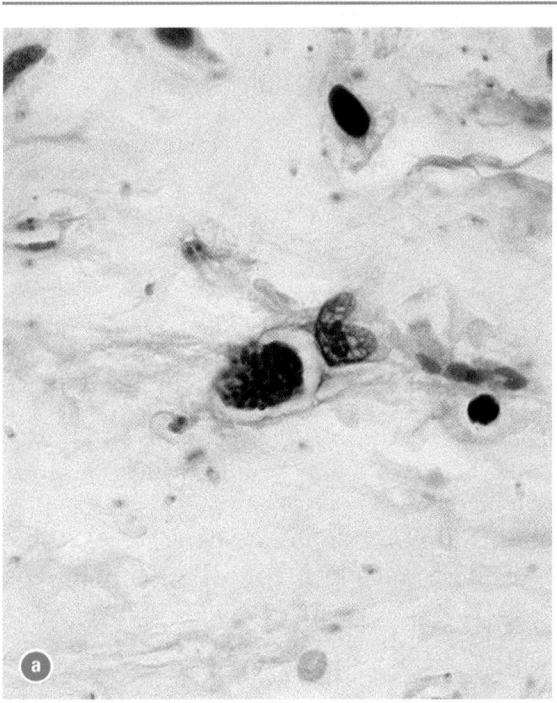
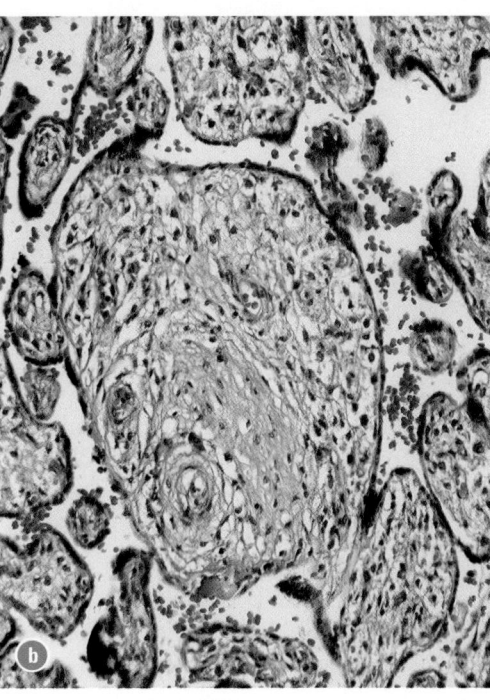

Fig. 34.11 Infections associated with IUGR or fetal/neonatal death. (a) Toxoplasmosis present in Wharton's jelly. (b) Syphilis, present as hypercellular villi with mild mononuclear infiltrate and onion-skinning around villous capillaries.

Continued

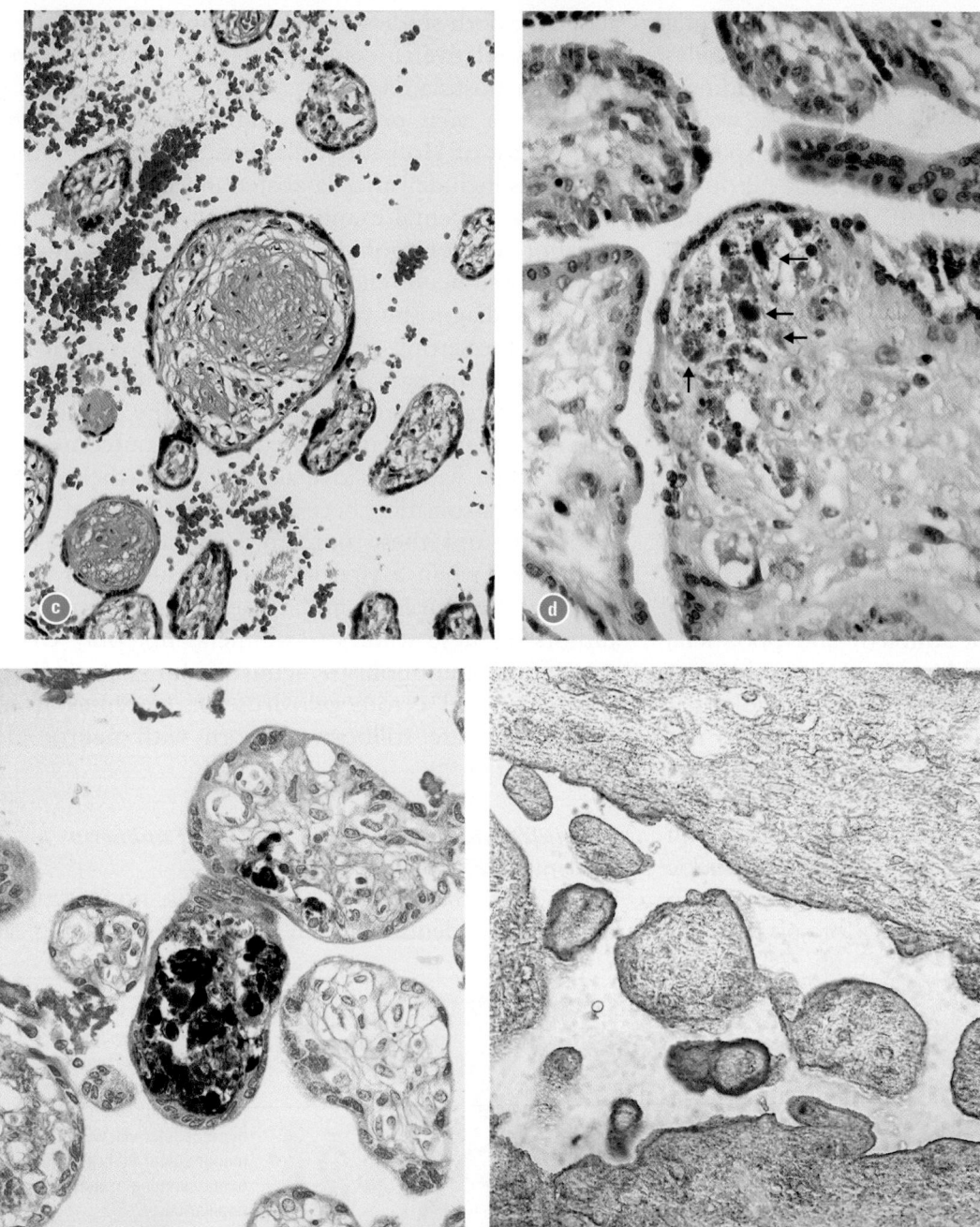

Fig. 34.11 Cont'd (c) Vascular obliterations seen in terminal villi in a case of syphilis. (d) Chronic cytomegalovirus villitis with eosinophilic debris and subtle inclusions (arrows). (e) The virus is highlighted by immunostaining. (f) Immunohistochemical staining for enterovirus in a placenta associated with fetal death. (Courtesy of Dr Gerard Nuovo, Ohio State University Medical Center.)

abnormalities or of fetal death. Such cases fall into the category villitis of unknown etiology, or VUE. VUE is found in 5 to 10% of placentas examined and has a recurrence rate of approximately 20%.[74] VUE should be suspected in cases of growth-restricted neonates and recurrent abortions or fetal death. The possibility remains that an as-yet-unidentified infectious agent (for example, RNA viruses or other such viruses that are hard to identify by routine histologic or electron microscopic means) is responsible for some or all cases of VUE; however, recent data point toward an alternative theory (see below).

Gross examination may show a small placenta, which is stiff due to increased fibrin content, although the majority of VUE placentas are grossly unremarkable.[1] Microscopically, VUE shows a wide spectrum of lesions, including marked intervillous accumulation of histiocytes and lymphocytes ('intervillositis'), avascular villi, necrotizing villitis and deciduitis, fetal vascular thrombosis and placental infarction (Fig. 34.12a,b).[1] Fluorescent *in situ* hybridization has been used to demonstrate that the intravillous and perivillous chronic inflammatory cells of VUE are mostly maternal in origin.[75] This, along with the helper T cell/histiocytic predominance of the inflammation and the high probability of recurrence, has led to the hypothesis that VUE may have

an immunologic etiology, akin to placental 'rejection'.[76] In fact, VUE is more prevalent in placentas from women with autoimmune disorders, such as systemic lupus erythematosus.[77] The associated thrombosis is thought to be secondary to the cytokines released by the maternal inflammatory cells, which in turn increase endothelial tissue factor, leading to activation of coagulation through the extrinsic pathway.[76,78]

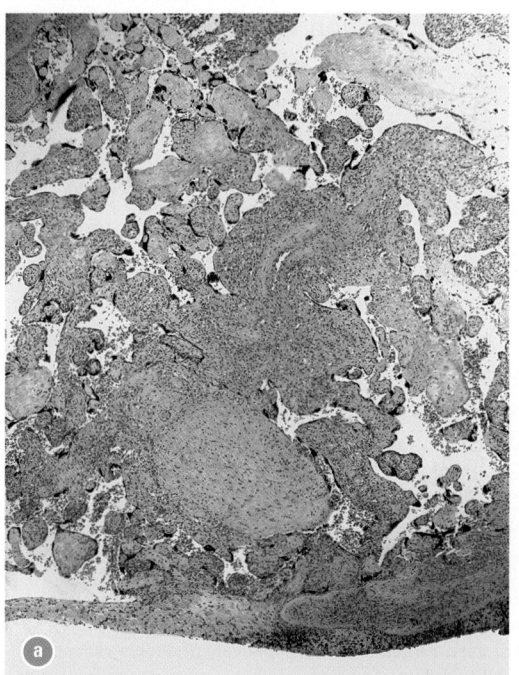

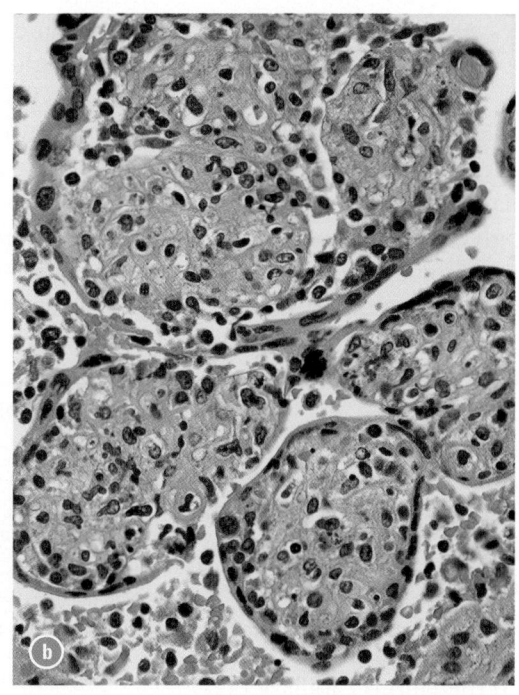

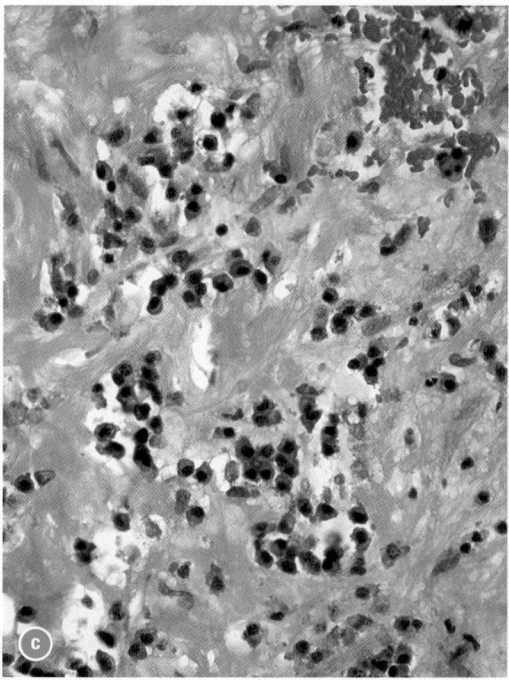

Fig. 34.12 Non-infectious villitis (of unknown etiology) associated with IUGR. (a) Lower power illustrating darker areas containing extensive mononuclear infiltrates. (b) Higher-power magnification showing increased number of mononuclear cells in villous parenchyma. (c) Chronic deciduitis. This is often associated with IUGR and some infections such as syphilis, but is non-specific.

Chronic deciduitis

Chronic inflammatory changes in the decidua (deciduitis) have been associated with a range of conditions leading to poor fetal outcome, including syphilis, VUE, infectious mononucleosis and others (Fig. 34.12c).[79–81] The significance of chronic lymphoplasmacytic deciduitis by itself is not certain and occasional plasma cells are not uncommon in the decidua or fallopian tubes in normal pregnancies. Nevertheless, their presence is worth noting in the context of IUGR.

MATERNAL DIABETES

Background

Gestational diabetes is defined as carbohydrate intolerance with onset and recognition during pregnancy.[82] The principal morbid sequelae include macrosomia, birth trauma, neonatal hypoglycemia, hypocalcemia, hyperbilirubinemia and polycythemia.[83] However, the extent of these complications relative to the control population is less pronounced. Approximately 80% of macrosomic infants are born to non-diabetic mothers.[84]

Placental findings

In maternal diabetes, several placental disorders have been classically described (Table 34.9).[85,86] Additional findings associated with diabetes include preferential deposition of fibrin-like fibrinoid at sites of epithelial (trophoblast) loss and damage suggesting an alteration in hemostasis.[87] Another study reported greater complexity of capillary branching in the villous capillary bed of diabetic placentas.[88] Poor control of blood glucose levels has been associated with fibrin thrombi, villous edema and basement membrane thickening in the placenta.[89,90]

Despite the above, in our experience, many of these characteristic placental features are often not found in the placentas of diabetic mothers. This is possibly related to 'tight diabetic' control and early delivery, both of which may minimize the development of characteristic placental findings.[91] At the current time, the most frequently observed histologic abnormalities in diabetic placentas are mild decidual vasculopathy, including vascular wall thickening and hyalinization, a mild increase in nucleated fetal RBCs and, occasionally, fetal vascular thrombosis.

IMMUNE AND NON-IMMUNE HYDROPS

Hemolytic disease of the newborn with immune hydrops (erythroblastosis fetalis) has recently declined to an incidence of 1 to 6 cases per 1000 live births.[92] This is largely due to administration of RhoGAM (Rho(D) immunoglobulin). In the occasional cases of erythroblastosis (Rh, Kell, Duffy, etc.) that do arise, management with intrauterine transfusion is successful in 90% of cases. Most cases of placental and fetal hydrops are now of the 'non-immune' variety (Table 34.10). The histologic features include villous enlargement (Fig. 34.13). These disorders, as a group, herald a poor prognosis and most can be classified into one of the following five etiologies:[93] (1) Fetal cardiovascular disease has been reported in 26% of cases of fetal hydrops and consist principally of cardiac anomalies that increase right atrial pressure or volume overload.[94] Additional causative

Table 34.10 *Causes of the hydropic fetus*

Immune hydrops (erythroblastosis fetalis)
Non-immune hydrops
  Fetal cardiovascular disease
    Early closure of ductus arteriosus, foramen ovale or ductus venosus
    High-output cardiac failure
    Arrhythmias
    Myocarditis
    Cardiomyopathy
  Chromosomal/genetic abnormalities
    Down syndrome
    Turner's syndrome
  Fetal thoracic abnormality
    Diaphragmatic hernia
    Congenital cystic adenomatoid malformation (CCAM)
    Pulmonary sequestration
  Twins
    Twin–twin transfusion syndrome
    Acardiac twinning
  Fetal tumors in the heart, lungs, abdomen or pelvis
  Fetal anemia
    α-Thalassemia
    Parvovirus B19
    Glucose-6-phosphate dehydrogenase deficiency
  Fetal–maternal hemorrhage
  Arterio-venous fistulas
  Placental anomalies
    Umbilical cord lesions, vascular abnormalities
  Other
    Nephrotic syndrome, hepatic necrosis.

Adapted from Sosa.[93]

Table 34.9 *'Classic' placental pathology in maternal diabetes*

Large, heavy placenta (>90th percentile)
Dysmaturity (admixture of mature and immature villi)
Fetal vascular thrombosis
Mild maternal decidual vasculopathy (thickening/hyalinization – not dilated)
Chorangiosis[86]
Single umbilical artery
Nucleated fetal RBCs

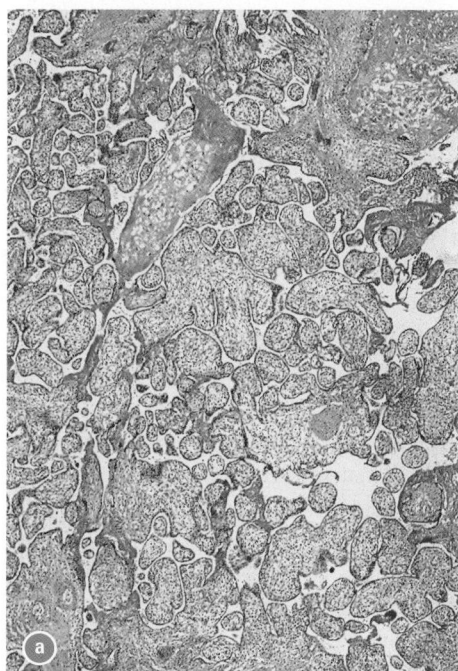 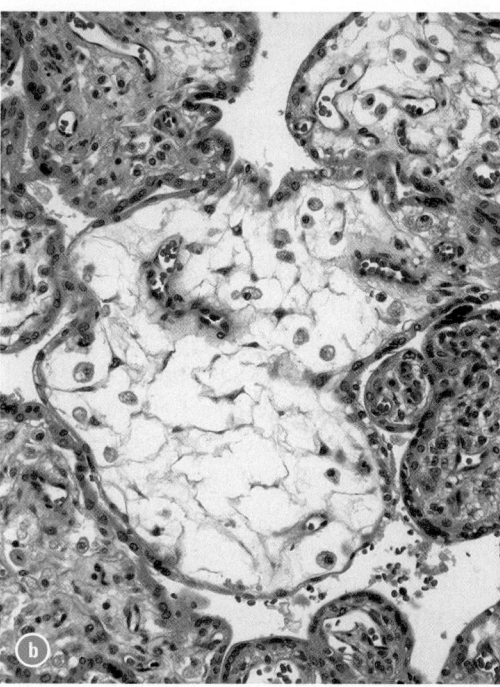

Fig. 34.13 (a) Extensive villous hydrops associated with erythroblastosis. (b) Focal non-immune villous hydrops.

factors include cardiac arrhythmias, failure, neoplasms, myopathies, infections, inflammatory lesions, infarction and arterial calcifications.[94] In one study, 40% of fetuses presenting at late gestation with tachycardia were hydropic and two-thirds could be controlled pharmacologically.[95] In contrast, fetal bradycardias carry a worse prognosis.[95] (2) Fetal chromosomal (abnormalities include most often Down syndrome (trisomy 21) or Turner's syndrome. (3) Fetal thoracic anomalies, including diaphragmatic hernia, congenital cystic adenomatoid malformation, etc.) have been reported. (4) Twinning, specifically twin-twin transfusion syndrome, can precipitate hydrops (see below). (5) Fetal anemia caused by parvovirus B19 infection, thalassemia and other disorders, is also a cause of hydrops.[96] When present in hydropic placentas, nucleated red blood cells are evidence of fetal anemia. Nucleated fetal red blood cells (nRBCs) are not found in great numbers in normal placentas after 20 weeks of gestation, although an occasional one might be seen. A good place to evaluate the number of nRBCs in fetal blood is the lumen of a large cord/chorionic plate vessel. Abundant nRBCs in non-hydropic placentas after 20 weeks reflects subacute to chronic fetal hypoxia.[97]

One specific cause of fetal anemia is infection with parvovirus B19, a perinatal pathogen which does not cause villitis. Parvovirus infects fetal erythroblasts, resulting in hemolysis, severe anemia, hydrops fetalis and possible stillbirth. The placenta may be heavy and hydropic, with edema of stem and terminal villi. Large numbers of nRBCs and erythroblasts are found in the fetal vessels, similar to the picture of Rh erythroblastosis. Parvoviral intranuclear inclusions are readily found in nRBC precursors in fetal (autopsy) tissue: nuclei are enlarged with a thin peripheral rim of chromatin surrounding a central glassy, pink-purple homogeneous inclusion. Such inclusions are very prominent in fetal tissues, especially liver and marrow, but are not easily observed in placental villi, even when large numbers of nucleated RBCs are present.

Fetal ascites is sometimes seen in non-immune hydrops and is associated with any of the above disorders, including gastrointestinal and genitourinary abnormalities.[98]

Much lesser degrees of villous swelling may be seen in the second and third trimesters in the absence of a hydropic gestation and are usually of no consequence. However, conspicuous villous hydrops has been associated with poor fetal outcome and correlates with fetal acidosis.[30]

FETAL DISTRESS

In cases of fetal distress, such as asphyxia or low neonatal Apgar scores, the placenta is usually sent for examination to determine whether the pathology explains the clinical scenario. Certain placental disorders such as abruptio placentae, cord prolapse and ruptured vasa previa are highly associated with fetal asphyxia (Table 34.11). In some of these conditions, however, pathologic findings may be minimal or absent (i.e. cord prolapse or very acute abruptio). One placental pathologic feature associated with antepartum asphyxia (as well as fetal anemia) is an increase in the number of fetal nucleated red blood cells (see Ch. 33). More commonly, meconium passage is present with clinical fetal distress. However, some stillborn fetuses have not passed meconium and meconium passage may sometimes be a physiologic process, not necessarily indicative of fetal compromise. Despite the caveats, a relationship may exist between meconium passage and asphyxia. The extent and location of meconium staining may reflect timing of its passage (Table 34.12).

A slimy, green appearance grossly suggests meconium staining, a finding most common in term or post-term placentas; gross meconium staining begins at 1–2 hours and is maximal by 3–6 hours after meconium exposure (Table 34.12) (Fig. 34.14a).[99] Histologically, meconium in chorioamniotic tissues appears as a pale gold, iron stain-negative, pigmentation within cytoplasm of stromal cells and macrophages (Fig. 34.14b). With meconium exposure, the amniotic epithelium takes on a damaged appearance, with disorganization, pseudostratification and necrosis (Fig. 34.14c). The stromal tissue frequently displays a bluish appearance due to myxoid degeneration. *In vitro* studies have demonstrated meconium

pigment within amniotic macrophages within 1 hour post-exposure and within chorionic macrophages by 3 hours; the amniotic epithelial degenerative changes usually appear within 1 hour of exposure.[99] Meconium-induced vascular necrosis is a recently described, important pathologic finding associated with prolonged, severe meconium exposure and a poor perinatal outcome.[100] Histologically, meconium vasonecrosis consists of individual necrobiotic smooth muscle cells, with dark eosinophilic cytoplasm and pyknotic nuclei, found in the outer media of fetal arteries and veins of the umbilical cord and chorionic plate. There is always extensive meconium pigmentation and occasionally a small amount of acute inflammation. Prolonged meconium exposure of at least 16 hours' duration can cause not just such tissue necrosis but also linear fissures and ulcerations of the umbilical cord. When such prolonged and severe meconium exposure is suspected, extra sampling of the umbilical cord and the chorionic plate is indicated to look for such meconium-induced changes.

The placenta in the setting of the malformed fetus

BACKGROUND

About 3% of live-born infants have congenital malformations; this rate is higher in stillborns and aborted fetuses. For most congenital malformations, no specific placental abnormalities are recognized. However, certain anomalies (listed in Table 34.13)[101] are associated with

Table 34.11 Placental findings associated with fetal distress/asphyxia

Meconium-stained membranes
Abruptio placentae
Cord prolapse
Chronic placental compromise (small size, infarcts, villitis, fibrosis, extensive fibrin)
Fetal normoblastemia
Fetal vascular thrombosis

Table 34.12 Duration of meconium exposure[99,100]

Within minutes:
    amniotic epithelial change
    disorganized, reactive, necrotic amnion
    meconium macrophages in amnion
    minimal gross staining of placenta and cord
Within hours:
    maximal gross staining of placenta and cord
    meconium macrophages in chorion
Within days:
    umbilical ulcers/fissures
    meconium-induced vascular necrosis (umbilical and chorionic plate vessels)
    associated acute inflammation in necrotic vessel wall

Table 34.13 Placental abnormalities associated with specific congenital malformations.

Placental abnormality	Fetal malformation
Single umbilical artery	Renal abnormalities; sirenomelia[101]
Short umbilical cord	Gastroschisis
Amnion nodosum	Lethal renal anomalies:
	Renal agenesis
	Renal dysplasia
	Bladder outlet obstruct
Early amnion rupture:	Amniotic band syndrome:
Umbilical cord stricture	Amputations
Umbilical 'sheath'	Tethering
No amnion on chorion	Constriction rings
Reactive chorionic stroma	Bizarre body wall defect
'vernix granulomas'	Bizarre cranial deformity
Monochorionic twins, anastomoses	TTTS
	Hydranencephaly
Partial hydatidiform mole	Syndactyly, etc.
Marked hydrops (cavitation)	Beckwith-Wiedemann syndrome

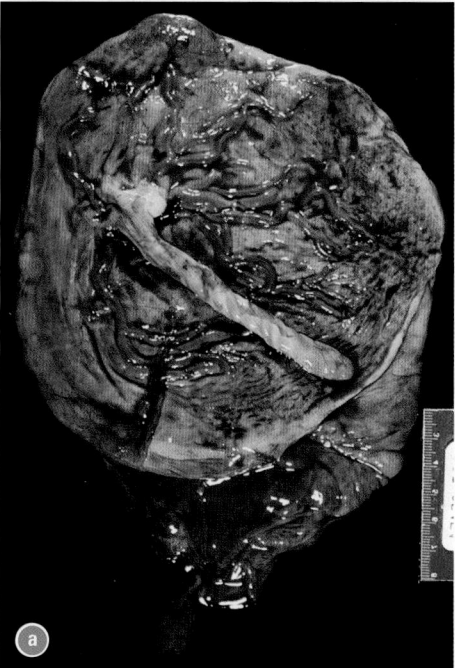

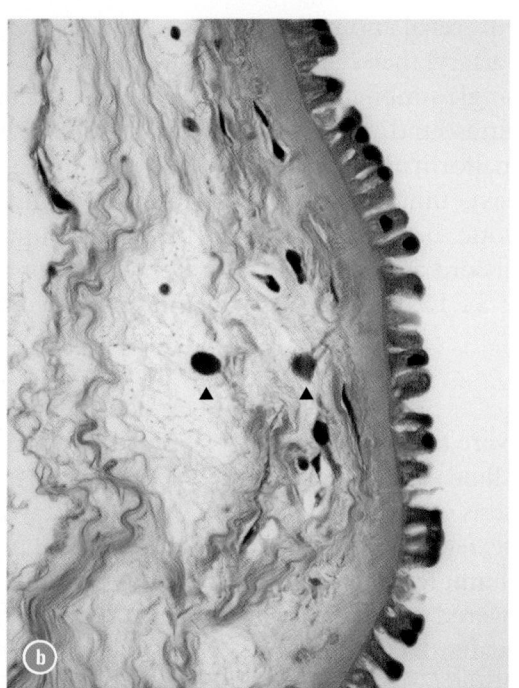

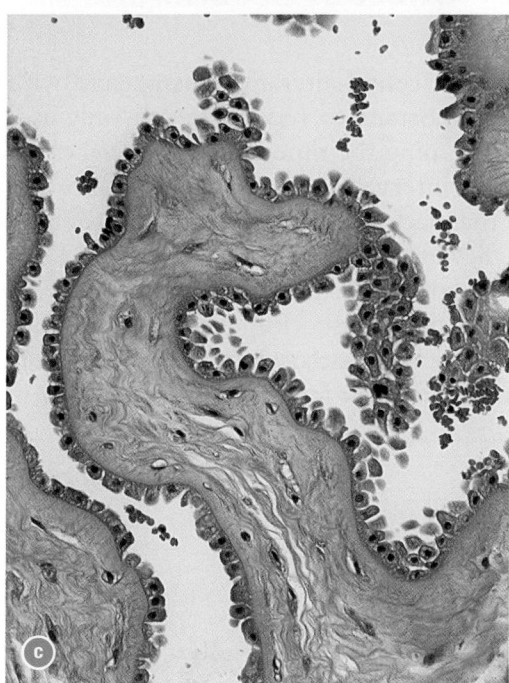

Fig. 34.14 (a) Meconium-stained membranes. (b) Meconium within macrophages in the amnion (arrowheads). (c) Stratification of the amnion epithelium ('dysplasia'), following meconium exposure.

specific placental disorders. Among these associations, several unusual placental abnormalities (such as amnion nodosum and amniotic bands) are highly linked with particular malformations; in contrast, other more common placental disorders (fetal thrombosis, single umbilical artery) are less frequently associated with specific fetal malformations. Fetal thrombosis and the pathology of amniotic band syndrome are discussed elsewhere in this chapter.

SINGLE UMBILICAL ARTERY

Single umbilical artery of the umbilical cord occurs, on average, in approximately 1% of term births (0.3–1.5%).[101,102] This finding is associated with increased rates of stillbirth, neonatal death, congenital anomalies and chromosomal anomalies. It is an important pathologic diagnosis because it alerts the pediatrician to assess the neonate for possible associated congenital anomalies (Fig. 34.15a). Using ultrasound,

Leung and Robson detected 'silent' renal anomalies in 19% of cases with single umbilical artery; they suggested that all live-born infants with a single umbilical artery should be screened with renal ultrasound.[101,102] Additional cord anomalies linked to malformations include *short umbilical cord* (gastroschisis), umbilical sheath (amnion) associated with amniotic band syndrome and, rarely, velamentous umbilical cord associated with congenital hip dislocation (Table 34.13).

AMNION NODOSUM

Amnion nodosum results from severe oligohydramnios (reduction in volume of amniotic fluid) and is most frequently caused by fetal renal agenesis or renal dysplasia. With reduced amniotic fluid, the fetus has increased contact with the amniotic epithelium, leading to small amniotic epithelial ulcerations covered by eosinophilic debris from the fetal vernix; usually, fetal squamous cells are embedded within the debris. Grossly, amnion nodosum can be differentiated from squamous metaplasia in that nodules of amnion nodosum can be peeled off the placental surface, while plaques of squamous metaplasia are adherent (Fig. 34.15b).

The placenta in fetal death

Placental pathologic changes associated with fetal death are divided into primary placental disorders leading to fetal death and placental pathology secondary to fetal death.

PRIMARY PLACENTAL DISORDERS

Specific placental pathology seen at time of fetal autopsy can provide either the primary cause of death or important clues to a process which could have contributed to fetal death (Table 34.14). Examples of the former include abruptio placentae, cord obstruction due to tight knots or rupture of cord vessels (see Fig 33.11), multiple placental infarcts, or ruptured vasa previa. The latter category includes such findings as chronic villitis, which interferes with fetal oxygenation and nutrient exchange and may indicate an infectious process. Similarly, chorioamnionitis hints at the predisposition to fetal sepsis, intervillous thrombi suggest possible transplacental hemorrhage and severe villous edema suggests fetal hydrops. Table 34.14 provides a list of the most common such placental findings which explain, or provide clues to, the cause of fetal death.

PLACENTAL PATHOLOGY SECONDARY TO FETAL DEATH

The non-specific placental alterations associated with fetal death are important to recognize not only as a rough guide concerning the time of fetal death (i.e. the death-to-delivery interval) but also as post-mortem artifacts rather than factors which may have contributed to fetal death. Several findings, listed in Table 34.15, can be used to roughly determine the death-to-delivery interval.[103] Most changes used for 'timing' fetal death involve the fetal placental vessels, which undergo gradual, progressive alterations after fetal death. Fetal vessels in

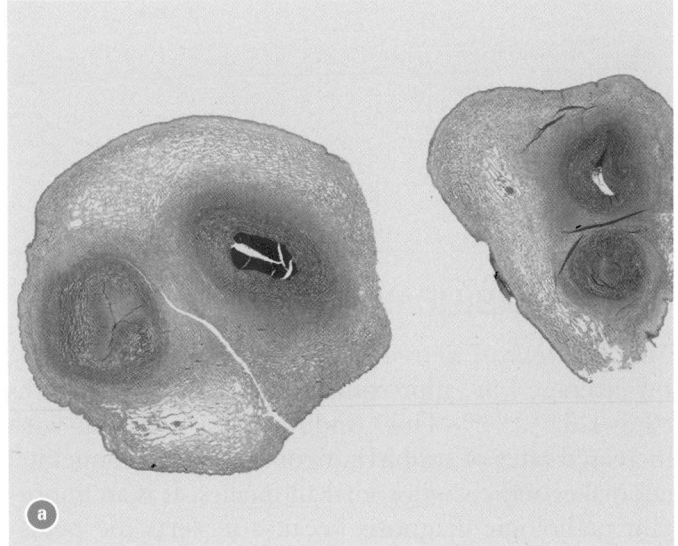

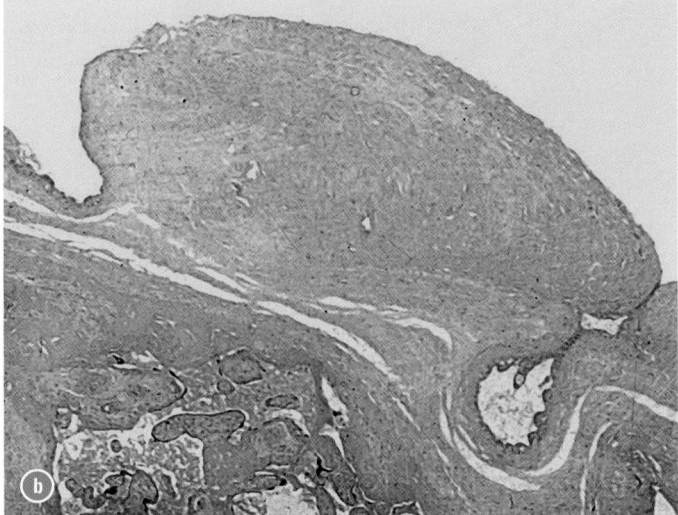

Fig. 34.15 Placental findings associated with fetal anomalies (see also Ch. 33). (a) Single umbilical artery (often associated with cardiovascular or renal anomalies). (b) Amnion nodosum (oligohydramnios, renal anomalies).

Table 34.14 *Primary placental disorders causally related to fetal death*

Chorionic villi
  acute villitis
  chronic villitis (infectious, VUE)
  villous edema (fetal hydrops)
  intervillous thrombi/hematoma (transplacental hemorrhage)
  large/multiple placental infarcts
  abruptio placentae
Umbilical cord
  knots
  thrombosis or rupture of cord vessel (vein)
  velamentous (membranous) cord insertion
    rupture of membranous vessels
    vasa previa (rupture during labor associated with fetal
      exsanguinetion)
Membranes
  chorioamnionitis (possible fetal sepsis)

VUE, villitis of unknown etiology.

Table 34.15 *Placental changes secondary to fetal death*

>6 hours	Brown/red gross discoloration umbilical cord Intravascular karyorrhexis in fetal chorionic villous vessels
>2 days	Multi luminal bridges in stem villous arteries and veins
>2 weeks	Widespread luminal bridges or luminal occlusions in stem villous arteries and veins Loss of capillary lumens in >25% terminal villi

Non-specific changes, reflect duration from death to delivery, not cause of fetal death.

non-placental locations (i.e. systemic and umbilical cord vessels) do not develop these progressive alterations; this suggests that post-mortem changes of fetal placental vessels require maternal oxygenation of the placenta after fetal death.

The placenta in multiple gestations

ESTABLISHING CHORIONICITY

The vast majority of twin placentas are submitted to establish chorionicity. There are two types of twin placentation, namely monochorionic and dichorionic. Dichorionic placentas are always diamnionic (DiDi), whereas monochorionic placentas can be either diamnionic (DiMo) or monoamnionic (MoMo). The expected proportions of these types of placentas in monozygotic (MZ or identical) and dizygotic (DZ or fraternal) twins are summarized in Table 34.16.[104] In general, it can be stated that all monochorionic placentas come from MZ twins, but that not all MZ twins have monochorial placentas.[1]

On gross examination, a DiDi placenta can sometimes be differentiated from a DiMo placenta by the opacity of the dividing membranes in the former; however, microscopic examination is always recommended for confirmation. The best section for such examination is a 'T section' from the site of insertion of the membranes on the placental disc (see also Ch. 33) (Fig. 34.16a,b).

Overall, morbidity is higher in twin gestation, with a fetal loss rate at 24 weeks of over 10% and a perinatal/infant mortality of 41 and 33 per 1000 live births.[105] The rates are higher in monochorionic versus dichorionic twin pregnancies. In one study the frequency of neurologic morbidity (in the form of cerebral palsy or impaired development) was seven-fold higher in monochorionic gestations.[106] The risk is even higher in monoamnionic gestations. In a small series of seven prospectively managed monoamnionic twin pairs, Sau et al. recorded two twin pairs (4) losses prior to 20 weeks. Of the remaining 10, nine were born alive and seven survived.[107] Complications of monochorionic twinning are summarized in Table 34.17.

Table 34.16 *Chorionicity and zygosity*

	Prevalence	DZ/MZ (%)
DiDi	80%	90% DZ (fraternal) 10% MZ (identical, TTT not expected)
DiMo	19%	100% MZ (anastomoses common, TTT possible)
MoMo	<1%	100% MZ (umbilical cord entanglement, IUFD possible)

DiDi, diamnionic, dichorionic; DiMo, diamnionic, monochorionic; MoMo, monochorionic, monoamnionic; DZ, dizygous; MZ, monozygous; TTT, twin-twin transfusion syndrome; IUFD, intrauterine fetal death. Based on Cameron.[104]

Table 34.17 *Complications of monochorionic gestations*

Cord entanglement or cord compression/disruption (accident) (MoMo)
Congenital anomalies
Twin-twin transfusion syndrome (MoDi)
Intrauterine growth restriction
Pre-term delivery
Intrauterine fetal death

MoMo, monochorionic, monoamnionic; MoDi, monochorionic, diamnionic.

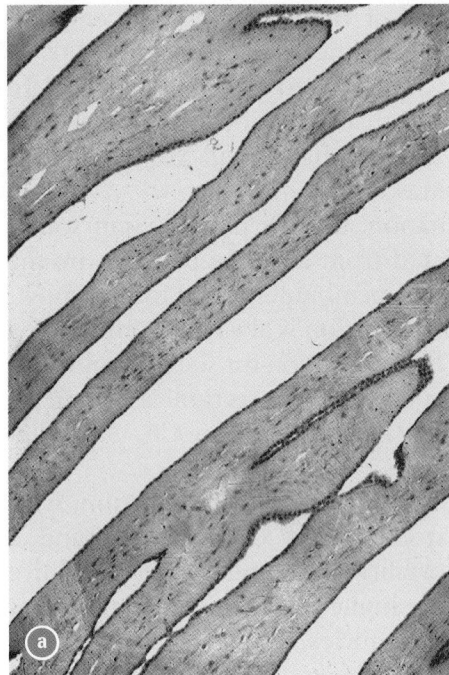
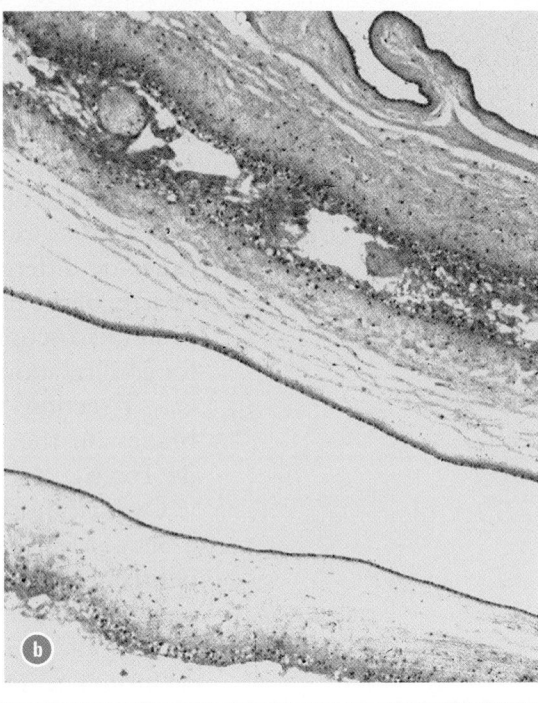

Fig. 34.16 Establishing chorionicity by examination of the dividing membrane. (a) Diamnionic, monochorionic gestation. (b) Diamnionic, dichorionic gestation. The dividing membrane displays intervening chorion.

TWIN-TWIN TRANSFUSION SYNDROME

Twin-twin transfusion syndrome complicates between 4 and 35% of monozygotic twin pregnancies and contributes to adverse outcome.[108] It can be subdivided into two components. The rarest and most profound is acardiac twinning. More common is a disparity in fetal size due to variable degrees of twin-twin transfusion.

Acardiac twin

Acardiac twins result from reversed arterial perfusion, in which significant anastomoses lead to dominance of the circulation by one twin early during development. Ultimately, this results in absence of, or severe restriction in, cardiac development in the recipient and in turn a profound defect in somatic and neural development (Fig. 34.17). This has been termed the TRAP (twin reversed arterial perfusion) sequence.[108] Mortality to the normal (pump) twin varies. In one study 9 of 10 survived with delivery at 34 weeks.[109] Others have reported higher mortality.[108]

Twin-twin transfusion syndrome

In monochorionic placentas, superficial anastomoses connect vessels with similar pressures (artery to artery or vein to vein), minimizing shunting due to the equality of pressures. In contrast, 'deep' anastomoses connect vessels of unequal pressure (artery and vein), allowing shunting to occur through the intervening capillary bed. If multiple deep shunts exist in both directions (A-to-V and V-to-A), the intertwin exchange may balance and blood volume shift may be minimal. However, when such deep shunts are unbalanced or unidirectional, particularly when only one deep shunt is present, blood

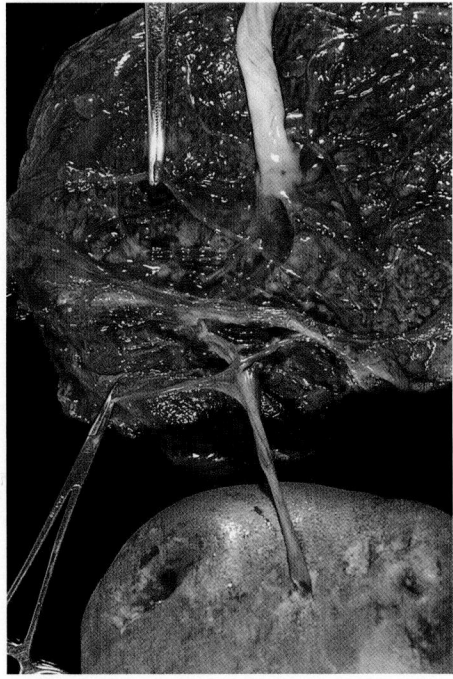

Fig. 34.17 Acardiac twin, seen as an amorphous mass tethered to the placenta by an attenuated umbilical cord. The cord of the normal twin is seen above.

volume will gradually shift from one twin to the other. This gradual shift in blood volume produces chronic twin-to-twin transfusion syndrome (chronic TTTS). In chronic TTTS, either or both twins may die from sequelae of severe volume contraction or volume overload. Twin-twin transfusion is a major cause of intrauterine death of one twin. In a study of 972 twin births, Aslan et al. reported the death of one twin in 32 (3.3%), a quarter of which were attributed to twin-twin transfusion syndrome.[110] Also, half of neonatal deaths in the other twin occurred in the setting of TTTS. TTTS is first suspected when acute hydramnios develops around mid-gestation. Currently, Doppler ultrasound is highly accurate in prenatal diagnosis of this syndrome; however, the diagnosis can be confirmed, or the extent of anastomoses determined, by postnatal examination of placental vasculature through injection of various dyes.

Most often, chronic TTTS results in a small, pale, growth-restricted 'donor' twin, with oligohydramnios and oliguria due to volume contraction and a larger, plethoric, hydropic 'recipient' twin, with polyhydramnios due to polyuria (Fig. 34.18). The placenta is almost always found to be monochorial. Usually, the donor twin's placenta is pale (from low blood volume) and hydropic (due to fetal CHF and anemia) (Fig. 34.19). The donor twin usually has smaller organs, including decreased brain weight, partially due to periventricular encephalomalacia, and suffers from anemia and hypoglycemia. An increased incidence of velamentous cord insertion has also been seen in the donor twin.[111,112]

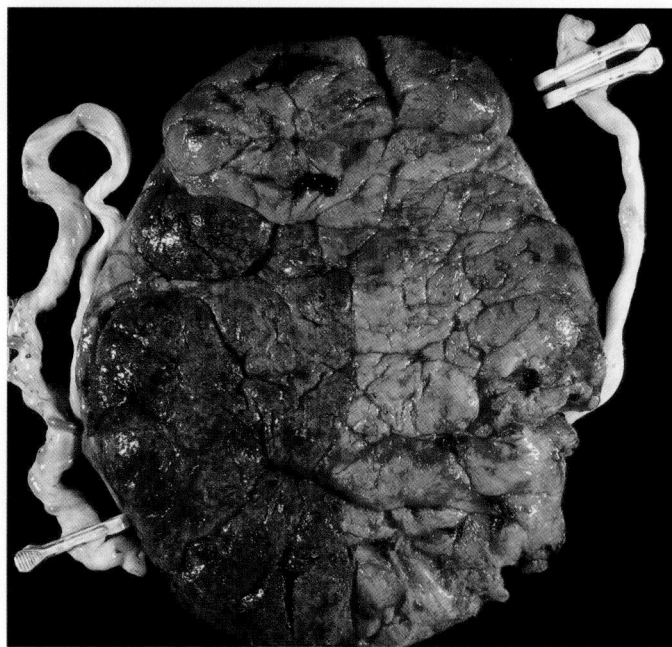

Fig. 34.19 Discordant placental perfusion in twin-twin transfusion syndrome (donor right, recipient left). (Courtesy of Dr Julie Reimann, Brigham and Women's Hospital.)

The recipient twin, on the other hand, usually has a congested placenta, larger organs, including a heart showing hypertrophic changes and kidneys with glomerular hyperplasia and tubular dilatation, and suffers from hyperbilirubinemia and polycythemia. Indeed, due to the latter entity, an increased risk of thrombosis exists in recipient twins, resulting in gangrenous extremities and intracranial hemorrhage. Increased numbers of nucleated RBCs may be found in either circulation.

Immediately before one twin dies, a preterminal drop in blood pressure may allow rapid shunting through large surface AA or VV shunts from the other twin; such rapid shunting from the surviving to the dying co-twin has been termed acute TTTS. Acute TTTS provides a plausible mechanism to account for brain infarcts and other abnormalities, including cerebral palsy, in surviving twins after death of the co-twin.

TTTS has a poor prognosis, particularly when diagnosed before 28 weeks of gestation. In case of natural death of one twin (and development into a fetus papyraceous, see below), the hydramnios may cease and the other twin may reach term. Based on such cases, induced abortion of one twin, in most cases the donor, has been attempted in cases of severe TTTS, with good outcome in the remaining twin.[113] Amnioreduction has also been tried for treatment of TTTS, but the results have been variable, with questionable improvement in

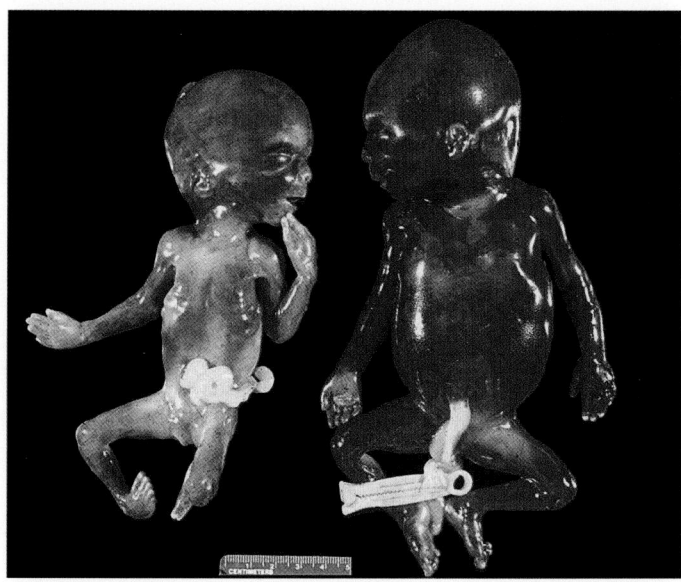

Fig. 34.18 Discordant twin growth in twin-twin transfusion syndrome (donor left, recipient right).

overall survival. Most recently, fetoscopic laser therapy of all vascular anastomoses has been favored. After a thorough review of clinical studies and therapeutic outcomes, van Gemert et al. suggest that laser therapy offers significantly improved survival rates in severe TTTS, diagnosed before 26 weeks of gestation, but that amnioreduction or delivery may be just as efficacious in mild TTTS, diagnosed after 26 weeks.[114]

OTHER COMPLICATIONS OF TWINNING

Aside from TTTS, twin gestations still exhibit significantly increased perinatal morbidity and mortality compared with singleton gestations (reviewed by Sherer, in Table 34.18).[115] Rates of stillbirth are significantly higher in twin pregnancies.[116,117] In fact, antepartum death of a single fetus complicates 2–5% of all twin pregnancies and may be associated with the development of fetus papyraceous (Fig. 34.20). In such cases, there is increased risk of morbidity and mortality in the surviving twin, including defects in CNS, liver, spleen and kidneys, as well as an absent ear or pulmonic stenosis.[1] Perinatal mortality is usually higher in the second-born twin, although this may be an artifact imposed by the fact that the dead twin is usually delivered second.[118]

Twin gestations are also at increased risk for discordant growth, with one twin's growth below the 10th percentile, which by itself is associated with a higher adverse outcome.[119] There is also an increased risk of prematurity, small-for-gestational age fetuses and fetal growth restriction, the latter complicating up to 47% of multiple gestations.[120] Chorionicity also affects perinatal morbidity and mortality, with monochorionic monoamnionic twins having the highest risk. Aside from increased risk of TTTS and acardiac twinning, monochorionic gestations also have an increased frequency of abnormal umbilical cord insertion. Marginal and velamentous insertions occur in 21 and 16% of dichorionic pregnancies, respectively, but in 33% of monochorionic pregnancies.[121]

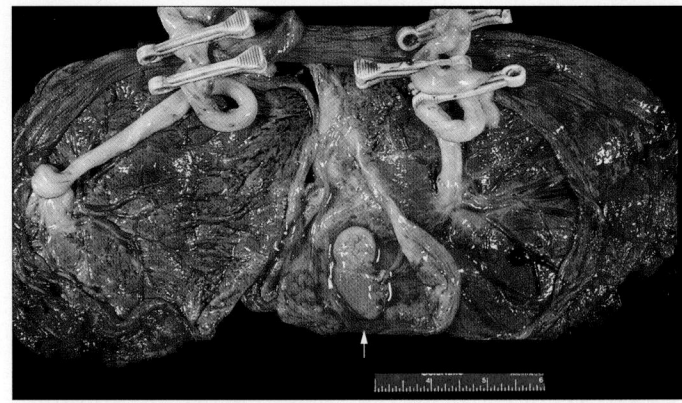

Fig. 34.20 Fetus papyraceous, seen here between two normal placentas of the remaining twin gestation (arrow).

Interestingly, twinning may impose a lower risk of preeclampsia in subsequent pregnancies. In one study, the recurrence risk of preeclampsia in second pregnancy was approximately one half (7.3 vs 14.1%) if the prior pregnancy was a twin versus singleton pregnancy.[122]

Tumors in the placenta seen at term

All of the entities discussed below are detailed in Chapter 33, under examination of the placenta. They are not associated with specific clinical findings and are revisited for completion.

CHORANGIOMA

Chorangiomas are hemangiomas of the chorionic stroma, occurring in about 1% of placentas. They usually present as solitary masses adjacent to the fetal chorionic plate, usually contiguous with the chorionic plate or large stem villi. This distinguishes them from infarcts, which are usually basally oriented. On cross-section, chorangiomas have a firm, gelatinous, myxoid consistency with a tan, to dark red, to variegated color, occasionally with necrosis or calcification (Fig. 34.21a). Sometimes, however, they have a uniformly dark red appearance, grossly resembling an old blood clot. Chorangiomas can range from microscopic to over 20 cm. When very small in size, these benign tumors are insignificant. In contrast, large chorangiomas (>5 cm) have resulted in fetal congestive heart failure, hydrops, consumptive coagulopathy and

---

Table 34.18 Placental pathology and multiple gestation

Placental findings more common in twins than singletons
   Marginal cord insertion
   Velamentous (membranous) cord insertion
   Single umbilical artery
   Chorangioma
Placental findings specific to multiple gestation
   Fetus papyraceous
   Acardiac twin
   Vascular anastomoses (restricted to monochorionic placentas)

death. Chorangiomas can be associated with fetal cutaneous or visceral hemangiomas.[123] They are also highly associated with the placentas of multiple gestations, for unclear reasons.

CHORIOCARCINOMA

Choriocarcinoma arising in a term placenta is very rare, with a few reported cases in the literature (discussed in Ch. 33). These tumors are not likely to be suspected clinically but should be excluded when infarcts are identified grossly and examined histologically (Fig.

34.21b). Intraplacental choriocarcinomas are at risk for systemic dissemination and can rarely metastasize to the fetus; thus their identification has important clinical consequences.[124]

PLACENTAL SITE TROPHOBLASTIC TUMOR

This has been discussed in detail in Chapter 33. A small percentage of PSTTs follow term pregnancy and may be detected months and years following delivery. Prognosis is closely linked to the interval between delivery and detection of the tumor.[125]

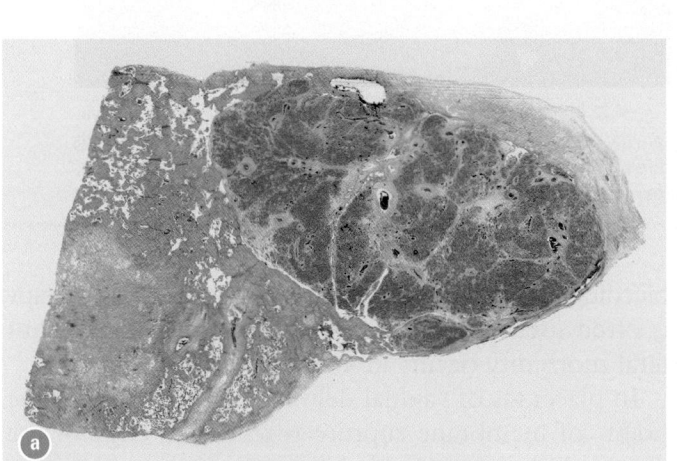

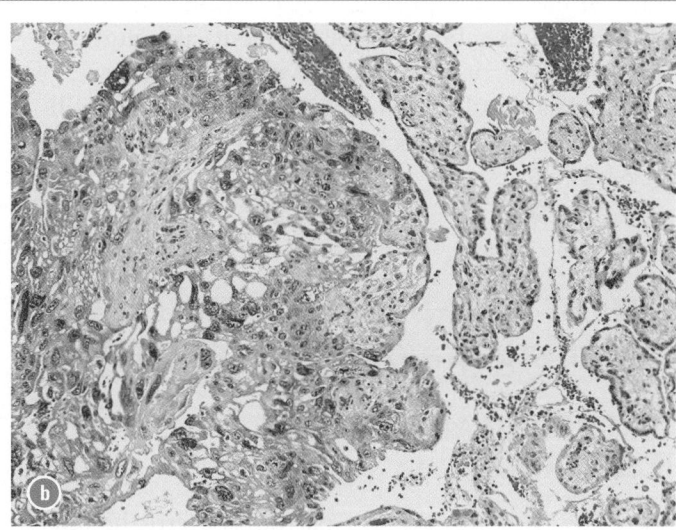

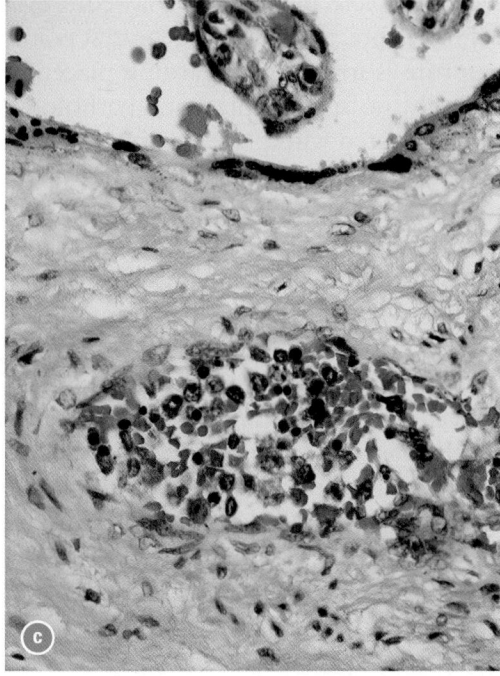

Fig. 34.21 Tumors seen in the term placenta. (a) Chorangioma. (b) Intraplacental choriocarcinoma. (c) Fetal leukemia, seen here as myeloid precursors and normoblasts within a stem villous vessel lumen.

METASTATIC CARCINOMA

Metastatic cancer in the placenta, from mother or fetus, is rare.[126] Melanoma is the most frequent maternal metastatic tumor in the placenta and the only maternal metastatic tumor which characteristically crosses the placenta and metastasizes to the fetus.[126] The second most common metastatic maternal tumor in the placenta is breast carcinoma. Fetal neuroblastoma can also metastasize to the placenta.

CONGENITAL LEUKEMIA

Congenital leukemia is rare and carries a much more ominous prognosis than its counterpart later in childhood.[127] It has been reported in association with Down syndrome and may be acute or transient, although the latter scenario carries the risk of eventual recurrence.[128] The diagnosis should be excluded in the setting of stillbirth, particularly in association with Down syndrome (Fig. 34.21c).

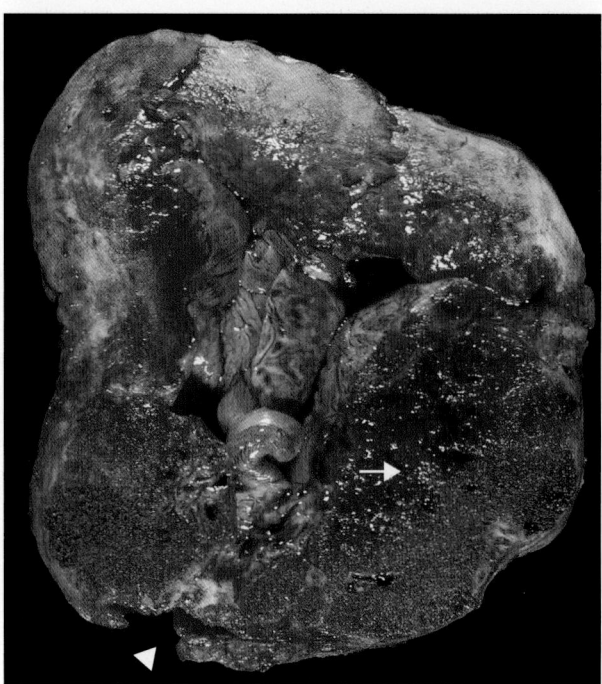

Fig. 34.22 Hemisectioned uterus with placenta extending to the cervix (previa; arrowhead). The placenta is still within the uterus and extends through the entire wall of the lower uterine segment and myometrium (percreta; arrow).

Peri- or post-partum hemorrhage (including gravid hysterectomy)

BACKGROUND AND CLINICAL PRESENTATION

Massive intra-partum and post-partum obstetric hemorrhage is a major cause of maternal morbidity and necessitates hysterectomy in 2–5 cases per 1000. The most common causes are placenta previa, uterine atony and/or uterine rupture and placenta accreta. Maternal morbidity in cases of emergency hysterectomy is high, both in the extent of blood loss and other complications, including disseminated intravascular coagulopathy, wound infection and ureteral damage. Despite these complications, most studies report no or few (0–5%) maternal deaths, which were linked to the severity of the underlying condition.[129–133]

PLACENTA PREVIA

Placenta previa is defined as implantation within the lower uterine segment or the cervix and may be associated with accreta (see below) (Fig. 34.22). Management involves the exclusion of digital vaginal examination and delaying delivery until either the fetus has achieved pulmonary maturity or 36 weeks gestation.[133] Because bleeding is associated with contractions, tocolytic therapy is often used. Maternal morbidity is uncommon, but fetal morbidity occurs in 4–8% of cases.[133]

In placentas of vaginal deliveries, when the 'nearest point' of membrane rupture reaches the edge of the placental disc, a marginal placenta previa should be suspected. However, complete placenta previa requires a Cesarean delivery; therefore, analysis of the 'nearest point' of membrane rupture is irrelevant regarding placental position. Surprisingly, no specific placental pathologic abnormalities are associated with placenta previa, which can be remarkably 'normal' both by gross and histologic assessment. Retroplacental blood clots and maternal surface disruption are sometimes present in cases of placenta previa. Other somewhat non-specific findings occasionally seen in placenta previa include regional thinning or infarction and maternal surface fragmentation. When a placenta previa is diagnosed in a patient who has had a prior Cesarean section, there is a high risk of a placenta accreta; in this setting, a Cesarean hysterectomy is sometimes performed. Even if the placenta has been removed by the surgeon, the diagnosis of placenta previa can be confirmed in a hysterectomy specimen when placental implantation site is histologically documented surrounding the internal os (i.e. involving both the anterior and posterior lower uterine segments).

CRETA

Placenta accreta defines implantation without an intervening buffer of decidua. Depending on the extent of the abnormality, it may be termed accreta (when the placental tissue is adherent to the superficial myometrium), increta (when villi invade the deep myometrium) and percreta (when the villi are transmural) (Fig. 34.23a–c). The greatest risk factors for accreta are prior curettage, submucosal leiomyoma, uterine surgery and prior pregnancy or Cesarean section, which have been associated with 80% of case.[130,134]

The gross findings in placenta accreta vary. Accreta may be suspected if the placenta is focally fragmented or myometrium is identified at the maternal surface (Fig. 34.23a). In instances where the uterus is removed, the pathologist should carefully examine the endometrial surface for retained placenta and liberally sample the endomyometrium in areas of suspected implantation. If villi are identified in direct contact with the myometrium, a diagnosis of accreta is made. If implantation bed fibrin is identified in direct continuity with the myometrium, with the absence of decidua, a diagnosis of accreta is justified (Fig. 34.23b). Documentation of accreta is important to verify the cause of bleeding.

Management of accreta includes manual removal of the placenta, focal hemostasis with endometrial sutures, artery ligation, methotrexate in some studies and ultimately hysterectomy. Ota et al. reported hysterectomy in 30% of cases, endometrial sutures in 20% and manual removal of the placenta in 50%.[134]

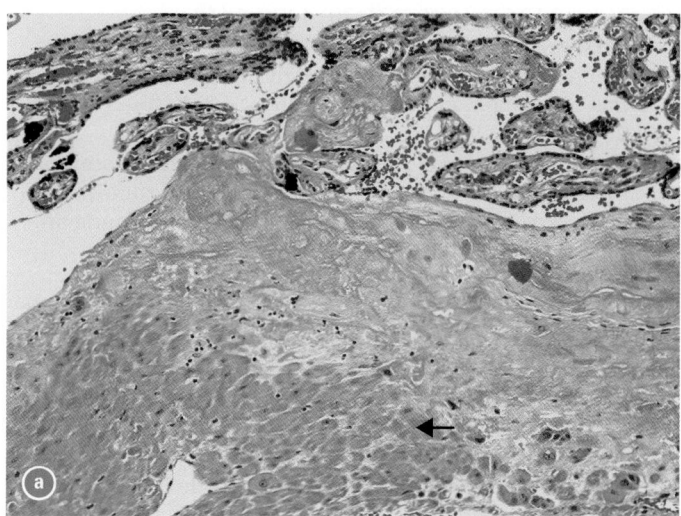

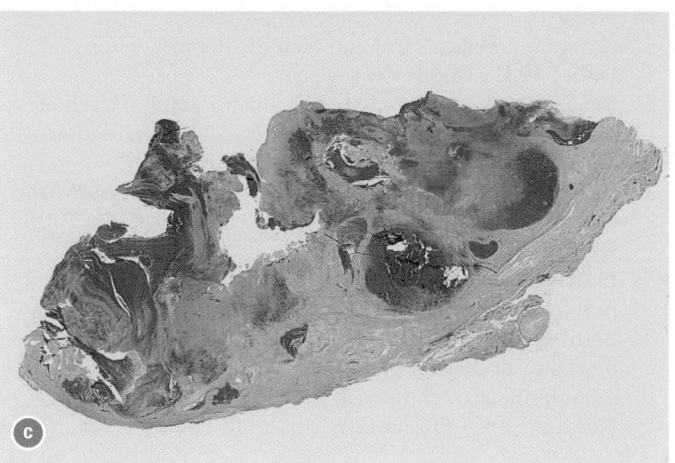

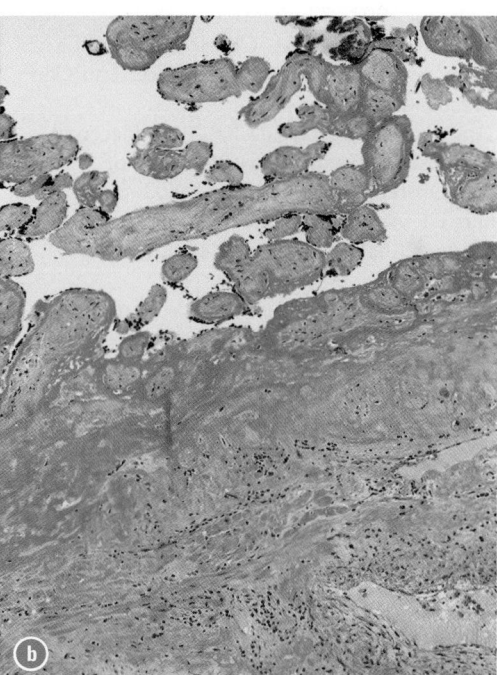

Fig. 34.23 (a) Placenta accreta diagnosed by the presence of myometrial fibers at the maternal surface of the placenta (arrow). (b) Juxtaposition of myometrium and placenta in a curetting for retained products of conception. (c) Placenta increta, seen in this myometrial section as villi and blood clot extending well into the uterine wall.

References

1 Benirschke K, Kaufmann P. Pathology of the human placenta, 4th edn. New York: Springer-Verlag; 2000.

2 Genest DR, Granter S, Pinkus GS. Umbilical cord 'pseudo-vasculitis' following second trimester fetal death: a clinicopathological and immunohistochemical study of 13 cases. Histopathology 1997; 30(6):563–569.

3 Muraskas JK, McDonnell JF, Chudik RJ, et al. Amniotic band syndrome with significant orofacial clefts and disruptions and distortions of craniofacial structures. J Pediatr Surg 2003; 38:635–638.

4 Craven C, Ward K. Placental causes of fetal malformation. Clin Obstet Gynecol 1996; 39:588–606.

5 Hameed C, Tejani N, Verma UL, Archbald F. Silent chorioamnionitis as a cause of preterm labor refractory to tocolytic therapy. Am J Obstet Gynecol 1984; 149:726–730.

6 Naeye RL, Ross SM. Amniotic fluid infection syndrome. Clin Obstet Gynaecol 1982; 9:593–607.

7 Miller RB, Camp SD Van, Barnum DA. The effects of intra-amniotic inoculation of Hemophilus somnus on the bovine fetus and dam. Vet Pathol 1983; 20:574–583.

8 Elst CW van der, Lopez Bernal A, Sinclair-Smith CC. The role of chorioamnionitis and prostaglandins in preterm labor. Obstet Gynecol 1991; 77:672–676.

9 Madan E, Meyer MP, Amortegui A. Chorioamnionitis: a study of organisms isolated in perinatal autopsies. Ann Clin Lab Sci 1988; 18:39–45.

10 Pankuch GA, Appelbaum PC, Lorenz RP, et al. Placental microbiology and histology and the pathogenesis of chorioamnionitis. Obstet Gynecol 1984; 64:802–806.

11 Zhang JM, Kraus FT, Aquino TI. Chorioamnionitis: a comparative histologic, bacteriologic and clinical study. Int J Gynecol Pathol 1985; 4:1–10.

12 American College of Obstetricians and Gynecologists. ACOG Practice Bulletin. Cervical insufficiency. Obstet Gynecol 2003; 102(5):1091–1099.

13 Andersen HF, Nugent CE, Wanty SD, Hayashi RH. Prediction of risk for preterm delivery by ultrasonographic measurement of cervical length. Am J Obstet Gynecol 1990; 163(3):859–867.

14 Rust OA, Atlas RO, Meyn J, et al. Does cerclage location influence perinatal outcome? Am J Obstet Gynecol 2003; 189:1688–1691.

15 Rush RW, Isaacs S, McPherson K, et al. A randomized controlled trial of cervical cerclage in women at high risk of spontaneous preterm delivery. Br J Obstet Gynaecol 1984; 91:724–730.

16 Medical Research Council/Royal College of Obstetricians and Gynaecologists multicentre randomised trial of cervical cerclage. Final report of the MRC/RCOG Working Party on Cervical Cerclage. Br J Obstet Gynaecol 1993; 100(6):516–523.

17 Duley L. Pre-eclampsia and the hypertensive disorders of pregnancy. Br Med Bull 2003; 67:161–176.

18 Genbacev O, Krtolica A, Kaelin W, Fisher SJ. Human cytotrophoblast expression of the von Hippel-Lindau protein is downregulated during uterine invasion in situ and upregulated by hypoxia in vitro. Dev Biol 2001; 233:526–536.

19 Zhou Y, Fisher SJ, Janatpour M, et al. Human cytotrophoblasts adopt a vascular phenotype as they differentiate: a strategy for successful endovascular invasion? J Clin Invest 1997; 99:2139–2151.

20 Zhou Y, Damsky CH, Fisher SJ. Preeclampsia is associated with failure of human cytotrophoblasts to mimic a vascular adhesion phenotype. One cause of defective endovascular invasion in this syndrome? J Clin Invest 1997; 99:2152–2164.

21 Khong TY, Wolf F De, Robertson WB, Brosens I. Inadequate maternal vascular response to placentation in pregnancies complicated by pre-eclampsia and by small-for-gestational age infants. Br J Obstet Gynaecol 1986; 93(10):1049–1059.

22 Waite LL, Atwood AK, Taylor RN. Preeclampsia, an implantation disorder. Rev Endocr Metab Disord 2002; 3(2):151–158.

23 Zhou Y, McMaster M, Woo K, et al. Vascular endothelial growth factor ligands and receptors that regulate human cytotrophoblast survival are dysregulated in severe preeclampsia and hemolysis, elevated liver enzymes and low platelets syndrome. Am J Pathol 2002; 160(4):1405–1423.

24 Ferris TF. Pregnancy, preeclampsia and the endothelial cell. N Engl J Med 1991; 325(20):1439–1440.

25 Chavarria ME, Lara-Gonzalez L, Gonzalez-Gleason A, et al. Prostacyclin/thromboxane early changes in pregnancies that are complicated by preeclampsia. Am J Obstet Gynecol 2003; 188(4):986–992.

26 Maynard SE, Min JY, Merchan J, et al. Excess placental soluble fms-like tyrosine kinase 1 (sFlt1) may contribute to endothelial dysfunction, hypertension and proteinuria in preeclampsia. J Clin Invest 2003; 111:649–658.

27 Thadhani R, Mutter WP, Wolf M, et al. First trimester placental growth factor and soluble fms-like tyrosine kinase 1 and risk for preeclampsia. J Clin Endocrin Metab 2004; 89:770–775.

28 Levine RJ, Maynard SE, Qian C, et al. Circulating angiogenic factors and the risk of preeclampsia. N Engl J Med 2004; 350:672–683.

29 Labarrere CA. Acute atherosis. A histopathological hallmark of immune aggression? Placenta 1988; 9:95–108.

30 Naeye RL. Functionally important disorders of the placenta, umbilical cord and fetal membranes. Hum Pathol 1987; 18:680–691.

31 Salafia CM, Vintzileos AM, Silberman L, et al. Placental pathology of idiopathic intrauterine growth retardation at term. Am J Perinatol 1992; 9:179–184.

32 Redline RW, Pappin A. Fetal thrombotic vasculopathy: the clinical significance of extensive avascular villi. Hum Pathol 1995; 26(1):80–85.

33 Lin CC. Intrauterine growth retardation. Obstet Gynecol Annu 1985; 14:127–221.

34 Bernstein IM, Horbar JD, Badger GJ, et al. Morbidity and mortality among very-low-birth-weight neonates with intrauterine growth restriction. The Vermont Oxford Network. Am J Obstet Gynecol 2000; 182:198–206.

35 Kraus FT. Cerebral palsy and thrombi in placental vessels of the fetus: insights from litigation. Hum Pathol 1997; 28:246–248.

36 Naeye RL. Maternal floor infarction. Hum Pathol 1985; 16(8):823–828.

37 Andres RL, Kuyper W, Resnik R, et al. The association of maternal floor infarction of the placenta with adverse perinatal outcome. Am J Obstet Gynecol 1990; 163:935–938.

38 Katzman PJ, Genest DR. Maternal floor infarction and massive perivillous fibrin deposition: histological definitions, association with intrauterine fetal growth restriction and risk of recurrence. Pediatr Dev Pathol 2002; 5:159–164.

39 Desmonts G, Couvreur J. Congenital toxoplasmosis. A prospective study of 378 pregnancies. N Engl J Med 1974; 290:1110–1116.

40 Popek EJ. Granulomatous villitis due to *Toxoplasma gondii*. Pediatr Pathol 1992; 12:281.

41 Foulon W, Naessens A, Catte L de, Amy J-J. Detection of congenital toxoplasmosis by chorionic villus sampling and early amniocentesis. Am J Obstet Gynecol 1990; 163:1511–1513.

42 Fricker-Hidalgo H, Pelloux H, Racinet C, et al. Detection of *Toxoplasma gondii* in 94 placentae from infected women by polymerase chain reaction, *in vivo* and *in vitro* cultures. Placenta 1998; 19:545–549.

43 Schulz KF, Cates W Jr, O'Mara PR. A synopsis of the problems in Africa in syphilis and gonorrhoeae during pregnancy. Afr J Sex Transmi Dis 1986; 2(2):56–57.

44 Nagot N, Meda N, Ouangre A, et al. Review of STI and HIV epidemiological data from 1990 to 2001 in urban Burkina Faso: implications for STI and HIV control. Sex Transm Infect 2004; 80(2):124–129.

45 Larkin JA, Lit L, Toney J, Haley JA. Recognizing and treating syphilis in pregnancy. Medscape Women's Health 1998; 3:5.

46 Lukehart SA, Godornes C, Molini BJ, et al. Macrolide resistance in *Treponema pallidum* in the United States and Ireland. N Engl J Med 2004; 351:154–158.

47 Genest DR, Choi-Hong SR, Tate JE, et al. Diagnosis of congenital syphilis from placental examination: comparison of histopathology, Steiner stain and polymerase chain reaction for *Treponema pallidum* DNA. Hum Pathol 1996; 27(4):366–372.

48 Sheffield JS, Sanchez PJ, Wendel GD Jr, et al. Placental histopathology of congenital syphilis. Obstet Gynecol 2002; 100:126–133.

49 Casper C, Fenyo EM. Mother-to-child transmission of HIV-1: the role of HIV-1 variability and the placental barrier. Acta Microbiol Immunol Hung 2001; 48:545–573.

50 Toth FD, Bacsi A, Beck Z, Szabo J. Vertical transmission of human immunodeficiency virus. Acta Microbiol Immunol Hung 2001; 48:413–427.

51 Behbahani H, Popek E, Garcia P, et al. Upregulation of CCR5 expression in the placenta is associated with human immunodeficiency virus-1 vertical transmission. Am J Pathol 2000; 157:1811–1818.

52 Arias RA, Munoz LD, Munoz-Fernandez MA. Transmission of HIV-1 infection between trophoblast placental cells and T-cells take place via an LFA-1 mediated cell-to-cell contact. Virology 2003; 307:266–277.

53 Soilleux EJ, Coleman N. Transplacental transmission of HIV: a potential role for HIV binding lectins. Int J Biochem Cell Biol 2003; 35:283–287.

54 Pohlmann S, Soilleux EJ, Baribaud F, et al. DC-SIGNR, a DC-SIGN homologue expressed in endothelial cells, binds to human and simian immunodeficiency viruses and activates infection in trans. Proc Natl Acad Sci 2001; 98:2670–2675.

55 Doyle M, Atkins JT, Rivera-Matos IR. Congenital cytomegalovirus infection in infants infected with human immunodeficiency virus type 1. Pediatr Infect Dis J 1996; 15:1102–1106.

56 Moore JM, Ayisi J, Nahlen BL, et al. Immunity to placental malaria, II: placental antigen-specific cytokine responses are impaired in human immunodeficiency virus-infected women. J Infect Dis 2000; 182:960–964.

57 Muhlemann K, Miller RK, Metlay L, Menegus MA. Cytomegalovirus infection of the human placenta: an immunocytochemical study. Hum Pathol 1992; 23:1234–1237.

58 Ozono K, Mushiake S, Takeshima T, Nakayama M. Diagnosis of congenital cytomegalovirus infection by examination of the placenta: application of polymerase chain reaction and in situ hybridization. Pediatr Pathol Lab Med 1997; 17:249–258.

59 Overall JC Jr. Herpes simplex virus infection of the fetus and newborn. Pediatr Ann 1994; 23(3):131–136.

60 Hyde SR, Giacoia GP. Congenital herpes infection: placental and umbilical cord findings. Obstet Gynecol 1993; 81(5):852–855.

61 Schwartz DA, Caldwell E. Herpes simplex virus infection of the placenta. The role of molecular pathology in the diagnosis of viral infection of placental-associated tissues. Arch Pathol Lab Med 1991; 115(11):1141–1144.

62 Benirschke K, Robb JA. Infectious causes of fetal death. Clin Obstet Gynecol 1987; 30(2):284–294.

63 Bendon RW, Perez F, Ray MB. Herpes simplex virus: fetal and decidual infection. Pediatr Pathol 1987; 7(1):63–70.

64 Basso NG, Fonseca ME, Garcia AG, et al. Enterovirus isolation from foetal and placental tissues. Acta Virol 1990; 34(1):49–57.

65 Satosar A, Ramirez NC, Bartholomew D, et al. Histologic correlates of viral and bacterial infection of the placenta associated with severe morbidity and mortality in the newborn. Hum Pathol 2004; 35(5):536–545.

66 Genen L, Nuovo GJ, Krilov L, Davis JM. Correlation of *in situ* detection of infectious agents in the placenta with neonatal outcome. J Pediatr 2004; 144(3):316–320.

67 Euscher E, Davis J, Holzman I, Nuovo GJ. Coxsackie virus infection of the placenta associated with neurodevelopmental delays in the newborn. Obstet Gynecol 2001; 98(6):1019–1026.

68 Parry S, Holder J, Strauss JF 3rd. Mechanisms of trophoblast-virus interaction. J Reprod Immunol 1997; 37(1):25–34.

69 Petignat P, Vial Y, Laurini R, Hohlfeld P. Fetal varicella-herpes zoster syndrome in early pregnancy: ultrasonographic and morphological correlation. Prenat Diagn 2001; 21(2):121–124.

70 Matovina M, Husnjak K, Milutin N, et al. Possible role of bacterial and viral infections in miscarriages. Fertil Steril 2004; 8:662–669.

71 Chow KC, Lee CC, Lin TY, et al. Congenital enterovirus 71 infection: a case study with virology and immunohistochemistry. Clin Infect Dis 2000; 31:509–512.

72 Rhone SA, Magee F, Remple V, Money D. The association of placental abnormalities with maternal and neonatal clinical findings: a retrospective cohort study. J Obstet Gynaecol Can 2003; 25(2):123–128.

73 Incerpi MH, Miller DA, Samadi R, et al. Stillbirth evaluation: what tests are needed? Am J Obstet Gynecol 1998; 178(6):1121–1125.

74 Redline RW, Abramowsky CR. Clinical and pathological aspects of recurrent villitis. Hum Pathol 1985; 16:727–731.

75 Redline RW, Patterson P. Villitis of unknown etiology is associated with major infiltration of fetal tissue by maternal inflammatory cells. Am J Pathol 1993; 143:473–479.

76 Labarrere CA, McIntyre JA, Faulk WP. Immunohistologic evidence that villitis in human normal term placentas is an immunologic lesion. Am J Obstet Gyn 1990; 162:515–522.

77 Labarrere CA, Catoggio LJ, Mullen EG, Althabe OH. Placental lesions in maternal autoimmune diseases. Am J Reprod Immunol 1986; 12:78–86.

78 Labarrere CA, Carson SD, Faulk WP. Tissue factor in chronic villitis of unestablished etiology. J Reprod Immunol 1991; 19(3):225.

79 Russell P, Atkinson K, Krishnan L. Recurrent reproductive failure due to severe placental villitis of unknown etiology. J Reprod Med 1980; 24(2):93–98.

80 Ornoy A, Crone K, Altshuler G. Pathological features of the placenta in fetal death. Arch Pathol Lab Med 1976; 100(7):367–371.

81 Lee WK, Schwartz DA, Rice RJ, Larsen SA. Syphilitic endometritis causing first trimester abortion: a potential infectious cause of fetal morbidity in early gestation. South Med J 1994; 87(12):1259–1261.

82 Oats JJ. Fourth International Workshop-Conference on Gestational Diabetes Mellitus. Overview and commentary on first session. Diabetes Care 1998; 21(Suppl 2):B58–B59.

83 Cousins L. Pregnancy complications among diabetic women: review 1965–1985. Obstet Gynecol Surv 1987; 42(3):140–149.

84 Vidaeff AC, Yeomans ER, Ramin SM. Gestational diabetes: a field of controversy. Obstet Gynecol Surv 2003; 58(11):759–769.

85 Driscoll JJ, Gillespie L. Obstetrical considerations in diabetes in pregnancy. Med Clin North Am 1965; 49:1025–1034.

86 Chorangiosis AG. An important placental sign of neonatal morbidity and mortality. Arch Pathol Lab Med 1984; 108(1):71–74.

87 Mayhew TM, Sampson C. Maternal diabetes mellitus is associated with altered deposition of fibrin-type fibrinoid at the villous surface in term placentae. Placenta 2003; 24(5):524–531.

88 Jirkovska M, Kubinova L, Janacek J, et al. Topological properties and spatial organization of villous capillaries in normal and diabetic placentas. J Vasc Res 2002; 39:268–278.

89 Younes B. Baez-Giangreco A, al-Nuaim L, et al. Basement membrane thickening in the placentae from diabetic women. Pathol Int 1996; 46:100–104.

90 al-Okail MS, al-Attas OS. Histological changes in placental syncytiotrophoblasts of poorly controlled gestational diabetic patients. Endocr J 1994; 41(4):355–360.

91 Clarson C, Tevaarwerk GJ, Harding PG, et al. Placental weight in diabetic pregnancies. Placenta 1989; 10:275–281.

92 Moise KJ Jr. Management of rhesus alloimmunization in pregnancy. Obstet Gynecol 2002; 100(3):600–611.

93 Sosa ME. Nonimmune hydrops fetalis. J Perinat Neonatal Nurs 1999; 13(3):33–44.

94 Knilans TK. Cardiac abnormalities associated with hydrops fetalis. Semin Perinatol 1995; 19:483–492.

95 Simpson LL. Fetal supraventricular tachycardias: diagnosis and management. Semin Perinatol 2000; 24(5):360–372.

96 Machin GA. Hydrops revisited: literature review of 1,414 cases published in the 1980s. Am J Med Genet 1989; 34:366–390.

97 Fox H. Abnormalities of the foetal stem arteries in the human placenta. J Obstet Gynaecol Br Commonw 1967; 74:734–738.

98 Zelop C, Benacerraf BR. The causes and natural history of fetal ascites. Prenat Diagn 1994; 14:941–946.

99 Miller PW, Coen RW, Benirschke K. Dating the time interval from meconium passage to birth. Obstet Gynecol 1985; 66:459–462.

100 Altshuler G, Arizawa M, Molnar-Nadasdy G. Meconium-induced umbilical cord vascular necrosis and ulceration: a potential link between the placenta and poor pregnancy outcome. Obstet Gynecol 1992; 79:760–766.

101 Byrne J, Blanc WA. Malformations and chromosome anomalies in spontaneously aborted fetuses with single umbilical artery. Am J Obstet Gynecol 1985; 151:340–342.

102 Leung AK, Robson WL. Incidence and associations of single umbilical artery. Am J Med Genet 1993; 46(2):248–249.

103 Genest DR. Estimating the time of death in stillborn fetuses: II. Histologic evaluation of the placenta; a study of 71 stillborns. Obstet Gynecol 1992; 80(4):585–592.

104 Cameron AH. The Birmingham twin survey. Proc R Soc Med 1968; 61:229–234.

105 Glinianaia SV, Rankin J, Wright C, et al. Northern Region Perinatal Mortality Survey Steering Group. A multiple pregnancy register in the north of England. Twin Res 2002; 5(5):436–439.

106 Adegbite AL, Castille S, Ward S, Bajoria R. Neuromorbidity in preterm twins in relation to chorionicity and discordant birth weight. Am J Obstet Gynecol 2004; 190:156–163.

107 Sau AK, Langford K, Elliott C, et al. Monoamniotic twins: what should be the optimal antenatal management? Twin Res 2003; 6(4):270–274.

108 Sohi I, Chacko B, Masih K, Choudhary S. A case of TRAP sequence: acardiac twin. Indian J Pathol Microbiol 2003; 46:664–665.

109 Sullivan AE, Varner MW, Ball RH, et al. The management of acardiac twins: a conservative approach. Am J Obstet Gynecol 2003; 189:1310–1313.

110 Aslan H, Gul A, Cebeci A, et al. The outcome of twin pregnancies complicated by single fetal death after 20 weeks of gestation. Twin Res 2004; 7:1–4.

111 Boyd JF. Disseminated fibrin thrombo-embolism in stillbirths: a histological picture similar to one form

of maternal hypofibrinogenaemia. J Obstet Gynaecol Br Commonw 1966; 73:629–639.

112 Fries MH, Goldstein RB, Kilpatrick SJ, et al. The role of velamentous cord insertion in the etiology of twin-twin transfusion syndrome. Obstet Gynecol 1993; 81:569–574.

113 Baldwin VJ, Wittmann BK. Pathology of intragestational intervention in twin-to-twin transfusion syndrome. Pediatr Pathol 1990; 10:79–93.

114 Gemert MJC van, Umur A, Tijssen JGP, Ross MG. Twin-twin transfusion syndrome: etiology, severity and rational management. Curr Opin Obstet Gyn 2001; 13:193–206.

115 Sherer DM. Adverse perinatal outcome of twin pregnancies according to chorionicity. Am J Perinatol 2001; 18:23–37.

116 Dodd JM, Robinson JS, Crowther CA, Chan A. Stillbirth and neonatal outcomes in South Australia, 1991–2000. Am J Obstet Gynecol 2003; 189:1731–1736.

117 Skeie A, Froen JF, Vege A, Stray-Pedersen B. Cause and risk of stillbirth in twin pregnancies: a retrospective audit. Acta Obstet Gynecol Scand 2003; 82:1010–1016.

118 Fakeye O. Perinatal factors in twin mortality in Nigeria. Int J Gynaecol Obstet 1986; 24(4):309–314.

119 Amaru RC, Bush MC, Berkowitz RL, et al. Is discordant growth in twins an independent risk factor for adverse neonatal outcome? Obstet Gynecol 2004; 103:71–76.

120 Sherer DM, Divon MY. Fetal growth in multifetal gestation. Clin Obstet Gynecol 1997; 40:764–770.

121 Malinowski W. Umbilical cord complications in twin pregnancies. Ginekol Pol 2003; 74:1208–1212.

122 Trogstad L, Skrondal A, Stoltenberg C, et al. Recurrence risk of preeclampsia in twin and singleton pregnancies. Am J Med Genet 2004; 126a:41–45.

123 Sepulveda W, Alcalde JL, Schnapp C, Bravo M. Perinatal outcome after prenatal diagnosis of placental chorioangioma. Obstet Gynecol 2003; 102:1028–1033.

124 Jacques SM, Qureshi F, Doss BJ, Munkarah A. Intraplacental choriocarcinoma associated with viable pregnancy: pathologic features and implications for the mother and infant. Pediatr Dev Pathol 1998; 1(5):380–387.

125 Kim SJ. Placental site trophoblastic tumour. Best Pract Res Clin Obstet Gynaecol 2003; 17(6):969–984.

126 Potter JF, Schoeneman M. Metastasis of maternal cancer to the placenta and fetus. Cancer 1970; 25:380–388.

127 Isaacs H Jr. Fetal and neonatal leukemia. J Pediatr Hematol Oncol 2003; 25(5):348–361.

128 Robertson M, Jong G De, Mansvelt E. Prenatal diagnosis of congenital leukemia in a fetus at 25 weeks' gestation with Down syndrome: case report and review of the literature. Ultrasound Obstet Gynecol 2003; 21(5):486–489.

129 Engelsen IB, Albrechtsen S, Iversen OE. Peripartum hysterectomy–incidence and maternal morbidity. Acta Obstet Gynecol Scand 2001; 80:409–412.

130 Castaneda S, Karrison T, Cibils LA. Peripartum hysterectomy. J Perinat Med 2000; 28:472–481.

131 Zaideh SM, Abu-Heija AT, El-Jallad MF. Placenta praevia and accreta: analysis of a two-year experience. Gynecol Obstet Invest 1998; 46:96–98.

132 Hamsho MA, Alsakka M. Emergency obstetric hysterectomy in Qatar – a 20-year review. Int J Fertil Women's Med 1999; 44:209–211.

133 Mabie WC. Placenta previa. Clin Perinatol 1992; 19:425–435.

134 Ota Y, Watanabe H, Fukasawa I, et al. Placenta accreta/increta. Review of 10 cases and a case report. Arch Gynecol Obstet 1999; 263:69–72.

Appendix I

Tumor, Nodes, Metastases (TNM)* and FIGO** staging of reproductive tract tumors***

Note: The use of staging classifications may vary according to practice. Each pathologist should ensure that the classification they use is accurate and conforms to local practice standards.
*American Joint Committee on Cancer (AJCC)/International Union Against Cancer (UICC);
**International Federation of Gynecology and Obstetrics (FIGO).
***See AJCC Cancer Staging Manual, 6th edition, Springer Verlag, New York 2002.

Carcinoma of the cervix

Category	FIGO Stage	Primary tumor (T)
TX		Primary tumor cannot be assessed
T0		No evidence of primary tumor
Tis		Carcinoma *in situ*
T1	I	Cervical carcinoma confined to uterus
T1a	IA	Preclinical invasive carcinoma diagnosed by microscopy
T1a1	IA1	Minimal microscopic stromal invasion
T1a2	IA2	Tumor invades 5 mm or less in depth by 7 mm or less in length
T1B	IB	Tumor larger than T1a2
T2	II	Cervical carcinoma invades beyond the uterus but not to the pelvis or the lower third of the vagina
T2a	IIA	Tumor does not involve the parametrium
T2b	IIB	Tumor involves the parametrium
T3	III	Tumor extends to the pelvic wall and or involve the vagina and/or causes hydronephrosis or non-functioning kidney
T3a	IIIA	Tumor involves the lower-third of the vagina, no extension to pelvis
T3b	IIIB	Tumor extends to pelvic wall and/or causes hydronephrosis or non-functioning kidney
T4	IVA	Tumor invades mucosa of bladder or rectum and/or extends beyond the true pelvis

Category	Lymph node (N)
NX	Regional lymph nodes cannot be assessed
NO	No regional lymph node metastases
N1	Regional lymph node metastases

Carcinoma of the cervix *(Continued)*

Category	Distant metastases (M)
MX	Presence of distant metastases cannot be assessed
MO	No distant metastases
M1	Distant metastases

FIGO Stage	Grouping	(AJCC /	UICC)
0	Tis	NO	MO
IA	T1a	NO	MO
IB	T1b	NO	MO
IIA	T2a	NO	MO
IIB	T2b	NO	MO
IIIA	T3a	NO	MO
IIIB	T1	N1	MO
	T2	N1	MO
	T3b	Any N	MO
IVA	T4	Any N	MO
IVB			

Carcinoma of the *Corpus Uteri*

Category	FIGO Stage	Primary tumor (T)
TX		Primary tumor cannot be assessed
T0		No evidence of primary tumor
Tis		Carcinoma *in situ*
T1	I	Tumor confined to *corpus uteri*
T1a	IA	Tumor confined to the endometrium
T1b	IB	Tumor invades through up to one-half of the myometrial thickness
T1c	IC	Tumor invades through greater than one half of the myometrial thickness
T2	II	Tumor invades cervix but does not extend beyond the uterus
T2a	IIA	Endocervical mucosal involvement only
T2b	IIB	Cervical stromal invasion
T3	III	Local and/or regional spread as specified below
T3a	IIIA	Tumor involves serosa and/or adnexae (direct extension or metastasis) and/or cancer cells in ascites or peritoneal wash.
T3b	IIB	Vaginal involvement (direct extension or metastasis)
N1	IIIC	Metastasis to pelvic or para-aortic lymph nodes
T4	IVA	Tumor invades bladder or bowel mucosa
M1	IVB	Distant metastases (excluding vagina, parametrium or adnexae; includes metastasis to intraabdominal lymph nodes, other than para-aortic or inguinal lymph nodes)

Carcinoma of the *Corpus Uteri* (Continued)

Category	Lymph node (N)
NX	Regional lymph nodes cannot be assessed
N0	No regional lymph node metastasis
N1	Regional lymph node metastasis

Category	Distant metastasis
MX	Presence of distant metastasis cannot be assessed
M0	No distant metastasis
M1	Distant metastasis

FIGO Stage	Grouping	(AJCC /	UICC)
0	Tis	N0	M0
IA	T1a	N0	M0
IB	T1b	N0	M0
IC	T1c	N0	M0
IIA	T2a	N0	M0
IIB	T2b	N0	M0
IIIA	T3a	N0	M0
IIIB	T3b	N0	M0
IIIC	T1	N1	M0
	T2	N1	M0
	T3a	N1	M0
	T3b	N1	M0
IVA	T4	Any N	M0
IVB	Any T	Any N	M1

Carcinoma of the ovary

Category	FIGO Stage	Primary tumor (T)
TX		Primary tumor cannot be assessed
T0		No evidence of primary tumor
T1	I	Tumor limited to the ovaries
T1a	IA	Tumor limited to one ovary; intact capsule no surface involvement; no malignant cells in washings or ascites
T1b	IB	Tumor limited to both ovaries; capsules intact, no surface involvement. No malignant cells in washings or ascites.
T1c	IC	Tumor limited to one or both ovaries and one of the following: capsular rupture, surface involvement, malignant cells in ascites or washings.
T2	II	Tumor involves one or both ovaries with extension to the pelvis.

Carcinoma of the ovary (Continued)

Category	FIGO Stage	Primary tumor (T)
T2a	IIA	Extension and/or implants on uterus and/or tube(s). No malignant cells in ascites or peritoneal washings.
T2b	IIB	Extension to other pelvic tissues. No malignant cells in peritoneal washings.
T2c	IIC	Pelvic extension (2a or 2b) with malignant cells in ascites or peritoneal washings.
T3	III	Tumor involves one or both ovaries with microscopic peritoneal metastasis outside the pelvis and/or N1 and/or lymph node metastasis.
T3a	IIIA	Microscopic peritoneal metastasis beyond pelvis
T3b	IIIB	Macroscopic peritoneal metastasis beyond pelvis (<2 cm).
T3c	IIIC	Peritoneal metastasis beyond pelvis more than 2 cm in greatest dimension and/or regional lymph node and/or N1 metastasis.
M1	IV	Distant metastasis (excludes peritoneal metastasis)

Category	Lymph node (N)
NX	Regional lymph nodes cannot be assessed
N0	No regional lymph node metastasis
N1	Regional lymph node metastasis

Category	Distant metastasis (M)
MX	Presence of distant metastasis cannot be assessed
M0	No distant metastasis
M1	Distant metastasis (excludes peritoneal metastasis)

FIGO Stage	Grouping	(AJCC /	UICC)
IA	T1a	N0	M0
IB	T1b	N0	M0
IC	T1c	N0	M0
IIA	T2a	N0	M0
IIB	T2b	N0	M0
IIC	T2c	N0	M0
IIIA	T3a	N0	M0
IIIB	T3b	N0	M0
IIIC	T3c	N0	M0
	Any T	N1	M0
IV	Any T	Any N	M1

Carcinoma of the vagina

Category	FIGO Stage	Primary tumor (T)
TX		Primary tumor cannot be assessed
T0		No evidence of primary tumor
Tis	0	Carcinoma *in situ*
T1	I	Tumor confined to the vagina
T2	II	Tumor invades paravaginal tissue but not to the pelvic wall
T3	III	Tumor extends to the pelvic wall
T4	IVa	Tumor invades mucosa of bladder or rectum and/or extends beyond the true pelvis

Category	Lymph node (N)
NX	Regional lymph nodes cannot be assessed
N0	No regional lymph node metastasis

Category	Upper two-thirds of vagina
N1	Pelvic lymph node metastasis

Category	Lower one-third of vagina
N1	Unilateral inguinal lymph node metastasis
N2	Bilateral inguinal lymph node metastasis

Category	Stage	Distant metastasis (M)
MX		Presence of distant metastasis cannot be assessed
M0		No distant metastasis
M1	IVb	Distant metastasis

FIGO Stage	Grouping	(AJCC /	UICC)
0	Tis	N0	M0
I	T1	N0	M0
II	T2	N0	M0
III	T1	N1	M0
	T2	N1	M0
	T3	N0	M0
	T3	N1	M0
IVA	T1	N2	M0
	T2	N2	M0
	T3	N2	M0
	T4	Any N	M0
IVB	Any T	Any N	M1

Carcinoma of the Vulva

Category	FIGO Stage	Primary tumor (T)
TX		Primary tumor cannot be assessed
T0		No evidence of primary tumor
Tis	0	Preinvasive carcinoma (carcinoma *in situ*)
T1	I	Tumor confined to the vulva or to the vulva and perineum, 2 cm or less
T2	II	Tumor confined to the vulva or vulva an perineum more than 2 cm
T3	III	Tumor involves any of the following: lower urethra, vagina, anus
T4	IV	Tumor invades any of the following: bladder mucosa, upper vaginal mucosa, rectal mucosa, or fixed to bone

Category	Lymph node (N)
NX	Regional lymph nodes cannot be assessed
N0	No regional lymph node metastasis
N1	Unilateral regional lymph node metastasis
N2	Bilateral regional lymph node metastasis

Category	Distant metastasis (M)
MX	Presence of distant metastasis cannot be assessed
M0	No distant metastasis
M1	Distant metastasis (pelvic LN metastasis is M1)

FIGO Stage	Grouping	(AJCC /	UICC)
0	Tis	N0	M0
I	T1	N0	M0
II	T2	N0	M0
III	T1	N1	M0
	T2	N1	M0
	T3	N0	M0
	T3	N1	M0
IVA	T1	N2	M0
	T2	N2	M0
	T3	N2	M0
	T4	Any N	M0
IVB	Any T	Any N	M1

Carcinoma of the anal canal

Category	FIGO Stage	Primary tumor (T)
TX		Primary tumor cannot be assessed
T0		No evidence of primary tumor

Carcinoma of the anal canal *(Continued)*

Category	FIGO Stage	Primary tumor (T)
Tis	0	Tumor 2 cm or less in dimension
T1	I	Carcinoma in situ
T2	II	Tumor >2 cm and <5 cm
T3	III	Tumor >5 cm
T4	IV	Tumor of any size involving adjacent organs, including vagina, urethra, bladder (excludes sphincter muscle alone)

Category	Lymph node (N)
NX	Regional lymph nodes cannot be assessed
N0	No regional lymph node metastases
N1	Metastasis in perirectal lymph node(s)
N2	Metastasis in unilateral iliac and/or inguinal lymph node(s)
N3	Metastasis in perirectal and inguinal lymph nodes and/or bilateral iliac and/or inguinal lymph nodes

Category	Distant metastasis (M)
MX	Distant metastasis cannot be assessed
M0	No distant metastasis
M1	Distant metastasis

FIGO Stage	Grouping	(AJCC /	UICC)
0	Tis	N0	M0
I	T1	N0	M0
II	T2	N0	M0
	T3	N0	M0
IIIA	T1	N1	M0
	T2	N1	M0
	T3	N1	M0
	T4	N0	M0
	T4	N1	M0
	Any T	N2	M0
	Any T	N3	M0
IV	Any T	Any N	M1

Carcinoma of the fallopian tube

Category	FIGO Stage	Primary tumor (T)
TX		Primary tumor cannot be assessed
T0		No evidence of primary tumor
Tis	0	Carcinoma *in situ*

Carcinoma of the fallopian tube *(Continued)*

Category	FIGO Stage	Primary tumor (T)
T1	I	Tumor limited to the fallopian tube(s)
T1a	IA	Tumor limited to tube without penetrating serosa, no ascites
T1b	IB	Tumor limited to both tubes without penetrating serosa, no ascites
T1c	IC	Tumor extends onto or through serosa or malignant cells in washings
T2	II	Tumor extends to pelvis
T2a	IIA	Uterus and or ovaries
T2b	IIB	Other pelvic structures
T2c	IIC	Above and malignant cells in washings
T3/N1	III	Implants beyond pelvis and/or positive nodes
T3a	IIA	Microscopic extra pelvic mets
T3b	IIIB	Macroscopic less than 2 cm
T3c	IIIC	Macroscopic greater than 2 cm and/or pos nodes
N1		
M1	IV	Distant metastasis

Category	Lymph node (N)
NX	Regional lymph nodes cannot be assessed
N0	Negative
N1	Positive

Category	Distant mets (M)
MX	Distant metastases cannot be assessed
M0	No distant metastases
M1	Distant metastases

FIGO Stage	Grouping	(AJCC	/	UICC)
0	Tis	N0		M0
IA	T1a	N0		M0
IB	T1b	N0		M0
IC	T1c	N0		M0
IIA	T2a	N0		M0
IIB	T2b	N0		M0
IIC	T2c	N0		M0
IIIA	T3a	N0		M0
IIIB	T3b	N0		M0
IIIC	T3c	N0		M0
	Any T	N1		M0
IV	Any T	Any N		M1

Appendix II

Common diagnostic terms in use in the Division of Women's and Perinatal Pathology, Brigham and Women's Hospital

Note: These diagnostic terms are used routinely at Brigham and Women's Hospital and are intended to illustrate one approach used in practice. They may or may not apply to other practices. The use of any diagnostic term should be made with a clear understanding of its clinical impact in a given practice locale.

Vulva

Code	Diagnosis
LSA	Lichen sclerosus
LSC	Lichen simplex chronicus
FIBPOL	Fibroepithelial stromal polyp
CONDY	Condyloma acuminatum
CONDYS	Condylomata acuminata
CONDYSK	Condyloma with features of seborrheic keratosis
LOVIL	Low-grade squamous intraepithelial lesion (condyloma/VIN1)
HIVIL2	High-grade squamous intraepithelial lesion (VIN2)
HIVIL3	High-grade squamous intraepithelial lesion (VIN3)
DVIN	Vulvar intraepithelial neoplasia, differentiated type
DVIN NOTE	Differentiated VIN occurs in the setting of inflammatory vulvar disease (LSA or LSC) and confers an increased risk of vulvar squamous carcinoma. Conservative excision and follow-up are advised.

Vagina

Code	Diagnosis
BSM	Benign squamous mucosa
CONDY	Condyloma acuminatum
LOVAIL	Low-grade squamous intraepithelial lesion (condyloma/VAIN1))
HIVAIL2	High-grade squamous intraepithelial lesion (vaginal intraepithelial neoplasia 2)
HIVAIL3	High-grade squamous intraepithelial lesion (vaginal intraepithelial neoplasia 3)

Cervix

Code	Diagnosis
MSE	Mature squamous epithelium
MSM	Mature squamous metaplasia
SM	Squamous metaplasia
WSM	with squamous metaplasia
CI	Chronic inflammation
ACI	Acute and chronic inflammation
SCI	Severe chronic inflammation
FOC	Follicular cervicitis
FC NOTE	Follicular cervicitis, although not specific, may be associated with chlamydia infection (clinical correlation advised)
PK	Parakeratosis
ULCER	Ulceration
GT	Granulation tissue
ACAN	Acanthosis
HK	Hyperkeratosis
NSPC	No significant pathologic change
MC	Mucus (Nabothian) cyst
ECP	Endocervical polyp
ECPS	Endocervical polyps
REP	Reparative epithelial changes
REACT	Reactive epithelial changes
MGH	Microglandular change
EC	Endocervix
PORTIO	Cervical portio (exocervix) only
FOBE	Fragments of benign endocervix
LSILCONDY	Squamous intraepithelial lesion, low-grade (exophytic condyloma)
LSILI	Squamous intraepithelial lesion, low-grade (immature condyloma)
LSIL	Squamous intraepithelial lesion, low-grade (condyloma/CIN1)
HSIL	Squamous intraepithelial lesion, high-grade (CIN II/CIN III)
GLINV	With gland (crypt) involvement
SONE	Fragments of neoplastic squamous epithelium
SONE1	One fragment of neoplastic squamous epithelium
CONH	Consistent with a high-grade squamous intraepithelial lesion.
CONL	Consistent with a low-grade squamous intraepithelial lesion.
QSIL	Squamous intraepithelial lesion, not amenable to precise grading (CIN1–CIN2)
ACIS	Adenocarcinoma *in situ*
SMILE	Stratified mucin producing intraepithelial lesion

Cervix *(Continued)*

Code	Diagnosis
SMILE NOTE	*Comment:* This lesion exhibits features of both HSIL and adenocarcinoma *in situ.* Cone biopsy is advised (where appropriate)
NOSIL	No evidence of squamous intraepithelial lesion
ECZ	Blood, mucus and scant endocervical epithelium
TIFD	No tissue identified
SCANT	Scant specimen
BC	Blood clot
NTZ	No transformation zone seen
LE	Levels examined
CAUT	Specimen distortion and cautery artefact preclude assessment of margins
FREE	Margins are uninvolved by the lesion

Endometrium

Code	Diagnosis
Benign cyclic	
PE	Proliferative endometrium
16d	16-day endometrium
16note	*Comment:* Although this pattern may reflect recent ovulation, it is not specific and may not be caused by estrogen alone.
SE	Secretory endometrium
SED	Secretory endometrium, day ——
OME	Menstrual endometrium (ovulatory)
BEF	Benign endometrial fragments
WSB	With stromal breakdown
EARLY	Early proliferative endometrium with residual stromal breakdown (late menstrual endometrium)
CANT	*Note:* ovulation cannot be confirmed in the late stage of endometrial shedding
LUS	Lower uterine segment
EM	Endometrium
Benign non-cyclic	
CE	Chronic endometritis
ACE	Acute and chronic endometritis
PILL	Endometrial gland and stromal changes consistent with oral contraceptive effect
DRUG	Altered endometrium with gland and stromal changes consistent with progestin therapy
ANOV	This pattern is consistent with anovulatory cycle

Endometrium *(Continued)*

Code	Diagnosis
SBUN	*Comment:* It is impossible morphologically to distinguish between ovulation, anovulation, and other causes of stromal breakdown in this sample
PFOC	Proliferative endometrium with alterations in gland architecture consistent with anovulation
MIX	Altered endometrium with a mixed proliferative and secretory pattern
MIXCOM	*Comment:* This pattern is consistent with anovulatory cycles with superimposed ovulation or progestin therapy
AGLAND	Fragments of aglandular functionalis suggestive of underlying submucosal leiomyoma
HRT	Benign endometrium with alterations in glands and stroma consistent with hormonal replacement therapy
EMP	Endometrial polyp
EMPS	Endometrial polyps
ESTRO	*Comment:* this pattern is consistent with unopposed or poorly opposed estrogen effect (clinical correlation advised)

Endometrial intraepithelial neoplasia

Code	Diagnosis
EIN	Endometrial intraepithelial neoplasia (atypical complex hyperplasia)
	Adequacy
EMZ	Scant fragments of surface endometrium and glands
NODATE	Secretory endometrium, insufficient for precise dating
NOFUN	There is insufficient functionalis present for precise dating

Myometrium

Code	Diagnosis
LEIO	Leiomyoma
LEIOS	Leiomyomata
AMYOS	Adenomyosis
IM	Intramural
SS	Subserosal
SUM	Submucosal

Fallopian tube

Code	Diagnosis
NPO	Negative portion of oviduct
CCS	Complete cross-section

Fallopian tube *(Continued)*

Code	Diagnosis
TUBES	Specimen designated 'right fallopian tube segment':
	Negative portion of oviduct (complete cross-section)
	Specimen designated 'left fallopian tube segment':
	Negative portion of oviduct (complete cross-section)
CS	Chronic salpingitis
SIN	Salpingitis isthmica nodosum
TA	Peritubal adhesions
POA	Periovarian adhesions
TOAD	Tubo-ovarian adhesions
FOS	Follicular salpingitis
HS	Hydrosalpinx
PYO	Pyosalpinx
EMOS	Endometriosis
PTC	Paratubal cysts

Ovaries

Code	Diagnosis
POA	Periovarian adhesions
CF	Cystic follicles
CICS	Cortical (mesothelial) inclusion cysts
EMOMA	Endometrioma
UNDET	Hemorrhagic cyst of undetermined origin
CL	Corpus luteum

Early gestation

Code	Diagnosis
Identification (early spontaneous/therapeutic abortuses)	
EMBRYO	Intact embryo (specify crown-rump length)
FREM	Fragments of embryonic tissue (i.e. less than 10 weeks and 3 cm)
FRFT	Fragments of fetal tissue (i.e. greater than 10 weeks and 3 cm
FRIP	Fragments of immature placenta
WVS	With villous sclerosis
WVE	With villous edema

Early gestation (Continued)

Code	Diagnosis
IS	Placental implantation site
DE	Decidualized endometrium

Trophoblastic neoplasia

Code	Diagnosis
PM	Partial hydatidiform mole
CM	Complete hydatidiform mole
MIS	Molar implantation site

Ectopic (exclude/confirm)

Code	Diagnosis
NOVIL	No villi or trophoblast present
ROECT	Ectopic pregnancy cannot be excluded on the basis of this examination
TECTOP	Ectopic tubal gestation

Placenta

Code	Diagnosis

Cord

Code	Diagnosis
SUA	Single umbilical artery
MARGUC	Marginal insertion of umbilical cord
MEMUC	Membranous insertion of umbilical cord
UCV	Umbilical cord vascular inflammation

Membranes

Code	Diagnosis
MOMO	Monochorionic, monoamnionic twin placenta
MODI	Monochorionic, diamnionic twin placenta
DIDI	Diamnionic, dichorionic twin placenta
ACA	Acute chorioamnionitis
SUBC	Subchorionitis
DV	Decidual vasculopathy
PLMMEC	Pigment-laden macrophages in membranes
PLMHEM	Hemosiderin laden macrophages in membranes.
VASC	Decidual vasculopathy may be associated with maternal conditions such as pre-eclampsia, hypertension, diabetes mellitus and collagen vascular disease, among others

Chorionic plate and villi

Code	Diagnosis
MP	Mature placenta
IP	Immature placenta
SIP	Slightly immature placenta (for above, specify large/small and greater/less than —— percentile for —— weeks)

Placenta *(Continued)*

Code	Diagnosis
RETRO	Retroplacental hematoma (specify recent or old)
IVT	Intervillous thrombus (specify size)
PLIN	Placental infarct (specify recent, old, single, multiple, size)
DEADV	Villous vascular changes consistent with fetal death
CV	Chronic villitis
VNOTE1	Although chronic villitis is sometimes associated with fetal infection with 'TORCH' organisms, no viral inclusions were identified in histologic sections

General statements, recommendations and adequacy

CLINCO	Clinical correlation is advised
FRAG	Fragmentation of the specimen precludes optimal evaluation
ZYGO	Zygosity cannot be determined by placental examination in dichorionic placentation
MONO	Monochorionic placentation equals monozygosity
THEFOL	The following organs were identified and appear appropriate for gestational age: (specify)

Appendix III

Diagnostic variables commonly reported in resected genital tract neoplasms

1. **Vulvar squamous carcinoma**
   Size in two dimensions (if grossly visible)
   Length (if microscopic)
   Grade (optional)
   Depth of invasion or thickness
   Tumor-stromal interface (blunt *vs* infiltrative)
   Presence or absence of capillary-lymphatic space invasion
   Presence or absence of associated VIN
   Margins (deep and radial)

2. **Vulvar Melanoma**
   Size in two dimensions (if grossly visible)
   Breslow thickness (from granular cell layer or surface if mucosa)
   Clark anatomic level (for tumors involving skin)
   Margins (deep and radial)
   Ulceration (measured)
   Regression
   Mitotic rate per mm^2
   Presence or absence of brisk tumor infiltrating lymphocytes
   Vascular/lymphatic invasion
   Microscopic satellites
   Cell type (epithelioid, spindle, etc.)
   Coexisting nevus or precursor lesion
   Presence or absence of vertical growth phase (Nests of cells in the dermis exceeding size of the intra-epidermal nests; or mitotic activity)

3. **Cervical squamous carcinoma**
   Size in two dimensions (if grossly visible)
   Length (if microscopic)
   Grade (optional)

Depth of invasion from the highest epithelial-stromal interface, or thickness if normal epithelium is not identified adjacent to the tumor

Tumor-stromal interface (blunt *vs* infiltrative)

Presence or absence of capillary-lymphatic space invasion

Presence or absence of associated SIL

Margins

4. Endometrial carcinoma

Size in two dimensions (if grossly visible)

Length (if microscopic)

Tumor type (endometrioid, serous, etc.)

Grade (endometrioid)

Depth of invasion, measured and percent myometrial thickness

Pattern of invasion (blunt *vs* infiltrative)

Presence or absence of capillary lymphatic space invasion

Presence or absence of associated EIN

Presence or absence of cervix involvement

Depth of cervix involvement, if present

5. Leiomyosarcoma

Size

Grade

Mitoses per 10 HPF (50 HPF counted)

Tumor necrosis

Percent myometrial thickness occupied by tumor

Presence or absence of capillary-lymphatic space invasion

Involvement of serosa

6. Carcinoma of the fallopian tube

Size

Location

Extent (mucosa, muscularis, serosa)

Presence or absence of co-existing intraepithelial carcinoma

Presence or absence of capillary lymphatic space invasion

7. Borderline epithelial tumor of the ovary

Tumor size in three dimensions

Number of sections examined (optimal 1/cm of maximum tumor width)

Presence or absence of surface involvement

Presence or absence of implants

Type of implant (epithelial noninvasive, desmoplastic non invasive, or invasive)

8. Adenocarcinoma of the ovary

Tumor size in three dimensions

Tumor type

Tumor grade

Presence or absence of co-existing benign or borderline cystadeno(fibro)ma

Presence or absence of surface involvement

Presence or absence of capillary-lymphatic space invasion

Appendix IV

Sample reports from Brigham and Women's Hospital

Note: These examples of reporting are used routinely at Brigham and Women's Hospital and are intended to illustrate one approach used in practice. They may or may not apply to other practices. The use of any diagnostic reporting scheme should be made with a clear understanding of its clinical impact in a given practice locale.

Specimen labeled (or designated) 'VULVAR BIOPSY':

HIGH-GRADE SQUAMOUS INTRAEPITHELIAL LESION (VIN2/3)

Margins are free of lesion

Specimen labeled 'VULVAR BIOPSY':

VULVAR INTRAEPITHELIAL NEOPLASIA, differentiated type, see *Comment*

Margins are free of lesion

Comment: Differentiated VIN occurs in the setting of inflammatory vulvar disease (LSA or LSC) and confers an increased risk of vulvar squamous carcinoma. Conservative excision and follow-up are advised

Specimen labeled (or designated) 'VULVAR MASS':

LEIOMYOSARCOMA (8 cm)

Necrosis is present

Mitoses number up to 15 per 10 HPF

The tumor was removed piecemeal

Specimen labeled 'CERVICAL BIOPSY AT 12 O'CLOCK':

HIGH-GRADE SQUAMOUS INTRAEPITHELIAL LESION (CIN2)

Specimen labeled (or designated) 'ENDOCERVICAL CURETTING':

STRIPS OF NEOPLASTIC EPITHELIUM consistent with high-grade squamous intraepithelial lesion (CIN2/3).

Specimen labeled 'LEEP (CONE) BIOPSY':

SQUAMOUS INTRAEPITHELIAL LESION, high-grade (CIN2/3) with gland (crypt) involvement, see *Comment*.

Margins are free of lesion.

Comment There are mild irregularities in the epithelial-stromal interface, however, the criteria for invasion are NOT met. Follow-up is advised

Specimen labeled 'LEEP (CONE) BIOPSY':

SUPERFICIALLY INVASIVE SQUAMOUS CELL CARCINOMA, see *Comment*.

SQUAMOUS INTRAEPITHELIAL LESION, HIGH-GRADE, see *Comment*.

Comment   The invasive carcinoma measures 6.0 mm in length by 2.5 mm in greatest depth (or thickness)

Capillary-lymphatic space invasion is NOT identified

Margins are free of both intraepithelial and invasive neoplasia (specify if margins are less than 1.0 mm)

Specimen labeled 'ENDOMETRIAL CURETTAGE':

Early proliferative endometrium with residual stromal breakdown.

Comment   Ovulation cannot be confirmed in the late stage of endometrial shedding

Specimen labeled 'ENDOMETRIAL CURETTAGE':

Proliferative endometrium

Strips of aglandular functionalis suggestive of submucosal leiomyoma

Specimen labeled 'ENDOMETRIAL CURETTAGE':

ENDOMETRIAL INTRAEPITHELIAL NEOPLASIA (atypical complex hyperplasia), see *Comment*.

Comment   The lesion consists of a single focus involving an endometrial polyp. Follow-up sampling is advised to excluded residual disease

Specimen labeled 'UTERUS, TUBES AND OVARIES':

Uterus (250 g)

Cervix	Squamous metaplasia
Endomyometrium	ENDOMETRIAL ADENOCARCINOMA, endometrioid type, grade 1 (of 3), with squamous (morular) differentiation
	The tumor invades 5mm in depth and through approximately 35% of the myometrial thickness
	The tumor exhibits a blunt pattern of invasion
	Capillary-lymphatic space invasion is NOT identified
Serosa	Adhesions
Right fallopian tube	No significant pathologic change
Left fallopian tube	Paratubal cyst
	Serosal keratin granulomas, no tumor identified
	Peritubal adhesions
Right ovary	Cortical stromal hyperplasia
Left ovary	Cortical stromal hyperplasia
	Cortical inclusion cysts

Specimen labeled 'UTERUS, TUBES AND OVARIES':

Uterus (200 g)

Cervix	Squamous metaplasia
Endomyometrium	UTERINE PAPILLARY SEROUS CARCINOMA
	The tumor invades 2 mm in depth through approximately 15% of the myometrial thickness
	The tumor exhibits an infiltrative pattern of invasion
	Capillary-lymphatic space invasion is present
	The tumor is diffusely immunopositive (>70%) for p53, consistent with the above diagnosis
Serosa	Adhesions
Right fallopian tube	No significant pathologic change
	Entire specimen submitted
Left fallopian tube	PAPILLARY SEROUS CARCINOMA, confined to the mucosa, see *Comment*
	Entire specimen submitted
Right ovary	Atrophy
	Entire specimen submitted
Left ovary	Atrophy
	Cortical inclusion cysts
	Entire specimen submitted

Comment The tumor in the tubal mucosa is interpreted as a metastasis from the endometrial carcinoma

Specimen labeled 'RIGHT FALLOPIAN TUBE AND OMENTAL BIOPSY':

Ovary:	SEROUS BORDERLINE TUMOR WITH COMPLEX (MICROPAPILLARY) ARCHITECTURE (12 cm), see *Comment*
	The tumor is present within a cyst
	Stromal invasion is not identified
	No surface involvement is identified
Fallopian tube:	MICROSCOPIC NON-INVASIVE SEROSAL IMPLANTS OF SEROUS NEOPLASIA, see *Comment*
Omental biopsy:	Microscopic, non-invasive implants of serous neoplasia, see *Comment*

Comment The ovarian tumor contains focal architectural complexity, but is not accompanied by stromal invasion or sufficient cellular atypia to warrant a diagnosis of serous carcinoma. Complex (micropapillary/cribriform) architecture in an ovarian serous borderline tumor has been linked to a higher overall risk of adverse outcome than conventional borderline serous tumors. However, based on the available literature, the risk is not increased in the absence of invasive peritoneal implants.

Specimen labeled 'MYOMECTOMY' (300 g):

UTERINE LEIOMYOSARCOMA, 10 cm

Mitoses number up to 12 per 10 HPF

Necrosis is present

Specimen labeled 'PLACENTA':

Small hypermature placenta (240 g); less than 10th percentile for 36 weeks gestation

Focally increased syncytial knots

Decidual vasculopathy

Placental infarcts (1.0 and 0.5 cm), multiple, recent and old

Comment   The above findings are consistent with uteroplacental insufficiency

Clinical   Pre-eclampsia toxemia

Specimen labeled 'PLACENTA':

Slightly immature placenta (360 g)

Retro-membranous hemorrhage, old, with hemosiderin laden macrophages in the chorion, consistent with prior abruption (clinical correlation is advised)

Clinical   Vaginal bleeding prior to delivery, rule out abruption

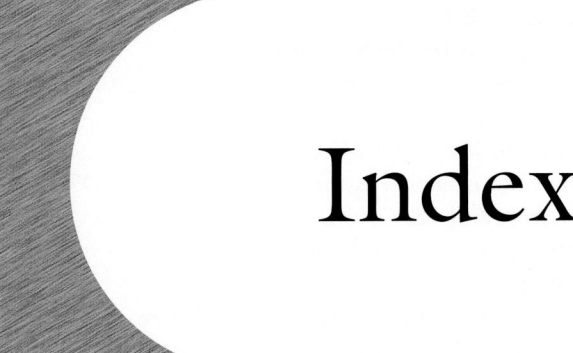

Index

Page references to significant material in figure legends and tables have only been given in the absence of its concomitant mention in the text referring to that illustration. 'vs' indicates the differentiation of two or more conditions.

abdominal cavity *see* peritoneal and abdominal cavity
ablation, endometrial 485
abortion 1001-5, 1013-15, 1084-7
  complications following 1013-15
  induced/elective (legal and illegal) 1013-14
    late 1087
  spontaneous (miscarriage) 996, 1001-5
    early/sporadic 1001-4
    gross pathology 998-1000
    histology indicative of specific mechanism of 1003
    late 1084-7
    prior, as risk factor for gestational trophoblastic disease 1016
    recurrent/habitual, and their causes 455, 996, 1004-5
    risk factors 1001
abruptio placentae *see* placenta
abscesses
  anal 206
  periclitoral 84-5
acantholysis
  differential diagnosis in 41, 124
  in Hailey—Hailey disease 42, 43
  in melanoma 171
  in Paget's disease 171
  in pemphigus vulgaris 41
  vulvocrural *see* vulvocrural area
acanthosis
  with altered differentiation, vulval 128
  in condyloma acuminatum 112, 115
  in eczematous dermatitis 27

acanthosis—cont'd
  lichen sclerosus with 127
  in lichen simplex chronicus 28
  see also hyperandrogenic—insulin-resistant—acanthosis nigricans syndrome
acardiac twin 1110
acetic acid staining, vagina 247
acral-type melanoma 169, 170
actin, smooth muscle (SMA), peritoneal mesenchymal tumors and 764
actinic-like lesions vs vulval intraepithelial neoplasia 124
actinomycosis, IUD-associated 470-2
adenocarcinoma
  anus
    anal canal 221
    anal margin 222
    in fistula 222
  cervical 373-402
    benign mimics 391-8
    cytologic findings 358-60
    diagnostic pitfalls 360-4, 514-15
    early invasive/microinvasive 373-5
    management and prognosis 399-402
    metastases (from other sites) 390-1
    metastatic spread of 399
    types 377-91
  endometrial 546-89
    clinical parameters for risk assessment 551-2
    differential diagnosis 482, 505, 511, 513, 537, 540-1, 567-8, 594
    exclusion 583
    histopathology 552-71
    laboratory studies 574-87
    management 588-9
    outcome 588-9
    outcome-associated parameters 587
    ovarian metastases 978

adenocarcinoma—cont'd
  ovarian stromal hyperthecosis co-existing with 740
  risk factors and epidemiology 546-51
  endometrioid *see* endometrioid adenocarcinoma
  minimal deviation *see* minimal deviation adenocarcinoma
  ovarian
    embryonal carcinoma vs 935
    endometriosis-associated 757-8
    granulosa cell tumor vs 959-60
  peritoneal metastases 780
  tubal 697
  vaginal 256, 257-8
  vulval 150-4
    Bartholin's gland 157
adenocarcinoma in situ (AIS), cervical 356, 366-73
  concept of 356
  diagnosis 366-73
    criteria 357
    differential 369-73
  false-negatives 360-1
  false-positives 361-4
  high-grade squamous intraepithelial neoplasia presenting as 306
  histology 366-7
  incidence relative to squamous carcinoma 356
  treatment 373
adenofibroma
  endometrioid 853
  ovarian 844-5, 857
    as cancer precursor, pre-existing 800
    clear cell 880
    endometrioid 870
    mucinous 857, 888
    papillary 834, 844-5, 853
    serous 844-5
  uterine 658-9
  uterine tube 696
adenoid basal carcinosarcoma, cervical 424
adenoid basal cell carcinoma
  cervical 387-9
    differential diagnosis 398-9, 423-4
  vulval 157
adenoid cystic carcinoma
  Bartholin's gland 155-7
  cervix 387-9
adenoid cystic carcinosarcoma, cervical 424
adenoma
  Bartholin's gland 106-7
  villous, cervix 399
adenoma malignum *see* minimal deviation adenocarcinoma

adenomatoid tumors
  peritoneal 780
  uterine and tubal 656-7, 695-7
adenomyoma
  cervical 420, 422
  uterine/endometrial 464, 597-8, 655, 659
adenomyomatous polyps (endometrial) 464, 597-8, 656
adenomyosis 655-6
  adenocarcinoma involving 580-1
  fallopian tube 685
adenosalpingitis (salpingitis isthmica nodosum) 685-6
adenosarcoma, Müllerian
  cervical 421-2
    differential diagnosis 420, 422, 425
  ovarian 877
    gross examination 878
    microscopic examination 878
  peritoneal 759-62
    polypoid endometriosis vs 759
  uterine 464-5, 657-8
    cervical involvement 422
    clinical presentation 657-8
    definition 657
    differential diagnosis 464-5, 592-3
    histopathology 658
    prognosis and management 659-60
  vaginal 256-7
    metastatic 236
adenosis, vaginal 18-19, 234
adenosquamous carcinoma
  cervical 381-3
  vulval skin appendages 150
adenosquamous carcinoma in situ, endocervical 367
adhesions
  periovarian *see* ovaries
  tubal/paratubal 681-3, 685
  vaginal, in Stevens—Johnson syndrome 241
adnexae/appendages
  anus
    benign tumors 208-9
    intraepithelial neoplasia 213
  female adnexal tumors of Wolffian origin 964-5
  vulva
    benign tumors 105-7, 144
    carcinomas 150, 154
    intraepithelial neoplasia involving 119
adolescence
  abnormal uterine bleeding in, causes 442
  pelvic inflammatory disease 690
adrenal hyperplasia, congenital 19
adrenal neuroblastoma, ovarian metastases 989
adrenal rests 679
adrenogenital syndrome 13

age
  abnormal uterine bleeding etiology related to 442,
      457-8
  cervical cancer and
      age at presentation influencing outcome 340
      age as risk factor 273
  endometrial carcinoma risk related to 546-7, 551
  gestational, assessment 1005
  ovarian tumor type and 822-4, 915, 947
  vulval melanoma risk and 166, 168
  see also older and elderly women
agenesis
  ovarian 10
  uterine/cervical 14
  vaginal 18
AIDS see HIV disease
ALK-1 768
allergic contact dermatitis 26
alpha-fetoprotein, yolk sac tumor 931
Alport syndrome 626
alveolar—glandular yolk sac tumor 932
alveolar rhabdomyosarcoma 988
alveolar soft-part sarcoma 425-6
amelanotic melanoma
  ovarian metastatic, theca-lutein hyperplasia
      of pregnancy vs 727
  vulva 169
amnion
  absence 1051
  cysts 1049
  nodules 1049-50, 1108
  normal gross appearance 1048
  space between chorion and 1061
amniotic band syndrome 1051, 1087
amniotic fluid infection see chorioamnionitis
ampulla of fallopian tube 676
amyloidosis
  cervical 434
  tubal 695
anal canal
  anatomy 201-3
  malignancy see malignant tumors
anal duct carcinoma 217-18
anal gland carcinoma 222
anal intercourse as risk factor for anal squamous
      intraepithelial lesions 209-10
anal lesions see anorectum; perianal region
anaplastic carcinoma see undifferentiated carcinoma
anaplastic lymphoma kinase-1 gene 768
anastomoses, vascular, twin placenta 1058-9, 1110
anemia, fetal 1105
angiofibroma, cellular 185-6
  differential diagnosis 180, 186

angiokeratoma 192
angioleiomyoma, vulvovaginal 189
angiomatosis, bacillary 88-90
angiomyofibroblastoma 182
  differential diagnosis 180, 182
angiomyoma, uterine 630
angiomyxoma 182-5
  aggressive 182-4
      clinical presentation 181, 182-3
      differential diagnosis 180, 181, 182, 183-4
      histopathology 183
      prognosis and management 184
  superficial 184-5
      clinical presentation 184
      differential diagnosis 180, 185
      histopathology 184-5
      prognosis and management 185
anisokaryosis, squamous intraepithelial neoplasia 304
annular tubules, sex cord tumor with 966-7
anorectum 199-228
  anatomy (gross and histologic) 201-3
  embryology 200
  lesions 199-228
      developmental 19, 200-1
      neoplastic 208-24
      non-neoplastic 203-8
anovulation (ovarian failure) 457, 458, 460, 477-8
  ovulation following 477-8
  premature (POF) 730-1
      autoimmune causes 731-2
  therapy 455, 475-6, 477-8
antibiotics
  bacillary angiomatosis 89-90
  bacterial vaginosis 71
  chancroid 82
  granuloma inguinale 84
  lymphogranuloma venereum 83
  syphilis 80
  tuberculosis 88
antifungal drugs
  candidiasis 69
  tinea cruris 70
antihelminthics 85-6
antiprotozoals, trichomoniasis 73
antivirals, HSV 77-8
Antoni A and B areas 771
anus see anorectum; perianal region
apocrine miliaria see Fox—Fordyce disease
apoptotic bodies, adenocarcinoma in situ 367
appendages see adnexae
appendix epiploica, infarcted 783
appendix veriformis tumors (incl. carcinoma) 981
  mucinous 866, 981

arcuate uterus 16-17
Arias—Stella reaction 371, 484, 512, 998
  curettings 1009
  differential diagnosis 482, 636, 1011
  papillary 573
Arias—Stella-like patterns 484
aromatase and endometriosis 737
arteritis 695
artery-to-artery anastomoses, twin placenta 1058
artery-to-vein anastomoses, twin placenta 1058
asbestos and malignant mesothelioma 780
assisted reproduction, ectopic pregnancy risk 1007
atopic dermatitis 26
atretic follicles 720
atrophic vaginitis 231-2
atrophy
  cervical/endocervical 363-4
    atypical squamous cells associated with 283-4
    high-grade squamous intraepithelial neoplasia
      309-10
  endometrial, postmenopausal 480-1
  ovarian 738-9
  vaginal, radiation-induced 35
atypia (nuclear and cytologic)
  anal squamous intraepithelial lesions
    high-grade 212-13
    low-grade 211
  cervical glandular
    adenocarcinoma 357
    adenocarcinoma in situ 366-7
    not fulfilling criteria for classic adenocarcinoma in
      situ 367-9
    viral infection-associated 373
  in cervical squamous intraepithelial neoplasia 304
  endometrial carcinoma 571, 572
  endometrial epithelial, benign 482-7
    categories 472
  ovarian intestinal-type borderline mucinous tumor
    with atypia only 858-9
  uterine leiomyoma 647
  uterine leiomyosarcoma 632-3, 635, 647
  vulval lesions
    dysplastic nevus 167-8
    pigmented 164
    verruciform 115, 119, 124
atypical glandular cells see glandular lesions
atypical hyperplasia, complex (endometrial) 494
atypical squamous cells see squamous cells
atypical stromal change/stromal
  cervix 435
  endometrium, with polyps 465
autoimmune ovarian failure 731-2
AutoPap 279

bacillary angiomatosis 88-90
bacterial infections
  amniotic fluid 1089
  fallopian tube, causative organisms 690-1, 693-4, 694
  lower genital tract 70-2
    immunosuppressed persons 87-92
    sexually-transmissible 78-84
  uterine, IUD-related risk 470-2
  see also microbiology
Bartholin's gland (and its ducts)
  carcinoma 155-7
  cyst 100-1
    hidradenoma vs 106
  nodular hyperplasia and adenoma 106-7
Bartonella henselae and B. quintana infection 88-90
basal cell (and basal cell layer/basalis)
  cervix 291, 292, 293
  endometrium 465
    development 520
basal cell carcinoma
  adenoid see adenoid basal cell carcinoma
  anal margin 221
  cervical 387-9, 398-9
  perianal 219
  vulval 143-4
    adenoid 157
    differential diagnosis 143-4, 157
basal surface of placenta see maternal surface
basaloid carcinosarcoma, cervical 424
basaloid squamous cell carcinoma
  anal 217
  cervical 338-9
Beckwith—Wiedemann syndrome, placenta in 1026-7
Behçet's disease 48-9, 241
Bethesda 2001 system 265
  atypical glandular lesions 365
  atypical squamous lesions 279, 285
bicornuate uterus 15
biliary tract carcinoma, ovarian metastases 981-2
biopsy
  cervical/endocervical 290-310
    biomarkers in management of 313
    discordant with Pap smear results 314-15
    endometrial carcinoma 575-7
    follow-up of squamous intraepithelial neoplasia
      proven by 316
    HPV testing 317
    invasiveness assessed by 328
    practical considerations before performing 290-1
    superficially invasive squamous carcinoma 333
  endometrial 575-7
    carcinoma 575-7
    dating 445, 455

biopsy—cont'd
    intraepithelial neoplasia 497
    in luteal phase defect 454-5
  vulval, melanocytic lesions 163
birth *see* delivery
bladder, urinary, endocervicosis 756
blastocyst 996
bleeding, uterine
  abnormal (AUB) 442, 456-8, 459-79
    causes related to age 442, 457-8
    causes related to frequency 442
    clinical work-up 458
    definitions 443
    management 487-8
    patterns associated with 459-79
    postmenopausal *see* older and elderly women
  dysfunctional (DUB) 457, 459-79
    definition 443, 457
    patterns associated with 459-79
    stromal breakdown in 448
  menstrual/cyclical 456-7
    normal vs abnormal 443
  see also hemorrhage
bleeding disorders, inherited, abnormal uterine
    bleeding in 457
blistering disorders *see* bullous disorders
blood
  clot, retroplacental 1052-3
  fetal 1068
  loss *see* bleeding; hemorrhage
  maternal, intervillous space 1066, 1076-7,
    1084-5
blood vessels *see* vascular space; vasculature
bone, ectopic
  cervix 434
  endometrium 543
borderline tumors
  ovaries (in general) 800, 840-1
    age and 823
    concept 840-1
    frequencies 822
  ovaries, clear cell tumors
    general and clinical aspects 879
    gross examination 880
    microscopic examination 880
  ovaries, endometrioid tumors
    general and clinical aspects 869
    gross examination 869
    microscopic examination 870-1
    pathology-based management 909
  ovaries, mixed epithelial 853
    general and clinical aspects 890-1
    gross examination 891

borderline tumors—cont'd
  ovaries, mucinous tumors 803, 826, 827
    endocervical-like 853, 860, 861, 868, 891, 892
    general and clinical aspects 855
    gross examination 856
    microscopic examination 857-60
    pathology-based management 910
  ovaries, serous tumors 800, 826, 827
    general and clinical aspects 842
    gross examination 843
    microscopic features 845-51
    pathology-based management 907-8
  ovaries, transitional cell and Brenner tumors
    etiology/genetics/biomarkers 888
    general and clinical aspects 884
    gross examination 884
    microscopic examination 885
  tubal serous cystadenoma 696
bowel cancer *see* colon cancer; intestinal cancer;
    small bowel carcinoma
Bowen disease 211-12
bowenoid papulosis 119, 211
BRCA1/BRCA2
  ovarian and breast/ovarian cancer and 802-3,
    812
    familial 698-701, 801, 802, 812, 843, 844
    sporadic 802-3
  papillary serous carcinoma and 762
breast, ectopic tissue in vulva 103-4
  carcinoma arising in 154
breast cancer (primarily carcinoma) 982-5
  metastases from 982-5
    in cervix 391
    in endometrium 601
    in ovary 825, 982-5
    in vulva 160-1
  ovarian and
    familial *see* familial syndromes
    presentation with independent lesions 984-5
  vulvar Paget's disease and risk of 153-4, 155
Brenner tumor 829, 830
  differential diagnosis 887-8, 892
  general and clinical aspects 884
  gross examination 884
  malignant 884-5, 886-7, 888, 888-9, 892
  microscopic examination 885-7
Breslow depth 171, 172
broad ligament
  tumors 696-7
  vasculitis 695
Brues' mole 1051, 1085
bullous (blistering) disorders 39-42, 240
  differential diagnosis 38, 42, 43

Burkitt's lymphoma, ovarian 989
Buschke—Löwenstein tumors *see* giant condylomata

CA125, ovarian cancer and 855
  management of 911
  screening of 814
calcifications
  tubal 689
  villous stromal 1072-3
calcifying fibrous tumor 766-7, 768
caldesmon (H-caldesmon)
  endometrial stromal tumors 622
  peritoneal mesenchymal tumors 764
  uterine leiomyoma 644
Call—Exner bodies 876
Calymmatobacterium granulomatis 82-4
canal of Nuck, hydrocele 103
cancer *see* malignant tumors
candidiasis
  amniotic fluid 1089
  umbilical cord 1059
  vulvovaginal
    differential diagnosis 32, 125
    HIV infection and 87
    vulvodynia 59-60
capillary
  fetal, microscopic appearance 1073
  proliferation *see* chorangiomas; chorangiosis
capillary space invasion
  cervical cancer 329-30, 332-3
  endometrial adenocarcinoma 587
carboplatin-based chemotherapy, tubal carcinoma
  705
carcinoembryonic antigen, minimal deviation cervical
  adenocarcinoma 379
carcinogenesis
  cervical 268
  ovarian *see* ovarian cancer
carcinoid syndrome 415
carcinoid tumor
  cervical 412
    atypical 412
  ovarian 887-8, 921-4
    differential diagnosis 868, 887-8, 960
    metastatic 924, 980-1
    mucinous/goblet cell 868, 923
    Sertoli—Leydig cell tumors containing elements
      of 966
    struma ovarii co-existing with 919-20, 964
carcinoma (sites)
  anal 216-22
    anatomy relating to spread of 203
    risk factors 203

carcinoma (sites)—cont'd
  appendiceal *see* appendix veriformis
  biliary, ovarian metastases 981-2
  breast *see* breast cancer
  cervical 267-402, 412-18
    ovarian metastases 979
    pitfalls in diagnosis 321
  colonic *see* colon cancer
  endometrial/uterine 546-89, 598-601, 825
    clinical parameters for risk assessment 551-2
    histopathology 552-71
    intraepithelial neoplasia and risk of 498-9, 549-51
    laboratory studies 574-87
    outcome-associated parameters 567-8, 581-2, 588
    ovarian metastases 854, 874-5, 978
    ovarian tumor concurrent with 824
    rarer forms 598-601
    risk factors and epidemiology 546-51
  endometrial/uterine, differential diagnosis 571-3
    altered surface epithelial changes 484-5
    Arias—Stella effect 482
    intraepithelial neoplasia 494, 498, 504, 511
    mucinous metaplasia 534
    tubal metaplasia 537
  gastric *see* Krukenberg tumor
  ovarian 793-993
    age and 823
    co-existing with endometrial carcinoma 585
    in cystic teratomas 916, 918
    development 793-809
    gross appearances 827, 830
    histologic grading/types 803-5, 841-2, 873
    pathology-based management 907-10
    risk factors 811-19
    staging 906-7
    see also specific types
  ovarian metastatic
    gross appearance 830
    theca-lutein hyperplasia of pregnancy vs 727
  pancreatic, ovarian metastases 867, 981-2
  peritoneal
    primary 910
    secondary (metastases) 780, 783
  renal cell, metastatic 883, 985-6
  thyroid, in ovary 920-1
  tubal 697, 702-7
    adenomatoid tumor vs 696
    co-existing with endometrial carcinoma 585
    epithelial pseudoneoplasia associated with
      salpingitis vs 689
    metastatic 705-7
    ovarian metastases 979
    primary 702-5

carcinoma (sites)—cont'd
  urothelial, vulval extension 152
  vaginal 253-8
  vulval 130-43, 154-62
    benign rests vs 103, 104-5
carcinoma (types)
  adenoid cystic *see* adenoid cystic carcinoma
  adenosquamous *see* adenosquamous carcinoma
  basal cell *see* basal cell carcinoma
  clear cell *see* clear cell carcinoma
  embryonal *see* embryonal carcinoma
  endometrioid *see* endometrioid adenocarcinoma
  Merkel cell 158-9
  mesonephric *see* mesonephric carcinoma
  mucinous *see* mucinous carcinoma
  neuroendocrine *see* neuroendocrine carcinoma
  serous *see* serous carcinoma
  serous intraepithelial *see* serous intraepithelial
      carcinoma
  small cell *see* small cell carcinoma
  squamous cell *see* squamous cell carcinoma
  sweat gland 104
  transitional cell *see* transitional cell carcinoma
  undifferentiated *see* undifferentiated carcinoma
  verrucous *see* verrucous carcinoma
  see also adenocarcinoma; choriocarcinoma
carcinoma in situ, *see also* intraepithelial neoplasia
carcinosarcoma (malignant mixed Müllerian tumors;
    MMMTs)
  cervical (primary) 422-5
    mesonephric carcinoma vs 390
  endometrial (primary) 589-97, 660
    clinical presentation 590
    differential diagnosis 592, 594, 659
    outcome/prognosis 592-4, 594
    pathogenesis 590
    pathology 590-4
    risk factors 590
    staging 594-5
    therapy 595-7
  metastatic
    to cervix 236, 425
    from corpus or ovary 425
    to endometrium 592
    from vagina 236
  ovarian 877
    differential diagnosis 878-9, 937
    gross examination 878
    microscopic examination 878
  peritoneal 759-62
  tubal 707
carcinosarcomatous mural nodules in ovarian mucinous
    tumors 866

cardiovascular disease, fetal 1104
Carney's complex 164
cartilage
  ectopic
    cervix 434
    endometrium 543
  Sertoli—Leydig cell tumors with 867, 966
β-catenin and endometrioid carcinoma 877
cautery artifact, endocervix 372
CD10
  endometrial carcinoma invading myometrium vs
      involving adenomyosis 580-1
  endometrial stromal tumors 622, 623, 973
  endometriosis (ovarian) 737
  peritoneal mesenchymal tumors 764
  uterine leiomyoma 644
cdx-2 867
cellularity
  leiomyoma 643-5
  peripheral nerve sheath tumor
    malignant 771
    schwannoma 771
cervicitis 372-3
  ligneous 434
cervix 267-439
  developmental and acquired childhood disorders 14-17
  ectopic pregnancy 1012
  endometrial tumors involving 582-3
    epithelial 575, 577, 582-3
    mesenchymal 422
  endometriosis *see* endometriosis
  incompetence 1093
  pregnancy-related epithelial changes 371
  smears (Pap smears) 278-9, 574-5
    discordant with biopsy results 314-15
    endometrial cancer and 574-5
    expectations in cancer prevention 278-9
    glandular lesions 356, 357-66, 574
    HPV testing as adjunct to 319-20
    in malignancy prediction 320-1
    squamous lesions 278-9, 287-90
  tumors 267-354
    endometrial invasion by 582
    glandular *see* glandular neoplasia
    metastatic 390-1, 425, 601
    ovarian metastases 979
    pathogenesis 268
    risk factors 268-78
    squamous *see* squamous lesions
  see also endocervix
cesarean section in placental previa 1114
chancre 78, 79
chancroid 81-2

chemotherapy
  cervical cancer
    adenocarcinoma 399-402
    neuroendocrine carcinoma 417-18
    squamous carcinoma 341-2
  endometrial adenocarcinoma, adjuvant 589
  endometrial carcinosarcoma 595-6
    adjuvant 595
  gestational trophoblastic disease
    complete mole 1025-6
    placental site trophoblastic tumor 1036
  inflammatory myofibroblastic tumor 768
  ovarian cancer
    adjuvant (postoperative) 910
    immature teratoma 938
    neoadjuvant 911
    yolk sac tumor 934
  peritoneal papillary serous carcinoma 762
  tubal carcinoma 705
chickenpox 92
childbirth *see* delivery
children
  genital warts 117
  ovarian and tubal disorders 13-14, 16
  placental abnormality-associated disorders in 1042
Chlamydia trachomatis
  cervical neoplasia and 275
  in cervical samples 294
  pelvic inflammatory disease and 690-1, 693
  see also lymphogranuloma venereum
chocolate cyst *see* endometriotic cyst
chorangiomas (placental capillary hemangioma)
      1112-13
  gross appearance 1050, 1055, 1112
  microscopic appearance 1068
chorangiosis 1073
chorioamnionitis, acute 1085, 1089-91
  cause and clinical presentation 1089
  pathology 1089-91
    gross appearance 1045, 1085, 1089
    microscopic appearance 1066, 1085, 1089-91
choriocarcinoma 935-6, 1028-33
  clinico-radiologic features 1016, 1028-9
  diagnosis/exclusions 936, 1017, 1029-31, 1033
  gross features 935, 1016, 1029
  histopathology 935-6, 1017, 1029
  intraplacental 1031-3
  management and outcome 936, 1033
  presentation
    signs and symptoms 935
    at term 1031-2, 1113
  risk factors 935
  vaginal metastases 258

chorion 1062-5
  cysts 1049
  space between amnion and 1061-2
  surface nodules 1049-51
  villi *see* villi
chorionic gonadotrophin, human *see* human chorionic
      gonadotrophin
chorionic membrane 996
chorionic plate 1001-6
chorionic sphere 996, 997
chorionic trophoblasts 1020
chorionic vessels 1062, 1065-6
  thrombosis 1046, 1065
chorionicity 1056, 1057, 1109-10
chromosome abnormalities *see* cytogenetic abnormalities
cicatricial pemphigoid 39, 40, 240
  differential diagnosis 40, 43
cilia, cervical/uterine 535-6
ciliated cell, fallopian tube 676
ciliated cell differentiation *see* tubal/ciliated cell differentiation
ciliated cysts 101-2
ciliated metaplasia 541-2
cisplatin-based chemotherapy
  cervical squamous carcinoma 341-2
  endometrial carcinosarcoma 595-6
  tubal carcinoma 705
clear cell adenosquamous carcinoma 382-3
clear cell carcinoma/adenocarcinoma
  cervical 384-5, 390
  endometrial 547, 559, 568-9
    differential diagnosis 482, 569
  intestinal, ovarian metastases 876, 981
  ovarian 805, 854, 876
    differential diagnosis 882-3, 933, 963-4
    etiology/genetics/biomarkers 883-4
    general and clinical aspects 879, 880
    gross examination 880
    microscopic examination 881
  vaginal 257-8
clear cell cytoplasm in non-clear cell endometrial
      adenocarcinoma 559
clear cell leiomyoma 628-9
clear cell tumors, ovarian 879-84
  malignant *see* clear cell carcinoma
  pathology-based management 909
clitoris
  abscess in area around 84-5
  squamous cell carcinoma involving 142
cloacal development 200
  anomalies 19, 201
cloacogenic neoplasms
  vagina 258
  vulva 159-60

cloacogenic polyps, inflammatory 205-6
cloacogenic squamous cell carcinoma, anal 217
clomiphene 455, 477
    ovarian cancer risk 813
clonal events leading to mixed pattern endometrium 479
clonality
    leiomyoma 625-6
    leiomyomatosis 654
clot, blood, retroplacental 1052-3
CMV *see* cytomegalovirus
colitis, ulcerative, anal disease 207
colon, ovarian cancer extending into 824
colon (and colorectal) cancer
    hereditary non-polyposis (Lynch syndrome II)
        endometrial carcinoma risk 548
        endometrial intraepithelial neoplasia risk 496
        ovarian cancer risk 812
    ovarian metastases 824, 828, 876, 979
color
    placental 1044
        sectioned surface 1053-4
    placental membranes 1048
    umbilical cord 1047
colposcopy 320-1
    adenocarcinoma in situ, limitations 366
    endocervical sampling at initial colposcopy 314
    indications 247
    malignancy prediction 320-3
columnar cells
    transformation zone, differentiation 291, 292, 293, 294
        in squamous carcinoma 339
        in stratified intraepithelial lesions 306
    vaginal, postmenopausal 234
compound nevus 165
conception, retained products 1014
condyloma(ta), cervical 338
    flat 297, 300
    immature 296-7, 300-2, 338
    see also giant condylomata; warts
condylomatous cervical carcinomas 336-8
cone biopsy
    in assessment of invasion 328
    superficially invasive squamous carcinoma 333
congenital adrenal hyperplasia 19
congenital anomalies/malformations *see* developmental
        anomalies
contact dermatitis 25-6
contraceptive 473-5
    hormonal
        emergency 473
        oral *see* oral contraceptives
    intrauterine device *see* intrauterine contraceptive device
copper IUD 470

cord *see* umbilical cord
corps rond(s) 44
corps rond-like structures 44
corpus luteum 718, 720-2
    clinical complications 722
    deficient development 455
    differential diagnosis 721-2
        cystic follicles 719
    of pregnancy 723
    recent 720-2
    regressing/degenerating 443, 720-2
        gross appearance 720-1, 826
cortex, ovarian
    endometriosis 737
    fibromatosis 741-2
    in hysterectomy specimens, incidental findings 716-22
    structure 714-15
Cowden's syndrome
    endometrial carcinoma in 549
    endometrial intraepithelial neoplasia in 496
coxsackie virus 1101
crab lice 66-7
cribriform architecture
    endometrial lesions 538
    ovarian serous cervical borderline tumors 847-8
Crohn's disease, vulval 50-2
    differential diagnosis 46, 49, 51-2, 88
    fistulas 50, 206
crypts (endocervical)
    invasion originating from 331-2
    involvement in cervical cancer 326, 327
cultures, placental tissue 1043-4
curettage, endocervical (ECC) and endometrial
        (and sample interpretation)
    cervical specimens 317-18
        squamous intraepithelial neoplasia 313-14
        choriocarcinoma vs residual matter (post-molar)
            1030-1
    ectopic pregnancy 1008-11
    endometrial carcinoma 575-7
    endometrial intraepithelial neoplasia 497
    endometrial stromal tumors 620-1
    trophoblastic neoplasia 1016
cyclin E
    cervical squamous lesions and 312
    endometrial receptivity to implantation and 456
cyst(s)
    endocervical 391
    ovarian/para-ovarian 716-18
        age and function cyst occurrence 823
        dermoid cyst *see* cystic teratoma, mature/benign
        endometriotic cysts *see* endometriotic cyst
        epidermoid cyst *see* epidermoid cyst

cyst(s)—cont'd
    gross appearance 826-7
    inclusion cysts *see* inclusion cysts
    perianal 203-4
    peritoneal, serous cysts 778
    placental septal 1055
    placental surface 1049
    tubal/paratubal 679-83
        gross appearance 826
    ultrasound evaluation 816, 817
    vulvovaginal 100-3, 234-6
cystadenofibroma, ovarian 844-5, 870
    pathology-based management 909
cystadenoma
    ovarian 844-5
        borderline 800, 880, 909
        gross appearance 826, 827, 856
        microscopic appearance 844-5, 856, 880
        mucinous 844-5, 856, 857
        pathology-based management 909
    rete 853
    tubal 680-1, 696
        adenofibromatous component 696
cystic adhesions, tubal/paratubal 681-3, 685
cystic carcinoma *see* adenoid cystic carcinoma
cystic endosalpingiosis, florid 394
cystic follicles (follicle cysts) 719-20, 743
    cystic granulosa cell tumors vs 720
    in hyperreactio luteinalis 728
    solitary luteinized 728-9
cystic glandular change in dysfunctional uterine
    bleeding 457, 460
cystic granulosa cell tumors 720
cystic masses of ovary, gross examination 825-7
cystic mesothelioma 697, 777-8
    periovarian adhesions vs 715-16
cystic ovarian mucinous tumors 856-7
cystic teratoma (ovarian) 836, 915-24
    mature/benign (dermoid cyst) 830-1, 915-17
        gross pathology 915-16
        histopathology 916
        intraoperative evaluation 915-16
        management and outcome 917
        monodermal and malignant variants, *see subheading*
           below
        presenting signs 915
        risk factors 823, 915
    monodermal and malignant 918-24
        risk factors 918
cystic yolk sac tumor 931
cytogenetic (karyotypic/chromosomal) abnormalities
    endometrial stromal sarcoma 765
    ovarian serous carcinoma vs borderline serous tumor 800

cytogenetic (karyotypic/chromosomal) abnormalities—
    cont'd
    peritoneal malignant mesothelioma 782
    peritoneal mesenchymal tumors
        desmoplastic small round cell tumor 776
        liposarcoma 775
    pregnancy
        elective abortion 1084, 1087
        hydatidiform mole 1016-17, 1026
        placental samples (in general) 1044
        placental site trophoblastic tumor 1035
        spontaneous abortion 1000, 1001, 1004-5
    uterine smooth muscle tumors
        leiomyoma (benign metastasizing form) 655
        leiomyoma (classic form) 626-7, 629-30
        leiomyosarcoma 631-2
        lipoleiomyoma 630
        quasi-malignant 652
    vulvovaginal dermatofibroma protuberans 187
    see also genetics; molecular genetics
cytokeratins, ovarian mucinous carcinoma 868
    metastatic 867
cytology
    anal, in HPV-infected women 210
    cervical 278-86
        atypical glandular cells 357-66, 574
        in malignancy prediction 320-3
        neuroendocrine carcinoma 412
        squamous lesions 278-86, 287-90
    endometrium
        adenocarcinoma 574-5
        intraepithelial neoplasia 503-4
    peritoneal, endometrial carcinoma 583-4
cytomegalovirus (CMV) infection
    endocervical glandular atypia associated with 373
    endometrial 467
    placental villous 1070, 1100
cytotrophoblast (cells and layer) 996, 1017
    in gestational trophoblastic disease 1017
        choriocarcinoma 935, 936, 1029
        complete mole 1017, 1021
        partial mole 1026

Darier's disease 43-4
    differential diagnosis 42, 44, 45
death, embryo/fetal (intrauterine) 1084, 1086-7
    histology findings indicative of specific mechanism
        of 1003
    placental changes in 1001, 1108-9
    second trimester 1086-7
    twin 1112
    in villous fibrosis 1072
    see also abortion; fetus papyraceus

decidua 482, 1077-8
  absence in placenta creta 1079-80, 1115
    ectopic (deciduosis)
      cervix 434
      endometrium 482
      ovary 722, 729-30
      peritoneal cavity 754
      tubal mucosa 678
    hemorrhage 1078-9
    inflammatory/reactive change 1011
    plasma cells in 467-8
    vasculopathy in pre-eclampsia 1096
decidualized endometrioma 746
deciduitis 1078
  chronic 1104
dediduoid mesothelioma 754, 782
dedifferentiated liposarcoma 774-5
degeneration
  cervical atypical squamous cells 284
  endometrial surface epithelial 529
  hyaline, mimicking implantation site 482
  uterine leiomyoma 640
delivery
  induced see induced delivery
  operative 1093-106
  premature or accelerated 1088-93
demographics
  anal squamous cell carcinoma 216-17
  endometrial adenocarcinoma 546-7
dentate line 201
Depo-Provera 475
dermatitis
  eczematous see eczematous dermatitis
  seborrheic 32
  spongiotic see spongiosis
dermatofibroma 186-7
  differential diagnosis 186, 187
dermatofibroma protuberans 187-8
  differential diagnosis 186, 187-8
dermatophytoses 69-70
dermis
  melanoma involving 169
  nevus involving 166
dermoid cyst see cystic teratoma, mature/benign
desmin
  endometrial stromal tumors 622
  peritoneal mesenchymal tumors and 764
  uterine leiomyoma 644
  uterine perivascular epithelioid cell tumor 660
desmoid fibromatosis 773-4
  clinical features 773
  differential diagnosis 764, 768, 770, 773-4, 783
  pathology 773-4

desmoplastic implants of ovarian serous borderline
    tumors 849, 850
desmoplastic small round cell tumors
  abdominal 775-6
  ovarian metastatic 988
desquamative inflammatory vaginitis 240
development
  anogenital (incl. embryology) 2-9, 200, 946
    anorectal 200
    vulvodynia and 58
  placental 996-8
developmental anomalies (congenital/anatomical
    malformations)
  fetus
    elective abortion for 1084, 1087
    placenta and 1106-7
  woman 9-20
    abortion due to 1004
    anorectal 19, 200-1
diabetes, maternal 1104
diaphragm-related lesions 238
dichorionic placenta 1056, 1057, 1109
didelphic uterus 15
dietary factors, ovarian cancer 813
diethylstilbestrol (DES) exposure 17, 18-19
  clear cell adenocarcinoma of vagina and 257-8
differentiation, endometrial, altered see metaplasia
differentiation-specific pathways, ovarian cancer 794,
    795, 803-5
diffuse laminar endocervical glandular hyperplasia 393
diffuse mesonephric hyperplasia 397
digital examination, anal canal 203
dimensions see size
discs, placental 1061
  conditions 1061
  twin gestation 1056-7
disseminated intravascular coagulation in eclampsia
    1093, 1094
DNA mismatch repair genes and endometrial cancer
    548, 549
donovanosis 82-4
dpc4 867
drug-related lesions, endometrial intraepithelial
    neoplasia 496
ductal carcinoma of breast, ovarian metastases 984
ductal mesonephric hyperplasia 397
dysesthesia, vulva 58, 59
dysgenesis, ovarian 10
dysgerminoma 924-31
  differential diagnosis 930
    clear cell carcinoma 883
  gross appearance 830
  gross pathology 926

dysgerminoma—cont'd
  histopathology 926-30
  management and outcome 930-1
  presenting signs/symptoms 925
  risk factors 924-5
dyskeratoma, warty, differential diagnosis 42, 45
dysmenorrhea, membranous 445
dysmorphic villi 1003
dysplasia
  glandular see glandular dysplasia
  ovarian 799-800
  vaginal, post-radiation 253
dysplastic nevus 167-8
  genital-type nevus vs 166

EBV 86-7
eclampsia 1093, 1094
ectoparasites 66-8
ectopia/heterotopia/implants
  bone and cartilage see bone; cartilage
  breast tissue in vulva see breast
  decidua see decidua
  glial tissue see glia
  pregnancy 996, 1005-13
    clinical diagnostic algorithm 1008
    clinical presentation 1007-8
    co-existing intrauterine pregnancy 1011
    curettings, examination 1008-9
    examination of fallopian tubes 1011-12
    extra-tubal sites 1012
    management 1008
    risk factors 693, 1005-7
  prostate 397-9
eczematous dermatitis 24-7
  differential diagnosis 27, 29, 31, 45
edema
  massive ovarian 747, 825
  villous see villi
elderly see older and elderly women
embryo
  death see death
  development see development
  specimens in recurrent abortion 1005
embryonal carcinoma 934-5
  yolk sac tumor vs 933, 935
embryonal rhabdomyosarcoma (sarcoma botryoides)
    191-2, 988
  differential diagnosis 181, 191-2
embryonal tumors 924-39
embryonic disc 997
emphysematous vaginitis 241-2
EMSY and sporadic breast and ovarian cancer 802-3
endocervical glandular hyperplasia 393

endocervical mesenchyme, metaplasia 434
endocervical polyps see polyps
endocervical-type adenocarcinoma (mucinous
    adenocarcinoma) 377-80
  endometrial intraepithelial neoplasia vs 514-15
endocervical-type adenocarcinoma in situ 367
endocervical-type adenomyoma 420, 422
endocervical-type mucinous/Müllerian tumors of ovary
    borderline 853, 860, 861, 868, 891, 892
    carcinoma 863-4, 891, 892
endocervicosis 394, 756
endocervix (and endocervical cells)
  atrophy see atrophy
  atypical cells, HPV testing 365-6
  biopsy/curettage see biopsy; curettage
  reactive changes, adenocarcinoma and
      adenocarcinoma in situ vs 360, 361, 363, 372-3
endocrine disease, autoimmune 731
  see also entries under hormone
endodermal elements, Sertoli—Leydig cell tumor with 966
endodermal sinus tumor see yolk sac tumor
endometrioid (adeno)carcinoma 380-1, 804-5, 910
  cervical 380-1
    mesonephric carcinoma vs 390
    metastatic 391
  endometrial/uterine
    endometrial intraepithelial neoplasia vs 513
    estrogen stimulation (chronic) and risk of 546-7
    grading 569-70, 580
    histopathology 552-60
    mixed with serous component 563-8
    molecular genetics 549
    precursor lesions 549-50
    villoglandular 559-60, 565-6, 573
  ovarian 804-5
    differential diagnosis 854, 867, 882-3, 892, 963-4
    etiology/genetics/biomarkers 876-7
    general and clinical aspects 869
    gross examination 869
    microscopic examination 871-4
    misclassification 835
    pathology-based management 909-10
    precursors 804-5
  tubal 703
endometrioid adenocarcinoma in situ 367
endometrioid adenofibroma 853
endometrioid glands, endometrial stromal tumor with
    617, 659
endometrioid stromal sarcoma see stromal sarcoma
endometrioid tumors, ovarian 868-79
  differential diagnosis 874-6
  etiology/genetics/biomarkers 876-7
  general and clinical aspects 868-9

endometrioid tumors, ovarian—cont'd
  gross examination 869
  microscopic examination 870-4
endometrioid yolk sac tumor 876, 933
endometrioma *see* endometriotic cyst
endometriosis
  anal/perianal 207
  cervical 370-1
    gland-poor 436
  extra-ovarian (in general), carcinoma arising in
      256-7, 705, 910
  management 746
  ovarian 736-7, 743-6
    cancer and 743, 757-8, 795, 876-7, 890,
        909
  peritoneal 756-9
    polypoid 758-9
  tubal 683
    carcinoma occurring within 705
  vaginal 236
    primary tumor arising in 256-7
  vulval 105
endometriotic/chocolate cyst (endometrioma) 737,
    743-6, 826
  early carcinoma arising in, management 909-10
  gross appearance 743-4, 826
endometritis 466-70
  chronic (plasmacytic) 466-70
    differential diagnosis 452, 468
  granulomatous 467
  lymphocytic 468
endometrium (and endometrial cells) 411-610
  ablation 485
  artifacts 482-7
  benign lesions 459-87
    intraepithelial neoplasia vs 504, 505-8
  in cervical smear samples 574-5
    resembling adenocarcinoma in situ 361-2
  cyclical 442-52
    classification 443
    menstrual *see* menstrual phase
  histiocytes, in cervical smear 574
  hyperplasia *see* hyperplasia
  intraepithelial neoplasia *see* intraepithelial
      neoplasia
  mixed pattern 477-9
    causes 472
  postmenopausal 480-1
  receptivity to implantation, biomarkers in assessment
      of 455-6
  sampling
    biopsy *see* biopsy
    in endometrial intraepithelial neoplasia 497-8

endometrium (and endometrial cells)—cont'd
  stroma *see* stroma
  thickening, assessment 552
  tumors 545-610
    epithelial *see* epithelial tumors
    malignant *see* malignant tumors
    mesenchymal *see* mesenchymal tumors
    polycystic ovarian syndrome-related risk 735-6
    stromal *see* stromal tumors
endosalpingiosis 681, 716
  florid cystic 394
  omental 849
  ovarian 716
  peritoneal 754-5
endotoxin toxic shock syndrome toxin-1 239
enterovirus 1101
eosinophilic folliculitis 72
eosinophilic metaplasia 538
ependymoma, ovarian 876
epidermal inclusion cyst *see* inclusion cyst
epidermoid cyst 914-15
  etiology 890
  gross examination 889
  microscopic examination 889
epiploic appendage, infarcted 783
epithelial implants (in peritoneal cavity) of ovarian
    serous borderline tumors 849-50
epithelial inclusion cyst *see* inclusion cyst
epithelial membrane antigen (EMA)
  and mesothelial hyperplasia 777
  and ovarian tumors 801
epithelial—mesenchymal tumors, mixed *see* mixed
    tumors
epithelial metaplasia *see* metaplasia
epithelial proliferation of fallopian tube, benign 687-9
epithelial pseudoneoplasia associated with salpingitis
    688-9
epithelial tumors (and epithelial—stromal tumors)
  borderline *see* borderline tumors
  endometrial 545-610
    classification 553
  ovarian 839-912
    pathology-based management 905-12
    sex cord-stromal tumors, differential diagnosis 950,
        951
    staging *see* staging
    terminology and classification 840
    uni- vs bilateral 824
epithelioid cell tumor, uterine perivascular 660-1
epithelioid leiomyoma
  uterine 628-9
  vulvovaginal 190
epithelioid leiomyosarcoma 637

epithelioid trophoblastic tumor 1035
epithelioma, spindle cell, vaginal 261
epithelium
　amniotic, disorganization or erosion 1061
　cervical pregnancy-related changes 371
　endometrial
　　altered surface changes 484-5
　　repair *see* repair
　ovarian surface
　　carcinogenesis and the 795-8, 799-800
　　hysterectomy specimens, incidental findings
　　　715-16
　　structure 714
　vaginal 230
　　older women, benign changes 230-2
　vulval Paget's disease and extent of spread to 153
Epstein—Barr virus 86-7
epulis-like mural nodules in ovarian mucinous tumors
　865-6
erosive lichen planus 36-7, 37
erythroblastosis fetalis 1104
estrogen therapy
　in atrophic vaginitis 232
　excess/persistent effect (with continuous unopposed
　　estrogen) 481, 506
　endometrial carcinoma risk 546-7, 548
ethnicity (RACE)
　and endometrial carcinoma 547-8
　and endometrial carcinosarcoma 590
　and trophoblastic disease 1105-6
Ewing's sarcoma (peripheral/primitive
　　neuroectodermal tumor)
　cervical 429-30
　ovarian 973, 988-9
　peritoneal 776
　see also EWS-WT-1 protein
EWS-WT-1 protein 776
excisional biopsy, melanocytic lesions of vulva 163
exfoliation artifacts, endometrial 482-3
exophytic cervical adenocarcinoma 375

fallopian tube *see* tube
familial (inherited) syndromes
　endometrial intraepithelial neoplasia risk 496
　ovarian and breast/ovarian cancer 801, 802, 812
　　prophylactic surgery *see* oophorectomy
　　tubal component 698-701
families wishes, obstetric tissue samples 996
fasciitis
　necrotizing, vulval 90-2
　nodular 768, 774
female pseudohermaphroditism 11, 13
feminization, testicular 10-11

fertility problems
　drug therapy, ovarian cancer risk associated with 813
　ovarian conditions 730-7
　salpingitis/pelvic inflammatory disease 693, 694
fetal differentiation, germ cell tumors with 924-39
fetal surface of placenta, gross appearance 1048-51
fetiform teratoma 915
fetus
　blood 1068
　death *see* death
　distress 1105-6
　growth restriction *see* intrauterine growth restriction
　in fetu, vs benign cystic teratoma 915
　malformations *see* developmental anomalies
　metastatic tumor 1068
　specimens in recurrent abortion 1005
　vasculature
　　capillaries, microscopic appearance 1073
　　thrombosis *see* thrombosis
fetus papyraceus 1050, 1057
FH and leiomyoma 626
fibrin (placenta) 1055-6
　extensive deposits 1055-6
　inter-/perivillous 1033, 1075-6
　localized deposits 1055
　Nitabuch's 1077, 1078
　subchorionic *see* subchorionic fibrin
fibroadenoma, vulval 103
fibroepithelial mucosal (stromal) polyps
　anal 205
　cervix, atypical stromal cells in 435
　vulvovaginal 179-80, 236-7
　　clinical presentation 180
　　differential diagnosis 112, 180, 181, 191-2
　　histopathology 180-1, 236-7
　　prognosis and management 181
fibroepithelial papilloma 112
fibrohistiocytic tumors 186-8
fibroids *see* leiomyoma
fibroma
　ovarian 829, 949-52
　　cellular 952-5
　　definition 949-51, 952-3
　　differential diagnosis 951-2
　　gross features 951
　　histopathology 951, 953-4
　　management and outcome 952, 954-5
　　risk factors 951
　vulval, prepubertal 19-20
fibromatosis
　cortical 741-2
　desmoid *see* desmoid fibromatosis
fibrosarcoma, ovarian 830, 952-5

fibrosis, villous 1072

fibrothecoma, ovarian 879, 949, 951
   unclassified tumors similar to 968

fibrous histiocytoma 186-7

fibrous stroma in uterine papillary serous carcinoma 562

fibrous tumor
   calcifying 766-7, 768
   solitary 765-6

FIGO (International Federation of Gynaecology and
      Obstetrics)
   grading
      endometrioid carcinoma 569-70, 580
      ovarian carcinoma 841
   staging
      cervical adenocarcinoma 375-6, 399
      cervical squamous carcinoma 320, 328
      endometrial carcinoma 579
      ovarian carcinoma 906-7
      tubal carcinoma 703
      vaginal carcinoma 255
      vulvar carcinoma 140

filiform mucosal excrescences of vagina 302-3

fissures, anal 206

fistulas
   anal 206
      adenocarcinoma in 222
   Crohn's disease 50, 206

fixation
   endometrial, artifacts 482-3
   placental 1043

flexural psoriasis 30

flexural-type nevus 165-6

florid cystic endosalpingiosis 394

5-fluorouracil, vaginal intraepithelial lesions 253

follicle(s), ovarian
   atretic 720
   cystic see cystic follicles
   development 3, 718
   differential diagnosis of follicular changes 720
   graafian 718-19
   primary 718
   primordial 3, 718
   secondary 718

follicle-stimulating hormone and the cyclical
      endometrium 443

follicular phase see proliferative phase

follicular salpingitis 685, 692
   chronic 685
   salpingitis isthmica nodosum vs 686

follicular thyroid carcinoma in struma ovarii 920

folliculitis 71-2

foot length, gestational age assessment 1005

Fordyce spots 45

foreign bodies, vaginal 237

Forkhead transcription factor and premature ovarian
      failure 731

Fox—Fordyce disease (apocrine miliaria) 45
   differential diagnosis 45, 46, 106

FOXO3 and premature ovarian failure 731

fragmentation, placental 1051, 1084

friable ovarian tumor 828

frozen sections of ovarian tumors, intraoperative 831

FSH and the cyclical endometrium 443

fumarate reductase gene and leiomyoma 626

fungal infections 68-70
   differential diagnosis of various forms 29, 31, 32, 68,
      69

funisitis 1059

Gartner's duct cyst 235

gastric carcinoma see Krukenberg tumor

gastrointestinal cancer
   endometrial metastases 601
   ovarian metastases 876, 979-81

gastrointestinal epithelium, heterologous, Sertoli—Leydig
      cell tumor with 867-8, 966

gastrointestinal stromal tumor (GIST) 764, 768-70
   differential diagnosis 764, 770

genetics (and genetic factors)
   abortion (recurrent) 1004
   endometrial carcinoma 548-9
   endometrial intraepithelial neoplasia 495-6, 499
   of genital tract development 2, 6, 7-10
   ovarian tumors/cancer 801
      clear cell tumors 883-4
      endometrioid tumors 876-7
      mucinous tumors 876
      serous tumors 854-5
      transitional cell tumors 887-8
   uterine leiomyoma 626
   vulvodynia 60
   see also cytogenetic abnormalities; molecular genetics

genital ridge see gonadal ridge

genital tract
   development see development
   lower/external 6-9
      acquired childhood disorders 19, 19-20
      ambiguous genitalia 14, 19
      developmental anomalies 18-19, 19
      infections see infections

genomic instability
   leiomyoma 646
   leiomyosarcoma 632, 646

geographic necrosis in uterine smooth muscle tumors
   with classification difficulties 648
   leiomyosarcoma 636-7, 637

germ cell(s), development 3
germ cell tumors, ovarian 913-43
  children 14
  common 914-17
  malignant 918-36
    age and 823
    uni- vs bilateral 824
  mixed 937, 938-9
  rare 924-39
gestational age assessment 1005
gestational sac
  masquerading as cavitated villous 1028
  sonographic evaluation 998
gestational trophoblastic disease *see* trophoblastic disease
giant-cell carcinoma
  endometrial 599
  vulval 136
giant condylomata (Buschke—Löwenstein tumors)
  anal 218-19
  cervical 336
  vulva 134-5
gingival lesions in lichen planus 37
gitterinfarct 1056, 1076
glands (endocervical) *see* crypts
glands (endometrial)
  artifactual displacement 506
  cystic change in dysfunctional uterine bleeding 457, 460
  in endometrial cancer 571, 572
    endometrioid adenocarcinoma 553
    papillary serous carcinoma 562
  in endometrial precancer 502-3
  in endometrial stromal tumor, endometrioid 617, 658, 659
  inspissated material 484
  progesterone-related changes 475-6
glandular dysplasia
  endocervical 367-9
  endometrial 550-1
glandular hyperplasia, endocervical 393
glandular lesions/cells
  Bartholin's gland 106-7
  cervical, atypical 547-56, 558
    cytology 357-66, 574
    of undetermined significance 364-6
glandular neoplasia
  cervix 355-410
    categories 378
    identification of at-risk women 356-7
  vagina 256-8
  vulva 149-62
glandular yolk sac tumor 932-3
glassy cell adenosquamous carcinoma 382-3

Gleevec®, gastrointestinal stromal tumor therapy 770
glia, ectopic
  cervix 434
  endometrium 543
  peritoneal cavity (gliomatosis) 785, 937
goblet cell carcinoids, ovarian 868, 923
gonad(s), developmental and childhood acquired disorders 9-20
gonadal ridge (genital ridge) 2-3
  and transitional metaplasia 888
gonadotrophin, human chorionic, dysgerminoma and 928, 929-30
gonadotrophin-dependent precocious puberty 13-14, 16
gonadotrophin-releasing hormone, cyclical endometrium and 443
gonadotrophin-releasing hormone analogs, leiomyoma 625
gonorrhea *see Neisseria gonorrhoeae*
graafian follicle 718-19
grading
  anal intraepithelial neoplasia *see* intraepithelial neoplasia, anal
  anal squamous intraepithelial lesions *see* squamous intraepithelial lesions, anal
  cervical intraepithelial neoplasia 316
  cervical squamous carcinoma 334-9
  endometrial carcinoma 569-71, 580
    endometrioid carcinoma with squamous differentiation 556
    intraoperative 577, 577-8
    outcome and 589
  ovarian carcinomas 803-5, 841-2, 873
  uterine leiomyosarcoma, prognostic importance 638-9
granular cell tumor
  anal 209
  vulvovaginal 193-4
granulation tissue, vaginal, post-hysterectomy 232
granulocytes, endometrial stromal, in secretory phase 452
granulocytic sarcoma
  cervical 431-3
  ovarian 973-4, 990-1
granuloma(ta)
  keratin 585
  in syphilis 79
  vulval
    Crohn's disease 51
    other causes 51
granuloma inguinale 82-3
granulomatous endometritis 467
granulomatous salpingitis 694
granulomatous vulvitis 51

granulosa cell(s) (and granulosa cell layer) 718
  luteinization 721
  in pregnancy 725
granulosa cell tumors, ovarian 957-62
  clinical features 958
  cystic 720
  definition 957-8
  differential diagnosis 720, 875, 879, 883, 887-8,
      893, 934, 956-7, 959-60
  gross appearance 830, 958
  histology 958-9
  juvenile 823, 883, 934, 959
  management and outcome 960-2
  unclassified tumors similar to 968
granulosa-theca cell tumor 957-62
  gross appearance 830
group B streptococcus 238
Grover's disease vs acantholytic dermatosis of vulvocrural
    area 45
growth restriction, intrauterine see intrauterine growth
    restriction
gumma 79
guttate psoriasis 31
gynandroblastoma 966

H-caldesmon see caldesmon
Haemophilus ducreyi 81-2
Hailey—Hailey disease (benign familial pemphigus) 42-3
  differential diagnosis 42, 43, 45
hair, benign cystic teratoma 830-1, 915
HAIR-AN (hyperandrogenic—insulin-resistant—
    acanthosis nigricans) syndrome 733-4
hamartoma, myxoid 782-3
HE4 and ovarian tumors 801
heart, congenital absence in twin 1110
helminths 84-6
hemangiomas, placental see chorangioma
hemangiopericytoma 765-6
hematoma see hemorrhage
hematopoietic tumors 973-4, 989-91
  cervix 431-3
  fetal/congenital 1068, 1114
  ovary 973-4, 989-91
hemorrhage (and hematoma)
  decidual 1078-9
  intervillous 1066, 1076-7, 1084-5
  intravillous 1073, 1085
  peri-/postpartum 1114-15
  retroplacental 1052-3
  subchorionic 1050-1, 1066
  see also bleeding
hemorrhagic ovarian cysts, gross appearance 826
hemorrhoids 204-5

hepatoid yolk sac tumor 932, 934
heredity see familial syndromes; genetics
hermaphrodites 11-13
herpes simplex virus (HSV) infection 74-8
  cervical samples 294
  HIV patients 92
  placental villous 1100-1
herpes zoster (shingles) 92
  vulval intraepithelial neoplasia vs 119-20
herpesviruses
  endocervical glandular atypia associated with 373
  type-8 89
HHV-8 89
hidradenitis suppurativa 45-6, 206
hidradenoma, papillary (hidradenoma papilliferum)
    105-6, 208-9
  differential diagnosis 104, 106, 157, 209
  perianal 208-9
  vulvovaginal 105-6
hilus, ovarian
  in hysterectomy specimens, incidental findings 722
  structure 715
hilus cell 722
  hyperplasia 740-1
hilus cell tumor, gross appearance 830
histiocytes, endometrial, in cervical smear 574
histiocytoma, fibrous 186-7
histocompatibility antigens (HLA) and cervical
    neoplasia 273
histone acetyltransferase gene, cellular leiomyoma 645
HIV disease/AIDS
  anal carcinoma and 216, 217
  anal squamous intraepithelial lesions and 209, 210, 213
  cervical neoplasia and HPV in 273-4
  infection predisposition 87-94
  pregnancy and 1100
  seborrheic dermatitis in 32
  syphilis and 81
HLA and cervical neoplasia 273
HMB-45, uterine perivascular epithelioid cell tumor 660-1
HMGA1/HMGA2
  leiomyoma 626-7, 629
  lipoleiomyoma 630
hobnail metaplasia 538
Hodgkin's lymphoma, anorectal 223
hormonal (endocrine) factors/pathophysiology
  abortion (recurrent) 1004
  endometrial intraepithelial neoplasia 495, 499
  uterine leiomyoma 625
hormone replacement therapy (estrogen replacement
    ± progestogen) 477
  cervical neoplasia and 356
  extra-ovarian adenocarcinoma and 758, 813

hormone replacement therapy (estrogen replacement ± progestogen)—cont'd
  ovarian cancer risk 758, 813
  see also estrogen therapy
hormone therapy 472-7
  in atrophic vaginitis 232
  see also specific (types of) hormones and their analogs
hormone-producing ovarian tumors and precocious puberty 14
HPV (human papilloma virus) infection
  anal carcinoma and 216, 217, 220, 221
  anal squamous intraepithelial lesions and 209, 210, 211, 213
  in cervical cancer therapy and prevention, vaccines against 342-4
  cervical glandular neoplasia and 356
  cervical neuroendocrine carcinoma and 416
  cervical squamous neoplasia and 268-73
    and age of presentation 340
  classification of types 270
  endometrial squamous cell carcinoma and 598
  immunosuppressed patients 93-4
  respiratory papillomatosis and 118
  testing for/markers of 130, 276-7, 319-20
    with atypical glandular or endocervical cells 365-6
    cervical biopsies 317
    HIV-positive women 210
  vaginal intraepithelial lesions and 246
  vulval adenosquamous carcinoma and 150
  vulval carcinoma and 255
  vulval intraepithelial neoplasia and 118-19, 119
  vulval squamous cell carcinoma and
    early invasive 142
    growth patterns of 132, 133, 134
    invasion by 132
  vulvodynia and 60
  warts and 93-4, 112, 117
HSV *see* herpes simplex virus
human chorionic gonadotrophin (hCG) levels
  dysgerminoma 928, 929-30
  trophoblastic neoplasia 1016, 1018
    complete mole 1025
human herpes virus type-8 89
human immunodeficiency virus *see* HIV
human leucocyte antigens (HLA) and cervical neoplasia 273
human papilloma virus *see* HPV; warts
hyaline degeneration mimicking implantation site 482
hydatid of Morgagni 679-80
hydatidiform mole *see* mole
hydrocele of canal of Nuck 103
hydropic abortus *see* villi, edema
hydropic degeneration, leiomyoma 641

hydrops
  fetal 1104-5
  villous *see* villi
hydrosalpinx 691, 826
hymen, imperforate 18
hyperandrogenic—insulin-resistant—acanthosis nigricans syndrome 733-4
hyperandrogenism in polycystic ovarian syndrome 733, 734
hypercalcemic-type small cell ovarian carcinoma 970-1
  age and 823
hypercellularity
  leiomyoma 643, 644
  leiomyosarcoma 644
  malignant peripheral nerve sheath tumor 771
  parabasal, in low-grade squamous intraepithelial neoplasia 303
hyperchromatic clumped groups of cells 321
hyperinsulinemia in polycystic ovarian syndrome 733
hyperkeratosis, condyloma acuminatum 112, 115
hyperplasia
  adrenal, congenital 19
  Bartholin's gland, nodular 106-7
  endocervical glandular 393
  endometrial
    complex atypical 494
    pregnancy-related 1004
    WHO diagnostic criteria 495
  mesonephric 389, 397-8
  mesothelial 777
  microglandular 363, 395-7
  ovarian
    hilus cell hyperplasia 740-1
    stromal hyperplasia 739, 825, 879
  pseudoepithelial 136, 194, 213, 219
  theca-lutein, of pregnancy 724-7, 825
  trophoblastic, benign 1033
hyperreactio luteinalis 727-8
hyperthecosis, stromal 739-40
hypertrophic lichen planus 36
hypertrophic scar tissue vs desmoid fibrosis 773
hypertrophy, labial 20
hypogonadotropic hypogonadism, autoimmune 731
hypoplasia
  lower genital tract 19
  of Müllerian duct development 14
  ovarian 10
hypothalamic—pituitary axis
  in abnormal uterine bleeding, disorders of 457
  in menstrual cycle 444
hysterectomy
  benign vaginal lesions following 232-3
  cervical adenocarcinoma 399

hysterectomy—cont'd
  cervical adenosarcoma 422
  cervical squamous carcinoma 341, 342
    superficially invasive 333
  endometrial assessment 574
    carcinoma grading 577
  gravid 1114, 1115
  ovarian assessment 715-29
  ovarian cancer 906
    dysgerminoma 931
    endometrioid 909
    mucinous 910
  ovarian remnants 748-9
  placental site trophoblastic tumor 1036
  pregnancy following 1012
  tubes attached, specimen examination 678-89
  uterine smooth muscle tumors
    leiomyosarcoma 639
    of uncertain malignant potential 649
  vaginal carcinoma 254-5
hysteroscopy
  in abnormal uterine bleeding 458
    diagnostic 458
    therapeutic 458, 488
  endometrial cancer 552
  endometrial intraepithelial neoplasia 496-7, 498

iatrogenic trauma see trauma
ichthyosis uteri 525
ifosfamide + cisplatin, endometrial carcinosarcoma
    595-6
imaging, ovarian cancer screening 815-16
imatinib (Gleevec®), gastrointestinal stromal tumor
    therapy 770
imiquimod
  condyloma acuminatum 94
  vulval intraepithelial neoplasia 122
immune factors
  abortion (recurrent) 1004
  vulvodynia 60
immune hydrops 1104
immunoassays
  HSV 75, 76
  lymphogranuloma venereum 84
  syphilis 79, 80
immunobullous disorders see bullous disorders
immunosuppressed subjects
  anal squamous intraepithelial lesions 210
  cervical neoplasia risk 273-4
  vulvar infections 87-94
  see also HIV disease
implantation, endometrial receptivity to, biomarkers in
    assessment of 455-6

implantation site, placental
  in ectopic pregnancy diagnosis/exclusion
      (in curettings) 1009-10, 1011
    mimics 482, 1011
  exaggerated reaction 1003
  old 482, 996-8, 1003
    nodule 435, 482, 1010
  recent 482
  squamous intraepithelial neoplasia vs 308-9
  trophoblastic disease/tumors (PSTT) 435, 1010-11,
      1031, 1033-6, 1113
    biomarkers 1035
    clinico-radiologic features 1016, 1033
    diagnosis/exclusions 1017, 1031, 1035
    gross pathologic presentation 1016
    histology 1017, 1031, 1033-5
    management and outcome 1018, 1035-6
    metastases 258, 1033
    molecular studies 1035
    risk factors 1033
implantation site trophoblast 1019, 1020
implanted tissue see ectopia
inclusion cysts, epidermal/epithelial
  ovarian cortical (CICs) 716-18, 737
    as cancer precursor 795, 796-7, 799-800
  vagina 235
  vulva 102
induced delivery 1093-106
  premature 1088-93
infarction
  appendix epiploica 783
  ovarian 825
  placental 1055
    maternal floor 1056, 1078
    in pre-eclampsia 1096
infections
  abortion as cause of 1015-16
  abortion due to
    late 1084
    recurrent 1004
  amniotic fluid see chorioamnionitis
  anal 207-8
  cervical samples (other than HPV) 294
  fungal see fungal infections
  lower genital tract 65-97, 238-41
    immunosuppressed persons 87-94
    vulvodynia associated with 59-60
  ovarian 742-3
  placental villous 1070, 1099-100
  Reiter's syndrome-predisposing 47
  sexually-transmitted see sexually-transmitted
      diseases
  tubal 689-94

infections—cont'd
  umbilical cord 1059
  uterine/endometrial
    causing endometritis 466, 467
    IUD-related risk 470-2
  villous 1099-101
  see also microbiology *and specific pathogens and*
    diseases
infertility *see* fertility problems
infiltration *see* invasion
inflammation, vulvodynia with 60
  see also reactive change *and specific inflammatory*
    disorders
inflammatory bowel disease, anal involvement 206-7
inflammatory cells
  amnion 1061
  chorion 1062-5
  granulomatous endometritis 468
inflammatory cloacogenic polyps 205-6
inflammatory disorders/dermatoses
  vaginal, of unknown etiology 240-1
  vulval 23-56
    carcinoma risk 29, 35, 42, 46, 110
inflammatory myofibroblastic tumor 767-8
  calcifying fibrous tumor and 767, 768
  differential diagnosis 768, 783
infliximab, Crohn's disease 52
infundibulum of fallopian tube 676
inheritance *see* familial syndromes; genetics
injection studies, twin placenta 1058
injury *see* trauma
INK4 *see* p16
insular carcinoids 922
  granulosa cell tumor vs 960
insulin resistance and polycystic ovarian syndrome 733
intercalated cells of fallopian tube 676
interferon therapy
  melanoma 174
  viral warts 94
International Federation of Gynaecology and Obstetrics
    see FIGO
intersex 11-13
intervillositis, chronic 1005, 1076-7
intervillous space 1074-7
  fibrin 1033, 1075-6
  maternal blood in 1066, 1076-7, 1084-5
  thrombi 1055, 1075
intestinal cancer, ovarian metastases 820, 824, 876,
    979-81
  see also colon cancer; small bowel carcinoma
intestinal differentiation, yolk sac tumor 932-3
intestinal metaplasia of endometrium 456-7
intestinal-type cervical adenocarcinoma 381

intestinal-type cervical adenocarcinoma in situ 367
  pregnancy-related changes vs 371
intestinal-type ovarian borderline mucinous tumor
    857-9, 861
intraepithelial carcinoma
  endometrial 494, 550, 563
  ovarian intestinal-type mucinous borderline tumors
    with 859
  tubal 703
intraepithelial glandular neoplasia, cervical (CIGN)
    367, 368
intraepithelial lesions
  anal, squamous *see* squamous intraepithelial lesions,
    cervical
  cervical *see* squamous intraepithelial lesions
  vaginal 246-53
    histology 247-50
    management 251-3
    patient examination 247
    post-radiation high-grade 253
  vulval (other than VIN) 126-8
    squamous (SIL) 129
intraepithelial neoplasia
  anal (AIN)
    grade 1 (AIN1) 210-11
    grade 2/3 (AIN2/3) 210-14
  cervical *see* squamous intraepithelial lesions, cervical
  endometrial 493-518
    biomarkers 499
    cancer risk 498, 549-51
    definition 494
    diagnostic criteria 501-5
    differential diagnosis 494, 526
    historical background 494, 504-7
    interpretive problems in diagnosis 508-13
    management/treatment 501, 515-16
    non-endometrioid 511
    pathology 498-504
    preoperative diagnosis of, significance 576-7
    risk factors 495-6
  tubal 677
  vaginal (VAIN) 246-53
    natural history 246-7
  vulval (VIN) 118-26, 129-30
    classic 118-21, 129
    differentiated (simplex) 122-6, 130, 144
    pagetoid *see* pagetoid vulval intraepithelial neoplasia
    squamous cell carcinoma coexisting with 142
intrauterine contraceptive device 468-72
  ectopic pregnancy risk 1007
  pelvic inflammatory disease risk 690
intrauterine growth restriction 1097-104
  one twin in twin-twin transfusion syndrome 1111

intravenous leiomyomatosis 651
intravillous hemorrhage 1073, 1085
invasion and microinvasion (local spread)
  anal carcinoma, anatomy relating to 203
  cervical carcinoma 321-33
    clinical detection 321
    diagnosis/assessment 323-33
    percent of high-grade squamous intraepithelial
      neoplasia associated with 321
    reporting 339
    risk following high-grade squamous intraepithelial
      neoplasia treatment 321
  endometrial carcinoma 584-7
    intraoperative assessment 577
    postoperative assessment 570-1
  endometrial carcinosarcoma 595
  hydatidiform mole *see* mole, invasive
  ovarian borderline tumors
    endometrioid 870-1
    mucinous intestinal-type 859
    serous 846-7, 908
  ovarian immature teratoma 937
  uterine smooth muscle tumors 647-8
  vulval tumors
    melanoma, depth of invasion and microinvasion
      173
    in Paget's disease diagnosis, exclusion 152-3
    squamous cell carcinoma, diagnostic criteria 130-2
  see also specific tissues
inverse psoriasis 30
irradiation *see* radiation
irritant contact dermatitis 25-6
ischemia, villous 1096
isthmus of fallopian tube 676

JAZF1—JJAZ1 fusion and endometrial stromal tumors
  619, 765
junctional nevus 165-6

Kaposi's sarcoma, differential diagnosis 89
karyotypic abnormalities *see* cytogenetic abnormalities
keratin, peritoneal mesenchymal tumors 764
keratin granuloma 585
keratinizing lesions
  cervix 321
    high-grade squamous intraepithelial neoplasia 306
  vulval squamous carcinoma 132, 134
keratoacanthoma 136-8
keratosis, seborrheic, vulval condylomata resembling
  113, 119-20
Ki-67 (and detection with MIB-1) 3, 8
  anal squamous intraepithelial lesions 213-14
  cervical dysplasia 368

Ki-67 (and detection with MIB-1)—cont'd
  cervical squamous lesions 312
  non-HPV vs HPV related lesions 116
  ovarian development 3, 8
  uterine smooth muscle tumors 650
    leiomyoma 646
    leiomyosarcoma 639
  vaginal intraepithelial lesions 249-50
  vulval intraepithelial neoplasia 120
kidney, ovarian metastases from 883, 985-6
c-kit and gastrointestinal stromal tumor 769-70
knotted cord 1047
koilocytes and koilocytosis 112
  carcinoma and 321
  squamous intraepithelial neoplasia and
    high-grade 306, 321
    low-grade 288
Krukenberg tumor (incl. gastric carcinoma) 979
  clear cell carcinoma vs 883
  Sertoli—Leydig cell tumors vs 964

labium majus enlargement 20
labium minus hypertrophy 20
lamina propria, tubal 676
laminar endocervical glandular hyperplasia, diffuse
  393
large bowel cancer *see* colon cancer
large cell neuroendocrine carcinoma 412, 414,
  415-16
large cell patterns in uterine/endometrial carcinomas
  papillary serous carcinoma 562
  undifferentiated carcinoma 599
Laugier—Hunziger disease 164
leiomyoblastoma 628-9
leiomyoma (fibroids)
  broad ligament 697
  cervical 427-8
  ovarian 829
    thecoma vs 957
  peritoneal 762-4
    differential diagnosis 764, 773-4
  uterine 464, 623-31, 639-48
    clinical considerations 624-5
    epidemiology 612
    leiomyosarcoma compared with 633, 634
    management 624-5, 642-3
    pathobiology 625-9
    submucosal 472
    variant forms 639-48
  vulvovaginal 189, 190
leiomyomatosis 652-4
  disseminated peritoneal 652-3
  intrauterine 654

leiomyomatosis—cont'd
  intravenous 651
  vulvovaginal 190
leiomyosarcoma 631-9
  cervical 428
  peritoneal 762-4
    differential diagnosis 764, 770, 773-4
  uterine 631-9
    clinical considerations 630-1
    diagnostic strategy 637
    management 639
    myxoid 638, 641
    pathobiology/histology 631-8, 644
    prognosis 638-9
length see size
lentiginosis 165
leukemia
  acute myelogenous, gynecological lesions see
      granulocytic sarcoma
  fetal/congenital 1068, 1114
  ovarian 973-4, 990-1
levonorgestrel-coated IUD 469-70
Leydig cell 946
Leydig cell tumor 969
  see also Sertoli—Leydig cell tumors
LH see luteinizing hormone
Lhx9 6
lice, pubic 66-7
lichen planus 36-8
  differential diagnosis 37-8, 40
lichen sclerosus (et atrophicus) 32-6
  differential diagnosis 34-5, 124, 125-6
  melanocytic lesions coexisting with 170
lichen sclerosus with acanthosis 127
lichen simplex chronicus 28-9
  differential diagnosis 29, 31, 124, 125-6
  superimposed on dermatitis 25, 27
  verruciform 128
ligation, tubal see sterilization
ligneous cervicitis 434
lipoleiomyoma 630
  adenomatoid tumor vs 696
lipoma
  broad ligament 697
  vulvosarcoma 188-9
  vulvovaginal 188
liposarcoma 774-5
  intra-abdominal 774-5
  vulva 188-9
liquid-based cervical cytology 279
  glandular abnormalities 365
lobular carcinoma of breast, ovarian metastases 984
lobular endocervical glandular hyperplasia 393

lobular mesonephric hyperplasia 397
loop electroexcision procedure (LEEP)
    cervical, specimen interpretation 317-18
    vaginal intraepithelial neoplasia 253
louse, pubic 66-7
Lugol's solution, vagina 247
lung cancer see pulmonary carcinoma
luteal phase see secretory phase
luteinization, granulosa cell layer 721
luteinized granulosa cell tumors 958, 960
luteinized thecoma 956
luteinizing hormone (LH)
    cyclical endometrium and 443
    in polycystic ovarian syndrome 733
luteoma
    pregnancy 725-7
    stromal 968-9
lymph node metastases
    anal carcinoma 203
    cervical squamous carcinoma, reporting
        presence/absence 339
    endometrial adenocarcinoma 586-7
    ovarian serous borderline tumors 848
    vulvar melanoma, sentinel node evaluation 173-4
    vulvar squamous carcinoma (early invasive) 140, 142
        sentinel node evaluation 142-3
lymphangioma, cervical 434
lymphangioma circumscriptum 193
    differential diagnosis 106, 193
lymphatic space invasion
    cervical cancer 329-30, 332-3
    endometrial adenocarcinoma 587
    endometrial carcinosarcoma 595
lymphocytic endometritis 468
lymphoepithelial-like carcinoma of cervix 334
lymphogranuloma venereum 84
    differential diagnosis 46
lymphohistiocytic malignant mesothelioma 781-2
lymphoma 973, 989-90
    anorectal 223
    cervical 431
    endometrial 468
    ovarian 989-90
        gross appearance 830
    peritoneal 783
    tubal 707
lymphovascular malformations 19-20
Lynch syndrome II see colon cancer, hereditary non-polyposis

macrocystic yolk sac tumor 931
macrophages
    amniotic 1061
    chorionic 1062

macule, genital melanotic 164-5
magnetic resonance guided focused ultrasound
     treatment, leiomyoma 642
malakoplakia
  cervical 434-5
  vaginal 239-40
male partner and HPV infection and cervical neoplasia
     274-5
male pseudohermaphroditism 11, 13
malformations *see* developmental anomalies
malignant tumors (cancers)
  anal/anal canal 216-24
     anatomy relating to spread of 203
  cervical 320-44, 373-402, 421-7, 428, 429-30, 431,
        431-3
     diagnosis and management 320-44
     expectations from cytology in prevention of 278-9
     HPV variants and risk of 272-3
     ovarian metastases 979
     relationship with cervical intraepithelial neoplasia I
        and 316
  endometrial 546-97, 598-602
     ovarian metastases 854, 874-5
     squamous metaplasia vs 528-9
     vaginal metastases 258
  fallopian tube *see* tube
  lesions with risk of development *see* premalignant
        lesions
  myometrial 631-9
  ovarian *see* ovarian cancer
  peritoneal, primary 910
  spread of *see* invasion; metastases
  vaginal 253-61
     natural history 246-7
  villous area 1073
  vulval 130-43, 149-62, 168-75, 188-9
     benign rests vs 103, 104-5
  vulvovaginal, children 19
  see also borderline tumors *and specific histological types*
mammary-type vulval carcinoma vs benign rests 104-5
maternal blood, intervillous space 1066, 1076-7, 1084-5
maternal disorders, operative or induced delivery for
     1093-106
maternal surface (basal surface) of placenta
  gross appearance 1051-3
  infarcts 1056, 1078
  microscopic appearance 1077-80
maternal tissues in spontaneous abortion 1003-4
meconium staining, placenta in 1106
  gross appearance incl. color 1045
  microscopic findings 1060-1, 1061-2, 1065-6
medication risk factors for endometrial intraepithelial
     neoplasia 496

medulla, ovarian, structure 715
megestrol 476
melanocytic lesions
  cervix 430-1
  vulva 163-78
melanoma
  anorectal 223
  cervical 431
  ovarian metastatic 825, 987-8
     theca-lutein hyperplasia of pregnancy vs 727
  placental metastatic 1114
  vaginal 258-60
  vulval 168-75
     age and diagnosis of 166, 168
     clinical features 168-9
     differential diagnosis 152, 166, 170-1, 188
     histologic features 169-70
     laboratory management/staging/prognosis 171-4
     risk factors 168
melanosis, genital 164-5
melanotic schwannoma 771
membranes, placental
  gross appearance 1048
  microscopic appearance 1059-61
membranous dysmenorrhea 445
men *see* male
menopausal status *see* older and elderly women
menopausal status and endometrial carcinoma risk 551
menorrhagia 457
  unexplained 458
menstrual cycle 442-52
  endometrium in *see* endometrium
  prototypical 443
  schematic events 444
menstrual phase, endometrium in 445
  adenocarcinoma in situ mistaken for 361, 362-3
  variations 445
mental retardation, childhood, placental abnormalities
     associated with 1042
Merkel cell carcinoma, vulval 158-9
mesenchymal differentiation patterns, carcinosarcoma
     591
mesenchymal—epithelial tumors of cervix, mixed *see*
     mixed tumors
mesenchymal metaplasia
  endocervical 434
  endometrial 543
mesenchymal (soft tissue) tumors
  anal 233-4
  cervical 425-30
  ovarian sex cord-stromal tumors (pure mesenchymal)
     949-57
     differential diagnosis 949

mesenchymal (soft tissue) tumors—cont'd
  peritoneal 762-76
  uterine 611-72
    at-risk patient identification 612
    clinical features 612-13
    definitions 612
  vulvovaginal 179-97
mesenteritis, sclerosing 783
mesodermally-derived tumors *see* mesenchymal tumors
mesonephric carcinoma/adenocarcinoma, cervical 389-90
  spindle cell component 424
mesonephric cysts 235-6
mesonephric duct (Wolffian duct) tumors *see* Wolffian
  duct tumors
mesonephric hyperplasia 389, 397-8
mesonephric tumors vs Sertoli—Leydig cell tumors 964-5
mesothelial cysts, tubal 681-3
mesothelial lesions/proliferations
  ovarian surface 716
  peritoneal cavity 777-82
mesothelin and ovarian tumors 801
mesothelioma 779-80, 780-2, 966
  cystic *see* cystic mesothelioma
  fibrous 765-6
  malignant 780-2
    clinical features 780
    differential diagnosis 754, 766, 777, 778, 781-2,
      854, 966
    epidemiology 780
    ovarian metastatic 989
    ovarian primary 854
    pathology 780-2
    transformation of papillary mesothelioma into 779
  papillary 779-80, 966
mesothelium 795
  and ovarian carcinogenesis 795-8
metabolic syndrome and polycystic ovarian syndrome
  734
metaplasia
  cervical/endocervical
    atypical immature squamous metaplasia 283, 308
    mesenchyme 434
    papillary immature metaplasia (=immature
      condyloma) 296-7, 300-2, 338
  endometrial 519-44
    adenocarcinoma and adenocarcinoma in situ vs
      361, 369-70, 399
    assessment algorithm 539-42
    classification and outcome 525
    intraepithelial neoplasia vs 511, 526
    non-epithelial 543
    repair and 529-31
    risk factors 525

metaplasia—cont'd
  in endometrioma 746
  fallopian tube 678-9, 687-8
  morular *see* squamous morules
  Müllerian 795
  ovarian 795-6
    smooth muscle metaplasia 729
  vestibular glands 61
metaplastic phenotype, immature squamous cells with
  321
metastases (distant sites) 977-93
  from anal melanoma 223
  from cervix 399
  to cervix 391, 425, 601
  from endometrium 258, 854, 874-5, 978
  to endometrium 585, 593, 601-2
  from fallopian tubes 258, 978
  to fallopian tubes 705-7
  from fetus 1068
  in gestational trophoblastic (disease, in staging 1026
  to intervillous space 1076
  from ovaries
    carcinoma 258, 585
    carcinosarcoma 425
    dysgerminoma 930
    Sertoli—Leydig cell tumors 966
  to ovaries 824-5, 825, 828, 830, 867, 977-93
    carcinoids 924, 980-1
    endometrial carcinoma 854, 874-5, 978
    intestinal tumors 820, 824, 876, 979-81
    mucinous carcinoma 867, 978
    renal cell carcinoma 883, 985-6
    squamous carcinoma 890
    theca-lutein hyperplasia of pregnancy vs 727
    uni- vs bilateral 824
    urothelial carcinoma 888, 986-7
    uterine stromal sarcoma 879, 978-9
  from peritoneal liposarcoma 775
  to peritoneal cavity 780, 783
  to placenta 1114
  of placental site trophoblastic tumor 258, 1033
  of smooth muscle tumors
    from uterine benign metastasizing leiomyoma
      654-5
    from vulvovaginal sites 190
  from uterus 425, 978
  to vagina 258
  from vulva 160-1
metastases (regional lymph nodes) *see* lymph node
  metastases
metatypical basal cell carcinoma 144
MIB-1 *see* Ki-67
Michaelis—Gutmann bodies 412

microbiology (incl. bacteriology; virology), placental samples 1043-4
  amnion 1061
  chorion 1066
  stem villi 1068
microcystic papillary serous carcinoma of uterus 562-3
microcystic yolk sac tumor 931
microglandular change of cervical origin in endometrial curetting 534
microglandular hyperplasia, cervical 363, 395-7
microinvasion *see* invasion and microinvasion
micropapillary architecture
  endometrial adenocarcinoma 573
  ovarian serous borderline tumor 847-8, 908
micropapillary ovarian carcinoma (=low-grade serous carcinoma) 800-1, 803
micropapillomatosis, ovarian 716
microsatellite instability and endometrial cancer/precancer 499
miliaria, apocrine *see* Fox—Fordyce disease
milk-line nevus 165-6
minimal deviation adenocarcinoma (adenoma malignum) 378-80, 391, 420
  endometrioid type 381
  sex cord tumors and 967
miscarriage *see* abortion
mismatch (DNA) repair genes
  endometrial cancer 548, 549
  endometrioid ovarian carcinoma and 877
mitoses
  cervical adenocarcinoma in situ 367
    compared with other lesions 370
  uterine leiomyoma 645-6
  uterine leiomyosarcoma 634-5, 638-9
mixed tumors
  cervical epithelial—mesenchymal 419-25
  malignant Müllerian *see* carcinosarcoma
  ovarian 890-3
    borderline *see* borderline tumors
    differential diagnosis 892-3
    epithelial—mesenchymal mixed tumors, differential diagnosis 950
    general and clinical aspects 890-1
    germ cell tumors 937, 938-9
    gross examination 891-2
    microscopic examination 892
  uterine epithelial—mesenchymal 612, 657-60
  vaginal 261-2
MLH1
  endometrial cancer 549
  endometrial intraepithelial neoplasia and 499
  endometrioid ovarian carcinoma and 877

mole, hydatidiform (molar pregnancy) 996, 1021-8
  choriocarcinoma vs 1033
  complete 1015, 1021-6
    classic (late) 1021
    clinico-radiologic features 1016
    differential diagnosis and biomarkers 1022-3, 1026
    early 1021-2
    gross pathologic presentation 1016
    histologic classification/diagnosis/exclusions 1017
    management and outcome 1018, 1025-6
    trophoblast types in 1017, 1018, 1021
  ectopic pregnancy vs 1011
  invasive 1023-5
    clinico-radiologic features 1016
    gross pathologic presentation 1016
    management and outcome 1018
  molecular pathogenesis 1016-17
  partial 1026-8
    classification/diagnosis/exclusions 1017
    clinico-radiologic features 1016, 1026
    differential diagnosis 1026
    gross pathologic presentation 1016
    histology 1017, 1026
    management and outcome 1018, 1028
    molecular studies 1026
    trophoblast types in 1018-19, 1026
  recurrence risk 1016
molecular genetics and molecular profiling
  endometrial adenocarcinoma 588
  endometrial carcinoma 549
  endometrial intraepithelial neoplasia 499
  endometrial stromal tumors 618-20, 765
  gestational trophoblastic disease
    partial mole 1026
    placental site trophoblastic disease 1035
  ovarian cancer 795, 802-3, 805
  uterine leiomyoma 626-7
  uterine leiomyosarcoma, prognostic value 639
  see also cytogenetic abnormalities; genetics
molecular risk factors for cervical neoplasia 276-8
molluscum contagiosum 73-4
  disseminated 94
monochorionic placenta 1056, 1057-8, 1109
MORF, cellular leiomyoma 645
Morgagni's hydatid 679-80
morphology, placental 1044-5
morules, squamous *see* squamous morules
MSH2/MSH6 and endometrial cancer 549
mucinous carcinoid (goblet cell carcinoid), ovarian 868, 923
mucinous carcinoma/adenocarcinoma
  endocervical *see* endocervical-type adenocarcinoma
  endometrioid adenocarcinoma 556
  ovarian 803

mucinous carcinoma/adenocarcinoma—cont'd
    differential diagnosis 867-8, 875, 888
    etiology/genetics/biomarkers 868
    general and clinical aspects 855
    metastatic 867, 978
    microscopic examination 861-5
    pathology-based management 910
mucinous cystadenoma, ovarian, gross appearance 827
mucinous differentiation, endometrioid
    adenocarcinoma 556-8
    metastatic, ovarian mucinous carcinoma vs 867
mucinous intraepithelial lesions of cervix, stratified
    (SMILEs) 306
mucinous metaplasia
    endometrial 524, 525, 531-5, 541-2
    tubal 687-8
mucinous tumors
    appendiceal 866, 981
    ovarian
        borderline *see* borderline tumors
        carcinoids arising in association with 924
        differential diagnosis 867-8, 875, 888
        etiology/genetics/biomarkers 868
        general and clinical aspects 855
        gross examination 855-7
        microscopic examination 857-65
        misclassification 835, 836
        uni- vs bilateral 824
    see also seromucinous tumors
mucosa, tubal 676
mucosal disorders, vulval 24-46
    fibroepithelial polyps *see* fibroepithelial mucosal polyps
mucosal excrescences of vagina, filiform 302-3
mucous cysts
    vaginal 235
    vulvar 101-2
Müllerian adenosarcoma *see* adenosarcoma
Müllerian cysts
    ovarian 718
    paratubal 679-80
    vaginal 235
Müllerian-derived peritoneal lesions 754-62
Müllerian duct (paramesonephric duct)
    development 3, 6, 200
        disorders 14
    fallopian tube formed from 676
Müllerian epithelium 795
Müllerian metaplasia 795
Müllerian papilloma
    cervical 394-5
    vaginal 258
Müllerian seromucinous tumor 826
Müllerian sites, tubal metastases from 644

Müllerian tumors
    endocervical-like mucinous ovarian *see* endocervical-
        type mucinous/Müllerian tumors
    mixed 893
        malignant *see* carcinosarcoma
    peritoneal 759-62
multilocular cyst 683
multiple (incl. twin) pregnancy 1056-9, 1109-12
    with complete mole and normal gestation 1027-8
    fetus papyraceus 1050, 1057
    placenta in 1056-9, 1109-12
mural nodules, mucinous ovarian tumors with 864-5
muscle tumors
    cervical 427-8
    vulvovaginal 189-92
muscularis, tubal 676
Mycobacterium tuberculosis and *M. bovis* infection *see*
    tuberculosis
myelogenous leukemia, acute (granulocytic sarcoma),
    ovarian 973-4
myelogenous leukemia, acute, gynecological lesions *see*
    granulocytic sarcoma
myofibroblastic tumor, inflammatory *see* inflammatory
    myofibroblastic tumor
myomectomy 624
myometrium
    tumors invading
        endometrial carcinoma 580-1
        endometrial carcinosarcoma 595
    tumors of 623-57
        definition and classification 623-4
myxohyaline leiomyoma, vulvovaginal 190
myxoid hamartoma 782-3
myxoid leiomyosarcoma 638, 641
myxomatous yolk sac tumor 932

nabothian cysts 391
necrosis (tumor cell)
    ovarian tumor, types 828
    uterine smooth muscle tumors
        leiomyoma 640, 641
        leiomyosarcoma 636-7, 637
        problematic tumors 648
necrotizing fasciitis, vulval 90-2
Neisseria gonorrhoeae 78
    pelvic inflammatory disease 690
neoplasms *see* malignant tumors; tumors *and specific*
    types of benign and malignant tumors'
nerve sheath tumors, peripheral 770-3, 770-3
    cervical 428-9
    malignant (MPSNT) 771-2
        clinical features 771
        differential diagnosis 764, 772

nerve sheath tumors, peripheral—cont'd
  epidemiology 770
    treatment and prognosis 772-3
  peritoneal 770-3
  vulvovaginal 193
neural pathways in vulvodynia 60
  treatment aimed at 62
neural tumors
  cervical 428-9
  vulvovaginal 193-4
  see also nerve sheath tumor; neuroectodermal tumor
neuroblastoma 776
  adrenal, ovarian metastases 989
  fetal 1068
neuroectodermal tumor
  ovarian 876
  peripheral/primitive *see* Ewing's sarcoma
neuroendocrine carcinoma
  Bartholin's gland 157
  cervical 412-18
    classification 412-14
    definition 412
    diagnosis 412-14
    differential diagnosis 414-16
    management and outcome 417-18
  ovarian
    non-small cell type 893
    small cell type 972-3
neurofibroma, vulvovaginal 193
neurofibromatosis, vulvovaginal 193
neurologic disease, childhood, placental abnormalities
    associated with 1042
neutrophils
  amniotic 1061
  amniotic-chorionic cleft 1061
  chorionic 1062-5, 1066
nevus
  dysplastic *see* dysplastic nevus
  flexural-type/genital-type/milk-line 165-6
Nitabuch's fibrin 1077, 1078
nodular fasciitis 768, 774
nodular hyperplasia, Bartholin's gland 106-7
nodular theca-lutein hyperplasia of pregnancy
    (NTLHP) 725, 727
nodule(s)
  amniotic 1049-50, 1108
  chorionic surface 1049-51
  endometrial stromal 613-14, 621
  mural, mucinous ovarian tumors with 864-5
  placental site 435, 482, 1010
non-Hodgkin's lymphoma *see* lymphoma
Norwegian scabies 94
Nuck's canal, hydrocele 103

nucleus
  atypia *see* atypia
  grade, endometrial adenocarcinoma 588
nulliparity and risk of gestational trophoblastic disease 1016
nummular dermatitis 26-7

obesity
  endometrial intraepithelial neoplasia and 496
  ovarian cancer and 813
Oct-3/4 3-4, 8
older and elderly (perimenopausal/postmenopausal/
    over-50s) women
  abnormal uterine bleeding in, causes 442, 458
    endometrial carcinoma 551-2
  cervical squamous atypia 303
  endometrial cancer risk 546-7, 551
  endometrium of 480-1
  melanoma 166, 168
  ovarian benign conditions 737-41
  vaginal epithelial changes 230-2
  see also age
omental involvement, ovarian cancer 824
omentum, endosalpingiosis 849
oncogenesis *see* carcinogenesis
oocyte development 3
oogonia 3
oophorectomy (or salpingo-oophorectomy)
  in familial breast/ovarian cancer, prophylactic 814
    specimens 698-701, 843-4
  ovarian tumors
    dysgerminoma 931
    endometrioid tumors 909
    mucinous tumors 910
    serous tumors 908
    yolk sac tumor 934
oophoritis 692, 742
oral contraceptives 473-5
  cervical premalignancy/malignancy risk and 275, 356
  endometrial pathology risk and 473-5
  ovarian cancer risk reduction with 813-14
oral lesions in lichen planus 37
ovarian cancer 793-819
  children 14
  differential diagnosis 853-4, 867-8, 874-6, 878-9,
    882-3, 888
  endometrial carcinoma co-existing with 585
  endometriosis-associated 743, 757-8, 795, 876-7,
    890, 909
  etiology/genetics/biomarkers 854-5, 868, 876-7,
    888-9
  familial *see* familial syndromes
  general and clinical aspects 842, 855, 869, 877-8,
    879, 880, 884

ovarian cancer—cont'd
  germ cell origin *see* germ cell tumors
  gross examination 843, 855-7, 869, 878, 880, 994-5
    in differentiation of primary from secondary 978
  management based on pathology 905-12
  metastases from *see* metastases
  metastatic *see* metastases (to distant sites)
  microscopic findings 851-3, 861-5, 871-4, 878, 881,
    886-8
  pathogenesis/carcinogenesis 793-810
    divergent pathways 805
    integrated pathways 806
  presenting signs/symptoms 816
  risk-increasing factors 812-13
  risk-reducing factors 813-14
  screening 814-16
ovarian cycle 444
ovarian failure *see* anovulation
ovarian hormones in menstrual cycle 444
ovarian remnant syndrome 748-9
ovarian tumors 793-993
  clinical history 822-4
  epithelial—stromal *see* epithelial tumors
  germ cell *see* germ cell tumors
  gross evaluation in differentiation of primary from
    secondary 978
  intraoperative evaluation 815-16
    benign cystic teratoma 915-16
    diagnostic pitfalls 834-6
    frozen sections 831
    gross examination 825-31
  malignant *see* ovarian cancer
  pediatric 14, 16
    hormone-producing, and precocious puberty 14
  peritoneal implants of teratoma 785
  relative frequencies 822
  sex cord *see* sex cord (stromal) tumor
  synchronous and metachronous, with endometrial
    cancer 548-9
ovaries 713-52, 793-993
  adhesions, connecting with tubes 685
  anatomy 714-15
  benign conditions 713-52
    causing enlargement 743-8, 825
  childhood acquired disorders 13-14, 16
  development 2, 3-6
    disorders 9-13
  ectopic pregnancy 1012
  hysterectomy specimens, incidental findings 715-29
  infections 742-3
  infertility-related conditions 730-7
  peri-/postmenopausal women 737-41
  in pregnancy 722-9

ovaries—cont'd
  salpingitis involving 692
  tumors *see* ovarian cancer; ovarian tumors
ovulation
  anovulation followed by 477-8
  in cancer causation 796-7
  defined as day 14 of cycle 448
  failure *see* anovulation
  induction 455
oxyphilic clear cell carcinoma 881
oxyphilic endometrioid carcinoma 876
oxyphilic metaplasia (eosinophilic metaplasia) 538

p16 (INK4)
  cervical glandular atypia 368
  cervical squamous lesions 312-13
  vulval intraepithelial neoplasia 119-20, 126
p53
  anal squamous carcinoma and 220
  anal squamous intraepithelial lesions and 214
  endometrial carcinoma and 549
    mixed serous—endometrioid form 563-5
  endometrial intraepithelial neoplasia and 499
  homologue p63 *see* p63
  ovarian cancer and 854
    breast cancer and 802
  tubal specimens of prophylactic salpingo-oophorectomy
    701
  uterine leiomyosarcoma and 639
  uterine papillary serous carcinoma 485
  vulval intraepithelial neoplasia (differentiated form) 126
p63 (p53 homologue)
  cervical metaplasia and 522
  cervical squamous vs neuroendocrine carcinoma and
    415
  in cervical and uterine development 520, 521
  cloacal anomalies and null mutants of 201
  ovarian development and 4
  trophoblastic expression
    normal 1020
    in placental site trophoblastic tumor 1035
pagetoid vulval intraepithelial neoplasia 119
  melanoma vs 171
  Paget's disease vs 152, 171
Paget's disease (extramammary)
  anal/perianal 213, 222-3
  vulval 150-4
    melanoma vs 152, 171
pancreatic carcinoma, ovarian metastases 867, 981-2
Pap smears *see* cervix, smears
papillary adenofibroma 834, 844-5, 853
papillary clear cell carcinoma of ovary 854
papillary hidradenoma *see* hidradenoma

papillary immature metaplasia, cervix (=immature condyloma) 296-7, 300-2, 338
papillary lesions
　cervical, exceeding morphologic limits of immature condyloma 304-5
　endometrial 538, 571, 573
　　poorly-differentiated tumors 598
　　squamous metaplasia vs 542
papillary mesothelioma 779-80, 966
papillary serous carcinoma
　cervical metastases 391
　ovarian, pathogenesis 799
　peritoneal 760, 762
　　biomarkers 762, 766
　　pathology 760
　　treatment and prognosis 762
　uterine 484-5, 514, 547, 560-8
　　histopathology 560-8
　　precursor lesions 550
papillary serous tumors, peritoneal 759-62
papillary squamo-transitional carcinoma, cervical 336
papillary squamous cell carcinoma
　cervical 332-3
　vulval 135-6
papillary squamous neoplasms, cervical 336
papillary syncytial metaplasia 530, 538
papillary thyroid carcinoma in struma ovari 919, 920
papillary yolk sac tumor 932
papilloma
　fibroepithelial 112
　Müllerian see Müllerian papilloma
　squamous, cervical (=immature condyloma) 296-7, 300-2, 338
　tubal 687
　see also micropapillomatosis
papillomatosis, respiratory 118
papulosis
　bowenoid 119, 211
　pseudobowenoid 114, 119
para-aortic node metastases, endometrial adenocarcinoma 586
parabasal hypercellularity in low-grade squamous intraepithelial neoplasia 303
parakeratotic cells, atypical (in cervical samples) 282-3
paramesonephric duct see Müllerian duct
parametrial spread of endometrial adenocarcinoma 586
parasites 72-3, 84-6
　external 66-8
parity and risk of gestational trophoblastic disease 1016
parvovirus B19 1105
PEComa 660-1
pectinate line 201
pediatrics see children

pediculosis pubis 66-7
pelvic examination, ovarian cancer screening 814-15
pelvic inflammatory disease 689-94
pelvic mass, suspected, ultrasound evaluation 816-17
pelvic node metastases, endometrial adenocarcinoma 586-7
pemphigoid 39-41
　bullous 39-41, 42, 43, 240
　cicatricial see cicatricial pemphigoid
　differential diagnosis 40-1, 42, 43
pemphigus, benign familial see Hailey—Hailey disease
pemphigus vegetans 41-2
　differential diagnosis 42, 45
pemphigus vulgaris 41-2, 241
　differential diagnosis 42, 43
perforation, endometrial introduction of tissue via 486-7
perianal region/skin
　basal cell carcinoma 219
　cysts 203-4
peripheral nerve sheath tumors see nerve sheath tumors
peripheral neuroectodermal tumor see Ewing's sarcoma
peritoneal and abdominal cavity 753-92
　carcinoma see carcinoma
　ectopic pregnancy 1012
　in endometrial carcinoma
　　cytology 583-4
　　mimics of 584
　　spread 583-4
　implants/deposits and spread 783-5
　　endometrial carcinoma 583-4
　　ovarian endometrioid carcinoma 874
　　ovarian immature teratoma 785, 937
　　ovarian serous borderline tumors 848-50
　leiomyomatosis disseminata 652-3
　mesenchymal lesions 762-76
　mesothelial lesions 777-82
　Müllerian-derived lesions 754-62
peritonitis, sclerosing, luteinized thecoma and 956
perivascular epithelioid cell tumor, uterine 660-1
pessary-related lesions 238
Peutz—Jeghers syndrome, sex cord tumor with annular tubules 966, 967
photography, placental samples 1044
Phthirus pubis 66-7
pigment deposition, amniotic stromal 1061
pigmented chorionic macrophages 1062
pigmented vulval lesions 163-78
piles (hemorrhoids) 204-5
Pipelle instrument, endometrial intraepithelial neoplasia 497
pituitary hormones in menstrual cycle 444
　see also hypothalamic—pituitary axis
placenta 1041-119
　abruption 1052, 1084-5, 1091-3

placenta—cont'd
    cause and clinical presentation 1091
    pathology 1084-5, 1091-3
  development 996-8
  evaluation 1041-81
    gross 1044-59
    microscopic 1059-80
    multiple gestations 1056-9, 1109-12
    rationale 1042
    selection of placentas for 1042
    technical aspects 1043-4
  gross identification in early abortion specimens 998-9
  implantation site see implantation site
  in toxemia of pregnancy 1094-6
  tumors seen at term 1031-3, 1112-14
placenta creta (accreta and percreta) 1051-2, 1079-80, 1115
placenta previa 1114-15
plaque-type psoriasis 31
plasma cell(s), in endometrial samples 467-8
plasma cell vulvitis see Zoon's vulvitis
plasmacytic deciduitis 467
plasmacytic endometritis see endometritis
platinum-based chemotherapy
  cervical squamous carcinoma 341-2
  endometrial carcinosarcoma 595-6
  ovarian cancer, postoperative 910
  tubal carcinoma 705
pleomorphic carcinoma, endometrial 599
pleomorphic mural nodules in ovarian mucinous
    tumors 865-6
plexiform leiomyoma 628-9
ploidy
  early spontaneous abortion 1001
  hydatidiform mole 1016, 1026
polycystic ovarian syndrome 732-6, 825
polyembryoma 935
polyglandular disease, autoimmune 731
polymerase chain reactions, HSV detection 75
polyp(s)
  endocervical 419-20
    atypical 422
  endometrial 461-5
    adenomyomatous 464, 597-8, 656
    adenosarcoma vs 659
    intraepithelial neoplasia in 509, 510
    intraepithelial neoplasia vs 507
    papillary serous carcinoma associated with 563
    plasma cells in 467
  fibroepithelial see fibroepithelial mucosal polyps
  inflammatory cloacogenic 205-6
polypoid adenomyoma
  endocervical-type 420
  endometrial, atypical (APA) 464, 597-8, 655, 658, 659

polypoid endometriosis
  peritoneal 758-9
  vaginal 236
polyvesicular yolk sac tumor 932
poorly-differentiated carcinoma
  uterine/endometrial
    papillary serous carcinoma 562
    transitional cell 598
  vulval squamous cell carcinoma 132
poorly-differentiated Sertoli—Leydig cell tumor 965
poorly-differentiated small round cell ovarian tumors
    970-4
postmenopausal women see older and elderly women
postpartum period
  endometrium 481-2
  hemorrhage 1114-15
  placental tumors seen in 1031-3, 1112-14
precancer see premalignant lesions
precocious puberty 13-14, 16
predecidua 451-2, 482
pre-eclampsia (toxemia of pregnancy) 1093-6
  twins and 1112
pregnancy 995-1119
  cervical cancer in 340
    safety of delaying treatment 340
  cervical epithelial changes 371
  early 995-1039
    complications 995-1039
    gross examination 998-1000
    sonography 998
  ectopic see ectopia
  ectopic decidua 434
  endometrium following 481-2
  loss see abortion
  molar see mole
  ovaries in 722-9
    sex cord stromal tumor in 968
    theca-lutein hyperplasia 724-7, 825
  toxemia of see pre-eclampsia
  trophoblastic disease see trophoblastic disease
  twin see multiple pregnancy
premalignant lesions
  cervix
    connection with cancer 356
    oral contraceptives and 356
  endometrium 493-518, 549-51, 598
  ovary 795-805
  vulva 29, 35, 42, 46, 110, 118-30
    diagnostic terminology 129-30
  see also specific lesions
premature delivery 1088-93
primitive neuroectodermal tumor see Ewing's sarcoma
primordial follicles 3, 718

proctitis, ulcerative, anal disease 207
progestogens/progestins (and progesterone)
    IUCD coated with 469-70
    therapeutic use (and its effects) 476, 509, 512-13
        in abnormal endometrial bleeding 487
        in anovulation 455, 476
        in endometrial intraepithelial neoplasia 509,
            512-13, 516
    see also hormone replacement therapy
prolapse
    fallopian tube, post-hysterectomy 232-3
    urethral 102-3
    vaginal 230-1
proliferative/follicular phase (endometrium in) 442,
        443-4, 445-8
    early 445-8
    stromal breakdown 445-8, 460
prostate, ectopic 397-9
protozoan infections 72-3
Provera 476
pseudobowenoid papulosis 114, 119
pseudocyst, xanthomatous 722, 746
pseudodecidua with progestogens 476
pseudoepithelial hyperplasia 136, 194, 213, 219
pseudohermaphrodites 11-13
pseudo-Meigs' syndrome 627
pseudomyxoma peritonei 783-5
    ovarian mucinous tumors 857, 866, 981
pseudoneoplasia/pseudotumor
    epithelial, associated with salpingitis 688-9
    xanthomatous (=xanthomatous pseudocyst) 722,
        746, 826
pseudopuberty 14
pseudoxanthomatous salpingitis 683-4
psoriasis 29-32
    differential diagnosis 29, 31, 32, 48, 125
psychological disturbances, childhood, placental
        abnormalities associated with 1042
PTEN
    endometrial carcinoma and 498, 549
    endometrial intraepithelial neoplasia and 495, 496,
        499, 499-500
    endometrioid ovarian carcinoma and 877
Pthirus (Phthirus) pubis 66-7
puberty, precocious 13-14, 16
pubic lice 66-7
puerperium see postpartum period
pulmonary carcinoma
    cervical metastases 391
    ovarian metastases 825, 985
pulmonary-type ovarian small cell carcinoma 972-3
pustular psoriasis 31
pyoderma gangrenosum 49-50

pyometra 467
pyosalpinx 691

race see ethnicity
RAD51B and uterine leiomyoma 626-7
radiation-induced changes/lesions
    cervical/endocervical cells 310, 372
    endometrial cancers 547, 590
    vagina 253, 358
    vulval lichen sclerosus vs 35
radiation therapy
    cervical cancer
        adenocarcinoma 399-401
        neuroendocrine carcinoma 417-18
        squamous carcinoma 341, 342
    endometrial adenocarcinoma, preoperative
        (neoadjuvant) and (postoperative) adjuvant 589
    endometrial carcinosarcoma 596
    placental site trophoblastic tumor 1036
    vaginal carcinoma 254-5
ras mutations
    endometrial intraepithelial neoplasia 499
    ovarian mucinous carcinoma 868
    ovarian serous carcinoma 854
reactive change
    cervical/endocervical cells
        adenocarcinoma and adenocarcinoma in situ vs
            360, 361, 363, 372-3
        squamous intraepithelial neoplasia lesions vs 303,
            308
    decidua see deciduitis
    endometrial, intraepithelial neoplasia vs 506
    endometrioma 746
rectum see anorectum
Reed syndrome 626
Reiter's syndrome 46-8
    differential diagnosis 31
renal cell carcinoma, metastatic 883, 985-6
repair (surface epithelium)
    cervical, atypical 283
    endometrial 484-5
        metaplasia and 529-31
reproductive tract see genital tract
reserve cells and reserve-type cells
    cervix 291, 292
    endometrium 520-4
respiratory papillomatosis 118
rests, benign
    fallopian tube 678-9
    vulva 103-5
retained products of conception 1014
rete cystadenoma 853
retiform Sertoli—Leydig cell tumor 853, 934, 965-6

retroviral drugs and anal squamous intraepithelial lesions 213
rhabdomyoma, genital 190-1
rhabdomyosarcoma 776
    alveolar 988
    embryonal *see* embryonal rhabdomyosarcoma
ringworm (tinea), groin 69-70
Rokitansky's tubercle 915

salpingitis 466, 683-5
    endometriosis and, relationship between 683
    epithelial pseudoneoplasia associated with 688-9
    follicular *see* follicular salpingitis
    granulomatous 694
    oophoritis and 692, 742
    pseudoxanthomatous 683-4
    xanthogranulomatous 684-5
salpingitis isthmica nodosum 685-6
salpingo-oophorectomy *see* oophorectomy
sarcoma
    cervical 425, 431-3
    endometrial, undifferentiated 617-18, 622
    endometrial stromal *see* stromal sarcoma
    endometrioid stromal *see* stromal sarcoma
    Ewing's *see* Ewing's sarcoma
    granulocytic *see* granulocytic sarcoma
    Kaposi's, differential diagnosis 89
    ovarian 973-4
        endometrioid stromal *see* stromal sarcoma
        metastatic 988
    synovial, differential diagnosis 766, 772
    tubal 707
    vulvovaginal 89, 188-9
    see also adenosarcoma; carcinosarcoma; fibrosarcoma; liposarcoma; rhabdomyosarcoma
sarcoma botryoides *see* embryonal rhabdomyosarcoma
sarcomatoid mesothelioma, ovarian 989
sarcomatoid Sertoli—Leydig cell tumor 965
sarcomatoid squamous carcinoma *see* spindle cell squamous carcinoma
sarcomatous component, ovarian tumors with 877-9
sarcomatous mural nodules in ovarian mucinous tumors 866
sarcomatous transformation, angiomyofibroblastoma 182
Sarcoptes scabiei 67-8
scabies (*Sarcoptes scabiei* var *hominis* infection) 67-8
    Norwegian/crusted 94
scar tissue, hypertrophic, vs desmoid fibrosis 773
schistosomiasis 84-6
schwannoma
    cervical 428-9
    peritoneal 771

schwannoma—cont'd
    clinical features 770-1
    differential diagnosis 764, 770, 772
    epidemiology 770
    treatment and prognosis 772
    vulvovaginal 193
sclerosing mesenteritis 783
sclerosing peritonitis and luteinized thecoma 956
sclerosing stromal tumor 970
screening
    HPV infection 276-7
    ovarian cancer 814-16
seborrheic dermatitis 32
seborrheic keratosis, vulval condylomata resembling 113, 119-20
secretory (luteal) phase 442, 450-2
    defects/disturbances/inadequacy 453-6, 478-9
    endometrial intraepithelial neoplasia vs endometrium in 506-7
    exhaustive (mid) phase of 450-1, 506-7
    predecidual (late) phase of 451-2, 506-7
    vacuole (early) phase of 450
secretory cells of fallopian tube 676
secretory differentiation, endometrial adenocarcinoma 558-9
secretory metaplasia 538
sentinel node evaluation
    vulval melanoma 173-4
    vulval squamous carcinoma 142-3
septal (placental) cysts 1055
septate uterus 15-16
septate vagina 18
septic abortion 1015-16
serologic tests
    HSV 76
    syphilis 79
seromucinous tumors, ovarian 891
    carcinoma 864, 891, 892
    Müllerian 826
serous carcinoma
    cervical 385-6, 390
    endometrial
        mixed with endometrioid component 563-8
        molecular genetics 549
        ovarian metastases 854
    ovarian 803
        differential diagnosis 853-4, 882
        etiology/genetics/biomarkers 854-5
        gross examination 843
        high-grade 803
        low-grade 800-1, 803
        microscopic findings 851-3
        pathogenesis 799
        pathology-based management 908-9

serous carcinoma—cont'd
  papillary *see* papillary serous carcinoma
  tubal origin 703
    evidence for 697
serous cystadenoma
  ovarian, gross appearance 826
  tubal 680-1, 696
    borderline 696
serous cysts, peritoneal 778
serous intraepithelial carcinoma
  endometrial 494, 550, 563
  tubal 703
serous tumors
  ovarian 842-55, 907-8
    borderline *see* borderline tumors
    differential diagnosis 853-4, 882
    etiology/genetics/biomarkers 854-5
    general and clinical aspects 842
    gross examination 842-3
    microscopic examination 844-53
    misclassification 836
    pathology-based management 907-10
  peritoneal papillary 759-62
  see also seromucinous tumors
Sertoli cell 946
Sertoli cell tumors 962-6
  differential diagnosis 874, 875
  gross appearance 830
Sertoli—Leydig cell tumors 962-6
  clinical features 962
  differential diagnosis 853, 867-8, 874, 879, 934,
      963-4, 965, 965-6
  gross features 962-3
  with heterologous elements 867-8, 966
  histology 963-6
  juvenile 823
  retiform 853, 934, 965-6
  unclassified tumors similar to 968
sex chromosomes *see* X chromosome; Y chromosome
sex cord-like elements, endometrioid stromal sarcoma
    with 879
sex cord (stromal) tumor 946-70
  broad ligament 697
  ovarian 946-70
    with annular tubules 966-7
    classification/categories (histologic) 949-70
    frequency and clinical significance 946
    histogenesis 946
    intermediately-differentiated, differential diagnosis 950
    pure mesenchymal, differential diagnosis 949
    risk factors 946-9
    unclassified 967-8
    uni- vs bilateral 824

sex cord (stromal) tumor—cont'd
    uterine tumor resembling (UTROSCT) 390, 616-17
    well-differentiated, differential diagnosis 951
sex determination 3-6
  abnormalities 11-13
sex determining region (SRY) 3, 9
sexual abuse and genital warts 117
sexual intercourse, anal, risk factor for anal squamous
      intraepithelial lesions 209-10
sexual partners and cervical neoplasia risk
  female 275-6
  male 274-5
sexually-transmitted diseases (STDs) 72-8
  common 72-8
  common infections not typically linked to 68-72
  immunosuppressed persons 87
  pelvic inflammatory disease with 690
  uncommon 78-84
SGO staging of cervical squamous carcinoma 328
shape, placental 1044-5
Shh 7-8
shingles *see* herpes zoster
sickled maternal RBCs 1076
signet-ring carcinoma
    adenomatoid tumor vs 696
    gastric *see* Krukenberg tumor
signet-ring stromal tumor 970
size/dimensions
    cervical tumor 328-9
    endometrial intraepithelial neoplasia 504
    umbilical cord 1046
    uterine leiomyosarcoma, prognostic importance 639
skeletal muscle, Sertoli—Leydig cell tumors with 867, 966
skeletal muscle tumors, vulvovaginal 190-2
Skene's duct cyst 100, 101
skin
  appendages *see* adnexae
  disorders
    perianal *see* perianal region
    vaginal 240-1
    vulval 24-46
small bowel carcinoma, ovarian metastases 876, 980-1
small cell carcinoma
  ovarian
    age and 823
    differential diagnosis 893, 960
    gross appearance 830
    hypercalcemic-type *see* hypercalcemic-type small
        cell ovarian carcinoma
    pulmonary-type 972-3
  peritoneal 776
small cell neuroendocrine carcinoma 412, 413-14, 415-16
small cell undifferentiated endometrial carcinoma 599

small round blue cell tumors 988-9
  immunoprofile 776
small round cell tumors
  desmoplastic *see* desmoplastic small round cell tumors
  poorly-differentiated, ovarian 970-4
smoking and cervical neoplasia 275
smooth muscle actin (SMA), peritoneal mesenchymal
    tumors and 764
smooth muscle metaplasia, ovarian 729
smooth muscle tumors
  cervical 427-8
  ovarian, thecoma vs 957
  peritoneal 762-4
  uterine 623-57
    biomarkers 649-50
    classification problems 648-9
    mixed endometrial stromal and 615-16
    quasi-malignant 650-5
    tumors mimicking 655-7
    of uncertain malignant potential (STUMP) 648,
      649
  vulvovaginal 189-90
Society of Gynecologic Oncologists' staging of cervical
    squamous carcinoma 328
soft-part sarcoma, alveolar 425-6
soft tissue tumors *see* mesenchymal tumors
somatic elements in ovarian tumors 830-1, 915
sonic hedgehog gene 7-8
sonography *see* ultrasound
spindle cell differentiation in smooth muscle tumors
    637
  classification 637
  vulvovaginal leiomyoma 190
spindle cell epithelioma, vaginal 261
spindle cell (sarcomatoid) mesothelioma, ovarian 989
spindle cell (sarcomatoid) squamous carcinoma
  cervical 334-6, 422, 423-4, 425
  vulval 136, 188
spiral arteries/arterioles, pathology 1078
  in pre-eclampsia 1096
spongiosis in eczematous dermatitis 27
  vulval intraepithelial neoplasia vs 125
spread of tumor *see* invasion; metastases
squamo-columnar junction 291
squamo-transitional carcinoma
  cervical papillary 336
  vaginal 256
squamous cell(s), cervical
  atypical
    postmenopausal 303
    of undetermined significance (ASCUS) 279-86
  differentiation 291, 294
  immature, with metaplastic phenotype 321

squamous cell carcinoma (squamous cancer), anal 216-21
  clinical presentation 217
  demographics 216-17
  differential diagnosis 219
  histology 217-19
  risk factors 203
  therapy and outcome 219-21
squamous cell carcinoma (squamous cancer), cervical
    320-44
  differential diagnosis 415
  high-grade squamous intraepithelial neoplasia
      preceding 317
  incidence relative to adenocarcinoma 356
  invasion by, diagnosis 323-8
  low-grade squamous intraepithelial neoplasia and,
      uncommon association 316-17
  pathology 334-9
  spindle cell (sarcomatoid) 334-6, 422, 423-4, 425
  superficially invasive (microinvasive) 330-1
    management 333-4
  treatment and outcome 339-44
squamous cell carcinoma (squamous cancer),
    endometrial 598
squamous cell carcinoma (squamous cancer), ovarian
  in cystic teratoma 918
  differential diagnosis 889-90
  etiology 890
  general and clinical aspects 899
  gross examination 889
  microscopic examination 889
squamous cell carcinoma (squamous cancer), vaginal
    253-5
  variants 255-6
squamous cell carcinoma (squamous cancer), vulval 110,
    130-43
  Bartholin's gland 155
  invasive 130-43
    clinical presentation 130
    diagnostic criteria for invasion 130-2
    differential diagnosis 136-8, 170-1, 194
    growth patterns 132-6
    management 110
  precursor lesions 29, 35, 42, 46, 110
  superficially invasive (microinvasive) 138-43
    definition 139-40
    natural history 140-2
squamous cell tumors, ovarian *see* epidermoid cyst;
    squamous cell carcinoma
squamous differentiation, endometrioid
    adenocarcinoma 553-6
  in grading 571
  see also squamous metaplasia
squamous epithelium, vaginal 230

squamous intraepithelial lesions (SILs), anal 209-14
  clinical presentations 210, 211-12
  definition 209, 210, 211-12
  differential diagnosis and diagnostic pitfalls 211
  epidemiology/risk factors 209-10
  examination 210
  high-grade (HSIL) 210, 211-14
  histology 210-11
  low-grade (LSIL) 210-11
  natural history 211
squamous intraepithelial lesions (SILs), cervical
    (squamous CIN) 268-320, 333
  definitions 268, 294
  high-grade (HSIL; CIN II/III) 288-90, 305-10
    on biopsy, vs LSIL on smear 314
    cytology 288-90
    differential diagnosis 306-10
    histology 305-10
    HPV 16 variants and risk of 272
    invasion risk following treatment 321
    invasive carcinoma preceded by 317
    microinvasion by 321
    mistaken for adenocarcinoma in situ 364
    on smear, vs LSIL on biopsy 314-15
    stromal invasion portended by features in 322-3
  intermediate to low and high-grade 303-4
  low-grade (LSIL; CIN I) 287-8, 298-303
    on biopsy, vs HSIL on smear 314-15
    cancer risk 316
    cytology 287-8, 290
    differential diagnosis 302-3
    histology 298-303
    on smear, vs HSIL on biopsy 314
    subtypes 300-2
  ovarian squamous carcinoma etiology and 890
  therapeutic options 315-20
squamous intraepithelial lesions (SILs), vulval 129
squamous lesions
  cervix 267-354
    biomarkers and diagnosis and classification 310-13
    cytology 278-86, 287-90
  vulval 109-48
  Paget's disease and 151
squamous metaplasia 525-8
  cervical, atypical immature 283, 308
  endometrial 520, 525, 525-8, 540
  in endometrioid adenocarcinoma 553, 571
  placental surface 1050
  vestibular glands 61
squamous morules (morular metaplasia) 509, 511,
    525-7
  in endometrioid adenocarcinoma 553
    grading and 571

squamous papilloma of cervix (=immature condyloma)
    296-7, 300-2, 338
staging
  anal squamous carcinoma 221
  cervical adenocarcinoma 375-6, 399-400
  cervical squamous carcinoma 320, 328
  endometrial carcinosarcoma 594-5
  gestational trophoblastic disease 1025
  ovarian epithelial tumors (and subsequent
      management) 906-7, 910
    endometrioid tumors 909-10
    mucinous tumors 910
    serous borderline tumors 907-8
  tubal carcinoma 703
  vaginal carcinoma 255
  vulval carcinoma 140
  vulval melanoma 171-4
Staphylococcus aureus and toxic shock syndrome 239
steatocystoma multiplex 106
Stein—Leventhal (polycystic ovary) syndrome 732-6, 825
stem villi 1066-8
sterilization, tubal (via ligation) 677-8
  ectopic pregnancy risk 1006
  ovarian cancer risk reduction 814
  reversal 678
    ectopic pregnancy risk 1006
steroid-producing cells
  autoantibodies to 731
  hyperplasia 742
  neoplasia 968-70
Stevens—Johnson syndrome, vaginal adhesions 241
STI-571, gastrointestinal stromal tumor therapy 770
stomach carcinoma *see* Krukenberg tumor
storage disorders 1068
stratified-type adenocarcinoma in situ 367
streptococcus
  group A (incl. S. pyogenes), and toxic shock
      syndrome 239
  group B 238
stroma, amniotic, pigment deposition 1061
stroma, cervical
  atypical cells 435
  invasion
    papillary lesions without 332-3
    portended by features of high-grade squamous
        intraepithelial neoplasia 322
stroma, endometrial
  breakdown 460-1
    differential diagnosis 448, 508
    in proliferative phase 445-8, 460
    stratified syncytial epithelial changes with 529
  in endometrial intraepithelial neoplasia 502-3
  granulocytes in, in secretory phase 452

stroma, endometrial—cont'd
  nodule 613-14, 621
  in papillary serous carcinoma 562
  polyps with atypical change in 465
stroma, ovarian
  hyperplasia 739, 825, 879
  hyperthecosis 739-40
  invasion
    by endometrioid borderline tumor 870-1
    by serous borderline tumor 846-7
  structure 714-15
stroma, villous
  calcification 1072-3
  fibrosis 1072
stromal polyps, fibroepithelial see fibroepithelial mucosal
    polyps
stromal sarcoma
  endometrial/uterine 425, 615, 973
    adenosarcoma vs 658
    in classification schemes 613
    high-grade 618
    intra-abdominal 764-5
    low-grade 615, 621-2
    ovarian metastases 879, 978-9
  endometrioid ovarian 877-8, 878, 879
    with sex cord-like elements 879
stromal tumors
  endometrial 613-22
    biomarkers 622-3
    clinicopathologic features 613-20
    curettings, interpretation 620-1
    definition and classification 613
    differential diagnosis 622-3
    management and prognosis 621-3
    resembling ovarian sex cord tumor (UTROSCT)
        390, 616-17
  gastrointestinal see gastrointestinal stromal tumor
  ovarian 946-70
    epithelial see epithelial tumors
  sex cord see sex cord (stromal) tumor
  vulvovaginal 179-86
stromatosis 436
structural anomalies see developmental anomalies
struma ovarii 919-20
  carcinoids coexisting with 919-20, 964
  clear cell carcinoma vs 883
  gross appearance 830
  Sertoli—Leydig cell tumors vs 964
  thyroid tissue in 919-20
strumosis 785
subchorionic fibrin 1066
  absence 1051
subchorionic hematoma 1050-1, 1066

subchorionic maternal blood/hematoma 1066, 1085
submucosal leiomyoma 472
surgery (incl. excision)
  anal intraepithelial neoplasia 214
  cervical adenocarcinoma 399
  cervical adenosarcoma 422
  cervical squamous carcinoma 341, 342
    superficially invasive 333-4
  cervical squamous intraepithelial neoplasia,
      and follow-up 317-20
  endometrial assessment during 574
  endometrial bleeding 458, 488
  endometrial carcinoma
    postoperative evaluation 577-8
    preoperative adjuvant therapy 589
    preoperative evaluation 579-81
  endometrial intraepithelial neoplasia diagnosed
      before, significance 575-6
  ovarian neoplasia 907-10
    cystic teratoma 917
    dysgerminoma 931
    evaluation at see ovarian tumors
    postoperative management 910
  peritoneal lesions
    desmoid fibromatosis 774
    papillary serous carcinoma 762
  placental site trophoblastic tumor 1036
  tubal carcinoma 705
  uterine smooth muscle tumors
    intraoperative examination 650
    leiomyoma 625
    leiomyosarcoma 639
    of uncertain malignant potential 649
  vaginal carcinoma 254-5
  vaginal intraepithelial lesions 253
  vaginal melanoma 260
  vulval lesions
    angiomyxoma (aggressive form) 184
    dermatofibroma 186-7
    intraepithelial neoplasia 122
    melanoma 171
  see also specific procedures
sweat gland carcinoma vs benign rests 104
"swiss cheese" endometrium 487
syncytial epithelial changes with breakdown, stratified 529
syncytial metaplasia 525, 530, 538
  papillary 530, 538
syncytiotrophoblast (cells and layer) 996, 1017-18
  in gestational trophoblastic disease 1018
    choriocarcinoma 935, 936, 1029
  complete mole 1018, 1021
  partial mole 1026
synovial sarcoma, differential diagnosis 766, 772

syphilis (*T. pallidum* infection) 78-84, 1100
  congenital 1100
  Zoon's vulvitis vs 39
syringoma 106
systemic disorders
  tubal 695
  vulval 46-52

tags, anal 205
talc exposure and ovarian cancer 813
tamoxifen 477
  endometrial carcinoma risk 548
  endometrial carcinosarcoma risk 590
  endometrial intraepithelial neoplasia risk 496
  endometrial thickening with 552
  uterine mesenchymal tumor risk 612
teratoma, broad ligament 697
teratoma, ovarian 785, 915-17
  cystic *see* cystic teratoma
  immature 936-8
    differential diagnosis 836, 878-9, 915-16, 937
    peritoneal gliomatosis 785, 937
terminal villi 1068-73
testicular feminization 10-11
theca cell(s) 718
theca cell tumor (thecoma) 955-7
  gross appearance 830, 956
  see also fibrothecoma; granulosa-theca cell tumor
theca-lutein hyperplasia of pregnancy 724-7, 825
ThinPrep (cervix) 279
  glandular lesions 365
thrombosis (fetoplacental)
  chorionic vessel 1046, 1065
  fetal 1067-8, 1097-9
    growth restriction due to 1097-9
  intervillous 1055, 1075
thyroid tissue, ovarian tumors containing 919-20
tinea cruris 69-70
TORCH syndrome 1099
torsion
  ovarian 747-8, 825
  tubal 695
toxemia of pregnancy *see* pre-eclampsia
toxic shock syndrome 238-9
toxoplasmosis 1099-100
  chorionic stroma 1066
  villous 1099-100
  Wharton's jelly 1059
  see also TORCH syndrome
trabecular carcinoids 922
trachelectomy, squamous carcinoma 333-4
transcription factors in ovarian development 3-4
transformation zone 291

transitional cell carcinoma
  endometrial 598
  ovarian
    differential diagnosis 888, 892, 986-7
    etiology/genetics/biomarkers 888-9
    general and clinical aspects 884
    gross examination 885
    microscopic examination 887
  tubal 703
  urinary tract, ovarian metastases 888, 986-7
  see also squamo-transitional carcinoma
transitional cell tumors
  ovarian 854, 884-9
    differential diagnosis 887-8
    etiology/genetics/biomarkers 887-8
    general and clinical aspects 884
    gross examination 884-5
    microscopic examination 885-7
translocations, chromosomal
  dermatofibroma protuberans 187
  endometrial stromal tumors 619, 620, 765
  uterine smooth muscle tumors
    leiomyoma 627
    quasi-malignant 652
transvaginal ultrasound *see* ultrasound
trauma (iatrogenic)
  anal region 208
  fetal capillary 1073
  neoplastic epithelium displaced into spaces by 136
  umbilical cord vessel 1048
  vaginal 237-8
Treponema pallidum infection *see* syphilis
trichomoniasis 72-3
triploid hydatidiform mole 1016, 1026
trisomies, early spontaneous abortion 1001
trophoblast 996
  benign hyperplasia 1033
  contaminating curettings, and suspected ectopic
    pregnancy 1009-11
  histologic classification/diagnosis/exclusion
    of trophoblastic disease 1017
  intermediate/extra-villous 996, 1019-20
    in gestational trophoblastic disease 1019-20, 1029
  previllous, early gestation vs choriocarcinoma 1030
trophoblastic differentiation, endometrial carcinoma 601
trophoblastic disease/lesions, gestational 1015-36
  cervix 435
  clinico-radiologic features 1016
  definitions 1015
  gross pathologic features 1016
  management and outcome 1018
  placental site *see* implantation site
  risk factors 1015-16, 1018

trophoblastic disease/lesions, gestational—cont'd
  target tissues 1017-20
  see also specific lesions
tubal/ciliated cell differentiation 537
  cervical adenocarcinoma in situ 367
  endometrial adenocarcinoma 537
tubal metaplasia
  cervical adenocarcinoma and adenocarcinoma in situ
      vs 361, 369-70
  endometrial 524, 525, 535-7
tube(s), fallopian 611-48
  anatomy and histology 676-7
  benign tumors 695-7
  cancer 697-709
    adenomatoid tumor vs 696
    endometrial co-involvement 585
    epithelial pseudoneoplasia associated with
        salpingitis vs 689
    ovarian metastases 979
    vaginal metastases 258
  childhood acquired disorders 13-14
  development 2
  ectopic pregnancy in *see* ectopia
  in ectopic pregnancy
    in causation 1005-6
    examination 1011-12
  infections 689-94
  ligation *see* sterilization
  prolapse, post-hysterectomy 232-3
  regional and systemic disorders 695
  specimens, approaches 677-89
  see also oophorectomy (or salpingo-oophorectomy);
      salpingitis
tuberculosis (*M. tuberculosis* and *M. bovis* infection)
  ovarian 742-3
  vulvovaginal 87-8, 240
tuboendometrial metaplasia, cervical adenocarcinoma
    and adenocarcinoma in situ vs 361, 369-70, 399
tubo-ovarian adhesions 685
tubules, annular, sex cord tumor with 966-7
tumors
  anorectal 208-24
  cervical *see* cervix
  endometrial *see* endometrium
  ovaries *see* ovarian tumors
  placental, seen at term 1031-3, 1112-14
  tubal
    benign 695-7
    salpingitis vs 692
  vaginal 245-65
    childhood 19
  see also malignant tumors; metastases *and specific types
    of benign and malignant tumors*

tunnel clusters 391-2
Turner syndrome (45,XO) 10
  premature ovarian failure 730
twin pregnancy *see* multiple pregnancy
twin-twin transfusion syndrome 1110-12
twisted cord 1046

ulcer(s)
  anal 206
  vulvovaginal 240
    Behçet's disease 48
    chancroid 81, 82
    Crohn's disease 49, 50
    differential diagnosis 77
    HSV-associated 76
    pyoderma gangrenosum 49-50
    syphilitic (=chancre) 78, 79
    tampon-related 237
ulcerative colitis, anal disease 207
ultrasound (transvaginal)
  in abnormal uterine bleeding 458
    endometrial polyp 462
  complete mole 1021
  early pregnancy 998
  endometrial intraepithelial neoplasia 496-7
  endometrial thickness 552
  ovarian cancer
    in risk assessment 816-17
    in screening 815-16
ultrasound treatment, focal, leiomyoma 642-3
umbilical artery, single 1107-8
umbilical cord
  gross appearance 1046-8
    twin gestation 1056
  microscopic appearance 1059
undifferentiated (anaplastic) carcinoma
  cervix 418
  choriocarcinoma vs 1031
  endometrial 599
  ovarian
    differential diagnosis 893
    general and clinical aspects 891
    gross examination 892
    microscopic examination 892
    mural nodules with 865
undifferentiated sarcoma, uterine 617-18, 622
unicornuate uterus 14-15
urethral prolapse 102-3
urinary bladder, endocervicosis 756
urinary tract transitional cell carcinoma, ovarian
    metastases 888, 986-7
urogenital sinus, vulvar cysts originating from 101-2
urorectal septum, embryology 200

urothelial carcinoma, vulval extension 152
uterine artery embolization 625, 641-2
uterine tube *see* tube
uterus
  bleeding from *see* bleeding
  carcinoma *see* carcinoma, endometrial/uterine
  development 2, 6
    anomalies 14-17
  endometrial carcinoma involving lower segment
    of (LUS) 581-2
  mesenchymal tumors 611-72
    adenosarcoma involving cervix 422
    carcinosarcoma metastatic to cervix 425
    definition 442
    tumor resembling ovarian sex cord tumor
      (UTROSCT) 390, 616-17
  neck of *see* cervix
  see also endometrium; myometrium

vaccines, cervical cancer prevention and therapy 342-4
vagina
  acquired childhood lesions 19
  benign lesions 229-44
  development 2, 6
    disorders 18-19
  neoplasms *see* tumors
  see also vulvovaginal lesions
vaginitis
  atrophic 231-2
  desquamative inflammatory 240
  emphysematous 241-2
vaginosis, bacterial 70-1
varicella-zoster virus 92-3
  see also herpes zoster
vascular endothelial growth factor in pre-eclampsia 1094
vascular leiomyoma 630
vascular space invasion
  cervical cancer 329-30, 332-3
    conditions mimicking 330
    reporting 339
  endometrial adenocarcinoma 587
  endometrial carcinosarcoma 595
  hydatidiform mole 1023-4
  leiomyomata 650
  vulval squamous carcinoma 142
vascular tumors (and tumor-like lesions)
  cervical 434
  ovarian, yolk sac tumor vs 933
  vulvovaginal 192-3
vasculature, fetoplacental
  distribution 1046
  microscopic changes 1060, 1062, 1065-6
  number of vessels 1047-8

vasculature, fetoplacental—cont'd
  patency 1048
  thrombosis *see* thrombosis
  trauma 1048
  twin gestation, anastomoses 1058-9, 1110
  see also specific (types of) vessels
vasculitis 695
vasculopathy, spiral arteries *see* spiral arteries
VEGF in pre-eclampsia 1094
vein-to-vein anastomoses, twin placenta 1058
venous spaces, leiomyomatosis 650
verruciform lesion of vulva, differential diagnosis 115
verruciform lichen simplex chronicus 128
verrucopapillary cervical neoplasms 336
verrucous carcinoma
  anal 218-19
  cervical 336
  vaginal 255-6
  vulval 134
    giant condylomata of Buschke—Löwenstein vs 134-5
villi (placental/chorionic) 996, 1066-73
  in curettings, ectopic pregnancy diagnosis/exclusion
    1009, 1011
  dysmorphic 1003
  edema (and fetal hydrops/hydropic abortus) 1002,
    1071-2
    diagnosis/exclusion 1017, 1026
    histology 1017, 1071-2
  fibrin deposition in region of 1033, 1075-6
  hydropic 999-1000
    gestational sac masquerading as 1028, 1030
  ischemia 1096
  stem villi 1066-8
  terminal villi 1068-73
  trophoblastic disease 1017
  see also intervillositis; intervillous space; intravillous
    hemorrhage
villitis 1070, 1099-103
  acute 1070, 1091
  chronic 1070, 1099-103
  of unknown etiology 1070, 1101-2
villoglandular adenocarcinoma
  cervical 383-4
  endometrioid 559-60, 565-6, 573
villous adenoma, cervix 399
villous intermediate trophoblast 1019-20
viral infections 86-7
  endocervical glandular atypia associated with 373
  immunosuppressed patients 92-4
  in pregnancy 1100-1
  sexually-transmissible 73-7
  villous 1070
  see also microbiology

vitiligo vs lichen sclerosus 34-5
Volgstein-type model of ovarian cancer development
   794
vulva 23-197
  acquired childhood anomalies 19-20
  cysts 100-3
  development 2
    anomalies 19-20
  folliculitis 71-2
  glandular malignancies 149-62
  immunosuppression-associated infections 87-94
  inflammatory disorders *see* inflammatory disorders
  malignant tumors *see* malignant tumors
  melanocytic/pigmented lesions 163-78
  mucosal disorders *see* mucosal disorders
  necrotizing fasciitis 90-2
  pain *see* vulvodynia
  rests (benign) 103-5
  squamous lesions *see* squamous lesions
  systemic disorders 46-52
  see also vulvovaginal lesions
vulvitis
  granulomatous 51
  plasma cell/Zoon's *see* Zoon's vulvitis
vulvocrural area, 44-5
  acantholysis, differential diagnosis 42, 45
vulvodynia (localized) 57-64
  etiology 58-60
  histopathology 60-2
  terminology 58-9
  treatment 62
vulvovaginal candidiasis *see* candidiasis
vulvovaginal lesions
  benign cysts/rests/adnexal tumors 99-108, 234-6
  soft tissue 179-97
vulvovaginal—gingival syndrome of lichen planus 37
VZV 92-3
  see also herpes zoster

Walthard cell rests 678-9
wart(s), genital (condyloma acuminatum) 93-4, 112-18,
   210-11
  biomarkers and diagnosis 115-16
  cervical 296-7, 300
  clinical presentation 93, 112
  differential diagnosis 115, 119, 219
  endometrial 598
  histopathology 112-14
  immunosuppressed patients 93-4
  management 93-4, 117-18
  natural history 117-18
  risk factors 112
warty carcinoma 134

warty dyskeratoma, differential diagnosis 42, 45
weight
  ovarian tumor 825
  placental 1044
Wharton's jelly, toxoplasmosis 1059
WHO *see* World Health Organization
Wilms' tumor, cervical and endometrial 424
Wilms' tumor gene *see* WT-1
Wolffian development 3
Wolffian duct tumors 707
  ovarian 876, 964-5
  tubal endometrioid carcinoma resembling 703-4
World Health Organization (WHO)
  classification
    anal tumors 208, 221
    endometrial stromal tumors 613
    ovarian borderline tumors 840, 841
    ovarian steroid cell tumors 968
  diagnostic criteria for endometrial hyperplasias 495
  grading of ovarian carcinomas 841
WT-1 (protein and gene)
  ovarian serous carcinoma 854
  peritoneal malignant mesothelioma 782
  peritoneal mesenchymal lesions 762, 766, 776, 777

X chromosome
  in hydatidiform mole, karyotype 1016
  inactivation
    leiomyoma 626
    leiomyomatosis 654
xantho(granulo)matous pseudocyst/pseudotumor 722,
   746, 826
xanthogranulomatous salpingitis 684-5
45,XO *see* Turner syndrome

Y chromosome
  in hydatidiform mole, karyotype 1016
  sex determining region (SRY) 3, 9
yellow ovarian tumors 830
yolk sac 997
yolk sac (endodermal sinus) tumor, ovarian 931-4
  differential diagnosis 876, 883, 930, 933-4, 966
  endometrioid 876, 933
  as endometrioid carcinoma component 874
  gross pathology 931
  histopathology 931-3
  management and outcome 934
  presenting signs/symptoms 931
Yupze regimen 473

Zoon's vulvitis 38-9
  differential diagnosis 38, 39, 80-1
zygosity in twin placenta, establishing 1056, 1109